JIPMER
20 Authors

JIPMER
20 Authors

Chief Editors

Abirami
MBBS MD

J Magendran
MBBS MD
Associate Professor
Department of Forensic Medicine
Saveetha Medical College
Chennai, Tamil Nadu, India

Rajamahendran R
MS MRCS (Edinburgh) FAMS MCh (SGE)
Long and Short Cases in Surgery
Founder/Director
KONCPT PG Medical Coaching Centre
Chennai, Tamil Nadu, India

Antan Uresh Kumar T
MS FMAS MCh Urology
Founder Faculty of KONCPT PG Medical Coaching Centre
Laparoscopic, Endoscopic and Transplant Surgeon
Assistant Professor in Urology
Madras Medical College
Chennai, Tamil Nadu, India

Foreword
Rajamahendran R

JAYPEE *The Health Sciences Publisher*
New Delhi | London | Panama | Philadelphia

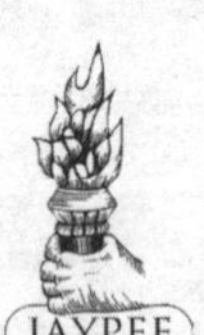

Jaypee Brothers Medical Publishers (P) Ltd

Headquarters

Jaypee Brothers Medical Publishers (P) Ltd.
4838/24, Ansari Road, Daryaganj
New Delhi 110 002, India
Phone: +91-11-43574357
Fax: +91-11-43574314
Email: jaypee@jaypeebrothers.com

Overseas Offices

J.P. Medical Ltd.
83, Victoria Street, London
SW1H 0HW (UK)
Phone: +44-20 3170 8910
Fax: +44-(0)20 3008 6180
Email: info@jpmedpub.com

Jaypee-Highlights Medical Publishers Inc.
City of Knowledge, Bld. 237, Clayton
Panama City, Panama
Phone: +1 507-301-0496
Fax: +1 507-301-0499
Email: cservice@jphmedical.com

JP Medical Inc.
325 Chestnut Street, Suite 412
Philadelphia, PA 19106, USA
Phone: +215-713-7181
Email: joe.rusko@jaypeebrothers.com

Jaypee Brothers Medical Publishers (P) Ltd.
17/1-B, Babar Road, Block-B, Shaymali
Mohammadpur, Dhaka-1207, Bangladesh
Mobile: +08801912003485
Email: jaypeedhaka@gmail.com

Jaypee Brothers Medical Publishers (P) Ltd.
Bhotahity, Kathmandu, Nepal
Phone: +977-9741283608
Email: Kathmandu@jaypeebrothers.com

Website: www.jaypeebrothers.com
Website: www.jaypeedigital.com

Inquiries for bulk sales may be solicited at: jaypee@jaypeebrothers.com

JIPMER 20 Authors

First Edition: 2016

ISBN: 978-93-5250-054-3

Printed at Rajkamal Electric Press, Plot No. 2, Phase-IV, Kundli, Haryana.

Dedicated to

Our Dear Friend

(Late) Dr S Karthikeyan MD Anesthesia

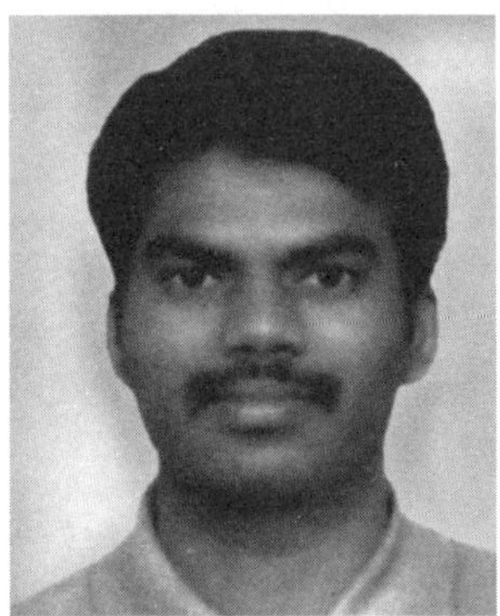

Dr SK — Another name for Enthusiasm, Dedication and Energy

Contributors

Abirami MD

J Magendran MD (Forensic Medicine)
Associate Professor
Department of Forensic Medicine
Saveetha Medical College
Chennai, Tamil Nadu, India

Rajamahendran R MS MRCS (Edinburgh) FAMS MCh (SGE)
Long and short cases in surgery
Founder/Director
KONCPT PG Medical Coaching Centre
Chennai, Tamil Nadu, India

Antan Uresh Kumar T MS FMAS MCh (Urology)
Gold Medalist in Surgery
Founder/Faculty
KONCPT PG Medical Coaching Centre
Laparoscopic, Endoscopic and Transplant Surgeon
Assistant Professor in Urology
Madras Medical College
Chennai, Tamil Nadu, India

K Arumugam MD (Anatomy)
Assistant Professor
Department of Anatomy
Tirunelveli Medical College
Tirunelveli, Tamil Nadu, India

B Vinodh Kumar MD (Biochemistry)
Consultant Clinical Biochemist
Sundaram Medical Foundation
Chennai, Tamil Nadu, India

J Suria Kumar MD FHM FCIP
Senior Assistant Professor
Institute of Microbiology
Madurai Medical College
Madurai, Tamil Nadu, India

Marquess Raj MD Dip MB NB F (Cytopath)
Head of Laboratory Medicine
Fortis Malar Hospital
Chennai, Tamil Nadu, India

Ravindra MD Pharmacology (JIPMER)

A Balaji MD DIH MIPHA
Associate Professor
Research Analyst
Advisory Member
National IFSMA
Author and Reviewer of National and International journals

VJ Vikram MS ENT DLO

R Anjana MS (Ophthalmology)
Madras Medical College
Chennai, Tamil Nadu
India

Suthantira Kannan S MD
Junior Resident
Calicut Medical College
Kozhikode, Kerala
India

Anuradha Dhanasekharan DNB OBG DOL
Consultant in OBG
MedWay Medical Centre
Chennai, Tamil Nadu
India

Subramani Seenivasan MD (Paed)
Fellowship in Pediatric Intensive Care
Assistant Professor
Government Hospital for Women and Children
Madras Medical College
Chennai, Tamil Nadu
India

Prem Kumar MD DA DNB
Associate Professor
Department of Anesthesia
Saveetha Medical College and Hospital
Chennai, Tamil Nadu
India

M Garthick Arivudainambi Dip (Derma)

K Vino Bharath DMRD DNB FRCR
Consultant Radiologist
Deepam Hospital
Deepam Kidney Stone Centre and Urology Clinic
Chennai, Tamil Nadu, India

P Selvaraj MS (Ortho) DNB (Ortho)
Assistant Professor
Government Villupuram Medical College
Chennai, Tamil Nadu
India

K Raman MD (Psy) PDFCAP (CMC, Vellore)
Associate Professor
Department of Psychiatry
Saveetha Medical College and Hospital
Chennai, Tamil Nadu
India

Foreword

With the extreme success of the TNPG 20 authors (TNPG Entrance book by the KONCPT 20 authors' team), the authors have released another book for the JIPMER entrance examination. JIPMER examination is always a high-standard examination with questions taken from the nooks and corners of the various textbooks. But, however, every year, about 50 percent questions get repeated from the previous JIPMER Question Banks. Also, the questions should cover the recent concepts and updated points. Keeping this in mind, the authors/contributors of the book have worked with utmost sincerity and dedication to give perfect explanation to the questions being previously asked. The students would always sit up for the preparation of JIPMER in the last one month after finishing their AIPG entrance examination. So, the students will crave for a book which will help them brush up the important topics and read the MCQs so that they can memorize the topics in a very easy manner.

To help the students in their study, this book is designed to cover the following important topics. Salient points have been given first followed by the important questions and then finally followed by the authenticated explanatory answers from the standard textbooks by the topmost 20 authors, who are also the faculties in many PG Entrance Coaching Centres.

The chief coordinating authors – Dr Abirami and Dr Magendran have put in a lot of efforts in bringing this book to live up to the expectations of the JIPMER-PG aspirants.

All the best for your exams!!

Rajamahendran R

Preface

As the JIPMER PG entrance examinations always pose a great challenge to the candidates all over the country, it has been a long-felt need of the PG aspirants for a compact and comprehensive book to help them get through the crisis. This book is a step towards this endeavor.

The book is integrative in its approach, allowing the students to have a broad general understanding of even difficult concepts that have been repeatedly asked in the JIPMER examinations. The uniqueness of this book is the spirit of collective responsibility evinced by its 20 authors, who are well-versed in their subjects of specialization.

The authors have made their best and sincere efforts in introducing the easiest possible approach to go through the previous years' JIPMER questions and answers with appropriate explanations in a more lucid and simple manner. All the subjects have been updated with the latest references.

We hope the students will find this book clear, cogent, and enjoyable to read.

We are very grateful to our publishers, Jaypee Brothers Medical Publishers (P) Ltd. for their editorial assistance.

We would sincerely appreciate the critical appraisal of this book and suggestions for its improvement in future.

"I would like to thank Dr Antan Uresh Kumar T and Dr Rajamahendran R from the bottom of my heart for their constant support and motivation. This book would not have seen the light of the day without their encouragement and guidance."

The difference between ordinary and extraordinary is that little EXTRA....

I am sure this book will provide you that little extra edge above others, which can help you streak ahead of competition and succeed in the forthcoming JIPMER examinations.

Wishing you all the success!!

Abirami

Acknowledgments

First and foremost, I am thankful to the Almighty, my parents, and my dear brother for what I am today.

I extend my heartfelt gratitude to Dr Antan Uresh Kumar T for encouraging my interest in teaching and bringing out the best in me. His confidence in me has always propelled me to work harder.

I express my sincere thanks to Dr Rajamahendran R for his useful suggestions and immense support throughout this project.

I wish to pay my deepest regards to JIPMER 20 authors' team. This book is just the reflection of the hard work and knowledge of all the 20 authors. I would like to thank my co-editor Dr Magendran for his support throughout the preparation of this book.

I would always remain grateful and obliged to all my teachers for their immense inspiration and guidance.

I am thankful to the KONCPT PG Medical Coaching Centre team for their constant support.

Special thanks to all my friends, especially Dr Brinda Angel and Dr Rajeshwari for their constant encouragement and motivation.

Thanks to our publishers, Jaypee Brothers Medical Publishers (P) Ltd, New Delhi, India, especially Shri Jitendar P Vij (Group Chairman), Ms Chetna Vohra (Associate Director), and Ms Payal Bharti (Project Manager) for their remarkable editorial and production support.

I would like to thank my parents-in-law, who have always blessed me with their love and affection. I would also thank my sister-in-law and brother-in-law for their love and care.

Behind every successful woman there is a man. Yes, I would love to thank the man behind my dreams and success—My Husband, who has been an unending source of moral support and help not only with this book but also with my life.

Abirami

From the Publisher's Desk

We request all the readers to provide us their valuable suggestions/errors (if any)

at: jppgmee@gmail.com

so as to help us in further improvement of this book in the subsequent edition.

Contents

Chapter

1

Anatomy

K Arumugam

SKIN

Epidermis: Ectoderm
Dermis: Mesoderm
Melanocytes: Yellow, brown or black colors.

Sweat glands

- 3 million in no
- Greatest concentration: Palm, sole, face
- Absent: Glans penis, tympanic membrane, margin of the lips.

Types

- Eccrine (Epicrine or Merocrine): Secretions by exocytosis—No loss of cytoplasam.
- Apocrine: Apical part of cell shed off to discharge secretion—partial loss of cytoplasm.
- Holocrine: Entire cell distentegrate to discharge the secretion—Whole cytoplasm lost.

Apocrine Glands

Examples: Atypical sweat glands: Axilla, areola of breast, Anal region (3 A'S) and Mammary glands.

- Odorless secretion
- Under control of sex hormones

Holocrine glands ex-sebaceous glands: Seen in relation with hair follicles

- Absent palms and soles. Montgomery tubercles around the areola are sebaceous glands.
- Ducts open directly on the skin suface (modified sebaceous glands) male and female genitalia, lip, papillae of breast, labia minora, Tarsal gland (meibonian gland).

Subcutaneous Tissues

- Panniculus adiposus: Blanket of fat beneath the skin.
- Panniculus carnosus: Flat sheet of muscle in panniculus adiposus.

Examples,

- Platysma, plamaris brevis, scalp muscles, scrotum: Dartos, subareolar muscle of nipple corrugator cutis ani, facial muscles.

Deep Fascia

- Absent: Face, ischioanal fossa, anterior abdominal wall

Ligaments Types

- White fibrous: Unstretchable, nonelastic
- Yellow elastic: Ligmantum flava, capsular ligament of joints of auditory ossicles.

CARTILAGE

- Nonvascular tissue and no nerves present in the cartilage
- Nutrition: Diffusion
- Most abundant cartilage: Hyaline cartilage
- Most durable cartilage: Fibrocartilage
- Largest yellow elastic cartilage: Cartilage of auricle
- Largest hyaline cartilage: Thyroid cartilage
- Perichondrium present in hyaline and elastic cartilage, but absent in fibrocartilage
- Growth of the cartilage: Interstitial and appositional
- Articular cartilage: Four Zones: Zone 1–Tangential stratum, Zone 2–Transitional stratum, Zone 3–Radiate stratum and Zone 4–calcified matrix.

Type	Nourishment	Calcification	Examples
Hyaline	Diffusion	Yes	All typical synovial joints articular surface, growing bones end. Broncial, Laryngeal, Articular, Costal, Embryonic, Tracheal cartilage (BLANKET)–Laryngeal cartilage except apex of arytenoids, corniculate, cuneiform and epiglottis. Articular cartilage are not covered by the perichondrium.
Elastic 3 Es	Diffusion	Never	Eustachian tube, external ear, epiglottis and corniculate, cuneiform
Fibro-cartilage	Sparse blood supply	No	Menici of knee joint, Intervertebral disks, labrum of shoulder joint and hip joint and symphysis-(MILS) at clavicle and mandible (articular surfaces) tendon to bony epiphysis attachment.

Bone

- *Intramembranous* (no cartilage precursor): Vault of skull, Clavicle
- *Intracartilaginous:* Base of skull, long bones

  Secondary cartilage: Special type of cartilage that develops in growing membrane bones (head of mandible, clavicle end)

  Sharpey's fibers: Inner layer of periosteum attached to cortex.

Law of Ossification

- The secondary center which appears first fuses last and that extremity of bone is growing end [Growing end is in opposite direction to nutrient foramen]
- In upper limb nutrient foramina directed towards elbow. In lower limb they are directed away from knee joint.

Fibula violates law of ossification

Metaphysis

- Muscles are mostly inserted here
- Vascularity is great
- More prone to pathological conditions.

Primary centre of ossification

The site where bone first forms. For example, in long bones diaphysis.

	Compact bone	Cancellous bone
Site	Shaft (Diaphysis)	Epiphysis
Lamallae	Haversian system +	No haversian system
Bone marrow	Yellow stores fat after puberty	Red produce RBC, WBC, Platlets
Nature	Hard and Ivory	Spongy

Bone of fetus and young child is red and then it become yellow. Red marrow persist thought life in the following sites sternum, ribs, iliac crest, vertebrae and skull bones

Woven Bone: Newly formed bone. Abnormal persist of woven bone is a feacture of Paget's disease.

Sesamoid bone: Seed like

Constant site: Patella, flexor pollicis brevis (hand and foot)

Skeletal Muscle

- The upper attachment is usually origin and lower attachment is insertion, exception—rectus abdominis, popliteus
- Insertion of tendon is usually at epiphysis except adductor magnus.

Nerve Supply

As a matter of morphological fact, limb nerves do not pierce muscles at all, but pass actually in planes between distinct morphological masses.

Exception: Coracobrachialis, supinator, sternocleidomastoid.

Blood Vessels

Smallest vessel capillaries

Layer	Artery	Vein
Tunica intima	Internal elastic lamina +	Present, no internal elastic lamina
Tunica media	Present	Thin
Tunica adventitia	External elastic lamina	Present

- IVC: No tunica media
- Umbilical arteries (2 in number)
  - Media—two layers
  - No elastic lamina

Venous Valves

No true valves: **PVC–SHHIP**

Pulmonary veins Vertebral veins Cardiac veins	SVC Head and neck veins Hepatic vein IVC Pelvic vein Portal vein

Muscles

Pennate muscle	–	Feather like
Unipennate	–	Extensor digitorum longus, Flexor pollicis longus, Tibialis posterior, peroneus tertius
Bipennate	–	Rectus femoris, flexor digitorum longus
Multipennate	–	Tibialis anterior, middle part of deltoid, Soleus, Flexor hallucis longus

Ephithelium type	Example
Simple squamous	Endothelium, mesothelium, endocardium
Simple cuboidal	Surface of ovaries-germinal epithelium,duct of gland, choroid plexuses, inner surface of lens and pigment layer of retina.
Simple columnar	Stomach, large intestine, cervical canal of uterus

Contd...

Contd...

Ephithelium type	Example
Pseudostratified columnar	Upper respiratory tract, distal part of ductus deferens and membranous and penile urthera
Stratified squamous-non-keratinized. Keratinized	Buccal cavity, esophagus, vagina and cornea. Skin
Stratified columnar	Longer ducts of gland
Transitional epithelium	Urinary tract

Mucous membrane of respiratory tract and GIT secrete mucus, but not most of urinary tract mucosa.

End arteries: Liver, spleen, kidney, lung, retina, medullary branches of CNS, straight branches of mesenteric arteries.

Lymphatic vessels: Superficial lymphatics follow veins while deep lymphatics follow arteries except tongue.

Hilton's law

The motor nerve to a muscle tends to give a branch of supply to the joint which the muscle moves and another branch to skin over the joint, e.g. nerve to quadratus femoris—Hip joint

Histology of Pancreas

- Exocrine and endocrine part
- **Exocrine part:** Secretory elements are called as pancreatic acini (Long tubular)
- Lining cells are serous with basophilic cytoplasm with eosinophilic granules at the apical part of the cell.
- **Centroacinar cells:** Intercalated ducts—cells in the centre part of the acinus that are invaginated into secretary elements.
- **Endocrine part:** Numerous collection of the cells embended within the exocrine part called as Islets of Langherhans neumerous in the tail of the pancreas.
- **Cells of Ilets of Langerhans are** 1. Alpha cells (A2) 2. Beta cells 3. Delta cells (A1) Type III cells

Alpha cells	Beta cells	Delta cells
Situated cortical part Stain with acid fusion	Medullary part Stain with aldehyde fusion	Periphery part Stain with silver salts with black so called as argyrophile
Smaller granules	Large electron dense granules	Round or ovoid less electron dense
Secrete glucagon	Secrete insulin	Secrete gastrin and somatostatin.
It form 20% of the total cells	It forms 70% of the cells	

EMBRYOLOGY

Tympanic membrane (All three dermal derivatives)

1. Tympanic membrane is formed by apposition of the tubotympanic recess and the first ectodermal cleft
2. These two structures form the inner endodermal and outer ectodermal epithelial linings
3. The intervening mesoderm forms the connective tissue

Tongue

- Starts at-approximately 4 weeks of embryo.

Anterior two-third (body of the tongue):

- Develops from first pharyngeal arch: two lateral lingual swellings and one medial swelling, the tuberculum impar.
- Lateral lingual swellings increase in size and merges with tuberculum impar, forming body of the tongue
- **Sensory innervation:** Mandibular branch of the trigeminal nerve.

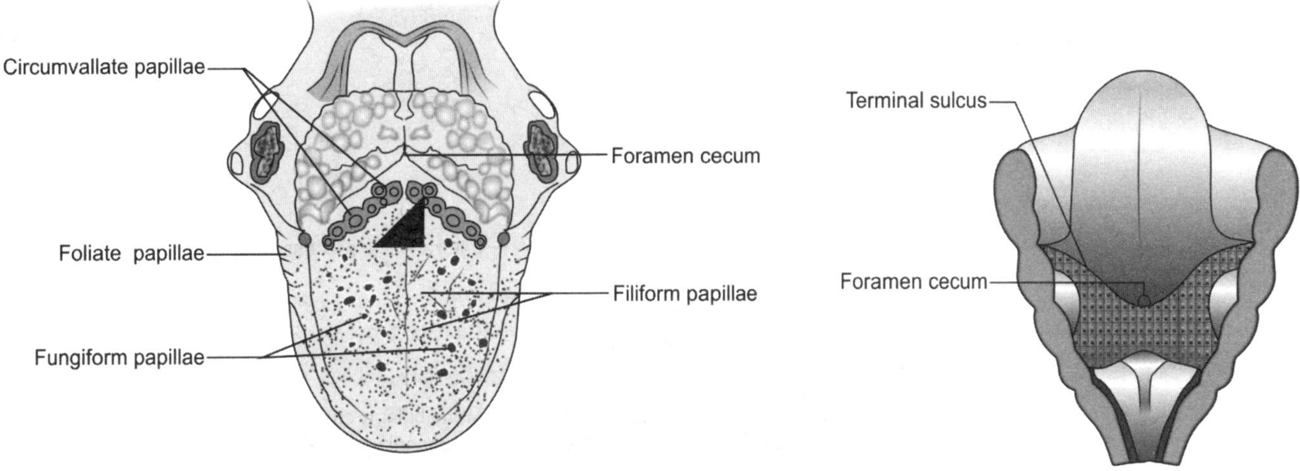

Fig. 1.1: Dorsal surface of the tongue

Posterior one Third (root of the tongue)

- A **second median swelling,** the **copula of His** or **hypobranchial eminence** is formed by mesoderm of the second, third, and part of the fourth arch
- **Sensory innervations: Glossopharyngeal nerve.**

Epiglottis

The epiglottis and the extreme posterior part of the tongue develop from the fourth arch as a **third median swelling** and are innervated by the **superior laryngeal nerve**

Tongue muscles: Intrinsic and Extrinsic muscles of tongue are derived from myoblasts that migrate into region of tongue from occipital somites. Motor innervations is by Hypoglossal nerve.

Origins of the craniofacial muscles

Mesodermal origin	Muscles	Innervations
Somitomeres 1, 2	Superior, medial, inferior recti	Oculomotor (III)
Somitomeres 3	Superior oblique	Trochlear (IV)
Somitomeres 4	Muscles of 1st pharyngeal arch	Mandibular nerve
Somitomeres 5	Lateral rectus	Abducens (VI)
Somitomeres 6	Jaw opening other 2nd arch	Facial (VII)
Somitomeres 7	Stylopharyngeus	Glossopharyngeal (IX)
Somites 1, 2	Intrinsic laryngeals	Vagus (X)
Somites 3–5	Tongue	Hypoglossal (XII)

Somites 3–5 constitute the occipital group (somite 1 degenerates for the most part).

Thyroid Gland

Derived: Foregut as thyroid diverticulum

Foramen cecum: Former site of thyroglossal duct

Face

5 processes → 1. Frontonasal process. V_1

2. A Pair of maxillary process. V_2
3. A pair of Mandibular arches. V_3

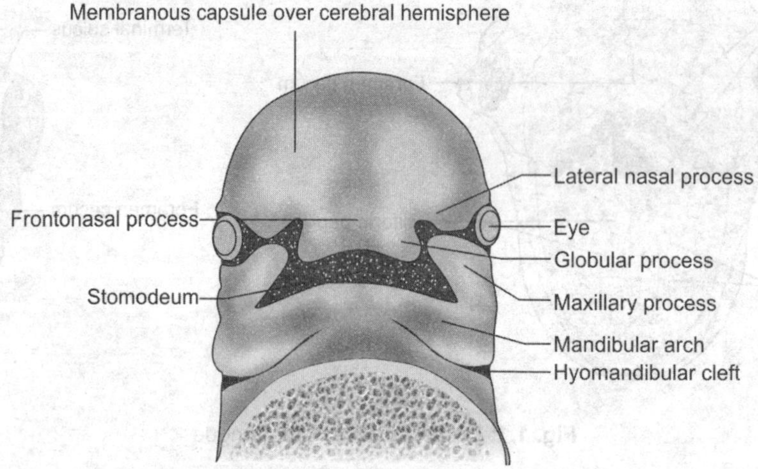

Fig. 1.2: Development of face

Structures contributing to formation of the face:

Prominence		Structures Formed
Frontonasal	Unpaired	Forehead, bridge of nose, medial and lateral nasal prominences
Maxillary	Paired	Cheeks, lateral portion of upper lip
Medial nasal	Paired	Philtrum of upper lip, crest and tip of nose
Lateral nasal	Paired	Alae of nose
Mandibular	Paired	Lower lip

Palate

Intermaxillary Segment and Primary Palate

Intermaxillary segment forms when two medial nasal prominences fuse together at midline. It gives rise to philtrum of lip, four incisor teeth and primary palate (anterior to incisive foramen).

Secondary Palate

Formed by outgrowth of maxillary prominences called palatine shelves

Primary and secondary palate fused at incisive foramen to form definitive palate

Development of alimentary system

Foregut	Midgut	Hindgut
Artery: Celiac trunk	**Artery: Sup. Mesenteric. A**	**Artery: Inf. Mesenteric. A**
Part of floor of the mouth, including tongue, Pharynx and Respiratory system Thyroid and various derivates of pharyngeal pouches esophagus, Stomach, Duodenum: Whole of the first part and upper half of the descending part (up to the major duodenal papilla)/ Ampulla of Vater Liver and extrahepatic biliary system, Pancreas	Duodenum: Part distal to major papilla Jejunum, Ileum cecum, appendix Ascending colon Right two-thirds of transverse colon	Left 1/3rd of transverse colon Descending and Sigmoid colon, Rectum Upper part of anal canal Parts of the urogenital system derived from the primitive urogenital sinus

Spleen: The spleen develops in the dorsal mesentery of the stomach (dorsal mesogastrium) and its mesodermal in origin.

Stomach: Left vagus nerve supplies the antreosuperior surface and right vagus nerve supplies posteroinferior surface of the stomach because stomach rotates to right through an angle of 90° rotation.

Secondary Retroperitonealization

Parts of the gut tube (most of the duodenum, ascending colon, descending colon, part of rectum) fuse with the body wall by way of fusion of visceral peritoneum with parietal peritoneum and secondary retroperitonealized.

Rotations of the Gut

The abdominal foregut rotates 90 degrees around its own long-axis such that the dorsal side rotates to the left and the ventral side rotates to the right. This results in the spleen being on the left. The communication between the lesser sac and the greater sac is the Epiploic foramen (of Winslow).

- Midgut: Herniates into the umbilical cord
  - Rotates 270 degrees (marked by the superior mesenteric artery), counterclockwise rotation,
  - Causes the colon to assume the shape of an **inverted 'U'**

Derivatives of:

Dorsal mesogastrium	Ventral mesogastrium
Greater Omentum, Gastrosplenic ligament, Gastrophrenic ligament and Lieno Renal ligament	Lesser Omentum, Falciform ligament, Coronary ligament, Right and left Triangular ligament

Meckel's Diverticulum

- Represents the persistent proximal part of the vitlline duct.
- It is present in 2% of population, situated in the antimesenteric border, usually 2 inches long and 2 feet from the Ileocecal valve. It has all the 3 coats of the intestinal wall and has its own blood supply.
- Derived from midgut.

Embryology of The Reproductive System

- Mesonephric duct/Wolffian duct is the main genital duct of males
- Paramesonephric duct/Mullerian duct is the main genital duct of females.

Fate of the structures derived from undifferentiated genital system

	Male	Female
Gondal/genital ridge	Testes, seminiferous tubules, rete testes	Ovary, follicles, rete ovary
Gubernacular cord	Gubernaculums testis	Proximal: Ovarian ligament Distal: Round ligament of uterus
Mesonephros (Wolffian body)	Appendix of epididymis Efferent ductules Lobules of epididymis	Appendices vesiculosae Epoophoron tubules Paroophoron tubules
Mesonephric duct (Wolffian duct)	Appendix of epididymis, Epididymis, Ductus Deferens, Seminal vesicle, Ejaculatory duct, Prostate. Remnants: – Superior aberrant tubule – Inferior aberrant tubule – Paradidymis	Remnants: – Paroophoron (Equivalent to paradidysmis in males) – Epoophoron/Gartner's duct (Equivalent to ductus deferens in males)
	Collecting tubule, Calyces, Pelvis, Ureter, trigone of bladder, Posterior wall of urethra	*Collecting tubule, Calyces, Pelvis, Ureter, trigone of bladder, Posterior wall of urethra*
Paramesonephric duct (Mullerian duct)	Appendix of testis Prostatic utricle	Uterine tube Uterus Vagina
Allantoic duct	Urachus	Urachus
Cloaca (Two parts)	Divided by Urorectal septum	

Contd...

Contd...

	Male	Female
Dorsal part (Anorectal canal)	Rectum and upper part of anal canal	Rectum and upper part of anal canal
Ventral part (Urogenital sinus)	Most of bladder Part of prostatic urethra Prostatic urethra distal to utricle Bulbourethral glands Rest of urethra to glands	Most of bladder and the Urethra Greater vestibular glands Vestibule, lower 1/3rd of vagina
Urogenital folds	Ventral penis	Labia minora
Genital tubercle	Glans penis	Clitoris
Labioscrotal swellings	Scrotum	Labia majora

The urorectal septum divides the cloaca into the anorectal canal and the urogenital sinus by week 7.

- Appendix of tests: Hydatid of morgagni
- Appendix of epididymis: Pedunculated hydatid of morgagni
- Paradidymis: Organ of girlades
- Epoophoron/organ of rosenumuller: Proximal tubules of mesonephric duct, at mesosalphinx
- Paraoophoron: Distal tubles of mesonephric duct, at base of broad ligament
- Gartner's duct: Remnant of Wolffian duct runs parallel and below the fallopian tube in the mesosalpinx and opens into lateral fornix of vagina.

Testis descent

- 4th month: Iliac fossa
- 7th month: Deep inguinal ring
- 7th and 8th month: Inguinal canal

Ectodermal derivatives:

- **Neuroectoderm:** CNS PNS, spinal, cranial and autonomic ganglia
- Neural crest: During neural plate formation, some cells at the junction between the neural plate and the rest of the ectoderm become specialized to form neural crest
- These cells soon become free by losing the property of cell to cell adhesion and migrate to different parts of the body.

Structures Derived from Neural Crest

- Connective tissue and bones of the face and skull
- Glial cells
- Arachnoid and pia mater (leptomeninges)
- Spinal (dorsal root) ganglia
- Cranial nerve ganglia [5, 7, 9, 10]
- Odontoblasts
- Dermis in face and neck
- C cells of the thyroid gland/parafollicular cells
- Conotruncal septum in the heart
- Sympathetic chain and preaortic ganglia of GIT
- Adrenal medulla
- Schwann cells
- Melanocyte, APUD, paraganglia, para aortic body.

Applied Aspects in Neural Crest

- Cleft-lip and cleft palate
- Frontonasal dysplasia

- Hirchsprung's disease
- Cardiac-septal defects (Aorticopulmonary)
- Tumors of adrenal medulla
- Albinism.

Surface Ectoderm: Epidermis, and its appendages, pituitary, mammary gland, cornea epithelium, conjunctiva, lacrimal gland, lens and retina, muscle: Iris muscles, erector pili and epithelial lining of oral cavity and terminal part of anal canal and urethra.

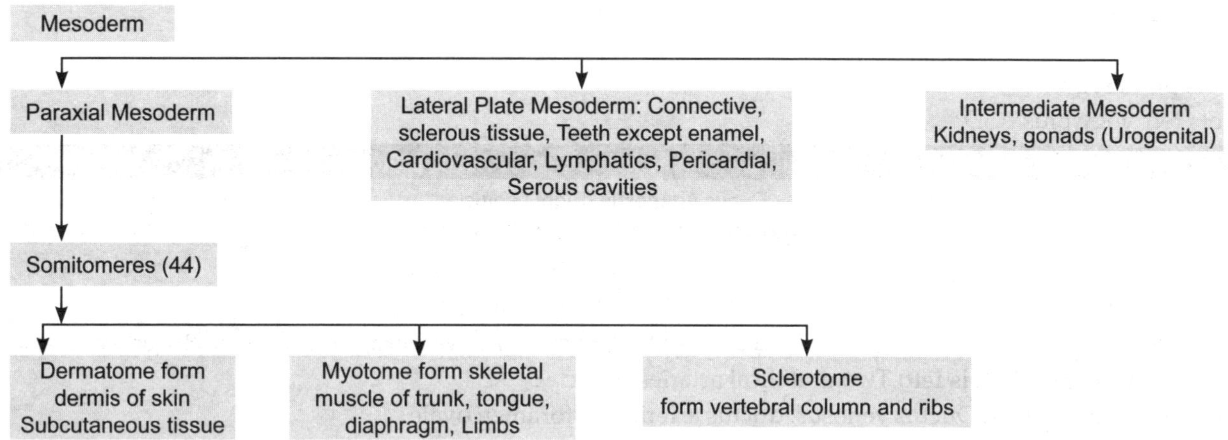

HEART EMBRYOLOGY

Development of Heart: Dextral rotation occurs

Intraembryonic coelom	Dorsal mesocarium	Somatopleuric mesoderm	Myocardium and epicardium	Endocardium
Pericardial cavity	Transverse pericardial sinus	Parietal pericardium	Myoepicardial mantle	Endothelial lining lateral plate mesoderm, primitive heart tube

Epicardium: Mesoderm from coelomic wall

Endothelial tube divided into 5 parts:

1. Sinus venosus
2. Primitive atrium
3. Primitive ventricle
4. Bulbus cordis
5. Truncus arteriosus

Left horn and body of the sinus venosus forms coronary sinus

Dextral rotation occurs during development

Interatrial septum from 3 sources:

1. Septum primum: Floor of fossa ovalis.
2. Septum secundum: Limbus fossa ovalis.
3. Septum intermedium.

Interventricular septum from

- Muscular part of ventricle
- Septum intermedium: Membranous part
- Proximal bulbar septum

Fallots tetralogy

- Pulmonary stenosis
- Displacement aortic orifice to right to override ventricular septum
- RV hypertrophy
- Patent interventricular foramen.

Fallots trialogy

- Pulmonary stenosis
- RV hypertrophy
- ASD

Fallots pentalogy

Fallots tetrology plus ASD

Truncus arteriosus	Aorta, pulmonary trunk
Bulbus cordis	Conus Arteriosus (Right ventricle) Aortic vestibule (Aortic outflow Tract)
Primitive ventricle	Trabeculated part of Rt. and Lt. ventricle
Primitive atrium	Trabeculated part of Rt. and Lt. atrium
Sinus venosus	Smooth part of Rt.atrium (sinus venerum),coronary sinus, oblique V of Lt.atrium

One umbilical vein (Left is left) Two umbilical arteries–VAA

Fetal circulation shunts: Ductus venosus, ductus arteriosus, foramen ovale

- Common arterial trunk: Truncus arteriosus—6 pairs of aortic arches appear 1st, 2nd and 5th arches disappear.

First artery to appear in embryo: Right and left primitive aorta.

DEVELOPMENT OF VENOUS SYSTEM

Superior vena cava	From right anterior cardinal vein and right common cardinal vein	
Inferior vena cava	**Segment**	**From**
	Hepatic	Right hepatic vein
	Prerenal	Right subcardinal vein
	Renal	Right subcardinal and supracardinal anastomosis
	Postrenal	Right supracardinal vein
	Lower end	Right posterior cardinal vein

Vein	Developed from
Superior mesenteric vein	Anterior limb of anastomosis between the two infrahehatic vitelline veins
Trunk portal vein	Dorsal anastomosis between the two vitelline veins and the right vitelline vein
Terminal part of IVC	Suprahepatic part of right vitelline vein
Cavernous sinus	Primary head vein medial to the trigeminal ganglion.
Sigmoid sinus	Communicating channel between the middle and posterior dural stems including posterior dural stem
Transverse sinus	Communicating channel between the middle and anterior dural stems
Superior petrosal sinus	Middle dural stem
Superior ophthalmic vein	Primitive maxillary vein
Left brachiocephalic vein	Oblique cross communication between both anterior cardinal veins caudal to subclavian vein
Right brachiocephalic vein	Right anterior, cardinal vein between subclavian and oblique channel

Contd...

Contd...

Vein	Developed from
Internal jugular vein	Anterior cardinal vein cephalic to subclavian vein
SVC	Right anterior cardinal vein below the oblique connection and right common cardinal vein (Duct of cuvier)
Ligament of left vena cavae and left superior intercostals vein	Caudal part of left anterior cardinal vein
Oblique vein of left atrium	Left common cardinal vein
Arch of azygos vein	Cephalic part of right posterior cardinal vein
Vertical part of azygos vein	Right azygos venous line
IVC	Caudal part of right posterior cardinal vein Right supracardinal vein Anatomosis between right supracardinal and right subcardinal vein Upper part of right subcardinal vein New vessel arise from right subcardinal veingrows dorsal to liver with the common hepatic vein Common hepatic vein suprahepatic part of right vitelline vein

Vestigeal

Remnant of	Structure
Ductus arteriosus	Ligamentum arteriosum
Ductus venosus	Ligamentum venosus
Left umbilical vein	Ligamentum teres of liver
Right umbilical vein	Disappears
Urachus	Median umbilical ligament
Foramen ovale	Fossa ovalis
Proximal part of umbilical A	Internal iliac and superior vesical artery
Distal part of umbilical A	Medial umbilical ligament
Left common cardinal vein/cuvier's duct	Oblique vein of left atrium
Vitellointestinal duct	Meckel's diverticulum

1. **Left gonadal vein drain into**
   a. IVC
   b. Left renal vein
   c. Left common iliac vein
   d. Left internal iliac vein
   Ans. **b.**
2. **Right gonadal vein drain into**
   a. IVC
   b. Right Renal vein
   c. Right common iliac vein
   d. Right internal iliac vein
   Ans. **a.**
   The anastomosis between the left subcardinal vein and left supracardinal vein which receive left gonadal vein developed into left renal vein. This part on the right side developed into part of postrenal segment of IVC.
   Embryology of Diaphragm
   Septum transversum: Central tendon
   Pleuroperitoneal membrane: Tendinous part
   Dorsal mesentry of esophagus: Crus
   Body wall: Musculature
   Applied: Congenital Hernia/posterolateral opening: Bochdalek

DEVELOPMENT OF SKIN

- Epidermis and its appendages, pilo sebaceous unit, nail and sweat glands: surface ectoderm
- Melanocyte and Merkel cells: Neural crest
- Langerhan's cells: Bone marrow
- Dermis in limbs and trunks: Somatopleuric mesenchyme
- Dermis in face, head and neck: Neural crest.

Extra Points

- The major growth-promoting factor during development before and after birth is insulin like **growth factor–I (IGF–I), which has mitogenic and anabolic effects**.
- Fetal tissues express IGF: I and serum levels are correlated with fetal growth
- Mutations in the IGF: I gene result in IUGR and this growth retardation is continued after birth
- In contrast to the prenatal period, postnatal growth depends upon growth hormone (GH).

UPPER LIMB

Brachial Plexus

- Named as posterior, medial and lateral cord w.r.t. relation to axillary artery lying under pectoralis minor.
- In the axilla, the lateral and posterior cords of the brachial plexus are lateral to the first part of the axillary artery, and the medial cord is behind the artery. The cords surround the second and third part of the artery, their names indicating their relationship. *Ref: Gray's 40/e ch46*
- Roots–C5, C6, C7, C8, T1
- **Site:** Roots (scalene anterior muscle, prevertebral muscle) The roots usually pass through the gap between the anterior and the middle scalene muscles with the subclavian artery *Ref: Keith & more p774*
- The subclavius, although not of major importance as a muscle, affords some protection to the underlying neurovascular structures when the clavicle is (commonly) fractured in its middle third. *Ref: Keith & more p775*
- The roots lie between the anterior and middle scalene muscles. The trunks traverse the posterior triangle of the neck. The divisions lie behind the clavicle. The cords lie in the axilla. *Ref: Harold Ellis 11/e p190*

Only exception for 3, 5, 5 rule is branch from trunk—suprascapular nerve 10% are prefixed, 10% are post fixed.

Supraclavicular part

Roots: Dorsal scapular nerve (rhomboids) C5
Long thoracic nerve of Bell C5, 6, 7
Nerve to scalene and longus colli C5, C6, C7, C8
Branch to phrenic nerve C5

Trunks: suprascapular nerve (C5, C6) and N to Subclavis (C5, C6).

Infraclavicular Part

Lateral cord

- Lateral pectoral nerve: Pectoralis major and minor
- Lateral root of median nerve (Direct continuation of lateral cord)
  - Musculocutaneous nerve (C5–7): Coracobrachialis, Biceps, Branchialis, Lateral cutaneous nerve of forearm. The musculocutaneous nerve arises from the lateral cord (C5–7), opposite the lower border of pectoralis minor. It pierces coracobrachialis. The branch to coracobrachialis is given off before the musculocutaneous nerve enters the muscle: its fibers are from the seventh cervical ramus and may branch directly from the lateral cord. Branches to biceps and brachialis leave after the musculocutaneous has pierced coracobrachialis. *Ref: Gray's 40/e ch46*

Medial cord: (4MU)

- Medial pectoral nerve: Pectoralis major and minor (Pierces pectoralis minor)
- Medial root of median nerve
- Medial cutaneous nerve of arm (smallest and most medial of all branches)
- Medial cutaneous nerve of forearm
- Ulnar nerve (largest branch of medial cord) (C7, C8, T1): Direct continuation of medial cord is ulnar nerve. The ulnar nerve arises from the medial cord (C8, T1) but often receives fibres from the ventral ramus of C7. It runs distally through the axilla medial to the axillary artery, between it and the vein. *Ref: Gray's 40/e ch46*
- The median nerve has two roots from the lateral (C5, 6, 7) and medial (C8, T1) cords, which embrace the third part of the axillary artery, and unite anterior or lateral to it. *Ref: Gray's 40/e p46*

Posterior cord: (ULNAR)

- Upper subscapular nerve: Subscapularis muscle
- Lower subscapular nerve: Subscapularis muscle, teres major
- Nerve to lattismus dorsi (thoracodorsal nerve)
- Axillary nerve: Deltoid, teres minor, upper lateral cutaneous nerve of arm
- Radial nerve (largest branch of whole plexus) (C5–8,T1): Direct continuation of posterior cord. The radial nerve is the largest branch of the brachial plexus. It arises from the posterior cord (C5, 6, 7, 8, (T1) and descends behind the third part of the axillary artery and the upper part of the brachial artery, anterior to subscapularis and the tendons of latissimus dorsi and teres major. *Ref: Gray's 40/e ch46*

Brachial Plexus Injury

Erb's palsy–C5 C6 Upper trunk

Upper plexus

- **M**usculocutaneous nerve
  - **B**iceps, **B**rachialis, **C**oracobrachialis
- **A**xillary nerve
  - Deltoid and Teres minor
- **S**uprascapular nerve
  - Supraspinatus and Infraspinatus

Causes: Fall on the shoulder, obstetric complication.

Effects

- Forearm: Extended (Biceps) and Pronated (biceps)
- Arm: Adducted (Deltoid and Supraspinatus) and Medially rotated (Infraspinatus and teres minor)
- Shoulder: Loss of intrinsic muscles
- Waiter's tip
- Loss of sensation: Lower part of Deltoid
- Nerve arises from Erb's point: Suprascapular nerve and Nerve to subclavius (Sometimes)

A superior brachial plexus injury may produce muscle spasms and a severe disability in hikers (backpacker's palsy) who carry heavy backpacks for long periods. *Ref: Keith & more p780*

Klumpke's Paralysis: Lower Trunk Involved

Causes

Pancoast tumor, CA of breast, Cervical rib

- Root: C8, T1
- Nerves: Ulnar, median
- Ape thumb, claw hand
- Include horner's syndrome

- Caused by: Excessive abduction of shoulder
- Cutaneous anesthesia and analgesia in a narrow zone along the ulnar border of forearm and hand

Root Damage

Serratus anterior also paralyzed

Terminal nerves and motor supply

Musculocutaneous N	Biceps brachii, Coracobrachialis and medial part of Brachialis
Axillary N	Deltoid and Teres minor
Radial N	Posterior muscles of arm and forearm

Innervation of upper limb

- All muscles of anterior compartment of arm: **Musculocutaneous nerve**
- Muscles in the anterior compartment of the forearm, except the flexor carpi ulnaris (ulnar nerve) and medial half of the flexor digitorum profundus (ulnar nerve): **Median nerve**
- Most intrinsic muscles of the hand: **Ulnar nerve,** except thenar muscles and two lateral lumbrical muscles (median nerve)
- All muscles in the posterior compartments of the arm and forearm: **radial nerve.**

Collateral Nerves

Long thoracic N	Serratus anterior
Medial pectoral N	Pectoralis major and minor
Lateral pectoral N	Pectoralis major and minor
Upper subscapular N	Subscapularis
Lower subscapular N	Subscapularis and Teres major
Thoracodorsal N	Lattismus dorsi
Suprascapular N	Supraspinatus and Infraspinatus
Dorsal scapular N	Rhomboids

Segmental innervation of muscles

- Proximal: Distal gradient
- C5—C6: Shoulder
- C8—T1: Hand

Important Root Values

- Median nerve: C5, 6, 7, 8 and T1
- Radial nerve: C5, 6, 7, 8 and T1
- Axillary nerve: C5, 6
- Thoracodorsal nerve: C6, C7 and C8
- Musculocutaneous nerve: C5, C6 and C8
- Upper and lower subscapular nerve: C5 and C6.

1. Which of the following nerve end as Pseudoganglion?

a. Radial nerve

b. Musculocutaneaous nerve

c. Median nerve

d. Axillary nerve

Ans. **d.** *Ref: AK Dutta 4/e p52*

Axillary nerve: Root value C5, C6.
Leaves the axilla and enters the arm through the quadrangular space along with posterior circumflex vessels.
Anterior branch supplies Deltoid muscle.
Posterior branch supplies Teres minor.
Posterior branch ends as pseudoganglion.
Nerves forming pseudoganglion: Axillary nerve, lateral branch of deep peroneal nerve and posterior interossseous nerve.

2. **What is Ulnar collateral nerve?**
   a. Medial cutaneous nerve of forearm
   b. Medial cutaneous nerve of arm
   c. Nerve to medial head of ticeps
   d. All the above

Ans. **c.** *Ref: Gray's 40/e p46*

Radial nerve: Continuation of posterior card of brachial plexus.
Root value C5, C6, C7, C8 and T1
Leaves the axilla through the lower triangular space accompanied with the profunda brachii artery. Enters the upper part of front of arm behind the Brachial artery.
Enter the spiral groove by passing between longhead of triceps and medial head of triceps. Then passing between lateral and medial head of triceps.
Again enter the front of lower part of arm by piercing lateral intermuscular septum along with radial collateral artery.
Medial muscular branches arise from the radial nerve on the medial side of the arm. They supply the medial and longheads of triceps; the branch to the medial head is a long, slender filament which, lying close to the ulnar nerve as far as the distal third of the arm, is often termed the ulnar collateral nerve. A large posterior muscular branch arises from the nerve as it lies in the humeral groove. It divides to supply the medial and lateral heads of triceps and anconeus. Lateral muscular branches arise in front of the lateral intermuscular septum; they supply the lateral part of brachialis, brachioradialis and extensor carpi radialis longus.

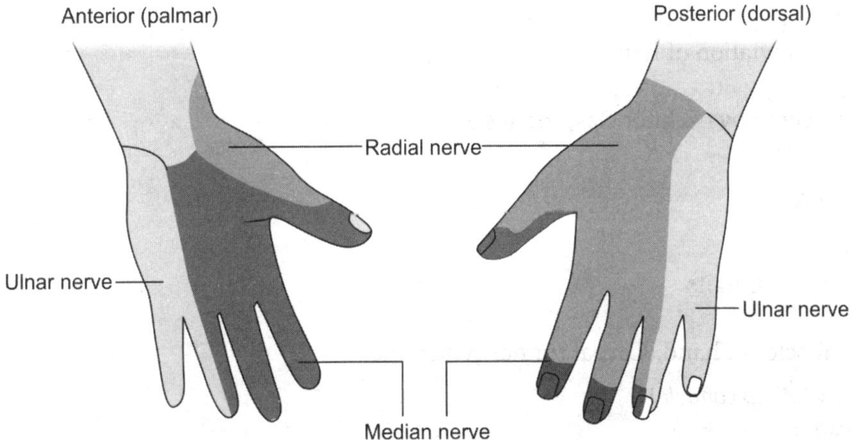

Fig. 1.3: Innervation of palmar and dorsal surface of the hand

Radial Nerve Innervation

- **B**rachioradialis, **E**xtensors Carpi Radialis longus, **A**nconeus and **T**riceps. All other posterior compartment muscles are supplied by posterior interosseus nerve.

Radial nerve injury: Axilla

- Saturday night palsy
- **Extensors loss**: At elbow, wrist, digits

- Weakened extensors: Shoulder
- Weakened supination
- **Anesthesia**: Posterior arm, forearm and hand, **Wrist drop**
- Autonomous Zone for radial nerve is dorsum of first space

Radial nerve injury: Elbow

Radial tunnel syndrome is an entrapment neuropathy of the radial nerve near the elbow, where four structures can potentially cause compression of the nerve. These are fibrous bands (which can tether the radial nerve to the radiohumeral joint); the sharp tendinous medial border of extensor carpi radialis brevis; a leash of vessels from the radial recurrent artery as it passes to supply brachioradialis and extensor carpi radialis longus; **the arcade of Frohse, which is the free aponeurotic proximal edge of the superficial part of supinator.** *Ref: Gray's 40/e ch49*

- Extensors loss: Wrist, digits
- Anesthesia: Posterior forearm and hand
- Fracture of shaft of humerus
- **Wrist drop.**

Radial nerve injury–wrist

- Only sensory loss posterior hand (1st web space)

Median Nerve Injury: Elbow

Pronator syndrome

This is an uncommon entrapment neuropathy of the median nerve occurring in the elbow region. Entrapment can occur typically at four sites. The first occurs at the site of the ligament of Struthers. The nerve may also be trapped as it passes deep to the bicipital aponeurosis; the aponeurotic edge of the deep head of pronator teres muscle; or the tendinous aponeurotic arch forming the proximal free edge of the radial attachment of flexor digitorum superficialis. *Ref: Gray's 40/e ch48*

- Ape thumb deformity or Simian hand
- Claw hand
- Loss of pronation
- Wrist flexion: Ulnar deviation of hand
- Sensory loss
- Pointing Index (detected by oschner clasping test)
- Pen test.

Median Nerve Injury–Wrist

- Ape thumb
- Claw hand: 2nd and 3rd digits
- Sensory loss
- Loss of intrinsic muscles of hand, Carpal tunnel syndrome

Ulnar Nerve Injury–Elbow (Ml. epicondyle)

Cubital tunnel syndrome

Typically the ulnar nerve can be compressed in the tunnel formed by the tendinous arch connecting the two heads of flexor carpi ulnaris at their humeral and ulnar attachments. Other local causes of compression and neuritis at this site include trauma, inflammatory arthritis, compression by the medial head of the triceps. *Ref: Gray's 40/e ch48*

- Claw hand
- Sensory loss
- Forearm Muscles: Deinnervation.

Ulnar nerve injury: Wrist

- Claw hand
- Sensory loss

- Ulnar tunnel syndrome is an entrapment neuropathy of the ulnar nerve as it passes through Guyon's canal at the wrist. Causes of compression at this site include a ganglion, trauma, and proximity of aberrant or accessory muscles. The symptoms include pain in the hand or forearm and sensory changes in the palmar aspect of the little and ulnar half of the ring fingers, however sensation on the ulnar aspect of the dorsum of the hand is normal. In addition there may be weakness and wasting of the intrinsic muscles of the hand supplied by the ulnar nerve, with clawing posture in extreme cases. *Ref: Gray's Anatomy 40/e ch50*
- In low ulnar palsy, forearm muscles are spared by clawing will be more (**ulnar paradox).**

Nerves passing through

- Median N: Pronator teres
- Ulnar N: Flexor carpi ulnaris
- Posterior interosseus N: Supinator
- Musculocutaneous N pierces: Coracobrachialis.

Axillary nerve injury

Axillary nerve injury: Bandage like sensory loss over lower part of the deltoid called Regimental bandage. **(BDC)**

- Fracture surgical neck of humerus
- Loss of abduction of arm
- Sensory loss: Lower half of Deltoid (egg shaped anesthesia).

Speciality	Ulnar nerve	Radial nerve	Median nerve
Passes between	Two heads of flexor carpii ulnaris	Posterior interosseus nerve between 2 heads of Supinator	Two heads of pronator teres
Relation to forearm muscle	Under cover of flexor carpii ulnaris	Under cover of brachioradialis	Deep to flexor digm. Superficialis
Vessels	Ulnar artery lies radially	Radial artery lies medially	Crosses ulnar artery and lies between ulnar artery and FDS (flexor digm superficialis)
Flexor retinaculum	Superficial to it		Deep to it
	Guyons canal		Carpal tunnel
Branches	Superficial and deep branch	Posterior interosseus nerve	Anterior interosseus nerve

Martin–Gruber connection

Multiple communicating branches between the median nerve (and sometimes the anterior interosseous nerve) arise proximally and pass medially between flexors digitorum superficialis and profundus, present in 17% of individuals. *Ref: Gray's 40/e ch49*

- **Muscles and the nerves related**

Between two heads of Pronator teres	Median N
Between two heads of Flexor carpi ulnaris	Ulnar N
Supinator muscle (pierced)	Posterior interosseus N
Coracobrachialis (pierced)	Musculocutaneous N

Fractures and Nerve Injury

Surgical neck of humerus	Axillary nerve
Inferior dislocation of shoulder	Axillary nerve, radial N
Spiral groove fracture	Radial N
Medial epicondyle: Humerus	Ulnar nerve

Contd...

Contd...

Supracondylar fracture	Median nerve
Radius neck fracture	Posterior interosseus nerve
Hook of hamate	Ulnar
Lunate dislocation	Median nerve

TESTS TO DETECT ULNAR PLASY

- Book test **(Froment sign)**
- Card test (to test Palmar interossei) adduction of fingers (PADI)
- **Egawa's test** (to test dorsal interossei) adduction of fingers (DAB)
- Ulnar claw hand (main en grifee)
  - Tip of little finger is the autonomous zone for ulnar N.
  - Entrapment of ulnar N leads to cubital tunnel syndrome
  - Involvement beneath flexor carpi ulnaris: less claw hand

Nerve paralysis	Muscle transplanted	
Radial nerve	Pronator teres	Posterior compartment
Median nerve	Brachioradialis	Into Flexor pollicis longus

Know it

- Most commonly injured nerve at high up (upper limb): Radial nerve
- Most commonly injured nerve behind elbow or at wrist: Ulnar
- Most commonly injured nerve at wrist by cuts or compression: Median
- Only autonomus area of median nerve supply: Pulp pad of index and middle finger
- Web of thumb: Sensory innervations by radial nerve
- Musculocutaneous nerve gives lateral cutaneous nerve of forearm
- Crutch pressing in axilla: Radial nerve palsy
- The lateral two (1st and 2nd) lumbricals are unipennate muscles
- The medial two (3rd and 4th) lumbricals are bipennate.

Movements of pectoral girdle

Elevation : Trapezius, levator scapula
Depression : Pect. minor, serratus anterior
Protract : Serratus Anterior and pectoralis minor
Retraction : Trapezius, Rhomboids.

Mammary Gland

Modified sweat gland

Apocrine gland

Extent: mid line to mid axillary line, 2nd to 6th rib

Mammary tissue does not extend beyond areola

Milk line: Axilla to groin, develops 4th week of intrauterine life.

Foramen of langer: Defect in axillary fascia through which breast tissue extends into axilla

Axillary tail of Spence: Breast tissue extending into axilla in superficial plane (mostly)

Coopers ligament: Suspensory ligament

Nipple

4 Intercostal space in nulliparaous

15–20 lactiferous duct opening

Areola has sebaceous gland

Tubercles of montgomery: Modified sebaceous gland in the areola enlarged during pregnancy and lactation.

Ref: Gray's anatomy 40/e ch54

Capsule of breast

Behind the breast superficial fascia condensed to form a posterior capsule

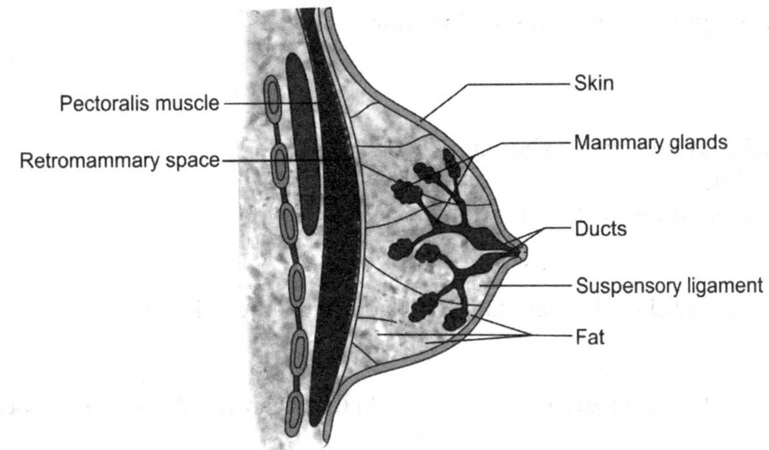

Fig. 1.4: The female breast

Retromammary space

- Space between capsule of breast and fascia over pectoralis major
- This is the space in which breast prosthesis are inserted
- Avascular space
- Contains lymphatics called as **Lake of Marelli.** (TSR)

Suspensory ligaments of cooper (fibrous tissues connects dermis to Capsule of breast)

Blood supply

- Main supply lateral thoracic artery
- Internal thoracic artery: 2nd and 3rd space vessels are largest
- Drainage to axillary v. tributaries
- Some drainage to posterior intercostal vein (main link for vertebral venous system).

Lymphatics

- Most lymph drains into axilla
- There are no valves in intramammary lymphatic channels
- Axillary nodes: 35 to 50 in number
- Rotters node: Interpectoral node

Pectoral group or Anterior axillary most

75% axillary (pectoral, subscapular, central, apical)

Deep node apical

Medial parasternal

Nerves: Intercostal 2 to 6 sensory and Sympathetic.

Pectoralis major

- Origin sternal head: Clavicular head
- Insertion: Lateral lip of bicipital groove
- Supply: Medial and lateral pectoral nerve
- The muscle is only one in upper limb to be supplied by all five segments of brachial plexus
- The degree of paralysis of pectoralis major may be helpful in gauging the extent of a brachial plexus injury

- Action: Medial rotator of arm, adductor of arm (Along with latissimus)
- Poland syndrome absent pectoralis major.

Pectoralis minor

- Inserted into coracoids process
- By both pectoral nerves
- Action: Protraction of scapula along with serr. Anterior
- Depression of shoulder.

Rectus sternalis

- Derivative of superficial layer of rectus abdominis
- Supplied by intercostal nerves
- Fused with sternal tendon of sternocleidomastoid.

Subclavius muscle

Prevents jagged end of fractured clavicle from damaging adjacent subclavian vein.

Clavi pectoral fascia

Forms costocoracoid ligament, suspensory ligament of axilla (between 1st rib coracoid process).

Structures piercing

- **C:** Cephalic vein
- **A:** Acromiothoracic vessels thoracoacromial vein joins the cephalic vein before it pierces the clavipectoral fascia. So only artery pierces the fascia not vein *Ref: Datta 4/e vol 1 p42*
- **L:** Lateral pectoral nerve
- **L:** Lymphatics
- Axillary abscess incised pus drained at axillary base.

Trapezius

- Most superficial muscle of upper part of back

Action

- Retract the scapula (pull it towards midline)
- Turning wing nut

Lattismus dorsi

- Adductor of arm (along with pectoralis major)
- Climbing muscle
- Accessory muscle of expiration
- Only muscle of upper limb to have a pelvic attachment

Triangle of auscultation:

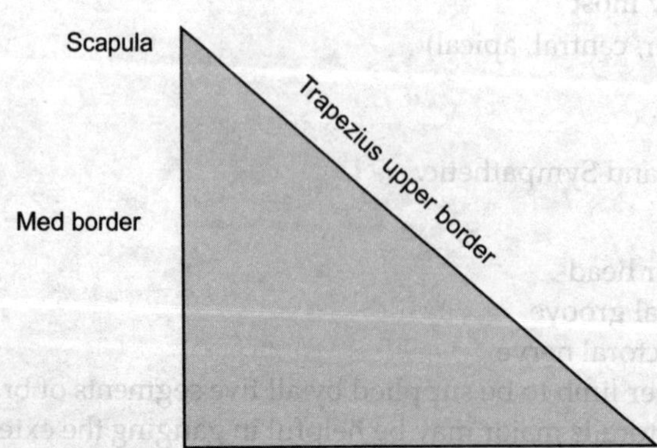

Triangle of auscultation	
Medially	Lateral border of trapezius
Laterally	Medial border of Scapula
Inferiorly	Upper border of Latissimus dorsi
Floor	6th and 7th intercostals space, 7th rib, Rhomboideus major

Importance

- Left side: Cardiac orifice of stomach during preradiological days, splash of swallowed liquids was timed in cases of esophageal obstruction.

Levator scapulae

Forms floor of posterior triangle.

Serratus anterior

- Upper eight ribs: Origin as eight digitations
- Punching and pushing action.

Quadrangular space

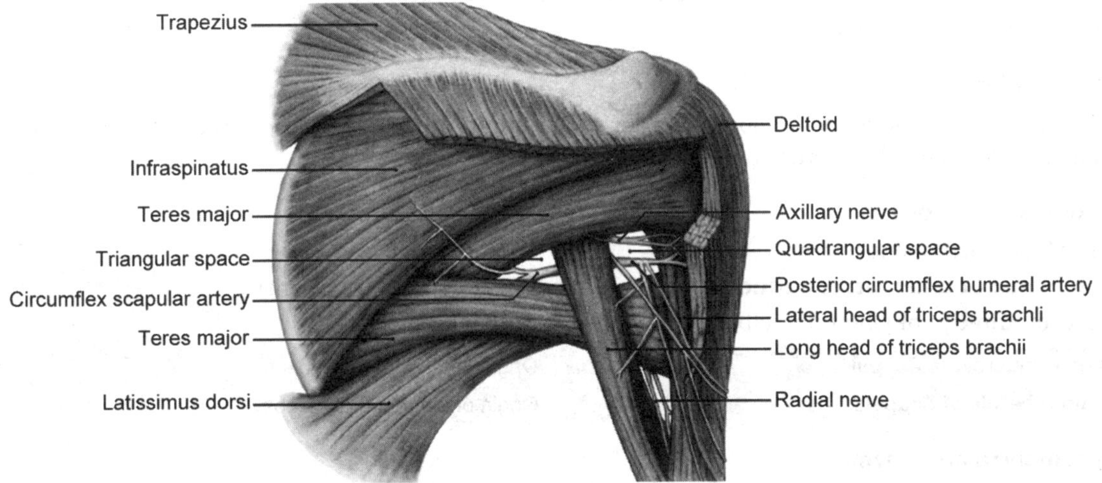

Fig. 1.5: Section shows quadrangular and triangular spaces

- Lateral: Humerus surgical
- **Superior: Subscapularis, teres minor, capsule of shoulder**
- Inferior: Teres major
- Medial: Longhead of triceps.

Contents: Axillary nerve, posterior circumflex humeral vessels.

Triangular space

- Lateral—Humerus
- Superior—Teres major
- Medial—Longhead of triceps.

Contents: radial nerve, profunda brachii artery.

Triceps

Heads of origin: Longhead, medial head, lateral head.

Longhead of triceps: Stabilise shoulder joint during abduction (lower part of the shoulder joint–weakest part of joint)

Articularis cubiti or subanconeus: Fibers of triceps attached to the capsule of the elbow joint. It prevent nipping the capsule of elbow joint.

Attachment to lesser tuberosity

- Subscapularis muscle.

Attachment to greater tuberosity

- Supraspinatous, infraspinatous, teres minor.

Lateral rotator of humerus

- Intraspinatous
- Teres minor.

Medial rotator

- Subscapularis
- Teres major.

Rotator cuff

- Supraspinatous
- Infraspinatous
- Teres minor
- Subscapularis.

It gives strength to the capsule of shoulder joint all around **except inferiorly**

No rotator action for supraspinatous.

Intramuscular Injection

Should not be more than 4 cm below lower border of acromion process, axillary nerve curls forwards round the back of humerus 5–6 cm below acromion.

Anterior compartment of arm

- Nerve: Musculocutaneous.

Coracobrachialis: Counterpart of adductors of thigh, struthers ligament (remnant)

Biceps: Acts on three joint (shoulder, elbow, proximal radioulnar).

Supraglenoid tubercle of Scapula	Origin of longhead of biceps
Infraglenoid tubercle of Scapula	Origin of longhead of triceps

Posterior compartment of arm:

Triceps: Medial, long, lateral head

Innervations by radial before it gets into spiral groove—medial and longhead, lateral head, and medial head is supplied behind the humerus.

Applied: Fracture humerus will spare triceps innervations.

Septum of arm

Medial intermuscular septum	Pierced by ulnar nerve and ulnar collateral artery
Lateral intermuscular septum	Pierced by radial nerve and profunda brachii artery

Carrying angle

Definition: Extended ulna makes with the humerus an angle of about 170 degree

Most of carrying angle at elbow is formed by obliquity of shaft of ulna to its curved ridge (Which joins the prominence of coronoid process and olecranon, the ridge fits groove in the trochlea of humerus)

Arm and the forearm forms an obtuse angle which opens on the lateral side. This angle prominent on extended elbow and supinated forearm. Cause Medial edge of the trochlea projecting below the lateral edge and the obliquity of the superior articular surface of the coronoid process. *Ref: Datta 4/e p118*

Anterior compartment of forearm:

Superficial	Deep
Pronator teres Flexor carpi radialis Flexor digitorum superficialis Palmaris longus Flexor carpi ulnaris	Pronator quadrates Flexor pollicis longus Flexor digitorum profondus

Pronator teres

- Supplied by first (highest) branch of median nerve
- Median nerve lies between its two heads
  1. *Flexor carpi radialis tendon:*
     - The radial artery lies lateral to the tendon and the median nerve lies medial to it
     - Important stabilizer of wrist in finger and thumb movements.
  2. *Flexor carpi ulnaris tendon:*
     - Ulnar artery pulsation is felt lateral to tendon of flexor carpi ulnaris just above pisiform bone.

Palmaris longus

- Absent in 13% of arms
- Short belly and long tendon
- Mistaken for median nerve
- Go in front of flexor retinaculum.

Flexor carpi ulnaris

- Ulnar nerve enters between two heads
- The pisiform is morphologically a sesamoid bone in the tendon.

Cubital fossa

- Triangular area between pronator teres, branchioradialis and a line joining the humeral epicondyles
- Contents: (Medial to Lateral) **MBBS**—Median Nerve, Branchial Artery, Biceps tendon, farther laterally–superficial branch of radial nerve.
- **Boundaries of cubital fossa:**

Boundary	Content	Boundary	Content
Lateral	Brachioradialis	Apex	Joining of medial and lateral walls
Medial	Pronator teres	Floor	Brachialis, supinator
Base	Line joining epicondyles	Roof	Median cubital vein, lateral and medial cutaneous nerve of forearm, Antebrachial fascia, Bicipital aponeurosis

Deep Fascia of the Forearm

This deep fascia, together with the interosseous membrane and fibrous intermuscular septa, divide the forearm into a number of compartments. These are the superficial and deep flexor (anterior) compartments, the extensor (posterior compartment) and a proximolateral compartment known as the **mobile wad (encompassing brachioradialis and extensors carpi radialis longus and brevis)** *Ref: Gray's anatomy 40/e ch49*

Flexor digitorum superficialis or sublimus:

- Oblique origin of FDS: Upper limit of space of Parona
- Median nerve plastered to its deep surface.

Flexor digitorum profundus (FDP)

- Most powerful and bulkiest muscle
- Dual supply median nerve and ulnar nerve

- Great gripping muscle
- Lumbricals arises from tendon of FDP.

Brachioradialis

- Flex elbow
- Weak pronating action from fully supine position to midpronation–no supination action.

Anconeus

- Pronator of ulna
- Small amount of extension and abduction of ulna during pronation
- Tensor of elbow capsule
- Screwing movement.

Spaces of upper limb

- Forearm space of parona–Rectangular space (Superficial to pronator quadratus and deep to flexor tendon of fingers. Limited proximally by Flexor Digitorum Superficialis)
- Midpalmar space (Kanavel's space)—Triangular shaped
- Thenar space–Triangular shaped
- Pulp space (infection of this space—whitlow or felon).

Dorsal subscutaneous space will receive lymph from the palmar aspect of the hand. Thus a hand-infection can easily result in swelling on posterior aspect of the hand, in which case it would be lymph—not pus—so do not incise it.

Speciality	Thenar space	Midpalmar space
Floor	Adductor pollicis, first dorsal interosseus	3rd and 4th metacarpal spaces
Contain	1 Lumbrical	2, 3, 4 Lumbricals
Also	Flexor tendon of Index finger	

Posterior compartment of forearm

- All muscle are innervated by posterior interosseous nerve except brachioraidalis, anconeus, extensor carpii radialis longus
- Powerful supinator of forearm: Biceps (Spurt muscle) in elbow flexed. When elbow extended position only supinator, supinates forearm.
- **Listers tubercle:** Dorsal tubercle of radius forming a boundary for anatomical snuff box
- *There is no extensor expansion on the thumb*
- *Posterior interosseous nerve has no cutaneous branches*
- **Hammer thumb:** In colles fracture, anterior interosseous artery which supplies the extensor pollicis longus tendon is occluded and lead to necrosis and spontaneous rupture of tendon.

Extensor retinaculum

- Thickening of deep fascia of forearm
- Not attached to ulna, < 2.5 cm wide
- Attached to radius (laterally) and pisiform, triquetral (medially)
- Six compartments.

Flexor retinaculum

Attachments → Ulnar—pisiform and hook of hammate → Radial—scaphoid and trapezium

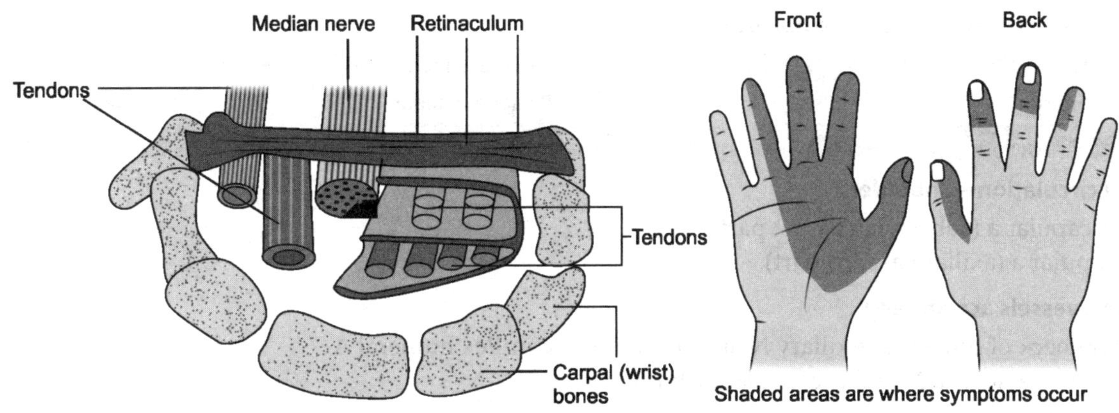

Fig. 1.6: Carpal tunnel and the areas of involvement carpal tunnel syndrome

Carpal tunnel (between flexor retinaculum and lunate)

Contents (Structures passing through carpal tunnel (deep to flexor retinaculum)

- Four tendons of Flexor digitorum superficialis
- Flexor digitorum Profundus
- Flexor pollicis longus
- Median nerve.

Structures passing superficial to flexor retinaculum

- Ulnar nerve and vessels
- Palmaris longus tendon
- Superficial branch of radial artery
- Palmar cutaneous branches of ulnar and median nerve.

PAD and DAB: *Palmar interossei adducts and dorsal interossei abduct. If dorsal and ventral interosseous act together only no adduction or abduction but results in flexion of MCP (metacarpophalangeal joint) and extension at IP (interphalangeal joint).*

Lumbricals action: *Flexion of MCP (metacarpophalangeal joint) and extension at IP (interphalangeal joint).*

Rarely: *Median nerve may have muscular branch in arm to pronator teres. (usually branch comes at forearm).*

Extensor Expansion or Dorsal Digital Expansion

- Lumbricals, interosseous (dorsal and ventral) attaches to it
- Long extensors of fingers
- Index and little finger receives extensor indicis and extensor digiti minimi also.

Axillary artery (Between outer border of 1st rib—Teres major)

Enters the axilla behind midpoint of clavicle

- Pectoralis minor divides it into 3 parts
- Covered by sheath (axillary) derived from prevertebral fascia.

Branches (SAL-SAP)

Superior thoracic A

Acromiothoracic A

Lateral thoracic A

Subscapular a **(largest branch)**

Anterior and

Posterior circumflex humeral a (surgical neck of humerus, along with axillary nerve)

Axillary vein has no axillary sheath into its 1st part cephalic vein joins

Division of major vessels into three parts by

Axillary artery	Pectoralis minor
Subclavian artery	Scalene anterior
Maxillary artery	Lateral pterygoid muscle

Collateral circulation—shoulder

- Suprascapular a (subclavian a—1st part)
- Subscapular a (axillary a—3rd part).

Nerves and vessels accompany

- Surgical neck of humerus: Axillary N and posterior circumflex humeral A
- Spiral groove: Radial N and profunda brachii A

Axillary sheath

- Derived from prevertebral fascia
- Covers axillary artery and brachial plexus
- Axillary vein not covered.

Brachial artery

- Profunda brachii A: Largest branch
- Nutrient A to humerus.

Ulnar artery

- Common interosseous A: Anterior and posterior interosseous
- Superficial palmar arch
- Hockey stick shaped, incomplete arch
- May be completed by superficial branch of radial artery
- Thumb and thumb side of index finger are not supplied by superficial palmar arch, but by radial artery itself.

Radial artery

- Radial artery appears to be direct continuation of brachial artery
- Enters palm between two heads of adductor pollicis.

Deep palmar arch

- Lies deep to the flexor retinaculm. This is formed by the radial artery, and it anastomoses with the terminal ulnar artery. It gives off the 3 Palmar Metacarpal Arteries
- Thumb is supplied by radial artery.

Posterior carpal arch

- Anastomosis between radial, ulnar and anterior interosseous artery
- Gives dorsal metacarpal arteries.

Venous drainage

- Most of blood from palm passes through superficial network of dorsum
- Preaxial vein of upper limb: Cephalic vein drains in to axillary vein
- Axial artery of fetal limb: Anterior interosseous artery
- Postaxial vein of upper limb: Basilic vein continues as axillary vein
- Median cephalic vein is less movable: Use in intravenous theraphy.

Nutrient artery

- Clavicle: Suprascapular artery
- Humerus: Profunda brachii
- Ulna: Anterior interosseous artery
- Radius: Anterior interosseous artery.

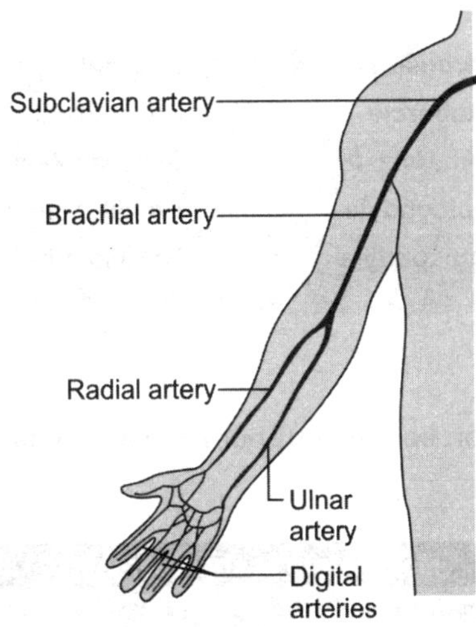

Fig. 1.7: Superficial palmar arch and its branches

Vessel of flexor compartment

- Radial artery usually appears to be direct continuation of brachial artery
- Ulnar artery continuous as superficial palmar arch
- Deep palmar arch: Formed by terminal branch of radial artery, anastomosis with deep branch of ulnar artery
- Ulnar artery gives common interosseous artery which divides into anterior interosseous and posterior interosseous artery
- Anterior interosseous artery gives nutrient branch to radius and ulna
- Most of blood from palm of hand drains by superficial venous network
- Median nerve is nourished by median artery (Branch of anterior interosseous artery).

Attachment of coracoids process

- Pectoralis minor
- Shorthead of biceps
- Coraco brachialis.

Clavicle

- Only bone which lies horizontally
- Only long bone with membranous ossification
- First bone of the skeleton (ossify between 5th and 6th week of intrauterine life)
- Only long bone which has two primary centers of ossification
- No medullary cavity and it is subcutaneous throughout
- Fractured at the junction of its lateral and middle one-third, for this is weakest part.

Carpal bones:

Scaphoid is largest in the proximal row	Boat shaped	Mostly fractured
Lunate	Semilunar	Mostly dislocated
Capitate	Ossifies first in carpal (1st year)	Largest carpal
Pisiform	Ossifies last (10th year)	Smallest bone
1st metacarpal		Most mobile bone of palm
5th metacarpal		2nd Most mobile bone of palm

- The carpal bones are usually cartilaginous at birth
- The first carpal bone to ossify is the capitate and the last to ossify is pisiform
- The first metacarpal is shortes and stoutes, second metacarpal is the longest, third metacarpal has a styloid process.

Muscles of humerus:

Insertion muscles (upper humerus)	**Intertubercular sulcus**	Pectoralis major, Latissmus dorsi and Teres major
	Greater tubercle	Supraspinatus, Infraspinatus and Teres minor
	Lesser tubercle	Subscapularis
Origin muscles (lower humerus)	**Medial epicondyle**	Pronator teres, common flexor origin
	Lateral epicondyle	Brachioradialis, extensor carpi radialis longus, common extensor origin and anconeus

Joints

Sternoclavicular joint: Only communication between upper limb and axial skeleton

Shoulder Joint

Movements at shoulder joint		
Abductors	Supraspinatus (<15°) initiation Deltoid (15–90°) Serratus anterior and trapezius (overhead abduction)	
Adductors	Pectoralis major latissmus dorsi	**Accessory Muscles:** Teres major Coracobrachialis Shorthead of biceps Longhead of triceps
Flexion	Pectoralis major Deltoid (anterior fibers), coracobrachialis	
Extension	Deltoid (posterior fibres) and teres major Latissums dorsi [for flexion from extended position]	
Medial rotation	Pectoralis major Deltoid (anterior fibers) Teres major Latissmus dorsi	
Lateral rotation	Deltoid (posterior fibers) Teres minor Infraspinatus	

- Coracoid process takes no part in formation of shoulder joint
- **Strong coracoclavicular ligament** attaches the clavicle and scapula to each other and the clavicle is anchored to first costal cartilage by **costoclavicular ligament**. Forces of upper limb are normally transmitted to axial skeleton through these ligaments
- In 180 degree of abduction about 120 degree takes place at shoulder joint remaining 60 degree is provided by scapular rotation.

Longhead of biceps: Strong support over head of humerus (Intracapsular).

Longhead of triceps: Give stability to abducted humerus.

Elbow joint

Capsule not attached to radius.

Wrist joint

Distal radius: Scaphoid, Lunate, Triquetral

Adduction of wrist joint by:

Flexor and extensor carpi ulnaris simultaneous action.

Muscles producing flexion at the wrist joint:

- Flexor carpi radialis (Median N)
- Flexor carpi ulnaris (Ulnar N)
- Palmaris longus (Median N)

Pronation	Supination
Median nerve	Median nerve, Posterior interosseous nerve
Pronator quadratus,	Biceps brachii
Pronator teres	Supinator muscle

Pronation and supination is produced by movement of radius around immobile ulna.
Pronator quadrates is more powerful than pronator teres in its action.

Joints	Type	Movements
Sternoclavicular	Atypical synovial-sellar	Passive
Acromioclavicular	Atypical synovial-plane	Passive
Shoulder	Ball and socket	Abduction, adduction flexion, extension, rotation (Internal and External), Circumduction
Elbow	Hinge	Flexion, extension
Radioulnar joint	Pivot	Pronation, supination
Wrist	Synovial	Flexion, extension, abduction, adduction, circumduction
Carpometacarpal joint of thumb	Saddle joint	
Metacarpophalangeal joint	Synovial Biaxial (Ellipsoid)	Flexion, extension, abduction, adduction
Interphalangeal joint	Hinge	Flexion, extension

Important Things

- Serratus anterior: No of digitations–8
- Preaxial vein of upper limb: **Cephalic vein**
- Postaxial vein of upper limb: **Basilic vein**
- Largest bursa in body: Subacromial bursa
- Deltoid: Multipennate muscle
- *Ligament of struthers*: Represent remains of 3rd head of coracobrachialis, goes to medial epicondyle, under which median nerve/brachial artery might get compressed
- Axilla: Lower limit 4th rib, virtually does not exist when arm is fully abducted
- Nerve supply of flexor pollicis brevis subject to more variation than that of any other muscle in body
- Intercostobrachial nerve–T2, skin over shoulder–C4
- Medial cutaneous nerve of forearm is used as nerve graft
- *Digital arteries and nerve*: Swap places palm—artery superficial, nerve deep. Digits: Nerve superficial, artery deep.
- Vinculum: Flexor tendon over phalanges have vascular synovial fold. Type–long (vascular), Short
- Most superficial muscle of upper part of back: Trapezius
- *Guyons canal*: Content–ulnar nerve and ulnar artery
- Pisiform is only carpal bone to give attachments to both flexor and extensor retinaculum
- Structure passing though **tarsal tunnel is posterior tibial** nerve
- Commonly injured in cut injury at flexor retinaculum–Median Nerve
- Commonly gets involved in entrapment neuropathy (carpal tunnel syndrome)–Median Nerve
- Angle of humeral torsion is 164 degree (Angle of femoral torsion is–15°)

- Most common cause of nerve root compression in neck: cervical spondylosis
- **Natatory ligament** (Superficial transverse metacarpal ligament)
- The transverse fibres of the palmar aponeurosis (**fibres of Skoog)**
- There is a discrete interval between the inferior margin of Radioscaphocapitate ligament and the palmar horn of the lunate which is known as the space of Poirier
- *Space of parona compression:* Vines are subject to compression when swelling or fluid buildup occurs in any potential space. This causes blood to back flow.
- *Coracobrachialis syndrome:* Loss of the Musculocutaneous nerve where it runs through the coracobrachialis Muscle. If the muscle dies, then nerve dies with it.
- *Supinator channel syndrome*: Compression of the deep br. of Radial N between the superficial and deep heads of Supinator, and Lateral Epicondyle or due to compression of posterior interosseous N.
- *Arcade of frosh*: Occurs in 20–30% of population, where one head of the supinator is actually a sharp tendon inserting on the lateral epicondyle. This can also lead to Radial N. damage.
- *Supracondylar syndrome:* Entrapment of the median. Beneath the ligament of struthers, which connects the supracondylar process to the medial epicondyle.
- *Pronator teres syndrome:* Entrapment of Median N. passing between the deep and superficial heads of the pronator teres.
- *Martin-gruber anastomosis:* Connection between the Median and Ulnar nerves in the nerves in the palm of the hand, in about 30% of population. When the connection is there, it is mainly a motor connection.
- *Fracture of distal phalanx of middle finger is commonest:* It is treated by splinting the injured phalanx to the adjacent normal phalanx **(buddy splint)**
- Growing end of the humerus is the upper end; (femur—lower end)
- The humerus and scapula ossify from one primary end seven secondary centres (P7S)
- *Painful are syndrome/Impingement syndrome:* Most vulnerable structures are supraspinatus tendon, longhead of biceps and subacromian bursa, when humerus is abducted, flexed and internally rotated.
- *Horseshoe infection:* Infection spreading from little finger to thumb or vice versa, as a consequence of the communication between the radial and ulnar bursae

NO NO NO NO.., NO NO NO………,

- No palmar aponeurosis extension reaches the thumb
- *There is no extensor expansion on the thumb*
- No muscles crosses wrist, only tendon crosses it
- *Posterior interosseous nerve and anterior interosseous nerve has no cutaneous branches*
- *No branches for ulnar and median nerve in arm*
- *No motor supply for radial nerve in palm*
- No palmar interosseous for middle finger and thumb
- No dorsal interosseous for little finger and thumb
- Annular ligament has no attachment to radius
- Capsule of wrist joint has no attachment to radius.

LOWER LIMB

Thigh

Anterior compartment	: Femoral nerve
Adductor group	: Obturator nerve
Posterior compartment	: Tibial part of sciatic nerve
(Exception short head of biceps by common peroneal nerve)	
Gluteal medius, minimus, tensor fascia lata	: Superior gluteal nerve
Gluteal maximus	: Inferior gluteal nerve

Contd...

Contd...

Adductor magnus	: Tibial part + obturator nerve
Flexor compartment of leg	: Tibial nerve
Intrinsic muscles of foot	: Plantar branch—tibial nerve
Peroneal or lateral compartment	: Superficial—peroneal nerve
Extensor or anterior compartment	: Deep peroneal nerve

Lumbar Plexus

- Lies in the posterior part of the psoas major, anterior to the lumbar transverse processes
- Formed by the anterior rami of spinal nerves L1 through L4 and some fibers from T12.

Branches

- Femoral nerve
- Obturator nerve
- Lumbosacral trunk (L4, L5)
- Ilioinguinal and iliohypogastric nerves (L1)
- Genitofemoral nerve (L1, L2)
- Laeral femoral cutaneous nerve (L2, L3).

SACRAL PLEXUS

- Lies immediately inferior to the lumbar plexus
- Formed by the anterior rami of spinal nerves L4, L5, and S1 through S4
- Contain fibers from the nerves of the lumbar plexus through the lumbosacral trunk; hence the two plexuses are described collectively as the lumbosacral plexus
- Main branch is sciatic nerve (L4, L5, S1, S2, S3).

Lumbosacral Plexus

The lumbosacral plexus is formed by the anterior rami of spinal nerves T12 through S4. The innervation of the lower limb arises from segments L2 through S3.

The tibial nerve and common peroneal nerve travel together through the gluteal region and thigh in a common connective tissue sheath and together are called the sciatic nerve.

Course of Femoral Nerve

- Enters the femoral triangle by passing behind the inguinal ligament lateral to the femoral artery. It lies in the groove between the iliacus and the psoas major, outside the femoral sheath.

Terminal nerves of lumbosacral region

Nerve	Origin	Muscles innervated
Femoral nerve (Largest branch of lumbar plexus)	L2 through L4 posterior divisions	Anterior compartment of thigh [quadriceps femoris (largest muscle in body), Sartorius (Longest muscle in body), pectineus] Saphenous nerve—sensory Cutaneous innervations: To the anterior and lateral thigh and the medial leg and foot
Obturator nerve	L2 through L4 anterior divisions	Medial compartment of thigh (gracilis, adductor longus, adductor brevis, anterior portion of adductor magnus), pectineus and obturator externus Cutaneous innervations: To the medial thigh
Tibial nerve	L4 through S3 anterior divisions	Posterior compartment of thigh (semimembranosus, semitendinosus, longhead of biceps femoris, posterior portion of adductor magnus) Popliteus muscle

Contd...

Contd...

Nerve	Origin	Muscles innervated
		Posterior compartment of leg (gastrocnemius, soleus, flexor digitorum longus, flexor hallucis longus, tibialis posterior) Plantar muscles of foot
Tibial nerve	Terminate as	Medial plantar nerve Lateral plantar nerve
Common peroneal nerve	L4 through S2 posterior divisions	Shorthead of biceps femoris The common peroneal nerve is easily injured at the fibular neck
Superficial peroneal nerve		Lateral compartment of leg (peroneus longus, peroneus brevis)
Deep peroneal nerve or Anterior tibial nerve		Anterior compartment of leg (tibialis anterior, extensor hallucis, extensor digitorum, peroneus tertius)

- Sciatic nerve: Thickest nerve in the body and largest branch of sacral plexus
- Nerve to Vastus medialis: **Largest of muscular branches of femoral nerve**
- The saphenous nerve is the longest cutaneous branch of the femoral nerve
- Medial femoral cutaneous nerve branch of anterior division of femoral nerve crosses the femoral artery at the apex of femoral triangle from medial to lateral
- Saphenous nerve branch of posterior division of femoral nerve crosses the femoral artery at the middle of Hunter's canal from lateral to medial
- Articular branch to hip joint arises from nerve to rectus femoris
- Articular branch to knee joint arises from nerve to vastii
- Infrapatellar plexus: Formed by infrapatellar branch of saphenous nerve, medial, lateral, and intermediate femoral cutaneous nerves.
- Subsartorial pluxus: Formed by saphenous nerve, medial femoral cutaneous nerve and anterior division of obturator nerve.

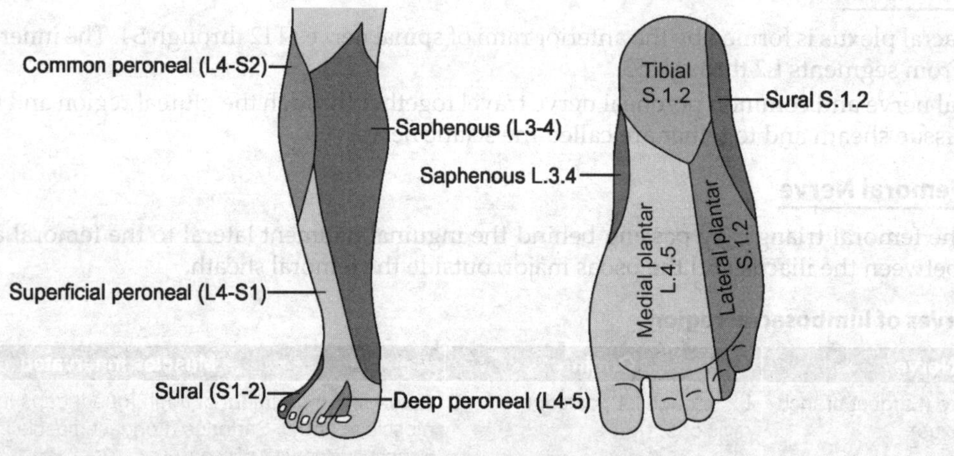

Fig. 1.8: Sensory innervations of leg and foot

Saphenous L3 L4	Femoral nerve	Medial side of leg, Ball of great toe
Sural nerve L5 S1 S2	Tibial nerve	

Salient Points

- The sciatic nerve in the buttock lies deep to the gluteus maximus muscle, midway between the greater trochanter and the ischial tuberosity. Because of its position, the sciatic nerve is of tremendous clinical importance
- A posterior dislocation of the hip joint will generally injure the sciatic nerve
- A herniated disk or pressure from the uterus during pregnancy may damage the nerve roots, resulting in a condition called sciatica

- An improperly administered injection into the buttock may injure the sciatic nerve itself
- Sciatic nerve does not give any branches in the gluteal region.

Saphenous nerve

- The saphenous nerve is the longest cutaneous branch of the femoral nerve
- Forms peripatellar plexus and subsartorial plexus
- It descends along the medial tibial border with the long saphenous vein
- The saphenous nerve connects with the medial branch of the superficial peroneal nerve
- The nerve maybe subject to an entrapment neuropathy as it leaves the adductor canal.

Cutaneous Innervation of Thigh: Lumbar Plexus

Nerve	Root	Supplies
Ilioinguinal nerve	**L1**	Root of penis
Iliohypogastric nerve	**L1**	Upper part of buttock, Hypogastric region
Genitofemoral nerve	**L1, L2**	– Divides lateral to the common and external iliac arteries into femoral and genital branches – Genital branch: Supplies cremaster, skin over scrotum and labium majus – Femoral branch: Supplies skin over femoral triangle
Femoral cutaneous nerve (Medial, Lateral, Intermediate)	**L2, L3**	Lateral femoral cutaneous nerve (Entrapment—Meralgia paresthetica)
Obturator nerve	**L2, L3, L4**	Medial side of thigh

Know it again

Muscle	Action
Gluteous maximus	Chief extensor of thigh at hip joint
Psoas major and iliacus	Flexors of hip
Gluteous medius and gluteous minimus	Powerful abductors of thigh
Gluteous medius and gluteous minimus, tensor fascia lata	Medial rotators of thigh short
Obturator internus and externus, glamelli and quadratus femoris	Lateral rotators of thigh
Tibialis anterior	Powerful dorsi flexor of foot
Gastronemius and soleus	Powerful plantar flexor of foot
Tibialis posterior and Tibialis anterior	Invertor of foot
Peroneous longus and brevis	Evertor of foot
Hamstrings	Flexors of knee, Extensor of hip
Semitendinosus and semimembranosus	Medial rotator of tibia
Biceps femoris	Lateral rotator of tibia
Popliteus	Rotate the knee (unlocking of knee joint)

Articularis genu

- Flat ribbon muscle
- Derived from vastus intermedialis
- Inserted into suprapatellar bursa.

Adductor magnus

- Composite muscle (fusion of adductor and hamstrings muscle).

Riders bone

- Adductor longus, upper end is round tendon.

Custodies virginatis

- Pair of gracilis muscle, whimsical name

OS peronium: Sesamoid bone over peroneous

Gluteal fold: Formed by horizontal skin crease of hip joint, not the inferior fold of gluteus maximus muscle

Short head of biceps: Not a true hamstrings

Femoral triangle: (Scarpa's Triangle)

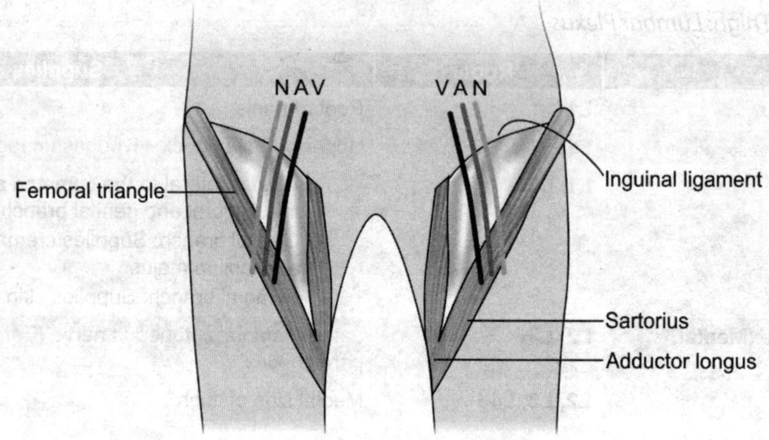

Fig. 1.9: Femoral triangle

Floor: Iliacus, pectineus, psoas

Geometric triangle: Floor of the femoral triangle without adductor longus is called as Geometric triangle. But with the adductor longus is called as anatomic triangle. *Ref: AK Datta 4/e p167 and Grant's Anatomy*

Arrangment of structures at the apex of the femoral triangle from anterior to posterior are femoral artery, femoral vein, profudafemoris vein and profundafemoris artery. The saphenous nerve and nerve to vastus medialis pass through the apex. *Ref: Neeta Kulkarni 2/e p847*

Within the triangle are the femoral sheath (containing the femoral artery and vein) and the femoral nerve (which is outside of the femoral sheath).

Passing under the inguinal ligament (from lateral to medial) are the: Femoral nerve, femoral artery, femoral Vein, an empty space within the femoral sheath called the femoral canal, and an inguinal lymph node (node of Cloquet or Rosenmuller) within the femoral canal. The femoral canal is the site of femoral hernias.

Anterior compartment of the thigh contains the anterior thigh muscles, the flexors of the hip and extensors of the knee. The anterior thigh muscles include the pectineus, iliopsoas, sartorius, and quadriceps femoris.

Ref: Keith and Moore p591

Sartorius

- Part of guy rope (stabilizes pelvis)
- Tailor's muscle
- Most superficial muscle of thigh.

The sartorius, the longest muscle in the body, acts across two joints. It flexes the hip joint and participates in flexion of the knee joint. *Ref: K.L. Moore p592*

Bursa ansernia: Bursa between the tendinous insertion of the sartorius and gracilis and semitendinosus.

Ref: Neeta Kulkarni 2/e p853

Iliacus

- Attached to lesser trochanter

- Innerved by femoral nerve
- Has iliac bursa
- Thigh muscle which ascends up
- Powerful flexor of hip
- Attached to femoral shaft just below lesser trochanter.

Psoas

- Attached to lesser trochanter
- By L1, L2, L3 nerve
- Body wall muscle descends down
- Powerful flexor of hip, also flexes lumbar vertebrae
- Attached to lesser trochanter.

Psoas major, arise from the iliac fossa and lumbar vertebrae, respectively. Thus it is the only muscle attached to the vertebral column, pelvis, and femur. Concentric contraction of the iliopsoas typically moves the free limb, producing flexion at the hip to lift the limb and initiate its forward swing during walking or to elevate the limb during climbing. The iliopsoas is also a postural muscle, active during standing in maintaining normal lumbar lordosis. Unilateral weakness or spasticity maybe a factor in the development of scoliosis.

Ref: KL Moore p591, 592

Pectineus

- Femoral vein and femoral canal lies on the surface of the muscle
- Dual nerve supply by femoral nerve and obturator nerve. Composite muscle
- Key muscle of femoral triangle
- Adductor brevis lies behind it.

Because of the dual nerve supply and the muscle's actions (the pectineus adducts and flexes the thigh and assists in medial rotation of the thigh), **it is actually a transitional muscle between the anterior and the medial compartments.** *Ref: KL Moore p591*

The **patellar ligament (L. ligamentum patellae),** attached to the tibial tuberosity (Fig. 5.1 5B), is the continuation of the quadriceps tendon in which the patella is embedded. The patella is thus the largest sesamoid bone in the body. The medial and lateral vasti muscles also attach independently to the patella and form aponeuroses, the medial and lateral patellar retinacula. *Ref: KL Moore p593*

Because of its attachments to the hip bone and tibia, the rectus femoris crosses two joints; hence it is capable of flexing the thigh at the hip joint and extending the leg at the knee joint. The rectus femoris is the only part of the quadriceps that crosses the hip joint. *Ref: KL Moore p593*

The rectus femoris, the kicking muscle. *Ref: KL Moore p593*

Chondromalacia patellae (runner's knee) is a common knee problem for marathon runners. Such overstressing of the knee can also occur in running sports such as basketball. The soreness and aching around or deep to the patella results from quadriceps imbalance. Chondromalacia patellae may result from a blow to the patella or extreme flexion of the knee (e.g., during squatting when power lifting). *Ref: KL Moore p595*

Gluteus maximus	3 bursa
Gluteus medius	1 bursa

Muscle	Shape
Tensor fascia lata, Adductor brevis	Triangular
Pectineus	Quadrilateral
Quadrates femoris	Rectangular
Semimembranosus	Hollow ground razor

Femoral sheath

- Funnel shaped prolongation of extraperitoneal fascia
- Transversalis fascia in front psoas fascia behind
- Three components: Femoral canal (medial), femoral vein, femoral artery (lateral) with genito femoral nerve.

Femoral ring

- Anterior: Inguinal ligament
- Medially: Lacunar ligament
- Posterior: Pectineal ligament
- Laterally: Vein-femoral
- Femoral canal: Lymph nodes of cloquet

Midingunial point: Femoral artery

Midpoint of inguinal ligament: Deep inguinal ring.

Femoral Nerve

- Posterior divisions of L2, L3, L4
- Gives saphenous nerve, medial and intermediate cutaneous nerve and nerve to quadriceps femoris.

Quadriceps femoris

- Largest muscle in the body
- Includes rectus femoris and three vastus muscle (Bipennate).

Vastus lateralis is preferred for intramuscular injection in neonates. *Ref: Neeta Kulkarni 2/e p853*

Rectus femoris muscle consists of reflected and sright head. Reflected head arises from the groove above the actabulum. This head represents the Primary attachment of the muscle.

Straight head arises from upper part of anterior inferior iliac spine above the attachment of iliofemoral ligament. This head represent as secondary attachment of rectus femoris. *Ref: AK Datta 4/e p177*

Vastus medialis oblique: The part of vastus medialis attached the medial margin of the patella. *Ref: Neeta Kulkarni 2/e p853*

Patellofemoral complex: Combination of quadriceps tendon, patella and ligamentum patellae. *Ref: Neeta Kulkarni 2/e p853*

Q angle or Quadriceps angle: Valgus angle between the oblique line of quadriceps muscle and the straight line of patellar ligament. Normally it is about 10–12 degree. It is increased in females due to wider pelvis and more oblique femur. If Q angle is more than 15 degree, there will be lateral displacement of patella. *Ref: Neeta Kulkarni 2/e p854*

Medial Compartment of Thigh

Gracilis: Most superficial muscle of medial side of thigh.

Riders bone: Ossified part of adductor longus tendon.

Adductor magnus: Composite muscle (fusion of adductor and hamstring muscle).

All are supplied by obturator nerve in addition to this adductor magnus is also supplied by tibial part of sciatic nerve.

Custodes virginitatis: Older name for pair of gracilis muscle.

The adductor hiatus is an opening or gap between the aponeurotic distal attachment of the adductor part of the adductor magnus and the tendinous distal attachment of the hamstring part. The adductor hiatus transmits the femoral artery and vein. *Ref: KL Moore p600*

Pulled groin or groin injury these terms mean that a strain, stretching, and probably some tearing of the proximal attachments of the anteromedial thigh muscles has occurred. The injury usually involves the flexor and adductor thigh muscles. *Ref: KL Moore p600*

Deep to the inguinal ligament, the **subinguinal space** (created as the inguinal ligament spans the gap between the two bony prominences to which it is attached, the ASIS and public tubercle).

The passageway posterior to the ligament is divided into two compartments, or lacunae, by a thickening of the iliopsoas fascia, the **iliopectineal arch.**

Lateral to the arch is the **muscular lacuna**, through which the iliopsoas muscle and femoral nerve pass from the greater pelvis into the anterior thigh; medial to the arch, the **vascular lacuna** allows passage of the major vascular structures (veins, artery, and lymphatics)

Structures Through Greater Sciatic Foramen

- Piriformis
- Above piriformis: Superior gluteal vessels and superior gluteal nerve
- Below piriformis:
  - Inferior gluteal nerve, inferior gluteal vessels,
  - Sciatic nerve,
  - PIN structures—pudendal nerve, Internal pudendal vessels, Nerve to obturator internus.

  Posterior cutaneous nerve of thigh, nerve to quadratus femoris

  (pain from pelvic disease is referred over the distribution posterior femoral cutaneous nerve over thigh and calf muscle)

Structures through lesser sciatic foramen

Pudendal nerve, internal pudendal vessels, nerve to obturator internus and tendon of obturator internus

Segmental Innervation to Muscles of Lower Limb

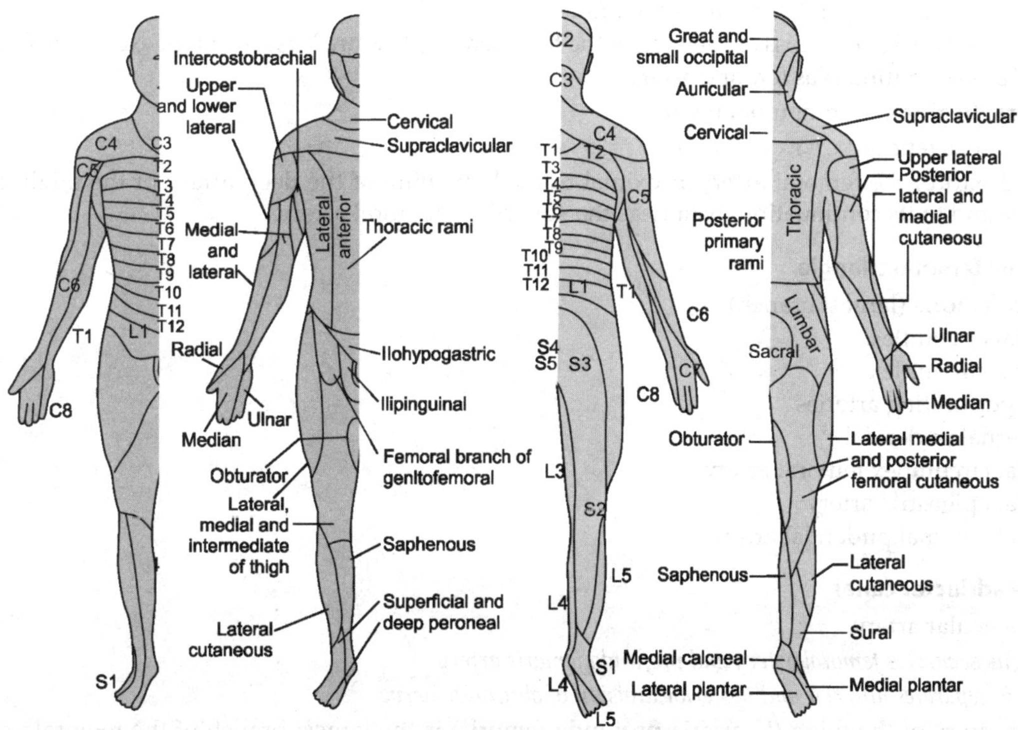

Fig. 1.10: Various dermatomes distribution

The **segmental innervation** to the muscles of the lower limb has a **proximal-distal gradient,** i.e., the more proximal muscles are innervated by the higher segments and the more distal muscles are innervated by the lower segments.

- The muscles that cross the **anterior** side **of the hip** are innervated by L2 **and** L3
- The muscles that cross the **anterior** side **of** the **knee** are innervated by L3 **and** L4
- The muscles that cross the **anterior side** of **the** ankle are innervated by L4 and L5
- The muscles that cross the **posterior** side **of the hip** are innervated by L4 **and** L5
- The muscles that cross the **posterior side of the knee** are innervated by L5 and S1
- The muscles that cross the **posterior side of the ankle** are innervated by S1 **and** S2.

NERVE INJURIES AND ABNORMALITIES OF GAIT

Superior gluteal nerve: Causes loss of abduction of the limb; impairment of gait; patient cannot keep pelvis level when standing on one leg. Sign *is* 'Trendelenburg gait.'

Inferior gluteal nerve: Produces a weakened hip extension; patient has difficulty rising from a sitting position or climbing stairs.

Femoral nerve: Induces weakened hip flexion; loss of extension of the knee. Sensory loss occurs on the anterior thigh, medial leg, and foot.

Obturator nerve: Causes a loss of adduction of the thigh as well as sensory loss on medial thigh.

Sciatic nerve: Brings about a weakened extension of the thigh; loss of flexion of the knee; and loss of function below the knee. Sensory loss on the posterior thigh, leg (except medial side), and foot is also observed. Sciatic nerve divides into tibial nerve, common peroneal nerve at apex of popliteal fossa.

Tibial nerve only: Causes a loss of flexion of the knee and digits; loss of plantar flexion; weakened inversion and sensory loss on the leg (except medial) and plantar foot.

Common peroneal nerve

Produces a combination of deficits of lesion of the deep and superficial peroneal nerves. Sign is 'foot drop.'

- Deep peroneal nerve: Weakened inversion; loss of extension of the digits; loss of dorsiflexion 'foot drop.' Sensory loss on anterolateral leg and dorsum of the foot.
- Superficial peroneal nerve: Loss of eversion of the foot. Sensory loss on dorsum of foot except the first web space.

External iliac artery continues as femoral artery

Femoral artery: Begins at midinguinal point

Lies over psoas tendon

The initial part of the femoral artery, proximal to the branching of the deep artery of the thigh, the common femoral artery and to its continuation distally as the superficial femoral artery. *Ref: KL Moore p603*

Branches in the femoral triangle

- **Profunda femoris** (largest branch)
  - Medial circumflex
  - Lateral circumflex
  - Four perforating arteries
- Deep external pudendal
- Superficial circumflex femoral artery
- Superficial epigastric artery
- Superficial external pudendal artery.

Branch in the adductor canal

Desending genicular artery.

Adductor longus separates femoral artery and profunda femoris artery

Adductor brevis separates anterior and posterior division of obturator nerve.

The deep artery of the thigh (L. arteria profunda femoris) is the largest branch of the femoral artery and the chief artery to the thigh. *Ref: KL Moore p603*

Popliteal artery

- Anterior tibial A: Dorsalis pedis 1st dorsal metatarsal A
- Posterior tibial A: Medial and Lateral plantar A (Terminal branches)
- Peroneal artery (largest branch of posterior tibial)
- Plantar arterial arch: Dorsalis pedis and Lateral plantar artery
- Only one plantar arch.

Obturator artery

- Branch of internal iliac (supplies head of femur).

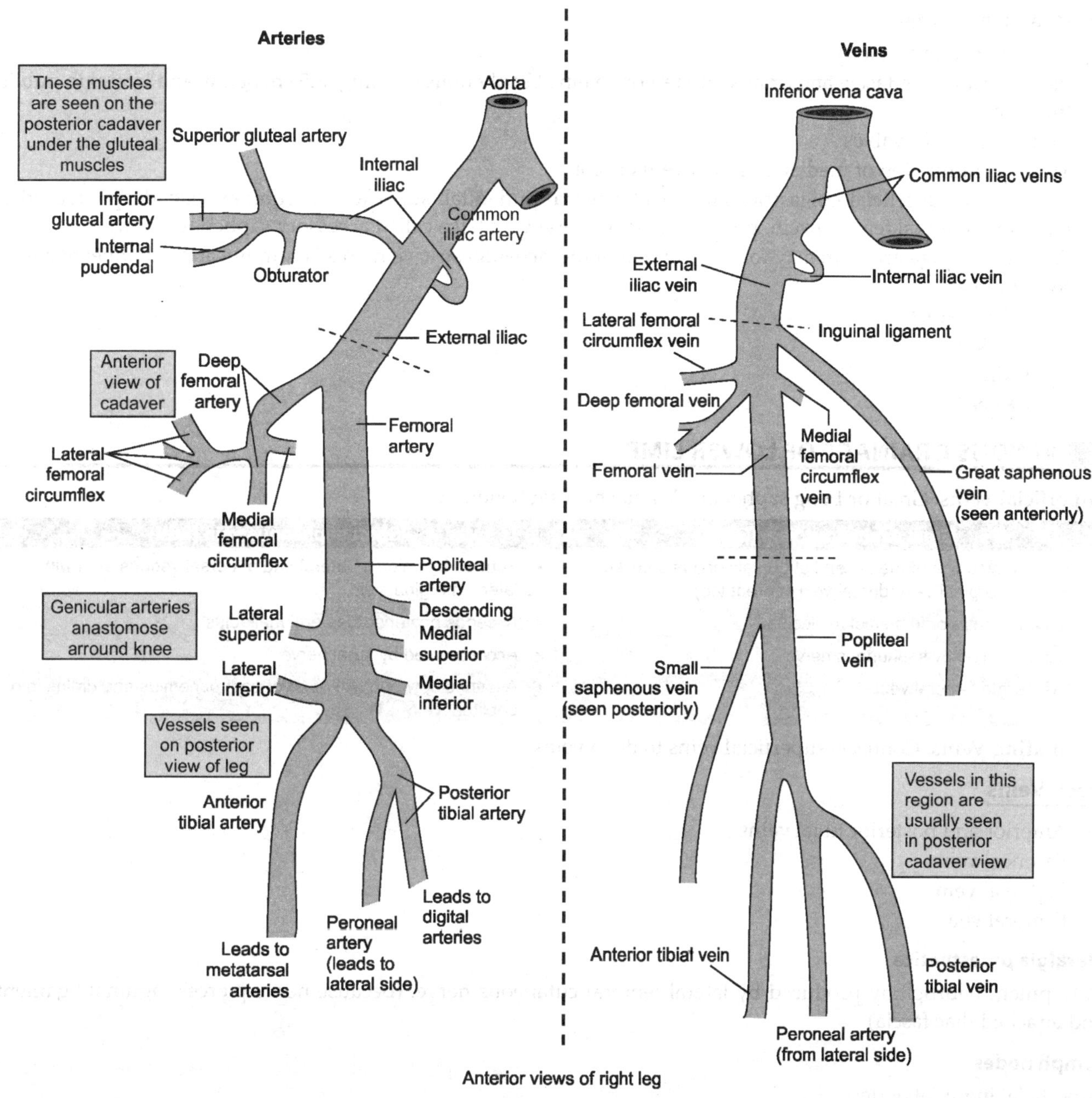

Fig. 1.11: Arterial supply and major anastomoses

Abnormal obturator A

An enlarged pubic branch of the inferior epigastric artery either takes the place of the obturator artery (replaced obturator artery) or joins it as an accessory obturator artery in approximately 20% of people. Closely related to the neck of a femoral hernia. Consequently, this artery could be involved in a strangulated femoral hernia.

- Normal Obturator artery gives a pubic branch which anastomoses with the pubic branch of the inferior epigastric Artery.
- Occasionally, this anastomosis is large and then the obturator then appears to be a branch of inferior epigastric Artery. (Abnormal obt. A).

Companion artery to Sciatic nerve or Artery of Sciatic nerve is a branch of Inferior gluteal artery *(remnant of original axial artery of limb).*

Great saphenous vein

- Longest vein in the body
- Pierces cribriform fascia and drains into femoral vein at saphenous opening (3.5 cm below and lateral to public tubercle)
- Contain up to 20 valves
- This is continuation of medial marginal vein of foot
- Tributaries: Superficial epigastric, superficial external pudendal, superficial circumflex iliac, deep circumflex iliac, anterolateral femoral vein, posteromedial femoral vein (also called accessory saphenous vein).
- Superficial epigastric vein may form lower end of thoracoepigastric vein, this is commucation channel between SVC and IVC
  - 5 Perforators
  - 3 Ankle
  - 1 Midhunter
  - 1 Knee

VENOUS DRAINAGE OF LOWER LIMB

Superficial veins: Great or Long saphenous V and short saphenous V

Great saphenous vein (GSV)	Short saphenous vein (SSV)
• Formed by union of medial end of dorsal venous arch with medial marginal vein (dorsal vein of great toe)	• Formed by union of lateral end of dorsal venous arch with lateral marginal vein
• Ascends anterior to medial malleolus	• Ascends posterior to lateral malleolus
• Accompanied by saphenous nerve	• Accompanied by sural nerve
• Drains into femoral vein	• Ascends between two head of gastrocnemius and drains into popliteal vein

Perforating Veins: Connects superficial veins to deep veins

Deep Veins

- Anterior and posterior tibial veins
- Peroneal vein
- Popliteal vein
- Femoral vein.

Meralgia paresthetica

Entrapment neuropathy produced by lateral femoral cutaneous nerve. (Because nerve pierces inguinal ligament and attached iliac fascia)

Lymph nodes

Superficial inguinal nodes

- 20 in number
- Arranged in T shaped pattern

Deep inguinal lymph nodes: Around femoral vessels glans penis/clitoris.

Fascia lata

- Deep fascia of thigh
- Encloses the thigh like stocking.

Iliotibial tract

- Thickening of facial lata
- Attached to lateral condyle of tibia

- Gluteus maximus and tensor fascia lata inserted into iliotibial tract
- Assist quadriceps
- Saphenous opening: Oval opening in fascia lata, lies 4 cm below and lateral to pubic tubercle.

Tensor fascia latae

- Triangular muscle attached to iliotibial tract
- Action is to pull the iliotibial tract. (so assisting gluteus maximus in extending the knee joint).

Popliteal Fossa

Diamond-shaped region

Boundaries

Biceps femoris superolaterally semimembranosus and semitendinosus superomedially, two heads of the gastrocnemius inferolaterally and inferomedially.

Floor (from superior to inferior) popliteal surface of the femur, the knee joint capsule, and the popliteus muscle.

Within the fossa (from posterior to anterior) are the tibial nerve, popliteal vein, and popliteal artery.

Note that the artery is the deepest structure and closest to the femur. It may be endangered by a fracture of the supracondylar region of the femur.

The common peroneal nerve is in the lateral part of the fossa and lies against the tendon of the biceps femoris. As the tendon of the biceps femoris inserts on the head of the fibula, the common peroneal nerve wraps around the lateral surface of the fibular neck. In this location, the nerve may be damaged by trauma to the fibular head or neck.

In popliteal fossa, popliteal vein lies between popliteal artery and tibial nerve at all levels.

Nutrient artery

Femur	Second perforating artery
Tibia	Posterior tibial artery (largest single nutrient A)
Fibula	Peroneal artery

Sole of foot

- 4 layers
- Neurovascular bundle lies between I and II layer
- Segmental nerve supply of all muscle S2
- Plantar aponeurosis give 5 slip, in each of 5 toes.

Four Phases of walking

- Heel strike
- Support (weight bearing)
- Toe–off

Last part to leave the ground is anterior pillar of medial longitudinal arch and medial 3 digits.

Shock Absorbing

Muscle tibialis anterior

Bones and joint

Longest and strongest bone in body	Femur
Largest sesamoid bone in body	Patella
Largest nutrient artery in body	Tibia-posterior tibial A
Largest tarsal bone	Calcaneum
Longest metatarsal	Second

Contd...

Contd...

Shortest, thickest, stoutest metatarsal	First
Largest cuneiform	Medial cuneiform
Largest and complex joint in body	Knee joint
March fracture	2nd metatarsal

Joint	Type	Movements
Hip joint	Ball and socket	Flexion, Extension, Abduction, Adduction, Circumduction, Medial and Lateral Rotation

HIP: Ball and Socket joint

The hip joint is formed by the **head of the femur** and the **acetabulum.**

The fibrous capsule of the hip joint is reinforced by three ligamentous thickenings: **Iliofemoral ligament (Ligament of Bigelow or inverted V shaped), ischiofemoral ligament**, and **pubofemoral ligament.**

Ligament	Nature
Ligament of Bigelow	Strongest ligament of hip
Ischiofemoral ligament	Weakest ligament of hip
Ligament of head of femur	Ligamentum teres (contain obturator artery)

Most of the blood supply to the head of the femur (arising mostly from the medial femoral circumflex artery) ascends along the neck of the femur. Capsule (Trochanteric anastomosis)

Fracture of the femoral neck can compromise this blood supply and lead to **avascular necrosis of the head of the femur.**

Knee joint: Compound synovial joint

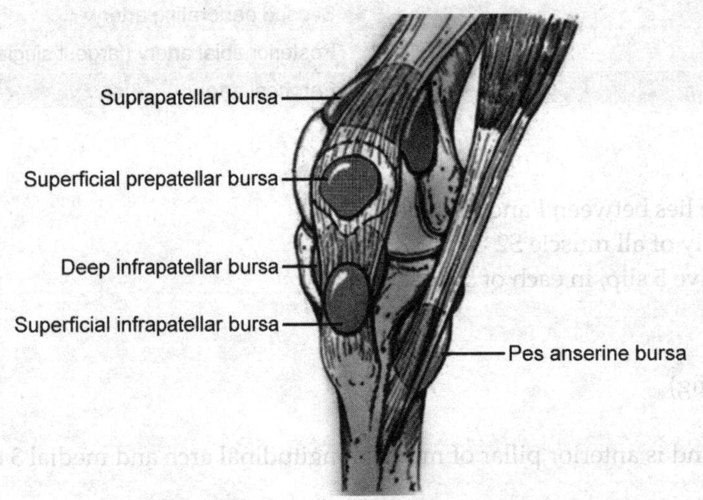

Fig. 1.12: Bursae around the knee joint

The largest synovial joint in the body

Capsule of the knee joint has two gaps

- Popliteus tendon
- Suprapetellar bursa

The knee joint is formed by the articulations of the medial and lateral femoral condyles, the medial and lateral tibial condyles, and the patella.

Medially and laterally, the knee joint capsule is strengthened by the medial and lateral collateral ligaments. These ligaments resist abduction and adduction, respectively.

There are two major intracapsular ligaments: the anterior and posterior cruciate ligaments. They are pain sensitive. These are named according to the site of inferior attachment of the ligament on the tibia, i.e. the anterior cruciate ligament attaches to the tibia anterior to the posterior cruciate ligament. These ligaments prevent anterior and posterior displacement of the tibia on the femur, respectively.

The poplieal tendon and cruciate ligaments are intra-articular and extrasynovial.

Attachment of structure on the Tibia: Intercondylar Area

M–Ant born of med. Menisus

A–Ant. Cruciate Ligament

L–Ant. horn of Lat meniscus

L–Posthorn of Lat meniscus

M–Posthorn of med. Meniscus

P–Postcruciate Ligament

The tests for the integrity of these ligaments are the anterior and posterior drawer signs (**anterior** drawer sign indicates damage to the **anterior** cruciate ligament).

The medial and lateral menisci are wedge-shaped fibrous and fibrocartilaginous structures between the femoral condyles and the tibial plateaus.

The medial meniscus is comma shaped, more firmly anchored to the tibia, and attached to the medial collateral ligament.

The lateral meniscus is C-shaped, less firmly anchored to the tibia, and not attached to the lateral collateral ligament.

Therefore, the medial meniscus is more commonly injured than the lateral meniscus.

The 'triad' knee injury is composed of tears of the medial collateral ligament, medial meniscus, and anterior cruciate ligament.

Vastus medialis: Most important for final degree of complete extension. (Medial rotation or locking of joint), indispensable to stability of patella.

Lateral rotation or unlocking of joint must precede flexion produced by popliteus.

Bursa around knee–13 bursae each

Prepatellar bursa = housemaids knee = Miners beat knee

Subcutaneous infrapatellar bursa = clergymans knee

Inferior tibia fibular joint: Fibrous joint

Ankle joint: Dorsiflexion and Plantar flexion

Subtalar: Anterior **talocalcaneonavicular joint,** Posterior: **Talocalcaneal joint**

Inversion and Eversion (some extent)

Midtarsal (Calcaneocuboid and Talonavicular) joint: fore-foot adduction and abduction. Inversion and Eversion (some extent).

Muscles acting at ankle joint and subtalar joint

Movement	Main muscle	Accessory muscle
Plantar flexion	Gastrocnemius, Soleus	Plantaris, Tibialis posterior, Flexor Hallucis Longus (FHL), Flexor Digitorum Longus (FDL)
Dorsiflexion	Tibialis anterior	Peroneus tertius, EHL, FDL
Inversion	Tibialis anterior, Tibialis posterior	FHL/FDL
Eversion	Peroneus longus, Peroneus brevis	Peroneus tertius

Ligament	Represents
Patellar ligament	Tendon of quadriceps femoris
Medial collateral ligament	Adductor magnus muscle
Lateral collateral ligament	Peroneous longus muscle

Contd...

Contd...

Oblique popliteal ligament	Semimembranosus (Pierced by middle genicular vessels) In locked position, limits rotation–extension.
Long plantar ligament	Gastrocnemius muscle

The **bifurcate ligament** is a strong Y-shaped band. It is attached by its stem proximally to the anterior part of the upper calcaneal surface, and distally it divides into calcaneocuboid and calcaneonavicular parts.

Ref: Gray's anatomy 40/e ch84

The **long plantar ligament** is the longest ligament associated with the tarsus. *Ref: Gray's anatomy 40/e ch84*

Lisfranc's ligament: Interosseous cuneometatarsal ligament passes from the lateral surface of the medial cuneiform to the adjacent angle of the second metatarsal known as **Lisfranc's ligament**, it is crucial to the stability of the tarsometatarsal joint complex. Disruption of this ligament can lead to instability and deformity and subsequent degenerative changes. *Ref: Gray's anatomy 40/e ch84*

Spring ligament: Plantar calcaneonavicular ligament

Lateral longitudinal arch: Most important factor is peroneus longus tendon

Medial longitudinal arch: Maintained by plantar aponeurosis (Number 1), Spring ligament (Number 2)

Important features

Holdens line: Membranous layer of superficial of thigh attached to deep fascia of thigh near inguinal ligament horizontally. (otherwise its loosely adherent) Importance: this prevents urinary extravasation into thigh in urethral injury.

Thickest nerve in body: Sciatic nerve

Guy ropes: Sartorius, Gracilis and Semitendinosus. Stabilizes pelvis on femur

Anserine bursa: Separates tendons of Sartorius, Gracilis and Semitendinosus

Brodies bursa: Medial head of gastronemius

Flabella: Sesamoid bone in lateral head of gastronemius

Number of layers in foot four

Spring ligament: Plantar calcaneonavicular ligament—maintains medial arch of foot

Talus bone does not have any muscular attachment.

Sural nerve: Cutaneous branch of Tibial nerve, accompanies short saphenous vein.

Os Trigonum

During ossification of the talus, the secondary ossification center, which becomes the lateral tubercle of the talus, occasionally fails to unite with the body of the talus.

Os perineum: Sesamoid bone within the peroneus longus tendon on the plantar aspect of cuboid.

Os vesalis: Sesamoid bone within the peroneus brevis tendon at the base of the 5th metatarsal bone.

THORAX

Skeletal elements

Sternum

Manubrium I and 2 rib

Body 3 to 7 ribs (Mesosternum)

Xiphoid–cartilaginous at birth, 40 years ossifies

Ribs

True ribs – 1 to 7

False ribs – 8 to 10

Floating ribs – 11, 12

Costal groove – Inferior border

Typical ribs – 3 to 9
Atypical ribs – 1, 2, 10, 11, 12
Cervical rib – behind

Costal groove: Inner surface along lower border for lodgement of intercostals nerves and vessels.

First Rib

- Strongest, flattest and most curved of all ribs
- Shaft has upper and lower surface: Upper surface has Scalene tubercle gives attachment of scalene anterior two grooves—Anterior lodges subclavian vein and Posterior lodges subclavian artery
- No costal groove in the lower surface.

Intercostal Spaces

- 11 in number
- Typical: 3rd, 4th, 5th and 6th
- **Boundaries**
  Above: Sharp lower margin of rib, Below: Blunt upper margin of rib, In front: Lateral border of sternum, and Behind: Bodies of thoracic vertebrae
- **Contents: Inrecostal muscles, nerves and vessels.**

Muscles

External intercostal m: 11 pairs
Internal intercostal m: 11 pairs
Innermost intercostal m: (Intercostal intimus), Subcostalis and Sternocostalis. (Transversus thoracis)
Neurovascular bundle passes between Internal intercostal m and Innermost intercostal m.

Intercostal structures

Ventral spinal rami (12th thoracic)
Nerves: 11 intercostal, 1 subcostal
Typical intercostal nerves: 3 to 6

Intercostobrachial nerve: Undivided lateral cutaneous branch of second intercostals nerve on the medial side of arm and armpit.

Branches Communicating: Ganglionic and adjacent intercostals nerves

Distributing: Collatcral and lateral cutaneous.

Peculiarities of first intercostals nerve

- Larger upperbranch joins C8 to form lower trunk of brachial plexus and smaller lower branch continue as 1st intercostals nerve
- Passes between Intercostal inturnus and costal pleura
- Runs along lower surface devoid of costal groove
- No collateral and Lateral branch
- Relation of structures from above downwards reversed as Nerve, Artery and Vein. (NAV)

Arteries

Anterior intercostal–Two in No
 1 to 6: Internal mammary
 7 to 9: Musculophrenic
No anterior intercostals in last two spaces
Posterior intercostals–One in No
 1 to 2: Superior intercostal
 3 to 11: Descending thoracic aorta.

Internal Thoracic (Mammary) Artery

- Branch of first part of subclavian artery
- Branches
  - Pericardiophrenic
  - Mediastinal
  - Pericardial
  - Sternal
  - Upper 6 anterior intercostals arteies.
  - Perforating arteries: 2nd to 4th supplies mammary gland
  - Terminal branches: Musculophrenic and Superior epigastric.

Main muscle of inspiration is diaphragm. Others are intercostals muscles, errector spinae, scalene group of muscles, sternocledomastoid, pectoral, serratus and quadratus lumborum.

Muscle of Expiration: Passive elastic recoil of lungs and thoracic cage.

Forced expiration: Anterior abdominal muscles and Latissmus dorsi.

Mechanism of Respiration

- Increased AP diameter: Pump handle movement
- Increased transverse diameter: Bucket handle movement
- Increased vertical diameter: Piston movement.

Pleura

- Visceral
- Parietal: Costal, Diaphramatic, cervical and mediastinal.

Surface anatomy

	Bottom of lung	Bottom of pleura
MCL	6 Rib	8 Rib
MAL	8	10
Paravertebra	10	12

Surface Markings of Parietal Pleura

Level	Left pleura	Right pleura
Apex	About 4 cm superior to middle of clavicle	About 4 cm superior to middle of clavicle
4th costal cartilage	Midline (anteriorly)	Midline (anteriorly)
6th costal cartilage	Lateral margin of sternum	Midline (anteriorly)
8th costal cartilage	Midclavicular line	Midclavicular line
10th rib	Midaxillary line	Midaxillary line
11th rib	Line of inferior angle of scapula	Line of inferior angle of scapula
12th rib	Lateral border of erector spinae to T12 spinous process (slightly lower level than right pleura)	Lateral border of erector spinae to T12 spinous process

Surface Markings of Lungs Covered with Visceral Pleura

Level	Left lung	Right lung
Apex	About 4 cm superior to middle of clavicle	About 4 cm superior to middle of clavicle
2nd costal cartilage	Midline (anteriorly)	Midline (anteriorly)

Contd...

Contd...

Level	Left lung	Right lung
4th costal cartilage	Lateral margin of sternum	Lateral margin of sternum
6th costal cartilage	Follows 4th costal cartilage, turns inferiorly to 6th costal cartilage in the midclavicular line (cardiac notch)	Midclavicular line
8th rib	Midaxillary line	Midaxillary line
10th rib	Line of inferior angle of scapula to T10 spinous process	Line of inferior angle of scapula to T10 spinous process

Supraplural Membrane (Sibson's Fascia)

- Musculofacial expansion protect the apex of lung
- Muscle: Scalenes minimus, Fascia: Endothoracic fascia.
- Attachment behind: Transverse process of C7, In front: Inner border of 1st rib
- Continuous as pretracheal fascia.

Pleural Recesses (Dead space)

Costodiaphragmatic (Phrenico-costal sinus): Right is in surgical app of rt. Kidney—Most dependent part of pleural sac, pleural fluid collect first in this space.

Costomediastinal

Pulmonary ligament: Allows pulmonary vein to expand

Extends from esophagus to lung.

Pleural innervation

Diaphragmatic pleura and mediastinal pleura: Phrenic nerve

Rest of pleura: Intercostal nerve

Lungs

Presenting parts: Apex, base, costal and medial surfaces and anterior, posterior and inferior

Surfaces: Costal, medial mediastinal and vertebral

Lobes: Right three, left two

Apex (cupola): Crossed by subclavian vessels in front, covered by suprapleural membrane

Fissures: Horizontal and oblique

Right lung is divided into three lobes (upper, middle and lower) by two fissures, oblique and horizontal

Left lung is divided into two lobes by the oblique fissure.

Division of bronchus

- Twenty-third generations of division beyond main bronchi, of which first 16 are conducting airways (principal bronchus to terminal bronchioles.
- Principal bronchi: Secandary bronchi, tertiary bronchi, terminal bronchioles, respiratory bronchioles, respiratory bronchioles, alveolar duct, atria, air saccules and alveoli.
- Cilia disapear: beyond respiratory bronchiole
- **Pulmonary or lung unit:** The area of the lung supplied by one terminal respiratory bronchiole. Respiratory part of lung-exchange of gas take place here.

Bronchopulmonary Segments

Portion of lung aerated by the tertiary bronchi is called Bronchopulmonary segments

- 10 right/10 left (medial basal absent)
  - Pyramidal shaped, apex points towards hilum, base toward surface
  - Pulmonary vein lies between two segments intersegmental
  - Each segment has own pulmonary artery
  - Bronchovascular unit: Area of lung drained by intersegmental tributary of pulmonary vein.

Right	Left
Upper lobe: Apical Posterior Anterior	**Upper lobe:** Apicoposterior Anterior Upper lingular Lower lingular
Middle lobe: Lateral Medial	
Lower lobe: Apical Medial basal (Cardiac) Anterior basal Lateral basal Posterior basal	**Lower lobe:** Apical Anterior basal Lateral basal Posterior basal

Hilum of lung corresoponds: Triangular nonplural impression of lung through which the structures of root enter or leave the organ.

- 3rd and 4th costal cartilages
- T5, 6, 7 vertebrae

Oblique fissure: Begins from the mediastinal surface above and behind the hilum, cut the posterior border about 2.5 cm lateral to junction of T3 and T4, extend along the costal surface coinsiding with the 5th intercostals space in mid-axillary line cut the inferior border at 6th costochondral Jn 7.5 cm lateral to midline plane of cleavage.

Horizontal fissure from oblique horizontally at mid-axillary line up to 4th costochondral Jn.

Contents of Root of the lung

- Principal bronchus on the left side, eparterial and hyparterial bronchi on the right side
- One pulmonary artery and two pulmonary veins superior and inferior
- Bronchial arterial, one on the right side, two on the left and bronchial veins
- Anterior and posterior pulmonary plexus of nerves
- Lymphatics of the lungs
- Bronchopulmonary lymph nodes
- Areolar tissue.

Structures related to the mediastinal surfaces:

- **Right lung**
  - Azygos vein arches above hilum
  - Cardiac impression below the hilum
  - Terminal part of IVC along with right phrenic nerve in posteroinferior to cardiac impression
  - Groove above the Cardiac impression lodges SVC lower part and Rt Brachiocephalic vein in the upper part
  - Above arch of azygos vein behind Rt Brachiocephalic vein, lodges
  - Brachcephalic trunk
  - Behind the Brachcephalic trunk present Trachea and Rt vagus
  - Vertical groove behind hilum lodges Rt side of esophagus.
- **Left lung**
  - Cardiac impression below the hilum more deeply concave.
  - Arch of aorta lodges above hilum between arch of aorta and the lung following structures present. They are left phrenic N, superior and inferior cervical cardiac branch, left vagus, left superior intercostals vein.
  - Descending thoracic aorta behind the hilum continues as arch
  - Vertical groove extend from arch contain left subclavian artery and infront of it lodges left Brachiocephalic vein.

- Behind arch contain left edge of esophagus and thoracic duct.
- Shallow groove behind descending thoracic aorta contain left edge of esophagus. So **esophagus related twice with the left lung.**

- **Lobe of wrisberg (Lobe of azygos vein):** One percent upper lobe of Rt lobe split in to medial and lateral by vertical fissure, the bottom of which contain arch of azygos vein suspended by plural septum-mesoazygos. The medial part forms lobe of azygos vein.

ARRANGEMENT OF STRUCTURES IN THE ROOT

From before backwards: (Similar on Both Sides)

- Superior pulmonary vein
- Pulmonary artery
- Bronchus and bronchial vessels

From above downwards

Right side	Left side
Eparterial bronchus Pulmonary artery	Pulmonary artery bronchus
Hyparterial bronchus Inferior pulmonary vein	Inferior pulmaonry vein

Differences between right and left lungs

Right lung	Left lung
2 fissures and 3 lobes	Only one fissure and 2 lobes
Anterior border is straight	Anterior border interrupted by cardiac notch
Larger and heavier (700 g)	Smaller and lighter (600 g)
Shorter and broader	Longer and narrower
Absence of lingual	Present
Cardiac impression shallow	Deep
Single bronchial artery	Two bronchial artery

Histology

Bronchi: Pseudostratified ciliated columnar epithelium
Alveolar ducts: Cuboidal epithelium
Alveoli lining: Squamous cells or Type I pneumocytes
Type II pneumocytes: Secretory cells surfactant

Arterial supply

Left Bronchial artery (two) Thoracic aorta
Bronchial vein Azygos vein
Right Bronchial artery (Two) 3rd Posterior intercostal artery (Br of thoracic aorta)

Lymphatic drainage

Pulmonary node deep parenchyma
Bronchopulmonary node superficial

Mediastinum

Superior
Inferior: Anterior, Middle (Widest), Posterior (Longest)
Division: Sternal angle to T4/T5 junction.

Superior mediastinum	Inferior mediastinum		
	Anterior mediastinum	**Middle mediastinum**	**Posterior mediastinum**
• Sternohyoid, Sternothyroid • Vagus, phrenic, Left recurrent laryngeal • Aortic arch and its branches • SVC, Left superior intercostals vein • Thymus • Internal thoracic arteries • Brachiocephalic veins	• Fat • Sternopericardial ligaments • Retrosternal lymph nodes • Mediastinal branch in internal thoracic artery	• Pericardium • Phrenic nerve and Pericardio-phrenic vessels • Heart • Ascending Aorta and Pulmonary trunk • Lower half of SVC and arch of azygos • Four pulmonary veins • Bifurcation of trachea and Deep cardiac plexus	(Dates) Descending aorta Azygos vein Thoracic duct Esophagus Splanchinic nerves, Vagus nerve Posterior mediastinal nodes Post. intercostal vessels,Termination of Sup and Inf hemiazygos vein.

Thoracic duct Elongated lymphatic trunk conveys chyle and most of lymph of body into bloodstream.

From cisterna chyli T12

Crosses to left T5

Passes through aortic hiatus

Passes through the posterior mediastinum in the lower part and above T5 passes through superior mediastinum.

Azygos vein

Formed: Union of Rt. subcostal V., Rt. ascending lumbar V., lumbar azygus or arises as lumbar azygus vein.

At T4: Joins SVC. Main communication between SVC and IVC

Tributaries: Posterior intercostals vein on right side except first, Rt. subcostal V., Rt. ascending lumbar V (First tributary), Hemiazygos and accessory azygos vein and Rt bronchial vein (Last tributary).

Hemiazygos

- Union of Lt. Subcostal V., Lt. ascending lumbar V
- **Communicate below with the renal vein**
- Enters the thorax by piercing the left crus
- Receives lower 4 posterior intercostals veins and ends in the azygos vein at T8.

Accessory azygos vein

- Continuation of left fourth posterior intercostals vein
- Receives 5th, 6th and 7th left posterior intercostals veins
- Terminate in the azygos vein opposite to T7.

Diaphragm

Origin

Lumbar

Two crura

Medial arcuate ligament

Lateral arcuate ligament

Costal: Lower 6 ribs

Sternal

Nerve supply: Phrenic nerve motor supply

Vessels of the diaphragm:

	Superior surface	Inferior surface
Arteries	• Periardicophrenic and musculophrenic arteries (branches of internal thoracic. A) • Superior phrenic arteries (Br. of thoracic aorta)	• Inferior phrenic arteries, (the first branches of the abdominal aorta however; they may arise from the celiac trunk).

Contd...

Contd...

	Superior surface	Inferior surface
Veins	• Percardiacophrenic and musculophrenic veins (tributaries of the internal thoracic vein)	• The right inferior phrenic vein drains to the IVC • The left inferior phrenic vein is often double, anterior branch ending in the IVC • Posterior branch ending in the left renal or suprarenal vein. • The two vein may anastomose with each other

- Invariably there is a communicating artery between the left gastric and inferior phrenic arteries
- Right phrenic artery passes through IVC opening of diaphragm
- Left phrenic artery passes through esophageal opening of diaphragm.

Heart: Intrafibrous and Extraserous

Pericardium Fibrous: Structures pierces are Ascendind aorta, SVC, IVC, Rt and Lt Pulmonary artery and four Pulmonary veins.

- Serous: Parietal, visceral (epicardium)
- **Transverse sinus:** Passage between two tubular reflections of serous pericardium lined by Visceral layer only Intervisceral space above and in front of Lt atrium.
- **Boundaries:** In front ascending aorta and pulmonary trunk, behind upper margin of Lt atrium, Above: Bifurcation of Pulmonary trunk, below upper surface of Lt atrium
- **Oblique sinus:** Sac behind Left atrium and is closed except below: Within the limbs of J shaped attachment of serous sac between Parietal and Visceral Parietovisceral space.
- **Fold of marshall (Fold of IVC):** Triangular fold of serous pericardium extend from left pulmonary artery to upper left pulmonary vein-remnant of left duct of cuvier.

Borders

Right: Extend from opening of SVC and IVC accompanies sulcus terminalis correspond with crista terminalis

Left (Margo obutus): Lt. auricle to apex accompanies marginal branch of left coronary artery.

Inferior (Margo acutus): Opening of IVC to apex accompanies marginal branch of left coronary artery.

Apex: Lt. Ventricle

Surfaces

Base: 2/3 Lt. Atrium and 1/3 Rt atrium

Left: Lt. ventricle and partly left atrium

Anterior (Sternococtal): Rt. Ventricle 2/3 and Lt ventricle 1/3

Inferior Diaphramatic: Lt. Ventricle 2/3 and Rt ventricle 1/3

Atrioventricular groove

Anterior-Right: Trunk of right coronary artery

Left: Trunk and circumflex branch of left coronary artery, termination of great cardiac vein and commencement of coronary sinus.

Posterior: Coronary sinus and anastomosis between Rt and Lt coronary artery.

Interventricular groove

Anterior: Anterior interventricular branch of left coronary artery and great cardiac vein

Posterior: Posterior interventricular branch of right coronary artery and middle cadiac vein and anastomosis of interventricular branches of both coronary artery.

Right Atrium

- **Rt auricle:** Conical muscular projection from anterosuperior part to upwards and left towards ascending aorta. Site for thrombosis.

- **Interior**
  - Smooth posterior part: Sinus venorum and rough anterior part: Atrium proper
  - Crista terminalis separate the above two and correspond to sulcus terminalis.
  - Sinus venorum: Developed from Rt horn of sinus venosus and Atrium proper developed from right half of Primitive atrium.
  - **Sinus venorum**
    - SVC opening: Not guarded by valve
    - IVC opening: Guarded by Eustachian valve—Rt horn continuous with lower end of crita treminalis, Lt horn anterior limb of fossa ovalis. Eustachian valve developed from Rt sinus valve and sinus septum
    - Opening of Coronary sinus: Guarded by thebesian valve which developed from lower part of sinus valve.
    - Openings of foramina minimarum
    - Sometimes anterior cardiac vein and Rt marginal vein open into Rt atrium through foramina minimarum
    - Intervenous tubercle: Small conical projection below the opening of SVC.
  - **Atrium proper**
    - Crista terminalis remnant of upper part of sinus valve
    - Musculi pectinati
    - **Rt side of interatrial septum**
    - Fossa ovalis: Above and left of opening of IVC—Floor formed by septum premium
    - Limbus fossa ovalis (Annulus ovalis): Surround upper, anterior and posterior margin of fossa developed from lower free margin of septum secundum
    - **Triangle of Koch:** Site of AV node.

Septal cusp of tricuspid valve: In front

Opening of coronary sinus: Behind

Tendon of Todaro: Above

Tendon of Todaro

- Present in right atrium
- Palpable in subendocardial tissue from central fibrous body to the left horn of valve of IVC
  - Torus aorticus: Elevation in anterosuperior part of the septum caused by right posterior coronary sinus.

Right Ventricle

- **Interior**
  - Rough in-flow part (ventricle proper) and smooth outflow part (infundibulum or conus arteriosus)
  - In flow part developed from Rt part of primitive ventricle and outflow part developed from right part of bulbus cardis
  - Superoventricular crest intervene between both parts
  - In flow part tricupid valve complex: It includes AV orifice, tricuspid annulus, tricuspid leafts, Chordae tendineae and Papillary muscles
  - Septal cusps anterior, septal and posterior. Three zone rough, clear and basal
  - Chordae tendineae true: Connecting apical third of pappilar muscle to free margin
  - Ventricular surface
  - **Trabeculae carneae:** Superoventricular crest: Remnent of bulboventricular ridge. Septomarginal trabecula: Modrrator band bidges extends from Rt side of ventricular septum to the base of anterior papillary muscles
  - Papillary muscle-2–anterior and posterior.

Outflow Part

- Pulmonary orifice guarded by three cusps-semilunar valve two in front and one posterior
- Pulmony sinus: Dilated pulmonary trunk above the cusps
- During diastole opposed cusps Triradiate appearance and Systole cusps assume triangle in outline.

Left Atrium

- Left auricle projects from anterosuperior aspect of left atrium upwards and medially towards the pulmonary trunk
- Musculi pectinati found in the left auricle
- Posterior wall receives the openings of four pulmonary veins
- Left AV orifice: Bicuspid valve (Mitral valve)
- Semilunar fold present on septal wall: Lunate impression above this fold
- Posterior part developed from endocardial cushion of single pulmonary vein which split into four and Anterior part developed from left half of primitive atrium.

Left Ventricle

- Three times thicker than the right
- In flow part (ventricle proper): Left AV orifice, mitral valve complex, Mitral annulus, mitral leaflets, Anterior and Posterior, trabeculae carneae, more prominent than the Rt papillary muscles (anterior and posterior)
- Outflow part, aortic vestibule, semilunar valve
- Subaortic curtain and anterior leaflet of mitral valve separate the above two parts
- The shape of mitral orifice is cresentric during systole as leaflets tightly apposed
- Aortic sinus of valsava: Dilatation of ascending aorta above the aortic cusp
- Supravalvular ridge: Upper limit of aortic sinus
- During ventricular systole aortic cusps stretched as straight line and aortic opening assumes triangular outline.
- During ventricular diastole, nodules of center of cusps meet to form triradiate form.

Character	SA Node	AV Node	Bundle of His
Nature	Specially differentiated atrial muscle fibers		Only muscular connection between atria and ventricle
Site	In right atrium–to right of SVC opening	In right atrium (Medial wall) Subendocardial – 1 cm above of opening of coronary sinus – Behind basal attachment of septal cusp of tricuspid valve	Right bundle – Passes through posterior limb of Septomarginal band (Moderator band) and reaches right ventricular apex Left bundle – 3 major branches (Anterior, Septal and Posterior)
Size	15 × 7 × 1 mm	7 × 3 × 1 mm	2–3 cm long

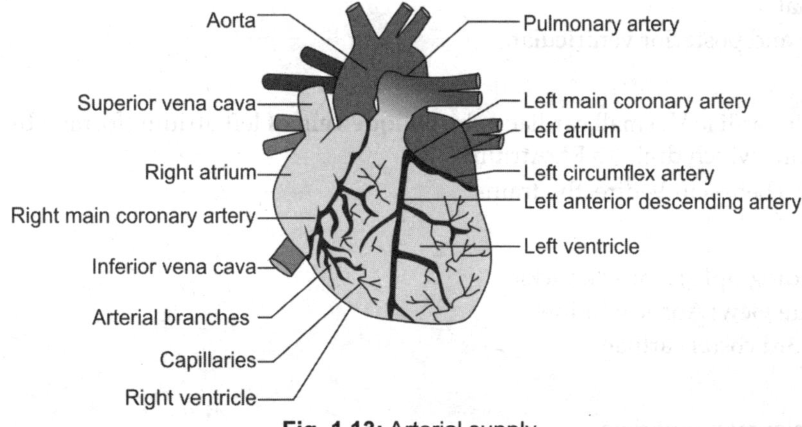

Fig. 1.13: Arterial supply

Right Coronary A

- Arise from anterior aortic sinus of ascending aorta
- Runs in right anterior coronary sulcus (or right Atrioventricular groove) then in posterior AV groove (coronary sulcus) and anastomose with LCA in posterior interventricular groove)
- Area of distribution
  - Rt atrium
  - Ventricular
    Most of the Rt. Ventricle except the area adjoining the anterior interventricular groove
    Small part of it ventricle adjoining posterior interventricular groove
  - Posterior part of interventricular septum
  - Whole conducting system except
    - Right Bundle Branch (RBB)
    - Part of it branch of AV bundle
    - SA node in 60%
- Branch
  - Rt Marginal
  - Posterior interventricular (descending), in 90% cases
  - Rt. infundibular
  - Nodal (in 65% cases)
  - Atrial, anterior and posterior ventricular.

Left Coronary A

- Arise from left posterior aortic sinus of ascending aorta
- Gives anterior descending (interventricular) br. which runs in interventricular groove; further continuation is k/a circumflex artery which runs in it anterior coronary (atrioventricular) sulcus then in it. Post. AV groove
- Area of distribution
  - Lt. atrium
  - Ventricles
    - Most it ventricle except area adjoin posterior interventricular groove
    - Small part of Rt. Ventricular adjoining anterior interventricle groove
  - Anterior part of inter ventricular septum
  - Right Bundle Branch (RBB), part of left branch of AV bundle and SA node in 35%
- Branch
  - Anterior inter ventricular (descending)
  - Circumflex artery
  - Left diagonal
  - Obtuse marginal
  - Atrial, anterior and posterior ventricular.

Venous drainage

Great cardiac V., middle cardiac V., small cardiac vein, oblique vein of left atrium (formed by left common cardinal vein) joins coronary sinus which drain to Rt. Atrium

Anterior cardiac V and Thebesian V. directly drains

Aoric arch

- Anteroposterior radiographs: Aortic knuckle
- Left anterior oblique view: Aortic window
- SVC: Rt. atrium at 3rd costal cartilage.

Important words

Sibsons facia or suprapleural membrane

Scalenous minimus or pleuralis: Morphologically
Foramen of morgagni or larrys space
Sternum shape sword

Important measurements

Trachea: 10 to 15 cm length, 12 mm lumen
Esophagus: 25 cm
Thoracic duct: 45 cm
The thoracic inlet bounded by first thoracic vertebra, medial borders of first rib and costal cartilage, superior border of manubrium.

ABDOMEN

Surface Anatomy

Linea Alba

The linea alba is a shallow groove that runs vertically in the median plane from the xiphoid to the pubis. It separates the right and left rectus abdominis muscles.

Linea Semilunaris

The linea semilunaris is a curved line defining the lateral border of the rectus abdominis, a bilateral feature.

Inguinal Groove

The inguinal groove indicates the site of the inguinal ligament, the rolled-over, free border of the external oblique aponeurosis. It separates the abdomen superiorly from the lower limb inferiorly. **The inguinal ligament extends from the ASIS to the pubic tubercle.**
Planes and regions
There are four planes to define nine regions

Transpyloric plane of Addison L1

- Between jugular notch and pubic symphysis
- Cuts costal margin at tip of ninth costal cartilage
- Passes through pylorus of stomach, hilum of kidney, fundus of gallbladder, origin of superior mesenteric artery and lower border of L1 vertebrae
- Supracolic compartment lies above this plane
- Splenic vein passes transversely at this plane
- Neck of pancreas
- Spinal cord ends as conus medullaris.

Subcostal Plane

- The subcostal plane (horizontal) passes through the inferior margins of the 10th costal cartilages and body of vertebra L3.

Transtubercular Plane

- The transtubercular plane (horizontal) passes through the iliac tubercles and the body of vertebra L5 near its upper border.

Midclavicular Lines

The midclavicular lines (vertical) are the two planes that pass from the midpoint of the clavicle to the midpoint of the inguinal ligament on each side.

Regions of the Abdomen

The nine regions between the vertical and horizontal planes present three zones. They are upper, middle and lower. Upper zone consists of epigastric region in the middle and right and left hypochondric region.

Middle zone consists of umbilical in the middle and right and left lumbar regions on each side.

Lower zone consists of hypogastric in the middle and right and left lumbar regions on each side.

Umbilicus

Cicatritical dense fibrous tissue and represent the attachment of fetal end of the umbilical cord.

Level: Usually at the level of the disk between L3 and L4 (In newborn lower level due to poor development of anterior abdominal wall and in old age also lower level due to reduced tone of abdominal muscles.

Watershed line: A horizontal line across the umbilicus

Above the line lymphatics drain into axillary nodes and below the line lymphatics drain into superficial inguinal nodes.

T10 supplies at this level (both somatic and autonomic)

Pain in the umbilicus may be local in origin or referred from inflamed appendix or from gonads because of similarity of segmental nerve supply.

Fascial layers

Superficial Fascia

Two layer of superficial fascia seen in lower abdomen beloew the line connecting the both ASIS

Camper fascia subcutaneous and variable in thickness (presence of fat)

Scarpa fascia

- Deeper membranous layer devoid of fat
- Fuses to the fascia lata of the thigh below the inguinal ligament
- Continuous with the dartos fascia of the scrotum or the labia majora, and colles fascia of the perineum.
  - Structures passing between the two layers of superficial fascia are:
    - Superficial epigastric artery
    - Superficial circumflex artery
    - Superficial external pudendal artery.

Deep Fascia

The deep fascia is the investing fascia of the abdominal musculature.

Fundiform ligament: In the midline fascia scarpa continues in front of pubic symphysis as findiform ligament.

Superficial inguinal space: Potential space in the anterior abdominal wall between the fascia of scarpa band the external oblique aponeurosis. Extravasated urine appears in this space from superficial perineal pouch.

Layers of anterior abdominal wall

- Skin
- Superficial fascia
- Aponeurosis of external oblique
- External oblique muscle
- Aponeurosis of internal oblique
- Internal oblique muscle
- Aponeurosis of transversus abdominis
- Fascia transversalis
- Extraperitoneal tissue
- Parietal peritoneum.

Muscles

External Oblique

Arises by eight digitations

The fibers run anteriorly and inferiorly (i.e. the hands-in-pockets direction like the external intercostal layer in the thorax).

Structures passing through the pelvifemoral space (Space between hip bone and inguinal ligament)

- Lateral femoral cutaneous nerve

- Iliacus muscle
- Femoral nerve
- Psoas tendon
- Femoral artery
- Femoral branch of genitor-femoral nerve
- Femoral vein
- Pectineus muscle
- Accessory obturator nerve
- Lymphatics communicate deep inguinal and external iliac nodes.

Internal Oblique

The fibers run posteriorly and inferiorly at right angles to those of the external oblique like those of the internal intercostal layer in the thorax.

Transversus Abdominis

The muscle fibers run horizontally. As the fibers pass medially, they become aponeurotic and contribute to the posterior rectus sheath.

Inferiorly, the fibers join with those of the internal oblique to form the conjoint tendon. (Falx inguinalis)

Rectus Abdominis

The fibers run vertically between the pubic symphysis and the xiphoid process.

The right and left recti muscles are separated medially by the linea alba

Typically three tendinous intersections: One at umbilicus, Xiphisternum and between two intersections occupies only superficial part. The muscle is formed by fusion of mesodermal somites

Rectus Sheath

- Aponeurotic envelope for rectus abdominis on each side of linea alba.
- Principle of formation: Splitting of internal oblique aponeurosis at the lateral border of rectus abdominis between costal margin to midway between umbilicus to symphysis pubis.
  - **The arcuate line or semicircular line of douglas** is located midway between the umbilicus and pubis. It is a landmark for the change in disposition of the aponeurotic fibers. Above the arcuate line, posterior and anterior layers of the rectus sheath have equal thickness; below it, all aponeurotic fibers run anterior to the rectus abdominis.

Rectus Sheath Formation

Site	Anterior wall	Posterior wall
Above the costal margin	External oblique aponeurosis	5th to 7th costal cartilages
From costal margin to midway between umbilicus and symphysis pubis	Anterior lamella of internal oblique and external oblique aponeurosis	Posterior lamella of internal oblique and transverses abdominis aponeurosis
Below the above point	Fusion of three aponeurosis	Thickend fascia transversalis (Ilio-pubic crest)

Medial margin Linea alba Expansions: Suspensory ligament of penis (Superficial fibers in front of symphysis and attached to dorsal surface of body of penis) and Adminiculum linea alba (Deep fibers of linea alba attached to pubic crest passes behind rectus).

Lateral margin: Linea semilunaris

Contents

Muscles: Rectus and pyramidalis

Vessels: Superior and inferior epigastric

Nerves: Lower 5 intercostal nerves and subcostal nerve.

Contents of Rectus Sheath

Rectus abdominis and pyramidalis
Inferior and superior epigastric artery
Subcostal and lower five intercostals nerves

Pyramidalis

- Arises from pubic crest and symphysis pubis
- Inserted into linea alba midway between umbilicus and symphsis pubis
- Supplied by subcostal nerve
- Tensor of linea alba
- Sometimes absent in one or both sides.

Transversalis fascia

The transversalis fascia lines the abdominal cavity. It forms the posterior layer of the rectus sheath below the arcuate line and the internal spermatic fascia of the spermatic cord.

The deep inguinal ring begins as an outpouching of transversalis fascia just lateral to where the inferior epigastric vessels intersect the inguinal ligament.

The transversalis fascia is separated from the peritoneum by a layer of fatty areola connective tissue.

Nerves, blood vessels, and lymphatics

Innervation of the skin and musculature of the anterior abdominal wall is via branches of the ventral primary rami of the lower six thoracic spinal nerves (includes the subcostal nerve T 12), plus the iliohypogastric and ilioinguinal branches of the ventral primary rami of L1.

The major arterial blood supply: Superior epigastric branch of the internal thoracic artery, inferior epigastric and the deep circumflex iliac branches of the external iliac artery.

Venous drainage from the anterior wall is to the superficial epigastric, the lateral thoracic veins superiorly, and the great saphenous vein inferiorly.

Lymph from tissues of the anterior wall drains to axillary nodes superiorly above umbilicus and to superficial inguinal nodes inferiorly.

There are no lymph nodes in the abdominal wall correspond to intercostal nodes of thoracic wall

Action: Rectus abdominis most powerful flexor, oblique muscles: Abductors and rotators of trunk.

Conjoint tendon (Falx inguinalis)

- Fusion of aponeuroses of internal oblique and transverses abdominis
- 2/3 formed by transverses abdominis and 1/3 formed by internal oblique
- Forms medial half of posterior wall of inguinal canal
- Infront related to reflected part of inguinal ligament, spermatic cord
- Behind related to fascia transversalis, extraperitoneal tissue and peritoneum.
- Interfovelar ligament: Fibrous band extends from lateral free margin of conjoint tendon to superior ramus of pubis.

Cremastric Muscle

- Well developed in male
- Derived from internal oblique or both internal oblique and transverses abdominis
- Anterolateral superficial part and Posteromedial deep part
- Superficial part arises from middle one-third of inguinal ligament and deep part attached to pubic tubercle, pubic crest and conjoint tendon
- Supplied by genital branch of genitor-femoral nerve L2
- Actions: Cremastric plug ball valve action and cremastric reflex and thermoregulation.

Extraperitoneal tissue

- Composed of fibroareolar tissue
- Structures traversed through this from medial to lateral
  - Inferior epigastric artery
  - Obiliterated umbilical artery
  - Median umbilical ligament—extends from apex of the bladder to umbilicus.

Parietal peritoneum

Below umbilicus

Five folds and six fossae

Folds

- Median umbilical fold contains median umbilical ligament
- Pair of medial umbilical fold containing obliterated umbilical artery
- Pair of lateral umbilical fold containing inferior epigastric artery.

Fossae

- Pair of supravesical fossae: Between median and medial umbilical fold
- Pair of medial inguinal fossae: Between medial and lateral umbilical fold
- Pair of lateral inguinal fossae: Outside the lateral umbilical fold.

Hessalbachs triangle

Lateral border: Inferior epigastric vessels

Medial border: Rectus abdominis,

Inferior border: Inguinal ligament.

Injury to ilioinguinal nerve and iliohypogastric nerve during appendicectomy leads to direct inguinal hernia due to paralysis of conjoint tendon, but injury in inguinal canal leads to sensory loss alone.

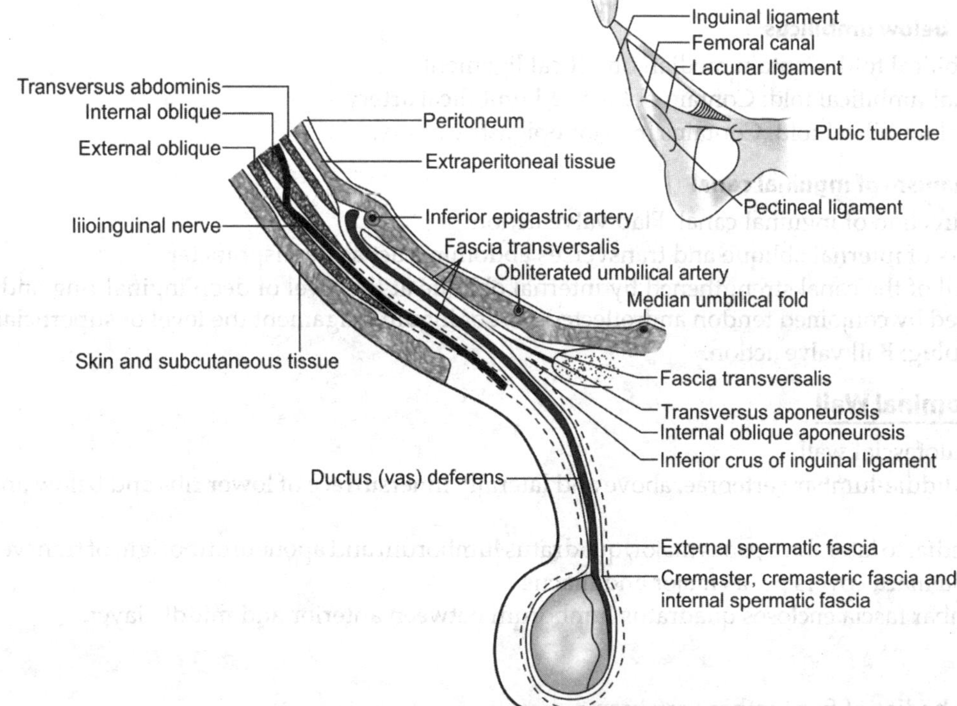

Fig. 1.14: Inguinal canal

Contents

Female: Round ligament and ilioinguinal nerve.

Male: Spermatic cord and ilioinguinal nerve.

Spermatic cord includes: Spermatic fascias testicular artery, pampiniform venous plexus and Vas deferens (ductus deferens), artery to ductus (Branch of superior or inferior vesical artery).

All above structure passes through deep inguinal ring except ilioinguinal nerve.

Boundaries of the Inguinal Canal

Roof

Internal abdominal oblique and the transverse abdominus muscles.

Anterior wall

- Entirely: Skin, superficial fascia and aponeurosis of the external abdominal oblique and the internal abdominal oblique muscle on lateral one third
- Superficial inguinal ring: V-shaped opening in external oblique aponeurosis
- Deep inguinal ring: Defect in fascia transversalis, lies at midpoint of inguinal ligament.

Floor

Inguinal ligament, medially lacunar ligament.

Posterior wall

- Entirely transversalis fascia (weak area) and conjoint tendon medial half and medial one fourth by the reflected part of the inguinal ligament
- The conjoint tendon reinforces the medial part of the posterior wall
- The conjoint tendon is formed by the aponeuroses of the internal oblique and transversus abdominus muscles
- Interfoveolar ligament: Transversalis fascia in posterior wall is strengthened by muscular fibers derived from transverse abdominis
- Inferior epigastric artery: Divides into pubic branch and cremasteric branch.

Peritoneal folds below umbilicus

- Median umbilical fold: Contain median umbilical ligament
- Pair of medial umbilical fold: Contain obliterated umbilical artery
- Pair of lateral umbilical fold: Contains inferior epigastric artery.

Defensive mechanism of inguinal canal

- Obliquity direction of inguinal canal: Flap valve action
- Arched fibers of internal oblique and transverses abdominis act as demisphincter
- Anterior wall of the canal strengthened by internal oblique at the level of deep inginal ring and posterior wall strengtehened by conjoined tendon andreflected part of inguinal ligament the level of superficial inguinal ring.
- Cremastric plug: Ball valve action.

Posterior Abdominal Wall

- Osseomusculofascial wall
- Bony part: Middle-lumbar vertebrae, above and laterally innersurface of lower ribs and below and laterally alae of sacrum
- Muscles: Medial to lateral are psoas major, quadratus lumborum and aponeurotic origin of transverse abdominis.
- Fascia: Fascia iliaca covers psoas major and iliacus
  Thoracolumbar fascia encloses quadratus lumborum between anterior and middle layer.

Psoas major

- Origin from bodies of five lumbar vertebrae
- Inserted into anterior surface of the tip of lesser trochanter of femur

- Nerve supply ventral rami of L2 and L3
- Action
  - Acting from above chief flexor of hip joint
  - Acting from below flexes the trunk at the hip joint
  - When foot is on the ground medial rotator of hip joint
  - When foot is off the ground lateral rotator of hip joint.

Quadratus Lumborum

- Origin from posterior one third of inner lip of iliac crest
- Inserted to anterior surface of transverse process of upper 4 lumbar vertebrae
- Nerve supply ventral rami of upper 3 or 4 lumbar nerves
- Action
  - Acting on one side act as lateral flexor of the trunk
  - Acting on both sides act as extensor of vertebral column.

Fascia iliaca

Covers both psoas major and iliacus

2 parts Iliac and psoas part-Iliac part covers iliacus and psoas and psoas part covers psoas muscle only.

Septum extends from ilac fascia to capsule of hip joint separates the space between inguinal ligament and hip bone into lateral lacuna musculorum and medial lacuna vasculorum.

Medial arcuate ligament: Thickened psoas part of fascia iliaca attached medially body of 1st lumbarvertebrae and laterally its transverse process.

Structures piercing fascia iliaca

- In front genitofemoral nerve
- Laterally Iliohypogastric, Ilioinguinal nerve and 4th lumbar artery
- Meadially lumbosacral trunk, Iliolumbar artery and Obturator nerve.

Thoraclumbar fascia (Lumbar fascia)

- Three layers anterior, middle and posterior
- Encloses two muscles quadrates lumborum between anterior and middle layer
  - Erector spinae between middle and posterior layer.
- Lateral arcuate ligament: Thickened anterior layer of thoracolumbar fascia extends transverse process of L1 to lower border of 12th rib.
- **Anterior layer** covers anterior surface of the quadrates lumborum—attached above thickened to form lateral arcuate ligament, below posterior part of iliac crest, medially anterior surface of transverse process and laterally blends with middle layer.
- **Middle layer** Covers the posterior surface of quadrates lumborum attached above to the lower border of 12th rib and extend to its head. Below posterior part of iliac crest, medially tip of transverse process of lumbar vertebrae, laterally blends with anterior layer at lateral border of quadrates lumborum and posterior layer at lateral border of erector spinae in an X manner.
- **Posterior layer** covers the posterior surface of erretor spinae—attached to spine and supraspinous ligament so lumbar vertebrae, laterally blends with middle layer, above enters the thorax and blends with investing layer of deep cervical fascia and below dorsal surface of sacrum and dorsal segment of the ilac crest.
- **Muscles attached to thoracolumbar fascia**
  - Anterior layer diaphragm
  - Fusion of anterior and posterior layer: Transversus abdominis and internal oblique
  - Posterior layer: Latissmus dorsi, serratus posterior inferior and few fibers of gluteus maximus

PERITONEUM

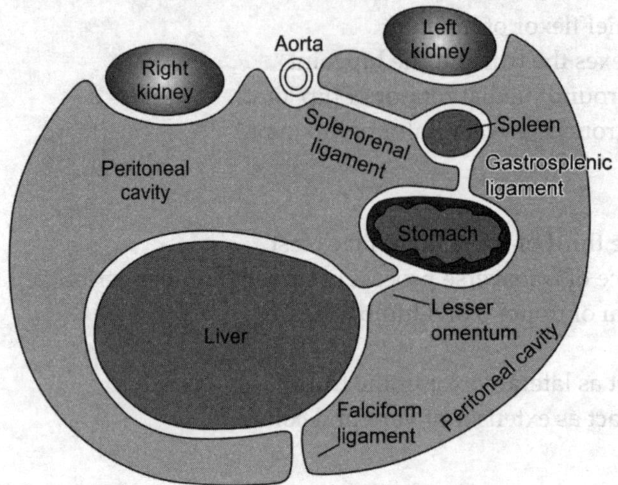

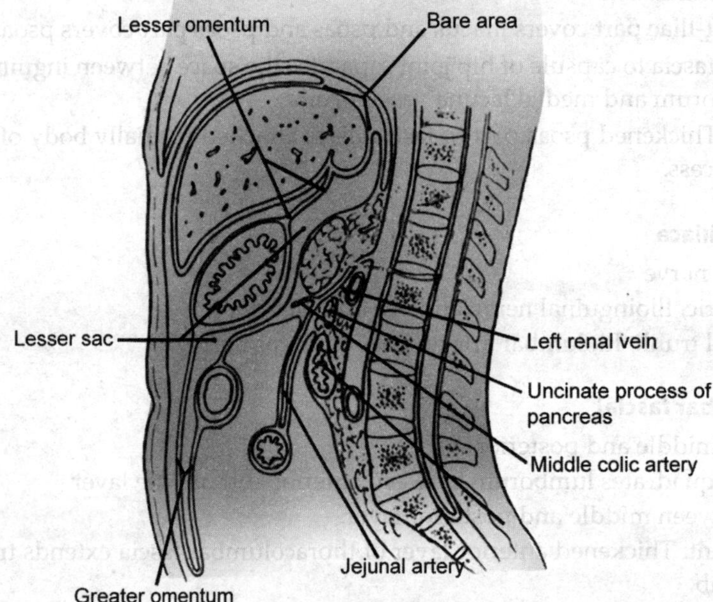

Fig. 1.15: Peritoneal reflection

Parietal layer: The parietal layer lines the body wall and covers the retroperitoneal organs. Developed from somatopleuric layer of lateral plate of mesoderm and supplied by somatic vessels and nerves.

Visceral layer: Develped from splanchnopleuric layer of lateral plate of mesoderm.

Mesogastrium: Suspend from the body wall to endodermal gut tube. (Midgut and Hindgut having only dorsal mesentry).

Ventral and Dorsal Mesogastrium

Derivatives of ventral mesogastrium

Lesser omentum

Falciform ligament

Derivatives of dorsal mesogastrium

- Gastrophrenic ligament
- Gastrosplenic ligament
- Lineorenal ligament
- Greater omentum.

Peritoneal cavity: Potential space filled with capillary fluid between parietal and visceral layer.

Two intercommunicating sacs, Greater and Lesser sac.

Greater sac: Main abdominal cavity surround the majority of abdominal and pelvic viscera.

Lesser sac: (Omental bursa)—Sac behind the stomach and lesser omentum and in front of the pancreas and retroperitoneum.

Greater sac communicate with the lesser sac through the epiploic foramen (Aditus to lesser sac or Foramen of Winslow).

Abdominal organs covered with peritoneum of lesser sac are

- Caudate lobe of liver
- Posteroinferior surface of stomach
- Posterior surface of proximal half of first part of duodenum
- Anterosuperior surface of transverse colon
- Anterior surface of neck, body and tail of pancreas
- Gastric area of left kidney
- Anterior surface of left suprarenal gland

Peritoneal fold	Structures present
Superior or left gastropancreatic fold	Left gastric artery
Inferior or right gastropancreatic fold	Hepatic artery
Paraduodenal fold	Inferior mesenteric vein
Inferior ileocecal fold	Bloodless fold of treves

Blood supply of GIT

Blood supply to foregut: Celiac trunk.

Blood supply to Midgut: Superior mesenteric artery.

Blood supply to Hindgut: Inferior mesenteric artery.

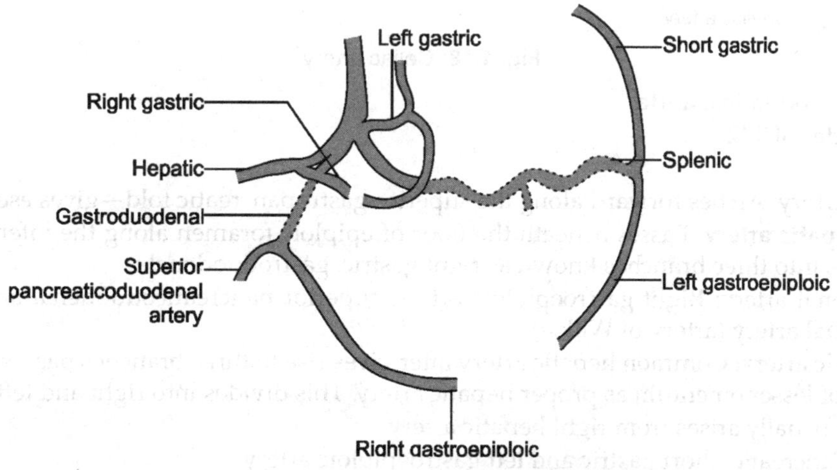

Fig. 1.16: Celiac trunk

Superior Mesenteric Artery

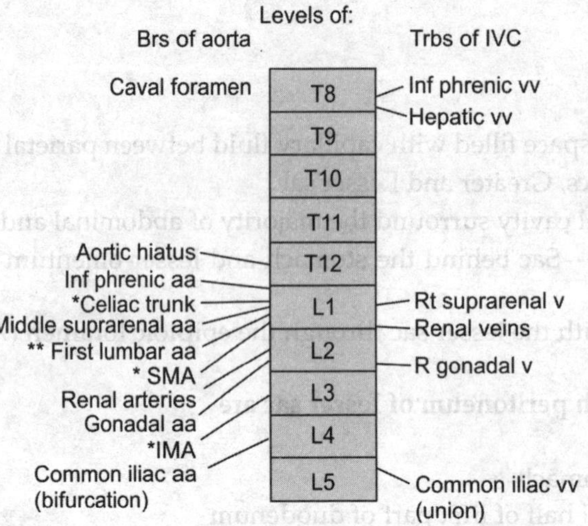

Fig. 1.17: Levels of brs. of aorta and trbs. of IVC

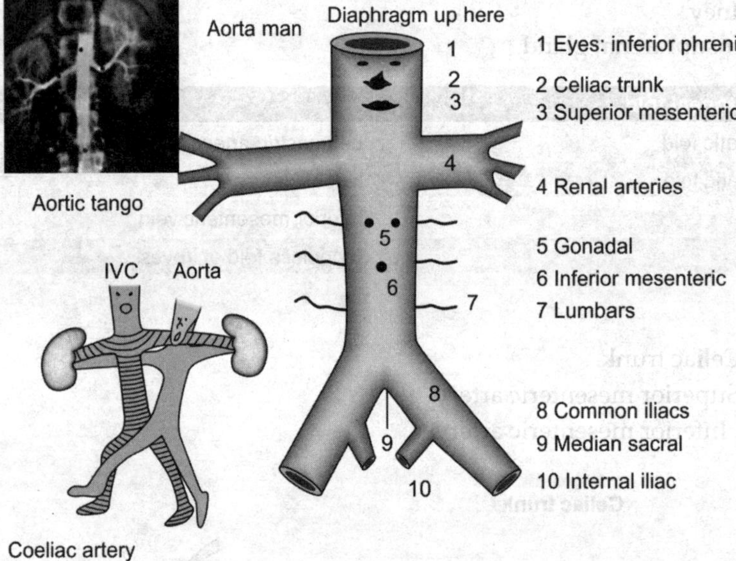

Fig. 1.18: Celiac artery

- Ventral branch of abdominal aorta
- Level–lower border of T12
- **Branches:**
  - **Left gastric artery:** Arches forward along the superior gastropancreatic fold—gives esophageal branches
  - **Common hepatic artery**: Passes beneath the floor of epiploic foramen along the inferior gastropancreatic fold—divides into three branches known as right gastric, gastroduodenal.

    Gastroduodenal artery: Right gastroepiploic artery, superior pancreaticoduodenal artery and sometimes Supraduodenal artery (artery of Wilkie)

    Proper hepatic artery: Common hepatic artery after gives rise to three branches passes upwards within the free margin of lesser omentum as proper hepatic artery. This divides into right and left hepatic artery.

    Cystic artery usually arises from right hepatic artery.
- **Splenic artery**: Pancreatic, short gastric and left gastroepiploic artery.

There is no gastroduodenal vein but there is small prepyloric vein of Mayo

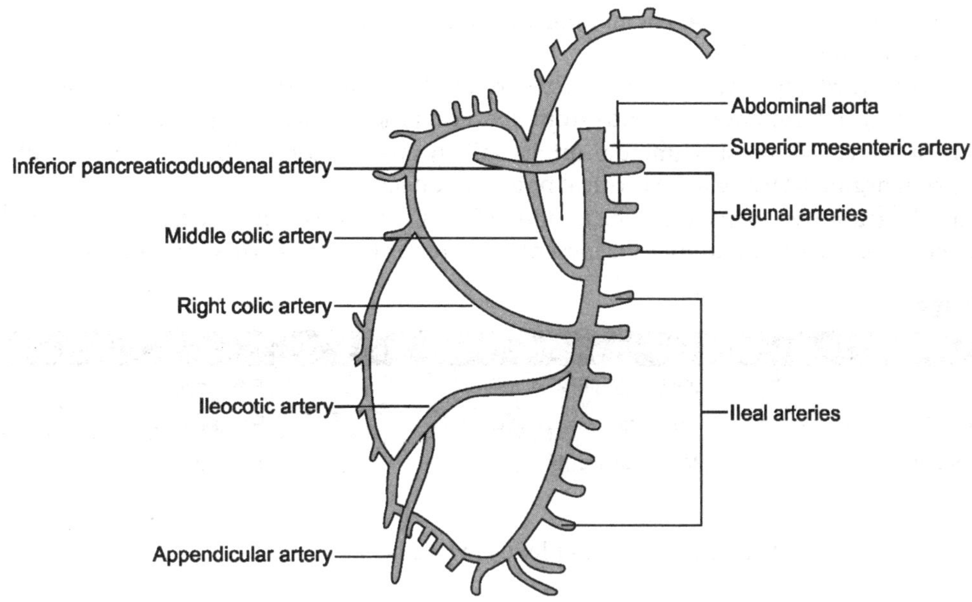

Fig. 1.19: Superior mesentric artery and its branches

- Ventral branch of abdominal aorta
- Level–lower border of L1
- **Branches**
  - **From concave right side**: Inferior pancreaticoduodenal artery, middle colic, right colic artery and ileocolic artery. (Ileocolic gives rise to anterior, posterior cecal and appendicular artery.)
  - **From convex right side:** 12 to 15 jejunal and ileal arteries. Jejunal 1 or 2 arterial arcades and ileal 2 or 3 arterial arcades—Vasa recta straight branches of terminal arcades—End arteries.
- Supplies entire small intestine except proximal part of duodenum up to ampulla of water and large intestine up to the junction of right one third and left two third

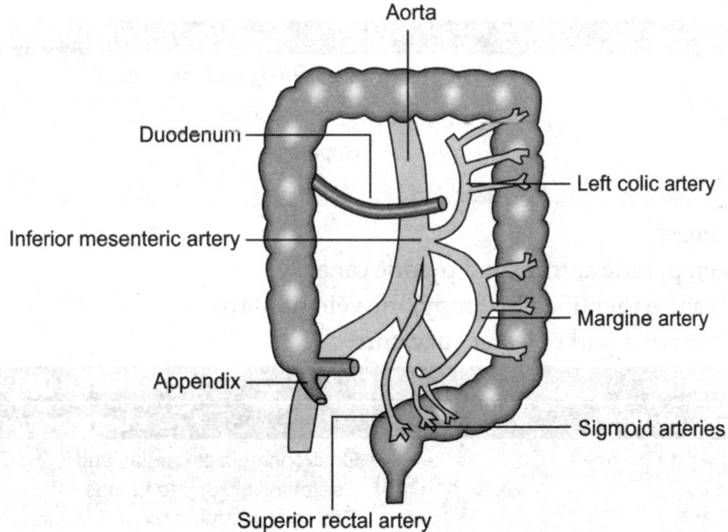

Fig. 1.20: Inferior mesenteric artery

- Ventral branch of abdominal aorta
- Level L3
- Branches: Left colic artery, sigmoid artery and continues as superior rectal artery

- Supplies left one third of transverse colon, descending colon, sigmoid colon, rectum and upper part of anal canal up to pectinate line
- Marginal artery of Drummond: Anastomoses between colic branches of superior and inferior mesenteric arteries form marginal artery of Drummond extends from ileocecal junction to rectosigmoid junction
- Critical point of sudeck: Lowest sigmoidal artery fail to anastomoses with inferior mesenteric artery and discontinuity of marginl artery called as critical point of Sudeck.
- Arc of riolan: Anastomoses between middle and left colic arteries fail to occur. In these situation direct anastomoses between superior and inferior mesenteric arteries occurred. This is called as arc of riolan.

Lymphatic drainage

Gut	Small bowel	Large bowel
Margin of gut	Juxta intestinal	Paracolic
Along blood vessel	Preaortic	Preaortic
External surface of gut	**No equivalent**	Epicolic

Nervous system

Enteric: Myenteric plexus (Auerbach), Submucous plexus (Meissner).

Viscera

Viscera are classified as:

Peritoneal organs: Have a mesentery and are almost completely enclosed in peritoneum. These organs are mobile.

Retroperitoneal organs: Are partially covered with peritoneum and are immobile or fixed organs.

Note: Cecum is sometimes peritoneal and sometimes secondarily retroperitoneal.

Stomach

- Shape: Sickle shaped in cadavers and livings J shaped
  - Sthenic: Longer J limb and slightly oblique
  - Hypersthenic: Very oblique (Steer-horn stomach)
  - Hyposthenic or Asthenic: Vertical.

Cardiac orifice	Pyloric orifice
2.5 cm left of the midline	1.25 cm right of the midline
Under left the costal cartilage-T7	Opposite to L1
Deeply placed	Superficial
Immobile	Movable

Pylorus: Gate keeper of stomach

Sulcus intermedius: Between pyloric antrum and pyloric canal

Living individual pylorus can be identified by Prepyloric vein of Mayo

Incisura angularis: Most depended part of lesser curvature.

Curvature	Peritoneal fold attached
Lesser curvature	**Lesser omentum**
Greater curvature	Gastrophrenic at cardiac end Gastrosplenic opp to fundus Greater omentum rest of cuvature

Structures related to anterosuperior surface

- Gastric impression of left lobe of liver
- Left costal margin, diaphragm, left pleura, base of left lung and 6th to 9th costal cartilages
- Anterior abdominal wall and in empty state transverse colon

Gastric canal (Magenstrasse)

Mucosal gutter extends from cardiac orifice to pyloric antrum along the lesser curvature.

Stomach bed structures

- Left crus of diaphragm
- Left suprarenal
- Anterior surface of left kidney
- Spleenic artery
- Anterior surface of pancreas
- Anterior layer of transverse mesocolon
- Gastric impression of spleen.

Blood supply

- Left gastric artery
- Right gastric artery
- Short gastric artery
- Left gastroepiploic
- Right gastroepiploic
- Posterior gastric from splenic artery.

Mode of arterial supply

- Forming subserosal, intermuscular and submucosal plexuses and from this plexuses long mucosal arteries arises and supply.
- These sort of plexuses are not present along the lesser curvature and so there is frequent formation of peptic ulcers in the region.

Venous drainage

- Right and left gastric vein drain into portal vein
- Short gastric and left gastroepiploic veins drain into splenic vein
- Right gastroepiploic veins drain into superior mesenteric vein.

Lymphatic drainage

- From left of the vertical line from cardiac orifice drain in to pancreaticosplenic nodes along the upper border of body and tail of pancreas.
- From right upper two third of the vertical line from cardiac orifice drain into left gastric nodes.
- From right lower one third of the vertical line from cardiac orifice drain into right gastroepiploic nodes and from thereto pyloric nodes.
- From the pyloric part to Hepatic, Pyloric and left gastric nodes.

  At the cardiac orifice esophageal and gastric lymphatics are continues. So carcinoma of stomach extends to esophagus.

  At the pyloric orifice gastric lymphatics are not continues with the duodenum due to

  - *Circular muscle of stomach not continues with duodenum*
  - *Presence of connective tissue septum in the submucosa of the pylorus.*
  - *Longitudinal muscle fibers turn inwards and join the pyloric sphincter.*

  So carcinoma of stomach does not extend to duodenum.

Nerve supply

- Sympathetic–lateral horn cells of T6–T9 Carries paiful sensation from stomach. (GSA)
- Parasympathetic–Vagus–Anterior vagal trunk from left vagus and posterior vagal trunk from right vagus. Carries nausea, distension and hunger sensation. (Visceral sensations–GVA)
- Anterior vagal trunk–Hepatic and Gastric branches (Nerve of Latarjet)
- Hepatic divides into ascending and descending (Pyloric)
- Posterior vagal trunk–Gastric (Nerve of Latarjet) and celiac branches.
- Nerve of Grassi–Branch from posterior vagal trunk at gastroesophageal junction to supply the fundus of stomach.

Duodenum

- Lies opposite of first, second, and third lumbar vertebra
- Development: Partly from foregut and midgut. The opening of the bile duct into the second part of duodenum represents the junction
- **Parts:**
  - 1st (superior) part–5 cm long, proximally free, distally fixed
  - 2nd (descending) part–7.5 cm long, fixed throughout
  - 3rd (Horizontal) part –10 cm long, fixed throughout
  - 4th (Ascending) part–2.5 cm long, terminal part is free.

First Part

- Begins at the pylorus, passes backwards, upwares and to the right to meet the second part at the superior duodenal flexure
- **Relations:**

Peritoneal	Visceral			
	Anterior	Posterior	Superior	Inferior
Proximal 2.5 cm: Movable and attached to the greater and lesser omentum Distal 2.5 cm: Fixed and retroperitoneal and covered with peritoneum only in its anterior aspect	Quadrate lobe of liver Gall bladder	Gastroduodenal. A A Bile duct Portal Vein	Epiploic foramen	Head and neck of pancreas

Peculiarities of 1st part of duodenum

- Most movable part and behaves like stomach
- Supplied by end arteries
- Affected by peptic ulcers
- Devoid of circular mucosal fold
- Duodenal cap or bulb in the barium meal due to 1st part.

  Arterial supply of 1st part of Duodenum
  - Upper 1/3rd of posterior and upper 2/3rd of anterior surface–Gastroduodenal artery
  - Part of posterior surface: Retroduodenal artery branch of gastroduodenal artery
  - Lower margin: Infraduodenal artery branch of right gastroepiploic artery.

Second Part

- Begins at the superior duodenal flexure, passes downwards to reach the lower border of L3
- **Relations:**

Peritoneal	Visceral			
	Anterior	Posterior	Medial	Lateral
Retroperitoneal and fixed anterior surface is covered with peritoneum except in the middle where it is directly related to the colon	• Right lobe liver • Transverse colon • Root of transverse mesocolon Small intestine	• Anterior surface of the right kidney • Right renal vessels • Right edge of IVC • Right psoas major	Head of pancreas Bile duct	Right colic flexure

- **Interior of 2nd part of duodenum**
  - Plica circularis–circular folds
  - Major duodenal papillae–10 cm distal to pylorus-posteromedial wall
  - Minor duodenal papillae: 2 cm above and ventral to above
  - Plica semicicularis
  - Plica longitudinalis: Intradudenal part of the bile duct
- Most protected part of duodenum from external injury as behind the curvature of vertebral column.

Third Part

- Begins at the inferior duodenal flexure on the right side of the lower border of L3, passes horizontally and slightly upwards in front of the IVC and ends by joining the fourth part in front of the abdominal aorta.
- **Relations:**

Peritoneal	Visceral			
	Anterior	Posterior	Superior	Inferior
Retroperitoneal and fixed Anterior surface is covered with peritoneum except in the median plane where it is crossed by the superior mesenteric vessels and by the root of mesentery	Superior mesenteric vessels Root of mesentery	Right ureter Right psoas major Right testicular/ovarian vessels IVC Abdominal aorta with the origin of Superior Mesenteri Artery	Head of the pancreas with uncinate process	Coils of jejunum

Fourth Part

- Runs upward immediately to the left of aorta, up to L2
- **Relations:**

Peritoneal	Visceral				
	Anterior	Posterior	To the right	To the left	Superior
Retroperitoneal and covered with peritoneum in the Ant surface	Transverse colon Transverse mesocolon lesser sac Stomach	Left sympathetic chain Left psoas major Left renal vessels Left testicular vessels Inferior mesenteric vein	Attachment of the upper part of root of mesentery	Left kidney Left ureter	Body of pancreas

Blood Supply

- Up to the level of the opening of the bile duct, the duodenum is supplied by the superior pancreaticoduodenal artery (Br. of Gastroduodenal. A from celiac trunk)
- Below it by the inferior pancreaticoduodenal. A (Br. Of superior mesenteric Artery)
- Venous drainage: splenic, superior mesenteric and portal vins.

PERITONEAL FOSSAE (RECESSES)

Small pockets of peritoneal cavity enclosed by small, inconstant folds peritoneum. **They are classified as:**

- **Lesser sac**
- **Duodenal fossae/recesses**
  - Superior duodenal recess: present in 50%. Situated at the level of L2. Its orifice looks downwards.
  - Inferior duodenal recess: present in 75%. Situated at the level of L3. Its orifice looks upwards
  - Paraduodenal recess: present in 20%. It orifice looks to the right. The inferior mesenteric vein lies in the free edge of the fold of peritoneum
  - Retroduodenal recess: largest of the duodenal recesses, present occasionally, orifice looks to the left
  - Duodenojejuna/mesocolic recess: present in 20%. Its orifice looks downwards to the right
  - Mesentericoparietal fossa of Waldeyer's: 1%, orifice looks to the left. The superior mesenteric vessels lie in the fold of peritoneum covering this fossa.

All the Duodenal Recesses are in Relation to the Fourth Part of Duodenum

- **Cecal fossae:**
  - Superior ileocecal recess: Formed by a vascular fold present between the ileum and the ascending colon
  - Inferior ileocecal recess: Covered by the fold of Trieves, inflamed by retrocecal appendix
  - Retrocecal recess: Lies behind the Cecum and often contains the appendix.

- Intersigmoid recess: Disappears in advance of age, lies behind the apex of the sigmoid mesocolon. Contains left ureter and bifurcation of left common iliac artery.

Duodenum	Rest of small intestine
Fixed	Mobile
Supplied by two rows of vasa recta	Single row of vasa recta
Brunner's gland present in the submucosa	Absence of brunner's glands

Jejunum	Lieum
Wider	Narrower
Thicker	Thinner
More vascular	Less vascular
Proximal 2/5th of small intestine	Distal 3/5th of small intestine
Occupies umbilical region	Occupies hypogastric and pelvic region
One or two arterial arcades and longer	3 or more and shorter
Fat confined along the root of mesentry. Translucent windows between vasa recta.	Fat uniformly distributed and no translucent windows.
Internal features Larger and thickly present mucosal folds Longer villi Scanty payer's patches	Smaller and widely separated mucosal folds Smaller villi Numerous peyer's patches

Meckel's diverticulum

- Arises from the antimesentric border
- Two ft proximal to the iliocecal junction
- Two inches in length
- Present in 2% of population
- It causes peptic ulceration, inflammation and intestinal obstruction. When meckel's diverticulum enters the hernia sac, it is known as Littre's hernia.
  Mesentery See Question no 4
  Large intestine

Characteristic features

- Teniae coli-absent in appendix and rectum
- Sacculations and haustrations
- Appendices epiploicae: Peritoneal pouches of fat absent in cecum, appendix and rectum.

Small intestine	Large intestine
Long and narrower (6.5 meters) and movable	1.5 mt long and wider and fixed
Villi present	Villi absent
Paneth cells present in the crypts of lieberkuhn.	No paneth cells
Numerous peyer's patches	Less payer's patches
Not present	Teniae coli, sacculations and haustrations and appendices epiploicae present.
Supplied by vasa recta arise from terminal arterial arcades.	Supplied by marinal artery of drummond.

Cecum

Types

- Fetal type: 2% Conical;
- Infantile(Quadrate): 3% Quadrate in shape

- Normal adult: 90% Rt saccule enlarge more than left
- Exaggerated: 4 to 5% Rt saccule hugely enlarge and Lt atrophies.

Topography

Trinagular area bounded above transtubercular plane, below lateral half of inguinal ligament (fold of groin) and medially by right lateral plane.

Arterial supply

Anterior and posterior cecal artery

Venous drainage

Drain into ileocolic vein and into superior mesenteric vein.

Lymphatic drainage

Ileocolic nodes

Nerve supply

Sympathetic–T10–L1
Parasympathetic–Vagus

Interior of cecum

- Ileocecal orifice: Posteromedial wall at the junction with ascending colon represented at the intersection of transtubercular and right lateral plane.
- Appendicular orifice: 2 cm below the above guarded by Vale of Gerlach.

Peritoneal recess around the Ileocecal junction

- Superior ileocecal recess
- Inferior ileocecal recess
- Retrocecal recess.

APPENDIX

- Suspended by peritoneal fold mesoappendix.
- Surface anatomy: Base of appendix is 2 cm below the intersection between transtubercular and right lateral plane.
- Mc Burney's point: Junction of medial two-third and lateral one-third of a line connecting the umbilicus and the anterior superior iliac spine.
- **Various positions of appendix are**
  - Subcecal: 11 o'clock 2%
  - Retrocecal: 12 o'clock 60% commonest
  - Left paracecal: 10'clock
  - Splenic: 2 o'clock 1–2%
  - Promontoric: 3 o'clock Rare type
  - Pelvic: 4 o'clock 30% second commonest type
  - Midinguinal 6 o'clock

Arterial supply: Appendicular branch of inferior division of the ileocolic artery end artery
Artery of Seshachalam: Accessory appendicular artery branch on posterior cecal artery.
Venous drainage: Drain into superior mesenteric vein
Lymphatic drainage: Superior mesenteric nodes via ileocolic nodes
Nerve supply: Parasympathetic vagus
Sympathetic: Superior mesenteric plexus

LIVER

- Largest gland in the body, covered by glisson's capsule
  External features:
  Surfaces (5) Anterior, Posterior, Superior, Inferior, Right;
- Lobes (2) m Right and left (Right lobe occupies 5/6th of the liver has all the 5 surfaces and presents the caudate lobe and quadrate lobe.

Relations of the Liver

Anterior	Posterior surface	Superior	Inferior surface	Right
– Xiphoid process – Ant-Abd wall – Diaphragm (each side) Falciform Lig. Gets Attached to this surface	• Bare area of liver – Related to left Suprarenal gland- upper pole and diaphragm • Groove for IVC – Lodges IVC • Caudate lobe – Diaphragmatic crura – Right Inferior phrenic. A – Celiac trunk • Fisure for ligamentum venosum • Esophageal impression	– Cardiac Impression – Dome of the diaphragm	– Gastric impression – Omental tuberosity or tuber omentale – Fissure for ligamentum teres – Quadrate lobe: • Leser omentum • Pylorus • 1st part of duodenum – Fossa for gall-bladder – Impressions of • Hepatic flexure • Right kidney • 2nd part of duodenum	Upper 1/3 Diaphragm Pleura Lung Middle 1/3 Diaphragm Pleura, 9th and 10th ribs Lower 1/3 Diaphragm

Peritoneal relations: Most of the hepatic surface is covered by peritoneum except:

- Bare area
- Groove for IVC
- Fossa of Gallbladder
- Coronary ligament
- Lesser Omentum

Lobes are divided by:
- Attachment of falciform lig: Anteriorly and Superiorly
- Fissure for the ligamentum teres: Inferiorly
- Fissure for the ligamentum venosum: Posteriorly

Blood supply: 20% → from hepatic artery 80% Portal vein

Venous drainage: Hepatic veins then into IVC

- Couinand's classification is based on hepatic vein mainly and portal vein
- Each Couinad Segment contains portal vein, Bile duct and a branch of hepatic artery
- Liver biopsy is done through Right 8th intercostals space.

Extra points

The liver is divided into two lobes of unequal size by the falciform ligament.
Liver is divided functionally by plane passing through Gallbladder and IVC (Canties line).
The quadrate and caudate lobes are anatomically part of the right lobe but functionally part of the left.
Hepatic vein and IVC supports the Liver. (Hepatic vein has no extrahepatic course)
The hepatic artery divides as 'Y' shaped and Portal vein divides as 'T' shaped.

Gallbladder

The gallbladder lies in a fossa on the visceral surface of the liver to the right of the quadrate lobe.
Globular or Pear shaped, 50 ml volume.

Hartmanns pouch is not a normal feature of GB

Cystic artery is a branch of right hepatic artery, thrombosis of which does not usually lead to ischemia of GB, because supply from GB bed is adequate.

Spiral valve of Heister: Mucosal arrangement in neck of GB.

Structure	Length/diameter	Speciality
Common hepatic duct	4 cm/4 mm	
Bile duct	8 cm/8 mm	3 parts–Supraduodenal, Retroduodenal, Paraduodenal

Bile Duct

- Two hepatic ducts forms common hepatic duct and runs near the liver, with the hepatic artery proper and portal vein in the free margin of the lesser omentum
- The bile duct lies to the right of the hepatic artery proper and usually of the right of, and anterior to, the portal vein in the free margin of the lesser omentum
- The omental foramen is posterior to these structures at this point.

Relations

Supra duodenal	Retroduodenal	Infraduodenal	Intraduodenal
Anterioraly: liver Posteriorly: portal vein and epiploic foramen To the left: Hepatic. Art	Anteriorly: Ist part of duodenum Posteriorly: IVC To the left: Gastroduodenal. Art	Anteriorly: posterior surface of head of pancreas Posteriorly: IVC	

- Bile duct joins the pancreatic duct at an angle of about 60 degree at hepatopancreatic ampulla of Vater.
- Most of blood supply to supraduodenal part of Bile duct comes from below.

Pancreas

The ventral pancreatic diverticulum becomes the major pancreatic duct (of Wirsung), and the dorsal pancreatic diverticulum becomes the minor pancreatic duct (of Santorini).

Most of the pancreas is secondarily retroperitoneal, but the distal part of the tail of the pancreas remains peritoneal in the splenorenal ligament. The tip of the tail of the pancreas reaches the hilus of the spleen.

Both pancreatic ducts open into the second portion of the duodenum.

The main vessel supplying it is splenic vessel.

The neck, body and tail of the pancreas receive their blood supply from the splenic artery.

The head of the pancreas receives its blood supply from the superior and inferior pancreaticoduodenal arteries. This region is an important region for collateral circulation because there are anastomoses between these branches of the celiac trunk and superior mesenteric artery.

Length is 15 cm, retort shaped.

Spleen

Spleen is largest lymphoid organ. **It is not a endodermal derivative.** A lymphoid aggregate forms it. So it is a mesoderm derivative.

The spleen is a peritoneal organ in the upper left quadrant that is related to the left 9th, 10th and 11th ribs. Fracture of these ribs may lacerate the spleen.

In as much as the spleen lies above the costal margin, a normal-sized spleen is not palpable. An enlarged spleen may be palpated below the left costal margin.

The splenic artery and vein reach the hilus of the spleen by traversing the splenorenal ligament.

The odd numbers 1, 3, 5, 7, 9, 11, is related to it by measuring 1 × 3 × 5, weighing 7 Oz and lies between 9th and 11th rib

Pedicle of spleen: Gastrosplenic and Linorenal ligament

Suspensory ligament of spleen: Lienophrenic (Phrenicosplenic) ligament
Sustentacular liensis: Phrenicocolic ligament
Clinical angle of spleen: Anterior basal angle

Linorenal ligament contains

Tail of pancreas, Splenic vessels, nerves and lymphatics.

Sites of accessory spleen are

Hilum of spleen, Gastro-splenic lig and left spermatic cord.

GER (Gastroesophageal reflux) prevented by

- Right crus of diaphragm
- Lower esophageal muscle fibers–sphincteric action
- Mucosal flap produced by stomach
- Cecum like prosate have width greater than length.

Organs	Length
Cecum 6 × 7.5 cm	
Ascending colon	15 cm
Transverse colon	45 cm
Descending colon	30 cm
Sigmoid colon	45 cm
Rectum	12 cm
Anus	4 cm
Male urethra	20 cm
Female urethra	4 cm
Female urethra during birth (vaginal stretching)	10 cm
Uterine tube	10 cm
Ureter	25 cm
Duodenum	25 cm
Esophagus	25 cm
Vagina	10 cm
Kidney	12 cm
Testes	4 × 3 × 2 cm
Prostate	3 × 4 × 2 cm

Transverse mesocolon

Peritoneal fold suspends transverse colon from the posterior abdominal wall.

Contents

- Transverse colon
- Anastomosis between middle colic and ascending branch of left colic artery forming marginal artery of Drummond.
- Nerves and lymphatics
- Loose areolar tissue.

Sigmoid colon

- Continuation of descending colon and end at the rectosigmoid junction at the level of S3.
- Suspended from posterior abdominal wall by sigmoid mesocolon which is inverted 'V'shaped and apex in front of the bifurcation of left common iliac artery and left ureter enters the pelvic cavity. Intersigmoid recess behind the apex. Left limb extends from left pelvic brim to junction of descending and sigmoid colon. Right limb extends from left sacroiliac jt to middle of S3.

- **Contents of sigmoid mesocolon**
  - Sigmoid colon
  - Sigmoid branches of inferior mesenteric artery
  - Branch from superior rectal artery
  - Nerves and lymphatics
  - Loose areolar tissue.
- **Arterial supply**
  - 3 or 4 sigmoid branches of inferior mesenteric artery
  - Recurrent branch from superior rectal artery.
- **Venous drainage**
  - Drain into portal vein via inferior mesenteric vein

  Lymphatic drainage

  Inferior mesenteric nodes and preaortic nodes.

  Nerve supply

  Sympathetic: Superior hypogastric plexus–from L1–L2
  Parasymphathetic: Pelvic splanchinic nerve–S1, S2, S3

Rectum

- Continuation of sigmoid colon at the level of S3 and extends up to anus at anorectal ring 2–3 cm in front and below the tip of coccyx corresponds I male apex of prostate.
- Rectus–Straight.
  Originally named in monkey.
- The superior one-third of the rectum is covered by peritoneum anteriorly and laterally.
- Three valves of Houston: Allow the flatus to pass.
  Three lateral curves: Upper and lower curves convex to right, middle curve convex to left.
  Two anteroposterior curve–Sacral curve–convex backwards and Perineal curve–convex backwards.
- **Specialities of Rectum–No Tenia coli, No Appendices epiploicae, No Sacculations**
- Rectouterine pouch (female) 5.5 cm from anal margin
- Rectovesical pouch (male) 7.5 cm from anal margin
- Denonvilliers facia: Rectovesical fascia (connective tissue condensation)
- Waldeyers fascia: Attachment to sacrum by connective tissue extends from anorectal junction to the coccyx. Thickened pelvic fascia
- Lateral ligament of rectum: Retroperitoneal tissue around middle rectal vessels
- Superior rectal artery is direct continuation of Inferior mesenteric artery
- **Spaces related to rectum**
  Upper 1/3–Pararectal fossae
  Middle 1/3–Pelvic rectal space
  Lower 1/3–Ischiorectal space.
- Longitudinal muscles of rectum continues above as teniae and below at anorectal junction lends with puborectalis and levator ani to forms conjoind fibroelastic sheath.
- Rectourethral muscle (Muscle of Roux): Some longitudinal muscle fibers attached to urethra called recturethral muscle.
- Houston's valves
  Permanent mucosal folds 4 in number
  First at anorectal junction
  Second at 2.5 cm above 3rd along the concavity of upper lateral curve.
  Third along the concavity of middle lateral curve: Most important and constant valve.
  Fourth 2.5 cm below the 3rd along the concavity of lower lateral curve.

- **Arterial supply**
  Superior rectal artery: Principal artery of rectum—Continuation of inferior mesenteric artery.
  Midle rectal artery: Branch of andterior division of internal iliac artery.
  Inferior rectal artery: Branch of internal pudendal artery.
- **Venous drainage**
  Superior rectal vein drain into inferior mesenteric vein
  Middle rectal vein drain into internal iliac vein
  Inferior rectal vein drain into internal puddendal vein
  Importance of rectal veins
  - **Impotant communication between portal and systemic**
  - Superior rectal vein devoid of valves
  - Superior rectal vein pierces the posterior rectal wall.
- **Lymphatic drainage**
  - Upper part: Left common iliac nodes
  - Middle part: Internal iliac nodes
  - Lower part up to anal valves: Internal iliac nodes
  - Below the anal valves: Superficial inguinal nodes
- **Nerve supply**
  - Sympathetic: Superior hypogastric plexus from L1–L2
  - Parasymphathetic: Pelvic splanchnic nerve S1, S2, S3

Anal canal

Hilton's and Pectinate line divide the interior of anal canal into three parts

- Upper area: Above the pectinate line 15 mm
  - Anal column (Column of morgagni) 6–8 in number
  - Anal valves: Crescentric mucosal folds connecting the lower end of the anal columns. The position of valve is indicated by pectinate or dentate line.
  - Anal papillae: Projection of epithelial process from the free margin of the anal valve.
  - Anal recess: Recess above the valves and in between the anal column
  - Anal glands: Tubular glands.
- Intermediate area: Between pectinate and Hilton's line 15 mm
  Lined by nonkeratinized stratified squamous epithelium.
- Lower area: Anal verge 8 mm
- Corrugator cutis ani: Longitudinal muscles of rectum attached to perianal skin by piercing the subcutaneous part of external anal sphincter.

Pectinate line

- Mucocutaneous junction
- Corresponds with the position of anal valves
- Middle of internal sphinter
- Divides the anal canal into upper and lower area
- Upper area developed from endoderm and lower area developed from ectoderm
- Upper area supplied by superior rectal artery and lower area supplied by inferior rectal artery.
- Upper area drained into portal vein and lower area drained in to systemic vein via inferior rectal vein.
- Upper area drained into internal iliac nodes and lower area drained into superficial inguinal nodes. Pectinate line is the Watershed line of anus.
- Upper area supplied by autonomic nerves and lower area supplied by spinal nerves inferior rectal nerve.

Hilton's line

- Represented by anal intersphincteric groove at the lower end of internal anal sphincter
- Anal and Lunate fascia extend up to this line

- Intermuscular septum attached at this line carrying the fibers of levator ani and longitudinal muscles of rectum
- Ischiorectal abscess opens at or below this line.

Anorectal ring

- Responsible for continence of anus
- Muscular ring at the anorectal junction
- Formed by upper part of internal anal sphincter, deep part of external anal sphincter and puborectalis part of levator ani muscle.

Internal anal sphincter

- Involuntary muscle
- Thickening of circular muscle of the lower part of rectum
- Separated from the mucosa by internal venous plexus
- Supplied by sympathetic from superior hypogastric plexus and parasympathetics from pelvic splanchnic nerves.

External anal sphincter

- Voluntary muscle three parts subcutaneous, superficial and deep
- Subcutaneous: Separated from skin by external plexus.
- Superficial: Arises from tip of coccyx from anococcygeal raphe and inserted into perineal body.
- Deep part: Surrounds anorectal junction no bony attachments-inserted into perineal body continuous opposite superficial transverse perineal muscle.
- Supplied by inferior rectal branch of pudendal nerve and 4th sacral nerve.

Kidneys and Ureter

The kidneys are a pair of bean-shaped organs approximately 12 cm long. They extend from vertebral level T12 to L3 when the body is in the erect position. The right kidney is positioned slightly lower than the left because of the mass of the liver.

Kidney moves with respiration about 2 cm vertically.

Coverings of the kidney (From within outwards)

True capsule

Perinepheric fat

Perirenal fascia

Paranephric fat

Perirenal fasia: Anterior layer—Fascia Zukerkandel Gerota

Posterior layer: Fascia Lateral conal fasia—Above two layers fuses at the lateral border of kidney and form lateral conal fasica.

Presenting parts

Upper pole, lower pole

Medial border and lateral border

Anterior and posterior surface.

Kidney's relation to the posterior abdominal wall

Both kidneys are in contact with the diaphragm, Costodiaphragmatic recess, psoas major and iliopsoas fascia, quadratus lumborum and anterior layer of thoracolubar fascia and transverses abdominis and fascia transversalis.

Right kidney: Contacts the above structures and the 12th rib.

Left kidney: Contacts the above structures and the 11th and 12th ribs.

Anterior Relations

Left kidney	Right kidney
• Suprenal gland • Small Intestine (jejunum) and Stomach • Spleen and Its vessels, Splenic flexure • Descending colon, Pancreas	• Suprarenal gland • Jejunum • Second part of duodenum • Hepatic flexure of colon and Liver

Posterior Relations (of both kidneys)

Muscles (4)	Nerves (3)	Ligaments (2)	Vessels and rib (each 1)
• Diaphragm • Psoas major • Quadrates lumborum • Transverses abdominis	• Subcostal N • Iliohypogastric N • Ilioinguinal N	• Medial arcuate • Lateral arcuate	• Subcostal Vessels • 12th rib-upper pole of right kidney • Left kidney is also related to 11th rib

Ureter's Relation to the Posterior Abdominal Wall

The ureter lies on the anterior surface of the psoas major.

Applications

The most common sites of ureteral constriction susceptible to blockage by renal calculi are, where the renal pelvis joins the ureter, where the ureter crosses the pelvic inlet, where the ureter enters the wall of the urinary bladder Most important of all posterior relation is costodiaphragmatic recess.

Renal pelvis

- Funnel shaped
- Capacity less than 5 ml
- Pacemaker wall of minor calyces
- Hilum of kidney **VAP:** Renal **V**ein, renal **A**rtery and **P**elvis (front to back).

Internal structure

Outer renal substance and inner renal sinus.

Renal substance: Outer cortex and inner medulla

Cortex: Contains renal column and cortical arches. Renal coloumn in between the adjacent pyramids Traversed by interlobar vessels.

Cortical arches intervenes between the base of pyramid and the surface of the kidney. Each arch contains medullary rays and convoluted parts. Interlobular vessels pass on either side of arches.

Lobule of kidney

Area of cortical arches bounde on each side interlobular vessels with central axis of medullary ray known as lobule of the kidney.

Convoluted part (Cortical labyrinth): In between medullary rays and contain renal corpuscles and convoluted portion of nephron.

Medulla contains 8–18 pyramids which contains loop of henle, collecting tubules and duct of Belini.

Lobe of kidney: One pyramid capped with a joining cortex known as Lobe of kidney.

Renal Sinus

Cavity within the kidney and communicates outside through the hilum.

Contents of renal sinus

- Renal blood vessels, lymph vessels and nerves
- Perinephric fat
- Minor, Major calyces and Renal pelvis: Minor 7–13, Major 2–3

The apex of each pyramid ends as a papilla where collecting ducts open.

Calyces: The minor calyces receive one or more papillae and unite to form major calyces, of which there are two to three per kidney.

Renal pelvis: The dilated upper portion of the ureter that receives the major calyces.

Arterial supply

- The paired renal arteries are branches of the abdominal aorta
- Interlobar arteries travel in renal columns in the cortical areas between pyramids
- Arcuate arteries run parallel to bases of pyramids
- Interlobular arteries are branches of arcuate arteries
- Afferent arterioles lead to capillary tufts of glomeruli.

Venous drainage

Follows the same pattern as the arteries:

- The right renal vein enters the inferior vena cava.
- The left renal vein receives the left gonadal vein, the left suprarenal vein, and the left inferior phrenic vein, and may receive a root of the hemiazygos vein before crossing anterior to the aorta to join the inferior vena cava.

Lymphatic drainage

The kidneys drain to the lumbar nodes.

Innervation

Primarily sympathetic with postganglionic cell bodies located in the renal plexus.

- Preganglionic sympathetic fibers are from T10–L1. This accounts for referred pain in the renal colic from loin to groin and inner side of thigh.
- Parasympathetics: Vagus.

Ureters

Ureters are fibromuscular tubes, whitish cord, nonpulsatile with peristalsis.

Three parts

- Pelvis of ureter
- Abdominal part
- Pelvic part

Relations of the Ureter

Abdominal part of ureter

Anteriorly		Posteiorly	Medially
Right side	Left side	• Psoas major • Tips of transverse process • Genitofemoral nerve	Right side IVC
Third part of duodenum Peritneum Right colic vessels Ileocolic vessels Gonadal vessels Root of mesentery Terminal part of ileum	Peritoneum Gonadal artery Left colic vessels Sigmoid colon Sigmoid mesocolon		Left side Left gonadal vein Inferior mesenteric vein

Pelvic part of ureter

Three parts

First part Vertical part: Extends from lateral pelvic wall along the anterior margin of greater sciatic notch up to ischial spine

Second part Oblique part: From the ischial spine to superolateral border of bladder above the levator ani muscle

Third part (Intravesical part): Within the bladder wall

In its downward course		
Posteriorly	**Laterally**	**Anterior**
• Internal Iliac. A and its anterior division • Internal Iliac. V • Lumbosacral trunk • Sacroliac joint	Obliterated umbilical aretry • Inferior vesical A • Obturator N • Obturator A • Obturator V • Uterine and Vaginal arteries. • Middle Rectal A	Male Peritoneum **Female** Ovarian fossa. Ovary and uterine tube

In its forward course	
In males	**In females**
• Ductus deferens crosses from lateral to medial side • Seminal vesicle lies below and behind the urter • Vesical veins surround its terminal part	• Ureter lies in lower and medial part of broad ligament • Uterine A lies first above and in front and then crosses it from lateral to medial side • Ureter lies 2 cm lateral to the supravaginal protion of cervix and runs above the lateral fornix • The terminal portion lies anterior to vagina

Blood Supply

- Upper part: Renal artery, common iliac and internal iliac
- Middle part: Aorta
- Pelvic part: Vesical, middle rectal or uterine vessels.

Nerve supply

- Sympathetic T10–L1
- Parasympathetic S2–S4

Constrictions on Ureter

- At the pelvis-ureteric junction
- At the brim of the lesser pelvis
- At its passage through the bladder wall [narrowest]

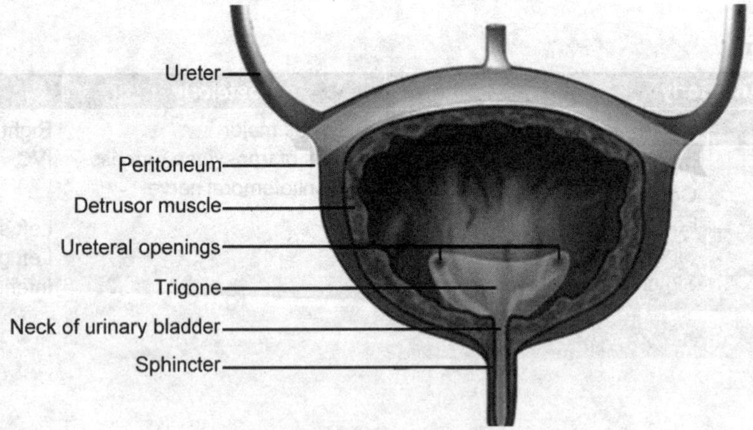

Fig. 1.21: Urinary bladder

- In children abdominopelvic organ
- Adults pelvic organ
- Shape: Tetrahedral in empty stage and ovoid in distended stage.

- Presenting parts: Apex, base (Posteroinferior surface or fundus), Superior surface and inferolateral surface.
- Apex gives attachment of median umbilical ligament
- Base upper part covered by peritoneum: The nonperitoneal area of the base called external trigone.
- **Space of retizius**
  - Potential space between the anterolateral pelvic wall and the sides of the bladder.

Boundaries

In front: Symphysis and body of pubis
Behind and on each side: Posterior true ligament of bladder
Above: Paravesical fossa
Below: Puboprostatic and pubovesical ligament
Medially: Inferolateral surface of the bladder.
Laterally: Fascia covering levator ani and obturator intenus.
Contents: Retropubic fat and Vesical plexus of veins.

- Neck of the bladder: The lowest point of the bladder from which urethra begins.

True ligaments 9	False ligaments 7
Condensation of fascia around the neck and base of the bladder	Folds of peritoneum
Lateral true ligament 2 Lateral puboprostatic ligament (females: lateral Pubovesical ligament) 2 Medial puboprostatic ligament (females: medial Pubovesical ligament) 2 Median umbilical ligament 1 Posterior true ligament of bladder 2	Lateral false ligament 2 Posterior false ligament: the sacrogenital fold 2 Media (2) l and Median umbilical folds (1)

- **Bladder bed**
  - Structures upon which bladder rests
  - Symphysis pubis, Fascia of levator ani and obturator internus, Ampulla of rectum, Anterior vaginal wall, Base of prostate and superior fascia of uro genital diaphragm.

  Trigone of bladder (Internal trigonum or trigonum vesicae)
  - Equilateral triangle on the inner aspect of the base of the bladder where the mucous membrane is tense and glistening due to absence of submucous coat.

  Boundaries
  - Apex: Internal urethral orifice
  - Base: Interureteric ridge (Mercier's bar)
  - Posterolateral angle: Ureteric orifice
  - Sides: Urethrourteric lines

  Structures of trigone
  - Mucous membrane of transitional epithelium
  - Trigonal muscle of bell
  - Loose areolar sheet known as fascia of waldeyer
  - Detrusor muscle.
- **Importance of trigone**
  - Most fixed and dependent part
  - Richly supplied by vessels and nerves
  - Developed from mesoderm.

Blood supply

The bladder is supplied by vesicular branches of the internal iliac arteries. The vesicular venous plexus drains to internal iliac veins.

Lymphatics

Drain to the external and internal iliac nodes.

Innervation

Parasympathetic innervation is from sacral segments S2, S3, and S4. (Nervi erigentes) The preganglionic parasympathetic fibers travel in pelvic splanchnic nerves to reach the detrusor muscle.

Sympathetic innervation is through preganglionic fibers, which are derived from T11 through L2. Stimulates sphincter vesicae and inhibits detrusor (Nerve of filling).

Urethra

- Male urethra: 18–20 cm
- Female urethra: 4 cm

Urethra (3 parts)

Prostatic urethra	Membranous urethra	Spongy/penile urethra
• 3–4 cm • Wides 7 Most dilatable • Shows Urethral creast • Colliculus seminalis (Verumontanum)- rounded elevation in the middle of urethral crest into which prostatic utericle (correspons to vagina so it is called Vaginus masculinus) in the center and ejaculatory duct on either sides open • Prostatic sinuses: Mucosal gutters on each side of the crest, receive ducts of prostatic glands • Transverse section is semilunar	• 1.5 cm • Shortest portion of urethra • Narrowest and least dilatable part of male urethra, except the urethral orifice • Transverse section is stellate • Bulbourethral glands are situated	• 10–15 cm • Longest portion passes through the bulb, body and glans penis. • Two dilatations: intrabulbar fossa in the bulb and navicular fossa in the glans. • External urethral orifice is the narrowest part • Blubourethral glands open here

Posterior urethra: Prostatic and Membranous urethra

Anterior urethra: Penile urethra (Bulbar and Pendular part)

Features of spongy urethra

- Urethral glands (Littre's gland)
- Urethral lacunae: Largest lacunae called lacunae magnaguarded by valve of Guerin.

Arterial supply

Inferior vesical, middle rectal, internal puddendal artery

Lymphatic drainage

Internal and external iliac nodes

Nerve supply

Sympathetic: Superior hypogastric plexus–L1 and L2, Parasympathetic–Pelvic splanchnic nerves S1, S2 and S3

Name of valve	Site
Valve of Guerin	Spongy urethra
Valve of Gerlach	Appendicular orifice
Valve of Houston	Rectum
Spiral valve of Heister	Cystic duct
Valve of Hasner	Nasolacrimal duct

Female urethra

- **Glands around the female urethra**
  - Urethral glands: Simple tubular mucosal gland present around entire urethra.

- Paraurethral glands: Corresponds with prostatic glands in male. Present close to external urethral orifice. Tubular mucosal gland
- Greater vestibular gland: Compound racemose gland. Situated behind the bulb of the vestibule. Corresponds to bulbourethral glands of male.

- **Urethral lacunae**

Male counterpart	Female counterpart
Penis	Clitoris
Prostate	Paraurethral glands of skeene
Bulbourethral glands	Grater vestibular glands
Testis	Ovary

Testis

- Pair of male reproductive gland ellipsoid in form suspended into scrotum by corresponding spermatic cord.
- Left testis 1 cm lower than the right
- **Presenting parts**
  - Upper end overlapped by head of epididymis and connected by efferent ductules. **Upper end gives attachment of sessile fibrofatty body known as Appendix of testis which is remnant of cephalic part of Mullarian duct.**
  - Lower end connected to tail of epididymis
  - Anterior border
  - Posterior border
  - Medial surface
  - Lateral surface related posteriorly epididymis, which is separated from the testis by semilunar recess called **sinus of epididymis.**
- **Coverings of the testis**
  - Outside to inwards
  - Visceral layer of tunica vaginalis
  - Tunical albuginea: Project in the posterior border into the testis called mediastinum of testis and from the anterior surface of mediastinum fibrous septa extends and divide into lobules of the testis.
  - Tunica vasculosa: Vascular membrane lines the individual lobules.

Epididymis

- Comma shaped
- Head: Coiled efferent ductules called lobule of the epididymis. **Head gives attachment of sessile or pedunculated mass known as Appendix of epididymis which is the remnant of cephalic part of mesonephros.**
- Body and tail: Coiling of single tube called canal of epididymis.
- **From the tail canal of epididymis continues as vas deferens.**
- **Store house of spermatazoa head and body of epididymis.**

Arterial supply of testis

- Testicular artery branch of abdominal aorta
- Artery to vas branch of either superior or inferior vesical artery
- Cremastric artery branch of inferior epigastric artery.

Venous drainage

- Fifteen to twenty veins from testis and epididymis join to form pampniform plexus content of spermatic cord.
- At superficial inguinal ring plexus join to form four veins.
- At deep inguinal ring joins to form two veins.

- Finally join to form single vein at the posterior abdominal wall and right drain into IVC and left drain into left renal vein.

Lymphatic drainage
- Preaortic and para-aortic nodes.

Nerve supply
- Sympathetics T10 and T11

Vas deferens
- Length 45 cm
- Principal content of spermatic cord: Placed posteriorly accompanied by pair of testicular veins and artery to vas.
- Join with duct of seminal vesicle at the base of prostate and form ejaculatory duct
- Ampulla: Behind the base of bladder dilated portion known as Ampulla.
- Storage of semen: Bulk of semen produced by the seminal vesicle.

Prostate

Conical fibromuscular gland around the proximal part of male urethra

Seminal vesicle semen	Prostate semen
Forms the bulk amount	Forms considerable amount
Alkaline	Acidic
Rich in fructose, PG, vesiculase enzyme	Contain acid phosphatase, fibrinolysin, PG and zinc (protection of spermatozoa against the spermiophagic cells in the female genital tract and role in chronic inflammation.

Coverings of the prostate

True capsule: Condensation of the fibrous stroma

False capsule: Visceral layer of pelvic fascia

Between these two prostatic venous plexus present.

Presenting parts

Apex

Base

Posterior surface: 4 cm above the anus palpable per rectum diveded by transverse groove into smaller upper part and lower larger part. Upper part is Median lobe and lower part divided by median sulcus into two lateral lobe.

Anterior surface: Separated from symphysis pubis by retropubic fat, prostatic venous plexus and deep dorsal vein of penis.

Inferolateral surface

Lobes of prostate

Anatomically: 3 lobes median and lateral lobes.

Surgically: 5 lobes Median, Anterior, Posterior and two lateral.

Median lobe forms vulva vesicae at apex of trigone: Fibromuscular impregnated with mucosal glands-commonly enlarged in benign hypertrophy of prostate.

Two lateral lobes separated superficially median sulcus and deeply continuous as posterior lobe. Lateral lobes covers the side of urethra.

Isthmus of prostate: Infront of urethra lateral lobe connected by fibroumuscular isthmus. In fetal life it contains glands called anterior lobe–Anterior lobe persis up to the age of 6.

Now only Zones of prostate: By Mc Neal
- Peripheral zone (70%)
- Central zone
- Transitional and periurethral zone

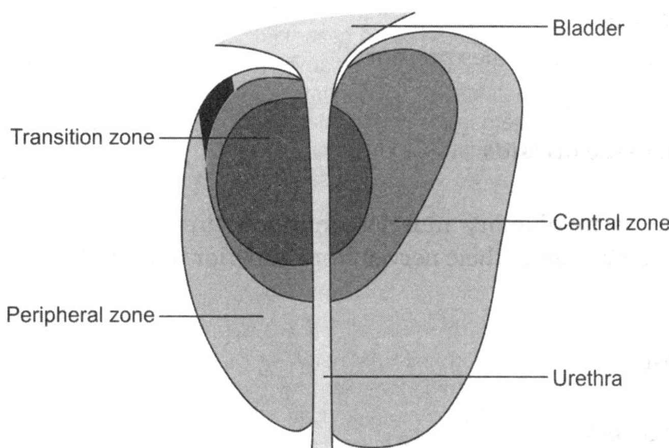

Fig. 1.22: Prostate zones

Structures traversing the prostate

- Prostatic urethra
- Ejaculatory duct
- Prostatic utericle

Arterial supply

Inferior vesical, middle rectal and internal pudendal artery.

Venous drainage

Prostatic venous plexus Vesical venous plexus Internal iliac vein
Internal vertebral venous plexus (Paravertebral veins of Batson) This is the route of vertebral metastasis in prostatic cancer.

Lymphatic drainage

Internal and External iliac and sacral nodes.

Nerve supply

Sympathetics–L1 and L2
Parasympathetics–Pelvic splanchnic nerves S1, S2 and S3

Spermatic cord

- Length–7.5 cm
- Extends from upper posterior border of testis to deep inguinal ring.
- **Coverings of spermatic cord**
  - Internal spermatic fascia from fascia transvesalis at deep inguinal ring
  - Cremastric muscle and cremastric fascia from internal obilique
  - External spermatic fascia derived from external obilique aponeurosis at superficial inguinal ring
- Contents of spermatic cord
  - Vas deferens
  - Pampniform venous plexus
  - Testicular artery, artery to vas and cremastric artery.
  - Lymphatics from testis and epididymis.
  - Genital branch of genitorfemoral nerve supplies cremaster and testicular plexus of sympathetic from T10 and T11
  - Loose connective tissue.

- Vestige of process vaginalis.
- Accessory suprarenal tissue sometimes present.

Scrotum

Coverings of scrotum from outside inwards

- Skin
- Dartos muscle–Subcutaneous involuntary muscle continuous in front with fascia camper and scarpa and behind fascia colles-supplied by sympatheic nerves from superior hypogastric plexus subcutaneous fat absent in the scrotum
- External spermatic fascia
- Cremastric muscle and fascia
- Internal spermatic fascia
- Parietal layer of tunica vaginalis.

Arterial supply

Superficial and deep external pudendal artery branch of femoral artery.
Posterior scrotal branch of internal pudendal artery.

Venous drainage

Partly great saphenous and partly internal iliac veins.

Lymphatic drainage

Horizontal group of inguinal nodes

Nerve supply

Anterior third–ilioinguinal and genitorfemoral nerve conveying the fibers of L1
Posterior third Posterior scrotal branch from pudendal nerve and perineal branch from posterior femoral cutaneous nerve derived fibers from S4.

Penis

- Two parts Root and Body
- **Root or Radix**
  - Situated in the superficial perineal poch
  - Consists of diverging crura and bulb
  - Each crus attached to the inner aspect of everted ischiopubic ramus
  - Covered superficially and sides by ischiocavernosus
  - Deep artery of penis traverses this crus
  - Two crura united as corpora cavernosa on the dorsal aspect
  - Bulb is covered by bipennate bulbospongiosus
  - Bulb continuous as Corpora spongiosum on the ventral aspect
  - Urethra traverses the bulb.

Body of penis

- Pendulous structure directed downwards and forwards and makes an angle with the root
- Distal expanded portion is called glans penis.
- Prepuce or Foreskin–Fold of skin covering the glans
- Corona glandis–Raised margin at the base of glans penis
- Corona glandis contain sebaceous gland which secrete smegma
- Preputial sac–Potential space between prepuce and glans
- Frenulum–Undersuface of the glans connected to the prepuce by median fold

- Body of penis composed of paired corpora cavernosa on the dorsal surface and unpaired corpora spongiosa on the ventral surface. Both of which separated by sptum pectiniformis
- Erection of penis is purely vascular.

Coverings of the penis

- Skin
- Superficial fascia (Fascia penis)–contain superficial dorsal vein of penis
- **Structures deep to fascia penis are:**
  - Unpaired deep dorsal vein of penis middle
  - Pair of dorsal arteries of penis on each side of vein
  - Pair of dorsal nerves of penis lateral to artery
- Tunica albuginea–covers separately the corpora cavernosa and corpora spongiosum.

Ligaments of penis

- Fundiform ligament
- Suspensory ligament of penis-Apex attached to symphysis of pubis and the base blends with the fascia peni on the dorsal surface.

Arterial supply

Three paired arteries artery to bulb, dorsal artery of penis and the deep artery of penis branches of terminal branches of internal pudendal artery.

Venous drainage

- Superficial dorsal veins of penis from prepuce–Great saphenous vein
- Deep dorsal vein of penis–Prostatic venous plexus.

Lymphatic drainage

- Prepuce and the skin of the penis–Superficial inguinal nodes.
- Glans penis–Deep inguinal nodes and sometimes external iliac nodes.

Nerve supply

- Somatic nerves–Dorsal nerve of penis branches of pudendal nerve.
- Parasympathetics–Pelvic splanchnic nerves (Nervi erigentes–S2, S3, S4)
- Sympathetics–From L1-Vasocontrictors.

Uterine tubes (Ovi ducts or Fallopian tube)

- Paired length 10 cm
- Four parts namely intramural, isthmus, ampulla and infundibulum.
- **Arterial supply**
  - Both ovarian and uterine artery
- **Venous drainage**
  - Ovarian vein
- **Lymphatic drainage**
  - Preaortic and lateral aortic nodes
  - Intramural portion drain into superficial inguinal nodes through round ligament of the uterus.
- **Nerve supply**
  - Sympathetics–T10–L2
  - Parasympathetics–vagus.

Uterus

- Parts (Fundus)-Part of uterus above the attachment of uterine tube.
- Body–Extends from fundus to isthmus corresponds with internal os of the cervical canal.

- Cervix–Part below the isthmus divided into supravaginal and vaginal portion.
- Axes of uterus–Anteversion and antiflexion. It is maintained by 1. Forward pull of the fundus by the traction of the round ligament of uterus 2. Backward pull on the cervix by traction of the uterosacral ligament. 3. Intrinsic growth of uterine maculature.
- Angle between cervix and the vagina is 90 degree.
- Angle between body of uterus and cervix is 125 degree.
- Mucous membrane is called endometrium.
- Lateral border of body of uterus gives attachment of broad ligament and related to tortuous uterine vessels.
- Lateral angle or cornua gives attachment of following structures
  - Uterine tube
  - Proximal part of round ligament below and in front
  - Ligament ovary below and behind.
- **Cervix**–2.5 cm in length supravaginal and vaginal part

Vaginal part cervix surrounded by gutter of vaginal canal and divided into anterior, posterior and two lateral vaginal fornix. Posterior fornix is the deepest and is covered by peritoneum of rectouterine pouch. Lateral fornix gives attachment of Mackenrodt's ligament and crossing of ureter and uterine artery.

Arbor vitae uteri: Median logitutinal fold in the anterior and posterior wall of cervix and palmate folds spread laterally from the median fold resembling branches of tree.

Ovula Nebothi: Tubular or branched glands in the cervix which are blocked and retained secretion produce cystic dilatation called Ovula Nebothi.

Functional isthmus: Upper one-third of cervical canal and internal os.

Ligaments of cervix:

- Pair of Mackenrodt's ligament posteriorly
- Pair of Uterosacral ligaments posteriorly
- Pair of Pubocervical ligaments anteriorly.

Arterial supply of uterus

Uterine artery and ovarian artery

Anastomosis between the above arteries take place in the broad ligament close to the lateral angles of the uterus.

Uterine artery–Coronary or arcuate artery Radial artery form stratum vasculare in the middle layer of muscle coat Basal and spiral artery spiral artery supplies the functional zone of endometrium and basal supplies the basal portion of endometrium.

Venous drainage

Uterine and ovarian veins

Lymphatic drainage

From fundus and upper part of uterus–Preaortic and lateral aortic nodes some drain into superficial inguinal nodes.

From the lower part of uterus–External iliac nodes

From the cervix–External iliac, internal iliac, obturator and lateral sacral nodes.

Nerve supply

Sympathetics–T12–L1

Parasympathetics–S2–S3

Ligaments of Uterus

True ligaments	False ligaments
Round ligament of uterus (Ligamentum teres uteri)-Lateral angle of uterus through deep inguinal ring, inguinal canal inserted in the subcutaneous tissue of labium majus-Remnant of distal part of gubernaculums testis	Uterovesical fold (Anterior false ligament)

Contd...

Contd...

True ligaments	False ligaments
Mackenrodt's ligament (Transverse cervical ligament) from cervicovaginal junction to fascia covering levator ani. Related above crossing ureter and uterine artery and loer attachment of brad ligament-Cardinal ligament of uterus.	Rectovaginal fold (Posterior false ligament)
Uterosacral ligament Cervix to 3rd sacral vertebrae.	Pair of rectouterine fold
Pubocervical ligament-Cervix to pubic bone	Pair of Broad ligament–Peritoneal fold extends from lateral border of uterus to lateral pelvic wall. **Contents:** • Uterine tube • Proximal part of round ligament • Ligament of ovary • Ovarian vessels • Uterine vessels • Tubules and duct of epoophoron • Tubles of paraophoron • Lymphatics.

Pouch of Douglas (Rectouterine pouch)

Boundaries

In front–Supravaginal part of cervix and posterior fornix of vagina.

Behind–Middle one-third of rectum.

On each sides–Rectouterine fold.

Floor–Rectovaginal fold 5.5 cm above anus and 7.5 cm above vagina.

Support of uterus

- **Structural supports**
  - Mackenrodt's, round and uterosacral ligaments and pubocervical ligaments
  - Muscles–Levator and muscles and perineal body (Gynecological perineum)
  - Visera–Slanting posterior wall of vagina and anorectal flexure, upper surface of urinary bladder, sigmoid colon.
- Peritoneal investments
- Maintaining anteversion and anteflexion position of uterus.

Vagina

- Arterial supply–branches from vagina, uterine, internal pudendal and middle rectal artery. Azygos vaginal artery–Longitudinal anastomosis between uterine and vaginal artery.
- Venous drainage–Internal iliac vein.
- Lymphatic drainage:
  - Upper third–External iliac nodes
  - Middle third–Internal iliac nodes
  - Lower third–Superficial inguinal nodes.
- Nerve supply Sympathetics–L1, L2
  Parasympathetics–S2, S3, S4

Ischiorectal fossa

- Space on each side of the anal canal between inferior surface of the pelvic diaphragm and pelvic surface of ischium.
- Wedge shaped
- **Boundaries**
  - Laterally–Obturator internus and obturator fascia and ischial tuberosity.
  - Medially–Levator and muscle covered by anal fascia and sphincter ani externus.

- In front–Transversus perinea superficialis and profundus.
- Behind–Sacrotuberous ligament covered by lower fibers of gluteus maximus.
- Apex–Fusion of anal fascia and obturator fascia.
- Base–Skin and superficial fascia.

- **Recess**–Anterior and posterior
- Fascia–Lunate fascia
- **Alcocks or pudendal canal**–Fascial tunnel situated in lateral wall of the fossa 2.5 cm above the ischial tuberosity- Contents are internal pudendal vessels and pudendal nerve which divides in the canal into dorsal nerve of penis and perineal nerve.
  Arrangement above downwards are dorsal nerve of penis, internal pudendal vein, artery and perineal nerve.
- **Tegmentum:** Summit of the lunate fascia.
- **Subdivisions of ischiorectal fossa**
  - Suprategmental space
  - Ischiorectal space
  - Perianal space.
- **Contents of ischiorectal fossa**
  - Internal pudendal vessels and pudendal nerve
  - Inferior rectal nerve and vessels
  - Posterior scrotal vessels and nerves
  - Perineal branch of 4th sacral nerve
  - Perforating branches of 2nd and 3rd sacral nerves
  - Pad of fat.
- Hiatus Schawlbe–Failure of origin of levator ani from obturator fascia.
  Structures piercing the fascia colles are:
  - Perineal branch of posterior femoral cutaneous nerve
  - In female urethra and vagina.

  Superficial perineal pouch
  Boundaries
  - Above–Perineal membrane
  - Below–Fascia colles
  - Each sides–Inner surface of ischiopubic ramus
  - Behind–Fusion of perineal membrane and fascia colles
  - In front–Open continuous as superficial inguinal space.

Contents

- Muscles–Ischiocavernous, transverse perinea superficialis and Bulbospogiosus
- Vesssels–Two posterior scrotal branches, Transverse perineal vessels.
- Nerves–Two posterior scrotal nerves, Perineal branches of posterior femoral cutaneous nerve
- Crus penis or clitoris, male bulb of penis, female urethra, vagina, bulb of the vestibule and greater vestibular gland.

Structures piercing of perineal membrane (Inferior fascia of urogenital diaphragm)

- Two posterior scrotal vessels and nerves
- Deep artery of penis
- Dorsal artery of penis
- Urethra
- Male–Duct of bulbourethral gland and artery to the bulb
- Female–Vagina behind urethra.

ABDOMINAL VASCULATURE

Branches of abdominal aorta

Ventral branches	Lateral branches	Dorsal branches	Terminal branches
Celiac trunk Superior mesenteric A Inferior mesenteric A	Inferior phrenic A Middle superarenal A Renal A Testicular/ovarian A	Lumbar arteries-4 paired Median sacral artery-unpaired	Common iliac A

Arterial supply abdominal aorta

The most common site for an abdominal aneurysm is in the area between the renal arteries and the bifurcation of the abdominal aorta.

The most common site of atherosclerotic plaques is at the bifurcation of the abdominal aorta.

Common Iliac Artery

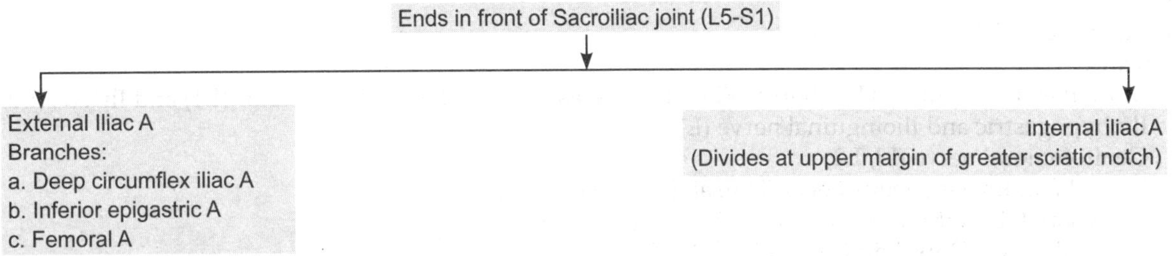

Branches of Internal Pudendal A

- Inferior rectal A
- Perineal A
- Artery of penis/clitoris
- Urethral A

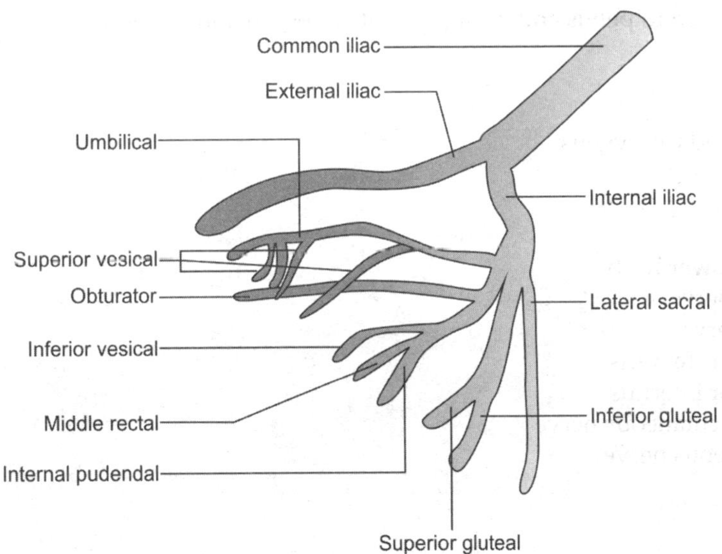

Fig. 1.23: Internal iliac artery

Anterior division	Posterior division
Obliterated umbilical artery Superior vesical artery Inferior vesical artery Middle rectal artery	Iliolumbar artery Superior gluteal artery Lateral sacral artery

Contd...

Contd...

Anterior division	Posterior division
Obturator artery Uterine artery Vaginal artery Inferior gluteal artery Internal pudendal artery	

Lumbar Plexus

- Formed in the substance of Psoas major.
- Formed by the union of the ventral ramus of upper three lumbar nerves and larger ascending part of ventral ramus of the fourth lumbar nerve.
- Lumbosacral trunk–Descending smaller part of fourth lumbar and fifth lumbar nerve join to form lumbosacral trunk.
- Nervus furcalis–L4
- **Branches**
  - Muscular–To Quadratus lumborum (T12–L4), Psoas major (L2–L4), Psoas minor (L1) and Iliacus (L2, L3)
  - Iliohypogastric and Ilioinguinal nerve (L1)
  - Genitofemoral nerve (LI, L2)
  - Lateral femoral cutaneous nerve (Dorsal division of L2, L3)
  - Accessory Obturator nerve (Ventral division of L3, L4)
  - Femoral nerve (Dorsal division of L2, L3, L4)
  - Obturator nerve (Dorsal division of L2, L3, L4).

Sacral plexus

- Formed by the ventral rami of the L4, L5, S1, S2, S3 and S4.
- Sacral plexus in front of the piriformis and behind the pelvic vessels.
- **Branches**
  12 in numbers–5 confined to pelvis and 7 supply gluteal region and lower limb.

Pelvis

- Nerve to piriformis
- Nerve to levator ani and Coccygeus
- Perineal branch of S4 nerve
- Pelvic splanchnic nerve S2, S3, S4
- Pudendal nerve

  Gluteal region and lower limb
  - Superior gluteal nerve
  - Inferior gluteal nerve
  - Nerve to quadratus femoris
  - Nerve to obturator internus
  - Posterior femoral cutaneous nerve
  - Perforating cutaneous nerve
  - Sciatic nerve.

Coccygeal plexus

- Formed by the union of the ventral rami of the fourth sacral, fifth sacral and the coccygeal nerves.
- Anococcygeal nerve arises from the coccygeal plexus pierces the sacrotuberous ligament and supply the skin close to the tip of coccyx.

In females, Uterine. A comes as a seventh branch of ant division of internal iliac A. And Inferior Vesicular A is replaced by Veginal A Thus,

Superior rectal A → Continuation of inferior mesenteric A
Middle Rectal A → Branch of ant division of int iliac A
Inferior Rectal A → Branch of internal Pudendal A

Internal iliac artery

- First and highest branch of anterior division–Superior vesical artery
- Largest of all branches–Superior gluteal artery
- Inferior vesical artery gives prostatic artery.

Venous Drainage

The drainage of the inferior vena cava and its tributaries

Blood Supply of Git

Celiac trunk artery of foregut	Superior mesenteric artery of midgut	Inferior mesenteric. artery of hindgut
• Left gastric A • Splenic A – Left gastroepiploic A – Short gastric A – Pancreatic A • Hepatic A – Right gastric A – Right and left Hepatic A – Cystic. A [Br. of Right hepatic A] – Gastro-duodenal A – Rt. Gastro epiploic A – Superior pancreatico duodenal A	• Inf. Pancreatico Duodenal A • Middle Colic A • Right Colic A • Ileocolic A – Supperior and Inferior Branch – Anterior Cecal A – Posterior Cecal A (Appendicular) – Jejunal and Ileal A	• Superior Rectal A • Sigmoid A • Left colic A

- Right gastroepiploic A is a br. of Gastroduodenal A but left gastroepiploic A is a br. of Splenic A
- Right gastric A is a br. of Hepatic A and left gastric A is a br. of celiac A
- Superior pancreaticoduodenal is a br. of Gastroduodenal. A when as inferior is a br. of superior mesenteric A

HEAD AND NECK ANATOMY

Neck

General features

Cutaneous Innervation

Lesser Occipital–C2 cervicogenic headache

Great auricular–C2 C3

Transverse cervical Number of neck C2 C3

Supraclavicular–C3 C4 Sternoclavicular joint

Neck is divided into two compartments anterior and posterior. Anterior or visceral compartment and posterior or vertebral compartment.

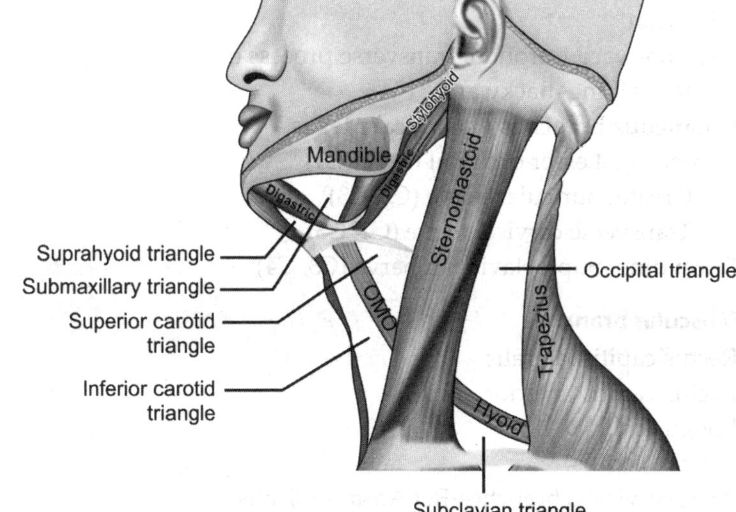

Fig. 1.24: Triangles of the neck

Posterior triangle

Bounded by Trapezius, sternocleidomastoid and clavicle.

Floor above downwards semispinalis capitis, splenius capitis, levator scapulae, scaleneus medius and scalenus posterior.

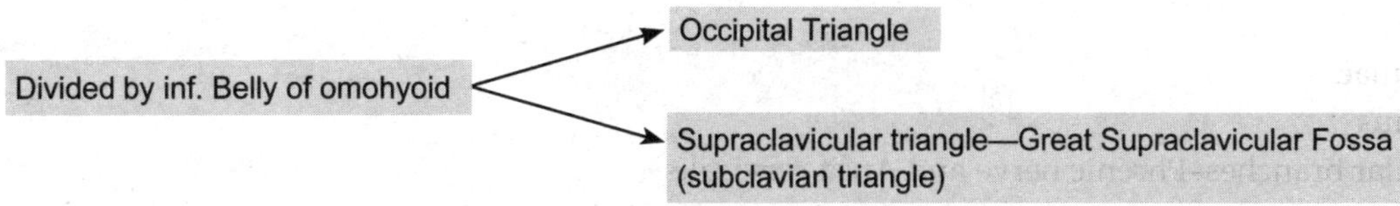

Contents of occipital triangle:
- Sinal accessory nerve
- 3rd and 4th cervical nerve
- Dorsal scapular nerve
- Cutaneous branches of cervical plexus-lesser occipital nerve, greater auricular nerve, tranverse cervical nerve and supraclavicular nerve.
- Upper trunk of brachial plexus
- Superficial cervical artery
- Occipital artery.

Contents of supraclavicular triangle:
- Third part of subclavian artery
- Subclavian vein
- Trunks of brachial plexus and branches of root and trunk.
- Terminal part of external jugular vein
- Superficial cervical, Suprascapular and Dorsal scapular artery.
- Supraclavicular lymph nodes.

What is accessory phrenic nerve?

Twing from nerve to subclavius to phrenic nerve (mainly from C5)

Anterior triangle

Bounded by anterior border of sternocleidomastoid, anterior midline and body of mandible, Apex manubrium sterni. Divided into digastric, submental, Muscular and carotid by omohyoid and digastric.

Contains 5 pairs of strap muscles, Submandibular gland, common carotid artery, internal carotid artery, external carotid artery and parts of cranial nerves X and XII.

Cervical plexus

Formation C1 to C4 ventral rami and situated behind sternocleidomastoid on the scalenus medius and levator scapulae behind the prevertebral fascia.

Loops 3 C1 and C2, C2 and C3, C3 and C4

Direction

First–Forward infront of transverse process of atlas

Remaining–Backwards

Cutaneous branches of cervical plexus

Ascending–Lesser occipital nerve (C1)

Greater auricular nerve (C2, C3)

Transverse cervical nerve (C2, C3)

Decending–Supraclavicular nerve (C3, C4)

Muscular branches

Rectus capitis lateralis

Rectus capitis anterior

Longus colli

Longus capitis

Ansa cervicalis branches-Ref Ansa cervicalis

Phrenic nerve

Sternocleidomastoid

Trapezius

Levator scapulae

Sclenus medius

Major muscular branches–Phrenic nerve and Ansa cervicalis

Infrahyoid Muscles (Ribbon muscles) Rectus cervicis

Superficial–Sternohyoid and Omohyoid.

Deep–Sternothyroid and Thyrohyoid. Segmental innervations by C1, C2 and C3 Like rectus adominis

All are depressor of hyoid

Suprahyoid muscles–Digastric, styloid, mylohyoid and geniohyoid

Larynx downwards–For low notes Sternothyroid

Larynx upwards–For high notes Thyrohyoid

Infrahyoid muscles morphologically correspond with Rectus abdominis so they are called Rectus cervici.

Suprahyoid muscles: Digastric, stylohyoid, mylohyoid and geniohyoid.

Carotid triangle

Boundaries

In front and above - Posterior belly of digastrics and Stylohyoid. In front and below–Superior belly of omohyoid. Behind-Sternocledomastoid Floor–Thyrohyoid, Hyoglossus, Inferior and middle pharyngeal constrictor.

Contents

- Common carotid artery and internal and external carotid artery
- Internal jugular vein
- Spinal accessory nerve
- Hypoglossal nerve
- Vagus nerve
- Cervical part of sympathetic chain
- Parotid gland
- Jugulodigastric and Jugulo-omohyoid nodes.

Most significant artery of external carotid is middle meningeal artery, a branch of maxillary artery. Injury in trauma produces epidural hematoma.

ECA 5 branches in carotid triangle

- Superior thyroid
- Lingual
- Facial
- Asc. Pharyngeal
- Occipital

Digastric triangle: Bounded above body of mandible, below and behind posterior belly of digastrics, below and behind Anterior belly of digastrics and floor mylohyoid, hyoglossus and middle constrictor.

The structure which divides the digastrics triangle is stylomandibular ligament.

Contents

- Submandibular glang
- Facial vein
- Submandibular lymph nodes
- Facial artery
- Mylohyoid nerve and vessels
- Hypoglossal nerve
- Lower part of parotid gland
- External carotid artery
- Carotid sheath and its contents.

Submental triangle: Bounded by base-body of hyoid bone, Side-Anterior belly of digastrics, Apex-Lower border of symphysis menti and floor-Mylohyoid.

Contents: Submental lymph node

Cervical Rib

7th cervical vertebra compresses brachial plexus and subclavian artery

SCM (Sternocleidomastoid)

Supply–spinal accessory, cervical rami-proprioception

Action–both-head forwards, raises head from supine, forced inspiration.

Branchial cyst–At the junction of upper and middle third of SCM, through carotid bifurcation ends in pharyn Constrictor.

Branchial Fistula–Lower border of SCM connection between 2nd pouch and cervical sinus.

Enters into tonsillar fossa → opens into pharynx.

Stylohyoid Ligament Styloid process–lesser horn

Deep cervical fascia

Suprasternal space of Burn's (Interclavicular space) contents–Anterior jugular veins, jugular venous arch, sternal heads of SCM, Lymph node and interclavicular lig.

Stylomandibular ligament–thickening of deep fascia.

Infec tissue spaces–Infratemp fossa, mediastinum below

Above hyoid–Subnandibular, submental, pharyngeal spaces, prevertebral (near base of skull)

Below hyoid–Pretracheal infront of esophagus

Retrovisceral–Behind oesophagus

Prevertebral–Between Ver. Column and Pre Ver. Fascia extends–post. mediastinum.

Cellulitis of neck–Mandibular molar teeth (3rd Molar)–Lingual plate of mandible–Extends into

Submandibular, Sublingular space } Anteriorly

Parapharyngeal space, Pterygoid space } Posteriorly

1. **Content of Lesser triangle is:**

   a. Linual nerve b. Lingual artery
   c. Hypoglossal nerve d. Lingual node

   Ans. b

Lesser triangle Above–Hypoglossal nerve
  Below–Diverging digastric tendon

Content: Lingual artery

2. **Structure piercing the sphenomandibular lig:**

   a. Mylohyoid nerve b. Lingual nerve
   c. Facial artery d. ECA

   Ans. a

   Sphenomandibular lig–Extend from spine of sphenoid to the Lingula of the mandible
   Structure piercing the sphenomandibular lig–Mylohyoid nerve and vessels
   Stylomandibular lig–Extend from tip of styloid process and the angle of the mandible
   Structure piercing the Stylomandibular lig–Facial artery

Carotid Body (Chemo)–Adventitia at its bifurcation contains → Glomus (I), Sustentacular cells (II)

Developmental Arch 3rd–gives rise to ICA. Glossopharyngeal nerve supplies carotid body and sinus.

Subclavian Artery–Scalenus Anterior–3 Parts

Subclavian Vein–anteroinferior to subclavian artery

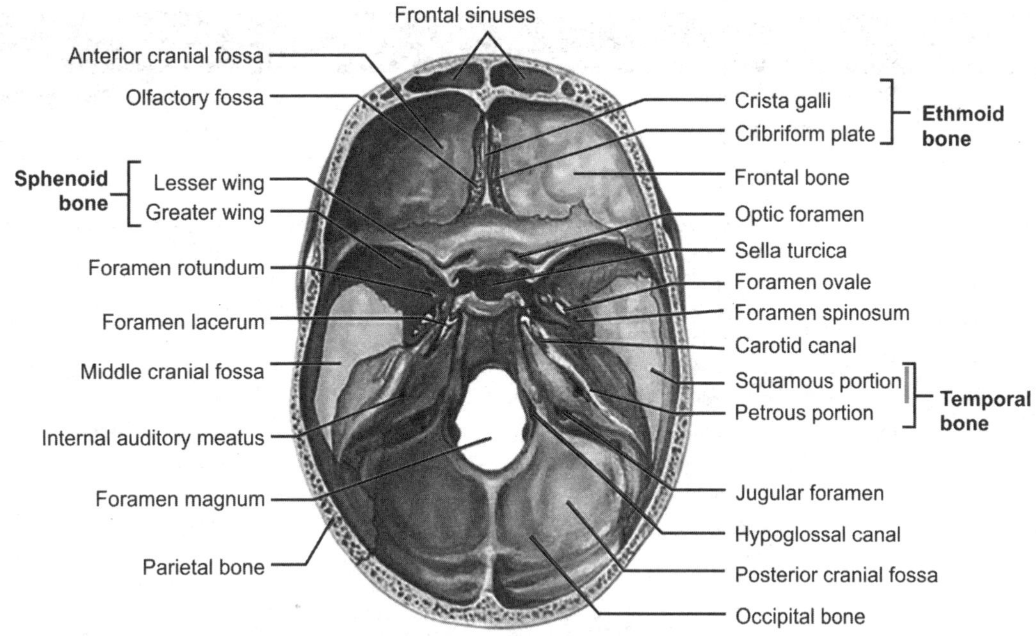

Fig. 1.25: Cranium

Base of skull openings

Foramen magnum	– Meninges, ant and post spinal arteries, membrana tectoria, apical ligament of dens, Vertebral arteries
Hypoglossal canal	– XII nerve
Jugular foramen	– IX, inferior petrosal sinus (anterior compartment), X, XI nerve (middle compartment), Jugular vein (posterior compartment)
Internal acoustic meatus	– VII , VIII nerve
Foramen spinosum	– Middle meningeal artery
Foramen ovale	– Mandibular nerve, accessory middle meningeal artery, lesser petrosal nerve, emissary veins. **(Male)**
Foramen rotandum	– Maxillary nerve
Superior orbital fissure	– III, IV, V–Ophthalmic nerve, VI nerve, Ophthalmic veins
Optic canal	– II nerve and Ophthalmic artery
Cribriform plate	– I nerve
Petrotymp fissure	– Chordotympani, anterior malleolar ligament

Speciality of cranial nerves

Speciality	Cranial nerve
Longest intracranial course	Abducent nerve
Longest subarachnoid course	Trochlear nerve
Longest cranial nerve in body	Trigeminal nerve
Smallest nerve (Slender)	Trochlear nerve
Only nerve emerges dorsally from brainstem	Trochlear nerve
Only nerve decussate within brainstem	Trochlear nerve
Only nerve emerges from pons	Trigeminal nerve
Shortest nerve	Mandibular nerve

CN	Name	Type	Function	Lesions	Exits-Enter cranium	Region innervated
I	Olfactory	Sensory	Smells	Anosmia	Cribriform plate	Nasal cavity
II	Optic	Sensory	Sees	Anopsia Loss of light reflex with III,	Optic canal	Orbit
III	Occulomoto Nuclear Edinger westpal nucleus	Motor	Moves eyeball in all direction Adduction most important action Constricts pupil Accommodation(ciliary muscle) Raises eyelid (LPS)	Diplopia Dilated pupil Drooping of eyelid	Superior orbital fissure	Orbit
IV	Trochlear (Only nerve arises dorsally)	Motor	Superior oblique–depresses and abduction of eyeball Intorsion	Trouble in going downstairs	Superior orbital fissure	Orbit
V	Trigeminal Ophthalmic V1 Maxillary nerve V2 Mandibular nerve V3 Four nucleus Meckels cave: lodges Gasserian ganglion	Mixed	General sensation of forehead/scalp/cornea General sensation of nasal cavity, palate, maxillary face and maxillary teeth General sensation in skin over mandible, mandibular teeth, tongue-anterior two third, Motor to muscles of mastication, digastic- antr belly mylohyoid, tensor tympani and palati	V1–loss of sensation in affected side Loss of blink reflex V2–loss of general sensation in skin over maxilla and maxillary teeth Loss of general sensation in skin over mandible, mandibular teeth, tongue, weakness in chewing, Jaw deviation toward weak side	V1–Superior orbital fissure V2–Foramen rotandum V3–Foramen ovale	Orbit and Scalp Pterygopalatin fossa Infratemporal fossa
VI	Abducens (Dorellos canal)	Motor	Lateral rectus–abduction	Diplopia Pseudoptosis	Superior orbital fissure	Orbit
VII	Vestibulocochlear	Sensory	Hears Linear acceleration (gravity) Angular acceleration (head turning)	Sensorineural hearing loss Loss of balance Nystagmus	Internal auditory meatus	Inner ear
VIII	Facial	Mixed	To muscles of facial expression, stylohyoid, stapedius Posterior belly of digastric Anterior two-third of tongue Salivates (submandibular and sublingual gland) Tears (lacrimal gland) Makes mucus (nasal and palatine gland)	Deviation of mouth to opposite side, loss of blink reflex Hyperacusis Loss of taste (Ageusia) Dry eye Bells palsy	Internal auditory meatus	Face, Nasal and oral cavity Branches leave skull at stylomastoid foramen
IX	Glossopharyngeal	Mixed	Stylopharyngeous muscle–motor Senses and tastes posterior one-third of tongue Salivates (parotid) Senses carotid sinus and body	Loss of gag reflex with X	Jugular foramen	Neck, pharynx and tongue

Contd...

Contd...

CN	Name	Type	Function	Lesions	Exits-Enter cranium	Region innervated
X	Vagus nerve	Mixed	To all muscles of palate and pharynx for swallowing except tensor palati (V) and stylopharyngeus (IX) To all muscles of larynx Senses larynx and laryngopharynx and GI tract to GI tract smooth muscle and glands in foregut and midgut	Uvula pointing away from affected side Nasal speech, nasal regurgitation Dysphagia, palate droop Hoarseness and fixed vocal cord Loss of gag reflex with XI Loss of cough reflex	Jugular foramen	Neck, pharynx, larynx, thorax Abdomen
XI	Accessory	Motor	Turns head to opposite (SCM) chin to same side Elevates and rotate scapula (Trapezius)	Weakness in head turning Shoulder droops	Jugular foramen	Neck
XII	Hypoglossal	Motor	All muscles of tongue except palatoglossus (X nerve)	Deviation of tongue to affected side	Hypoglossal canal	Tongue
XIII	Sympathetics to head	Motor	Raises eyelid (LPS) Dilates pupil Innervates sweat gland Constricts blood vessel	Horners syndrome Ptosis Miosis Anhydrosis Enophthalmus	Carotid canal on internal carotid artery	Orbit Face Scalp

Specialities

Optic nerve: Has 3 layers of meninges, 4 cm. It is a tract, not a nerve, as it cannot regenerate.

Cavernous sinus

- Either side of body of sphenoid
- 3rd, 4th, 5th trigeminal nerve lies laterally.
- Abducent nerve passes inferolateral along with internal carotid artery
- Superior ophthalmic vein communicates with anterior facial vein resulting in pass of infection from face to sinus resulting in cavernous sinus thrombosis.

Pituitary gland

- Rathkes pouch anterior lobe. Circle of willis lies above.
- Enlargement causes bitemporal hemianopia.

Orbit

- Tendon of Zinn
- Superior oblique muscle–Longest muscle
- Medial rectus–Largest muscle
- Superior rectus insertion–Farthest from limbus
- Medial rectus insertion–Nearest to limbus
- Spiral line of Tillaux–Line connecting insertion of recti
- Mullers muscle–LPS smooth muscle
  - Danger space of Scalp–Loose areolar tissue
  - Danger area of face–Area around the mouth and lower part of nose

Because facial vein communicates to cavernous sinus via–superior ophthalmic and supraorbital veins and with pterygoid plexus via–deep facial vein.

Venous drainage of face

Supratrochlear vein + supraorbital vein = Anterior facial vein

Superficial temporal vein + maxillary vein = Retromandibular vein (divides into anterior and posterior division)

Anterior division + anterior facial vein = Common facial vein

Posterior division + Posterior auricular vein = External jugular vein

Internal jugular vein–continuation of sigmoid sinus

Facial muscle	Action
Buccinator	Whistling
Zygomaticus major	Laughing
Risorius	Grinning

Important words

- Meckels cave–Gasserian ganglion Trigeminal nerve
- Dorellos canal–Abducent nerve
- Valve of Hesner–Nasolacrimal duct.

Submandibular gland

- J-shaped gland
- Divided into superficial and deep part by Mylohyoid muscle (Diaphragm of oral cavity)
  - Sup. Sali Nucleus → Facial → chordatympani → lingual nerve → Posterior root → submandibular ganglion → post gang directly → Submandibular gland
  - Via anterior root to Lingual nerve → sublingual gland.
- Facial artery closely related.

Thyroid

- Extent–C5 to T1, Ligament of Berry (posteromedial condensation of pretracheal fascia)
- Capsules of Thyroid–True (Close to gland), False (pretracheal fascia–superficial to true capsule)
- In between true and false
  - Parathyroid
  - Anastomosis of arteries
- No significant sex difference in gland volume from 8 months to 15 years
- Posteromedial aspects of the lobes are attached to the side of the cricoids cartilage by a lateral thyroid ligament
- A fibromuscular band, the hyoid to the isthmus or pyramidal lobe.

Relations

- The convex lateral (superficial) surface is covered by sternothyroid
- Anteriorly: Sternohyoid and the superior belly of Omohyoid
- Inferiorly: Overlapped by the anterior border of sternocleidomastoid
- Medial surface: Adapted to the larynx and trachea, contacting the inferior pharyngeal constrictor, posterior part of Cricothyroid and the external laryngeal nerve
- Medial Relations: Inferiorly trachea and, more posteriorly the recurrent laryngeal nerve and esophagus (which is closer on the left)
- Posterolateral surface: Close to the carotid sheath, and overlaps the common carotid artery
- Anterior border of the gland: Near the anterior branch of the superior thyroid artery
- Posterior border: Inferior thyroid arery and its anastomosis with the posterior branch of the superior thyroid artery, the parathyroid glands and thoracic duct.
- Isthmus: Covered by sternothyroid, sternohyoid, the anterior jugular veins, fascia and skin
- The superior thyroid arteries anastomose along its upper border and the inferior thyroid veins leave the gland at its lower border

- Blood vessels of thyroid located deep to true capsule.
- Lobes–Till oblique line of thyroid cartilage
- Levator glandular thyroidea–Detached part of infrahyoid muscles
- Pyramidal lobe–Left side
- Arteria thyroideaima–Branch from arch of aorta/brachiocephalic trunk
- Medial relationship of lobes of thyroid–2 tubes of trachea/esophagus 2 muscle–Inferior Constrictor/Cricothyroid, 2–nerve–ELN, RLN
- Artery–Supthyroid–Close ext laryngeal N, Inferior Thyroid A–Recurrent laryngeal N
- Vein of Kocher between middle and inferior thyroid vein drains into Internal jugular vein
- Supeior and middle thyroid vein drains–IJV
- Inferior thyroid vein–BCV

Lymphatic Drainage

Periglandular → Prelaryngeal (Delphian) → Pretracheal → Paratracheal (along RLN) → Brachiocephalic (sup mediastinum) → Deep cervical → Thoracic duct

Tc99 m–Ectopic thyroid

Divisions

- C 4–Common carotid bifurcates
- T 4–Arch of aorta divides
- L 4–Abdominal aorta bifurcates

Paranasal sinuses

Maxillary-largest, Ethmoid, Frontal and Sphenoid–functional endoscopic sinus surgery (FESS), fron, max, eth–Occip

Openings of air sinus

Inferior meatus–Nasolacrimal duct

Middle meatus–Frontal sinus, maxillary sinus, anterior and middle ethmoidal sinus

Superior meatus–Posterior ethmoidal sinus

Nasal cavity Ant part–Keratinized stratified squamous epithelium

- Nonkeratinized stratified squam pseudostratified coeliated (respiratory) + olfactory conchae meatuses floor, roof.

Kiesselbach's area (little's area)

Anteroinferior part of nasal septum. Formed by Sphenopalatine artery and facial artery (septal br sup labial)

- All muscles of palate are innervated by pharyngeal plexus except tensor palati which is being innervated by V3 (Mandibular nerve).
- All muscles of pharynx are being innervated by cranial accessory via pharyngeal plexus except stylopharyngeous which is being innervated by Glossopharyngeal nerve.
- All muscles of Tongues are being innervated by Hypoglossal nerve except palatoglossus which is being innervated by pharyngeal plexus.
- Taste buds present in all papillae except filiform
- Taste salty, sweet, sour, bitter, metallic umami.

Larynx

Extent–C3 To C6 From upper border of epiglottis to lower boder of circoid cartilage.

Laryngeal cartilages–3 paired-Arytenoid, Corniculate and Cuneiform.

3 unpaired-Thyroid, Circoid and Epiglottis.

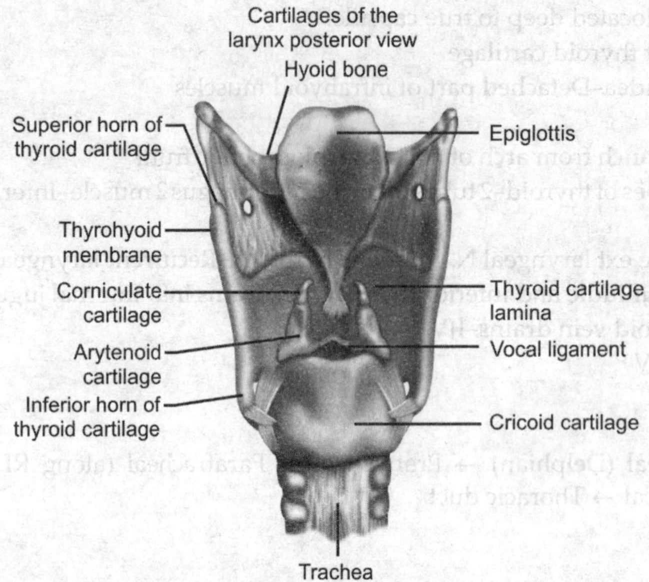

Fig. 1.26: Laryngeal cartilages

1. All the following laryngeal cartilages are hyaline except:

a. Apex of arytenoids
b. Thyroid cartilage
c. Circoid cartilage
d. Body of arytenoid.

Ans. a (Explanation ref histology cartilage)

- Cricoid cartilage–Malform subglottic stenosis
- Tritiate–Posted of thyrohyoid membrane-Fibrocartilage type.

All muscles of larynx are being innervated by recurrent laryngeal nerve except cricothyroid muscle which is being innervated by external laryngeal nerve.

The only unpaired intrinsic muscle of larynx is transverse arytenoideus. It has dual nerve supply from both recurrent and external laryngeal nerve.

Sensory innervation above vocal fold by internal laryngeal nerve, below the vocal fold is being innervated by Recurrent laryngeal nerve.

Safety muscle of Larynx: Posterior cricoarytenoid (only abductor of larynx)

Vocal fold: Extends between Thyroid cartilage and Arytenoid cartilage

Ligam–Ext–Thyrohyoid memb, Hyo and thyroepiglottic lig., cricotracheal lig.

Structures piercing the thyrohyoid membrane are internal laryngeal nerve and superior laryngel artery.

Structure piercing the circothyroid membrane is recurrent laryngeal nerve.

Ligam–Int–Quadrate Memb–Lower border thickened as vestibular fold.

Cricivocal memb–Upper thickened border as Vocal fold.

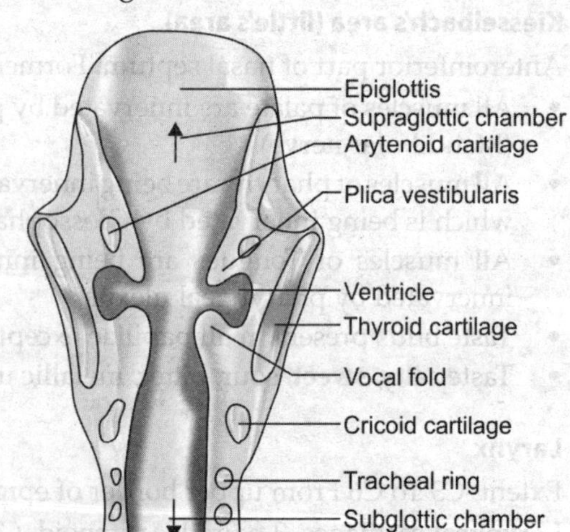

Fig. 1.27: Laryngeal cartilages

Laryngeal Cavity

- Mucous folds–Aryepiglottic fold, vestibular fold and vocal fold.
- Aryepiglottis contains both aryepiglottis and thyroepiglottis muscles.
- Aryepiglottis is the upward continuation of oblique arytenoideus.
- Larygeal inlet–Space between the artepiglottic folds.
- Rima vestibulai (False vocal cord)–Space between the vestibular folds.

- Rima glottidis (True vocal cord)–Space between the vocal folds. Water shed line.
- Vocal cord–Pearly white, lined by nonkeratinized stratified squamous epithelium, devoid of submucosa and sound production.
- Vestibule–Extends from aryepigollic folds to vestibular folds.
- Sinus of larynx–Extends from vestibular folds to vocal folds.
- Infraglottic part–Below the vocal folds.
- Lining epithelium of larynx–Ciliated psedostratified epithelium except anterior and upper part of epiglottis, vocal card and aryepigltis fold.
- Vocal cords Nodules
  - Ant 1/3 and post 2/3
  - Singer's nodes/clergyman's nodes
  - Lower part–subglottis, Laryngoscopic
  - Spaces–pre epiglottic space
  - Paraglottic
  - Subglottic space

Cartlilage	Speciality
Thyroid	Largest laryngeal cartilage
Cricoid	Signet ring
Epiglottis	Elastic cartilage,Oblong shape

- One side recurrent laryngeal nerve palsy–paramedian position of vocal cord on the same side
- Both sides recurrent nerve palsy–vocal cord paramedian position on both sides lead onto aphonic
- Both recurrent laryngeal and external laryngeal nerve palsy–vocal cord cadaveric position
- Joints of larynx—Circothyroid jt, Circoaryteniod jt and Arytenocorniculate jt. All the joint are plain variety of synovial joint
- The nerve related posterior to circothyroid jt is recurrent nerve.

Ear

Tympanic membrane

Oval, Oblique 55 degree, UMBO-most convex part, pars flaccida, pars tensa Auditory canal–3.6 cm–Outer 1/3rd cartilaginous, Inner 2/3rd bone

Eustachian tube–4 cm–Outer 2/3rd cartilaginous, inner 1/3rd bony.

External Ear

Cryptotia: Upper part of auricle buried in temporal skin.

Stahls deformity: Pointing of ear reversal of concavity of scaphoid fossa

Ext. Acous meatus: 2.5 cm Cartilagenous 8 mm, Osseous–16 mm

Palate: Palatine aponeurosis tensor veli palatini

Pillars of fauces–Palatoglossal arch post between these tonsillar sinus

Snoring–Palate and pharynx muscles tone increased

Uvulopalatopharyngoplasty: Length of soft palate

All muscles of palate supplied by cranial part of accessory nerve via phary plexus except tensor veli palatini Supplied by Mandibular nerve via N. To medial pterygoid

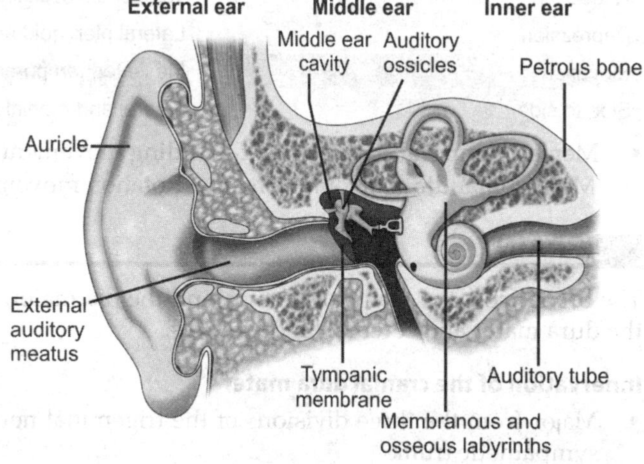

Fig. 1.28: Parts of ear

Paltopharyngeus muscles passavanti muscle passavant's ridge change from respiratory to stratified squam Epi occurs along this ridge. Muscle HT in complete cleft palate.

Pharyngeal Plexus

- Glossopharygeal
- Vagus
- Sup. Cervical Sym. Ganglia

Swallowing Oral phase/Pharyngeal phase/esophageal phase

Pharyngostomy: Alternative feed throu' piriform fossa

Eye

Tenons capsule—covers sclera, all extraocular muscle gets attached to it. Weakest part of eyeball—sclerocorneal junction

Deep cervical fascia

Layer	Ends
Investing layer	Suprasternal notch (space of Burns)
Pretracheal	Fibrous pericardium
Prevertebral	Diaphragm

Temporomandibular Joint

- Condylar variety of the synovial joint.
- Articular process are anterior articular part of the mandibular fossa and articular tubercle above and head of the mandible below.
- Articular disk divide the joint into upper meniscotemporal and lower meniscomandibular compartments. **Joints divided by articular disk are TM joint, Acromioclavicular joint Sternoclavicular joint and Knee joint.**
- Articular disk represents the degenerated primitive insertion of lateral pterygoid. Parts of the articular disk are Anterior extension, anterior thick, intermediate band, posterior thick and bilamellar region. Articular disk is the fibrocartilage.
- Sphenomandibular ligament—Extend from the spine of the sphenoid to the lingual of the mandible and developed from fibrous envelope of the Meckel's cartilage of the first branchial arch. This is pierced by the mylohyoid nerve and vessels.
- Stylomandibular ligament is the thickened deep cervical fascia extends from the tip of the styloid process of the temporal bone to the angle of the mandible which separates the parotid from submandibular gland.

Movements	Muscles responsible
Protrusion	Medial and Lateral pterygoid
Retraction	Temporalis assisted by deep fibers of masseter, Digastric and geniohyoid.
Depression	Lateral pterygoid and assisted by geniohyoid, mylohyoid and digastric
Elevation	Masseter, temporalis and medial pterygoid
Side to side	Lateral and medial pterygoid of one side alternately with the other side.

- Meniscotemporal compartment—Gliding movement
  Meniscomandibular compartment—Rotation movements.

BRAIN

The brain itself, the arachnoid mater, and the pia mater, does not contain sensory endings. These are restricted to the dura mater and cerebral blood vessels.

Innervation of the cranial dura mater

- Major from the three divisions of the trigeminal nerve, the first three cervical spinal nerves, and the cervical sympathetic trunk
- Minor meningeal branches from the vagus, hypoglossal, facial and glossopharyngeal nerves

Nerve	Innervates
Meningeal branches of the anterior and posterior ethmoidal. N	Dura of anterior cranial fossa
Anterior filaments of the meningeal rami of the maxillary (nervus meningeus medius) and mandibular (nervus spinosus) trigeminal divisions	Dura of anterior cranial fossa, but largely distributed to the dura of the middle cranial fossa, which also receives filaments from the trigeminal ganglion
Recurrent tentorial nerve (branch of ophthalmic division of the trigeminal. N)	Tentorium cerebella
Ascending meningeal branches of the upper cervical nerves, Meningeal branches of vagus from the superior vagal ganglion	Dura in the posterior cranial fossa
Meningeal branches from the hypoglossal nerve	Diploe of the occipital bone, the dural walls of the occipital and inferior petrosal sinuses, and musch of the floor and anterior wall of the posterior cranial fossa

Nervus Spinosus

- Re-enters the cranius through the foramen spinosum with the middle meningeal artery
- Also contains sympathetic postganglionic fibers from the middle meningeal plexus
- The anterior branch communicates with the meningeal branch of the maxillary N
- The posterior branch supplies the muscous lining of the mastoid air cells

Cerebral hemisphere–One hemisphere usually left in right handed person is slightly larger than other one, constitutes dominant hemisphere.

Fissure of Rolando (Central sulcus)—Separates frontal and parietal lobe

Fissure of Sylvius (Lateral sulcus)—Separates frontal and temporal lobe

Calcarine sulcus—Great importance because of associated visual area of cortex

Largest mass of cells in each hemisphere is **Thalamus**

Structure	Shape
Caudate nucleus	Comma
Lentiform nucleus	Lens
Putamen	Quadrilateral
Globus pallidus	Conical
Hippocampus	Knuckles of clenched fist
Lateral ventricle	C shaped

Geniculate bodies lateral: Concerned with visual pathways

Geniculate bodies medial: Concerned with auditory pathways

Ventricles:

Cerebrospinal fluid

Produced by: Choroidal epithelial, choroid plexus in the lateral 3rd and 4th ventricle

Circulation: Lateral ventricle Interventricular formina 3rd ventricle cerebral aqueduct 4th ventricle through foramina of magendie and luschka in the roof of 4th ventricle enters subarachnoid space and circulates over cerebral hemispheres around spinal cord (up to S2 vertebral)

Absorption: CSF absorption into venous system is through arachnoid villi and arachnoid granulations

Lateral ventricles–**Interventricular foramen of Monro** 3rd Ventricle **Aqueduct of Sylvius** 4th Ventricle

Foramen of Magendie: Median aperture by which CSF escapes into cerebellomedullary cistern

Foramen of Luschka: Lateral aperture by which CSF escapes into pontine cistern

Fifth ventricle–Septum Pellucidum (Misnomer) cavity is lined with pia mater, not ependyma

Lateral ventricle–contains 1. Anterior horn 2. Body 3. Posterior horn 4. Inferior horn (Largest)

Most of nuclei of medulla are below the floor of fourth ventricle.

Blood brain barrier:

Formed by Abundant tight junction between endothelial cells

Structures outside the blood brain barrier are SOAP

- Subfornical organ
- Organum vesculosum of lamina terminalis
- Area postrema
- Posterior pituitary and ventral part of pineal gland of hypothalamus.

Brain sand: 1. Calcification of pineal body (Corpora Arenacea) 2. Calcification in choroid plexus

Congenital aneurysms

Most frequent sites–Anterior cerebral A with Anterior communicating A. **(Tunica media is weakest)**

The largest and most direct branch of internal carotid Artery → Middle cerebral A (**Most subject to embolism)**

Largest branch of Vertebral A → Posterior inferior cerebellar A (One of most tortuous artery in body)

Artrery of Cerebral hemorrhage: Branch of Middle cerebral Artery as lateral striate branch

Recurrent artery of Heubner: Branch of Anterior cerebral A supplying posterior part of internal capsule

Artery of Adamkiewicz: Arteria radicularis magna is at T10 or T11 roots, injury will cause grave damage to cord.

Vascular Supply of Brain

2 ICA and 2 vertebral arteries

Forebrain except Occipital lobe ICA

Veretebral artery → Occip lobe, Brainstem, cerebellum

Arteries lie in Subarachnoid space.

ICA parts	Branches
• Cervical • Petrous • Cavernous	No Branch Caroticotympanic artery – Cavernous branches – Meningeal – Hypophyseal arterie
• Cerebral	• Ophthalmic – Posterior Comm. Artery – Anterior choroidal → choroid plexus of Lat Ventricle Basal ganglia, postr. Limb of Int. Capsule – Anterior cerebral $A_1 A_2 A_3$ - A_1 → ICA–Ant. Comm Ar. - A_2 → Ant Com A–Origin of callosomarginal - A_3 → Distal to callosomarginal.
Cortical branches → Motor/Somato sens area of Lower Limb Central → Medial striate artery	

- Middle Cerebral artery
  M_1 → ICA → bifurcation Sphenoidal reg. Insular Operator
  M_2 → Sylvian fissuse
  M_3 → Out of sylvian fissure
  M_4 → Cortical
  Supply Cortical → Motor/Somatic Sensory area other than lower limb, Auditory area insula
  Central → Lat Striate/Lenticulo striate.

Vertebral artery branches

- Ant spinal artery
- PICA → Largest branch of VA
  → Choroid plexus of 4th ventricle, postspinal artery.

Basilar artery

- Pontine branch
- Labyrinthine–or (AICA) Origin.

- AICA
- Superior Cerebellar artery → chor. Plexus of 3rd ventricle.
- Postcerebral arteries
  P_1 → Bifurcation to junc. post comm. artery
  P_2 → Post comm. A–perimesenceph. Cistern
  P_3 → Portion in calcrine fissure
- Cortical → Visual area and Visual pathway Structures
- Central → Post chordidal br. Supply–Inf. Horn of Lat. Ventricle
- **Circle of willis** → Inter peduncular fossa.

Polygon of Willis

Communication between internal carotid system and vertebral system

Formation

Basilar A → **Posterior cerebral A.** → **Posterior communicating A** → Internal carotid A → **Anterior cerebral A** → **Anterior communicating A**

Aneurysm ICA → Compression of optic chiasma → 3rd N. Palsy

Venous drainage Does not follow arterial pattern

Great cerebral vein of Galen:

Two internal cerebral vein forms Great cerebral vein–joined by basal veins

Great cerebral vein + Inferior sagittal sinus → Straight sinus → Transverse sinus

VENOUS DRAINAGE OF CEREBRUM

External cerebral veins:

- **Superior cerebral vein**
  - 6–12 in number
  - Drain the superolateral surface of the hemisphere
  - Drains into superior sagittal sinus.
- **Superficial middle cerebral vein**
  - Drain the area round the posterior ramus of lateral sulcus

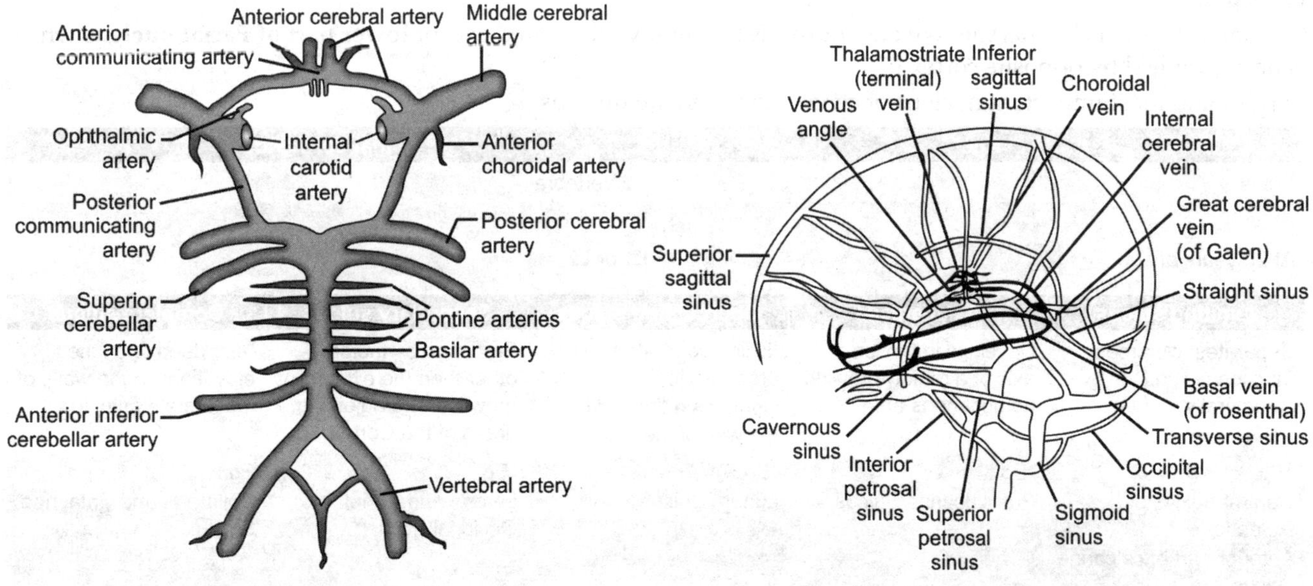

Fig. 1.29: Circle of willis

Fig. 1.30: Venous drainage of brain

- Drains into cavernous sinus or rarely into sphenoparietal sinus
- Also communicates with the deep middle cerebral vein.

- **Deep middle cerebral vein**
  - Drains the surface of insula
  - Terminates into the basal vein.
- **Inferior cerebral veins**
  - Several in number, divided as orbital and tentorial V
  - Orbital Veins terminate in superior cerebral veins
  - Tentorial veins drain in the cavernous sinus
- **Anterior cerebral veins**
  - Drains corpus callosum
  - Terminate in the basal vein
- **Internal cerebral veins**
  - One vein on each side
  - Formed by the union of thalamo-striate and choroidal veins
  - Situated at the apex of teal choroideo of IIIrd ventricle
  - The right and left veins unite together to form the great cerebral vein of galen below the splenium of corpus callosum

Terminal veins:

Great cerebral vein (vein of galen):

Terminates in the Straight sinus. Tributaries are basal Veins and the Veins from

- Pineal body
- Colliculi
- Cerebellum
- Occipital lobes of cerebrum

Basal vein

- One vein on each side
- Formed at the anterior perforated substance by the union of deep middle cerebral vein and striate vein

Note: ultimately all veins drain into the various cranial venous sinuses which, in turn drain into the internal jugular vein.

Extra points

Cranial nerves which innervate skeletal muscle is bilaterally innervated except **lower part of Facial nucleus** which is only supplied by opposite cortex

Largest and most important nucleus of cerebellum–dentate nucleus

Age	Spinal cord ends
Fetus	S2 vertebra
At birth	L3
At 20 years of age	L1 or L2

Limiting sulcus	Axial sulcus	Operculated sulcus	Secondary sulcus	Complete sulcus
Separates two areas functionally and Structurally	Develops in the long axis of a rapidly growing homogenous area	Its lips separate two areas and Contains a third area in the wall of the sulcus	Produced by factors other than the exuberant growth in the adjoining areas of the Cortex	Very deep to cause elevations in the walls of the lateral ventricle
*Eg.: Central Sulcus of Rolando Anterior part of calcarine sulcus	*Eg.: Postcalcarine Sulcus	*Eg.: Lunate Sulcus	*Eg.: Lateral and Parieto-Occipital Sulci	Eg.: Collateral and Calacrine Sulci

Procencephalon (Forebrain)		Mesencephalon (Midbrain)	Rhombancephalon (Hindbrain)		
Diencephalon Thalmus, Metathalamus Epithalamus, Subthalamus, Caudal part of hypothalamus, Caudal part of IIIrd ventricle.	**Telancephalon** Rostral part of hypothalamus, Rostral part of IIIrd ventricle, Lateral ventricle, Corpus striatum.	Cerebral peduncle, Tegmentum, Tectum, Aqueduct.	**Mylencephalon** Medulla oblongata, Caudal part of IVth ventricle and Inferior cerebellar peduncle.	**Metencephalon** Pons, Cerebellum, Middle cerebellar peduncle, Middle part IVth Ventricle	**Isthmus rhombencephali** Rosral part of IVth ventricle, Superior cerebellar peduncle and Anterior medullary velum.

PONS

Ref: AK Datta 4/p p128–136

Middle part of the brainstem connecting the midbrain with the medulla. Literally 'pons' means 'bridge'.

1. **Pontine nuclei are developed from:**
   a. Neuar tube　　b. Neral cleft
   c. Neral pore　　d. Rhombic lip

   Ans. d

   Other structures developed from rhombic lip and migrated ventally are:
   a. Arcuate nuclei　　b. Pontobulbar body.

2. **The cranial nerve related to the ventral surface of pons**
   a. 6th nerve　　b. 7th nerve
   c. 5th nerve　　d. 8th nerve.

   Ans. c

   Trgeminal nerve attached at the junction of vental surface with middle cerebellar peduncle.
   Ventral surface at the pontomedullary junction from medial to lateral 6, 7 and 8th cranial nerves attached.

3. **Facial colliculus produced by what structure?**
   a. Inferior colliculus　　b. Facial nuclei
   c. Abducent nuclei　　d. All

   Ans. d

   Dorsal surface of pons at the level of superior fovea the medial eminence shows rounded elevation called facil colliculus produced by the underlying abducent nuclei and the internal genu of the facial nerve around the nucleus.

4. **Which neurotransmitter present in the Locus ceruleus?**
   a. Acetylcholine　　b. Noradrenalin
   c. Dopamine　　d. GABA

   Ans. b

   Parts of midbrain
   Dorsally–Tectum
   Ventrally–Cerebellar peduncle which includes tegmentum dorsally and crus cerebri ventrally.
   Substantia nigra pigmented nerve cells which separate tegmentum and crus cerebri.
   Imaginary line at the level of aqueduct divide tegmentum ventrally and tectum dorsally.

   Structures traversing crus cerebri are:
   - Optic tract
   - Basal vein
   - Posterior cerebral artery
   - Superior cerebellar artery

   Oculomotar nerve emerges through medial sulcus (which separates crus cerebri from interpedugular fossa) between posterior cerebral and superior cerebellar artery.
   Trochlear nerve emerges in the interval between the cerebral peduncle and the temporal lobe.

   Bounderies of interpeduncular fossa
   Anterior–Caudal boder of Optic chiasma.

Anterolateral–Optic tract.
Posterolateral–Crus cerebri.
Posterior–Cranial border of Pons.

Contents

Infundibular stalk and tuber cinereum, Median eminence, Mamillary bodies and Posterior perforated substance.

Corpra Quadrigemina

Dorsal suface of midbrain (Tectum) contains pairs of Superior and Inferior colliculi called Corpora Quadrigemina.

Substantia Nigra

Afferents: Strio-nigral-contain GABA
Efferents: Nigro-striate-Contain Dopamine.

Trigeminal nerve sensory nuclei

- Spinal nucleus of Trigeminal nerve–Second order neuron –Site–2nd cervical segment to ponto-medullary junction.
- Chef (Principal) sensory nucleus–Second order neuron–Site–Upper part of Pons
- Mesencephalic nucleus–First order neuron–Site–Midbrain at the level of inferior olliculli

Locus cerulieus- dorsal part of pons sulcus limitans rostrally flattened to form bluish greypigmented nerve cells known as substantia ferruginea rich in noradrenalin.

S No	Site	Neurotransmitter
1.	Parasympathetic ganglia	Acetylcholine
2.	Substantia nigra	Dopamine
3.	Raphe nuclei	Serotonin
4.	Hypothalamus	Histamine
5.	Postganglonic sympathetic neurons	Noradrenalin
6.	Adrenal edulla	

Neurotransmitters *Ref:* AK Datta 4/p p15

Two types

Excitatory: Glutamate and Aspartate. Present in the projection fibres from cortex to thalamus, tectum, substantia nigra,pontine nuclei,central pathway of trigeminal and auditory nerves and terminals of parallel fibres of cerebellum ending Purkinji neurons.

Inhibitory GABA-Gamma amino butyric acid-present in thenerons of brainstem, spinal cord (Renshaw loop), Purkinji neurons of cerebellum.
Glycine and Taurine

Pigments in various parts of brain *Ref:* AK Datta 4/p p7

S No	Site/Age	Pigment
1.	Substantia nigra	Neromelanin
2.	Old age	Lipochrome and Lipofusion (Senility pigment)

Metals in various parts of brain

S No	Site	Metals
1.	Locus ceruleus	Copper
2.	Hippocampus	Zinc
3.	Oculomotor nucleus	Iron

Int. Capsule

Lateral Striate → AL/genu/Major part of PL of IC
Charcots Artery of Cerebral Hemorrhage–Lat striate of MCA

Arterial Supply of the Cerebral Cortex

Anterior cerebral A	Middle cerebral A	Posterior cerebral A
• A strip of about 2 cm wide along the Superomedial border from the frontal Pole to the Parieto Occipital Sulcus • Medial Surface of the brain • Medial Part of orbital surface • Areas that represent for leg areas	• Greater Part of the Superolateal surface except – A 2 cm wide strip from frontal Pole to the Parieto-occipital Sulcus – Area belonging to Occipital lobe – Inferior temporal gyrus • Lateral Part of orbital Surface • Temporal pole • Main Somatic motor and Sensory areas except in their uppermost Parts (leg areas) • Auditory cortex	• Occipital lobe • Inferior temporal gyrus • Tentorial Surface • Visual cortex

Cerebellar Peduncle	Afferent tract	Efferent tract
Superior cerebellar peduncle	Tecto-crebellar Trigemino-cerebellar Ventral Spino-cerebellar	Cerebellorubral Dentatothalmic
Middle Cerebellar Peduncle	Pontocerrebellar (part of cortico-pontocerebellar pathway)	No efferents
Inferior cerebellar peduncle	Mnemonic 'VC-SPORT' Vestibulocerebellar Cuneocerebellar Spinal (Posterior)–cerebellar Par Olivocerebellar Olivocerebellar Reticulocerebellar Rostro Spinocerebellar. Striae medullaris Anterior external arcuate fibers	Cerebellovestibular/Olivary/Reticular

Middle cerebellar peduncle has only afferent tract (pontocerebellar tract)

Archicerebellum	Paleocerebellum	Neocerebellum
Phylogenetically, oldest part	Next to develop	Newest part to develop
Made up of flocculonodular lobe and the lingual	Made up of anterior lobe (without lingual) and the pyramid and uvula)	Made up of the middle lobe (largest part of cerebellum) without pyramid and uvula
Chiefly vestibular in Connections	Connections are chiefly Spinocerebellar	Rubrospinal
Controls the axial musculature and bilateral movements (used for locomotion and equilibrium)	Controls tone, posture and crude movements of the limbs	Concerned with the regulation of fine movements
Output passes directly to brainstem	Output to brainstem passes through Emboliform fast igial or globose nuclei	Output goes to Venterolateral nucleus of thalamus through dentate nucleus

Ref: AK Datta 4/p p159–172

Cerebellar nuclei: From medial to lateral Fastigus, Globusus, Emboliformis and Dentatus. Fastigus nuleus present over the roof of the fourth ventricle so it is called as Roof nucleus. Dentate nucleus is the largest nucleus.

Fissures in the cerebellum: Posterolateral First to appear.

Present on the inferior surface separating Flocculonodular lobe from corpus cerebella.

Fissura primi–V shaped present on the superior surface cutting the superior vermis at the junction of anterior two-third and posterior one third and divide corpus cerebella into anterio and posterior lobe.

Horizontal fissure–Along the lateral and posterior margin of the cerebellum marks the junction between superior and inferior surface.

Secondary fissure–Between pyramid and uvula.

Cells in the cerebellum

- Purkinje cells–Inhibitory
- Granule cells–Excitatory
- Golgi cells–Inhibitory
- Stellate cells–Inhibitory
- Basket cells–Inhibitory

Cerebellum

Lobe	Vermis	Hemispher/Lteral extension
Anterior Lobe	Lingula	—
	Central lobule	Alae
	Culumen	Quadrangular lobe.
Posterior Lobe	Declive	Lobulus simplex
	Folium vermis	Superior semilunarlobule.
	Tuber vermis	Inferior semilunar lobule.
	Pyramid	Biventral lobule.
	Uvula	Tonsil.
	Nodule	Flocculus

Synaptic glomerulus

- Rosette of mossy fibres
- Claw like of dentrites of granule cells
- Axon terminals of golgi cells
- Entire glomerulus is ensheathed by Bergmann glial cells.

Sensory fibres of cerebellum

Two types. They are Mossy and Climbing fibers.

Mossy fibers	Climbing fibers
All the afferents omming to the cerebellum except those coming from inferior olivary nucleus.	Fibres coming from inferior olivary and accessory Nuclus
Excite the single Purkinje	Excite the thousand Purkinje

Ref: AK Datta 4/p p158-166

Pineal gland: Only part of brain receive nerve supply from outside brain-from postganglionic sympathetic fibres from superior cervical ganglion-Nervi conarii.

Only part of brain which has no nerve cells.

- Small, conical organ situated between the 2 superior colliculi, consisting of the body and a stalk (Peduncle).
- Composed of pinealocytes and neuroglial cells
- Calcareous concretions are constantly present in the pineal after the 17th year of life and may from aggregations **(brain sand)**
- Sometimes, referred as 'THE THIRD EYE'
- Produces hormones that may have an important regulatory influence on may other endocrine Organs.
- The best known hormone is melatonin (hormone of darkness) which causes changes in the skin color

Functional areas of the cerebral cortex

Lobe	Area	Location	Function	Effect of lesion
Frontal Lobe	Motor area 4	Precentral gyrus and Paracentral lobule Paracentral lobule	Controls voluntary activities of the opposite half of body	Contralateral Paralysis and jacksonian fits
	Pre motor area 6	Posterior parts of superior, middle and inferior frontal gyri	Controls extrapyramidal system	Often mixed with pyramidal effect

Contd...

Contd...

Lobe	Area	Location	Function	Effect of lesion
	Frontal eye field 6,8	Posterior parts of middle frontal gyri	Controls the spoken speech	Horizontal conjugate movements are lost
	Motor speech area (Broca's area) 44, 45	Pars triangularis and pars opercularis	Controls the spoken speech	Aphais (motor)
	Preforntal area	The remaining large, anterior part of frontal lobe	Controls emotin, concentration, attention and judgment	Loss of orientation
Parietal lobe	Sensory (somesthetic) area 3, 1, 2	Postcentral gyrus and paracentral lobule	Perception of exteroceptive (touch, pain and temperature) and proprioceptive impulses	Loss of appreciation of the impulses received
	Parietal area	Between sensory and visual areas	Stereognosis and sensory speech	Astereognosis and sensory aphasias
Occipital lobe	Visuo sensory area or striate area 17	In and around the postcalcarine sulcus	Reception and perception of the isolated visual impressions of colour, size, Form motion, illumination and transparency	Homonymous hemianopia with macular sparing
	Visuopsychic area para striate and peristriate areas 18, 19	Surround the striate area	Correlation of visual impulses with past memory and recognition of objects seen and also the depth	Visual agnosia
Temporal lobe	Auditosensory area 41, 42	Posterior par to fsuperior temporal gyrus and anterior transverse temporal gyrus	Reception and perception of isolated auditory impressions of loudness, quality and pitch	Impaired hearing
	Auditopsychic area 22	Rest of the superior temporal gyrus	Correlation of auditory impressions with past memory and identification (interparetation) of to he sounds heard	Auditory agnosia

Cerebrum

Allocortex

- Three layers- Molecular,Pyramidal and Polymorphous.
- **Parts**
  - Archipallium–Hippocampus and Dentate gyrus
  - Paleopallium–Uncus and part of parahippocampus
  - Mesocortex (or) Juxta allocortex–Cinguli gyrus,part of Hippocampus and Sibiculum.
- **Isocortex (or) Neopallial cortex**
  - Six layers–Molecular layer, outer granular, outer pyramidal layer, inner granulr layer, inner pyramidal layer and Polymorphous (or) Pleomorphic layer
- **Sulcus-i** First sulcus appear is Lateral sulcus
  - Primary sulcus–All the sulci belong to primary except Lateral and parieto-occipital sulcus.
  - Secondary sulci–Lateral and parieto-occipital sulcus.
  - Axial sulcus–Posterior part of Calcarine sulcus
  - Limiting sulci–Central sulcus and Anterior part of Calcarine sulcus
  - Operculated sulcus–Lunate sulcus
  - Complete sulcus–Depth of sulci produce elevationin the wall of Lateral Ventricle
  - Anterior part of Calcarine sulcus and Collateral sulcus. *Ref: AK Datta 4/Part p40–41*

Island of Reil (Insula) or Central Lobe

Submerged pyramidal cortex along the stem and posterior ramus of lateral sulcus.

Structures beneath the Insula are

Clastrum, External capsule and Lentiform nucleus. *Ref: AK Datta 4/p p43*

Area number	Functional area
4	Primary motor area
6 and 8	Pre motor area
8	Frotal eye field
Upper part of area 6	Writing centre
9 and 12	Pre frontal area
3, 1, 2	Primary somesthetic area
Lower part of post central gyrus 43	Taste receptive area
MsI	Primary motor area
MsII	Supplementary motor area
Posterior part of medial frontal gyrus	Supplementary motor area
44, 45	Broca's area
SmI	3, 1, 2 or primary somesthetic area
SmII	Supplementary somesthetic area (Upper lip of posterior ramus of lateral sulcus
40	Supramargianal gyrus-sterieognosis
17, 18 and 19	Primary visual area
39	Angular gyrus (Higher visual association area)
18, 19	Occipital eye field
22	Wernicke's area
41	Anretior transverse temporal gyrus Heschl's
Paracentral lobule	Cortical centre of micturition and defecation

Ref: AK Datta 4/p p55–61

Cells in the cerebral cortex

- Pyramidal cells
- Stellate cells
- Cells of Martinotti
- Horizontal cells of cajal
- Granular cells

Granular cortex–Area 3, 1, 2, Area 17, 18, 19 and Area 41, 42

Agranular cortex–Area 4, 6, 8 and 44 *Ref: AK Datta 4/p p53–55*

Thalamus

Hypothalamic sulcus–Extent from interventricular foramen to aqueduct of midbrain

It divide Diencephalaon in to dorsl and ventral part. Dorsal part includes thalamus, epithalamus and metathalamus. Ventral part includes hypothalamus and subthalamus.

Thalamic nuclei

- **Anterior**
  - Anterior ventral
  - Anterior dorsal
  - Anterior medial
- **Medial or dorsomedial**
  - Magnocellular
  - Parvocellular

- **Lateral**

  Ventral tier
  - Ventral anterior
  - Ventral lateral
  - Ventral posterior

  Dorsal tier
  - Lateral dorsal
  - Lateral posterior
  - Pulvinal
- **Intralaminar**
  - Centromedian
  - Parafascicular
- Mid-line
- Reticulár thalamic

Ref: AK Datta 4/p p99–100

White fibers of cerebrum

↓

Association fibres Projection fibers Commissural fibers

↓

(Itinerant fibers)

↓

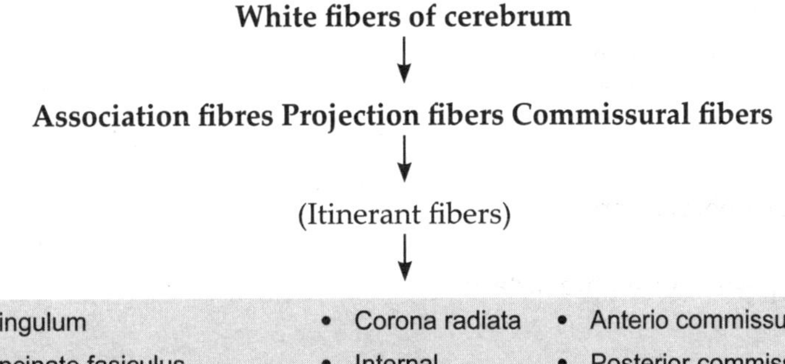

Association fibres	Projection fibers	Commissural fibers
• Cingulum	• Corona radiata	• Anterio commissure
• Uncinate fasiculus (Arcuate)	• Internal capsule	• Posterior commissure
• Superior longitudinal fasiculus	• Hippocampus	• Habunular commissure
• Inferior longitudinal fasiculus		• Hippocampal commissure
• Fronto-occipital fasiculus		• Corpus callosum

Internal capsule

Main highway for input and output fibres of cerebrum

Bounded medially by head of caudate nucleus and laterally by lentiform nucleus

Parts are Anreior limb, Genu, Posterior limb, Sublentiform and Retrolentiform

Anterior limb

- Frontopontine
- Anterior Thalamic radiation
- Medial fore brain bundle
- Pathway of Papez circuit
- Corticostriate fibers

Genu

- Corticonuclear
- Corticoreticular

Posterior limb

- Corticospinal tract
- Corticorubral
- Corticostriate
- Frontopontine, Parietipontine
- Superior thalamic radiation

Sublentiform
- Auditary radiation
- Meyer's loop of optic radiation
- Temporo-pontine and Parieto-pontine

Retrolentiform
- Optic radiation
- Posterior thalamic radiation
- Parieto-pontine and Occipitopontine

Blood supply of internal capsule

Anterior limb
- Striate branch of anterior cerebral artery
- Recurrent branch of anterior cerebral artery (Artery of Heubner)
- Striate branch of middle cerebral artery

Genu
- Recurrent branch of anterior cerebral artery
- Striate branch of middle cerebral artery
- Internal carotid artery

Posterior limb
- Striate branch of middle cerebral artery
- Anterior choroidal artery
- Posterolateral branch of posterior cerebral artery

Sublentiform
- Anterior choroidal artery
- Posterior cerebral artery

Retrolentiform

Posterolateral branch of posterior cerebral artery

QUESTIONS

1. Which is not a true arterial anastomosis? (2014)
a. Uterine and ovarian arteries
b. Intercostals artery
c. Labial artery
d. Cerebral cortical arteries

2. Which of the following joint is a syndesmosis? (2011)
a. Superior tibiofibular joint
b. Inferior tibiofibular joint
c. Talocalcaneal joint
d. Calcaneocuboid joint

3. Hassal corpuscles are seen in: (2011)
a. Thymus
b. Thyroid
c. Parathyroid
d. Spleen

4. The type of joint between epiphysis and diaphysis? (2010)
a. Syndesmosis
b. Synchondrosis
c. Fibrous joint
d. Plain synovial joint

5. The following are present in seminiferous tubules except: (2009)
a. Sertoli cells
b. Leydig cells
c. Spermatid
d. Spermatogonia

6. True regarding epithelial cells are: (2014)
a. Upper respiratory tract is lined by keratinized epithelium
b. Abundant goblet cells are present in ureter epithelium
c. Sebaceous glands appear from epithelium in scalp
d. Epithelium is surrounded by single layered membrane

7. **Hassal corpuscles are seen in: (2008)**
   a. Thymus
   b. Thyroid
   c. Parathyroid
   d. Spleen
8. **All the following are Secondary lymphoid organs except: (2007)**
   a. Spleen
   b. Lymph node
   c. Bone marrow
   d. MALT
9. **Which of the following joint is a syndesmosis?**
   a. Superior tibiofibular joint (2007)
   b. Inferior tibiofibular joint
   c. Talocalcaneal joint
   d. Calcaneocuboid joint
10. **Lymphatic follicles are not seen in: (2006)**
    a. Thymus
    b. Tonsil
    c. Lymph node
    d. Spleen
11. **Collecting duct develops from which of the following? (2014)**
    a. Mesonephros
    b. Metanephros
    c. Ureteric bud
    d. Paramesonephric duct
12. **Differentiation of gonads in human fetus is complete by: (2013)**
    a. 9 weeks
    b. 12 weeks
    c. 20 weeks
    d. 25 weeks
13. **Which of the following is a 3rd pharyngeal pouch derivative? (2013)**
    a. Thyroid
    b. C-cells
    c. Thymus
    d. Superior Parathyroids
14. **Which organ develops from both ectoderm and mesoderm? (2012)**
    a. Adrenal
    b. Pancreas
    c. Kidney
    d. Spleen
15. **The cranial end of wolffian duct forms: (2012)**
    a. Epoophoron
    b. Paraophoron
    c. Gartners duct
    d. Yterine Canal
16. **Fetal heart septum is formed at: (2011)**
    a. 5–8 weeks
    b. 8–9 weeks
    c. 10–12 weeks
    d. 3–4 weeks
17. **All the following develops from wolffian duct except: (2011)**
    a. Eoophoron
    b. Paraooporon
    c. Gartner duct
    d. Bartholin duct
18. **Umbilical cord contains: (2011)**
    a. 1 vein and 2 arteries
    b. 2 veins and 1 artery
    c. 1 vein and 1 artery
    d. 2 veins and 2 arteries
19. **Cause of Renal Agenesis is: (2011)**
    a. Defective ascent of metanephron
    b. Defective ureteric bud and Mesonephros
    c. Defective formation of nephritis tissue
    d. All the above
20. **All are derivatives of urogenital sinus except:**
    a. Bladder (2010)
    b. Ejaculatory duct
    c. Prostatic urethra
    d. Membranous urethra
21. **All are the following arise from mesonephric duct except: (2010)**
    a. Ductus deferens
    b. Seminal vesicles
    c. Epididymis
    d. Rete testic
22. **Cranial end of wolfian duct forms: (2010)**
    a. Epoophoron
    b. Paraepoophoron
    c. Gartner cyst
    d. Bartholin cyst
23. **Vestibular anus is classified under which of the following anorectal anomalies? (2009)**
    a. Imperforate anus
    b. High anorectal
    c. Low anorectal
    d. Mid anorectal
24. **Which organ develops from both ectoderm and mesoderm? (2009)**
    a. Adrenal
    b. Pancreas
    c. Kidney
    d. Spleen

25. All the following organs are developed from endoderm except: (2009)
a. Liver
b. Kidney
c. Pancreas
d. Urinary bladder

26. All the following develops from wolffian duct except: (2009)
a. Eoophoron
b. Paraoophoron
c. Gartner duct
d. Bartholin duct

27. Bulbourethral glands in males develops from: (2007)
a. Urogenital sinus
b. Mesonephric duct
c. Paromesonephric duct
d. Phallus

28. Following is not a derivative of first arch: (2006)
a. Stapes
b. Malleus
c. Maxilla
d. Mandible

29. Common carotid artery is derived from: (2006)
a. Third arch
b. Second arch
c. Fourth arch
d. Sixth arch

30. Lens is derived from: (2006)
a. Surface ectoderm
b. Neuroectoderm
c. Mesoderm
d. Endoderm

31. One of the following is not derived from the endoderm: (2006)
a. Kidney
b. Urinary bladder
c. Liver
d. Pancreas

32. Omphalocoele is associated with: (2006)
a. Spinal bifida
b. Cardiac defects
c. Chromosomal abnormalities
d. Malignancies

33. Epoophoron is a remnant of:
a. Wolffian duct
b. Paramesonephric duct
c. Wolffian body
d. Allantoic duct

34. Pressure on hook of hamate when hand is hyperextended will damage? (2015)
a. Ulnar nerve
b. Superficial branch of ulnar nerve
c. Median nerve
d. Musculocutaneous nerve

35. Wrist is more adducted than to be abducted because (2015)
a. Ulnar styloid process extends far more distally
b. Radial styloid process extends far more distally
c. Radial styloid process is bulky and prevents muscle action
d. Ulnar styloid process is thin and moves more medially

36. Superficial branch of ulnar nerve supplies: (2013)
a. Abductor pollicis
b. Palmaris brevis
c. Abductor digitiminimi
d. Oppenenspollicis

37. Median nerve supplies all except (2012)
a. Adductor pollicis
b. Abductor pollicis
c. Opponens pollicis
d. Flexor pollicis brevis

38. Short head of biceps attached to: (2011)
a. Coracoids process
b. Supraglenoid tubercle
c. Acromion process
d. Bicipital groove

39. Superficial branch of ulnar nerve supplies: (2010)
a. Palmaris brevis
b. Abductor pollicis
c. Biceps brevis
d. Flexor carpi radialis

40. Which is not a branch of posterior cord of branchial plexus? (2010)
a. Long thoracic nerve
b. Axillary nerve
c. Thoracodorsal nerve
d. Radial nerve

41. Short head of biceps attached to? (2010)
a. Coracoids process
b. Supraglenoid tubercle
c. Acromino process
d. Bicipital groove

42. Anatomical snuff box not formed by: (2010)
a. Extensor pollicis longus
b. Extensor pollicis brevis
c. Abductor pollicis longus
d. Abductor pollicis brevis

43. One of the following is supplied by median nerve (2009)
a. 1st and 2nd lumbricals
b. Hypothenar muscle
c. Palmar interossei
d. Dorsal interossi

44. The following muscles are supplied by radial nerve below the spiral groove except: (2009)
a. Brachialis
b. Brachioradialis
c. Extensor carpiradialis longus
d. Anconeus

45. False statement regarding adductor pollicis muscle: (2008)
a. Has 2 heads
b. Supplied by Median nerve
c. Causes Adduction of thumb
d. Arterial supplies is from Arteria priceps pollicis

46. False regarding Klumpke's paralysis is: (2008)
a. Claw hand deformity
b. Intrinsic muscles of hand involved
c. Horner's syndrome
d. Upper trunk of branchial plexus involved

47. A lesion involving the C8 nerve root will affect:
a. Extensors of fingers and wrist (2007)
b. Flexors of fingers and wrist
c. Small muscles of hand
d. None of above

48. Dorsal scapular nerve supplies: (2007)
a. Levator scapulae and rhomboids
b. Supraspinatus and infra spinatus
c. Lattismus dorsi
d. Serratus anterior

49. Longhead of biceps attached to: (2007)
a. Coracoids process
b. Supraglenoid tubercle
c. Acromion process
d. Bicipital groove

50. Posterior cord of brachial plexus contains all except: (2006)
a. Long thoracic nerve of Bell
b. Axillary
c. Radial
d. Upper subscapular

51. Major branches of popliteal artery are: (2015)
a. Genicular, anterior tibial and deep femoral arteries
b. Genicular artery only
c. Genecular, anterior and posterior tibial artery
d. Genicular and circumflex tibial artery

5 1a. Cruciate ligament of knee prevents: (2015)
a. Gliding of femur on tibia during flexion
b. Locking of knee
c. Extension of knee joint
d. Rotational movements of knee joint

52. Spring Ligament refers to: (2011)
a. Plantar Calcaneonavicular Ligament
b. Short planatar ligament
c. Long Plantar Ligament
d. Both b and C

53. Nerve supply of tensor facial lata is: (2010)
a. Superior gluteal nerve
b. Inferior gluteal nerve
c. Femoral nerve
d. Sciatic nerve

54. Which of the following is not a content of adductor canal? (2010)
a. Femoral artery
b. Femoral vein
c. Saphenous nerve
d. Nerve to vastus lateralis

55. Scarpa's fascia merges with: (2010)
a. Inguinal ligament
b. Conjoint tendon
c. Tensor fascia lata
d. Public crest

56. Nutrient artery to tibia arises from which of the following arteries? (2008)
a. Popliteal artery
b. Anterior tibial artery
c. Peroneal artery
d. Posterior tibial artery

57. Angle formed by the shaft and the neck of the femur is—degrees: (2007)
a. 115
b. 125
c. 135
d. 145

58. With foot off the ground and knee flexed, medial rotation of tibia is brought about by (2007)
a. Popliteus
b. Gastrocnemius
c. Vastus medialis
d. Adductor magnus

59. Oblique popliteal ligament attaches to: (2006)
a. Semimembranosus
b. Semitendinosus
c. Sartorius
d. Adductor magnus

60. A patient with recurrent chest infections present to the emergency department. He was ordered for an X-ray. The patient says that he has an 'azygos lobe' diagnosed few years back. What is the locationof azygos lobe? (2015)

a. Right Upper lobe
b. Left upper lobe
c. Right lower lobe
d. Left lower lobe

61. Pleura that continues into the neck as cervical pleura is: (2014)

a. Costal pleura
b. Diaphragmatic pleura
c. Visceral pleura
d. Mediastinal pleura

62. Right superior intercostals vein drains into: (2008)

a. Right brachiocephalic vein
b. Azygos vein
c. Hemiazygos vein
d. Accessory hemiazygos vein

63. Not a tributary of portal vein: (2015)

a. Inferior phrenic vein
b. Spenic vein
c. Cystic vein
d. Superior mesenteric vein

64. A patient present with hematemesis. On esophagogastroduodenoscopy, bleeding in lesser curvature was noted. The artery of bleed is (2015)

a. Right gastric artery
b. Left gastro omental artery
c. Anterior gastric artery
d. Posterior gastric artery

65. The major support for the liver to be held in position is: (2015)

a. Peritoneal ligaments
b. Pressure exerted by the abdominal muscles and their tone
c. Attachment of hepatic vein to Inferior vena cava
d. Suction force given by the diaphragm

66. True regarding biliary anatomy: (2015)

a. Normal diameter of common bile duct is 10 mm.
b. Gall bladder is innervated by sympathetic nerve
c. 1–2 litres of bile is secreted by the liver daily and it is 10 fold concentrated by the gall bladder
d. Right and left hepatic ducts join to form common bile duct

67. Root of mesentery crosses all except: (2015)

a. Second part of duodenum
b. IVC
c. Abdominal aorta
d. Right ureter

68. Deep inguinal ring is a defect in: (2015)

a. Fascia transversalis
b. Rectus sheath
c. External oblique aponeurosis
d. Pelvic fascia

69. Which of the following is NOT true about ligament of Treitz? (2014)

a. Suspends duodenojejunal flexure
b. Radiological investigation for malrotation
c. Contains suspensory ligament of duodenum
d. Contains duodenal mesentery

70. Which of the following is not a constituent of mesorectum? (2014)

a. Pararectal lymph nodes
b. Inferior rectal artery
c. Middle rectal vein
d. Inferior mesenteric plexus

71. Smallest cross-section of large bowel is seen at: (2014)

a. Descending colon
b. Ascending colon
c. Transverse colon
d. Sigmoid colon

72. False regarding anatomy of cervix is: (2014)

a. Cervix is 2 times longer in size than uterus in children
b. Cervix size is equal to uterus size in puberty
c. Fundus of uterus is drained by para-aortic lymph nodes
d. Uterine artery is lateral to cervix and passes anterior ureter

73. Which of the following muscle is attached to perineal body? (2013)

a. Pubocervical
b. Bulbospongious
c. Ischoicavernous
d. Ischoococcyeus

74. Root of mesentry is crossed by all except: (2013)

a. Inferior vena cava
b. Right ureter
c. 2nd part of duodenum
d. Abdominal aorta

75. Waldeyer's fascia is formed between: (2012)

a. Sacrum and rectum
b. Lateral pelvic wall and rectum
c. Bladder and rectum
d. Prostate and rectum

76. Aortic opening in diaphragm is found at the level of: **(2012)**
a. T 12
b. T 10
c. T 8
d. L1

77. Internal anal sphincter is formed by: **(2012)**
a. Puborectalis
b. Circular muscle fibres
c. Longitudinal muscle fibres
d. Deep peroneal muscle

78. Posterior gastric artery is a branch of: **(2011)**
a. Splenic artery
b. Hepatic artery
c. Left gastric artery
d. Right Gastric artery

79. Medial boundary of Inguinal Ring is formed by: **(2011)**
a. Lacunar ligament
b. Pectineal ligament
c. Inguinal ligament
d. Fascia lata

80. Cortex of ovary consist of all the following except: **(2011)**
a. Graffian follicle
b. Hilus
c. Primordial follicle
d. Corpus luteum

81. All are true about portal vein except: **(2011)**
a. Formed behind neck of pancreas
b. Bile duct lies anterior to PV
c. Gastroduodenal artery lies left to PV
d. Ascends behind the second part of duodenum

82. Duct of Bellini are seen in: **(2011)**
a. Kidney
b. Lung
c. Submandibular salivary gland
d. Parotid gland

83. Superficial inguinal ring is a defect in: **(2010)**
a. External oblique aponeurosis
b. Internal oblique aponeurosis
c. External oblique abdominis
d. Internal oblique abdominis

84. Left posterosuperior invagination of peritoneal cavity is known as: **(2010)**
a. Lesser Sac
b. Hepato Renal Pouch
c. Upper end of supra colic compartment
d. Morrison's pouch

85. The afferent impulses of cremastric reflex are transmitted through: **(2010)**
a. Genitofemoral nerve
b. Ilioinguinal nerve
c. Pudenal nerve
d. Iliohypogastic nerve

86. Milky spots' present in the greater omentum consists of: **(2009)**
a. Macrophages
b. Neutrophils
c. Lymphocytes
d. Langerhans cells

87. Morrison pouch is: **(2009)**
a. Right subphrenic space
b. Right subhepatic space
c. Right infracolic space
d. Right extraperitoneal space

88. True statement regarding bare area of liver:
a. Covered by visceral peritoneum **(2008)**
b. Supplied by phrenic nerve
c. Present in the left lobe of liver
d. Attached to the diaphragm

89. Which of the following artery gives rise to posterior gastric artery? **(2008)**
a. Left gastric artery
b. Right gastric artery
c. Splenic artery
d. Left gastroepiploic artery

90. The opening transmitting Azygos vein in the diaphragm is at the level of: **(2008)**
a. T 10
b. T 12
c. T 6
d. T 8

91. Which of the following is not a content of the pudendal cannal? **(2008)**
a. Pudendal nerve
b. Internal pudendal artey
c. Internal pudendal vein
d. Nerve to obturator internus

92. Internal anal sphincter is formed by: **(2007)**
a. Puborectalis
b. Circular muscle fibers
c. Longitudinal muscle fibers
d. Deep peroneal muscle

93. All of the following are features of flat type of pelvis except: **(2007)**
a. Narrow subpubic angle
b. Short concave sacrum
c. Divergent side walls
d. Wide sciatic notch

94. Waldeyer's fascia is between? **(2006)**
a. Rectum and urinary bladder
b. Rectum and sacrum

c. Bladder and uterus
d. Pubis and bladder

95. Prostate is supplied by: (2006)
a. Sympathetic + Parasympathetic
b. Parasympathetic
c. Sympathetic
d. None

96. The ligament that maintains the stability of atlanto axial joint is: (2015)
a. Alar ligament
b. Apical ligament
c. Transverse ligament
d. Tectorial ligament

97. Eustachian tube opens into which part of tympanic cavity? (2014)
a. Medial
b. Lateral
c. Anterior
d. Posterior

98. Which of the following is not a part of ethmoid bone? (2014)
a. Crista galli
b. Agar nassi
c. Inferior turbinate
d. Uncinate process

99. Inferior tympanic artery is a branch of which of the following? (2014)
a. Posterior occipital artery
b. Posterior auricular artery
c. Ascending pharyngeal artery
d. Middle meningeal artery

100. Which of the following muscle produces abduction of vocal cord? (2014)
a. Posterior cricoarytenoid
b. Lateral cricoarytenoid
c. Cricothyroid
d. Oblique arytenoids

101. Retropharyngeal space extends up to which of the following level? (2014)
a. Base of skull to C6 vertebra
b. Base of skull to bifurcation of trachea
c. Base of skull to the level of diaphragm
d. Base of skull to cricoids cartilage

102. All the following are true regarding 5th cranial (Trigeminal) nerve except: (2014)
a. Arises from midbrain
b. Innervate muscles of mastication
c. Carries parasympathetic fibres to salivary glands
d. Provides sensory innervations to face

103. All are true about chorda tympani nerve except:
a. Supplies anterior 2/3rd tongue (2013)
b. Sensory supply of face
c. It is a branch of facial nerve
d. It joints with lingual nerve

104. All the following veins drain into internal jugular vein except: (2013)
a. Facial vein
b. Lingual vein
c. Superior thyroid vein
d. Retromandibular vein

105. Hardest substance in teeth: (2013)
a. Cementum
b. Enamel
c. Pulp
d. Dentin

106. Medical wall of orbit is formed by all except:
a. Lesser wing of sphenoid (2013)
b. Ethmoid bone
c. Frontal process of maxilla
d. Lacrimal bone

107. Closing of jaw is brought about by all the following muscles except: (2013)
a. Mylohyoid
b. Medial pterygoid
c. Temporalis
d. Masseter

108. Retropharyngeal space extends from: (2013)
a. Skull base to tracheal bifurcation
b. Skull base to circoid
c. Skull base to thoracic inlet
d. Skull base to thyroid

109. True statement regarding parotid gland is all except: (2013)
a. Facial nerve divides into 5 branches within parotid gland
b. Mucinous gland
c. Covered by a dense capsule
d. Surrounded by investing layer of deep cervical fascia

110. Abductor of vocal cord is: (2013)
a. Posterior circoarytenoid
b. Lateral cricoarytenoid
c. Cricothyroid
d. Oblique arytenoids

111. One of the following does not form hypopharynx:
a. Epiglottis (2012)
b. Pyriform fossa
c. Posterior pharyngeal wall
d. Post cricoids region

112. Secretomotor innervations to Parotid gland relays in: (2012)
a. Otic ganglion
b. Geniculate
c. Ptergopalatine
d. Ciliary

113. All the following muscles are innervated by oculomotor nerve except: (2011)
a. Superior rectus
b. Inferior rectus
c. Lateral rectus
d. Medial rectus

114. All the following structures are related to carotid sheath except: (2010)
a. Sympathetic trunk
b. Vagus nerve
c. Internal carotid artery
d. Internal jugular vein

115. Which is not a branch of ophthalmic artery?
a. Dorsal nasal artery (2010)
b. Superificial temporal artery
c. Supraorbital artery
d. Supratrochlear artery

116. Scala tympani and vestibule is drained by:
a. Aqueduct of cochlea (2010)
b. Perilymphatic duct
c. Enolymphatic duct
d. Cochlear lymphatics

117. Muscle not supplied by ansa cervicalis? (2010)
a. Stylohyoid
b. Sternothyroid
c. Sternohyoid
d. Omohyoid

118. Which of the following is not present at birth?
a. Malleus (2010)
b. Incus
c. Stapes
d. Petrous temporal bone

119. Middle ear cavity is connected anteriorly to:
a. Nasal cavity (2010)
b. Nasopharynx
c. Mastoid antrum
d. Mastoid air cells

120. Which is not a branch of facial nerve? (2010)
a. Chorda tympani
b. Lingual nerve
c. Greater superficial petrosal nerve
d. Branch to stylohyoid muscle

121. Which is true regarding central retinal artery?
a. Supplies optic nerve (2010)
b. End artery
c. Branch of ciliary artery
d. Course similar to central retinal vein

122. Skin over the angle of mandible and parotid area is supplied by: (2009)
a. Auriculotemporal nerve
b. Posterior auricular nerve
c. Great auricular nerve
d. Facial nerve

123. Abductor of vocal cord is (Repeat): (2009)
a. Posterior cricoarytenoid
b. Lateral cricoarytenoid
c. Cricothyroid
d. Oblique arytheniods

124. All the following are true about trochlear nerve except: (2009)
a. Purely motor
b. Only nerve emerging from ventral aspect of brain stem
c. Originates from mibdbrain at level of inferior colliculus
d. Supplies only the superior oblique muscle

125. Hypoglossal nerve supplies all the following muscles except: (2008)
a. Styloglossus
b. Hyoglossus
c. Palatoglossus
d. Genioglossus

126. All the following extra ocular muscles are supplied by 3rd nerve except: (2008)
a. Lateral rectus
b. Medial rectus
c. Superior rectus
d. Inferior oblique

127. Which of the following muscle produces abduction of vocal cord? (2008)
a. Transverse arytenoids
b. Posterior cricoarytenoid
c. Lateral cricoarytenoid
d. Oblique arytenoids

128. All are true regarding tensor tympani muscle except: (2008)
a. Origin from cartilaginous part of auditory tube
b. Innervated by facial nerve
c. Related to processus trochleariformis
d. Inserted on handle of malleus

129. Vocalis is a part of which of the following: (2008)
a. Thyroarytenois
b. Cricoarytenoid
c. Transverse arytenoids
d. Posterior cricoarytenoid

130. All are true about Chorda tympani nerve except:
a. Supplies anterior 2/3rd tongue (2008)
b. Sensory supply of face
c. It is a branch of facial nerve
d. It joins with lingual nerve

131. All the following veins drain into internal jugular vein except: (2008)
a. Facial vein
b. Lingual vein
c. Superior thyroid vein
d. Retromandibular vein

132. True regarding trigeminal nerve: (2007)
a. Supplies muscles of mastication
b. Sensation of neck
c. Mandibular division of trigeminal nerve supply angle of mandible
d. Mandibular division of trigeminal nerve pass through foramen rotundum

133. Tongue is protruded by which of the following muscle: (2007)
a. Hyoglossus
b. Palatoglossus
c. Myelohyoid
d. Genioglossus

134. All the following muscles are innervated by oculomotor nerve except: (2007)
a. Superior rectus
b. Inferior rectus
c. Superior oblique
d. Medial rectus

135. Which is not a branch of facial nerve? (2007)
a. Chorda tympani
b. Lingual nerve
c. Greater superficial petrosal nerve
d. Brach to stylohyoid muscle

136. All are branches of mandibular nerve except:
a. Auriculotemporal (2006)
b. Zygomatic
c. Inferior alveolar nerve
d. Lingual

137. Not a branch of external carotid artery: (2006)
a. Superior thyroid artery
b. Lingual artery
c. Ascending pharyngeal artery
d. Ophthalmic artery

138. Nasolacrimal duct opens into: (2006)
a. Inferior meatus
b. Superior matus
c. Middle meatus
d. Sphenoethmoidal recess

139. The parasympathetic supply to otic ganglion comes from: (2006)
a. 7th cranial nerve
b. 8th cranial nerve
c. 9th cranial nerve
d. 3rd cranial nerve

140. All the following glands are supplied by facial nerve except: (2006)
a. Parotid
b. Submandibular
c. Lacrimal nasal

141. Stylopharyngeus is supplied by: (2006)
a. Glossopharyngeal nerve
b. Oculomotor nerve
c. Accessory nerve
d. Abducent nerve

142. Upper 1st molar is supplied by: (2006)
a. Superior alveolar nerve
b. Inferior alveolar nerve
c. Mental nerve
d. Lingual nerve

143. Myelination begins at: (2015)
a. 20 weeks
b. 25 weeks
c. 30 weeks
d. 35 weeks

144. Which of the following occupy field H2 of Forel?
a. Ansa lenticularis (2014)
b. Fasciculus thalamicus
c. Fasciculus subthalamicus
d. Fasciculus lenticularis

145. Cerebellar Myelination in newborn is completed by: (2013)
a. 3 months
b. 1 months
c. 12 months
d. 6 months

146. 'Induseum griseum' is found in: (2012)
a. Association fibres of corpus callosum
b. Lateral fibres of corpus callosum
c. Medial fibres of corpus callosum
d. Dorsal surface of corpus callosum

147. Which of the following cranial nerve nuclei is not related to the floor of 4th ventricle? (2011)
a. Abducent nerve
b. Facial nerve
c. Hypoglossal nerve
d. Vagus nerve

148. **Lower end of spinal cord in adults?** **(2011)**
a. Lower border of L1 vertebra
b. Lower border of L3 vertebra
c. Lower border of L2 vertebra
d. Upper border ofL3 vertebra

149. **Sinus located in falx cerebelli is:** **(2010)**
a. Sigmoid sinus
b. Straight sinus
c. Occipital sinus
d. Inferior petrosal sinus

150. **Red nucleus is present in:** **(2009)**
a. Upper pons
b. Lower pons
c. Midbrain
d. Medulla

151. **All the following are general visceral efferent except:** **(2008)**
a. Nucleus ambiguous
b. Dorsal nucleus of vagus
c. Salivatory nucleus
d. Edinger Westphal nucleus

152. **Red nucleus is present in:**
a. Upper pons
b. Lower pons
c. Midbrain
d. Medulla

153. **Type of neuron present in the autonomic ganglion:** **(2006)**
a. Unipolar
b. Bipolar
c. Multipolar
d. Apolar

ANSWERS AND EXPLANATIONS

1. **Ans. d. Cerebral cortical arteries** *Ref: Gray's Anatomy, 39/e p303, 2008*

In general, long branches traverse the cortex and penetrate the subjacent white matter for 3 or 4 cm without communicating. Short branches are confined to the cerebral cortex, and form a compact network in the middle zone of the grey matter.

Arterial anastomoses

Arteries can be joined to each other by an anastomosis

Types

- An **end-to-end anastomosis** occurs when two arteries communicate directly, e.g. the uterine and ovarian arteries, the right and the left gastroepiploic arteries, the ulnar artery and the superficial palmar branch of the radial artery.
- Anastomosis by **convergence** occurs when two arteries converge and merge, as happens when the vertebral arteries form the basilar artery at the base of the brain.
- A **transverse anastomosis** occurs when a short arterial vessel links two large arteries transversely, e.g. the anastomoses between the two anterior cerebral arteries; the posterior tibial artery and the fibular artery; and the radial and ulnar arteries at the wrist.

2. **Ans. b. Inferior tibiofibular joint** *Ref: Grays Anatomy 40/e p101*

Classifiaction of Joints

- **Fbrous joint**
  - Sutures
    - Plane–Internasal sutures
    - Serrate–Interparietal suture
    - Squamous–Temporo-parietal suture
    - Denticulate–Lamdoid suture
    - Schindysis–Between rostrum of sphenoid and upper border of the vomer
  - **Sydesmosis**–Inferior tibio-fibular joint
  - **Gomphosis–Peg and socket joint**—Root of the tooth in the socket.
- **Cartilagenous joints**
  - **Primary cartilaginous joint**–ex Joint between epiphysis and diapysis, Spheno-occipital, 1st Condrosternal, Costochodral joints
  - **Secondary cartel; agenous joint**–ex Symphysis pubis, Manubriosternal joint and Intervertebral joint.

- **Synovial joint**
  - **Plane**–ex Inter carpal jt, Inter tarsal jt, Circothyroid jt, Circoarytenoid jt, Superior tibiofibular jt, Interchodral jt, Costovertebral jt, Costotransvers jt, Carpometocarpal jt (except 1st), Tarsometatarsal jt, Intermetacarpal jt, Intermetatarsal jt, Chodraosternal jt (except 1st) and sacroiliac jt.
  - **Hinge joint**–ex Elbow jt, Ankle jt, Interphalangeal jt
  - **Pivot joint**–ex Superior and Inferior radio-ulnar jt, Median atlantao-axial joint
  - **Condylar joint**–ex Knee jt and Rt and Lt Tempor-mandibular joint
  - **Ellipsoid joint**–Ex Wrst jt, Metocarpophalangeal jt and Atlanto-occipital jt
  - **Saddle joint(Sellar)** –Ex 1st Carpmetacarpal joint, Sternoclavicular jt, Calcaneocuboid jt, Incudomalleolar jt and Femoro-pallar jt
  - **Ball and Socket joint (Spheroidal)–**Ex Shouder jt, Hip jt, Talo-calcaneonavicular joit and Incudostapedial jt

3. Ans. a. Thymus *Ref: Grays Anatomy 40/e p939*

Histology of thymus

- Made-up of lymphoid tissue arranged in the form of distinct lobules. No Lymphatic follicles. The presence of lobules enables easy distinction of the thymus from other lymphoid organs.
- The lobules separated each other by the connective tissue septae.
- Each lobule outer darkly stained cortex in which densely packed lymphocytes and inner lightly stained medulla in which the cells are diffuse.
- Medulla contains pink staining rounded masses called the Hassall corpuscles.
- Hassall corpuscles has central core of degenerated epithelial cells. These cells ultimately form pink hyaline mass. Around this mass concentrically arranged epithelial cells. Central mass also contain degenerating macrophages. The functional significance of the Hassell corpuscles is not known.

4. Ans. b. Synchondrosis (Primary cartilaginous joint) *Ref: Grays Anatomy 40/e p101*

5. Ans. b. Leydig cells *Ref: Wheater's Fucntional Histology: A Text and Colour Atlas, 5/p348 and 349*

Semniferous Tubules

- Present in the lobule of the testis
- Each lobule contains 2 or 3 semniferous tubules and Interstitial cells of Leydig
- Semniferous tubules supports internally by Spertogenic and supporting Sertoli cells.
- Spermatogenic cells arranged in to 3 zones. Outer consists spermatogonia, Intermediate consists of Primary and secondary spermatocytes and Inner consists of Spermatids.
- Sertoli cells–Tight junction between them divide the intercellular space in to basal and adluminal compartments. Basal compartment contain spertogonia and adluminal compartment contain primary and secondary spertocytes.
- **Functions of sertoli cells**
  - Support
  - Form the blood-testis barrier
  - Phagocytic
  - FSH activates to secrete Androgen Binding Protein (ABP)
  - Secretes Anti-Mullerian hormone promote regression of the mullarian ducts

Interstitial cells of Leydig

- Polyhedral cells situated within the lobules of the testis and external to seminiferous tubules
- Abundent in the foetal testis, disappear after birth
- Reappear at puberty and persists throughout life
- Rich in Vit C, lipid droplets and cholesterol
- Secrete Testosteron and probably estragen
- Stimulate the growth of the secondary sex characters.

6. Ans. c. Sebaceous glands appear from epithelium in scalp

Ref: The developing human clinically oriented embryology, 8/e p441 and Histology A text and Altlas, Michael H. Ross, 6/e p134, 666 and 725

- Sebaceous glands develop as buds from the sides of developing epithelial root sheaths of hair follicles

- The glandular buds grow in to the surrounding connective tissue and branch to form the primordial of several alveoli and their associated ducts
- The central cells of the alveoli break down forming an oily secretion (sebum), which is released in to the hair follicle and passes to the surface of the skin,where it mixes with desequmated peridermal cells to form vernix caseosa.

7. **Ans. a. Thymus** *Ref: Grays Anatomy 40/e p939, 2008*
8. **Ans. c. Bone marrow** *Ref: Grays Anatomy 40/e p127*

Primary lymphoid organs: Generate and/or mature and educate cells of the immune system.
Bone marrow Bcells and Thymus Tcells.

Secondary lymphoid organs: Site where mature immunocompetent lymphocytes are exposed to antigen.
Lymph node, Spleen and Mucosa associated with lymphoid organs (MALT—Tonsils. Payer patches and adenoids)

9. **Ans. b. Inferior tibiofublar joint–Ref 2nd question** *Ref: Grays Anatomy 40/e p101*
10. **Ans. a. Thymus** *Ref: Juinquera textbook of histology*
Ref: 8th Question
11. **Ans. c. Ureteric bud** *Ref: Langman's Medical Embryology, 9/e p321–327, 2013*

Kidney development

Ureteric bud	Metanephric blasema
Ureter, Renal pelvis, Major and minor calyces, and collecting duct	Nephrons, PCT, Henles loop and DCT

Renal development is characterized by three successive, slightly overlapping kidney systems

Pronephros–Disappears

Mesonephros

Mesonephric tubules function temporarily and degenerate by the beginning of the third month.

Metanephros

During week 5, the metanephros, or permanent kidney, develops from two sources: the ureteric bud, a diverticulum of the mesonephric duct, and the metanephric mass, from intermediate mesoderm of the lumbar and sacral regions.

Ascent

- The kidneys develop in the pelvis but appear to ascend into the abdomen as a result of fetal growth of the lumbar and sacral regions.
- With their ascent, the ureters elongate, and the kidneys become vascularized by lateral splanchnic arteries, which arise from the abdominal aorta.

Paramesonephric duct or Mullarian duct

- Developed as a longitudinal groove like of invagination of coelomic epithelium on lateral side of mesonephric ridge in the 6th week.

Divided into three parts

1. Cephalic part–Vertical part lateral to mesonephric duct opens to coelomic cavity.
2. Intermediate horizontal part–Passes medially ventral to mesonephric duct.
3. Caudal vertical part–Bulges blindly in the dorsal wall of the urogenital sinus.

Derivatives of paramesonepric duct

Female	Male
• Cephalic vertical and most of the horizontal parts–Uterine tubes. • Caudal vertical parts of both sides fuse to form utero-vaginal canal. Cranial part of the cannal developed into uterus. • Caudal part of the canal forms vagina.	• Most of the duct degenerated. • Cephalic part persists as Appendix of testis a sessile body attached to the upper pole of the testis. • United caudal part forms prostatic utricle homologous to vagina.

12. Ans. a. 9 weeks *Ref: Langmann embryology 11/e*

- Gonads appear as longititudinal ridge called as Genital or Gonadal ridge.
- Primordial germ cells developed from the epiblast during the 2nd week and migrate through the primitive dorsal mesentry during the 4th week and appear in the gonads at the end of 5th week.
- The gonads do not acquire male or female characteristics until 7th week of intrauterine life.

13. Ans. c. Thymus *Ref: Langman's Medical Embryology 9/e p384–385; IBS Human Embryology 7/e p119–120*

Derivatives of pharyngeal pouches

1st pouch	2nd pouch	3rd pouch	4th pouch	5th pouch
• Tubotympanic recess- • Medial portion-Auditary tube • Lateral portion-Tympanic cavity	• Dorsal wing–forms tubotympanic recess • Ventral wing–Tonsilar pits and crypts.	• Dorsal wing–Parathyroid III (Inferior parathyroid) • Ventral wing–Thymic rudiment	• Dorsal wing—Parathyroid IV (Superior parathyroid) • Ventral wing—Caudal pharyngeal complex (Thymic element, Lateral thyroid element and Ultimo-branchial body)	Rudimentary

14. Ans. a. Adrenal *Ref: Langman's Embryology 11/e*

Development of adrenal gland

Cortex–Developed from mesoderm.

- Developed from the suprarenal ridge which is the proliferation of the mesothelial cells lining the coelomic cavity—appears at 2nd month of IUL-Extends from the T6–T12.
- Medulla–Developed from neuroectoderm—the ventral sympathochromoffin masses of the primitive spinal ganglia which migrate and invade the dorsomedial side of the suprarenal ridge.

Development of Pancreas

- Developed at 4th week of IUL from the endoderm of the duodenal segment of the foregut.
- Dorsal pancreatic bud arises from the dorsal wall of the primitive duodenum cephalic to the hepatic bud. This gives rise to entire pancreas except the lower part of the head.
- Ventral pancreatic bud—develops from the commencement of the primitive bile duct at the junction of the foregut and midgut. This give rise to lower part of the head including the uncinate process.
- After the axial rotation of the 2nd part of the duodenum the ventral pancreatic bud winds around the posterior surface of the duodenum and appears on the posteromedial aspect and meet the dorsal pancreatic bud.

Development of Spleen

Spleen developed from mesoderm within the dorsal mesogastrium. Appears at first number of lobules which join together to form a single mass.

15. Ans. a. Epoophoron *Ref: Langman's Embryology 11/e*

Mesonephric tubules 26 in numbers

- Male–**1 or 2 proximal tubules** form **Superior aberrant ductules**
- Successive **12–15 tubules** form **Efferent ductules** of testis
- Caudal tubules persist as **Inferior aberrant ductules** of the testis

Some disconnected from mesonephric duct to form discrete tubules of the **paradidymis**

Female–Proximal 12 to 15 form the **Tubules of Epoophoron**

Distal tubules persist as the **tubules of paroohoron** between the ovary and the uterus.

Mesonephric duct

- **Male**–Persist cranocaudally as Canal **of epididymis, Ductus deferens and the ejaculatory duct.**
- **Female**–Proximal persist as **duct of epoohoron (Duct of Gartner)**
- Rest of the duct disappears.
- Sometimes traces of the ducts persist in the wall of the cervix, lateral wall of vagina and hymenal orifice. These remnants undergoes abnormal dilatation to produce **Gartner's cyst.**

16. Ans. a. 5–8 weeks *Ref: Grays Anatomy 40/e p1013*

Period	Important events development
Early part of 3rd week	Intraembryonic blood cells and vessels
Later part of 3rd week	Intraembryonic blood vessels

Contd...

Contd...

Period	Important events development
2nd–3rd week	Paired lateral endothelial tubes
3rd week	Fusion of paired lateral endothelial tubes into single tube
22nd–24th day	Primitive Heart starts to beat
4th week	Bulboventricular loop
5th–8th week	Septation of definitive heart
After birth	Foramen ovale closes

17. Ans. d. Bartholin duct *Ref: Grays Anatomy 40/e p1305, 101*

18. Ans. a. 1 vein and 2 arteries *Ref: Grays Anatomy 40/e p167*

Umbilical cord

- Tubular cord like structure enveloped by the glistening membrane
- One end attached to the center of the anterior abdominal wall of the fetus and the other end attached to the fetal surface of the placenta
- Formed by the primary mesoderm of the connecting stalk
- 50 cm in length
- **Contents**
  - Umbilical arterie and veins–Two artery and one vein
  - Wharton's jelly–Mucoid degeneration of mesodermal cells
  - Distal part of the allantoic diverticulum fibrosed to urachus
  - Vitellointestinal duct.

19. Ans. a. All of the above *Ref: Grays Anatomy 40/e p1305*

Renal agenesis due to

- Failure to develop the ureteric bud on one side.
- Failure of separation of metenephric blastema which is capped the first order of ureteric bud.

20. Ans. b. Ejaculatory duct *Ref: Grays Anatomy 40/e*

Cloaca (Two parts)	Divided by Urorectal septum	
	Male	Female
Dorsal part (anorectal canal)	Rectum and upper part of anal canal	Rectum and upper part of anal canal
Ventral part (urogenital sinus)	• Most of bladder • Part of prostatic urethra • Prostatic urethra distal to utricle • Bulbourethral glands • Rest of urethra to glands	Most of bladder and the urethra Greater vestibular glands Vestibule, lower 1/3rd of vagina

Ejaculatory duct develops from the mesonephric duct.

21. Ans. d. Rete testis *Ref: Grays Anatomy 40/e*

Fate of the structures derived from undifferentiated genital system

	Male	Female
Gonadal/genital ridge	Testes, seminiferous tubules, rete testes	Ovary, follicles, rete ovary
Mesonephros (Wolffian body)	Appendix of epididymis Efferent ductules Lobules of epididymis	Appendices vesiculosae Epoophoron tubules Paroophoron tubules
Mesonephric duct (Wolffian duct)	Appendix of epididymis, epididymis, ductus deferens, seminal vesicle, ejaculatory duct, Prostate. Remnants: • Superior aberrant tubule	Remnants: • Paroophoron (Equivalent to paradidysmis in males) • Epoophoron/Gartner's duct (Equivalent to ductus deferens in males)

Contd...

Contd...

	Male	Female
	• Inferior aberrant tubule • Paradidymis *Collecting tubule, calyces, pelvis, ureter, trigone of bladder, posterior wall of urethera*	*Collecting tubule, calyces, pelvis, ureter, trigone of bladder, posterior wall of urethera*
Paramesonephric duct (Mullerian duct)	Appendix of testis Prostatic utricle	Uterine tube Uterus Vagina
Labioscrotal swellings	Scrotum	Labia majora

22. Ans. a. Epoophoron *Ref: Grays Anatomy 40/e p101*

23. Ans. b. High anorectal *Ref: Keith L Moore and TVN Persaud The Developing Human Clinically Oriented Embryology, 8/e p240, 2008*

High rectal anomaly

- Rectum ends superior to puborectalis
- Associated with rectovesical or recto-urethral fistula in male and Recto-uterine fistula nad rectovaginal fistula or recto-vestibular fistula.
- Diagnosis presence of muconium in the vestibule of vagina
- Embryological cause is incompete separation of cloaca by the uro-rectal septum.

24. Ans. a. Adrenal *Ref: Langman's Embryology, 11/e, Grays Anatomy 40/e p939*

25. Ans. a. Kidney *Ref: Keith L Moore and TVN Persaud The Developing Human Clinically Oriented Embryology, 8/e p2219, 244–252 and 257, 2008*

Kidney development: From the intermediate mesoderm

Pancreas (Endoderm–foregut)

Ventral bud: The inferior portion of the head of the pancreas and the uncinate process

Dorsal bud: Superior portion of the head and the neck, body, and tail of the pancreas

Liver

Endodermal diverticulum from the terminal part of the forgut at the ventral border of primitive duodenum. Heaptic bud grows ventrally and headwards within ventral mesogastrium and reaches the septum transversum where divides into right and left branch and each branch give rise to hepatic cylinders.

Urinary bladder

Entire mucosa of the urinary bladder except the trigone is developed from the endoderm of vesicourethral part of cloaca.

Apex is derived from the absorption of the proximal part of the allantoic diverticulum.

Trigone of the bladder is developed from mesoderm by the incorporation of the caudal part of the mesonephric ducts.

26. Ans. d. Bartholin duct *Ref: Grays Anatomy 40/e p1305, 2008, 101*

	Male	Female
Mesonephric duct (Wolffian duct)	Appendix of epididymis, Epididymis, Ductus Deferens, Seminal vesicle, Ejaculatory duct, Prostate. Remnants: Superior aberrant tubule Inferior aberrant tubule Paradidymis *Collecting tubule, Calyces, Pelvis, Ureter, trigone of bladder, Posterior wall of urethera*	Remnants: Paroophoron (Equivalent to paradidysmis in males) Epoophoron/Gartner's duct (Equivalent to ductus deferens in males) *Collecting tubule, Calyces, Pelvis, Ureter, trigone of bladder, Posterior wall of urethera*

27. Ans. a. Urogenital sinus *Ref: Grays Anatomy 40/e p101*

Derivatives of paramesonepric duct

Female	Male
• Cephalic vertical and most of the horizontal parts–Uterine tubes. • Caudal vertical parts of both sides fuse to form utero-vaginal canal. Cranial part of the cannal developed into uterus. • Caudal part of the canal forms vagina.	• Most of the duct degenerated. • Cephalic part persists as appendix of testis a sessile body attached to the upper pole of the testis. • United caudal part forms prostatic utericle homologous to vagina.

Mesonephric duct or Wolffian duct	Genital tubercle rudementary phallus
Male–Canal of epididymis, vas deferens, seminal vesicle, and Ejaculatory duct Female–Duct of Epoophron (Duct of Gartner)	Penis and Clitoris

28. Ans. a. Stapes *Ref: Grays Anatomy 40/e p596*

Derivatives of pharyngeal arches

Number of pharyngeal arch	Arteries	Nerves	Muscles	Bones and Ligaments
1st arch	Maxillary artery	Mandibular–Pretrematic and Chordatympani nerve- Post-trematic	Tensor tympani,Tensor veli palatine, Mylohyoid, Muscles of mastication and Anterior belly of digastrics. (T2 M2 A)	Dorsal–Maxillary process-upper lip, jaw and palate Ventral-Malleus, Incus, Anterior ligament of malleus, Sphenomandibular ligament, body of the mandibile
2nd arch	Stapedial artery	Facial nerve	Stapedius, stylohyoid, posterior belly of digastrics, muscles of facial expression, platysma, auricular muscles and epicranius.	Reichert's cartilage- Stapes, Styloid process of temporal bone, Stylohyoid ligament, smaller cornu of the hyoid and superior part of the body of the hyoid.
3rd arch	Ventral part–Common carotid artery Dorsal part-Stem of Internal carotid artery	Glossopharyngeal nerve	Stylopharyngeus	Greater cornu of the hyoid, Lower part of body of hyoid.
4th arch	Rt–Rt Subclavian artery Lt–Part of arch of aorta	Superior laryngeal nerve	Circothyroid	Thyroid cartilage
5th arch	Disappears	Disappears	Disappears	Disappears
6th arch	Rt–Rt pulmonary artery Lt–ventral part–Lt pulmonary artery and Dorsal part–Ductus arteriosus	Recurrent laryngeal nerve	All the intrinsic muscles of larynx except circothyroid.	Circoid and Arytenoid cartilage.

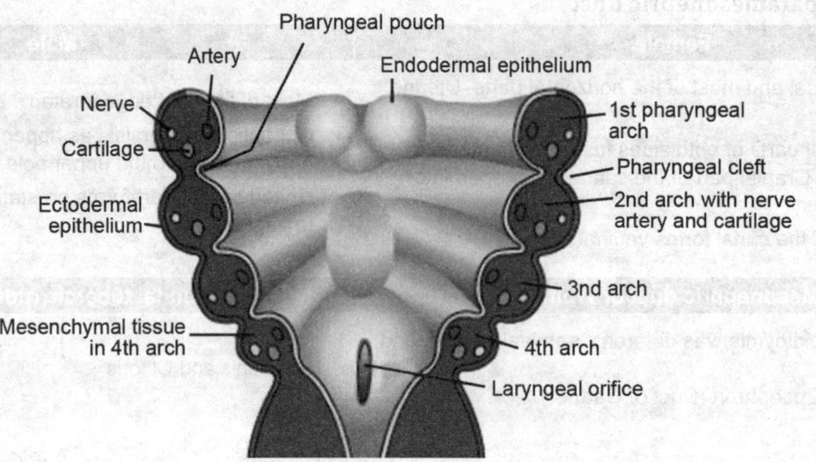

Fig. 1.31: Pharyngeal arches

29. Ans. a. Third arch *Ref: Grays Anatomy 40/e p399*

Embryonic Structure	Adult structure
Remnant of first aortic arch	Maxillary Artery, may form External Carotid Artery
Remnant of 2nd aortic arch	Hyoid and stapedial arteries
Bud from 3rd Arch Artery	External Carotid artery
Ventral part of3rd aortic arch	Common carotid artery
Dorsal part of 3rd aortic arch, dorsal aorta, cranial to ductus caroticus	Internal carotid artery
Dorsal aorta between 3rd and 4th aortic arch	Ductus caroticus
Left limb of aortic sac, left dorsal aorta and left 4th aortic arch	Arch of Aorta
Left dorsal Aortal do fused dorsal Aorta	Descending Aorta
Right Horn of Aortic sac	Brachiocephalic. A
Right 4th Arch artery, right dorsal aorta and 7th Cervical Intersegmental artery.	Right subclavian. A
Left 7th Cervical Intersegmental. A	Left Subclavian
Ventral Part of 6th arch (pulmonary arch) artery	Pulmonary Artery
Dorsal Part of left 6th arch artery	Ductus arteriosus
Dorsal Part of right 6th arch artery	Regressed.

30. Ans. a. Surface ectoderm *Ref: Grays Anatomy 40/ e p700*

- Optic vesicle forms as out pouching of the forebrain which comes in contact with surface ectoderm
- The optic vesicle invaginate to form optic cup.
- The cells of surface ectoderm contact with the optic vesicle begin to elongate to form lens placode which develops in to lens vesicle.
- The lens develop from the lens vesicle.

31. Ans. a. Kidney *Ref: Langmann Embryology, 11th edition*

Derivatives of Ectoderm

Lining Epithelia	Glands	Others
• Skin and Pigment cells • Mucus membranes • Lower part of anal canal • Terminal part of male urethra	Exocrine: Sweat glands Sebaceous glands Parotid glands	Hair Nails Enamel of teeth Lens of eye

Contd...

Contd...

Lining Epithelia	Glands	Others
• Labia majora and outer labia minora • Anterior epithelium of Cornea, epithelium of Conjunctiva, Iris and ciliary body	Mammary glands Lacrimal gland Endocrine Pituitary, Adrenal Medulla	+ All derivatives of neural crest

Derivatives of Endoderm

Epithelium of	Glands
• Part of mouth, palate, tongue, tonsil, Respiratory tract, pharynx and GIT up to upper part of anal canal • Eustachian tube, middle and Inner ear, gall bladder, extrahepatic and pancreatic ducts • Greater part of Vagina, Vestibule and inner surface of labia minora	**Exocrine:** Liver, Pancreas Glands in walls of GIT Prostate (except glandular Zone)

Derivatives of Mesoderm

- All Connective tissues-fascia, tendons, ligaments
- Dermis of skin and Dentine of teeth
- Adipose tissue, cartilage, Bone
- All muscle sexcept that of iris
- Heart, blood vessels, lymphatics
- Kidneys, ureters, glandular zone of Prostate
- Ovary, Uterus, tubes, vagina (upper part)
- Adrenal Cortex
- Testes, epididymis, ductus deferens, Seminal Vesicles and ejaculatory duct
- Meninges and Microglia

32. **Ans. b. Cardiac defects** *Ref: Langmann Embryology, 11/e*

Omphalococele

- Ventral body wall defect.
- Due to the midgut loop fails to return to the abdominal cavity
- Associated with cardiac abnormalities and neural tube defects.
- Chromosomal abnormalities present 15% of cases
- Increases Aipha feto protein.

Exaomphalos

- Ventral wall defect with mid-line herniation of the intra-abdominal contents to the base of the umbilical cord.

33. **Ans. c. Wolffian body** *Ref: Grays Anatomy 40/e p1305, 101*

34. **Ans. b. Superficial branch of ulnar nerve** *Ref: Gray's Anatomy 40/e p897*

The superficial terminal branch supplies palmaris brevis and the medial palmar skin. It divides into two palmar digital nerves, which can be palpated against the hook of the hamate bone.

35. **Ans. b. Radial styloid process extends far more distally** *Ref: Gray's Anatomy 40/e*

Adduction of the hand is considerably greater than abduction, perhaps due to the more proximal site of the ulnar styloid process.

Most adduction occurs at the radiocarpal joint.

36. **Ans. b. Palmaris brevis** *Ref: Grays Anatomy 40/e p589*

Ulnar nerve–(Musicians Nerve)

- Branch of medial cord–C8 and T1
- Axilla—Between third part of axillary artery and axillary vein–more posterior plane. No branches in the axilla.
- Arm—Accompanied by medial cutaneous nerve of forearm and medial to Brachial artery–Pierces the medial intermuscular septum at the middle of arm–Lies in the groove on the posterior surface of medial epicondyle. No branches except to twings to Elbow joint.

- Forearm–Enters by passing between two heads of Flexor carpi ulnaris. Upper half–coverd by Flexor carpi ulnaris– Lower half–Sub fascial lateral to Flexor carpi ulnaris and related Ulnar artery on radial side. Related radial side of Pisiform bone
  - Branches–Flexor carpi ulnaris, and Flexor digitorum profundus (ulnar ½)–Palmar ctaneous branch arises near the middle of forearm and supplies the skin over the hypothenar eminence.
- Enters the palm by passing superficial to Flexor retinaculum
  - Branches–3rd and 4th lumbricals
  - Adductor pollicis
  - All interosseus muscle–palmar and dorsal
- All hypothenar muscle
  - Abductor digiti minimi
  - Flexor digiti minimi brevis
  - Opponens digiti minimi
- Palmaris brevis–only muscle supplied by superficial branch of ulnar nerve.
- **Cutaneous innervations of palm**

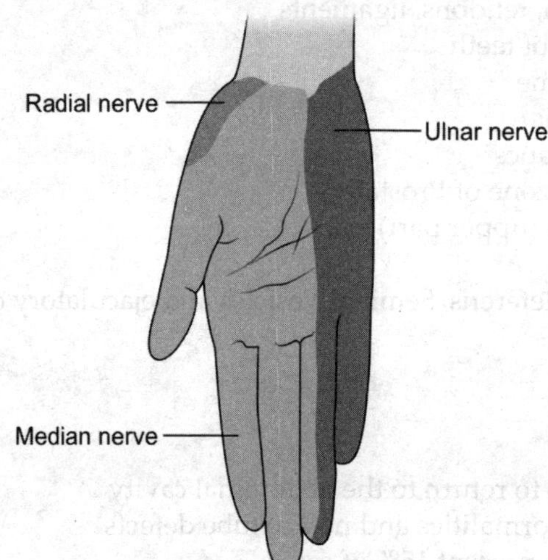

Fig. 1.32: Sensory innervation of palm

- **Cutaneous innervations of dorsum**

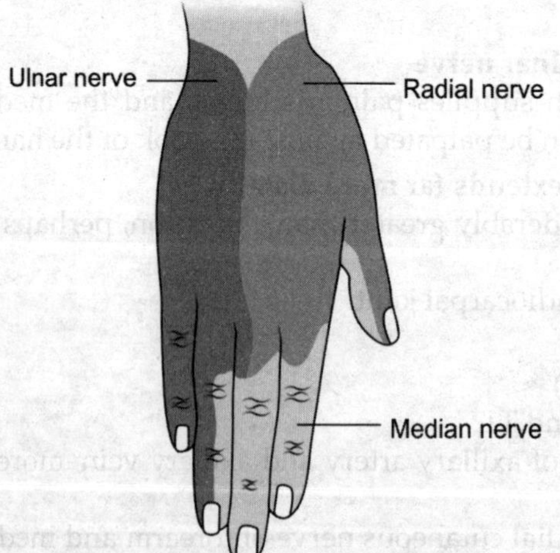

Fig. 1.33: Sensory innervation of dorsum of hand

- Lesions
  - **Cubital tunnel syndrome**–Causes–a. Compressed behind the tendinous arch connecting two heads of Flexor carpi ulnaris b. Trauma c. Fractured medial epicondyle

    Deformities–Claw hand–Medial two fingers extended at MP jt and Partially flexed at IP jt, Wasting of hypothenar muscles.

    Ulnar paradox–More proximal injury at elbow joint produce lesser degree of claw hand than at wrist. This is due to sparing nerve to Flexor digitorum profundus at the injury at wrist.

37. Ans. a. Adductor pollicis *Ref: Grays Anatomy 40/e*

Median nerve

- 2 Roots- Lateral–continuation of lateral cord (C5, C6 and C7), Medial–derved from medial cord (C8 and T1)
- Labourers nerve
- No branches in the axilla.
- Arm –Relation with Brachial artery–Upper part-Lateral, Middle part–In front, Lower part–Medial
- Branches in the arm–Nerve to Pronator teres.
- Enters the forearm by passing between the two heads of Pronator teres.
- In the forearm it crosses Ulnar artery from medial to lateral side and separated from Ulnar artery by ulnar head of Pronator teres.
- Passes under the tendinous arch between two heads of Flexor digitorum superficialis.
- Plastered posterior surface of Flexor digitorum superficialis.
- Branches- All mucles of forearm–anterior compartment except Flexor carpi ulnaris and ulnar½ of flexor digitorum profundus
- Anterior interosseous nerve arises distal Pronator teres–Supplies Flexor pollicis longus, Flexor digitorum profundus and Ponator quadrates. Accompanied by Anterior interosseous artery.
- Palmar cutaneous branch passes superficial to Flexor retinaculum and supplies skin of thenar eminence and centre palm.
- Enter palm by passing deep to Flexor retinaculum.
- Branches in palm to 1st and 2nd Lumbricals, Thenar muscles.

Sensory innervations of Palm

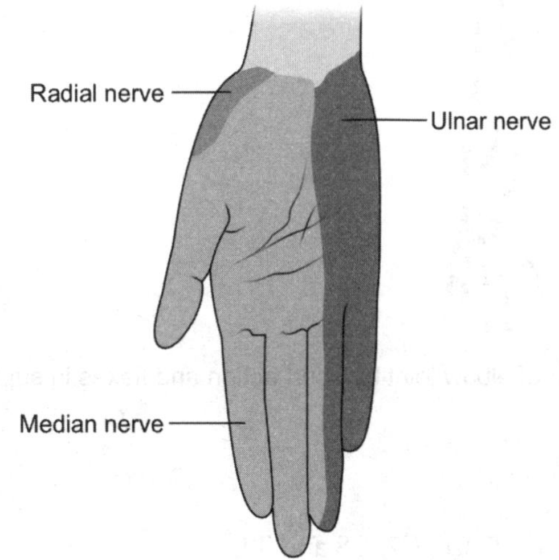

Fig. 1.34: Sensory innervation of palm

- **Lesions**
  - **Pronator syndrome**–Causes–(a) Under Struther ligament (b) Under Bicipital aponeurosis (c) Aponeurotic edge of deep head of Pronator teres (d) Under tendinous arch connecting Flexor digitorum superficialis.
  - **Anterior interosseous syndrome**–Causes–(a) Pronator syndrome (b) External pressure in the form of Saturday night palsy (c) Tight grip in association with pronation.

- **Carpal tunnel syndrome**–Causes–(a) Rheumatoid arthritis (b) Myxedema (c) Pregnancy (d) Obesity (e) Anterior dislocation of Lunate (f) Acromegaly
- Defomities Ape like hand, Pointing index finger (Lesion at the middle of forearm branch of Flexor digitorum superficialis to Index finger is involved)

38. Ans. a. Coracoids process *Ref: Grays Anatomy 40/e p825*

Biceps (Supinator longus)

- Acts on three joint (shoulder, elbow, proximal radioulnar)
- Bicepital aponeurosis (Lacertus fibrosus)–Fibrous expansion from medial border of bicep tendon to upper subcutaneous posterior border of Ulna. Superficial to brachial artery and median nerve.

Supraglenoid tubercle of Scapula	Origin of longhead of biceps
Infraglenoid tubercle of Scapula	Origin of longhead of triceps

- Short head of biceps–Tip of the coracoid process along with the coracobrachialis on its medial side.
- Insertion–Posterior part of the radial tuberosity.
- Both heads join 7 cm above the elbow joint.
- Nerve supply Musculucutaneous nerve
- Action–Powerful supinator of forearm

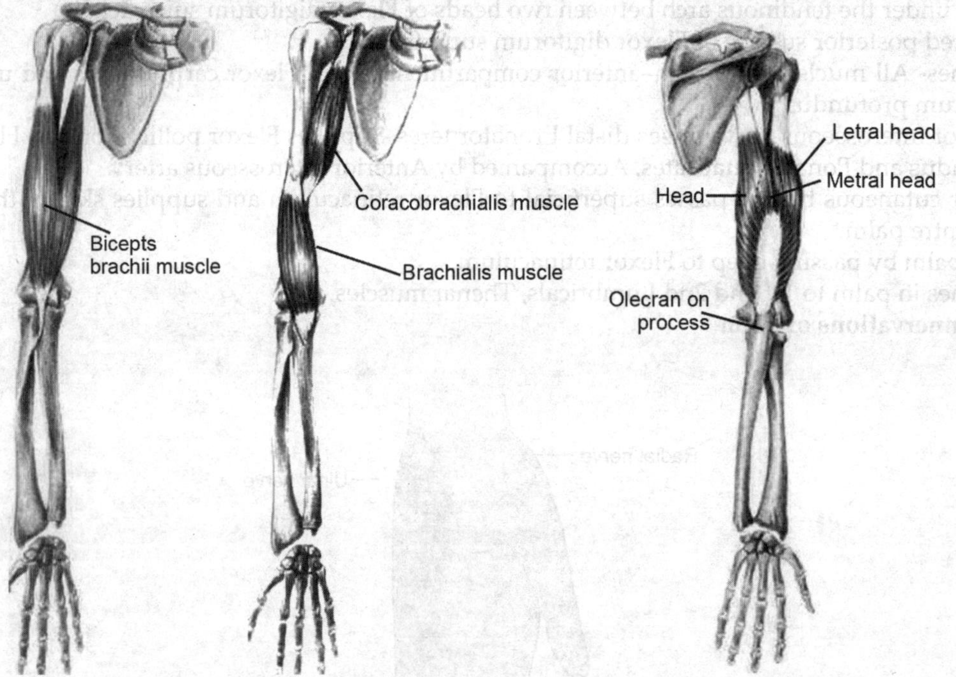

Fig. 1.35: Flexor of elbow joint by spurt action and flexes in supinated position

39. Ans. a. Palmaris brevis *Ref: Grays Anatomy 40/e p939*

40. Ans. a. Long thoracic nerve *Ref: Grays Anatomy 40/e*

Brachial plexus

- Formed by the ventral rami of C5, C6, C7, C8 and T1
- Prefixed–C4 joins C5. Postfixed–T2 joins with T1.
- Parts–Root, Trunk, Division, Cords and Branches.
- Roots and Trunk–Lower part of posterior triangle of neck. Division–Apex of axilla (behind clavicle). Cords and Branches–Axilla.

Supraclavicular part

Roots: Dorsal scapular nerve (rhomboids) C5-Pierces the Scleneus medius.

Long thoracic nerve of Bell C5, 6, 7

Muscular branches to Longus colli and scalene

C5 root gives accessory phrenic nerve.
Trunks: Suprascapular nerve C5 C6
Nerve to subclavius–C5 C6 (Gives accessory phrenic nerve)
Infraclavicular part:
Lateral cord:
Lateral pectoral nerve–pectoralis major and minor
Lateral root of median nerve (Direct continuation of lateral cord)
Musculocutaneous nerve–(C 5–7) coracobrachialis, Biceps, Branchialis, Lateral cutaneous nerve of forearm
Medial cord: (4MU) (Money Makes Many Man Unhappy)
Medial pectoral nerve–pectoralis major and minor (Pierces pectoralis minor)
Medial root of median nerve
Medial cutaneous nerve of arm (smallest and most medial of all branches)
Medial cutaneous nerve of forearm
Ulnar nerve (largest branch of medial cord) (C7, C8, T1)–direct continuation of medial cord is ulnar nerve
Posterior cord: (ULNAR)
Upper subscapular nerve–subscapularis muscle
Lower subscapular nerve–subscapularis muscle, teres major
Nerve to lattismus dorsi (thoraco dorsal nerve)
Axillary nerve–Anterior branch-deltoid, Posterior branch-teres minor, forms Pseudoganglion. Upper lateral cutaneous nerve of arm
Radial nerve (largest branch of whole plexus) (C5-8, T1)–direct continuation of posterior cord

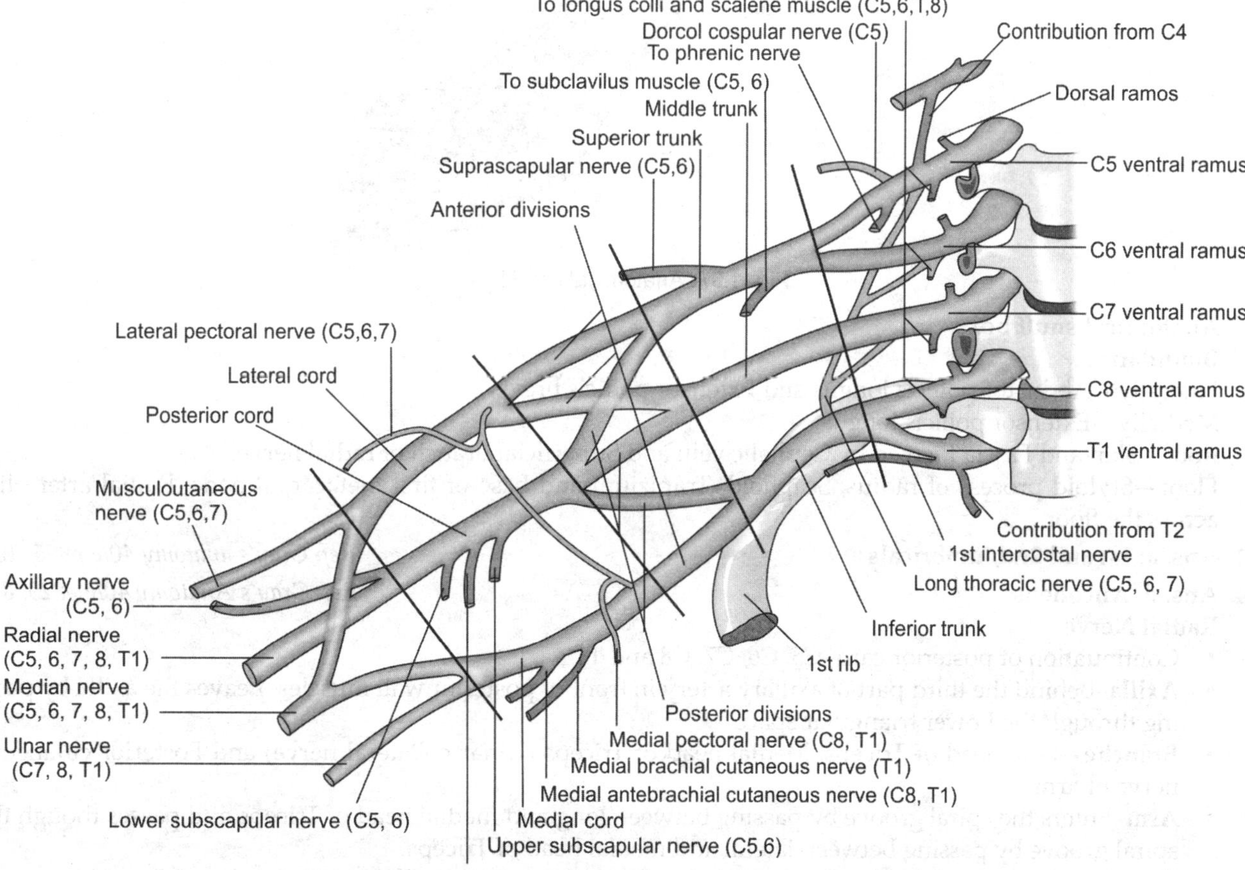

Fig. 1.36: Brachial plexus and its branches

41. Ans. a. Coracoid process *Ref: Grays Anatomy 40/e*

Ref: Wheater's Fucntional Histology: A Text and Colour Atlas, 5/p348 and 349

42. Ans. d. Abductor pollicis brevis *Ref: Grays Anatomy 40/e*

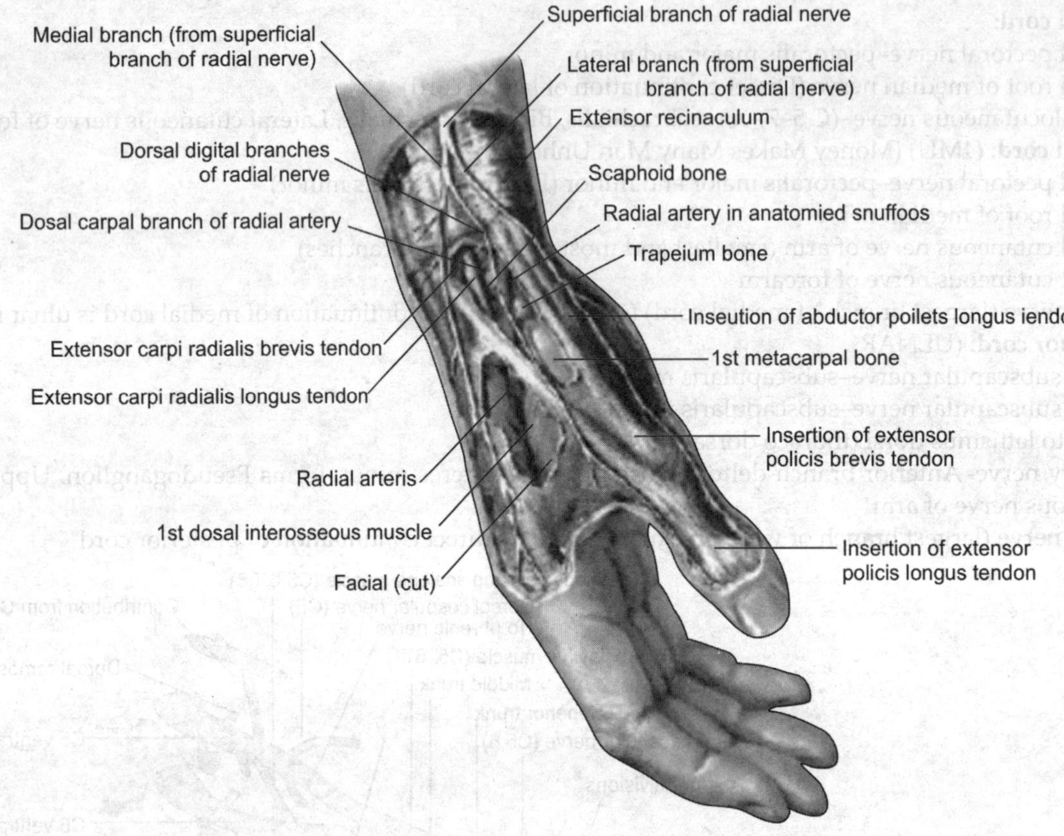

Fig. 1.37: Anatomical snuff box

Anatomical snuff box

Boundaries

Laterally—Abductor pollicis longus and Extensor pollicis brevis

Medially—Extensor pollicis longus

Roof—Skin and Fascia Pierced by Cephalic vein and Superficial branch of radial nerve.

Floor—Styloid process of radius, Scaphoid, Trapizium and base of first metacarpal bone. Radial artery lies across the floor.

43. Ans. a. 1st and 2nd lumbricals *Ref: Gray's anatomy 40/e p895, 101*

44. Ans. d. Anconeus *Ref: Gray's Anatomy 40/e p829, 837*

Radial Nerve

- Continuation of posterior card–C5, C6, C7, C8 and T1
- **Axilla**–Behind the third part of axillary artery in front of posterior wall muscles. Leaves the axilla by passing through the Lower triangular space.
- **Branches**–Longhead of Triceps, Medial head of Triceps (Ulnar collateral nerve) and Posterior cutaneous nerve of arm.
- **Arm**–Enters the spiral groove by passing between long and medial head of Triceps and passes though the spiral groove by passing between lateral and medial head of Triceps.
- **Branches**–Lateral and Medial head of Triceps, Lower lateral cutaneous nerve of arm and Posterior cutaneous nerve of forearm. The nerve to medial head of Triceps at arm supplies Anconeus.
- After spiral groove it gives branches to Brachialis, Brachioradialis and Extensor carpi radialis longus.

- By piercing lateral intermuscular septum, reach in front of lateral epicondyle where divide in to Superficial and Deep branches.
- About 7 cm above wrist, curves laterally and enters dorsum of hand.

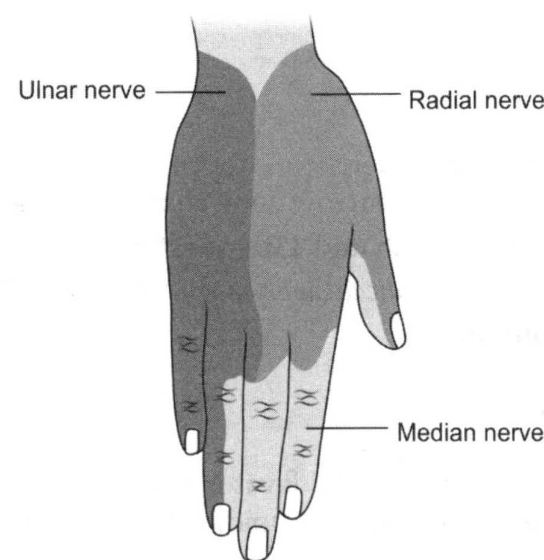

Fig. 1.38: Cutaneous innervations of superficial branch on dorsum of hand

Deep branch (Posterior interosseous nerve)

- Enters forearm by passing between two strata of Supinator
- Branches–Before passing between Supinaor–Give branch to Extensor carpi radialis brevis and Supinator. After passing between Supinaor–All other. extensors
- End in pseudoganglion
- Lesions
  - Injury in axilla
    Causes–(a) Crutch palsy (b) Fracture of upper end of humerus (c) Downward dislocation of shoulder joint.
  - Spiral groove–Saturday night palsy
  - **Radial tunnel syndrome**–(a) Sharp medial border of Extensor carpi radialis brevis
  - **Arcade of Frohse**–Free aponeurotic proximal edge of superficial part of Supinator.
  - **Wartenberg's syndrome**–Entrapment of radial nerve due scissoring effect of Brachioradialis and Extensor carpi radialis brevis as it emerges 6 cm above styloid process.
- **Deformity**–Wrist drop.

45. Ans. b. Supplied by Median nerve *Ref: Grays Anatomy 40/e p918, 2008*

Adductor pollicis

- It has two heads. Oblique and Tranverse heads.
- Oblique head–origin–Capitate and 2nd and 3rd metacarpal base and Transverse head–Origin–palmar surface of 3rd metacarpal
- Insertion–ulnar side of the base of the proximal phalanx of thumb.
- Nerve supply–Deep branch of ulnar nerve
- Blood supply–Arteria princeps pollicic and arteria radialis indicis and branches of deep palmar arch.

Intrinsic muscles of palm

- **Thenar muscles**–Abductor pollicis brevis, Flexor pollicis brevis and Opponens pollicis
  - Supplied by recurrent branch of median nerve.
- **Hypothenar muscles**–Abductor digiti minimi, Flexor digiti minimi and Opponens digiti minimi.
  - Supplied by deep branch of Ulnar nerve.
- **Lumbricals**–four in number, Counted lateral to medial, 1st and 2nd–Unipennate and supplied by median nerve. 3rd and 4th–Bipennate and supplied by deep branch of Ulnar nerve, Link muscles.
- Interosseous–Palmar–Unipannate, Dorsal bipennate–supplied by deep branch of ulnar nerve
- Adductor pollicis–supplied by deep branch of ulnar nerve.
- Palmar brevis–Superficial branch of ulnar nerve.

46. Ans. d. Upper trunk of brachial plexus involved *Ref: Grays Anatomy 40/e p848, 2008*

Klumpkes paralysis–Lower trunk involved

Causes

Pancoast tumor, CA of breast, Cervical rib

- Root–C8, T1
- Nerves–Ulnar, Median
- Ape thumb, Claw hand
- Include horners syndrome
- Caused by–Excessive abduction of shoulder
- Cutaneous anesthesia and analgesia in a narrow zone along the ulnar border of forearm and hand

47. Ans. b. Flexors of fingers and wrist—Ref 7th and 13th questions. *Ref: Grays Anatomy 40/e p791, 939, 2008*

Ref: Langman's Medical Embryology 9/e p384–385; IBS Human Embryology 7/e p119–120

48. Ans. a. Levator scapulae and rhomboids *Ref: Grays Anatomy 40/e p791*

Dorsal scapular nerve

- Also called as nerve to rhomboids.
- Arises from the root C5.
- Pierces the scalenus medius,passes behind the levator scapulae which supplied it and rus with the deep branch od the dorsal scapular artery to the rhomboids which it supplies.

49. Ans. b. Supraglenoid tubercle *Ref: Grays Anatomy 40/e*

Ref: Wheater's Fucntional Histology: A Text and Colour Atlas, 5/p348 and 349

50. Ans. a. Long thoracic nerve of Bell *Ref: Grays Anatomy 40/e p820, 939, 2008*

51. Ans. c. Branches of popliteal artery *Ref: Gray's Anatomy 40/e 9th chapter*

- Genicular branches–Superior medial, Superior lateral, Inferior medial and Inferior lateral
- Terminal branches–Anterior and Posterior tibial artery.

Or

51a. Ans. a. Gliding of femur on tibia during flexion *Ref: Snell's Clinical Anatomy 8/e*

The anterior cruciate ligament prevents posterior displacement of the femur on the tibia. With the knee joint flexed, the anterior cruciate ligament prevents the tibia from being pulled anteriorly.

The posterior cruciate ligament prevents anterior displacement of the femur on the tibia. With the knee joint flexed, the posterior cruciate ligament prevents the tibia from being pulled posteriorly

52. Ans. a. Plantar calcaneonavicular ligament

Plantar calcaneonavicular ligament

- Attachments–plantar surface of the navicular and sustentaculum tali of calcaneus
- Medially continuous with superficial fibres of deltoid ligament
- Laterally continuous with short plantar ligament.
- Lower surface related to tibialis posterior tendon and tendon of flexor digitorum longus.
- Resist the downward displacement of the head of talus.
- Stretched and lessens the height of the medial longitudinal arch when the foot is on the ground and when the foot is off the ground the arch restored to the original position. So it is called as spring ligament.

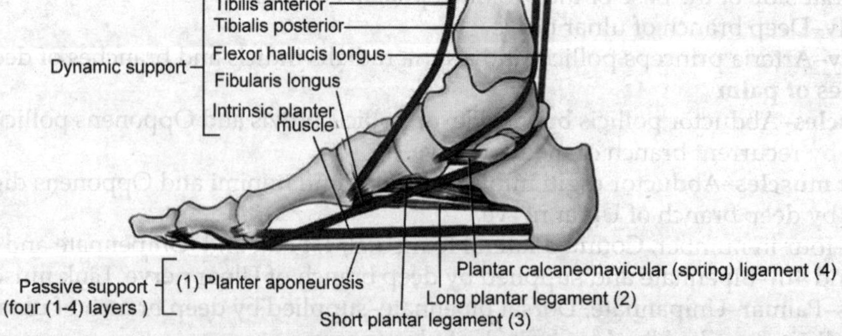

Fig. 1.39: Ligaments of foot

53. Ans. a. Superior gluteal nerve *Ref: Grays Anatomy 40/e*

Nerve	Spinal components	Innervations
Superior gluteal	Dorsal branch of ventral rami of L4, L5, S1	Abductor muscles of thigh (gluteus miniums, gluteus medius, tensor fasciae late)
Inferior gluteal	Dorsal branch of ventral rami of L5 to S2	Extensor muscle of hip joint (gluteus maximus)
Nere to piriformis	S1, S2	Abductor and rotator of thigh (piriformis)
Nerve to quadratus femoris	Ventral branch of ventral rami of L4, L5, S1	Rotators of thigh (gemellus inferior, quadrates femoris)
Nerve to internal obturator	Ventral branch of ventral rami of L5 toS2	Rotators of thigh (gemellus superior, internal obturator)
Perforating cutaneous	S2, S3	Skin over lower medial surface of buttock
Posterior cutaneous femoral	Dorsal branch of S1, S2 andVentral branch of S2, S3	Skin over lower lateral surface of buttock, anal region, upper posterior surface of thigh, upper aspect of calf, scrotum in male and labia major in female
Sacral muscular	S4	Levator ani, External anal sphincter
Sacral visceral	S2, S4	Pelvic splanchnic nerve
Pudendal	Ventral branch of ventral rami of S2 to S4	Skin of penis and scrotum in male and skin of clitoris, labia majora, labia minora, and lower vagina in female; muscles of perineum

No cutaneous innervations by superior and Inferior gluteal nerve

54. Ans. d. Nerve to vatus lateralis *Ref: Grays Anatomy 40/e*

Adductor canal (Hunter's canal) (Subsartorial canal)

Gutter shaped

Bounded: Floor-adductor longus above and adductor magnus below and anterolaterally vastus medialis Roof–Fascia over the adductor longus and adductor magnus and the Sartorius muscle and the subsartorial plexus intervene between them.

Roof is pierced by the saphenous nerve and the saphenous branch of the descending genicular artery.

Contents: femoral artery, femoral vein, saphenous nerve, nerve to vastus medialis, Posterior division of Obturator nerve and terminal part of Profunda femoris vessels.

55. Ans. c. Tensor fascia lata *Ref: Grays Anatomy 40/e*

Superficial fascia of abdomen—superficial fatty layer–fascia campor and deep membranous layer–fascia scarpa which extends to thigh and attached to the fascia lata.

Tensor fascia lata

- Arises from the outer lip of the iliac crest from the anterior superior iliac spine to the tubercle if the iliac crest and inerted to the upper part of the ilio-tibial tract which is the thickened lateral part of the fascia lata.
- It is supplied by the superior gluteal nerve (L4, L5, S1-dorsal branches of ventral rami)
- Action–Abducts the hip joint and maintain the extended position of the knee joint.

56. Ans. d. Posterior tibial artery *Ref: Grays Anatomy 40/e p1493, 2008*

- **Posterior tibial artery**
  - Larger terminal branch of Popliteal artery
  - Ends by dividing in to Medial and Lateral plantar artery.
  - Branches–Circumflex fibular, Peroneal, Medial malleolarbranch, Calcaneal branch, Medial plantar, Lateral plantar, Nutrient artery to tibia, Communicating branch to peroneal artery.
  - Nutrient artery to fibula from Peroneal artery.

57. Ans. b. 125 *Ref: Grays Anatomy 40/e p1349*

Femoral Neck Angle

- Femoral neck extends inferolaterally from head to meet shaft at angle of about 125 degree
- Angle varies with age, stature and width of pelvis being less in adult, in persons with short limbs and in women.

- When this angle is > 135 degree–Coxa valga
- When the angle is > 120 degree–Coxa vara
- Femoral neck is not parallel to frontal plane or plane of femur.
- Head is anterior to midline of the shaft of the femur and thus is said to be anteverted.

58. Ans. a. Popliteus *Ref: Grays Anatomy 40/ e p1393*

Popliteus

- Intracapsular origin
- Arises from the anterior part of the groove on the lateral surface of the lateral femoral condyle and inserted posterior surface of the tibia above the soleal line.
- Articular muscle–Few fibres attached to the posterior part of the lateral meniscus.
- Action–Popliteus rotates the tibia medially on femur and rotates femur laterally on the tibia when the tibia is fixed.
- Unlocks the knee joint and initiates the flexion of fully extended knee.
- Its connection with the arcuate popliteal ligament, Fibrous capsule and lateral meniscus, retract the posterior horn of the lateral meniscus during lateral rotation of the femur and flexion of the knee joint and thus protecting the meniscus from being crushed between femur and the tibia during movements.
- Main function is provision of dynamic stability to the posterolateral part of the knee by preventing excessive rotation of the tibia partly by direct action, but more by the tensing the popliteofibular ligament.

59. Ans. a. Semimembranosus *Ref: Grays Anatomy 40/e p1393*

Oblique Popliteal Ligament

- Expansion of semimembranosus which blends with the posterior capsule.
- It is pierced by middle genicular nerve and vessels
- Terminal part of posterior division of obturator nerve also pierces the oblique popliteal ligament.
- It attached to the intercondylar line and lateral femoral condyle.

Expansion of the semimebranosus

- Oblique popliteal ligament
- Few fibres extend downward and laterally through the fasia covering the popliteus to the soleal line of the tibia.
- Tuberculum tendinum–slip attached to the tubercle on the back of medial condyle of the tibia.

Some fibres attached to the upper part of the tibia behind the tibial collateral ligament.

60. Ans. a. Right upper lobe *Ref: Gray's Anatomy 40/e 7th chapter*

The medial part of the right upper lobe is partially separated by a fissure of variable depth which contains the terminal part of the azygos vein, enclosed in the free margin of a mesentery derived from the mediastinal pleura, and forming the 'lobe of the azygos vein'.

61. Ans. a. Cervical pleura *Ref: Gray's Anatomy 40/e*

- Continuation of costal pleura.
- Covers the apex of the lung
- Suprapleural membrane protects the cervical pleura.

62. Ans. b. Azygos vein *Ref: Grays Anatomy 40/e p966, 2008*

Intercostal veins
Anterior–Internal thoracic 1–6
Musculophrenic 7–9
Posterior –Right–1st–Right brachiocephalic vein
2nd and 3rd–Right superior intercostals vein–Arch of azygos vein.
5th to 11th–Vertical part of azygos vein.
Left–1st–Left brachiocephalic vein
2nd and 3rd–Left superior intercostals vein–Left brachiocephalic vein
5th to 7th–Superior hemiazygos vein (Acessory –azygos vein)–Opposite T7
8th to 11th–Inferior hemiazygos vein (Hemiazygos vein)–Opposite T8

63. Ans. a. Tributaries of portal vein are *Ref: AK Datta 1/p p255*

- Superior mesenteric vein
- Splenic vein

- Right and left gastric vein
- Cystic vein
- Paraumbilical vein
- Infrior mesenteric vein
- Right gastroepiploic vein
- Prepyloric vein of Mayo

64. Ans. a. Right gastric artery *Ref: Gray's Anatomy 40/e*

- The left gastric artery is the smallest branch of the coeliac axis. In its course along the lesser curvature, it gives off multiple branches that run onto the anterior and posterior surfaces of the stomach and anastomose with the right gastric artery in the region of the incisura angularis.
- The left gastroepiploic artery is the largest branch of the splenic artery. It lies between the layers of peritoneum close to the greater curvature, running inferiorly to anastomose with the right gastroepiploic artery.
- Posterior gastric artery arises from the splenic artery in its middle section posterior to the body of the stomach. It ascends behind the peritoneum of the lesser sac towards the fundus and reaches the posterior surface of the stomach in the gastrophrenic fold.
- The right gastric artery arises from the hepatic artery. It runs between the peritoneal layers of the lesser omentum just above the medial end of the lesser curvature, passes superiorly along the lesser curvature, giving off multiple branches onto the anterior and posterior surfaces of the stomach, and anastomoses with the left gastric artery.

65. Ans. c. Three-tier classification of the anatomical factors: *Ref: Gray'S Anatomy 50/e*

- The suspensory attachments at the posterior abdominal wall to the inferior vena cava, hepatic veins, coronary and triangular ligaments (primary factors);
- The support provided by the right kidney, right colonic angle and duodenopancreatic complex (secondary factors);
- The attachment to the anterior abdominal wall and diaphragm by the falciform ligament (tertiary factors).

66. Ans. c. 1–2 litres of bile is secreted by the liver daily and it is 10 fold concentrated by the gall bladder *Ref: Gray's Anatomy 40/e*

The main right and left hepatic ducts emerge from the liver and unite near the right end of the porta hepatis as the common hepatic duct.

The common bile duct is formed near the porta hepatis, by the junction of the cystic and common hepatic ducts and is usually between 6 and 8 cm long. Its diameter tends to increase somewhat with age but is usually around 6 mm in adults.

Gall bladder is innervated by both sympathetic and parasympathetics from celiac plexus.

67. Ans. a. Mesentery *Ref: Gray's Anatomy 40/e*

- Peritoneal fold suspends jejunum and ileum from the posterior abdominal wall and conveys nutrition to small intestine.
- 2 borders–Root or Vertebral border and Free or iIntestinal border.
- Extends from left side of L3 vertebra at the duodenojejunal junction to right sacroiliac joit at ileocaecal junction.
- **Structures crossed by the roor of mesentery are:**
  - 3rd duodenum
  - Abdominal aorta
  - IVC
  - Right gonadal vessels
  - Right ureter and rt psoas
  - Rt genitorfemoral nerve
  - Rt sacroiliac joint

Contents of mesentery

- Jejunum and ileum
- Jejunal and ileal branches of superior mesenteric artery
- Intestinal lymphatics called as Lacteals and mesenteric nodes

- Loose areolar tissue
- Fat
- Occasionally Suspensory muscle of duodenum, accessory suprarenal tissue andtip of appendix

68. Ans. a. Fascia transversalis *Ref: Gray's Anatomy 40/e*

The deep inguinal ring begins as an outpouching of transversalis fascia just lateral to where the inferior epigastric vessels intersect the inguinal ligament–1.25 cm above the midinguinal point.

69. Ans. d. Contains duodenal mesentery *Ref: Gray's Anatomy, 39/e p1165, 2008*

Ligament of Treitz

- Superior and inferior surfaces of the 4th part of duodenum covered by the peritoneum and suspended from retroperitonem by double fold called ligament trietz.
- Start at the duodenojejunal flexure.
- Contain suspensory muscle of the duodenum–contains the skeletal muscle run from the left crus of the diaphragm to connective tissue around the celiac axis and smooth muscle that run from the celiac axis. Its function not known.
- Important landmark in the radiological diagnosis of incomplete rotation and malrotation of the small intestine.
- Ligament of treitz does not form part of the duodenal mesentry because the vascular supply to the 4th part of the duodenum continues to enter its wall from the posteromedial aspect.

70. Ans. b. Inferior rectal artery *Ref: Gray's Anatomy, 39/e p1201–1203, 2008*

Mesorectum (Mesentery of the rectum)

- Related to the rectum down to the level of levator ani.
- It contains
  - Superior rectal vein and its tributaries
  - Superior rectal artery
  - Branches of inferior mesenteric plexus
  - Lymphatic vessels and nodes
  - Loose connective tissue
  - Branches of middle rectal artery and veins–Lateral rectal ligaments are branches of middle rectal artery and veins ensheathed with mesorectum. They are not visualized on MRI or CT scan.

Mesorectal Fascia

- Viseral peritoneum encloses the mesorectum.
- It is also called as Viseral fascia of mesorectum or Fascia propria of the rectum or Presacral wing of the hypogastric sheath.
- Bounds the mesorectum posteriorly and lies anterior to the retrorectal space and presacral fascia.
- **Tracings**
  - **Superiorly**–Blends with the sigmoid mesentery.
  - **Laterally**–extends around the rectum and mesorectum and continuous with rectovesical fascia of Denovillier in males and rectovaginal septum in females.

71. Ans. d. Sigmoid colon

Ref: Gray's Anatomy, 40/e ch67 and Shackelford's surgery of the alimentary tract, vol. 1, 6/e ch133

Part	Diameter
Ascending colon	5 cm
Transverse colon	5 cm close to rt end and 3.5 cm to 4 cm at lt end
Descending colon	3.5 cm
Sigmoid colon	3.5 cm

72. Ans. b. Cervix size is equal to uterus size in puberty

Ref: Clincially oriented anatomy, keith L Moore, 5/e p418, 2006 and Shaw's textbook of Gynecology, 15/e p8

Cervix Corpus Ratio

Children–2 : 1

At puberty–1 : 2

Reproductive period–1 : 3

The arterial supply to the uterus comes from the uterine artery. This arises as a **branch of the anterior division of the internal iliac artery.**

It is the **homolog to the artery to the ductus deferens in the male.**

The uterine artery **crosses the ureter anteriorly in the broad ligament from lateral to medial** side before branching as it reaches the uterus at the level of the cervicouterine junction.

The relationship of ureter to artery is often remembered by the phrase water (urine) passes under the bridge (uterine artery).

On reaching the side of the cervix, the uterine artery divides into a smaller descending vaginal branch, which supplies the cervix and vagina, and a larger ascending branch, which runs along the lateral margin of the uterus, supplying the body and fundus of the uterus.

Lymphatic drainage of the uterus

Part of uterus	Draining nodes
Fundus and upper part of the body Lateral angle of the uterus along the round ligament of uterus	Preaortic and para-aortic nodes. Horizontal groups of Superficial inguinal nodes
Lower part of the body	External iliac nodes
Cervix	External iliac, Obturator, Parcervical nodes Internal iliac nodes Sacral nodes

73. Ans. b. Bulbospongious *Ref: Gray's Anatomy 40/e p1083*

Perineal Body

Pyramidal fibromuscular node intervening between anal canal and urogenital canal.

Formed by 9 muscles.

They are Pair of superficial and deep transverse perinii muscle, external and internal anal sphincter, sphincter urethrae, Pubococcygeus and Illiococcygeus part of levatoe ani and Bulbospongiosus.

Bulbospongiosus covering the bulb of the penis and Ischiocavernosus covering the crus of the penis.

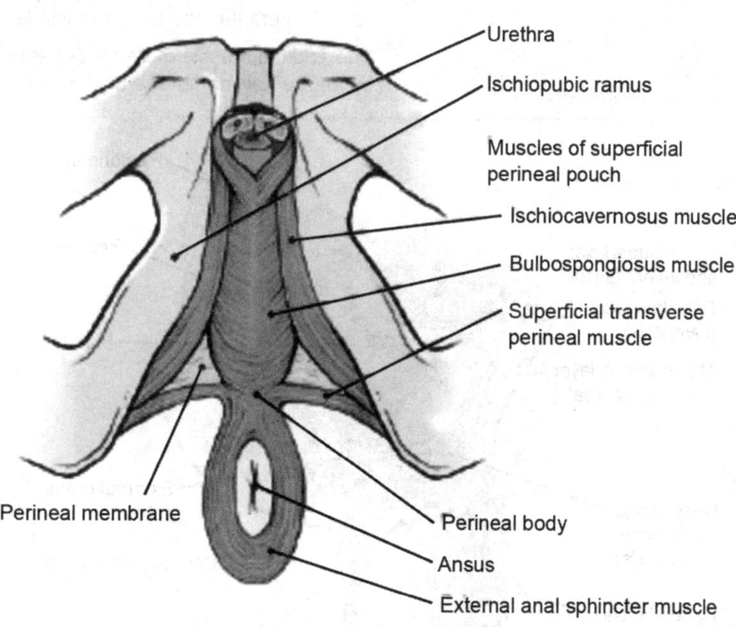

Fig. 1.40: Muscles of perineal body

74. Ans. c. 2nd part of duodenum. Ref question no 4 *Ref: Grays Anatomy 40/e p1104*

76. Ans. a. Sacrum and rectum *Ref: grays Anatomy 40/e Thickening of the Pelvic Fascia.*

Waldeyer's Fascia

- Thickening of the pelvic fascia.
- Extends from the anorectal junction to the coccyx
- Behind the rectum in the midline.

Fascia	Name of the fascia
Fascia of the penis	Buck's fascia
Renal fascia	Fascia Gerota
Anterior renal fascia	Fascia Toldt
Posterior renal fascia	Fascia Zukerkandle
Extension of external aponeurosis	External spermatic fascia
Extension of fascia transversalis	Internal spermatic fascia
Extension of internal oblique and transverse abdomins	Cremastic fascia
Fascia covering saphenous opening	Fascia cribrosa
Superficial fatty layer of abdomen between umbilicus and pubis	Fascia Camper
Deep membranous layer of abdomen between umbilicus and pubis	Fascia Scarpa
Extension of Fascia Scarpa in the perineum	Fascia Colles
Rectovesical fascia	Fascia Denovillers
Deep fascia of the thigh	Fascia lata
Fascia extends from the anorectal junction to the coccyx	Fascia of Waldeyer
Supraplural membrane	Sibson's fascia
Endoabdominal fascia	Transversalis fascia
External obliquefascia	Gallaudt's fascia
Fascia Lunata	Fascia of ischiorectal fossa forming medial wall of the Alcock's canal covers the obturator's fascia laterally.
Fascia Waldeyer	The Triginal muscle of Bell is separated from the detrusor muscle by an areolar membrane called as Fascia Waldeyer.

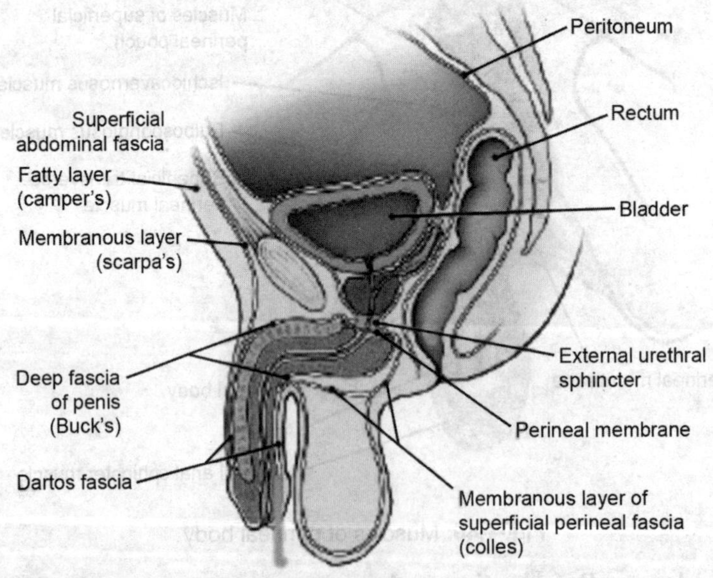

Fig. 1.41: Sagittal section of male pelvis

76. Ans. a. T 12 *Ref: Grays Anatomy 40/e*

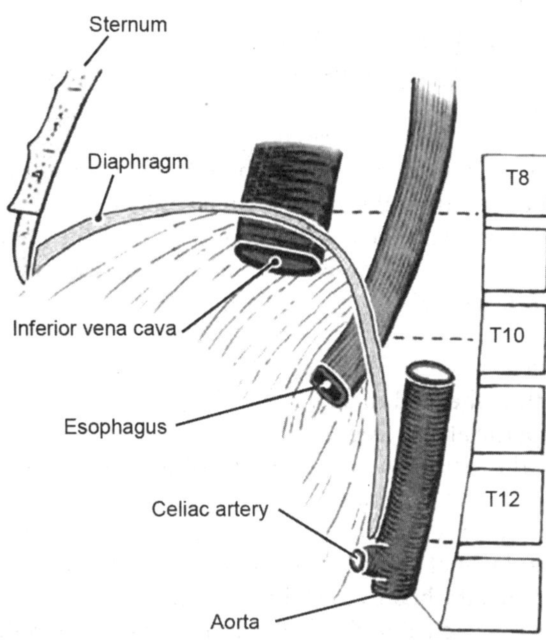

Fig. 1.42: Openings of diaphragm

Name	Level	Shape	Position
Vena caval (Inferior)	T8	Square	Slightly to right of median plane
Esophageal	T10	Oval	Slightly to left of median plane
Aortic	T12	Round	Central

Structures traveling between the thorax and abdomen pass through diaphragm or between the diaphragm and its peripheral attachments:

Opening	Level	Portion of diaphragm	Structures passing through
Vena caval (V)	**T8**	**Central tendon (highest)**	Inferior vena cava, right phrenic nerve
Esophageal (O)	**T10**	**Muscular portion of Right crus**	Esophagus, Esophageal br. of left gastric Artery, Vagus nerve [Gastric nerves], lymphatics
Aortic (A)	**T12**	**Aponeurosis between right and lateral crus [lowest and posterior]**	Aorta, thoracic duct, azygos vein, lymph trunks

Remover: VOA (voice of Aminjaikarai (8/10/12))
Sternocostal hiatus–Supr. Epigastric Vessel

Diaphragmatic Openings

Opening	Location	Structures passing
Medial lumbocostal arch	Behind medial arcuate ligament	Sympathetic chain
Lateral lumbocostal arch	Behin arcuate ligament	Subcostal nerve and vessels
Foramen of Morgagni/Larry's space	Between xiphoid and costal margin of diaphragm	Superior epigastric vessels, lymphatics

- Greater and lesser splanchnic vessels pierce both the diaphragmatic crura
- Hemiazygos vein pierces the left crus
- Musculophrenic vessels pierce the diaphragm at the level of 9th costal cartilage

77. Ans. b. Circular muscle fibres *Ref: Grays Anatomy 40/e*

Internal anal Sphincter

- Involuntary sphincter.
- Thickened circular muscleof the loer part of the rectum.
- Lower end of internal anal sphincter corresponds to the white line of Hilton and Mid sphincter corresponds to the pectinate line.
- Surround the upper threefourth of the anal canal.
- Internal anal sphincter separated from the mucosa by internal venous plexus.
- Internal anal sphincter separated from the external anal sphincter by a conjoint sheath derived from union of puborectalis part of levtor ani with the longitudinal muscle of the rectum at the ano-rectal junction.
- Nerve supply–autonomic–Sympathetic derived from superior hypogastric plexus and parasympathetic derived from pelvi splanchnic nerve.

External Sphincter

- Voluntary sphincter muscle.
- Surrounds the entire length of the anal canal.
- 3 parts–Subcutaneous, Superficial and Deep.
  - Longitudinal muscle of the rectumblends with the puboretalis part of levator ani muscle and form conjoint fibro elastic sheath.
  - It pass downwards between internal and external anal sphincter around the anal canal.
  - At the lower end of internal anal sphincter it splits in to a number of septa. Medial most interseptum is anal intermuscular septum attached to the Hilton's white line.
  - Some longitudinal muscle attached to the urethra called as Rectourethral muscle (Muscle of Roux) and some attached to the coccyx called as recto–coccygeus muscle.

Parts of Levetor Ani Muscle are

Iliococcygeus

Pubococcygeus–Pubococcygeus proper, Puborectalis, Puboanalis and Pubovesicalis or Puboanalis.

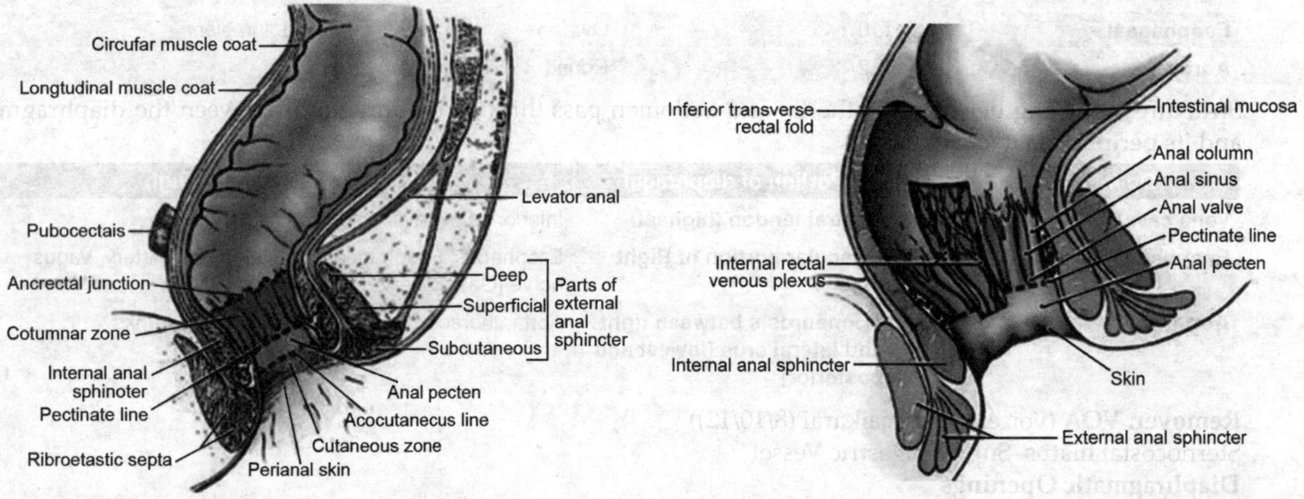

Fig. 1.43: Interior of anus

Fig. 1.44: Interior of anus

78. Ans. a. Splenic artery and **c.** Left gastric artery

Ref: Grays Anatomy 40/e p111 and Loukas M, Wartmann CT, Louis RG Jr, Tubbs RS. Ona M. Curry B et al. The clinical anatomy of the posterior gastric artery revisited. Surg Radiol Anat. 2007 Jul; 29(5):361–6.

Posterior gastric artery

- Branch of splenic artery
- Supplies the posterior surface of the fundus of the stomach through the gastrophrenic ligament.

Hepatic artery–Branch of celiac axis

Left gastric artery is the branch of celiac axis

Right gastric artery is the branch of proper hepatic artery which is the continuation of the common hepatic artery.

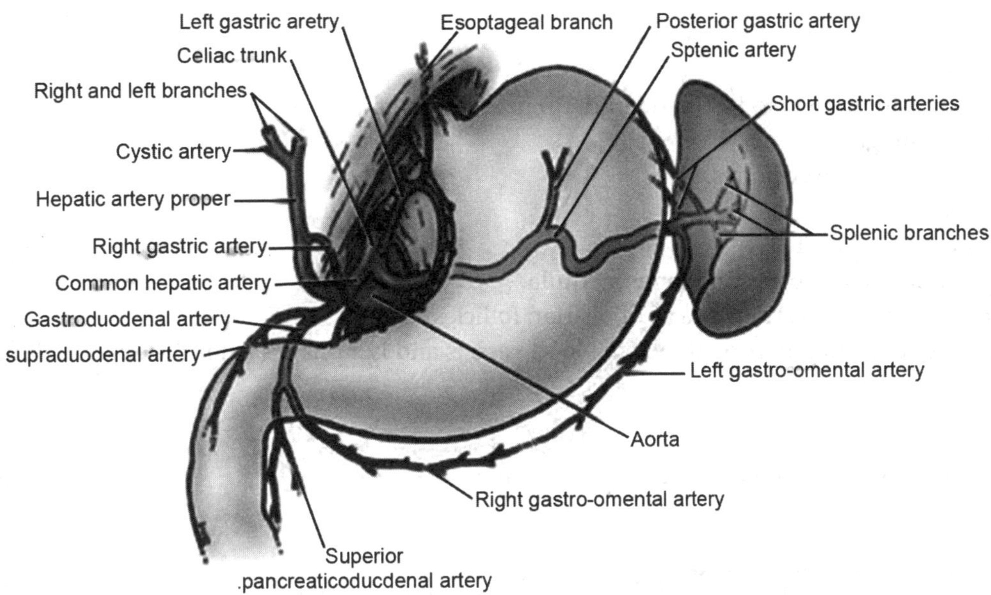

Fig. 1.45: Blood supply of stomach

79. Ans. a. Lacunar ligament *Ref: Grays Anatomy 40/e p1055*

Femoral ring:

Anterior–Inguinal ligament

Medially–Lacunar ligament

Posterior–Pectineal ligament

Laterally–Vein-femoral

Inguinal ligament (Fallopian ligament)

Inferiorly, the free border of the external oblique aponeurosis forms the inguinal ligament **(Pouparts lig ament),** in which fascia lata of thigh attached.

Lacunar ligament (Gimber nats ligament): Pectinal part of inguinal lig–From medial end of inguinal ligament extends backward to pectineal line and forms medial margin of femoral ring.

Reflected part of inguinal lig (Colles lig): Third crus of superficial ring–Forms medial ¼ of posterior wall of inguinal canal-reflected upwards and medially from pubic tubercle in front of conjoint tendon and inserted in to linea alba.

Astley cooper ligament: Pectinal ligament of cooper-extends from base of lacunar ligament to pecten pubis and ilio pubic eminence.

80. Ans. b. Hilus *Ref: Grays Anatomy 40/e p1279*

Ovary

- Intraperitoneal organ-lined by cuboidal epithelium.
- Presenting parts–Tubal end –related to uterine tube, attachment of ovarian fimbria and Suspensory ligament of ovary (Connecting uterine tube, ovary to the pelvic brim.

  Uterine end–connected to the uterine angle of tube by ligament of ovary.

  Anterior border (Mesovarian)- attached to posterior layer of broad ligament by a fold acts as hilum of ovary through which ovarian vessels and nerves passes.

  White line of Furre–Transition between mesothelium of broad ligament and germinal epithelium of ovary.

  Free posterior border–related to uterine tube, ureter and internal iliac vessels.

Medial surface–related to uterine tube from which separated by Bursa ovarica.

Lateral surface–ovarian fossa.

Arterial supply

Ovarian artery branch of abdominal aorta.

Venous drainage

Right ovarian vein drain in to IVC and left drain in to left renal vein.

Lymphatic drainage

Preaortic and lateral aortic nodes.

Nerve supply

Sympathetic nerve–T10, T11

- Ovary contain outer cortex and inner medulla.
- Outer cortex contain various stages of ovarian follicles
- Medulla contains hilum through which blood vessels and lymphatics enter the ovary. Hilum contain hilus cells.

81. Ans. d. Ascends behind the second part of duodenum *Ref: Grays Anatomy 40/e p1163*

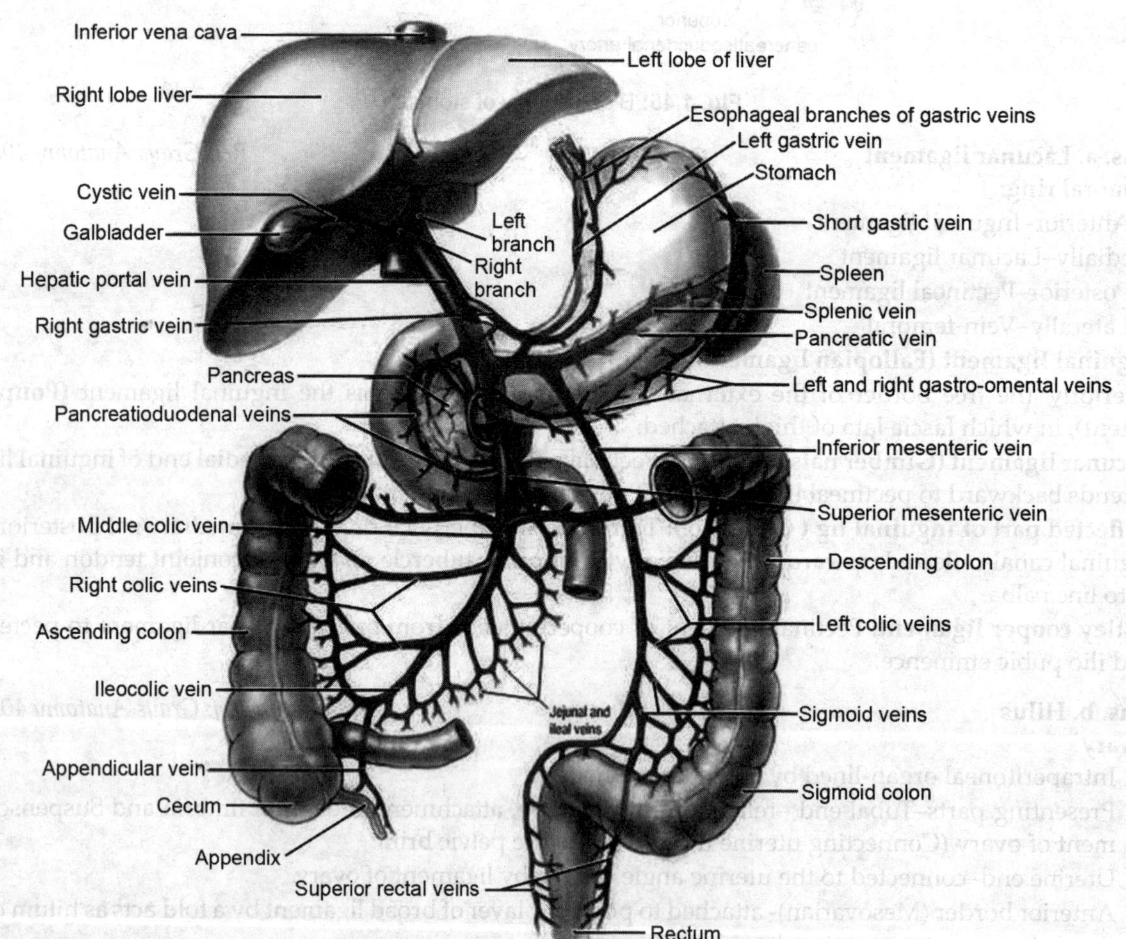

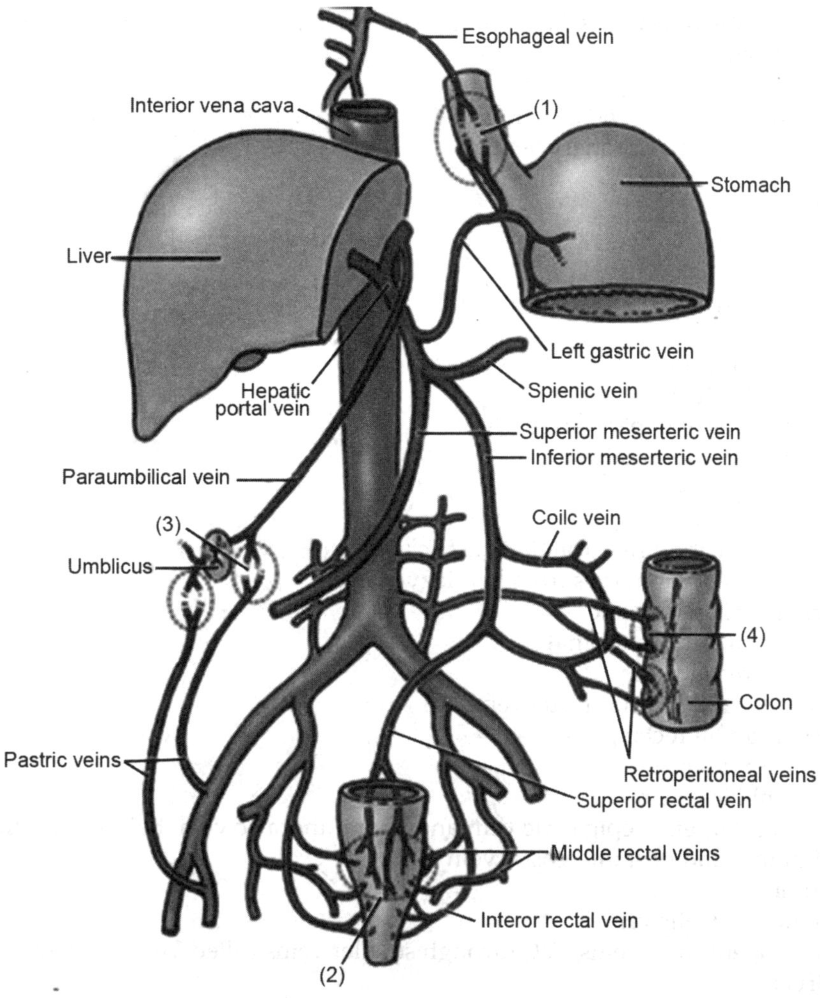

Fig. 1.46: Porto-caval communications

Portal vein

Peculiarities of Portal vein

- Devoid of valves.
- Begins like vein and end like artery
- Conveys blood and products of digested food
- Reservoir of blood
- Blood from SMV to right branch of portal vein.
  Blood from Splenic vein to leftt branch of portal vein.
- Portal pressure is 8 mm of Hg to 10 mm of Hg.

Formation of portal vein–Union of splenic and superior mesenteric vein

Site: Behind the neck of pancreas. At the level of L2 and in front of IVC.

Relations

Infraduodenal part–In front–Neck of pancreas, Behind–IVC and Right–Bile duct

Retroduodenal part–In front–1st part of duodenum separated by bile duct on right side and gastroduodenal artery on left side and Behind–IVC.

Supra-duodenal part–In front and right–Bile duct, infront and left–Hepatic artery and Behind–IVC

Porta hepatis–From before backwards Rt and Lt hepatic duct, Rt and Lt branches of hepatic artery and Rt and Lt branches of portal vein.

Tributaries
- Formative tributaries–Splenic and Superior mesenteric vein
- Right and Left gastric vein (Coronary vein)
- Cystic vein
- Paraumbilical vein
- Inferior mesenteric vein
- Right gastroepiploic vein
- Prepyloric vein of Mayo.

At porta hepatis
- From before backwards are
- Right and left hepatic duct
- Right and left branches of hepatic artey
- Right and left branches of portal vein

Portacaval anastomosis sites
- **Lower end of Esophagus**
  - Portal–esophageal tributaries from left gastric vein
  - Systemic–esophageal tributaries from hemiazygos vein
  - Clinical sign–esophageal varix
- **Lower end of rectum and Anal canal**
  - Portal–Superior rectal vein
  - Systemic–Middle and Inferior rectal vein.
  - Clinical sign–Internal rectal piles
- **At Umbilicus**
  - Portal–Para-umbilical vein
  - Systemic–above- Superior epigastric vein and lateral thoracic vein. Below superficial and in epigastric vein side–Lumbar and post intercostal vein
- **Retroperitonium**
  - Portal–Splenic and Colic vein
  - Systemic–Retroperitoneal veins, IVC through smaller veins called Veins of Retzius.
- **Bare area of liver**
  - Portal–Portal radicals
  - Systemic–Diaphragmatic veins
- **Falciform ligament** (Accessory portal system of Sappy)
  - Portal–Paraumbilical vein
  - Systemic–Diaphragmatic veins
- **Ligamentum venosus** Present in foetal life
  - Portal–Left branch of portal vein
  - Systemic–IVC
- **Posterior vaginal wall**
  - Portal–Superior rectal vein
  - Systemic–Vaginal vein
- **Beneath the rectouterine pouch**
  - Portal–Superior rectal vein
  - Systemic–Uterine vein

82. Ans. a. Kidney *Ref: Grays Anatomy 40/e p1225*

Internal structure of Kidney

Outer renal substance and inner renal sinus.

Renal substance–outer cortex and inner medulla

Cortex—contains renal column and cortical arches. Renal column in between the adjacent pyramids–Traversed by interlobar vessels.

Cortical arches intervenes between the base of pyramid and the surface of the kidney. Each arch contains medullary rays and convoluted parts. Interlobular vessels pass on either side of arches.

Lobule of kidney

Area of cortical arches bounded on each side interlobular vessels with central axis of medullary ray known as lobule of the kidney.

Convoluted part (Cortical labyrinth)–In between medullary rays and contain renal corpuscles and convoluted portion of nephron.

Medulla contains 8–18 pyramids which contains loop of henle, collecting tubules and duct of Belini (papillary or collecting duct)

Lobe of kidney–One pyramid capped with a joining cortex known as Lobe of kidney.

Renal sinus

Cavity within the kidney and communicates outside through the hilum.

Contents of renal sinus

- Renal blood vessels,lymph vessels and nerves
- Perinephric fat
- Minor, Major calyces and Renal pelvis. Minor 7–13, Major 2–3

The apex of each pyramid ends as a papilla where collecting ducts open.

Calyces—the minor calyces receive one or more papillae and unite to form major calyces, of which there are two to three per kidney.

Renal pelvis—the dilated upper portion of the ureter that receives the major calyces.

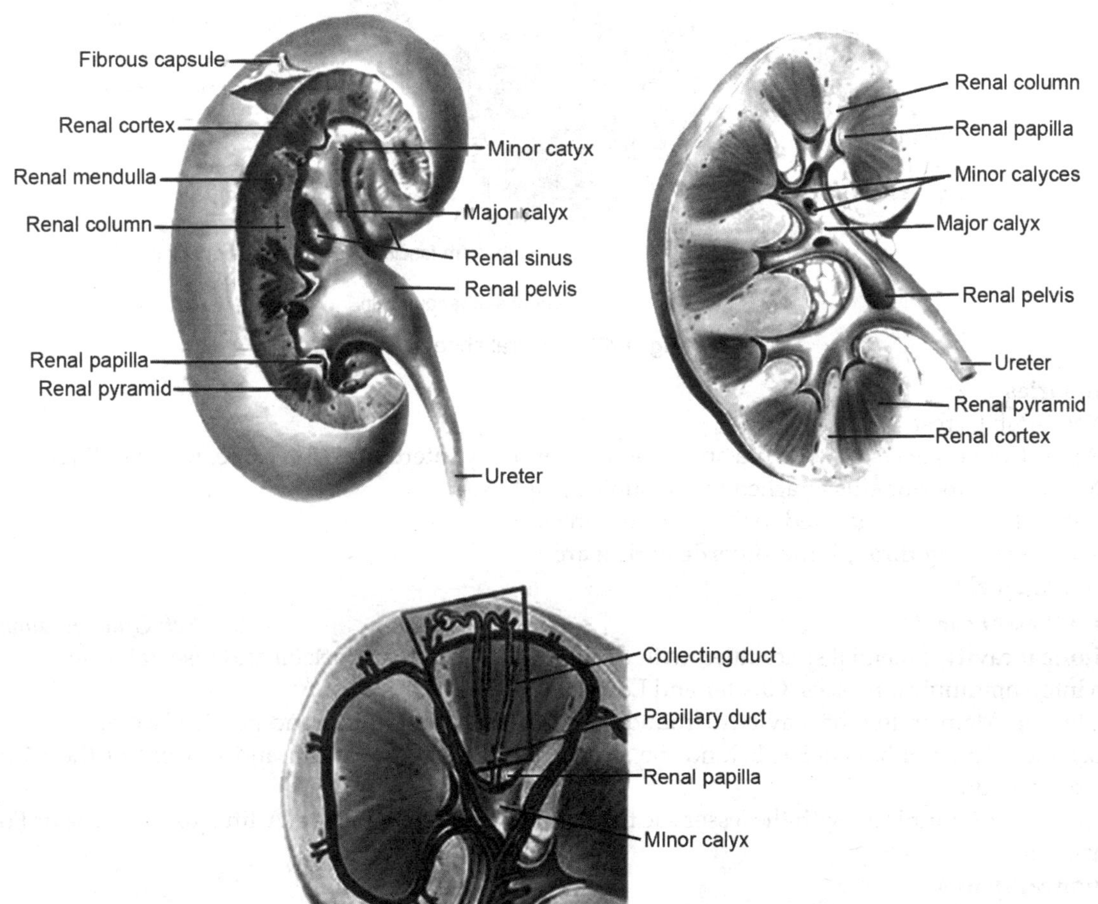

Fig. 1.47: Interior of kidney

83. Ans. a. **External oblique aponeurosis** *Ref: Grays Anatomy 40/e*

- Superficial inguinal ring–Triangular gap in the external aponeurosis above the pubic crest.

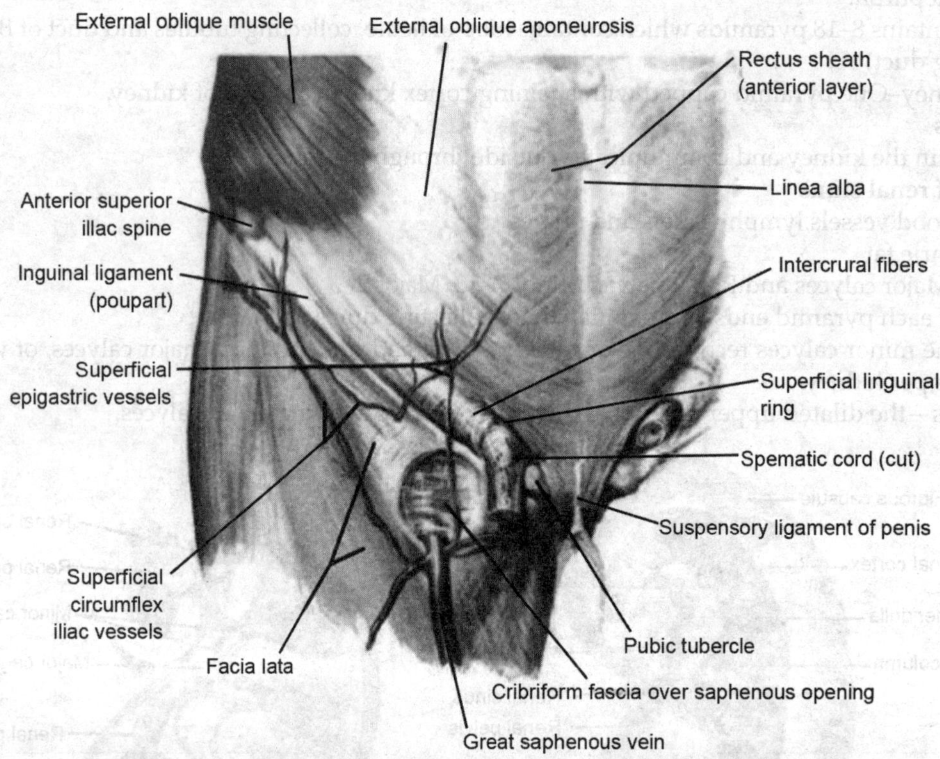

Fig. 1.48: Femoral sheath

Boundaries

- Base–Pubic crest.
- Apex–Convergence of two crura and kept in position by intercrural fibres of external oblique.
- Medially–Superior crus attached to the pubic symphysis.
- Laterally–Inferior crus fixed to the pubic tubercle.

Structures passing through the superficial ring are

- Ilioinguinal nerve

84. Ans. a. Lesser sac *Ref: Grays Anatomy 40th ed*

Peritoneal cavity: Potential space filled with capillary fluid between parietal and visceral layer

Two intercommunicating sacs, Greater and Lesser sac.

Greater sac–Main abdominal cavity surround the majority of abdominal and pelvic viscera.

Lesser sac–(Omental bursa)–Sac behind the stomach and lesser omentum and in front of the pancreas and retroperitoneum..

Greater sac communicate with the lesser sac through the epiploic foramen (Aditus to lesser sac or Foramen of Winslow)

Peritoneal spaces

Two main compartments–Supramesocolic and Infracolic compartment by transverse colon and mesocolon

Supramesocolic compartment

- **Right**
  - Right subphrenic space (Suprahepatic)
  - Right subhepatic space (Heapatorenal recess)

- **Left**
  - Left subphrenic space (Suprahepatic) (Left anterior intraperitoneal)
  - Left subhepatic space (Left posterior intraperitoneal or Lesser sac)

Inframesocolic compartment
- Right infracolic
- Left infracolic

Lesser sac–Anterior wall–peritoneum covering caudate lobe, posterior layer of lesser omentum, peritoneum coverings of posteroinferior surface of stomach and the second layer of greater omentum

Posterior wall–3rd layer of greater omentum, peritoneum covering the antero superior surface of transverse colon, upper layer of tranverse mesocolon and peritoneum covering anterior surface of body of pancreas, part of left suprarenal and left kidney and undersurface of the diaphragm

Upper margin–Reflexion of peritoneum from the diaphragm to the upper end of caudate lobe of liver.

Lower margins–Fused 2nd and 3rd layer of greater omentum.

Right margin –right free margin of greater omentum, peritoneal reflexion from neck of pancreas to posterior surface of 1st part of duodenum

Left margin–left free margin of greater omentum, inner layer of gastrosplenic and lienorenal ligament and gastrophrenic ligament.

Epiploic foramen (Foramen Winslow)
- Communication between lesser sac and hepatorenal pouch of grater sac.
- 3 cm slit at the level of T12
- Bounded–In- front–Right free margin of lesser omentum containing bile duct, hepatic vein, and portal vein
  - Behind–IVC
  - Above–Caudate process of liver
  - Below–1st part of duodenum.

85. Ans. a. Genitofemoral nerve *Ref: Grays Anatomy 40th ed*

Cremastric muscle
- Well developed in male
- Derived from internal oblique or both internal oblique and transverses abdominis.
- Anterolateral superficial part and Posteromedial deep part
- Superficial part arises from middle one third of inguinal ligament and deep part attached to pubic tubercle, pubic crest and conjoint tendon.
- Supplied by genital branch of genitofemoral nerve L2
- Actions–Cremastric plug ball valve action and cremastric reflex and Thermoregulation.
- Cremasteric reflex–Elicited by lightly stroking the superior and medial aspect of the thigh in a downward direction.
- Normal response is the contraction of cremater and pulls the testis on the side stroked.
- Afferent–femoral branch of genitorfemoral nerve
- Efferent–Genital branch of genitorfemoral nerve.

86. Ans. a. Macrophages *Ref: Grays Anatomy 40/e p1132, 2008*

Milky spots
- Dense, oval or round visible spots in the greater omentum (Policeman of abdomen)
- Milky spots contains numerous fixed macrophages
- Other areas where milky spots present–Plura.

87. Ans. b. Right subhepatic space *Ref: Grays Anatomy 40/e p1135, 2008*
Ref questions 2010

Hepatorenal space of Morison (right subhepatic space or right posterior intraperitoneal space)

Boundaries

In front–Inferior surface of the right lobe of the liver

Behind–Anterior surface of the right kidney

Above–Inferior layer of coronary ligament

Below–Communicates with the infra-colic compartment

Left side–Communicates with the lesser sac through the epiploic foramen
Right side–Diaphragm communicates with the right anterior intra-peritoneal recess around the free margin of right triangular ligament
This is themost dependent part of the peritoneal cavity.

88. Ans. d. Attached to the diaphragm *Ref: Grays Anatomy 40/e p1222, 2008*

Bare area of the liver

- Present in the posterior surface of the right lobe of the liver.
- Not covered by the peritoneum.
- Boundaries–Above–Superior layer of coronary ligament, Below–Inferior layer of coronary ligament, Apex–Right triangular ligament and Base–Groove for IVC.
- This area related to upper part of right kidney and right suprarenal gland.
- This is attached to the diaphragm by aerolar tissue.

89. Ans. c. Splenic artery. Ref 15th question *Ref: Grays Anatomy 40/e p1147, 2008*

90. Ans. b. T 12 *Ref: Grays Anatomy 40/e p1007*
Langman's Medical Embryology 9/e p384–385; IBS Human Embryology 7/e p119–120

91. Ans. d. Nerve to obturator internus *Ref: Grays Anatomy 40/e p1140*

Alcock's canal or Pudendal canal

- Fascial canal situated in the lateral wall of the ischiorectal fossa 2.5 cm above ischial tuberosity.
- Formed by the splitting of the obturator fascia or separation between lunate and obturator fascia or splitting of the perianal fascia.
- **Contents**
  - Internal pudendal vessels, pudendal nerve which divides within the canal in to dorsal nerve of penis and perineal nerve.

92. Ans. c. Longitudinal muscle fibers *Ref: Grays Anatomy 40/e, Langman's Embryology 11/e*

Deep perineal pouch

Boundaries

Above–Superior fascia of urogenital diaphragm.
Below–Perineal membrane.
In front–Transverse perineal ligament.
Behind–Fusion of Superior fascia of urogenital diaphragm and Perineal membrane.
Each sides–Inner surface of ischiopubic ramus.

Contents

- Muscles–Sphincter urethrae and Tranverse perinea profundus.
- Veesels–Internal pudendal artery-divides to 3 terminal branches namely dorsal artery of penis, deep artery of penis and Artery to bulb
- Dorsal nerve of penis
- Membranous urethra.
- Male bulbourethral glands
  - Female–vagina, behind urethra
- Longitudinal muscles of rectum continues above as taeniae and below at anorectal junction lends with puborectalis and levator ani to forms conjoind fibroelastic sheath.

93. Ans. a. Narrow subpubic angle *Ref: Grays Anatomy 40/e p1329*

GynecIod	Android	Anthropoid	Platypaloid
• Rounded • Transverse diameter being widest • Anterior and posterior segments ard wide • More than 50% belongs to this type	• Heart shaped • Posterior segment is more than the anterior segment since sacral promontory projects forwards • There is the difficulty in parturition	• Oval • Anteroposterior diameter is more than the transverse diameter. • Neonates of both sexes have this type • This is retained in Negro people	• Flat Transversely oval • Transverse diameter is disproportionally wider than the anterioposterior diameter • Associated with the rickets and vitamin D deficiency

94. Ans. b. Rectum and sacrum *Ref: Grays Anatomy 40/ e p1139*

Fascia of Waldyer

Extends from theanorectal junction to the coccyx.

Formed by the thickening of the pelvic fascia.

95. Ans. a. Sympathetic + Parasympathetic *Ref: Grays Anatomy 40/e p1245*

Sympathetic—superior hypogastric plexus—derived from L1 and L2

Para-sympathetics—pelvic splanchnic nerves—S2, S3, S4

96. Ans. c. Transverse ligament *Ref: AK Datta part 25/e p204*

- Transverse ligament extends between the tubercles on the medial side of the lateral mass of the atlas. This ligament keep the dens in the position.
- Alar ligament extends from the tip of the dens to the tubercles on the medial surface of occipital condyles This ligaments are stretched during flexion and relaxed on extension and also check the excessive rotation at the atlantoaxial joint.
- Apical ligament connect the tip of the dens to the dorsal surface of the basilar part of the occipital bone close to the foramen magnum.
- Membrana tectoria is the extension of the upward continuation of the posterior longitudinal ligament. It extends from the posterior surface of the body of axis to the upper surface of the basilar part of the occipital bone.

97. Ans. c. Anterior *Ref: Gray's Anatomy for Students, 2007, page 859*

Eustachian tube (Pharyngotympanic tube)

- Osseocartilaginous tube connecting the anterior wall of the tympanic cavity to the lateral wall of the nasopharynx.
- 36 mm in length, lateral one third 12 mm bony and medial two third 24 mm is cartilage which is elastic in type.
- Its apex is attached by fibrous tissue to the bony part of the tube between the petrous part of the temporal bone and the greater wing of the sphenoid, and its base is under the mucosa of the lateral nasopharyngeal wall, forming a tubal elevation (torus tubarius; eustachian cushion) behind the pharyngeal orifice of the tube.
- Junction of the two parts the isthmus.
- Bony part starts from the anterior tympanic wall and ends at the junction of the squamous and petrous parts of the temporal bone.
- The carotid canal lies medially.
- Near the pharyngeal orifice lymphoid mass called the tubal tonsil.
- At birth the pharyngotympanic tube is about half its adult length, it is more horizontal and its bony part is relatively shorter
- **Muscles attached to the Eustachian tube are**
  - Salpingoopharyngeus
  - Levator veli palatine medial lamina of the tube
  - Tensor veli palatine lateral lamina of the tube (the part of fibers attached to the lateral lamina of the cartilage and to the fibrous part are called dilator tube since by its contraction it opens the tube.
- Blood supply—ascending pharyngeal artery, middle meningeal artery and artey to pterygoid canal. Venous drainage to pterygoid venous plexus.
- Innervetion—typanic plexus and pheryngeal branch from pterygopalatine ganglion.

Features of the tympanic cavity

Medial wall (Labyrinthine wall)	Lateral wall (Membranous wall)	Posterior wall (Mastoid wall)	Anterior wall
• Promontory (Produced by basal turn of cochlea) • Fenestra vestibuli (Fenestra ovalis)–Closed	Tympanic membrane	• Opening the aditus to the mastoid antrum • Fossa incudis-short process of incus is	• Upper part- canal for tensor tympani muscle • Lower canal –for bony part of the auditory tube.

Contd...

Contd...

Medial wall (Labyrinthine wall)	Lateral wall (Membranous wall)	Posterior wall (Mastoid wall)	Anterior wall
by base of stapes and annular ligament. • Fenestra cochleae (Fenestra rotunda)-closed by tympanic membrane. • Sinus tympani–position of the ampulla of the posterior semicircular canal. • Oblique part of the facial nerve • Processus trochlearisformis-backward extension of the bony partition between canals for the tensor tympani and the auditory tube.		suspended from the fossa. • Vertical bony canal for facial nerve • Pyramidal eminence-contains Stapidius muscle and its nerve supply.	

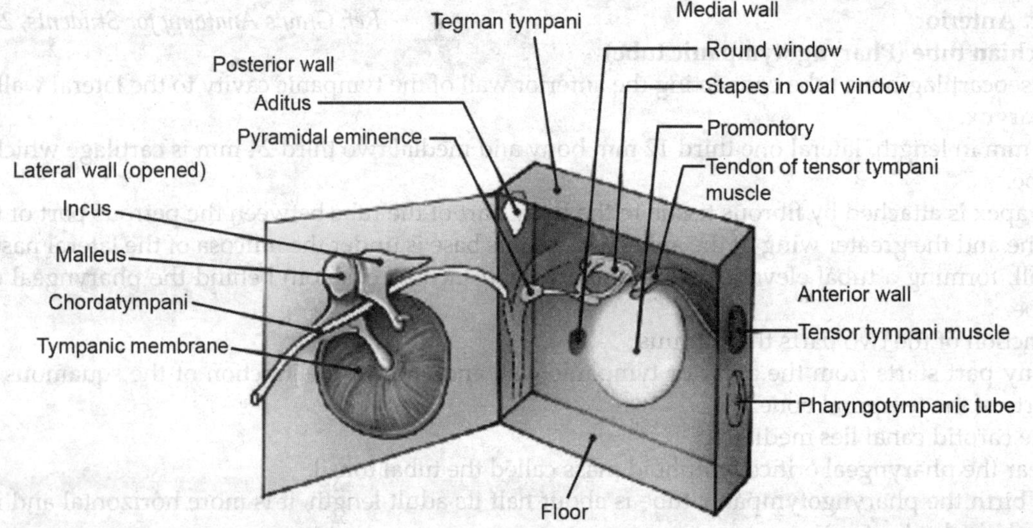

Fig. 1.49: Schematic drawing of the walls of the tympanic cavity. Right ear in lateral view with the lateral wall opened

98. Ans. c. Inferior turbinate *Ref: Gray's Anatomy, 39/e p 474–476, 2008*

Ethmoid bone contains

- Cribriform plate–**Upper surface**
  - Crista galli–Posterior border gives attachment of falx cerebri and anterior border–alae
  - Perforated plate on each side of crista galli–supports Gyrus rectus of frontal lobe and olfactory bulb
  - Laterally—foramen for anterior ethmoidal nerves and vessels

Lower surface—perpendicular plate–anterior border articulate with nasal spine of the frontal bone, posterior border articulate with sphenoidal crest in the upper part and vomer in the lower part and inferior border receives septal cartilage.

- Labyrinths–contains anterior, middle and posterior air cells.
  Orbital plate–forms medial wall of the orbit
  Nasal plate forms the lateral wall of the nasal cavity. It contains
  - Middle concha
  - Middle meatus having

- Uncinate process
- Bulla etmoidalis produced by middle ethmoidal air cells.
- Hiatus semilunaris–maxillary air cells open floor.
- Ethmoidal infundibulum–receives anterior ethmoidal air cells and Frontal air sinus opens in the tip
- Atrium–depression in the anterior part
- Aggar nasi–mucosal ridge limiting the atrium above

– Superior nasal concha
– Superior meatus–receives posterior ethmoidal air cells

Inferior nasal concha is the separate bone

99. Ans. c. Ascending pharyngeal artery

Tympanic branch	Branch of
Anterior tympanic artery	1st part of maxillary artery
Superior tympanic artery	Middle meningeal artery
Posterior tympanic artery	Stylomastoid branch of posterior auricular artery
Inferior tympanic artery	Ascending pharyngeal artery

100. Ans. a. Posterior cricoarytenoid *Ref: Gray's Anatomy, 39/e p642, 2008*

Action	Laryngeal muscles
Oblique Artytenoid,Transverse ary	Adduction of Aryepiglottic fold
PCA	Open glottis, abduction of the vocal cord
LCA	Rotates Arytenoid cartilage closes glottis Adduction of the vocal cord
Cricothyroid	Tensor of vocal cord lengthens vocal lig
Thyroarytenoid, vocalis	Relaxor
Thyroepiglotticus	Widens inlet of larynx

101. Ans. b. Base of skull to bifurcation of trachea *Ref: Gray's Anatomy, 39/e p626, 2008*

Retropharyngeal space

Potential space behind the pharynx and acts as bursa to allow expansion of pharynx during deglutition.

Boundaries

In front–Buccopharyngeal fascia covering the constrictors of the pharynx

Behind–Prevertebral fascia, Pre and Paravertebral muscles

On each side–Carotid sheath and its contents.

Above–Base of the skull

Below–Open and continuous with superior mediastinum.

Contents

- Retropharyngeal lymph nodes
- Loose areolar tissue
- Pharyngeal vessels and nerves.

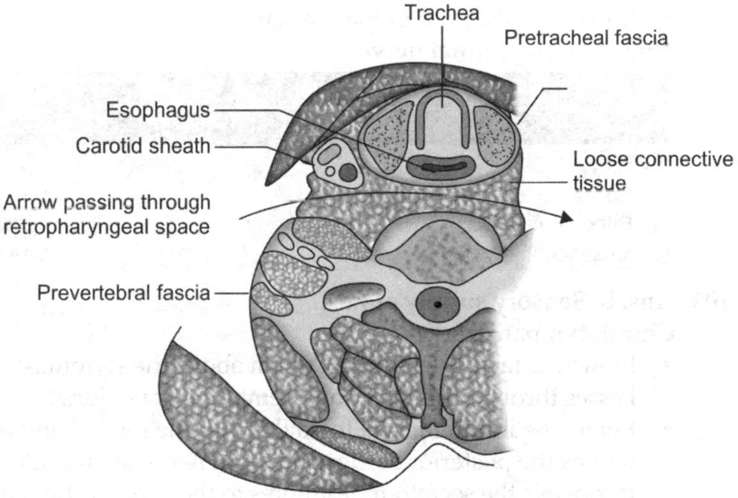

Fig. 1.50: Tracings of deep cervical fascia

102. Ans. a. Arises from midbrain *Ref: Clinical Neuroanatomy, Richard Snell, 7/e p341-344*

The trigeminal nerve emerges near the midpontine level. It has a small superomedial motor root and a large inferolateral sensory root.

The large sensory root expands to form the crescent-shaped trigeminal ganglion, which lies within a pouch of dura mater called the trigeminal or Meckel cave.
The **ophthalmic, maxillary, and mandibular** nerves arise from the anterior border of the ganglion.
The **ophthalmic nerve** (V1) contains **only sensory fibers** and leaves the skull through the **superior orbital fissure** to enter the orbital cavity.
The maxillary nerve (V2) also contains **only sensory fibers** and leaves the skull through the **foramen rotundum.**
The **mandibular nerve (V3)** contains **both sensory and motor fibers** and leaves the skull through the **foramen ovale. It supplies the muscles of the mastication.**
Trigeminal nerve carries the parasympathetic fibres to the salivary glands.
Parasympathetic ganglia are

Name of the ganglia	Topographically related	Functionally related	Supplies
Otic	Mandibular nerve	Glossopharygeal nerve	Parotid gland
Pterygopalatine ganglion	Maxillary nerve	Greater petrosal branch of facial nerve	Lacrimal gland, Nasal, Palatine and Pharyngeal glands.
Submandibular ganglion	Lingual nerve branch of mandibular nerve	Facial and its chordatympanic branch	Submandibular and sublingual gland
Ciliary ganglian	Nasociliary branch of Opthalmic branch	Oculomotor nerve	Ciliaris and Sphincter papillae through parasympathetic and dilator papillae through sympathetic.

Mandibular nerve sensory supply
- Teeth and Gums of the mandible
- Skin in the temporal region
- EAM and Tympanic membrane
- Lower lip
- Lower part of the face
- Mucosa over anterior 2/3 of the tongue
- Mucosa of the floor of the oral cavity.

Nuclei of Trigeminal nerve

Type of nuclei	Site
Motor	**Pons medial to principal sensory nuclus**
Sensory • Spinal nucleus of trigeminal nerve • Principal nucleus • Mesencephalic nucleus	 In the pons caudal to Principal nucleus to C2–C3 In the pons lateral to the motor nucleus Central grey matter of mid brain on each side of the aqueduct.

103. Ans. b. Sensory supply of face *Ref: Grays Anatomy 40/e p543*
Chordotympani nerve
- Branch of facial nerve about 6 mm above the stylomastoid foramen.
- Passes through the tympanic membrane at the junction of pars flaccid and Pars densa.
- Enters the infratemporal fossa through the medial end of the pterygotympanic fissure.
- It joins the posterior border of lingual nerve at an acute angle.
- It conveys the secreto-motor fibres to the submandibular and sublingual glands and taste fibres of anterior two thirds of the tongue.

104. Ans. d. Retromandibular vein *Ref: Grays Anatomy 40/e p400*
Internal jugular vein
- Begins the continiuation of the sigmoid sinus at the base of the skull.
- Superior bulb–dilatation at the commencement lodges in the jugular fossa of the temporal bone in the floor of the tympanic cavity.
- Termination–behind the medial end of the clavicle it unites with the subclavian vein to form the brachio-cephalic vein.

- Inferior bulb–Dilatation at the termination–present in lesser supraclavicular space which is the a triangular interval between the sternal and clavicular heads of the sternomastoid muscle.
- **Tributaries**–Inferior petrosal sinus (1st tributaries)
  - Pharyngeal veins
  - Common facial vein
  - Lingual vein
  - Superior thyroid vein
  - Middle thyroid vein
  - Occipital vein
  - Thoracic duct on left side or right lymphatic duct.

Retromandibular vein

- Formed the union of superficial temporal vein and the maxillary vein.
- Retromandibular vein divides into anterio and posterior division.
- Anterior division joins with the facial vein and form common facial vein which finally drain into internal jugular vein.
- Posterior division joins with the posterior auricular vein to form external jugular vein which in turn drain into subclavian vein.

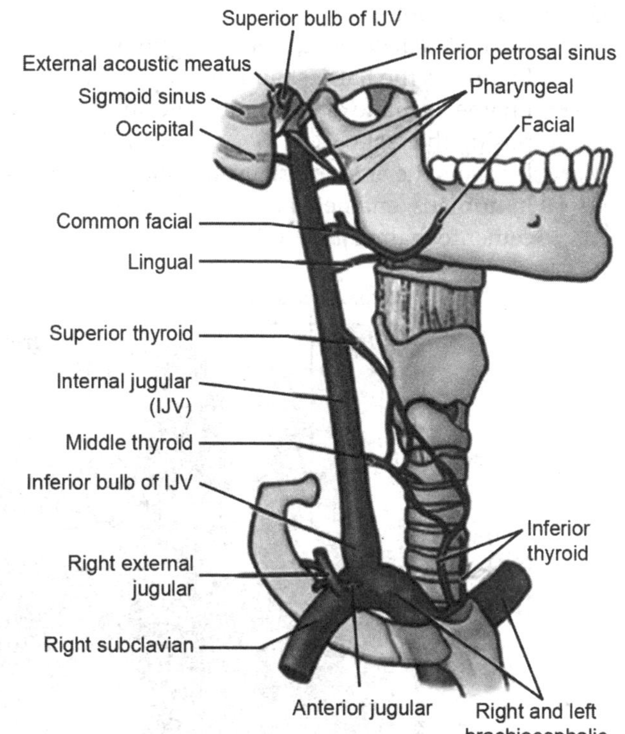

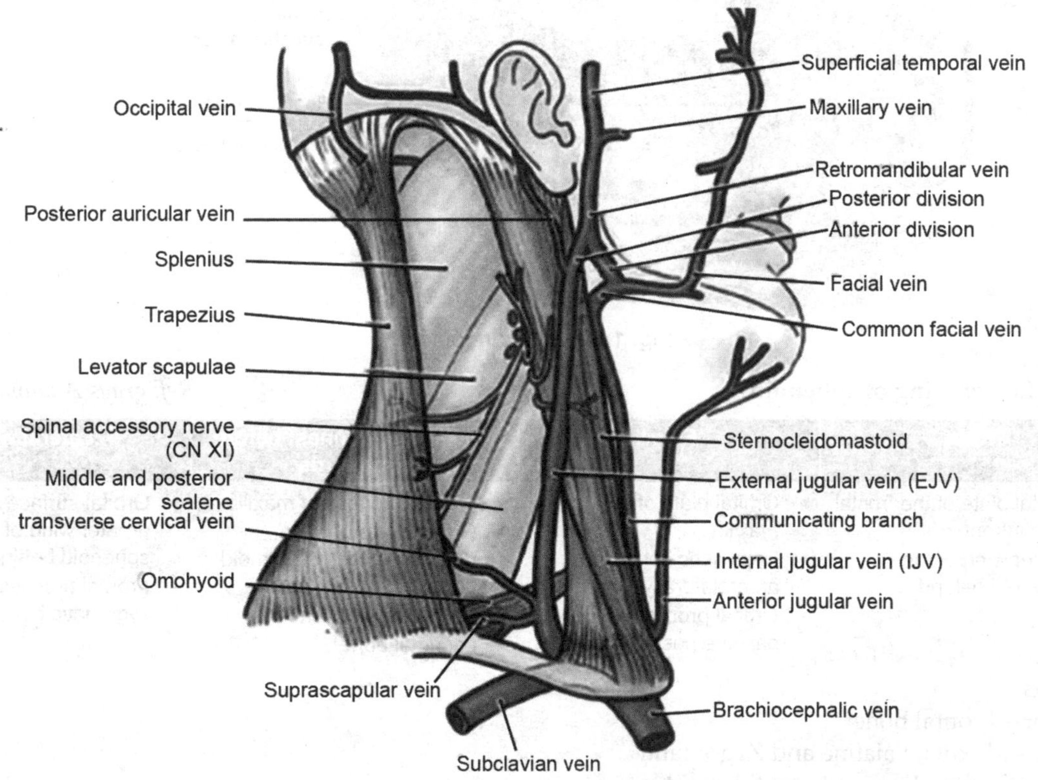

Fig. 1.51: Posterior triangle of neck

105. Ans. b. Enamel *Ref: grays Anatomy 40/e p509, histology ross pawlina 6/e p536*

- Enamel is developed from the ameloblast and the dentine is developed from the odendoblast.
- Enamel is the hardest and the most highly mineralized substance in the human body.
- Enamel is made of 96% inorganic mineral (Calcium hydroxyapatite) with water and organic material composing the rest.
- It covers the anatomical crown and must be supported by the underlying dentine.
- In humans, enamel varies in thickness over the surface of the teeth, thickest at the cusp and thinnest at the cementoenamel junction.

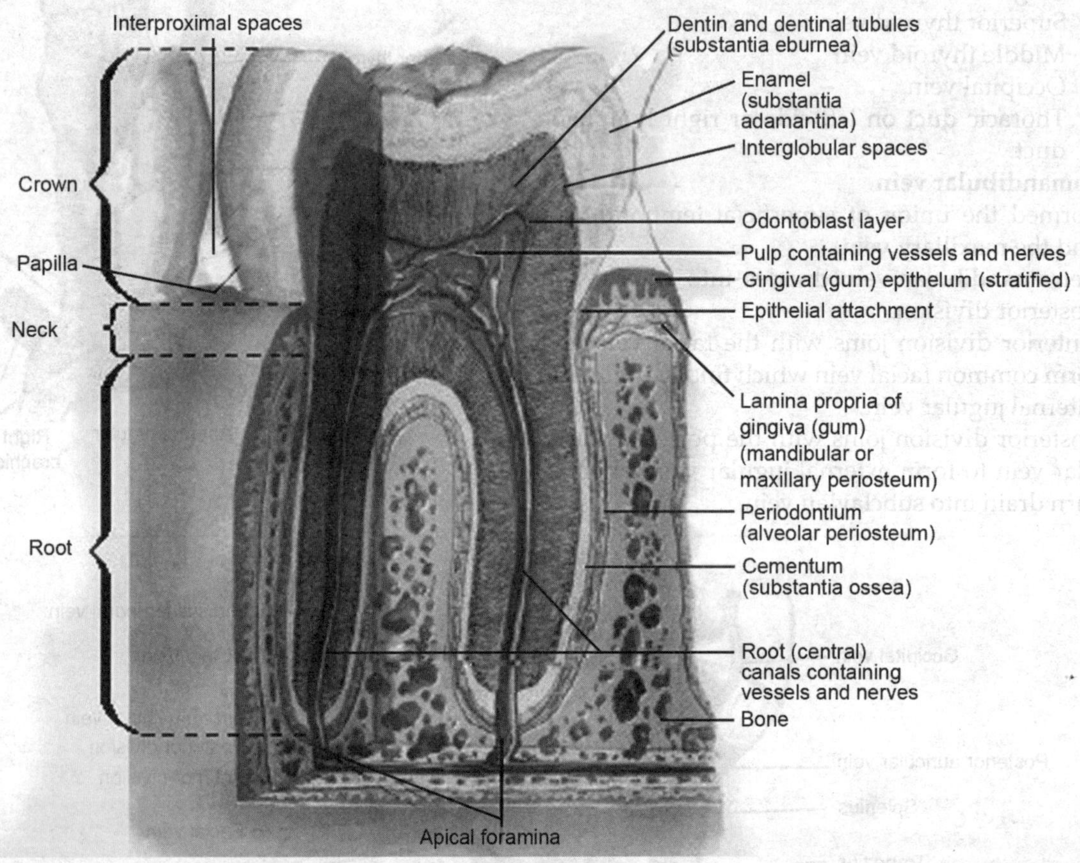

Fig. 1.52: Structure of tooth

106. Ans. a. Lesser wing of sphenoid *Ref: grays Anatomy 40/e p243*

Roof	Floor	Medial wall thinnest before backwards	Lateral wall
• Orbital plate of the frontal bone infront • Lesser wing of the sphenoid behind	• Orbital plate of the maxilla • Zygomatic bone anterolaterally • Orbital process of the palatine posteromedially	• Frontal process of maxilla • Orbital plate (lamina papyracea) of the ethmoid bone • Body of the sphenoid • Lacrimal bone	• Orbital surface of the greater wing of the sphenoid behind • Frontal process of the zygomatic bone infront

Margins

Superior—Frontal bone
Inferior—Maxilla, Palatine and Zygomatic
Medial—Frontal, Lacrimal and Ethmoid
Lateral—Sphenoid and Zygomatic

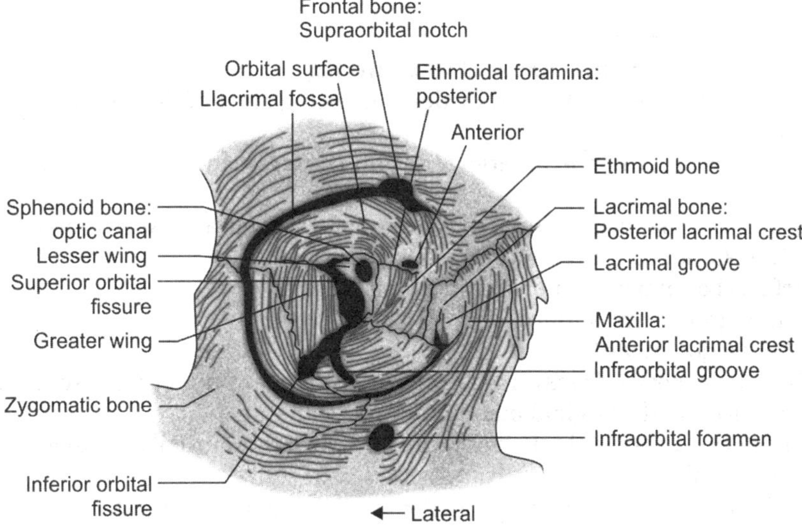

Fig. 1.53: Orbital cavity

107. Ans. b. Medial pterygoid *Ref: Grays Anatomy 40/e p534*

Temporomandibular joint

Movements	Muscles responsible
Protrusion	Medial and lateral pterygoid
Retraction	Temporalis assisted by deep fobres of masseter, digastric and geniohyoid.
Depression (Opening the mouth)	Lateral pterygoid and assisted by geniohyoid, mylohyoid and digastric
Elevation (closing the mouth)	Masseter, temporalis and Medial pterygoid
Side to side	Lateral and medial pterygoid of one side alternately with the other side.

108. Ans. a. Skull base to tracheal bifurcation *Ref: Grays Anatomy 40/e p568*

- **Retropharyngeal space**
  - Extends from the base of the skull to the tracheal bifurcation
  - The space is divided in to two lateral compartments (space of gillette) by a fibrous raphe. Each lateral space contains retropharyngeal nodes which usually disappear at 3–4 years.
  - Infection of this space can pass down behind the esophagus in to posterior mediastinum.

Boundaries

In front—buccopharyngeal fascia covers the constrictors of pharynx.

Behind—prevertebral fascia covers the cervical vertebrae, prevertebral and paravertebral muscles.

On each side—carotid sheath and its contents.

Above—base of the skull

Below—continuous with the superior mediastinum.

Contents—loose areolar tissue and pharyngeal plexus of vessels and nerves.

109. Ans. b. Mucinous gland *Ref: grays Anatomy 40/e p495*

Salivary glands

Gland	Type	Duct	Opening
Parotid (Largest)	Serous	Stensons	Upper 2nd molar
Submandibular	Mixed	Whartons 5cm	Sublingual papillae
Sublingual (smallest)	Mucous	Rivinus 8–20 ducfs	Floor of buccal cavity (sublingual fold)

Parotid gland

- Largest of the three salivary glands.
- Coverings–true capsule–Condensation of fibrous stroma.
  - False capsule (Parotid sheath)–formed by deep investing layer of deep cervical fascia.
- **Presenting parts**

Apex–Cervical branch of facial nerve, anterior division of retromandibular vein and formation of external jugular vein.

Base–Temporal branch of facial nerve, Supaerficial temporal vessels and Auriculotemporal nerve.

Anteromedial surface–Grooved for ramus of the mandible.

Posteromedial surface–Facial nerve enters through this surface

External carotid artery groove this surface.

Anterior border–Above downwards

Zygomatic branch of facial nerve, Transverse facial vessels, Upper buccal, Accessory parotid gland and duct, Parotid duct, Lower buccal and Marginal mandibular nerve.

Posterior border–Posterior auricular branch of facial and posterior auricular vessels.

Medial border–Pharyngeal border

Accessory parotid gland present between zygomatic arch and main parotid duct.

Process of the parotid gland

Facial process–Triangular projection superficial to the masseeter along the parotid duct.

Pteygoid process–Between ramus of the mandible and medial pterygoid muscle.

Glenoid process–Between external meatus and capsule of TM joint.

Pre and Post styloid process.

Structures passing through the gland

- Facial nerve and its branches.
- Retromandibular vein.
- External carotid artery.

The parotid gland is divided in to superficial and deep by the facial nerve and its branches. Pateys plane–plane between superficial lobe and deep lobe.

Secretomotor of parotid gland

Inferior salivatory nucleus → Tympanic branch of glossopharyngeal nerve → Tympanic plexus → Lesser petrosal nerve → Otic ganglion → Auriculotemporal nerve → Parotid gland.

Hilton's method–Parotid abscess drained by the horizontal incision to avoid injury to branches of facial nerve.

Frey's syndrome–Complication during the recovery of the penetrating wound of the parotid gland.

110. Ans. a. Posterior cricoarytenoid *Ref: grays Anatomy 40/e p580*

Action	Laryngeal muscles
Oblique Artytenoid Transverse ary	Adduction of Aryepiglottic fold
PCA	Open glottis, abduction
LCA	Rotates Arytenoid cartilage closes glottis
Cricothyroid	Tensor of vocal cord lengthens vocal lig
ThyroArytenoid vocalis	Relaxor
Thyroepiglotticus	Widens inlet of larynx

Semon's Law → Abductors are paralysed first followed by other muscles due to the abductors are supplied by thickly myelinated nerve fibres which are more vulnerable to oxygen lack.

Nerve supply of larynx

Sensory	Motor	Secreto-motor
Above the vocal folds Internal laryngeal nerve **Below the vocal folds** Recurrent laryngeal neve	All the muscles supplied by the recurrent laryngeal nerve except the circothyroid which is supplied by the external laryngeal nerve	Recurrent laryngeal nerve.

111. Ans. a. Epiglottis *Ref: Grays Anatomy 40/e Dhingra PL's ENT*

Pharynx

Interior divided in to 3 parts they are 1. Nasopharynx (Epi-pharynx) 2. Oropharynx (Mesopharynx) 3. Laryngopharynx (Hypopharynx)

Hypopharynx

- Extends from the upper border of epiglottis to the lower border of the circoid cartilage. Behind C4–C6
- Anterior wall presents laryngeal inlet. Bounded above and in front—upper margin of the epiglottis, below and behind—inter-arytenoid fold and on each side—aryepiglottic fold.
- On each side—piriform fossa bounded medially aryepiglottic fold, laterally—mucosa covering the medial surface of the lamina of the thyroid cartilage.

Nasopharynx

- Situated behind the nasal cavity and above the soft palate.
- **Features**
  - Roof and posterior wall has 1. Nasopharyngeal tonsil 2. Pharyngeal bursa (Pouch of Luschka) 3. Paryngeal hypophysis
  - Floor pharyngeal isthmus–bounded in front by the posterior surface and free margin of the soft palate, behind–Passavant's ridge formed by palate-pharyngeal sphincter and on each side by the palate-pharyngeal fold
  - Laterally–Pharyngeal opening, Tubal elevation, Pharngal recess (Fossa rosenmuller)

Oropharynx

- Behind the oral cavity
- Lateral wall presents palatine tonsils and Tonsilar fossa which is bounded in front by palate-glossal arch, behind by palate-pharyngeal fold, apex soft palale where both arches meet, base by dorsal surface of the posterior 1/3 of the tongue and lateral wall superior constrictor and styloglossus muscles covered by pharygo-basilar fascia.

112. Ans. a. Otic ganglion *Ref: Grays Anatomy 40/e*

Secretomotor of parotid gland

Inferior salivatory nucleus → Tympanic branch of glossopharyngeal nerve → Tympanic plexus → Lesser petrosal nerve → Otic ganglion → Auriculotemporal nerve → Parotid gland.

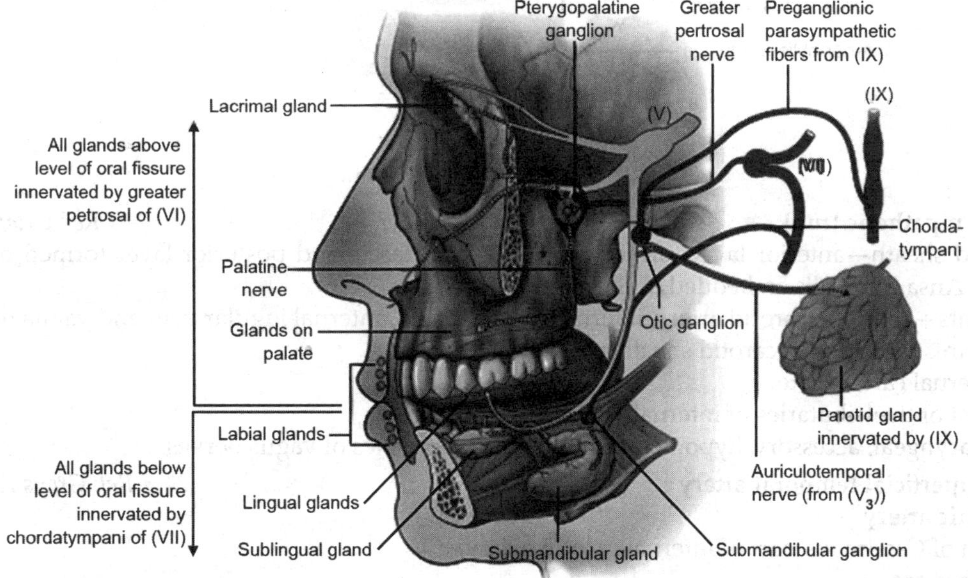

Fig. 1.54: Secretomotor pathway of lacrimal, parotid and salivary glands.

113. Ans. c. Lateral rectus *Ref: Grays Anatomy 40/e p655*

Muscles of orbit

Muscles	Nerve supply
Voluntary muscle	
• Superior rectus	Oculomotor nerve
• Medial rectus	Oculomotor nerve
• Inferior rectus	Oculomotor nerve
• Inferior oblique	Oculomotor nerve
• Lateral rectus	Abducent nerve
• Superior oblique	Trochlear nerve
• Levator palpebrae superioris	Oculomotor nerve
Involuntary muscle	
• Superior tarsal	Sympathetic fibers from superior cervical ganglion
• Inferior tarsal	
• Orbitalis	

LR66 and SO_4–Lat rectus supplied by 6th cranial nerve abducent nerve and superior oblique is supplied by 4th cranial nerve Trochlear nerve and all other muscles are supplied by 6th nerve.

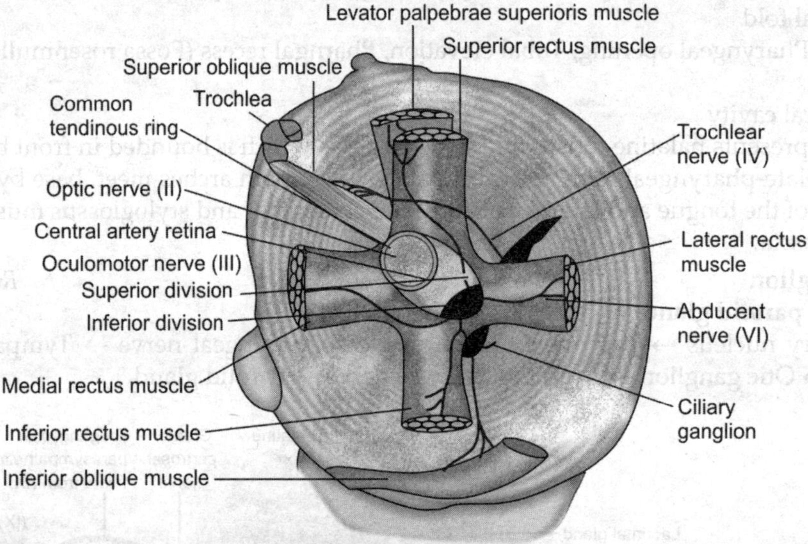

Fig. 1.55: Rectal muscles

114. Ans. a. Sympathetic trunk *Ref: Grays Anatomy 40/e*

- Carotid sheath—anterior layer formed by pretracheal fascia and posterior layer formed by prevertebral fascia. Ansa cervicalis embedded in the anterior wall.
- Contents—common carotid artery, internal carotid artery, internal jugular vein and vagus nerve.
- Structures piercing the carotid sheath are
  - External carotid artery
  - Most of the tributaries of internal jugular vein

Glossopharyngeal, accessory, hypoglossal and cervical branches of vagus nerves

115. Ans. b. Superficial temporal artery *Ref: Grays Anatomy 40th ed*

Ophthalmic artery

- Branch of Cavernous part of Internal carotid artery.
- **Branches are**
  - Central artery of retina
  - Posterior ciliary arteries–2 pairs of long ciliary and 2 pairs of short ciliary arteries

- Anterior ciliary arteries
- Lacrimal artery
- Posterior ethmoidal artery
- Anterior ethmoidal artery
- Medial palpebral arteries
- Supraorbital and Supratrochlear arteries
- Dorsal nasal artery

• Superficial temporal artery is the branch of Smaller terminal branch of the External carotid artery.

ECA–Origin–Upper border of Thyroid cartilage, C3–C4 vertebra

Branches Sister Lucy Powdered Face Often Attract Medical Student

Lingual artery

- Opposite–Tip of greater Cornu
- Hyoglossus divides into 3 parts.
- Rests on the middle constrictor
- Branches–1st part–Crossed by the hypoglossal nerve-suprahyoid artery.
  - 2nd part–Between Hyoglossus laterally and middle constrictor and Stylohyoid lig medaially. Dorsal lingual artery.
  - 3rd part–(Arteria profunda linguae)–Sublingual artery

Superior thyroid

- Below greater cornu
- Superior laryngeal artery accompanies internal laryngeal nerve and pierces thyrohyoid membrane
- Accompany with the external laryngeal nerve which is posteromedial to it and close to the thyroid gland separated from the nerve and superficial to the gland.
- Branches—infrahyoid, superior laryngeal, circothyroid, sternomastoid and glandular.

Facial Artery

- Above greater cornu
- Branches in neck ascending palatine, tonsillar, submental, glandular (TAGS)
- Branches in the face—superior labial, inferior labial and lateral nasal artery.

Occipital artery

- Arises from—opposite to the facial artery
- Branches—Sternomastoid, mastoid, menigeal, muscular, descending, occipital and auricular branches.
- Sternomastoid—upper branch—accompanies the spinal part of accessory nerve
  - Lower branch—hypoglossal nerve loop around this.

Posterior auricular artery

- Arises from the posterior aspect above the origin of occipital artery.
- Branches—stylomastoid, auricular and occipital.
- Posterior tympanic artery arises from the stylomastoid branch.

Ascending pharyngeal artery

- First smallest artery arises from the medial side
- Branches—pharyngeal, Inferior tympanic and meningeal

Artery	Branch
Superior tympanic	Middle meningeal artery
Inferior tympanic	Ascending palatine artery
Anterior tympanic	1st part of Maxillary artery
Posterior tympanic	Stylomastoid branch of posterior auricular artery

Superficial temporal artery

- Smaller terminalbranch of External carotid artery in the parotid gland.
- Branches—Transverse facial artery (arises within the parotid), anterior auricular, zygomatico-orbital, middle temporal, anterior or frontal and posterior or parietal.

Maxillary artery

- Larger terminal branch of external carotid artery in the parotid gland.
- Divided in to three parts by the lower head of lateral pterygoid muscle.

ICA parts	Branches
• Cervical	No Branch
• Petrous	Caroticotympanic artery
• Cavernous	• Cavernous branches • Meningeal • Hypophyseal arterie
• Cerebral	• Opthalmic • Posterior Comm. Artery • Anterior choroidal → choroid plexus of Lat Ventricle Basal ganglia, postr. Limb of Int. Capsule • Anterior cerebral • Middle Cerebral artery

116. Ans. b. Perilymphatic duct *Ref: Grays Anatomy 40/e*

Perilymph

- Fills the bony labyrinth (Scala tympani and scala vestibule)
- Resembles the extra-cellular fluid and CSF
- Na^{++} being higher than K^{+} ion
- It communicates with CSF through the cochlear canaliculus.
- It is drained via perilymphatic duct.
- Perlymph derived from
  - A transudate from the surrounding blood vessels
  - The tissue fluids from the sheaths of the vestibule-cochlear nerve
  - Flow of the CSF through the cochlear nerve

Endolymph

- Fills the membranous labyrinth
- Has high K^{+} and low Na^{++} similar to intracellular fluid
- It is drained via endolymphatic duct.

117. Ans. a. Stylohyoid *Ref: Grays Anatomy 40/e*

Superior root (descendens hypoglossi)—A branch from the loop between C1 and C2 carrying fibers of C1 joins with hypoglossal. From this superior root arises and supplies Superior belly of Omohyoid.

Inferior root (descendens cervicalis)—carries fibers of C2 and C3–spiral around the internal jugular vein and forms loop, ansa cervicalis in front of carotid sheath supplies sternohyoid, sternothyroid and inferior belly of omohyoid.

Ansa cervicalis in front of the carotid sheath.

Stylohyoid supplied by facial nerve.

Fig. 1.56: Ansa cervicalis

118. Ans. d. Petrous part of temporal bone *Ref: Grays Anatomy 40th ed*

Ear ossicles completely developed before birth.

In neonate, petrous and squamous parts of temporal bone are usually partially separated by the petro-squamous fissure.

This opens directly in to the mastoid antrum of the middle ear.

The fissure remains open till 20 years in 20–40% individuals.

119. Ans. b. Nasopharynx *Ref: Grays Anatomy 40/e, question 2014*

Middle ear cavity

Medial wall separates it from the internal ear

Lateral wall separetes from the external ear

Anterior wall—upper canal for tensor tympani and lower canal for auditory tube which communicates with the nasopharynx.

Posterior wall communicates with the mastoid antrum through additus.

120. Ans. b. Lingual nerve *Ref: Grays Anatomy 40th ed*

Branches of facial nerve

Communicating branches

- In the internal acoustic meatus–with the vestibulocochlear nerve
- **At the geniculate ganglion**
  - Branch from the geniculate ganglion greater petrosal nerve carries the preganglionic secretomotor fibers of lacrimal, glands of nasl mucosa and the soft palate-joins the pterygopalatine ganglion.
  - Lesser petrosal nerve branch joins with otic ganglion.
  - Branch from the geniculate ganglion coonect with the branch from the sympathetic plexus around the middle meningeal artery known as external petrosal nerve
- **Facial canal:** communicate with the auricular branch of vagus nerve which conveys the cutaneous sensation from the concha
- Below the stylomastoid foramen communicate with the glossopharyngeal, vagus, auriculotemporal and greater auricular nerve.
- Behind the ear communicate with the lesser occipital nerve
- In the face communicate with the trigeminal nerve
- In the neck communicate with the transverse cervical cutaneous nerve

Branches

Facial canal

- Nerve to stapedius
- Chordatympani nerve

Below the stylomastoid foramen

- Posterior auricular nerve
- Nerve to posterior belly of digastrics
- Nerve to stylohyoid muscle

In the face

- Temporal
- Zygomatic
- Buccal
- Marginal mandibular
- Cervical

121. Ans. b. End artery *Ref: Grays Anatomy 40/e*

Central artery of the retina

- Branch of Opthalmic artery below the optic nerve
- Piersces the optic nerve infero-medially about 1.25 cm behind the eye ball
- Reaches the optic disc through the central part of the nerve
- Supplies the optic nerve and the inner six or seven layers of the retina
- Typical end artery
- Obstruction lead to total blindness.

122. Ans. c. Great auricular nerve *Ref: Grays Anatomy 40/e p515*

Greater auricular nerve

- Branch of cervical plexus
- Ventral rami of C2 and C3
- Winds around the posterior border of the sternomastoid and ascends obliquely across the muscle on to the parotid where divides in to anterior and posterior branches. Anterior supplies the skin the faces over the angle of mandible and the posterior branch supplies over the mastoidprocess and the cranial and lateral surface of the auricle including the concha and the lobule.
- Accompany the upper half of the external jugular vein.

Auriculotemporal nerve
- Branch of the posterior division of the mandibular nerve
- Arises by two roots which encircle the middle meningeal artery.
- Passes under the lateral pterygoid muscle between the neck of the mandible and the spheo-mandibular ligament.
- Lies the first part of the maxillary artery.
- Provides auricular branches, supperficial temporal branches and articular branches.
- Recieves the communicating branch from the otic ganglion convey the postganglionic seretomotor fibers of the parotid gland.

Posterior auricular nerve
- Branch of facial nerve below the stylomastoid foramen
- Supplies auricularis posterior and occipital belly of occipitofrontalis

123. Ans. a. Posterior cricoarytenoid *Ref: Grays Anatomy 40/e p508*
Ref: Langman's Medical Embryology 9/e p384–385; IBS Human Embryology 7/e p119–120

124. Ans. b. Only nerve emerging from ventral aspect of brain stem
Ref: Gray's Anatomy: Anatomical basis of Clinical Practice by Susan Standring, Churchill Livingstone: 40/e p666

Trochlear nerve
- 4th cranial nerve
- Supplies the superior oblique muscle.
- Most of the fibres are somatomotar.
- Nucleus situated at the periaqueductal grey matter of the midbrain along the floor of the aqueduct at the level of the inferior colliculus.
- The nerve arising from the nucleus at first pass dorsolaterally around the central grey matter medial to the mesencephalic nucleus of the trigeminal nerve and exten caudally to decussate in the superior medullary velum with similar fibres of the opposite nerve and finally emerges caudal to the inferior colliculus by the side of the frenulum veli.
- Peculiarites
  - Only cranial nerve emerges through the dorsal aspect of the brainstem.
  - Only cranial nerve undergoes complete decussation with the opposite side.

*It is related to thelateral wall of the cavernous sinus with oculomotor nerve above and ophthalmic and maxillary nerve below.
*It passes through the lateral compartment of the supraorbital fissure and passes forward and medially above the levator palpebrae superioris.

125. Ans. c. Palatoglossus *Ref: Grays Anatomy 40/e p628*

Innerevation of the tongue

Motor			Sensory			
Somatomotor	Seretomotor	Vasomotor	Anterior 2/3	Posterior 1/3	Vallecula	Proprioception
All the musceles by hypoglossal except Palato-glossal which is by cranial part of accessory nerve through pharyn-geal plexus	Sup.saliva-tory nucleus-facial, chordotympanic andlingual nerves-submandibular ganglion-Lingual glands through lingual nerve.	Sympatheti plexus around lingual artery	Genral sense-Ligual nerve Special sense-chordotym-panic nerve.	Both-Glosso-pharyngeal nerve.	Internal laryngeal nerve	Through hypo-glossal, Lin-gual, trigeminal ganglion without interruption to mesencephalic nucleus of tri-geminal nerve.

126. Ans. a. Lateral rectus *Ref: Grays Anatomy 40/e p693*

Muscles of orbit

Muscles	Nerve supply
Voluntary muscle	
• Superior rectus	Oculomotor nerve
• Medial rectus	Oculomotor nerve

Contd...

Contd...

Muscles	Nerve supply
• Inferior rectus	Oculomotor nerve
• Inferior oblique • Lateral rectus • Superior oblique • Levator palpebrae superioris	Oculomotor nerve Abducent nerve Trochlear nerve Oculomotor nerve
Involuntary muscle • Superior tarsal • Inferior tarsal • Orbitalis	Sympathetic fibres from superior cervical ganglion

127. Ans. b. Posterior cricoarytenoid *Ref: Grays Anatomy 40/e p642, 2008, Ref: Langman's Medical Embryology 9/e p384–385; IBS Human Embryology 7/e p119–120*

128. Ans. b. Innervated by facial nerve *Ref: Grays Anatomy 40/e p658, 2008*

Tensor tympani

- Arises from the cartilaginous part of the auditory tube and from sulcus tubae.
- Passes through the canal for auditory tube along the medial wall of the tympanic cavity.
- Turns laterally around the processus trochleariformis.
- Inserted in to the root of the handle of the malleus.
- Supplied by the trunk of the mandibular nerve through the otic ganglion without relay and conveys the fibres from the nerve to the medial pterygoid.
- Action—draws the handle of malleus medially and tightens the medial pterygoid.

129. Ans. a. Thyroarytenoid *Ref: Grays Anatomy 40/e p642, 2008*

Muscles of the larynx

- Lateral ciroarytenoideus—Arises from the outer lip of the upper border of the circoid cartilage and inserted into anterior surface of the muscular process of the arytenoids cartilage of corresponding side.
- Circothyroid—arises from the outer surface of the anterior arch of circoid cartilage and inserted into lower border of the thyroid lamina. (Stright part—pars recta and oblique part—pars oblique)
- Posterior circoarytenoideus—arises from lateral area of the posterior surface of the thyroid cartilage and inserted into posterior surface of the muscular process of the corresponding arytenoids cartilage.
- Transverse arytenoideus—posterior surface of both arytenoids are connected each other—only unpaired muscle.
- Oblique arytenoideus—paired muscle behind the transverse arytenoideus. Extends from the muscular process of one arytenoids to the apex of the opposite arytenoids cartilage.
- Thyroarytenoideus—posterior surface of the thyroid angle lateral to vocalis and medial to throepiglotticus and inserted in to vocal process of arytenoids above and behind the vocalis.
- Vocalis–arises from the medial part of the posterior surface of the thyroid angle and inerted into the vocal process of arytenoids just lateral to vocal ligament. Part of the thyroarytenoideus.
- Aryepiglotticus—present within the aryepiglottic fold and as a continuation of oblique arytenoids.
  - Action: Laryngeal muscles
  - Oblique artenoid transverse ary: Adduction of aryepifold
  - PCA: Open glottis, Abduction
  - LCA: Rotates arytentenoid cartilage closes glottis and adduction.
  - Cricothyroid: Tensor of vocal cord lengthens vocal ligament
  - Thyroarytenoid vocalis: Relaxor
  - Thyroepiglotticus: Widens inlet of larynx.
  - Vocalis—Differential tension of vocal cord.

130. Ans. b. Sensory supply of face *Ref: Grays Anatomy 40/e p543, 939, 2008*

131. Ans. d. Retomandibular vein *Ref: Grays Anatomy 40/e p400, 127*

132. Ans. a. Supplies muscles of mastication *Ref: Grays Anatomy 40/e p535, The developing human clinically oriented embryology, 8/e p441 and Histology A text and Altlas, Michael H. Ross, 6/e p134, 666 and 725*

133. Ans. d. Genioglossus *Ref: Grays Anatomy 40/e p499*

Tongue

Muscle	Action
Genioglossus	Protrusion
Palatoglossus	Retraction
Styloglossus and Hyoglossus	Depression
Styloglossus	Up and backwards

Mylohyoid muscle

- Arises from the myelohyoid line on inner surface of the mandible extends from the last molar teeth to the symphysis menti.
- Insertion—posterior one third to body of the hyoid bone. Anterior ¾ to the median fibrous raphe extends from symphysis menti to hyoid bone.
- The two sides of the mylohyoid muscle together forms diaphragma oris.
- Nerve supply—nerve to mylohyoid branch of inferior alveolar nerve
- Action—elevates the floor of the mouth and tongue.

134. Ans. c. Superior oblique *Ref: Grays Anatomy 40/e p655*
Ref: 28/Question

135. Ans. b. Lingual nerve *Ref: Grays Anatomy 40/e*
Ref: 23rd Question

- Lingual nerve is the branch of posterior division of the mandibular nerve.
- It receives the chordatympani nerve from behind at an angle.
- Emerges from the lower border of the lateral pterygoid
- Direct contact with the mandible medial to the 3rd molor tooth and intervene between the superior constrictors and mylohyoid muscle. Palpable against the mandible about 1 cm below and behind the 3rd molor tooth.
- Provides the general sense to the pre-sulcul part of the tongue and the floor of the mouth and mandibular gum.

136. Ans. b. Zygomatic *Ref: Grays Anatomy 40/e p535*

Mandibular nerve

- Largest of the three divisions of the trigeminal nerve.
- Mixed nerve. Sensory derived from the trigeminal ganglion and motor from motor nucleus of trigeminal at pons.
- Nerve of 1st branchial arch
- Leaves the cranial cavity through the foramen ovale and below the foramen both roots unites to form trunk of mandibular nerve which is between the tensor veli palatine medially and lateral pterygoid laterally.
- Otic ganglion between the trunk and the tensor veli palatine.
- Divides into anterior and posterior division
- Branches–From the trunk–1. Meningeal (Nervous spinosus) and 2. Nerve to medial pterygoid which supplies apart from medial pterygoid also supplies Tensor veli palatine and tympani.
  - From anterior division–3 motor and 1 sensory. Massetric, deep temporal, nerve to lateral pterygoid and Buccal
  - From posterior division–3 sensory auriculotemporal, lingual and inferior alveolar (Dental).
  - Inferior alveolar nerve gives motor root as mylohyoid nerve which supplies mylohyoid and anterior belly of digastic muscle. Mylohyoid nerve pierces sphenomandibular ligament.

Branches of Inferior alveolar nerve are

- Branches to molar and premolar teeth
- Incisive branch
- Mental
- Mylohyoid

Lingual nerve

- Receives Chordotympani nerve at angle of mandible.
- Medial to the 3rd molar tooth.
- Conveys the secretomotor fibres to the submandibular and sub-lingual glands.

Maxillary nerve

- Second division of the Trigeminal nerve.
- Purely sensory.
- Arises from the convex border of the trigeminal ganglion and traverses middle cranial fossa in the lateral wall of the cavernous sinus with ophthalmic, trochlear and oculomotar nerve above and leave the cranial cavity through the foramen rotundum and enters the pterygopalatine fossa. Then enters the orbit as infra orbital nerve.
  - Infraorbital nerve passes through the infra orbital groove, infraorbital canal and foramen.
- **Branches**
  - **Middle cranial fossa**
  - Meningeal
  - **Pterygopalatine fossa**
  - Ganglionic, Zygomatic and Posterior superior alveolar nerve
  - **Infra orbital canal**
    - Middle superior alveolar nerve and Anterior superior alveolar nerve
    - **Face**
    - Palpebral, Nasal and Superior labial branches.

137. Ans. d. Oppthalmic *Ref: Grays Anatomy 40/e p399, 167*

138. Ans. a. Inferior meatus *Ref: Grays Anatomy 40/e p550*

Paranasal sinuses

Maxillary–largest, ethmoid, frontal and sphenoid–functional endoscopic sinus surgery (FESS), fron, max, eth–occip

Openings of air sinus

Inferior meatus—Nasolacrimal duct
Middle meatus—Frontal sinus, Maxillary sinus, Anterior and middle ethmoidal sinus
Superior meatus—Posterior ethmoidal sinus

139. Ans. c. 9th cranial nerve *Ref: Grays Anatomy 40/e p495*

Parasympathetic ganglia are

Name of the ganglia	Topographically related	Functionally related	Supplies
Otic	Mandibular nerve	Glossopharygeal nerve	Parotid gland
Pterygopalatine ganglion	Maxillary nerve	Greater petrosal branch of facial nerve	Lacrimal gland, Nasal, Palatine and Pharyngeal glands.
Submandibular ganglion	Lingual nerve branch of mandibular nerve	Facial and its chordatympanic branch	Submandibular and sublingual gland
Ciliary ganglian	Nasociliary branch of Opthalmic branch	Oculomotor nerve	Ciliaris and Sphincter papillae through parasympathetic and dilator papillae through sympathetic.

140. Ans. a. Parotid *Ref: Grays Anatomy 40/e p700*

Secretomotor of parotid gland

Inferior salivatory nucleus → Tympanic branch of glossopharyngeal nerve → Tympanic plexus → Lesser petrosal nerve → Otic ganglion → Auriculotemporal nerve → Parotid gland.

Submandibular and Sublingual gland

- Sup. Sali Nucleus → Facial → chorda tympani → lingual nerve → Posterior root → submand ganglion → post gang directly → Submandibular gland
- Via anterior root to Lingual nerve → sublingual gland.

- Lacrimal gland
  Superior salivatory nucleus
  ↓
  Nervus intermedius
  ↓
  Trunk of facial nerve
  ↓
  Geniculate ganglion
  ↓
  Greater petrosal nerve
  ↓
  Nerve of pterygoid canal
  ↓
  Pterygo-palatine ganglion
  ↓
  Maxillary nerve
  ↓
  Zygomatic branch → Zygomatico-temporal → Lacrimal branch → Lacrimal gland
  For nasal and palatine glands through the greater palatine nerve.

141. Ans. a. Glossopharyngeal nerve *Ref: Grays Anatomy 40/e p546*

- All muscles of palate are innervated by pharyngeal plexus except Tensor palati which is being innervated by V3 (Mandibular nerve).
- All muscles of pharynx are being innervated by cranial accessory via pharyngeal plexus except stylo-pharyngeous which is being innervated by Glossopharyngeal nerve.
- All muscles of Tongues are being innervated by Hypoglossal nerve except palatoglossus which is being innervated by pharyngeal plexus.
- All the muscles of the larynx are supplied by the recurrent laryngeal nerve except circothyroid which is supplied by external laryngeal nerve.
- All the muscles of the face are supplied by facial nerveexcept levator palpebrae superioris which is supplied by upper ramus of oculomotor nerve.

142. Ans. a. Superior alveolar nerve *Ref: Grays Anatomy 40/e p500*

- Anterior superior alveolar nerve—innervate all incisor teeth,premolars and buccal root of the first molar nerve.
- Posterior superior alveolar nerve—innervates 2nd and 3rd molar teeth
- Middle superior alveolar nerve—innervates sinus mucosa,roots of the maxillary premolars

143. Ans. a. 20 Weeks *Ref: Gray's Anatomy 40/e*

Myelination commences during the 16–20th week of prenatal life, around the axons of CNS of about 1 μm diameter and around the axons of the peripheral nerves of about 1.5 μm diameter.

Myelin sheath of peripheral nerves are derived from Schwann cells and those of CNS derived from Oligodendrocytes

144. Ans. d. Fasciculus lenticularis *Ref: Essentials of Neuroanatomy, AK Datta, 3/e p81–82*

- Zona increta—grey matter between ventral nuclei of thalamus and subthalamic nucleus.
- Field H1 forel—between ventral nuclei of thalamus and zona increta. Contain thalamic fasiculus comprising fasicularis lenticularis, ansa lenticularis and dento-rubro-thalamic fibres.
- Field H2 Forel—between subthalamic nucleus and zona increta. Contain fasicularis lenticularis,
- Prerubral or field H3 forel—caudal margin of zona increta. Contain fasicularis lenticularis, ansa lenticularis.

145. Ans. b. 1 months *Ref: Internet Source: http://radiopaedia.org/normal-myelination*

Myelination of brain

- Cranial nerves–6th month motor nerves earlier than the sensory nerves. Optic nerve later at about full term.
- Medial longitudinal bundle–6th month

- Vestibulo-spinal, tecto-spinal and reticulo-spinal tract–7th month
- Spinothalamic and spinocerebellar tract–8th month
- Brain stem, cerebellum and posterior limb of internal capsule–at term
- Anterior limb of internal capsule–2nd month
- Splenium of corpus callosum–3rd month
- Genu of the internal capsule–6th month

Myelination of the spinal cord

- Inter-segmental tracts–4th month
- Ventral and dorsal nerves–5th month
- Posterior finiculi–6th month
- Spinothalamic and spinocerebellar tracts–7th month
- Corticospinal tract starts at 9th month and ends 2 or 3 years.

146. Ans. d. Dorsal surface of corpus callosum *Ref: Grays Anatomy 40/e*

Corpus callosum

Parts

From backward to forward Splenium, Body (Trunk), Genu, Rostrum

Upper convex margin–Thin seet of grey matter called as indusium grisum continues in front with upper end of paraterminal gyrus and behind as gyrus fasiolaris over the spleenium and continuous as dentate gyrus on the para-hippocampal gyrus.

Two pairs of longitudinal fibres, medial and lateral longitudinal fibres embedded in the indusium griseum.

Indusium grisum and longitudinal striae are remnant of upper part of hippocampal formation–Rhinocephalon.

Lower concave surface

Posterior part contact with the crura of the fornix and in front is separated from the body of the fornix by an interval occupied by the neural tissue called as septum pellucidum

Arrangment fibers in corpus callosum

Rostrum–connect orbital surfaces of both hemispheres

Genu–Forceps minor- connect medial and lateral surfaces of the frontal lobes.

Trunk–Projected bilaterally wide areas of the cerebral cortex and bisected by the corona radiate. Some fibres called tapetum forms roof and lateral wall of posterior horn and lateral part of the roof of the inferior horn.

Splenium–Forceps major connect the occipital lobes.

147. Ans. b. Facial Nerve *Ref: Grays Anatomy 40/e p237*

Floor of the IVth ventricle (Rhomboid fossa)

- Divided into two halves by median sulcus
- Each halves divided by sulcus limitans in to medial eminence and lateral vestibular area
- In the widest intermediate area presents depression known as superior fovea.
- At the level of superior fovea presents Folliculus colliculus beneath which the abducent nucleus encircled by the motor rootn of the facial nerve.
- Rostrally sulcus limitants flattened to form bluish Locus ceruleus rich in nor-adrenalin concerned with Paradoxical sleep.
- Caudally sulcus limitants present another depression known as inferior fovea.
- Opposite to inferior fovea in the medial eminence triangular elevation known as Hypoglossal trigone contains hypoglossal nucleus medially and intercalates nucleus laterally.
- Lateral to the sulcus limitants presents Vestibular area containing 4 vestibular nuclei superior,inferior lateral and medial.
- Below the inferior fovea between the hypoglossal trigone and the vestibular area vagal trigone present containing dorsal vagal nucleus.
- Ependymal thickening known as Funiculus separans separate the vagal trigone and the inferolateral area known as Area postrema which is related to the vomiting and respiratory centers.
- Striae medullaris–Nerve fibers extend horizontally across the vestibular area and the medial eminence. These fibres derived from arcuate nuclei.

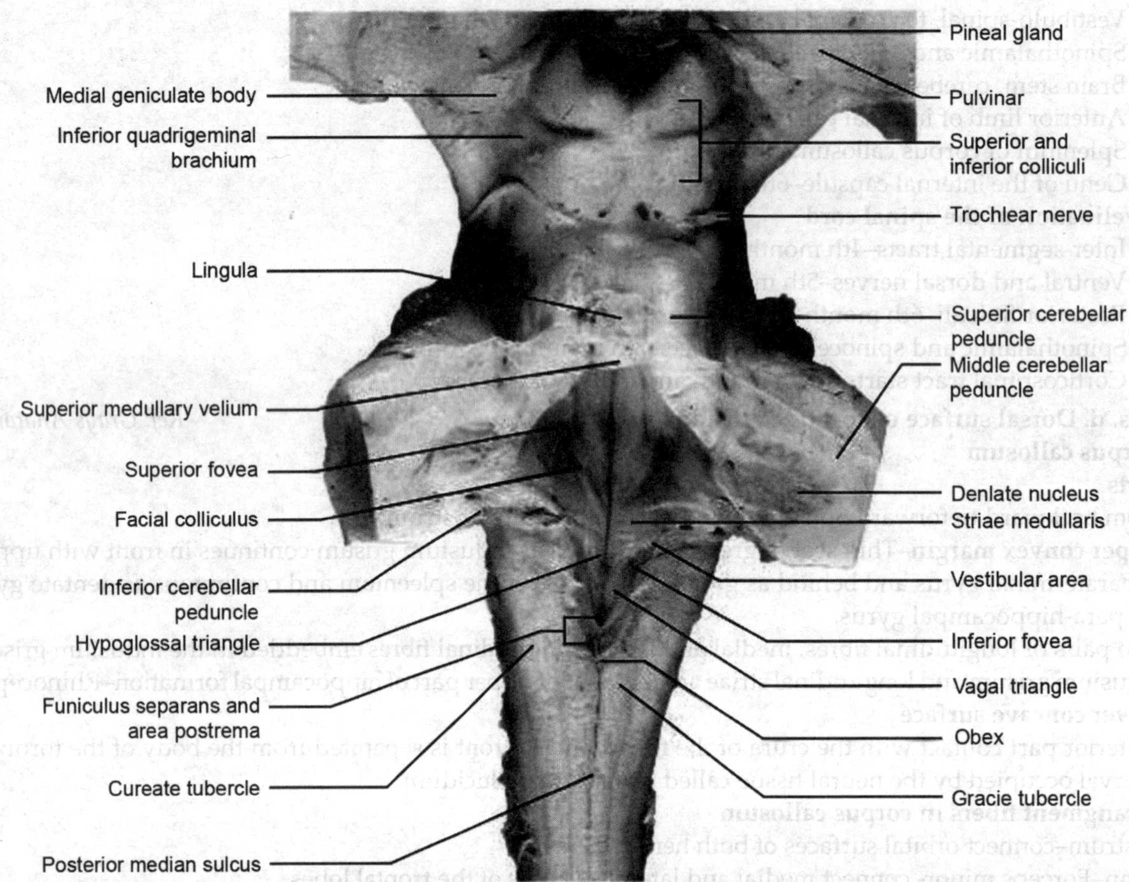

Fig. 1.57: Dorsal surface of brain stem

148. Ans. a. Lower border of L1 vertebra *Ref: Grays Anatomy 40/e p225*

Spinal cord

- Extent—Continuation of the medulla oblongata below the imaginary horizontal plane rostral to the 1st pair of cervical nerves along the upper border of the atlas meets the middle of the odontoid process of the axis to lower border of L1 in adult and lower border of L3 in the newborn.
- Conus medullatier—Tappering lower end of spinal cord.
- Length–45 cm
- Enlargements–Cervical and Lumbosacral.
  - Cervical–C4–T2 and Lumbo-sacral–L2–S3
- Spinal nerves–31 pairs–Cervical 8 pairs, Thoracic–12 pairs, Lumbar–5 pairs, Sacral–5 pairs and Coccygeal–1 pair.
- Cervial spinal nerves leave the intervertebral foramen above the pedicle the corresponding vertebrae and 8th leave above the pedicle of the T1 vertebrae.
- Spinal or coed segment (Neuromere)–The part of the spinal cord giving attachment of the spinal nerve are called spinal or core segment.
- Cauda equine–Bunches of spinal nerves extend from the lower end of the cord around the filum terminale.
- Filum terminale–Pial non-nervous filament extend from the tip of the conus medullaris of the spinal cord to 1st coccyx.

149. Ans. c. Occipital sinus *Ref: Grays Anatomy 40/e*

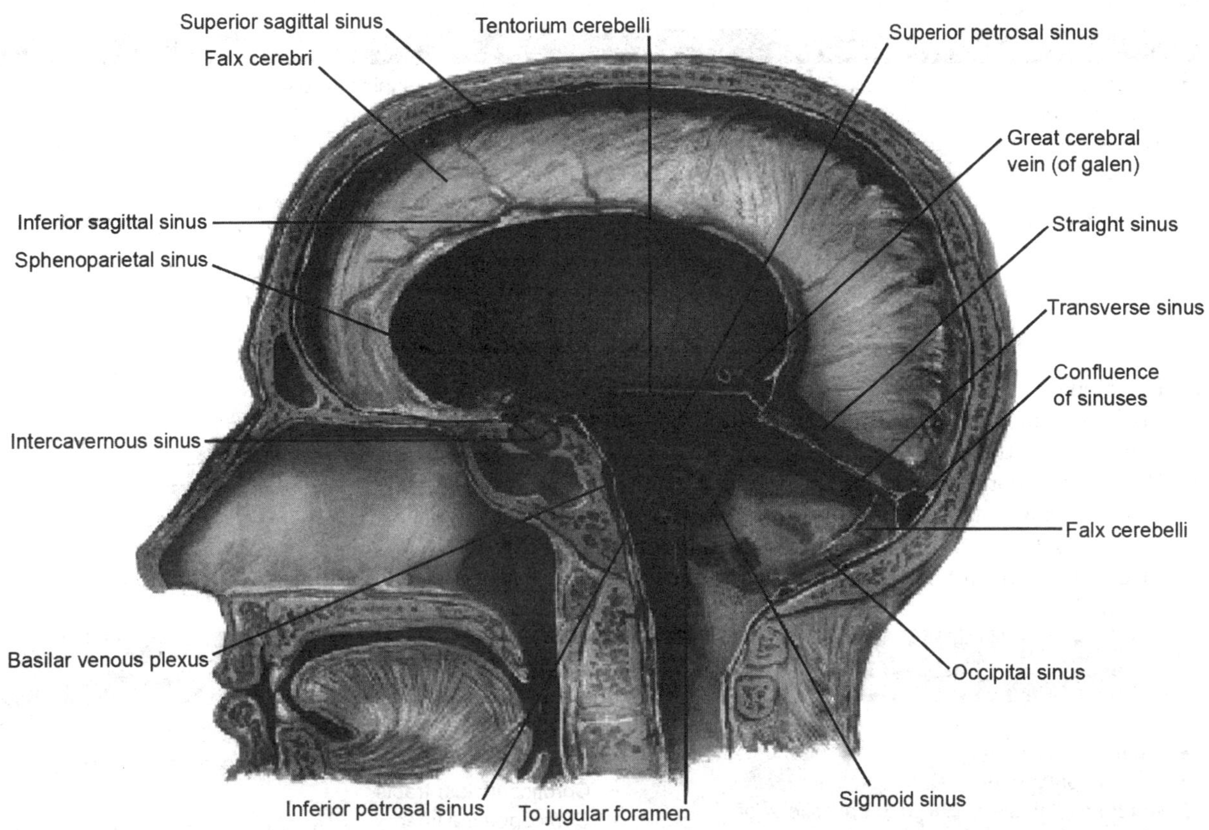

Fig. 1.58: Dural folds and sinuses

Falx cerebelli
- Small midline fold of dura matter
- Sickle shaped fold below the tentorium
- Extends from the internal occipital crest to the posterior cerebellar notch
- Base attached to the inferior surface of the tentorium
- Apex attached to the posterior margin of the foramen magnum
- This contains occipital sinus.

150. Ans. c. Midbrain *Ref: Grays Anatomy 40/e p280, 2008*

Structures present in the Midbrain at the level of Superior colliculi

Grey matter	White matter
Oculomotar nerve nuclei.	• Median Logitudinal fassiculus • Dorsal tegmental decussation (Efferents from Superior colliculi. • Red nucleus • Ventral tegmental decusstion (efferents from • Medial, Trigeminal (Ventral trigeminal tract) and Spinal lemniscus. • Central tegmental tract • Dorsal trigeminal tract • Superior colliculli • Pretectal nuclei.

Structures present in the Midbrain at the level of Inferior colliculi

Grey matter	White matter
• Trochlear nerve nuclei. • Mesencephalic nuclei • Dorsal tegmental nuclei • Nucleus of Darkschewitch	• Median Logitudinal fassiculus • Ventral tegmental nuclei • Tectospinal tract • Rubrospinal tract • Decussation of Superior cerebellar peduncle • Medial, Trigeminal (Ventral trigeminaln tract), Spinal and Lateral lemniscus. • Central tegmental tract • Dorsal trigeminal tract • Inferior colliculli

Red nucleus

- Present as pair in the rostral tegmentum of midbrain.
- Ovoid 5 mm diameter.
- Rich in iron content
- Caudal–Magnocellular part and Rostral–Parvocellular part.
- **Afferents**–Cerebellorubral, Cortico-rubral, Tectorubral fibers.
- **Efferents**–Ventral tegmental decussation of Forel and descend as Rubrospinal, Rubrobulbar and rubroreticular fibers.

Basilar part of pons		
Grey matter	White matter	
• Pontine nuclei • Arcuate nucleus • Pons to bular body Fibers from all these nuclei go to opposite ½ of cerebellum	Longitudinal fibers	Transverse fibers
	• Corticospinal tracts • Coroticonuclear tracts • Corticopontine fibers	Ponto cerebellar fibers

Tegmentum in the lower Part of Pons	
Grey matter	White matter
• Sixth nerve nucleus (beneath facial Colliculus) • Seventh nerve nucleus (in reticular formation of Pons) • Vestibular and Cochlear nuclei (in relation of Inferior Cerebellar Peduncle) • Spinal nucleus of the Trigeminal nerve • Salivatory nuclei and Lacrimatory nuclei Nucleus of corpus trapezoideum, Superior olivary nucleus.	• Trapezoid body (Ventral Part of Pons) • Medial lemniscus. Trigerminal lemniscus, spinal lemniscus, lateral lemniscus. • Inferior cerebellar peduncle

Tegmentum in the upper part of pons	
Grey matter	White matter
• Motor and Superior Sensory nuclei of the Trigeminal nerve	• Medial lemniscus, trigeminal lemniscus, Spinal lemniscus, lateral lemniscus • Superior cerebellar peduncle • Medial longitudinal bundle

Several nuclei are seen in the upper part of the medulla (floor of the fourth ventricle). They are:

- Hypoglossal nucleus
- Dorsal nucleus of vagus (lateral to XII nerve nucleus).
- Nucleus of tractus solitaries (Ventro lateral to the dorsal nucleus of vagus)
- Inferior and medial vestibular nuclei
- Nucleus ambiguous-lies deep in the reticular formation-gives origin to motor fibres for carnial nerves IX, X and XI.
- Dorsal and ventral cochlear nuclei

- Nucleus of the spinal tract of the trigeminal nerve
- Inferior Olivary nucleus (largest mass of grey matter at this level, responsible for the producing the elevation of the olive)
- Arcuate nucleus

151. Ans. a. Nucleus ambiguous *Ref: Grays Anatomy 40/e p225*

Functional coloumn	Nuclei
Somatic efferents (Somatomotor)	Oculomotor, Trochlear, Abducent and Hypoglossal nuclei
Special visceral efferents (Branchiomotor)	Nucleus ambiguous
Genral visceral efferents (Secretomotor)	Edinger-Westphal nucleus of oculomotor,Superior salivatory nucleus of facial, Inferior salivatory nucleus of the glossopharyngeal and dorsal nucleus of the vagus.
Genral visceral afferents	Nucleus solitaries
Special visceral afferents	Nucleus solitaries
Genral somatic afferents	Spinal nucleus, Principal sensory and mesencephalic nuleus of trigeminal nerve.
Special somatic afferents	Cochlear and vestibular nuclei of vestibulocochlear nerve

Functional component	General function	Cranial nerves
General somatic afferent	Perception of touch, pain, temperature	V, VII, X
General visceral afferent	Sensory input form viscera	IX, X
Special afferent	Smell, taste, vision, hearing and balance	I, II, VII, VIII, IX, X
General somatic efferent	Motor innervations to skeletal (voluntary) muscles	III, IV, VI, XII
General somatic efferent	Motor innervations to smooth muscle, heart muscle and glands	III, VIII, IX, X,
Branchial efferent	Motor innervations to skeletal muscles derived from pharyngeal arch mesoderm	V, VII, IX, X, XI

152. Ans. c. Midbrain *Ref: Grays Anatomy 40/e p280, 939, 2009*

153. Ans. c. Multipolar *Ref: Grays Anatomy 40/e p225*

Unipolar neurons	Bipolar neurons	Multipolar neurons
Dorsal root ganglion, Sensory ganglia of 5, 7, 9, 10th cranial nerves	Scarpa's ganglion, Cochlear ganglion and Olfactory ga, Bipolar cells of retina.	Autanomic ganglion

QUESTIONS 2015

1. Musculocutaneous from which cord of brachial plxs?
a. Lateral cord
b. Posterior cord
c. Trunk
d. Medial

2. Transpyloric plane of addison is a horizontal line halfway between the jugular notch and the upper border of the pubic symphysis. It cuts through:
a. Bifurcation of Aorta
b. Inferior vena cava pierces through diaphragm
c. Ureters enter bladder
d. Superior Mesentric artery arises from abdominal aorta

3. Patient with tonsilitis had otalgia reffered pain through which nerve?
a. Glossopharynegeal
b. Vagus
c. Internal laryngeal nerve
d. Auriculotemporal nerve

4. Horizontal line from angle of louis to t4 vertebrae divide mediatinum to:
a. Superior and inferior
b. Anterior and posterioir
c. Anterior and middle
d. Middle and posterior

5. Abductor of vocal cord:
a. Postcricoarytenoid
b. Lateral circoarytenoid
c. Transverse arytenoid
d. Circothyroid

6. Posterior to 1st part of duodenum:
a. Portal vein
b. Superior mesentric vessels
c. Spleenic vein
d. IVC

7. Swelling in the midline of neck due to:
a. Thyroid cartilage
b. Cricoid
c. Arytenoid
d. Epiglottis

8. Abdominal viscera in infant protuding through abdomen wall covered by sac:
a. Exomphalos
b. Gastrochisis
c. Volvulus
d. Diverticulum

9. Nerve injured while extracting third molar:
a. Inf Alv Nerve
b. Marginal mandibular
c. Mental nerve
d. Mandibular nerve

10. Bronchopulmonary segment in right lung:
a. 10
b. 9
c. 8
d. 11

11. True abt femoral artery:
a. Crossed by cutaneous nerve of thigh
b. Medial to femoral vein

12. Rotator cuff attachment all except:
a. Teres minor
b. Subclavius
c. Supraspinatus
d. Inraspinatus

13. Which is true?
Ureteric bud develops collecting tubules, a part of metanephros fundus of bladder develops from mesonephros

14. True abt female urethra:
a. Homologous to male prostatic urethra.
b. Embedded in or related to posterior vaginal wall

15. True?
a. Female has both X-chromosome active
b. Turner 1 extra X-chromosome
c. Klinefelter is male wd extra Y-chromosome.
d. ??

ANSWERS AND EXPLANATIONS

1. Ans. a. Lateral cord *Ref: Gray's Anatomy 40th ed*

Lateral pectoral nerve–pectoralis major and minor
Lateral root of median nerve (direct continuation of lateral cord)
Musculocutaneous nerve–(C 5–7)coracobrachialis, Biceps, branchialis, lateral cutaneous nerve of forearm

Medial cord: (4 MU) (Money Makes Many Man Unhappy)
Medial pectoral nerve–pectoralis major and minor (pierces pectoralis minor)
Medial root of median nerve
Medial cutaneous nerve of arm (smallest and most medial of all branches)
Medial cutaneous nerve of forearm
Ulnar nerve (largest branch of medial cord) (C7, C8, T1)—direct continuation of medial cord is ulnar nerve
Posterior cord: (ULNAR)
Upper subscapular nerve–subscapularis muscle
Lower subscapular nerve–subscapularis muscle, teres major
Nerve to lattismus dorsi (thoracodorsal nerve)
Axillary nerve–anterior branch–deltoid, posterior branch-teres minor, forms pseudoganglion. Upper lateral cutaneous nerve of arm
Radial nerve (largest branch of whole plexus) (C5–8, T1)–direct continuation of posterior cord

2. **Ans. d. Superior Mesentric artery arises from abdominal aorta** *Ref: A.K. Datta Human Anatomy 5/e p1*
Structures present in this plane pylorus of stomach, Hilum of kidney, fundus of gall bladder, Origin of superior mesenteric artery, Neck of pancreas, Splenic vein passes transversely at this plane, Spinal cord ends as conus medullaris and lower border of L1 vertebrae.

3. **Ans. a. Glossopharynegeal** *Ref: Gray's Anatomy 40/e*
The glossopharyngeal nerve lies immediately lateral to the muscular wall of the tonsillar fossa. It is at risk if the wall is pierced, and is commonly temporarily affected by oedema following tonsillectomy.

4. **Ans. a. Superior and inferior** *Ref: A.K. Datta Human anatomy 5/e p1*
Mediastinum
Superior
Inferior–anterior, middle (widest), posterior (longest)
Division–sternal angle to T4/T5 junction

5. **Ans. a. Postcricoarytenoid** *Ref: A.K. Datta 5/e p2*

Action	Laryngeal muscles
Oblique Artytenoid transverse ary	Adduction of Aryepiglottic fold
PCA	Open glottis, abduction
LCA	Rotates Arytenoid cartiage closes glottis
Cricothyroid	Tensor of vocal cord lengthens vocal lig
Thyroarytenoid vocalis	Relaxor
Thyroepiglotticus	Widens inlet of larynx

6. **Ans. a. Portal vein** *Ref: A.K. Datta Human Anatomy 5/e p1*
   - Ist part Relations:

Peritoneal	Visceral			
• Proximal 2.5 cm: movable and attached to the greater and lesser omentum	Anterior	Posterior	Superior	Inferior
• Distal 2.5 cm: fixed and retro peritoneal and covered with peritoneum only in its anterior aspect	Quadrate lobe of liver Gallbladder	Gastroduodenal. A A Bile duct Portal Vein	Epiploic foramen	Head and neck of pancreas

7. **Ans. a. Thyroid cartilage**

8. **Ans. b. Gastrochisis** *Ref: Langman's Medical Embryology 11/e*
Omphalocele involves herniation of abdominal viscera through an enlarged umbilical ring.
Gastroschisis is a herniation of abdominal contents through the body wall directly into the amniotic cavity.

9. **Ans. a. Inf Alv Nerve** *Ref: Gray's Anatomy 40/e*
In the mandibular canal, the inferior alveolar nerve runs downward and forward, generally below the apices of the teeth until below the first and second premolars where it divides into terminal incisive and mental branches. The incisive branch continues forward in a bony canal or in a plexiform

10. **Ans. a. 10**
Bronchopulmonary segments
    - 10 Right/10 Left (medial basal absent)

11. **Ans. a. Crossed by cutaneous nerve of thigh**

12. **Ans. b. Subclavius**
Codman's Musculotendinous rotators cuff
Supraspinatus, Infraspinatus, Subscapularis and Teres minor

14. **Ans. a. Homologous to male prostatic urethra**
Kidney development:

Ureteric bud	Metanephric blasema
Ureter, Renal pelvis, Major and minor calyces, and collecting duct	Nephrons, PCT, Henles loop and DCT

15. **Ans. a. Female has both X-chromosome active**

Chapter

2

Physiology

Abirami

GENERAL PHYSIOLOGY—HIGH YIELD TOPICS

The Nobel Prize in Physiology or Medicine

Year	Laureates	Citation
2014	**John O'Keefe, May-Britt Moser and Edvard I. Moser**	**'For their discoveries of cells that constitute a positioning system in the brain'**
2013	James E. Rothman, Randy W. Schekman and Thomas C. Südhof	'for their discoveries of machinery regulating vesicle traffic, a major transport system in our cells'
2012	Sir John B. Gurdon and Shinya Yamanaka	'for the discovery that mature cells can be reprogrammed to become pluripotent'

The Foundation of Physiology

- **WB Cannon** coined the term **homeostasis**
- **Claude Bernard**-concept of ***milieu intérieur***

Control Systems and Feedback

- Basically designed to maintain a controlled variable at a set point
- Effectiveness of a control system assessed using gain
- **Gain = Correction/Error**
- Higher the gain, higher the accuracy of regulation
- For body temperature control system, gain is –33

Negative Feedback

- A pathway in which response opposes or removes the signal
- Most control systems of the body act by negative feedback
- Stabilize the variable being regulated
- Examples-ACTH secretion, Aldosterone-potassium, Glucose regulation, Growth hormone secretion, BP regulation

Positive Feedback

- Response reinforces rather than decrease or removes it. Leads to vicious cycle.
- Examples: **Clotting, Calcium entry into sarcoplasmic reticulum, LH surge during ovulation, Action potential (Hodgkin's cycle), Parturition (Ferguson reflex), Shock (Mnemonic: CLAPS)**

Feedforward Control

- Allows the body to anticipate change and maintain stability
- Example: Salivation reflex-sight, smell, thought of food leads to salivation-anticipation of food

Total body water (60% of body weight, for a 70 kg man) is 42 liters		
Intracellular fluid	Extracellular fluid	
2/3rd of TBW i.e., 40% Body weight (28 liters)	1/3rd of TBW. i.e., 20% Body weight (14 liters)	
	Interstitial fluid	Plasma
	75% or 3/4th of ECF or 15% of body weight (10.5 litres)	25% or 1/4th of ECF or 5% of body weight (3.5 litres)

- In the average young adult male, **18%** of the body weight is **protein** and related substances, **7%** is **mineral**, and **15%** is **fat**
- Daily intake of water–2300 ml
- Output: Insensible—skin 350 ml and lungs 350 ml
- Others: Sweat 100 ml, Feces 100 ml, Urine 1400 ml
- Transcellular fluid (1–2 L): Synovial, peritoneal, pericardial, intraocular spaces, cerebrospinal fluid

	ECF	ICF
Most abundant cation	Na^+	K^+
Most abundant anion	Cl^-	Phosphates > Proteins

Measurement of Body Fluid Volumes

- Measurement of fluid volumes in the different body fluid compartments is by **The Indicator-Dilution Principle: Volume =Amount/concentration**
- Total body water: ^2H_2O (Deuterium oxide), ^3H_2O (Tritium Oxide), Antipyrine (Mn:TAD)
- Extracellular fluid: ^{22}Na, ^{125}I-Iothalamate, Thiosulfate, Inulin, Sucrose (Mn: NITIS)
- Intracellular fluid: Calculated as Total body water–Extracellular fluid volume
- Plasma volume: ^{125}I-Albumin, Evans blue dye (T-1824) (Mn:PIE)
- Blood volume: ^{51}cr-labeled red blood cells, or calculated as blood volume = Plasma volume/ (1–Hematocrit)
- Interstitial fluid: (calculated as extracellular fluid volume–Plasma volume)

Osmolarity and Osmolality

- A mole is the gram molecular weight of a substance or molecular weight of a substance in grams
- Each mole consists of 6×10^{23} molecules
- One osmole equals the gram molecular weight of a substance divided by the number of freely moving particles that each molecule liberates in solution
- Osmolarity—number of osmoles per litre of solution
- Osmolality—number of osmoles per kg of solvent. Serum osmolality-285-295 mOsm/kg H_2O
- Osmolality is not affected by changes in volume of solution or by temperature
- Most accurate way of finding out osmolality is by **Freezing point depression**
- Approximate formula is Osmolality (mOsm/L) = 2 [Na^+] (mEq/L) +0.055 [Glucose] (mg/dL) + 0.36 [BUN] (mg/dL)
- Vant Hoff Law-used to calculate osmotic pressure-
  $\Pi = \sigma$ (nCRT)
  σ **Reflection coefficient**
  Π–osmotic pressure
  N = number of dissociable particles
  R = Gas constant
  T = Temperature (K)
- The pressure necessary to prevent solvent migration to the more concentrated solution is the osmotic pressure of the solution
- Osmotic pressure depends on the number rather than the type of particles in a solution (colligative property)

Tonicity

- Used to describe the osmolality of a solution relative to plasma
- Same osmolality as plasma-isotonic (0.9% NaCl)

Plasma Protein	Molecular Weight (Daltons)	Concentration	Contribution to osmotic pressure
Albumin	69, 000	3.5–5 g%	80%
Globulin	1, 40, 000	2 g%	20%
Fibrinogen	4, 00, 000	0.3 g%	0%

Nonionic diffusion
- Substances cannot cross the membrane in charged form but cross in undissociated form
- Example: Ammonia transport in GIT/Kidney

CELLULAR PHYSIOLOGY—HIGH YIELD TOPICS

Electrophysiology of the Cell

Resting Membrane Potential (RMP)
- Every cell shows a potential difference with the inside being negative.
- Due to diffusion of K^+ and sodium potassium ATPase (5–10%)

Structure	RMP (mv)
Neuron	– 70
Skeletal muscle	– 90
SA node	– 30 to–40
Ventricle	– 90
Smooth muscle	– 30 to–40
RBC	– 10

Cell organelle	Function
Nucleolus	• Site of synthesis of ribosomes
Ribosomes	• Site of protein synthesis
Rough/granular endoplasmic reticulum	• Synthesis of proteins
Smooth/agranular endoplasmic reticulum	• Synthesis of lipids and steroid
Golgi bodies	• Processing/packaging of proteins, • Synthesizing certain carbohydrates that cannot be formed by ER (eg; hyaluronic acid and chondroitin sulphate) • Lysosome formation
Lysosomes	• Formed by breaking off from the Golgi apparatus • Also called intracellular digestive system • Contains hydrolases to digest proteins, carbohydrates, lipids • Contains bactericidal agents lysozyme and lysoferrin
Peroxisomes	• Physically similar to lysosomes, but contain oxidases instead of hydrolases • Proteins are directed to peroxisomes by protein chaperones called peroxins
Mitochondria	• Formation of ATP

Cell Membrane	• Current concepts of membrane physiology is based on fluid and Mosaic model proposed by **Singer and Nicolson, 1972**
Membrane lipids	• Has both hydrophilic and hydrophobic properties (Amphipathic) • Has phospholipids, and glycolipids • Sterols-Cholesterol • Membrane fluidity changes with temperature: Temperature at which the membrane undergoes ordered to disordered (melts) is the transition temperature (Tm) • Cholesterol modifies fluidity: Below Tm-Increases fluidity, Above Tm-Limits fluidity and that's why is called as Fluidity Buffer • Membrane lipids are asymmetrically distributed: Outer Membrane-Lecithin and sphingomyelin • Inner leaflet- Phosphotidyl serine, phosphotidylethanolamine
Membrane Proteins	• Integral proteins (Glycophorins in RBC) • Peripheral proteins (Spectrin in RBC) • Examples of GPI anchored proteins: Alkaline Phosphatase, CAMs, proteins that Combat Cell lysis by complement • Functions as 1. CAMs 2. Pumps 3. Carriers 4. Receptors 5. Enzymes (Mn: PCR-E. Coli)

Cell Cycle

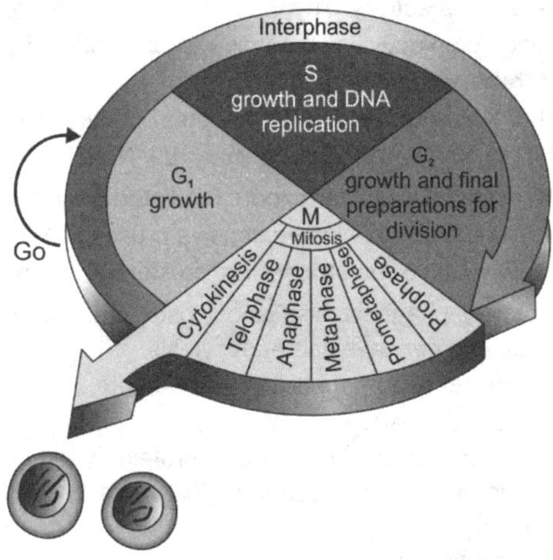

Fig. 2.1: Cell cycle

- G1 (first gap) phase: Cells grow in size and synthesise RNAs and proteins required for DNA synthesis
- S (synthesis) phase: Cells actively replicate their chromosomes
- G2 (second gap) phase: After progressing through a second gap phase, the cells enter the M (mitotic) phase
- Interphase: G1, S, G2 phase together are called interphase
- Most nonproliferating cells in vertebrates leave the cell cycle in G1 and enter G0 phase (resting phase). Some G0 cells can return to the cell cycle and resume replicating

Transport Across Cell Membrane

Passive Processes	**Diffusion:** • No energy is expended directly • Net flux of solute particles from areas of high to areas of low concentration • Fick's law of diffusion: $J = -DA\,\Delta C/\Delta X$, where J is the net rate of diffusion, D is the diffusion coefficient, A is the area, and $\Delta C/\Delta X$ is the concentration gradient **Facilitated Diffusion:** • Carrier proteins move substances in the direction of their chemical or electrical gradients, no energy input is required. • Has a transport maximum (it is saturable), can be inhibited competitively and noncompetitively • Example: Glucose transport by GLUT
Active Processes	**Primary active transport:** • Energy is used and substances transported against gradient. • Energy derived directly by hydrolysis of ATP (Na^+ K^+ ATPase) **Sodium potassium ATPase pump** • Discovered by Jens Skou-1997 nobel prize in chemistry • Accounts for about 24% of the energy utilized by cells, and in neurons it accounts for 70% • Has an alpha and beta subunit **Alpha subunit:** • Intracellular: Na^+ binding site, Phosphorylation site, ATP binding site • Extracellular: K^+ binding site, Ouabain binding site **Beta subunit:** • Extracellular glycosylation site • Extrude three Na^+ from the cell and take two K^+ into the cell for each molecule of ATP hydrolyzed (electrogenic) • Activity is inhibited by ouabain, digitalis

Active Processes	**Regulation of Na, K ATPase:** • Agents Increasing pump activity: Thyroid hormones, Aldosterone, Insulin (MN:ThAI) • Agents decreasing pump activity: Dopamine, causes natriuresis **Secondary active transport:** • Active transport of Na^+ is coupled to the transport of other substances • Examples: $Na^+K^+Cl^-$, Na-Glucose, Na-aminoacids. Na-bile salts, Na-choline uptake
Exocytosis	• For vesicles containing material for export, mediated through v-SNARE and t-SNARE • Non constitutive (regulated) pathway-extensive processing occurs before exocytosis. Ex-insulin release • Constitutive pathway-little or no processing, no storage. Ex-mucus release into GI lumen
Endocytosis	• Various types namely phagocytosis, pinocytosis, clathrin-mediated endocytosis, caveolae-dependent uptake, and nonclathrin/noncaveolae endocytosis • Pinocytosis-cell drinking and phagocytosis-cell eating • Clathrin mediated endocytosis: – Involves clathrin (triskelion), GTP binding protein dynamin – Examples: Internalisation of receptors for nerve growth factor, low density lipoprotein receptor, Transferrin (Iron) • Caveolae mediated endocytosis: – Involves Rafts-rich in cholesterol and sphingolipids and caveolae (flask-shaped membrane depression) and caveolin. Examples-Folate receptor (Folate) • Emeiocytosis: Insulin release from stored granules, requires calcium
Transcytosis	• Combines both exocytosis and endocytosis. • The transport mechanism makes use of coated vesicles that appear to be coated with caveolin • Otherwise called as cytopempsis

Coats and vesicle proteins
- Assembly protein 1 (AP-1): Vesicles from transgolgi to lysosomes
- Assembly protein 2: Endocytic vesicles to endosomes
- COP I and COP II: Vesicles that transport between the endoplasmic reticulum and the golgi

Ion channels
- Specific for K^+, Na^+, Ca^{2+}, and Cl^- as well as nonselective
- Examples-Amiloride sensitive epithelial sodium channels (ENaC)
- Cl^- channels-$GABA_A$, Glycine receptors, Cystic fibrosis transmembrane conductance regulator (CFTR)

Cytoskeleton

- Maintains structure, allows the cells to change shape and move
- Made up of microtubules, intermediate filaments, and microfilaments

Microtubules (25 nm)	• Dynamic portion of cytoskeleton, provide the tracks that moves transport vesicles, organelles • Made up of alpha, beta and gamma tubulins • γ-tubulin-production of microtubules by centrosomes [Microtubule Organising centres (MTOCs)]
Intermediate filaments (8–14 nm)	• Form a flexible scaff olding for the cell and help it resist external pressure • Keratin (epithelia), Vimentin (fibroblasts), Desmin (muscle), GFAP, Peripherin, Neurofilaments, Nestin, Lamin (Mn:DVL-GP-KPN)
Microfilaments (4–6 nm)	• Made up of ACTIN-most abundant protein in mammalian cells • Found in microvilli (GIT) and lamellipodia (Crwaling) • Involves in cytokinesis during cell division

Molecular Motors

There are three super families of molecular motors: **kinesin, dynein,** and **myosin.**
Kinesin-move its cargo toward the '+' ends of microtubules
Dyneins-move particles and membranes to the '–' end of the microtubules.
Myosin- for contraction of muscle and cell migration

Intercellular Connections

- Hold cells together: Tight junctions (zonula occludens), gap junction, desmosome and zonula adherens
- Attach cells to their basal lamina-hemidesmosome and focal adhesions

Tight junctions	Gap junctions
Intestinal mucosa, the walls of the renal tubules, and the choroid plexus Proteins-occludin, junctional adhesion molecules (JAMs), and claudins Helps maintain cell polarity-prevent the movement of proteins in the plane of the membrane Determines the degree of leakiness (paracellular pathway	3 nm gaps lined up with Connexons (Cx) 6 subunits of connexins =1 connexon Permit the rapid propagation of electrical activity from cell to cell diseases: X-linked Charcot-Marie-Tooth disease (Cx32), cataract (Cx46 and Cx50), Clouston syndrome (Cx 30), myoclonic epilepsy (Cx36), arteriosclerosis (Cx37), idiopathic atrial fibrillation (Cx40), erythrokeratoderma variabilis (Cx30.3 and Cx31), inherited deafness (Cx26, Cx30, Cx31)

- **Zonula adherens**: Major site of attachment for intracellular microfilaments, contains cadherins
- **Hemidesmosomes**: Connected to intermediate filaments. Contains cadherins

Aging (Senescence)

Cellular and molecular mechanisms of aging:

1. Oxidative stress (Free radical theory)-widely accepted theory of aging. Damage to the macromolecules by H_20_2, OH, superoxide anion radical
2. Glycation hypothesis of aging: Due to formation of advanced glycation end products from Amadori product
3. Mitochondrial theory of aging: Damage to mitochondria leads to reduced synthesis of ATP
4. DNA damage theory of aging: Accumulated DNA damage interferes with DNA replication and transcription
5. DNA repair theory of aging: DNA repair declines with advancing age
6. Hayflick limit: Cells could divide only a limited number of times

NERVE MUSCLE PHYSIOLOGY—HIGH YIELD TOPICS

Glial Cells

- Two types: Microglia and microglia
- Microglia: Derived from macrophages, physiologically and embryologically unrelated to other neural cell types
- Macroglia: Oligodendrocytes, Schwann cells, and astrocytes

Neurons

- The human central nervous system (CNS) contains about 10^{11} (100 billion) neurons
- Site of action potentials generation: The initial segment in spinal motor neurons, the initial node of Ranvier in cutaneous sensory neurons
- Location of cell body: Dendritic zone end of the axon (most common). Within the axon (e.g., auditory neurons), Attached to the side of the axon, (e.g. cutaneous neurons)
- Action potentials can be recorded in dendrites
- Dendritic spines: Dynamic structures, produce proteins, which alters the effects of input from individual synapses. Implicated in motivation, learning, and long-term memory

Myelin

- Protein-lipid complex formed by Schwann cells in PNS and oligodendrocytes in CNS
- Sphingomyelin-excellent electrical insulator
- Formed by protein zero (P_0) -mutations in P_0 causes peripheral neuropathies
- Envelops the axon except at nodes of Ranvier (periodic 1-µm constrictions about 1 mm apart)

- Schwann cell forms the myelin between two nodes of Ranvier but oligodendrocytes emit multiple processes that form myelin on many neighboring axons
- Loss of myelin: Multiple sclerosis caused due to the autoimmune attack of myelin leads to leakage of K^+ through voltage-gated channels, hyperpolarization, and failure to conduct action potentials

EXCITATION AND CONDUCTION

- Nonpropagated potentials: Synaptic, generator or electrotonic potentials
- Propogated: Action potentials
- Resting membrane potential in nerve is usually about –70 mV, which is close to the equilibrium potential for K^+
- Intracellular and extracellular K^+ concentrations are the prime determinants of the resting membrane potential

Nerve Action Potential

Action potential	Feature
Depolarization	Na^+ influx
Firing level	After initial 15 mV of depolarization (the threshold) the rate increases. This is firing level
Upstroke phase	Rapid depolarization phase caused by rapid Na^+ influx
Overshoot	Part of action potential in which the membrane potential is positive (above of mV)
Repolarization or down stroke phase	Rapid return of membrane towards RMP. It is due to a. Closing of Na^+ channels; b. Opening of K^+ channels
Hyperpolarization	Membrane potential becomes more -ve than its initial RMP due to late closure of K channels.
After hyperpolarization	Result of K^+ channels remaining open, allowing the continued efflux of K^+ ions

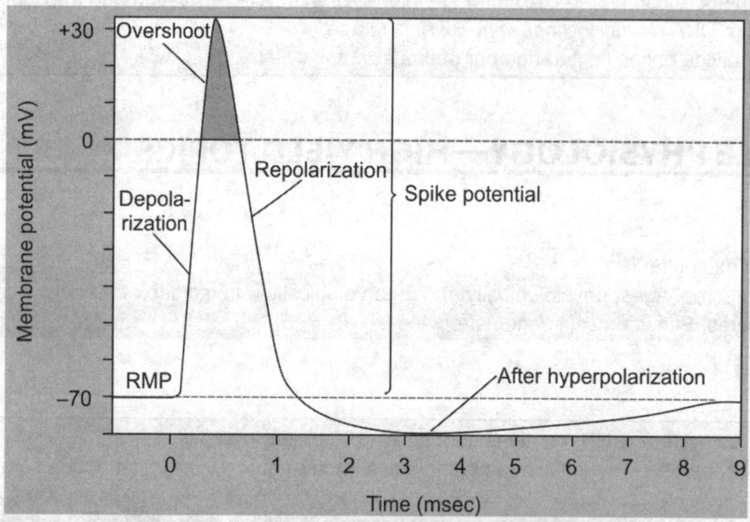

Fig. 2.2: Action potential

- Hyperkalemia: Resting potential moves closer to the threshold for eliciting an action potential (more excitable)
- Hypokalemia: Membrane potential is reduced, neuron hyperpolarized
- Hypocalcemia: Increases the excitability by decreasing the amount of depolarization necessary to initiate action potential
- Hypercalcemia: Stabilize the membrane by decreasing excitability

All or None Character of Action Potential

- Increase in the intensity of a stimulus produce no increment or other change in the action potential as long as the other experimental conditions remain constant
- Constant amplitude and form regardless of the strength of the stimulus if the stimulus is at or above threshold intensity

Saltatory Conduction

'Jumping' of depolarization from node to node in myelinated axons for rapid conduction

Safety Factor for Propagation of Action Potential

- For continued propagation of an impulse to occur, the ratio of action potential to threshold for excitation must be at all times greater than 1
- This 'greater than 1' requirement is called the safety factor for propagation

Neurotrophins

- Produced by astrocytes and transported both anterogradely and retrogradely
- The first neurotrophin to be characterized was NGF- growth and maintenance of cholinergic neurons in the basal forebrain and the striatum
- NGF reduce apoptosis of neurons thereby enhancing survival
- p75 NTR- binds all four neurotrophins with equal affinity. Has a role in apoptosis

Other Growth Factors Trophic to Neurons

- Ciliary neurotrophic factor (CNTF)
- Glial cell line-derived neurotrophic factor (GDNF)
- Leukemia inhibitory factor (LIF)
- Insulin-like growth factor I (IGF-I)
- Transforming growth factor (TGF)
- Fibroblast growth factor (FGF)
- Platelet-derived growth factor (PDGF)

Skeletal Muscle

Structure of Skeletal Muscle

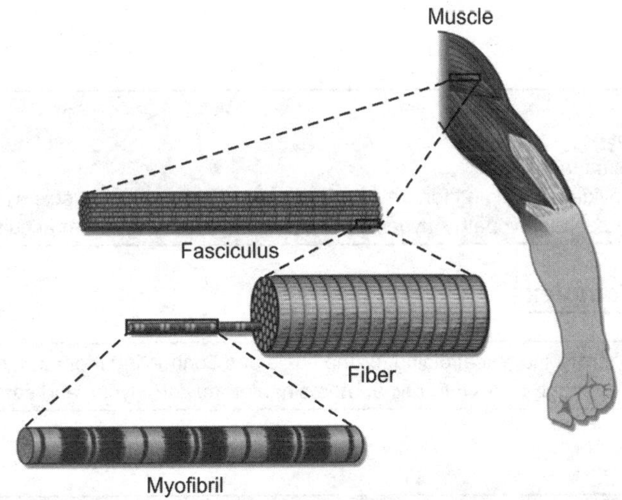

Fig. 2.3: Skeletal muscle structure

- Each muscle is composed of numerous cells called **muscle fibers.**
- A connective tissue layer called the **endomysium** surrounds each of these fibers.
- Each skeletal muscle fiber contains bundles of filaments, called **myofibrils,** running along the axis of the cell.
- Individual muscle fibers are then grouped together into **fascicles,** which are surrounded by another connective tissue layer called the **perimysium.** Within the perimysium are the blood vessels and nerves that supply the individual muscle fibers.
- Finally, fascicles are joined together to form the muscle. The connective tissue sheath that surrounds the muscle is called the **epimysium.**

Skeletal muscle

- Have two types of filaments (thick and thin).
- **Thick-**made of Myosin-II proteins (Two heads and single long tail). The head contains ATP ase activity). Each myosin filament is surrounded by six actin filaments.
- **Thin-**made of Actin, Troponin and Tropomyosin
- TROPONIN: Has 3 sub units-I, T, C.
- TROP-I: Inhibits the interaction of myosin with actin
- TROP-C: Contains the binding sites for the Ca^{2+} that helps to initiate contraction
- TROP-T: Binds troponin components to tropomyosin
- Z line: Divides each myofibril into compartments. The protion of myofibril between two Z line is a sarcomere
- I band: Formed by thin filament mainly actin
- A band: Overlapping of actin and myosin
- H zone: Narrow lighter area at the middle of A band, no actin in this zone
- M line: Transverse line in the middle of H zone. Site of the reversal of polarity of the myosin molecules

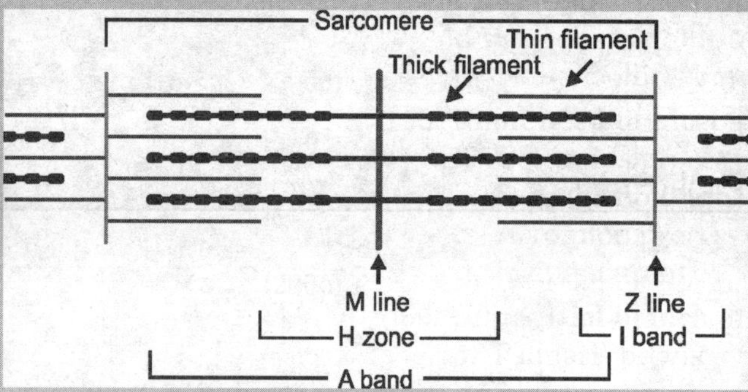

Other Structural Proteins

- Actinin, titin and desmin
- Actinin binds actin to the Z lines
- Desmin-binds Z line to the plasma membrane
- **Titin**-largest known protein, provides scafolding for the sarcomere and also provide muscle with its elasticity
- Mutations in titin leads to dilated cardiomyopathy, hypertrophic cardiomyopathy, tibialis muscular dystrophy

Dystrophin-Glycoprotein Complex

- Adds strength to the muscle by providing a scaffolding for the fibrils and connecting them to the extracellular environment
- Comprises of dystrophin, beta-dystroglycan, syntrophins, merosin, alpha-dystroglycan and sarcoglycan

Sarcotubular System

- Made up of a T system and a sarcoplasmic reticulum
- Triads- arrangement of the central T system with a cistern of the sarcoplasmic reticulum on either side

- **'I' (transverse) tubules:** Penetrate the muscle and opens to the ECF: responsible for rapid transmission of AP
- **'L' (longitudinal) tubules:** Extends throughout the sarcoplasm, no connection to exterior: storage house of Ca^{2+}

Electrical Characteristics of Skeletal Muscle

- The resting membrane potential of skeletal muscle is about–90 mV
- Action potential lasts 2–4 ms
- Conduction velocity–5 m/s
- Absolute refractory period is 1–3 ms

Cardiac Muscle

Has numerous mitochondria, and a high content of myoglobin

35% of the caloric needs of the human heart are provided by carbohydrate, 5% by ketones and amino acids, and 60% by fat

Intercalated disks (occur at Z lines) -helps in effective transfer of contractile force along the axis

Presence of Gap junctions (Functional syncytium)

The T system in cardiac muscle is located at the Z lines (skeletal muscle at A-I junction)

The resting membrane potential of individual mammalian cardiac muscle cells is about –80 mV

Smooth Muscles

- Lacks cross striations. Contains **dense bodies** (Attaches α-actinin to actin) in place of Z lines
- Contains tropomyosin, but lacks troponin
- Has different isoforms of actin and myosin
- Has less extensive sarcoplasmic reticulum and few mitochondria
- Two types—Unitary and multiunit smooth muscles
- Unitary type—Has Many gap junctions (Syncytium). Present in intestine, the uterus, and the ureters
- Multiunit type—few or no gap junctions. Present in iris of the eye. Able to display fine and discrete contraction patterns
- Blood vessels has both types of smooth muscles
- No true RMP. varies between –20 to –65 mV
- Main source of calcium—Extracellular
- Ca^{2+} binds to calmodulin-activates **calmodulin-dependent myosin light chain kinase-** phosphorylates myosin on serine at position 19, increasing its ATPase activity (myosin based)
- Regulation is through **myosin light chain phosphatase**—dephosphorylates myosin (relaxation)
- Relaxation also occurs through endothelium derived relaxating factor (Nitric Oxide)
- Latch bridge mechanism—myosin cross-bridges remain attached to actin for some time after the cytoplasmic Ca^{2+} concentration falls leading to sustained contraction with little expenditure of energy
- Plasticity—If an Unitary smooth muscle is stretched-at first there is increase in tension but the tension gradually decreases, if the muscle is held at the greater length after stretching
- Norepinephrine-decreases the spikes and acetyl choline-increases the spikes in unitary smooth muscles

SYNAPTIC TRANSMISSION

- **Synapse:** The junctions where the axon or some other portion of one cell (the **presynaptic cell**) terminates on the dendrites, soma, or axon of another neuron, muscle or gland
- **Synaptic cleft:** Space between presynaptic and postsynaptic neuron
- **Postsynaptic density:** Ordered complex of specific receptors, binding proteins, and enzymes induced by postsynaptic effects
- **Synaptic vesicles:** Three types—small, clear vesicles-acetylcholine, glycine, GABA, or glutamate; small vesicles with a dense core-catecholamines; and large vesicles with a dense core-neuropeptides
- **Active zones:** Site of discharge of small vesicles. Calcium channels arranged in rows

- Proteins that hold synapses together: **Neurexins**
- Proteins involved in exocytosis of vesicles: **v-snare** protein **synaptobrevin** and t-snare protein **syntaxin**
- Toxins blocking neurotransmitter release: Tetanus toxin and botulinum toxin
- Tetanus toxin: Attaches to **gangliosides** and blocks release of inhibitory transmitters glycine and GABA leading to spastic paralysis
- Botulinum toxin: Toxins A, B, and E-toxic to humans. Toxins A and E cleave synaptosome-associated protein **(SNAP-25)** -a presynaptic membrane protein needed for fusion of synaptic vesicles containing acetylcholine to the terminal membrane. Toxin B-cleaves **synaptobrevin** ultimately leading to flaccid paralysis. BOTOX (botulinum toxin) clinically useful in achalasia and to remove wrinkles in face

EPSP (Extitatory postsynaptic potential)	IPSP (Inhibitory postsynaptic potential)
• Transient partial depolarization • The excitability of the neuron to other stimuli is increased • Due to opening of Na^+ or Ca^{2+} channels	• Transient hyperpolarization • The excitability of the neuron to other stimuli is decreased • Due to opening of Cl^- channels, opening of K^+ channels

- Slow EPSP—due to decreases in K^+ conductance. Latency is 100–500 ms
- Slow IPSPs are due to increases in K^+ conductance. Latency is 100–500 ms
- Presynaptic inhibition—Mediated by GABA acting through $GABA_A$- increases Cl^- conductance and $GABA_B$- increases K^+ conductance
- Renshaw cell inhibition—Neurons inhibiting themselves through negative feedback mechanisms. Neurotransmitter involved is Glycine

Neuromuscular Transmission

- Impulse arriving in the end of the motor neuron—increases the permeability of its endings to Ca^{2+}–Exocytosis of acetylcholine—containing synaptic vesicles—acetylcholine binds to nicotinic cholinergic (NM) receptors—Increases Na^+ and K^+ conductance—End plate potential
- Average human end plate contains about 15–40 million acetylcholine receptors
- On arrival of nerve impulse---Ach released from 60 synaptic vesicles. Each vesicle contains 10, 000 molecules of Ach. This amount is enough to activate about 10 times the number of NM receptors needed to produce a full end plate potential (10-fold safety factor)
- Miniature end plate potential (MEEP): At rest, small quanta (packets) of acetylcholine are released randomly---produces MEEP of 0.5 mV amplitude. size of the quanta of acetylcholine released varies directly with the Ca^{2+} concentration and inversely with the Mg^{2+} concentration

Myasthenia Gravis

- Caused by the formation of circulating antibodies to the muscle type of nicotinic cholinergic **receptors**
- Affected muscles have 70–90% decrease in the number of receptors per end plate

Lambert Eaton Syndrome

- Due to autoimmune attack of the voltage-gated Ca^{2+} channels
- Use of **aminoglycoside antibiotics** also produces a similar syndrome

Denervation supersensitivity: When the motor nerve to skeletal muscle is cut and allowed to degenerate, the muscle gradually becomes extremely sensitive to acetylcholine. This is called denervation hypersensitivity or supersensitivity

NEUROPHYSIOLOGY—HIGH YIELD TOPICS

Dermatomes

- In adults, a given **dorsal root ganglion** supplies a specific cutaneous region, which is called as **dermatome**

For easy Understanding, Dermatomes Represented in Quadrupedal Position

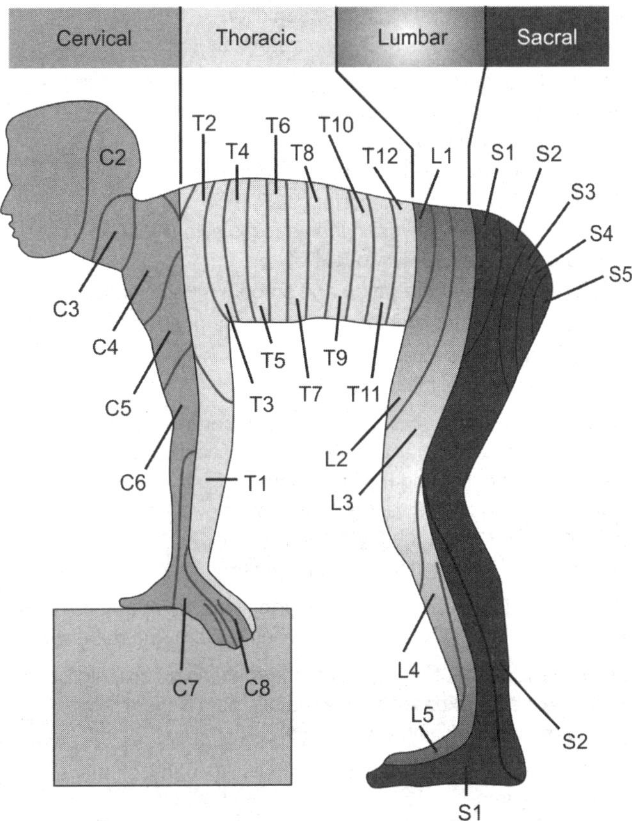

Fig. 2.4: Dermatomes represented in quadrupedal position

Neurotransmitters

Acetylcholine	• Transmitter at—neuromuscular junction, in autonomic ganglia, and in postganglionic parasympathetic, basal forebrain complex, pontomesen-cephalic cholinergic complex • Involved in regulation of sleep-wake states, learning, and memory • Removal—by acetylcholinesterase in the synaptic cleft • Receptors: 2 types i. Muscarinic: (M_1, M_4, and M_5-CNS), (M_2-Heart), (M_3-glands and smooth muscles) ii. Nicotinic: (N_M- neuromuscular junction), (N_N- CNS and autonomic ganglia)
Norepinephrine and epinephrine	• Location- locus coeruleus, spinal cord, cerebellum, paraventricular, supraoptic, and periventricular nuclei of the hypothalamus, the thalamus, the basal telencephalon, neocortex • Synthesised from Tyrosine • Rate limiting enzyme: Tyrosine hydroxylase (subject to feedback inhibition by dopamine and norepinephrine) • Nor-epinephrine-only small-molecule transmitter that is synthesized in synaptic vesicles instead of being transported into the vesicle after its synthesis • phenylethanolamine-N-methyltransferase (PNMT) -Converts Nor epinephrine to epinephrine • Catabolism-Enzymes involved are monoamine oxidase (MAO), catechol-O-methyltransferase (COMT) • MAO isoenzyme form locations: • MAO-**A** in: **A**drenergic peripheral structures, **A**limentary mucosa • MAO-**B** in: Brain, **B**lood platelets • Urinary metabolites- vanil-lylmandelic acid (VMA), 3-methoxy-4-hydroxyphenylglycol (MHPG)

Dopamine	• Location: **Nigrostriatal system** (midbrain substantia nigra to the striatum in the basal ganglia) and **mesocortical system** (ventral tegmental area to nucleus accumbens and limbic subcortical areas • Involved in reward behavior and addiction • Receptors: D_1, D_2, D_3, D_4, D_5 (All are metabotropic).
Serotonin	• Present in highest concentration in blood platelets and in the gastrointestinal tract • Also in midline raphé nuclei • Synthesized from tryptophan • Rate limiting enzyme: Tryptophan hydroxylase • Reuptake: Serotonin transporter (SERT) • Urinary metabolite-5-hydroxyindoleacetic acid (5-HIAA) • Receptors-7 types (5-HT_1 to 5-HT_7) • 5-HT_{2A}— platelet aggregation and smooth muscle contraction • 5-HT_3— gastrointestinal tract and the area postrema-related to vomiting • 5-HT_4— facilitate secretion and peristalsis • 5-HT_6 and 5-HT_7—limbic system
Histamine	• Location—gastric mucosa, mast cells, tuberomammillary nucleus of the posterior hypothalamus • Formed by decarboxylation of the amino acid histidine • Receptors—H_1, H_2, and H_3, H_4 • Involved in—arousal, sexual behavior, blood pressure, drinking, pain thresholds, regulation of anterior pituitary hormone secretion • H_4- regulating cells of the immune system
ATP	• Colocalized in nor-adrenergic postganglionic sympathetic neurons • Neurotransmitter in autonomic nervous system and habenula
Substance P	• Location: Primary afferent neurons in the spinal cord, nigrostriatal system, hypothalamus • Responsible for axon reflex, peristalsis, pain transmission • Receptors: Neurokinin receptors (NK_1-NK_3)
Glutamate	• Secreted by the presynaptic terminals in many of the sensory pathways entering the central nervous system • Responsible for 75% of the excitatory transmission in the CNS • Excitotoxicity—excessive levels of glutamate during ischemia, anoxia, hypoglycemia, or trauma-Death of neurons (massive Ca^{2+} influx) • Involved in learning and memory—synaptic plasticity, long-term potentiation • Receptors—AMPA, Kainate, NMDA, mGLUR
GABA	• Secreted by nerve terminals in the spinal cord, cerebellum, basal ganglia, and many areas of the cortex • Vesicular GABA transporter (VGAT) - transports GABA and glycine into secretory vesicles • Receptors- $GABA_A$, $GABA_B$, and $GABA_C$
Glycine	• Secreted mainly at synapses in the spinal cord • Facilitate pain transmission by NMDA receptors in the dorsal horn • Acts by increasing Cl–conductance (Like GABA)
Gas neurotransmitters	• Nitric oxide and carbon monoxide • They do not bind to receptors, but they activate enzymes involved in second messenger systems

Sensory Physiology

Modality	Stimulus Energy	Receptor Cell Types
Touch	Tap, flutter 5–40 Hz	Meissner corpuscles
Touch	Motion	Hair follicle receptors
Touch	Deep pressure, vibration 60–300 Hz	Pacinian corpuscles
Touch	Touch, pressure	Merkel cells
Touch	Sustained pressure	Ruffini corpuscles

Contd...

Contd...

Modality	Stimulus Energy	Receptor Cell Types
Proprioception	Stretch	Muscle spindles
Proprioception	Tension	Golgi tendon organ
Temperature	Thermal	Cold and warm receptors
Pain	Chemical, thermal, and mechanical	Polymodal receptors or chemical, thermal, and mechanical nociceptors
Vision	Light	Rods, cones
Hearing	Sound	Hair cells (cochlea)
Balance	Angular acceleration	Hair cells (semicircular canals)
Balance	Linear acceleration, gravity	Hair cells (otolith organs)
Smell	Chemical	Olfactory sensory neuron
Taste	Chemical	Taste buds

Pain Physiology

Pain	• **First pain (epicritic pain)**—Activation of Aδ fibers, which release **glutamate,** is responsible for this • **Slow pain (protopathic pain)**—Activation of C fibers, which release a combination of glutamate and **substance P,** is responsible for this • Receptor channels: 1. **Transient receptor potential** (TRP) channels. **TRPV1**—activated by intense heat, acids, and chemicals such as capsaicin. **TRPA1** receptors-activated by Noxious mechanical, cold, and chemical stimuli 2. **Acid sensing ion channel (ASIC) receptors**—activated by pH changes **Purinergic receptors**—ATP acts on it 3. **Tyrosine receptor kinase A (TrkA)—activated by nerve growth factor (NGF)** • Hyperalgesia: Exaggerated response to a noxious stimulus • Allodynia: Sensation of pain in response to a normally innocuous stimulus • **Two components of pain pathways:** 1. From VPL nuclei in the thalamus, fibers project to SI and SII. Pathway responsible for the **discriminative** aspect of pain—the **neospinothalamic tract** 2. **Paleospinothalamic tract**—the pathway that includes synapses in the brain stem reticular formation and centrolateral thalamic nucleus projects to the frontal lobe, limbic system, and insula. This pathway mediates the **motivational-affect** component of pain.
Modulation of pain transmission	1. **Gate-control mechanism:** – Proposed by Melzack and wall – Simultaneous activation of innocuous cutaneous mechanoreceptors—reduce the responsiveness of dorsal horn neurons to their input from nociceptive afferent terminals – This is the rationale behind the use of transcutaneous electrical nerve stimulation (TENS) 2. **Opiod peptides:** – Endogenous opioid peptides—enkephalin, endorphin and dynorphin – Action on postsynaptic opioid receptors—increase in K^+ conductance – Action on presynaptic opioid receptors—decrease in Ca^{2+} influx, resulting in a decrease in release of glutamate and substance P 3. **Endogenous analgesic system:** – Periaqueductal gray (PAG)—projects to nucleus raphé magnus and rostral ventromedial medulla – Neurons in both of these regions project to the dorsal horn of the spinal cord—release serotonin and norepinephrine which inhibits the activity of dorsal horn neurons that receive input from nociceptive afferent fibres – Locus coeruleus—Releases norepinephrine which modulates pain transmission
Stress induced analgesia	• Release of endogenous cannabinoids such as 2-arachidonoylglycerol (2AG) and anandamide • acts on CB_1 and CB_2 receptors • CB_1—accounts for the euphoric actions of cannabinoids • CB_2—expressed in activated microglia. Resposible for analgesia

Vision:

Rods (RoD: Dim light), Photopigment-Rhodopsin
Cones (Cones: Colour), Photopsin (vision in bright light)

Phototransduction in Rods and Cones

Incident light → Structural change in the retinal of photopigment → Conformational change of photopigment → Activation of transducin → Activation of phosphodiesterase → Decreased Intracellular cGMP → Closure of Na^+ channels → Hyperpolarization → Decreased release of Synaptic transmitter (Glutamate) → Response in bipolar cells and other neural elements

Neural Functions of Retina

Horizontal cells	• Lateral inhibition to enhance visual contrast is the primary function • The outputs of the horizontal cells are always inhibitory
Bipolar cells	• Two types – Depolarising bipolar cell – Hyperpolarising bipolar cell • Provides second mechanism for lateral inhibition, in addition to horizontal cell mechanism • Provides a mechanism for seperating contrast borders in the visual image
Amacrine cells	• Transmits signals from bipolar cells to ganglionic cell • Respond to movement of a spot across the retina in a specific direction and said to be directional sensitive • Help analyze visual signals before they ever leave the retina
Ganglion cells	• These are the only output neuron of the retina, their axons form the optic nerve
Interplexiform cell	• Transmits signals in the retrograde direction from the inner plexiform layer to the outer plexiform layer • These signals are inhibitory • Their role may be to help control the degree of contrast in the visual image

Melanopsin

- Few retinal ganglion cells contain melanopsin rather than rhodopsin or cone pigments
- Project to the suprachiasmatic nuclei of the hypothalamus
- Involved in circardian rhythms

Lateral geniculate body	• Fibres from ipsilateral hemiretina—ends in lamina 2, 3, 5 • Fibres from contralateral nasal retina—ends in lamina 1, 4, 6
From lateral geniculate nucleus to visual cortex	• Two pathways • Magnocellular pathway—From layer 1 and 2. Carries signal for detection of movement, depth and flickers • Parvocellular pathway—From layers 3, 4, 5, 6. Carries signals for color vision, texture, shape and fine details
Blobs and the visual pathway	• Layers 2 and 3 contain a high concentration of 'cytochrome oxidase' called as blobs and are concerned with colour processing

Types of cones: Short wave/blue sensitive, Medium wave/green sensitive, Long wave/red sensitive

Sense of Hearing

External ear	Pinna, external auditory meatus, tympanic membrane
Middle ear	• Auditory ossicles—malleus, incus, and stapes • Communicates with the nasopharynx by the eustachian tube, allowing air pressure to be equalized on both sides of the tympanic membrane

	• Functions of middle ear – Impedance matching to amplify sound – Attenuation reflex- caused by contraction of the tensor tympani and stapedius muscle to protect cochlea from loud sounds. This reflex reduces the intensity of lower frequency sound transmission by 30–40 decibels – Efficient transmission-critical damping of tympanic membrane to mask low frequency sounds and effectively transmit sounds in the vocal frequency range
Inner ear '**Outer** cells are **Out of the brain. Inner** cells are Into the Brain' Outer hair cells are motor efferents to amplify signal Inner hair cells are sensory afferents that actually pick up the sound	• Comprises of the utricle, saccule, semicircular canals and the cochlear duct • Endolymph-fluid inside the vestibular labyrinth. Rich in K^+ • Perilymph- fluid outside the vestibular labyrinth. Rich in Na^+ • Organ of Corti- located in the basilar membrane and contains inner and outer hair cells • Prestin-motor protein of outer hair cells. • Spiral ganglion- contains cell bodies of the auditory nerve whose peripheral axons innervate hair cells on the organ of corti • High-frequency sound waves cause maximum displacement of the basilar membrane and stimulation of hair cells at the base of the cochlea • Low-frequency sound waves maximally stimulate hair cells at the apex of the cochlea
Auditory transduction	• E-eighth nerve • C-cochlear nuclei • O-olivary complex • L-lateral lemniscus • I-Inferior colliculi • M-medial geniculate body • A-auditory cortex – Auditory cortex -located on the superior temporal gyrus of the temporal lobe – Planum temporal-located between Heschl's gyrus (transverse temporal gyrus) and the sylvian fissure. This area is larger in the left than in the right. involved in language-related auditory processing

Vestibular Apparatus

- Utricle: One of the vestibular organs that responds to movements of the head in the horizontal plane
- Saccule: One of the vestibular organs that responds to movements of the head in the vertical plane
- Semicircular canals: A set of 3 semicircular canals, which are part of the vestibular system, and respond to rotational movements in 3 planes
- Maculae: Sensory organs of the utricle and saccule for detecting orientation of the head with respect to gravity.

Central connections of the vestibular system

- The vestibular nerve carries information from the utricle, saccule and semi-circular canals to the brain stem, after passing through Scarpa's ganglion in the internal auditory canal
- These vestibular afferents connect with the vestibular nucleus in the brain stem, which has 4 parts: the lateral (Deiter's nucleus), medial (Schwalbe's nucleus), superior (Bechterew's nucleus), descending (spinal vestibular nucleus).

Smell

Olfactory epithelium	• Comprises of: – Bipolar olfactory sensory neurons – Supporting (sustentacular) cells – Basal stem cells – Bowman glands (mucus secreting) – Odorant-binding proteins (OBP): concentrate the odorants and transfer them to the receptors, sequester odorants-for clearance
Olfactory sensory neuron	• Contains 6–12 cilia • Contains odorant receptors

Olfactory bulb	• Contains excitatory neurons: Mitral and tufted cells (glutamate • Inhibitory neurons (periglomerular cells and granule cells (GABA) • Anatomically discrete synaptic units called as olfactory glomeruli
Olfactory cortex	• Anterior olfactory nucleus, olfactory tubercle, piriform cortex, amygdala (for emotional response), entorhinal cortex (for olfactory memory) • Cortical representation of olfaction is asymmetric (greater on right)

Taste

Taste buds	• Contains 4 types of cells: – Basal cells – Dark cells (type I) – Light cells (type II) – Intermediate cells (type III) • Has between 50 and 100 taste cells • Receptors couple to the heterotrimeric G protein, gustducin • Fungiform papillae- most numerous near the tip of the tongue • Circumvallate papillae- arranged in a V on the back of the tongue • Foliate papillae-Back of tongue
Taste modalities	1. Sweet: T1R3 family of GPCR 2. Salt: ENaC Channels 3. Sour: Enac channels, HCN, a hyperpolarization-activated cyclic nucleotide-gated cation channel 4. Bitter: T2R family 5. Umami: mGluR4
Taste pathways	• Anterior 2/3rd of tongue-chorda tympanic branch of facial nerve • Posterior third-Glossopharyngeal nerve • Pharynx-Vagus nerve • Unite in the gustatory portion of the nucleus of the tractus solitarius (NTS) → Thalamus → anterior insula and the frontal operculum in the ipsilateral cerebral cortex

Motor System

Muscle spindles	• Intrafusal muscle fibers-pure sensory function • Extra fusal fibres-the regular contractile units of the muscle • Two types of intrafusal fibers- nuclear bag fiber (dynamic and static) and nuclear chain fiber
Sensory endings in spindle	• There are 2 kinds of sensory endings in each spindle. A single primary (group Ia) ending and up to eight secondary (group II) endings • The Ia afferent fiber wraps around the center of the dynamic and static nuclear bag fibers and nuclear chain fibers • Group II sensory fibers are located adjacent to the centers of the static nuclear bag and nuclear chain fibers; these fibers do not innervate the dynamic nuclear bag fibers • Dynamic response: Ia afferents are very sensitive to the velocity of the change in muscle length during a stretch • Static response: Activity of group Ia and II afferents provide information on steady-state length of the muscle
Motor nerve supply	• γ-motor neurons (constitute about 30% of the fibers) • Two types of γ-motor neurons: dynamic-supplies the dynamic nuclear bag fibers and static- supply the static nuclear bag fibers and the nuclear chain fibers • Activation of dynamic γ-motor neurons increases the dynamic sensitivity of the group Ia endings • Activation of the static γ-motor neurons increases the tonic level of activity in both group Ia and II endings, decreases the dynamic sensitivity of group Ia afferents, and can prevent silencing of Ia afferents during muscle stretch
α–γ **co-activation**	• Both α- and γ-motor neurons are activated- In response to descending excitatory input • Intrafusal and extrafusal fibers shorten together, and spindle afferent activity can occur throughout the period of muscle contraction • Responsible for reflexively adjustment of α-motor neuron discharge

Reflexes

- Monosynaptic reflexes: The simplest reflex arc with a single synapse between the afferent and efferent neuron. The best known example; the stretch reflex
- Polysynaptic reflexes: Reflex arcs in which interneurons are interposed between the afferent and efferent neurons

Withdrawal Reflex

- Typical polysynaptic reflex that occurs in response to a noxious stimulus to the skin or subcutaneous tissues and muscle
- The response is flexor muscle contraction and inhibition of extensor muscles, so that the body part stimulated is flexed and withdrawn from the stimulus
- Withdrawal reflexes are **prepotent**, that is, they pre-empt the spinal pathways from any other reflex activity taking place at the moment

Crossed Extensor Response

- When a strong stimulus is applied to a limb, the response includes not only flexion and withdrawal of that limb but also extension of the opposite limb. This is called Crossed extensor response and is properly part of the withdrawal reflex

Inverse Stretch Reflex

- The relaxation response to strong stretch is called the inverse stretch reflex
- The receptor is the - **Golgi tendon organ** (net like collection of knobby nerve endings among the fascicles of a tendon). There are 3–25 muscle fibers per tendon organ
- Regulates muscle force (or tension)

Postural Reflexes

Reflex	Stimulus	Receptor	Centre
Stretch reflex	Stretch	Muscle spindle	Spinal cord, medulla
Positive supporting reaction	Contact with palm or sole	Proprioceptors in extensors	Spinal cord
Negative supporting reacting	Stretch	Proprioceptors in extensors	Spinal cord
Tonic labyrinthine reflex	Gravity	Otolith organs	Medulla
Tonic neck reflex	Head turned to side/up/down	Neck proprioceptors	Medulla
Labyrinthine righting reflex	Gravity	Otolitth organs	Midbrain
Neck righting reflex	Stretch of neck muscles	Muscle spindle	Midbrain
Body on head righting reflex	Pressure on side of body	Exteroceptors	Midbrain
Body on body righting reflex	Pressure on side of body	Exteroceptors	Midbrain
Optical righting reflex	Visual cues	Eyes	Cortex
Vestibular placing reactions	Linear acceleration	Receptors in utricle and saccule	Cortex
Visual placing reactions	Visual cues	Eyes	Cortex
Hopping reactions	Lateral displacement while standing	Muscle spindle	Cerebral cortex

- All righting reflexes are integrated at midbrain except **optical righting reflex,** which is integrated at cortex

Motor Cortex

Primary motor cortex	• In precentral gyrus of the frontal lobe • Cortical representation of body parts- **motor homunculus** • Executes the movements • Representation of each body part is proportional in size to the skill with which the part is used in fine, voluntary movement • The areas involved in speech and hand movements are especially large

Supplementary motor area	• In superior bank of the cingulate sulcus • Projects to the primary motor cortex • Involved primarily in organizing or planning motor sequences
Premotor cortex	• Located anterior to the precentral gyrus • Receives input from sensory regions of the parietal cortex and projects to M1, the spinal cord, and the brain stem reticular formation • Concerned with setting posture at the start of a planned movement and with getting the individual prepared to move • Involved in control of proximal limb muscles needed to orient the body for movement

Cerebellum

Structure	• Weighs only 10% as much as the cerebral cortex, but its surface area is about 75% of that of the cerebral cortex • Superior cerebellar peduncle-fibers from deep cerebellar nuclei--project to the brain stem, red nucleus, and thalamus • Middle cerebellar peduncle-afferent fibers from the contralateral pontine nuclei • Inferior cerebellar peduncle-afferent fibers from the brain stem and spinal cord and efferent fibers to the vestibular nuclei
Organisation	• Four deep nuclei: **D**endate, **G**lobose, **E**mboliform, **F**astigial (Mn. **DEFG**) • Globose and Emboliform nuclei together are known as the interpositus nucleus
Divisions of cerebellum	• **Anatomical division** – Flocculo-nodular lobe – Anterior lobe – Posterior lobe • **Phylogenetic division** – Archicerebellum – Paleocerebellum – Neocerebellum • **Functional division** – Vestibulocerebellum – Spinocerebellum – Cerebrocerebellum (Neocerebellum)
Histology	• **Layers** – External molecular layer – Middle Purkinje cell layer – Internal granule cell layer • **Cell types (Mn. SPB-G^2)** – **P**urkinje cell – **G**ranule cell – **B**asket cell – **S**tellate cell – **G**olgi cell
Input to the cerebellar cortex	• **Climbing fibres** – Arise from the region of inferior olivary nucleus in medulla. – They make synaptic connections with Purkinje cells. – Climbing fibres produce high frequency bursts or complex spikes. – They play a major role in motor learning. – Carry proprioceptive impulses from all over the body • **Mossy fibres** – Arise from different centres in brainstem and spinal cord. – They make synaptic connection with Purkinje cells. – They produce simple spikes.

	– They also synapse with granule cells. – Axons of granule cells bifurcate. They excite the Purkinje cells through parallel fibres. – Carry proprioceptive input from all parts of the body and cerebral cortex
Output from cerebellar cortex	• Output of the cerebellar cortex is from Purkinje cells. These outputs are always inhibitory. • The output projects to deeper cerebellar nuclei and vestibular nucleus. • The inhibitory inputs influence the output from the cerebellum to regulate range, direction and rate of movement. • Gamma aminobutyric acid (GABA) is the neurotransmitter
Functions	**Vestibulo cerebellum** (Archi cerebellum) • It is concerned with maintenance of balance and equilibrium. • It is responsible for regulating the stability of head and body in space. • It adjusts the tone of the trunk muscle. • Controls the ocular movements and other postural reflexes. **Spino cerebellum** (Paleocerebellum) • Maintains the posture and helps in execution of gross movements. • It controls the interplay between the agonist and antagonist group of muscles • It is essential for the control of rapid muscular activities like running and talking **Cerebro cerebellum** (Neocerebellum) • Controls fine, highly precise and coordinated movements. • It is involved in programming of voluntary and skilled movements. • It plays a major role in the timing of the motor activities and rapid progression from one movement to the next
Effects of cerebellar lesions	• Ataxia • Hypotonia or atonia • Dysmetria • Dysdiadokokinesia • Decomposition of movement • Staccato speech or slurring speech. • Pendular knee jerk • Intention tremors • Nystagmus

Basal Ganglia

Structure	Deep telecephalic nuclei (noncortical gray matter): • Caudate and putamen = striatum • Globus pallidus (also known as 'paleo-striatum') Associated nuclei: • Diencephalon: ventral anterior thalamic nucleus, ventral lateral, thalamic nuc, central median nuc, subthalamic nuc • Mesencephalon: substantia nigra
Connections	Caudate and putamen: • Caudate = projections mostly from prefrontal, temporal, parietal assoc areas • Putamen = from motor, somatosensory cortices • Inhibitory to Globus pallidus (GABAergic) Globus pallidus: • External segment (GPe) - inhibitory (GABA) to subthalamic nucleus • Internal segment (GPi) - inhibitory (GABA) to VL/VA, CM of thalamus (balances excitatory input from dentate nucleus to cerebellum) Subthalamic nucleus: • Excitatory to internal globus pallidus (GPi) (inhibits thalamus → cortex) • Receives strong excitatory projection from motor cx (net inhibition of cortex)

	Substantia nigra pars compacta- Dopaminergic efferents to caudate/putamen • D1 = excitatory, D2 = inhibitory • Projects to pallidum
Pathways	Direct pathway: • Net excitatory effect on cortex Indirect pathway: • Net inhibitory effect on cortex
Applied aspects	Damage to basal ganglia—classical symptoms: • Increased motor tone—rigidity • Dyskinesias-tremors, other involuntary movement • Bradykinesia/Akinesia-slowing/ almost absent voluntary movement Hemiballismus • Damage to subthalamic nucleus or its connections to GPi (unilateral) • Involuntary, irregular flinging of contralateral extremity (usually upper) Huntington's disease • Early degeneration of the striatum • Involuntary movements 'choreiform'- writhing Parkinson's disease • Damage to SNpc (depletion of DA in striatum) • Rigidity and tremor, brady/akinesia • Reflects disruption of cortical-basal ganglia-cortical loop: 1. Direct pathway: loss of DA1 → decrease inhibition of GPi. . . less net excitation of cortex 2. Indirect pathway: loss of DA2 → more inhibition less net excitation of cortex 3. Result is akinesia – Imbalance of excitatory (D1) and inhibitory (D2) effects of pathway→ treat by restoring balance: - Increasing efficacy of dopamine release (administer L- DOPA) - Lesions to block GPi/STN activity - Transplant dopaminergic neurons

Cerebral dominance	
Dominant (categorical) hemisphere	**Representational hemisphere**
Functions: • Understanding and expression of speech and ideas • Categorization • Symbolization	**Functions:** • Spatio-temporal relations • Identification of form of objects • Recognition of faces • Recognition of musical themes
Lesions: Language disorders	Lesions: Asterognosis and Agnosia

- Hemispheric specialization is related to handedness
- Handedness appears to be genetically determined

Right-handed individuals

- 96%—left hemisphere is dominant
- 4%—right hemisphere is dominant.

Left-handed individuals

- 70%—left hemisphere is dominant
- 15%—right hemisphere is dominant
- 15%—no clear lateralization.

Hypothalamus

Functions	Integrating area of hypothalamus
Increased ECF osmolarity (thirst)	Osmoreceptors-Anterior hypothalamus
Response to heat	Anterior hypothalamus
Response to cold	Posterior hypothalamus
Emotion	Dorsal and posterior hypothalamus
Circadian rhythm	Suprachiasmatic nucleus
Gn RH secretion	Arcuate nucleus
TSH (vai TRH secretion)	Paraventricular and neighboring nuclei
Prolactin via PRH and PIH	Arcuate nucleus
Oxytocin release	Paraventricular nucleus (mainly)
ADH release	Supra optic nucleus (mainly)
Satiety centre	Ventro medial nucleus
Feeding centre	Lateral nucleus
Sexual behaviour	Anterior ventral hypothalamus plus, in the male, piriform cortex

CIRCUMVENTRICULAR ORGANS (Mn-SOAP-M)

- Posterior pituitary
- Median eminence
- Area postrema
- Organum vasculosum of the lamina terminalis
- Subfornical organ

- The circumventricular organs surround the cerebral ventricles and lack a blood–brain barrier
- The subfornical organ and the organum vasculosum are involved in thirst

Reciprocal Inhibition

- When a stretch reflex excites one muscle, it often simultaneously inhibits the antagonist muscles
- This is the phenomenon of reciprocal inhibition, and the neuronal circuit that causes this reciprocal relation is called reciprocal innervation

Cord 'Righting' Reflexes

- When a spinal animal is laid on its side, it will make uncoordinated movements trying to raise itself to the standing position. This is called the Cord 'Righting' Reflex
- Such a reflex demonstrates that some relatively complex reflexes associated with posture are integrated in the spinal card

Decerebration

- The elimination of cerebral function by cutting across the brain stem

Sherringtonian Rigidity

- Decerebration by cutting across the brain stem at the level of the superior colliculi

Ischemic Rigidity

- Decerebration by blocking or ligating the basilar arteries

Motor Homunculus

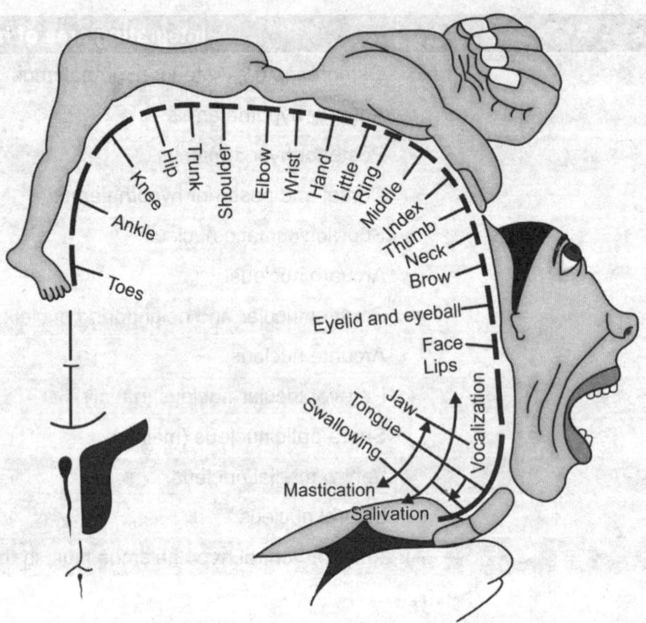

Fig. 2.5: Motor homunculus

CARDIOVASCULAR PHYSIOLOGY-HIGH YIELD TOPICS

Location of SA node	Junction of the superior vena cava with the right atrium
Location of AV node	Right posterior portion of the interatrial septum
Fibres connecting SA node to AV node	Anterior, middle (tract of Wenckebach), and posterior (tract of thorel) tracts Bachmann's bundle- connects the right and left atria
Cardiac output	5 L/min
Stroke volume	70 ml
Cardiac index	3.2 L/min/m^2
End-diastolic ventricular volume	130 ml
End-systolic ventricular volume	50 ml
Ejection fraction	Percentage of the end-diastolic Ventricular volume that is ejected with each stroke, is about 65%
Total electromechanical systole (QS_2)	QS_2 is the period from the onset of the QRS complex to the closure of the aortic valves
Left ventricular ejection time (LVET)	Period from the beginning of the carotid pressure rise to the dicrotic notch
Preejection period (PEP)	Difference between QS_2 and LVET and represents the time for the electrical as well as the mechanical events that precede systolic ejection
PEP/LVET ratio	0.35
Normal arm to tongue circulation time	15 s

Properties of ventricular myocyte	Pacemaker potentials
• Resting membrane potential is –90 mV • Action potential phases:	• Resting membrane potential fluctuates between –60 and –40 mV • Initial part of pacemaker potential-due to the channel activated following hyperpolarization (h channel), also called as 'funny current' (permeable to both Na^+ and K^+)

Contd...

Contd...

Properties of ventricular myocyte	Pacemaker potentials
1. Rapid depolarization (phase 0) - rapidly opening Na^+ channels 2. Rapid repolarization (phase 1) - inactivation of Na^+ channels 3. Plateau (phase 2) - Ca^{2+} influx through more slowly opening Ca^{2+} channels 4. Return to the resting membrane potential (phase 4) - net K^+ efflux	• Later part- (I_{Ca}) due to opening of T channels completes the prepotential, and I_{Ca} due to opening of L channels produces the impulse • Repolarisation-K^+channels • The action potentials in the SA and AV nodes are largely due to Ca^{2+}, with no contribution by Na^+ influx • Reduced slope of the prepotential- after vagal stimulation via M_2 muscarinic receptors which increases the K^+ conductance • Increased spontaneous discharge- after sympathetic stimulation. Norepinephrine via β_1 receptors resulting in the increase in intracellular cAMP which facilitates the opening of L channels

Conduction speeds in cardiac tissue: Purkinje system **(Highest)** - Conduction Rate 4 m/s

Tissue	Rate of impulse generation
S. A. Node	70–80/min
A. V. Node	40–60/min
Bundle of His	40/min
Purkinje fibres	24/min

First of the heart to be depolarized: left endocardial surface of the inter ventricular septum

Last part of the heart to be depolarized:

- Postero basal portion of left ventricle
- Pulmonary conus
- Upper most portion of the septum

	Depolarization	Repolarization
Single ventricular muscle fiber	From endocardium to epicardium	From endocardium to epicardium
Whole heart	From endocardium to epicardium	From epicardium to endocardium

Electrocardiogram (ECG)

Intervals	Normal duration in secs		Events in the heart
	Average	Range	
P wave			Atrial depolarization
PR interval	0.18	0.12–0.20	Atrial depolarization and conduction through AV node
QRS interval	0.08	0.08–0.10	Ventricular depolarization and atrial repolarization
QT interval	0.40	0.40–0.43	Ventricular depolarization and ventricular repolarisation
AT interval	0.32		Ventricular repolarization

Einthoven's law:	Lead II = lead I + lead III
Kirchoff's law	Lead I + lead II + lead III=0
Normal cardiac axis	Between–30 degrees to +110 degrees
Standard limb leads (bipolar)	Lead I, II and III
Augmented limb leads (unipolar)	aVR, aVL, aVF
Chest leads (unipolar)	V_1, V_2, V_3, V_4, V_5, V_6

Generalizations for Leads in Normal ECG

aVR	All the deflections are negative
aVL/aVF	Predominantly positive or biphasic
V1, V2	No Q wave, deep S wave
V3, V4	Biphasic
V5, V6	Small Q wave, Tall R wave
Lead I, II, III	All positive deflection, largest in lead II

His Bundle ECG

- Studying the electrical events of AV node, Bundle of His and Purkinje system in a patient with heart block by placing catheter with electrode through a vein

Wave	Significance	Interval	Significance	Duration
A wave	AV node activation	PA	Conduction time from the SA node to the AV node	27 ms
H spike	His bundle transmission	AH	AV nodal conduction time	92 ms
V deflection	Ventricular depolarization	HV	Conduction in the bundle of his and the bundle branches	43 ms

Heart Block

Incomplete heart block	• First-degree heart block- all the atrial impulses reach the ventricles but the PR interval is abnormally long • Second-degree heart block- not all atrial impulses are conducted to the ventricles. PR interval lengthens progressively until a ventricular beat is dropped **(Wenckebach phenomenon).**
Complete heart block	• Third degree heart block- conduction from the atria to the ventricles is com-pletely interrupted • Ventricles beat at a low rate **(idioventricular rhythm)** -as low as 15 beats/min leads to Stokes–Adams syndrome- cerebral ischemia causes dizziness and fainting

Electrolyte Abnormalities

Hyponatremia	• Low-voltage electrocardiographic complexes
Hyperkalemia	• The appearance of tall peaked T waves, prolongation of the QRS complexes, heart stops in diastole
Hypokalemia	• Prolongation of the PR interval, prominent U waves, T wave inversion
Hypercalcemia	• Plasma calcium level is rarely high enough to affect the heart • Heart stops in systole **(calcium rigor)**
Hypocalcemia	• Prolongation of the ST segment and QT interval

Cardiac Cycle

- The cardiac events that occur from the beginning of one heartbeat to the beginning of the next are called the cardiac cycle

Phase	Ventricle	Atrium	Total duration of cardiac cycle 0.8 Sec
Systole	0.27 sec	0.1 sec	
Diastole	0.53 sec	0.7 sec	

Atrial systole	• Duration-0.1 s • Follows impulse generation in the S. A. node • Proples 30% of additional blood into the ventricles

Ventricular systole	• Duration-0.27 s 1. Isometric contraction: 0.05 sec: - Ventricles contract and the pressure exceeds the arterial pressure - Closure of AV Valves → first heart sound - Bulging of AV valves into the atrium 2. Ventricular systole proper: (0.25 sec) - Rapid ejection phase: (0.1 sec) - 2/3rd of the stroke volume is ejected, Intra ventricular pressure rises to the maximum, AV valves come back to original position and a sharp fall in atrial pressure occurs - Slow ejection phase (0.15 sec)
Ventricular diastole	• Duration-0.5 s 1. Proto diastole: (0.04 sec): Ventricular pressure drops more rapidly. Closure of semilunar valves → second heart sound 2. Isometric relaxation: (0.08 sec): Initial part of ventricular diastole. Intraventricular pressure drops, ventricular muscle continues to relax without change in the ventricular volume 3. Ventricular diastole proper: passive filling of ventricles (70%) 4. Initial rapid filling phase: opening of AV valves and continued relaxation of ventricles 5. Slow filling phase (diastasis): continuous venous return filling both atrium and ventricles
Atrial Diastole	• Duration-0.7 • Atrial muscle relaxes and the pressure gradually increases due to venous return

Valvular events	Cardiac events	ECG	JVP
Opening of AV valve	End of isometric relaxation phase	End of T wave	V-Y descent
Closure of AV valve	End of diastole	Later half of R wave	End of X descent
Opening of semilunar valve	End of isometric contraction	ST segment	Peak of C wave
Closure of semilunar valve	Beginning of diastole	Later half of T wave	

Arterial Pulse

Rate of travel:

- Aorta: 4 m/s
- Large arteries: 8 m/s
- Small arteries: 16 m/s

Waves in arterial pulse	
Ascending limb/Anacrotic or primary limb	Rise in pressure during systole
Descending limb/Catacrotic limb	Fall in pressure during diastole
Percussion wave (P wave)	Ejection phase of ventricular systole
Tidal wave (T wave)	Falling blood column during slow ejection phase
Dicrotic notch (N)	Closure of Aortic valve, marks the end of ventricular systole
Dicrotic wave (D)	Rebound of blood column from closed aortic valve

Waves in JVP	
A wave	**A**trial systole
C wave	Bulging of tricuspid valve into the right atrium during isovolumic ventricular **c**ontraction
V wave	Filling of the right atrium by **v**enous return
X decent	Atrial relaxation and downward displacement of closed tricuspid valve during ventricular contraction
Y descent	Blood flow from RA to RV

Various Pressures

	Diastole	Systole
Right Atrium	0	5 mm Hg
Right Ventricle	0–5 mm Hg	15–30 mm Hg
Pulmonary Artery	10 mm Hg	15–30 mm Hg
Left Atrium	4 mm Hg	12 mm Hg
Left Ventricle	4–12 mm Hg	90–140 mm Hg
Aorta	60–90 mm Hg	90–140 Hg

Heart Sounds

First Heart Sound	Second Heart Sound	Third Heart Sound	Fourth Heart Sound
Due to closure of AV valves	Due to closure of semilunar valves	Due to vibration of the ventricle and turbulence of blood flow	Produced by atrial systole
Marks the onset of ventricular systole	Marks the onset of ventricular diastole	Rapid filling phase of ventricle	Due to ventricular filling
• Continuous sound • Lasts 0.14–0.17 sec • Audible better at tricuspid and mitral areas • Coincides with 'R' wave of ECG • Dull, prolonged, soft, low-pitched sound (LUB)	• Split sound • Last 0.1 to 0.14 sec • Audible better at aortic and pulmonary areas • Coincides with end of 'T' wave of ECG • Short, sharp, high-pitched sound (DUB)	• Low pitched sound • Lasts < 0.1 sec • **Audible In** – 30% of normal population – MI and -Heart filure – Cardiomyopathy – Ventricular hypertrophy	• Also called atrial sound • Low-pitched sound • **Audible in** – MI – Heart failure

Methods of Measuring Cardiac Output

Direct method	Indirect method
• Electromagnetic flow meter	• Fick's principle • Indicator dilution principle/Thermodilution technique • Doppler echocardiogram

- **Fick's Principle:** Amount of a substance taken up by an organ (or by the whole body) per unit of time is equal to the arterial level of the substance minus the venous level (A-V difference) times the blood flow
- Factors controlling cardiac output:
  - Changes in heart rate (controlled primarily by the autonomic nerves, with sympathetic stimulation increasing the rate and parasympathetic stimulation decreasing it)
  - Changes in stroke volume

Preload	• The degree to which the myocardium is stretched before it contracts
Afterload	• Resistance against which blood is expelled
Frank-Starling law	• 'Energy of contraction is proportional to the initial length of the cardiac muscle fiber' • For the heart, the length of the muscle fibers, (i.e. the extent of the preload) is proportional to the end-diastolic volume
Frank-Starling curve	• The relation between ventricular stroke volume and end-diastolic volume
Heterometric regulation	• When cardiac output is regulated by changes in cardiac muscle fiber length
Homometric regulation	• Regulation due to changes in contractility independent of length
Pericardial sac	• Contains 5–30 mL of clear fluid

Effect of Various Conditions on Cardiac Output

No change	Increase in CO	Decrease in CO
• Sleep • Moderate change in temperature	• Anxiety, eating, exercise • Hyperthermia • Pregnancy, Epinephrine	• Rapid cardiac arrhythmias • Heart disease • Sitting/standing from lying posture

Factors That Depress Myocardial Contractility

- Hypercapnia
- Hypoxia
- Acidosis
- Drugs such as quinidine, procainamide, and barbiturates
- Acute heart failure (myocardial hibernation)

Oxygen Consumption by the Heart

- Basal O_2 consumption-2 mL/100 g/min
- O_2 consumption by the beating heart-9 mL/100 g/min
- Determined by:
  1. Intramyocardial tension
  2. Contractile state of the myocardium
  3. Heart rate
- 'Increase in afterload causes a greater increase in cardiac O_2 consumption than does an increase in preload'

Characteristics of Human Red Cells

RBC indices	Normal value
Mean corpuscular volume (MCV) = Hematocrit /Number of red cells	80–94 cubic microns (μ_3)
Mean corpuscular hemoglobin (MCH) = Blood hemoglobin (g/L) /Red ell count (cells/L)	27–32 Picograms (pg)
Mean corpuscular Hb concentration (MCHC) = Hb (g/L) /hematocrit	33%
Colour Index (CI) = %of Hb/% of RBC	0.9–1.1%
Mean cell diameter (MCD) (µm) = mean diameter of 500 cells in smear	7.5

Hemoglobin

Adult human haemoglobin:	Fetal hemoglobins:
• Hemoglobin A ($\alpha_2\beta_2$)	• Hemoglobin F ($\alpha_2\gamma_2$) • In young embryos there are, in addition, ζ and ε chains forming, – Gower 1 hemoglobin ($\zeta_2\varepsilon_2$) – Gower 2 hemoglobin ($\alpha_2\varepsilon_2$)

ABO System

Blood Type	Agglutinins in Plasma	Frequency in India (%)	Plasma Agglutinates Red Cells of Type
O	Anti-A Anti-B	40	A, B, AB
A	Anti-B	22	B, AB
B	Anti-A	33	A, AB
AB	None	5	None

Clotting Factor	Other Names	Deficiency Clinical Syndrome	Cause
I	Fibrinogen	Afibrinogenemia	Depletion during pregnancy with premature separation of placenta; also congenital (rare)
II	Prothrombin	Hypoprothrombinemia (hemorrhagic tendency in liver disease)	Decreased hepatic synthesis, usually secondary to vitamin K deficiency
III	Thromboplastin		
IV	Calcium		
V	Proaccelerin, labile factor, accelerator globulin	Parahemophilia	Congenital
VII	Proconvertin, SPCA, stable factor	Hypoconvertinemia	Congenital
VIII	Antihemophilic factor (AHF), antihemophilic factor A, antihemophilic globulin (AHG)	Hemophilia A (classic hemophilia)	Congenital defect due to various abnormalities of the gene on X chromosome that codes for factor VIII; disease is therefore inherited as a sex-linked characteristic
IX	Plasma thromboplastic component (PTC), Christmas factor, antihemophilic factor B	Hemophilia B (Christmas disease)	Congenital
X	Stuart-Prower factor	Stuart-Prower factor Deficiency	Congenital
XI	Plasma thromboplastin antecedent (PTA), antihemophilic factor C	PTA deficiency	Congenital
XII	Hageman factor, glass factor	Hageman trait	Congenital
XIII	Fibrin-stabilizing factor, Laki-Lorand factor		

Proteins Synthesized by Liver

Name	Principal Function	Binding Characteristics
Albumin	Binding and carrier protein; osmotic regulator	Hormones, amino acids, steroids, vitamins, fatty acids
Orosomucoid	Uncertain; may have a role in inflammation	
α_1-Antiprotease	Trypsin and general protease inhibitor	Proteases in serum and tissue secretions
α-Fetoprotein	Osmotic regulation; binding and carrier proteina	Hormones, amino acids
α_2-Macroglobulin	Inhibitor of serum endoproteases	Proteases
Antithrombin-III	Protease inhibitor of intrinsic coagulation system	1:1 binding to proteases
Ceruloplasmin	Transport of copper	Six atoms copper/molecule
C-reactive protein	Uncertain; has role in tissue Inflammation	Complement C1q
Fibrinogen	Precursor to fibrin in hemostasis	
Haptoglobin	Binding, transport of cell-free Hemoglobin	Hemoglobin 1:1 binding
Hemopexin	Binds to porphyrins, particularly heme for heme recycling	1:1 with heme
Transferrin	Transport of iron	Two atoms iron/molecule
Apolipoprotein B	Assembly of lipoprotein particles	Lipid carrier
Angiotensinogen	Precursor to pressor peptide angiotensin II	
Proteins, coagulation factors II, VII, IX, X	Blood clotting	

Contd...

Contd...

Name	Principal Function	Binding Characteristics
Antithrombin C, protein C	Inhibition of blood clotting	
Insulinlike growth factor I	Mediator of anabolic effects of growth hormone	IGF-I receptor
Steroid hormone-binding	Carrier protein for steroids in	Steroid hormones
Globulin	Bloodstream	
Thyroxine-binding globulin	Carrier protein for thyroid hormone in bloodstream	Thyroid hormones
Transthyretin (thyroid-binding prealbumin)	Carrier protein for thyroid hormone in bloodstream	Thyroid hormones

Arteries	1. Large Elastic Arteries: – **Windkessel vessel,** e.g. Aorta and its main branches – Smooth muscles arranged spirally – More elastic 2. Large Muscular Arteries: – Smooth muscle content is high – Few elastic fibres are present 3. Arterioles (stop cocks of circulation): – Seat of maximum peripheral resistance – Lacks elastic fibres – Rich in smooth muscle-arranged in circular fashion
Veins	1. Large Veins: – Thin walled – Large than largest arteries – Elastin content is less – Capacitance vessels (hold maximum blood) 2. Venules: – Thin-walled but larger than arterioles – Less elastin content than arterioles
Capillaries	• Small vessels guarded by precapillary sphincter • Modified smooth musles (pericytes) are present • Has single layer of endothelium • Types: 1. Continuous - Seen in heart, lung, brain and skeletal muscle 2. Fenestrated - Seen in the endocrinal glands and renal glomeruli 3. Discontinuous (sinusoids) - Seen in red bone marrow and liver - Highly permeable

Blood Flow

The probability of turbulence is given by **Reynolds's number**: $Re = \frac{\rho DV}{\eta}$

ρ is the density of the fluid; D is the diameter of the tube

V is the velocity of the flow; η is the viscosity of the fluid

- The higher the value of Re, the greater the probability of turbulence
- Flow is usually not turbulent is Re is less than 2000
- When Re is more than 3000, turbulence is almost always present.

Critical closing pressure: The pressure at which flow ceases. Value is not zero but above zero

Poiseuille-Hagen formula	• $F = (P_A - P_B) \times (\pi/8) \times (1/ή) \times (r^4/L)$ Where, F = flow $P_A - P_B$ = pressure difference between two ends of the tube ή = viscosity r = radius of tube L = length of tube
Bernoulli's principle	• The sum of the kinetic energy of flow and the potential energy is constant
Newtonian fluid	• Viscosity is independent of the rate of shear. Examples—Plasma, saline
Non Newtonian fluid	• Viscosity changes with changes in shear rate. Example—Blood

Blood Pressure

- Cardiac output × peripheral resistance

Mean arterial pressure = Diastolic BP + 1/3 (Pulse Pressure)
= Diastolic BP + 1/3 (Systolic-Diastolic)

Regulation of Blood Pressure

Short-term regulation of BP	Long-term regulation of BP
• Baroreflex • Chemoreflex • CNS Ischaemic Response • Hormonal Mechanisms – Catecholamine Release – Renin-Angiotensin Mechanism • Intrinsic Vascular Mechanism – Capillary Fluid Shift – Stress Relaxation	• Blood Volume (Fluid Balance) • ADH, Renin-Angiotensin System, Atrial Natriuretic Peptide

Cardiovascular Regulation

Medulla	Vasomotor area (rostral ventrolateral medulla): • Neurotransmitter-Glutamate • **Direct stimulation of RVLM:** 1. CO_2 2. Hypoxia • **Excitatory inputs to RVLM:** 1. Cortex via hypothalamus 2. Mesencephalic periaqueductal gray 3. Brain stem reticular formation 4. Pain pathways 5. Somatic afferents (somatosympathetic reflex) 6. Carotid and aortic chemoreceptors • **Inhibitory inputs to RVLM:** 1. Cortex via hypothalamus 2. Caudal ventrolateral medulla 3. Caudal medullary raphé nuclei 4. Lung inflation afferents 5. Carotid, aortic, and cardiopulmonary baroreceptors
Baroreceptors (Carotid **S**inu**S**: measures pressure. Carotid b**O_2**dy measures **O_2**)	• Carotid sinus and aortic arch receptor (Buffer Nerves) • Afferent from carotid sinus-Glossopharyngeal nerve • Afferent from aortic arch-Vagus

	Increased blood pressure → buffer nerves → nucleus tractus solitarius • Tract 1: NTS → excitatory glutaminergic neurons → caudal and intermediate ventrolateral medulla → stimulate GABA ergic neurons → rostal ventrolateral medulla (RVLM), the VMC → inhibition of VMC → decreased sympathetic activity • Tract 2: NTS → dorsal motor nucleus and nucleus ambiguous → vagal neurons Baroreflex: • Increased BP → Stimulation of baroreceptors → vagal stimulation + inhibition of VMC (↓ sympathetic activity) → Vasodilatation, ven dilatation, ↓BP, bradycardia, ↓ cardiac output
Chemoreflex	• When MAP falls below 80 mm Hg → fall in blood flow to chemoreceptors → corresponding reduction in oxygen delivery (hypoxia) and an accumulation of CO_2 and H^+→ detected by chemoreceptors located in the carotid and aortic bodies → excites the vasomotor centre • Not a powerful arterial pressure controller until pressure falls below 80 mm Hg
Atrial stretch receptors	• Type-A: discharge primarily in atrial systole • Type-B: discharge primarily in late atrial diastole • The response is vasodilatation, fall in BP and increase in heart rate
Cushing's reflex (CNS Ischemic Response/Last Ditch Sand)	• Increase in Intracranial tension → hypoxia and hypercapnia of VMC → direct simiulation of VMC → increased sympathetic activity → intense vasoconstriction → increase in BP • Doesn't become significant until pressure falls below 60 mm Hg • Greatest degree of stimulation at 15 to 20 mm Hg • Elevate mean arterial pressure for as long as 10 minutes and as high as 250 mm Hg
Bainbridge reflex:	• Rapid perfusion of blood saline stimulates the atrial stretch receptors and results in increased heart rate if the initial HR is low
Bezold-Jarisch reflex (coronary chemoreflex)	• Serotonin and chemicals like nicotine in the coronary or pulmonary arteries can stimulate the receptors of the left ventricle resulting in profound bradycardia, hypotension, and a brief period of apnea followed by rapid shallow breathing • Activation of chemosensitive vagal C fibers

Autoregulation

- Ability of an organ to regulate its blood flow with changes in perfusion pressure. Seen in brain, kidney, skeletal muscle, heart, liver etc... (Not in skin)

Theories of autoregulation

- **Myogenic theory:** Pacemaker cells in the smooth muscles of blood vessels possess basal myogenic tone, which responds to change in blood pressure
- **Metabolic theory:** Accumulation of metabolites increases the blood flow by vasodilatation
- **Nutrient lack theory:** Lack of oxygen → vasodilatation

Factors Affecting the Caliber of the Arterioles

Vasoconstriction	Vasodilation
Local factors	
• Decreased local temperature • Autoregulation	• Increased CO_2 and decreased O_2 • Increased K^+, adenosine, lactate • Decreased local pH • Increased local temperature

Endothelial products	
• Endothelin-1 • Locally released platelet • Serotonin • Thromboxane A_2	• Nitric oxide • Kinins • Prostacyclin
Circulating neurohumoral agents	
• Epinephrine (except in skeletal muscle and liver) • Norepinephrine • Arginine vasopressin • Angiotensin II • Endogenous digitalis-like substance • Neuropeptide Y • Urotensin-II	• Epinephrine in skeletal muscle and liver • Calcitonin G-related protein • Substance P • Histamine • Atrial natriuretic peptide • Vasoactive intestinal polypeptide
Neural factors	
• Increased discharge of sympathetic nerves	• Decreased discharge of sympathetic nerves • Activation of sympathetic cholinergic vasodilator nerves to vasculature of skeletal muscles of the limbs

Coronary circulation	• Metabolic factors (hypoxia) are more potent regulators than neural factors • Only organ in which the blood flow is decreased during systole • The coronary arterioles contain α-adrenergic receptors, which mediate vasoconstriction, and β-adrenergic receptors, which mediate vasodilation • However, norepinephrine increases the heart rate and the force of cardiac contraction, and the vasodilation is due to production of vasodilator metabolites in the myocardium secondary to the increase in its activity

Regulation of Coronary Blood Flow

Physical Factors	Metabolic Factors	Neural Factors
Arterial BP: Diastolic BP influences the rate of coronary blood flow Coronary vascular resistances Extracoronary vascular pressure	Hypoxia (**most potent**) CO_2, H^+, K^+, lactate, prostaglandins, adenine nucleotides and adenosine	Sympathetic Vasodilatation (β-receptors) Vasoconstriction (α–receptors)

Cerebral circulation	• Exhibits autoregulation • Most important vasodilator-CO_2 • Sympathetic nerves play a minor role
Cutaneous circulation	• Temperature regulation is the principal function • Has extensive sympathetic innervations • Triple response: 1. Redness- due to capillary dilation 2. Wheal-increased permeability of the capillaries and postcapillary venules 3. Flare-due to arteriolar dilation • When the skin needs to **CONS**erve heat, the blood vessels of the skin **CONS**trict

Circulation Through Special Regions

	Blood flow			Arteriovenous Oxygen Difference (mL/L)	Oxygen Consumption		Resistance (R units)	Percentage of Total		
Region	Mass (kg)	mL/min	mL/100g/min		mL/min	mL/100g/min	Absolute	Per kg	Cardiac Output	Oxygen Consumption
Liver	2.6	1500	57.7	34	51	2.0	3.6	9.4	27.8	20.4
Kidneys	0.3	1260	420.0	14	18	6.0	4.3	1.3	23.3	7.2
Brain	1.4	750	54.0	62	46	3.3	7.2	10.1	13.9	18.4
Skin	3.6	462	12.8	25	12	0.3	11.7	42.1	8.6	4.8
Skeletal muscle	31.0	840	2.7	60	50	0.2	6.4	198.4	15.6	20.0
Heart muscle	0.3	250	84.0	114	29	9.7	21.4	6.4	4.7	11.6
Rest of body	23.8	336	1.4	129	44	0.2	16.1	383.2	6.2	17.6
Whole body	63.0	5400	8.6	46	250	0.4	1.0	63.0	100.0	100.0

Overall (ml/min)	
Blood flow	O_2 consumption
Liver > Kidney > Skeletal muscle > Brain > Skin > Heart	Liver > Skeletal muscle > Brain > Heart

Per unit mass (ml/100g/min)	
Blood flow	O_2 consumption
Kidney > Heart > Liver	Heart > Kidney > Brain

Resistance	
Absolute	Per Kg
Heart-Max Liver-Min	Skeletal muscle-Max Kidney-Min

Av O_2 difference
Heart-Max
Kidney-Min

	Systemic circulation	Pulmonary circulation
Blood flow (liters/min)	5	5
Percentage of blood volume	84	9
Arterial blood pressure (mmHg)	120/80	25/8
Oxygen content of the arteries (pO_2; mmHg)	100	40

RESPIRATORY PHYSIOLOGY-HIGH YIELD TOPICS

Conducting Zone	• First 16 generations • Comprises of trachea, bronchi, bronchioles and terminal bronchioles
Respiratory Zone	• Last 7 generations • Comprises of Respiratory bronchioles, alveolar ducts and alveolar sacs

Conduction Zone to Respiratory Zone Transition Events

- Secretory glands are absent from the epithelium of the bronchioles and terminal bronchioles
- Smooth muscle-more prominent
- Cartilage-absent
- Clara cells, Basal cells- serve as progenitor cells after injury

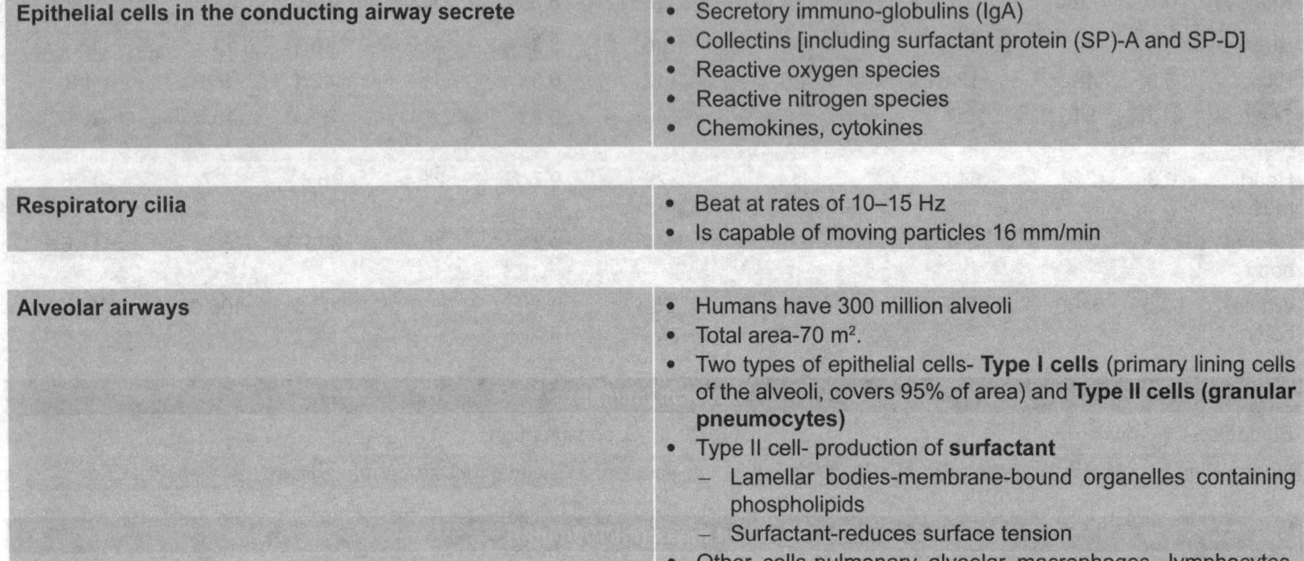

Epithelial cells in the conducting airway secrete	• Secretory immuno-globulins (IgA) • Collectins [including surfactant protein (SP)-A and SP-D] • Reactive oxygen species • Reactive nitrogen species • Chemokines, cytokines

Respiratory cilia	• Beat at rates of 10–15 Hz • Is capable of moving particles 16 mm/min

Alveolar airways	• Humans have 300 million alveoli • Total area-70 m^2. • Two types of epithelial cells- **Type I cells** (primary lining cells of the alveoli, covers 95% of area) and **Type II cells (granular pneumocytes)** • Type II cell- production of **surfactant** – Lamellar bodies-membrane-bound organelles containing phospholipids – Surfactant-reduces surface tension • Other cells-pulmonary alveolar macrophages, lymphocytes, plasma cells, neuroendocrine cells, and mast cells

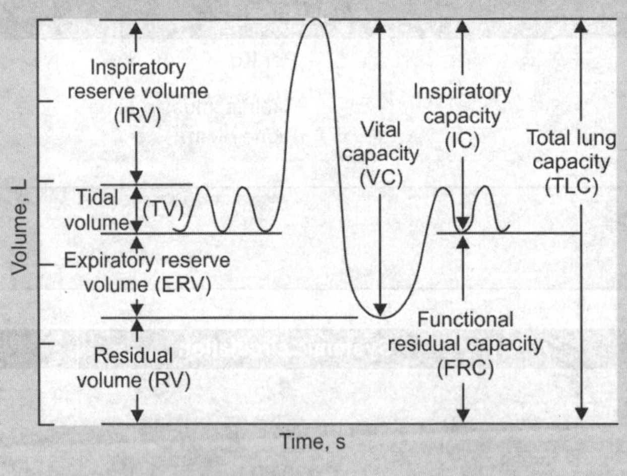

Fig. 2.6: Respiratory volumes and capacities

Respiratory Volumes		
Measurement	**Typical value**	**Definition**
Tidal volume (TV)	500 mL	Amount of air that enters or leaves lungs during one inspiration or expiration (respiratory cycle)
Inspiratory reserve volume (IRV)	3000 mL	Maximum volume of air that can be inspired over the normal TV
Expiratory reserve volume (ERV)	1200 mL	Extra volume of air expired by forceful expiration after the end of normal tidal expiration

Contd...

Contd...

Measurement	Typical value	Definition
Respiratory Volumes		
Residual volume (RV)	1200 mL	Amount of air left in lungs after forced exhalation
Closing volume		Lung volume above the residual volume at which the alveoli of lung bases begin to close off
Respiratory Capacities		
Vital capacity (VC)	4700 mL	IRV + TV + ERV, maximum amount of air that can be exhaled after a maximum inspiration
Inspiratory capacity (IC)	3500 mL	TV + IRV, maximum amount of air that can be inhaled after a normal expiration
Functional residual capacity (FRC)	2400 mL	RC + ERV, amount of air remaining in the lungs after a normal tidal expiration
Total lung capacity (TLC)	5900 mL	RV + VC, maximum volume to which the lungs can be expanded
Closing capacity		RV + The volume expired between the beginning of airway closure and the RV

Dead Space
- Anatomical: Volume of air occupying the conducting zone (not participating in gaseous exchange). (150 ml), measured by Bohr's method
- Roughly equal to body weight in pounds or twice the body weight. in kgs
- Alveolar dead space-volume of gas not equilibrating with blood, 'Wasted Ventilation', Physiological dead space = Anatomical dead space + alveolar dead space
- Under normal conditions, alveolar dead space is zero. Hence both anatomical and physiological DS are equal

- **Spirometer**: measures all volumes and capacities except RV, FRC and TLC
- Methods to measure RV and FRC:
  - Helium dilution technique
  - Plethysmography
  - Nitrogen washout method

- Obstructive disorders-marked decrease in both FVC and FEV 1/FVC
- Restrictive disorders result in a loss of FVC without loss in FEV 1 /FVC

Surfactant
- Mixture of dipalmitoylphosphatidylcholine (DPPC), other lipids, and proteins
- Surfactant deficiency-infant respiratory distress syndrome (Prolonged immaturity of the epithelial Na^+ channels (ENaCs)
- Overproduction/dysregulation of surfactant proteins-Pulmonary alveolar proteinosis (PAP)

Diffusion Across Alveolocapillary Membrane

- Substances passing from the alveoli to the capillary blood reach equilibrium in the 0.75 s
- N_2O- not limited by diffusion but by the amount of blood flowing through the pulmonary capillaries (Perfusion-limited)
- Carbonmonoxide- taken up by hemoglobin in the red blood cells at such a high rate, equilibrium is not reached in the 0.75 s (not limited by perfusion at rest -**diffusion-limited)**
- Oxygen-Intermediate. Taken up by hemoglobin, but much less avidly than CO, reaches equilibrium with capillary blood in about 0.3 s (Perfusion limited)
- Diffusing capacity- directly proportional to the surface area of the alveolocapillary membrane and inversely proportional to its thickness
- Diffusing capacity for CO (D_{LCO}) - measured as an index of diffusing capacity because its uptake is diffusion-limited
- $D_{LCO} = V_{CO}/P_{ACO}$
- Normal value of D_{LCO} at rest-25 mL/min/mm Hg
- Normal value of diffusing capacity for O_2 at rest-25 mL/min/mm Hg

Ventilation-Perfusion Ratio

- For the whole lung at rest is about 0.8
- Ventilation, as well as perfusion in the upright position, declines in a linear fashion from the bases to the apices of the lungs
- Gravity affects perfusion much more than it affects ventilation
- Ventilation/perfusion ratios are high in the upper portions of the lungs
- At apex-Intrapleural pressure more negative, greater transmural pressure, large alveoli (more underperfused than underventilated)

Respiratory Exchange Ratio

- The ratio of carbon dioxide output to oxygen uptake is called the Respiratory Exchange Ratio
- R = rate of carbon dioxide output/rate of oxygen uptake
- During hyperventilation, R rises because CO_2 is being blown off
- During strenuous exercise, R may reach 2.00 because CO_2 is being blown off and lactic acid from anaerobic glycolysis is being converted to CO_2.
- In metabolic acidosis, R rises because of respiratory compensation for the acidosis causes the amount of CO_2 expired to rise
- In metabolic alkalosis, R falls
- During secretion of gastric juice, the stomach has a negative R because it takes up more CO_2 from the arterial blood than it puts into the venous blood.

Agents Affecting Smooth Muscle in Pulmonary Arteries and Veins

Constriction	Relaxation
1. Adrenergic (α_1)	1. Adrenergic (α_1, β_2)
2. Purinergic (P_{2x})	2. Muscarinic (M_3)
3. Tachykinin (NK_2)	3. Purinergic (P_{2Y})
4. Adenosine (A_1)	4. Tachykinin (NK_1)
5. Angiotensin II (AT_1)	5. VIP
6. Endothelin (ET_A)	6. CGRP
7. Serotonin (5-HT_1)	7. Adenosine (A_2)
8. Thromboxane (TP)	8. ANP
	9. Bradykinin
	10. Endothelin (ET_B)
	11. Histamine (H_1, H_2)
	12. Serotonin (5-HT_C)
	13. Vasopressin (V_1)

Biologically Active Substances Metabolized by the Lungs

Synthesized and used in the lungs
Surfactant
Synthesized or stored and released into the blood
Prostaglandins
Histamine
Kallikrein
Partially removed from the blood
Prostaglandins
Bradykinin
Adenine nucleotides
Serotonin
Norepinephrine
Acetylcholine
Activated in the lungs
Angiotensin I → angiotensin II

- **Oxygen Hemoglobin Dissociation curve -** Relates percentage saturation of the O_2 carrying power of hemoglobin (SaO_2) to the pO_2
- The point where 50% of Hb is saturated with O_2 is called the P50 → 27 mmHg
- Hemoglobin-tense (T) configuration- reduced the affinity for O_2
- Relaxed (R) configuration- exposes more O_2 binding sites
- When fully saturated, each gram of normal hemoglobin contains 1.34 mL of O_2
- 1 dL of blood contains 20.1 mL (1.34 mL × 15) of O_2 bound to hemoglobin when the hemoglobin is 100% saturated

Arterial Blood	Venous Blood
PO_2 95 mm Hg; PCO_2 40 mm Hg; Hb 97% Saturated	**PO_2 40 mm Hg; PCO_2 46 mm Hg; Hb 75% Saturated**

FACTORS AFFECTING THE AFFINITY OF HEMOGLOBIN FOR OXYGEN

Shift to the Right (Release/tissues)	Shift to the left (Lungs/binding)
• Increased pCO_2 • Increased temperature • Increased 2, 3-DPG • Growth hormone • Exercise • Hypoxia • High altitude • Anemia • Acidosis (decreased pH) • Sickle cell anemia • Adult Hb	• Decreased pCO_2 • Decreased temperature • Decreased 2, 3-DPG • Alkalosis (increased pH) • Fetal Hb (poor binding of 2, 3-DPG by the γ polypeptide chains) • Stored blood (2, 3-DPG level falls)

- Hb**F** binds **F**orcefully to oxygen
- Stored blood is **SOS**: **S**tored blood Hb binds to **O**xygen **S**trongly because of decrease in 2, 3 BPG
- 2, 3 BPG binding site is **BBC**: **B**PG binds to **B**eta **C**hain of Hb

Bohr Effect

- The decrease in O_2 affinity of hemoglobin when the pH of blood falls
- Curve shifts to the right

Haldane Effect

- Increased capacity of deoxygenated hemoglobin to bind and carry CO_2

Chloride Shift

When the HCO_3^- ions move out of red blood cells into the plasma, to maintain the electrolytic equilibrium the chloride ions move into the red blood cells from plasma. This is called chloride shift and this is why the chloride content of the red cells in venous blood is significantly greater than that in arterial blood.

- This process is mediated by anion exchanger 1 (also called Band 3) a major membrane protein in the red blood cell

Myoglobin

- Iron-containing pigment found in skeletal muscle
- Binds 1 mol of O_2 per mole protein (Hb binds 4)
- Dissociation curve- a rectangular hyperbola
- Higher affinity for O_2 (Leftward shift in curve)
- Its utmost purpose is utilised during exercise (O_2 is released only at low pO_2 values)
- During exercise- it continues to provide O_2 under reduced blood flow and/or reduced pO_2 in the blood
- Myoglobin binding strength is **MOM**: **M**yoglobin binds **O**xygen **M**ore strongly than Hb

Acid Base Balance

Plasma pH, HCO_3^-, and pCO_2 values in various typical disturbances of acid-base balance:

	Arterial Plasma			
Condition	pH	HCO_3^- (mEq/L)	pCO_2 (mm Hg)	Cause
Normal	7.40	24.1	40	
Metabolic	7.28	18.1	40	NH_4Cl ingestion
Acidosis	6.96	5.0	23	Diabetic acidosis
Metabolic	7.50	30.1	40	$NaHCO_3$ ingestion
Alkalosis	7.56	49.8	58	Prolonged vomiting
Respiratory	7.34	25.0	48	Breathing 7% CO_2
Acidosis	7.34	33.5	64	Emphysema
Respiratory Alkalosis	7.53	22.0	27	Voluntary hyper-ventilation
	7.48	18.7	26	Three-week residence at 4000-m altitude

Anion Gap

- The difference between the concentration of cations other than Na^+ and the concentration of anions other than Cl^- and HCO_3^- in the plasma
- Comprises of proteins in anionic form, HPO_4^{2-}, SO_4^{2-}, and organic acids normal value-12 mEq/L
- Increased:
  1. When the plasma concentration of K^+, Ca^{2+}, or Mg^+ is decreased
  2. When the concentration of plasma proteins is increased
  3. When organic anions such as lactate or foreign anions accumulate in blood
  4. In metabolic acidosis due to ketoacidosis, lactic acidosis
- Decreased:
  - When cations are increased
  - When plasma albumin is decreased

Graphic Analysis of pH Disturbances can be Done Using

- The Davenport Diagram
- The Siggard-Anderson nomogram

Hypoxia: O_2 Deficiency at the Tissue Level

Type	Causes	Mechanism	PaO_2	PaO_2	O_2 content	A-V difference
Hypoxic/Anoxic	High altitude and pneumonia	• Poor availability of O_2 for diffusion • Decreased partial pressure of O_2 in arterial blood	↓	↓	↓	±
Anemic	Anemia CO poisoning	• Decreased O_2 carrying capacity	±	±	↓	±
Stagnant/ Ischemic/ Hypoperfusion	Cardiogenic shock	O_2 content of the blood is exhausted due to reduction in blood velocity	±	±	±	↑
Histotoxic	Beriberi HNC poisoning	Tissue cannot make use of available O_2	±	±	±	↓

Best test for Hypoxia

- Hypoxic hypoxia (Anoxic/Arterial): partial pressure of arterial O_2, treated by oxygen therapy
- Anemic hypoxia-oxygen content (Hb%)
- Stagnant hypoxia- A-V difference (increased)
- Histotoxic hypoxia- A-V difference (decreased) or pO_2 of venous blood (increased)

Neural Control of Respiration

- Voluntary system-located in the cerebral cortex and sends impulses to the respiratory motor neurons via the corticospinal tracts
- Automatic system-pacemaker cells in the medulla-activate motor neurons in the cervical and thoracic spinal cord that innervate inspiratory muscles

Medullary system:	Pontine and vagal influences:
Pre-Botzinger complex: • Rhythm of respiration (pace maker of respiration) • Has NK1 receptors, μ-opioid receptors and $5HT_4$ receptors • Substance P stimulates and opioids inhibit respiration • 5HT 4 agonists blocks the inhibitory effect of opiates **Dorsal respiratory group (DRG):** • Nucleus tractus solitaries (NTS) • Site of origin of rhythmic inspiratory discharge. (**Inspiratory ramp signals)** **Ventral respiratory group (VRG):** • Nucleus retro ambigualis (NRA) • Both inspiratory and expiratory control	Switching between inspiration and expiration **Pneumotaxic centre:** • Medial parabrachial and Kölliker-Fuse nuclei • Inhibitory effect on apneustic centre **Apneustic centre:** • Lower pons • Has an intrinsic rhythm, promotes prolonged inspirations when active **Vagus:** Stretching of lungs during inspiration ↓ Stimulates afferent pulmonary vagal fibres ↓ Inhibit inspiratory discharge

Chemical Control of Respiration

Peripheral chemoreceptors:	Central chemoreceptors:
Carotid and aortic bodies: • Two types of cells, type I and type II cells • Type-I (glomus) cells – Are closely associated with cup like endings of the afferent nerves – Resemble adrenal chromaffin cells and have dense-core granules containing catecholamines that are released upon exposure to hypoxia and cyanide – Excited by hypoxia-Neurotransmitter-Dopamine (D_2 receptor) – Have O_2 sensitive K^+ channels- conductance is reduced in proportion to the degree of hypoxia • Type II-Glia like cells, surrounds four to six type I cells • Blood flow per unit of tissue is so enormous- 2000 mL/100 g of tissue/min • Afferents from the carotid bodies ascend to the medulla via the carotid sinus and glossopharyngeal nerves and fibers from the aortic bodies ascend in the vagi • Respond to $\downarrow pO_2 \uparrow pCO_2$ and H^+ of arterial blood • Hypoxia is the potent stimulus • Carotid bodies more effective than aortic bodies	• Location: ventral surface of the medulla, solitary tract nuclei, the locus ceruleus, and the hypothalamus • CSF (H^+) is the potent stimulus to central chemoreceptor. • Effects of CO_2– mainly due to its movement into the CSF and brain interstitial fluid and increases the H_+ concentration • The magnitude of the stimulation is proportional to the rise in H^+ concentration.

Abnormal Respiratory Patterns

Pattern	Cause	Mechanics
Cheyne-stokes respiration	• Opium poisoning • Uremia and CCF • hypoxia	Periodic breathing due to rhythmic alteration of apnea and hyperpnea Waxing and waning tidal volume
Biot's breathing (Irregularly irregular breathing)	Meningitis	Periodic breathing with one or more large tidal volumes separated by apnea
Kussmaul's respiration hunger	• DKA • Uremia	Rapid and deep breathing
Ondine's curse		Loss of spontaneous breathing with only voluntary control

Minute Respiratory Volume (Minute Ventilation)

- Total amount of new air moved into the respiratory passages each minute, which is normally ~6 L/min
  Minute respiratory volume (minute ventilation) = Tidal volume × Respiratory rate
  = 500 ml × 12/min
  = 6000 ml/min or 6 L/min

Alveolar Ventilation

- The rate at which new air reaches the alveoli, alveolar sacs, alveolar ducts, and respiratory bronchioles
- Normal value is ~4200 ml/min
- It does not include the dead space air

Maximum Voluntary Ventilation (MVV)

- It is the largest volume of air that an individual can breathe into and out of the lungs in 1 minute with maximum voluntary effort
- Normal values range from 140-180 L/min for healthy adult males

Breathing Reserve

- It is the difference in MVV and the maximal ventilation measured during exercise
- Breathing reserve (L/min) = MVV - Maximum ventilation during exercise
- The normal value is between 20% and 50% if the MVV

GASTROINTESTINAL PHYSIOLOGY—HIGH YIELD TOPICS (SPECIALIZATIONS OF GI EPITHELIUM)

- Villi (fingerlike projections): Maximizes the surface area available for nutrient absorption.
- Crypts-Infoldings between villi. Base of the crypts contains Stem Cells that give rise to both crypt and villus epithelial cells
- Microvilli- dense glycocalyx (the brush border) that protects the cells from digestive enzymes. contains brush border enzymes

Salivary Secretion

- Saliva-Produced from three pairs of salivary glands (the **parotid, submandibular,** and **sublingual glands**)
- **1000–1500** mL of saliva per day is secreted
- Hypotonic and alkaline
- Parasympathetic-increases the secretion
- Sympathetic-increase protein content of saliva has little effect on volume
- Antibacterial agents in saliva- immunoglobulin A and lysozyme and thiocyanate ions
- The buffers in the saliva help to maintain the oral pH at about 7.0
- Saliva contains especially large quantities of potassium and bicarbonate ions. Conversely, the concentrations of sodium and chloride are several times less in saliva than in plasma

Source	Enzyme	Activator	Substrate	Catalytic Function or Products
Salivary glands	Salivary α-amylase	Cl^-	Starch	Hydrolyzes 1:4 α linkages, producing α-limit dextrins, maltotriose, and maltose

Gastric Secretion

- About 2.5 L per day
- Cephalic phase accounts for nearly 30% of total acid secretion
- Gastric phase accounts for 50–60% of total gastric acid secretion
- Intestinal phase accounts for 5–10% of total gastric acid secretion
- **Parietal (oxyntic) cells-**secrete hydrochloric acid and intrinsic factor (absorption of vitamin B_{12})
- **Chief (zymogen, peptic) cells**-pepsinogens and gastric lipase ('**Chief** of **Pepsi**': **Chief cells of stomach produce Pepsin**.
- Trefoil peptides- stabilize the mucus-bicarbonate layer

Contents of normal gastric juice (fasting state)
Cations: Na^+, K^+, Mg^{2+}, H^+ (pH approximately 3.0)
Anions: Cl^-, HPO_4^{2-}, SO_4^{2-}
Pepsins
Lipase
Mucus
Intrinsic factor

Three Primary Stimuli of Gastric Secretion

1. Gastrin
   - Comes from G cells in antrum. Releasing factors- gastrin releasing peptide (GRP) or bombesin, oligopeptides
   - Binds to receptors in parietal cells-to activate secretion and also enterochromaffin-like cells (ECL cells) -release histamine
2. **Histamine**-H_2 histamine receptors (triggers secretion)
3. **Acetylcholine**

'*Gastrin and acetylcholine promote secretion by elevating cytosolic free calcium concentrations, whereas histamine increases intracellular cyclic adenosine 3′, 5′-monophosphate (cAMP)* '

Synergistic-greater than additive effect on secretion rates when histamine plus gastrin or acetylcholine, or all three, are present simultaneously

Somatostatin: inhibits gastric secretion by inhibiting both G and ECL cells

Source	Enzyme	Activator	Substrate	Catalytic function or products
Stomach	Pepsins (pepsinogens)	HCl	Proteins and polypeptides	Cleave peptide bonds adjacent to aromatic amino acids
	Gastric lipase		Triglycerides	Fatty acids and glycerol

Pancreatic Secretion

- Exocrine cells (secrete enzymes) and duct cells (secrete bicarbonate)
- Composition-Cations: Na^+, K^+, Ca^{2+}, Mg^{2+} (pH approximately 8.0), Anions: HCO_3^-, Cl^-, SO_4^{2-}, HPO_4^{2-}, digestive enzymes and other proteins
- About 1.5 L per day

Source	Enzyme	Activator	Substrate	Catalytic Function or Products
Exocrine pancreas	Trypsin	Enteropeptidase	Proteins and polypeptides	Cleave peptide bonds on carboxyl side of basic amino acids (arginine or lysine)
	Chymotrypsins	Trypsin	Proteins and polypeptides	Cleave peptide bonds on carboxyl side of aromatic amino acids
	Elastase	Trypsin	Elastin	Cleaves bonds on carboxyl side of aliphatic amino acids

Contd...

Contd...

Source	Enzyme	Activator	Substrate	Catalytic Function or Products
	Carboxypeptidase A	Trypsin	Proteins and polypeptides	Cleave carboxyl terminal amino acids that have aromatic or branched aliphatic side chains
	Carboxypeptidase B	Trypsin	Proteins and polypeptides	Cleave carboxyl terminal amino acids that have basic side chains
	Colipase	Trypsin	Fat droplets	Binds pancreatic lipase to oil droplet in the presence of bile acids
	Pancreatic lipase		Triglycerides	Monoglycerides and fatty acids
	Cholesteryl ester hydrolase		Cholesteryl esters	Cholesterol
	Pancreatic α-amylase	Cl^-	Starch	Hydrolyzes 1:4α linkages, producing α-limit dextrins, maltotriose, and maltose
	Ribonuclease		RNA	Nucleotides
	Deoxyribonuclease		DNA	Nucleotides
	Phospholipase A	Trypsin	Phospholipids	Fatty acids, lysophospholipids

Regulation of Pancreatic Secretion

Secretin	CCK
Acts on the pancreatic ducts to cause copious secretion of a very alkaline pancreatic juice that is rich in HCO_3^- and poor in enzymes	Acts on the acinar cells to cause the release of zymogen granules and production of pancreatic juice rich in enzymes but low in volume
Acts by increase in intracellular cAMP	Mediated by phospholipase C

BILE

- About 500 mL is secreted per day
- Only route by which the body can dispose of cholesterol
- Alkaline electrolyte solution that resembles pancreatic juice
- The most potent stimulus for causing the gallbladder contractions is the hormone cholecystokinin
- Composition of bile- water, bile salts, bilirubin, cholesterol, fatty acids, lecithin, Na^+, K^+, Ca^{++}, Cl^-, HCO_3^-

Bile acids	
Bile acids	• Primary-cholic acid and chenodeoxycholic acid • Secondary-deoxycholic, lithocholic, and ursodeoxycholic acids • Synthesized from cholesterol • Reduce surface tension, emulsification of fat • Amphipathic • Form cylindrical disks called micelles • Absorbed from terminal ileum by Na^+ —bile salt cotransport system (ABST) • Normal rate of bile acid synthesis-0.2–0.4 g/d • Total bile acid pool-3.5 g • Recycles- 6–8 times per day via enterohepatic circulation

Daily Water Turnover (mL) in the Gastrointestinal Tract

A. Ingested-2000
B. Endogenous secretions-7000
   - Salivary glands-1500
   - Stomach-2500

- Bile-500
- Pancreas-1500
- Intestine-1000

Total input (A + B) -9000

Reabsorbed-8800 (98%)

- Jejunum-5500
- Ileum-2000
- Colon-1300

Balance in Stool-200

- Secretion-largely driven by the active transport of chloride ions into the lumen
- Colon-has ENaC channels for sodium absorption (expression increased by aldosterone)
- Cl^- enters enterocytes through Na^+ –K^+–$2Cl^-$ cotransporters and secreted into lumen through the cystic fibrosis transmembrane conductance regulator (CFTR) channel which is activated by protein kinase A and cAMP
- Cholera toxin (A^1 peptide) - binds to GM-1 ganglioside receptors-inhibits GTPase activity of α subunits leading to increase in the intracellular cAMP concentration. Function of NHE (Sodium/Hydrogen Exchanger) transporter for Na^+ is reduced leading to increased sodium chloride excretion

Gastrointestinal Hormones

Gastrin	• Produced by G cells in the antral portion of the gastric mucosa • Three forms- G 34, G 17, and G 14 gastrins • G 17 is the principal form • **Stimuli that increase gastrin secretion:** Peptides, amino acids (phenylalanine, tryptophan), distention, gastrin releasing peptide, calcium, epinephrine • **Stimuli that decrease gastrin secretion:** Acid, somatostatin, secretin, GIP, VIP, glucagon, calcitonin • Acts via CCK-B receptor • Actions- stimulation of gastric acid and pepsin secretion and stimulation of the growth of the mucosa of the stomach and small and large intestines **(trophic action)**
Cholecystokinin	• Secreted by I cells in the mucosa of the upper small intestine • Also found in nerves in the distal ileum, colon and brain • Acts via CCK-A receptor • Functions in gut-stimulation of pancreatic enzyme secretion, contraction of the gallbladder and relaxation of the sphincter of Oddi • Functions in brain-regulation of food intake, the production of anxiety and analgesia • Other actions-augments the action of secretin, inhibits gastric emptying, exerts a trophic effect on the pancreas, increases the synthesis of enterokinase • Releasing factors that activate CCK secretion-CCK-releasing peptide (intestinal mucosa) and monitor peptide (pancreas) • **Stimuli that increase CCK secretion:** Peptides and amino acids, fatty acids (more than 10 carbon atoms)
Secretin	• First hormone identified by Bayliss and Starling • Secreted by S cells (mucosa of the upper portion of the small intestine) • Increases the secretion of bicarbonate by the duct cells of the pancreas and biliary tract (watery, alkaline juice) • Augments the action of CCK, decreases gastric acid secretion • Stimuli that increase secretin secretion: Products of protein digestion, acid

GIP

- Produced by K cells in the mucosa of the duodenum and jejunum
- Secretion is stimulated by glucose and fat in the duodenum
- Stimulates insulin secretion-called as glucose-dependent insulinotropic peptide

VIP

- Stimulates intestinal secretion of electrolytes, water
- Relaxes intestinal smooth muscle, including sphincters; dilation of peripheral blood vessels; and inhibits of gastric acid secretion
- Potentiates the action of acetylcholine in salivary glands

Motilin

- Secreted by enterochromaffin cells and Mo cells in the stomach, small intestine, and colon
- Contracts smooth muscle in the stomach and intestines in between meals

Somatostatin

- Produced by D cells in the pancreatic islets and intestinal mucosa
- Inhibits the secretion of gastrin, VIP, GIP, secretin, and motilin
- Inhibits-pancreatic exocrine secretion, gastric acid secretion and motility and gallbladder contraction
- Inhibits the absorption of glucose, amino acids, and triglycerides
- ACID in lumen-main stimulus for somatostatin secretion

Ghrelin

- Produced in stomach
- Has a role in central control of food intake
- Stimulates growth hormone secretion

Gastrin Releasing Peptide (Bombesin)

- Neurotransmitter producing vagally mediated increases in gastrin secretion

Guanylin

- Binds guanylyl cyclise leading to increase in cGMP- causes increased secretion of Cl^- into the intestinal lumen
- *E. coli* has a structure very similar to guanylin and activates guanylin receptors in the intestine (Molecular mimickry)

Peptide YY

- Stimulated by presence of fat. Inhibits gastric acid secretion and motility

- Choleretics-stimulate bile secretion. Bile salts are most potent. Others are secretin and vagal stimulation
- Cholagogues-increases bile flow by GB contraction. Mainly CCK. Others are fatty acids and amino acids

Enteric Nervous System

- **Myenteric plexus** (Auerbach's plexus) -present between the outer longitudinal and middle circular muscle layers. Concerned primarily with motor control (**M**yenteric: **M**otility)
- **Sub mucous plexus** (Meissner's plexus) -present between the middle circular layer and the mucosa. Primarily involved in the control of intestinal secretion. Innervates the glandular epithelium, intestinal endocrine cells, and submucosal blood vessels (**S**ubmucosal: **S**ecretion and blood flow)
- Parasympathetic-increases intestinal smooth muscle activity
- Sympathetic-decreases intestinal smooth muscle activity—sphincters constrict
- Intestinal blood vessels-Dual innervations. Extrinsic-noradrenergic and intrinsic-NO and VIP (responsible for the increase in local blood flow **(hyperemia)** that accompanies digestion of food)
- Sphlanchnic circulation-receives about 30% of the cardiac output

Neurotransmitters:

- Norepinephrine, serotonin, GABA, ATP, nitric oxide, carbon monoxide

Absorption of Iron

- Regulated by three factors-1. Dietary intake of iron, 2. State of the iron stores in the body, 3. state of erythropoiesis in the bone marrow
- Amount of iron absorbed is normally about 3–6% of the amount ingested
- Dietary form- ferric (Fe^{3+}) and absorption form is ferrous (Fe^{2+})
- Role of stomach in iron absorption: Gastric secretions dissolve the iron and permit it to form soluble complexes with ascorbic acid and other substances that aid its reduction to the Fe^{2+} form
- Maximum absorption occurs in duodenum
- Transport of Fe^{2+} into the enterocytes-divalent metal transporter 1 **(DMT1)** and basolateral transporter named **ferroportin 1**
- **Hephaestin (Hp)** - facilitates basolateral transport (not a transporter by itself)
- Transport form- Transferrin. Has two iron-binding sites. Normally 35% saturated with iron
- HFE gene- normally inhibits expression of the duodenal transporters that participate in iron uptake. HFE mutations (short arm of chromosome 6) leads to hereditary forms of hemochromatosis

Lengths of Various Segments of the Gastrointestinal Tract

Segment	Length (cm)
Pharynx, Esophagus, and stomach	65
Duodenum	25
Jejunum and ileum	260
Colon	110

Neurotransmitters and Hormones that Influence Feeding and Satiety Centers in the Hypothalamus

Decrease Feeding (Anorexigenic)	Increase Feeding (Orexigenic)
• Melanocyte-stimulating hormone (a-MSH) • Leptin • Serotonin • Norepinephrine • Corticotropin-releasing hormone • Insulin • Cholecystokinin (CCK) • Glucagon-like peptide (GLP) • Cocaine- and amphetamine-regulated transcript (CART) • Peptide YY (PYY)	• Neuropeptide Y (NPY) • Agouti-related protein (AGRP) • Melanin-concentrating hormone (MCH) • Orexins A and B • Endorphins • Galanin (GAL) • Amino acids (glutamate and g-aminobutyric acid) • Cortisol • Ghrelin

Gastrointestinal Motility

- Smooth muscle of the GIT- membrane potential fluctuates between about –65 and –45 mV
- Interstitial cells of Cajal:
  - Stellate mesenchymal pacemaker cells
  - Location: stomach and the small intestine-the outer circular muscle layer near the myenteric plexus. In colon-submucosal border of the circular muscle layer
  - Initiates the basic electrical rhythm (BER)
  - Rate of BER: 4/min in the stomach, 12/min in the duodenum, 8/min in the distal ileum, 2/min at the cecum, 6/min at the sigmoid

Migrating Motor Complex (MMC)

- Has 3 phases

Phase I	Quiescent period
Phase II	Period of irregular electrical and mechanical activity
Phase III	Burst of regular activity

- Initiated by motilin, circulating level of this hormone increases at intervals of approximately 100 min in the interdigestive state.
- Migrate aborally at a rate of about 5 cm/ min
- Aids in clearing the stomach and small intestine of luminal contents in preparation for the next meal
- Erythromycin-binds to motilin receptors, useful in treating patients with reduced GI motility

Lower Esophageal Sphincter

- Tonically active but relaxes on swallowing
- Tone of the LES-under neural control: acetylcholine (Contracts the sphincter) and NO and VIP (Relaxation of sphincter)
- Achalasia cardia- myenteric plexus of the esophagus is deficient at the LES and release of NO and VIP is defective

Gastric Motility

- Receptive relaxation- fundus and upper portion of the body relax and accommodate the food with little if any increase in pressure
- Antral systole- contraction of the distal stomach, last up to 10 s
- Fastest emptying-meal rich in carbohydrates
- Slowest emptying-meal rich in fats
- Hyperosmolality of the duodenal contents-sensed by duodenal osmoreceptors and decrease gastric emptying

Transit Time in the Intestine and Colon

Segment	Time
Cecum	4 hrs
First third of the colon	6 hrs
Second third of the colon	9 hrs
Sigmoid colon	12 hrs

Hirschsprung Diseases

- Also called aganglionic megacolon
- Due to congenital absence of the ganglion cells in both the myenteric and submucous plexus in colon (failure of the normal cranial-to-caudal migration of neural crest cells)
- Endothelins-acts on endothelin B receptor necessary for normal migration of certain neural crest cells
- Mutations in endothelin B receptor is one cause of congenital aganglionic mega colon

RENAL PHYSIOLOGY—HIGH YIELD TOPICS

Parameters	Dimension
No. of nephrons in each kidney	1 million
Glomerulus	200 µm in diameter
Filtration slits	25 nm wide
Free passage of neutral substances across glomerulus	Up to 4 nm
Total area of glomerular capillary endothelium for filtration	0.8 m^2
Length of proximal convoluted tubule	15 mm
Distal convoluted tubule	5 mm long
Collecting ducts	20 mm long
Total length of the nephrons	45 to 65 mm
Volume of blood in the renal capillaries	30–40 mL
Renal blood flow	1.2–1.3 per minute
Effective renal plasma flow (ERPF)	625 mL/min
Glomerular capillary pressure	45 mm Hg

Contd...

Contd...

Parameters	Dimension
Peritubular capillary pressure	8 mm Hg
Pressure in the renal vein	4 mm Hg
Cortical blood flow	5 mL/g of kidney tissue/min
Medullary blood flow	Outer medulla (2.5 mL/g/min) Inner medulla (0.6 mL/g/min)
Arteriovenous oxygen difference for the whole kidney	14 mL/L of blood
pO_2 of the cortex	50 mm Hg
pO_2 of the medulla	15 mm Hg
GFR	125 mL/min is 7.5 L/h, or 180 L/d
Amount of protein in the urine	< 100 mg/day
Filtration fraction	0.16–0.20
Filtration coefficient (K_f)	4.2 ml/min/mm Hg
Peristaltic contractions in ureter	1–5 times/min
Half life of vasopressin	18 min

Renal Medullary Interstitial Cells (RMICs)

- Cells in the interstisial tissue of the medulla that appear to have a secretory function
- Specialized fibroblast like cells
- Major site of cyclooxygenase 2 (COX-2) and prostaglandin synthase (PGES) expression
- Synthesize PGE_2

Regulation of Renal blood Flow

- Vasoconstrictors- Norepinephrine, Angiotensin II
- Vasodilators-Dopamine, acetylcholine
- Prostaglandins- increase blood flow in the renal cortex and decrease blood flow in the renal medulla
- Norepinephrine-acting through β_1-adrenergic receptors increases renin secretion and increases Na^+ reabsorption
- Mediator for tubuloglomerular feedback-Adenosine

Filtration Fraction

- The ratio of the GFR to the RPF (renal plasma flow)
- Normally 0.16–0.20

Juxta Glomerular Apparatus

- Comprises of JG cells, Macula Densa and Lacis cells

JG cells	• Also known as Granular cells • Secrete Renin • Located in media of afferent arterioles as they enter glomeruli
Macula densa	• Morphologically distict region of thick ascending limb • Senses sodium chloride concentration via Na^+–K^+–2Cl– cotransporter
Lacis cells	• Also known as extraglomerular mesangial cells • Located at the junction between afferent and efferent arterioles

- **Counter-current multipliers-** loops of henle
- **Counter-current exchangers-** vasa recta

Mesangial Cells

- Support the entire glomerular tuft
- Secrete mesangial matrix
- Are contractile
- Are phagocytic
- Capable of proliferation

Agents Causing Contraction or Relaxation of Mesangial Cells

Contraction	Relaxation
• Endothelins • Angiotensin II • Vasopressin • Norepinephrine • Platelet-activating factor • Platelet-derived growth factor • Thromboxane A_2 • PGF_2 • Leukotrienes C_4 and D_4 • Histamine	• ANP • Dopamine • PGE_2 • cAMP

Transport proteins involved in the movement of Na^+ and Cl^- across the apical membranes of renal tubular cells:

Site	Apical Transporter	Function
Proximal tubule	Na/glucose CT	Na^+ uptake, glucose uptake
	Na^+/P_i CT	Na^+ uptake, P_i uptake
	Na^+ amino acid CT	Na^+ uptake, amino acid uptake
	Na/lactate CT	Na^+ uptake, lactate uptake
	Na/H exchanger	Na^+ uptake, H^+ extrusion
	Cl/base exchanger	Cl^- uptake
Thick ascending limb	Na–K–2Cl CT	Na^+ uptake, Cl^- uptake, K^+ uptake
	Na/H exchanger	Na^+ uptake, H^+ extrusion
	K^+ channels	K^+ extrusion (recycling)
Distal convoluted tubule	NaCl CT	Na^+ uptake, Cl^- uptake
Collecting duct	Na^+ channel (ENaC)	Na^+ uptake

Transport Maximum (Tm):

Renal active transport systems have a maximal rate at which they can transport a particular solute

Glucose T_{m} = 375 mg/min

Proximal convoluted tubule:

Reabsorption:

- Water-67% of filtered load
- NaCl-67% of filtered load
- K^+–67% of filtered load
- Ca^{2+}–70% of filtered load
- Pi-80% of filtered load
- HCO_3–80% of filtered load
- Protein–100% of filtered load
- Urea-67% of filtered load

Henle's loop:
Reabsorption:
- Water-15% of filtered load (thin descending limb only)
- NaCl-25% of filtered load
- K^+–20% of filtered load
- Ca^{2+}–20% of filtered load
- HCO_3–10% of filtered load

Secretion:
- Urea-thin descending limb only

Distal tubule:
Reabsorption:
- NaCl-5% of filtered load
- Ca^{2+}–9% of filtered load
- HCO_3–6% of filtered load
- Pi-10% of filtered load
- Water-variable depending on presence of ADH, ANP

Collecting Duct:
Reabsorption:
- Water-variable depending on presence of ADH, ANP
- NaCl-3% of filtered load
- K^+–normally zero
- HCO_3–4% of filtered load`
- Urea-variable depending on presence of ADH

Secretion:
- K^+–0% to 70% of the filtered load

Monogenic Renal Diseases Involving Transport Proteins

Diseases	Mode of inheritance	Gene	Transport protein	Nephron segment	Phenotype
Cystinuria type I	AR	SLC3A1	Basic amino acid transporter (rBAT)	Proximal tubule	Increased excretion of basic amino acids, nephrolithiasis (kidney stones)
Proximal renaltubular acidosis	AR	SLC4A4	Na^+ –HCO_3^- cotransporter	Proximal tubule	Hyperchloremic metabolic acidosis
Bartter syndrome	AR	SLC12A1 (type I)	Na^+–K^+–$2Cl^-$ transporter (furosemide sensitive)	TAL	Hypokalemia, metabolic alkalosis, hyperal-dosteronism
		KCNJ1 (type II)	Potassium channel		
		CLCNKB (type III)	Chloride channel		
X-linked nephrolithiasis (Dents disease)	XLR	CLC5	Chloride channel (C1C-5)	Distal tubule	Hypercalciuria, nephrolithiasis (kidney stones)
Hypomagnesemia-Hypercalciuria syndrome	AR	PCCLN-1	Paracellin-1	TAL	Hypomagnesemia, hypercalciuria, nephrolithiasis
Gitelman syndrome	AR	SLC12A3	Thiazide-sensitive cotransporter	Distal tubule	Hypomagnesemia, hypokalemic metabolic alkalosis, hypocalciuria, hypotension
Liddle syndrome	AD	SCNN1B SCNN1G	α, β, and γ subunit of amiloride-sensitive Na^+ channel	Collecting duct	Decreased excretionof Na^+, hypertension

Hormones that Regulate NaCl and Water Absorption

Hormone	Major stimulus	Nephron site of action	Effect on transport
Angiotensin II	↑Renin	PT	↑NaCl and H_2O reabsorption
Aldosterone	↑Angiotensin II, ↑ $[K^+]_p$	TAL, DT/CD	↑NaCl and H_2O reabsorption
ANP	↑ECV	CD	↓H_2O and NaCl reabsorption
Urodilatin	↑ECV	CD	↓H_2O and NaCl reabsorption
Sympathetic nerves	↓ECV	PT, TAL, DT/CD	↑NaCl and H_2O reabsorption
Dopamine	↑ECV	PT	↓H_2O and NaCl reabsorption
ADH	↑P_{osm}, ↓ECV	DT/CD	↑H_2O reabsorption

Major Functions of the Various Collecting-duct Cells

Principal Cells

- Reabsorb sodium (stimulated by aldosterone)
- Secrete potassium (stimulated by several signals, including aldosterone)
- Reabsorb water (stimulated by antidiuretic hormone)

Type A Intercalated Cells

- Secrete hydrogen ions, which effect reabsorption of bicarbonate and excretion of titratable acid (stimulated by increased pCO_2 and decreased extracellular pH)
- Reabsorb potassium

Type B Intercalated Cells

- Reabsorb chloride (stimulated by chloride depletion)
- Secrete bicarbonate (stimulated by increased extracellular pH)

Aquaporins

- In 2003, Dr Peter Agre received Nobel prize in chemistry for its discovery
- To date, 13 aquaporins have been identified

Aquaporin subtype	Location
AQP-1	Apical and basolateral membranes of proximal tubule and distal thin limb of Henle
AQP-2	Apical side of principal cells in collecting tubule (Levels regulated by ADH)
AQP-3 and AQP-4	Basolateral side of principal cells in collecting tubule
AQP-4	Blood brain barrier

'Free Water Clearance' (C_{H_2O})

- To quantitate the gain or loss of water by excretion of a concentrated or dilute urine
- Difference between the urine volume and the clearance of osmoles

$$CH_2O = V - \frac{U_{Osm} V}{P_{Osm}}$$

(V is the urine flow rate and U_{Osm} and P_{Osm}, the urine and plasma osmolality respectively)

- C_{H_2O} is negative when the urine is hypertonic and positive when the urine is hypotonic.

Vasopressin

Receptor	Characteristics
V_{1A}	• Acts by increasing the intracellular Ca^{2+} concentration • Mediate the vasoconstrictor effect • Also found in the liver and the brain • Decrease in cardiac output (**area postrema)** • Glycogenolysis in the liver
V_{1B} (also called V_3 receptors)	• Unique to the anterior pituitary • Acts by increasing the intracellular Ca^{2+} concentration • Increase secretion of adrenocorticotropic hormone (ACTH) from the corticotropes
V_2 receptors	• Acts through cAMP • Insertion of aquaporin 2 into the apical membranes of the principal cells of the collecting ducts

Stimuli Affecting Vasopressin Secretion

Vasopressin Secretion Increased	Vasopressin Secretion Decreased
Increased effective osmotic pressure of plasma	Decreased effective osmotic pressure of plasma
Decreased ECF volume	Increased ECF volume
Pain, emotion, stress, exercise	Alcohol
Nausea and vomiting	
Standing	
Clofibrate, carbamazepine	
Angiotensin II	

Vasopressin Escape

- Prolonged exposure to elevated levels of vasopressin can lead eventually to down-regulation of the production of aquaporin-2
- To limit the degree of hyponatremia in SIADH

- **AV3V region**- neuronal area important in controlling osmolarity and ADH secretion. Lesions of this region cause multiple deficits in the control of ADH secretion, thirst, sodium appetite and blood pressure

Renin

- Renin is a glycoprotein synthesised and stored in an inactive form called prorenin in the juxtaglomerular cells of the kidneys.
- Renin itself is an enzyme, not a vasoactive substance. Renin acts enzymatically on another plasma protein, a globulin called renin substrate (or angiotensinogen), to release angiotensin 1

Angiotensinogen

- Synthesized in the liver
- Its circulating levels is increased by glucocorticoids, thyroid hormones, estrogens, several cytokines, and angiotensin II

Angiotensin Converting Enzyme

- Converts angiotensin I to angiotensin II
- Inactivates bradykinin
- Increased tissue bradykinin produced when ACE is inhibited acts on B_2 receptors to produce the cough that is an annoying side effect in up to 20% of the patients treated with ACE inhibitors

Angiotensin-II

Receptor	Characteristics
AT_1	• Acts by increasing the cytosolic free Ca^{2+} level
AT_2	• Coded in X chromosome • Open K^+ channels • Increases the production of nitric oxide • More plentiful in fetal and neonatal life

Actions of Angiotensin II

- One of the most potent vasoconstrictors known
- Arteriolar constriction-rise in systolic and diastolic blood pressure
- Increase the secretion of aldosterone
- Facilitation of the release of norepinephrine
- Contraction of mesangial cells
- Increase Na^+ reabsorption
- Actions in brain-decrease the sensitivity of the baroreflex (area postrema), increase the secretion of vasopressin and ACTH (subfornical organ (SFO) and the OVLT)

Angiotensin III

- 40% of the pressor activity of angiotensin II
- 100% of the aldosterone-stimulating activity

Conditions that Increase Renin Secretion

- Na^+ depletion
- Diuretics
- Hypotension
- Hemorrhage
- Upright posture
- Dehydration
- Cardiac failure
- Cirrhosis
- Constriction of renal artery or aorta
- Various psychologic stimuli

Natriuretic Peptides

- Three types-Atrial Natriuretic Peptide (ANP), brain natriuretic peptide (BNP), C-type natriuretic peptide (CNP)
- Actions:
  1. Dilating afferent arterioles and relaxing mesangial cells-increase Na^+ excretion, inhibit Na^+ reabsorption
  2. Increase in capillary permeability
  3. Relax vascular smooth muscle in arterioles and venules (CNP has a greater dilator effect on veins)
  4. Inhibit renin secretion
  5. In the brain-effects are opposite to those of angiotensin II, involved in lowering blood pressure and promoting natriuresis

Na, K ATPase Inhibiting Factor

- Probably OUABAIN-comes from adrenal gland
- Produces natriuresis

Erythropoietin

- Glycoprotein-165 amino acid residues and 4 oligosaccharide chains
- Increases the number of erythropoietin-sensitive committed stem cells in the bone marrow- converted to red blood cell precursors

• Receptor-has tyrosine kinase activity, inhibits apoptosis of red cells • Source-85% from kidney (interstitial cells in the peritubular capillary bed) and 15% from Liver (perivenous hepatocytes) • Also produced in the brain- protective effect against excitotoxic damage triggered by hypoxia

Stimulators of erythropoietin secretion	1. Hypoxia 2. Cobalt salts 3. Androgens 4. Alkalosis at high altitude 5. Catecholamines via a β-adrenergic mechanism

Micturition

Innervation of bladder	• Degree of stretch–parasympathetic afferents (S_2, S_3 and S_4) • Micturition reflex - parasympathetic efferents (S_2, S_3 and S_4) • Relaxation of external sphincter–pudendal Nerve. • Sense of fullness, pain–sympathetic hypogastric plexus
Micturition centers	• Sacral micturition center (S_2-S_4) • Pontine micturition centre (Barrington's center) -Facilitatory • Posterior hypothalamus- Facilitatory • Mid brain-inhibitory • Cerebral cortex-Detrusor motor area located in medial frontal lobe (superior frontal gyrus)
Micturition abnormalities	**Sensory denervated bladder (Atonic bladder):** • Occurs due to lesions of sacral posterior nerve roots • Stretch impulses are not transmitted to the center, leading to over distension and overflow dribbling (overflow incontinence) • Bladder is thin walled, flaccid, distended and hypotonic **Denervated bladder (Autonomous bladder):** • Both afferent and efferent fibers are interrupted and the bladder is isolated from the spinal cord • Initially the bladder is flaccid and distended. Later becomes active and partially expel its contents • Bladder gets shrunken and atrophied • For Example Cauda equina lesion or section of pelvic nerves **Uninhibited neurogenic bladder:** • In lesions in which the corticospinal inhibitory fibres are damaged, leaving the facilitatory fibres intact • There is increased frequency with voiding of small quantities

ENDOCRINE PHYSIOLOGY AND REPRODUCTIVE PHYSIOLOGY—HIGH YIELD TOPICS

• The term endocrine was coined by Starling • The first hormone to be discovered–'secretin' in 1902 by Starling and Bayliss

Five Major Classes of Hormones

1. Amino acid derivatives---dopamine, catecholamine 2. Small neuropeptides ---GnRH, TRH 3. Large proteins---insulin, PTH 4. Steroid hormones ---Cortisol, estrogen 5. Vitamin derivatives---Vit-A, Vit-D

Receptors for Hormones

Membrane Receptors 1. Seven transmembrane GPCRs 2. Tyrosine kinase receptors (Insulin, IGF-1) 3. Cytokine receptors (Growth hormone, prolactin)	Nuclear Receptors Has various domains: • AF_1-also known as modulator region and involved in activating transcription

4. Serine kinase receptors (Activin. TGF-beta)	• DBD-C domain, binds to hormone responsive elements (DNA sequences) • LBD-Ligand binding domain which binds ligand • Hinge region-permits flexibility • AF_2-interacts with coactivators and facilitates transactivation Receptors for 1. Glucocorticoids 2. Mineralocorticoids 3. Androgen 4. Estrogen 5. Progestin 6. Thyroid hormones 7. Vitamin D
Receptors are dynamic structures Can be down regulated or up regulated	Down regulation through 1. Receptor mediated endocytosis 2. Internalization 3. Desensitization
First messenger	Extracellular ligands
Second messenger	Intracellular mediators

Three Major Families of G-proteins

G_s • b-adrenergic receptor • ACTH receptor • FSH receptor	• Couples to adenylate cyclase • Stimulates AC activity • Increases cAMP • Activates protein kinase A
G_i • a_2-adrenergic receptor • M_2 muscarinic receptor	• Couples to adenylate cyclase • Inhibits AC activity • Decreases cAMP • Inhibits protein kinase A
G_q • a_1-adrenergic receptor • M_1, M_3 muscarinic receptors • Angiotensin receptor	• Couples to phospholipase C • Increases diacylgyclerol (DAG) • Increases IP3 • Increases intracellular Ca^{2+} • Activates protein kinase C

G proteins and their Receptor Abnormalities

Site	Type of mutation	Disease
	Receptor	
Cone opsins	Loss	Colour blindness
Rhodopsin	Loss	Congenital night blindness; two forms of retinitis pigmentosa
V_2 vasopressin	Loss	X-linked nephrogenic diabetes insipidus
ACTH	Loss	Familial glucocorticoid Deficiency
LH	Gain	Familial male precocious puberty
TSH	Gain	Familial nonautoimmune hyperthyroidism
TSH	Loss	Familial hypothyroidism
Ca^{2+}	Gain	Familial hypercalciuric Hypocalcemia
Thromboxane A_2	Loss	Congenital bleeding

Contd...

Contd...

Site	Type of mutation	Disease
Receptor		
Endothelin B	Loss	Hirschsprung disease
G protein		
$G_s \alpha$	Loss	Pseudohypothyroidism type 1a
$G_s \alpha$	Gain/loss	Testotoxicosis
$G_s \alpha$	Gain (mosaic)	McCune-Albright syndrome
$G_s \alpha$	Gain	Somatotroph adenomas with acromegaly
$G_i \alpha$	Gain	Ovarian and adrenocortical tumors

Hormones that use the Adenylyl Cyclase–cAMP Second Messenger System (Mn-FLAGSHiP-CCTV$_2$-CASh)

- Adrenocorticotropic hormone (ACTH)
- Angiotensin II (epithelial cells)
- Calcitonin
- Catecholamines (b receptors)
- Corticotropin-releasing hormone (CRH)
- Follicle-stimulating hormone (FSH)
- Glucagon
- Human chorionic gonadotropin (hCG)
- Luteinizing hormone (LH)
- Parathyroid hormone (PTH)
- Secretin
- Somatostatin
- Thyroid-stimulating hormone (TSH)
- Vasopressin (V2 receptor, epithelial cells)

- **cAMP is constantly inactivated by phosphodiesterase**
- Theophylline blocks the phosphodiesterase

Hormones that use the Phospholipase C Second Messenger System (V$_1$ GOT AC)

- Angiotensin II (vascular smooth muscle)
- Catecholamines (a receptors)
- Gonadotropin-releasing hormone (GnRH)
- Growth hormone–releasing hormone (GHRH)
- Oxytocin
- Thyroid-releasing hormone (TRH)
- Vasopressin (V1 receptor, vascular smooth muscle)

Calcium-Calmodulin dependent protein kinases (Mn-MCG)
- Myosin Light Chain Kinase
- Glycogen Phosphorylase Kinase

Guanylate Cyclase Receptors (Mn. NAG)

Transmembrane Guanylate Cyclase Receptor	Activated by peptide hormones (Atrial natriuretic peptide/factor ANP)
Soluble Guanylate Cyclase Receptor	Activated by Nitric Oxide (NO)

Pituitary Gland

- The pituitary gland weighs approx. 600 mg
- Folliculostellate cells- release paracrine factors
- Pluripotent stem cells-responsible for plasticity in pituitary.

Anterior Pituitary

- Originates from Rathke's pouch
- Cell types—Somatotrope (GH), Lactotrope (prolactin), Corticotroph (ACTH), Thyrotroph (TSH), Gonadotrophs (FSH, LH)
- Maximum (30-40%) percentage of secretory cells-Somatotrope
- 20% of secretory cells-Corticotrophs
- Minimum percentage of secretory cells-Thyrotroph
- Acidophilic cells-Prolactin, Growth hormone (Mn. Parle-G)

Posterior Pituitary

- Originates from a neural tissue outgrowth from the hypothalamus and this explains the presence of glial-type cells in this gland
- Composed mainly of glial-like cells called pituicytes (modified astrocytes)
- Pituicytes do not secrete hormones but they act as a supporting cells
- Posterior pituitary hormones are initially synthesized in the cell bodies of the supraoptic and paraventricular nuclei and are then transported in combination with carrier proteins called neurophysins down to the nerve endings in the posterior pituitary gland.

Proopiomelanocortin (POMC)

- Intermediate lobe cells of pituitary, if present, and corticotropes of the anterior lobe both synthesize a large precursor protein that is cleaved to form a family of hormones. After removal of the signal peptide, this prohormone is known as **Proopiomelanocortin (POMC)**
- It is also synthesized in the hypothalamus, the lungs, the gastrointestinal tract, and the placenta
- In corticotrophs- POMC hydrolysed to ACTH, beta lipoprotein and beta endorphins
- In the Intermediate lobe cells, POMC is hydrolyzed to corticotropin-like intermediate-lobe peptide (CLIP), γ-LPH, β-endorphin, α and β-MSH
- α and β-MSH do not circulate in adult humans
- ACTH binds to melanotropin-1 receptors (pigmentation in addison's disease)

Human Growth Hormone

1. Present in long arm of human chromosome 17
2. Half life is 6-20 minutes
3. Daily growth hormone output- 0.5 to 1 mg/day in adults
4. 50% bound to protein—provides reservoir
5. Receptor - cytokine receptor superfamily
6. Acts through JAK2-STAT pathway
7. Ghrelin-marked growth hormone-stimulating activity

Factors that Stimulate or Inhibit Secretion of Growth Hormone

Stimulate Growth Hormone Secretion	Inhibit Growth Hormone Secretion
• Decreased blood glucose • Decreased blood free fatty acids • Starvation or fasting, protein deficiency • Trauma, stress, excitement • Exercise, pyrogen • Testosterone, estrogen • Deep sleep (stages II and IV) • Growth hormone–releasing hormone • Glucagon • Ghrelin	• Increased blood glucose • Increased blood free fatty acids • Obesity • Aging • Growth hormone inhibitory hormone (somatostatin) • Growth hormone (exogenous) • Somatomedins (insulin-like growth factors) • REM sleep • Cortisol

Effects of Growth Hormone

Effect on growth	• Epiphyses not yet closed---chondrogenesis is accelerated, as the cartilaginous epiphysial plates widen they lay down more bone matrix at the ends of long bones • Epiphyses closed---linear growth is no longer possible • Increased deposition of protein by the chondrocytic and osteogenic cells that cause bone growth • Increased rate of reproduction of chondrocytic and osteogenic cells • A specific effect of converting chondrocytes into osteogenic cells, thus causing deposition of new bone
Effects on protein metabolism	• Protein anabolic hormone • Positive nitrogen and phosphorus balance • Fall in blood urea nitrogen and amino acid levels
Effect on electrolytes	• GI absorption of Ca^{2+} increased • Na^+ and K^+ excretion is reduced • Excretion of the amino acid 4-hydroxyproline is increased
Effect on carbohydrate metabolism	• Anti insulin effect in muscles • Diabetogenic-increase hepatic glucose output
Effect on fat metabolism	• Ketogenic • Increases circulating free fatty acid (FFA) • Provides a ready source of energy during hypoglycaemia, fasting and stress
Effect on organs and soft tissues	• Increases the growth of all internal organs and soft tissues

Somatomedins (Insulin-like Growth Factors)

- Polypeptide growth factors secreted by the liver and other tissues
- The effects of growth hormone on growth, cartilage, and protein metabolism depend on an interaction between growth hormone and somatomedins
- Somatomedin C-otherwise known as IGF-1
- IGF-1: Mediates the insulin like activity, antilypolytic activity, protein synthesis, epiphyseal growth actions of growth hormone
- IGF-2-otherwise known as multiplication stimulating activity.

Growth Hormone Disorders

In children (excessive growth hormone before the epiphysis of long bones have fused with the shafts)	Gigantism • In 10% of giants, full blown diabetes mellitus eventually develops
In adults (excessive growth hormone after the epiphysis of long bones have fused with the shafts)	Acromegaly • Greatly enlarged hands and feet • Vertebral changes attributable to osteoarthritis • Soft tissue swelling, hirsutism • Protrusion of the brow and jaw • Abnormal growth of internal organs
Laron Dwarfism (growth Hormone insensitivity)	• Reduced plasma IGF-1 • GH levels normal or high
• Hypersecretion of growth hormone is accompanied by hypersecretion of prolactin in 20–40% of patients with acromegaly • About 25% of patients have abnormal glucose tolerance tests, and 4% develop lactation in the absence of pregnancy	

Prolactin

1. Weakly homologous to GH and human placental lactogen (hPL)
2. Normal levels--10–25 g/L in women and 10–20 g/L in men
3. Secretion is pulsatile
4. Highest peaks occurring during rapid eye movement sleep
5. Half life is 20 minutes
6. Inhibited by Dopamine (D2), Glucocorticoids, Thyroid hormones
7. Stimulated by thyrotrophin releasing hormone, vasoactive intestinal peptide
8. Serum PRL levels rise transiently after
   - Exercise, meals
   - Sexual intercourse
   - Minor surgical procedures
   - General anesthesia
   - Chest wall injury
   - Acute myocardial infarction

Prolactin levels increase markedly during pregnancy and lactation, in the breast, the lobuloalveolar epithelium proliferates

- Functions of prolactin:
  1. Decrease reproductive function
  2. Suppress sexual drive
  3. Promotes lactation---causes milk secretion from the breast after estrogen and progesterone priming
  4. In females---hypoestrogenism and anovulation
  5. In males---decreased spermatogenesis, low testosterone

Thyroid Gland

- One of the largest of the endocrine glands weighing 15–20 gms in adults
- Blood flow—160 ml/100 g/min
- Maintain the level of metabolism in the tissues
- Stimulate O_2 consumption by most of the cells
- Secretes T3, T4 and calcitonin
- Thyrocytes express receptors for
  TSH
  IGF-I
  EGF
  IGF-I and EGF promote growth
  Interferon γ and tumor necrosis factor inhibit growth
- Lodine-the raw material for thyroid hormone synthesis
  Dietary Iodide-absorbed from intestine
  Minimal daily requirement-150 μg in adults
  20% enters thyroid gland
  80% excreted by kidney
  Salivaryglands, mammaryglands, placenta-extrathyroidal
- Binding proteins
  - Albumin
  - A prealbumin called transthyretin (formerly called thyroxine binding prealbumin)
  - Thyroxine-binding globulin (TBG)
- Albumin--largest capacity to bind T4
- TBG--largest affinity to bind T4
- A protein called **pendrin** (chloride-iodide ion counter-transporter) helps to transport iodide out of the thyroid cells into the follicle
- Sodium-iodide symporter- A type of secondary active transport protein that cotransports one iodide ion along with two sodium ions across the basolatreal (plasma) membrane into the cell

T4 vs T3

Characteristics	T4	T3
Half life	Long (6 days)	Short (2 days)
Max binding	TBG	Albumin
In colloid	More (25%)	Less (7%)
Potency	Less	More (3–5 times)
Action	Slower	Much rapid
Binding to nuclear receptors	Less	More

Thyroid Stimulating Hormone (TSH)

1. Glycoprotein
2. Alpha chain-chromosome 6, beta chain-chromosome 1
3. Half life 60 min
4. Secretion is pulsatile, peaks at midnight
5. Average plasma level-2 µg/ml
6. Increases iodine trapping, synthesis of t3, t4, secretion of thyroglobulin, endocytosis of colloid
7. Inhibited by stress, dopamine, somatostatin, thyroid hormones

Physiologic Effects of Thyroid Hormones

Heart	Chronotropic and Inotropic	• Increased number of β-adrenergic receptors • Enhanced responses to circulating catecholamines • Increased proportion of α-myosin heavy chain (with higher ATPase activity)
Adipose tissue	Catabolic	• Stimulates lipolysis
Muscle	Catabolic	• Increased protein breakdown
Bone	Developmental	• Promote normal growth and skeletal development
Nervous system	Developmental	• Promote normal brain development
Gut	Metabolic	• Increased rate of carbohydrate absorption
Lipoprotein	Metabolic	• Formation of LDL receptors
Other	Calorigenic	• Stimulated oxygen consumption by metabolically active tissues (exceptions: **t**estes, **u**terus, **l**ymph nodes, **s**pleen, **an**terior pituitary (Mn. LUSTAN) • Increased metabolic rate

Wolf-Chaikoff Effect	Intake of iodide exceeds 2 mg/day --Iodide suppresses NADPH oxidase activity and the NIS and TPO genes --Inhibits hormone biosynthesis
Jod-Basedow Phenomenon	Lodine-induced hyperthyroidism, typically presenting in a patient with endemic goiter

Endocrine Pancreas

- The islet of Langerhans are Scattered throughout the pancreas, but they are more plentiful in the tail than the body and head

The cells in the islets can be divided into types on the basis of their staining properties and morphology-

- A cell- make up 20% of the total, surrounds the B cells and secrete glucagon
- B cell- most common, 60% of the total, located in the centre of each islet and secrete insulin
- D cell- less common, secrete somatostatin and gastrin
- F cell- less important in humans, secrete pancreatic polypeptide

Insulin

- Has an alpha and beta chain
- Transcription factors-hepatocyte nuclear factor-4 and pancreatic and intestinal homeobox-1
- Zinc bound crystals

- Insulin synthesis
  - Initially preproinsulin is formed in the ribosomes
  - Preproinsulin is then cleaved in the endoplasmic reticulum to form a proinsulin which consists of 3 chains of peptides, A, B and C
  - Most of the proinsulin is further cleaved in the golgi apparatus to form insulin (composed of the A and B chain) and the C chain peptide (called connecting peptide or C peptide)
  - The insulin and C peptide are packaged in the secretory granules and secreted in equimolar amounts
- C peptide binds to a membrane structure activates sodium potassium ATPase and endothelial nitric oxide synthase
- Measurements of C peptide in the blood--quantify endogenous insulin production in patients receiving exogenous insulin
- Glucokinase-rate limiting step in insulin secretion
- Biphasic insulin release-early phase-preformed insulin, late phase-newly formed
- Half life-5 min
- Degraded by Insulinase in liver
- Otherwise called' Hormone of abundance'

Principal Actions:

- Rapid-Increases transport of glucose amino acids and potassium into insulin sensitive cells.
- Intermediate-stimulates protein synthesis, Inhibits protein breakdown, activation of glycolytic and inhibition of gluconeogenic enzymes
- Delayed-Increases formation of mRNA for lipogenic action

Effects of insulin on various tissues:

Adipose tissue

- Increased glucose entry
- Increased fatty acid synthesis
- Increased glycerol phosphate synthesis
- Increased triglyceride deposition
- Activation of lipoprotein lipase
- Inhibition of hormone-sensitive lipase
- Increased K^+ uptake

Muscle

- Increased glucose entry
- Increased glycogen synthesis
- Increased amino acid uptake
- Increased protein synthesis in ribosomes
- Decreased protein catabolism
- Decreased release of gluconeogenic amino acids
- Increased ketone uptake
- Increased K^+ uptake

Liver

- Decreased ketogenesis
- Increased protein synthesis
- Increased lipid synthesis
- Decreased glucose output due to decreased gluconeogenesis, increased glycogen synthesis, and increased glycolysis

General

- Increased cell growth

Glucagon

- Human preproglucagon is found in pancreatic A cells, in L cells of the lower GIT, and in the brain.
- In A cells, it is processed primarily to glucagon and major proglucagon fragment
- In L cells it is processed primarily to glicentin, glucagon-like polypeptides 1 and 2, and oxyntomodulin
- Glicentin has some glucagon activity
- GLP-1 (7–36), is a potent stimulator of insulin secretion
- GLP-2 lowers food intake
- Oxyntomodulin-inhibits gastric acid secretion

Actions of glucagon:

- Glycogenolytic, gluconeogenic, lipolytic, and ketogenic
- Does not cause glycogenolysis in muscle

- Positively inotropic effect on the heart
- Stimulates the secretion of growth hormone, insulin and pancreatic somatostatin
- Half life-5–10 min

Somatostatin

- Growth hormone inhibiting hormone
- Secreted by D cells of pancreas and by similar D cells in the gastrointestinal mucosa
- Inhibit the secretion of insulin, glucagon, and pancreatic polypeptide—paracrine
- Inhibits secretion of gastrin, VIP, GIP, secretin, motilin
- Decreases gastric acid secretion and motility
- Inhibition of CCK secretion
- Increased by several of the same stimuli that increase insulin secretion

Pancreatic Polypeptide

- Secreted by F cells in the islets
- Secretion is under cholinergic control
- Increased by a meal containing protein and by fasting, exercise, and acute hypoglycemia
- Secretion is decreased by somatostatin and intravenous glucose
- Slows the absorption of food in humans

Other Factors Affecting Carbohydrate Metabolism

- Exercise-insulin independent increase in the number of GLUT 4
- Epinephrine-glycogenolysis, increase hepatic glucose output, decrease peripheral use
- Thyroid hormones-Hyperglycemia, metathyroid diabetes, enhances GI glucose absorption
- Cortisol-Gluconeogenic (Permissive)
- GH-Anti-insulin effect, increase hepatic glucose output

Adrenal Gland

- Adrenal Cortex
  {Mneumonic: Layers- ***GFR***
  Their secretions can be remembered as ***salt, sweet and sex*** for Mineralocorticoid, Glucocorticoids and androgens respectively
  - Zona glomerulosa-Mineralocorticoid (15%). Also involved in formation of new cortical cells
  - Zona fasciculata-Glucocorticoids (50%)
  - Zona reticularis-Adrenal androgens (7%)
- Adrenal Medulla (18%)
  - Epinephrine (90% cells, larger, less dense granules)
  - Nor epinehrine (10% cells, smaller dense granules)
  - Dopamine
- In the adrenal medulla, norepinephrine and epinephrine are stored in granules with ATP. The granules also contain substance called chromogranin A
- Adrenomedullin - a vasodepressor polypeptide found in the adrenal medulla
- Paraganglia- small groups of cells resembling those in the adrenal medulla, are found near the thoracic and abdominal sympathetic ganglia

Effects of Epinephrine and Norepinephrine:

1. Glycogenolysis in liver and skeletal muscle
2. Mobilization of free fatty acids (FFA),
3. Increased plasma lactate
4. Stimulation of the metabolic rate
5. Increases secretion of insulin and glucagon (Beta) and decreases the same (Alpha)
6. Intial increase in K^+, then prolonged fall (beta 2)

Effects of Dopamine:

1. Renal and mesentric vasodilation
2. Elsewhere-Vasoconstriction

3. Positive inotropic effect-use in cardiogenic, traumatic shock
4. Natriuresis by inhibiting renal sodium potassium ATPase

Adrenal cortical hormones:
- Derivatives of cholesterol
- Has cyclopentanoperhydrophenanthrene nucleus

Aldosterone

- Increase the reabsorption of Na^+ from the urine, sweat, saliva, and the contents of the colon
- In kidney they primarily act on principal cells (P cells) producing K^+ diuresis and urinary acidity
- Genomic action—through serum- and glucocorticoid-regulated kinase (sgk)
- Nongenomic action---increases the activity of membrane Na^+–K^+ exchangers

Aldosterone Escape:
- Whenever aldosterone is increased, Na^+ ions are retained in the body.
- This causes osmotic absorption of water. Therefore ECF volume increases.
- Increase in ECF leads to increase in arterial pressure causing excretion of salt and water by pressure diuresis, natriuresis (ANP)
- This secondary increase in water and salt excretion by the kidneys is called **aldosterone escape**.

Aldosterone Excess:
- **Primary Hyper Aldosteronism (Conn's syndrome):**
  - Caused by an adenoma of the zona glomerulosa, adrenal carcinoma
  - Renin secretion is depressed
- **Secondary Hyper Aldosteronism**
  - Caused by cirrhosis, heart failure, and nephrosis
  - High renin

Apparent Mineralocorticoid Excess (AME)
1. 11 -hydroxysteroid dehydrogenase type 2 deficiency
2. Due to intake of licorice containing glycyrrhetinic acid
3. Hyperaldosteronism, hypertension

Glucocorticoid-Remediable Aldosteronism (GRA):
1. Autosomal dominant disorder
2. ACTH-sensitive aldosterone synthase
3. Suppressed by administrating cortisol

Addison's disease: Primary adrenal insuffiency due to disease process that destroy the adrenal cortex
- Loss of sodium and chloride ions
- Excess of potassium ions
- Fluid and blood volume decreases
- Diminished cardiac output
- Shock like state
- Death in 3 days to 2 weeks
- Highly susceptible to stress and infections.
- Pigmentation of skin and mucus membrane
- Mineralocorticoid is life saving hormone of adrenal gland

Secondary adrenal insuffiency: Caused by pituitary diseases that decrease ACTH secretion

Tertiary adrenal insuffiency: Caused by hypothalamic disorders disrupting CRH secretion

Pseudohypoaldosteronism: Produced when there is resistance to the action of aldosterone

Addisonian crisis:
- A person with Addison's disease succumbs to stress. This condition is called addisonian crisis. They need extra amounts of glucocorticoids

Glucocorticoids-Cortisol

- This is a C21 steroid produced mainly from zona fasciculata
- It combines with cortisol binding globulin
- 96% of the cortisol is transported in bound form. Only 4% is transported in free form
- It stays in circulation for 1 to 2 hours
- It is degraded in the liver and conjugated to form glucuronides. It is excreted in urine
- About 75% of the daily production of cortisol occurs between 4 am and 10 am

Functions of Cortisol

On carbohydrate metabolism	• It stimulates gluconeogenesis by the liver by increasing glucose-6-phosphatase • It decreases rate of glucose utilization by the peripheral tissues by inhibiting phosphorylation (anti-insulin action) —Adrenal Diabetes • Increases glycogen synthesis in liver by increasing activity of glycogen synthase
On protein metabolism	• It causes protein breakdown in skeletal muscles • Cortisol enhances amino acid uptake by the liver cells and enhances transamination - (AA synthesis), deamination–(glucose formation) • Hence proteins like plasma proteins produced by liver are increased
On fat metabolism	• It causes fatty acid mobilization from adipose tissue increasing free fatty acids in plasma • It stimulates absorption of lipids from the intestine • It causes redistribution of fats in the body
Water and mineral metabolism	• Mild mineralocorticoid activity–retains Na^+ and excretes K^+ retains • Increases angiotensinogen synthesis in liver leading to Na retention via aldosterone • Provides adequate GFR via anti-ADH activity
Anti-inflammatory effect	• Cortisol inhibits all aspects of inflammation. • It reduces leucocyte margination, chemotaxis, phagocytosis of bacteria. • Aggregation of monocytes is also inhibited. • Cortisol inhibits the synthesis and release of chemical mediators of inflammation like prostaglandins and arachidonic acid
Effect on blood cells	• Causes eosinopenia-sequestration of it in lungs and spleen, increased destruction • Lymphopenia–due to reduced formation and increased destruction • Basopenia • Neutrophilia -increased release from bone marrow, decreased margination and escape to the tissues • Polycythemia by stimulation of erythropoiesis
Permissive action	• On glucagon and catecholamines to exert calorigenic action • On catecholamines to exert lipolytic effect and glycogenolytic effect • On catecholamines to exert pressor response and bronchodilation
On bone	• It causes demineralization of bone • Retards development of cartilage • Thinning of epiphyseal plate • Breaks down bone matrix • Decreases calcium deposition • Increases calcium excretion • Decreases calcium absorption from GIT • Results in osteoporosis and tetany

Abnormalities of the Adrenal Cortex

Cushing's syndrome	• Excess secretion of glucocorticoids **Causes** • Adrenocortical tumours • Anterior pituitary tumours • Ectopic ACTH producing tumour • Prolonged glucocorticoid therapy – Cushing's syndrome caused due to tumors of anterior pituitary is called **Cushing's disease**
21-Hydroxylase deficiency	• Adrenal and gonads • Most common form of congenital adrenal hyperplasia (80-90%) • Signs and symptoms: – Dehydration, hyperkalemia, hyponatremia – Genital ambiguity (XX) – Advanced somatic development – Short adult stature

11 β-hydroxylase deficiency	• Adrenals • 10–20% cases of congenital adrenal hyperplasia • 11-deoxycorticosterone accumulation • Signs and symptoms: – Hypertension – Genital ambiguity (XX) – Advanced somatic development – Short adult stature
3 β-hydroxysteroid dehydrogenase deficiency	• Adrenals and gonads • Signs and symptoms: – Dehydration – Hyperkalemia, hyponatremia – Ambiguous genitalia (hypospadia, undescended testis, cliteromegaly)
Lipoid adrenal hyperplasia	• Steroidogenic acute response protein (StAR) mutation • Adrenal and gonads • Signs and symptoms: – Dehydration – Alkalosis, hyperkalemia, hyponatremia – Female external genitalia regardless of genetic sex (male pseudohermaphroditism in XY individuals) – Undescended testis
17 α-hydroxylase deficiency	• Adrenal and gonads • Increased corticosterone, deoxycorticosterone • Decreased sex hormones, cortisol • Signs and symptoms: – Hypertension – Episodic vomiting, headache – Female external genitalia – Undescended testis
Adrenogenital syndrome	• An adrenocortical tumour secretes excess amounts of androgens causing intense masculanizing effects. • Females develop virile characteristics like growth of beard, deep voice, baldness, masculine distribution of hair and growth of clitoris. • Prepubertal male has rapid development of sexual organs (precocious puberty). • In an adult male, it is difficult to diagnose the condition because the signs are obscured by normal virilizing characteristics of testosterone.

Hormones Involved in Calcium Homeostasis

- 1, 25 Dihydrocholecalciferol
- Parathyroid hormone
- Calcitonoin
- Parathyroid hormone related protein { PTHrP}
- Miscellaneous hormones:
  - Glucocorticoids, growth hormone, estrogen

Parathormone

- Four parathyroid glands located behind the thyroid gland
- 6 × 3 × 2 mm
- Two types of cells:
  1. Chief cells
  2. Oxyphil cells
- Normal plasma PTH-10-55 pg/mL
- Half life–10 mins
- Magnesium is required to maintain normal parathyroid secretory responses

Actions of PTH:
- Increases calcium and phosphate absorption from the bones
- Decreases excretion of calcium by the kidneys
- Increases the excretion of phosphate by the kidneys (inhibits NaPi cotransporter) (Phosphate Terminating Hormone)
- Increases intestinal absorption of calcium and phosphate

All these actions leads to increased plasma calcium

Abnormalities of PTH Secretion

Primary hyperparathyroidism	• Tumors–adenoma of parathyroid glands • Extreme osteolytic resorption • Increase in calcium and decrease in phosphate levels
Secondary hyperparathyroidism	• Increased levels of PTH is the result of compensatory mechanism to hypocalcemia • Due to chronic renal disease or deficiency of vitamin D_3
Familial benign hypocalciuric hypercalcemia	• Inactivating mutation in calcium receptor (CaR)
Familial hypercalciuric hypocalcemia	• Gain of function mutation (CaR)
Pseudohypoparathyroidism	• 50% reduction of the activity of G_s occurs

Parathormone Related Peptide (PTHrP)

As a paracrine signal	• In cell differentiation and survival
Physiological endocrine role	• In pregnancy-increases placental calcium transport • During lactation-maintains adequate calcium levels for lactation
Pathological	• Hypercalcemia of malignancy

PTHrP is also found in keratinocytes in the skin, in smooth muscle, and in the teeth, where it is present in the enamel epithelium that caps each tooth. In the absence of PTHrP, teeth cannot erupt.

Vitamin D:

Promotes intestinal calcium absorption by
1. Formation of calcium binding protein (calbindin)
2. Formation of calcium stimulated ATPase
3. Formation of alkaline phosphatase

Decreases renal excretion of calcium and phosphate

Increases both bone resorption and bone mineralization

1. ***Bone Resorption*** by stimulating PTH

Calcitriol receptors are present in osteoblasts

Receptor–calcitriol complex–stimulate osteoblasts --- activation and differentiation of osteoclasts

2. ***Bone Mineralization***–by stimulation osteoblasts and alkaline phosphatase secretion

- Vitamin D Resistant Rickets:
  - Mutations in the gene coding for the enzyme
  - 1 α hydroxylase
  - 1, 25-dihydroxycholecalciferol receptor (type II vitamin D-resistant rickets)

Calcitonin and its Actions

- Secreted by C cells of thyroid
- Helps in calcium absorption during pregnancy and lactation
- Decreases osteoclasts number and activity

Fibroblast Growth Factor 23 (FGF 23)

- Secreted by osteoblasts
- Inhibits vitamin D

- Inhibits PTH
- Promotes calcium and phosphate excretion
- Mutation in PHEX-X-linked hypophosphatemia, FGF23 levels increase

Role of Other Hormones in Calcium Homeostasis

Glucocorticoids	• Lowers plasma calcium by inhibiting osteoclasts. • Over long periods–osteoporosis • Inhibit protein synthesis in osteoblasts, thereby synthesis of organic matrix • Inhibit absorption of calcium and phosphate from the gut and facilitate its excretion in the kidneys.
Growth hormone	• Increases intestinal absorption of calcium 'positive calcium balance'
IGF–I	• Stimulates protein synthesis in bone
Thyroid hormone	• Hypercalcemia, hypercalciuria and osteoporosis
Estrogens	• Prevents osteoporosis by inhibiting certain cytokines
Insulin	• Increases bone formation

REPRODUCTIVE PHYSIOLOGY—HIGH YIELD TOPICS

Genetic Sex	44XY and 44XX…presence or absence of Y chromosome
Gonadal Sex	Testis in male and ovary in female
Phenotypic Sex	Based on internal and external genital organs

The SRY Gene:

- Located on the Y chromosome, is the primary determinant of sexual development
- If a developing embryo has a **functional** SRY gene in its cells, it will develop as a male (Testis). And, if there is no functional SRY, the embryo develops as female

Female	Bipotential structure	Male
Clitoris	Genital tubercle	Glans penis
Labia minora	Urethral folds and groove	Shaft of penis
Labia majora	Labioscrotal swellings	Scrotum
Forms ovary	Gonad (cortex)	Regresses
Regresses	Gonad (medulla)	Forms testis

Functions of Sertoli cells:

1. Forms a blood-testes barrier
2. Mechanical support for maturing gametes
3. Provides nutrition to developing spermatozoa
4. Helps in maturation of sperms
5. Phagocytes damaged germ cells
6. Participates in spermiation
7. Provides driving force for conveying sperm from testes to epididymis
8. Produces various substances
   - H-Y antigen
   - Anti Mullerian hormone/MIS
   - Androgen binding protein (ABP)
   - Inhibins
   - Aromatase → Testosterone to estrogen

Peritubular Myoid cells:

- Have contractile effects on tubules and vasculature
- Secretes paracrine regulatory products

Reflex pathway for erection (Parasympathetic-Points)	• Afferent → Pudendal nerve • Efferent → Pelvic splanchnic neve/nervi erigenti (Parasympathetic) • Neurotransmitter → Ach, VIP, and Nitric Oxide
Emission (Sympathetic-Shoots)	• Movement of semen into urethra, by contraction of vas deferens, epididymis, ejaculatory ducts and seminal vesicles. • Sympathetic response (T_{12}-L_2)
Ejaculation	• Expulsion of semen out of urethra by contraction of bulbocavernous muscle and smooth muscles at the base of penis • It is also a spinal reflex

Spermatogensesis	Oogenesis
Spermatogonium (2n) ↓ Mitosis Primary spermatocyte (2n) ↓ Meiosis Two secondary spermatocytes (n) ↓ Two spermatids (n) from each ↓ Spermatozoa (n) ***1 primary spermatocyte gives rise to 4 spermatids** *1 Spermatogonium gives rise to 512 spermatids *It takes 74 days for the spermatogonium to become spermatozoa	**Oogonia** (2n), ↓ Ist meiotic division in embryonic ovary, arrested in the stage of late prophase **Primary Oocyte** (2n) ↓ completion of Ist meiotic division, Just before ovulation **Secondary Oocyte** (n) + Ist polar body ↓ IInd meiotic division, arrested at metaphase **Oozoa (n)** +IInd polar body The second meiotic division is completed only after the entry of sperm in to ovum **1 primary Oocyte gives rise to one ovum**

- The arrest in metaphase is due, at least in some species, to formation in the ovum of the protein PP39mos, which is encoded by the C-mos protooncogene. When fertilization occurs, the PP39mos is destroyed within 30 min by calpain, a calcium-dependent cysteine cysteine protease
- Matured spermatozoa are released from Sertoli cells and stored, matured and gains motility in epididymis
- The ability of the sperm to move forward (progressive motility), which is acquired in the epididymis, involves activation of a unique sit of proteins from the **CatSper** family, which are localized to the principal piece of the sperm tail
- Capacitation occurs in female genital tract
- The membrane of late spermatids and spermatozoa contain a special small form of angiotensin converting enzyme called **germinal angiotensin converting enzyme (gACE).** The full function of gACE has yet to be elucidated
- Spermatozoa express olfactory receptors, and ovaries produce odorant-like molecules. Recent evidence indicates that these molecules and their receptors interact, fastering movement of the spermatozoa toward the ovary (chemotaxis)

Soon after cell division has started during embryonic development, one of the two X chromosomes of the somatic cells in normal females becomes functionally inactive. In normal cells, the inactive X chromosome condenses and can be seen near the nuclear membrane as the **Barr Body** also called **sex chromatin**

Composition of Semen:

- Color → white, opalescent.
- Specific gravity → 1028
- pH → 7.35-7.5
- Composition:
  - Sperms → 5%
  - Prostate → 20%
  - Seminal vesicle → 60%
- Sperm count → about 50–100 million/ml.
- Volume → 2.5-3.5 ml/ejaculate.
- Sperm movement → 3 mm/min in female tract
- Maximal duration of fertilising capacity in female tract is 24-48 hours, motility persists for 48-60 hours
- Reaction of semen is alkaline

Prostate gland constituents:
- Citrate, Calcium, Zinc, Spermine, Cholesterol, Phospholipids, Fibrinolysins, Fibrinogenase, Acid Phosphatase.

Seminal vesicle constituents:
- Fructose, Phosphoryl choline, Ergothioneine, Ascorbic acid, Flavins, Prostaglandins

Capacitation:
- Continuation of sperm differentiation in female genital tract.
- Function: Prepares the sperm plasma membrane for acrosome reaction.
- Time taken → 1-4hours

Changes:
- Changes in motility pattern.
- Loss of adsorbed surface proteins, decapacitation factors.
- Loss of lipid and sterol components and redistribution of surface proteins.
- Increased permeability to calcium.
  - Ca^{++} influx into head → acrosome reaction.
  - Ca^{++} influx into mitochondria → changes in motility.

Acrosome reaction:
- Involves distinct structural changes in plasma membrane and outer acrosomal membrane.

Ca^{++} dependent

Changes in sperm after acrosome reaction:
- Conversion of inactive enzymes into active enzymes.
- A new surface, inner acrosomal membrane which contains proteins is exposed.
- Activation of sperm enzymes.
- Increased membrane fluidity

Actions of Testosterone:

On foetal life:
- Foetal differentiation
- Development of male brain
- Development of external and internal genitalia
- Descent of testes

At puberty:
- Initiation of spermatogenesis
- Growth of external and internal genitalia

Secondary sexual characterstics:
- Deepening of voice
- Moustache, beard, pubic hair, body hair& acne
- Masculine pattern of fat distribution
- Male body contour → broad thoracic cage and shoulders, narrow pelvis
- Mental changes → aggressive behaviour

In adult life:
- Maintenance of spermatogenesis
- Maintenance of accessory sex organs
- Maintenance of libido

Other actions
- Hyperglycemic
- Increases levels of LDL's and decreases levels of HDL's
- Accumulation of upper body, abdominal and visceral fat
- Increases protein synthesis
- Reabsorption of Na^+ from kidneys
- Promotes bone growth
- Causes enlargement of muscle mass
- Stimulates synthesis of erythropoietin, so increase in RBC mass

Ovarian Hormones

Oestrogen	Oestrone: more in postmenopause Oestradiol: Most potent; Oestriol: least potent, ↑ed during pregnancy Synthesized by Theca interna, granulose cells, corpus luteum
Progesterone	Synthesized in Corpus luteum • Suppresses ovulation and menstruation in pregnancy • Thermogenic effect

Inhibin	Secreted by sertoli cells in males and granulose cells in females. Inhibits FSH secretion
Relaxin	Secreted by corpus luteum and placenta Relaxes the pelvis during pregnancy and helps in cervical ripening
Activin	Secreted by sertoli cells in males and granulosa cells in females Stimulates FSH secretion

Estrous Cycle

- Mammals other than primates do not menstruate and their sexual cycle is called an estrous cycle
- No episodic vaginal bleeding occurs but the underlying endocrinal mechanisms are essentially the same as those in the menstrual cycle
- In other species ovulation is induced by copulation (reflex ovulation)

Ovarian cycle: Follicular enlargement → dominant follicle (6th day) → secreted oestrogen → graafian follicle → maturation of ovum → follicular rupture and release of ovum into the peritoneal cavity (ovulation) → remnants of graafian follicle forms corpus luteum → secretes progesterone > oestrogen → lysis of corpus luteum 2 days before menstruation leaving a fibrous scar called corpus albicans

Menstrual Cycle

Phase	Other names	Period	Endometrial changes
Proliferative phase (oestrogen)	Preovulatory/Post menstrual/follicular phase	6th day–14th day	Endometrial glands enlarge and proliferates Increased vascularity and coiled arteries Thickness: 2–3 mm
Secretory phase (progesterone)	Post ovulatory/premenstrual/ luteal/pro gestational phase	15th day –27th day	Endometrial glands hypertrophies and distended with mucus ↑ in no. of coiled arteries, ↑ blood flow *Thickness: 5–6 mm
Menstrual phase	Destructive phase/blooding phase	1-5th day	Vasoconstriction of spiral arteries → ischemic changes → necrosis of endometrium → shedding; Bleeding: 75% arterial

Endometrial Cycle

Endometrium		
Characteristics	**Proliferative Phase**	**Secretory Phase**
Thickness	Increases due to cell division and cell growth. 0.5 mm to 3.5–5 mm.	Slightly increases and becomes edematous.
Stromal cells	Proliferate and increase in size thus increasing thickness.	Stromal proliferation and cell growth continues.
Glands	Straight tubular glands form lined with columnar epithelial cell. Produce and store large amount of glycogen.	Becomes increasingly tortous and spiralised, produce great amount of mucus.
Spiral arteries	Increasingly vascularised and spiral arteries elongate	Becomes increasingly tortous and spiralised
Myometrium	Increase in excitability and contractility and increase sensitivity to oxytocin.	Decrease in excitability and decreases contractility.
Fallopian tubes	Increase ciliary activity and motility and secretory activity of cells.	Increases ciliary activity and sensitivity and decreases motility
Cervix	Cervical mucus is thin and become crystalline, forming channels that facilitate the passage of sperm into uterus, Alkaline in nature. Shows ferning like effect, i.e. arborisation on drying.	Cervical mucus is thick and sticky, tenacious and cellular. Does not show ferning effect.

Hormonal Influence of Menstrual Cycle

- FSH-early development of G Follicle
- Final maturation of ovum-FSH&LH
- LH-ovulation, formation and maintenance of C Luteum

- A surge in LH secretion triggers ovulation, and ovulation normally occurs about 9 h after the peak of the LH surge at midcycle
- The LH surge begins about 24-36 hours before ovulation and reaches its peak about 8-10 hours before ovulation. It is this surge that acts to trigger ovulation

Actions of Estrogen

On Ovary
- Increases size of ovary and stromal cells.
- Initiates oogenesis and development and maintainence of follicles.
- Brings cyclical changes in ovary

On Uterus
- Increases size of uterus, fallopian tubes, cervix.
- Increases excitability of smooth muscle.
- Increases blood supply to myometrium.
- Causes changes in endometrium & onset of menarche.
- Increases no. of oxytocin receptors on myometrium in pregnant uterus

On Fallopian Tubes:
- Increase ciliary activity and motility and secretory activity of cells.

On Cervix:
- Cervical mucus is thin and become crystalline, forming channels that facilitate the passage of sperm into uterus, Alkaline in nature.
- Shows ferning like effect, i.e. arborisation on drying.

On Vagina:
- Lined with stratified squamous epithelium
- Vaginal secretions are increased.

On Breast:
- Promotes ductal growth.
- Causes pigmentation of areola.
- Promotes deposition of fat.

On Metabolisms
- Carbohydrate $\rightarrow$ Hyperglycemic
- Protein $\rightarrow$ Anabolic and Protein synthesis
- Fat $\rightarrow$ Plasma Cholesterol
- Mineral and H_2O $\rightarrow$ Reabsorption of Na^+
  Water retention and Weight. gain

On Bone:
- The epiphyseal growth centers are more sensitive to estradiol than testosterone, they close sooner

Actions of Progesterone

Principal Target Organs:
- Uterus
- Breast
- Brain

Endometrium:
- Thickness slightly increases
- Makes edematous
- Promotes stromal cell growth & proliferation
- Glands–Tortous and spiralised, mucus secretion increases
- Spiral arteries–Tortous and spiralised

Myometrium
- Decrease excitability
- Decreases contractility

On Cervix
- Cervical mucus becomes thick and sticky, tenacious and cellular
- No Ferning effect

Calorigenic Action
- Thermogenic
- Responsible for rise in basal body temperature at time of ovulation

On Respiration
- Stimulates Respiration
- Decreases Alveolar pCO_2

On Kidneys
- Large doses–Natriuresis by blocking the action of Aldosterone

Lactation

- Oestrogen-proliferation of mammary ducts
- Progesterone-Lobuloalveolar development
- Prolactin-initiation of milk secretion and maintenance (**PRO**lactin-**PRO**duce milk)
- **O**xytocin-Milk ejection (**O**oze milk)
- Breast feeding stimulates prolactin secretion
- Prolactin- inhibits the action of GnRH on the pituitary, and antagonizes the action of gonadotropins on the ovaries

Oxytocin (Paraventricular Nucleus-Parturition)

- Acts primarily on the breasts and uterus and involved in luteolysis
- It triggers increase in intracellular Ca^{2+} levels
- The milk ejection Reflex
  a. Contraction of the myoepithelial cells in the ducts of breast resulting in milk ejection
  b. Milk ejection is a neuroendocrine reflex. The receptors involved are the touch receptors, Impulses generated are relayed from the somatic touch pathways to the supraoptic and paraventricular nuclei
  c. In lactating women, genital stimulation and emotional stimuli also produce oxytocin secretion
- The sensitivity of the uterine musculature to oxytocin is enhanced by estrogen and inhibited by progesterone
- Act on the nonpregnant uterus to facilitate sperm transport
- Circulating oxytocin increases at the time of ejaculation in males, and it causes increased contraction of the smooth muscle of the vas deferens, propelling sperm toward the urethra

MISCELLANEOUS TOPICS

Energy Balance

Law of Hess–As long as the final products are the same, the amount of energy released will be the same, independent of the pathaway followed

Components of 24 hour Energy Expenditure

Basal metabolic rate	~ 60%
Energy used for physical activity	~ 25%
Energy used for nonexercise activity	~ 7%
Thermogenic effect of food	~ 8%

Basal Metabolic Rate

- Normally averages about 65–70 calories per hour in an average 70 kg man

Determinants of Basal Metabolic Rate

Hormones	Thyroid hormones increase BMR Testosterone increases BMR Growth hormone increases BMR Catecholamines increase BMR
Muscle mass	BMR increases with increase in muscle mass
Body size	BMR increases proportional to body size
Age	BMR decreases with age due to loss of muscle mass

Nonshivering Thermogenesis

- Process that is stimulated by sympathetic nervous system activation, which releases norepinephrine and epinephrine, which in turn increases metabolic activity and heat generation

Body Temperature

- The average normal core temperature is generally considered to be between 98.0° and 98.6°F when measured orally and about 1°F higher when measured rectally

Fever

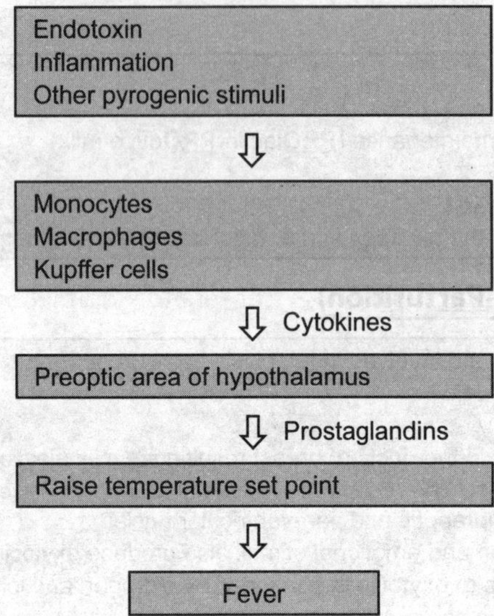

Pyrin–periodic fevers also occur in humans with mutations in the gene for pyrin (protein found in neutrophhils)
Interleukin 1–one of the most important cytokines in causing fever. It is also called as ***leukocyte pyrogen*** *or* ***endogenous pyrogen***.

QUESTIONS

1. Not a cell adhesion protein: (2014)
a. Anchorin
b. Integrin
c. Selectins
d. Cadherin

2. Transport of molecules in simple diffusion is not determined by: (2013)
a. ATP usage
b. Size of molecule
c. Lipid solubility
d. Number of channels

3. Function of ubiquitin in the cell is: (2008, 2011)
a. Degradation of intracellular protein
b. Endocytosis
c. Exocytosis
d. Plays an important role in acute inflammation

4. The differences in total body water (TBW) between males and females is minimal at: (2011)
a. Less than 1 years
b. 10–20 years
c. 20–40 years
d. > 60 years

5. Equilibrium potential of potassium is: (2008)
a. + 90 mV
b. – 90 mV
c. + 70 mV
d. – 70 mV

6. Major cation in intracellular space: (2008)
a. Proteins
b. Potassium
c. Sodium
d. Chloride

7. All are true about Gap junction except: (2006)
a. Permits amino acids upto 1000 Da mol wt
b. Opening of gap junction does not depend on trans membrane voltage
c. Halothane closes gap junction reversibly
d. Gap junction is made up of connexon is made up of six identical connexins

8. True statement regarding skeletal muscle is: (2013)

a. When myosin binds with ADP, Pi and calcium will be released
b. ATP divides into ADP and Pi in myosin head
c. Troponin I and calcium displace tropomyosin
d. When ATP depletes, myosin detaches from actin

9. Type 2 skeletal muscle fibers are rich in: (2009, 2012)

a. Mitochondria
b. ATPase activity
c. Anaerobic glycolysis
d. Oxidation

10. True regarding action potential is all except: (2012)

a. Upstroke is due to opening of voltage gated sodium channels
b. Down stroke is due to opening of voltage gated potassium channels
c. After hyperpolarisation is due to closure of potassium channels
d. During upstroke, the nerve is completely refractory

11. Efferent neuron for skeletal muscle: (2011)

a. Alpha motor neuron
b. Gamma motor neuron
c. Ia fibre
d. Ib fibre

12. Magnitude of action potential in neuron, is determined by: (2010)

a. Na^+
b. Mg^{2+}
c. K^+
d. Ca^{2+}

13. Action potential is transmitted in myofibrils via: (2009)

a. Terminal cisterns
b. T-Tlubules
c. Longitudinal
d. Sarcomere

14. Calmodulin acts through all except: (2006)

a. MLCK
b. Calcium-calmodulin kinase
c. Phosphorylase kinase
d. Phosphodiesterse

15. A standing person lies down. Which of the following physiological change occurs immediately? (2014)

a. Increased heart rate
b. Decreased blood flow to the apices of the lung
c. Immediate increase in venous return
d. Increase in blood pressure

16. Which of the following is a better predictor of vagal tone? (2013)

a. Basal heart rate
b. Ejection fraction
c. Stroke volume
d. LVET

17. All are true regarding ECG except: (2013)

a. Heart block causes increase in PR interval
b. QRS wave represents ventricular repolarization
c. T wave represents ventricular repolarization
d. Ventricular depolarization and repolarization happen during QT interval

18. Neutrophils increase in number after exercise due to: (2013)

a. Increased colony stimulating factor levels
b. Reduction in ECF
c. Demargination
d. Epithelial destruction

19. Under physiological conditions, stimulation of chemoreceptors result in: (2012)

a. Vasodilation and mild tachycardia
b. Vasoconstriction and bradycardia
c. Vasodilation and bradycardia
d. Vasoconstriction and tachycardia

20. Biconcave shape of RBC is useful in all aspects except: (2011)

a. Helps in passing through capillaries
b. Helps in cellular metabolism
c. Increased surface area diffusion of gases
d. Prevent osmotic lysis

21. Changes in cardiac output is minimal during: (2011)

a. Sleep
b. From supine to standing position
c. Exercise
d. Arrhythmias

22. Which of the following parameters does not change with age? (2011)

a. Hematocrit
b. Creatinine clearance
c. FEV1
d. Stress induced tachycardia

23. Which of the following causes decrease in diastolic blood pressure? (2010)

a. Sympathetic stimulation
b. Inhibition of vasomotor center
c. Stimulation of vagal center
d. Stimulation of vasomotor enter

24. The normal AV nodal delay is due to: (2010)

a. Junctional fibres are very small in size

b. Decrease in amplitude of firing
c. Resistance offered by myocytes
d. Lack of tight junctions

25. Decrease in BP causes: (2010)
a. Inhibition of vasoconstrictor center
b. Dis-inhibition of vasoconstrictor center
c. Increased stimulation of cardiac inhibitory enter
d. Increased vagal stimulation

26. Preload of the heart depends on: (2010)
a. End diastolic volume
b. End systolic volume
c. Stroke volume
d. Cardiac output

27. True regarding blood pressure measurement with sphygmomanometer in comparison with intra-arterial pressure monitoring is: (2010)
a. Less than intravascular pressure
b. Equal to intravascular pressure
c. Depends on velocity of flow
d. Greater than intravascular pressure

28. Carotid body baroreceptor is most sensitive to: (2009)
a. Mean blood pressure
b. Diastolic blood pressure
c. Systolic blood pressure
d. Pulse pressure

29. The incisura of arterial pulse corresponds with: (2008)
a. S1
b. S2
c. Opening snap
d. S3

30. Phase 2 of the action potential in cardiac muscle is due to: (2008)
a. Opening of Ca^{2+} channels
b. Opening of Na^{+} channels
c. Opening of K^{+} channels
d. Closure of NA^{+} channels

31. Ejection fraction of the ventricle refers to the ratio of: (2008)
a. Amount of blood received/amount of blood ejected
b. Stroke volume/end-diastolic volume
c. End-systolic volume/end diastolic volume
d. Stroke volume/end-systolic volume

32. To cause hemorrhagic shock, volume of blood loss should be: (2006)
a. 30%
b. 40%
c. 20%
d. 50%

33. Fick's principle is used to calculate: (2006)
a. Cardiac output
b. Pulse pressure
c. Cardiac axis
d. LVET

34. Partial pressure of CO_2 is lowest in: (2014)
a. Arterial blood
b. End tidal air
c. Expired air
d. Venous blood

35. In exhaled air, normal pCO_2 pressure is: (2014)
a. 36 mm Hg
b. 27 mm Hg
c. 40 mm Hg
d. 17 mm Hg

36. About O_2 dissociation curve, true is: (2014)
a. Affinity of O_2 with Hb decreases as Hb attaches to O_2 in linear fashion
b. 1 Hb attaches to 2 molecules of 2, 3 DPG
c. O_2 affinity will be equal in both HbF and HbA in the absence of 2, 3 DPG
d. Carboxy Hb increases release of O_2 in blood (shifts O_2 dissociation curve to right)

37. True statement regarding CO_2 in venous blood is: (2013)
a. Is carried only by hemoglobin
b. Is converted into bicarbonate in lung by carbonic anhydrase
c. Mainly carried as bicarbonate ions
d. Does not cross blood brain barrier

38. Venous air embolism during surgery is seen in position: (2012)
a. Supine
b. Sitting
c. Prone
d. Standing

39. Carbon monoxide poisoning is type of: (2006, 2011)
a. Anemic hypoxia
b. Histotoxic hypoxia
c. Hypoxemic hypoxia
d. Stagnant hypoxia

40. Respiratory causes of hypoxemia are all except: (2011)
a. Hypoventilation
b. Physiological shunt
c. VP mismatch
d. Dead space ventilation

41. Partial pressure of oxygen in room air at 760 mm of at mospheric pressure: (2010)
a. 160 mm Hg
b. 240 mm Hg

c. 580 mm Hg
d. 760 mm Hg

42. In plasma, carbon-dioxide is mainly transported as: (2007)
a. Dissolved CO_2
b. HCO_3^-
c. Carboxy hemoglobin
d. Carbamino hemoglobin

43. Pnemotaxic centre is situated in: (2006, 2007)
a. Medulla
b. Pons
c. Midbrain
d. Reticular activating system

44. All the following factors shift the oxygen dissociation curve to the right except: (2007)
a. ↑ CO_2
b. ↑ temperature
c. ↑ 2, 3 DPG
d. ↑ pH

45. Shock causes:
a. Stagnant hypoxia
b. Anemic hypoxia
c. Hypoxic hypoxia
d. Histotoxic hypoxia

46. Sensation of propiroception is transmitted by: (2014)
a. A alpha
b. A beta
c. A gamma
d. A delta

47. True regarding lateral spinothalamic tract is: (2014)
a. Transmits contralateral touch
b. Transmits ipsilateral pain
c. Crosses brain at thalamus
d. Lower most fibres are lateral

48. Example of electrical synapse: (2014)
a. Tight junction
b. Gap junctions
c. Anchoring junction
d. Neuromuscular junction

49. Blood nerve barrier is formed by: (2014)
a. Perineurium
b. Schwann cells
c. Epineurium
d. Endoneurium

50. Which of the following matches regarding receptors is not true? (2014)
a. Merkel's disk is seen in non-hairy skin
b. Pacinian corpuscle are fast adapting
c. True meissner in hairy skin
d. Hair end receptors detect motion

51. Claudius cells are seen in:
a. Canal of schlemn
b. Organ of corti
c. Parenchyma of parathyroid gland
d. Alveoli

51. All are true regarding withdrawal reflex except: (2008, 2013)
a. Hal long latency
b. Poly synaptic
c. Carried by 1a fibers
d. Has after-discharge

53. True statement about cerebrospinal fluid is: (2013)
a. Maximum secreted by choroid plexus
b. Flows from lateral ventricles to 3rd ventricle through aqueduct of sylvius
c. More in ventricle than in subarachnoid space
d. CSF formation and absorption are equal at 68 mm CSF pressure

54. Advantages of myelination of nerve are all except: (2013)
a. Acts as protective covering to axon
b. Allows faster conduction of impulse
c. Decreases energy expenditure from neuron
d. Helps in fast anterograde axoplasmic transport

55. All results from sympathetic nervous stimulation, except: (2013)
a. Vasodilation of cutaneous blood vessel
b. Bronchodilatation
c. Dilator papillae contraction
d. Rennin secretion

56. Ventral posteromedial nucleus of thalamus transmits: (2012)
a. Spinothalamic tract
b. Medial lemniscus
c. Lateral lemniscus
d. Trigeminothalamic tract

57. Electrical synapse will be seen: (2012)
a. NM junction
b. Gap junction
c. Tight junction
d. Adherens junctions

58. Amplification of intensity of sound occurs in: (2012)
a. Ear ossicles
b. Scala media
c. Tympanic membrane
d. Medial geniculate body

59. All are true about brain cells except: (2012)
a. Oligodedrocytes-myelination
b. Astrocytes-provide mechanical support
c. Astrocytes-provide nutrition
d. Ependymal cells-macrophage

60. Cerebral blood flow will be decreased in: (2012)
a. Increased ICT
b. Metabolic acidosis
c. Decreased viscosity of blood
d. Hypecapnia

61. In postnatal period the greatest growth in the CNS is of? (2011)
a. Cell body
b. Axon
c. Dendrite
d. Perikaryon

62. Receptor for stretch reflex is: (2009, 2011)
a. Muscle spindle
b. Golgi tendon organ
c. Proprioceptors
d. Paccinian corpuscle

63. Which of the following tract is not involved in maintenance of posture? (2011)
a. Reticulospinal tract
b. Rubrospinal tract
c. Tectospinal tract
d. Vestibulospinal

64. Which of the following tracts does not carry proprioceptive impulses? (2011)
a. Olivo cerebellar tract
b. Tecto cerebellar tract
c. Spino cerebellar tract
d. Cuneo cerebellar tract

65. Circadian rhythm is influenced by: (2010)
a. Supra optic nuclei
b. Ventrolateral nucleus
c. Posterolateral nucleus
d. Supra chiasmatic nucleus

66. Stimulation of bipolar cells results in all except:
a. Depolarization **(2010)**
b. Hyperpolarisation
c. Neurotransmitter release
d. Action potentials

67. Dopamine causes all, except: (2010)
a. Decreases splanchnic circulation
b. Increases cardiac output
c. Decreases peripheral resistance
d. Increases heart rate

68. Gamma efferent motor neuron is influenced by:
a. Corticospinal tract **(2010)**
b. Tectospinal tract
c. Vestibule spinal tract
d. Reticulospinal tract

69. Vestibulo-Ocular Reflex mediated by: (2010)
a. Flocculonodular lobe
b. Vermal portion of spinocerebellum
c. Neocerebellum
d. Paravermal region of spinocerebellum

70. Waves on EEG during stage 4-NREM period of sleep is: (2009)
a. Alpha
b. Beta
c. Delta
d. Theta

71. 'A' wave of electroretinogram corresponds to activity in: (2009)
a. Rods and cones
b. Pigment epithelium
c. Ganglion cell layer
d. Nerve fiber layer

72. . Which of the following parts of brain contains dopaminergic neurons? (2008)
a. Locus ceruleus system
b. Cerebellum
c. Nigro striatal system
d. Midline raphe nucleus

73. Most important sensory organ in the ampulla is:
a. Organ of corti **(2008)**
b. Macula
c. Otolith
d. Crista

74. Instrumental conditioning in learning was introduced and demonstrated by: (2008)
a. Pavlov
b. Skinner
c. Freud
d. Watson

75. Endothelium derived relaxation factor is supposed to be: (2008)
a. Nitric oxide
b. Angiotensin
c. Serotonin
d. Norepinephrine

76. All the following are involved in the control of posture except: (2008)
a. Anterior corticospinal tract
b. Lateral corticospinal tract
c. Tectospinal
d. Vestibulospinal

77. Which of the following sensations is not converging on thalamus? (2007)
a. Smell
b. Fine touch
c. Hearing
d. None of the above

78. **A 5-year-old obese boy has persistent food-seeking and aggressive behavior. A hypothalamic nuclei lesion is being suspected. What is the probable site of the lesion? (2007)**
   a. Lateral
   b. Supraoptic
   c. Suprachiasmatic
   d. Ventromedial

79. **Deafferentation of muscle explains: (2006)**
   a. Influence of vesibulo spinal tract on alpha fibers
   b. Influence of vestibule spinal tract on gamma fibers
   c. Influence of reticulo spinal tract on alpha fibers
   d. Influence of reticulo spinal tract on gamma fibers

80. **Touch and pressure sensation are carried by: (2006)**
   a. Alpha fibers
   b. Beta fibers
   c. Gamma fibers
   d. Delta fibers

81. **Sleep spindle and K complexes are seen in: (2006)**
   a. REM
   b. NREM stage II
   c. NREM stage III
   d. NREM stage IV

82. **Brunner's glands are seen in: (2007, 2012)**
   a. Duodenum
   b. Stomach
   c. Esophagus
   d. Colon

83. **Pepsin is activated by: (2007, 2011)**
   a. HCl
   b. Enterokinase
   c. Uropepsinogen
   d. Tripsinogen

84. **Receptor for vitamin B_{12}-intrinsic factor complex is located in: (2011)**
   a. Ileum
   b. Colon
   c. Jejunum
   d. Duodenum

85. **Enterohepatic circulation is necessary for the secretion of: (2011)**
   a. Bile
   b. Gastric fluid
   c. Intestinal secretions
   d. Pancreatic secretions

86. **Vitamin B_{12} and folic acid absorption are: (2010)**
   a. Na^+ dependent process in colon
   b. Na^+ independent process in colon
   c. Na^+ dependent process in ileum
   d. Na^+ independent process in ileum

87. **Meissner's plexus are present in: (2009)**
   a. Mucosa
   b. Submucosa
   c. Muscularis layer
   d. Serosa

88. **Intrinsic factor is secreted by: (2006)**
   a. Parietal cells
   b. Chief cells
   c. Mucus cells
   d. G cells

89. **Intestinal motility is enhanced by all except: (2006)**
   a. CCK
   b. Motilin
   c. Secretin
   d. Gastrin

90. **Which of the following will not decrease glomerular filtration rate (GFR) ? (2009, 2013)**
   a. Increased hydrostatic pressure in tubule
   b. Increased capillary oncotic pressure
   c. Hypoproteinemia
   d. Mesangial cell contraction

91. **Effectiverenalplasmaflow(ERPF)iscaldculatedby: (2013)**
   a. DTPA
   b. MAG 3
   c. Inulin
   d. Hippurate I 131

92. **Which of the following regarding dopamine is true? (2012)**
   a. Relaxes mesangial cells in kidney
   b. Decreases splanchnic blood flow
   c. Decreases renal blood flow
   d. Decreases GFR

93 **Renal blood flow contributes what % of the cardiac output? (2011)**
   a. 15%
   b. 25%
   c. 45%
   d. 50%

94 **Each kidney contains about_nephrons: (2008)**
   a. One million
   b. Two million
   c. Four million
   d. Half million

95. **Substance causing mesangial relaxation: (2006)**
   a. Histamine
   b. cAMP
   c. ADH
   d. Angiotensin II

96. Secretory phase of endometrium is due to which hormone? (2014)
a. Estrogen
b. Progesterone
c. Prolactin
d. Pregnendiol

97. Most common progesterone metabolite in urine is: (2014)
a. Pregnenolone
b. 17 hydroxy pregnenolone
c. Pregnanetriol
d. Pregnanediol

98. Testis is not the source for which of the following?
a. Testosterone (2013)
b. Dehydroepiandrosterone
c. Androstenodione
d. Dihydrotestosterone

99. Thyroid peroxidase will help in all the following except: (2012)
a. Iodide trapping
b. Iodide to iodine
c. Binding thyroglobulin
d. Secretion of thyroglobulin into colloid

100. cAMP is inhibited by: (2012)
a. Nor-epinephrine via alpha 2 receptor
b. ADH via V2 receptor
c. Nor-epinephrine via beta 1 receptor
d. ADH via V1 receptor

101. Least cell type in anterior pituitary: (2012)
a. Corticotroph
b. Gonadotroph
c. Lactotroph
d. Thyrotroph

102. All are true about epinephrine, except: (2012)
a. Increases insulin secretion
b. Increases glucagon secretion
c. Vasoconstriction in skeletal circulation'
d. Increases gluconeogenesis

103. All are true regarding estrogen, except: (2012)
a. Pre-ovulatory LH surge
b. Negative feedback on FSH
c. Secreted by granulose cells
d. Secreted by theca cells

104. Sertoli cells secrete: (2009, 2012)
a. FSH
b. Androgen binding protein
c. Testosterone
d. LH

105. Which is false regarding hCG? (2012)
a. It is a glycopeptides
b. Synthesized by syncytio-trophoblast
c. hCG α subunit is similar to α subunit of LH, FSH, TSH
d. Inhibits progesterone synthesis

106. Prolactin is secreted by: (2011)
a. Chromophobe cells
b. Acidophilic cells
c. Basophilic cells
d. Folliculostellate cells

107. Testosterone secreted by: (2010)
a. Leydig cells
b. Sertoli cells
c. Cowper's gland
d. Intermediate cells

108. Pituitary stalk damage can decrease the levels of all the following hormones except: (2010)
a. Prolactins
b. Growth hormone
c. Vasopressin
d. Follicular stimulating hormone

109. Inhibin secreted by: (2010)
a. Granulose cell
b. Theca cell
c. Corpus leuteum
d. Deciduas

110. Inhibition of prolactin is caused by: (2009)
a. Dopamine
b. Dobutamine
c. TRH
d. AT-II

111. Following is true of hormone leptin except: (2009)
a. It is found in increased levels in obese
b. Site of action is hypothalamus
c. It is produced by adipose all
d. Ii increases appetite

112. Which of the following hormones increase during sleep? (2009)
a. Insulin
b. ACTH
c. GH
d. Gluocorticoid

113. Which of the following has least half-life? (2009)
a. Norepinephrine
b. Insulin
c. Calcitonin
d. PTH

114. Most common cell type in anterior pituitary is:
a. Corticotroph (2008)
b. Gonadotroph
c. Lactotroph
d. Somatotrope

115. Which of the following has least effect on the metabolic rate: (2007)
a. TSH
b. TRH
c. TBG
d. Free T4

116. All are true about inhibin except: (2006)
a. It is a steroidal compound
b. FSH stimulates the secretion of inhibin B
c. Secreted by sertoli cells
d. Inhibin B inhibitis FSH secretion

117. Melatonin is secreted by: (2006)
a. Mammillary body
b. Pineal gland
c. Posterior pituitary
d. Hypothalamus

118. Function of thyroid hormones: (2006)
a. Inhibits beta myosin heavy chain
b. Increases cholesterol
c. Inhibits ovulation
d. Increases diastolic blood pressure

119. Major adrenocortical hormone in blood is: (2006)
a. Cortisol
b. Corticosterone
c. Aldosterone
d. Deoxy corticosterone

120. Protein present in brown adipose tissue: (2011)
a. Thermogenin
b. Dinitroprotein
c. Spectrin
d. Adiponectin

121. Function of brown fat is: (2009)
a. Glycogenosis
b. Gluconeogenesis
c. Glycogenolysis
d. Thermogenesis

122. Hardy-Weinberg law is used to predict inheritance of which of the following type: (2007)
a. Autosomal dominant
b. Autosomal recessive
c. X-linked dominant
d. X-linked recessive

123. Blood flow changes are least during exercise in:
a. Brain
b. Heart
c. Skin
d. Kidney

124. The main fuel used by brain, during starvation is:
a. Free fatty acids
b. Amino acids
c. Glucose
d. Ketone body

125. Neutrophils increase in number after exercise due to:
a. Increased colony stimulating factor leverls
b. Reduction in ECF
c. Demargination
d. Epithelial destruction

ANSWERS AND EXPLANATIONS

1. Ans. a. Anchorin

Ref: Ganong, 24/e, Walter F Boron Medical Physiology 2/e p18, Expression of Anchorin CII (Cartilage Annexin V) in Human Young, Normal Adult, and Osteoarthritic Cartilage-Journal of Histochemistry and Cytochemistry

Cell adhesion molecules (CAM)

- Cells are attached to the basal lamina and to each other by CAMs
- CAMs not only fasten cells to their neighbours, but also transmit signals into and out of the cell
- Found to be important in
  - Embryonic development and formation of the nervous system. Neurons migrate to their correct anatomical position in the brain with the help of adhesion molecules
  - In holding tissues together in adults
  - In inflammation and wound healing
  - In metastasis of tumors.
- Loss of cell to cell and cell to extracellular matrix adhesion is a hallmark of metastatic tumor cells
- CAMs pass through the cell membrane and are anchored to the cytoskeleton inside the cell
- Some bind to like molecules on other cells (homophilic binding)
- Others bind to non self molecules (heterophilic binding)
- Many bind to laminins, a family of large cross shaped molecules with multiple receptor domains in the extracellular matrix.

Family of CAMs

Integrins	• Heterodimers that bind to various receptors • Integrins are examples of matrix receptors or cell matrix adhesion molecules (attaches cell to the extracellular matrix) • Growing axons express integrins at their surface that bind laminin and fibronectin. As a result, growing axons move together in fascicles
Adhesion molecules of the IgG superfamily of immunoglobulins	Calcium independent neural cell adhesion molecules
Cadherins	Calcium dependent molecules that mediate cell-to-cell adhesion by homophilic reactions
Selectins	Have lectin–like domains that bind carbohydrates

Anchorin

- Cartilage annexin V is called anchorin CII
- In its tissue-specific function as a collagen receptor of chondrocytes, anchorin CII occupies a key position in the organization of the cell extracellular matrix junction for the tissue
- The general role of anchorin CII in other tissues suggests involvement in cellular secretory processes and in regulation of apoptosis.

2. Ans. a. ATP usage *Ref: GK Pal Textbook of Medical Physiology p32, 33*

Simple diffusion is a type of **passive transport** that **does not require ATP** usage.

Transport processes

Active Transport	Passive Transport
Transport against the electrochemical gradient (uphill)	Transport along the electrochemical gradient (down hill)
Requires energy from ATP	Does not require energy from ATP
Exhibits saturation kinetics	Not seen

Types of passive transport

- Simple diffusion
- Facilitated diffusion
- Osmosis
- Filtration
- Bulk flow
- Solvent drag

Simple diffusion

Diffusion is the process of passive transport in which molecules move from the area of higher concentration to the area of lower concentration. Example–O_2, CO_2, urea, ammonia

Factors that determine rate of diffusion
- Properties of the substance
- Properties of the membrane

Properties of the substance

- Effect of concentration and electrical gradients–usually substances move along both the electrical and chemical gradients
- Permeability of the substance: Permeability refers to the ease at which the substances pass through the membrane. The factors that determine the permeability are,

Lipid solubility	As the membrane is a lipid bilayer, the permeability is proportional to the lipid solubility of the substance
Molecular size	For water soluble substances like ions that pass through aqueous channels, permeability is inversely proportional to their molecular size
Charge on the molecule	Since membrane is polarized with its negative interior, cations easily enter from outside into the cell and anions in the opposite direction

Temperature	Rate of diffusion is high at higher body temperature as temperature facilitates motion of molecules in the solution
Distribution of channels in the membrane	The number of protein channels for the substance in the membrane determines the permeability of the substance through the membrane
Pressure gradient	Diffusion is more from high pressure to low pressure, as the pressure causes greater number of molecule to hit the membrane

Properties of the membrane

- In addition to the concentration gradient of the substance across the membrane, the cross sectional area and thickness of the membrane influence diffusion.
- According to Fick's law of diffusion, the rate of diffusion of a molecule through a membrane is proportional to the surface area available for diffusion, and inversely proportional to the thickness of the membrane

3. Ans. a. Degradation of intracellular protein

Ref: Berne and Levy Physiology 6/e, The ubiquitin system by Avram Hershko and Aaron Ciechanover published in Annu Rev Biochem. 1998; 67:425-79.

Ubiquitin

- Ubiquitin is a small peptide that is covalently attached to lysine groups in proteins
- Conjugation of proteins to the 74 amino acid polypeptide ubiquitin marks them for degradation
- This polypeptide is highly conserved and is present in species ranging from bacteria to humans
- The process of binding ubiquitin is called ubiquitination, and in some instances, multiple ubiquitin molecules bind (polyubiquitination)
- Ubiquitination of cytoplasmic proteins, including integral proteins of the endoplasmic reticulum, can mark the proteins for degradation in proteasomes
- Ubiquitination of membrane proteins, such as the growth hormone receptors, also marks them for degradation, however these can be degraded in lysosomes as well as via the proteasome
- Ubiquitin-mediated degradation of regulatory proteins plays important roles in the control of numerous processes, including cell-cycle progression, signal transduction, transcriptional regulation, receptor down-regulation, and endocytosis.
- The ubiquitin system has been implicated in the immune response, development, and programmed cell death.
- Abnormalities in ubiquitin-mediated processes have been shown to cause pathological conditions, including malignant transformation.

4. Ans. a. Less than 1 years *Ref: GK Pal Textbook of Medical Physiology p47*

Body Fluids

- In the average young adult male, 18% of the body weight is protein and related substances, 7% is mineral, and 15% is fat. The remaining 60% is water.
- The total body water (TBW) as percentage of body weight on average is about 60% in adult males, which is about 10% more than adult females.
- In females, TBW is less than males due to relatively greater amount of adipose tissue (subcutaneous fat) in them
- In infants and children, though TBW as percentage of body weight is more than in adults their absolute water content is significantly less
- In elderly people in both the sexes, TBW is about 10% less that their adult counterparts

Total body water as % of body weight

Age	Males	Females
Infants	65–70	65–70
Children (upto 9 yrs)	60–65	59–62
10–17 yrs	58–60	55–58
18–39 yrs	58–64	48–55
40–59 yrs	52–58	45–50
60 years and above	50–55	42–48

5. Ans. b. –90 mV *Ref: Ganong's Review of Medical Physiology 24/e p10, Walter F Boron Medical Physiology 2/e p112*

- To calculate equilibrium potential of a single ion: Nernst Equation

$$E_x = -\frac{61.5\ \text{mV}}{Z_x} \log \frac{[X]_I}{[X]_o}$$

E_x is the Nernst Equilibrium potential
Z_x is the valence of the ion
$[X]_I$ is the concentration of X inside the cell
$[X]_o$ is the concentration of X outside the cell.

Ions	Equilibrium potential (mV)
Na^+	+ 60
K^+	– 90
Cl^-	– 70
Ca^{++}	+ 125

6. Ans. b. Potassium *Ref: Guyton and Hall Textbook of Medical Physiology 2013, p51*

- ECF: Most abundant cation-**Na^+**
  Most abundant anion-**Cl^-**
- ICF: Most abundant cation-**K^+**
  Most abundant anion-**Phosphates**

Osmolar substances in extracellular and intracellular fluids

	Plasma (mOsm/L of H_2O)	Interstitial (mOsm/L of H_2O)	Intracellular (mOsm/L of H_2O)
Na^+	142	139	14
K^+	4.2	4	140
Ca^{++}	1.3	1.2	0
Mg^{++}	0.8	0.7	20
Cl^-	108	108	4
HCO_3^-	24	28.3	10
$HPO_4^=$, $H_2PO_4^-$	2	2	11
$SO_4^=$	0.5	0.5	1
Phosphocreatine			45
Carnosine			14
Aminoacids	2	2	8
Creatine	0.2	0.2	9
Lactate	1.2	1.2	1.5
Adenosine triphosphate			5
Hexose monophosphate			3.7
Glucose	5.6	5.6	
Protein	1.2	0.2	4
Urea	4	4	4
Others	4.8	3.9	10
Total mOsm/L	301.8	300.8	301.2
Corrected osmolar activity mOsm/L	282.0	281.0	281.0
Total osmotic pressure at 37°C (mm Hg)	5443	5423	5423

7. **Ans. b. Opening of gap junction does not depend on transmembrane voltage**

Ref: Ganong's Review of Medical Physiology 24/e p43

Walter F Boron Medical Physiology 2/e p51, Effects of Anesthetics Heptanol, Halothane and Isoflurane on Gap Junction Conductance in Crayfish Septate Axons; Journal of Membrane Biology 1991

Mechanism and Selectivity of the Effects of Halothane on Gap Junction Channel Function-circulation research

Gap junctions

- The gap junctions form a cytoplasmic 'tunnel' for diffusion of small molecules (<1000 Da) between 2 neighbouring cells
- The functional unit of the gap junction is the connexon
- A connexon is composed of 6 integral membrane protein subunits called connexins
- Gap junctions facilitate the passage of inorganic ions and small molecules such as Ca^{++} and cAMP, from the cytoplasm of one cell into the cytoplasm of an adjacent cell
- Excellent pathways for the flow of electrical current between adjacent cells, playing a critical role in cardiac and smooth muscle
- The permeability of gap junctions rapidly regulated by
  - Changes in cytosolic concentrations of Ca^{++}, cAMP, and H^+
  - The voltage across the cell membrane or membrane potential (V_m)
- Gap junction permeability can be reduced by a variety of treatment including cell damage, inhibition of metabolism, acidification, hypoxia, exposure to anesthetics like halothane
- Halothane gates gap junction channels to the closed state in a dose-dependent manner.

8. **Ans. b. ATP divides into ADP and Pi in myosin head**

Ref: Ganong's Review of Medical Physiology 24/e p102-104; Guyton and hall Textbook of Medical Physiology 2013 p90

Skeletal muscle contraction

- Sliding filament theory/walk along theory/ratchet theory, **proposed by AF Huxley and H.e. Huxley**

Steps in contraction

- Discharge of motor neuron
- Release of transmitter (ACH) at motor end plate
- Binding of ACH to nicotinic ACH receptors
- Increased Na^+ and K^+ conductance in end plate membrane
- Generation of end plate potential
- Generation of action potential in muscle fibers
- Inward spread of depolarization along T tubules
- Release of Ca^{2+} from terminal cisterns of sarcoplasmic reticulum and diffusion to thick and thin filaments
- Binding of calcium to troponin C, uncovering myosin binding sites on actin
- Formation of myosin-actin cross bridges
- ADP released, causing a conformational change in the myosin head that moves the thin filament relative to the thick filament–power stroke
- ATP quickly binds to the free site on the myosin head, which leads to detachment of the myosin head from the thin filament
- ATP is hydrolysed and inorganic phosphate (Pi) released, causing recocking of the myosin head and completing the cycle

Steps in relaxation

- Ca^{2+} pumped back into sarcoplasmic reticulum
- Release of Ca^{2+} from troponin
- Cessation of interaction between actin and myosin

Option a–before contraction begins, the heads of the myosin cross bridges bind with ATP. The ATPase activity of the myosin head immediately cleaves the ATP into ADP and phosphate

Option c–Troponin C and calcium displace tropomyosin

Option d–when ATP depletes, there is no separation of the myosin cross-bridges from the actin and hence muscle remains in a contracted state (basis of Rigor mortis)

9. Ans. b. ATPase activity and C. Anaerobic glycolysis *Ref: Ganong's Review of Medical Physiology 24/e p107*

Skeletal muscle fibers

- Skeletal muscle fibers can be classified as Type 1 and Type 2
- Type 2 fibers are divided into Type 2A and Type 2B

Classification of fiber types in Skeletal Muscles

	Type 1	Type 2A	Type 2B
Other names	Slow, oxidative	Fast, oxidative, glycolytic	Fast, glycolytic
Color	Red	Red	White
Myosin ATPase activity	Slow	Fast	Fast
Ca^{2+} pumping capacity of sarcoplasmic reticulum	Moderate	High	High
Diameter	Small	Large	Large
Glycolytic capacity	Moderate	High	High
Oxidative capacity	High	Moderate	Low
Associated motor unit type	Slow	Fast Resistant to fatigue	Fast Fatigable
Oxidative capacity	High	Moderate	Low

- Both type 2A and type 2B are rich in ATPase activity and anaerobic glycolysis

10. Ans. c. After hyperpolarisation is due to closure of potassium channels

After hyperpolarisation - Result of K^+ channels remaining open, allowing the continued efflux of K^+ ions

11. Ans. a. Alpha motor neuron *Ref: Berne and Levy Physiology 6/e p157*

The basic circuit that underlies a reflex is called reflex arc. A reflex arc can be divided into 3 parts

- An afferent limb (sensory receptors and axons) that carries information to the CNS
- A central component (synapses and interneurons within the CNS)
- An efferent limb (motor neurons) that causes the response

Somatic motor neurons (efferent) → α motor neurons; γ motor neurons

- Skeletal muscle fibers are innervated by large neurons, called α motor neurons in the ventral horn of the spinal cord or in cranial nerve nuclei
- A motor unit is an α motor neuron and all of the skeletal muscle fibers that its axon supplies
- Each skeletal muscle fiber in mammals is supplied by just one α motor neuron
- However, a given α motor neuron may innervate a variable number of skeletal muscle fibers
- When an α motor neuron discharges under normal circumatances, all the muscle fibers of the motor unit contract
- Another type of motor neuron is called the γ motor neuron
- γ motor neurons do not supply ordinary skeletal muscle fibers. Instead they synapse on specialized striated muscle fibers, the intrafusal muscle fibers, that are found within muscle spindles
- Contraction of intrafusal fibers does not directly cause significant changes in muscle tension or length, however, γ motor neurons, by adjusting the level of tension in these fibers, influence the sensitivity of the muscle spindle to stretch

Sensory receptors responsible for eliciting spinal reflexes (afferent)

- Muscle spindle - Ia fibers are related to muscle spindle primary endings
- Golgi tendon organs - Ib fibers are related to golgi tendon organs

12. Ans. a. Na^+ *Ref: Ganong's Review of Medical Physiology 24/e p88*

- The rapid upstroke in the action potential is due to opening of voltage gated Na^+ channels
- The opening of voltage gated K^+ channels contributes to the repolarization
- Mg^{2+} and Ca^{2+} do not have much significant role in the generation of action potential in a neuron

13. Ans. b. T-Tubules *Ref: Ganong's Review of Medical Physiology 24/e p98; Berne and Levy Physiology 6/e p234*

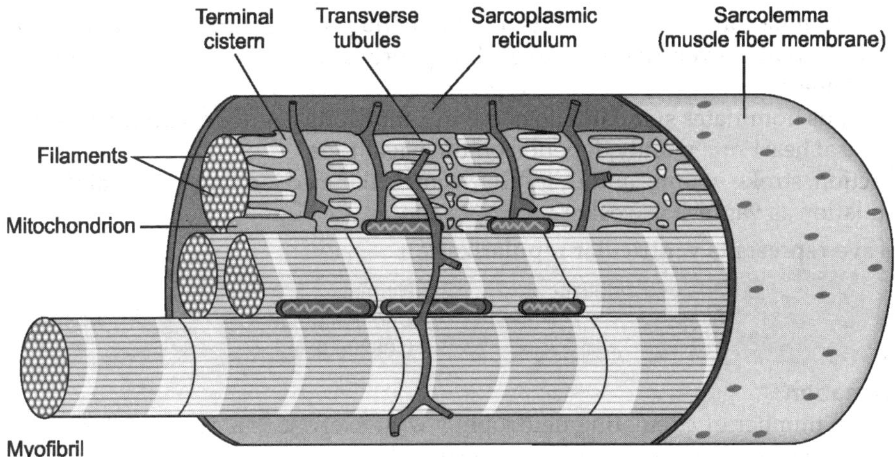

Fig. 2.7: Structure of a single muscle fiber showing individual myofibrils

Sarcotubular system

- The muscle fibrils are surrounded by the sarcotubular system, which is made up of a T system and a sarcoplasmic reticulum
- The T system, which is continuous with the sarcolemma, provides a path for the rapid transmission of the action potential from the cell membrane to all the fibrils in the muscle
- The sarcoplasmic reticulum is an important store of Ca^{2+} and also participates in muscle metabolism
- The portion of the sarcoplasmic reticulum nearest the T tubule is called the terminal cisternae, and it is the site of calcium release, which is critical for the contraction of skeletal muscle

14. Ans. d. Phosphodiesterase *Ref: Ganong's Review of Medical Physiology 24/e p56-58*

Calmodulin

- Calcium binding protein
- Has four Ca^{++} binding domains
- When calmodulin binds Ca^{++}, it is capable of activating 5 different calmodulin–dependent kinases
  1. Myosin light chain kinase
  2. Phosphorylase kinase
  3. Ca^{++} /calmodulin kinase I
  4. Ca^{++} /calmodulin kinase II
  5. Ca^{++} /calmodulin kinase III
- Myosin light chain kinase–phosphorylates myosin and brings about contraction in smooth muscle
- Ca^{++} /calmodulin kinase I and Ca^{++} /calmodulin kinase II–concerned with synaptic function
- Ca^{++} /calmodulin kinase III–concerned with protein synthesis
- Another calmodulin-activated protein is calcineurin, a phosphatase that inactivates Ca^{++} channels by dephosphorylating them.

15. Ans. c. Immediate increase in venous return

Ref: Guyton, 12/e and A Textbook of Practical Physiology by CL Ghai

- Standing to lying position
- Decreased peripheral vascular resistance
- Increased venous return to heart
- Rise in HR followed by slowing of heart
- The rise and fall in HR is due to changes in vagal tone

16. Ans. a. Basal heart rate

- Right vagus mainly innervates the SA node, right atrium and left vagus innervates left atrium, AV node and bundle of His.
- Hence, vagal stimulation strongly inhibits heart rate thus strong negative chronotropic effect
- Vagal innervations of the ventricle is sparse. Thus poorly affects force of contraction and hence weak negative inotropic effect
- Moreover, vagus dominates sympathetic nerve in controlling SA node activity at rest
- Therefore, basal heart rate mainly depends on the vagal tone
- Ejection fraction, stroke volume and LVET (left ventricular ejection time) are mainly influenced by sympathetic stimulation as vagus has weaker inotropic effect

17. Ans. b. QRS wave represents ventricular repolarization

QRS interval	Average duration 0.08	Normal Duration range 0.08–0.10	Ventricular depolarization and atrial repolarization

18. Ans. c. Demargination

- Increase in the number of circulating neutrophils with exercise is a result of demargination of cells from endothelial tissues (mediated by catecholamines) and bone marrow (mediated by cortisol)

19. Ans. d. Vasoconstriction and mild tachycardia *Ref: Berne and Levy Physiology 6/e*

Effects of stimulation of peripheral arterial chemoreceptors

- They are primarily activated by a reduction in partial pressure of oxygen, but they also respond to an increase in the partial pressure of carbon dioxide and pH
- The intrinsic cardiovascular effects of hypoxia on the peripheral chemoreceptors include vasoconstriction and bradycardia
- However, it is not easy to demonstrate this primary reflex bradycardia, indeed, it is observed only during forced apnea
- Under real life conditions, hypoxia causes tachycardia.
- Hypoxia through the peripheral chemoreceptors, normally stimulates the medullary respiratory centers, which in turn stimulate ventilation. Increased ventilation has 2 effects
  1. It stretches the lungs, which in turn stimulates pulmonary stretch receptors. Afferent impulses from these pulmonary stretch receptors ultimately inhibit the cardiainhibitory center, causing reflex tachycardia
  2. Increased alveolar ventilation caused by hypoxia lowers systemic pCO_2, raising the pH of the brain extracellular fluid and inhibiting the cardioinhibitory centre. Again the net effect is tachycardia. Hypoxia also produces increased catecholamine secretion from the adrenal medulla, which produce tachycardia and an increase in cardiac output
  3. Thus, the physiological response to hypoxia is tachycardia

20. Ans. b. Helps in cellular metabolism *Ref: Pal GK Red Blood Cells. In: Textbook of Medical Physiology*

Advantages of biconcavity of RBCs

- Withstand lysis when exposed to hypotonic environment
- Better exchange of gas
- Easy movement through capillaries

21. Ans. a. Sleep *Ref: Ganong's Review of Medical Physiology 24/e p546*

- Sleep causes no change in cardiac output
- Heart disease, rapid arrhythmias, sitting from supine cause decrease in cardiac output
- Exercise increases cardiac output

22. Ans. a. Hematocrit *Ref: Pal GK Cardiac Output. In: Textbook of Medical Physiology*

The Effect of Age on Creatinine clearance in Men: a Cross-sectional and Longitudinal Study. Rowe JW, Andres R, Tobin JD, Norris AH, Shock NW, Decline of FEV1 by age and smoking status: facts, figures, and fallacies HA Kerstjens, B Rijcken, JP Schouten, and DS Postma

- Hematocrit does not change with age
- Creatine clearance decreases with age
- FEV1 Decreases with age

23. Ans. b. Inhibition of Vasomotor center

Ref: Pal GK Blood pressure and its regulation. In: Textbook of Medical Physiology 80:643

- Diastolic pressure is mainly decided by peripheral resistance, which is mainly controlled by sympathetic system (remember-NO parasympathetic nerve supply to blood vessel)
- Vasomotor center (rostral ventrolateral medulla) is the higher center for sympathetic system. Inhibition of VMC, results in reduced vasoconstrictor tone (reduced sympathetic activity) which in turn reduces diastolic BP

24. Ans. a. Junctional fibres are very small in size

Ref: Anatomy and Physiology for Health Professionals- by Jahangir Moini, Professor Eastern Florida State College Jahangir Moini

AV Node

- The SA node impulse passes along junctional fibers of the conduction system to a mass of specialized tissue called the atrioventricular node (AV node), located in the inferior interatrial septum, beneath the endocardium
- The AV node provides the only normal conduction pathway between the atrial and ventricular syncytia
- Impulses are slightly delayed for 0.1 second because of the small diameter of the junctional fibers

25. Ans. b. Disinhibition of vasoconstrictor center

Ref: Pal GK Blood Pressure and its Regulation. In: Textbook of Medical Physiology

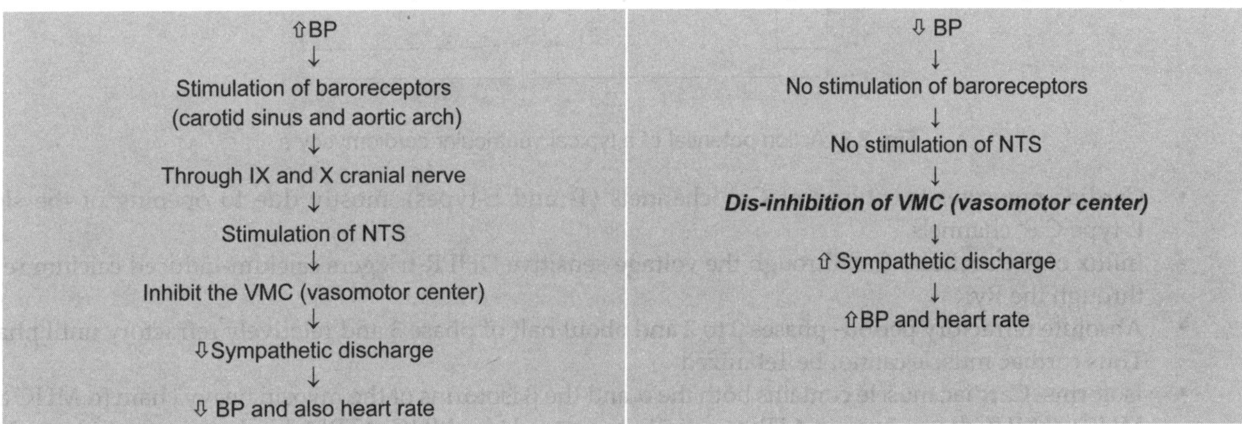

26. Ans. a. End diastolic volume *Ref: Berne and Levy Physiology 6/e p320*

- Contraction of cardiac muscle is influenced by both preload and afterload
- Preload refers to the force that stretches the relaxed muscle fibers. In left ventricle, for example, the bloos filling and thus stretching the wall during diastole represents the preload
- Afterload refers to the force against which the contracting muscle must act. Again from the perspective of the left ventricle, afterload is the pressure in the aorta that must be overcome by the contracting left ventricular muscle to open the aortic valve and eject the blood
- Preload can be increased by greater filling of the left ventricle during diastole (ie; increasing end-diastolic volume)

27. Ans. a. Less than intravascular pressure *Ref: Comparison of Performance of Various Sphygmomanometers with Intra-arterial Blood-pressure Readings. Br Med J. 1978 July 15; 2 (6131): 159-162*

28. Ans. d. Pulse pressure *Ref: Berne and Levy Physiology 6/e p387*

- The baroreceptors (or pressoreceptors) are stretch receptors located in the carotie sinuses and in the aortic arch
- The carotid sinus baroreceptors are more sensitive than those in the aortic arch
- Baroreceptors regulate blood pressure in the pressure range of 50–200 mm Hg
- Baroreceptors are very sensitive to changes in the pulse pressure

29. Ans. b. S2

The incisura corresponds to the aortic valve closure

30. Ans. a. Opening of Ca^{2+} channels

Action potential of a typical ventricular cardiomyocyte:

- Initial rapid depolarization and the overshoot (phase 0) -opening of voltage-gated Na^+ channels.
- The initial rapid repolarization (phase 1) -closure of Na^+ channels and opening of one type of K^+ channel.
- Prolonged plateau (phase 2) -slower but prolonged opening of voltage-gated Ca^{2+} channels.
- Final repolarization (phase 3) to the resting membrane potential (phase 4) -closure of the Ca^{2+} channels and a slow, delayed increase of K^+ efflux through various types of K^+ channels.

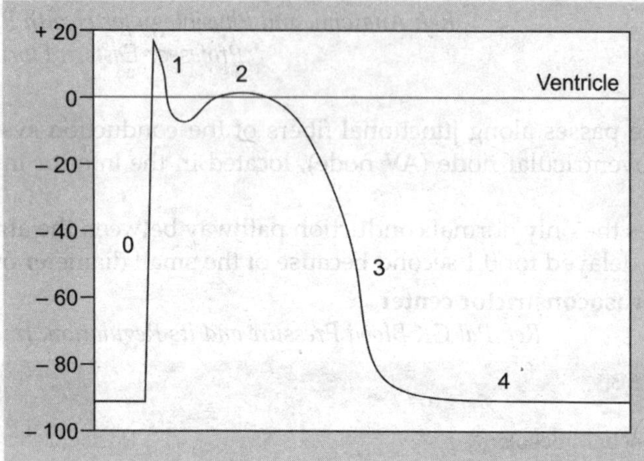

Fig. 2.8: Action potential of a typical ventricular cardiomyocyte

- Cardiac myocytes-two types of Ca^{2+} channels (T- and L-types), mostly due to opening of the slower L-type Ca^{2+} channels.
- Influx of extracellular Ca^{2+} through the voltage-sensitive DHPR-triggers calcium-induced calcium release through the RyR
- Absolute refractory period- phases 0 to 2 and about half of phase 3 and relatively refractory until phase 4. Thus cardiac muscle cannot be Tetanized
- Isoforms- Cardiac muscle contains both the α and the β isoforms of the myosin heavy chain (α MHC and β MHC). β MHC-lower myosin ATPase activity compared to α MHC. ATRIA-has both isoforms but α MHC. Ventricles-has β MHC

Long QT syndrome-due to mutations in voltage gated K^+ channel genes (KCNQ1 or KCNH2), voltage-gated Na^+ channels (eg, SCN5A), Ca^{2+} channels (e.g., CACNA1C). K^+ or Mg^{2+} deficiencies should be corrected in these patients. Therapy with β-blockers-to reduce the risk of cardiac arrhythmias

31. Ans. b. Stroke volume/end-diastolic volume

Ejection fraction

- Percentage of the end-diastolic ventricular volume that is ejected with each stroke, is about 65%
- Stroke volume/end-diastolic volume

32. Ans. c. 20% *Ref: Internet*

Stages of hypovolemic shock

- Stage 1
  - Up to 15% blood volume loss (750 mL)
  - Blood pressure maintained
- Stage 2
  - 15–30% blood volume loss (750–1500 mL)
  - Blood pressure cannot be maintained by arterial constriction
- Stage 3
  - 30–40% blood volume loss (1500–2000 mL)
  - Systolic BP falls to 100 mmHg or less

- Stage 4
  - Loss greater than 40% (>2000 mL)
  - Significantly decreased systolic blood pressure of 70 mmHg or less

33. Ans. a. Cardiac output

Fick's Principle
- Used to calculate cardiac output
- Amount of a substance taken up by an organ (or by the whole body) per unit of time is equal to the arterial level of the substance minus the venous level **(A-V difference)** times the blood flow

34. Ans. c. Expired air *Ref: Berne and Levy Physiology 6/e p445*

Guyton and Hall Textbook of Medical Physiology 2013, p354

Capnography-McHenry Western Lake County McHenry Western Lake County EMS

- The partial pressure (measured in mm Hg or kPa) - is the pressure that a particular gas exerts in a gas mixture
- Atmospheric pressure at sea level is approximately 760 mm Hg
- Oxygen constitues 21% of the atmosphere, so its partial pressure in atmospheric air is 21% of 760 = 159 mm Hg
- Carbon dioxide constitutes only 0.04%, so its partial pressure in atmospheric air is 0.04% of 760 = 0.3 mm Hg

Partial pressures of respiratory gases in mm Hg as they enter and leave the lungs (at sea level)

	Atmospheric air	Moist tracheal air	Alveolar air	Systemic arterial air	Mixed venous blood	Expired air
pO_2	159	150	104	90	40	120
pCO_2	0.3	0	40	40	46	27

- $ETCO_2$ (end tidal CO_2) is the level of carbon dioxide released at the end of expiration
- Normal $EtCO_2$ range is 35–45 mm Hg

35. Ans. b. 27 mm Hg *Ref: Previous Question*

36. Ans. c. O_2 affinity will be equal in both HbF and HbA in the absence of 2, 3DPG

Ref: Berne and Levy Physiology 6/e p462, 463

- Presence of 2, 3-DPG shifts the oxyhemoglobin dissociation curve to the right, because the affinity of Hgb for O_2 decreases as 2, 3-DPG increases. Binding of 2, 3-DPG creates an allosteric effect that inhibits the binding of O_2
- Decreased levels of 2, 3-DPG are observed in stored blood samples and thus may present a problem to transfusion recipients because of the greater affinity of Hgb for O_2, which inhibits the unloading of O_2 to tissues
- Normal adults have 2α globulin chains and 2β globulin chains (HgbA), whereas children younger than 1 year have fetal hemoglobin (HgbF) consisting of 2α globulin chains and 2γ chains
- This difference in the structure of HgbF increases its affinity for O_2 and aids in the transport of O_2 across the placenta
- HgbF is not inhibited by 2, 3-DPG, thus further enhancing O_2 uptake
- Hence in the absence of 2, 3-DPG, O_2 affinity will be equal in both HbF and HbA
- Option A-The oxygen carrying capacity of blood is enhanced about 65 times by its ability to bind to Hgb
- Option B-One molecule of DPG interacts with one molecule of Hb
- Option C-in the presence of CO, the affinity of Hgb for O_2 is enchanced-this shifts the dissociation curve to the left

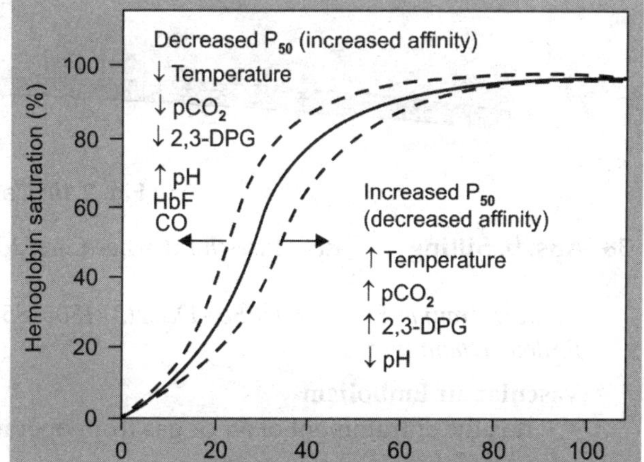

Fig. 2.9: Oxygen hemoglobin dissociation curve

37. Ans. c. Mainly carried as bicarbonate ions *Ref: Berne and Levy Physiology 6/e p465, 466*

The major transport mechanism of O_2 in blood is within the red blood cell bound to Hgb

The major transport mechanism of CO_2 is within the red blood cells in the form of HCO_3^-

CO_2 transport

- In blood CO_2 is transported in red blood cells primarily as bicarbonate, but also as dissolved CO_2 and as carbamino protein complexes (CO_2 binds not only to Hgb but also to plasma proteins)
- Once CO_2 diffuses thorough the tissue and enters plasma, it quickly dissolves
- The reaction of CO_2 with H_2O to form carbonic acid provides the major pathway for the generation of HCO_3^- in red blood cells. This reaction being catalyzed by carbonic anhydrase
- The blood brain barrier is relatively impermeable to H^+ and HCO_3^- ions, but it is very permeable to CO_2

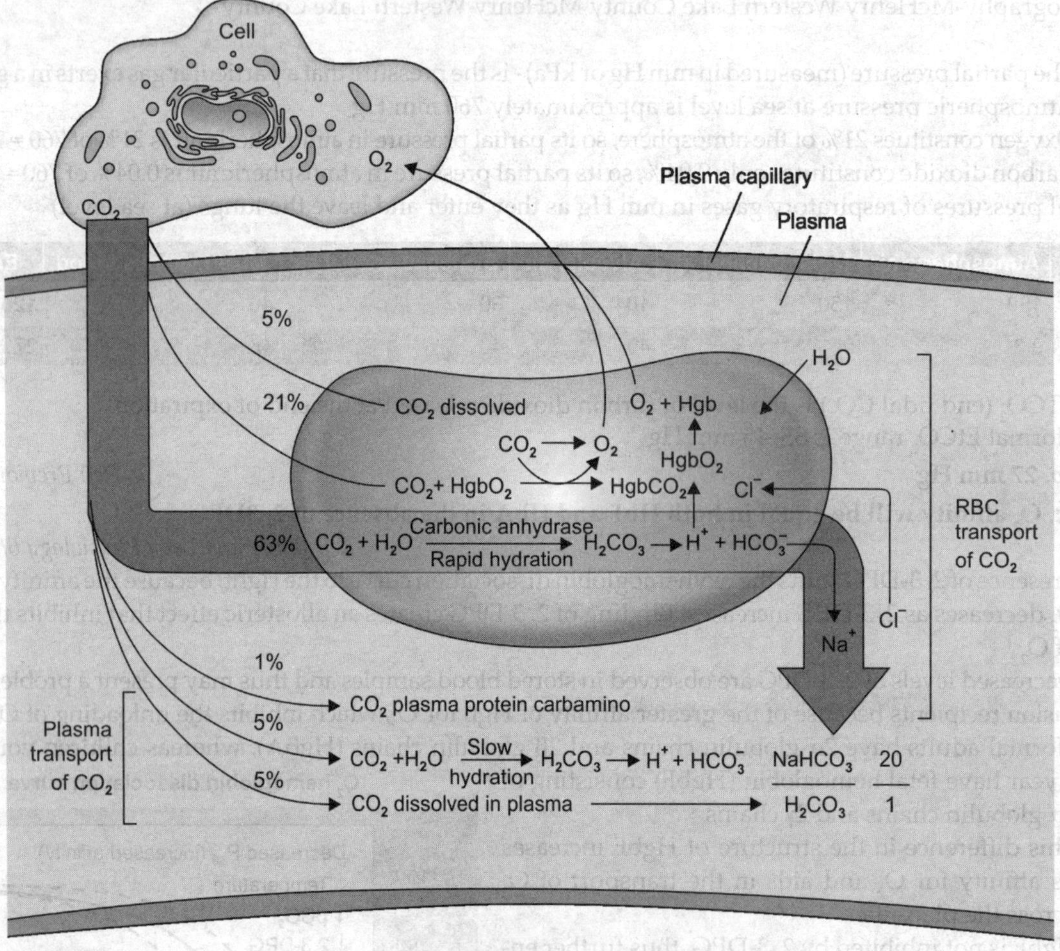

Fig. 2.10: Carbondioxide transport

38. Ans. b. Sitting *Ref: Anaesth Intensive Care. 2005 Jun; 33(3):323-31–Anaesthesia for Neurosurgery in the Sitting Position: A Practical Approach-Domaingue CM1*

J Emerg Trauma Shock. 2009 Sep-Dec;2(3):180–185. Acute management of vascular air embolism-Nissar Shaikh and Firdous Ummunisa

Vascular air Embolism

- It is the entrainment of air or gas from operative field or other communications into the venous or arterial vasculature
- High risk surgeries for VAE are ***sitting position*** and posterior fossa neurosurgeries, cesarean section, laparoscopic, orthopedic surgeries, pulmonary overpressure syndrome, and decompression syndrome

- The transesophgeal echocardiography is the most sensitive device which will detect smallest amount of air in the circulation
- Neurosurgery in the sitting position offers advantages for certain operations
- However, the approach is associated with potential complications, in particular venous air embolism
- As the venous pressure at wound level is usually negative, air can be entrained
- This air may follow any of four pathways.
  - Most commonly it passes through the right heart into the pulmonary circulation, diffuses through the alveolar-capillary membrane and appears in expelled gas
  - It may pass through a pulmonary-systemic shunt such as a probe patent foramen ovale (paradoxical air embolism)
  - It may collect at the superior vena cava-right atrial junction
  - Rarely it may traverse through lung capillaries into the systemic circulation.
  - Treatment of VAE is to prevent further entrainment of air, reduce the volume of air entrained and hemodynamic support
  - Various manoeuvres, including neck compression and volume loading, are also useful in reducing the incidence of venous air embolism

39. Ans. a. Anemic hypoxia *Ref: Berne and Levy Physiology 6/e p464*

Type of hypoxia	Pathology	Causes
Hypoxic hypoxia	Caused by diseases that result in decreased PaO_2 and O_2 content of arterial blood with a subsequent decrease in the delivery of O_2 to tissues	COPD, pulmonary fibrosis, neuromuscular diseases
Circulatory or stagnant hypoxia	Caused by reduced blood flow to an organ	Vascular disease, arteriovenous shunt Heart failure, shock
Anemic hypoxia	Caused by an inability of blood to carry sufficient O_2	CO poisoning, anemia
Histotoxic hypoxia	Caused by poisons that block the electron transport system in mitochondria and prevent the utilization of O_2 by the cell	Cyanide poisoning, sodium azide, some pesticides

40. Ans. d. Dead space ventilation *Ref: Berne and Levy Physiology 6/e p454*

Arterial hypoxemia

Defined as an arterial pO_2 less than 80 mm Hg in an adult who is breathing room air at sea level

Causes of hypoxemia

Cause	Arterial pO_2	$AdDO_2$	Arterial pO_2 Response to 100% O_2
Anatomic shunt	Decreased	Increased	No significant change
Decreased FiO_2	Decreased	Normal	Increased
Physiological shunt	Decreased	Increased	Decreased
Low ventilation-perfusion ratio	Decreased	Increased	Increased
Diffusion abnormality	Decreased	Increased	Increased
Hypoventilation	Decreased	Normal	Increased

Alveolar to arterial oxygen pressure difference - **$AaDO_2$**

Dead space ventilation

Ventilation to airways that do not participate in gas exchange

41. Ans. a. 160 mm of Hg *Ref: Berne and Levy Physiology 6/e p444*

Partial pressure

- The partial pressure of a gas is equal to the fraction of that gas in the gas mixture times the total or ambient (barometric) pressure (P_b).
- Ambient air is composed of N_2 and O_2, with minute quantities of CO_2, argon, and inert gases

- Ambient air is composed of approximately 21% O_2 and 79% N_2. Therefore, the partial pressure of O_2 in ambient air (pO_2) is

$pO_2 = FO_2 \times P_b$
$= 0.21 \times 760$ mm Hg
$= 159$ mm Hg

Therefore, partial pressure of oxygen in room air at 760 mm of atmospheric pressure is approximately 160 mm Hg

42. Ans. b. HCO_3^- *Ref: Question No 4*

43. Ans. b. Pons *Ref: Ganong's Review of Medical Physiology 24/e p658; Guyton and Hall Textbook of Medical Physiology 2013 p372; Walter F Boron Medical Physiology 2/e p731*

Respiratory Center

The respiratory center is composed of several groups of neurons located bilaterally in the medulla oblongata and pons. It is divided into 3 major collections of neurons

1. A dorsal respiratory group
2. A ventral respiratory group
3. The pneumotaxic center

	Dorsal group	Ventral group		
		Rostral	Intermediate	Caudal
Location	Dorsal medulla	Midway between dorsal and ventral surfaces of medulla		
Major component	Nucleus tractus solitarii	Nucleus retrofacialis or Botzinger complex	Pre-Botzinger complex, nucleus ambiguus and nucleus para-ambigualis	Nucleus retroambigualis
Dominant activity	Inspiratory	Expiratory	Inspiratory	Expiratory

Pneumotaxic center

- Located in the medial parabrachial and kolliker-fuse nuclei of the ***dorsolateral pons***
- Transmits signals to the inspiratory area
- The primary effect of this center is to control the 'switch- off' point of the inspiratory ramp, thus controlling the duration of the filling phase of the lung cycle
- The function of pneumotaxic center is to limit inspiration
- This has a secondary effect of increasing the rate of breathing because limitation of inspiration also shortens expiration and the entire period of each respiration
- A strong pneumotaxic center can increase the rate of breathing to 30–40 breaths per min, whereas a weak pneumotaxic signal may reduce the rate to only 3–5 breaths per minute
- When this area is damaged, respiration becomes slower and tidal volume greater

44. Ans. d. ↑ pH *Ref: Berne and Levy Physiology 6/e p462*

Oxyhemoglobin dissociation curve

- The oxyhemoglobin dissociation curve illustrates the relationship between pO_2 in blood and the number of O_2 molecules bound to Hgb
- The S shape of the curve demonstrates the dependence of Hgb saturation on pO_2, especially at partial pressures lower than 60 mm Hg.
- The clinical significance of the flat portion of the oxyhemoglobin dissociation curve (> 60 mm Hg) is that a drop in pO_2 over a wide range of partial pressures (100 to 60 mm Hg) has only minimal effect on Hgb saturation, which remains at 90% to 100%, a level sufficient for normal O_2 transport and delivery.
- The clinical significance of the steep portion (< 60 mm Hg) of the curve is that a large amount of O_2 is released from Hgb with only a small change in pO_2, which facilitates the release and diffusion of O_2 into tissue.
- The point on the curve where 50% of Hgb is saturated with O_2 is called the P_{50}, and it is 27 mm Hg in normal adults

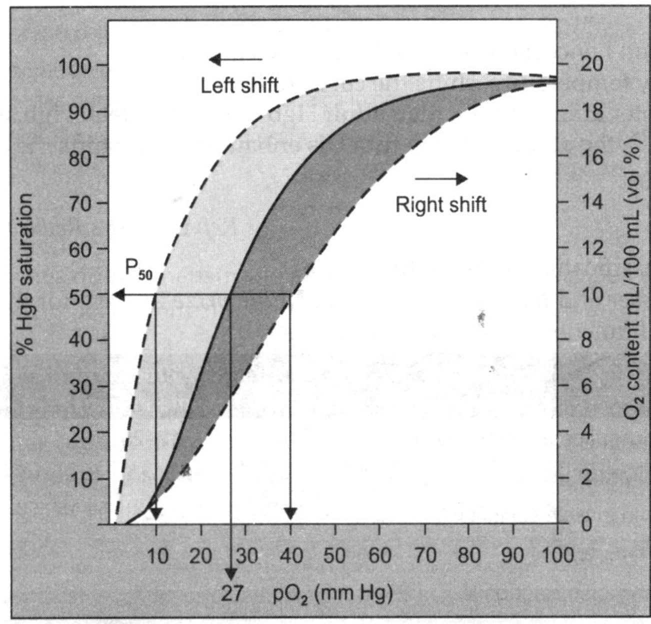

Fig. 2.11: Oxyhemoglobin dissociation curve

Physiological factors that shift the oxyhemoglobin dissociation curve

Shift to right:

- The curve is shifted to right when the affinity of Hgb for O_2 decreases, which enhances O_2 dissociation
- An increase in CO_2 production by tissue and release into blood results in the generation of hydrogen ions and a decrease in pH
- This shifts the dissociation curve to the right, which has a beneficial effect by aiding in the release of O_2 from Hgb for diffusion into tissues
- The shift to the right in the dissociation curve is due to the decrease in pH an due to the direct effect of CO_2 on Hgb
- This effect of CO_2 on the affinity of Hgb for O_2 known as Bohr effect, and it serves to enhance O_2 uptake in the lungs and delivery of O_2 to tissues
- Increased body temperature, such as during exercise, shifts the oxyhemoglobin curve to the right and enables more O_2 to be released to tissues where it is needed because the demand increases
- Presence of 2, 3-DPG shifts the oxyhemoglobin dissociation curve to the right, because the affinity of Hgb for O_2 decreases as 2, 3-DPG increases

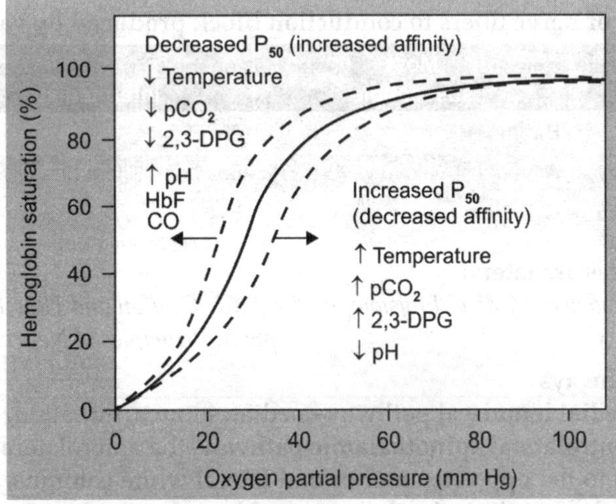

Fig. 2.12: Oxyhemoglobin dissociation curve

Shift to left:

- Decrease in pCO_2, and hence increase in pH shifts the curve to left
- Decrease in the body temperature, shifts the curve to left
- Fetal Hgb has a greater affinity for O_2 than adult Hgb does. Thus fetal Hgb shifts the curve to left
- In the presence of CO, the affinity of Hgb for O_2 is enhanced. This shifts the curve to the left

45. Ans. a. Stagnant hypoxia *Ref: Question No 6*

46. Ans. a. A alpha *Ref: Ganong's Review of Medical Physiology 24/e p92*

Erlanger and Gasser classification of nerve fibre types

- ***Herbert Spencer Gasser*** and ***Joseph Erlanger*** won ***Noble prize*** in 1944 'for their discoveries relating to the highly differentiated functions of single nerve fibres'

Fiber Type	Function	Fiber Diameter (μm)	Conduction Velocity (m/s)
Aα	Proprioception; somatic motor	12–20	70–120
Aβ	Touch, pressure	5–12	30–70
Aγ	Motor to muscle spindles	3–6	5–30
Aδ	Pain, temperature	2–5	12–30
B	Preganglionic autonomic	< 3	3–15
C, Dorsal root	Pain, temperature	0.4–1.2	0.5–2
C, Sympathetic	Postganglionic sympathetic	0.3–1.3	0.7–2.3

- In general, the greater the diameter of a given nerve fiber, the greater is its speed of conduction
- Type A fibers are the typical large and medium sized myelinated fibers of spinal nerves
- Type C fibers are the small unmyelinated nerve fibers that conduct impulses at low velocities
- Type C fibers constitute more than one-half of the sensory fibers in most peripheral nerves, as well as all the post ganglionic autonomic fibers

Numerical classification of sensory nerve fibers:

Number	Origin	Fiber Type
Ia	Muscle spindle, annulospiral ending	Aα
Ib	Golgi tendon organ	Aα
II	Muscle spindle, flower-spray ending; touch, pressure	Aβ
III	Pain and cold receptors; some touch receptors	Aδ
IV	Pain, temperature, and other receptors	Dorsal root C

Relative susceptibility of nerve fibers to conduction block produced by various agents (Mn. HPL is BACk)

Susceptibility	Most susceptible	Intermediate	Least susceptible
Hypoxia	B	A	C
Pressure	A	B	C
Local anesthetics	C	B	A

47. Ans. d. Lower most fibres are lateral

Ref: Ganong's Review of Medical Physiology 24/e p167, Guyton and Hall Textbook of Medical Physiology 2013 p693, Principles of Neural Science by Eric R. Kandel 5/e p492

Ascending sensory pathways

- **Dorsal coloumn medial lemniscal pathway**–mediates touch, vibration, proprioception
- **Anterolateral or ventrolateral spinothalamic pathway**–the anterolateral fibers cross in the anterior commissure of the cord to the opposite anterior and lateral white columns, where they turn upward toward the brain by way of the anterior spinothalamic and lateral spinothalamic tracts

Anterolateral pathway
Pain
Thermal sensations, including both warmth and cold sensations
Crude touch and pressure sensations
Tickle and itch sensations
Sexual sensations

Lateral Spinothalamic Tract

- Mediates ***pain and temperature***
- These sensory fibers terminate in the dorsal horn projections from there cross the midline ascend in the ventrolateral quadrant of the spinal cord VPL (ventral posterior lateral) nucleus of the thalamus primary somatosensory cortex
- The fibers in the spinothalamic tract are arranged somatotopically. Fibers originating in the ***lumbar and sacral segments are located laterally,*** whereas those from the ***cervical spinal segments are positioned medially*** (as shown in the diagram)

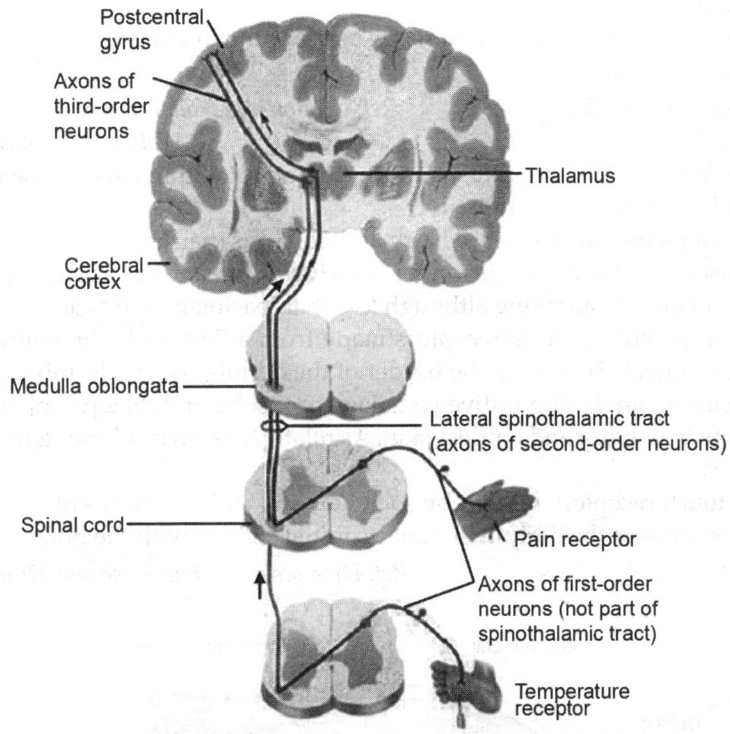

Fig. 2.13: Lateral spinothalamic tract

48. Ans. b. Gap junction *Ref: Berne and Levy Physiology 6/e p37, 83*

Types of Synapses

- Electrical synapse
- Chemical synapse

Electrical synapse

- In electrical synapses, the membranes on the presynaptic and postsynaptic neurons come close together and gap junctions form between the cells
- ***A gap junction is the morphological correlate of an electrical synapse***
- Electrical synapses are fast (essentially no synaptic delay) and bidirectional (i.e. current generated in either cell can flow across the gap junction to influence the other cell)
- Each gap junction channel is formed by 2 hemichannels (called connexons), one contributed by each cell. Each connexon is a hexamer of connexin protein subunits

- Recently, a second family of proteins that form gap junctions, the pannexins, has also been identified
- The permeability of gap junctions is regulated by cytosolic [Ca^{++}], [H^{+}], and cAMP and by the membrane potential
- Gap junctions also allow the cells to be electrically coupled

Chemical synapse

- At chemical synapses, a synaptic cleft separates the terminal of the presynaptic cell from the post synaptic cell
- An impulse in the presynaptic axon causes secretion of chemical intermediates known as neurotransmitters that diffuses across the synaptic cleft and binds to receptors on the surface of the postsynaptic cell
- Unlike the electrical synapses, at chemical synapses there is no direct communication between the cytoplasm of the two cells

49. Ans. a. Perineurium *Ref: Histology, Volume 518 by Ray C Henrikson, Joseph E Mazurkiewicz*

- Perineurium is a sleeve like of connective tissue that sharply defines nerve bundles
- The perineurium is formed by an epithelioid arrangement of flattened cells that are joined by tight junctions. The perineural layer is usually stratified
- The perineurium appears to have a blood nerve barrier function in establishing a intrafascicular environment for axons and Schwann cells

50. Ans. c. True meissner in hairy skin *Ref: Guyton and Hall Textbook of Medical Physiology 2013 p688, Walter F Boron Medical Physiology 2/e p402*

- ***Pacinian corpuscle adapts very rapidly***, hair receptors adapt within a second or so, and some joint capsule and muscle spindle receptors adapt slowly
- Two major types of mammalian skin are hairy and glabrous (hairless)
- ***Meissner's corpuscles*** are located in the ridges of ***hairless skin*** and are about one tenth the size of pacinian corpuscle. They are rapidly adapting although less than pacinian corpuscles
- ***Merkel's disks*** are slowly adapting receptors made from a flattened, non neural epithelial cell that synapses on a nerve terminal. They lie at the border of the dermis and epidermis of glabrous ***(hairless) skin***
- Ruffini's corpuscles resemble diminutive pacinian corpuscles and, like pacinian corpuscles occur in subcutaneous tissue of both hairy and hairless skin. As relatively slowly adapting receptors, they respond best to low frequencies
- ***Hair end organ***–touch receptors formed by each hair and its basal nerve fiber. Detects mainly ***movement*** of objects on the surface of the body. Also detects initial contact with the body

51. Ans. b. Organ of Coti *Ref: Diseases of the Ear, Nose and Throat by PL Dhingra, 5/e 2010*

Organ of corti

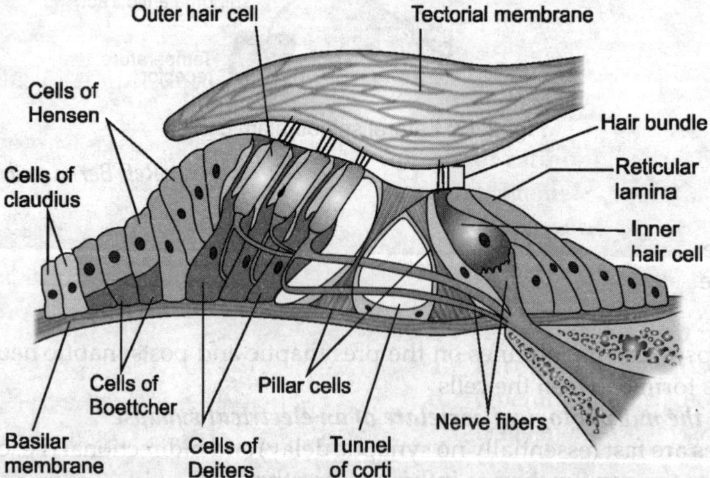

Fig. 2.14: Organ of corti

- Those cells continuing onto the pars pectinata of the basilar membrane are known as cells of Claudius.
- In parts of the cochlea, polyhedral cells separate the Claudius cells and the basilar membrane and are known as cells of Boettcher.
- The organ of Corti is composed of two types of cells, supporting and hair cells. The supporting cells are tall, slender cells extending from the basilar membrane to the free surface of the organ of Corti.
- The supporting cells include the outer and inner pillars, inner and outer phalangeal cells, and cells of Hensen.
- The inner tunnel within the organ of Corti is bounded below by the basilar membrane and above by the outer and inner pillar cells.

52. Ans. c. Carried by 1a fibers *Ref: Ganong's Review of Medical Physiology 24/e p234; http://www. kumc. edu/ AMA-MSS/Study/neuro3. htm*

Reflexes

- Monosynaptic reflexes–the simplest reflex arc with a single synapse between the afferent and efferent neuron. The best known example; the stretch reflex
- Polysynaptic reflexes–reflex arcs in which interneurons are interposed between the afferent and efferent neurons

Withdrawal Reflex

- Typical polysynaptic reflex that occurs in response to a noxious stimulus to the skin or subcutaneous tissues and muscle
- The response is flexor muscle contraction and inhibition of extensor muscles, so that the body part stimulated is flexed and withdrawn from the stimulus
- Withdrawal reflexes are **prepotent**, that is, they pre-empt the spinal pathways from any other reflex activity taking place at the moment
- **C FIBERS:** Pain fibers initiate the reflex.
- Exhibit after-discharge. This is due to continued bombardment of motor neurons by impulses arriving by complicated and circuitous polysynaptic paths
- Exhibit fractionation and occlusion
- Fractionation–supramaximal stimulation of any of the sensory nerves from a limb never produces as strong a contraction of the flexor muscles as that elicited by direct electrical stimulation of the muscles themselves. This indicates that the afferent inputs fractionate the motor neurom pool.
- Occlusion–if all the sensory inputs are dissected out and stimulated one after the other, the sum of the tension developed by stimulation of each is greater than that produced by direct electrical stimulation of the muscle or stimulation of all inputs at once. This indicates that the various afferent inputs share some of the motor neurons and that occlusion occurs when all inputs are stimulated at once.

53. Ans. a. Maximum secreted by choroid plexus

Ref: Berne and Levy Physiology 6/e p61, Guyton and Hall Textbook of Medical Physiology 2013 p814, Ganong's Review of Medical Physiology 24/e p603

Cerebrospinal fluid

- In humans, the volume of CSF is about 150 mL
- CSF production
  - ***2/3rd originates from choroid plexuses***
  - Small amount secreted by the ependymal surfaces of all the ventricles and by the arachnoidal membranes
  - A small amount also from the brain itself through the perivascular spaces that surround the blood vessels passing through the brain
- Volume of CSF within the ***ventricles*** is approximately ***30 mL***
- Volume of CSF in the ***subarachnoid space*** is about ***125 mL***
- Rate of CSF production is about 550 mL/day
- CSF turn over = 3.7 times a day
- ***At pressure of 112 mm H_2O, which is the normal CSF pressure, filtration and absorption are equal***
- Below a pressure of approximately 68 mm H_2O, absorption stops

- **CSF flow**
  Lateral ventricle → foramen of monro → 3rd ventricle → ***aqueduct of sylvius*** → 4th ventricle → 2 lateral foramina of Luschka and a midline foramen of Magendie → Cistern magna → continuous with the subarachnoid space that surrounds the entire brain and spinal cord → arachnoidal villi → large sagittal venous sinus and other venous sinuses of the cerebrum

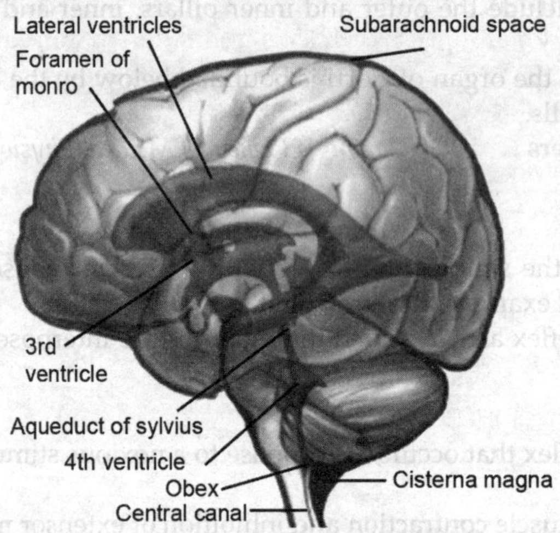

Fig. 2.15: CSF flow

Constituent	Lumbar CSF	Blood
Na^+ (mEq/L)	148	136-145
K^+ (mEq/L)	2.9	3.5-5
Cl^- (mEq/L)	120-130	100-106
Glucose (mg/dL)	50-75	70-100
Protein (mg/dL)	15-45	6.8×10^3
pH	7.3	7.4

54. Ans. d. Helps in fast anterograde axoplasmic transport

Ref: Berne and Levy Physiology 6/e p55, 74, 75, Ganong's Review of Medical Physiology 24/e p85-87

Myelin

- Myelin is a protein-lipid complex that is wrapped around the axon
- The myelin sheath ***envelops and protects the axon*** except at its ending and at the nodes of Ranvier
- A myelinated axon has much ***greater conduction velocity*** than an unmyelinated fiber of the same calibre because, the myelin sheath
  - Increases the length constant of the axon
  - Decreases the capacitance of the axon membrane
  - Restricts the generation of action potentials to the nodes of Ranvier
- **Saltatory conduction**–the sodium channels that bring generation of the action potential are highly concentrated at the nodes of Ranvier and are not found between them. Thus, the action potential is regenerated only at the nodes of Ranvier. This jumping of action potential from node to node is called saltatory conduction
- The action potentials of myelinated axons do not have a hyperpolarising after potential because they lack K^+ channels at their nodes. This increases the rate at which these fast conducting axons can fire
- Myelinated axons are more metabolically efficient then unmyelinated axons
- In myelinated axons, ionic currents are restricted to the small fraction of the membrane surface at the nodes of ranvier. For this reason, much ***less ion pumping and energy expenditure is required to maintain the gradients***

Types of Axonal transport	
Anterograde (orthograde) transport	Retrograde transport
From cell body towards the axon terminal	From the nerve ending to the cell body
Occurs along microtubules • Fast transport – 400 mm/day • Slow transport – 0.5 to 10 mm/day	Occurs along microtubules at about 200 mm/day
Involves dynein and kinesin	Involves dynein
Allows the replenishment of synaptic vesicles and enzymes responsible for the synthesis of neurotransmitters in synaptic terminals	This process returns recycled synaptic vesicle membrane to the soma for lysosomal degradation
Axonal transport requires metabolic energy and involves calcium ions	

55. Ans. a. Vasodilation of cutaneous blood vessel *Ref: Ganong's Review of Medical Physiology 24/e p260*

Effector organs	Parasympathetic nervous System	Sympathetic nervous system	
		Receptor type	Response
Eyes Radial muscles of iris Sphincter muscle of iris Ciliary muscle	 – Contraction (miosis) Contraction for near vision	 α_1	 Contraction (mydriasis) – –
Heart SA node Atria and ventricle AV node and purkinje	 Decreased heart rate Decreased atrial contractility Decreased conduction velocity	 β_1 β_1, β_2 β_1	 Increased heart rate Increased contractility Increased conduction velocity
Arterioles Skin, splanchnic vessels Skeletal muscle	 – –	 α_1 α_1/β_2 M	 Constriction Constriction/Dilation
Systemic veins	–	α_1, α_2/β_2	Constriction/Dilation
Bronchial smooth muscle	Contraction	β_2	Relaxation
Stomach and intestine Motility and tone Secretion Sphincters	 Increased Stimulation Relaxation	 α_1, α_2/β_2 – α_1	 Decreased – Contraction
Gallbladder	Contraction	β_2	Relaxation
Urinary bladder Detrusor Sphincter	 Contraction Relaxation	 β_2 α_1	 Relaxation Contraction
Uterus (pregnant)	–	α_1/β_2	Contraction/Relaxation
Male sex organs	Erection	α_1	Ejaculation
Skin Pilomotor muscles Sweat glands	 – –	 α_1 M	 Contraction Secretion
Liver	–	α_1, β_2	Glycogenolysis
Pancreas Acini Islet cells	 Increased secretion –	 α α/β_2	 Decreased secretion Decreased/increased secretion
Salivary glands	Profuse, watery secretion	α_1/β	Thick, viscous secretion/amylase secretion
Lacrimal glands	Secretion		–
Adipose tissue	–	β_3	Lipolysis

56. Ans. d. Trigeminothalamic tract *Ref: https://en. wikipedia. org/wiki/Anterior_trigeminothalamic_tract*

- The anterior trigeminothalamic tract (or ventral trigeminothalamic tract) serves as a proprioception, touch, and vibration pathway from the face, head and neck
- After receiving input from Meissner's and Pacinian corpuscles, first order neurons (of the trigeminal nucleus) enter the pons and synapse in the principal sensory trigeminal nucleus.
- Axons of the second order neurons cross the midline and terminate in the ventral posteromedial nucleus of the thalamus to mediate conscious sensation of proprioception, touch, and vibration from the face, head, and neck.
- The third order neuron in the thalamus then connects to the sensory cortex of the postcentral gyrus.

57. Ans. b. Gap junction *Ref: Questions No 48*

58. Ans. a and c Ear ossicles and Tympanic membrane

Ref: Textbook of Human Physiology for Dental Students- by Khurana

59. Ans. d. Ependymal cells-Macrophage

Ref: Ganong's Review of Medical Physiology 24/e p86, Berne and Levy Physiology 6/e p56

- The major cell types in nervous system are ***neurons*** and ***non neuronal elements called neuroglia***
- Neuroglial cells in the CNS include astrocytes and oligodendroglia. Microglia and ependymal cells are also considered to be central neuroglial cells
- Neuroglial cells in the PNS are Schwann cells and satellite cells

Oligodendroyctes	• Forms myelin in the CNS • Emit multiple processes that form myelin on many neighbouring axons
Astrocytes	2 subtypes Fibrous astrocytes and protoplasmic astrocytes • Fibrous astrocytes which contain many intermediate filaments, are found primarily in white matter • Protoplasmic astrocytes are found in gray matter and have a granular cytoplasm. • Both types send processes to blood vessels, where they induce capillaries to form the tight junctions making up the blood brain barrier • Help regulate the microenvironment of the CNS • Can actively take up K^+ ions and neurotransmitter substances, which they metabolize, biodegrade, or recycle • Buffer the extracellular environment of neurons • Cytoplasm of astrocytes contains glial filaments, which provide mechanical support for the CNS tissue
Microglia	• Latent phagocytes
Ependymal cells	• Form the epithelium lining the ventricular spaces of the brain that contain CSF • CSF is secreted in large part by specialized ependymal cells of the choroid plexuses located in the ventricular system
Schwann cells	• Form myelin in the PNS • Forms myelin between 2 nodes of ranvier on a single neuron
Satellite cells	• Encapsulate dorsal root and cranial nerve ganglion cells and regulate their microenvironment in a fashion similar to that used by astrocytes

60. Ans. a. Increased ICT

- Increase in the ICT causes compression of cerebral arteries and hence decreases the cerebral blood flow
- Metabolic acidosis, hypercapnea and hypoxia cause vasodilation. Hence increase the cerebral blood flow
- Decrease in viscosity will increase the flow. According to poiseille-hagen formula, blood flow varies inversely with viscosity

Flow = $(P_A - P_B) \times (\pi/8) \times (1/\acute{\eta}) \times (r^4/L)$

Where,

F = flow

$P_A - P_B$ = pressure difference between two ends of the tube

$\acute{\eta}$ = viscosity

r = radius of tube

L = length of tube

61. Ans. c. Dendrite *Ref: Dendritic Spine formation and stabilization Curr Opin Neurobiol 2009*

62. Ans. a. Muscle spindle *Ref: Ganong's Review of Medical Physiology 24/e p229*

Stretch reflex

- When a skeletal muscle with an intact nerve supply is stretched, it contracts
- This response is called the stretch reflex or myotatic reflex
- The stimulus that initiates this refled is stretch of the muscle, and the response is contraction of the muscle being stretched
- The sense organ is a small encapsulated spindle like or fusiform shaped structure called the muscle spindle, located within the fleshy part of the muscle
- The neurotransmitter at the central synapse is glutamate
- The stretch reflex is typified by the knee jerk reflex

63. Ans. b. Rubrospinal tract *Ref: Ganong's Review of Medical Physiology 24/e p240*

Medial brain stem pathways

- Pontine and medullary reticulospinal, vestibulospinal, and tectospinal tracts
- They control axial and proximal muscles
- Medial and lateral vestibulospinal tracts–involved in vestibular function, controls posture and balance
- Pontine and medullary reticulospinal tracts–maintenance of posture and in modulating muscle tone
- Tectospinal tract–control head and eye movements

Lateral brain stem pathway

- Rubrospinal tract
- Main control of distal muscles
- Excites flexor motor neurons and inhibits extensor motor neurons
- This pathway is not very prominent in humans, but it may play a role in the posture typical of decorticate rigidity

64. Ans. b. Tectocerebellar tract *Ref: Ganong's Review of Medical Physiology 24/e p250*

Functions of principal afferent systems to the cerebellum

Afferent tracts	Transmits
Vestibulocerebellar	Vestibular impulses from labyrinths, direct and via vestibular nuclei
Dorsal spinocerebellar	Proprioceptive and exteroceptive impulses from body
Ventral spinocerebellar	Proprioceptive and exteroceptive impulses from body
Cuneocerebellar	Proprioceptive impulses, especially from head and neck
Tectocerebellar	Auditory and visual impulses via inferior and superior colliculi
Pontocerebellar	Impulses from motor and other parts of cerebral cortex via pontine nuclei
Olivocerebellar	Proprioceptive input from whole body via relay in inferior olive

65. Ans. d. Supra chiasmatic nucleus

66. Ans. d. Action potentials *Ref: Ganong's Review of Medical Physiology 24/e p182*

- The eye is unique in that the receptor potentials of the photoreceptors and the electrical responses of most of the other neural elements in the retina are local, graded potentials, and it is only in the ganglion cells that all or none action potentials transmitted over appreciable distances are generated
- The responses of the rods, cones, and horizontal cells are hyperpolarizing
- The responses of the bipolar cells are either hyperpolarizing or depolarizing
- Amacrine cells produce depolarizing potentials and spikes that may act as generator potentials for the propagated spikes produced in the ganglion cells

67. Ans. d. Increases heart rate *Ref: KD Tripathi Essentials of Medical Pharmacology*

68. Ans. d. Reticulospinal tract *Ref: Question No 81, Ganong's Review of Medical Physiology 24/e p240*

- The medial brain stem pathways, are pontine and medullary reticulospinal, vestibulospinal, and tectospinal tracts
- The pontine and medullary reticulospinal tracts project to all spinal levels

- The pontine and medullary reticupospinal tracts are involved in the maintenance of posture and in modulating muscle tone, especially via an input to gamma motor neuron
- Pontine reticulospinal neurons are primarily excitatory
- Medullary reticulospinal neurons are primarily inhibitory
- Vestibulo spinal tract mainly influences alpha motor neuron.

69. Ans. a. Flocculonodular Lobe *Ref: Pal GK Textbook of Medial Physiology*

Vestibulo cerebellum/floculonodular lobe (Archi cerebellum)

- Connections with vestibular apparatus
- Concerned with equilibrium and learning induced changes in vestibule ocular reflex

Spino cerebellum (Paleocerebellum)

- Vermis–controls muscle movements of axial body
- Intermediate zone–controls muscle movements of limbs

Cerebro cerebellum (Neocerebellum)

- Overall planning programming of motor activities

70. Ans. c. Delta *Ref: Ganong's Review of Medical Physiology 24/e*

Sleep

- In a typical night of sleep, a young adult first enters NREM sleep, passes through stages 1 and 2, and spends 70–100 min in stages 3 and 4
- Sleep then lightens, and a REM period follows
- This cycle is repeated at intervals of about 90 min throughout the night
- **Beta wave** activity dominates in an awake, **aroused individual**
- In relaxed individuals with their eyes closed, the EEG is dominated by **alpha waves**

Non REM Sleep	Features
Stage 1	Alpha waves are interspersed with lower-frequency waves called theta waves
Stage 2	Sleep spindles K complexes
Stage 3	Delta waves
Stage 4	Delta waves

REM Sleep

- The low voltage, fast activity of REM sleep resembles that seen in an aroused subject
- Hence, REM sleep is also called **paradoxical sleep**
- **More dreaming** occurs during **REM** sleep
- Newborn children spend about half of their sleep time in REM sleep, whereas the elderly have little REM sleep
- About 20–25 % of the sleep of young adults is REM sleep.

71. Ans. a. Rods and cones *Ref: http://eyewiki. aao. org/Electroretinogram*

- The electroretinogram (ERG) is a diagnostic test that measures the electrical activity generated by neural and non-neuronal cells in the retina in response to a light stimulus
- ***a-wave***: initial corneal-negative deflection, derived from the cones and rods of the outer photoreceptor layers
- b-wave: corneal-positive deflection; derived from the inner retina, predominantly Muller and ON-bipolar cells
- c-wave: derived from the retinal pigment epithelium and photoreceptors

72. Ans. c. Nigrostriatal system *Ref: Guyton and Hall Textbook of Medical Physiology 2013 p828*

Neurohormonal systems in the human brain

- The locus cerulus–secretes norepinephrin
- The **nigrostriatal pathway**-dopaminergic pathway that connects the substantia nigra with the striatums, secretes dopamine
- Raphe nuclei–secretes serotonin
- Gigantocellular neurons of the reticular excitatory area–secretes acetylcholine

73. Ans. d. Crista *Ref: Berne and Levy Physiology 6/e p147*

The vestibular apparatus

- The ampulla of each of the semicircular canals contains a sensory epithelium
- The sensory epithelium in a semicircular canal is called a crista ampullaris, or ampullary crest

74. Ans. b. Skinner *Ref: Internet*

- Instrumental conditioning involves learning the association between a response and its consequences (what happens immediately after that response)
- BF Skinner was the most forceful and influential exponent of instrumental conditioning and its importance in everyday behavior. Skinner used the term operant conditioning, which is slightly different from instrumental conditioning, but the difference can be ignored.

75. Ans. a. Nitric oxide *Ref: Berne and Levy Physiology 6/e p225*

- Endothelium derived relaxing factor is nitric oxide
- Nitric oxide–relaxes vascular smooth muscle by stimulating guanylate cyclase and thereby increasing levels of cGMP, which inturn activates a cGMP-dependent protein kinase

76. Ans. b. Lateral corticospinal tract *Ref: Pal GK Textbook of Medial Physiology*

Lateral system pathways (regulation of skilled voluntary movements)

- Lateral corticospinal tract
- Rubrospinal tract

Medial system pathways (regulation of posture)

- Reticulospinal pathways
- Vestibulospinal pathways
- Tectospinal tract
- Anterior cortico-spinal tract
- Interstitiospinal tract.

77. Ans. d None of the above *Ref: Ganong's Review of Medical Physiology 24/e*

78. Ans. d. Ventromedial

- Satiety center is located in the ventromedial nuclei
- This opposes the desire for food
- When it is damaged bilaterally, satiety is lost. And therefore there is persistent food seeking and aggressive behaviour.

79. Ans. d. Influence of reticulospinal tract on gamma fibers

- De-afferentation causes abolition of input from muscle spindle to spinal cord
- Experimentally, even after deafferentation, influence of vestibule spinal tract on alpha fibers is not affected
- But, gamma motor neuron (which is controlled by the reticulospinal tract) mediated response in extra fusal fibers is lost
- Therefore, vestibulo spinal tract mainly influences alpha motor neuron and reticulospinal tract mainly influences gamma fibers

80. Ans. b. Beta fibers *Ref: Question No 1*

81. Ans. b. NREM stage II *Ref: Question No 25*

82. Ans. a. Duodenum *Ref: Gastroenterol Hepatol-2008-Brunner Gland Hamartoma*

Brunner's glands

- First described by Brunner in 1688
- Brunner glands are branched acinotubular glands in the submucosa of the duodenum
- They are located mainly in the duodenal bulb, proximal duodenum, and, with a progressive decrease in number and size, in the distal duodenum
- The Brunner glands, which empty into the crypts of Lieberkuhn, secrete an alkaline fluid composed of mucin, which exerts a physiologic anti-acid function by coating the duodenal epithelium, therefore protecting it from the acid chyme of the stomach
- Furthermore, in response to the presence of acid in the duodenum, these glands secrete pepsinogen and urogastrone, which inhibit gastric acid secretion.

83. Ans. a. HCl *Ref: Guyton and Hall Textbook of Medical Physiology 2013 p412*

Secretions from oxyntic (gastrin) glands of stomach

1. Mucous neck cells-secrete mucus
2. Peptic or chief cells-secrete pepsinogen
3. Parietal or oxyntic cells-secrete hydrochloric acid and intrinsic factor

Pepsinogen

- When pepsinogen is first secreted, it has no digestive activity
- As soon as it comes in contact with ***hydrochloric acid,*** it is activated to form ***active pepsin***
- Pepsin functions as an active proteolytic enzyme in a highly acidic medium, but above a pH of about 5 it has almost no proteolytic activity
- Hydrochloric acid is as necessary as pepsin for protein digestion in the stomach

84. Ans. a. Ileum *Ref: Medical Physiology-Walter F. Boron 2/e p971*

Transport of vitamin B_{12}

- Cobalamin reaches the stomach bound to proteins in ingested food. In the stomach, pepsin and the low gastric pH release the cobalamin from the ingested proteins.
- The now-free cobalamin binds to haptocorrin (formerly known as 'R' type binder), a glycoprotein secreted by the salivary and gastric glands.
- The parietal cells of the stomach secrete a second protein, intrinsic factor (IF), crucial for the absorption of cobalamin. However ***cobalamin and IF do not interact in the acidic milieu of the stomach***. Rather, ***gastric acidity enhances the binding of cobalamin to haptocorrin***.
- When this cobalamin-haptocorrin complex reaches the duodenum, the haptocorrin is degraded by pancreatic proteases.
- After the release of cobalamin from the cobalamin-haptocorrin complex in the proximal small intestine, both dietary cobalamin and cobalamin derived from bile bind to IF.
- The next step is the binding of the ***cobalamin-IF complex*** to specific ***receptors*** on the apical membranes of enterocytes in the ***ileum.***
- The enterocyte next internalizes the cobalamin-IF complex in a process that is energy dependent but has not been well characterized.
- Inside the cell, cobalamin and IF dissociate; lysosomal degradation may play a role here.
- Within the enterocyte, cobalamin binds to another transport protein—transcobalamin II—which is required for cobalamin's exit from the enterocyte. The cobalamin exits the ileal enterocyte across the basolateral membrane bound to transcobalamin II, possibly by an exocytotic mechanism.
- The transcobalamin II-cobalamin complex enters the portal circulation, where it is delivered to the liver for storage and for secretion into the bile.

85. Ans. a. Bile *Ref: Guyton and Hall Textbook of Medical Physiology 2013 p423*

Enterohepatic Circulation of Bile Salts

- About 94 percent of the bile salts are reabsorbed into the blood from the small intestine, about one half of this by *diffusion* through the mucosa in the early portions of the small intestine and the remainder by an *active transport* process through the intestinal mucosa in the distal ileum.
- They then enter the portal blood and pass back to the liver.
- On reaching the liver, on first passage through the venous sinusoids these salts are absorbed almost entirely back into the hepatic cells and then resecreted into the bile.
- In this way, about 94 percent of all the bile salts are recirculated into the bile, so on the average these salts make the entire circuit some 17 times before being carried out in the feces. .
- The small quantities of bile salts lost into the feces are replaced by new amounts formed continually by the liver cells.
- This recirculation of the bile salts is called the ***enterohepatic circulation of bile salts.***

86. Ans. d. Na^+ independent process in ileum *Ref: Ganong's Review of Medical Physiology 24/e p479, 485*

Vitamin B_{12} and folic acid absorption

- ***Vitamin B_{12} and folate absorption are Na^+–independent,*** but all 7 of the remaining water soluble vitamins-thiamin, riboflavin, niacin, pyridoxine, pantothenate, biotin and ascorbic acid–are absorbed by carriers that are Na^+ cotransporters

- Most vitamins are absorbed in the upper small intestine, but vitamin B_{12} is absorbed in the ***ileum***
- This vitamin binds to intrinsic factor, a protein secreted by the parietal cells of the stomach, and the complex is absorbed across the ileal mucosa

Absorption of	Small intestine			Colon
	Upper	Mid	Lower	
Sugars	++	+++	++	0
Aminoacids	++	++	++	0
Water-soluble and fat-soluble vitamins except vitamin B_{12}	+++	++	0	0
Long-chain fatty acid absorption and conversion to triglyceride	+++	++	+	0
Bile acids	+	+	+++	
Vitamin B_{12}	0	+	+++	0
Na^+	+++	++	+++	+++
K^+	+	+	+	Sec
Ca^{2+}	+++	++	+	?
Fe^{2+}	+++	+	+	?
Cl^-	+++	++	+	+
SO_4^{2-}	++	+	0	?

87. Ans. b. Submucos *Ref: Berne and Levy Physiology 6/e p488; Ganong's Review of Medical Physiology 24/e p456*

Organization of the wall of intestine

Mucosa

- The **mucosa** is the innermost layer of the GI tract. It consists of the **epithelium,** the **lamina propria,** and the **muscularis mucosae**
- The most abundant are cells termed absorptive **enterocytes,** which express many proteins important for the digestion and absorption of macronutrients
- **Enteroendocrine cells** contain secretory granules that release regulatory peptides and amines to help regulate GI function
- Throughout the small intestine, it is folded up into fingerlike projections called **villi**
- Between the villi are infoldings called crypts
- The crypt base contains Paneth cells, which secrete antimicrobial peptides, as well as stem cells that provide for continual turnover of the crypt and villus epithelium
- The epithelium turns over every 3–5 days in healthy adult humans
- The lamina propria immediately below the epithelium consists largely of loose connective tissue that contains collagen and elastin fibrils
- The lamina propria is rich in several types of glands and contains lymph vessels and nodules, capillaries, and nerve fibers
- The muscularis mucosae is the thin, innermost layer of intestinal smooth muscle

Submucosa

- The next layer is the **submucosa.** It consists largely of loose connective tissue with collagen and elastin fibril
- The submucosa contains a dense network of nerve cells called the submucosal plexus (**Meissner's plexus**)

Muscle Layers

- The **muscularis externa** or **muscularis propria** typically consists of two substantial layers of smooth muscle cells: an inner circular layer and an outer longitudinal layer.
- Between the circular and longitudinal layers of muscle lies the other plexus of the ENS, the **myenteric plexus**

Serosa

- The **serosa,** or **adventitia,** is the outermost layer of the GI tract and consists of a layer of squamous mesothelial cells.

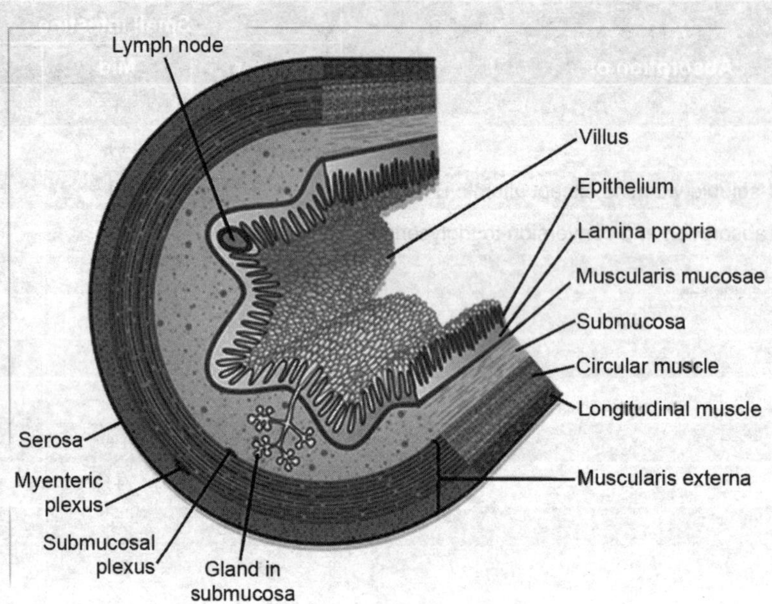

Fig. 2.16: Organization of wall of intestine

88. Ans. a. Parietal cells *Ref: Guyton and Hall Textbook of Medical Physiology 2013 p408*

Gastric secretions

Oxyntic glands	Pyloric glands
Secrete mainly Acid	Secrete mainly mucus
Located on the inside surfaces of the body and fundus of the stomach	Located in the antral portion of the stomach
Constitute 80% of the stomach	Constitute 20% of the stomach
Secretions • Mucous neck cells-mucus • Peptic or chief cells-pepsinogen • Parietal or oxyntic cells-hydrochloric acid and ***intrinsic factor***	Secretions • Mucous neck cells-mucus • Peptic or chief cells-pepsinogen • G cells-gastrin

89. Ans. c. Secretin *Ref: Ganong's Review of Medical Physiology 24/e p504; Guyton and Hall Textbook of Medical Physiology 2013 p448*

Small intestinal motility

- There are 3 types of smooth muscle contractions: peristaltic waves, segmentation contractions, and tonic contractions
- Peristalsis propels the intestinal contents (chyme) towards the large intestines. Peristaltic activity is increased by the gastroenteric reflex that is initiated by distention of the stomach
- Segmental contractions move the chyme to and fro and increase its exposure to the mucosal surface. These contractions are initiated by focal increases in Ca^{2+} influx
- Tonic contractions are relatively prolonged contractions that in effect isolate one segment of the intestine from another
- Intestinal motility is ***enhanced by gastrin, CCK, insulin, motilin, serotonin***
- Intestinal motility ***inhibited by secretin and glucagon***

90. Ans. c. Hypoproteinemia

Glomerular Filtration Rate:

GFR = K_f × Net filtration pressure

The net filtration pressure represents the sum of the hydrostatic and colloid osmotic forces that either favour or oppose filtration across the glomerular capillaries. These forces include

1. Hydrostatic pressure in the glomerular capillaries (P_G), which promotes filtration
2. Hydrostatic pressure in the Bowman's capsule (P_B), which opposes filtration
3. The colloid osmotic pressure of the glomerular capillary plasma proteins (π_G), which opposes filtration
4. The colloid osmotic pressure of the proteins in the Bowmans capsule (π_B), which promotes filtration
   - Hypoproteinemia causes decrease in the colloid osmotic pressure of the glomerular capillary plasma proteins, thereby increasing GFR

91. Ans. b. MAG 3 *Ref: J Nucl Med Allied Sci. 1990-99 mTc-MAG3 versus 131I-orthoiodohippurate in the routine determination of effective renal plasma flow*

92. Ans. a. Relaxes mesangial cells in kidney *Ref: KD Tripathi Essential of medical pharmacology*

Dopamine actions

- Low dose of dopamine dilates the renal and mesenteric blood vessels
- Relaxes the mesangial cells and increases GFR.

93. Ans. b. 25% *Ref: Ganong's Review of Medical Physiology 24/e p602*

Region	Mass (kg)	Blood flow		Percentage of total	
		mL/min	mL/100 g/min	Cardiac output	O_2 consumption
Liver	2.6	1500	57.7	27.8	20.4
Kidneys	0.3	1260	420	23.3	7.2
Brain	1.4	750	54	13.9	18.4
Skin	3.6	462	12.8	8.6	4.8
Skeletal muscle	31	840	2.7	15.6	20
Heart muscle	0.3	250	84	4.7	11.6
Rest of the body	23.8	336	1.4	6.2	17.6
Whole body	63	5400	8.6	100	100

94. Ans. a. One million *Ref: Ganong's Review of Medical Physiology 24/e p673; Guyton and Hall Textbook of Medical Physiology 2013 p462*

Nephron

- Each individual renal tubule and its glomerulus is a unit called nephron
- Each human kidney has approximately 1 million nephrons
- The kidney cannot regenerate new nephrons
- After the age of 40, the number of functioning nephrons usually decreases about 10% every 10 years
- Thus at age 80, many people have 40% fewer functioning nephrons than they did at age 40
- This loss is not life threatening because adaptive changes in the remaining nephrons allow them to excrete the proper amounts of water, electrolytes and waste products

95. Ans. b. cAMP *Ref: Ganong's Review of Medical Physiology 24/e p680*

Mesangial cells

- Support the entire glomerular tuft
- Secrete mesangial matrix
- Are contractile
- Are phagocytic
- Capable of proliferation

Agents causing contraction or relaxation of mesangial cells

Contraction	Relaxation
• Endothelins • Angiotensin II • Vasopressin • Norepinephrine • Platelet-activating factor • Platelet-derived growth factor • Thromboxane A_2 • PGF_2 • Leukotrienes C_4 and D_4 • Histamine	• ANP • Dopamine • PGE_2 • cAMP

96. Ans. b. Progesterone *Ref: Walter F Boron 2/e p1164-1167, Berne and Levy Physiology 6/e p777*

Hormonal influence on the endometrium during menstrual cycle

E-Estrogen, P-progesterone

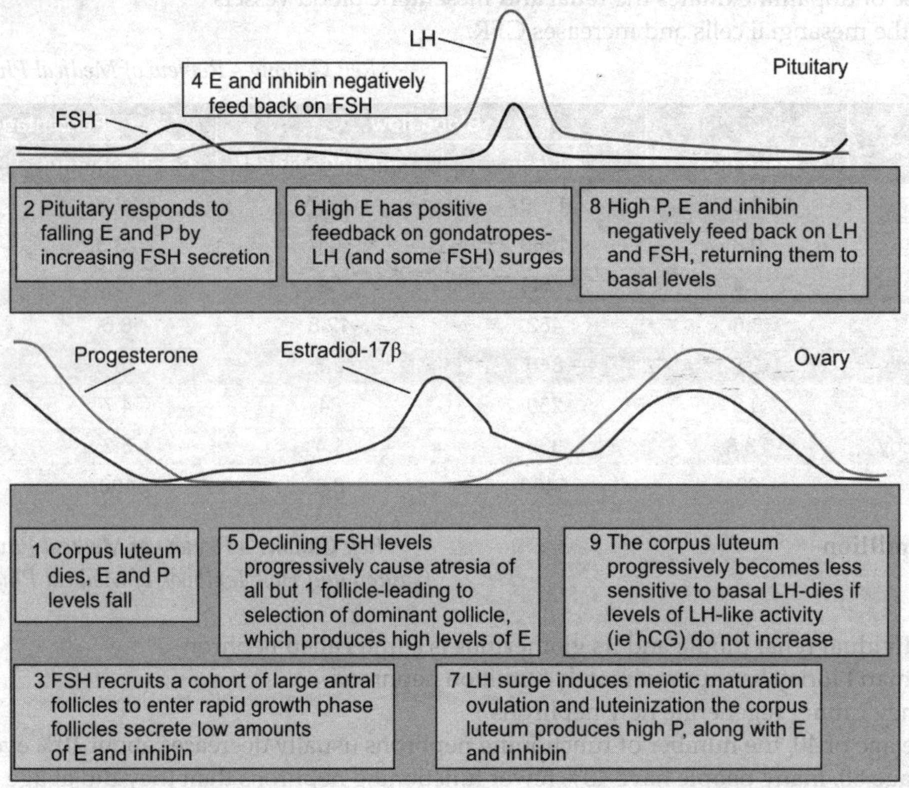

Fig. 2.17: Hormonal influence on endometrium during menstrual cycle

Menstrual phase (first 5 days)

- If the oocyte was not fertilized and pregnancy did not occur in the previous cycle, a sudden diminution in estrogen and progesterone secretion will signal the demise of the corpus luteum
- As hormonal support of the endometrium is withdrawn, the vascular and glandular integrity of the endometrium degenerated, the tissue breaks down, and menstrual bleeding ensues

Proliferative phase (6–14 days)

- Proliferation and differentiation of the endometrium are stimulated by estrogen that is secreted by the developing follicles

- Levels of estrogen rise early in the follicular phase and peak just before ovulation
- Levels of endometrial estrogen receptor are highest during the proliferative phase and decline after ovulation in response to the changing levels of progesterone
- Estrogen induces synthesis of growth factors such as the insulin-like growth factors, TGFs, and epidermal growth factor which are necessary for maturation and growth of the endometrium
- Estrogen causes the stromal components of the endometrium to become highly developed.
- Estrogen also induces the synthesis of progestin receptors in endometrial tissue.
- Levels of progestin receptors peak at ovulation, when estrogen levels are highest, to prepare the cells for the high progestin levels of the luteal phase of the cycle.
- Progesterone, in contrast, opposes the action of estrogen on the epithelial cells of the endometrium and functions as an antiestrogen. Although progesterone inhibits epithelial cell proliferation, it promotes proliferation of the endometrial stroma.

Secretory Phase (15–28 days)

- During the early luteal phase of the ovarian cycle, the antiestrogenic effects of progesterone halt the proliferative phase of the endometrial cycle
- The major products of the corpus luteum are progesterone and 17α-hydroxyprogesterone, although the corpus luteum also produces estradiol.
- Increased progesterone biosynthesis is characteristic of the midluteal phase
- The endometrium must be conditioned by estrogen for progesterone to act effectively.
- During the latter half of the menstrual cycle, progesterone induces final maturation of the uterine endometrium for reception and implantation of the fertilized ovum

97. Ans. d. Pregnanendol

Ref: Guyton and Hall Textbook of Medical Physiology 2013 p642, Berne and Levy Physiology 6/e p784

Ovarian sex hormones

- Estrogens and Progestins
- The most important of the estrogens is the hormone estradiol, and the most important progestin is progesterone
- The estrogens mainly promote proliferation and growth of specific cells in the body that are responsible for the development of most secondary sexual characteristics of the female.
- The progestins function mainly to prepare the uterus for pregnancy and the breasts for lactation.

Progesterone

- **Secretion of progesterone**
  - In the normal nonpregnant female, progesterone is secreted in significant amounts only during the latter half of each ovarian cycle, when it is secreted by the corpus luteum.
  - Large amounts of progesterone are also secreted by the placenta during pregnancy, especially after the fourth month of gestation.
- **Transport of progesterone in the blood**
  - Progesterone binds primarily to cortisol binding globulin (transcortin) and albumin
  - Because it has relatively low binding affinity for these proteins, its circulating half life is about 5 min
- **Fate of Progesterone**
  - Within a few minutes after secretion, almost all the progesterone is degraded to other steroids that have no progestational effect
  - The major end product of progesterone degradation is ***pregnanediol.***
  - About 10 percent of the original progesterone is excreted in the urine in this form. Therefore, one can estimate the rate of progesterone formation in the body from the rate of this excretion.
- **Functions of progesterone**
  - Progesterone Promotes Secretory Changes in the Uterus the latter half of the monthly female sexual cycle, thus preparing the uterus for implantation of the fertilized ovum
  - Progesterone decreases the frequency and intensity of uterine contractions, thereby helping to prevent expulsion of the implanted ovum

- Progesterone also promotes increased secretion by the mucosal lining of the fallopian tubes, which is necessary for nutrition of the fertilized, dividing ovum as it traverses the fallopian tube before implantation
- Progesterone promotes development of the lobules and alveoli of the breasts
- Progesterone (and pregnenolone) are used by the transitional zone of the fetal cortex to make cortisol late in pregnancy.

98. Ans. d. Dihydrotestosterone *Ref: Ganong's Review of Medical Physiology 24/e p423-426*

Testosterone synthesis

- Testosterone is the principal hormone of the testes
- Testosterone is synthesized from cholesterol in the leydig cells of testes
- In leydig cells, pregnenolone is hydroxylated in the 17th position and then subjected to side chain cleavage to form ***dehydroepiandrosterone***
- ***Androstenedione*** is also formed via progesterone and 17-hydroxyprogesterone, but this pathway is less prominent in humans
- ***Dehydroepiandrosterone and androstenedione*** are then converted to testosterone
- ***Dihydrotestosterone (DHT)*** - is a testosterone metabolite. Testosterone is converted to DHT by 5α reductase in some target cells
- Humans have two 5α reductases that are encoded by different genes. Type1 5α reductase is present in skin throughout the body and is the dominant enzyme in the scalp
- Type 2 5α reductase is present in genital skin, the prostate and other genital tissues.

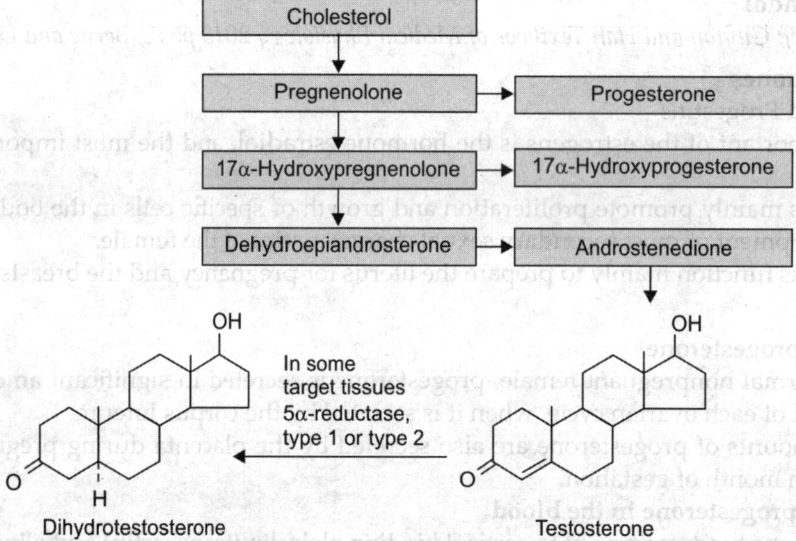

Fig. 2.18: Testosterone synthesis

99. Ans. a. Iodide trapping *Ref: Berne and Levy Physiology 6/e p727*

Iodide trapping

- Active transport of iodide into the gland against chemical and electrical gradients by a $2Na^{+}$-$1I^{-}$ symporter located in the basolateral membrane of thyroid epithelial cells
- This iodide trap requires the generation of energy by oxidative phosphorylation and displays saturation kinetics

Reactions catalyzed by thyroid peroxidase

- Oxidation of iodide to iodine
- Binding of iodine to thyroglobulin
- Coupling of two Diiodotyrosine to form T4, or one Monoiodotyrosine and one diiodotyrosine to form T3

100. Ans. a. Norepinephrine via alpha 2 receptor

- Hormones that act by increasing cAMP formation
- GHRH
- FSH
- LH
- GnRH
- CRH
- Norepinephrine via β1 receptor
- ADH via V2 receptor

Hormones that act by inhibiting cAMP formation

- Norepinephrine via α2 receptor
- Somatostatin

ADH via V1 receptor act by increasing IP 3, DAG

101. Ans. d. Thyrotoph *Ref: Ganong's Review of Medical Physiology 24/e p324*

Cell type of anterior pituitary	Hormones secreted	Percentage of total secretory cells
Somatotrope	Growth hormone	50
Lactotrope	Prolactin	10-30
Corticotrope	ACTH	10
Thyrotrope	TSH	5
Gonadotrope	FSH, LH	20

102. Ans. c. Vasoconstriction in skeletal circulation

Ref: Berne and Levy. Physiology Chapter 42 The Adrenal Gland p741; Ganong's Review of Medical Physiology 24/e p357

Effects of epinephrine

- Increases blood glucose by increasing hepatic glycogenolysis and ***gluconeogenesis***. Decreases glucose utilization
- **Increases insulin** and ***glucagon*** secretion (β_2)
- ***Dilates the blood vessels in skeletal muscle*** and the liver via β_2 receptors
- Increases lipolysis and calorigenesis
- Increases cardiac contractility, heart rate and conduction velocity (β_1)
- Mobilization of free fatty acids
- Increases plasma lactate
- Stimulation of metabolic rate.

Actions of Catecholamine Hormones

β: Epinephrine > Norepinephrine	α: Norepinephrine > Epinephrine
↑ Glycogenolysis	↑ Glycogenolysis (α_1)
↑ Gluconeogenesis (β_2)	↑ Gluconeogenesis (α_1)
↑ Lipolysis (β_3) (β_2)	
↑ Calorigenesis (β_1)	
↓ Glucose utilization	
↑ Insulin secretion (β_2)	↓ Insulin secretion (α_2)
↑ Glucagon secretion (β_2)	
↑ Muscle K^+ uptake (β_2)	
↑ Cardiac contractility (β_1)	↑ Cardiac contractility (α_1)
↑ Heart rate (β_1)	
↑ Conduction velocity (β_1)	
↑ Arteriolar dilation: ↓ BP (β_2) (muscle)	↑ Arteriolar vasoconstriction; ↑BP (α_1) (splanchnic, renal, cutaneous, genital)

Contd...

Contd...

β: Epinephrine > Norepinephrine	α: Norepinephrine > Epinephrine
↑ Muscle relaxation (β_2)	↑ Sphincter contraction (α_1)
Gastrointestinal	Gastrointestinal
Urinary	Urinary
Bronchial	
	↑ Platelet aggregation (α_2)
	↑ Sweating ('adrenergic')
	↑ Dilation of pupils (α_1)

103. Ans. d. Secreted by theca cells

Ref: Walter F Boron Medical Physiology 2/e p1154-1157, Williams Textbook of Endocrinology 12/e p606, Ganong's Review of Medical Physiology 24/e p406, Berne and Levy Physiology 6/e p777

Estrogens
- The naturally occurring estrogens are 17 β-estradiol, estrone and estriol
- Estradiol is the biologically potent estrogen
- Estradiol is secreted by granulosa cells of the dominant ovarian follicle

Secretion of estrogen
- In the follicular phase of the menstrual cycle, the follicle synthesizes estrogens whereas in luteal phase, the corpus luteum does the synthesis
- **Theca cells**–these cells can take up cholesterol and produce the adrenal androgens, but they do not have the aromatase necessary for estrogen production
- **Granulosa cells**–have aromatase to synthesize estradiol, but lack enzymes for making the adrenal androgens
- Therefore, Estradiol synthesis requires the contribution of both theca and granulosa cells

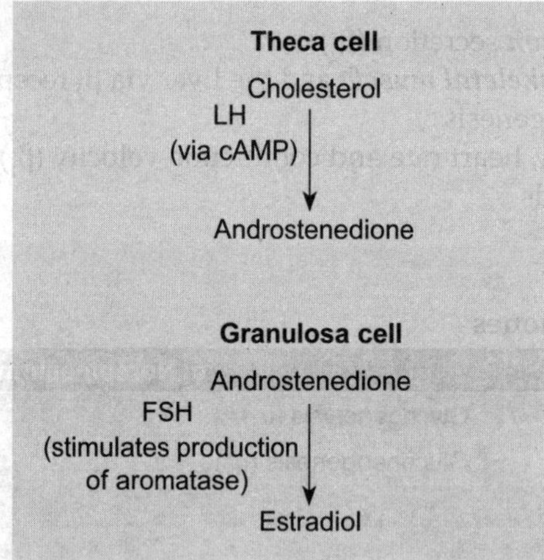

- 2% of secreted estrogen is free, and the remainder is bound to protein: 60% to albumin and 38% to gonadal steroid binding globulin

LH surge
- Abrupt rise in the LH level that occurs around 13th to 14th day of the follicular phase
- LH surge peaks 12 hours after its initiation and lasts for 48 hours
- Once the dominant follicle causes circulating estrogen levels to exceed 200 pg/mL, estrogen exerts a positive feedback on the gonadotrope to produce the LH surge
- The LH surge drives meiotic maturation, ovulation, and differentiation of granulose cells into progesterone-producing cells

Negative feedback by ovarian steroids
- Throughout most of the menstrual cycle, the estrogens and progestins feedback negatively on both the hypothalamus and the gonadotrophs of the anterior pituitary
- The net effect is to reduce the release of both LH and FSH
- The estrogens exert a negative feedback at both low and high concentrations, whereas the progestins are effective only at high concentrations

Positive feedback by ovarian steroids
- At the end of the follicular phase, the estrogens feedback positively on the hypothalamic pituitary axis
- One manifestation of this positive feedback is LH surge.

104. Ans. b. Androgen binding protein

Ref: Ganong's Review of Medical Physiology 24/e p419-421, Berne and Levy Physiology 6/e p762

Testis–made up of leydig cells and sertoli cells

Sertoli cells
- Lines the wall of the seminiferous tubules
- Tight junctions between adjacent sertoli cells near the basal lamina form a ***blood-testis barrier*** that prevents many large molecules from passing the interstitial tissue to the lumen
- Spermatids mature into spermatozoa in deep folds of the cytoplasm of sertoli cells. Mature spermatozoa are released from the sertoli cells and become free in the lumens of the tubules
- They do not synthesize androgens, but they contain aromatase (CYP19), the enzyme responsible for conversion of androgens to estrogens, and they can produce estrogens
- Perform phagocytic function by ***engulfing residual bodies*** (cytoplasm shed by spermatozoa during spermiogenesis).

Sertoli cell secretions	Functions
Androgen-binding protein	Maintains a high androgen level in the lumens of the seminiferous tubules
Antimullerian hormone (mullerian inhibitory substance)	Induces regression of the embryonic mullerian duct that is programmed to give rise to the female reproductive tract
Inhibin	Keeps FSH levels within a set point by inhibiting FSH (negative feedback)

Leydig cells
- Between the seminiferous tubules in the testes are nests of cells containing lipid granules, the interstitial cells of leydig
- Leydig cells secrets ***testosterone*** into the bloodstream
- These cells can synthesize cholesterol denovo.

105. Ans. d. Inhibits progesterone systhesis

Ref: Ganong's Review of Medical Physiology 24/e p414, Berne and Levy Physiology 6/e p788

Human chorionic gonadotropin
- hCG is a ***glycoprotein*** that contains galactose and hexosamine
- It is produced by the ***syncytiotrophoblast***
- It is made up of α and β subunits
- ***hCG- α is identical to the α subunit of LH, FSH and TSH***
- hCG is primarily luteinizing and luteotropic and has little FSH activity
- The primary action of hCG is to stimulate LH receptors on the corpus luteum. This prevents luteolysis and maintains a high level of luteal-derived ***progesterone production*** during the first 10 weeks
- The rapid increase in hCG is responsible for the nausea of morning sickness associated with early pregnancy
- A small amount of hCG enters the fetal circulation and stimulates fetal leydig cells to produce testosterone before the fetal gonadotropic axis is fully mature
- hCG also stimulates the fetal adrenal cortex during the 1st trimester
- It can be measured by radioimmunoassay and detected in the blood as early as 6 days after conception

- Its presence in urine in early pregnancy is the basis of the various laboratory tests for pregnancy, and it can sometimes be detected in the urine as early as 14 days after conception
- The serum hCG levels double every 2 days for the first 6 weeks and peak at about 10 weeks. Then declines to a constant level at about 50% of the peak value
- Antibodies used to detect hCG (in assays and pregnancy tests) are designed to specifically detect the β subunits
- hCG appears to act on the same receptor as LH
- It is not absolutely specific for pregnancy. Small amounts are secreted by a variety of gastrointestinal and other tumors in both sexes
- It also appears that the fetal liver and kidney normally produce small amounts of hCG.

106. Ans. b. Acidophilic cells *Ref: Berne and Levy Physiology 6/e p712*

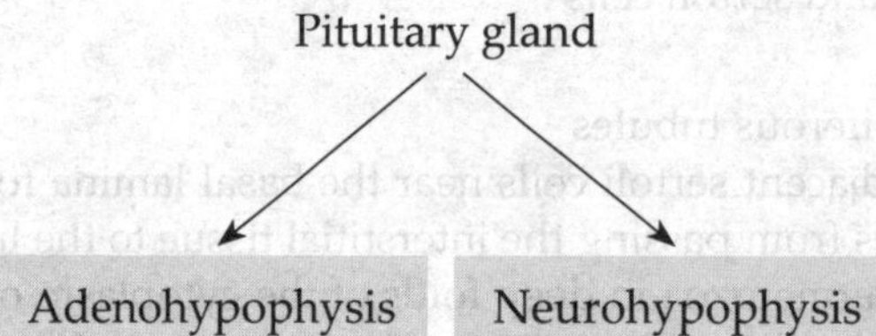

Cell types of the adenohypophysis

	Basophils			Acidophils	
	Corticotrope	Thyrotrope	Gonadotrope	Somatotrope	Lactotrope
Primary hypothalamic regulation	Corticotropin releasing hormone - Stimulatory	Thyrotropin releasing hormone - Stimulatory	Gonadotropin releasing hormone - Stimulatory	Growth hormone releasing hormone - Stimulatory, Somatostatin- Inhibitory	Dopamine - Inhibitory, PRL releasing factor– Stimulatory
Tropic hormone secreted	Adrenocortic-otropic hormone	Thyroid stimulating hormone	Follicle-stimulating hormone and luteinizing hormone	Growth hormone	Prolactin
Peripheral hormone involved in negative feedback	Cortisol	Triiodothyronine	Estrogen, progesterone, testosterone, and inhibin	IGF-1 GH (short loop)	None

107. Ans. a. Leydig cells *Ref: Question No 104*

108. Ans. a. Prolactins *Ref: Berne and Levy Physiology 6/e p723*

The Lactotrope

- The lactotrope produces the hormone **prolactin**
- PRL is structurally related to GH and hPL (Human Placental Lactogen)
- The lactotrope differs from the other endocrine cell types of the adenohypophysis in two major ways:
  1. The lactotrope is not part of an endocrine axis. This means that PRL acts directly on nonendocrine cells (primarily of the breast) to induce physiological changes
  2. Production and secretion of PRL are predominantly under inhibitory control by the hypothalamus. hus, disruption of the pituitary stalk and the hypothalamohypophysial portal vessels (e.g., secondary to surgery or physical trauma) results in an increase in PRL levels but a decrease in ACTH, TSH, FSH, LH, and GH.

109. Ans. a. Granulosa cell *Ref: Berne and Levy Physiology 6/e p762, Guyton and Hall Textbook of Medical Physiology 2013 p646, Walter F Boron Medical Physiology 2/e p1154*

Inhibin

- Glycoprotein heterodimers consisting of one α and one β subunit that are covalently linked
- Members of Transforming growth factor β gene family

Inhibin

In males	In females
Produced by sertoli cells of testes	Produced by ***granulosa cells*** of ovary (also to some extent by pituitary, brain, adrenal, kidney, bone marrow, corpus luteum, and placenta)
FSH stimulates inhibin production, which then negatively feeds back on gonadotropes to inhibit FSH production	Inhibin production stimulated by • FSH (most specific) • Estradiol • LH
Inhibin keeps FSH levels within a set point	Inhibin inhibits the secretion of FSH and to a lesser extent LH

110. Ans. a. Dopamine

Ref: Berne and Levy Physiology 6/e p724, Angiotensin II effects on second messengers involved in prolactin secretion are mediated by AT1 receptor in anterior pituitary cells - Mol Cell Neurosci 1994,

Prolactin secretion increased by	Prolactin secretion decreased by
• Prolactin - releasing factor • Dopamine antagonist • ***AT-II*** • Stress • Surgery, fear, stimuli causing arousal • Exercise • Sleep • ***TRH*** • Secretin • Glucagon • VIP • GIP	• ***Dopamine*** • Dopamine agonists (bromocriptine) • Somatostatin • TSH • GH

111. Ans. d. It increases appetite

Ref: Berne and Levy Physiology 6/e p690, Ganong's Review of Medical Physiology 24/e p399, Walter F Boron Medical Physiology 2/e p1040, Guyton and Hall Textbook of Medical Physiology 2013 p615, The role of leptin and ghrelin in the regulation of food intake and body weight in humans: a review - Obes Rev 2007

Leptin

- Leptin is an adipocyte derived protein that ***signals information to the hypothalamus*** about the degree of adiposity and nutrition, which in turn controls eating behavior and energy expenditure
- Leptin is ***secreted by mature adipocytes*** and is structurally related to cytokines. Thus it is sometimes referred to as an adipocytokine
- Leptin crosses the blood brain barrier and modulates specific neurons in the arcuate nucleus of the hypothalamus that control feeding behaviour
- ***Obese individuals already have elevated endogenous circulating levels of leptin*** and appear to have developed leptin resistance
- Diet induced obesity, advanced age and T2DM are associated with leptin resistance
- Leptin and insulin are anorexigenic (i.e., satiey) signals for the hyopothalamus
- ***Leptin suppresses food intake***
- Leptin has an important role in liporegulation in peripheral tissues. Leptin protects peripheral tissues (eg., liver, skeletal muscle, cardiac muscle, beta cells) from the accumulation of too much lipid by directing storage of excess caloric intake into adipose tissue
- Leptin also acts as a signal that the body has sufficient energy stores to allow reproduction and to enhance erythropoiesis, lymphopoiesis, and myelopoiesis. For example-in women suffering from anorexia nervosa, leptin levels are extremely low and result in low ovarian steroids, amenorrhea, anemia from low red blood cell production and immune dysfunction
- Leptin has a role in progression of puberty
- Leptin output is increased by insulin. Leptin decreases insulin secretion

- Leptin output is inhibited by fasting and weight loss and lipolytic signals (eg., increased cAMP, and β3 agonists)

112. Ans. c. GH *Ref: Berne and Levy Physiology 6/e p720, Ganong's Review of Medical Physiology 24/e p330*

Growth hormone secretion

- The somatotrope produces growth hormone
- GH is a protein that is similar to prolactin and human placental lactogen
- GH secretion shows diurnal rhythms.
- GH secretion is ***stimulated during sleep***, slow wave sleep (stages III and IV)
- GH secretion is lowest during the day. This rhythm is entrained to sleep-wake patterns rather than light-dark patterns, so a phase shift occurs in people who work night shifts
- GH secretion is pulsatile
- The GH receptor is a member of the cytokine/GH/PRL/erythropoietin receptor family and, as such, is linked to the JAK/STAT signaling pathway
- Human GH also act as an agonist for the PRL receptor
- Half life–20 min
- Liver and kidney are the major sites of GH degradation
- The hypothalamus predominantly stimulates GH secretion via the Growth hormone- releasing hormone
- The hypothalamus also inhibits GH synthesis and release via somatostatin
- GH secretion is also regulated by ghrelin, which is primarily produced by the stomach but is also expressed in the hypothalamus
- The primary negative feedback on the somatotrope is exerted by IGF-I
- GH also increases somatostatin release

GH secretion increased by	GH secretion decreased by
• Sleep	• Hyperglycemia
• Stress	• Increase in free fatty acids
• Acute hypoglycemia	• Obesity
• Some amino acids	• Cortisol
• Exercise	• Medroxyprogesterone
• Starvation	• Growth hormone and IGF-I
• Protein meal	
• Glucagon	
• Pyrogen	
• Lysine vasopressin	
• Estrogen	
• Androgen	
• Thyroid hormone	
• L-Dopa, α adrenergic agonists that penetrate the brain	
• Apomorphine and other dopamine receptor agonists	

ACTH–bursts are most frequent in the ***early morning***, and about 75% of the daily production of ***cortisol*** occurs between 4 am and 10 am

113. Ans. a. Norepinephrine *Ref: Ganong's Review of Medical Physiology 24/e p382, 384, 433, Norepinephrine kinetics and dynamics in septic shock and trauma patients- British journal of Anesthesia*

Half life

- PTH–10 min
- Calcitonin - < 10 min
- Insulin–5 min
- Norepineprine–2-2.5 min

114. Ans. d. Somatotrope *Ref: Question No 10*

115. Ans. c. TBG

- Thyroid hormones (T3 and T4) increase basal rate of metabolism
- THS and TRH stimulate thyroid gland for synthesis and release of thyroid hormones. Therefore influence basal rate of metabolism

- On entering the blood, more than 99% of the thyroxine and triiodothyronine combines immediately with several of the plasma protein, mainly with thyroxine-binding globulin and much less so with thyroxine –binding prealbumin and albumin. Thyroid hormones are functionally active only in free form, not in bound form (bound with TBG).
- Therefore, TBG has least effect on the metabolic rate among the given options

116. Ans. a. It is a steroidal compound *Ref: Question No 109*

117. Ans. b. Pineal gland

Melatonin

- Released from pineal gland
- Plays a role in sleep mechanisms
- The diurnal change in melatonin secretion may function as a timing signal to coordinate events with the light dark cycle
- Melatonin secretion is increased during the dark period and maintained at low level during daylight hours
- This diurnal variation is brought about by norepinephrine secreted by the postganglianic sympathetic nerves that innervate the pineal gland

118. Ans. a. Inhibitis beta myosin heavy chain *Ref: Ganong's Review of Medical Physiology 24/e p312*

Effects of thyroid hormones on cardiovascular system

- T3 is not formed from T4 in myocytes to any degree
- Circulatory T3 enters the myocytes, combines with its receptors, and enters the nucleus, where it promotes the expression of some genes and inhibits the expression of others

Genes enhanced	Genes inhibited
• Alpha myosin heavy chain • Sarcoplasmic reticulum Ca^{2+} ATPase • Beta adrenergic receptors • G proteins • Na K ATPase • Certain K^{+} channels	• Beta myosin heavy chain • Phospholamban • Two types of adenyl cyclase • T3 nuclear receptors • NCX- sodium calcium exchanger

- The net result is increased heart rate and force of contraction

119. Ans. a. Cortisol *Ref: Ganong's Review of Medical Physiology 24/e p354, 360*

Adrenal cortex	Adrenal Medulla (28%)
{Mneumonic: Layers- ***GFR*** Their secretions can be remembered as ***salt, sweet and sex*** for Mineralocorticoid, Glucocorticoids and androgens respectively • Zona glomerulosa (15%)–Secretes Mineralocorticoid (aldosterone). Also involved in Formation of new cortical cells • Zona fasciculata (50%)–Secretes Glucocorticoids (cortisol and corticosterone) • Zona reticularis (7%)–Secretes Adrenal androgens (dehydroepiandrosterone, androstenedione)	• 90% cells secrete epinephrine • 10% cells secrete nor epinephrine • Dopamine

Cortisol

- The major glucocorticoid hormone in humans - ***Cortisol***
- In humans, the ratio of secreted cortisol to corticosterone is approximately 7:1
- The average amount of cortisol secreted is 10 mg/24 hr
- The average plasma concentration of cortisol (free and bound)–13.9 microgram/dL
- Cortisol is bound in the circulation to an α globulin called transcortin or corticosteroid-binding globulin. A minor degree of binding to albumin also takes place

120. Ans. a. Thermogenin *Ref: Walter F Boron 2/e p1206*

Brown fat

- Brown fat differs from white fat in having a high density of mitochondria (the cytochromes in these mitochondria give the brown fat cells their color)

- Newborns have particularly high levels of brown fat in the neck and midline of the upper back
- In brown fat, the locally generated T_3 upregulates a protein called **uncoupling protein UCP1**, originally called ***thermogenin***
- Thermogenin is a H^+ channel located in the inner mitochondrial membrane
- Normally intracellular purine nucleotides (eg-ATP and GTP) inhibit thermogenin
- However, epinephrine, acting through cAMP pathway, activates the lipase that liberates Fatty acids from triglycerides
- These fatty acids relieve the inhibition of the H^+ channel and increase its conduction of protons
- Consequently, the protons generated by electron transport enter the mitochondria through UCP1, which dissipates the H^+ gradient needed by the H^+ translocating ATP synthase
- Thus, mitochondria in brown fat can produce heat without producing useful energy in the form of ATP
- The oxidation of fatty acids in brown fat generates 27 kcal/kg of body weight each day and contributes a large fraction of the neonate's high metabolic rate

121. Ans. d. Thermogenesis

122. Ans. b. autosomal recessive *Ref: https://medicalnotebook. wordpress. com/2012/12/12/ application-of-hardy-weinberg-principle-in-population-genetics/*

- The Hardy-Weinberg principle states that in a large randomly breeding population, allelic frequencies will remain the same from generation to generation assuming that there is no mutation, gene migration, selection or genetic drift.
- Application - If one knows the population frequency of an autosomal recessive disease, one can calculate the population frequency of carriers of this disease.

123. Ans. a. Brain *Ref: Internet Sources*

124. Ans. d. Ketone body *Ref: Guyton and Hall Textbook of Medical Physiology*

Starvation

- Even though the tissues preferentially use carbohydrates for energy over both fat and protein, the quantity of carbohydrate normally stored in the entire body is only a few hundred grams and it can supply energy only for first few hours of starvation
- Therefore, except for the first few hours of starvation, the major effects are progressive depletion of tissue fat and protein
- Protein undergoes 3 phases of depletion. Rapid depletion at first, then greatly slowed depletion, and finally, rapid depletion again shortly before death
- After the readily mobilized protein stores have been depleted during the early phase of starvation, the remaining protein is not so easily removed
- At this time, the rate of gluconeogenesis decreases to 1/3rd its previous rate
- The lessened availability of glucose then initiates a series of events that leads to excessive fat utilization and conversion of fat breakdown products to ketone bodies
- The ketone bodies can cross the blood brain barrier and can be used by the brain cells for energy
- Therefore, ***2/3rd of the brains energy is now derived from these ketone bodies***, principally from beta-hydroxybutyrate
- This sequence leads to atleast partial preservation of the protein stores of the body
- Then finally comes a time when the fat stores are almost depleted, and the only remaining source of energy is protein
- At that time, the protein stores once again enter a stage of repid depletion
- Because proteins are also essential for the maintenance of cellular function, death ordinarily ensues when the proteins of the body have been depleted to about half their normal level

125. Ans. c. Demargination

Increase in number of circulating neutrophils with exercise is a result of demargination of cells from endothelial tissues and bone marrow, or as part of the phagocytic and inflammatory response to exercise-induced tissue damage

Ref: Pal GK Practical physiology

Important laws and principles

Nernst Equation	To calculate equilibrium potential of a single ion
Gibbs Donnan Effect	The presence of non-diffusible ions across the cell membrane affects the concentration of diffusible ions. The negatively charged proteins and phosphates which are present inside the cell cannot diffuse across the membrane. This results in a greater permeability of chloride (a diffusible anion)
Goldman-Hodgkin-Katz Equation	• Involves multiple ions • Depends on concentration gradient and permeability of ions
Boyles law	At constant temperature, the volume of a given mass of gas is inversely proportional to the pressure exerted on it
Charle's law	At constant pressure, the volume is proportional to the absolute temperature i.e., $V \propto T$
Avogadro's law	Equal volumes of different gases at the same temperature and pressure contain the same number of molecules
Ideal gas law	PV = nRT P = the pressure in atmospheres, V = volume in liters, n = number of gram-moles of a gas, R = universal gas constant, T = temperature in Kelvin
Dalton's law	In a mixture of gases, the total pressure exerted is equal to the sum of the partial pressures of the individual component gases
Henry's law	At constant temperature, the amount of gas dissolved in a liquid will be directly proportional to the partial pressure of the gas with which the liquid is in equilibrium
Graham's law	In a gas phase, the rate of diffusion of a gas is inversely proportional to its moleculat weight
Fick's law of diffusion	The net diffusion rate of a gas through a membrane is proportional to the tissue area and the difference in partial pressure between the two sides, and is inversely proportional to the thickness
Laplace law	The tension (T) in the wall of a cylinder is equal to the product of the transmural pressure (P) and the radius (r) divided by the wall thickness (h) T = Pr/h,
The 'Place' Principle	• For determination of sound frequency
The 'Power' law	• For detection of changes in loudness

Labeled line principle	• The specificity of nerve fibres for transmitting only one modality of sensation is called the labeled line principle
Size principle	• The recruitment of motor units during muscle contraction is not random, rather it follows a general scheme, the size principle
Fenn effect	• Muscle uses extra energy in proportion to the work done
Frank starling law	• Within physiological limits, the force of contraction is directly proportional to the initial length of the muscle fiber (although commonly referred to as Frank-Starling law of the heart, this is applicable to skeletal muscle as well)

Few important One liners

- Apoptosis -programmed cell death
  - Initiated by activation of a family of proteases called caspases
- Vesicular traffic in golgi–controlled by small G proteins and SNAREs
- Patch clamp method–for recording ion current flow through single channels
- **Mitochondria** contain DNA similar to that found in the cell nucleus
- Transcription–assembly of the RNA chain from activated nucleotides using the DNA strand as template
- Translation–the process by which the genetic information of the messenger RNA is used to make proteins in the ribosome
- The sodium potassium pump moves 3 sodium ions to the exterior for every 2 potassium ions to the interior

- Total blood volume = $\frac{\text{Plasma volume}}{1\text{–hematocrit}}$
- Main source of Ca^{2+} for contraction in:
  - Skeletal muscle-SR
  - Cardiac and Smooth muscle-ECF
- A single action potential causes a brief contraction followed by relaxation. This response is called a **muscle twitch**
- The length of the muscle at which the active tension is maximal is usually called its **resting length**
- In mammals, fast axonal transport proceeds as fast rapidly as 400 mm/day, whereas slow axonal transport occurs at about 1mm/day
- **Synapse en passant**–characteristic of smooth muscle
- Absent Dystrophin-**Duchenne** muscular dystrophy
- Altered Dystrophin-**Becker** muscular dystrophy
- In neurons, the resting membrane potential is -70 mV, which is close to the equilibrium potential for potassium
- The resting membrane potential of skeletal muscle is about -90 mV
- In smooth muscle there is no true RMP. Varies between -20 to -65 mV
- **Rheobase -** Minimum strength of stimulus that can elicit a biological response
- **Chronaxie -** The duration that a stimulus twice the strength of rheobase needs to be applied in order to elicit a response
- **Nissel bodies** are stacks of endoplasmic reticulum
- All righting reflexes are integrated at midbrain except **optical righting reflex,** which is integrated at cortex
- Glutamate - Responsible for 75% of the excitatory transmission in the CNS
- Endogenous opioid peptides-enkephalin, endorphin and dynorphin
- Sound frequency is measured in cycles per second, or hertz
- The unit of sound pressure level is decibel
- The normal speech has an intensity of about 65 decibel
- Sounds that exceed 100 decibel can damage the peripheral auditatory apparatus, and those higher than 120 decibel can cause pain and permanent damage
- **Zeitgebers**–cyclical factors in the environment that help to synchronize biological rhyhms
- ***Bundle of Kent*** -In ***Wolff-Parkinson-White Syndrome*** - additional muscular or nodal tissue connection between the atria and the ventricles
- **Lown–Ganong - Levine syndrome**
  - Attacks of paroxysmal supraventricular tachycardia
  - Usually nodal tachycardia
  - Seen in individuals with short PR intervals and normal QRS complexes
- **Bathmotropy**–relating to excitability
- The arterial pressure during the first day after birth averages about 70 mm Hg systolic and 50 mm Hg diastolic
- **Cardiac reserve**–the maximum percentage that the cardiac output can increase above normal. In healthy adults, the cardiac reserve is 300 to 400 percent.
- **Cardiac index** is cardiac output per square meter of body surface area which approximately equals *3.2 L/min/m² of body surface area*
- **Phospholamban**–protein that inhibits the sarcoplasmic reticulum calcium ATPase
- The affinity of haemoglobin for carbon monoxide is **210 times** its affinity for oxygen
- Rhythmic respiration is initiated by a small group of synaptically coupled pacemaker cells in the pre-Botzinger complex
- The maximal colonic water absorptive capacity is between 4-5 L/day.
- *Folds of Kerckring* (valvulae conniventes) - folds in the small intestinal mucosa which increase the surface area of the absorptive mucosa about threefold.

- Somatostatin: inhibits gastric secretion by inhibiting both G and ECL cells
- Dent disease
  - Mutations in the gene for one of the renal chloride channels
  - Associated with Calcium containing kidney stones and hypercalciuria
- **Goldblatt or renal hypertention-** constriction of one renal artery causes a prompt increase in renin secretion and the development of sustained hypertension
- **Siggaard–Andersen curve nomogram**:
  - To plot the acid–base characteristics of arterial blood.
  - This nomogram has pCO_2 plotted on a log scale on the vertical axis and pH on the horizontal axis
- **Megalin and cubilin**–glycoproteins that mediate protein and peptide endocytosis in the proximal tubule
- **Alfa Klotho** - An anti aging protein
  - Recently been discovered to play important roles in calcium and phosphate homeostasis by its reciprocal effects on 1, 25-dihydroxycholecalciferol levels
- During fetal life, glucocorticoids accelerate the maturation of surfactant in the lungs
- **Transcortin**- approximately 90-95% of the cortisol in the plasma binds to plasma proteins, especially a globulin called cortisol-binding globulin or transcortin
- **Somatostatin** - Inhibit the secretion of insulin, glucagon, gastrin, VIP, GIP, secretin, motilin
- About 75% of the daily production of cortisol occurs between 4 am and 10 am.

QUESTIONS 2015

1. **Normal CSF volume:**
   a. 150 ml
   b. 100 ml
   c. 200 ml
   d. 250 ml
2. **Which of the following is correct for 70 kg person:**
   a. Plasma volume 5 L
   b. Total body fluid 42 L
   c. Interstitial volume 22
   d. None of the above
3. **Component present more in extra cellular compartment than intracellular:**
   a. Phosphate
   b. Protein
   c. Sodium
   d. Magnesium
4. **Oxygen dissociation curve shifts to right in:**
   a. Decrease in pH
   b. Decrease in temperature
   c. Decrease in 2, 3 DPG
   d. All the above
5. **The active form of vitamin D is produced in:**
   a. Distal tubule of kidney
   b. Proximal tubule of kidney
   c. Skin
   d. None of the above

ANSWERS AND EXPLANATIONS

1. **Ans. a. 150 ml**

Cerebrospinal fluid

- In humans, the volume of CSF is about 150 mL
- CSF production
  - 2/3 rd originates from choroid plexuses
- Volume of CSF within the ventricles is approximately 30 mL
- Volume of CSF in the subarachnoid space is about 125 mL
- Rate of CSF production is about 550 mL/day
- CSF turn over = 3.7 times a day.

2. Ans. b. Total body fluids is 42 L

Total body water (60% of body weight, for a 70 kg man) is 42 liters		
Intracellular fluid	**Extracellular fluid**	
2/3rd of TBW, i.e. 40% Body weight (28 liters)	1/3rd of TBW, i.e. 20% Body weight (14 liters)	
	Interstitial fluid	Plasma
	75% or 3/4th of ECF or 15% of body weight (10.5 Litres)	25% or 1/4th of ECF or 5% of body weight (3.5 Litres)

3. Ans. c. Sodium

4. Ans. a. Decrease in pH

5. Ans. b. Proximal tubule of kidney

- Cholecalciferol (vitamin D_3) is formed in the skin
- Cholecalciferol is converted to 25-hydroxycholecalciferol in the liver
- 25-hydroxycholecalciferol is converted to 1, 25-dihydroxycholecalciferol in the proximal tubules of kidney
- 1, 25-dihydroxycholecalciferol is by far the most active form of vitamin D because the previous products have less than 1/1000 of the vitamin D effect
- Therefore in the absence of kidney, vitamin D loses almost its effectiveness.

Chapter

3 Biochemistry

B Vinodh Kumar

CELL MEMBRANE

It is composed of:
- Protein: 55%E
- Phospholipid: 25%
- Cholesterol: 13%

Phospholipids		Proteins	
Along with cholesterol	Caveolae (Lipid rafts + caveolin-1)	Integral proteins (Channels, pumps, carrier)	Peripheral proteins
Maintains the fluidity of membrane	Involved in signal transduction	• Transmembrane proteins, Usually globular proteins • Span the lipid bilayer • Asymmetrical distribution	• Present embedded in either the inner or outer leaflet of the lipid bilayer • Weakly bound to the hydrophilic region

- Major Lipids in Membranes: Phospholipids, Glycosphingolipids, and Cholesterol
- Of the two major phospholipid classes present in membranes, phosphoglycerides are more common
- The simplest phosphoglyceride is phosphatidic acid, which is 1, 2-diacylglycerol 3-phosphate
- The second major class of phospholipids is composed of sphingomyelin
- A fatty acid is attached by an amide linkage to the amino group of sphingosine, forming ceramide
- The most common sterol in membranes is cholesterol
- In almost all the membranes of the body, proteins are either equal or exceed the quantity of lipids. The exception is MYELIN (high lipid content provides good insulation)
- Nucleus is the most prominent organelle and can occupy up to 10% of the space inside a cell
- The membrane is not a solid component. It floats like a gel (fluid mosaic theory)

Fraction	Enzymes
Plasma membrane	5 nucleotidase, Na-K ATPase
Nucleus	DNA, RNA polymerases
ER	Glucose-6 phosphatase
Golgi apparatus	Galactosyl transferase, manosidase
Lysosomes	Acid phosphatase
Mitochondria/Cytosol	Cytochrome oxidase, succinated dehydrogenase Lactate dehydrogenase Glucose-6 phosphate dehydrgenase

PROTEIN METABOLISM

Protein structure is studied at 4 levels:

1° structure

Linear sequence of amino acids linked by (C = O–NH) peptide bond.

Features of a peptide bond:

- It is a covalent bond with partial double-bond character.
- The adjacent atoms around the bond are in 'trans' configuration and are coplanar.
- No rotation (nonflexible) is possible around this bond, but is possible around other bonds of proteins.
- Peptide bonds make primary structure as the most stable one among all other types.

2° structures

α-helix

- Amino acid sequences form right- or left-handed helix.
- Stabilised by hydrogen bonds between carbonyl oxygen of 1st amino acid with peptidyl nitrogen atom of next 4th amino acid (intrachain H_2 bonds).

α-helix is destabilized by: Gly, Pro, Asp, Glu, Leu, Lys, Arg, Ser, Thr.

β-pleated sheet

- Two amino acid sequences lie adjacent to each other (parallel or antiparallel).
- Hydrogen bonds formed between the chains (interchain H_2 bonds) stabilize this structure.

Other 2° structures: β bends and turns.

- Bends and turns are rich in small amino acids like glycine and amino acids (proline).

2° structures are identified by:

- X-ray diffraction, optical rotatory dispersion
- Circular dichroism and NMR spectroscopy.

Tertiary structure

- This refers to three-dimensional arrangements of secondary structures of proteins.
- Stabilized by H_2 bonds, hydrophobic interactions, electrostatic interactions, ionic forces and van der Waals forces.
- Studied by X-ray crystallography.

Quaternary structure

- Refers to the association of several polypeptides or subunits.
- Forces stabilizing this structure: H_2 bonds, hydrophobic interactions (major forces), electrostatic interactions, disulfide bonds, ionic forces and van der Waals forces.

Protein denaturation

- Loss of protein structure sufficient enough to lead to loss of protein function.
- In this process, usually secondary, tertiary and quaternary structures of proteins are lost with the preservation of primary (peptide bond) structure.

Agents causing denaturation

Physical: Heat, UV light, high pressure, vigorous shaking.

Chemical: Acids, alkalies (extremes of pH), urea, detergents, etc.

Effects of denaturation

- Loss of biological function of proteins
- Reduction of solubility

- Increase in precipitability
- Increase in viscosity of the solution
- Increase in digestibility.

Reversible denaturation

- Certain proteins after denaturation will renaturate once the denaturating conditions are eliminated. Ex: Ribonuclease, Bence-Jones proteins.

Proteins which are elevated during inflammatory conditions are called Positive Acute Phase Reactants (Positive APR):

For example: C-reactive protein, α_1-acid glycoprotein, α_2-macroglobulin, ceruloplasmin

Proteins which are decreased during inflammatory conditions are called Negative Acute Phase Reactants (Negative APR):

For example: Albumin, Pre-albumin (Transthyretin), Transferrin

Electrophoresis:

- Electrophoresis is a process where charged molecules move under the influence of electrical field.
- Positively charged molecules (cations) move towards cathode and negatively charged molecules (anions) towards anode.
- Molecules are separated based on the difference in their rate of migration.

Rate of migration depends on:

- Size and shape of the molecules
- Charge on the molecule
- Electrical field strength
- Temperature
- Resistance offered by electrophoretic medium

Paper electrophoresis: (Filter paper or cellulose acetate paper is used)

- Used for Hb and lipoprotein separation and immunoelectrophoresis.

Agarose gel electrophoresis:

- For separation of big DNA molecules (based on size)
- For separation of plasma proteins (based on charge-mass ratio)

Sodium dodecyl sulfate-polyacrylamide gel electrophoresis (SDS-PAGE):

- SDS, an anionic detergent, imparts negative charges and removes all hydrophobic interactions present within the proteins. Hence, the proteins are separated only based on their molecular weight (size).

Applications

Separation of proteins and determination of molecular weight of proteins

Polyacrylamide gel electrophoresis (PAGE): It is used for:

- Separation of small DNA sequences
- Southern and northern blotting
- RFLP
- DNA fingerprinting
- DNA sequencing

Isoelectric Focusing (IEF):

- Electrophoresis is run on a gel with a pH gradient. pH gradient is generated using ampholytes.
- Molecules are separated based on their isoelectric point. It is also used to determine the pI of a protein.

Twodimensional (2D) electrophoresis

- Combines the resolving power of Isoelectric focusing (IEF) and SDS-PAGE.
- Initially proteins are separated based on their pI in IEF and then subjected to SDS-PAGE.

Chromatography

- Chromatography is a separation technique where mixtures of molecules are separated based on their differences in the distribution behavior between a mobile phase and a stationary phase.
- Components of a mixture may be interacting with the stationary phase based on charge, relative solubility, affinity or adsorption.

Based on stationary phase:

- Planar chromatography
- Column chromatography

Based on mobile phase:

- Gas based on stationary phase
- Liquid chromatography

Name	Stationary phase	Mobile phase	Principle
Paper chromatography	Water/Solvent coated onto the paper fibers	Organic solvents, water and additives	Partition between Stationary and mobile phase
Thin-layer chromatography	Silica, alumina gel pasted on glass	Solvent – Methanol, Acetic acid and Chloroform	Based on differential adsorption of solutes
Ion exchange chromatography	Cation/Anion exchange resins	Buffers with different pH gradient	Separation is based on charges
Gel filtration/ Size exclusion/ Molecular exclusion chromatography	Agarose, agar gel of different pore size	Buffers	Differential retention of solutes based on their size/ mass
Affinity chromatography	Specific ligands immobilized on cellulose/agarose/glass beads	Buffers	Molecules separated based on difference in affinity towards stationary phase

Glycine	Histidine	Glutamine	Phenylalanine/ Tyrosine
• Optically inactive • Simplest amino acid, helps in flexibility of proteins • Smallest amino acid • Lacks chirality • Synthesize creatine (with arginine and methionine) • Along with Succinyl CoA condenses to form heme	• Most stable at physiological pH • Acts as buffer at pH-7 • Protonate and deprotonate at neutral pH • Precursor of histamine	• Storage and transport form of ammonia • Major pathway for removal of NH_3 in brain • Precursor of purines and pyrimidines	• Phenylalanine is precursor of tyrosine • Tyrosine is a precursor of Catecholamines (Adr, NA, Dopamine), Thyroxine, Melanin
Cysteine	**Methionine**	**Tryptophan**	**Arginine**
• Sulfur containing amino acid • Two cysteines join to form cystine • Can be synthesized in body from methionine • Responsible for reducing action of glutathione • Taurine, a decarboxylated product of cysteine, is involved in bile acid conjugation	• Sulfur containing AAs • Methionine forms S-adenosyl methionine (SAM), a major methyl group donor in body • Precursor of homcysteine • associated with atherosclerotic vascular disease	• Precursor of niacin, melatonin, serotonin • 60 mg tryptophan yields 1 mg niacin	• Member of urea cycle • Precursor of nitric oxide

Specialized products from amino acids

Amino acid	Product
Glycine	Creatine, glutathione, heme, purines, conjugated bile acids
Tyrosine	Thyroxine, epinephrine, norepinephrine, dopamine, melanin
Tryptophan	NAD, NADP, serotonin, melatonin
Methionine	Creatine, epinephrine, polyamines
Cysteine	Glutathione, taurine, coenzyme-A, active sulfate
Histidine	Histamine
Arginine	Creatine, nitric oxide
Lysine	Carnitine
Glutamate	GABA, glutathione, gamma-carboxyglutamate
Glutamine	Purines, pyrimidines, amino sugars
Aspartate	Purines, pyrimidines,
Serine	Phosphatidyl serine, sphingomyelins, choline
β-alanine	Coenzyme-A

Classification of amino acids based on structure

ALIPHATIC	Monoamino monocarboxylic acids	**Simple AAs:** Glycine, Alanine **Branched chain AAs:** Valine, Leucine, Isoleucine **Hydroxyl AAs:** Serine, Threonine **Sulfurcontaining AAs:** Cysteine, Methionine **AAs with amide group:** Asparagine, Glutamine
	Monoamino dicarboxylic acids	Aspartic acid, Glutamic acid
	Dibasic monocarboxylic acids	Lysine, Arginine
AROMATIC	Phenylalanine, Tyrosine	
HETEROCYCLIC	Tryptophan, Histidine	
IMINO	Proline	
DERIVED AAs	Found in proteins	Hydroxyproline, hydroxylysine
	Nonprotein AAs	Ornithine, Citrulline, Homocysteine
	Nonalpha amino acids	GABA, Beta-alanine

Classification of Amino Acids on The Basis of Metabolism

Essential amino acids:

- Leucine
- Valine
- Lysine
- Isoleucine
- Threonine
- Phenylalanine
- Histidine (partially essential)
- Methionine
- Arginine (partially essential)
- Tryptophan

Ketogenic	Glucogenic	Both glucogenic and ketogenic
Leucine	Valine, Cysteine, Serine, Alanine, Histidine, Threonine, Arginine, Glycine, Glutamate, Proline/Hydroxyproline	Isoleucine, tyrosine Tryptophan, phenylalanine

Classification of amino acids on the basis of side chains

With aliphatic side chains	Glycine, alanine, valine, leucine, isoleucine
With side chains containing hydroxyl OH Groups	Serine, threonine, tyrosine
With side chains containing sulfur atoms	Cysteine, cystine, methionine
With side chains containing acidic groups or their amides	Aspartic acid, asparagine, glutamic acid, glutamine
With side chains containing basic groups	Arginine, lysine, histidine
With side chains containing aromatic rings	Histidine, phenylalanine, tyrosine, tryptophan

- Amino acids in living organisms are all a-amino acids (so called because the amino group is attached to the first carbon atom after the one in the–COOH group
- 300 AAs exist in nature, but only 20 are found in the structure of proteins → Standard amino acids
- While proteins contain only L-α-amino acids, microorganisms elaborate peptides that contain both D-and L-α-amino acids
- The alkyl group-R is what makes each of the twenty natural amino acids individual.

α amino acids	Non α amino acids
Ornithine, Citrulline, Arginosuccinic acids, T3, T4, S-Adenyl methionine, Homocysteine, Homoserine, 3, 4-Dihydroxyphenylalanine, Creatinine, Azaserine	B-Alanine, β-Aminoisobutyric acid, γ-Aminobutyric acid, δ-Aminolevulinic acid, Taurine

Classification of aminoacids based on side chain

Hydrophobic	Hydrophilic		
	Uncharged polar side chain	Acidic side chain (positive R chain)	Basic side chain (negative R chain)
Tryptophan Valine Methionine Leucine Isoleucine Alanine Phenylalanine Proline	Serine Asparagines Threonine Cysteine Tyrosine Tyrosine Glycine Glutamine	Aspartic acid Glutamic acid Tyrosine: mildly acidic	Histidine Arginine (most basic) Lysine

Catabolism of amino acids

- Amino acids that form Oxaloacetate: Asparagines (Aspartate)
- Amino acids that form Fumarate: Phenylalanine, Tyrosine
- Amino acids that form Succinyl CoA: Methionine, Isoleucine, Valine, Threonine
- Amino acids that form a-ketoglutarate: Glutamine, Proline, Arginine, Histidine
- Amino acids that form pyruvate: Alanine, Cystine, Serine, Threonine, Glycine
- Amino acids that form Acetyl CoA/Acetoacetyl CoA: Leucine, Tryptophan, Isoleucine, Phenylalanine, Lysine, Tyrosine.

Uses of amino acids

Amino acids	Uses
Glycine	Biosynthesis of Heme, Creatinine, Purines, and Glutathione, One-carbon metabolism. Conjugation of toxins and Bilirubin
	Neurotransmitter.
Tyrosine	T_3, T_4, Dopamine, Dopa, Norepinephrine, Epinephrine and Tyramine.
Methionine	Transmethylation reactions
Tryptophan	Nicotinic acid, Serotonin, Melatonin.
Histidine	Histamine, Buffering action in plasma.

Urea Cycle

- Urea is produced in liver and transported to kidneys for excretion
- First metabolic cycle to be elucidated–Hans Krebs and Kurt Henseleit (Krebs-Henseleit cycle)
- First two reactions in mitochondria and remaining enzymes in cytosol
- Synthesis of 1 mol of urea requires 3 mol of ATP plus 1 mol each of ammonium ion and of the a-amino nitrogen of aspartate
- Urea is the major end-product of nitrogen catabolism in humans
- Kidney and intestine contribute to most of body arginine because they possess all the urea enzymes except arginase
- Thus neither brain nor kidney can form urea in significant amount
- Glucose-Alanine cycle: Skeletal muscle transport NH_3 to liver in the form of alanine, resulting in reciprocal transfer of glucose to muscle. This cycle is called glucose-alanine cycle
- Condensation of CO_2 ammonia, and ATP to form carbamoyl phosphate is catalyzed by mitochondrial carbamoyl phosphate synthetase I (Rate-limiting enzyme of the urea cycle).
- Overall energetic:

  Ammonium + CO_2 + Aspartate + 3 ATP → Urea + Fumarate + 2ADP + 2Pi + AMP + PPi

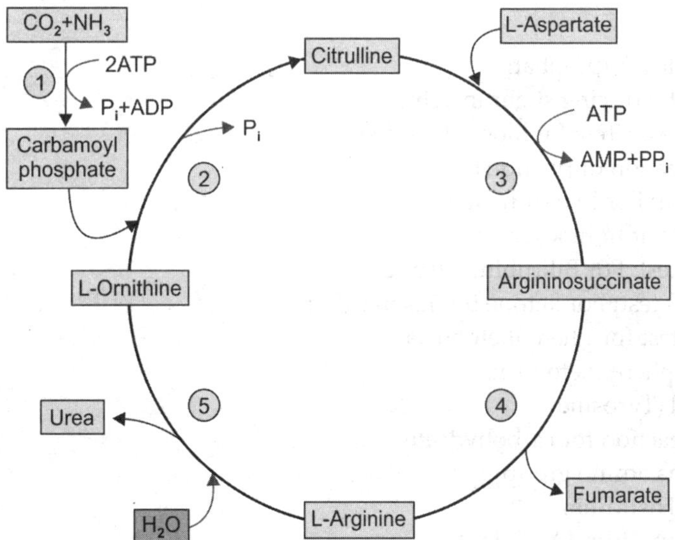

Key to enzymes (circled numbers)
1. Carbamoyl-phosphate synthase (ammonia)
2. Ornithine carbamoyltransferase
3. Argininosuccinate synthase
4. Argininosuccinate lyase
5. Arginase

Nitric oxide/endothelium-derived relaxing factor

Synthesis:

- NO is formed by the action of Cytosolic enzyme NO synthase in endothelial and neuronal cells
- Substrate: Arginine, O_2, NADPH
- Coenzyme: NADPH, FAD, FMN, Heme, Tetrahydrobiopterin
- Product: Citrulline, NO

Features:

- Reacts with oxygen and superoxide producing peroxynitrite which decomposes to from highly reactive free radical
- It stimulates guanyl cyclase (cGMP)

Functions:

- Relaxes smooth muscles
- Prevents platelet aggregation
- Functions as neurotransmitter in brain
- Mediates tumoricidal, bactericidal actions of macrophages
- Involved in penile erection; [sildenafil citrate (Viagra) affects this process by inhibiting a cGMP-dependent phosphodiesterase].

Subtype	Name	Comments	Result of Gene Knockout in Mice
1	nNOS	Activity depends on elevated Ca_2+ First identified in neurons Calmodulin-activated	Pyloric stenosis, resistance to vascular stroke Aggressive sexual behavior (males)
2	iNOS	Independent of elevated Ca_2+ prominent in macrophages	More susceptible to certain types of infection
3	eNOS	Activity depends on elevated Ca_2+ First identified in endothelial cells	Elevated mean blood pressure

Tests to be remembered

- Aldehyde test: For indole (Tryptophan)
- Benedict's test: To detect reducing sugar in urine
- Benzidine test (Adler's test): Test for blood, blood stains
- Biuret test: For determination of peptide bonds
- Bromosulfophthalein test: For liver function
- Cyanide-Nitroprusside: For homocystinuria
- Fouchet's test/Gmelin's test: For Bilirubin in urine
- Rothera's test/Gerhardt's test: For ketone bodies in urine
- Guthrie test: Screening test for Phenylketonuria
- Ferric chloride test: For phenylketonuria
- Millon's test: For phenol (Tyrosine)
- Molisch's test: A color reaction for carbohydrate
- Ninhydrin test: For alpha amino group
- Pauly's test: Imidazole (Histidine)
- Sakaguchi's test: For guanidium (Arginine)
- Schilling' test: Vitamin B_{12} deficiency
- Foulger's test/Seliwanoff's test: For fructose in urine
- Sulfur test: Sulfhydryl test (Cysteine and cystine)
- Xanthoproteic test: For benzene ring

Porphyrias:

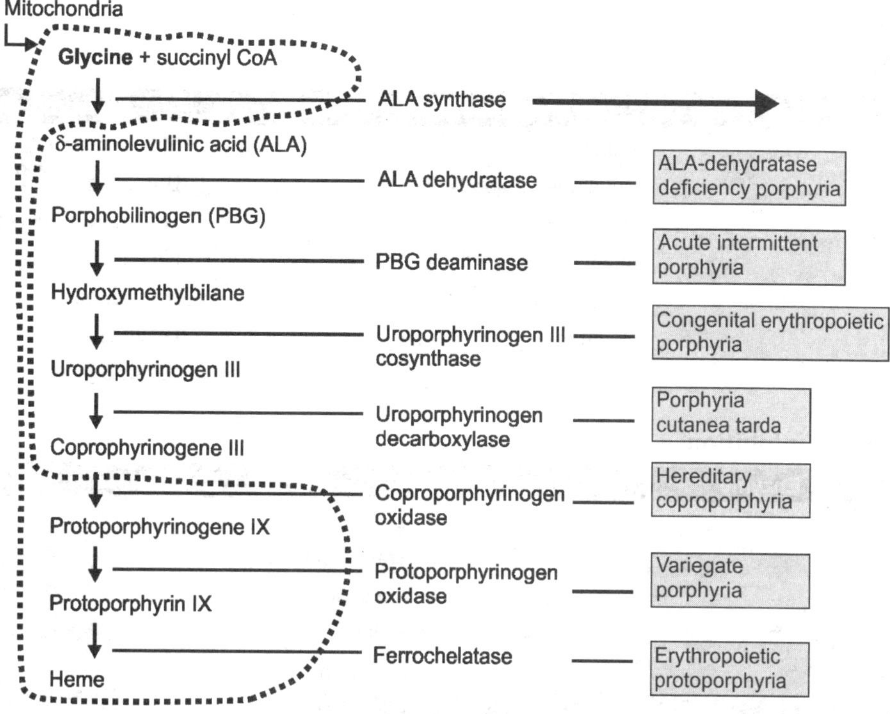

Fig. 3.1: Steps of heme synthesis and enzyme deficiencies in porphyrias

- Group of disorders due to abnormalities in the pathway of biosynthesis of heme, resulting in accumulation and increased excretion of porphyrins or its precursors
- Site of heme synthesis: Liver and bone marrow

Porphyria	Types	Deficient Enzymes	Photo Sensitivity	Features
Hepatic porhyria	Acute intermittent porphyria	Uroporphyrinogen I	–	Abdominal pain and neuropsychiatric symptoms
	Variegate porphyria	Protoporphyrinogen oxidase	+	
	Hereditary Copro porphyria	Coproporphyrinogen	+	
Erythropoietic porphyria	Erythropoietic protoporphyria	Ferrochelatase	+	Protoporphyrins accumulate in RBCs' bone marrow and plasma
	Congenital erythropoietic porphyria	Uroporphyrinogen III synthase	–	
Combined	Porphyria cutanea tarda	Uroporphyrinogen decarboxylase	+	Most common type

All porphyrias are AD disorders except congenital erythropoietic porphyria, which is AR

- Porphyrins and porphyrin derivatives exhibit a characteristic absorption spectrum in both the visible and the ultraviolet regions of the spectrum, e.g. absorption curve for a solution of porphyrin in 5% hydrochloric acid produces the sharp absorption band near 400 nm (Soret band).

ENZYMES

Enzyme Inhibition

	Competitive inhibition	Noncompetitive inhibition
Acting on	Active site	May or may not
Structure of inhibitor	Substrate analog	Unrelated
Inhibition is	Reversible	Generally irreversible
Excess substrate	Inhibition relieved	No effect
Km	Increased	No change
Vmax	No change	Decreased
Significance	Drug action	Toxicological

Examples of competitive inhibition

Enzyme	Competitive inhibitor
Lactate dehydrogenase	Oxamate
Aconitase	Trans-conitate
Succinate dehydrogenase	Malonate
HMG-CoA reductase	HMG
Dihydrofolate reductase	Amethopterin
Xanthine oxidase	Allopurinol
Folate reductase	Methotrexate, Trimethoprim, Pyrimethamine
Adenylosuccinate synthetase	6-Mercaptopurine
Thymidylate synthetase	5-fluorouracil
DNA polymerase	Cytosine arabinoside
Neuraminidase	Oseltamivir
Phosphoribosyl amidotransferase	Azaserine
Transpeptidase	Penicillin
Pteroyl synthetase	Sulfonamide
Monoamine oxidase (MAO)	MAO inhibitor like amphetamine
Acetylcholineesterase	Physostigmine
Thus, all competitive inhibitors are complex compounds and not simply metallic ions.	

Uncompetitive inhibition

In this type, inhibitor can bind only to enzyme-substrate complex (ES) and not to the isolated enzymes.

Vmax and Km: Both are decreased. Ex: Hydrazine-inhibiting aryl sulfatase.

REGULATION OF ENZYME ACTIVITY

- **Covalent modification:** A type of enzyme regulation where enzymatic activities are modulated by forming or breaking a covalent bond to the enzyme
  - *Reversible covalent modification:* Ex: phosphorylation and dephosphorylation of regulatory enzymes of carbohydrate and lipid metabolic pathways, tyrosine kinase activity of insulin receptor, etc
  - *Irreversible covalent modification:* Ex: proteolytic activation of protein-digesting enzymes, like pepsin, trypsin, chymotrypsin and rennin, etc.

- **Allosteric regulation**
  Allosteric enzymes:
  - Have an allosteric site and an active site
  - Mostly made up of multiple subunits
  - Exist in two states: T (inactive) and R (active) states
  - They exhibit co-operativity
  - Substrate saturation cure is sigmoidal in shape, explained by Hill's plot

Allosteric effects may be on Km or on Vmax

Alterations in Km or Vmax result from conformational changes at the catalytic site induced by binding of the allosteric effector at its site.

Two classes of allosteric-regulated enzymes:

K-series	V-series
• Kinetics are competitive in the sense that Km is raised without an effect on Vmax • The conformational change may weaken the bonds between substrate and substrate-binding residues	• The allosteric inhibitor lowers Vmax without affecting the Km • Primary effect of conformational change may be to alter the orientation or charge of catalytic residues, lowering Vmax

Allosteric Inhibition

- Mixed kind of inhibition where the inhibitor binds to enzyme at a site other than active (allosteric) site.
- Does not follow Michaelis-Menten hyperbolic kinetics. Instead it gives a sigmoid kinetics.

Examples of Allosteric Inhibiton

Enzyme	Allosteric Inhibitor	Allosteric Activator
1. Glutamate dehydrogenase	ATP, NADH	ADP
2. Hexokinase	ATP, G-6P	ADP
3. Pyruvate carboxylase	ADP	Acetyl CoA
4. Protein kinase	–	cAMP

- Feedback inhibition: Inhibition of an enzyme by an end-product of that pathway.

  Enz 1 Enz 2 Enz 3

  $A \rightarrow B \rightarrow C \rightarrow D$
- High concentrations of D inhibit the conversion of A to B.
- Generally, D binds at an allosteric site spatially distinct from the catalytic site of the target enzyme.
- Feedback inhibitors thus typically bear little or no structural similarity to the substrates of the enzymes they inhibit.
- In this example, the feedback inhibitor D acts as a negative allosteric effector of Enz 1:
  - **Activation of latent enzymes**
  - **Compartmentation of metabolic pathways**
  - **Control of enzyme synthesis**
  - **Enzyme degradation**
  - **Suicidal inhibition:**
    - A special class of irreversible inhibitors is the suicide inactivator.
    - A suicide inactivator undergoes the first few chemical steps of the normal enzymatic reaction, but instead of being transformed into the normal product, the inactivator is converted to a very reactive compound that combines irreversibly with the enzyme.
    - These compounds are also called mechanism-based inactivators, because they hijack the normal enzyme reaction mechanism to inactivate the enzyme.

- Suicide inactivator plays a significant role in rational drug design, a modern approach to obtaining new pharmaceutical agents in which chemists synthesize novel substrates based on knowledge of substrates and reaction mechanisms.

Isoenzymes

- Isoenzymes are the physically distinct forms of the same enzyme that catalyze the same reaction, and differ from each other structurally, electrophoretically and immunologically.
- They differ in their physical properties because of genetically determined difference in amino acid sequence.
- They are separated by electrophoresis as they have different electrophoretic mobility:
  They have different Km value LDH isoenzyme: Isoenzyme LDH-1 with four 'H' subunit predominates in cardiac tissue, since heart expresses the H subunit almost exclusively.

LDH Isoenzymes			
Type	Polypeptide chains	Electrophoretic mobility	Tissue rich in isoenzyme type
LDH-1	(H4) H H H H	Fast moving	Heart
LDH-2	(H3M) H H H M		
LDH-3	(H2M2) H H M M		
LDH-4	(HM3) H M M M		
LDH-5	(M4) M M M M	Slowest moving	Liver

Isoenzyme of lactate dehydrogenase (LDH)

- Lactate dehydrogenase is a tetrameric enzyme and consists of four subunits
- These subunits can occur in two isoforms: H-isoform (for heart)/M-isoform (for muscle)
- All these isozymes, though different physically, catalyze the same reaction of oxidation of LA to PA.
- In normal serum, LDH2 (H3M) is the most prominent isoenzyme. **Creatinine phosphokinase exists as three isoenzymes in a human tissue:**
  - CPK-1 or CPK-BB: Found in brain
  - CPK-2 or CPK-MB: Found in myocardium
  - CPK-3 or CPK-MM: Found in skeletal muscle

  Creatinine phosphokinase-1 is essentially found in brain and increased in brain ischemia.

Creatine Phosphokinase (CPK)-2-CPKM

Normally

- CPK-2 occurs in very small quantity accounting for as less as 2% of total CK activity of plasma.
- CKMB also exists in 2 forms: CK-MB1: Extracardiac form/CK-MB2: cardiac form.

Myocardial infarction

- Elevation of CK-MB isoenzyme occurs within 4 hours, maximum in 24 hrs, then falls rapidly.
- A ratio of CKMB1: CKMB2 above 1.5 is highly sensitive for the diagnosis of acute MI after 4–6 hours of onset of myocardial ischemia.

CARBOHYDRATE METABOLISM

Introduction

Carbohydrates are defined as polyhydroxy aldehydes or polyhydroxy ketones and other compounds which yield these aldehydes or ketones on their hydrolysis.

Trehalose is a disaccharide having two glucose residues linked by α-1–1 glycosidic linkage. Other physiologically important disaccharides:

Disaccharides	Sugars	Linkage
1 Lactose	Gal-Glu	β,1–4
2 Sucrose	Glu-Fru	α,1–2
3 Maltose	Glu-Glu	α,1–4
4 Isomaltose	Glu-Glu	α,1–6

Inulin is a homopolymer of D-fructose, present in tubers of Dahlia plants. It acts as a storage polysaccharide in these plants. Used to assess the glomerular filtration rate.

Proteoglycans

These are proteins with covalently attached glycosaminoglycans (GAG). Upto 95% of molecule is made of GAG and the protein portion is less.

For example: Syndecan, aggrecan, versican, biglycan, decorin, betaglycan, serglycan and fibromodullin.

Proteoglycans are rich in extracellular matrix. Since they are rich in anionic charges, they retain water and contribute to strength and turgor.

The GAG are attached to the proteins through two types of linkages:

- O-Glycosidic linkage: GAG form glycosidic bond with OH group of Ser or Thr residues
- N-Glycosidic linkage: GAG attached to amide N atom of asparagine.

GAG

They are linear and unbranched heteropolysaccharides.

Basically have repeating units of an amino sugar and an uronic acid.

GAG	Amino sugar	Acidic sugar
Hyaluronic acid	N acetyl glucosamine	Glucuronic acid
Chondroitin SO_4	N acetyl galactosamine	Glucuronic acid
Keratan SO_4	N acetyl glucosamine	Galactose
Dermatan SO_4	N acetyl galactosamine	Iduronic acid
Heparan SO_4	Glucosamine	Glucuronic acid
Heparin	Glucosamine	Iduronic acid

Exceptions

- GAG without uronic acid: Keratan SO_4
- GAG without SO_4: Hyaluronic acid
- Galactose containing GAG: Keratan SO_4
- GAG which is not attached covalently to proteins: Hyaluronic acid
- GAG with nonacetylated amino sugar: Heparan SO_4, Heparin

ISOMERS: Molecules having same molecular formula but different structure or spatial orientation of groups and different physical properties.

Classification of isomers

1. Structural isomers: Differ in structural organization
2. Stereoisomers: Differ in spatial orientation of groups.

- **Functional isomers:** Differ in functional groups—Aldoses and Ketoses
  For example: Glucose (CHO group) and fructose (C=O group)
- **Anomers:** Differ in spatial orientation of groups around the anomeric carbon atom.
  For example: α and β glucose.

- **Epimers:** Differ in spatial orientation of groups (OH and H) around a single asymmetric carbon atom other than anomeric C-atom
  For example: Glucose and mannose are epimers with respect to C_2
  Glucose and galactose are epimers with respect to C_4
- **Optical isomers:** Differ in rotating the plane polarized light.
  For example:
  - **d (+): Dextrorotatory: Rotates the plane polarized light to right.**
  - **l (–): Levorotatory: Rotates the light towards left.**
- **Enantiomers (D/L forms):** They differ in spatial orientation of OH group at the last asymmetric (penultimate C-atom of glucose) C-atom.
  For example:
  - D-Glucose: OH of C5 is at right side
  - L-Glucose: OH of C5 is at left side
- **Diastereomers:** They differ in spatial orientation of OH groups around the asymmetric carbon atoms but not forming mirror images.
  For example: Galactose and Mannose are diastereomers.

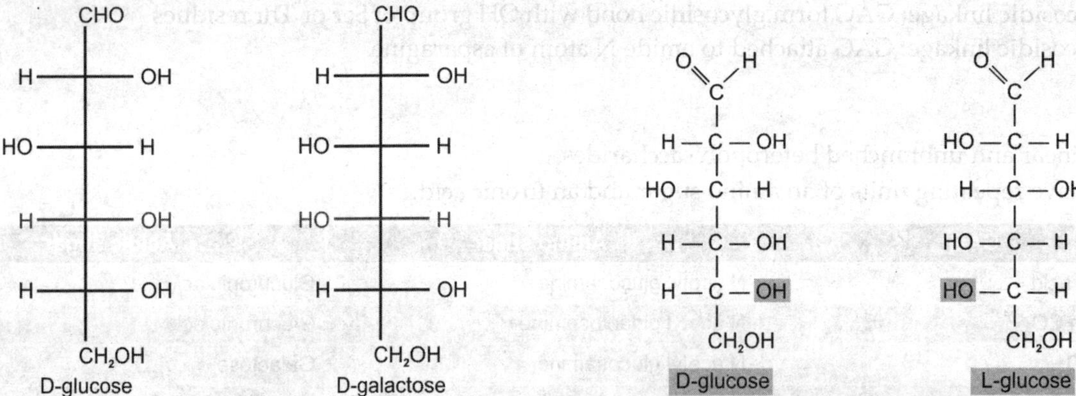

Fig. 3.2: Epimers **Fig. 3.3:** Enantiomers

van 't Hoff Rule

The total no. of possible isomers by any molecule = 2^n
Where n is the no. of asymmetric C-atoms.
∴ For glucose = $2^5 = 32$
So, glucose can form 32 isomers.

Monosaccharide	Reduction product
Glucose	Sorbitol
Galactose	Dulcitol/Galactitol
Fructose	Sorbitol and mannitol
Ribose	Ribitol

Glycerol is a derived lipid and not a carbohydrate.
- Molisch test: To detect the presence of carbohydrates
- Benedict's test: To detect reducing property of sugars
- Fehling's test: To detect reducing property of sugars
- Barfoed's test: To differentiate reducing monosaccharides from disaccharides
- Foulger's test and Seliwanof's test: To detect the ketosugars, e.g. fructose
- Iodine test: To detect the polysaccharides.

Osazones are crystals obtained during condensation of phenyl hydrazine with reducing sugars. The shapes of the crystals are characteristic of the sugar.

Sugars	Shape of osazones
• Glucose, fructose, mannose	Needle-shaped or hay-stack
• Lactose	Cotton ball shape
• Maltose	Sunflower shape

During osazone formation, phenyl hydrazine condenses with 1st and 2nd carbon atoms of the sugars.

Glycolysis

(Embeden Meyerhoff Pathway)

A process where a glucose molecule is split into two molecules of pyruvate (aerobic) or lactate (anerobic glycolysis).

Rate-limiting steps: (Irreversible steps also)

- Hexokinase or glucokinase
- Phosphofructokinase
- Pyruvate kinase.

Committed step:

- Phosphofructokinase.

Substrate level phosphorylation steps of glycolysis:

- Phosphoglycerate kinase and pyruvate kinase.

Energetics

	ATP consumed	ATP generated	Net ATP production
Aerobic	2	9	7
Anerobic	2	4	2

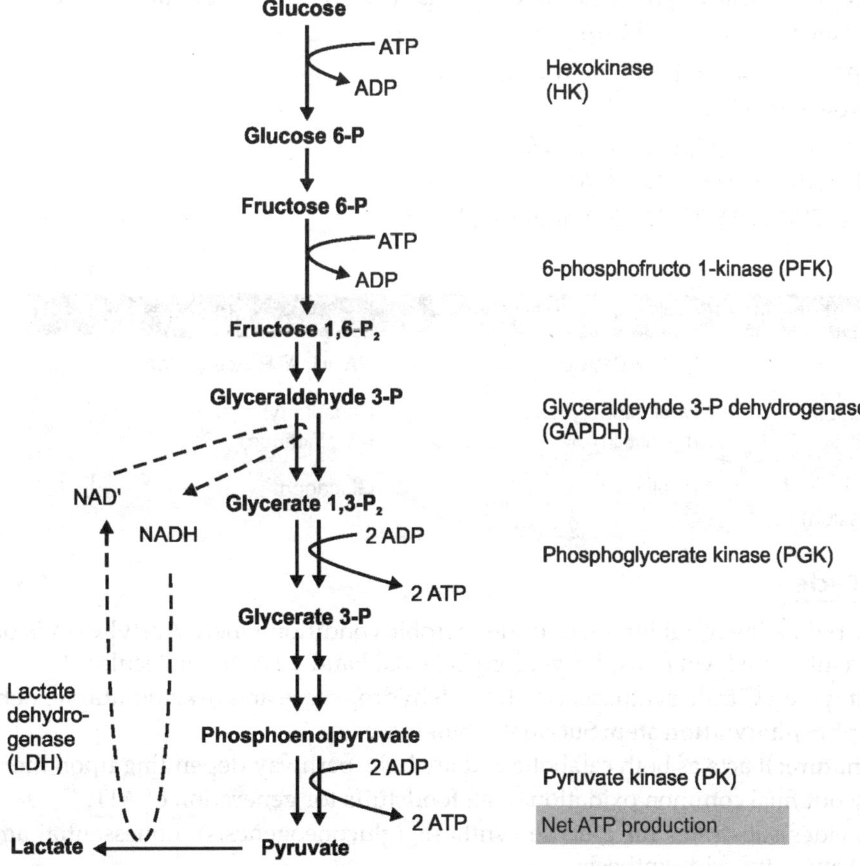

Fig. 3.4: Glycolytic pathway

Glucose to glucose-6-phosphate is converted by either glucokinase or hexokinase.

Glucokinase	Hexokinase
• Site: liver and β-cells of pancreas	All other peripheral tissues
• km: 10.0 mmol/l	0.5 mmol/l
• Affinity for glucose: low	High
• Function: Glucose storage and insulin stimulation	Usage by peripheral tissues
• Induced by insulin	Not inducible
• No product inhibition	Inhibited by Glu-6-P

Anerobic glycolysis

- In tissues where mitochondriae are absent (e.g. RBC) or whenever oxygen supply is less (hypoxic conditions), Substrate Level Phosphorylation of Anaerobic Glycolysis is the prime source of energy.
- 2, 3 bisphosphoglycerate and Phosphoenol pyruvate are the substrates which donate high energy phosphates by substrate level phosphorylation.
- **The main purpose of Anerobic Glycolysis is to regenerate NAD from NADH,** so that NAD can be reused for glyceraldehydes-3-phosphate dehydrogenase step for continuous Glycolysis to occur. When PO_2 is sufficient, the NADH will be taken up by electron transport chain to regenerate NAD.

Pasteur Effect: Inhibition of Glycolysis by excessive oxygen.

Crabtree Effect: With the constant supply of O_2, if the glucose concentration is increased, it will create a comparative anerobiasis.

Chemiosmotic Effect: Explains the oxidative phosphorylation.

Fate of Pyruvate Dehydrogenase: Pyruvate Dehydrogenase (PDH) is present in mitochondria where it oxidatively decarboxylates Pyruvate to form Acetyl CoA.

It is a multisubunit protein having 3 enzymatic activities:

- Pyruvate dehydrogenase (TPP)
- Dihydrolipoyl transacylase (Lipoic acid and CoA)
- Dihydrolipoyl dehydrogenase (FAD, NAD)

It requires 5 cofactors: TPP, FAD, NAD, CoA and lipoid acid.

Regulation of PDH:

Mode of regulation	Activator	Inhibitor
Allosteric	NAD, ADP, CoA, Ca^{++}	NADH, ATP, Acetyl CoA
Covalent modification	Dephosphorylation (by insulin)	Phosphorylation (by glucagon)
Hormonal (Induction/Repression)	Insulin	Glucagon

TCA or Citric Acid Cycle

- It is a mitochondrial pathway, taking place under aerobic condition where Acetyl CoA is oxidized to CO_2 and generates 1 ATP (substrate level phosphorylation), 3 NADH and 2 FADH molecules.
- **Rate-limiting enzymes:** Citrate synthase, isocitrate dehydrogenase and α-ketoglutarate dehydrogenase.
- **Substrate level phosphorylation step:** Succinate thiokinase
- **Amphibolic in nature:** It acts as both catabolic and anabolic pathway depending upon the need of the system.
- **Catabolic:** Carry out final common oxidation of all foodstuffs for generation of ATP.
- **Anabolic:** It provides substrates for glucose synthesis (gluconeogenesis), nonessential amino acid synthesis (transamination) and fatty acid synthesis.

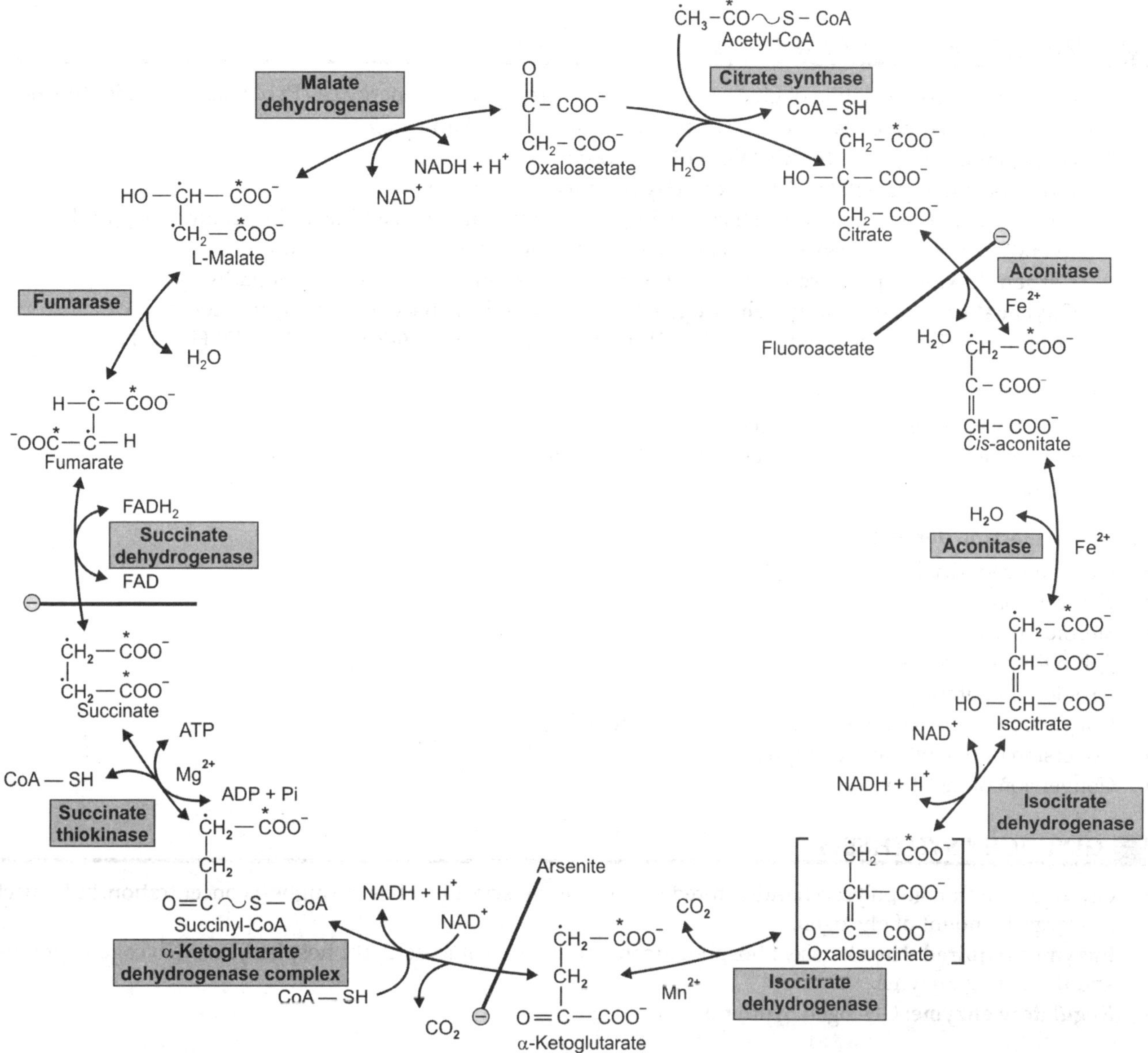

Fig. 3.5: Citric acid cycle/TCA cycle/Krebs cycle

Energetics of TCA cycle when Acetyl CoA is oxidized to CO_2.

Steps	Mode of energy liberated	No. of ATP generated
Isocitrate dehydrogenase	1 NADH	2.5 ATP
α-ketoglutarate dehydrogenase	1 NADH	2.5 ATP
Succinate thiokinase	1 ATP	1 ATP
Succinate dehydrogenase	1 FADH2	1.5 ATP
Malate dehydrogenase	1 NADH	2.5 ATP
		10 ATP
Pyruvate dehydrogenase	1 NADH	2.5 ATP

Total per mole of glucose under aerobic conditions: $(10 \times 2) + (2.5 \times 2) + 7$ 32 ATP

Total per mole of glucose under anerobic conditions: 2 ATP

HMP PATHWAY/PENTOSE PHOSPHATE PATHWAY

Alternative pathway for oxidation of glucose not meant for production of energy (ATP) but has two major functions:

- **Provides NADPH which is required for synthesis of fatty acid and steroids**
- **Provides pentose required for nucleic acid synthesis**
  - It occurs in the cytosol. **No ATP is directly produced or consumed**
  - It is **important in liver, adipose tissue, RBC, testes, adrenal cortex and lactating mammary gland**
  - In HMP shunt, two transketolation and one transaldolation reactions are involved
  - **Carbon dioxide is produced in this pathway, which is never produced in EM pathway**
  - **Oxygenation is achieved by dehydrogenation but NADP+ is used as hydrogen acceptor**
  - Overall reaction: 6 Glucose-6-P + 12 NADP + 7 H2O → 5 Glucose-6-P + Pi + 12 NADPH + 12 H+

Sources of NADPH

- HMP pathway: Main source of NADPH
- Malic enzyme/Malate Dehydrogenase: Pyruvate to Malate
- Isocitrate Dehydrogenase: Extramitochondrial

Used as an electron donor in:

- Extramitochondrial fatty acid synthesis
- Cholesterol synthesis
- Steroid synthesis
- Sphingolipid synthesis
- Uronic acid pathway
- Conversion of oxidized glutathione to reduced glutathione
- Coversion of phenylalanine to tyrosine
- Conversion of met-Hb to Hb

GLYCOGEN SYNTHESIS

- Glycogen is a storage polysaccharide, stored in liver and muscle. Liver has the highest concentration, but muscle has largest amount of glycogen.
- **Enzymes required:** Hexokinase, Phosphoglucomutase, UDP-Glucose Pyrophosphorylase, Glycogen Synthase and Branching Enzyme.
- **Regulatory enzyme:** Glycogen Synthase.

GLYCOGENOLYSIS

- Process of generating glucose from glycogen.
- **Enzymes involved:** Glycogen phosphorylase, Debranching enzyme (Glucan transferase, α, 1-6 glucosidase), Phosphoglucomutase and Glu-6-Phosphatase.
- **Regulatory enzyme:** Glycogen phosphorylase.

Liver glycogen content is the net result of rates of glycogen synthesis and glycogenolysis.

	Activators	Inhibitors
Glycogen synthase Glycogen phosphorylase	Insulin Glu-6-P Glucagon, epinephrine Ca^{++} (in muscle)	Glucagon, Epinephrine (c-AMP),Glycogen Insulin

- Insulin levels are controlled by serum glucose and dietary amino acids.
- Liver glycogen phosphorylase doesn't require pyridoxine, whereas muscle phosphorylase is pyridoxine-dependent.

GLUCONEOGENESIS

Formation of glucose or glycogen from noncarbohydrate sources

Substrates

- Glucogenic amino acids:
  - That forms pyruvate: serine, cysteine, glycine, threonine, tryptophan, alanine, hydroxyproline
  - That produces intermediate of TCA cycle:
    - Oxaloacetic acid and α-ketoglutarate
    - Lactate
    - Pyruvate
    - Glycerol: obtained from lipolysis of fat
    - Propionic acid (important in ruminants)
  - **Main pathway of gluconeogenesis is a reversal of glycolytic pathway** but thermodynamic 'barriers' prevent a simple reversal of glycolysis.
  - There are four such energy barriers which are irreversible:
    - Between pyruvate and phosphoenol pyruvate
    - Between fructose-1,6 bi PO_4 and fructose-6-P
    - Between glucose 6-P and glucose.

Phosphofructokinase (PFK)

- PFK-1: It takes part in glycolysis
- PFK-2: It is a bifunctional enzyme as it has fructose-2–6 phosphatase activity. It plays a unique role in regulation of both Glycolysis and Gluconeogenesis

  The overall summary of gluconeogenesis for the conversion of pyruvate to glucose is:

  2Pyruvate + 4ATP + 2GTP + 2NADH + 2H+ $+6H_2O \rightarrow$ Glucose + 2NAD+ +4ADP + 2GDP + 6Pi + 6H–

ATP formation in the catabolism of glucose (malate shuttle)			
Pathway	Reaction catalyzed by	Method of ATP formation	ATP per Mol of glucose
Glycolysis	Glyceraldehydes 3-phosphate dehydrogenase	Respiratory chain oxidation of 2 NADH	5
	Phosphoglycerate kinase	Substrate level phosphorylation	2
	Pyruvate kinase	Substrate level phosphorylation	2
			10
	Consumption of ATP for reactions of hexokinase and phosphorylation		–2
			Net 7
Citric acid cycle	Pyruvate dehydrogenase	Respiratory chain oxidation of 2 NADH	5
	Isocitrate dehydrogenase	Respiratory chain oxidation of 2 NADH	5
	α-Ketoglutarate dehydrogenase	Respiratory chain oxidation of 2 NADH	5
	Succinate thiokinase	Substrate level phosphorylation	2
	Succinate dehydrogenase	Respiratory chain oxidation of 2 FADH2	3
	Malate dehydrogenase	Respiratory chain oxidation of 2 NADH	5
			Net 25
	Total per mol of glucose under aerobic conditions		32
	Total per mol of glucose under aerobic conditions		2

- One mole of NADH yields 2.5 ATP whereas one mole of FADH yields 1.5 ATPs

  If the glycerophosphate shuttle is used, then only 1.5 ATP will be formed per mol of NADH.

Major fuel sources used in exercise:

Sprinter (100 m)	Marathon runner
Type II (glycolytic) fibers are used predominantly	Type I (oxidative) fibers are used predominantly
Creatine phosphate is the major energy source during the first 4-5 secs	ATP is the major source of energy throughout
Glucose from anerobic glycolysis of muscle glycogen	Blood glucose and free fatty acids are major fuel sources
Muscle glycogen is rapidly depleted	Muscle glycogen is slowly depleted

Duration of exercise	Energy supply
4 mins	Glucose in the blood
18 mins	Glycogen in the liver
70 mins	Glycogen in the muscle
4000 mins	Triacylglycerol in adipose tissue

LIPID METABOLISM

Classification of lipids:

- **Simple lipids**
  They are esters of fatty acids with alcohol (glycerol or other higher alcohols).
  They are subclassified as:
  - Triacylglycerol or triglycerides or neutral fats
  - Waxes
- **Compound lipids**
  They are esters of fatty acids with alcohols with additional compounds.
  Depending on these extra groups, they are subclassified as:
  - *Phospholipids* (containing phosphoric acid):
    With glycerol as alcohol (glycerophospholipids):
    - Phosphatidic acid (parent glycerophospholipid)
    - Phosphatidylcholine (lecithin)
    - Phosphatidylethanol amine (cephalin)
    - Phosphatidylserine
    - Phosphatidylinositol
    - Phosphatidylglycerol
    - Diphosphatidyl glycerol (cardiolipin)
    - Plasmalogens (Platelet-activating factor)

    With sphingosine as alcohol (sphingolipids):
    - Sphingomyelin
  - *Glycolipids:*
    - Cerebrosides (ceramide with monosaccharides)
    - Globosides (ceramide with oligosaccharides)
    - Gangliosides (ceramide + oligosaccharides + N-acetyl neuraminic acid)
  - *Others:*
    - Sulfolipids or sulfatides
- **Derived lipids**
  They are lipids derived on hydrolysis of simple, compound lipids or precursors of lipids.
  For example: Fatty acids, glycerol, cholesterol, steroids, prostaglandins, leukotrienes, fat-soluble vitamins and steroid hormones.

Omega Numbering System:

Omega (ω) numbering system: Starts from terminal methyl c-atom.

For example:

$^{\omega}{}_{n}CH_3–CH_2–CH_2–CH_2–CH_2$---------------$^{\gamma}{}_{4}CH_2–^{\beta}{}_{3}CH2–^{\alpha}{}_{2}CH_2–{}_{1}COOH$

Delta (Δ) numbering of a fatty acid: Starts from carboxyl end carbon atom as 1,2,3,------n. Carbon atom next to carboxyl group is called α-carbon atom. The next carbons are named as β, γ, δ, ε, etc. and the last carbon is called ω-carbon atom.

ω^3 Fatty Acids

- α-Linolenic acid
- Eicosapentaenoic acid (EPA)
- Docosahexaenoic acid (DHA)

ω^6 Fatty Acids

- Linoleic acid
- Eicosatetraenoic (arachidonic) acid
- γ-Linolenic acid

ω^9 Fatty Acids

- Oleic acid
- Eicosatrienoic acid

Essential Fatty Acids

- Cannot be synthesized by human bodies and must be provided in diet.
- The most important EFA → Linoleic acid (because it serves as a basis for the production of other EFAs).
- Docosahexanoic acid (DHA; ω3, 22:6), which is synthesized from α-linolenic acid or obtained directly from fish oils, is present in high concentrations in retina, cerebral cortex, testis and sperm.
- DHA is particularly needed for development of brain and retina and is supplied via the placenta and milk.
- Milk is the constant and continuous source of DHA as placenta is not present all the time.
- Patients with retinitis pigmentosa are reported to have low levels of DHA.

Essential fatty acid deficiency: Seen in:

- Infants receiving formula diets
- Patients maintained for long periods exclusively by IV nutrition
- Retinitis pigmentosa

Saponification number

- Index of molecular weight (chain length) of fatty acids
- Inversely proportional to mol. wt. of fatty acids

Iodine number

- Index of degree of unsaturation (number of double bonds) of fatty acids
- Directly proportional to the number of double bonds.

Ceramide

- It is a common content of all glycolipids (which contains sphingosine and a fatty acid) to which carbohydrate moieties will be attached.
- Ceramide is present in all the glycolipids, namely cerebrosides, globosides and gangliosides.

  For example:

  Glucosylcerebroside : Ceramide + Glucose
  Galactosylcerebroside : Ceramide + Galactose
  Ganglioside : GM_1 ganglioside

Ceramide–Glu–Gal–NANA
I
GalNAC–Gal

GM_2 Ganglioside
Ceramide–Glu–Gal–NANA
I
GalNAC

GM_3 Ganglioside
Cer–Glu–Gal–NANA

Lipoproteins

- Lipoproteins are compound lipids meant for transport of lipids in plasma. They are spherical particles made up of outer surface layer and inner core.
- The inner core contains: Cholesterol esters, TGL and fatty acids.

Outer surface layer contains: Amphipathic lipids (Phospholipids, Cholesterol) and apoproteins.

Four major groups of lipoproteins:

- Chylomicrons, derived from intestinal absorption of triacylglycerol and other lipids;
- Very low-density lipoproteins (VLDL, or pre-β-lipoproteins), derived from the liver for the export of triacylglycerol;
- Low-density lipoproteins (LDL, or β-lipoprioteins), representing a final stage in the catabolism of VLDL;
- High-density lipoproteins (HDL, or–α lipoproteins), involved in cholesterol transport and also in VLDL and chylomicron metabolism.

	Triacylglycerol	Protein	Phospholipids	Cholesterol and esters
Chylomicrons	90%	2%	3%	5%
VLDL	60%	5%	15%	20%
LDL	8%	20%	22%	50%
HDL	5%	40%	30%	25%

Diameter and lipid content

- Chylomicrons have the highest diameter and the highest lipid content
- HDL has the lowest diameter and has the least lipid content.

Density and protein content

- HDL has the highest density and has maximum protein content
- Chylomicrons have the least density.

Note:

- Triacylglycerol is the predominant lipid in chylomicrons and VLDL
- Cholesterol and phospholipids are the predominant lipids in LDL and HDL, respectively
- Lipoproteins are separated based on their electrophoretic properties into α, β and pre-β
- Endogenous (from liver): maximum VLDL
- Exogenous (from diet): maximum content in chylomicrons.

Apoproteins of various lipoprotein particles are:

Chylomicrons	: Apo B48, Apo A, Apo E, Apo C
VLDL	: Apo B 100, Apo E, Apo C
IDL	: Apo B 100, Apo E
LDL	: Apo B 100
HDL	: Apo A, Apo E, Apo C, Apo D

Apo B-48 and B-100 are two different proteins obtained from the same gene.

In the intestine, RNA editing system incorporates a stop codon once 48% of total Apo B m-RNA is translated and hence the protein synthesis will be stopped. This system is absent in liver and hence whole Apo B-100 is produced.

Lipoprotein(a)

- Lp(a) is an LDL particle attached with a special apoprotein called Apoprotein(a) through a disulfide linkage.
- Lp(a) has similar homology with plasminogen. Hence, it interferes with the action of plasminogen activators, thereby leading to the reduction of plasmin formation and hence reduced fibrinolysis. So, patients with high Lp(a) concentrations are more prone to develop thrombosis and its complications.

HDL

- Synthesized and secreted from both liver and intestine
- Synthesized in liver and are released into blood by exocytosis
- Remove free cholesterol from extrahepatic tissue and esterify it
- Esterified cholesterol is carried to liver where HDL is degraded and cholesterol is removed
- Protective in coronary disease (scavenging action)
- It has the highest electrophoretic mobility
- Apoproteins associated with HDL are Apo A, Apo C II, and Apo E
- Apo C and Apo E are synthesized in the liver and transferred from liver HDL to intestinal HDL
- The class B scavenger receptor B1 (SR-B1) → HDL receptor with a dual role in HDL metabolism
  - In the liver and in steroidogenic tissues, it binds HDL via Apo A-I
  - In the tissues, SR-B1 binds with cholesterol effluxed from the cells by HDL → transport it to the liver → excreted (reverse cholesterol transport).
  - Reverse cholesterol transport also involves the ATP-binding cassette transporters A1 (ABCA1) and G1 (ABCG1).
  - Pre β-HDL is the most potent form of HDL inducing cholesterol efflux from the tissues.

Chylomicrons

- Are assembled in intestinal mucosal cells and carry exogenous dietary TGs to peripheral tissues
- Clearance of chylomicrons from the blood is rapid
- Larger particles are catabolized more quickly than smaller ones
- Fatty acids originating from chylomicron triacylglycerol are delivered mainly to adipose tissue, heart, and muscle (80%), while about 20% goes to the liver
- The liver does not metabolize native chylomicrons or VLDL significantly
- Chylomicron remnants: taken up by the liver by receptor-mediated endocytosis
- Uptake is mediated by apo E, via the LDL (apo B-100, E) receptor and the LRP (LDL receptor-related protein).

VLDL

- Are produced in the liver
- Are composed predominantly of TG (also cholesterol ester and cholesterol)
- Carry endogenous TG from liver to peripheral tissue

LDL

- Contain high concentration of cholesterol and cholesterol esters (bad cholesterol)
- Provide cholesterol to the peripheral tissue
- LDL is a causative for coronary disease

Lecithin–cholesterol acyltransferase (LCAT)

- Plasma LCAT is responsible for virtually all plasma cholesteryl esters in humans.
- Its activity is associated with HDL containing apo A-I
- As cholesterol in HDL becomes esterified, it creates a concentration gradient and draws in cholesterol from tissues and from other lipoproteins, thus enabling HDL to function in reverse cholesterol transport.

Cholesteryl Ester Transfer Protein

- This protein, associated with HDL, is found in plasma of humans and many other species.
- It facilitates transfer of cholesteryl ester from HDL to VLDL, IDL, and LDL in exchange for triacylglycerol, relieving product inhibition of LCAT activity in HDL.

Lipoprotein lipase

- Located on the walls of blood capillaries, anchored to the endothelium by negatively charged proteoglycan chains of heparin sulfate.
- Found in heart, adipose tissue, spleen, lung, renal medulla, aorta, diaphragm, and lactating mammary gland, although it is not active in adult liver.
- It is not normally found in blood; however, following injection of heparin, lipoprotein lipase is released from its heparin sulfate-binding sites into the circulation.
- Both phospholipids and apo C-II are required as cofactors for lipoprotein lipase activity, while apo a-II and apo C-III act as inhibitors
- Triacylglycerol undergoes hydrolysis by a hormone-sensitive lipase to form free fatty acids and glycerol.

Hepatic lipase is bound to the sinusoidal surface of liver cells and is also released by heparin. This enzyme does not react readily with chylomicrons or VLDL but is involved in chylomicron remnant and HDL metabolism.

- There is an association between patients possessing the apo E4 allele and the incidence of Alzheimer's disease
- Apo E4 binds more avidly to β-amyloid found in neuritic plaques.

Type	Primary disease	Basic defect	Serum cholesterol	Serum TGs	Elevated lipoprotein
I	Familial lipoprotein lipase deficiency	Lipoprotein lipase deficiency	N	↑	↑↑Chylomicrons
II	Familial hyper Cholesterolemia (FHC)	Deficiency of LDL receptors	↑	N	↑LDL
III	Familial dys beta lipoproteinemia	Abnormal apo-E	↑	↑	↑VLDL remnant and chylomicron remnant
IV	Familial hyper triglyceridemia	Unknown	↑	↑	↑V LDL
V	Familial combined hyperlipidemia	Deficiency of Apo-C	N	↑	Chylomicrons and VLDL

- **Triglycerides are normal only in type II**
- **Cholesterol is increased only in type II and type III**
- **Both cholesterol and triglycerides are increased in type III**

Fatty Acid Synthesis

- It is a cytoplasmic process.
- Acetyl CoA is the substrate (building block).

Vitamins required for fatty acid biosynthesis are:

- Niacin ____________ in NADPH form
- Biotin ____________ cofactor for Acetyl coA carboxylase
- Pantothenate _______ used in the CoA form

Regulation of fatty acid biosynthesis

Key Enzyme: Acetyl coA Carboxylase (converts acetyl CoA to malonyl coA).

- Allosterically stimulated by citrate which signals high energy state
- Activated by dephosphorylation through insulin
- Induced by insulin

Regulation by Nutritional Status

- Increased in:
  - Well-fed state
  - High-carbohydrate diet
- Decreased in:
  - Fasting
  - Starvation
  - Low-carbohydrate diet
  - High-fat diet
  - Insulin-deficient status

Steps:

- 1st step–Transfer acetyl CoA from mitochondria to cytosol (citrate shuttle)
- Citrate lyase–acts on it to form acetyl CoA and Oxaloacetate
- Acetyl CoA is converted to Malonyl CoA by carboxylation.
- Carbon atoms added in 1st cycle is 4 and in the next successive cycles is 2.
- Fatty acid synthesis stops at palmitate (16C)

Reaction in a line:

- 8 acetyl CoA + 14 NADPH + 7ATP → Palmitic acid + 8 CO_2.....

Fatty acid synthase enzyme:

- 4 main activities: Condensation, reduction, hydratase, reduction
- Dimer
- Contains 7 enzymes and ACP
- Active sites of fatty acid synthesis:
  At ketoacyl synthase: Cys-SH: Accepts acetyl CoA
  At ACP: Pan-SH: Accepts malonyl CoA

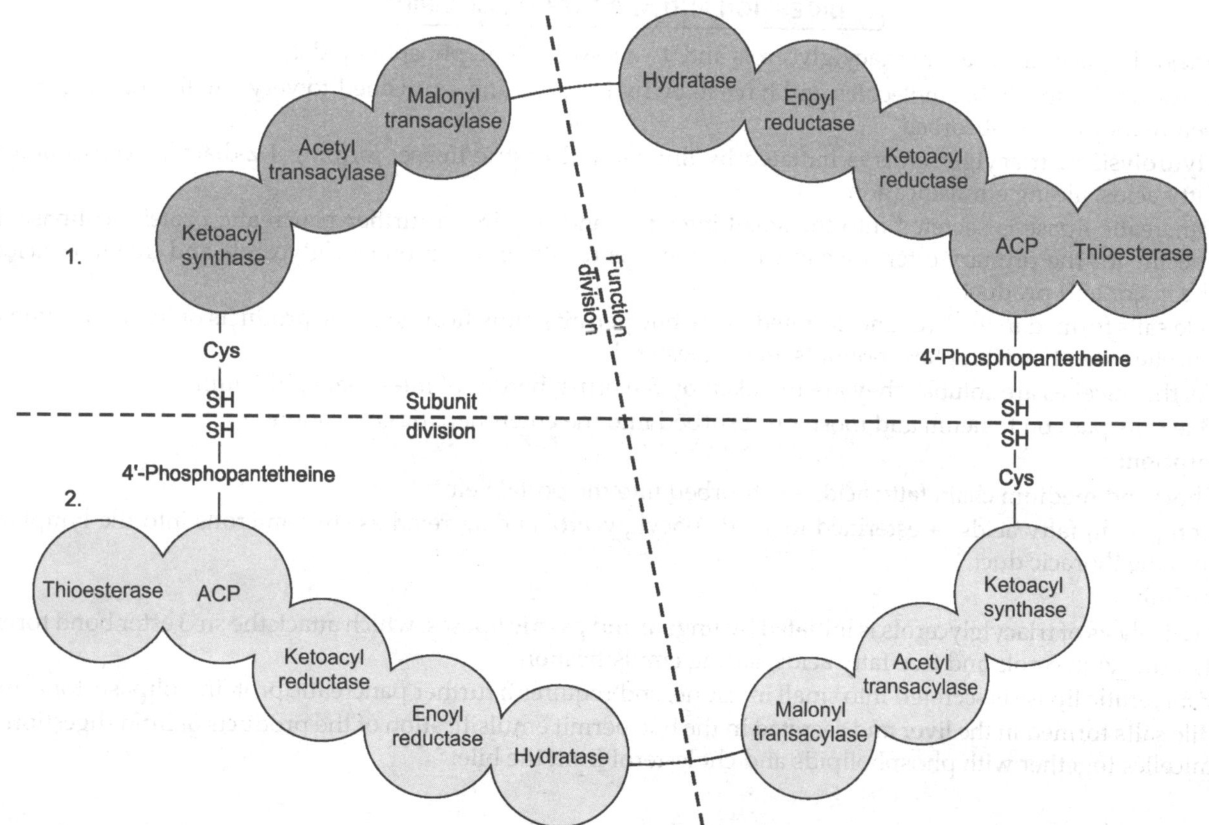

Fig. 3.6: Fatty acid synthase enzyme

Fatty acid chain elongation

Mitochondrial	Microsomal (ER)
Not a common pathway	Common pathway
Palmitoyl CoA is the starting molecule	**Acyl group acts as primer molecule**
Acetyl CoA(2c) directly incorporated into palmitoyl CoA	Acetyl moiety is added through malonyl CoA and not directly
NADPH is required Pyridoxal phosphate is needed	NADPH is required No need of pyridoxal phosphate
Operate under anerobic condition	Need oxygen

Cholesterol Synthesis

Step 1: Biosynthesis of Mevalonate:

- Two molecules of acetyl-CoA condense to form acetoacetyl-CoA catalyzed by cytosolic thiolase
- Acetoacetyl-CoA condenses with another acetyl-CoA catalyzed by HMG-CoA synthase to form HMG-CoA
- HMG-CoA is reduced to mevalonate by NADPH catalyzed by HMG-CoA reductase

Step 2: Formation of Isoprenoid Units:

- Mevalonate → phosphorylated and decarboxylated → isopentenyl diphosphate is formed

Step 3: Six Isoprenoid Units form Squalene:

- Isopentenyl diphosphate → dimethylallyl diphosphate → geranyl diphosphate → farnesyl diphosphate.
- Two molecules of farnesyl diphosphate condense at the diphosphate end to form squalene.

Step 4: Formation of Lanosterol.

Step 5: Formation of Cholesterol: From lanosterol takes place in the membranes of the endoplasmic reticulum.

Note: Farnesyl Diphosphate can also give rise to Dolichol and Ubiquinone.

DIGESTION AND ABSORPTION OF LIPIDS

The major lipids in the diet are triacylglycerols and, to a lesser extent, phospholipids:

- These are hydrophobic molecules and have to be hydrolyzed and emulsified to very small droplets (micelles) before they can be absorbed
- Hydrolysis of triacylglycerols is initiated by lingual and gastric lipase, forming 1,2-diacylglycerols and free fatty acids, aiding emulsification
- Pancreatic lipase is secreted into the small intestine, and requires a further pancreatic protein, colipase. It is specific for the primary ester links in triacylglycerols resulting in 2-monoacylglycerols and free fatty acids as the major end products
- Bile salts formed in the liver and secreted in the bile permit emulsification of the products of lipid digestion into micelles together with phospholipids and cholesterol
- As the micelles are soluble, they are up taken by the brush border of intestinal epithelium
- Bile salts pass on to ileum and most are absorbed into the enterohepatic circulation

Absorption:

- Short and medium chain fatty acids → absorbed into the portal vein
- Long chain fatty acids → esterified to yield triacylglycerol and secreted as chylomicrons into the lymphatics, into the thoracic duct

Digestion:

- Hydrolysis of triacylglycerols is initiated by lingual and gastric lipases, which attack the sn-3 ester bond forming 1, 2-diacylglycerols and free fatty acids, aiding emulsification.
- Pancreratic lipase is secreted into small intestine, and requires a further pancreatic protein, colipase, for activity.
- Bile salts formed in the liver and secreted in the bile permit emulsification of the products of lipid digestion into micelles together with phospholipids and cholesterol from the bile.

BILE ACIDS

Primary bile acids: synthesized in the liver from cholesterol

- Cholic and chenodeoxycholic acid
- Glycine and Taurine conjugate of cholic and chenodeoxycholic acid

Secondary bile acids: produced in intestines from primary bile acid by bacterial action

- Deoxycholic acid
- Lithocholic acid and their glycine and taurine conjugate

Formation of bile acids:

- Cholesterol is converted into 7-α hydroxyl cholesterol by the enzyme 7-α hydroxylase
- This is rate-limiting step. This step is catalyzed by NADPH, O_2, Vitamin C, and Cyt. P-450

Ketone Bodies:

Liver is the only organ which produces ketone bodies and adds to the blood, but it lacks the enzyme THIOPHORASE*—responsible for their degeneration and utilization. This is the reason why liver does not utilize ketone bodies.

Ketosis:

- Under certain metabolic conditions associated with high rate of fatty acid oxidation, liver produces ketone bodies, which is used as respiratory substrate (fuel) by extrahepatic tissues
- Ketone bodies are:
  - True ketone bodies → Acetone and Acetoacetate (possess keto group)
  - Beta hydroxybutyrate
- In a well-fed state, concentration of ketone bodies in blood does not exceed 1 mg/100 ml
- All ketone bodies are water-soluble except acetone

$H_3C-C(=O)-CH_2-C(=O)-SCoA$ (Acetoacetyl-CoA) + H_2O + $H_3C-C(=O)-SCoA$ (Acetyl-CoA) → (HMG-CoA synthase; HSCoA released) → $^{-}O-C(=O)-CH_2-C(OH)(CH_3)-CH_2-C(=O)-SCoA$ (Hydroxymethylglutaryl-CoA)

- HMG CoA synthase is the rate-limiting step for ketone synthesis.

MICRONUTRIENTS AND MINERALS

Selenium

- Constituent of aminoacid selenocysteine. Abundant in garlic
- Acts in synergism with vitamin E and prevents hepatic necrosis and muscular dystrophy
- Selenocysteine is present in the active sites of the enzymes Glutathione peroxidise, Thoredoxin reductase, Deiodinase
- Antioxidant and cancer-preventing property
- Impairments in human selenoproteins have been implicated in tumorigenesis and atherosclerosis and are associated with selenium deficiency cardiomyopathy (Keshan disease: Endemic cardiomyopathy in China)
- Kashin-Beck disease: Chronic endemic osteochondropathy in preadolescents in China.

Zinc

- Integral component of enzymes like Carbonic anhydrase, Alcohol dehydrogenase, Superoxide dismutase, Alkaline phosphatase
- Required for the synthesis and stabilization of DNA, RNA and proteins and for optimum immune function.
- Deficiency: Growth retardation, poor wound healing, loss of appetite, loss of taste sensation, impaired spermatogenesis, sexual infantilism, perioral pustular rash
- Zinc supplementation along with ORS decreases the duration and severity of acute and persistent diarrhea
- Severe maternal Zn↓: Spontaneous abortions and anencephaly; mild↓-LBW, IUGR, preterm delivery
- Acrodermatitis enteropathica-inherited metabolic disease of Zn deficiency. Autosomal recessive
- Excess: Anemia, weakness, neurological damage, ARDS, pulmonary fibrosis.

Copper

- Neutropenia is the best documented abnormality of Cu deficiency
- Ceruloplasmin is a copper-dependent ferroxidase, deficiency seen in Wilson's disease (hepatolenticular degeneration)
- Menkes kinky hair disease: X-linked recessive, mutation in ATP7A gene for copper-binding ATPase.
- Deficiency: Growth retardation, refractory hypochromic anemia, subperiosteal hematoma.

Chromium

- Lowers total serum cholesterol level, LDL and increases HDL
- Glucose tolerance factor, potentiator of insulin
- Unusual glucose tolerance curves are responsive to chromium
- Deficiency: hyperglycemia, glycosuria, peripheral neuropathy and encephalopathy.

Cobalt

- Compenent of vitamin B_{12}.
- Prolonged administration results in polycythemia due to increased EPO.

Molybdenum

- Component of xanthine oxidase and sulfite oxidase
- Excess: Bony deformities, growth retardation. Deficiency: mouth and esophageal cancer.

Manganese

- Present mainly in mitochondria and nucleus of cells.
- Required for synthesis of glycoproteins and glycosaminoglycans.
- Deficiency: Diminished activity of β-cells in pancreas, dermatitis, skeletal deformities. Toxicity: associated with Parkinsonism

Commonest clinical features of micronutrient disorders:

Micronutrient	Clinical Features	
Zinc	Deficiency	Acrodermatitis enteropathica, impaired spermatogenesis, perioral pustular rash
	Excess	Anemia, ARDS, pulmonary fibrosis
Copper	Deficiency	Growth retardation, refractory hypochromic anemia, neutropenia, subperiosteal hematoma
	Excess	Fanconi-like syndrome, hemolytic anemia
Manganese	Excess	Parkinsonism
Aluminum	Excess	Alzheimer's disease

MCQ Points

- Selenium deficiency, cobalt and iron excess causes cardiomyopathy
- Cadmium poisoning: Ouch-Ouch disease
- Arsenic and Thallium: Black foot disease

Enzyme Cofactors

Cofactors	Enzyme/Reaction
Zinc	Superoxide dismutase, Carbonic anhydrase, Glutamate dehydrogenase, Alcohol dehydrogenase, lkaline phosphatase, LDH (Lactate dehydrogenase), d-ALA synthase
Magnesium	Carboxylase, Transketolase, Phosphatase, Peptidase, Adenyl cyclase, Ribonuclease, Hexokinase, Phosphofructokinase, Glucose-6 phosphatase
Biotin	Carboxylase
Calcium	Lecithinase, lipase
Vitamin C	Hydroxylation
Copper	Tyrosinase, Cytochrome oxidase, Amine oxidase, Superoxide dismutase
Pyridoxine	Transamination
Molybdenum	Xanthine oxidase
Selenium	Glutathione peroxidase
Iron	Hemoglobin, cytochrome oxidase, Catalase, peroxidase, Xanthine oxidase, Aconitase
Manganese	Hydrolase, RNA polymerase, Glycosyl transferase, Pyruvate carboxylase, Superoxide dismutase

- **Holoenzyme:** Apoenzyme (protein part) + Coenzyme (nonprotein)
- **Cofactors:** Associated with enzymes needed for their activity
- **Abenzymes:** Catalytic antibodies (Ab + enzyme).

WATER-SOLUBLE VITAMINS

Vitamin B1 (Thiamine)

Sources

Whole grain cereals, pulses, oilseeds, nuts and yeast.

Functions

Cofactor for enzymes catalyzing:

- Oxidative decarboxylation of a keto acid:
  - Pyruvate dehydrogenase
  - α-ketoglutarate dehydrogenase
- Transketolase reaction

Diseases on deficiency

- Beriberi
  - High-output cardiac failure, Na+, H_2O retention
  - Biventricular failure
  - Wernicke-Korsakoff syndrome (most common in alcoholics)

Coenzyme form: Thiamine pyrophosphate

Its deficiency is detected by **decreased erythrocyte transketolase activity**

Vitamin B_2 (Riboflavin)

Sources

- Milk, meat, eggs, liver, kidney, cereals, fruits, vegetables and nuts.

Functions

FMN and FAD are coenzymes and electron carriers in oxidoreduction reaction in:
- Cytochrome C-reductase
- Warburg's yellow enzyme
- Fumarate dehydrogenase

Diseases on deficiency

- Seborrheic dermatitis
- Angular stomatitis
- Cheilosis, magenta tongue

Salient points

- Used as food additive because of its yellow color
- Deficiency detected by measuring RBC glutathione reductase.

Vitamin B_3 (Niacin)

(Pellagra Preventive factor of Goldberg)

Sources

Liver, yeast, whole grains, cereals, pulses, milk, fish, egg, vegetables.

Functions

- NAD and NADP are its active forms which operate as hydrogen and electron transfer agents.

Deficiency seen in

- Maize eaters
- Carcinoid syndrome
- Hartnup disease

Disease of deficiency

Pellagra:
- Diarrhea
- Dermatitis
- Dementia

Salient points

- Synthesized from tryptophan (60 mg tryptophan = 1 mg niacin)
- High doses used to treat hyperlipidemia
- Overdose causes cholestatic jaundice

Vitamin B_6 (Pyridoxine)

Sources

Egg yolk, fish, milk, meat, wheat, corn, cabbage, roots and tubers

Functions

Coenzyme in amino acid metabolism mainly in:
- Transamination reaction
- Deamination
- Decarboxylation
  (Involved in the transfer of amino groups).

Deficiency diseases

- Epileptiform convulsion in infants
- Sideroblastic anemia
- Deficiency can be induced by Isoniazide therapy (Increased kynurenine level in deficiency)

Salient points

- Required for synthesis of catecholamines and melanin
- Heme precursor (D-amino levulinic acid)
- In high does, causes sensory neuropathy
- B_6 is used in treatment of oxalate stone of kidney and homocystinuria
- Tryptophan loading test detects deficiency

Pantothenic Acid (Vitamin B_5)

Sources

- Egg, liver, meat, yeast, milk

Functions

- Formation of acetyl CoA and succinyl CoA
- Oxidation of fatty acid
  [As part of ACP (acyl carrier protein) in fatty acid synthesis].

Diseases

- Burning foot syndrome
- GI symptoms
- Changed sleep patterns.

Biotin (Vitamin B7/Vitamin-H/antiegg white injury factor)

Sources

- Liver, kidneys, egg yolk, milk, tomatoes, grains

Function

- Coenzyme in carboxylation reaction

Deficiency diseases

- Leiner's disease
- Exfoliative dermatitis

Salient features

- Large amounts of raw egg white (contains protein, avidin that binds biotin) induces biotin deficiency

Vitamin B_{12}

Sources

- Liver, kidney, eggs, pork and chicken.
- Curd is a better source than milk, due to the presence of lactobacillus (the only source for vegetarians is curd)

Cofactors for reactions

- Homocysteine → methionine
- Methyl malonyl CoA → succinyl CoA

Deficiency diseases

- Pernicious anemia (megaloblastic anemia)
- Homocystinuria

- Dementia
- SACD (subacute combined degeneration)

Salient features

- Found only in food of animal origin
- Absorption requires two binding protein
  - Intrinsic protein: Secreted by parietal cells of gastric mucosa
  - Cobalophillin: In saliva

Absorption of Vitamin B_{12}

- Contains cobalt
- Absorbed from the distal third of ileum and requires it to be bound to highly specific glycoprotein Intrinsic factor, secreted by parietal cells also called parietal factor.

Functions

- Catalyses the formation of Tetrahydrofolate from methyl H_4 folate
- Homocysteine is converted into methionine as the reaction proceeds.

Deficiency and Treatment

- **In deficiency of Vitamin B_{12}:** Trapping of folate as methyl H4 folate → Tetrahydrofolate is not synthesized and hence impaired purine and pyrimidine synthesis → impaired DNA synthesis → Prevent cell division and formation of nucleus of new RBCs → Accumulation of megaloblast in bone marrow → Megaloblastic anemia
- **Treatment:** Vitamin B_{12} and folic acid-increases DNA synthesis in bone marrow

Folic Acid

Source

- Green leafy vegetables, whole grain, liver, kidney, yeast and egg.
- Milk-poor source.

Function

- Tetrahydrofolate is a carrier of one carbon unit in synthesis of methionine, thymine and purine.

Deficiency diseases

- Megaloblastic anemia,
- Neural tube defect.

Salient feature reduces risk of neural tube defect and hyper homocystinemia

Other Vitamins Important from the Examination Point of View

Vitamin A

Structure

- Active forms are Retinol, Retinal and Retinoic acid
- Retinal is a component of visual pigment rhodopsin
- 1 mol β carotene yields 2 moles of retinal.

Dietary source	Functions	Deficiency
Liver, kidney, egg yolk, milk, cheese, butter, fish liver oil	• Vision • Maintenance of reproduction • Anti-infective, antioxidant, anti-carcinogenic	• Blindness • Xeropthalmia • Growth retardation

Hypervitaminosis A

- Liver damage
- Teratogenicity

- Hyperostosis, bone pains
- Increased intracranial pressure.

Vitamin C

- Not synthesized in humans, the guinea pigs, bats, passeriform birds, and most fish, due to deficiency of gulonolactone oxidase
- In animals: Synthesized from the uronic acid pathway
- Active form: Ascorbic acid.

Main functions

- Reducing agent in several different reactions
- Role as a coenzyme in hydroxylation of prolyl- and lysyl-residues of collagen
- Maintenance of normal connective tissue as well as for wound healing
- Proline and lysine hydroxylases are required for the postsynthetic modification of procollagen to collagen, and proline hydroxylase is also required in the formation of osteocalcin and the C1q component of complement.
- Aspartate β-hydroxylase is required for the postsynthetic modification of the precursor for protein C, the vitamin K-dependent protease that hydrolyzes activated factor V in the blood-clotting cascade
- Trimethyllysine and γ-butyrobetaine hydroxylases are required for the synthesis of carnitine
- Facilitates the absorption of dietary iron from the intestine.

Deficiency

- Scurvy, characterized by sore, spongy gums, loose teeth, fragile blood vessels, swollen joints, and anemia
- Scurvy: first disease identified due to dietary deficiency
- Symptoms due to deficiency in the hydroxylation of collagen, resulting in defective connective tissue.

Scurvy

Clinical features	Radiological features
• Swollen gums which bleed easily • Perifollicular and petechial hemorrhages • Ecchymoses, hemarthrosis • GI bleeding • Anemia • Poor wound healing	• Most commonly around knee • Pencil-thin cortex • Trummerfeld zone (metaphyseal lucency) • Frankel's white line • Pelkan's spur (lateral extension of white line) • Zone of rarefaction below white line • Wimberger's sign (small epiphysis)

Vitamin D

(Antirachitic or sunshine vitamin)

- Provitamins: Ergocalciferol (Vitamin-D2) and Cholecalciferol (Vitamin-D3) in diet and 7-dehydrocholesterol of skin.
- 7-dehydrocholesterol is converted into Cholecalciferol in the presence of sunlight (UV rays).
- Cholecalciferol undergoes hydroxylation in the liver to form 25 hydroxycholecalciferol.
- 25 hydroxycholecalciferol is converted in the kidney to 1,25 dihydroxycholecalciferol (active form) by the enzyme 1α hydroxylase.

Actions

- Increases absorption of Ca_2+ from gut and increased mineralization of bone
- It is a steroid hormone in the sense it binds to a nuclear receptor protein

Deficiency: Rickets (in children) and Osteomalacia (in adults)

Toxicity: Vitamin D is most toxic of all vitamins (Hypervitaminosis-D)

- Hypercalcemia and hyperphosphatemia
- Soft tissue calcification

- Hypertension
- Stupor and nausea

Vitamin K

- Abundant in cabbage, cauliflower, tomato, egg yolk, meat, liver, cheese and dairy products
- Occurs in 3 forms:
  - K1: Phylloquinone: Plants
  - K2: Menaquinone: Intestinal bacteria and animals
  - K3: Menadione and menodial acetate: Synthetic form.

Functions

- Post-translational modification of glutamate residue of precursor proteins to γ carboxyglutamate residue for the generation of clotting factor
- Vitamin K-dependent clotting factors are: Factor 2, 7, 9, 10 and Protein C and S
- Vitamin K along with Vitamin C is required for synthesis of osteocalcin
- Hemorrhagic disease of newborn (HDN) is seen in Vitamin K deficiency
- Vitamin K functions as a coenzyme for carboxylase enzyme responsible for post-translational modification of blood-clotting factor.

$$\text{Glutamate} \xrightarrow[\text{Pyruvate carboxylase, Vitamin K}]{CO_2} \gamma \text{ carboxyglutamate}$$

GENETICS

Functions and Uses of Purine and Pyrimidine Nucleotides:

ATP : Energy currency of the cell
Regulator of Electron Transport Chain
Helps in energy requiring biosynthetic reactions

c-GMP, c-AMP	: Second messengers
ATP, GTP	: Phosphorylation reactions
UDP-Sugars	: Glycoprotein, Proteoglycan synthesis
UDP-Glucuronic acid	: Conjugation of bilirubin and drugs
CDP-Acylglycerols	: Lipid biosynthesis
PAPS (Phosphoadenophosphosulfate)	: Sulfation of proteins and glycosaminoglycans
Coenzymes containing nucleotides	: SAM, NAD, NADP, FAD, CoASH.
Nucleic acid synthesis	: DNA and RNA

Plantderived nucleotides

Caffiene : 1, 3, 7 trimethylxanthine
Theophylline : 1, 3 dimethylxanthine
Theobromine : 3, 7 dimethylxanthine

Pharmacological uses

Anticancer drugs : Mercaptopurine, Cytarabine, 5-Fluorouracil
Antiviral drugs : Idoxuridine, Nucleoside protease inhibitors

In a nucleotide structure:

N_9 of purines is attached to Ribose through β-N glycosidic linkage.
N_1 of pyrimidines is attached to Ribose through β-N glycosidic linkage.

α-Phosphate is bound through phosphodiester bond, whereas 2nd and 3rd phosphates are attached through acid anhydride linkages.

Bases	Nucleosides	Nucleotides
Adenine	Adenosine	AMP
Guanine	Guanosine	GMP
Cytosine	Cytidine	CMP
Uracil	Uridine	UMP
Thymine	Thymidine	TMP
Hypoxanthine	Inosine	IMP
Xanthine	Xanthosine	XMP

Purine nucleoside

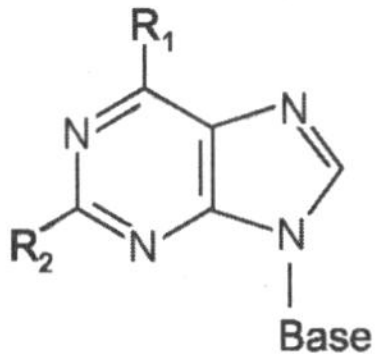

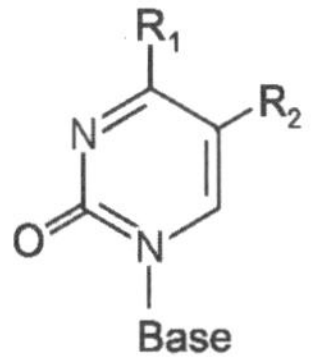

	R_1	R_2
Adenosine	NH_2	H
Guanosine	= O	NH_2

Pyrimidine nucleoside

	R_1	R_2
Cytidine	NH_2	H
Thymidine	= O	CH_3
Uracil	= O	H

DENOVO PURINE SYNTHESIS

- Derived from:
  - Amino acid, aspartic acid, glycine and glutamine
  - CO_2
  - Tetrahydrofolate derivatives

Purine synthesis:

- Ribose 5 phosphate ⟶ PRPP
  (PRPP synthase)
- Synthesis of 5′ phosphoribosylamine from PRPP. Glutamine is used for transamination.
  (Aminotransferase-ratelimiting step)
- The following steps utilizes 4 ATP′ to form inosine monophosphate *(parent purine nucleotide).*

**Uses methyl tetrahydrofolate (DHFR enzyme)*

Pharmacology:

- Sulfonamides: Competitively inhibit bacterial synthesis of folic acid. Since humans cannot synthesize FA and have to be taken in diet, it is not inhibited.
- Folic acid analogues (methotrexate) inhibit: DHFR enzyme, thus limiting the availability of THF in purine synthesis, and thus toxic to cells including cancer cells.

Salvage pathway:

- The hypoxanthine, adenine and guanine from uric acid metabolism are reutilized to form IMP, GMP and AMP. The enzyme used is ***HGPRTase*** (Hypoxanthine Guanine phosphoribosyltransferase)

  Deficiency leads to **LeschNyhan Syndrome***:* excessive production of uric acid + characteristic neurologic features (self-mutilation and involuntary movements)

Degradation of purine-catabolism:

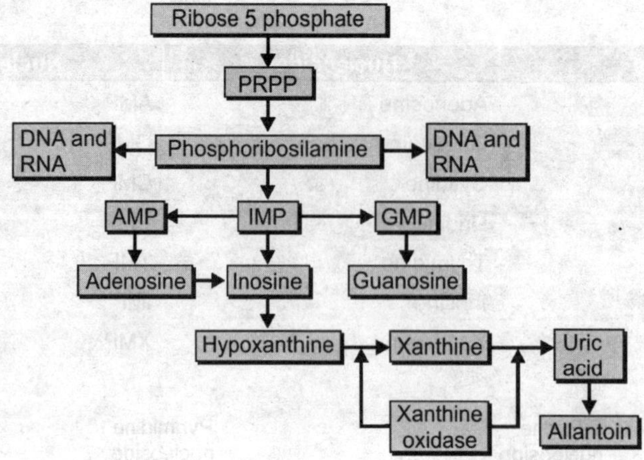

End products:

- **Human: Uric acid**
- **Mammals: Allantoin**
- **Animals: Urea and NH_3**

  Enzyme Deficiency:
  - **Adenosine deaminase deficiency:** Causes SCID and children die in less than 2 years of infection
  - **Gout:** Overproduction of uric acid crystals
  - **Primary gout:** Inborn error of uric acid metabolism
  - **Secondary gout:** Cancer, HGPRT, Renal failure

Pyrimidine synthesis:

- **Sources:**

  Glutamine

  CO_2

  Aspartic acid

  Committed step: Synthesis of carbamoyl phosphate by CPS-2 enzyme **(in cytosol)**

Ribonucleotide reductase:

- The nucleotides required for DNA synthesis are 2′ *deoxyribonucleotides* produced from ribonucleotide diphosphates.
- The enzyme playing here is Ribonucleotide reductase (contains 2 SH group).
- For the recovery of this enzyme (to recover the sulfhydryl group) another enzyme used is thioredoxin reductase.
- Thioredoxin is regenerated by NADPH.

DNA structure:

- **3′– 5′ phosphodiester bond forms the backbone of DNA.**
- Always written in 5′ $\rightarrow$ 3′ end.
- The 5′ end of one strand is paired with 3′ end of the other strand.
- The base of one strand forms hydrogen bond with opposite strand.
- *Adenine forms double bond with thymine*
- *Guanine forms triple bond with cytosine*
- Length of each turn: 3.4 nm
- There are 10 bases per turn
- Diameter: 2 nm
- Distance between each base = 0.34 nm

- According to **Chargaf's rule:**
  In a dsDNA'
  Number of A = T and number of G = C
  i.e; A + G = T + C
  Number of purines = Number of pyrimidines
- These hydrogen bonds and hydrophobic interactions stabilize the structure of double helix.
- *Denaturation is loss of double helical structure.*
- Can be done by altering pH or increasing temperature.
- DNA containing more of A and T will melt more easily at lower temperature than those with G and C, because of less hydrogen bonds.
- **The loss of helical structure can be monitored by measuring its absorbance at 260 nm.**

B FORM	A FORM	Z FORM
Resembles twisted ladder	Moderate dehydration of B form	
Right-handed helix	Right-handed helix	Left-handed helix
10 base pairs	11 base pairs	12 base pairs/turn
Bases are perpendicular to the backbone	20 degrees tilt to ribose phosphate backbone	Zig-zag backbone

DNA Replication

Step 1: Separation of two complementary DNA strands

Initiation of replication requires:

Prepriming complex:

- DNA A proteins
- SSB (single-stranded DNA-binding proteins)
- DNA helicases

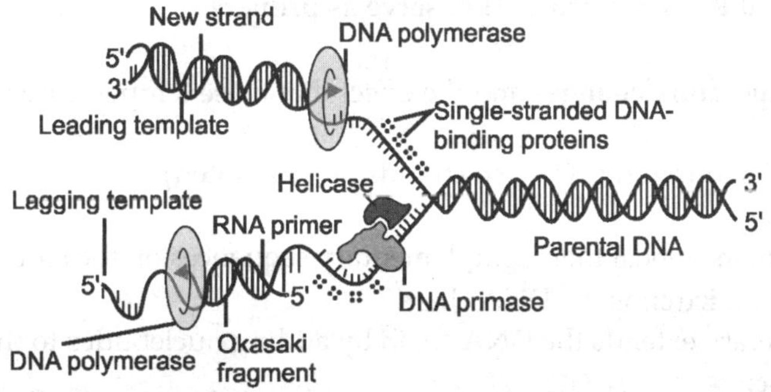

Fig. 3.7: Collaboration of proteins at the replication fork

DNA Topoisomerases

- The enzymes responsible for removing supercoils in the helix are called DNA topoisomerase.

Enzymes	Functions
DNA helicase	Requires ATP Used in replication fork
DNA topoisomerase I	Does not require ATP Negative supercoils in prokaryotes *Both negative and positive in eukaryotes*
DNA topoisomerase II	No need of ATP Releases both type of coils

Contd...

Contd...

Enzymes	Functions
DNA gyrase	A type II DNA topoisomerase in prokaryotes It requires ATP
DNA polymerase	
DNA ligase	
RNA primase	

The main enzyme in copying DNA template is **DNA polymerase.**
The copying process starts from 3′–5′ end and newly synthesized DNA formed from 5′–3′ end
The DNA polymerase requires a RNA polymerase called **RNA primase** which synthesizes short stretches of RNA.
On the leading strand: Only one stretch of RNA primer at origin of replication required.
On the lagging strand: RNA primer required at multiple sites.

E. coli	Eukaryotes	Functions
DNA polymerase I		Gap-filling following DNA replication, repair and recombination
DNA polymerase II	Beta Gamma	DNA repair Mitochondrial DNA synthesis
DNA polymerase III DnaG	**Epsilon** Alpha Delta	Processive, **leading** strand synthesis Primase Processive, **lagging** strand synthesis

PCR

Invitro version of DNA replication
The following components are needed to perform PCR in the laboratory:

1. DNA (DNA of interest)
2. A heat-stable **DNA polymerase**
3. All four nucleotide triphosphates
4. Buffers
5. **Two short, single-stranded RNA molecules that serve as primers**
6. Thermal cycler

- The bases of PCR are **temperature changes** and the effect that these temperature changes have on the DNA.
  - Step 1: **Denature** DNA
    At 95°C, the DNA is denatured (i.e. the two strands are separated)
  - Step 2: Primers **Anneal**
    At 40°C-65°C, the primers anneal their complementary sequences on the single strands of DNA
  - Step 3: DNA polymerase **Extends** the DNA chain
    At 72°C, DNA Polymerase extends the DNA chain by adding nucleotides to the 3′ ends of the primers.

Heat-stable DNA polymerase:

- Given that PCR involves very high temperatures, it is imperative that a heat-stable DNA polymerase be used in the reaction.
  - Most DNA polymerases would denature (and thus not function properly) at the high temperatures of PCR.
- **Taq DNA polymerase** was purified from the hot springs bacterium *Thermus aquaticus.*
- Taq has maximal enzymatic activity at 75 °C to 80 °C, and substantially reduced activities at lower temperatures.

Histones:

- DNA in eukaryotes is tightly bound to basic proteins called histones.
- 5 classes of histones: H1, H2A, H2B, H3, H4.
- Because of their **positive charge** due to abundance of basic amino acids arginine and lysine, they form ionic bonds with **negative DNA.**
- Mg 2+ ions help in this bond.
- **H1 is not involved in nucleosome core but binds to DNA chains.**

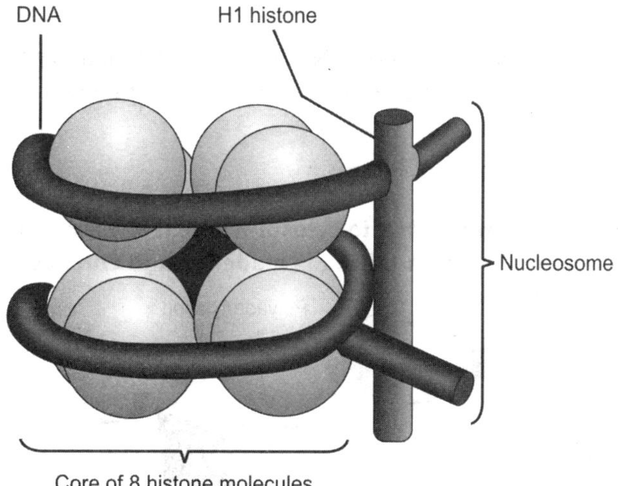

Fig. 3.8: Nucleosome

DNA Repair Mechanisms

1. **UV light damage:**

   Results in the formation of *thymidine dimers*

   These dimers prevent DNA polymerase replication.

   DNA Mismatch Repair Mechanism

   - UV-specific endonuclease (GATC endonuclease)
   - Exonuclease activity by DNA polymerase I
   - Defect repaired by DNA polymerase II

   Failure of this mechanism leads to colonic cancers (HNPCC)

2. **Base excision repair**

   Removal of abnormal bases by glycosylase

   Resulting in apyrimidine/apurine (AP) site

   The AP endonuclease identifies it and removes it

3. **Nucleotide excision repair**

   By exonucleases

   Defect: **Xeroderma pigmentosa**

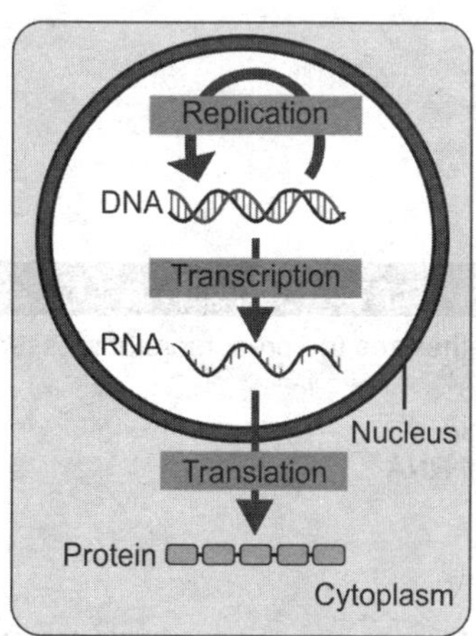

Fig. 3.9: Central dogma of biology

Transcription or RNA production:

- RNA molecules are produced by copying part of DNA into a complementary sequence of RNA
- This process is started and controlled by an enzyme called **RNA polymerase.**

mRNA:

- **Most heterogenous type of RNA.**
- **5% of RNA**
- **mRNA carries genetic information from DNA to cytosol where it is used as a template for protein synthesis.**
- **5′ end with capping and 3′ end with poly A tailing is made for it to enter cytosol.**

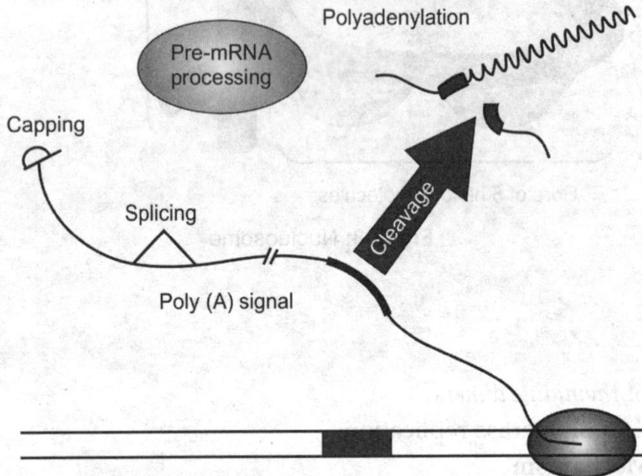

Fig. 3.10: Post-transcriptional processing of m-RNA

Ribosomal RNA:

- 80% of RNA in cell
- Eukaryotic RNA has **4 species:** 28 s, 18 s, 5.5 s, 5 s units.
- Prokaryotic RNA has ***3 subunits***- 23 s, 16 s, 5 s units

Transfer RNA

- Smallest of the three
- Adaptor molecule, 3′ end carries the amino acid.

Transcription:

- RNA is synthesized from 5′ end to 3′ end
- Antiparallel to its DNA template.

Steps involved:

1. Initiation
2. Elongation
3. Termination

RNA polymerase: Eukaryotes:

Type I	Type II	Type III
Synthesizes the large ribosomal RNA 28 s 18 s 5.8 s	Synthesizes the precursors of messenger RNA nRNA Viral RNA	Small RNA (5 s) Transfer RNA nRNA

Initiator:

Promoters:

TATA or GOLBERG HOGNESS box: 25 nucleotide upstream in the DNA to the start of transcription site for mRNA

CAAT box: 80 nucleotide upstream

Transcription factors:

1. Core enzyme: RNA polymerase
2. Holo enzyme: ρ subunit + RNA polymerase

Inhibitors:

- RNA polymerase II is inhibited by alpha amanitin- from poisonous mushroom
- Prokaryotic RNA polymerase beta subunit inhibited by rifampicin.

Elongation:

- Unlike DNA polymerase, the RNA polymerase doesn't need primer and has no endo- and exonuclease activity.
- Hence, there is no ability to repair the RNA.
- As it pushes away, it also creates the positive supercoils ahead and negative supercoils behind.
- *Positive coils are relaxed by DNA gyrase.*
- *Negative coils are relaxed by topoisomerase.*

Termination:

- **Rhoindependents:** Stable hair-pin bend that slows down the process of RNA polymerase.
  (*DNA palindrome:* Role in termination of RNA synthesis)
- **Rhodependent**: Rhodependent ATPase activity, helicase-like activity,

Post-translational modification:

- From the primary transcript:
  - tRNA: Modified
  - rRNA: Modified
  - Prokaryotic mRNA: Identical
  - Eukaryotic mRNA: Modified

Splicing:

From transcript mRNA:

- Removal of introns: Noncoding regions
- Exons: Coding sequences are then brought together
- Small nuclear (snRNA): Helps in this process
- *Antibodies to snRNA lead to SLE, muscular atrophy and beta thalassemia*

Protein Synthesis

(Translation)

Components needed:

- All the amino acids
- tRNA: Atleast one tRNA for one AA must be there. (Humans contain about 50 tRNA species.)
- mRNA: Template for protein synthesis
- **Amino acyl tRNA:** *Fidelity enzyme*: The enzyme needed for attachment of AA to their corresponding tRNAs at 3′ end. Requires ATP.
- Ribosomes
- Protein factors
- Sources of energy

Genetic Code:

- **Unambiguous:** Specific codon specifies only one AA
- **Universality:** Such thing in all species
- **Redundancy** (degeneracy of codons): Each codon has only AA coding. But each AA has many codons.
- Nonoverlapping or **commaless.**

Codons:

- Total = 64
- Coding = 61
- Initiator: AUG-methionine
- Termination: UAG, UGA, UAA.

Pro 30 s	Pro 50 s	Euk 40 s	Euk 60 s
16 s	23 s	18 s	28 s
21 proteins	5 s	30 proteins	5.8 s
	32 proteins		5 s
			50 proteins

Wobble Hypothesis:

- Atleast one tRNA must be there for one amino acid.
- Humans contain 50 species of tRNA. But total codons are 61. Then how do they adapt each?
- Wobble's hypothesis explain this is possible.

First 2 base pairs are specific for tRNA and third one wobbles

This wobble allows the single tRNA to recognize more than one codon.

Initiation:

- Assembly of 2 ribosome subunits
- mRNA to be translated
- Amino acyl tRNA
- GTP
- Initiation factors

In E. coli, a sequence of nucleotides located 6-10 bases upstream of the AUG: Initiator codon helps to fix and bind the position of mRNA called **Shine Dalgarno sequence.**

Elongation:

- Ribosomes moves from 5′ end to 3′ end of mRNA on elongation.
- **Peptidyl transferase** catalyzes the activity.
- This activity is intrinsic to the **23 s rRNA of the 50 s unit**; hence this enzyme is called **Ribozyme.** ***(28 s rRNA of the 60 s** ribosomal subunit in eukaryotes)*

QUESTIONS

1. Truth regarding GLP-1: **(2015)**

a. Acts at the satiety center
b. Inhibits glucose-induced insulin secretion
c. Secreted by alpha cells of pancreas
d. Release is inhibited by the presence of fatty acids.

2. Function of golgi apparatus: **(2015)**

a. Packs and sorts proteins
b. Synthesis of ATPs
c. Steroid synthesis
d. DNA replication

3. Pyridoxine is a coenzyme for: **(2015)**

a. Carboxylation
b. Transamination
c. Oxidation
d. Reduction

4. The vitamin whose RDA is related to protein intake is: **(2015)**

a. Pantothenate
b. Niacin
c. Pyridoxine
d. Thiamine

5. 55-year-old presents with bleeding gums. He is an alcoholic, has petechia. The vitamin deficiency associated with this condition is: **(2015)**

a. Vitamin B_1
b. Vitamin B_{12}
c. Vitamin C
d. Vitamin E

6. The common polymorphism in the gene for methylene-tetrahydrofolate reductase appears to influence the sensitivity of homocysteine levels due to the deficiency of: **(2015)**

a. Vitamin B_{12}
b. Folic acid
c. Vitamin A and D
d. Vitamin B_6

7. **Truth regarding metabolic acidosis: (2015)**
   a. Body shunts more glutamine from liver to kidneys
   b. Less ammonia is excreted in urine
   c. Urea synthesis is increased
   d. Liver glutaminase activity increases
8. **Impaired glucose tolerance is seen in deficiency of: (2015)**
   a. Selenium
   b. Chromium
   c. Manganese
   d. Molybdenum
9. **Divalent zinc ion is essential for: (2015)**
   a. Catalase
   b. Pancreatic lipase
   c. Alkaline phosphatase
   d. Salivary amylase
10. **Mucopolysaccharide not containing uronic acid is: (2015)**
    a. Heparin
    b. Heparan sulfate
    c. Keratan sulfate
    d. Chondroitin sulfate
11. **Lipoprotein-A is in structural homology to: (2015)**
    a. Albumin
    b. Prothrombin
    c. Collagen
    d. Plasminogen
12. **Injection of heparin releases: (2015)**
    a. Lipoprotein lipase
    b. Insulin
    c. Alkaline phosphatase
    d. Nitric oxide
13. **The rate-limiting enzyme of de novo purine biosynthesis pathway is: (2015)**
    a. Phosphoribosylpyrophosphate synthetase
    b. Phosphoribosylpyrophosphate amidotransferase
    c. Adenylosuccinate lyase
    d. Formyltransferase
14. **Function of pseudouridine arm of tRNA is: (2015)**
    a. Terminates translation
    b. Binding to tRNA to ribosomes
    c. Recognition of specific tRNA to add with specific amino acid
    d. Recognition of specific amino acid to be attached to the amino acid arm
15. **Polymerase chain reaction is used to amplify a small fragment of DNA for further analysis. To do this, DNA double helix must be split. This is done by: (2015)**
    a. DNA polymerase
    b. Centrifuge
    c. Alkali
    d. Heating around 100 °C.
16. **Northern blot detects: (2015)**
    a. RNA
    b. DNA
    c. Protein
    d. Antigens
17. **Ketone bodies are not utilized by: (2014)**
    a. Brain
    b. RBC
    c. Heart
    d. Skeletal muscle
18. **Which of the following enzymes is absent in muscle? (2014)**
    a. Glucose-1 phosphatase
    b. Glucose-6 phosphatase
    c. Glycogen phosphorylase
    d. Thiophorase
19. **Which is a reverse transcriptase? (2014)**
    a. Topoisomerase 2
    b. Telomerase
    c. RNA polymerase 2
    d. DNA polymerase alpha
20. **True statement regarding telomerase is: (2014)**
    a. It is a reverse transcriptase
    b. Active in somatic cells
    c. Involved in translation
    d. Helps in shortening of DNA
21. **Not a stimuli for insulin secretion: (2014)**
    a. Glucagon
    b. Hypokalemia
    c. Ketone bodies
    d. Amino acids
22. **The enzyme not involved in substrate level phosphorylation is: (2014)**
    a. Succinyl thiokinase
    b. Phosphofructokinase
    c. Pyruvate kinase
    d. Phosphoglycerate kinase
23. **Lipoprotein A shows homology with: (2014)**
    a. Plasminogen
    b. Albumin
    c. Prothrombin
    d. Plasmin
24. **False regarding electron transport chain is: (2014)**
    a. Cyanide inhibits electron transport, but not ATP synthesis
    b. Atractyloside inhibiting h+/ADP synthesis
    c. Oligomycin blocks H+ channel
    d. High dose aspirin acts as uncoupler

25. Insulin-dependent glucose transport occurs in all except: (2014)
a. Heart
b. Adipose tissues
c. Liver
d. Skeletal muscles

26. Which of the following is not true regarding iodine therapy? (2014)
a. Iodine inhibits release of thyroid hormones
b. Contraindicated in hyperthyroidism
c. Inhibits synthesis of mono-iodo- and di-iodotyrosine
d. It causes iodism

27. Which of the following is true about enzymes? (2014)
a. High km-high affinity
b. Low km-high affinity
c. Noncompetitive inhibition-decreased km
d. Noncompetitive inhibition-increased km

28. BMR is decreased in: (2014)
a. Cold temperature
b. Hyperthyroidism
c. Exercise
d. Hypothyroidism

29. Which one of the following is lyase enzyme? (2014)
a. Hexokinase
b. Pyruvate kinase
c. Proponyl CoA carboxylase
d. Aldolase B

30. The enzyme deficient in phenylketonuria is: (2013)
a. Phenylalanine dehydrogenase
b. Phenylalanine hydroxylase
c. Tyrosine hydroxylase
d. Dihydrobiopterin

31. Histamine causes: (2013)
a. Bronchodilation
b. Increased gastric secretion
c. Vasoconstriction
d. Papillary constriction

32. Most common enzyme deficient in urea cycle is: (2013)
a. Ornithine transcarbamoylase
b. Arginase
c. Carbamoyl phosphate synthase I
d. Argininosuccinate synthase

33. Pyridoxal phosphate is needed in: (2013)
a. Glucogenolysis
b. Fatty acid oxidation
c. Glycogenesis
d. Gluconeogenesis

34. Peptidyl transferase is: (2013)
a. Enzyme
b. Catalyst
c. Riboxyme
d. Elongation factor

35. All the following causes shift of oxygen dissociation curve to the left except: (2013)
a. Decreased pH
b. Hypothermia
c. Decreased 2, 3 DPG
d. Fetal hemoglobin

36. Enzyme deficiencies responsible for gout are all except: (2013)
a. PRPP synthase
b. Pseudogout enzyme
c. 5-phosphoribosyl amidotransferase
d. Glucose-6 phosphatase

37. Corticosteroid causes all the following except: (2013)
a. Inhibit immunoglobulin destruction
b. Increase glucose formation
c. Protein breakdown and amino acid mobilization
d. Increase lipolysis

38. All the following act via cyclic GMP except: (2013)
a. ANP
b. BNP
c. NO
d. None of the above

39. All are bile acids except: (2013)
a. Lithocholic acid
b. Taurocholic acid
c. Deoxycholic acid
d. Chenodeoxycholic acid

40. The most important function of 2,3 DPG is: (2013)
a. O_2 release
b. O_2 binding
c. Acid-base blance
d. Water electrolyte balance

41. True statement regarding insulin: (2013)
a. Produced by alpha cells of pancreas
b. Two polypeptide chains are bound by disulfide linkages
c. Shifts potassium outside the cell
d. Subcutaneous insulin t1/2 is 60 mins

42. All are true regarding prostaglandins except:
a. LT cause vasoconstriction and decreased vascular permeability (2013)
b. 20 carbon unsaturated fats
c. Prostacyclin inhibits platelet aggregation
d. Prostaglandins cause uterine muscle contraction and induce labor

43. Which is not an epigenetic modification? (2012)
a. Poly A tailing
b. Splicing
c. DNA methylation
d. Histone acetylation

44. Concentration of H+ ion is 1 × 10–9. What is the pH of the solution? (2012)
a. 9
b. 13
c. 4
d. 7

45. Most important polyunsaturated fatty acid:
a. Linolenic acid (2012)
b. Linoleic acid
c. Arachidonic acid
d. Eicosapentaenoic acid

46. All enzyme reactions are involved in substrate level phosphorylation except: (2012)
a. Phosphoglycerate kinase
b. Succinate thiokinase
c. Phosphofructokinase
d. Pyruvate kinase

47. Lesch-Nyhan syndrome is due to deficiency of:
a. HGPRTase (2012)
b. CPS I
c. CPS II
d. PRPP synthaese

48. GLUT-2 is seen in: (2012)
a. Pancreas
b. Adipose tissue
c. Skeletal muscles
d. Brain

49. All the following cause nonketotic hypoglycemia except: (2012)
a. Galactosemia
b. Fructose intolerance
c. Hyperinsulinemia
d. Alcohol intoxication

50. All are PUFAs except: (2012)
a. Linoleic acid
b. Linolenic acid
c. Palmitic acid
d. Arachidoic aid

51. Thiamine deficiency shows: (2012)
a. Reduced RBC transketolase activity
b. Reduced RBC transaminase activity
c. Increased excretion of urinary 4-pyridoxic aid
d. All of the above

52. Insulin-dependent glucose transport occurs in all except: (2012)
a. Skeletal muscle
b. Heart
c. Liver
d. Adipocytes

53. Insulin-mediated uptake of glucose into muscle is through: (2011)
a. GLUT 2
b. GLUT 4
c. GLUT 1
d. GLUT 3

54. Northern blot is used for: (2011)
a. RNA
b. DNA
c. Protein
d. cDNA

55. 7-Methyl guanosine cap is present in: (2011)
a. mRNA
b. tRNA
c. rRNA
d. DNA

56. Nitrogen content in 200 gm protein: (2011)
a. 8 g
b. 16 g
c. 32 g
d. 64 g

57. Toxicity due to ethanol is because of which pathological mechanism? (2011)
a. Increased NADH/NAD+
b. Decreased lactate/pyruvate
c. Inhibition of gluconeogenesis
d. Stimulation of fatty acid oxidation

58. Urea is formed by the action of the following enzyme: (2011)
a. Arginase
b. Ornithine transcarbamoylase
c. Aspartate carbamolyase
d. Citrulline synthase

59. False regarding von Gierke's disease is: (2011)
a. Metabolic acidosis
b. Hyperuricemia
c. Muscle atrophy
d. Hypertriglyceridemia

60. Aromatic enzyme complex is involved in the biosynthesis of: (2011)
a. Cholesterol
b. Adrenal hormones
c. Vitamin D_3
d. Estradiol/estrogens

61. Which of the following occurs in ischemic cardiac tissue? (2011)
a. Increased ATP
b. Increased anerobic glycolysis
c. Increased pH
d. Increased release of Ca

62. Stability of alpha helix is affected by which amino acid? (2011)
a. Tryptophan
b. Proline
c. Glutamate
d. Valine

63. HDL levels are increased by: (2011)
a. Exercise
b. 400 mg vitamin E daily
c. Aspirin
d. DHEA

64. Porphyrins absorb light in the wavelength of: (2011)
a. 340 nm
b. 400 nm
c. 540 nm
d. 670 nm

65. Which amino acid undergoes hepatic deamination? (2010)
a. Alanine
b. Glutamate
c. Aspartate
d. Glycine

66. Which of the following is a marker for peroxisomes? (2010)
a. Glutamate dehydrogenase
b. Glucose-6 phosphatase
c. 5′ nucleotidase
d. Uric acid oxidase

67. Acetyl CoA carboxylase is stimulated by: (2010)
a. Malonyl CoA
b. Citrate
c. Palmitoyl CoA
d. Acetoacetate

68. Which of the following is required for glycogen phosphorylase in glycogenolysis? (2010)
a. Thiamine pyrophosphate
b. Pyridoxal phosphate
c. FAD
d. Citrate

69. Insulin acts through all except: (2010)
a. Tyrosine kinase receptor
b. Inhibition of membrane Na K ATPase
c. Inducing hexokinase activity
d. Increased GLUT-4 in cell surface

70. Nitric oxide acts by: (2010)
a. cGMP
b. cAMP
c. Calcium
d. Kinase

71. Thyroid-binding proteins are increased by: (2010)
a. Androgens
b. Estrogens
c. Asparginase
d. Glucocorticoids

72. During starvation, which organ does not use ketone bodies? (2010)
a. Brain
b. RBC
c. Heart
d. Skeletal muscles

73. In starvation, the least common change seen is: (2010)
a. Depletion of buccal fat
b. Increased lipogenesis
c. Increased gluconeogenesis
d. Increased glycogenolysis

74. Which of the following is not a glycoprotein? (2010)
a. FSH
b. LH
c. TSH
d. ADH

75. Most stable amino acid at the physiological pH is: (2009)
a. Histidine
b. Lysine
c. Arginine
d. Glycine

76. All are polyunsaturated fatty acids except: (2009)
a. Linoleic acid
b. Linolenic acid
c. Palmitic acid
d. Arachidonic acid

77. All the following cause nonketotic hypoglycemia except: (2009)
a. Galactosemia
b. Fructose intolerance
c. Hyperinsulinemia
d. Alcohol intoxication

78. 7-Methyl guanosine cap is present in: (2009)
a. mRNA
b. tRNA
c. rRNA
d. DNA

79. During DNA replication, Okazaki fragments are seen in relation to: (2009)
a. Leading strand
b. Lagging strand
c. Both
d. Helicase

80. All enzyme reactions are involved in substrate level phosphorylation except: (2009)
a. Phosphoglycerate kinase
b. Succinate thiokinase
c. Phosphofructokinase
d. Pyruvate kinase

81. Lesch-Nyhan syndrome is due to deficiency of: (2009)
a. HGPRTase
b. CPS I
c. CPS II
d. PRPP synthetase

82. Pyridoxal phosphate is needed in: (2009)
a. Glucogenolysis
b. Fatty acid oxidation
c. Glycogenesis
d. Gluconeogenesis

83. Folic acid deficiency can be estimated by: (2008)
a. Histidine load test
b. Dexa suppression test
c. Isovaleric acid levels
d. Aminolevulinic acid levels

84. Solubility of cholesterol depends on: (2008)
a. Water
b. Phosphatidylcholine
c. Bile salts
d. Cholesterol

85. Enzyme catalyzing urea formation: (2008)
a. Arginase
b. Ornithine transcarbamylease
c. Carbamoyl phosphate synthetase
d. Argininosuccinate synthase

86. Marker of lysosome is: (2008)
a. Acid phosphatase
b. Lactate dehydrogenase
c. Oxidase
d. NaK, ATPase

87. Vitamin K is required for which of the following reactions? (2008)
a. Hydroxylation
b. Chelation
c. Transamination
d. Carboxylation

88. Fructose is absorbed by: (2008)
a. Simple diffusion
b. Facilitated diffusion
c. Cotransport
d. Symport

89. Enzyme deficiencies responsible for gout are all except: (2008)
a. PRPP synthetase
b. Pseudogout enzyme
c. 5-phosphoribosyl amidotransferase
d. Glucose6 phosphatase

90. In starvation, least common change seen is:
a. Depletion of buccal fat (2008)
b. Increased lipogenesis
c. Increased gluconeogenesis
d. Increased glycogenolysis

91. Following amino acid forms an integral part of collagen synthesis: (2008)
a. Lysine
b. Leucine
c. Arginine
d. Glutamic acid

92. Erythrocyte transketolase activity is inhibited in:
a. Pellagra (2007)
b. Beri-beri
c. Scurvy
d. Rickets

93. Oasthouse syndrome is due to malabsorption of:
a. Methionine (2007)
b. Valine
c. Cysteine
d. Tryptophan

94. In glycolysis, ATP is produced by the following enzyme: (2007)
a. Hexokinase
b. Phosphoglycerate kinase
c. Encolase
d. Phosphohexose isomerase

95. McArdle's disease is due to the deficiency of:
a. Glucose-1 phosphatase (2007)
b. Glucose-1, 6 diphosphatase
c. Glucose-6 phosphatase
d. Myophosphorylase

96. Reactive oxygen intermediates are released by:
a. NADPH oxidase (2007)
b. Superoxide dismutase
c. Catalase
d. Glutathione peroxidase

97. All are bile acids except: (2007)
a. Lithocholic acid
b. Taurocholic acid
c. Deoxycholic acid
d. Chenodeoxycholic acid

98. Stability of alpha helix is affected by which amino acid? (2007)
a. Tryptophan
b. Proline
c. Glutamate
d. Valine

99. Tay-Sach's disease is due to the deficiency of:
a. Hexoaminidase A (2006)
b. Sphingomyelinase
c. β-glucocerebrosidase
d. Galactocerebrosidase

100. Cirrhosis does not occur with: (2006)
a. Calcium
b. Copper
c. Alcohol
d. Iron

101. Following amino acid forms an integral part of collagen synthesis: (2006)
a. Lysine
b. Leucine
c. Arginine
d. Glutamic acid

102. Erythrocyte glutathione reductase deficiency is seen in deficiency of: (2006)
a. Riboflavin
b. Folic acid
c. Vitamin C
d. Vitamin E

103. Putrescine-a polyamine is formed by decarboxylation of: (2006)
a. Arginine
b. Ornithine
c. Citrulline
d. Adenine

ANSWERS AND EXPLANATIONS

1. Ans. a. Acts at the satiety center *Ref: Vasudevan DM, Sreekumari S, Textbook of Biochemistry 9/e p545*

GLUCAGON-LIKE PEPTIDES (GLP):

- Insulin production is 70% greater when glucose is administered orally than when similar blood concentrations were reached after intravenous administration of glucose; this increment is due to intestinal factors termed **incretins.**
- The most important incretins are **GLP1** and **GIP**. GLP1 and GLP2 are both secreted by enteroendocrine L cells in ileum, colon and central nervous system.
- GLP1 secretion is dependent on the presence of nutrients in the lumen of small intestine.
- It has an inhibitory effect on glucagon secretion and enhances glucose utilization after meals by stimulating insulin secretion.
- The incretin effect is by acting through second messengers in the beta cells to increase the sensitivity of these cells.
- GLP decreases food intake and its secretion is affected by oral ingestion of nutrients and vagal stimulation. Importantly, the incretin hormones also regulate the amount of nutrients ingested through their central action as satiety signals.
- Somatostatin has an inhibitory effect on GLP secretion.
- GLP is a good target for treating diabetes mellitus. GLP has a half-life of about 90 seconds, and newer drugs are being developed to increase the half-life to a few days.

2. Ans. a. Packs and sorts proteins *Ref: Vasudevan DM, Sreekumari S, Textbook of Biochemistry, 6/e p8*

Golgi Apparatus:

- The Golgi organelle is a network of flattened smooth membranes and vesicles. It may be considered as the converging area of endoplasmic reticulum.

- While moving through ER, carbohydrate groups are successively added to the nascent proteins. These glycoproteins reach the Golgi area.
- Golgi apparatus is composed of cis, medial and transcisternae. Glycoproteins are generally transported from ER to cis Golgi (proximal cisterna), then to medial Golgi (intermediate cisterna) and finally to trans-Golgi (distal cisterna) for temporary storage. Trans-Golgi are particularly abundant with vesicles containing glycoproteins. Newly synthesized proteins are sorted first according to the sorting signals available in the proteins. Then they are packed into transport vesicles having different types of coat proteins. Finally, they are transported into various destinations; this is an energy-dependent process.
- Main function of Golgi apparatus is proteinsorting, packaging and secretion.

3. Ans. b. Transamination

Ref: Vasudevan DM, Sreekumari S, Textbook of Biochemistry 6/e p396

Functions of Pyridoxal Phosphate:

- The pyridoxal phosphate (PLP) acts as a coenzyme for many reactions in amino acid metabolism.

(i) **Transamination:** These reactions are catalyzed by amino transferases (transaminases) which employ PLP as the coenzyme.
For example: Alanine + Alpha ketoglutarate → Pyruvate + Glutamic acid (Enzyme alanine transaminase).

(ii) **Decarboxylation:** All decarboxylation reactions of amino acids require PLP as coenzyme. A few examples are given below:
- Glutamate → GABA (gamma amino butyric acid). GABA is an inhibitory neurotransmitter, and, hence, in B6 deficiency, especially in children, **convulsions** may occur.
- Histidine → histamine, which is the mediator of **allergy** and anaphylaxis.
- 5-hydroxytryptophan → serotonin.

(iii) **Sulfur Containing Amino Acids**
PLP plays an important role in methionine and cysteine metabolism.
- Homocysteine + Serine → Cystathionine (Enzyme cystathionine synthase)
- Cystathionine → Homoserine + Cysteine (Enzyme cystathionase)

Both these reactions require PLP. Hence, in vitamin B6 deficiency, **homocysteine** in blood is increased. Homocysteine level is correlated with **myocardial infarction**. Therefore, pyridoxine is used to prevent homocysteinemia.

(iv) **Heme Synthesis:** ALA synthase is a PLP-dependent enzyme. This is the rate-limiting step in heme biosynthesis. So, in B6 deficiency, **anemia** may be seen.

(v) **Production of Niacin:** Pyridoxal phosphate is required for the synthesis of niacin from tryptophan (**one vitamin is necessary for synthesis of another vitamin**).
3-hydroxykynurenine → 3-hydroxyanthranilic acid (enzyme kynureninase).
Kynureninase is a PLPdependent enzyme. Hence, in vitamin B6 deficiency, niacin production is less. Moreover, kynurenine cannot be converted further, which is metabolized to xanthurenic acid and excreted through urine.

(vi) **Glycogenolysis: Phosphorylase** enzyme (glycogen to glucose-1-phosphate) requires PLP. In fact, more than 70% of total PLP content of the body is in muscles, where it is a part of the phosphorylase enzyme.

4. Ans. c. Pyridoxine

Ref: Vasudevan DM, Sreekumari S, Textbook of Biochemistry, 6/e p398

Requirement of B6

- Vitamin B6 requirements are related to protein intake and not to calorie intake.
- It is recommended that adults need 1 to 2 mg/day.
- During pregnancy and lactation, the requirement is increased to 2.5 mg/day.

Thiamine pyrophosphate is involved with carbohydrate metabolism.
Pyridoxal phosphate is involved in protein metabolism

5. Ans. c. Vitamin C *Ref: Vasudevan DM, Sreekumari S, Textbook of Biochemistry, 6/e p409*

Deficiency Manifestations of Vitamin C:

- **Scurvy**
  - Gross deficiency of vitamin C results in scurvy.
- **Infantile Scurvy (Barlow's Disease)**
  - In infants from 6 to 12 months of age (period in which weaning from breast milk), the diet should be supplemented with vitamin C sources. Otherwise, deficiency of vitamin C is seen.
- **Hemorrhagic Tendency**
  - In ascorbic acid deficiency, collagen is abnormal and the intercellular cement substance is brittle. So, capillaries are fragile, leading to the tendency to bleed even under minor pressure. Subcutaneous hemorrhage may be manifested as petechiae in mild deficiency and as ecchymoses or even hematoma in severe conditions. If a sphygmomanometer cuff is placed in the forearm, and the pressure is kept for 5 minutes, petechiae may be seen under the skin. This is a useful clinical test.
- **Internal Hemorrhage**
  - In severe cases, hemorrhage may occur in the conjunctiva and retina. Internal bleeding may be seen as epistaxis, hematuria or melena.
- **Oral Cavity**
  - In severe cases of scurvy, the gum becomes painful, swollen and spongy. The pulp is separated from the dentine and finally teeth are lost. Wound healing may be delayed.
- **Bones**
  - In the bones, the deficiency results in the failure of the osteoblasts to form the intercellular substance, osteoid. Without the normal ground substance, the deposition of bone is arrested. The resulting scorbutic bone is weak and fractures easily. There may be hemorrhage into joint cavities. Painful swelling of joints may prevent locomotion of the patient.
  - Vitamins C and B are essential nutrients to maintain bone density and bone quality. Recent literature clearly shows that vitamins C and B affect bone quality determinant "collagen cross-link formation". Mildly elevated plasma homocysteine levels induced by vitamin B insufficiency and methylenetetrahydrofolate reductase (MTHFR) deteriorate normal collagen cross-link formation.
- **Anemia**
  - In vitamin C deficiency, microcytic, hypochromic anemia is seen. Poikilocytosis and anisocytosis are also common in anemia due to deficiency of vitamin C. The reasons for anemia may be:
    - Loss of blood by hemorrhage
    - Decreased iron absorption
    - Decreased tetrahydrofolic acid
    - Accumulation of met-hemoglobin.

6. Ans. b. Folic acid *Ref: Mark's Textbook of Basic Medical Biochemistry, 3/e p755*

N5, N10-Methylene-Fh4 Reductase

- Folate deficiency during pregnancy has been associated with an increased risk of neural tube defects in the developing fetus. This risk is significantly reduced if women take folic acid supplements periconceptionally.
- The link between folate deficiency and neural tube defects was first observed in women with hyperhomocysteinemia brought about by a thermolabile variant of N5,N10-methylene-FH4 reductase.
- This form of the enzyme, which results from a single nucleotide change (C to T) in position 677 of the gene that encodes the protein, is less active at body temperature than at lower temperatures.
- This results in a reduced level of N5-methyl-FH4 being generated and, therefore, an increase in the levels of homocysteine.
- Along with the elevated homocysteine, the women were also folate-deficient. The folate deficiency and the subsequent inhibition of DNA synthesis lead to neural tube defects.
- The elevated homocysteine is one indication that such a deficit is present. These findings have led to the recommendation that women considering getting pregnant begin taking folate supplements before conception occurs, and for at least 1 month after conception.

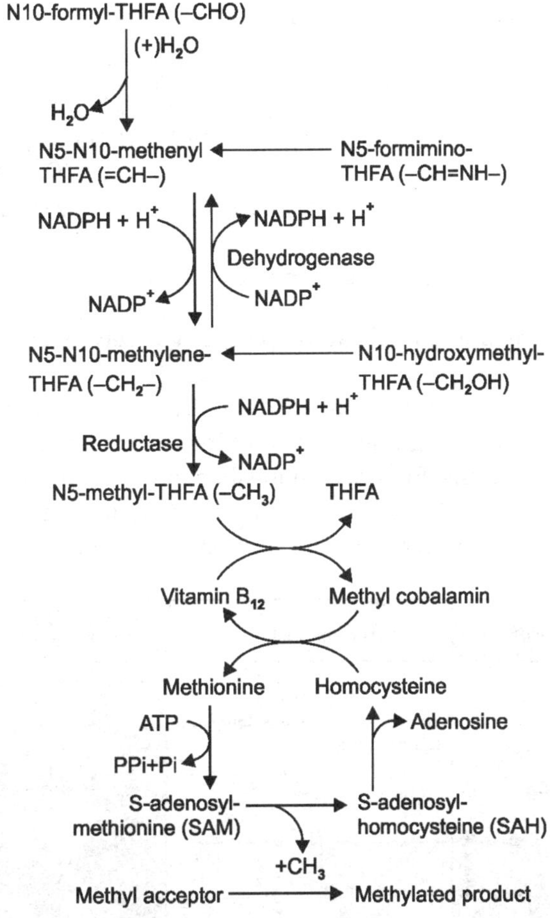

7. Ans. a. Body shunts more glutamine from liver to kidneys

Ref: Vasudevan DM, Sreekumari S, Textbook of Biochemistry, 6/e p345

Renal Regulation of pH:

- An important function of the kidney is to regulate the pH of the extracellular fluid. Normal urine has a pH around 6; this pH is lower than that of extracellular fluid (pH = 7.4). This is called **acidification of urine**. The pH of urine may vary from as low as 4.5 to as high as 9.8, depending on the amount of acid excreted. The major renal mechanisms for the regulation of pH are:
  - Excretion of H+
  - Reabsorption of bicarbonate (recovery of bicarbonate)
  - Excretion of titratable acid (net acid excretion)
  - Excretion of NH4+ (ammonium ions)

Excretion of Ammonium Ions:

- Predominantly occurs at the **distal convoluted tubules**. This would help to excrete H^+ and reabsorb HCO_3^-.
- This mechanism also helps to trap hydrogen ions in the urine, so that large quantity of acid may be excreted with minor changes in pH. The excretion of ammonia helps in the elimination of hydrogen ions without appreciable change in the pH of the urine.
- The **Glutaminase** present in the tubular cells can hydrolyze glutamine to ammonia and glutamic acid. The NH_3 (ammonia) diffuses into the luminal fluid and combines with H+ to form NH_4^+ (ammonium ion). The glutaminase activity in kidney is increased in acidosis. So, a large quantity of H+ ions is excreted as NH_4^+ in acidosis.

$$\text{Glutamine} + H_2O \xrightarrow{\text{Glutaminase}} \text{Glutamate} + NH_3$$

$$\text{Glutamate} + NAD^{\oplus} \xrightarrow{\text{Glutamate dehydrogenase}} \text{2-Oxoglutarate} + NADH + NH_4^{\oplus}$$

$$NH_4^{\oplus} \rightleftharpoons NH_3 + H^{\oplus}$$

- Since it is a positively charged ion, it can accompany negatively charged acid anions; so Na+ and K+ are conserved.
- Normally, about 70 mEq/L of acid is excreted daily; but in condition of acidosis, this can rise to 400 mEq/day. The enhanced activity of glutaminase and increased excretion of NH4+ takes about 3-4 days to set in under conditions of acidosis. But once established, it has high capacity to eliminate acid.
- Ammonia is estimated in urine after addition of formaldehyde. The titratable acidity plus the ammonia content will be a measure of acid excreted from the body. Maximum urine acidity reached is 4.4.

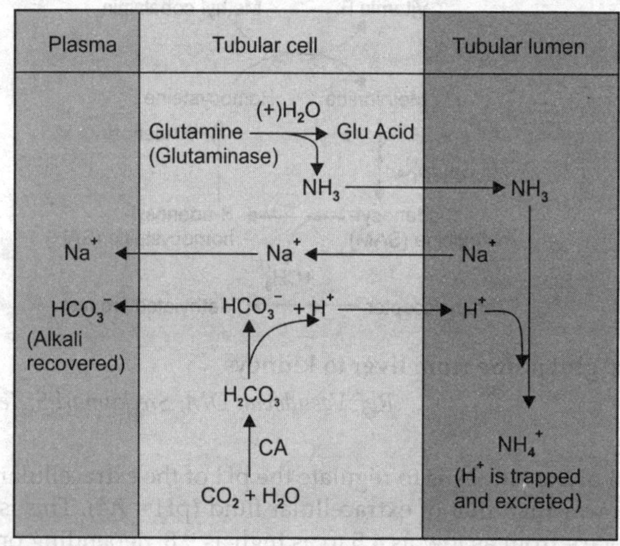

8. Ans. b. Chromium *Ref: Vasudevan DM, Sreekumari S, Textbook of Biochemistry, 6/e p431*

Chromium (Cr)

- Trivalent and hexavalent atoms of chromium are biologically active.
- Total body content of chromium is 6 mg, and this decreases with age.
- Daily requirement is 30 micrograms. Blood level of chromium is 25 nanogram/dl.
- Affinity of chromium for transferrin is the same as that of iron, and the two ions compete for binding to the protein.
- **In chromium deficiency, glucose tolerance is impaired. The efficiency of binding of insulin to its receptors on the peripheral cells is improved by chromium.**
- Deficiency also leads to impaired growth, decrease in fertility and sperm count.

9. Ans. c. Alkaline phosphatase *Ref: Vasudevan DM, Sreekumari S, Textbook of Biochemistry, 6/e p429*

ZINC (Zn):

- Total zinc content of body is about 2 g, out of which 60% is in skeletal muscles and 30% in bones. Highest concentration of zinc is seen in hippocampus area of brain and prostatic secretion.
- **Rich dietary sources** are grains, beans, nuts, cheese, meat and shellfish. Copper, calcium, cadmium, iron and phytate will interfere with the absorption of zinc. Zinc and copper will competitively inhibit each other's absorption. So, zinc is therapeutically useful to reduce copper absorption in Wilson's disease.

- In liver, zinc is stored in combination with a specific protein, **metallothionein**. Zinc is excreted through pancreatic juice and, to a lesser extent, through sweat.
- More than **300 enzymes** are zinc-dependent. Some important ones are carboxypeptidase, carbonic anhydrase, alkaline phosphatase, lactate dehydrogenase, alcohol dehydrogenase and glutamate dehydrogenase. RNA polymerase contains zinc and so it is required for **protein biosynthesis**. Extracellular superoxide dismutase is zincdependent and so zinc has an **antioxidant** activity.
- **Insulin** when stored in the beta cells of pancreas contains zinc, which stabilizes the hormone molecule. But the insulin released into the blood does not contain zinc. The commercially available preparation, protamin-zinc-insulinate (PZI) also contains zinc.
- Zinc containing protein, **Gusten**, in saliva is important for taste sensation.

Zinc-Deficiency Manifestations:

- Poor wound healing, lesions of skin, impaired spermatogenesis, hyperkeratosis, dermatitis and alopecia are deficiency manifestations of zinc.
- There is reduction in number of T and B lymphocytes. Macrophage function is retarded.
- Zinc deficiency leads to depression, dementia and other psychiatric disorders.
- Zinc binds with amyloid to form a plaque in **Alzheimer's** disease.

Acrodermatitis Enteropathica:

- It is a recessive condition where zinc absorption is defective and is characterized by acrodermatitis (inflammation around mouth, nose, fingers, etc.), diarrhea, alopecia (loss of hair in discrete areas), ophthalmoplegia and hypogonadism.

Requirement of Zinc:

- For adults is 10 mg/day; children 10 mg/day; in pregnancy and lactation 15-20 mg/day. Since iron inhibits absorption of zinc, when iron is supplemented, zinc is also given to prevent any deficiency.

10. Ans. c. Keratan sulfate

GAG:

They are linear and unbranched heteropolysaccharides.

Basically have repeating units of an amino sugar and an uronic acid.

GAG	Amino sugar	Acidic sugars
Hyaluronic acid	N acetyl glucosamine	Glucuronic acid
Chondroitin SO_4	N acetyl galactosamine	Glucuronic acid
Keratan SO_4	N acetyl glucosamine	Galactose
Dermatan SO_4	N acetyl galactosamine	Iduronic acid
Heparan SO_4	Glucosamine	Glucuronic acid
Heparin	Glucosamine	Iduronic acid

Exceptions:

- GAG without uronic acid: Keratan SO_4
- GAG without SO_4: Hyaluronic acid
- Galactose containing GAG: Keratan SO_4
- GAG which is not attached covalently to proteins: Hyaluronic acid
- GAG with nonacetylated amino sugar: Heparan SO_4, Heparin.

11. Ans. a. Plasminogen *Ref: Vasudevan DM, Sreekumari S, Textbook of Biochemistry 6/e p155*

Lipoprotein (a)

- Lipoprotein (a) is very strongly associated with myocardial infarction and is sometimes called the "little rascal".
- Lp (a), when present, is attached to apo-B-100 by a disulfide bond.
- In 40% population, there is no detectable level of Lp (a) in serum. In 20% of population, the Lp (a) concentration in blood is more than 30 mg/dl; and these persons are susceptible for heart attack at a younger age.
- Lp (a) is associated with heart attacks at the age of 30 or 40 years. Indians have a higher level of Lp (a) than western populations.

- **Lp (a) has significant homology with plasminogen. So, it interferes with plasminogen activation and impairs fibrinolysis. This leads to unopposed intravascular thrombosis** and possible myocardial infarction.

12. Ans. Lipoprotein lipase *Ref: Vasudevan DM, Sreekumari S, Textbook of Biochemistry, 6/e p153*

- The enzyme **lipoprotein lipase** (LpL) is located at the endothelial layer of capillaries of adipose tissue, muscles and heart; but not in liver.
- **Apo C-II** present in the chylomicrons activates the LpL.
- The LpL hydrolyzes triglycerides present in chylomicrons into fatty acids and glycerol. Muscle or adipose tissue cells take up the liberated fatty acids.
- Following injection of **heparin**, the LpL is released from the tissues and lipemia is thus cleared. This is called **post-heparin lipolytic activity.**
- Lack of C-II leads to decreased activity of LpL and consequent accumulation of chylomicrons and VLDL in blood.
- **Insulin** increases LpL activity.

13. Ans. b. Phosphoribosyl pyrophosphate amidotransferase

Ref: Lippincott Illustrated Reviews Biochemistry 4/e p293

Synthesis of Purine Nucleotides:

- The atoms of the purine ring are contributed by a number of compounds, including amino acids (aspartic acid, glycine, and glutamine), CO_2, and N10-formyltetrahydrofolate.
- The purine ring is constructed by a series of reactions that add the donated carbons and nitrogens to a preformed ribose 5-phosphate.

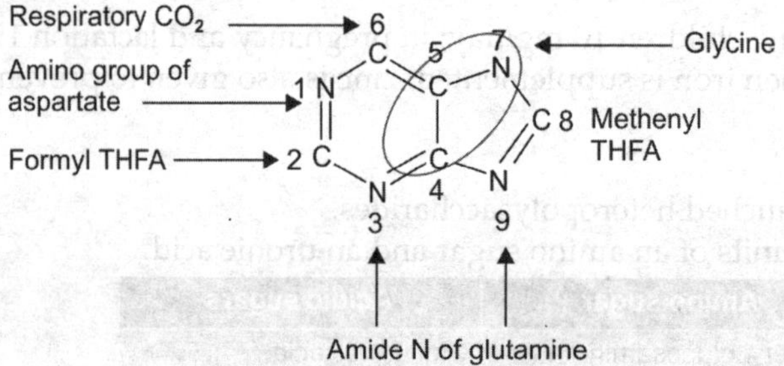

A. Synthesis of 5-Phosphoribosyl-1-Pyrophosphate (PRPP)

- PRPP is an "activated pentose" that participates in the synthesis and salvage of purines and pyrimidines.
- Synthesis of PRPP from ATP and ribose 5-phosphate is catalyzed by PRPP synthetase (ribose phosphate pyrophosphokinase).
- This X-linked enzyme is activated by inorganic phosphate and inhibited by purine nucleotides (end-product inhibition).

B. Synthesis of 5′-Phosphoribosylamine

- Synthesis of 5′-phosphoribosylamine from PRPP and glutamine. The amide group of glutamine replaces the pyrophosphate group attached to carbon 1 of PRPP.
- The enzyme, glutamine: phosphoribosyl pyrophosphate amidotransferase, is inhibited by the purine 5′-nucleotides AMP, GMP, and inosine monophosphate (IMP)—the end products of the pathway.
- **This is the committed step in purine nucleotide biosynthesis.** The rate of the reaction is also controlled by the intracellular concentration of PRPP.

14. Ans. b. Binding to tRNA to ribosomes *Ref: Vasudevan DM, Sreekumari S, Textbook of Biochemistry, 6/e p487*

Transfer RNA (tRNA) or (sRNA):

- They transfer amino acids from cytoplasm to the ribosomal protein synthesizing machinery; hence the name transfer RNA.
- Since they are easily soluble, they are also referred to as **soluble RNA** or sRNA. They are RNA molecules present in the cytoplasm.
- Each molecule is only 73–93 nucleotides in length; much shorter than mRNA molecules.
- When transcribed, the tRNA molecules are large and they undergo post-transcriptional modifications.

A. Structure of tRNA Molecule:

- The transfer RNAs show extensive internal base pairing and acquire **clover leaf**-like structure.
- They contain a significant proportion of **unusual bases**. These include dihydrouracil (DHU), pseudouridine and hypoxanthine. Moreover, many bases are methylated.

B. Acceptor Arm is at the 3′ End

- It carries the amino acid. This area has 7 base pairs. The end sequence is **CCA-3′**. The 3′ end hydroxyl group is forming an ester bond with the carboxyl end of amino acids.

C. Anticodon Arm of tRNA

- At the opposite side of the acceptor arm is the anticodon arm. It recognizes the triplet nucleotide codon present in mRNA. The specificity of tRNA resides in the anticodon site, which has base sequences complementary to that of mRNA codon.
- The tRNA molecule will show specificity in both aspects; in recognizing the mRNA codon as well as in accepting the specific amino acid coded by that codon. In this way, the tRNA molecules play a pivotal role in translation.
- The tRNAs act as **adapter molecules** between mRNA and the amino acids coded by it. The nucleotides of codons have no affinity for amino acids. So, the tRNA molecules act as mediators between the mRNA and amino acids.

D. DHU Arm of tRNA

- The D arm or DHU region is so named due to the presence of a **dihydrouridine** in that area. The DHU arm serves as the recognition site for the enzyme which adds the amino acid.

E. Pseudouridine Arm of tRNA

- The opposite arm is called pseudouridine arm, as it contains a pseudouridine. It is generally pronounced as "psi". It is involved in binding tRNA to ribosomes. About 75% of tRNA molecules possess a short extra arm, about 3 to 5 base pairs long and they belong to Class 1. The tRNA molecules belonging to Class 2 have a long extra arm, 13 to 21 base pairs in length.

15. Ans. d. Heating around 100 °C *Ref: Vasudevan DM, Sreekumari S, Textbook of Biochemistry, 6/e p616*

Polymerase Chain Reaction (PCR):

- PCR is an in vitro DNA amplification procedure in which millions of copies of a particular sequence of DNA can be produced within a few hours. The flanking sequences of the gene of interest should be known. Two DNA primers of about 20–30 nucleotides with complementary sequence of the flanking region can be synthesized. The reaction cycle has the following steps:

  Step 1: Separation (Denaturation):
  - DNA strands are separated **(melted)** by heating at 95°C for 15 seconds to 2 minutes.

  Step 2: Priming (Annealing):
  - The primers are **annealed** by cooling to 50°C for 0.5 to 2 minutes. The primers hybridize with their complementary single-stranded DNA produced in the first step.

  Step 3: Polymerization:
  - New DNA strands are synthesized by **Taq polymerase**. This enzyme is derived from bacteria *Thermus aquaticus* that are found in hot springs. Therefore, the enzyme is not denatured at high temperature. The polymerase reaction is allowed to take place at 72°C for 30 seconds in the presence of dNTPs (all four deoxyribonucleotide triphosphates). Both strands of DNA are now duplicated.

  4. The steps of 1, 2 and 3 are **repeated**. In each cycle, the DNA strands are doubled. Thus, 20 cycles provide for 1 million times amplifications. These cycles are generally repeated by automated instrument.
  5. After the amplification procedure, DNA hybridization technique or Southern blot analysis with a suitable probe shows the presence of the DNA in the sample tissue.

Clinical Applications of PCR

- **Diagnosis of Bacterial and Viral Diseases:**
  - In early phases of tuberculosis, the sputum may contain only very few tubercle bacilli, so that usual acid fast staining may be negative. But PCR could detect even one bacillus present in the specimen.

Any other bacterial infection could also be detected similarly. The specific nucleotide sequences of the bacilli are amplified by PCR and then detected by Southern blot analysis. If reverse PCR is done, living organisms could be detected. This technique is widely used in the diagnosis of viral infections like Hepatitis C, cytomegalovirus and HIV.

- **Medicolegal Cases:**
  - PCR allows the DNA from a hair follicle or a blood cell to be analyzed. The restriction analysis of DNA from the hair follicle from the crime scene is studied after PCR amplification. This pattern is then compared with the restriction analysis of DNA samples obtained from various suspects; the culprit's sample will perfectly match with that of PCR-amplified sample. The restriction analysis pattern of DNA of one individual will be very specific (DNA fingerprinting); but the pattern will be different from person to person. This is highly useful in forensic medicine to identify the criminal.
- Diagnosis of **genetic disorders**: The PCR technology has been widely used to amplify the gene segments that contain known mutations for diagnosis of inherited diseases, such as sickle cell anemia, beta thalassemia, cystic fibrosis, etc.
- PCR is especially useful for **prenatal diagnosis** of inherited diseases, where cells obtained from fetus by amniocentesis are very few.
- **Cancer detection:** PCR is widely used to monitor residual abnormal cells present in treated patients. Similarly, identification of mutations in oncosuppressor genes, such as p53, retinoblastoma gene, etc. can help to identify individuals at high risk of cancer (oncogenes and oncosuppressor genes).
- Fossil studies: DNA can be isolated and PCR amplified from fossils to be used to study evolution by comparing the sequences in the extinct and living organisms.

16. Ans. a. RNA *Ref: Harper's Illustrated Biochemistry 28/e p393*

Techniques	Used for
Northern blot	RNA analysis
Southern blot	DNA analysis
Western blot	Protein analysis

17. Ans. b. RBC *Ref: Lippincott's Biochemistry 4/e p196*

Ketone Bodies:

- **Liver mitochondria** have the capacity to convert acetyl CoA derived from fatty acid oxidation into ketone bodies.
- The compounds categorized as ketone bodies are **acetoacetate, 3-hydroxybutyrate (also called β-hydroxybutyrate), and acetone.**
- Acetoacetate and 3-hydroxybutyrate are transported in the blood to the peripheral tissues. There they can be reconverted to acetyl CoA, which can be oxidized by the TCA cycle.

  Ketone bodies are important sources of energy for the peripheral tissues because:
  - They are soluble in aqueous solution and, therefore, do not need to be incorporated into lipoproteins or carried by albumin as do the other lipids.
  - They are produced in the liver during periods when the amount of acetyl CoA present exceeds the oxidative capacity of the liver; and
  - They are used in proportion to their concentration in the blood by extrahepatic tissues, such as the skeletal and cardiac muscle and renal cortex. Even the brain can use ketone bodies to help meet its energy needs if the blood levels rise sufficiently. Thus, ketone bodies spare glucose.

Use of Ketone Bodies by the Peripheral Tissues: Ketolysis

- Although the liver constantly synthesizes low levels of ketone bodies, their production becomes much more significant during fasting when ketone bodies are needed to provide energy to the peripheral tissues.
- 3-Hydroxybutyrate is oxidized to acetoacetate by 3-hydroxybutyrate dehydrogenase, producing NADH.
- Acetoacetate is then provided with a CoA molecule taken from succinyl CoA by succinyl CoA: acetoacetate CoA transferase (thiophorase). This reaction is reversible, but the product, acetoacetyl CoA, is actively removed by its conversion to two acetyl CoAs.

- Extrahepatic tissues, including the brain but excluding cells lacking mitochondria (for example, red blood cells), efficiently oxidize acetoacetate and 3-hydroxybutyrate in this manner.
- In contrast, although the liver actively produces ketone bodies, it lacks thiophorase and, therefore, is unable to use ketone bodies as fuel.

Ketone bodies are not utilized by RBC because of the lack of mitochondria.

Substrate utilized for energy production:

Tissue	Fed	Fasting	Starvation
Brain	Glucose	Glucose	Ketone bodies
Heart	Fatty acids	Fatty acids	Ketone bodies
Liver	Glucose	Fatty acids	Amino acids
Muscle	Glucose	Fatty acids	Fatty acids

18. Ans. b. Glucose 6-phosphatase *Ref: Harper's Illustrated Biochemistry 26/e p153*

- The conversion of glucose 6-phosphate to **glucose is catalyzed by glucose 6-phosphatase.** It is present in liver and kidney but absent from muscle and adipose tissue, which, therefore, cannot export glucose into the bloodstream.

Thiophorase

- The liver actively produces ketone bodies. It lacks thiophorase and, therefore, is unable to use ketone bodies as fuel.

Glycogen Phosphorylase

- Glycogen phosphorylase catalyzes the rate-limiting step in glycogenolysis by promoting the phosphorylytic cleavage by inorganic phosphate (phosphorylysis; of hydrolysis) of the 1 → 4 linkages of glycogen to yield glucose 1-phosphate.
- The terminal glucosyl residues from the outermost chains of the glycogen molecule are removed sequentially until approximately four glucose residues remain on either side of a 1 → 6 branch.
- Another enzyme **glucan transferase**) transfers a trisaccharide unit from one branch to the other, exposing the 1 → 6 branch point. **Hydrolysis** of the 1 → 6 linkages requires the **debranching enzyme.**
- Further phosphorylase action can then proceed. The combined action of phosphorylase and these other enzymes leads to the complete breakdown of glycogen. The reaction catalyzed by phosphoglucomutase is reversible, so that glucose 6-phosphate can be formed from glucose 1-phosphate.
- In **liver** (and **kidney**), but not in muscle, there is a specific enzyme, **glucose 6-phosphatase**, that hydrolyzes glucose 6-phosphate, yielding glucose that is exported, leading to an increase in the blood glucose concentration.

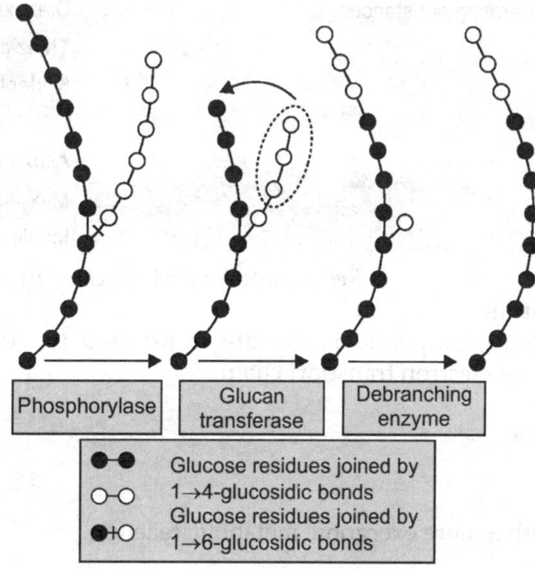

19. Ans. b. Telomerase *Ref: Vasudevan DM, Sreekumari S, Textbook of Biochemistry 6/e p480*

20. Ans. a. It is a reverse transcriptase *Ref: Vasudevan DM, Sreekumari S, Textbook of Biochemistry 6/e p480*

Telomere and Telomerase

- The replication always takes place from 5′ to 3′ direction in the new strand. The DNA polymerase enzyme is not able to synthesize the new strand at the 5′ end of the new strand. In other words, a small portion (about 300 nucleotides) in the *3′ ends of the parent strands could not be replicated.*
- This end piece of the chromosome is called **telomere**. Therefore, another enzyme, *telomere terminal transferase* or **telomerase** takes up this job of replication of the end piece of chromosomes.
- After the normal replication, there is only one single strand in this region; so this portion is degraded by exonucleases. This broken end leads to aberrant recombinations or end-to-end fusions. Unless there is some mechanism to replicate telomeres, the length of the chromosomes will go on reducing at each cell division (genes loss). The stability of the chromosome is thus lost.
- The shortening of telomere end is prevented by an enzyme *telomere terminal transferase* or **telomerase**. It contains an essential RNA component, which provides the template for telomerase repeat synthesis.
- ***Telomerase acts like a reverse transcriptase***. Telomerase recognises 3′ end of telomere, and then a small DNA strand is synthesized.
- Terminal restriction fragments from 70-year-old donors are shorter than those from 20-year-old ones. Thus, in **old age**, the telomerase activity is lost; leading to chromosome instability and cell death.
- **Cancer cells** have continued presence of telomerase, and the chromosome length equilibrium is maintained, leading to continued cell division. As cancer cells have increased and persistent activity of telomerase, the cancer cells become immortal. Premature shortening of telomeres is seen in some types of aplastic anemia.

21. Ans. b. Hypokalemia *Ref: Ganong's Physiology 24/e p441*

Factors Affecting Insulin Secretion	
Stimulators	**Inhibitors**
Glucose	Somatostatin
Mannose	2-Deoxyglucose
Amino acids (leucine, arginine, others)	Mannoheptulose
Intestinal hormones (GIP, GLP-1 [7–36], gastrin, secretin, CCK;)	-Adrenergic stimulators (norepinephrine, epinephrine)
-Keto acids	-Adrenergic blockers (propranolol)
Acetylcholine	
Glucagon	Galanin
Cyclic AMP and various cAMP-generating substances	Diazoxide
	Thiazide diuretics
-Adrenergic stimulators	K^+ depletion
Theophylline	Phenytoin
Sulfonylureas	Alloxan
	Microtubule inhibitors
	Insulin

22. Ans. b. Phosphofructokinase *Ref: Vasudevan DM, Sreekumari S, Textbook of Biochemistry 6/e p224.*

Substrate Level Phosphorylation

The energy from a high-energy compound is directly transferred to nucleoside diphosphate to form a triphosphate without the help of electron transport chain.

For example:

- Bisphospho glycerate kinase
- Pyruvate kinase
- Succinate thiokinase

ATP generation is coupled with a more exergonic metabolic reaction.

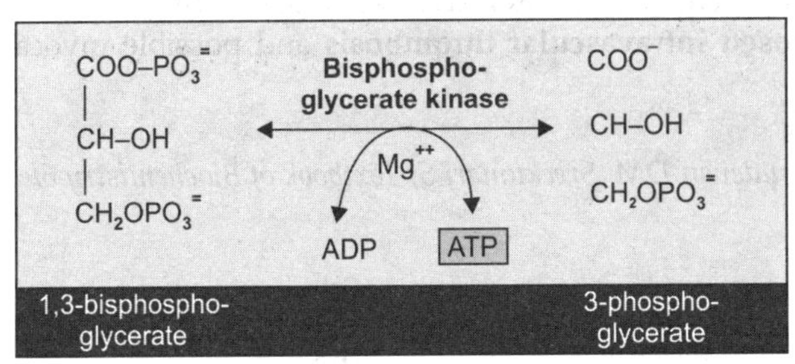

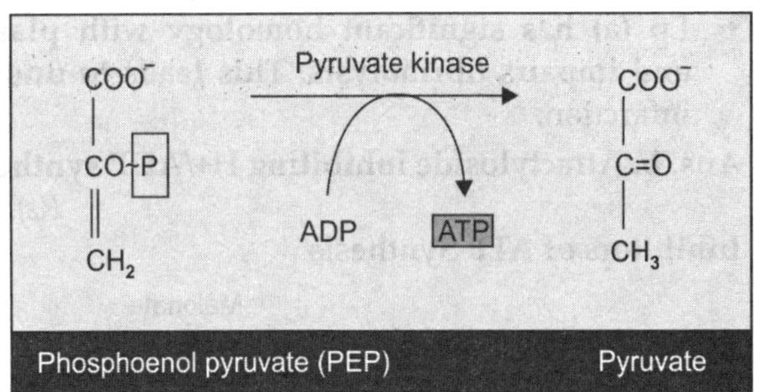

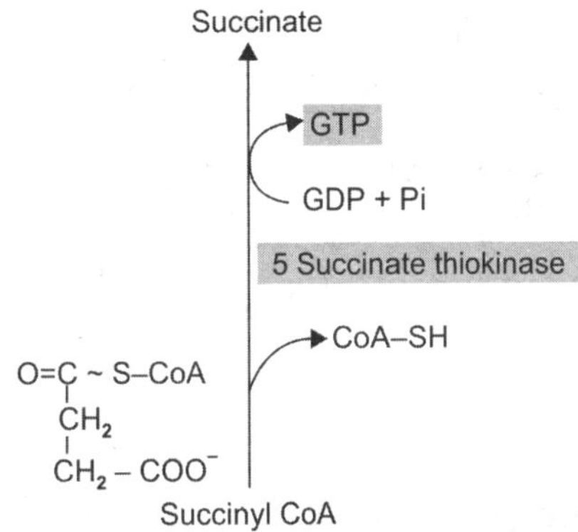

ATP Formation in the Catabolism of Glucose (Malate Shuttle)			
Pathway	**Reaction catalyzed by**	**Method of ATP formation**	**ATP per Mol of Glucose**
Glycolysis	Glyceraldehydes 3-phosphate dehydrogenase	Respiratory chain oxidation of 2 NADH	5
	Phosphoglycerate kinase	**Substrate level phosphorylation**	2
	Pyruvate kinase	**Substrate level phosphorylation**	2
			10
			–2
			Net 7
Citric acid cycle	Pyruvate dehydrogenase	Respiratory chain oxidation of 2 NADH	5
	Isocitrate dehydrogenase	Respiratory chain oxidation of 2 NADH	5
	α-Ketoglutarate dehydrogenase	Respiratory chain oxidation of 2 NADH	5
	Succinate thiokinase	**Substrate level phosphorylation**	2
	Succinate dehydrogenase	Respiratory chain oxidation of 2 FADH2	3
	Malate dehydrogenase	Respiratory chain oxidation of 2 NADH	5
			Net 25
	Total per mol of glucose under aerobic conditions		32
	Total per mol of glucose under aeroic conditions		2

23. Ans. a. Plasminogen *Ref: Vasudevan DM, Sreekumari S, Textbook of Biochemistry 6/e p155*

Lipoprotein (a)

- Lipoprotein (a) is very strongly associated with myocardial infarction and is sometimes called the "little rascal".
- Lp (a), when present, is attached to apo-B-100 by a disulfide bond.
- In 40% population, there is no detectable level of Lp (a) in serum. In 20% of population, the Lp (a) concentration in blood is more than 30 mg/dl; and these persons are susceptible to heart attack at a younger age.
- Lp (a) is associated with heart attacks at the age of 30 or 40 years. Indians have a higher level of Lp (a) than western populations.

- **Lp (a) has significant homology with plasminogen. So, it interferes with plasminogen activation and impairs fibrinolysis. This leads to unopposed intravascular thrombosis** and possible myocardial infarction.

24. Ans. b. Atractyloside inhibiting H+/ADP synthesis

Ref: Vasudevan DM, Sreekumari S, Textbook of Biochemistry 6/e p234

Inhibitors of ATP Synthesis

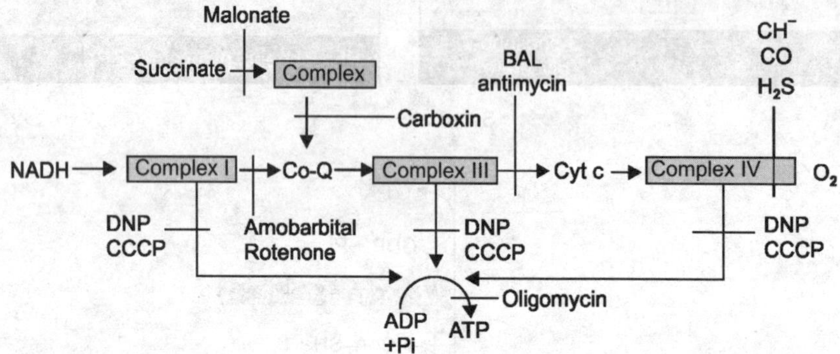

A. Site-specific Inhibitors

1. Complex I to Co-Q-specific inhibitors
- Alkylguanides (guanethide), hypotensive drug
- Rotenone, insecticide and fish poison
- Barbiturates (amobarbital), sedative
- Chlorpromazine, tranquilizer
- Piericidin, antibiotic

2. Complex II to Co-Q
- Carboxin

3. Complex III to cytochrome c inhibitors
- BAL (British anti-Lewisite), antidote of war gas
- Naphthoquinone
- Antimycin

4. Complex IV inhibitors
- Carbon monoxide, inhibits cellular respiration
- Cyanide (CN–)
- Azide (N3–)
- Hydrogen sulfide (H2S)

5. Site between succinate dehydrogenase and Co-Q
- Carboxin, inhibits transfer of ions from FADH2
- Malonate, competitive inhibitor of succinate DH

6. Inhibitors of oxidative phosphorylation
- Atractyloside, inhibits translocase
- Oligomycin, inhibits flow of protons through Fo
- Ionophores, e.g. Valinomycin

7. Uncouplers
- 2,4-dinitrophenol (2,4-DNP)
- 2,4-dinitrocresol (2,4-DNC)
- CCCP (chlorocarbonylcyanidephenyl hydrazone)

8. Physiological uncouplers
- Thyroxine, in high doses
- Thermogenin in brown adipose tissue

B. Inhibitors of Oxidative Phosphorylation

- **Atractyloside** inhibits the translocase where as **oligomycin** inhibits the Fo.
- Ionophores are lipid soluble compounds that increase the permeability of lipid bilayers to certain ions. There are two types of ionophores; mobile ion carries (e.g. **valinomycin**) and channel formers (e.g. **gramicidin**). Valinomycin allows potassium to permeate mitochondria and dissipate the proton gradient.
- The toxicity of cyanide is due to its inhibitory effect on the terminal cytochrome which brings cellular respiration to a standstill.

C. Uncouplers of Oxidative Phosphorylation

- Uncouplers will allow oxidation to proceed, but the energy instead of being trapped by phosphorylation is dissipated as heat. This is achieved by removal of the proton gradient. The uncoupling of oxidative phosphorylation is useful biologically. In hibernating animals and in newborn human infants, the liberation of heat energy is required to maintain body temperature.
- In brown adipose tissue, thermogenesis is achieved by this process. Thermogenin, a protein present in the inner mitochondrial membrane of adipocytes, provides an alternate pathway for protons. It is one of the uncoupling proteins (UCP). Thyroxine is also known to act as a physiological uncoupler.

25. Ans. c. Liver *Ref: Harper's Illustrated Biochemistry 28/e p171*

Glucose Transporters:

Major glucose transporters		
	Tissue Location	Functions
FACILITATIVE BIDIRECTIONAL TRANSPORTERS		
GLUT 1	Brain, kidney, colon, placenta, erythrocytes	Glucose uptake
GLUT 2	Liver, pancreatic cell, small intestine, kidney	Rapid uptake or release of glucose
GLUT 3	Brain, kidney, placenta	Glucose uptake
GLUT 4	Heart and skeletal muscle, adipose tissue	Insulin-stimulated glucose uptake
GLUT 5	Small intestine	Absorption of glucose
SODIUM-DEPENDENT UNIDIRECTIONAL TRANSPORTER		
SGLT 1	Small intestine and kidney	Active uptake of glucose against a concentration gradient

Glucose Transporter 4

- GluT4 is the major glucose transporter in **skeletal muscle and adipose tissue.**
- GluT4 is under the control of insulin. But other glucose transporters are not under the control of insulin.

Clinical application: Insulin induces the movement of intracellular GluT4 molecules to the cell surface and thus increases glucose uptake. In Type 2 **diabetes mellitus**, membrane GluT4 is reduced, leading to insulin resistance in muscle and fat cells. In diabetes, entry of glucose into muscle is only half of normal cells.

26. Ans. b. Contraindicated in hyperthyroidism

Ref: Harper, Vasudevan and Sreekumari; Textbook of Medical Biochemistry 6/e p539

"The thyroglobulin contains about 8 T4 residues per molecule. It is stored as colloid in the thyroid acini.The T4 is liberated by hydrolysis by specific proteases. This activity is markedly enhanced by TSH. This hydrolysis is depressed by **iodide** and, therefore, potassium iodide (Kl) is used as an adjuvant in hyperthyroidism."

"In normal individuals, large doses of iodide act directly on the thyroid gland to produce a mild and transient inhibition of organic binding of iodide and, hence, of hormone synthesis. This inhibition is called ***WOLF-CHAIKOFF EFFECT***."

- The thyroid hormones T3 and T4 are unique in that iodine (as iodide) is an essential component of both. In most parts of the world, iodine is a scarce component of soil, and for that reason, there is little in food.
- Thyroglobulin is the precursor of T4 and T3. It is a large iodinated, glycosylated protein with a molecular mass of 660 kDa. Carbohydrate accounts for 8–10% of the weight of thyroglobulin and iodide for about 0.2–1%, depending upon the iodine content in the diet.

- Thyroglobulin is composed of two large subunits. It contains 115 tyrosine residues, each of which is a potential site of iodination. About 70% of the iodide in thyroglobulin exists in the inactive precursors, monoiodotyrosine (MIT) and diiodotyrosine (DIT), while 30% is in the iodothyronyl residues, T4 and T3.
- When iodine supplies are sufficient, the T4:T3 ratio is about 7:1. In iodine deficiency, this ratio decreases, as does the DIT:MIT ratio.
- Thyroglobulin, a large molecule of about 5000 amino acids, provides the conformation required for tyrosyl coupling and iodide organification necessary in the formation of the diaminoacid thyroid hormones.
- Thyroid hormones is synthesized in the basal portion of the cell and moves to the lumen, where it is a storage form of T3 and T4 in the colloid; several weeks' supply of these hormones exists in the normal thyroid.
- Within minutes after stimulation of the thyroid by TSH, colloid re-enters the cell and there is a marked increase of phagolysosome activity.
- Various acid proteases and peptidases hydrolyze the thyroglobulin into its constituent amino acids, including T4 and T3, which are discharged from the basal portion of the cel. Thyroglobulin is thus a very large prohormone.

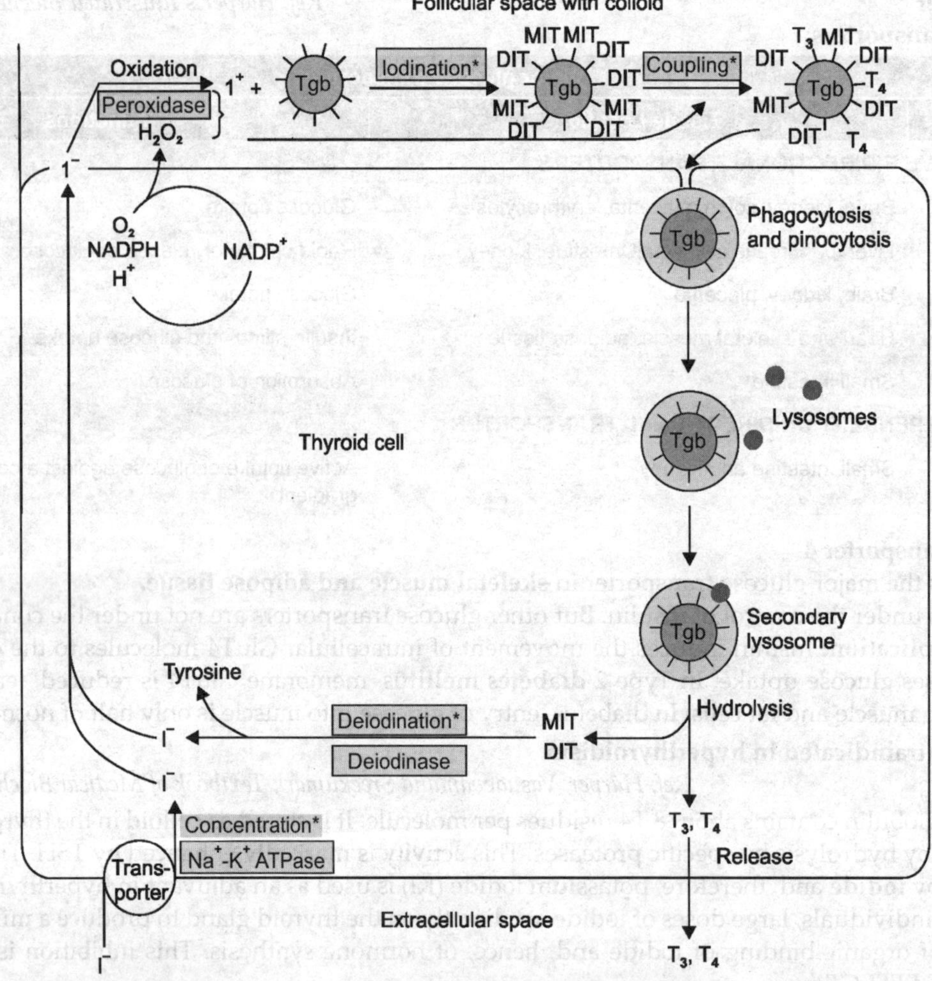

27. Ans. b. Low km-High affinity *Ref: Vasudevan DM, Sreekumari S, Textbook of Biochemistry, 6/e p50*

Salient features of Km:

- **Km value is substrate concentration** (expressed in moles/L) **at half-maximal velocity.**
- **It denotes that 50% of enzyme molecules are bound with substrate molecules at that particular substrate concentration.**

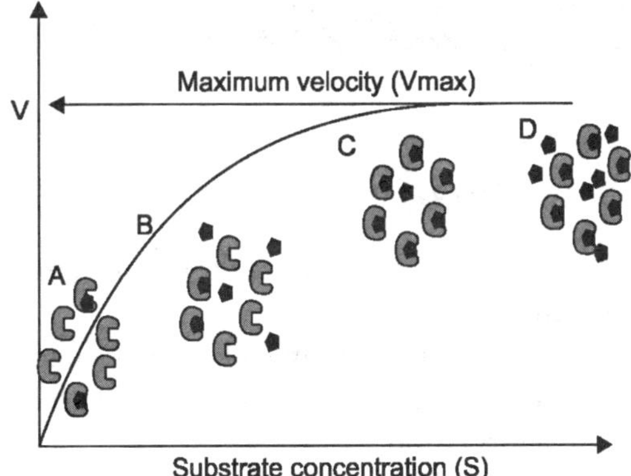

Enzyme molecules are shown as half-circles. Substrate molecules are red dots. (A) Substrate molecules are low; so only a few enzyme molecules are working and velocity is less. (B) At half-maximal velocity (Km), 50% enzyme molecules are bound with substrate. (C) As a lot of substrate molecules are available, all enzyme molecules are bound. (D) Further increase in the substrate will not increase the velocity further.

- **Km is independent of enzyme concentration.** If enzyme concentration is doubled, the Vmax will be double. But the Km will remain the exactly same. In other words, irrespective of enzyme concentration, 50% molecules are bound to substrate at that particular substrate concentration.

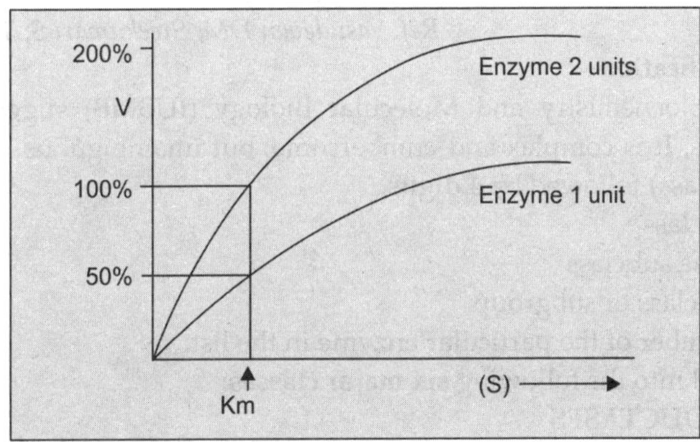

- **Km is the Signature of the Enzyme.** Km value is thus a constant for an enzyme. It is the **characteristic feature of a particular enzyme** for a specific substrate.
- The **affinity of an enzyme** towards its substrate **is inversely related** to the dissociation constant, Kd for the enzyme-substrate complex.

$$E+S \underset{K2}{\overset{K1}{\longrightarrow}} E\text{–}S \text{ complex} \overset{K3}{\longrightarrow} E+P$$

$$Kd = \frac{K2}{K1} \text{ and } Km = \frac{K2 + K3}{K1}$$

Therefore, the smaller the tendency for the dissociation of the complex, the greater is the affinity of the enzyme for the substrate.

- **Km denotes the affinity of enzyme for substrate.** The *lesser the numerical value of Km, the more the affinity of the enzyme for the substrate.*

Comparison of two types of inhibition		
	Competitive Inhibition	**Noncompetitive Inhibition**
Acting on	Active site	May or may not
Structure of inhibitor	Substrate analog	Unrelated molecule
Inhibition is	Reversible	Generally irreversible
Excess substrate	Inhibition relieved	No effect

Contd...

	Competitive Inhibition	Noncompetitive Inhibition
Km	Increased	No change
Vmax	No change	Decreased
Significance	Drug action	Toxicological

28. Ans. d. Hypothyroidism *Ref: Vasudevan DM, Sreekumari S, Textbook of Biochemistry, 6/e p540*

Metabolic Effects of Thyroid Hormones

- The hormone exerts action on every cell of the body. Calorigenic effect or thermogenesis is the major effect of thyroid hormone. One mg of T4 will produce an excess of 1000 kcal. This thermogenic effect is mediated by uncoupling of oxidative phosphorylation.
- Basal metabolic rate (BMR) is increased. Thyroxine increases cellular metabolism.
- Earliest effect of T4 is stimulation of RNA synthesis and consequent increase in protein synthesis. Higher concentration of T3 causes protein catabolism and negative nitrogen balance.
- Loss of body weight is a prominent feature of hyperthyroidism.
- Gluconeogenesis and carbohydrate oxidation are increased. Glucose tolerance test shows rapid absorption.
- Fatty acid metabolism is increased. Cholesterol degradation is increased and hence cholesterol level in blood is decreased, which is another hallmark of hyperthyroidism.

29. Ans. d. Aldolase B *Ref: Vasudevan DM, Sreekumari S, Textbook of Biochemistry, 6/e p41*

IUBMB System of Classification

International Union of Biochemistry and Molecular Biology (IUBMB) suggested the IUBMB system of nomenclature of enzymes. It is complex and cumbersome; but unambiguous. As per this system, the name starts with EC (enzyme class) followed by 4 digits.

First digit represents the class

Second digit stands for the subclass

Third digit is the sub-subclass or subgroup

Fourth digit gives the number of the particular enzyme in the list.

The enzymes are grouped into the following **six major classes:**

- **CLASS 1: OXIDOREDUCTASES**

  This group of enzymes will catalyze oxidation of one substrate with simultaneous reduction of another substrate or coenzyme. This may be represented as AH2 + BCC A + BH2; for example, Alcohol + NAD^+ Aldehyde + NADH + H^+

  The enzyme is **Alcohol dehydrogenase**; IUB name is Alcohol-NAD-oxidoreductase; Code number is EC.1.1.1.1. Oxidoreductases may also oxidize substrates by adding oxygen, e.g. oxidases, oxygenases and dehydrogenases.

  Other Examples: Lactate dehydrogenase (NAD); Glucose 6-phosphate dehydrogenase (NADP); Succinate dehydrogenase (FAD); dioxygenases.

- **CLASS 2: TRANSFERASES**

  This class of enzymes **transfers one group** (other than hydrogen) from the substrate to another substrate. This may be represented as A-R + B A + B-R, for example,

  Hexose + ATP Hexose 6-phosphate + ADP

  The name of enzyme is **Hexokinase**

- **CLASS 3: HYDROLASES**

  This class of enzymes can hydrolyze ester, ether, peptide or glycosidic bonds by adding water and then breaking the bond.

  Acetyl choline + H_2O choline + acetate

  The enzyme is **Acetyl choline esterase** or Acetyl choline hydrolase (systematic). All digestive enzymes are hydrolases.

- **CLASS 4: LYASES**
  These enzymes can remove groups from substrates or break bonds by mechanisms other than hydrolysis. For example,
  Fructose-1, 6-bisphosphate, Glyceraldehyde-3-phosphate + dihydroxyacetone phosphate
  The enzyme is **Aldolase.**
- **CLASS 5: ISOMERASES**
  These enzymes can produce optical, geometric or positional isomers of substrates. Racemases, epimerases, cistrans isomerases are examples.
  Glyceraldehyde-3-phosphate di-hydroxy-acetone-phosphate
  Enzyme is triosephosphate isomerase.
- **CLASS 6: LIGASES**
  These enzymes link two substrates together, usually with the simultaneous hydrolysis of ATP; for example,
  Acetyl CoA + CO_2 + ATP Malonyl CoA + ADP + Pi
  Enzyme is Acetyl CoA carboxylase.

30. Ans. b. Phenylalanine hydroxylase *Ref: Harper's Illustrated Biochemistry, 28/e p237*

Phenylketonuria

- CAUSES–Phenylalanine hydroxylase deficiency (classical/type-I)
- Inheritance–AR. Incidence-1:25,000 in india

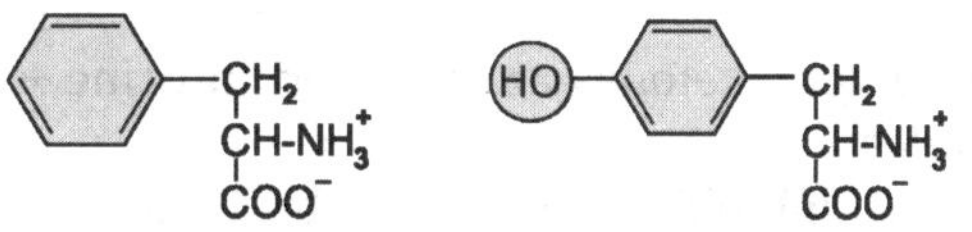

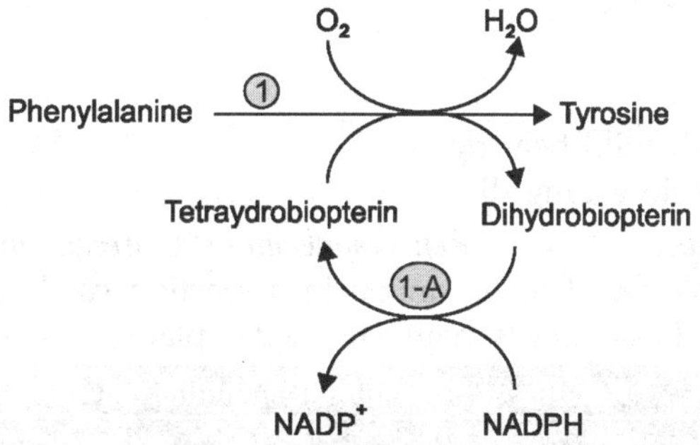

CH_2
$CH\text{-}NH_3^+$
COO^-
HO
CH_2
$CH\text{-}NH_3^+$
COO^-
O_2
H_2O
Phenylalanine
1
Tyrosine
Tetraydrobiopterin
Dihydrobiopterin
1-A
$NADP^+$
NADPH

1 = Phenylalanine hydroxylase;
1 – A = NADPH-dependent reductase

- **Types–Classical**
  Type I is the classical due to phenylalanine hydroxylase deficiency.
- **Nonclassical**
  Types II and III are due to deficiency of dihydrobiopterin reductase.
  Type IV and V are due to the deficiency of the enzyme-synthesizing biopterin. *Biopterin is synthesized from GTP.*

Clinical Features:

- Normal at birth
- Delay in developmental milestones
- Microcephaly
- Progressive impairment of cerebral function
- Mental retardation
- Hyperactivity, Agitation, Tremors, Seizures.

  Why mental retardation?
  – Elevated phenylalanine in brain interfers with the transport of other neutral amino acids into the brain.

Tyrosine–Epinephrine } Neurotransmitter precursors
Tryptophan–Serotonin

- Reduces the synthesis/increases the degradation of myelin.

- Mousy odor of skin, hair and urine (Phenylketone accumulation)
- ***Hypopigmentation***: (Due to defective melanin synthesis and excessive phenylalanine also inhibits tyrosinase)

Alternate Pathways in Phenylketonuria

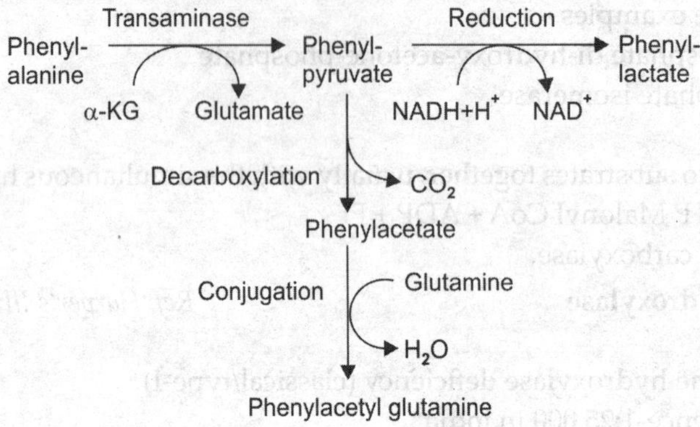

Diagnosis:

- ***Positive ferric chloride test:*** Phenylketones are excreted in urine + a drop of ferric chloride. Blue green colour–persists for 2–4 minutes.
- ***Positive Gutherie test***–Bacterial inhibition assay using bacillus subtilis.
- **Blood phenylalanine:** Normal level is 1 mg/dl. In PKU, the level is >20 mg/dl.

Treatment:

- Diet devoid of phenylalanine
- Till 6 years of age/lifelong/till child-bearing age
- Keep phenylalanine levles below 4 mg/dl

31. Ans. b. Increase gastric secretion *Ref: Vasudevan DM, Sreekumari S, Textbook of Biochemistry 6/e p202*

Histamine: Histidine is decarboxylated to histamine in a reaction catalyzed by histidine decarboxylase. The co-factor is pyridoxal phosphate. Histamine is mainly formed in platelets, mast cells, basophils, stomach and brain.

Actions of histamine: Histamine receptors			
Type	**Location**	**Actions**	**Antagonists**
H1 Receptor	*Smooth muscles*, vascular *endothelial cells*, heart mast cells, basophils, platelets	Vasodilatation Bronchospasm Mediation of allergic response	Chlorpheniramine Diphenylhydramine
H2 Receptor	Gastric mucosa	Secretion of HCl	Ranitidine
H3 Receptor	Presynaptic nerve endings	CNS-stimulant effects	

32. Ans. c. Carbamoyl phosphate synthetase I *Ref: Vasudevan DM, Sreekumari S, Textbook of Biochemistry 6/e p180*

Diseases	Enzyme defect	Features
Hyperammonemia type I	CPS-I	Very high NH_3 levels in blood. Autosomal recessive. Mental retardation. Incidence is 1 in 100,000
Hyperammonemia type II	(OTC) Ornithine transcarbamoylase	Ammonia level high in blood. Increased glutamine in blood, CSF and urine. Orotic aciduria due to channelling of carbamoyl phosphate into pyrimidine synthesis. X-linked
Hyperornithinemia	Defective ornithine transporter protein	Failure to import ornithine from cytoplasm to mitochondria. Defect in ORNT1 gene. Hyperornithinemia, hyperammonemia and homocitrullinuria are seen (**HHH syndrome**). Decreased urea in blood. Autosomal recessive condition

Contd...

Contd...

Diseases	Enzyme defect	Features
Citrullinemia	Argininosuccinate synthetase	Autosomal recessive inheritance. High blood levels of ammonia and citrulline. Citrullinuria (1–2 g/day)
Argininosuccinic aciduria	Argininosuccinate lyase	Argininosuccinate in blood and urine. Friable brittle tufted hair (Trichorrhexis nodosa). Incidence 3/200,000
Hyperargininemia	Arginase	Arginine increased in blood and CSF. Instead of arginine, cysteine and lysine are lost in urine. Incidence 1 in 100,000

33. Ans. a. Glucogenolysis *Ref: Vasudevan DM, Sreekumari S, Textbook of Biochemistry 6/e p396*

Functions of Pyridoxal Phosphate:

- The pyridoxal phosphate (PLP) acts as coenzyme for many reactions in **amino acid metabolism**
  - **Transamination:** These reactions are catalyzed by amino transferases (transaminases) which employ PLP as the coenzyme. For example: Alanine + Alphaketoglutarate → Pyruvate + Glutamic acid (Enzyme Alanine transaminase).
  - **Decarboxylation:** All decarboxylation reactions of amino acids require PLP as co-enzyme. A few examples are given below:
    - Glutamate → GABA (gamma amino butyric acid). GABA is an inhibitory neurotransmitter, and hence in B6 deficiency, especially in children, **convulsions** may occur.
    - Histidine → histamine, which is the mediator of **allergy** and anaphylaxis.
    - 5-hydroxy tryptophan → serotonin.
  - **Sulfur Containing Amino Acids:** PLP plays an important role in methionine and cysteine metabolism.
    - Homocysteine + Serine Cystathionine (Enzyme Cystathionine synthase)
    - Cystathionine Homoserine + Cysteine (Enzyme Cystathionase)

    Both these reactions require PLP. Hence, in vitamin B6 deficiency, **homocysteine** in blood is increased. Homocysteine level is correlated with **myocardial infarction**. Therefore, pyridoxine is used to prevent homocysteinemia.
  - **Heme Synthesis:** ALA synthase is a PLP-dependent enzyme. This is the rate limiting step in heme biosynthesis. So, in B6 deficiency, **anemia** may be seen.
  - **Production of Niacin:** Pyridoxal phosphate is required for the synthesis of niacin from tryptophan (**one vitamin is necessary for synthesis of another vitamin**).

    3-hydroxykynurenine 3-hydroxyanthranilic acid (Enzyme Kynureninase).

    Kynureninase is a PLP-dependent enzyme. Hence, in vitamin B6 deficiency, niacin production is less. Moreover, kynurenine cannot be converted further, which is metabolized to xanthurenic acid and excreted through urine.
  - **Glycogenolysis: Phosphorylase** enzyme (glycogen to glucose-1-phosphate) requires PLP. In fact, more than 70% of total PLP content of the body is in muscles, where it is a part of the phosphorylase enzyme.

34. Ans. c. Riboxyme *Ref: Vasudevan DM, Sreekumari S, Textbook of Biochemistry 6/e p485*

Ribozymes

- Enzymes made up of RNA are called ribozymes. Ribozymes or RNA enzymes are catalytic. RNA also exhibit Michaelis-Menten kinetics. Ribozyme cleave RNA phosphodiester bonds at specific sites in the RNA molecule, serving as ribonucleases and peptidyl transferase, the enzyme in protein synthesis that catalyzes the formation of peptide bond.
- **Peptidyl transferase** activity is done by **28s rRNA of 60S ribosomal subunit** present in ribosomes (used for protein biosynthesis). It is another example of ribozyme.
- **Spliceosomes** contain ribozymes as well as protein components which serve to stabilize the structure of ribozymes. **Small nuclear rnas (snRNAs)** are named as U1, U2, U4, U5, U6 and U7. The U stands for the uracil-rich nature of the snRNAs. They take part in the formation of spliceosomes. All of them are located in the nucleus. They complex with specific proteins, to form *small nuclear ribonucleoprotein particles (snRNPs)*. It is pronounced as "**Snurps**". Production of autoantibodies against "Snurps" cause **systemic lupus erythematosis** (SLE), a fatal autoimmune disease.

- **RNAse-P** is another ribozyme, which catalyzes the maturation of t-RNA by removing nucleotides from the 5'end of precursor t-RNA molecules.

35. Ans. a. Decreased pH *Ref: Vasudevan DM, Sreekumari S, Textbook of Biochemistry 6/e p256*

Binding of Oxygen to Myoglobin and Hemoglobin:

- Myoglobin can bind only one molecule of oxygen (O_2) because it contains only one heme group. In contrast, hemoglobin can bind four oxygen molecules—one at each of its four heme groups.

Oxygen Dissociation Curve:

- A plot of Y measured at different partial pressures of oxygen (pO_2) is called the oxygen dissociation curve. The curves for myoglobin and hemoglobin show important differences. The graph illustrates that myoglobin has a higher oxygen affinity at all pO_2 values than does hemoglobin. The partial pressure of oxygen needed to achieve half-saturation of the binding sites (P50) is approximately 1 mm Hg for myoglobin and 26 mm Hg for hemoglobin.

Myoglobin:

- The oxygen dissociation curve for myoglobin has a hyperbolic shape.

Hemoglobin:

- The oxygen dissociation curve for hemoglobin is sigmoidal in shape. Binding of oxygen to one of the subunits of hemoglobin enhances the binding of oxygen to other subunits. This phenomenon is called cooperativity. Sigmoid-shaped oxygen dissociation curve is due to cooperativity.

Factors Causing Shift to Right:	Factors Causing Shift to Left:
• Increased H+ (decreased pH)	Decreased H+ (increased pH)
• Increased pCO_2	Decreased pCO_2
• 2,3 BPG (bisphosphoglycerate)	Decreased 2,3 BPG
• Increased temperature	Decreased temperature
	Fetal hb (Hb F)

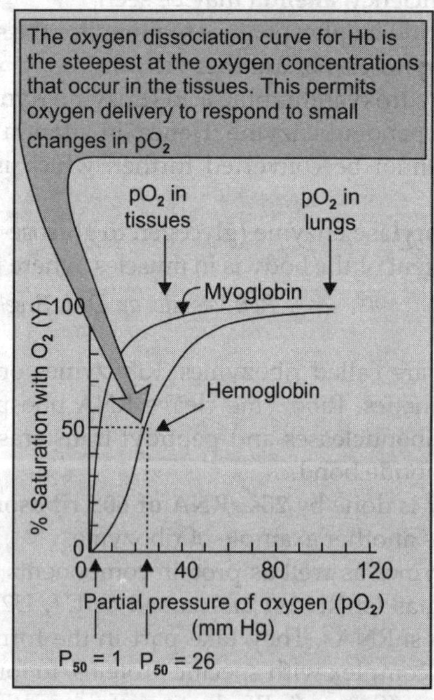

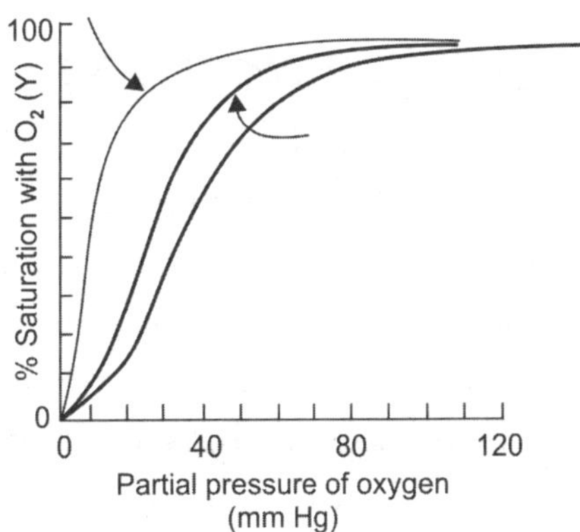

36. Ans. b. Pseudogout enzyme *Ref: Vasudevan DM, Sreekumari S, Textbook of Biochemistry 6/e p464*

GOUT:

- It is due to accumulation of urate crystals in the synovial fluid resulting in inflammation leading to acute arthritis.

Increased Formation of Uric Acid:

- ***Primary:***
  - Idiopathic
  - Due to enzyme defects in:
    - PRPP synthase
    - PRPP amidotransferase
    - HGPRTase deficiency (lesch-nyhan syndrome)
- ***Secondary:***
  - Excess purine intake
  - ↑ed nucleic acid turnover
  - Rapidly growing tumor–leukemias, lymphomas
  - Increased tissue breakdown after treatment
  - von Gierke's disease (glucose 6-phosphatase deficiency)

Decreased Excretion of Uric Acid:

- ***Primary:***
  - Idiopathic
- ***Secondary:***
  - Acute or chronic kidney disease
  - Increased renal reabsorption
  - Reduced secretion
  - Salicylate, thiazide diuretics
  - Diabetes mellitus
  - Metabolic acidosis
  - Lactic acidosis

37. Ans. a. Inhibit immunoglobulin destruction

Ref: Vasudevan DM, Sreekumari S, Textbook of Biochemistry 6/e p535

Effect of Glucocorticoids:

System	Effect
Carbohydrates	Activity of transaminases and gluconeogenic enzymes (PC, PEPCK, F-1,6-BPase and GPase) are stimulated, increasing gluconeogenesis. Glycolytic enzymes (GK, PFK and PK) are suppressed. Decreased glucose uptake by peripheral tissues. All of them lead to hyperglycemia.

Contd...

Contd...

System	Effect
Lipids	Increase lipid mobilization; facilitate lipolytic hormones leading to hyperlipidemia.
Proteins and nucleic acids	Catabolism of proteins and nucleic acids increased. Increase urea production.
Fluid and electrolytes	Promotes water excretion by increase in GFR and inhibition of ADH secretion.
Bone and calcium	Decrease serum calcium by inhibiting osteoblast function, leading to osteoporosis.
Secretory action	Stimulates secretion of gastric acid and enzyme. Induces acid peptic disease.
Connective tissue	Impaired collagen formation. Poor wound healing.
Immune system	Immunosuppressant. Lysis of lymphocytes. Anti-inflammatory and antiallergic

38. Ans. d. None of the above *Ref: Vasudevan DM, Sreekumari S, Textbook of Biochemistry 6/e p520*

General features of hormone classes		
	Group I	**Group II**
Types	Steroids, iodothyronines, calcitriol, retinoids	Polypeptides, proteins, glycoproteins, catecholamines
Solubility	Lipophilic	Hydrophilic
Transport proteins	Yes	No
Plasma half-life	Long (hours to days)	Short (minutes)
Receptor	Intracellular	Plasma membrane
Mediator	Receptor-hormone complex	cAMP, cGMP, Ca^{2+}, metabolites of complex phosphinositols, kinase cascades

Classification of hormones by mechanism of action
I. Hormones that bind to intracellular receptors
Androgens Calcitriol (1,25[OH]$_2$-D$_3$) Estrogens Glucocorticoids Mineralocorticoids Progestins Retinoic acid Thyroid hormones (T_3 and T_4)
II. Hormones that bind to cell surface receptors **A. The second messenger is cAMP**
α_2-Adrenergic catecholamines β-Adrenergic catecholamines Adrenocorticotropic hormone (ACTH) Antidiuretic hormone Calcitonin Chorionic gonadotropin, human (CG) Corticotropin-releasing hormone Follicle-stimulating hormone (FSH) Glucagon Lipotropin (LPH) Luteinizing hormone (LH) Melanocyte-stimulating hormone (MSH) Parathyroid hormone (PTH) Somatostatin Thyroid-stimulating hormone (TSH)

Contd...

Contd...

B. The second messenger is cGMP
Atrial natriuretic factor
Nitric oxide
C. The second messenger is calcium or phosphatidylinositols (or both)
Acetylcholine (muscarinic)
α1-Adrenergic catecholamines
Angiotensin II
Antidiuretic hormone (vasopressin)
Cholecystokinin
Gastrin
Gonadotropin-releasing hormone
Oxytocin
Platelet-derived growth factor (PDGF)
Substance P
Thyrotropin-releasing hormone (TRH)
D. The second messenger is a kinase or phosphatase cascade
Adiponectin
Chorionic somatomammotropin
Epidermal growth factor
Erythropoietin
Fibroblast growth factor (FGF)
Growth hormone (GH)
Insulin
Insulin-like growth factors I and II
Leptin
Nerve growth factor (NGF)
Platelet-derived growth factor
Prolactin

39. Ans. b. Taurocholic acid *Ref: Vasudevan DM, Sreekumari S, Textbook of Biochemistry 6/e p158*

Formation of Bile Acids:

- Bile acids are synthesized in the liver from cholesterol. They contain 24 carbon atoms. The reactions for synthesis of bile acids are summarized below:
  - Cholesterol hydroxylated at 3/7/12 positions. The **rate-limiting** step in bile acid synthesis is the introduction of this hydroxyl group by the enzyme **7-alpha-hydroxylase.**
  - Removal of 3-carbon unit, to make it 24 C
  - Conjugation with glycine/taurine
  - Secretion into intestinal canal
  - In the intestine, deconjugation and removal of hydroxyl groups.

Primary Bile Acids:

- Cholic acid
- Chenodeoxycholic acid

The primary bile acids are conjugated with either **glycine or taurine** to form bile acids. They are glycocholic acid, taurocholic acid, glycochenodeoxycholic acid and taurochenodeoxycholic acid

Secondary Bile Acids:

- Deoxycholic acid
- Lithocholic acid

Functions of Bile:

- The alkaline pH of the bile serves to neutralise the acidity of the gastric juice.
- The bile salts are efficient surfactants and detergents.
- Bile is the only route of excretion for bilirubin, the end product of heme catabolism.

- Bile salts facilitate the digestion of lipids. They can form molecular aggregates called micelle which bring about the absorption of lipids. Bile salt micelle also plays an important role in keeping the cholesterol in solution. It serves to excrete cholesterol, thus regulating the body cholesterol pool.
- Bile serves as the medium of excretion for several drugs, which are detoxified by the liver.

40. Ans. a. O_2 release *Ref: Lippincott's Biochemistry 5/e p31*

Effect of 2,3-Bisphosphoglycerate on Oxygen Affinity:

- 2,3-Bisphosphoglycerate (2,3-BPG) is an important regulator of the binding of oxygen to hemoglobin.
- It is the most abundant organic phosphate in the red blood cell, where its concentration is approximately that of hemoglobin.
- 2,3-BPG is synthesized from an intermediate of the glycolytic pathway (from 1,3-Bisphosphoglycerate).
- 2,3-BPG decreases the oxygen affinity of hemoglobin by binding to deoxyhemoglobin but not to oxyhemoglobin. This preferential binding stabilizes the taut conformation of deoxyhemoglobin.

Binding Site of 2,3-BPG:

- One molecule of 2,3-BPG binds to a pocket, formed by the two β-globin chains, in the center of the deoxyhemoglobin tetramer.
- This pocket contains several positively charged amino acids that form ionic bonds with the negatively charged phosphate groups of 2,3-BPG. 2,3-BPG is expelled on oxygenation of the hemoglobin.

Shift of the Oxygen Dissociation Curve:

- Hemoglobin from which 2,3-BPG has been removed has a high affinity for oxygen.
- However, as seen in the red blood cell, the presence of 2,3-BPG significantly reduces the affinity of hemoglobin for oxygen, shifting the oxygen-dissociation curve to the right.
- This reduced affinity enables hemoglobin to release oxygen efficiently at the partial pressures found in the tissues.
- Elevated 2,3-BPG levels lower the oxygen affinity of hemoglobin, permitting greater unloading of oxygen in the capillaries of the tissues. When there is a chronic tissue deprivation of oxygen, the level of 2,3-BPG increases.
- Such compensatory increase occurs in:
  - Individuals who live at high altitude.
  - Patients with chronic obstructive lung disease like emphysema.
  - Anemias and cardiac failure.

41. Ans. b. Two polypeptide chains are bound by disulfide linkages

Ref: Vasudevan DM, Sreekumari S, Textbook of Biochemistry 6/e p281

Structure of Insulin:

- Insulin is a protein hormone with 2 polypeptide chains.
- The A chain has 21 amino acids and B chain has 30 amino acids.
- These two chains are joined together by two interchain disulfide bonds, between A7 to B7 and A20 to B19.
- There is also an intrachain disulfide link in A chain between 6th and 11th amino acids. Species variation is restricted to amino acids 8,9 and 10 of A chain and C terminal of B chain.

Biosynthesis of Insulin:

- Insulin is a protein synthesized and secreted by the betacells of the islets of Langerhans of the pancreas.
- The insulin is synthesized as a larger precursor polypeptide chain, the **pre-pro insulin**. It has 109 amino acids. It is rapidly converted to pro-insulin in the endoplasmic reticulum by removal of leader sequence of 23 amino acid residues.
- The **proinsulin** with 86 amino acids is transported to Golgi apparatus where it is cleaved by a protease. Thus **C-peptide** or connecting peptide with 33 amino acids is removed. (The number of amino acids in C peptide may vary according to species). Insulin with 51 amino acids is thus formed.

Secretion of Insulin:

- Approximately 50 units of insulin are secreted per day.
- Normal insulin level in blood is 5–15 microunits/ml.
- Proinsulin contributes 5 to 10% of the total insulin measured in plasma. Proinsulin has about one-third biological activity as that of insulin.

- Insulin and C-peptide are synthesized and secreted in equimolar quantities.
- Therefore, measurement of C-peptide is an index of rate of secretion of insulin.
- Mutations causing changes in amino acid sequence at the cleavage points can lead to familial pro-insulinemia.

Factors Increasing Insulin Secretion:
- **Glucose:** Glucose is the major stimulant of insulin secretion. As blood glucose level increases, the insulin secretion also correspondingly increases. Glucose induces a biphasic response to insulin secretion. A discharge of insulin from the beta cell storage pool occurs during the initial rapid phase of insulin release within the first 2 minutes. The second phase of insulin release lasting for 5-10 minutes is of smaller magnitude and is due to discharge of newly synthesized hormone. The beta cells have **GluT 2 receptors**, through which glucose is absorbed. Glucose is oxidized so that more ATP is produced. ATP stimulates an **ATP Binding Cassette** protein (ABC protein) which is referred to as Sulfonyl Urea Receptor (SUR), **Simultaneously potassium channels are closed and calcium channels are opened**. Increased intracellular **calcium** causes the insulin secretion.
- **Gastrointestinal Hormones:** Insulin secretion is enhanced by secretin, pancreozymin and gastrin. After taking food, these hormones are increased.
- Proteins and amino acids: Leucine and arginine are stimulants.
- Parasympathetic and beta-adrenergic stimulation.
- Glucagon and growth hormone.
- Drug, Tolbutamide.
- **Incretin Hormones**: Glucose dependent insulinotropic polypeptide (GIP, 41 amino acids) and Glucagon like peptide 1 (GLP-1, 31 amino acids) are involved in the release of insulin following nutrient entry into stomach. They are both secreted by specialized cells in the gastrointestinal tract and have receptors located in islet cells. They have a very short half life. For treatment of diabetes, new drugs are being developed either to mimic or to target these hormones.

Degradation of Insulin:
- Insulin is rapidly degraded by the liver. Plasma half-life is less than 5 minutes. An insulin-specific protease (insulinase) is involved in the degradation of insulin.

42. Ans. a. LT cause vacoconstriction and decreased vascular permeability

Ref: Vasudevan DM, Sreekumari S, Textbook of Biochemistry 6/e p164

Eicosanoids: They are 20 C compounds derived from arachidonic acid. They are:
- Prostanoids, containing:
  - Prostaglandins (PGs);
  - Prostacyclins (PGIs);
  - Thromboxanes (TXs)
- Leukotrienes (LTs).

PROSTAGLANDINS (PGs):

Chemical Structure: All prostaglandins are considered to be derived from the 20 C cyclic saturated fatty acid, prostanoic acid. The five carbon ring is saturated.

Mechanism of Action: Prostaglandins are **local hormones.** They function through G-protein-coupled receptors. In most tissues, PGE increases cAMP (**cyclic AMP**) level. But in adipose tissue and in renal tubular cells, PGE lowers cAMP level. PGI activates adenylcyclase and TXA inhibits it.

BIOLOGICAL ACTIONS
- **Effects on Cvs: Prostacyclin** or PGI_2 is synthesized by the vascular endothelium. Major effect is **vasodilatation**. It also **inhibits platelet aggregation** and has a protective effect on vessel wall against deposition of platelets. But any injury to the vessel wall would inhibit PGI_2 synthesis so that platelet aggregation occurs to promote thrombus formation. **Thromboxane** (TXA2) is the main PG produced by platelets. The major effects are **vasoconstriction** and **platelet aggregation**. Prostacyclin and thromboxane are opposing in activity. Prostaglandins lower the blood pressure.

- **Effects on Ovary and Uterus:** PGF_2 stimulates the uterine muscles. Hence, PGF_2 may be used for medical **termination of pregnancy**. Yet another use is in **inducing labor** and arresting postpartum **hemorrhage**. PGs are involved in LH-induced ovulation.
- **Effects on Respiratory Tract:** PGF is a constrictor of bronchial smooth muscle; but PGE is a potent **bronchodilator**. PGE series are used in aerosols for relieving bronchospasm.
- **Effects on Immunity and Inflammation:** PGE_2 and D_2 produce inflammation by increasing capillary permeability. Erythema and wheal are produced at the site of injury. Moreover, PGE_2 reduces both T and B cell functions. PGE_2 is a sleep-promoting substance.
- **Effects on Gastrointestinal Tract:** PGs in general inhibit gastric secretion and increase intestinal motility. The inhibitory effect on gastric secretion is used therapeutically in the treatment of **acid peptic disease**. But diarrhea may be an unwanted side effect.

Leukotrienes (Lts): They are produced **from arachidonic acid**. LT B4 is produced in neutrophils; it is the most potent **chemotactic** agent. The **slow-reacting substance of anaphylaxis (SRS-A)** contains LTC_4, LTD_4 and LTE_4. They cause smooth muscle contraction, constrict the bronchioles, increase capillary permeability, activate leukocytes and produce vasoconstriction. SRS is the mediator of hypersensitivity reactions such as asthma.

Lipoxins: They are a group of compounds produced by leukocytes. They are conjugated tetraenes. They are formed by sequential action of 5 and 15-lipo-oxygenase. LXA_4 is the most common variety. It is anti-inflammatory and decreases immune response.

43. Ans. b. Splicing *Ref: Tietz Textbook of Clinical Chemistry and Molecular Diagnosis 5/e p1216*

Epigenetic Modifications: Epigenetics encompasses processes that alter gene function or its interpretation by mechanisms other than those that rely on DNA sequence change. Practically, epigenetics has evolved to include the study of:

- DNA methylation
- Genomic imprinting
- Histone modifications
- Chromatin remodeling

These epigenetic modifications control gene expression and changes are also inherited. This information is normally transferred from generation to generation with high fidelity.

DNA Methylation and Genomic Imprint:

- Genomic imprinting and gene dosage compensation of X-linked genes in females, termed as X-inactivation or lyonization, are also mediated by DNA methylation.
- Genomic imprinting refers to the phenomenon whereby the function of each of the two alleles of a gene is determined by its parental origin. Differential methylation of the imprinted locus from the time of germ cell development allows recognition of the parental origin of imprinted alleles by cellular processes. In Prader-Willi syndrome, a mutant gene is derived from father and in Angelman's syndrome, the mutant gene is from mother.
- The occurrence of 'large offspring syndrome' in cattle is attributed to exposure of embryos in vitro to environmental changes. A similar condition, 'Beckwith-Wiedemann syndrome', which is an imprinted disorder, was found to occur with increased frequency in children born by 'assisted reproductive technologies'. Therefore, environmental factors might cause epigenetic modification of DNA leading to alteration of 'imprinted gene expression'.

Histone Modifications:

- The amino termini of histone proteins can be modified posttranslationally by processes that include acetylation, methylation, phosphorylation, and ubiquitination. Acetylation of the lysines on amino termini of histones H_3 and H_4 by histone acetyltransferases decreases histone-DNA interaction and improves accessibility of DNA to transcriptional activation. On the contrary, histone deacetylation by histone deacetylases promotes the formation of compact nucleosomes, leading to repression of transcription.

Nucleosome Positioning and Remodeling:

- Besides histone modifications, the position of nucleosomes is known to affect the transcriptional activity of the corresponding region of DNA. It is now known that the positioning of histones is not an entirely random process. It has been demonstrated that nucleosome-free regions are present at the 5′ and 3′ ends of genes. The 5′ nucleosome-free region is thought to be the assembly point of the preinitiation complex for transcription, and the 3′ one is the location of transcription termination. A nucleosome unit is located just upstream to the 5′ nucleosome-free region, and another nucleosome is located just downstream to it, close to the transcription start site. It has been observed that the location of the nucleosome nearest to the transcription start site is predictable and consistent. Positioning of the nucleosomes further downstream through the gene, however, is shown to be more random. In summary, it seems that mechanisms control the positioning of nucleosomes, so that their presence will not be inhibitory to the initiation of transcription. Consequently, nucleosomes are dynamic structures that can be remodeled according to the transcriptional demands of the cell.

44. Ans. a. 9 *Ref: Vasudevan DM, Sreekumari S, Textbook of Biochemistry 6/e p339*

- pH is defined as Negative logarithm of hydrogen ion concentration.
- pH = $-\log_{10}$ (H+ conc)
- If H + conc. is 1×10^{-9}
- Then pH = $-\log_{10} (1 \times 10^{-9})$
- Hence, pH = 9

Relation between hydrogen ions, hydroxyl ions and pH of aqueous solutions. Ionic product of water = [H+] [OH–] = 10^{-14}

$[OH^-]$	$[H^+]$	log – log $[H^+]$			
mol/liter	ml/liter	$[H^+]$	= pH	pOH	Inference
1×10^{-13}	1×10^{-1}	– 1	1	13	Strong acid
1×10^{-10}	1×10^{-4}	– 4	4	10	Acid
1×10^{-7}	1×10^{-7}	– 7	7	7	Neutral
1×10^{-4}	1×10^{-10}	– 10	10	4	Alkali
1×10^{-1}	1×10^{-13}	– 13	13	1	Strong alkali

45. Ans. b. Linoleic acid *Ref: Vasudevan DM, Sreekumari S, Textbook of Biochemistry 6/e p76, 162*

Polyunsaturated Fatty Acids (PUFA)

The important polyunsaturated fatty acids are:

- Linoleic acid (18 C, 2 double bonds)
- Linolenic acid (18 C, 3 double bonds)
- Arachidonic acid (20 C, 4 double bonds)

They are present in good quantities in **vegetable oils** such as sunflower oil. They are used to esterify cholesterol, whereby the latter can be excreted. So, PUFAs in general are **anti-atherogenic.**

Significance of PUFA

- PUFAs are seen in vegetable oils.
- They are nutritionally essential; and are called Essential Fatty Acids.
- Prostaglandins, thromboxanes and leukotrienes are produced from arachidonic acid.
- PUFAs form an integral part of mitochondrial membranes. In deficiency of PUFA, the efficiency of biological oxidation is reduced.
- They are components of **membranes**. Arachidonic acid is 10-15% of the fatty acids of membranes.
- As double bonds are in cis configuration; the PUFA molecule cannot be closely packed. So, PUFAs will **increase the fluidity** of the membrane.
- As PUFAs are easily liable to undergo peroxidation, the membranes containing PUFAs are more prone to damage by free radicals.

- The production of DHA (docosahexaenoic acid) from alphalinolenic acid is limited. DHA is present in high concentrations in fish oils. DHA is present in high concentations in retina, cerebral cortex and sperms.

Clinical Significance of PUFA and EFA

- Persons with normal diet will not have any deficiency; but those who are on parenteral nutrition for long periods will have deficiency.
- PUFAs are used for esterification and excretion of cholesterol. PUFA will reduce serum cholesterol level.
- Deficiency of EFA causes acanthocytosis, hyperkeratosis, acrodermatitis and hypercholesterolemia.
- EFA deficiency is connected with acrodermatitis enteropathica, hepatorenal syndrome and CNS manifestations.
- Elevated PUFA levels are seen in Zellweger's syndrome.
- DHA levels in blood are low in patients with retinitis pigmentosa.
- Trans-fatty acids will compete with EFAs, and may increase the EFA deficiency and decrease fluidity of membranes.
- Trans-fatty acids decrease HDL-cholesterol and may cause atherosclerosis.

PUFA, in excess, may be harmful

- PUFA can definitely reduce cholesterol level. But there should be moderation. It is known that the diet should contain correct type and quantity; the optimum ratio of omega-6 to omega-3 fatty acids is 4:1.
- Very high intake of omega-6 oils will cause lowering of HDL, elevation of plasma triglycerides, and will promote platelet aggregation. Vegetable oils (sunflower oil) containing PUFA are rich in omega-6 variety; while ghee and butter are low in omega-6.
- Omega-3 group is present in fish oils.
- Normal Indian diet consisting of cereals, pulses and vegetables provides **'invisible oils'**, which contains about 10 g of PUFA/day (out of which about 2 g is omega-3 and the rest 8 g is omega-6). Further intake of omega-6 oils is unnecessary and may be harmful. The optimal **ratio for omega-6 to omega-3** in diet is 4:1.
- In an average Indian diet, this is about 30:1. In sunflower oil, this value is 160:1, and, therefore, unnecessary addition of such vegetable oils will further deteriorate the condition.
- Coconut oil, although contains saturated fatty acids, the omega ratio is 3:1, and, therefore, superior to sunflower oil in this respect.

46. Ans. c. Phosphofructokinase

Ref: Vasudevan DM, Sreekumari S, Textbook of Biochemistry 6/e p224. (Refer to question no. 6 in JIPMER 2014)

47. Ans. a. HGPRTase *Ref: Harper's illustrated Biochemistry 29/e p335,339 and 742*

Lesch-Nyhan Syndrome:

- Lesch-Nyhan syndrome, an overproduction hyperuricemia characterized by frequent episodes of uric acid lithiasis and a bizarre syndrome of self-mutilation, reflects a defect in **hypoxanthine-guanine phosphoribosyltransferase**, an enzyme of purine salvage. The accompanying rise in intracellular PRPP results in purine overproduction.
- Mutations that decrease or abolish hypoxanthine-guanine phosphoribosyltransferase activity include deletions, frameshift mutations, base substitutions, and aberrant mRNA splicing.

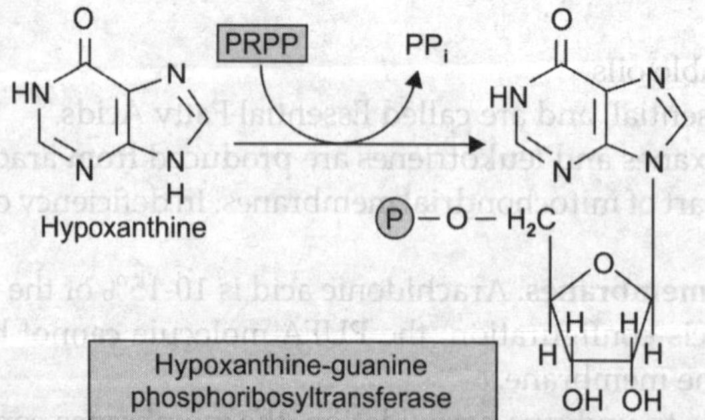

CPS-I and CPS-II

- One molecule of ammonia condenses with CO_2 in the presence of **two molecules of ATP** to form carbamoyl phosphate.
- The reaction is catalyzed by the mitochondrial enzyme carbamoyl **phosphate synthetase-I (CPS-I).**
- An entirely different cytoplasmic enzyme, carbamoyl phosphate synthetase-II, (CPS-II) is involved in pyrimidine nucleotide. CPS-I reaction is the **rate-limiting step** in urea formation. It is irreversible and allosterically regulated.

	CPS I	CPS II
1. Site	Mitochondria	Cytosol
2. Pathway of	Urea	Pyrimidine
3. Positive effector	NAG	Nil
4. Source for N	Ammonia	Glutamine
5. Inhibitor	Nil	CTP

48. Ans. a. Pancreas *Ref: Harper's Illustrated Biochemistry 28/e p171 (Refer to question no-9 in JIPMER 2014)*

49. Ans. d. Alcohol Intoxication: *Ref: Harper's Illustrated Biochemistry 29/e*

Ketoacidosis Results from Prolonged Ketosis

- Higher than normal quantities of ketone bodies present in the blood or urine constitute ketonemia (hyperketonemia) or **ketonuria**, respectively. The overall condition is called **ketosis**.
- The basic form of ketosis occurs in starvation and involves depletion of available carbohydrate coupled with mobilization of free fatty acids.
- This general pattern of metabolism is exaggerated to produce the pathologic states found in **diabetes mellitus, the type 2 form of which is increasingly common in Western countries; twin lamb disease; and ketosis in lactating cattle.**
- Nonpathologic forms of ketosis are found under conditions of high-fat feeding and after severe exercise in the postabsorptive state.
- Also seen in alcohol intoxication.
- Acetoacetic and 3-hydroxybutyric acids are both moderately strong acids and are buffered when present in blood or other tissues. However, their continual excretion in quantity progressively depletes the alkali reserve, causing **ketoacidosis**. This may be fatal in uncontrolled **diabetes mellitus**.
- Carnitine deficiency is another cause of nonketotic hypoglycemia along with Galactosemia, Fructose intolerance and Hyperinsulinemia.

Biochemical Alterations in Alcoholism

Both the oxidation steps of alcohol produce NADH, resulting in a high NADH/NAD+ ratio. As a result, several metabolic adaptations occur:

- In the cytoplasm, the high NADH level favors conversion of pyruvate to lactate, leading to **lactic acidosis**.
- Deficiency of pyruvate leads to inadequate formation of oxaloacetate. This results in depression of gluconeogenesis, leading to **hypoglycemia**.
- Reduced oxaloacetate, decreased pyruvate and high NADH level cause suppression of TCA cycle. So, acetyl CoA is accumulated, which favors **ketogenesis**.
- Increased level of acetyl CoA causes increased fatty acid synthesis; but fatty acid is not oxidized. So, fat is accumulated in liver, resulting in **fatty liver** and steatosis.
- Alcohol also increases the release of ROS, leading to mitochondrial damage and apoptosis.
- Lactic acidosis causes decreased excretion of uric acid, resulting in acute attack of gout.
- Alcohol causes **CNS depression** by inhibiting excitatory receptors (N-methyl aspartate receptors) and by potentiating inhibitory neurotransmitter (GABA) receptors.

50. Ans. c. Palmitic acid *Ref: Harper's Illustrated Biochemistry 29/e p142*

Fatty Acids are Aliphatic Carboxylic Acids: Fatty acids occur in the body mainly as esters in natural fats and oils, but are found in the unesterified form as **free fatty acids,** a transport form in the plasma. Fatty acids that occur in natural fats usually contain an even number of carbon atoms. The chain may be **saturated** (containing no double bonds) or **unsaturated** (containing one or more double bonds).

Saturated Fatty Acids

Common Name	Number of C Atoms	
Acetic	2	Major end product of carbohydrate fermentation by rumen organisms
Butyric	4	In certain fats in small amounts (especially butter). An end product of carbohydrate fermentation by rumen organisms
Valeric	5	
Caproic	6	
Lauric	12	Spermaceti, cinnamon, palm kernel, coconut oils, laurels, butter
Myristic	14	Nutmeg, palm kernel, coconut oils, myrtles, butter
Palmitic	16	Common in all animal and plant fats
Stearic	18	

51. Ans. a. Reduced RBC transketolase activity *Ref: Vasudevan DM, Sreekumari S, Textbook of Biochemistry, 6/e p392*

Thiamine is also called vitamin B_1.

Physiological Role of Thiamine:

- ***Pyruvate Dehydrogenase:*** The co-enzyme form is thiamine pyrophosphate (TPP). It is used in oxidative decarboxylation of alpha keto acids, e.g. pyruvate dehydrogenase catalyzes the breakdown of pyruvate to acetyl CoA and carbon dioxide.
- ***Alpha-Ketoglutarate Dehydrogenase:*** An analogous biochemical reaction that requires TPP is the oxidative decarboxylation of **alpha-Ketoglutarate** to succinyl CoA and CO_2.
  - **Transketolase:**
    - The second group of enzymes that use TPP as coenzyme are the transketolases, in the hexose monophosphate shunt pathway of glucose.
    - The main role of thiamine (TPP) is in **carbohydrate** metabolism. So, the requirement of thiamine is increased along with higher intake of carbohydrates.
    - In thiamine deficiency, blood thiamine is reduced, but pyruvate, alpha ketoglutarate and lactate are increased. Erythrocyte **transketolase** activity is reduced; this is the earliest manifestation seen even before clinical disturbances.

Deficiency Manifestations of Thiamine

- ***Beriberi:*** Deficiency of thiamine leads to beriberi. It is a Singhalese word, meaning 'weakness'. The early symptoms are anorexia, dyspepsia, heaviness and weakness. Subjects feel weak and get easily exhausted.
- ***Wet beriberi:*** Here cardiovascular manifestations are prominent. Edema of legs, face, trunk and serous cavities are the main features. Palpitation, breathlessness and distended neck veins are observed. Death occurs due to heart failure.
- ***Dry beriberi:*** In this condition, CNS manifestations are the major features. Walking becomes difficult. Peripheral neuritis with sensory disturbance leads to complete paralysis.
- ***Infantile beriberi:*** It occurs in infants born to mothers suffering from thiamine deficiency. Restlessness and sleeplessness are observed.
- ***Wernicke-Korsakoff syndrome:*** It is also called **cerebral beriberi**. Clinical features are those of encephalopathy (ophthalmoplegia, nystagmus, cerebellar ataxia) plus psychosis. It is seen only when the nutritional status is severely affected.
- ***Polyneuritis:*** It is common in chronic alcoholics. Alcohol utilization needs large doses of thiamine. Alcohol inhibits intestinal absorption of thiamine, leading to thiamine deficiency. Polyneuritis may also be associated with pregnancy and old age. Such thiamine deficiency in alcoholism may cause impairment of conversion of pyruvate to acetyl CoA. This results in increased plasma concentration of pyruvate and lactate, leading to **lactic acidosis.**

52. Ans. c. Liver *Ref: Harper's Illustrated Biochemistry 28/e p171 (Refer to question no. 9 in JIPMER 2014)*

53. Ans. b. GLUT4 *Ref: Harper's illustrated Biochemistry 28/e p171 (Refer to question no. 9 in JIPMER 2014)*

54. Ans. a. RNA *Ref: Harper's Illustrated Biochemistry 28/e p393, Ch39*

Techniques	Used for
Northern blot	RNA analysis
Southern blot	DNA analysis
Western blot	Protein analysis

55. Ans. a. mRNA *Ref: Vasudevan DM, Sreekumari S, Textbook of Biochemistry, 6/e p484*

Post-transcriptional Processing of mRNA:

- The mRNA formed and released from the DNA template is known as the **primary transcript**. It is also known as **heteronuclear mRNA** or hmRNA.
- In mammalian system, it undergoes extensive processing to become the **mature mRNA**.
  These modifications are:
  - Endonuclease cleavage
  - Poly-A tailing
  - Methylation
  - Removal of introns
  - Splicing of exons (connect together).

  These processings occur mainly in the nucleoplasm.
- In bacteria, mRNA is not changed; and translation of mRNA starts even before completion of transcription.
- Post-transcriptional processing is not only for mRNA but for tRNA and rRNA as well.

Poly-A Tailing At 3′ End:

- The 3′ terminus is polyadenylated in the nucleoplasm. This poly-A tail may be 20 to 250 nucleotides long. This tail protects mRNA from attack by 3′ exonuclease.

Capping At 5′ End:

- Eukaryotic mRNAs are all 'capped' at the 5′ terminus by **7-methyl guanosine triphosphate**. An unusual 5′ to 5′ triphosphate bridge is seen. This is also done inside the nucleus. The cap is useful in recognition of mRNA by the translating machinery.

Methylation:

- Methylation of N6 of adenine residue and 2′-hydroxyl group of ribose are common. These are mainly done in the cytoplasm.

56. Ans. c. 32 g *Ref: Vasudevan DM, Sreekumari S, Textbook of Biochemistry 6/e p38*

- Proteins on an average contain 16% nitrogen, the weight of nitrogen x 100/16, or nitrogen × 6.25 will give the value of proteins present in the original sample.
  Nitrogen content in 200 g protein = 200 × 16/100
  = 32 g.

57. Ans. a. Increased NADH/NAD+ *Ref: Vasudevan DM, Sreekumari S, Textbook of Biochemistry 6/e p121.*

Metabolism of Alcohol:

- An NAD + dependent **cytoplasmic** enzyme that oxidizes ethanol to acetaldehyde. Acetaldehyde is further oxidized to acetate by a **mitochondrial** NAD+ dependent enzyme.

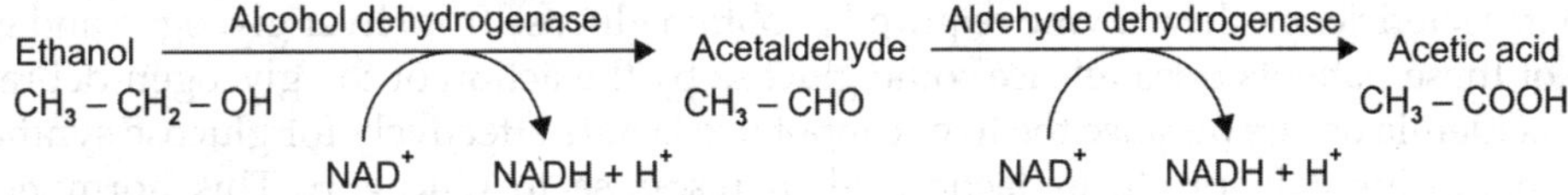

Biochemical Alterations in Alcoholism:

Both the oxidation steps of alcohol produce NADH, resulting in a high NADH/NAD+ ratio. As a result, several metabolic adaptations occur.

- In the cytoplasm, the high NADH level favors conversion of pyruvate to lactate, leading to **lactic acidosis**.
- Deficiency of pyruvate leads to inadequate formation of oxaloacetate. This results in depression of gluconeogenesis, leading to **hypoglycemia**.

- Reduced oxaloacetate, decreased pyruvate and high NADH level cause suppression of TCA cycle. So, acetyl CoA is accumulated, which favors **ketogenesis.**
- Increased level of acetyl CoA causes increased fatty acid synthesis; but fatty acid is not oxidized. So, fat is accumulated in liver, resulting in **fatty liver** and steatosis.
- Alcohol also increases the release of ROS, leading to mitochondrial damage and apoptosis.
- Lactic acidosis causes decreased excretion of uric acid, resulting in acute attack of gout.
- Alcohol causes **CNS depression** by inhibiting excitatory receptors (N-methyl aspartate receptors) and by potentiating inhibitory neurotransmitter (GABA) receptors.

58. Ans. a. Arginase *Ref: Vasudevan DM, Sreekumari S, Textbook of Biochemistry 6/e p178*

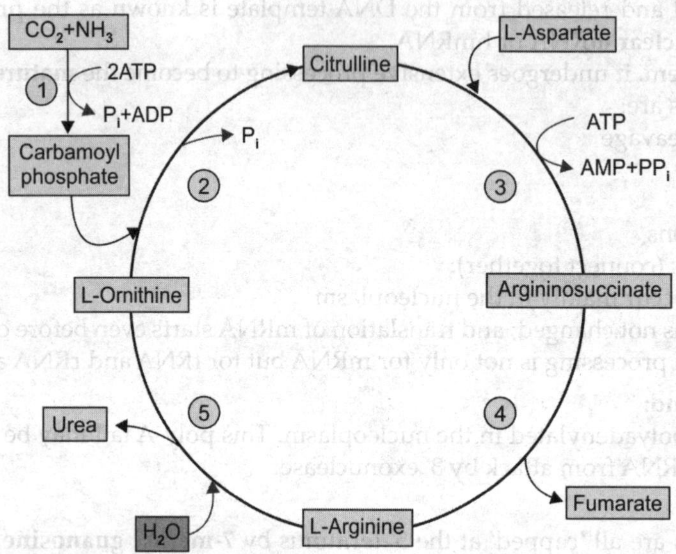

Key to enzymes (circled numbers)
1. Carbamoyl-phosphate synthase (ammonia)
2. Ornithine carbamoyltransferase
3. Argininosuccinate synthase
4. Argininosuccinate lyase
5. Arginase

59. Ans. c. Muscle atrophy *Ref: Thomas M. Devlin, Textbook of Biochemistry 4/e p317*

von Gierke's Disease:

- The most common glycogen storage disease, referred to as type I or von Gierke's disease, is caused by a deficiency of liver, intestinal mucosa, and kidney glucose 6-phosphatase.
- Patients with this disease can be further subclassified into those lacking the glucose 6-phosphatase enzyme per se **(type Ia)** and those lacking the glucose 6-phosphatase translocase **(type Ib).**
- A genetic abnormality in glucose 6-phosphate hydrolysis occurs in only about 1 person in 200,000 and is transmitted as an autosomal recessive trait.
- **Clinical manifestations** include ***fasting hypoglycemia, lactic acidemia hyperlipidemia, and hyperuricemia with gouty arthritis***. The fasting hypoglycemia is readily explained as a consequence of the glucose 6-phosphatase deficiency, the enzyme required to obtain glucose from liver glycogen and gluconeogenesis. The liver of these patients does release some glucose by the action of the glycogen-debranching enzyme. The lactic acidemia occurs because the liver cannot use lactate effectively for glucose synthesis. In addition, the liver inappropriately produces lactic acid in response to glucagon. This hormone should trigger glucose release without lactate production; however, the opposite occurs because of the lack of glucose 6-phosphatase. Hyperuricemia results from increased purine degradation in the liver; hyperlipidemia results because of increased availability of lactic acid for lipogenesis and lipid mobilization from the adipose tissue caused by high glucagon levels in response to hypoglycemia.
- The manifestations of von Gierke's disease can greatly be diminished by providing carbohydrate throughout the day to prevent hypoglycemia. During sleep, this can be done by infusion of carbohydrate into the gut by a nasogastric tube.

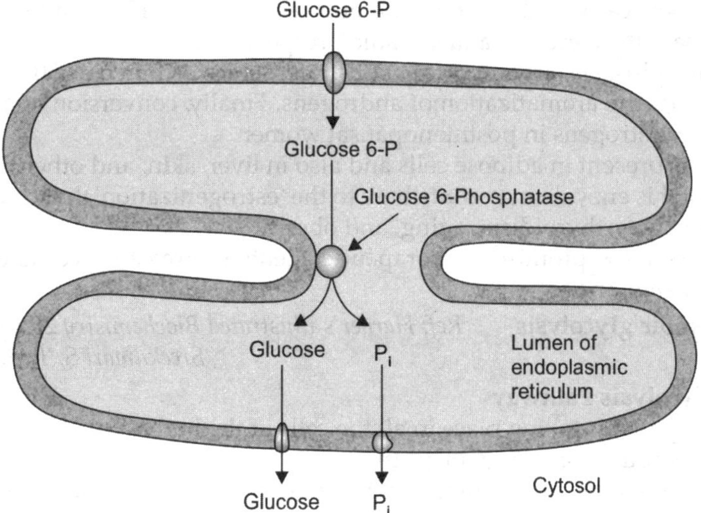

60. Ans. d. Estradiol/estrogens *Ref: Harper's Illustrated Biochemistry 28/e p431, Ch41*

Ovarian Steroidogenesis:

- The estrogens are a family of hormones synthesized in a variety of tissues. 17-β Estradiol is the primary estrogen of ovarian origin.
- In some species, estrone, synthesized in numerous tissues, is more abundant.
- In pregnancy, relatively more estriol is produced, and this comes from the placenta.
- Estrogens are formed by the aromatization of androgens in a complex process that involves three hydroxylation steps, each of which requires O_2 and NADPH.
- The aromatase enzyme complex is thought to include a P450 mono-oxygenase.
- Estradiol is formed if the substrate of this enzyme complex is testosterone, whereas estrone results from the aromatization of androstenedione.
- The cellular source of the various ovarian steroids has been difficult to unravel, but a transfer of substrates between two cell types is involved.

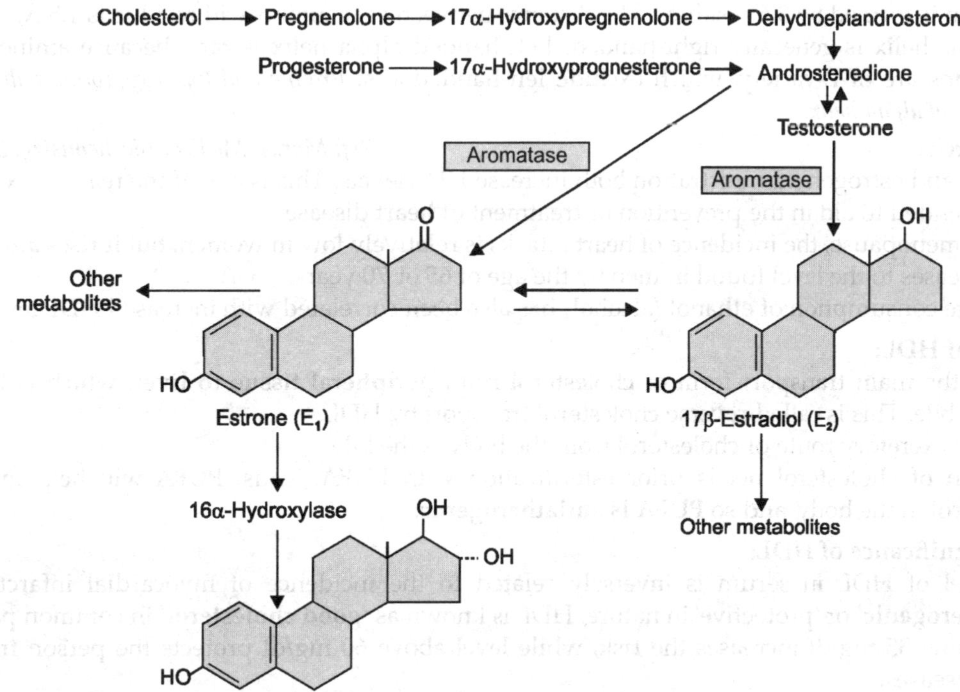

- Theca cells are the source of androstenedione and testosterone. These are converted by the aromatase enzyme in granulosa cells to estrone and estradiol, respectively.
- In females, adrenal androgens are important substrates, since as much as 50% of the E_2 produced during pregnancy comes from the aromatization of androgens. Finally, conversion of androstenedione to estrone is the major source of estrogens in postmenopausal women.
- Aromatase activity is present in adipose cells and also in liver, skin, and other tissues.
- Increased activity of this enzyme may contribute to the 'estrogenization' that characterizes such diseases as cirrhosis of the liver, hyperthyroidism, aging, and obesity.
- Aromatase inhibitors show promise as therapeutic agents in breast cancer and possibly in other female reproductive tract malignancies.

61. Ans. b. Increased anerobic glycolysis *Ref: Harper's Illustrated Biochemistry 28/e p151, Ch18; Vasudevan DM, Sreekumari S, Textbook of Biochemistry 6/e p93.*

Significance of the Glycolysis Pathway

- It is the only pathway that is taking place in all the cells of the body.
- Glycolysis is the only source of energy in erythrocytes.
- In strenuous exercise, when muscle tissue lacks enough oxygen, **anerobic glycolysis forms the major source of energy for muscles.**
- The glycolytic pathway may be considered as the preliminary step before complete oxidation.
- The glycolytic pathway provides carbon skeletons for synthesis of nonessential amino acids as well as glycerol part of fat.
- When oxygen is in short supply, mitochondrial reoxidation of NADH formed during glycolysis is impaired, and NADH is reoxidized by reducing pyruvate to lactate, so permitting glycolysis to proceed. While glycolysis can occur under anerobic conditions, this has a price, for it limits the amount of ATP formed per mole of glucose oxidized, so that much more glucose must be metabolized under anerobic than aerobic conditions.

62. Ans. b. Proline *Ref: Vasudevan DM, Sreekumari S, Textbook of Biochemistry 6/e p31*

Alpha Helix:

- The alpha-helix is the most common and stable conformation for a polypeptide chain. In proteins like hemoglobin and myoglobin, the alpha-helix is abundant, whereas it is virtually absent in chymotrypsin.
- The structure is stabilized by hydrogen bonds between NH and C=O groups of the main chain.
- Each turn is formed by 3.6 residues. The distance between each amino acid residue is 1.5 Å.
- The alpha-helix is generally right-handed. Left-handed alpha helix is rare, because amino acids found in proteins are of L-variety, which exclude left-handedness. *Proline and hydroxyproline will not allow the formation of alpha-helix.*

63. Ans. a. Exercise *Ref: Marks' Medical Biochemistry, 3/e p651, Ch34*

- Exercise and estrogen administration both increase HDL levels. This is one of the reasons exercise is often recommended to aid in the prevention or treatment of heart disease.
- Prior to menopause, the incidence of heart attacks is relatively low in women, but it rises after menopause and increases to the level found in men by the age of 65 or 70 years.
- Moderate consumption of ethanol (alcohol) has also been correlated with increased HDL levels.

Functions of HDL:

- HDL is the main transport form of cholesterol from **peripheral tissue to liver**, which is later excreted through bile. This is called reverse cholesterol transport by HDL.
- The only excretory route of cholesterol from the body is the bile.
- Excretion of cholesterol needs prior esterification with PUFA. Thus, PUFA will help in lowering of cholesterol in the body, and so **PUFA is antiatherogenic**.

Clinical Significance of HDL:

- The level of HDL in serum is inversely related to the incidence of myocardial infarction. As it is **'antiatherogenic'** or 'protective' in nature, HDL is known as **'good cholesterol'** in common parlance. HDL level below 35 mg/dl increases the risk, while level above 60 mg/dl protects the person from coronary artery diseases.

64. Ans. b. 400 nm *Ref: Vasudevan DM, Sreekumari S, Textbook of Biochemistry, 6/e p248*

Porphyrins and Absorption Bands

- In porphyrins (uroporphyrin, coproporphyrin and protoporphyrin), the 4 pyrrole rings are joined by methenyl (-CH=) bridges and they are colored compounds.
- The iron atom in the center of porphyrin is hexavalent and bonded to the 4 pyrrole nitrogens by coordinate valencies.
- The double bonds are resonating and, therefore, keep shifting their positions. When the ferrous iron (Fe++) in heme gets oxidized to ferric (Fe+++) form, **hematin** is formed, which loses the property of carrying the oxygen.
- Heme is red in color, but hematin is dark brown. When hemoglobin or porphyrin solutions are viewed through a spectroscope, the absorbed wavelengths are seen as dark bands. All porphyrins will have an absorption band near 400 nm; this distinguishing band is called the **Soret band**, after its discoverer.

Name of porphyrin	Alpha band	Beta band	Soret band
Uroporphyrin (UP)	594	552	406
Coproporphyrin (CP)	590	548	400
Protoporphyrin (PP)	598	554	408
Heme	580 to 575	560 to 540	Nil

65. Ans. b. Glutamate *Ref: Harper's Illustrated Biochemistry 26/e p244; Vasudevan DM, Sreekumari S, Textbook of Biochemistry 6/e p176*

Transdeamination

- The amino group of most of the amino acids is released by a coupled reaction, transdeamination, that is transamination followed by oxidative deamination.
- Transamination takes place in the cytoplasm of all the cells of the body; the amino group is transported to liver as glutamic acid which is finally oxidatively deaminated in the mitochondria of hepatocytes.
- Thus, the two components of the reaction are physically far away, but physiologically they are coupled. Hence, the term transdeamination.

Oxidative Deamination of Glutamate

- Only liver mitochondria contain glutamate dehydrogenase (GDH) which deaminates glutamate to alphaketoglutarate plus ammonia.
- So, all amino acids are first transaminated to glutamate, which is then finally deaminated (transdeamination). Amino acids are deaminated at the rate of about 50–70g per day.
- During the transamination reaction, the amino group of all other amino acids is funnelled into glutamate.
- Hence, the glutamate dehydrogenase reaction is the final reaction which removes the amino group of all amino acids. It needs NAD+ as co-enzyme. (NADP can also act as a coenzyme). It is an allosteric enzyme; it is activated by ADP and inhibited by GTP. The hydrolysis of glutamine also yields NH_3 but this occurs mainly in the kidney where the NH_{4+} excretion is required for acid base regulation.

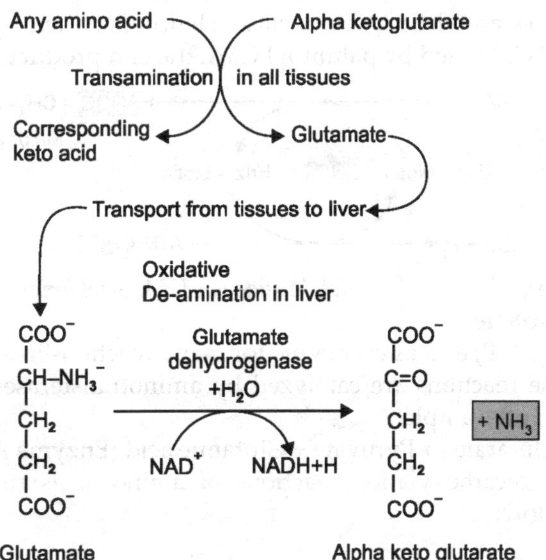

66. Ans. d. Uric acid oxidase *Ref: Vasudevan DM, Sreekumari S, Textbook of Biochemistry, 6/e p9*

Peroxisomes

- The peroxisomes have a granular matrix. They are of 0.3–1.5 m in diameter. They contain peroxidases and catalase. They are prominent in leukocytes and platelets.
- Peroxidation of **polyunsaturated fatty acids** *in vivo* may lead to hydroperoxide formation, ROOH → R-OO•. The free radicals damage molecules, cell membranes, tissues and genes.
- **Catalase and peroxidase** are the enzymes present in peroxisomes which will destroy the unwanted peroxides and other free radicals.

Peroxisomal Deficiency Diseases

- Deficiency of peroxisomal matrix proteins can lead to **adrenoleukodystrophy (ALD)** (Brown-Schilder's disease) characterized by progressive degeneration of liver, kidney and brain. It is a rare autosomal recessive condition. The defect is due to insufficient oxidation of very long chain fatty acids (VLCFA) by peroxisomes.
- In **Zellweger syndrome**, proteins are not transported into the peroxisomes. This leads to formation of empty peroxisomes or peroxisomal ghosts inside the cells.
- **Primary hyperoxaluria** is due to the defective peroxisomal metabolism of glyoxalate derived from glycine

Fraction	Enzymes
Plasma membrane	5 nucleotidase, Na, K-ATPase
Nucleus	DNA, RNA polymerases
ER	Glucose 6-Phosphatase
Golgi apparatus	Galactosyl transferase. Manosidase
Lysosomes	Acid phosphatase
Mitochondria	Cytochrome oxidase, Succinated dehydrogenase
Cytosol	Lactate dehydrogenase Glucose 6-Phosphate dehydrogenase

67. Ans. b. Citrate *Ref: Vasudevan DM, Sreekumari S, Textbook of Biochemistry, 6/e p139*

Acetyl CoA Carboxylase:

- The first step in the fatty acid synthesis is the carboxylation of acetyl CoA to form malonyl CoA.
- The acetyl CoA carboxylase is not a part of the multienzyme complex. But it is the **rate-limiting enzyme**.
- Biotin, a member of B complex vitamins, is necessary for this reaction.
- The enzyme is allosterically regulated, the major effectors being citrate (positive) and palmitoyl CoA (negative).
- **Acetyl CoA Carboxylase** is the **key enzyme**; citrate activates this enzyme. The citrate level is high only when both acetyl CoA and ATP are abundant. Covalent modification is another regulatory mechanism. Phosphorylation inactivates acetyl CoA carboxylase. Hence, fatty acid synthesis decreases when glucose level is low. The enzyme is inhibited by palmitoyl CoA, the end product.

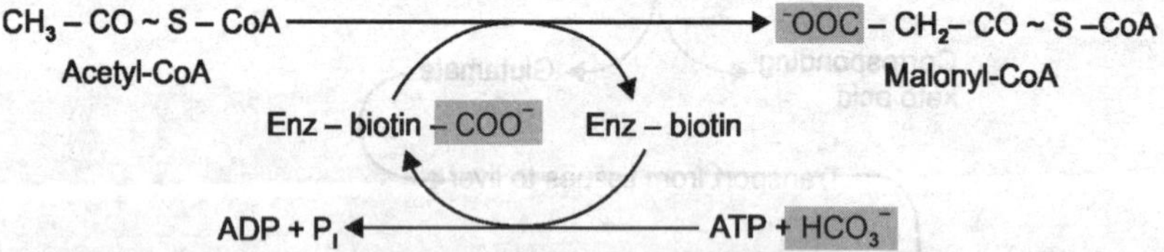

68. Ans. b. Pyridoxal phosphate *Ref: Vasudevan DM, Sreekumari S, Textbook of Biochemistry 6/e p396*

Functions of Pyridoxal Phosphate:

- The pyridoxal phosphate (PLP) acts as coenzyme for many reactions in amino acid metabolism:
  - **Transamination:** These reactions are catalyzed by aminotransferases (transaminases) which employ PLP as the coenzyme. For example:
    Alanine + Alpha ketoglutarate → Pyruvate + Glutamic acid (Enzyme Alanine transaminase).
  - **Decarboxylation:** All decarboxylation reactions of amino acids require PLP as coenzyme. A few examples are given below:

- Glutamate → GABA (gamma aminobutyric acid). GABA is an inhibitory neurotransmitter, and, hence in B_6 deficiency, especially in children, **convulsions** may occur.
- Histidine → histamine, which is the mediator of **allergy** and anaphylaxis.
- 5-hydroxy tryptophan → serotonin.

– **Sulfur-containing Amino Acids:** PLP plays an important role in methionine and cysteine metabolism.
- Homocysteine + Serine → Cystathionine. (Enzyme Cystathionine synthase)
- Cystathionine → Homoserine + Cysteine (Enzyme Cystathionase)

Both these reactions require PLP. Hence, in vitamin B_6 deficiency, **homocysteine** in blood is increased. Homocysteine level is correlated with **myocardial infarction**. Therefore, pyridoxine is used to prevent homocysteinemia.

– **Heme Synthesis:** ALA synthase is a PLP-dependent enzyme. This is the rate limiting step in heme biosynthesis. So, in B_6 deficiency, **anemia** may be seen.

– **Production of Niacin:** Pyridoxal phosphate is required for the synthesis of niacin from tryptophan (**one vitamin is necessary for synthesis of another vitamin**).
3-hydroxykynurenine → 3-hydroxyanthranilic acid (Enzyme Kynureninase).
Kynureninase is a PLP-dependent enzyme. Hence, in vitamin B_6 deficiency, niacin production is less. Moreover, kynurenine cannot be converted further, which is metabolized to xanthurenic acid and excreted through urine.

Glycogenolysis

Phosphorylase enzyme (glycogen to glucose-1-phosphate) requires PLP. In fact, more than 70% of total PLP content of the body is in muscles, where it is a part of the phosphorylase enzyme.

69. Ans. b. Inhibition of membrane Na, K-ATPase

Ref: Vasudevan DM, Sreekumari S, Textbook of Biochemistry, 6/e p282

MECHANISMS OF ACTION OF INSULIN

- **Insulin Receptors:**
  – Insulin acts by binding to a **plasma membrane receptor** on the target cells.
  – Insulin receptor is a glycoprotein with 4 subunits; 2 alpha and 2 beta subunits.
  – The alpha units are located on the extracellular side, to which insulin binds.
  – The beta subunits traverse the membrane and are exposed on the cytoplasmic side. Beta subunit has tyrosine kinase activity.
  – Insulin binds to the alpha subunit. This binding activates the tyrosine kinase activity of the beta subunit, leading to autophosphorylation of the beta subunit. This event, in turn, phosphorylates insulin receptor substrates (IRS).
- **Gene Transcription**
  Insulin acts at the transcriptional level to regulate synthesis of more than 100 proteins.
  2-A. Insulin **induces** the following enzymes:
  – Glucokinase
  – Pyruvate kinase
  – Phosphofructokinase
  – Acetyl CoA carboxylase
  2-B. Insulin **represses** the following enzymes:
  – Glucose 6-phosphatase
  – Phosphoenol pyruvate carboxykinase
  – Fructose 1,6-bisphosphatase
- **Activation of Enzymes**
  – Insulin activates the existing molecules of enzymes by covalent modification (phosphorylation or dephosphorylation). Insulin activates protein phosphatase I (PPI) which dephosphorylates enzyme proteins.
- **Glucose Uptake**
  – Insulin increases the recruitment of GluT4 in adipose tissue and skeletal muscle.

Metabolism	Key enzyme	Action of insulin on the enzyme	Direct effect	Overall effect
Carbohydrate	Translocase	stimulation	Glycolysis favored	Hypoglycemia
	Glucokinase	stimulation		
	Phosphofructokinase	stimulation		
	Pyruvate kinase	stimulation		
	Pyruvate carboxylase	inhibition	Gluconeogenesis depressed	
	PEPCK	inhibition		
	Fructose 1, 6-bisphosphatase	inhibition		
	Glucose 6-phosphatase	inhibition		
	Glycogen synthase	activation	Glycogen deposition	
	Glycogen phospharylase	inactivation		
	GPD	stimulation	Generation of NADPH	Glucose is used for lipogenesis;glucose, lowered
Lipid	Acetyl CoA carboxylase	stimulation	Lipogenesis favored	
	Glycerol kinase	stimulation		
	Hormone-sensitive lipase	inhibition	Lipolysis inhibited	Decreased ketogenesis
	HMG CoA reductase	stimulation	Cholesterol synthesis	
Protein	Transaminases	inhibition	Catabolism inhibited	General anabolism
	Ornithine transcarbamoylase	inhibition		
	RNA polymerase and ribosome assembly	favored	Protein synthesis favored	

70. Ans. a. cGMP

Ref: Vasudevan DM, Sreekumari S, Textbook of Biochemistry 6/e p520. (Refer to question no. 6 in JIPMER 2014)

71. Ans: B. Estrogens *Ref: Vasudevan DM, Sreekumari S, Textbook of Biochemistry, 6/e p541*

Transport of Thyroid Hormones

- Thyroid hormones are transported in plasma by proteins. The bound form is biologically inactive, but they can be rapidly released. Total protein bound iodine (PBI) is about 10 microgram/dl; out of which T4 constitutes 8 micrograms/dl. The thyroxine binding globulin (TBG) carries about 80% of T4 and 60% of T3. The rest of thyroid hormones are loosely bound with Transthyretin (TTR) (prealbumin) and albumin.
- The abnormalities in the level of binding proteins may be reflected as abnormal hormone on TBG; ***The binding proteins are increased in pregnancy when estrogen level is high.*** In malnutrition and nephrotic syndrome, binding proteins are low.

72. Ans. b. RBC *Ref: Harper's Illustrated Biochemistry 28/e*

Ketone Bodies:

- **Liver mitochondria** have the capacity to convert acetyl CoA derived from fatty acid oxidation into ketone bodies.
- The compounds categorized as ketone bodies are **acetoacetate, 3-hydroxybutyrate (also called β-hydroxybutyrate), and acetone.**
- Acetoacetate and 3-hydroxybutyrate are transported in the blood to the peripheral tissues. There they can be reconverted to acetyl CoA, which can be oxidized by the TCA cycle.
- Ketone bodies are important sources of energy for the peripheral tissues because:
  - They are soluble in aqueous solution and, therefore, do not need to be incorporated into lipoproteins or carried by albumin as do the other lipids;
  - They are produced in the liver during periods when the amount of acetyl CoA present exceeds the oxidative capacity of the liver; and
  - They are used in proportion to their concentration in the blood by extrahepatic tissues, such as the skeletal and cardiac muscle and renal cortex. Even the brain can use ketone bodies to help meet its energy needs if the blood levels rise sufficiently. Thus ketone bodies spare glucose.

Use of Ketone Bodies by the Peripheral Tissues: Ketolysis

- Although the liver constantly synthesizes low levels of ketone bodies, their production becomes much more significant during fasting when ketone bodies are needed to provide energy to the peripheral tissues.

- 3-Hydroxybutyrate is oxidized to acetoacetate by 3-hydroxybutyrate dehydrogenase, producing NADH.
- Acetoacetate is then provided with a CoA molecule taken from succinyl CoA by succinyl CoA: acetoacetate CoA transferase (thiophorase). This reaction is reversible, but the product, acetoacetyl CoA, is actively removed by its conversion to two acetyl CoAs.
- Extrahepatic tissues, including the brain but excluding cells lacking mitochondria (for example, red blood cells), efficiently oxidize acetoacetate and 3-hydroxybutyrate in this manner.
- ***In contrast, although the liver actively produces ketone bodies, it lacks thiophorase and, therefore, is unable to use ketone bodies as fuel.***

Ketone bodies are not utilised by RBC because of lack of mitochondria.

Substrate Utilized for Energy Production:

Tissue	Fed	Fasting	Starvation
Brain	Glucose	Glucose	Ketone bodies
Heart	Fatty acids	Fatty acids	Ketone bodies
Liver	Glucose	Fatty acids	Amino acids
Muscle	Glucose	Fatty acids	Fatty acids

73. Ans. b. Increased lipogenesis *Ref: Harper's Illustrated Biochemistry, 28/e*

Metabolic Fuel Reserves are Mobilized in the Fasting State:

- There is a small fall in plasma glucose in the fasting state, and then little change as fasting is prolonged into starvation.
- Plasma free fatty acids increase in fasting, but then rise little more in starvation; as fasting is prolonged, so the plasma concentration of ketone bodies (acetoacetate and 3-hydroxybutyrate) increases markedly.

Plasma Concentrations of Metabolic Fuels (mmol/L) in the Fed and Fasting States

	Fed	40 Hours Fasting	7 Days Starvation
Glucose	5.5	3.6	3.5
Free fatty acids	0.30	1.15	1.19
Ketone bodies	Negligible	2.9	4.5

In the fasting state, as the concentration of glucose in the portal blood falls, insulin secretion decreases, and skeletal muscle and adipose tissue take up less glucose. The increase in secretion of **glucagon** inhibits glycogen synthetase, and activates glycogen phosphorylase in the liver.

- The resulting glucose 6-phosphate is hydrolyzed by glucose 6-phosphatase, and glucose is released into the bloodstream for use by the brain and erythrocytes.
- Muscle glycogen cannot contribute directly to plasma glucose, since muscle lacks glucose 6-phosphatase, and the primary purpose of muscle glycogen is to provide a source of glucose 6-phosphate for energy-yielding metabolism in the muscle itself.
- However, acetyl-CoA formed by oxidation of fatty acids in muscle inhibits pyruvate dehydrogenase, leading to an accumulation of pyruvate.
- Most of this is transaminated to alanine, at the expense of amino acids arising from breakdown of 'labile' protein reserves synthesized in the fed state.
- The alanine, and much of the keto acids resulting from this transamination are exported from muscle, and taken up by the liver, where the alanine is transaminated to yield pyruvate.
- The resultant amino acids are largely exported back to muscle, to provide amino groups for formation of more alanine, while the pyruvate is a major substrate for gluconeogenesis in the liver.

- In adipose tissue the decrease in insulin and increase in glucagon results in inhibition of lipogenesis, inactivation of lipoprotein lipase, and activation of intracellular hormone-sensitive lipase.
- This leads to release from adipose tissue of increased amounts of glycerol (which is a substrate for gluconeogenesis in the liver) and free fatty acids, which are used by liver, heart, and skeletal muscle as their preferred metabolic fuel, therefore sparing glucose.
- Although muscle preferentially takes up and metabolizes free fatty acids in the fasting state, it cannot meet all of its energy requirements by beta-oxidation.
- By contrast, the liver has a greater capacity for beta-oxidation than it requires to meet its own energy needs, and as fasting becomes more prolonged, it forms more acetyl-CoA than can be oxidized.
- This acetyl-CoA is used to synthesize the **ketone bodies**, which are major metabolic fuels for skeletal and heart muscle and can meet some of the brain's energy needs.
- In prolonged starvation, glucose may represent less than 10% of whole body energy-yielding metabolism. Were there no other source of glucose, liver and muscle glycogen would be exhausted after about 18h fasting.
- As fasting becomes more prolonged, so an increasing amount of the amino acids released as a result of protein catabolism is utilized in the liver and kidneys for gluconeogenesis.

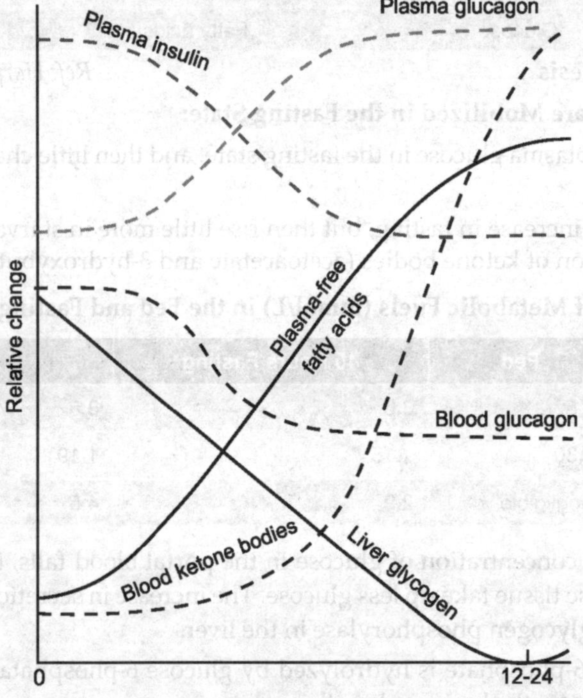

Summary of the Major Metabolic Features of the Principal Organs

Organ	Major pathways	Main substrates	Major products exported	Specialist enzymes
Liver	Glycolysis, gluconeogenesis, lipogenesis, beta-oxidation, citric acid cycle, ketogenesis, lipoprotein metabolism, drug metabolism, synthesis of bile salts, urea, uric acid, cholesterol, plasma proteins	Free fatty acids, glucose (in fed state), lactate, glycerol, fructose, amino acids, alcohol	Glucose, triacylglycerol in VLDL, ketone bodies, urea, uric acid, bile salts, cholesterol, plasma proteins	Glucokinase, glucose 6-phosphatase, glycerol kinase, phosphoenolpyruvate carboxykinase, fructokinase, arginase, HMG CoA synthase, HMG CoA lyase, alcohol dehydrogenase

Contd...

Contd...

Organ	Major pathways	Main substrates	Major products exported	Specialist enzymes
Brain	Glycolysis, citric acid cycle, amino acid metabolism, neurotransmitter synthesis	Glucose, amino acids, ketone bodies in prolonged starvation	Lactate, end products of neurotransmitter metabolism	Those for synthesis and catabolism of neurotransmitters
Heart	Oxidation and citric acid cycle	Ketone bodies, free fatty acids, lactate, chylomicron and VLDL triacylglycerol, some glucose	—	Lipoprotein lipase, very active electron transport chain
Adipose tissue	Lipogenesis, esterification of fatty acids, lipolysis (in fasting)	Glucose, chylomicron and VLDL triacylglycerol	Free fatty acids, glycerol	Lipoprotein lipase, hormone-sensitive lipase, enzymes of pentose phosphate pathway
Fast twitch muscle	Glycolysis	Glucose, glycogen	Lactate, (alanine and ketoacids in fasting)	—
Slow twitch muscle	Oxidation and citric acid cycle	Ketone bodies, chylomicron and VLDL triacylglycerol	—	Lipoprotein lipase, very active electron transport chain
Kidney	Gluconeogenesis	Free fatty acids, lactate, glycerol, glucose	Glucose	Glycerol kinase, phosphoenolpyruvate carboxykinase
Erythrocytes	Anerobic glycolysis, pentose phosphate pathway	Glucose	Lactate	Hemoglobin, enzymes of pentose phosphate pathway

74. Ans. d. ADH *Ref: Vasudevan DM, Sreekumari S, Textbook of Biochemistry, 6/e p528*

Oxytocin and Vasopressin (ADH) are nanopeptides; with 9 amino acids. They are secreted by posterior pituitary.

Antidiuretic Hormone (ADH/Vasopressin)

- Its main action is to prevent diuresis. So it reduces the urine output. ADH acts on the distal convoluted tubules of the kidney, producing reabsorption of water.
- ADH binds to membrane receptor and activates adenylate cyclase. The cyclic AMP thus produced will activate the protein kinase. This, in turn, phosphorylates proteins of the microtubules and microfilaments. The net effect is the reabsorption of water.
- The regulation of ADH secretion is through the osmolality of blood. Lowering of the osmolality (hemodilution) suppresses ADH secretion. Conversely, an increase in osmolality (hemoconcentration or dehydration) leads to stimulation of the secretion of ADH.
- Deficiency of ADH results in **diabetes insipidus.** It is characterized by excretion of large volumes of dilute urine. Hypernatremia and hypertonic contraction of extra cellular fluid volume are also seen. It is a very rare condition.
- Excess secretion of ADH often results from ectopic production of ADH by malignant tumors elsewhere, referred to as the **syndrome of inappropriate secretion of ADH** or SIADH. Here ADH is continuously secreted and is not subjected to any control mechanisms. There is hypotonic expansion of extracellular volume, with hyponatremia. Slow onset is mostly asymptomatic and goes unnoticed but those with acute onset will manifest the symptomatology of water intoxication (headache, confusion, anorexia, nausea, vomiting, coma and convulsions). Hyponatremia and impaired urinary dilution are seen.

75. Ans. a. Histidine *Ref: Textbook of Medical Biochemistry by Dinesh Puri, 3/e p49 Chapter 4*

- Histidine with imidazole ring functions as a general acid base catalyst.
- pKa range of histidine is 6.5 to 7.4, which ionizes within the physiological pH range.

76. Ans. c. Palmitic acid *Ref: Harper's Illustrated Biochemistry 29/e p142 (Refer to question no. 8 in JIPMER 2012)*

77. Ans. d. alcohol intoxication *Ref: Harper's Illustrated Biochemistry, 29/e p (Refer to question no 7 in JIPMER 2012)*

78. Ans. a. mRNA *Ref: Vasudevan DM, Sreekumari S, Textbook of Biochemistry, 6/e p484.*

Post-transcriptional Processing of mRNA:

- The mRNA formed and released from them DNA template is known as the **primary transcript**. It is also known as **heteronuclear mRNA** or hnRNA.
- In mammalian system, it undergoes extensive processing to become the **mature mRNA**.
  These modifications are:
  - Endonuclease cleavage
  - Poly-A tailing
  - Methylation
  - Removal of introns
  - Splicing of exons (connect together).

  These processings occur mainly in the nucleoplasm.
- In bacteria, mRNA is not changed; and translation of mRNA starts even before completion of transcription.
- Post-transcriptional processing is not only for mRNA but for tRNA and rRNA as well.

Poly-A Tailing At 3′ End:

- The 3′ terminus is polyadenylated in the nucleoplasm. This poly-A tail may be 20 to 250 nucleotides long. This tail protects mRNA from attack by 3′ exonuclease.

Capping At 5′ End:

- Eukaryotic mRNAs are all 'capped' at the 5′ terminus by 7-methyl guanosine triphosphate. An unusual 5′ to 5′ triphosphate bridge is seen. This is also done inside the nucleus. The cap is useful in recognition of mRNA by the translating machinery.

Methylation:

- Methylation of N6 of adenine residue and 2′-hydroxyl group of ribose are common. These are mainly done in the cytoplasm.

79. Ans. b. Lagging strand *Ref: Harper's Illustrated Biochemistry 29/e*

Ref: Lippincott Illustrated Reviews Biochemistry 4/e p403

- The DNA polymerases responsible for copying the DNA templates are only able to 'read' the parental nucleotide sequences in the 3′ → 5′ direction, and they synthesize the new DNA strands in the 5′ → 3′ (antiparallel) direction.
- Therefore, beginning with one parental double helix, the two newly synthesized stretches of nucleotide chains must grow in opposite directions—one in the 5′ → 3′ direction toward the replication fork and one in the 5′ → 3′ direction away from the replication fork. This feat is accomplished by a slightly different mechanism on each strand.
- **Leading Strand:** The strand that is being copied in the direction of the advancing replication fork is called the leading strand and is synthesized continuously.
- **Lagging Strand:** The strand that is being copied in the direction away from the replication fork is synthesized discontinuously, with small fragments of DNA being copied near the replication fork. These short stretches of discontinuous DNA, termed Okazaki fragments, are eventually joined to become a single, continuous strand. The new strand of DNA produced by this mechanism is termed the 'lagging strand'.

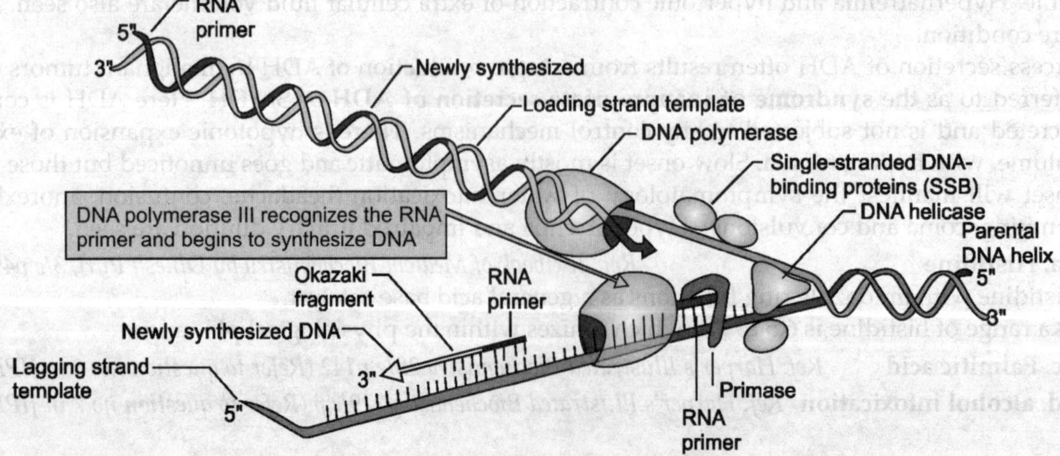

80. Ans. c. Phosphofructokinase

Ref: Vasudevan DM, Sreekumari S, text book of Biochemistry 6/e p224. (Refer to question no. 6 in JIPMER 2014)

81. Ans. a. HGPRTase *Ref: Harper's Illustrated Biochemistry 29/e p335, 339 and 742*

Lesch-Nyhan Syndrome:

- Lesch-Nyhan syndrome, an overproduction hyperuricemia characterized by frequent episodes of uric acid lithiasis and a bizarre syndrome of self-mutilation, reflects a defect in **hypoxanthine-guanine phosphoribosyl transferase**, an enzyme of purine salvage. The accompanying rise in intracellular PRPP results in purine overproduction.
- Mutations that decrease or abolish hypoxanthine-guanine phosphoribosyltransferase activity include deletions, frameshift mutations, base substitutions, and aberrant mRNA splicing.

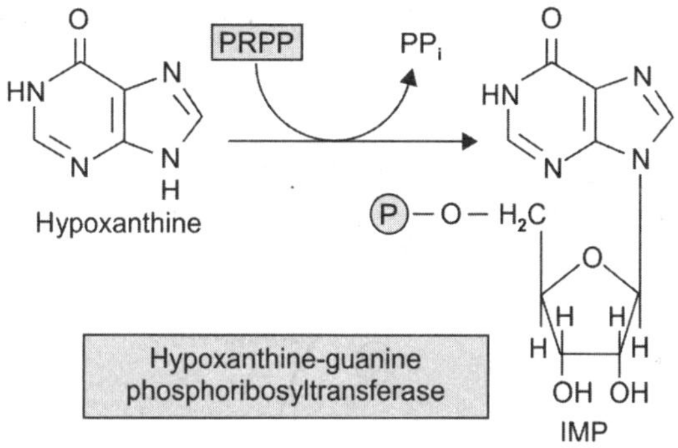

Hypoxanthine + PRPP → IMP + PP_i

Hypoxanthine

IMP

Hypoxanthine-guanine phosphoribosyltransferase

CPS-I and CPS-II:

- One molecule of ammonia condenses with CO2 in the presence of **two molecules of ATP** to form carbamoyl phosphate.
- The reaction is catalyzed by the mitochondrial enzyme **carbamoyl phosphate synthetase-I (CPS-I).**
- An entirely different cytoplasmic enzyme, carbamoyl phosphate synthetase-II, (CPS-II) is involved in pyrimidine nucleotide. CPS-I reaction is the **rate-limiting step** in urea formation. It is irreversible and allosterically regulated.

	CPS I	CPS II
1. Site	Mitochondria	Cytosol
2. Pathway of	Urea	Pyrimidine
3. Positive effector	NAG	Nil
4. Source for N	Ammonia	Glutamine
5. Inhibitor	Nil	CTP

82. Ans. a. Glucogenolysis

Ref: Vasudevan DM, Sreekumari S, Textbook of Biochemistry 6/e p396. (Refer to question no;4 in JIPMER 2013)

83. Ans. a. Histidine load test *Ref: Vasudevan DM, Sreekumari S, Textbook of Biochemistry, 6/e p202*

Assessment of Folate Deficiency

- **Blood Level:** Normal folic acid level in serum is about 20 nanogram/ml and about 200 microgram/ml of packed cells. The level is measured by radio-immuno-assay.
- **Histidine load test or FIGLU excretion test:** Histidine is normally metabolised to formimino glutamic acid (FIGLU) from which formimino group is removed by THFA. Therefore in folate deficiency, FIGLU is excreted in urine.
- **FIGLU Excretion Test:** It is a sensitive indicator for folic acid deficiency. About 5 g of histidine is given three times at 4- hourly intervals. Urine is collected for 24 hours after the initial dose. Normally less than 30 mg of FIGLU is excreted per day; the value is increased in folate deficiency.
- **AICAR Excretion:** In the purine nucleotide synthesis, the last step is the addition of C2 with the help of N10-formyl THFA. When this is blocked, the precursor, amino imidazole carboxamide ribosyl-5-phosphate (AICAR) accumulates and is excreted in urine.

84. Ans. c. Bile Salts *Ref: Vasudevan DM, Sreekumari S, Textbook of Biochemistry, 6/e p159*

Functions of Bile Salts:

- Bile salts facilitate the digestion of lipids.
- They can form molecular aggregates called micelle which bring about the absorption of lipids.
- Bile salt micelle also plays an important role in keeping the cholesterol in solution.

Solubilization of Cholesterol in Bile:

- The relative concentration of cholesterol in the bile favors the precipitation and resultant stone formation; it is referred to as lithogenic bile.
- Bile salts and phospholipids in the bile play a significant role in keeping the cholesterol in solution by forming mixed micelle.
- Infections of the gallbladder may predispose to stone formation. Dehydration may also lead to precipitation of cholesterol crystals.

85. Ans. a. Arginase *Ref: Vasudevan DM, Sreekumari S, Textbook of Biochemistry 6/e p178*

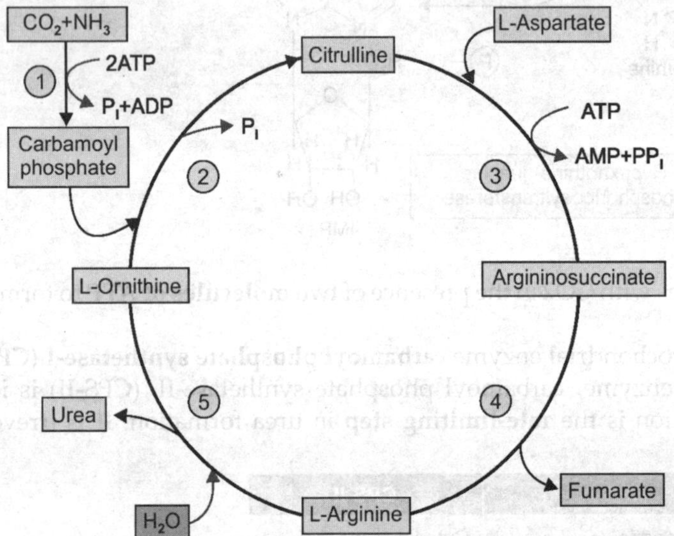

86. Ans. a. Acid Phosphatase *Ref: Vasudevan DM, Sreekumari S, Textbook of Biochemistry, 6/e p9*

Fraction	Enzymes
Plasma membrane	5 nucleotidase, Na-K ATPase
Nucleus	DNA, RNA polymerases
ER	Glucose 6-Phosphatase
Golgi Apparatus	Galactosyl transferase, Manosidase
Lysosomes	Acid phosphatase
Mitochondria	Cytochrome oxidase, Succinated dehydrogenase
Cytosol	Lactate dehydrogenase Glucose 6-Phosphate dehydrogenase

87. Ans. d. Carboxylation *Ref: Vasudevan DM, Sreekumari S, Textbook of Biochemistry, 6/e p389*

- Vitamin K1–Phylloquinone
- Vitamin K2–Menaquinone
- Vitamin K3–Menadione. It is water-soluble synthetic vitamin, widely used in clinical practice.

Biochemical Role of Vitamin K

- Vitamin K is necessary for coagulation. Factors dependent on vitamin K are Factor II **(prothrombin)**; Factor VII; Factor IX (Christmas factor); Factor X (Stuart-Prower factor).
- All these factors are synthesized by the liver as inactive zymogens. They undergo **post-translational** modification; gamma carboxylation of glutamic acid residues. These are the binding sites for calcium ions. The **gamma carboxyglutamic acid** (GCG) synthesis requires vitamin K as a cofactor.

- Vitamin Kdependent gamma carboxylation is also necessary for the functional activity of osteocalcin as well as structural proteins of kidney, lung and spleen. **Osteocalcin** is synthesized by osteoblasts and seen only in bone.

Vitamin K-dependent Carboxylase

- It is microsomal enzyme. It requires oxygen, CO_2, NADPH and reduced vitamin K. In this process, the vitamin passes through a cycle. This process is competitively inhibited by **warfarin and dicoumarol.**

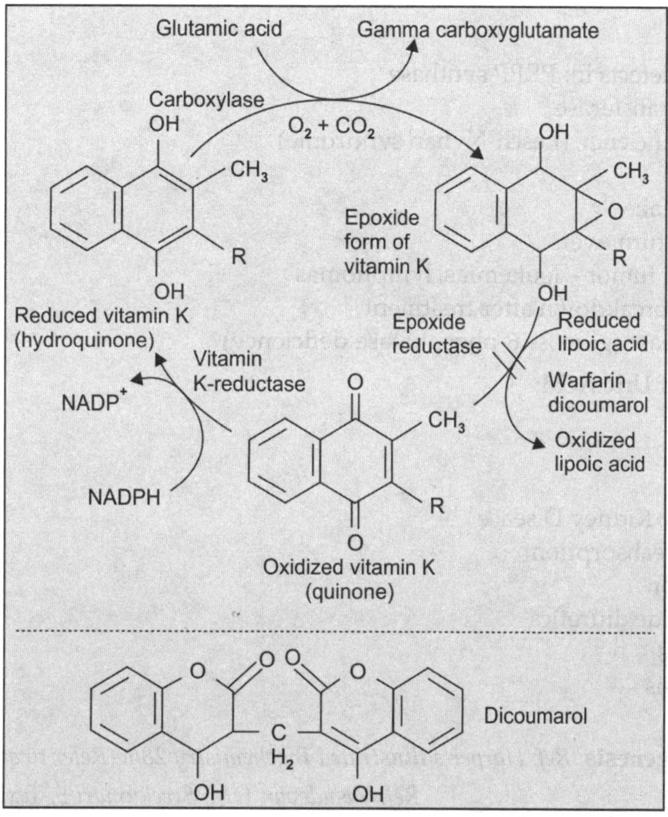

88 Ans. b. Facilitated diffusion *Ref: Vasudevan DM, Sreekumari S, Textbook of Biochemistry, 6/e p91*

- The GLUT 5 Na+ independent facilitative transporter allows fructose as well as glucose and galactose to be transported down their concentration gradients.
- Exit from the cell for all gugars is via the GLUT2 facilitative transporter.

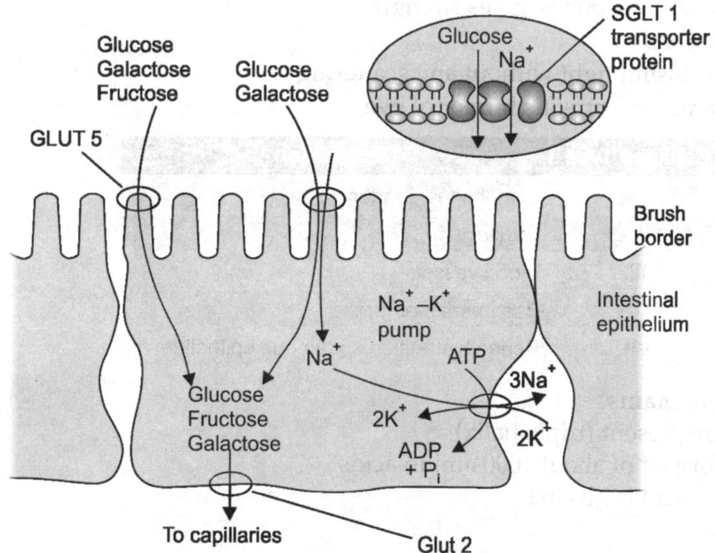

89. Ans. b. Pseudogout enzyme *Ref: Vasudevan DM, Sreekumari S, Textbook of Biochemistry 6/e p464*

GOUT:

- It is due to accumulation of urate crystals in the synovial fluid resulting in inflammation leading to acute arthritis.

Increased Formation of Uric Acid:

- ***Primary:***
  - Idiopathic
  - Due to enzyme defects in: PRPP synthase
    - PRPP amidotransferase
    - HGPRTase deficiency (Lesch-Nyhan syndrome)
- ***Secondary:***
  - Excess purine intake
  - ↑ed nucleic acid turn over.
  - Rapidly growing tumor – leukemias, lymphomas
  - Increased tissue breakdown after treatment
  - von Gierke's disease (glucose 6-phosphatase deficiency)

Decreased Excretion of Uric Acid:

- ***Primary:***
  - Idiopathic
- ***Secondary:***
  - Acute or Chronic Kidney Disease
  - Increased renal reabsorption
  - Reduced secretion
  - Salicylate, Thiazide diuretics
  - Diabetes mellitus
  - Metabolic acidosis
  - Lactic acidosis

90. Ans. b. Increased lipogenesis *Ref: Harper's Illustrated Biochemistry 28/e (Refer to question no. 9 in JIPMER 2010)*

91. Ans. a. Lysine *Ref: Vasudevan DM, Sreekumari S, Textbook of Biochemistry, 6/e p581*

Collagen

- Most abundant protein in the body (25% of proteins)
- Forms Extra-cellular framework
- Distributed throughout the body
- Fibres arranged at angles–bones–gives strength
- Parallel fibres–tendons
- Stacked–cornea–transmit light without any scattering
- Gel–extracellular matrix, vitreous humor of eye

Group	Collagen Type	Distribution
Fibril-forming	I	Skin, bones, tendon
	II	Cartilage
	III	Blood vessels
Network-forming	IV	Basement membrane
	VII	Beneath stratified squamous epithelium

Collagen Structure: α-chains

- Three α-chains are present (triple helix)
- Each α-chain is formed of about 1000 amino acids
- Every third amino acid is glycine

- Repeats of $(Gly\text{-}X\text{-}Y)_n$ is present
- X = mostly proline; can be any amino acid
- Y = mostly hydroxyproline; can be any amino acid
- Lysine and hydroxylysine are also present in position X and Y.
- Hydroxylation: helps in hydrogen bond formation and stabilizing the triple helix structure of collagen

Post-translational Processing of Collagen

Intracellular Alterations:

- Hydroxylation of proline and some lysine residues.
- Glycosylation of some of the hydroxylysine residues.
- Formation of intrachain and interchain disulphide bonds, mainly in the carboxy and amino terminal ends.
- Formation of triple helix.

Extracellular Alterations:

- Cleavage of 25–35 kDa portions at both carboxy and amino terminal ends
- Formation of quarter-staggered alignment
- Oxidative deamination of epsilon amino groups of lysine and hydroxylysine residues
- Formation of intra- and interchain crosslinks.

92. Ans. b. Beri-beri *Ref: Vasudevan DM, Sreekumari S, Textbook of Biochemistry, 6/e p392*

Thiamine is also called vitamin B1.

Physiological Role of Thiamine:

- *Pyruvate Dehydrogenase:* The coenzyme form is **thiamine pyrophosphate** (TPP). It is used in oxidative decarboxylation of alpha-keto acids, e.g. pyruvate dehydrogenase catalyzes the breakdown of pyruvate to acetyl CoA and carbon dioxide.
- *Alpha-Ketoglutarate Dehydrogenase:* An analogous biochemical reaction that requires TPP is the oxidative decarboxylation of **alpha-ketoglutarate** to succinyl CoA and CO_2.

  Transketolase:
  - The second group of enzymes that use TPP as co-enzyme are the transketolases, in the hexose monophosphate shunt pathway of glucose.
  - The main role of thiamine (TPP) is in carbohydrate metabolism. So, the requirement of thiamine is increased along with higher intake of carbohydrates.
  - In thiamine deficiency, blood thiamine is reduced, but pyruvate, alpha ketoglutarate and lactate are increased. Erythrocyte transketolase activity is reduced; this is the earliest manifestation seen even before clinical disturbances.

DEFICIENCY MANIFESTATIONS OF THIAMINE

- ***Beriberi:*** Deficiency of thiamine leads to beriberi. It is a Singhalese word, meaning "weakness". The early symptoms are anorexia, dyspepsia, heaviness and weakness. Subjects feel weak and get easily exhausted.
- ***Wet beriberi:*** Here cardiovascular manifestations are prominent. Edema of legs, face, trunk and serous cavities are the main features. Palpitation, breathlessness and distended neck veins are observed. Death occurs due to heart failure.
- ***Dry beriberi:*** In this condition, CNS manifestations are the major features. Walking becomes difficult. Peripheral neuritis with sensory disturbance leads to complete paralysis.
- ***Infantile beriberi:*** It occurs in infants born to mothers suffering from thiamine deficiency. Restlessness and sleeplessness are observed.
- ***Wernicke-Korsakoff syndrome:*** It is also called **cerebral beriberi**. Clinical features are those of encephalopathy (ophthalmoplegia, nystagmus, cerebellar ataxia) plus psychosis. It is seen only when the nutritional status is severely affected.
- ***Polyneuritis:*** It is common in chronic alcoholics. Alcohol utilization needs large doses of thiamine. Alcohol inhibits intestinal absorption of thiamine, leading to thiamine deficiency. Polyneuritis may also be associated with pregnancy and old age. Such thiamine deficiency in alcoholism may cause impairment of conversion of pyruvate to acetyl CoA. This results in increased plasma concentration of pyruvate and lactate, leading to **lactic acidosis.**

93. Ans. a. Methionine *Ref: Vasudevan DM, Sreekumari S, Textbook of Biochemistry, 6/e p192*

Hypermethioninemias

Causes of hypermethioninemia are:
- Impaired utilization
- Excessive remethylation of homocysteine
- Secondary to hepatic dysfunction.

Oasthouse syndrome is due to malabsorption of methionine. Such children excrete methionine, aromatic amino acids and branched chain amino acids in urine.

94. Ans. b. Phosphoglycerate kinase *Ref: Vasudevan DM, Sreekumari S, Textbook of Biochemistry, 6/e p97*

Energy Yield from Glycolysis:
- During **anerobic** (oxygen deficient) condition, when one molecule of glucose is converted to 2 molecules of lactate, there is a net yield of 2 molecules of ATP.
- 4 molecules of ATP are synthesized by the 2 substrate level phosphorylations (steps 6 and 9). But 2 molecules of ATP are used in the steps 1 and 3, hence the **net yield is only 2 ATP.**
- The whole reaction is summarized as:
  Glucose + 2 Pi + 2 ADP → 2 Lactate + 2 ATP
- But when **oxygen is in plenty**, the two NADH molecules, generated in the glyceraldehyde 3-phosphate dehydrogenase reaction (step 5), can enter the mitochondrial electron transport chain for complete oxidation. As each NADH provides 2.5 ATPs, this reaction generates 2.5 x 2 = 5 ATPs. Thus when oxygen is available, the net gain of energy from the glycolysis pathway is **7 ATPs.**
- Hence, the ATP yield from glycolysis is different in anaerobic and aerobic conditions.
- Pyruvate is later oxidatively decarboxylated to acetyl CoA, which enters into the citric acid cycle. Complete oxidation of glucose through glycolysis plus citric acid cycle will yield a **net 32 ATPs.**

ATP formation in the catabolism of glucose (malate shuttle)

Pathway	Reaction catalyzed by	Method of ATP formation	ATP per Mol of glucose
Glycolysis	Glyceraldehydes 3-phosphate dehydrogenase	Respiratory chain oxidation of 2 NADH	5
	Phosphoglycerate kinase	**Substrate level phosphorylation**	2
	Pyruvate kinase	**Substrate level phosphorylation**	2
			10
	Consumption of ATP for reactions of hexokinase and phosphorylation		–2
			Net 7
Citric acid cycle	Pyruvate dehydrogenase	Respiratory chain oxidation of 2 NADH	5
	Isocitrate dehydrogenase	Respiratory chain oxidation of 2 NADH	5
	α-Ketoglutarate dehydrogenase	Respiratory chain oxidation of 2 NADH	5
	Succinate thiokinase	**Substrate level phosphorylation**	2
	Succinate dehydrogenase	Respiratory chain oxidation of 2 FADH2	3
	Malate dehydrogenase	Respiratory chain oxidation of 2 NADH	5
			Net 25
	Total per mol of glucose under aerobic conditions		32
	Total per mol of glucose under aerobic conditions		2

95. Ans. d. Myophosphorylase *Ref: Vasudevan DM, Sreekumari S, text book of Biochemistry, 6/e p111*

Glycogen storage diseases:

Type	Name	Enzyme deficiency	Clinical features
Type 0	—	Glycogen synthase	Hyperglycemia, hyperketonemia, early death
Type I	von Gierke's disease	Glucose-6 phosphatase	Liver cells and renal tubule cells loaded with glycogen. Hypoglycemia, lactic academia, ketosis, hyperlipidemia, hyperuricemia
Type II	Pompe's disease	Lysosomal a 1 → 4 and 1 → 6-glucosidase (acid maltase)	Fatal accumulation of glycogen in lysosomes, heart failure
Type III	Forbes' or Cori's disease	Adebranching enzyme limit dextrinosis	Accumulation of a characteristic branched polysaccharide
Type IV	Amylopectinosis, Andersen's disease	Absence of branching enzyme	Accumulation of a polysaccharide having few branch points. Hepatosplenomegaly. Death due to cardiac or liver failure in first year of life
Type V	McArdle's syndrome	Muscle phosphorylase	Diminished exercise tolerance; muscles have abnormally high glycogen content (2.5-4.1%). Little or no lactate in blood after exercise
Type VI	Her's disease	Liver phosphorylase	High glycogen content in liver, tendency toward hypoglycemia
Type VII	Tarui's disease	Decrease of phosphofructokinase in muscle and erythrocytes	Features of McArdle's syndrome + possibility of hemolytic anemia
Type VIII	—	Liver phosphorylase kinase	Similar to Her's disease
Type IX	—	Liver and muscle phosphorylase kinase	Hepatomegaly; accumulation of glycogen in liver and muscle; mild hypoglycemia
Type X	—	C-AMP-dependent protein kinase	Hepatomegaly; accumulation of glycogen in liver

96. Ans. a. NADPH oxidase *Ref: Vasudevan DM, Sreekumari S, Textbook of Biochemistry, 6/e p236*

- A ***free radical*** is a molecule or molecular fragment that contains one or more unpaired electrons in its outer orbital.
- Free radical is generally represented by a superscript dot ($R^{\bullet}$). Oxidation reactions ensure that molecular oxygen is completely reduced to water.
- The products of partial reduction of oxygen are highly reactive and create havoc in the living systems. Hence, they are also called **Reactive oxygen species** or ROS.
  The following are members of this group:
  - Superoxide anion radical ($O_2^{-\bullet}$)
  - Hydroperoxyl radical ($HOO^{\bullet}$)
  - Hydrogen peroxide (H_2O_2)
  - Hydroxyl radical ($OH^{\bullet}$)
  - Lipid peroxide radical ($ROO^{\bullet}$)
  - Singlet oxygen
  - Nitric oxide ($NO^{\bullet}$)
  - Peroxy nitrite ($ONOO^{-\bullet}$).
- Out of this, hydrogen peroxide and singlet oxygen are not free radicals (they do not have superscript dot). However, because of their extreme reactivity, they are included in the group of reactive oxygen species.

GENERATION OF FREE RADICALS

- They are constantly produced during the normal oxidation of foodstuffs, due to leaks in the electron transport chain in mitochondria. About 1–4% of oxygen taken up in the body is converted to free radicals. Mitochondrial ROS production is modulated largely by the rate of electron flow through respiratory chain complexes.

- Some enzymes such as **xanthine oxidase** and aldehyde oxidase form superoxide anion radical or hydrogen peroxide.
- **NADPH oxidase** in the inflammatory cells (neutrophils, eosinophils, monocytes and macrophages) produces superoxide anion by a process of respiratory burst during phagocytosis. The superoxide is converted to hydrogen peroxide and then to hypochlorous acid (HClO) with the help of **superoxide dismutase** (SOD) and **myeloperoxidase** (MPO). The superoxide and hypochlorous ions are the final effectors of bactericidal action. This is a deliberate production of free radicals by the body. Along with the activation of macrophages, the consumption of oxygen by the cell is increased drastically; this is called **respiratory burst**.
  - In chronic granulomatous disease (CGD), the NADPH oxidase is absent in macrophages and neutrophils. In this condition, macrophages ingest bacteria normally, but cannot destroy them. However, streptococci and pneumococci themselves produce H_2O_2. Therefore, they are destroyed by the myeloperoxidase system of the macrophages. But staphylococci being catalase positive can detoxify H_2O_2 in the macrophages and therefore are not destroyed in such persons. Hence, recurrent pyogenic infection by staphylococci are common in chronic granulomatous disease.

FREE RADICAL SCAVENGER SYSTEMS

- ***Superoxide Dismutase (SOD)***
- The mitochondrial SOD is **manganese** dependent; cytoplasmic enzyme is **copper-zinc** dependent. SOD is a non-heme protein. A defect in SOD gene is seen in patients with amyotrophic lateral sclerosis (Lou Gehrig's disease).
- ***Glutathione Peroxidase***
- In the next step, the H_2O_2 is removed by glutathione peroxidase (POD). It is a selenium dependent enzyme.
- ***Glutathione Reductase***
- The oxidized glutathione, in turn, is reduced by the glutathione reductase (GR), in presence of NADPH. This NADPH is generated with the help of glucose 6-phosphate dehydrogenase (GPD) in HMP shunt pathway. Therefore in GPD deficiency, the RBCs are liable to lysis, especially when oxidizing agents are administered (drug-induced hemolytic anemia).
- ***Catalase***

When H_2O_2 is generated in large quantities, the enzyme catalase is also used for its removal. In such persons. Hence, recurrent pyogenic infection by staphylococci are common in chronic granulomatous disease.

$$2\,H_2O_2 \xrightarrow{\text{Catalase}} O_2 + 2\,H_2O$$

$$O_2^{\bar{\cdot}} + O_2^{\bar{\cdot}} + 2H^+ \xrightarrow{\text{SOD}} H_2O_2 + O_2$$

$$H_2O_2 \xrightarrow{\text{POD}} 2H_2O$$

2GSH → GS–SG (POD)

GS–SG → 2GSH (GR)

NADPH → $NADP^+$ (GR)

Glucose → NADPH (GPD)

97. Ans. b. Taurocholic acid *Ref: Vasudevan DM, Sreekumari S, Textbook of Biochemistry 6/e p158.*

FORMATION OF BILE ACIDS

- Bile acids are synthesised in the liver from cholesterol. They contain 24 carbon atoms. The reactions for synthesis of bile acids are summarized below:
  - Cholesterol hydroxylated at 3/7/12 positions. The **rate-limiting** step in bile acid synthesis is the introduction of this hydroxyl group by the enzyme **7-alpha-hydroxylase.**
  - Removal of 3-carbon unit, to make it 24 C

- Conjugation with glycine/Taurine
- Secretion into intestinal canal
- In the intestine, deconjugation and removal of hydroxyl groups.

PRIMARY BILE ACIDS

- Cholic acid
- Cheno deoxy cholic acid

The primary bile acids are conjugated with either **glycine or taurine** to form bile acids. They are glyco-cholic acid, tauro cholic acid, glyco chenodeoxycholic acid and tauro chenodeoxycholic acid

SECONDARY BILE ACIDS

- Deoxy cholic acid
- Lithocholic acid

FUNCTIONS OF BILE

- The alkaline pH of the bile serves to neutralise the acidity of the gastric juice.
- The bile salts are efficient surfactants and detergents.
- Bile is the only route of excretion for bilirubin, the end product of heme catabolism.
- Bile salts facilitate the digestion of lipids. They can form molecular aggregates called **micelle** which bring about the absorption of lipids. Bile salt micelle also plays an important role in keeping the cholesterol in solution. It serves to excrete cholesterol, thus regulating the body cholesterol pool.
- Bile serves as the medium of excretion for several drugs, which are detoxified by the liver.

98. Ans. b. Proline *Ref: Vasudevan DM, Sreekumari S, Textbook of Biochemistry 6/e p31*

ALPHA HELIX:

- The alpha-helix is the most common and stable conformation for a polypeptide chain.In proteins like hemoglobin and myoglobin, the alpha-helix is abundant, whereas it is virtually absent in chymotrypsin.
- The structure is stabilized by hydrogen bonds between NH and C=O groups of the main chain.
- Each turn is formed by 3.6 residues. The distance between each amino acid residue is 1.5 Å.
- The alpha-helix is generally right handed. Left handed alpha helix is rare, because amino acids found in proteins are of L-variety, which exclude left handedness. *Proline and hydroxy proline will not allow the formation of alpha-helix.*

99. Ans. a. Hexoaminidase A *Ref: Vasudevan DM, Sreekumari S, Textbook of Biochemistry, 6/e p169*

Examples of Sphingolipidoses

Disease	Enzyme deficiency	Clinical symptoms
Tay-Sachs disease	Hexosaminidase A	Mental retardation, blindness, muscular weakness
Fabry's disease	α Galactosidase	Skin rash, kidney failure (full symptoms only in males; X-linked recessive)
Metachromatic leukodystrophy	Arylsulfatase A	Mental retardation and psychologic disturbances in adults; demyelination
Krabbe's disease	β Galactosidase	Mental retardation; myelin almost absent
Gaucher's disease	β Glucosidase	Enlarged liver and spleen, erosion of long bones, mental retardation in infants
Niemann-Pick disease	Sphingomyelinase	Enlarged liver and spleen, mental retardation; fatal in early life
Farber's disease	Ceramidase	Hoarseness, dermatitis, skeletal deformation, mental retardation; fatal in early life

100. Ans. a. Calcium *Ref: Harper's Illustrated Biochemistry 28/e*

HEMOCHROMATOSIS:

- The key feature of hemochromatosis is an **increase of total body iron** sufficient to cause tissue damage.
- Total body iron ranges between 2.5 g and 3.5 g in normal adults; in hemochromatosis, it usually exceeds 15 g.
- A combination of hepatomegaly, skin pigmentation, diabetes mellitus, heart disease, arthropathy, and hypogonadism should suggest the condition.

- The finding of elevated levels of **transferrin saturation** and of serum **ferritin** are the most useful tests for **diagnosis.**
- Because **cirrhosis** is a major determinant of clinical outcome, a **liver biopsy** is important if the diagnosis of hemochromatosis is not made early in the course of the disease.
- It is critical to **diagnose the condition early** to prevent complications, such as cirrhosis and liver cancer. To achieve early diagnosis, a **high index of suspicion** is necessary.
- Hemochromatosis may be **hereditary** or **secondary** to a variety of causes (e.g. conditions requiring blood transfusions and dietary overload in parts of Africa where beer is brewed in iron pots).
- In hereditary hemochromatosis, **absorption** of iron from the small intestine is greatly increased. There is no pathway for disposing of excess iron and also the solubility of ferric iron is low. The accumulated iron damages organs such as the liver, pancreatic islets, and heart; it is thought to play an important role in tissue damage (e.g. cirrhosis), perhaps in part due to effects on free radical production. Melanin and various amounts of iron accumulate in the skin, accounting for the slate-blue color often seen. The precise cause of melanin accumulation is not clear. The frequent coexistence of diabetes mellitus (due to islet damage) and the skin pigmentation led to use of the term **bronze diabetes** for hereditary hemochromatosis.

ETHANOL ALSO CAUSES FATTY LIVER:

- **Alcoholic fatty liver** is the first stage in **alcoholic liver disease (ALD)** which is caused by **alcoholism** and ultimately leads to **cirrhosis.**
- The fat accumulation in the liver is caused by a combination of impaired fatty acid oxidation and increased lipogenesis, which is thought to be due to changes in the [NADH]/[NAD+] redox potential in the liver, and also to interference with the action of transcription factors regulating the expression of the enzymes involved in the pathways.
- Oxidation of ethanol by **alcohol dehydrogenase** leads to excess production of NADH.
- The metabolism of ethanol occurs mainly in the liver and involves two routes.
- The first and major route uses **alcohol dehydrogenase** and **acetaldehyde dehydrogenase,** converting ethanol via acetadehyde to acetate, which is then converted to acetyl-CoA. NADH + H+ are produced in both of these reactions.
- The intracellular **ratio of NADH/NAD+** can thus be increased appreciably by ingestion of large amounts of ethanol.
- In turn, this can affect the Keq of a number of important metabolic reactions that use these two cofactors.
- High levels of NADH favor **formation of lactate** from pyruvate, accounting for the lacticacidosis.
- This diminishes the concentration of pyruvate and thus **inhibits gluconeogenesis**. In severe cases, when liver glycogen is depleted and no longer available for glycogenolysis, **hypoglycemia** results.
- The second route involves a **microsomal cytochrome P450** (microsomal ethanol oxidizing system), also producing acetaldehyde.
- **Acetaldehyde** is a highly reactive molecule and can form adducts with proteins, nucleic acids, and other molecules.
- It appears likely that its ability to react with various molecules is involved in the causation of the toxic effects of ethanol.
- Ethanol also appears to be able to **interpolate into biologic membranes**, expanding them and increasing their fluidity.
- When the membranes affected are excitable, this results in alterations of their action potentials, impairs active transport across them, and also affects neurotransmitter release.
- All of these depress cerebral function and, if severe enough, can produce coma and death from respiratory paralysis.

Wilson's Disease is Due to Mutations in a Gene Encoding a Copper-binding P-type ATPase:

- Wilson disease is a genetic disease in which copper fails to be excreted in the bile and accumulates in liver, brain, kidney, and red blood cells.

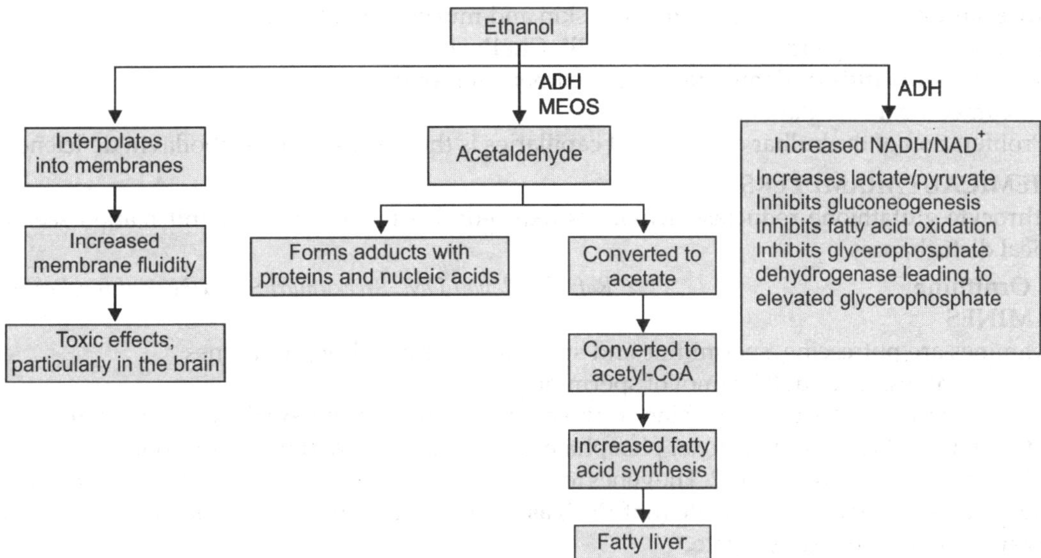

- It can be regarded as an inability to maintain a near-zero copper balance, resulting in copper toxicosis.
- The increase of copper in liver cells appears to inhibit the coupling of copper to apoceruloplasmin and leads to low levels of ceruloplasmin in plasma.
- As the amount of copper accumulates, patients may develop a hemolytic anemia, chronic liver disease (cirrhosis, hepatitis), and a neurologic syndrome owing to accumulation of copper in the basal ganglia and other centers.
- A frequent clinical finding is the Kayser-Fleischer ring. This is a green or golden pigment ring around the cornea due to deposition of copper in Descemet's membrane.

101. Ans. a. Lysine *Ref: Vasudevan DM, Sreekumari S, Textbook of Biochemistry, 6/e p581*

(Refer to question no. 9 in JIPMER 2008)

102. Ans. a. Riboflavin *Ref: Vasudevan DM, Sreekumari S, Textbook of Biochemistry, 6/e p393*

COENZYME ACTIVITY OF RIBOFLAVIN

- Riboflavin exists in tissues tightly bound (but not covalently) with enzymes. Enzymes containing riboflavin are called flavoproteins. The two coenzymes are FMN (flavin mononucleotide) and FAD (flavin adenine dinucleotide).
  - **A. FAD Accepts Hydrogen:** During the oxidation process, FAD accepts two hydrogen atoms from substrate. In turn, FAD is reduced to FADH2. The two nitrogen atoms of isoalloxazine nucleus accept the hydrogen atoms
  - **B. FMN-dependent Enzymes:**
    - During the **amino acid oxidation**, FMN is reduced. It is reoxidized by molecular oxygen to produce hydrogen peroxide.
    - In the **respiratory chain**, the NADH dehydrogenase contains FMN. The electrons are transported in the following manner:

      $NAD+ \rightarrow FMN \rightarrow CoQ$
  - **C. FAD-dependent Enzymes:**
    - Succinate to fumarate by succinate dehydrogenase.
    - Acyl CoA to alpha-beta unsaturated acyl CoA by acyl CoA dehydrogenase
    - Xanthine to uric acid by xanthine oxidase.
    - Pyruvate to acetyl CoA by pyruvate dehydrogenase
    - Alpha ketoglutarate to succinyl CoA by alphaketoglutarate dehydrogenase

    $FADH_2$ when oxidized in the electron transport chain will generate 1½ ATP molecules.

RIBOFLAVIN DEFICIENCY

- **Causes:** Natural deficiency of riboflavin in man is uncommon, because riboflavin is synthesized by the intestinal flora. Riboflavin deficiency usually accompanies other deficiency diseases such as beriberi, pellagra and kwashiorkor.

- **Manifestations:** Symptoms are confined to skin and mucous membranes.
  - **i. Glossitis. ii.** Magenta-colored tongue. **iii. Cheilosis**
  - **Angular stomatitis** (inflammation at the corners of mouth).
  - Circumcorneal vascularization.
  - Proliferation of the bulbar conjunctival capillaries is the earliest sign of riboflavin deficiency.

BIOCHEMICAL PARAMETERS

- Erythrocyte glutathione reductase activity is reduced; this is the earliest manifestation seen even before clinical disturbances.

103. Ans. b. Ornithine *Ref: Vasudevan DM, Sreekumari S, Textbook of Biochemistry, 6/e p199*

POLYAMINES

- Polyamines are putrescine, spermidine and spermine. The are aliphatic amines.
- Humans synthesize about 0.5 mmol of spermine per day.
- They are synthesized from Ornithine. Key enzyme of polyamine synthesis is ornithine decarboxylase (ODC) (step 4). It requires pyridoxal phosphate, and is induced by steroid hormones.
- ODC gene is on chromosome no. 2. The genes for the enzyme SAM decarboxylase (step 2) are on chromosomes 6 and X. This enzyme has pyruvate (not PLP) as the prosthetic group; it is the only mammalian enzyme, known to contain bound pyruvate.

COOH–CHNH$_2$–CH$_2$–CH$_2$–S–CH$_3$
Methionine
ATP
1
PPi + Pi
COOH–CHNH$_2$–CH$_2$–CH$_2$–S–CH$_3$
S-adenosyl-methionine (SAM)
Adenosine
2
CO_2
CH$_2$NH$_2$–CH$_2$–CH$_2$–S–CH$_3$
Decarboxy-SAM (DSAM)
Adenosine
3
CH$_2$NH$_2$–CH$_2$–CH$_3$
Amino propane (part added in reaction number 5 and 6)
CH$_3$–S–Adenosine (Methyl thioadenosine) (MTA)
COOH
Ornithine
4
CO_2
Putrescine
DSAM
5
MTA
Spermidine
DSAM
6
MTA
Spermine

Polyamine synthesis; 1 = methionine adenosyl transferase; 2 = SAM decarboxylase; 3 = reaction coupled with 5 and 6; 4 = Ornithine decarboxylase; 5 = Spermidine synthase; 6 = Spermine synthase. SAM = S-adenosyl methionine; DSAM = decarboxy-SAM; MTA = methyl thioadenosine

BIOCHEMICAL FUNCTIONS OF POLYAMINES

- Polyamines are required for protein biosynthesis.
- The translation initiation factor eIF-4D contains one **hypusine residue**, which is formed by addition of butylamine moiety from spermidine to lysine. IF-4D is the only known protein containing hypusine.
- Several roles are suggested for polyamines, e.g. cell proliferation, stabilisation of ribosomes and DNA, synthesis of DNA and RNA, protection of DNA against depurination, etc.
- Polyamine concentration is increased in **cancer** tissues.
- Polyamines are **growth factors** in cell culture systems. Methyl thio adenosine has growth inhibitory activity.

HIGH YIELD POINTS

- ***Olestra*** is an *artificial fat substitute* designed to allow individuals to obtain the taste and food constituency of fat without the calories from fat. It consists of sucrose molecules to which fatty acids are esterified to the hydroxyl group.
- ***PCNA*** is proliferating cell nuclear antigen which enhances the processivity of DNA polymerase enzyme in replication. It is clinically used as one of the diagnostic marker for proliferating cells.
- ***Perilipin*** are adipoctye phosphoproteins that bind to triacylglycerol droplets and regulate the accessibility of triacylglycerol to lipases.
- ***Abetalipoproteinemia*** is due to lack of microsomal triglyceride transfer protein (MTP) which contains two subunits namely protein disulfide isomerase (PDI) and triglyceride transfer activity subunit.
- ***Lysosomal acid lipase deficiency*** can lead to build up of fatty material in various organs includind liver, spleen, gut, in the walls of blood vessels.
- Early onset lysosomal acid lipase deficiency causes ***Wolman Disease.***
- Late onset lysosomal acid lipase deficiency causes ***Cholesterol Ester Storage Disease.***
- Glucose 1 phosphate is known as **Cori's Ester.**
- The optimal dietary ratio of omega-6 to omega-3 PUFA is 4:1.
- ***Malondialdehyde*** is formed by fatty acids with 3 or more double bonds and is used as a measure of lipid peroxidation.
- 1kcalorie = 4.18 KJ.
- ***Beta-2 microglobulin*** is found on the surface of all nucleated cells and can be used as a non specific marker of high cell turnover that is often observed in tumours.
- ***Fetal fibronectin*** is produced at the boundary between amniotic sac and deciduas which predicts the short term risk of premature delivery.
- ***Beta-trace protein***: Established as an accurate marker of CSF leakage and also as a promising marker in the diagnosis of perilymphatic fluid fistulas.
- There are two transferrin bands normally in CSF protein electrophoresis. The second transferring band is known as ***tau protein*** and is deficient in sialic acid content.
- All enzymes of TCA cycle are present in mitochondrial matrix except succinate dehydrogenase which is present in innr mitochondrial membrane.
- The ***placental lactogen*** secretion near term is 1–2 g/day, the largest of any known human hormone.
- Most common form of ***congenital adrenal hyperplasi*** is due to 21 alpha hydroxylase deficiency.
- Gaucher's disease of spleen is the only non-bone condition in which ***serum acid phosphatase*** (tartrate resistant) level is elevated.
- Amino acid that ***do not undergo transamination*** are lysine, threonine, proline and hydroxyproline.
- ***Garrods tetrad*** includes cystinuria, pentosuria, alkaptonuria and albinism.
- ***Glycoforms*** are glycoproteins with identical amino acid sequences but different oligosaccharide composition.
- In cells, multi-enzyme complex ensures efficient passage of the product of one enzyme reaction to the next enzyme in the pathway. Such complxes are called ***Metabolons.***
- ***Odor of urine*** in inborn errors of metabolism
  - Phenylketonuria–mousy odor
  - Maple syrup urine disease–burnt sugar odor.
  - Tyrosenemia type-1–cabbage like odor.
- **21st** amino acid is selenocysteine and 22nd amino acid is pyrrolysine.
- The end products of ***pyrimidine catabolism*** are ammonia, carbon dioxide, beta alanine and beta amino isobutyrate.
- ***Atkin's diet*** is low carbohydrate ketogenic high protein diet.
- The major function of ***hepcidin*** in iron metabolism is to downregulate DMT-1 and ferroportin, which are responsible for moving iron across cell membranes.

QUESTIONS 2015

1. **Normal volume of CSF is:**
   a. 150 ml
   b. 100 ml
   c. 200 ml
   d. 250 ml
2. **Which of the following is higher in CSF when compared to plasma:**
   a. Glucose
   b. Albumin
   c. Protein
   d. Chloride
3. **Northern blot is used for:**
   a. RNA
   b. DNA
   c. Protein
   d. cDNA
4. **Mousy odor of urine is seen in:**
   a. Phenylketonuria
   b. Tyrosenemia type-I
   c. Maple syrup urine disease
   d. Alkaptonuria
5. **All the following cause shift of oxygen dissociation curve to the left except:**
   a. Decreased pH
   b. Hypothermia
   c. Decreased 2,3 DPG
   d. Fetal hemoglobin
6. **Delta-Bilirubin is:**
   a. Unconjugated bilirubin
   b. Bilirubin monoglucuronide
   c. Bilirubin diglucuronide
   d. Conjugated bilirubin bound with albumin
7. **Which one of the following holds DNA strands together:**
   a. Phosphodiester bond
   b. Hydrogen bond
   c. Glycosidic bond
   d. Phosphate ester
8. **Angiotensin II causes all the following EXCEPT:**
   a. Inhibits rennin release
   b. Increased ADH secretion
   c. Vasodilatation
   d. Aldosterone secretion

ANSWERS AND EXPLANATIONS

1. **Ans. a. 150 ml** *Ref: Vasudevan DM, Sreekumari S, Textbook of Biochemistry, 7/e p422*

Cerebrospinal Fluid (CSF)

- The CSF is found within the subarachnoid space and ventricles of the brain, as well as around the spinal cord. The fluid originates in the choroid plexus and returns to the blood in the vessels of the lumbar region.
- The total volume of fluid is about 125 ml
- It is a transudate or ultrafiltrate of plasma.
- CSF has the chloride concentration higher than the plasma.

Disease	Color and appearance	Cell count	Protein	Sugar	Coagulation
Normal	Clear and colorless	0–4 × 10^6/L	10–30 mg/dL	50–70 mg/dL	Not seen
Bacterial meningitis (purulent meningitis)	Opalescent or turbid due to high cell content	Markedly increased polymorphs	Marked increase	Marked decrease	May clot on standing
Tuberculous meningitis	May be opalescent	Lymphocytes and mononuclear cells	Increased	Low but not very much decreased	Cobweb-type coagulation
Viral infection	Clear and colorless	Increased	Increased	Normal	Nil
Brain tumor	Clear and colorless	Within normal range	Increased	Low	Solidifies
Subarachnoid hemorrhage	Blood stained in fresh hemorrhage	RBCs and WBCs	Increased	Not significant	Nil

2. Ans. d. Chloride *Ref: Vasudevan DM, Sreekumari S, Textbook of Biochemistry 9/e p422*

CEREBROSPINAL FLUID (CSF)

- The CSF is found within the subarachnoid space and ventricles of the brain, as well as around the spinal cord. The fluid originates in the choroid plexus and returns to the blood in the vessels of the lumbar region.
- The total volume of fluid is about 125 ml.
- It is a transudate or ultrafiltrate of plasma.
- CSF has the chloride concentration higher than the plasma.

BIOCHEMICAL ANALYSIS OF CSF

- The protein concentration is usually 10–30 mg/dL, out of which about 20 mg/dL is albumin, and globulin is about 5–10 mg/dL.
- In **bacterial infections** of the meninges, the protein concentration is increased. But in such cases, the neutrophil cell count is also increased.
- In **viral infections,** the protein concentration is not significantly increased, but mononuclear cells are abundant.
- In **brain tumors**, albumin level is raised, but cell count is normal; this is called albuminocytological dissociation.

GLUCOSE LEVEL IN CSF

- Normal level of glucose in CSF is 50–70 mg/dL, which is lower than the plasma level. Hence, estimation of plasma glucose along with CSF glucose is always done to avoid misinterpretation due to a change in the plasma glucose.
- Elevated levels are seen in diabetes mellitus. In bacterial meningitis, however, the glucose level is far lower when compared to the plasma, because it is metabolized by bacteria.

3. Ans: a. RNA *Ref: Harper's Illustrated Biochemistry 28/e p393*

Techniques	Used for
Northern blot	RNA analysis
Southern blot	DNA analysis
Western blot	Protein analysis

4. Ans. a. Phenylketonuria *Ref: Harper's Illustrated Biochemistry, 28/e p237*

- ***Odor of urine*** in inborn errors of metabolism:
  - Phenylketonuria – mousy odor
  - Maple syrup urine disease–burnt sugar odor
  - Tyrosenemia type-1 – cabbage-like odor.

PHENYLKETONURIA

- **Causes**: Phenylalanine hydroxylase deficiency (classical/type-I)
- **Inheritance**: AR. **Incidence** 1:25,000 in india

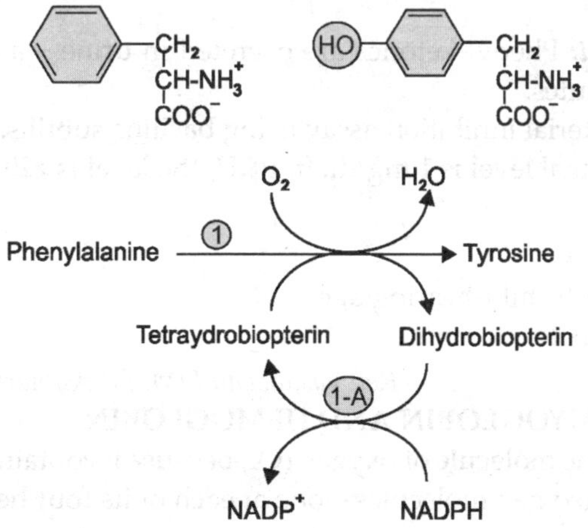

CH_2 $CH\text{-}NH_3^+$ COO^-

HO CH_2 $CH\text{-}NH_3^+$ COO^-

O_2 H_2O

Phenylalanine ① → Tyrosine

Tetraydrobiopterin Dihydrobiopterin

1-A

$NADP^+$ NADPH

1 = Phenylalanine hydroxylase;
1–A = NADPH-dependent reductase

- **TYPES–CLASSICAL**
  Type I is the classical due to phenylalanine hydroxylase deficiency.
- **NONCLASSICAL**

Types II and III are due to deficiency of dihydrobiopterin reductase.

Types IV and V are due to the deficiency of the enzyme synthesizing biopterin. *Biopterin is synthesized from GTP.*

CLINICAL FEATURES:
- Normal at birth
- Delay in developmental milestones
- Microcephaly
- Progressive impairment of cerebral function
- ***Mental retardation***
- Hyperactivity, Agitation, Tremors, Seizures
  Why mental retardation?
  I. Elevated phenylalanine in brain interfers with the transport of other neutral amino acids into the brain.
  Tyrosine–Epinephrine Neurotransmitter precursors
  Tryptophan–Serotonin
  II. Reduces the synthesis/increases the degradation of myelin.
- ***Mousy odor of skin,*** hair and urine (Phenylketone accumulation)
- ***Hypopigmentation***: (Due to defective melanin synthesis and excessive phenylalanine also inhibits tyrosinase)

ALTERNATE PATHWAYS IN PHENYLKETONURIA

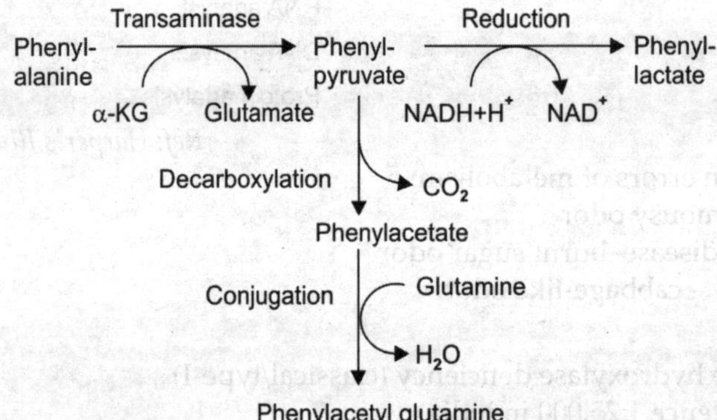

DIAGNOSIS:
- ***Positive ferric chloride test:*** Phenyl ketones are excreted in urine + a drop of ferric chloride. Blue green colour–persists for 2–4 minutes.
- ***Positive Gutherie test:*** Bacterial inhibition assay using bacillus subtilis.
- **Blood phenylalanine:** Normal level is 1 mg/dl. In PKU, the level is >20 mg/dl.

TREATMENT:
- Diet devoid of phenylalanine
- Till 6 years of age/lifelong/till child-bearing age
- Keep phenylalanine levels below 4 mg/dL

5. Ans. a. Decreased pH *Ref: Vasudevan DM, Sreekumari S, Textbook of Biochemistry, 9/e p256*

BINDING OF OXYGEN TO MYOGLOBIN AND HEMOGLOBIN
- Myoglobin can bind only one molecule of oxygen (O_2) because it contains only one heme group. In contrast, hemoglobin can bind four oxygen molecules—one at each of its four heme groups.

OXYGEN DISSOCIATION CURVE

- A plot of Y measured at different partial pressures of oxygen (pO_2) is called the oxygen dissociation curve. The curves for myoglobin and hemoglobin show important differences. The graph illustrates that myoglobin has a higher oxygen affinity at all pO_2 values than does hemoglobin. The partial pressure of oxygen needed to achieve half-saturation of the binding sites (P_{50}) is approximately 1 mm Hg for myoglobin and 26 mm Hg for hemoglobin.

MYOGLOBIN

- The oxygen dissociation curve for myoglobin has a hyperbolic shape.

HEMOGLOBIN

- The oxygen dissociation curve for hemoglobin is sigmoidal in shape.Binding of oxygen to one of the subunits of hemoglobin enhances the binding of oxygen to other subunits. This phenomenon is called cooperativity. Sigmoid shaped oxygen dissociation curve is due to cooperativity.

Factors Causing Shift to Right:	Factors Causing Shift to Left:
• Increased H^+ (decreased pH)	Decreased H+ (increased pH)
• Increased pCO_2	Decreased pCO_2
• 2,3 BPG (bisphosphoglycerate)	Decreased 2,3 BPG
• Increased temperature	Decreased temperature
	Fetal hb (Hb F)

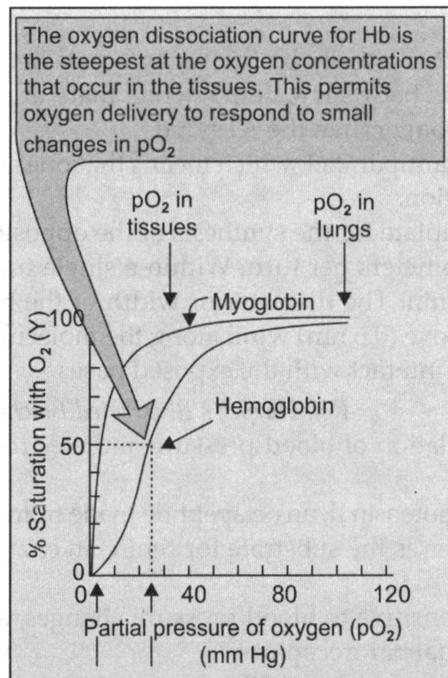

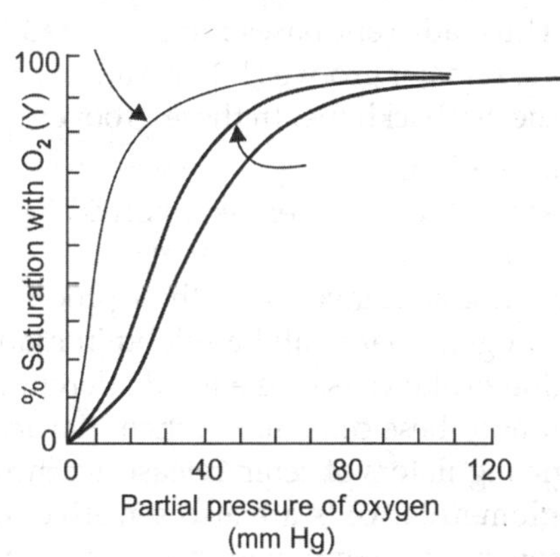

6. Ans. d. Conjugated bilirubin bound with albumin. *Ref: Harrison's Principle of Internal Medicine 18/e*

a. Alpha bilirubin – Unconjugated bilirubin
b. Beta bilirubin – Bilirubin monoglucuronide
c. Gamma bilirubin – Bilirubin diglucuronide
d. Delta bilirubin – Conjugated bilirubin bound with albumin.

- The albumin-linked bilirubin fraction (*delta fraction* or *biliprotein*) represents an important fraction of total serum bilirubin in patients with cholestasis and hepatobiliary disorders.
- Albumin-bound conjugated bilirubin is formed in serum when hepatic excretion of bilirubin glucuronides is impaired and the glucuronides are present in serum in increasing amounts.
- By virtue of its tight binding to albumin, the clearance rate of albumin-bound bilirubin from serum approximates the half-life of albumin, 12–14 days, rather than the short half-life of bilirubin, about 4 hours.

- The prolonged half-life of albumin-bound conjugated bilirubin explains two previously unexplained enigmas in jaundiced patients with liver disease:
  (1) that some patients with conjugated hyperbilirubinemia do not exhibit bilirubinuria during the recovery phase of their disease because the bilirubin is covalently bound to albumin and therefore not filtered by the renal glomeruli, and
  (2) that the elevated serum bilirubin level declines more slowly than expected in some patients who otherwise appear to be recovering satisfactorily. Late in the recovery phase of hepatobiliary disorders, all the conjugated bilirubin may be in the albumin-linked form. Its value in serum falls slowly because of the long half-life of albumin.

7. **Ans. b. Hydrogen bonds.** *Ref: Vasudevan DM, Sreekumari S, Textbook of Biochemistry, 9/e p470*

WATSON-CRICK MODEL OF DNA STRUCTURE

The salient features of Watson-Crick model of DNA structure are given below:

- **Right-handed Double Helix:** DNA consists of two polydeoxy ribonucleotide chains twisted around one another in a right handed double helix similar to a spiral stair case. The sugar and phosphate groups comprise the handrail and the bases jutting inside represent the steps of the staircase. The bases are located perpendicular to the helix axis, whereas the sugars are nearly at right angles to the axis.
- **The Base-pairing Rule:** Always the two strands are **complementary** to each other. So, the adenine of one strand will pair with thymine of the opposite strand, while guanine will pair with cytosine. The base pairing (**A with T; G with C**) is called **Chargaff's rule**, which states that the number of purines is equal to the number of pyrimidines.
- **Hydrogen-bonding:** The DNA strands are held together mainly by hydrogen bonds between the purine and pyrimidine bases. There are two hydrogen bonds between A and T while there are three hydrogen bonds between C and G. The GC bond is therefore stronger than the AT bond.
- **Antiparallel:** The two strands in a DNA molecule run antiparallel, which means that one strand runs in the 5′ to 3′ direction, while the other is in the 3′ to 5′ direction.
- **Other Features:** In the DNA, each strand acts as a template for the synthesis of the opposite strand during replication process. The spiral has a pitch of 3.4 nanometers per turn. Within a single turn, 10 base pairs are seen. Thus, adjacent bases are separated by 0.34 nm. The diameter or width of the helix is 1.9 to 2.0 nanometers. A major groove (1.2 nm) and a minor groove (0.6 nm) wind along the molecule, parallel to the phospho-diester backbone. In these grooves, proteins interact with the exposed bases.

8. **Ans. b. Vasodilatation.** *Ref: Harper's Illustrated Biochemistry 29/e p492*

- The renin-angiotensin system is involved in the regulation of blood pressure and electrolyte metabolism (through production of aldosterone).
- The primary hormone involved in these processes is angiotensin II, an octapeptide made from angiotensinogen
- Angiotensinogen, a large alpha$_2$-globulin made in liver, is the substrate for renin, an enzyme produced in the juxtaglomerular cells of the renal afferent arteriole.
- The position of these cells makes them particularly sensitive to blood pressure changes, and many of the physiologic regulators of renin release act through renal baroreceptors.
- The juxtaglomerular cells are also sensitive to changes of Na^+ and Cl^- concentration in the renal tubular fluid; therefore, any combination of factors that decreases fluid volume (dehydration, decreased blood pressure, fluid or blood loss) or decreases NaCl concentration stimulates renin release.
- Renal sympathetic nerves that terminate in the juxtaglomerular cells mediate the central nervous system and postural effects on renin release independently of the baroreceptor and salt effects, a mechanism that involves the beta-adrenergic receptor.
- Renin acts upon the substrate angiotensinogen to produce the decapeptide angiotensin I.
- Angiotensin-converting enzyme, a glycoprotein found in lung, endothelial cells, and plasma, removes two carboxyl terminal amino acids from the decapeptide angiotensin I to form angiotensin II in a step that is not thought to be rate-limiting.
- Various nonapeptide analogs of angiotensin I and other compounds act as competitive inhibitors of converting enzyme and are used to treat renin-dependent hypertension. These are referred to as **angiotensin-converting enzyme (ACE) inhibitors.**

- Angiotensin II increases blood pressure by causing vasoconstriction of the arteriole and is a very potent vasoactive substance. It inhibits renin release from the juxtaglomerular cells and is a potent stimulator of aldosterone production. This results in Na^+ retention, volume expansion, and increased blood pressure.
- In some species, angiotensin II is converted to the heptapeptide angiotensin III, an equally potent stimulator of aldosterone production. In humans, the plasma level of angiotensin II is four times greater than that of angiotensin III, so most effects are exerted by the octapeptide. Angiotensins II and III are rapidly inactivated by angiotensinases.
- Angiotensin II binds to specific adrenal cortex glomerulosa cell receptors. The hormone-receptor interaction does not activate adenylyl cyclase, and cAMP does not appear to mediate the action of this hormone. The actions of angiotensin II, which are to stimulate the conversion of cholesterol to pregnenolone and of corticosterone to 18-hydroxycorticosterone and aldosterone, may involve changes in the concentration of intracellular calcium and of phospholipid metabolites.

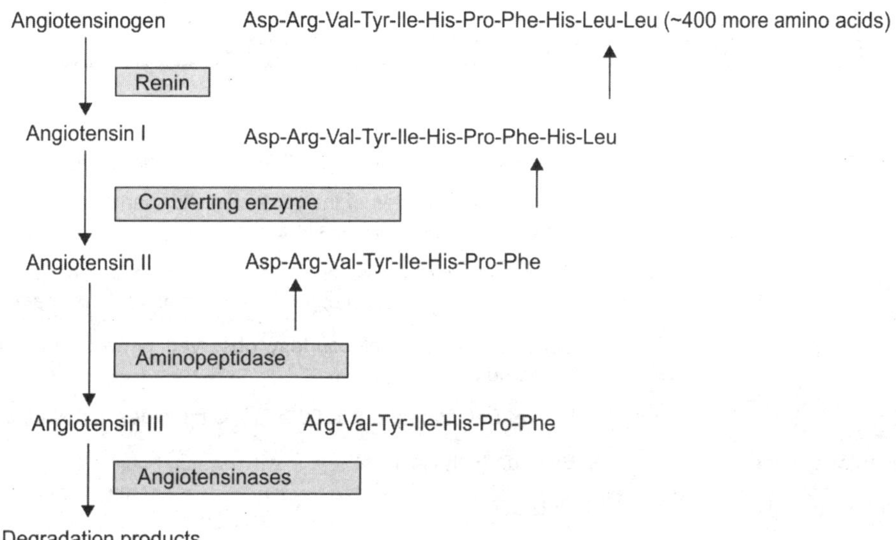

Chapter

4 Forensic Medicine

J Magendran

HISTORY, MEDICAL JURISPRUDENCE AND IDENTIFICATION

History of Forensic Medicine

Forensic or legal medicine	Application of medical knowledge to aid in the administration of justice
Medical jurisprudence	Legal responsibilities of the physician with particular reference to those arising from physician-patient relationship
Medical ethics	The moral principles which should guide members of the medical profession in their dealings with each other, their patients and the State
Medical etiquette	Conventional laws of courtesy observed between members of the medical profession
Code of Hammurabi	King of Babylon (about 2200 B.C.), is the oldest known medicolegal code
The first medicolegal autopsy done in	Bologna (Italy) in 1302
The founder of modern toxicology	Orifila

Legal Procedure

- Indian penal code (IPC) 1860: Defines offences and prescribe punishments
- Criminal procedure code (CrPC) 1973: Provides mechanism for punishment of offences, deals with police duties in arresting offenders, in production of documents, actual procedure in trials of criminal cases
- Indian Evidence Act (IEA) 1872.

Courts	Imprisonment	Fine	Location
Supreme Court	Any sentence	Any fine	National capital
High Court	Any sentence	Any fine	Capital of the state
Sessions Court	Any sentence Death sentence to be confirmed by High Court	Any fine	District
Assistant sessions	Up to ten years	Unlimited	
Chief Judicial Magistrate	Up to seven years	Unlimited	
I Class Judicial Magistrate	Up to three years	5000 rupees	
II Class Judicial Magistrate	Up to one year	1000 rupees	

- Supreme Court and High Court will hear only referrals not trials. Courts below the rank on Sessions Court cannot hear murder trials as they cannot award death sentence
- Any sentence awarded by a Court may be enhanced or decreased by a higher Court.
- The President of India has the power to grant pardons, remissions of punishments and commutation of death sentence.

INQUEST

- Police inquest
- Magistrate inquest
- Coroner's inquest (not in India)
- Medical examiners inquest (not in India).

Police inquest (S 174 CrPC)	Magistrate inquest (S 176 CrPC)
• Conducted usually by SI or Inspector, in the presence of two or more respectable persons (panchas) makes an investigation (S.175 CrPC) – The inquest report (panchanama) is then signed by the investigating police officer and by the witnesses	• Conducted by collector, Tahsildar, Deputy Commissioner, Revenue divisional officer – Death in police custody and while under police interrogation – Death due to police firing – Death in prisons, reformatories, Borstal school – Death in psychiatric hospitals – Dowry deaths – Exhumation

Coroner's Court	Cognizable offence	Conduct money
• Court of enquiry and not a court of trial, which has some judicial powers. • Type of inquest done in U.K., some States in U.S.A., and some other countries, but not in India	• Offence in which a police officer can arrest a person without warrant from the Magistrate, e.g., rape, murder	• Fee paid to a witness in civil cases, to meet the expenses towards attending the court

Dying Declaration vs Dying Deposition

Dying declaration	Dying deposition
Recorded by magistrate or doctor or Investigating officer	Recorded by magistrate
No oath is administered	Oath is administered
Inferior to dying deposition	Superior to dying declaration
Presence of accused or lawyer nor necessary	Recorded in presence of accused or lawyer
No cross examination	Cross examination is allowed
Has corroborative value if patient survives	Retains full legal value even if the person survives

- Witness
- Witnesses are of two types: (1) Common, and (2) Expert
- A doctor can be both a common and expert witness
- Hostile witness: one who purposefully makes statement contrary to facts
- Perjury: Willful utterance of falsehood by a witness under oath.

RECORD OF EVIDENCE IN A COURT OF LAW

Oath-child below 12 years is not required to take an oath

Examination in chief (Direct examination)	Cross examination
• Witness examined by public prosecutor and accused by defense lawyer • No leading questions • Leading questions may be asked if the witness is hostile	• Witness examined by defense lawyer and accused by public prosecutor • Leading Questions allowed • No time limit

Re-examination (Redirect examination)	Questions by the judge
• Similar to direct examination • No leading questions	• Can ask questions at any time of proceedings • Oral evidence is superior to documentary evidence because it is administered under oath and cross examined

Medical Council of India: Indian Medical Council Act 1956

First schedule	Second schedule	Third schedule part A	Third schedule part B
Medical degrees offered by different Universities in India, which are recognized by the Council	Medical degrees offered by different Universities outside India, which are recognized by the Council	Medical degrees conferred by Indian Universities, which are not mentioned in the 1st schedule	Standard medical qualifications of foreign countries, which are not mentioned in 2nd schedule

PENAL ERASURE/PROFESSIONAL DEATH SENTENCE

- Removal of the name of the doctor from the medical register
- Main cause: **Serious professional misconduct/Infamous conduct (conduct of the doctor that is regarded disgraceful and dishonorable)**
- Done by the **State Medical Council**
- Other instances of removal of name
  - After death
  - Name entered by fraud, impersonation.

Medical Negligence:
- Act of omission
- Act of commission.

Types:
- Civil Negligence
- Criminal Negligence.

Components of negligence	Duty, dereliction, direct causation, damage
Doctrine of res Ipsa loquitur	The things or facts speaks for itself. Example: Amputation of a wrong limb
Doctrine of calculated risk	Inherent risk of the procedure
Novus actus interveniens	Unrelated action intervening
Medical maloccurance	Inevitable accidents
Therapeutic misadventure	Mischance or disaster a person dies due to some unintentional act of doctor or hospital
Doctrine of respondent superior (Vicarious liability)	Let the master answer
Contributary negligence	Patient also responsible and contributed to the damage suffered
Corporate negligence	Failure in part of hospital management to provide adequate facilities

CONSENT

- Free and voluntary agreement compliance or permission given for specific purpose.
- Section 90 IPC defines consent in negative form. Not valid if given under fear, misconception, intoxication, unsound mind, less than 12 years of age.

Types
- Implied
- Expressed (Oral or verbal and written)

Exceptions to consent	Consent is not required	Consent of spouse must in
• Emergency, incompetence, therapeutic privilege, waiver	• Emergency, notifiable diseases, public Interest, court order, prisoner, immigrants, postmortem	• Termination of pregnancy, sterilization, artificial insemination, donation of sperm, any procedure hampers sexual activity

MEDICOLEGAL IMPORTANCE OF AGE

Time scale	Significance
4 months IUL	Sex can be recognized
> 7 months IUL	Infanticide
> 5 years	Criminal responsibility (Railways act)
< 7 years	Not guilty of crime (Sec 82 IPC)
7–12 years	Guilty of crime if sufficient maturity present (Sec.83 IPC)
< 12 years	Parents and guardians must given consent
< 14 years	Cannot be employed in factory jobs
14–15 years	Non-hazardous jobs in factories can be given
Boys < 16 years	Taking away without the onset of the parent/guardian is kidnapping
> 18 years	Valid consent, attainment of majority, minimum age to join government service, vote, consent for sexual intercourse, marriage age for girls
21 years	Marriage age for boys
> 25 years	Minimum age for a MP
35 years	Minimum age for president, VP, Governor

Race determination from skull: Cephalic Index = Max. breadth of Skull/Max. length of skull **X** 100

Stature

Estimation of stature or height of a person is subject to variations during life due to muscular relaxation and elasticity of intervertebral discs, but still is valuable.

Formulae for Stature Estimation

- Karl Pearson's formula
- Trotter and Gleser
- Dupertuis and Hadden

As a general rule, humerus is 20%, tibia is 22%, femur is 27% and spine is 35% of individual height.

Age in intrauterine life

HASSE'S Rule	Length of the fetus (crown-heel length) up to 25 cms SQUARE ROOT gives the age of the fetus in months
Morrison's Rule	Above 25 cms DIVIDED by 5 gives the age of the fetus in months

Dactylography

- First used in India: Sir William Herschel(1858). Systematized by Sir Francis Galton (1892)
- Types: Loops (60–70%) (most common), whorls (25-35%), Arch (6–7%), Composite (1–2%)
- In practice 16–20 points of comparison are accepted as proof of identity
- Fingerprint is absolutely individualistic (No two prints are like, even in twins)
- Most reliable method of identification
- Paternity cannot be proved from finger printing, but by DNA fingerprinting
- Brain finger printing invented by Dr Lawrence Farrel.

Conditions causing permanent impairment of finger prints

Leprosy	Radiation	Electrocution	Skin grafting

Poroscopy	Microscopic study of pores formed by mouths of ducts of subepidermal sweat glands
Cheiloscopy	Utilization of lip prints as a means of personal identification
Podogram	Study of foot prints
Bartillon system	Descriptive data, marks (moles) and body measurements for identification Useful above 21 years of age

Dentition

- Falling of temporary teeth starts at 6 years and eruption of permanent teeth starts at 6 years
- Age 6 to 12 years is the age of mixed dentition
- Superadded permanent teeth are those with do not have deciduous predecessors (*permanent molars*)
- Successional permanent teeth are those which erupt in the place of deciduous teeth.

Temporary Dentition	Age (months)
Lower central incisor 1st	6–8
Upper central incisor	7–9
Upper lateral incisor	7–9
Lower lateral incisor	10–12
Fist molar	12–14
Canine	17–19
Second molar last	20–30

Permanent dentition	Age (years)
First molar First	6–7
Central incisor	6–8
Lateral incisor	7–9
First premolar	9–11
Second premolar	10–12
Canine	11–12
Second molar	12–14
Third molar Last	17–25

Note: Premolars are absent in primary dentition.

Gustafson's Method

- Age estimation of adults > 21 years.
- Criteria used
  - Attrition
  - Paradentosis
  - Secondary dentin (2nd most reliable)
  - Cementum apposition
  - Root resorption
  - Root transparency (most reliable)—not seen up to 30 years.
- Anterior teeth are more suitable than posterior teeth, while 3rd molar is unsuitable for Gustafson's method.

Boyde Method

Most accurate age estimation method by incremental lines.

Age estimation by radiology

X-ray	Female	Male
Elbow	13–14	15–16
Wrist	16–17	18–19
Shoulder	17–18	19–20
Iliac crest	18–19	20–21
Ischial tuberosity	21–22	23–24
Clavicle medial end	21–22	23–24

Legal Sections

Some important sections of law

Sec 40 IPC	Cognizable offences
Sec 197 IPC	Punishment for issuing a false certificate
Sec 191 IPC	Perjury–willfully giving false evidence
Sec 192 IPC	Fabricating false evidence
Sec 193 IPC	Punishment for perjury–may extend to 7 years
Relevant sections of consent	
Sec 87 IPC	A person above 18 years can give a valid consent to suffer any harm, not known or intended to cause death or grievous hurt
Sec 89 IPC	A person below 12 years and an insane person cannot give a valid consent to suffer any harm
Sec 90 IPC	A consent given under fear of injury or misunderstanding or insane or intoxicated is not valid
Sec 92 IPC	Any harm caused to a person in good faith even without the consent, when it is impossible for the person to give consent is not an offence
Sec 52 IPC	Nothing is said to be done in good faith, which is done without care and attention
Relevant sections of injuries	
Sec 44 IPC	Injury–any harm what so ever caused illegally to any person in body, mind, reputation or property
Sec 299 IPC	Definition of culpable homicide
Sec 300 IPC	Definition of culpable homicide amounting to murder.
Sec 302 IPC	Punishment for murder–death or imprisonment for life
Sec 304 IPC	Culpable homicide not amounting to murder. Imprisonment for life or 10 years, and also fine
Sec 304-A IPC	Death caused by rash and negligent act–2 years
Sec 304-B IPC	Dowry death–death of a female within 7 years of marriage
Sec 306 IPC	Abetment of suicide–10 years, also fine
Sec 307 IPC	Attempt to murder–10 years
Sec 308 IPC	Attempt to commit culpable homicide– up to 10 years
Sec 319 IPC	Hurt–bodily pain, disease or infirmity
Sec 320 IPC	Grievous hurt–definition
Sec.323 IPC	Punishment for voluntarily causing hurt–1 year, with fine
Sec 324 IPC	Voluntarily causing hurt with dangerous weapon–3 years also fine
Sec 325 IPC	Voluntarily causing grievous hurt–7 years, also fine
Sec.326 I.P.C.	Voluntarily causing grievous hurt by dangerous weapon–10 years, also fine
Sec 351 IPC	Assault–offer of threat or attempt to apply force in a hostile manner
Sec 362 IPC	Abduction
Sec 498-A IPC	Punishment for harassment of dowry–3 years, also fine
Sec 82 IPC	Any act done by a child under 7 years of age is not an offence
Sec 83 IPC	Between 7 to 12 years of age, he is responsible if he understands the nature and consequences of his act
Sec 84 IPC	Mc Naughten Rule–Nothing is an offence, which is done by a person, who at the time of doing it, by reason of unsoundness of mind, is incapable of knowing the nature of the act, or that he is doing is either wrong or contrary to the law
Sec 375 IPC	Definition of Rape
Sec 376 IPC	1. Punishment for Rape 2. Custodial and Institutional Rape
Sec 377 IPC	Unnatural sexual offences

Contd...

Contd...

Relevant sections of injuries	
Sec 354 IPC	Indecent offence between two males, like mutual masturbation–2 years.
Sec 509 IPC	Indecent Assault–1 year
Sec 297 IPC	Necrophilia/Necrophagia.
Relevant sections of IEA	
Sec 61 to 90 IEA	Deals with documentary evidence
Sec 32 IEA	Dying declaration
Sec 118 IEA	All persons are competent to be witnesses, unless they are prevented from doing so
Sec 45 IEA	Expert witness
Sec 142 IEA	Leading question allowed in Examination-in-chief, if the witness is declared hostile
Sec 165 IEA	Questions by the judge.
Relevant sections of CrPC	
Sec 174 CrPC	Police Inquest
Sec 174 (4) and 176 CrPC	Magistrate Inquest
Sec 2 (n) CrPC	Cognizable offences
Sec 41 CrPC	In non-cognizable offences the accused may directly go to the doctor and get himself examined
Sec 53 CrPC	A male doctor can examine a female patient only in the presence of a female attendant
Sec 54 CrPC	An arrested person at his request, may be examined by a doctor to detect evidence in his favor
Sec 328 and 329 CrPC	Deals with provisions as to accused person of unsound mind

Grievous Hurt (Sec 320 IPC)

- Emasculation
- Permanent privation of sight of either eye
- Permanent privation of hearing of either ear
- Privation of any member or joint
- Permanent destruction of power of any member or joint
- Permanent disfiguration of head or face
- Fracture or dislocation of a bone or tooth
- Any hurt which **endangers life**, or which causes the victim to be in **severe bodily pain**, or **unable to follow his ordinary pursuits for a period of twenty days.**

Dowry Death (Sec 304-b IPC)

- Death within 7 years of marriage, caused by burns or other bodily injury or anyway other than normal
- Punishment not less than 10 years but may extend to life imprisonment
- Autopsy should be carried out by two doctors
- Sec 498-A IPC; Sec 113B IEA also death with dowry death.

Rape

Sec 375 IPC defines rape	• As per Criminal Law Amendment Bill 2013, the word rape has been replaced by 'Sexual Assault' as per Sec 375 IPC. • Penile penetration, inserting finger, manipulates the body part, applying the mouth to vagina or anus without the other person's consent all constitute the offence of sexual assault or rape
Sec 376 IPC (Punishment for sexual assault)	**Subsection 1:** Rigorous imprisonment for a term which shall not be less than 7 years (which may extend to life imprisonment) and liability to fine **Subsection 2** • Police officer • Public servant

Sec 376 IPC (Punishment for sexual assault)	• Member of armed forces • Management or staff of a jail, remand home or place of institution • Management or on the staff of a hospital • Relative, guardian or teacher • Pregnant women • Under 18 years of age • Person assaulted is incapable of giving consent • Person in social or economic dominance commits sexual assault on a person under such dominance • Sexual assault on a person suffering from mental or physical disability • Person causing grievous bodily harm or endangers the life of a person • Commits persistent sexual assault • Rigorous imprisonment for a term which shall not be less than 10 years which may extend to imprisonment for life
Sec 376–A	Punishment for causing death or resulting in persistent vegetative state of the victim–Imprisonment not be less than 20 years
Sec 376-B	Sexual assault by husband upon his wife during separation–Punishment–imprisonment for 2 years which may extend to 7 years
Sec 376 C	Sexual intercourse by a person in authority • Whoever in a position of authority or in fiduciary relationship • A public servant • Superintendent or manger of a jail, remand home or other place of custody or a women's or children institution • Being on the management of a hospital Rigorous imprisonment for 5 years which may extend to 10 years with fine
Sec 376 D	Sexual assault by gang Rigorous imprisonment which shall not be less than 20 years
Sec 376 E	Punishment for repeat offenders–Imprisonment for life or with death

Medicolegal Aspects of Poisons

- Sec 284 IPC deals with negligent conduct with respect to poisonous substances where punishment is up to 6 months
- Sec 324 and 326 IPC deals with hurt caused by corrosive substances and punishment up to 10 years
- Sec 328 IPC Whoever administers to any person any poison, or any stupefying intoxicating, or unwholesome drugs with the intent to cause hurt to such persons, shall be punished with imprisonment up to 10 years, and shall also be liable for fine
- Suspected articles of poison to be preserved. (noncompliance–Sec 201 IPC)
- Private practitioners are bound to inform the police in case of homicidal poisoning (Sec 39 Cr PC). Non compliance to be punished (Sec 176 IPC)
- If private practitioner if summoned by the investigative police officer, he is bound to divulge all information (Sec 175 Cr PC). If he conceals information, punishment according to Sec 202 IPC. If he furnishes wrong information, punishment according to Sec 193 IPC.

Drugs and cosmetic Act	1940 1964 (Amendment)
Drugs and cosmetic Rules Schedule H and L Drugs to be sold only on the prescription of RMP	1945
Narcotic and Psychotropic Substance Act	1985

THANATOLOGY (STUDY OF DEATH)

Death is of two types:

1. Somatic, systemic or clinical.

2. Molecular or cellular.

Somatic Death: It is the complete and irreversible stoppage of the circulation, respiration and brain functions.

Brain death is of three types:

Cortical or cerebral death-intact brainstem	Brainstem death	Whole brain death
• Vegetative state with normal respiration[Q]. • Cerebral hypoxia, widespread brain injury.	• The cerebrum may be intact, though cut off functionally by the stem lesion. This can be produced by raised intracranial pressure, cerebral edema, intracranial hemorrhage, etc.	• Combination of 1 and 2

The signs of death appear in the following order.

Immediate (Somatic death)	Early (cellular death)	Late (decomposition and decay)
1. Insensibility and loss of voluntary power 2. Cessation of respiration 3. Cessation of circulation	4. Pallor and loss of elasticity of skin 5. Changes in the eye 6. Primary flaccidity of muscles 7. Algor mortis (Cooling of the body) 8. Livor mortis (Post-mortem lividity) 9. Rigor mortis (Cadaveric rigidity)	10. Putrefaction 11. Adipocere formation 12. Mummification

Changes in the Eyes

Changes in anterior chamber	• Tache noir de la sclerotique within 3 to 4 • Intraocular pressure: Normal intraocular tension is 14 mm mercury Hg. Becomes zero by 2 hours after death • PUPILS: Dilated and fixed (no reaction to light), later becomes constricted
Changes in retina	• Pale- 1st two hours, optic disc: hazy- 6 hours, blurred in 7–10 hours • 'TRUCKING' Sign/Kevorkian's sign: fragmentation and segmentation of blood columns in retinal vessels, viewed by an ophthalmoscope, and interpreted by an expert ophthalmologist.
Changes in vitreous chamber	• There is a steady raise in the potassium level after death

Suspended Animation

- The vital functions of the body come down to a minimum level, just compatible with life
- The person appears apparently dead; seen in:
- Voluntarily produced by yoga practitioners (death trance)
- Involuntary suspended animation is seen in
  - New born infants
  - Drowning
  - Electrocution
  - Sunstroke
  - Cholera
  - Shock
  - Insanity
  - After anesthesia.

Brainstem Death

Irreversibly unconscious and irreversibly apneic

- Tests:
  - Brainstem Reflexes
  - *Apnea Test*

Test for Brainstem functions

Reflexes	Afferents	Efferents
Papillary reflex	II	III
Corneal reflex	V	VII
Grimace	V	VII
Vestibulo oculo reflex	VIII	III and VI
Gag or Cough reflex	IX	X

Board of Doctors to Certify Brainstem Death

- RMP treating the patient
- RMP in charge of the hospital
- Neurologist/Neurosurgeon nominated from the panel of names approved by the appropriate authority
- An independent Medical Specialist nominated from the panel of names approved by the appropriate authority.

RMP certifying death should not be a part of the transplantation team

- Organs are removed when the donor Heart is still beating–beating heart donor
- Kidneys are removed within 30 to 60 minutes and generally not stored for more than 12 hours
- Cornea–6 hours, skin–24 hours, bone–48 hours, blood vessels–72 hours.

Transplantation of Human Organs Act 1994

- Deals with the regulation of:
  - Removal, Storage,
  - Transplantation of Human Organs for therapeutic purposes, and
  - Prevention of commercial trade in Human Organs.
- The only organ which can be donated during life is kidney
- The donor must above 18 years of age.

Postmortem Changes-Signs of Death and Changes after Death

Algor Mortis (Cooling of the Body)

- Body loses heat by 2–3 °C in 1st hour, then 1–1.5 °C for each subsequent hour until the body reaches the environmental temperature
- When temperature is plotted against time, cooling represented by a sigmoid curve
- The body core temperature is obtained from intrahepatic/subhepatic temperature via abdominal stab (ideal site), Per rectum (except in cases of sodomy)
- Other sites—external auditory meatus, nasal cavity, peritoneal cavity
- Temperature measured using a chemical thermometer (thanatometer), graduated from 1 to 50 degrees centigrade, inserted 10 cms in to the rectum

$$\textbf{(Glaister equation)}\ \text{Time Since Death} = \frac{\text{Normal body temp–Rectal temperature}}{\text{Rate of fall of temp/hour}}$$

Postmortem caloricity

- The temperature of the body rises for the first few hours after death
- Disturbed regulation of heat production before death-sun stroke
- Increase in heat production in the muscles due to convulsions-tetanus, strychnine poisoning
- Excessive bacterial activity, as in septicemic conditions, cholera and other fevers.

Livor Mortis (Postmortem Staining, Postmortem Lividity, Postmortem Hypostasis, Suggillations, Vibices)

- Postmortem lividity begins as mottled patches ranging from 1 to 2 cms in diameter, which increase in size and coalesce with each other to form a uniform area of staining–2 to 3 hours.

- Lividity usually becomes fixed 6 to 8 hours after death
- It indicates the position of the body after death
- After fixation, the distribution of the pattern will not change even if the body's position is altered.

'Contact pallor or pressure pallor': Parts of the body which is in actual contact with the surface do not show staining

Lividity

Present in	Absent in
• Occurs in the dependent parts of the internal organs as well • Disappears with the onset of putrefaction–merges with that of the colour change of putrefaction	• If the body is tossed and turned continuously as seen in fast flowing water in rivers • Dark coloured individuals. • Profuse bleeding before death or severe anemia

Medicolegal Importance

- Helps in estimating the time of death
- Indicates the posture of the body at the time of fixation and death
- Sometimes the color may indicate the cause of death–poisoning

Etiology	Color	Mechanism
Normal	Blue purplish	Venous blood
Carbon monoxide Burn	Cherry red Bright red	CoHb
Cyanide	Bright Red	Excess oxygenated blood due to inhibition of cytochrome oxidase
Fluroacetate	Pink	Excess oxygenated blood due to inhibition of cytochrome oxidase
Hypothermia/ Refrigeration	Pink	Oxygen retention in cutaneous blood by cold air Left shifting of Hb-O_2 dissociation curve
NaCl/Nitrite/Nitrate/ aniline Potassium chlorate Phosphorous	Chocolate Brown Dark brown	Methemoglobin (meth Hb)
Septic abortion	Grayish brown Bronze	Due to Cl. Welchii
Hydrogen sulphide	Green	Sulfhemoglobin

PM Lividity vs Bruise

Criteria	Lividity	Bruise
Site	Dependant parts	Anywhere
Cuticle	Not injured	May be injured
Appearance	Not elevated	Elevated
Margin	Sharp/Well defined	Ill defined
Colour	Reddish purple uniform	Colour change with time
Cause	Capillo venous distension	Rupture vessels extravasation
Pressure effect	Appears pale	No effect
Cut section	Blood confined with in the vessel	Hemorrhage in the tissue
Enzymatic study	No change	Change in the level
MLI	Time of Death Position of the body	Nature of injury Weapon used

Rigor Mortis (Postmortem Rigor, Postmortem Rigidity, Postmortem Stiffening, Cadaveric Rigidity)

- Appears in both skeletal and smooth muscles; voluntary or involuntary muscles
- If the glycogen stores (muscle) is low before death (exhausted and starved)-rapid rigor develop like in individuals

- Rigor mortis is totally concerned with muscles and is independent of nervous system.
- Rigor mortis passes off in the same order of appearance in, which it develops.

Mechanism: (ATP depletion) *after death there is no synthesis of ATP. As long as there is ATP stores in the muscles the fibers remains relaxed; once the stores get exhausted then the muscle fibers goes in a for a permanent state of contraction*–called Rigor mortis. The level of ATP falls below a critical level (85% of the normal).

Order of appearance	• Occurs in proximodistal spread • Internally: Myocardium • Externally: First in the eyelids, muscles of the face, jaw, neck, upper limbs, chest, abdomen and lastly the lower limbs
Time of appearance	• (Rule of 12[Q]) • Starts in 3 to 6 hours, takes 12 hours to complete, stays for another 12 hours, disappears in next 12 hours, in the same order of appearance

Conditions altering the onset and duration of rigor mortis

Age	• Does not occur in a fetus of less than 7 months old
Muscular stage	• Onset is slow and duration is long in cases where muscles are healthy and at rest before death
Nature of death	• In deaths from diseases causing great exhaustion and wasting, the onset is early and duration is short
Atmospheric condition	• Onset is slow and duration is long in cold weather • Onset is fast and duration is short in hot weather

Conditions simulating rigor mortis

- Cadaveric spasm
- Heat stiffening: Due to coagulation of muscle protein
- Cold stiffening: Due to solidification of subcutaneous fat
- Gas stiffening: Due to gas accumulation under the skin and subcutaneous tissues, evolved from putrefaction.

Cadaveric spasm or instantaneous rigor

- The group of muscles which were at strenuous work during life (just before death) goes into a sudden state of stiffening, instead of passing to primary flaccidity after death
- Occurs especially in cases of sudden death, due to exhaustion and fear, etc.
- Reflects the last action of the individual at the time of death: firearm in the hands of victims in suicidal gunshot injuries, plants and weeds in the hands of victims in drowning, the weapon in the hands of victims in cut throat injuries, etc
- Cadaveric spasm cannot be mimicked.

Decomposition (Putrefaction)

It takes place in 2 steps-1) Autolysis 2) Putrefaction.

Autolysis: Aseptic process (maceration of dead fetus in the uterus[Q]).

Putrefaction

- The chief destructive agent of putrefaction is Clostridium welchii[Q]
- Lecithinase[Q] is the most important enzyme causing hemolysis, liquefaction of clots, gas formation and disintegration of tissue.

Stages of Putrefaction

Color changes	• 1st sign of decomposition -Greenish discolouration in the right lilac fossaQ; 12–24 hours in summer and 1 to 3 days in winter. • The superficial veins of the limbs, chest, abdomen and neck are stained greenish blue due to hemolysis of red cells and stain the walls of the vessels–MARBLING

Evolution of gases	• The main gases are ammonia, carbon dioxide, hydrogen sulphide, phosphorated hydrogen and methane • Abdomen gets distended due to accumulation of gases in the intestines • Diaphragm is pushed up compressing the lungs and heart; blood stained frothy fluid exudes from the mouth and nostrils (Postmortem purge) – Blisters 18–24 hours; first seen on the lower surface of trunk and thighs – Maggots 1–2 days – Skin slippage; anus and uterus prolapsed 2–3 days – Separation of skull sutures children 3–5 days – Postmortem luminescence is usually due to contamination by bacteria (Photobacterium fischeri) or fungi (Armillaria mellea)
Liquefaction of tissues	• Larynx and trachea • Stomach, intestines and spleen • Liver (foamy liver) lings • Brain • Heart • Kidneys, bladder • Prostate, uterus • Skin, muscle, tendon • Bones

Adipocere (Saponification)

- Commonly seen in **bodies immersed in water** or in damp warm environment
- Gradual **hydrolysis and hydrogenation of preexisting fats**, to form insoluble soaps
- These soaps being acidic in nature inhibit the putrefactive bacteria
- The body fat is converted into palmitic, **oleic, stearic and hydroxystearic acid** by the fat splitting enzyme **lecithinase**, produced by clostridia group of organisms, mainly **Clostridium perfringes**
- The water required for hydrolysis is obtained mainly from the body tissues.

Properities	Adipocere has a distinct offensive or sweetish smell
Distribution	• Any site, where fatty tissue is present • Face, buttocks, breast and abdomen are usual sites
Time required for adipocere formation	Shortest 3 weeks in summer, Complete conversion in an adult limb requires at least 3 to 6 months
Medicolegal Importance	• When involves face, the features are well preserved, helps to establish the identity • Cause of death–injuries are preserved • Time since death

Mummification (Modified Putrefaction)

- **Dehydration, drying and shriveling of the cadaver**
- Begins in exposed parts of the body–face, limbs then extends to the entire body including internal organs
- Mummified bodies if protected can be preserved for years; mummified bodies are practically odorless
- It takes 3 months to 1 year to develop
- Absences of moisture, continuous action of dry warm air are necessary for mummification
- **Chronic arsenic and antimony** poisoning favors the process of mummification.

Presumption of death	Presumption of survivorship
• Arise in connection with civil cases. • A person is presumed to be alive, if there is nothing to suggest the probability of his death within 30 years. But, if proof is presumed.	• Arise in connection with inheritance of Property. • When 2 or more persons DIE in a common Disaster. Example: Earth quake, Plane crash, etc. • The ouestion of who survived longer may arise. The case is decided on facts and evidence available.

Mechanical Injuries

Injuries by Blunt force:

Abrasions (SCRATCH, GRAZE, BRUSH BURNS, GRAVEL RASH)

- A **superficial injury,** not involving the full thickness of the skin, i.e. **confined to epidermis.**
- They are caused by a lateral rubbing, by a blow or a fall on a rough surface.
- Abrasions are simple injury, heals rapidly without leaving a *SCAR usually*

Types of Abrasion

• Scratch abrasion	• Nail marks
• Grazed abrasion (Brush Burn or Friction Burn)	• Produced by a scraping injury over a larger area in road traffic accidents
• Pressure abrasion (Crushing or Friction)	• Ligature marks in hanging and bite marks
• Impact abrasion (Contact, Imprint or Patterned Abrasion)	• Tyre marks and ligature marks are patterned
• Atypical abrasion	• Tiger skin abrasion

Age of an Abrasion

Abrasion heals from the **periphery by growth of new epithelial cells.**

Age of abrasion	Color
• Fresh	• Bright red
• 12–24 hours	• Bright scab
• 2–3 days	• Reddish brown scab
• 4–5 days	• Dark brown scab
• 5–7 days	• Black scab

Antemortem vs postmortem abrasions

• Features	• Antemortem abrasions	• Postmortem abrasions
• Site	• Anywhere on the body	• Bony prominences
• Oozing of lymph	• Present	• Absent
• Scab formation	• Present	• Absent
• Color changes	• Present	• Absent, mostly yellowish without any change
• Parchmentization	• Absent	• Present

Medicolegal Importance

- Abrasions are produced at the **site of impact**
- **Direction of force**: The torn layers of the epithelium are heaped up towards one end of the wound-indicating the direction of application of force/the direction of movement of the body
- **Relative position of the assailant and the victim**
- Patterned abrasions helps to **find out the object** causing the injury
- Example: Imprint of the tyre mark in a run over accident
- **Manner of injury** (accidental, suicidal, homicidal or fabricated)
- **Age of the injury** can be assessed which indicates the time of infliction of the injury.

Contusion (Bruise)

- Pinpoint contusions–Petechie
- Smaller than a few mm–Ecchymosis
- More than a few cms–Hematoma

Present not only in the skin, but also in internal organs–lung, brain or muscle.

- Usually there is no destruction of the skin[Q].

Color changes in a bruise

Age of the bruise	Color
Fresh	Red
1–2 days	Reddish blue (deoxyhemoglobin)
3–5 days	Reddish brown (Hemosiderin)
5–7 days	Green (Biliveridin)
7–10 days	Yellow (Bilirubin)
10–14 days	Gradually fades away

Bruise vs False bruise

Features	Bruise	False bruise
Site	Anywhere	Accessible
Margin	Diffused	Clear and sharply defined
Content	Blood	Acid serum
Redness, Inflammation	Not present	Present
Color changes	Occur as the age of the bruise progress	No color change
Cause	Mechanical force	Chemicals or plant juice
Extravasation of blood	Present in the subcutaneous tissue	Not present
Chemical test of skin scrapping	Detects nothing	Detects the chemical or the plant juice used

Bruises may not be evident

- When the offending weapon is yielding in nature and of flat surface like sand bag.
- Where the body surface to be hit is covered with thick rug, blanket, etc.
- Where the site of injury in yielding part such as anterior abdominal wall.
- In case of blow over sole of foot, palm of hand.

Laceration: The tissues are torn as result of forcible application of blunt force.

Types

- Split laceration
- Stretch laceration
- Avulsion/Grinding/Compression laceration
- Tearing laceration
- Cut laceration
- Lacerations of internal organs.

General features of laceration

Shape	Irregular
Edges	Ragged and may be undermined
Margins	Irregular, contused and abraded
Dimension	Length more than the breadth
Floor	Tags of tissue
Hemorrhage	Not pronounced due to crushing of lumen of blood vessels
Hair bulbs	Crushed

INCISED LIKE/INCISED LOOKING WOUNDS

- This injury will simulate closely an incised wound
- These are essentially lacerated wounds, easily detectable on examination with a magnifying lens
- Common Sites: Scalp, face, over the eyebrows, cheek, chin, lower jaw, iliac crest, shin.

Injuries by Sharp Force

Incised wound (Cut, Slash)

Margins	**Clean cut, regular and well defined,** usually no bruising
Length	It is the greatest dimension; does not have any relationship with the length of the blade
Depth and Direction	Deeper at the commencement of the wound; towards the termination, the cut becomes progressively shallow and is known as **-Tailing of the wound**
Hemorrhage	As blood vessels are clean cut, there will be free profuse bleeding with spurting

Beveled cuts	Hesitational cuts
• Usually homicidal	• Multiple, small, superficial, more or less parallel cuts noticed over the accessible body parts. • Sites-over throat, wrist, elbow, front of chest and abdomen. • Indicates suicidal nature of the wound

Stab Wound (Punctured Wound)

Stabwound produced with a pointed weapon

- Penetrating wound: terminates into the body cavities (Thorax and abdomen)
- Perforating wound: when the weapon enters the body through a cavity and exits, thus producing two surface wounds (Entry wound and Exit wound)

Features of a stabwound

A. Depth and Direction
   - Depth is the greatest dimension in stab injury
   - The depth of the wound (the length of the track), is a guide to the length of the blade.
   - Depth should be determined by dissecting the track of the wound in layers during operation or autopsy.

B. **Margins**

Features	Entry wounds	Exit wounds
Margins	Inverted	Everted
Size	Larger	Smaller

Langer's Line

- The pattern of fiber arrangement are the lines of cleavage of the skin and their linear representations on the skin are known as 'Langer's line of cleavage'
- A stab wound with long axis at right angles to the cleavage lines of Langer, will gape open with edges pulled apart
- A stab that runs parallel to these lines will appear slit-like or wedge shaped (dimension of blade is fairly accurate).

Defence/Protective Wound

It results from victim's spontaneous instinctive reaction towards self protection.

- A typical defence wound is seen in the web between the base of the thumb and index finger, when the blade is grasped
- The presence of defence wounds indicate homicidal nature of the injuries
- **Defence wound will be absent-**When the victim was unconscious due to drink, drug, or disease.

Self Inflicted and Fabricated Wounds

- Self inflicted wounds are those inflicted by a person on his own body
- Fabricated wounds (factious, forged or invented wounds) are inflicted by a person on his own body or by another with his consent
- Fabricated wounds are usually incised wounds and contusions; sometimes stab wounds and burns; lacerated wounds are rarely fabricated
- Clothes are not cut, and if cut are not compatible with the nature of the wounds
- The history of the assault in usually not compatible with the injuries present on the body.

Regional Injuries

Types of Skull Fractures

Type of fracture	Description	Type of force
Fissure #	Linear crack in inner table or outer table or both	Blows with an agent having a relatively broad striking surface or Forcible contact with a broad hard surface
Depressed # (Fracture ala signature)	Fracture pattern often resembles the weapon or agent which caused it	Heavy weapon with a small striking surface Example: Hammer, stone, chopper
Comminuted #	There are two or more intersecting lines of fracture, Which divide the bone into three or more fragments. When there is no displacement of fragments, it resembles a spider's web or mosaic	It is often a complication of fissured or depressed fracture.
Pond # (indented #)	Only in infants, as their skull bones are pliable	Obstetric forceps
Diastatic/sutural #	Separation of sutures In young persons	Blunt injury
Gutter #	Part of thickness of bone is removed	Oblique bullet wounds
Perforating #	Both tables are involved	Pointed sharp weapons like daggers, knives and axe
Ring or foramen #	It is a fissure fracture which runs at about 3-5 cm outside and around the foramen of magnum.	Fall from height on foot or buttocks

CONCUSSION OF BRAIN OR COMMOTIO CEREBRI OR 'STUNNING'

- State of temporary unconsciousness, due to head injury seen immediately after injury, and is always followed by amnesia and tends to recovery is spontaneous
- Patient recovers completely after few minutes followed by symptoms of **'Post-Concussional Syndrome'**.
- Recovery from concussion is often followed by complete loss of memory of recent events. **(Retrograde Amnesia)**
- As it may be associated with **Post-Traumatic Automatism.**

Intracranial Hemorrhages (Extradural/Epidural Hemorrhage)

- Mostly traumatic in origin
- Usually coup injury
- Rupture of middle meningeal artery/one of its branches
- It is due to fissured fracture of squamous part of temporal bone or parietal bone.

Lucid interval	Medicolegal importance
• Seen in insanity and epidural hemorrhage • It is the state of consciousness between the two states of unconsciousness • Early diagnosis and surgical intervention usually saves the patient	• Legally responsible for criminal acts • Make a valid will which can give valid evidence

Subdural Hemorrhage

- It is **invariably traumatic** in origin following a blow or fall.
- **May follow insignificant trauma** to head without loss of consciousness, even without any fracture of skull.

Causes of SDH

- **Rupture of the bridging veins**
- **Rupture of inferior cerebral veins, entering the sinuses at the base of the skull**
- **Rupture of dural venous sinuses following a blow**

According to the time of onset of symptoms after injury it is divided into three types.

Acute SDH (Immediately)	Subacute SDH (Several Days to 2–3 Weeks)	Chronic SDH (Pachymeningitis Hemorrhagica Interna)
Acute Subdural features simulate EDH but S/S does not appear before 2-4 hours of injury. It arises mostly from rupture of large bridging vein, rupture of one of the cortical arteries or cerebral lacerations	Occurs when bleeding is from smaller bridging veins. In this type the brain may or may not be damaged	It presents usually 3-6 weeks after the injury. After about a week chronic subdural hemorrhage begins to organize from the dural side. By 3–4 weeks the hematoma gets completely encapsulated

Subarachnoid Hemorrhage

Causes of Subarachnoid Hemorrhage

- Nontraumatic: due to rupture of minute developmental aneurysms of vessels of circle of Willis[Q].
- Traumatic Causes
  - **Commonly associated with traumatic head injuries.**
  - **Blow over jaw or side of upper part of neck may cause rupture of vertebral artery with basal SAH.**

Punch Drunk Syndrome/Traumatic Encephalopathy/Dementia Pugilistica

- State that occurs in old boxers due to the tiny hemorrhages in the brain.
- The patient suffers from post traumatic psychosis, loss of memory, tremor, dysarthria.
- Duration of boxing is more relevant than the severity of the blows.

Whip Lash Injury of Spinal Cord

- Sustained by occupant of a car
- Sudden hyperextension and hyperflexion
- Resulting in fatal contusion or laceration of spinal cord without fracture of spine.

Cardiac Temponade

Accumulation of 400-500 cc of blood in the pericardial sac will be sufficient to cause death.

FORENSIC BALLISTICS

Rifled Firearm

If **the barrel is grooved internally**, it is rifling.

Raised areas are called as 'lands' and depressed areas are called as 'grooves'.

Advantages

- Gives a spinning effect to the bullets
- Straight trajectory of the bullets
- Prevents 'wobbling' of bullets
- Increases penetrability.

Smooth Bored Firearm

No grooves.

Choking

This denotes to the constriction of a few cm. of bore in the muzzle end of the gun.

Advantages

- Pellets remain compact and there is less dispersion
- Increases the explosive forces of the pellets
- Increases the velocity of the pellets.

Paradox guns: If the barrel is partly smooth bored and partly rifled.

Caliber: Internal Dimension of barrel in decimals of inch or millimeters.

- In riffled firearms, caliber is measured between two opposite lands
- In shot guns, it is measured by the size of lead sphere that fits the diameter and denoted by the number of such sized spheres that can be made from 1 lb of lead (454 gm).

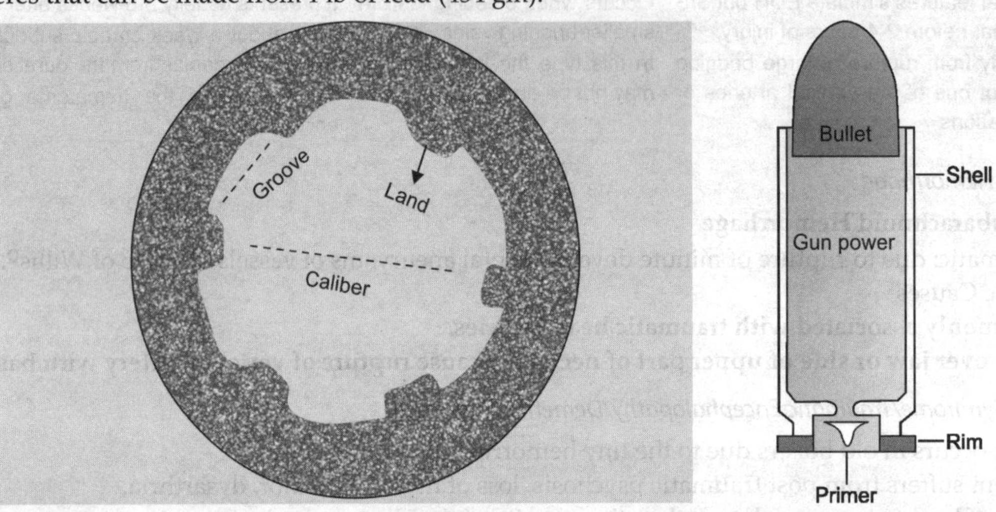

Fig. 4.1: Helixometer-instrument to examine the interior of the barrel

Sequence of Firing

- Pulling of trigger → Hammer release → Hitting percussion pin → Ignition of primer mixture →
- Production of flame → Ignition of gun powder → Ignition of gun powder → Gas production → Propelling of the shots/bullet/pellet → Reporting of fire.

Primer Mixture

Type–1	Type–2
• Mercury Fulminate • Antimony Sulfide • Potassium Chlorate	• Antimony Sulfide • Lead Styphanate • Lead Peroxide • Barium nitrate

Gun Powders

Black powder	Smokeless powder	Semi-Smokeless powder
Charcoal Potassium Nitrate Sulfur	Nitrocellulose Nitroglycerine	80% Black powder + 20% Smokeless powder

Range: The distance between the muzzle end of the firearm and the target.

Contact range	Close range	Near range	Distant range
The muzzle end is in contact with the body	The target is within the distance travelled by flame	Within the distance travelled by unburnt and partially burnt gun powder	Beyond the distance travelled by flame, smoke and gun powder

Wounds From Revolvers, Pistols, Rifles

Contact shot (Point black shot)	Close shot (Range of flame)	Near range (Range of gun power)	Long range (Beyond the range of gun power)
• Large wound, shows cavitation • Stellate or cruciate • Margins contused and everted • Singeing of hair present • Tattooing minimal or absent	• Circular wound • Singeing+ • Burning, blackening+ • Tattooing+ • Abrasion collar/grease collar/dirt collar+	• No burning, no blackening, tattooing • Round entrance wound • Abrasion collar	• Small circular wound smaller than the diameter of the bullet • Margins inverted • Burning, blackening, tattooing absent

	Shot guns	Revolvers and pistols	Rifles
Smoke	30 cm	30 cm	30 cm
Flame	45 cm	8 cm	15 m
Gun power (burnt and partially burnt)	60–90 cm	60 cm	75 cm
Cards	2 m	–	–
Wads	2–6 m	–	–

Components Causing Injury

Fire/Flame	Burning at entrance wound along with burning or singeing of hairs
Smoke	Blackening effect or smudging
Hot gases	Scorching effect
Unburnt gun powder	Tattooing effect, peppering or stippling effect
Felt wad	Minor abrasion and bruise
Bullet/Pellet	Puncture wound

Abrasion Collar

- Due to gyrating effect of bullet
- If contusion also present, contusion collar
- Grease collar or dirt collar is due to lubricants, gun oil or lead
- It will be round in shape if bullet has hit at right angle to body surface and oval if it hits at an angle
- The diameter of the entry wound together with the abrasion collar gives the approximate diameter of the bullet.

Test for firearms
• Harrison and Gilroy test • Neutron activation analysis • Atomic absorption spectroscopy (AAS) • Flameless AAS • Dermal nitrate (paraffin test)

Entry Wound vs Exit Wound

Character	Entry wound	Exit wound
Size	Smaller than the diameter of the bullet	Larger
Edges	Inverted	Everted
Abrasion collar and grease collar	Present	Absent
Scorching, smudging and tattooing	May be present	Absent
Bleeding	Less	More
Fat extrusion	Absent	May be present
Cherry red colour	May be present	Absent

Thermal Injuries

Thermal destruction of the skin results in severe local and systemic alterations.

Generalized effects of heat	Heat stroke, Heat cramps, Heat exhaustion
Localized effects of heat	Burns (Dry heat), Scalds (Wet heat)
Generalized effects of cold	Hypothermia
Localized effects of cold	Frost bite, Trench foot

Disorder	Body temperature	Skin	Mental status
Heat cramps	37 °C	Moist and cool	Normal
Heat exhaustion	40 °C	Sweating	Normal
Heat stroke	> 40 °C	Dry (anhydrosis) NO sweating	Impaired consciousness

Burns

Wilson's classification of burns

Epidermal burns	Dermoepidermal burns	Deep burns
• Patch of erythema with or without vesicle. • Blisters are painful and heal without scarring	• Burns involves the whole thickness of the skin • Extremely painful as they affect the sensory nerve endings • Heal with formation of scar	• Gross destruction of deeper tissues • The burnt areas may be completely charred • They are relatively painless, as the nerve endings are completely destroyed

Rule of nine

Area of the body	Percentage intended
Head and face	9%
Upper limbs	9%
Front of chest and abdomen	9%
Back of chest and abdomen	9%
Front of lower limbs	9%
Back of lower limbs	9%
Genitals	1%
Total	100%

Rule of thumb

In case of a scattered burn injury-Palm of hand rule → the surface area of a persons palm is roughly 1% of the total body surface.

Causes of death

Immediate	Delayed	Remote complications
• Primary or neurogenic shock • Asphyxia • Accidents and injuries • Vagal inhibition	• Secondary hypovolemic shock • Renal failure • Toxemia • Inflammatory complications	• Infection • Curling ulcer • Deep vein thombosis • Jaundice

Autopsy Findings

Specific findings indicative of antemortem burns	Nonspecific findings
• Soot in respiratory tract • Carboxy hemoglobin in blood • Line of redness • Albumin and chloride in vesicles • Increased enzymes • Healing granulation tissue • Infection	• Pugilistic attitude • Heat rupture • Heat hematoma

Respiratory passage	• Soot particles (burnt carbon particles) mixed with mucus adherent on to the congested mucosal surface of the larynx, trachea, primary and secondary bronchioles. • Blood is usually bright pink if death has occurred due to inhalation of CO. The level of cap is usually above 5%
Pugilistic attitude (universal flexion/boxers attitude)	• Due to coagulation of muscle proteins, when the body is exposed to sustained heat
Heat ruptures	• Multiple skin splits, seen over the extensor surfaces and joints • Absence of blood clots, absence of infiltration of blood vessels and intact blood vessels, help to differentiate from laceration or incised wounds
Heat fractures	• Prolonged exposure to heat may cause fracture of vault. • Occurs bilaterally above temple. Usually do not involve sutures

Antemortem vs Postmortem Vesicles

Antemortem vesicles	Postmortem vesicles
• It contains a serous fluid of albumin and chlorides • The base is inflamed and red with erythematous borders	• It contain traces of albumin and chlorides and more of gas • The base is dry, hard and yellow

Scalds

- Injury caused by moist heat; liquids above 60 °C
- No charring, carbonization or hair singeing in scalds as seen in dry heat

General features of scald injury

- Maximum damage at the point of commencement
- Evidence of splashing or trickling down of the liquid
- Restricted to exposed body parts or point of contact
- Inhalation of steam-scald the throat and air passage.

Electrocution

- Voltage is the fundamental force or pressure that causes electricity to flow through a conductor
- Electrocution is rare at less than 100 volts and most deaths occur at more than 200 volts
- Alternating current (AC) is 5 times as dangerous as an equal voltage of direct current (DC)
- Currents of 10 mA cause pain and muscle contractions and 100 mA is fatal.

Skin	Skeletal muscle	Bone
Joule burns (diagnostic of electricity) High voltage • Crocodile flash burns • Spark or flash burns Arc eye burn	• Zenkers degeneration	• Bone pearls or wax drippings • Zigzag micro fractures (Areas of bone necrosis)

Contd...

Contd...

Joule burn or endogenous burn	The electric burn at the point of entry is called Joule burn or endogenous burn
Spark burn or exogenous burn	Produced by intermittent contact and arcing of current from the conductor to the skin. There is an air gap between metal and skin
Crocodile flash burns	Multiple burnt or punched out lesions are produced due to an arc dancing over the body surface
Bone pearls or wax drippings	Heat generated by the current may melt the calcium phosphate, which is seen radiographically as round density foci

Lightening (Arborescent burns/Filigree burns/Lichtenberg's flowers)

- Superficial thin irregular tortuous markings on skin resembling branches of a tree
- Does not correspond to vascular channels
- Not associated with burning.

Asphyxia

Asphyxia literally means pulselessness.

Signs of asphyxia

Classical signs	Nonspecific signs
• Edema and congestion of organs • Petechial Hemorrhages • Cyanosis	• Abnormal fluidity of blood • Dilatation of right chambers of heart

Hanging

- Hanging is a form of asphyxia caused by suspension of the body by a ligature around the neck.
- The constricting force being the weight of the body.

Types of hanging

On the basis of the degree of suspension

Complete hanging	Partial hanging
When there is no contact with the ground	When any part of the body touches the ground

On the basis of the position of knot

Typical hanging	Atypical hanging
When the ligature passes symmetrically on both sides towards the point of suspension; i.e.–the knot is at the nape of the neck	When the knot is at any other place other than the back; i.e.–below the ears, below the chin, etc.,

Cause of death in hanging

- Asphyxia
- Venous congestion
- Combined asphyxia and venous congestion
- Cerebral Anemia
- Reflux vagal inhibition
- Fracture dislocation of cervical vertebra.

Post-mortem appearance

- Ligature mark (patterned abrasion)
- Post-mortem staining: Glove and stockings fashion
- Petechial Hemorrhages in the lower limbs if the body is suspended for a long time
- Salivary stains at the angle of mouth.

- If the knot presses on the cervical sympathetic ganglia, the eye on that side remains open, and the pupil dilated. [Le facie sympathique]
- The intima of the carotid arteries may show transverse splits with extravasation of blood in their wall.
- Hyoid bone in hanging
  Fracture is more common above the age of 40 years
  Abduction fracture [antero-posterior compression fracture]

Signs of antemortem hanging
Salivary dribbling Le facie sympathique

Frequency of hyoid bone fractures

Throttling > strangulation > hanging

Lynching

- It's a form of **homicidal hanging** where the person suspected to be involved in dacoit, murder or rape is overpowered by a mob, and hanged forcibly in public.

Strangulation

- Mode of violent asphyxial death accomplished by constricting the neck, **externally by hands (manual strangulation/throttling)** or by a **ligature (ligature strangulation)** or any other means **but without suspending the body.**

Features	Hanging	Strangulation by ligature
Ligature mark	Oblique Does not encircle the neck completely Below chin and above thyroid cartilage Base-pale, hard and parchment like	Transverse Encircles the neck completely At or below thyroid cartilage Base-soft and reddish
Bruising of neck muscles	Not common	Common
Neck	Stretched and elongated	Not common
Hyoid bone fracture	Common	Uncommon
Thyroid cartilage fracture	Less common	More common
Carotid intimal tears	Present	Absent
Salivary dribbling	Present	Absent
Bleeding from nose, mouth and ears	Uncommon	Common

Manual Strangulation (Throttling)

Autopsy findings: Signs of asphyxia more evident.

- Bruising of neck is seen due to assailants' fingers grasping the neck
- Abrasions (linear and crescentic)–by finger nails of assailant (victim in an attempt to get loosen the hand grip of assailant from the neck).

Auto-erotic Hanging	Victims usually males with masochism or transvestism enhance sexual pleasure by compressing neck by any means
Burking	Combination of smothering and traumatic asphyxia
Smothering	Occlusion of external air passages
Choking	Occlusion of internal air passages
Overlaying	Compression of chest, when mother shares bed with baby
Mugging	Neck is constricted by foot, knee and bend of elbow–compressing force
Bansdola	Neck is compressed in between two bamboo sticks
Garroting	When the victim is unaware, a ligature is put around the neck from behind and twisted fast; the victim losses consciousness very fast and the signs of resistance are absent

Drowning

- Type of asphyxial death caused by displacement of air from the lungs by any fluid, usually water Mechanism of Death.
- Fresh water drowning:

Water inhalation into the lungs → Blood → Circulatory overload

↓ Pulmonary edema ↕ Cardiac overload (Ventricular fibrillation)

Circulatory overload ↓ Hemodilution ↓ Hemolysis ↓ Increased extracellular potassium ↓ Cardiac toxicity

- Sea water drowning:

Water inhalation into the lungs ← blood

↓ Hemoconcentration ↓ Massive pulmonary edema

- Dry drowning:
  i. Laryngeal spasm–neither air nor water can enter into the respiratory tract.
  ii. Reflex cardiac arrest
  iii. Hyper stimulation of nerve endings all over the body by cold water

↓ (hydrocution) Ventricular fibrillation ↓ Death

Near drowning–recued but died within 24 hours

Secondary drowning–death after 24 hours due to complications.

POSTMORTEM FINDINGS

Specific signs of antemortem drowning	Nonspecific signs
External findings • Fine, copious persistent white leathery froth from mouth, nose and air passages, which increase on chest pressure • Weeds, grass mud, etc. in tightly clenched fist Internal findings • Water in stomach, intestine, middle ear • Diatoms in brain and bone marrow	• Cutis anserina or goose skin • Washer woman hand and feet • Paltaufs hemorrhage • Emphysema aquosum

Laboratory Tests

Medicolegal significance of Diatoms test
• Diatoms are unicellular algae with silica in its cell wall • Only a beating heart can transport the diatoms to distant organs • It indicates death due to drowning • Diatoms in bone marrow and brain is more reliable than any other organ • As diatoms resist putrefaction, it is valuable even in putrefaction • Diatoms are negative in dead bodies thrown in water or dry drowning

Gettler's Test

- Chloride content of the right and left chambers of heart is normally equal on both sides
- In fresh water drowning, 50% reduction in chloride concentration on the left side of heart

- In salt water drowning, 30–40% increase in chloride concentration on the left side of heart
- A 25% difference in chloride content considered significant.
  Other lab features
  - Serum strontium levels are raised in drowning
  - Plasma specific gravity on the left side of heart < right side (left > right in nondrowning cases)
  - Magnesium content of the left side of heart is 1.25 mg/ 100 ml > right side.

Sexual Jurisprudence

Hymen

- During sexual intercourse, Tearing usually occurs in the **4 or 8 o'clock position**, or in the middle
- Soon after the act, the margins of the torn hymen are sharp and red, which bleed on touch
- After 3 to 4 days, the edges are congested and swollen, which heal completely in 1 week.

Statutory rape	Marital rape
• Sexual intercourse with a girl below 18 years of age even with her consent. • It is neither violent nor physically coerced	• Forceful sexual intercourse with wife who is living separately from him, without her consent. • It is punishable with imprisonment up to two years provided the age of the wife is not <12 years

- Consent-A woman of 18 years and above can give valid consent for sexual intercourse
- Age of the accused-in India there is no age limit.

Non-habitual passive agent	Habitual passive agent
• Perianal abrasion and bruising • Anal laceration	• Perianal skin is thickened and keratinized from constant friction. • No pain or tenderness during examination • Lateral buttock traction test • Funnel shaped depression of the anus • Anus: Dilated and patulous • Loss of rugosity of mucus membrane

Sexual Perversions

Sodomy/Buggery	• Anal intercourse
Gerontophilia	• When the passive agent is an adult
Pederasty	• When the passive agent is a child (catamite)
Pedophile	• Adult who repeatedly engages in sexual activities with children
Eunuchs	• Male prostitutes in India, act as passive agents in sodomy
Lesbianism (Tribadism, Sapphism)	• Female homosexuality • Active lesbian is known as Butch or Dyke, while the usually passive agent is called Femme
Buccal coitus (sin of Gomorrah)	• Buccal-Penile intercourse is called Fellatio; the partner who performs the act is called the Fellator; and on whom it is performed is the Fellatee.
Bestiality	• Sexual intercourse by a human being with a lower animal
Incest	• Sexual intercourse by a man with a woman who is closely related to him by blood (prohibited degrees of relationship) e.g. daughter, sister, granddaughter, step sister • In India, incest as such, is not an offence
Uranism	• Sexual gratification by fingering, fondling, licking and sucking the genitalia of opposite sex
Paraphilias	• Unorthodox sex play by using objects or parts of the body
Sadism	• Sexual gratification obtained from acts of cruelty or infliction of pain on the partner
Lust murder	• Murder serves as a stimulus for sexual act

Contd...

Contd...

Necrophilia (S 297 IPC)	• Sexual intercourse with dead bodies
Necrophagia (S 297 IPC)	• Eating the flesh, drinking the blood of the victim to drive sexual pleasure
Masochism	• Opposite to sadism, asking the partner to inflict pain on himself for sexual pleasure
Bondage/Algolagnia	• Sadism + Masochism
Fetichism	• Sexual excitement by seeing undergarments of a woman
Transvestism/Eonism	• Desire to be identified as opposite sex
Scatalogia	• Obsence telephone calls
Fellatio	• Oral stimulation of male genitalia
Cunnilingus	• Oral stimulation of female genitalia
Exhibitionism (S 294 IPC)	• Exposure of genitalia in a public place to obtain sexual pleasure
Voyeurism/Scotophilia (Sec 354 C IPC)	• Whoever watches or captures the image of a women engaging in a private act and obtain sexual gratification–punishment for 1 year which may extend to 3 year
Stalking (Sec 354 D IPC)	• Whoever follows a person and contacts or attempts to contact such person to foster personal interaction repeatedly despite disinterest by such a person–Punishment-1 to 3 years
Frotteurism (S 290 IPC)	• Sexual satisfaction by rubbing his genitals against a female in crowd
Urolagnia	• Sexual pleasure by seen the act of urination
Pyromania	• Sexual pleasure by seeing flames and destruction of a building
Coprolaynia	• Sexual pleasure by urinating over the partner
Narcism	• Self love
Pygmalionism	• Falling in love with an object made by him
Bobbit syndrome	• Female amputates penis of her male partner
Troilism	• Sexual practice by involving 3 persons; 2 of one sex and one of the opposite sex
Mixoscopia	• Sexual satisfaction by the sight of others engaged in sexual intercourse
Edipus complex	• Sexual desire of son towards his mother
Electra complex	• Sexual desire of daughter towards her father
Pharoan complex	• Sexual desire of brother towards his sister
Onanism/Ipsation/Masturbation	• Self stimulation which effects sexual arousal
Indecent assault (S354 IPC)	• Any offence committed on a female with the intention to outrage her modesty

Impotence and Sterility

Impotence	Sterility	Frigidity
Inability to perform or take part in sexual intercourse	Inability to procreate by a male or conceive children in a female	Sexual unresponsiveness in females (Analogue of impotence in male)

Signs of Pregnancy

Presumptive signs	Probable signs	Positive signs
• Amenorrhea • Breast changes • Morning sickness • Quickening • Pigmentation of skin • Jackquemier's or Chadwick's sign (discoloration of vagina) • Urinary disturbances • Sympathetic disturbances	• Enlargement of abdomen • Hegar's sign • Goodell's sign (softening of cervix) • Braxton-Hick's sign (intermittent uterine contractions) • Ballottement • Uterine souffle. • Immunological tests	• Fetal parts and movements felt by placing the hands on the abdomen • Fetal heart sounds • Placental souffle • Umbilical souffle • X-ray diagnosis (not done now) • Ultrasound

Torture

Falanga	Canes or rods used to beat on the soles
Telefono	Repeated slapping on the side of head over ears
Wet submarine	Forced immersion of head in water contaminated with urine or feces
Dry submarine	Tying a plastic bag over the head until suffocation
Parrot's perch	Head down from a horizontal pole placed under the knees with wrists bound to ankle
Cattle prod	Electric shock especially over the genitals
Chapuwa	The legs and thighs are tied very tightly with bamboo sticks to induce severe pain
Ghotna	Rolling a wooden log over the things up and down, while the long is weighed by one or two policemen standing on it
Sham execution	Victim is blind folded and asked to stand before a wall and then threatened that a vehicle is going to hit him. He hears the sound of a vehicle very near to him, causing fear and shock
Dunking	Victim is immersed into water, taken out after some time and given chance to confess

Battered Baby Syndrome or Caffey's Syndrome

- Slightly more in male children; youngest or the eldest child
- **Repetitive physical injuries** as a result of **non-accidental violence**
- There may also be deprivation of nutrition, care and affection
- The classical feature of this lesion are discrepancy between the nature of injuries and the explanation offered by the guardian, delay between the injury and medical attention which cannot be explained
- Fractures and injuries will be at different stages of healing
- Most characteristic lesion-**laceration of mucosa inside the upper lip and often tear of frenulum noted**
- Nibbing fractures-multiple rib # in the posterior angle
- X-ray shows string of beads appearance in the para vertebral gutter after callus formation
- Infantile whiplash syndrome- shaking a child causes subdural hematoma and intraocular bleeding.

Tests for blood stains	Tests for seminal stains
• Benzidine test (Alder's test) • Phenolphthalein (Kastle Mayer test) • O-toluidine test • Leucomalachite green test • Luminal test • Hemin crystal test (Teichmann test) • Hemochromogen test (Takayama test) • Immunological test-precipitin test (To dientify the species) • Spectroscopy-most reliable	• Creatine phosphokinase test • Acid phosphatase test • Florence test • Barberio's test (crystals of spermin picrate)

Tests for Livebirth

- **Static or Fodere's test**-average weight of both lungs before respiration is 30–40 gms; after respiration is 60–66 gms. Not reliable
- **Plocquet's test**: The ratio of weight of lungs to weight of the body before respiration -1/70; after respiration-1/35. Not reliable
- **Hydrostatic test or Raygat's test**-the specific gravity of lungs before respiration: 1040–1050; after respiration: 940. Not of much value
- **Breslau's test or stomach bowel test-Air swallowed** into the stomach which floats
- **Wredin's test**-middle ear changes after birth
- **Vagitus uterinus:** Respiration (cry) of the fetus while in the womb after the rupture of membranes
- **Vagitus vaginalis:** Respiration while the head is in the vagina

Signs of live birth	• Viable child • Well expanded lungs • Vital reaction in the umbilical cord • Presence of milk in stomach

Suppositious children	Fictitious child claimed by a women as her own. DNA fingerprinting is confirmatory
Posthumous child	A child born after the death of the father
Spurious or phantom child (Pseudocyesis)	Seen in women nearing menopause or women whom intensely desire children Subjective symptoms of pregnancy may be present X-ray and clinical examination is confirmatory
Superfecundation	Fertilization of two ova released at the same time but impregnated by two acts of coitus at short intervals One fetus may be dead and flattened leading to fetus compressus or fetus papyaceus
Superfetation	Fertilization of a second ovum in a female who is pregnant Fertilization of two separate ova at different period of ovulation

FORENSIC PSYCHIATRY

Delusion

False belief in something which is not a fact. Delusion persists even after the falsity is clearly demonstrated.

Delusion-disorder of thought	Hallucination-False perception
• Grandeur or Exaltation • Persecution • Reference • Influence • Infidelity (Othello syndrome) • Self-Reproach • Nihilistic • Hypochondriacal • Erotomaniac (Cerambault's syndrome)	• Visual • Auditory • Olfactory • Gustatory • Tactile–Magnan's symptom–delirium tremens and chronic cocaine poisoning • Psychomotor

Phobia-Excessive fear	Impulse
• Claustrophobia: Fear of staying in a closed place • Nyctophobia: Fear of darkness. • Agoraphobia: Fear of open space • Acrophobia: Fear of height • Mysophobia: Fear of dirt • Hydrophobia: Fear of water	• Kleptomania: Irresistible desire to steal articles of little value • Pyromania:Irresistible desire to set fire • Mutilomania:Irresistible desire to mutilate animals • Dipsomania:Irresistible desire for alcoholic drinks at periodic intervals

Illusion

Illusion is a false interpretation by the senses of an external object or stimulus which has a real existence.

Lucid Interval

Symptoms	Insanity	Head Injury
History	Of Insanity +	Of Head Injury +
Preceding Symptoms	Of Insanity +	Symptoms of Concussion +
Following Symptoms	Of Insanity +	Cerebral Irritation and Brainstem Compression +
Occurrence	Frequent	Only Once

Alcoholism and Psychosis

Alcoholic blackouts	These are episodes of amnesia
Delirium tremens	1 or 2 days after sudden withdrawal-due to heavy drinking-Injuries, infection and shock as precipitating factors. Then he develops disorders of perception and coarse muscular tremors of face tongue and hands. He may commit suicide, murder or assault. Patient is not liable for his acts
Alcoholic hallucinosis	The patient may suffer from illusions and hallucinations

Symptoms	True insanity	Feigned insanity
Onset	Gradual	Sudden
Motive for the offence	No motive	Obvious motive
Predisposing factors	Of insanity-Present	Absent
Signs and symptoms	Uniform	Present only when observed by others
Face	Vacant look	Frequently changing
Insomnia and Exertion	Can withstand for a long time	Cannot withstand

Testamentary capacity	Mental ability of a person to make a valid will
Holograph will	Written by the testator in his own hand writing
Criminal Responsibility Sec 84 IPC	Nothing is an offence which is done by a person, who at the time of doing it, by reason of unsoundness of mind, is incapable of knowing the nature and consequences of the act, or that what he is doing is either wrong or contrary to law
Somnambulism	Sleep walking
Somnolentia	Sleep–drunkenness–midway between sleep and walking, he amy commit some crime due to confusion of the mind

Toxicology

General Considerations

Ideal poisons

Ideal homicidal poison	Ideal suicidal poison
• Organic compound of fluorine (used as rodenticide) and thallium • Arsenic and aconite	• Opium and barbiturates • Organophosphorus compounds and endrin

Poison Information Centers

- The 1st PI center in Netherlands in 1949
- Telephone answering service was introduced in Leeds, London in 1961.
- In India the National Poison Information Center was established at AIIMS, New Delhi, in December 1994.
- Other centers at Ahmedabad, MMC Chennai, Lucknow and AIMS Cochin
- The WHO has released its software (INTOX).

Confirmation by Subjecting the Viscera for Chemical Analysis

- Routine viscera: Stomach with its contents, upper 30 cm of the duodenum, 500 gms of liver and half of each kidney
- 100 ml of blood with sodium fluoride as preservative.

General Lines of Treatment

Decontamination: Emesis, gastric lavage, catharsis, activated charcoal, whole bowel irrigation.

Composition of universal antidote

Components	Quantity	Mechanism
Charcoal	2 parts	Adsorbs poisons
Magnesium oxide	1 part	Neutralizes acids
Tannic acid	1 part	Precipitates alkaloids, certain glycosides and metals

Smell of Poisons

Smell	Poison
Garlic like	Phosphorous, Arsenic
Sweet or fruity	Ethanol, Chloroform
Rotten egg	H_2S
Fishy	Zinc phosphide

Color of Postmortem Lividity

Poisons	Color of PM lividity
Carbon monoxide	Cherry Red
Cyanide	Bright Red
Hydrogen Sulfide	Greenish Blue
Phosphorus	Brown
Nitrobenzene, Potassium Chloride	Brownish Red
Aniline	Blue, Brown

Putrefaction changes: *Arsenic and Organophosphates* are said to delay putrefaction.

Preservatives

Saturated solution of common salt used in all except	Rectified spirit used in all except
• Corrosive acid • Mercuric chloride • Vegetable poison • Aconite	• Carbolic acid • Acetic acid • Paraldehyde • Phosphorous • Alcohol • Kerosene

Organophosphates and Organochlorine Poisoning

Organophosphorus poisons		Organochlorines
Alkyl phosphates	Aryl phosphates	
• HETP, TEPP, OMPA • Dimefox, isopestox • Malathion (kill bug, Bugs online) • Sulfotep, Demeton • Trichlorfon	• Parathion (Follidol, killphos) • Methyl parathion • Chlorthion • Paraoxon • Diazinon (Tik 20)	• DDT, BHC (lindane) • Aldrin, chlordane • Dieldrin, Endosulfan • Endrin (plant penicillin), mirex • Toxaphene paraquat

Mechanism of action-Inhibition of Acetylcholinesterase (AChE), true cholinesterase and pseudo-cholinesterase

Muscarinic symptoms	Nicotinic symptoms
• Bronchoconstriction • Increased bronchial secretions and pulmonary edema • Bradycardia, Miosis • Water loss due to sweating, salivation, lacrimation, micturition, diarrhea	• Fasciculation • Dyspnea and cyanosis due to respiratory paralysis

Intermediate syndrome	Delayed syndrome
• Due to inadequate treatment, sub-therapeutic administration of oximes and inadequate ventilation • It does not respond to oximes and atropine	• Peripheral neuropathy due to demyelination occurs 1-5 weeks after exposure • Rapidly progresses to a flaccid paresis which can ascent similar to Guillain-Barre syndrome

- Diagnosis
  - Cholinesterase determination in blood
  - Normal values 77–142 in red cells and 41–140 in the plasma
  - Plasma cholinesterase is more sensitive and fall more rapidly before that of red cells.
- Treatment
  - Antidote: Atropine
  - Specific antidote: Cholinesterase reactivators like diacetylmonoxime (DAM), pralidoxime (2-PAM)
- Chromolachryorrhea (red tears) due to accumulation of porphyearin in lacrimal glands.

Carbolc Acid/Carbolism

- Oxidized to **pyrocatechol and hydroxyquinone** whose excretion is the cause of green color urine (**carboluria**)
- Chronic poisoning (**Phenol marasmus**) causes pigmentation of skin of perforation is less
- PM appearances: gastric mucosa is swollen, grayish white, hardened (leather bottle stomach).

HCN (Prussic or sheele's acid or cyanogens)

- Smell of bitter almonds
- Cherry red postmortem staining
- Inhibits cytochrome oxidase and carbonic anhydrase
- Potassium ferrocyanide and ferricyanide are non poisonous
- Survivors of acute poisoning may develop delayed neurological sequeale in the form of parkinsonism
- Treatment
  - Amyl nitrite, sodium nitrite
  - Sodium thiosulfate
  - Hydroxyl cobalamine
  - Dicobalt EDTA

Alcohol

Absolute alcohol	Rectified spirit	Methylated spirit	Surgical spirit
99.95% alcohol	90–95% ethanol + 5–10% methanol + traces of castor oil	Methylated spirit -99% alcohol + 5% wood naptha	90–95% ethanol + 5–10% methanol

Beverage	% of alcohol
Vodka	60–65
Rum, liquor	50–60
Whisky, gin, brandy	40–45
Port, sherry	20
Wine, champagne	10–15
Beer	4–8

- Urine alcohol: blood alcohol=1.3:1
- Widmark's formula: a = pre (blood); a = 3/4 prq (urine)
- Henry's law: alveolar: blood alcohol = 2100:1.

Methods to find blood and urine alcohol levels

- Alcohol dehydrogenase method
- Kozelka and Hine test
- Gas chromatography (most specific)
- Breath analyzer
- Cavett test
  - Marchiafava syndrome-corpus callosum degeneration
  - **McEwan's sign** in alcoholic coma
  - This differentiates alcoholic coma from coma due to other causes
  - **Statutory limit for driving in India:** 30 mg% (S 185 of Motor Vehicles Act).

Cannabis (Indian Hemp)

- Principle component is cannabidiol which is inert, is converted to active isomer tetrahydrocannabinols (THC) on exposure to heat

- Chronic poisoning
  - Hashish insanity (running amok)
  - A motivation syndrome
  - Flash back phenomenon
- It does not produce physiological dependence or addiction,but psychological dependence and tolerance develop
- Various forms of cannabis.

Bang	Decoction from dried leaves and fruit shoots; 15% of active principle
Majoon	Sweet prepared from plant extract
Ganja	Leaves and flower tops of female plant; 15-25% of active principle
Charas or Hashish	Resin exuding from leaves and stems; 25-40% of active principle
Marijuana	Dried flowering tops crushed and smoked in a pipe
Sinsemilla	Seedless marijuana

Cocaine poisoning ('Coke', 'Snow', 'Cadillac', 'White lady')

- Acts as a CNS stimulant and local anesthetic with potent vasoconstrictor properties
- Speed ball–It is a combination of cocaine and heroin which is taken in the form of injection
- Chronic intoxication ('Cocainism'/Cocainophagia/Cocainomania)
  - Suspiciousness.
  - Visual and tactile hallucinations (Cocaine bugs)
  - Magnan's symptoms
- In pregnant woman: Incidence of abortion, abruption placenta and cerebrovascular disease
- Smoking of 'Crack' results in 'Crack babies'.

Arsenic

- Arsenious oxide or Arsenic trioxide is the most common form of arsenic used
- Regular, long-term arsenic exposure-cutaneous carcinomas as well as internal malignancies including bronchogenic carcinoma and hepatocellular carcinoma.
- **After ingestion**

After 2–4 weeks	Incorporated into hair, nails and skin-MEES LINES
After 4 weeks	Localize in the bone, where it substitutes for phosphate

- Chronic toxicity
  - Red velvety stomach
  - **Garlic odor** on breath, excessive perspiration
  - Peripheral vascular disease gangrene of feet–**Blackfoot disease**
  - Brittle nails with **Aldrich Mee's lines** (whitish transverse striate 1–2 mm-in the fingernails leukonychia). Also occurs in thallium poisoning
  - Subendocardial hemorrhage in the left ventricle
  - Hyperpigmentation of the skin of the face or extremities-**Rain drop type pigmentation**
  - Hyperkeratosis (wart like lesion) of palms and soles
  - Normochromic and normocytic anemia
  - Symmetrical sensorimotor polyoneuropathy, often resembling Guillain-Barre syndrome
  - **Arsenophagists**-some people take arsenic daily as tonic or aphrodisiac and acquire tolerance.

Lead

- Lead (Pb^{++}), competes with Ca^{++}, Fe^{++}
- Lead directly causes hemolysis of mature red cells. Affects erythropoiesis, myelopoiesis by depressing bone marrow → anemia, basophilc stippling of RBC's, thrombocytopenia
- ↓Uric acid excretion-↑ Blood urates–Saturnine gout
- Chronic lead poisoning called as plumbism or saturnism.

Signs and symptoms	Description
Facial pallor	Around the mouth Earliest sign
Blood	Anemia (Pb level 70–80 mg/100 ml) Reticulocytosis, poikilocytosis, anisocytosis, Nucleated RBCs. ↓polymorphs and platelets Punctate basophilia/ basophilic stippling of red cells
Lead line (burtonian line)	It is seen on the gums due to subepithelial deposits of granules at the junction within the teeth It is deposited in the dirty or caries teeth[Q] within a week of exposure, usually in the upper jaw
Colic and constipation	Late symptom Nocturnal colic of intestine, ureter, uterus Relieved by heavy pressure
Lead palsy	Late feature Affects muscle groups more prone to fatigue–extensor m's of wrist except supinator longus (wrist drop), extensor m's of foot except tibialis anterior (foot drop)
Lead encephalopathy	Common in children
Lead osteopathy	Lead is deposited beyond the epiphysis of the growing long bones Growth arrest lines, also known as lead bands, in bones of a child Lead lines are not observed in adults

Image Studies

- X-ray- radio opaque bands (lead lines) at the metaphyses of long bones in children
- The width of the lead lines is related to the duration of exposure
- Abdominal radiographs: Demonstrate the presence of radio-opacities throughout the GI tract.

Also, the presence of retained bullets.

Mercury Poisoning

- Chronic poisoning: Otherwise called as 'Hydragyrum'.
- Classic triad: Gingivitis, salivation and tremors.
- Signs and Symptoms:
  - Blue lines on gums
  - Tremors (Danbury tremors) which starts in hands and then progresses to other parts of the body. When generalized, it is called as 'Hatter's Shake', glassblowers shakes
  - Most severe form called as 'Concussion mercurialis' where no activity is possible.
  - 'Mercurial Erethism' which occurs in worker of mirror industry where there is development of psychological symptoms
  - 'Mercurialentis' is a peculiar eye change where brownish deposit of mercury seen on *anterior lens capsule* and this is due to exposure to mercury vapor. It has no effects on visual acuity
  - Acrodynia (Pink disease)
  - Idiosyncratic hypersensitivity reaction, seen in children
  - Generalized erythematous, eczematous papular type of lesions mostly in hands and feet, accompanied by thickening and peeling of the skin.

Copper

- Copper arsenite: Scheele's green
- Copper acetoarsenite: Paris green
- Copper sulfate (blue vitriol) and copper subacetate (verdigris) are poisonous

- Treatment: Stomach wash with 1% potassium ferrocyanide which is an effective antidote and chelation with penicillamine or BAL or EDTA
- Post mortem appearances-**Greenish blue froth at mouth and nostrils**
- Chronic inhalation of copper sulfate-**Vineyard sprayer's lung disease**
- Copper deposits in tissuses-**chalcosis**
- **Ptyalism** in chronic poisoning
- Chronic contact with swimming pool water containing algicidal copper chemical compounds may cause green hair discolouration.

Abrus Precatorius

- Seeds contain active principle **abrin**, a toxalbumen, which is similar to **viperine snake** venom
- Abrine, hemaglutinin, abralin are other toxins
- Sharp pointed needle like objects called suis are prepared from the paste of seeds, which are forced into the skin of animal or human for homicide (2 suis used to resemble fangs of viper).

Snakes

Poisonous snakes	Non-poisonous snakes
Head scales small (but large in pit viper)	Large
Belly scales-large and cover entire breadth	Small and do not cover entire breadth
Head usually triangular	Usually round or oval
Fangs-hollow like hypodermic needles	Short and solid
Teeth-two long fangs	Several small teeth
Tail-rounded or flattened	Always rounded
Habits-usually nocturnal	No variation

- Ophitoxemia is poisoning by snake venom
- Sutherland wrap is a modification of tourniquet used as a crepe bandage in snake bite cases

Cobra, krait	Neurotoxic
Viper	Vasculotoxic (hemotoxic)
Sea snakes	Myotoxic

Aconite/Monk's Hood

- Cardiac poison
- Root (most toxic part) mistaken for horse radish root
- **Hippus**-alternate constriction and dilation of pupil
- Ideal homicidal poison.

QUESTIONS

1. Bitten fruit is found at crime scene. Which of the following would be an ideal preservative? (2014)

a. NaCl
b. Formalin
c. Metabisulphite
d. Glacial acetic acid

2. Red velvety appearance of stomach mucosa is seen in the poisoning of: (2014)

a. Lead
b. Arsenic
c. Copper
d. Mercury

3. Magistrate inquest is done in all the following cases except: (2014)

a. Exhumation
b. Homicide
c. Lock up death
d. Alleged dowry death

4. Which of the following toxins have similar action to viper snake venom? (2014)

a. Yellow oleander
b. Semecarpus anacardium
c. Rauwolfia serpentina
d. Abrus precatorius

5. Last organ to putrefy after death is: (2014)

a. Heart
b. Prostate
c. Stomach
d. Brain

6. Alkaline dieresis for which poisoning? (2014)

a. Phencyclidine
b. Phenol barbitone
c. Amphetamine
d. Morphine

7. During postmortem no tattoo is visible, but according to deceased family, there was a tattoo present. What evidence can indicate the same? (2014)

a. Lymph node
b. Surrounding subcutaneous tissue
c. Adipose tissue
d. Adjacent skin

8. According to MTP Act, abortion can be done till: (2014)

a. 12 week
b. 20 weeks
c. 28 weeks
d. Till viability

9. Man hit by car is thrown up and hits road divider falls on the ground sustains head injury then run over by another car. Cause of head injury: (2014)

a. Primary impact injury
b. Secondary impact injury
c. Primary injury
d. Secondary injury

10. Florence test identifies which of the following? (2013)

a. Choline
b. Inositol
c. Spermine
d. Fructose

11. According to MCI, medical records of patients must be maintained by a Practitioner for a minimum period of: (2013)

a. 1 year
b. 2 years
c. 3 years
d. 5 years

12. In a macerated baby, ideal sample for genetic analysis is obtained from: (2012)

a. Clotted fetal blood
b. Placental Tissue
c. Fibroblast from skin
d. Fibroblast from Achiles tendon

13. 10 year imprisonment verdict can be given by: (2012)

a. Chief metropolitan magistrate
b. Metropolitan magistrate
c. Assistant sessions court
d. First class judicial magistrate

14. Ochronosis is caused by poisoning due to: (2012)

a. Carbolic acid
b. Mercury salts
c. Zine salts
d. Oxalic acid

15. Which of the following is not seen in aconite poisoning? (2012)

a. Hypertension
b. Tingling of lips
c. Hypersalivation
d. Hemoglobinuria

16. Which of the following is not present in datura? (2011)

a. Hyoscine
b. Hyoscyamine
c. Muscarine
d. Atropine

17. Most common type of primary Finger print pattern is: (2011)

a. Whorl
b. Loop
c. Arch
d. Composite

18. Filigree burns seen in: (2011)

a. Radiation
b. Electrical burn
c. Lightening
d. Vitriolage

19. Sample of spinal cord preserved in: (2011)

a. Oleander poisoning
b. War gases
c. Strychnine poisoning
d. Arsenic poisoning

20. Color of urine in phenol poisoning: (2011)

a. Red
b. Green
c. Yellow
d. Blue

21. When a doctor shows gross absence of skill and care during treatment resulting in death of patient is called: (2011)
a. Criminal negligence
b. Malpractice
c. Maloccurence
d. Misadventure

22. Metabolic acidosis and visual damage occurs in poisoning due to: (2010)
a. Methanol
b. Ethanol
c. Cocaine
d. Opium

23. Color of urine in phenol poisoning: (2010)
a. Red
b. Green
c. Yellow
d. Blue

24. Sample of spinal cord persevered in: (2010)
a. Strychnine poisoning
b. Arsenic poisoning
c. Yellow oleander poisoning
d. Nerve gas poisoning

25. A doctor leaves swab in abdomen during surgery under which doctrine will a criminal suit be filed against him? (2010)
a. Criminal negligence
b. Civil negligence
c. Res ipsa loquitur
d. Vicarious liability

26. A criminal negligence suit against a doctor must be filed within: (2010)
a. 6 months
b. 1 year
c. 2 years
d. 4 years

27. Incised looking lacerated wounds are seen in:
a. Hand (2010)
b. Thorax
c. Abdomen
d. Forehead

28. 'Hatter's shankes' are see in poisoning due to:
a. Mercury (2010)
b. Arsenic
c. Lead
d. Copper

29. Acrodynia is a feature of: (2010)
a. Iron deficiency anemia
b. Mercury poisoning
c. Copper poisoning
d. Zinc poisoning

30. Subpoena is a: (2009)
a. Legal document
b. Medicolegal document
c. Medical document
d. First information report (FIR)

31. Which of the following is most useful for sex determination? (2009)
a. Skull
b. Femur
c. Pelvis
d. Tibia

32. Which of the following is diagnostic of drowning? (2009)
a. Froth in the nostrils
b. Cutis anserine
c. Water in the stomach
d. Mud in the respiratory passages

33. Mummification refers to: (2009)
a. Hardening of muscle following death
b. Colliquative putrifaction
c. Saponification of subcuatenous fat
d. Desiccation of dead body

34. Rigor mortis start in: (2009)
a. Heart
b. Brain
c. Right iliac fossa
d. Left iliac fossa

35. MTP Act was introduced in: (2009)
a. 1961
b. 1971
c. 1981
d. 1991

36. The first permanent tooth to appear is: (2009)
a. 1st molar
b. Lateral incisor
c. Upper canine
d. 1st premolar

37. Which of the following is not present in datura?
a. Hyoscine (2009)
b. Hyoscyamine
c. Muscarine
d. Atropine

38. The lowest court that can give life imprisonment verdict is: (2009)
a. Chief metropolitan magistrate
b. Metropolitan magistrate
c. High court
d. First class judicial magistrate

39. Entry would shotgun from 30 to 60 cm is characterized by: (2008)
a. Abrasion collar
b. Abrasion rim
c. Tattooing
d. Cruciate shaped wound

40. Cephalic index of 80–85 is seen in: (2008)
a. Mongols
b. Chinese
c. European
d. Negroid

41. Medical Negligence is booked under which of the following IPC section? (2008)
a. 304 A
b. 300
c. 375
d. 320

42. Man commits rape even if he has sex with his wife when she is less than: (2008)
a. 15 years
b. 16 years
c. 14 years
d. 13 years

43. Leading questions are permitted only in: (2007)
a. Cross examination
b. Examination in chief
c. Re-examination
d. Dying Declaration

44. Green colored urine is seen after ingestion of: (2007)
a. Copper sulphate
b. Phenol
c. Organophosphaorus
d. Cyanide

45. Spalding sign is a feature of: (2007)
a. Prematurity
b. Postmaturity
c. Fetal death
d. Hydrocephalus

46. Most common organ to be injured in primary blast injuries is: (2007)
a. Liver
b. Spleen
c. Skin
d. Tympanic membrane

47. Which of the following is not characteristic of criminal negligence? (2006)
a. No specific violation of law needs to be proved
b. If found guilty, can be imprisoned
c. Gross negligence leading to death
d. Guilt should be proven beyond doubt in court

48. Heart blocks are caused by? (2006)
a. Yellow oleander poisoning
b. Organophosphorus poisoning
c. Phenol poisoning
d. Methyl alcohol poisoning

49. Methanol poisoning is treated by all except: (2006)
a. Ethanol
b. Fomepizole
c. Hemodialysis
d. Forced alkaline dieresis

ANSWERS AND EXPLANATIONS

1. Ans. b. or c. *Ref: (a) Fisher BAJ and Fisher DR, Techniques of Crime Scene Investigation, 8/e CRC Press, p239 (b) Nitul Jan. Textbook of Forensic Odontology, 1/e p140 and (c) Tekade pand Singh TRM, Forensic Dentistry: A Review, IJBPT 2011:2 (1): 265*

Bite marks:
- Human bites are usually semicircular or crescentic, caused by the front teeth (incisors and canines), with a gap at either side due to the separation of upper and lower jaw. Bite marks may be abrasions, contusions or lacerations or a combination of any two or three.
- In forcible bite, the appearance is of two 'bows' with their concavities facing each other, and a gap at each end.
- The sucking action reduces the air pressure over the Center and produces multiple petechial hemorrhages, due to rupture of capillaries and small venules in the subcutaneous tissues.
- Faint teeth marks should be when examined under ultraviolet light in a dark room.

In sexual offence cases:
- **Love bites** are usually seen on breast, neck, cheek, abdomen, arms, thighs and genitalia.
- In many such bites teeth marks are not seen.
- Swabs of the bite mark should be taken immediately, using a swab moistened with sterile water.
- **Self inflicted bite marks** are usually seen on the shoulders and arms.

Bite marks are useful in identification because the alignment of teeth is peculiar to the individual.

Preservation:

For bite marks in skin: By photographing or casting

For bite marks in fruits:

- Marks are preserved in 0.5% formalin solution.

Rudland's method:

- 5% glacial acetic acid + 40% formaldehyde solution + 70% ethanol in the ratio of 5:5:90 preserved apples for 10 years
- Campden solution-metabisulfite fluid

2. **Ans. b. Arsenic** *Ref: The Essentials of Forensic Medicine and Toxicology by KS Narayan Reddy, 29/e p482*
   - Red velvety mucosa: Seen in arsenic poisoning.
   - The mucosa is swollen edematous and red, especially in **pyloric region.**

   Mode of action: Arsenic interferes with cellular respiration by combining with the sulphydryl groups of mitochondrial enzymes.
   - Symptoms simulate those of cholera.

   Disadvantages of arsenic usage as poison:
   - It delays putrefaction
   - Can be detected in completely decomposed bodies.
   - Can be found in bones, hairs and nails for several years.
   - Can be detected in charred bones or ashes.
3. **Ans. b. Homicide** *Ref: The Essentials of Forensic Medicine and Toxicology by KS Narayan Reddy, 29/e 2010, p5*

   Magistrate inquest is not done in homicide/murder.

   Magistrate inquest is conducted in
   - Death in police custody and while under police interrogation
   - Death due to police firing
   - Death in prisons, reformatories, Borstal school
   - Death in psychiatric hospitals
   - Dowry deaths
   - Exhumation.
4. **Ans. d. Abrus precatorius**

   Ref: The Essentials of Forensic Medicine and Toxicology by KS Narayan Reddy, 29/e p497

	Abrus precatorius	Cerbera thevetia	Semicarpus anacardium
Other names	Indian liquorice, Rosary pea, Rati	Yellow oleander	Marking nut, Bhilawa
Active principle	Abrin (toxalbumen) Similar to viperine snake	Cerberine Thevetin Thevetoxin Nerifolin	Semicarpol, Bhilawanol
Clinical manifestations	Most poisonous: Seeds • Nausea, vomiting, diarrhea • Abdominal cramps, hematemesis and melena • Hemaglutination, hemolysis of red cells • Hypovolemic shock and direct toxic effect on kidneys lead to acute renal failure	Mode of action: Inhibit sodium-potassium ATPase • Negative chronotropic, positive inotropic effects • Bradyarrhythmias and tachyarrhythmias • Continuous ECG monitoring for 24 hours is essential	On External application • Bruise like painful lesions. • Marginal small blisters–black, raised and contain acrid serum. **On ingestion** • Burning pain in the throat with blister formation • Burning pain in abdomen • Dilated pupils • Rapid pulse, fall of BP
Treatment	• Gastric lavage • Activated charcoal • Anti-abrin • Oral sodium bicarbonate	• Induce emesis at home (ipecac) • Atropine 0.5 mg IV for bradycardia, repeated cardiac pacing for third degree heart block • Anti-digoxin Fab antibodies in severe cases	• Wash the contaminated skin • Demulcents

5. Ans. b. Prostate *Ref: The Essentials of Forensic Medicine and Toxicology by KS Narayan Reddy, 29/e p152*

- Larynx and trachea
- Stomach, intestines and spleen
- Liver (foamy liver) lings
- Brain
- Heart
- Kidneys, bladder
- Prostate, uterus
- Skin, muscle, tendon
- Bones
- Nulliparous uterus is the last organ to putrefy, gravid uterus and uterus soon after delivery putrefies rapidly
- In males, prostate is the last organ to putrefy
- Optimum temperature for putrefaction 21 °C
- Putrefaction arrested below 0 °C and above 48 °C.

Rapid putrefaction	Delayed putrefaction
• Peritonitis • Sepsis • Asphyxia • Clostridial infections • Intestinal obstruction • Abortion	• Anemia • Debility • Carbolic acid poisoning • Zinc chloride • Strychnine poisoning • Heavy metal poisoning • OPC poisoning

Putrefaction in water (CASPER DICTUM)-1: 2: 8 = Air: Water: Earth

6. Ans. b. Pheno barbitone

Ref: The Essentials of Forensic Medicine and Toxicology by KS Narayan Reddy, 29/e p527

Antidote	Indication
Theophylline	Adenosine poisoning
Atropine	Organophosphate and carbamate insecticide, mushrooms
Forced alkaline diuresis	Barbiturates
Calcium chloride	Black widow spider bites
Chelators such as EDTA, dimercaprol (BAL), penicillamine, and 2,3-dimercaptosuccinic acid (DMSA, succimer)	Heavy metal poisoning
Cyanide antidote (amyl nitrite, sodium nitrite, or thiosulfate)	Cyanide poisoning
Deferoxamine mesylate	Iron poisoning
Digoxin Immune Fab antibody (Digibind and Digifab)	Digoxin poisoning
Ethanol or fomepizole	Ethylene glycol poisoning and methanol poisoning
Flumazenil	Benzodiazepine poisoning
Glucagon	Beta blocker poisoning
100% oxygen or hyperbaric oxygen therapy (HBOT)	Carbon monoxide poisoning
Leucovorin	Methotrexate and trimethoprim
Methylene blue	Treatment of conditions that cause methemoglobinemia
Naloxone hydrochloride	Opioid overdose
N-acetylcysteine	Paracetamol (acetaminophen) poisoning
Octreotide	Oral hypoglycemic agents
Pralidoxime chloride (2-PAM)	Organophosphate insecticides, followed after atropine
Protamine sulfate	Heparin poisoning

Contd...

Contd...

Antidote	Indication
Prussian blue	Thallium poisoning
Physostigmine sulfate	Anticholinergic poisoning
Pyearidoxine	Isoniazid poisoning, ethylene glycol
Phytomenadione (vitamin K) and fresh frozen plasma	Warfarin poisoning and indanedione

7. Ans. a. Lymph node *Ref: The Essentials of Forensic Medicine and Toxicology by KS Narayan Reddy, 19/e p83*

Tattoo marks

- **Faint or disappeared tattoo marks can be made out on histological study of the regional lymph nodes.**
- In decomposed bodies, they are made visible by treating the area with *3% hydrogen peroxide.*
- Tattoo marks can be removed by surgical method or use of laser beams, without leaving any permanent mark.
- Apart from identification, tattoo marks may provide additional information like race, religion, nationality, language, mental make up, social status, etc.,
- Drug addicts often imprint tattoos over areas of multiple injection mark, in order to conceal the needle puncture marks.

Methods to demonstrate old or faint tatoos visible:

- Infrared photography
- UV lamp
- Magnifying glass
- High contrast photography.

8. Ans. b. 20 weeks *Ref: The Essentials of Forensic Medicine and Toxicology by KS Narayan Reddy, 29/e p381*

The MTP ACT-1971

Indications

- Therapeutic
- Eugenic
- Humanitarian
- Social
- Environmental.

Rules

- A doctor is qualified if he/she has assisted **25 cases of MTP in a recognized hospital**
- Consent of the husband **not** necessary
- Duration of pregnancy **< 12 weeks-one doctor** can perform
- **12–20 weeks-two doctors** must agree that there is an indication for MTP
- In case of emergency, can be performed by a single doctor, even without training, even after 20 weeks, even without consulting another doctor, even in a private hospital which is not recognized.

9. Ans. d. Secondary injury *Ref: Textbook of Forensic Medicine and Toxicology, Nageshwar Rao, p207*

Transportation injuries

Primary impact injuries	• Injuries are caused when the vehicle hits the victim (PEDESTRIAN). • Injuries are in the form of imprint abrasions or patterned bruises, Bumper fracture
Secondary impact injuries	• Injuries caused due to subsequent 2nd impact of same vehicle. • Injuries may be any of the hard blunt force injuries: abrasions, grazed abrasion, stretch lacerations
Secondary injuries	• Injuries caused by falling on the ground or on other stationary object. • Found on parts opposite to primary impact or head
Runover injuries	• Abrasions may be on two or more surfaces, avulsions.
Bumper #	• Fracture of femur or tibia, resulting from an impact of a vehicle against a pedestrian.
Motorcyclist #	• Hinge fracture of base of skull

10. Ans. a. Choline *Ref: The Essentials of Forensic Medicine and Toxicology by KS Narayan Reddy 29/e*

Methods applied for detection of seminal Stains are classified as:

- Physical examination
- Chemical examination
- Microscopic examination.

Physical examination:

- Include visual examination. To naked eye seminal stains generally appear translucent or opaque spots. also acquire stiffness due to dried semen.
- Seminal stains may appear to be fluorescent under ultraviolet light.

Chemical examination

Test	Principle	Inference	Significance
Florence Test	Detection of choline	Dark brown crystals of choline periodide, generally needle shaped	Non-specifics and false negative results are common.
Barberio Test	Spermine	Spermine picrate (needle shaped, rhombic and of yellow colour)	Non-specific
Acid Phosphatase Test	Presence of high percentage acid pohosphatase in semen	Blue colour	Conclusive in the absence of sperms
LDM Isoenzyme Method	Detection of Spermatozoa	Isoenzyme bands are revealed by staining	Specific biochemical detection of spermatozoa in semen in the presence of vaginal fluid, blood, nasal secretion, aaliva and urine
Creatinine Phosphokinase	Detection of creatinine phosphokinase	> 400 V of CPK/ml.	Enzyme is stable and can be demonstrated in old status of six months
Ammonium Molybdate Test	Phosphorus		
Semen Specific Glycoprotein test	Glycoprotein P30		

11. Ans. c. 3 years

Maintenance of medical records

- Inpatients-3 years
- Routine case records-6 years after completion of treatment and 3 years after death.
- Chance of litigation-25 years.
- Records of public interest transferred to public library; after 50 years. If confidential: It can be released after 100 years.

12. Ans. b. Placental tissue *Ref: Derom C et al. genotyping of macerated stillborn fetuses. Am J Obstet Gynecol. 1991 Mar; 164 (3): 797–800. and http://www2.marshfieldclinic.org/wissp/commonly.htm*

- In macerated babies, it is generally impossible to collect blood or to culture tissue from a macerated stillborn fetus. It is particularly important in these cases to sample fetal placenta since these cells tend to survive longer after fetal death.
- For non-placental samples, yield is less.

Dead born: This is a child, which has died in utero and shows one of the following signs after it is completely born:

- Rigor mortis at birth.
- Maceration:
  - This is aseptic autolysis and occurs when the child remains in the uterus for about 3–4 days immersed in liquor amnii but **devoid of air.**
  - **Earliest sign of maceration is skin slippage** and is seen in 12 hours of death in utero.
  - **Gas in aorta of fetus** indicates fetal death.
  - Other changes seen are red/purple skin, blebs, distended abdomen, flexible joints and bones, soft viscera, etc.
  - **Spalding sign**: Loss of alignment and overriding of skull bones of the cranial vault.

- Mummification.
- Putrefaction.

13. Ans. c. Assistant senssions court (Refer theory) *Ref: The Essential of Forensic Medicine, KS. Narayan Reddy. 24/e*

14. Ans. a. Carbolic acid *Ref: The Essentials of Forensic Medicine, KS. Naraya Reddy. 24/e*

Oochronosis:

Endogenous: Alkaptonuria is a rare autosomal recessive metabolic disorder caused by deficiency of homogentisic acid oxidase, the only enzyme capable of catabolizing homogentisic acid (HGA)

Exogenous: Exogenous ochronosis, in which bluish black pigmentation of cartilage is noted by exogenous agents, after exposure to noxious substances, including **phenol, trinitrophenol, benzene, and hydroquinone.**

15. Ans. d. Hemoglobinuria *Ref: The Essentials of Forensic Medicine, KS. Narayan Reddy, 24/e*

Aconite (Mitha Bish, Mitha Zahar, Bikh, Monk's Hood)

- All parts are poisonous, root is chiefly used as poison.
- Has no odor but sweetish in taste.
- Should be differentiated from Horseradish root.

Active principles:

- Aconitine
- Pseudoaconitine
- Aconine.

Mode of action:

- Stimulates the sensory nerve endings, producing **tingling and numbness** .
- The cardiotoxicity and neurotoxicity are due to their actions on the voltage-**sensitive sodium channels** of the cell membranes of excitable tissues, including the **myocardium, nerves, and muscles**

  Signs and symptoms
- Patients present predominantly with a combination of neurological, cardiovascular, and gastrointestinal features.

Neurological features can be sensory (paresthesia and numbness of face, perioral area, and the four limbs), motor (muscle weakness in the four limbs).

Cardiovascular features include hypertension, bradycardia, sinus tachycardia, ventricular arrhythmia

Gastrointestinal features include nausea, vomiting, abdominal pain, and diarrhea.

The main causes of death are refractory ventricular arrhythmias and asystole

Treatment

- Digitalis–To counter depressant action on heart.
- Atropine–For bradycardia.

16. Ans. c. Muscarine *Ref: The Essential of Forensic Medicine and Toxicology by KS Narayan Reddy. 29/e*

Datura

- Active principles: Hyoscine (Scopalamine) Hyoscyamine, Atropine
- Symptoms of Datura poisoning
- Dry hot skin
- Dilation of cutaneous blood vessels
- Dilation of pupils
- Diplopia
- Dryness of mouth, throat
- Delirium
- Dysphagia
- Drunken gait
- Dysuria
- Death.

17. Ans. b. Loop (Refer theory)

Ref: The Essentials of Forensic Medicine and Toxicology by KS Narayan Reddy 29/e p77

18. Ans. c. Lightening (Refer theory)

Ref: The Essentials of Forensic Medicine and Toxicology by KS Narayan Redy 29/e p298

19. Ans. c. Strychnine poisoning

Ref: The Essentials of Forensic Medicine and Toxicology by KS Narayan Reddy 29/e

Special organs has to be sent for specific poisons

Organs to be preserved	Poisons
Brain	Volatile and anesthetic poisons
Heart	Cardiac poisons
Spinal cord	Nervous poisons
Bile	Morphine poisoning
Skin and subcutaneous tissue	Injected poisons, drugs, venom
Hair, nail, and long bones	Heavy metal poisoning, especially arsenic
Add liquid paraffin on the top of blood sample	CO poisoning
Thigh muscles	In advanced decomposition in detection of poison

20. Ans. b. Green *Ref: The Essentials of Forensic Medicine and Toxicology by KS Narayan Reddy. 29/e p478*

Urine color	Conditions
Green color	• Phenol poisoning can lead to green or black urine due to carboluria • Carboluria is due to oxidation of phenol to hydroquinone and pyrocatechol
Red color	• Hematuria-microscopic examination of urine will demonstrate the present of RBCs • Myoglobinuria-there will be a brownish-red colour • Hemoglobinuria-with intravascular HEMOLYSIS • 'Pink diaper syndrome'-there is a pinkish discoloration on the diaper secondary to urate crystals in the urine
Vin rose color	• Use of deferoxamine will cause vin rose colored urine if serum Fe is elevated
Brown or black color	• Nitric acid poisoning • Hemoglobin • Nitrofurans • Alkaptonuria-on standing, the urine will turn a dark colour
Blue color	• Presence of indigo or of methylene blue (used as an antidote to certain types of poisoning)
Milky or cloudy Color	• Pus cells and bacteria in the urine • Chyluria

21. Ans. a. Criminal negligence

Ref: The Essentials of Forensic Medicine and Toxicology by KS Narayan Reddy 29/e p34

Criminal negligence

- Where the medical practitioner **is prosecuted in a criminal court** on the charge of having caused **death of his patient** because of **gross carelessness about his treatment.**
- **Examples of Criminal Negligence**
- Amputation of wrong part of body
- Leaving instruments or swabs inside the body
- Performing Criminal abortion
- Gross mismanagement during delivery
- Administration of wrong drug into the eye causing blindness

Legal liability: U/S 304 A, IPC

22. Ans. a. Methanol

Ref: The Essentials of Forensic Medicine and Toxicology by KS Narayan Reddy 29/e p521

- In the first step of methanol degradation, methanol is transformed into formaldehyde via the enzyme alcohol dehydrogenase (ADH). This reaction is slower than the next step, the transformation of formaldehyde into formic acid via the enzyme aldehyde dehydrogenase.
- Formaldehyde 33 times more toxic than methanol.
- Formic Acid is 6 times more toxic than methanol.

Metabolic acidosis:
- The metabolism of formic acid is very slow; thus, formic acid often accumulates in the body, which results in metabolic acidosis.

Visual damage:
- Vision loss is caused by interruption of mitochondrial function in the optic nerve, resulting in hyperemia, edema, and optic nerve atrophy.
- Optic nerve demyelination has been reported to be due to formic acid destruction of myelin.

23. Ans. b. Green (Refer previous discussion)

Ref: The Essentials of Forensic Medicine and Toxicology by KS Narayan Reddy 29/e

24. Ans. a. Strychnine poisoning (Refer previous discussion)

Ref: The Essentials of Forensic Medicine and Toxicology by KS Narayan Reddy 29/e

25. Ans. c. Res ispa loquitor

Ref: The Essentials of Forensic Medicine and Toxicology by KS Narayan Reddy 29/e p33

Doctrine of Res ipsa loquitur: 'The thing speaks for itself'.
- Patient is not obliged to prove negligence.
- It implies that
  - The damage could not have happened without negligent act of the doctor
  - No contributory negligence
  - Doctor had exclusive control over the procedure.

Examples:
- Giving over dosage of medicine.
- Failure to remove swabs and instruments.
- Transfusion of mismatched blood.
- Amputation of wrong body part.

26. Ans. c. 2 years

Ref: The Essentials of Forensic Medicine and Toxicology by KS Narayan Reddy 29/e

Limitation period: A suit for damages for negligence against the doctor should be filed within two years from the date of alleged negligence.

Defences against negligence:
- No duty owed to the plaintiff
- Duty discharged according to prevailing standards
- Misadventure
- Error of judgement
- Contributory negligence
- Res judicata *(S.* 300, Cr.P.c.). If a question of negligence against a doctor has already been decided by a Court, the patient will not be allowed to contest the same question in another proceeding
- Limitation. A suit filed after two years' will be dismissed as being beyond the period of limitation

27. Ans. d. Forehead *Ref: The Essentials of Forensic Medicine and Toxicology by KS Narayan Reddy 29/e p171*

Incised like/incised looking wounds
- When skin is closely applied to a bone with scanty subcutaneous tissue, blunt force injury will cause linear splitting of tissues under the site of impact.
- This injury will **simulate closely an incised wound** and called as incised looking wound/incised looking laceration.
- These are **essentially lacerated wounds**, easily detectable on examination with a magnifying lens.

Common sites:
- Scalp, face, over the eyebrows, cheek, chin, lower jaw, iliac crest, shin.

28. Ans. a. Mercury *Ref: The Essentials of Forensic Medicine and Toxicology by KS Narayan Reddy 29/e*

29. Ans. b. Mercury poisoning

Ref: The Essentials of Forensic Medicine and Toxicology by KS Narayan Reddy 29/e

Acrodynia (Pink disease)
- Caused by chronic mercury exposure.

- Idiosyncratic hypersensitivity reaction, seen in children.
- Generalized erythematous, eczematous papular type of lesions mostly in hands and feet, accompanied by thickening and peeling of the skin.

30. Ans. a. Legal document (Refer discussion)

Ref: The Essentials of Forensic Medicine and Toxicology by KS Narayan Reddy 29/e p7

31. Ans. c. Pelvis *Ref: The Essentials of Forensic Medicine and Toxicology by KS Narayan Reddy. 29/e p57-61*

According to Krogman, the degree of accuracy in sexing * by the examination of bones is:

Entire skeleton	– 100%
Pelvis + skull	– 98%
Pelvis	– 95%
Skull	– 90%
Long bones alone	– 80%

32. Ans. a. Froth in the nostrils D. Mud in the respiratory passages

Ref: The Essentials of Forensic Medicine and Toxicology by KS Narayan Reddy 29/e p328

33. Ans. d. Desiccation of dead body

Ref: The Essentials of Forensic Medicine and Toxicology by KS Narayan Reddy 29/e

Mummification: Drying and dessication of tissues
Adipocere: Saponification of fats
Colliquative putrefaction: Liquefaction of tissues.

34. Ans. a. Heart *Ref: The Essentials of Forensic Medicine and Toxicology by KS Narayan Reddy. 29/e*

- Occurs in proximodistal spread
- Internally: Myocardium
- Externally: First in the eyelids, muscles of the face, jaw, neck, upper limbs, chest, abdomen and lastly the lower limbs.

35. Ans. b. 1971 (Refer discussion)

Ref: The Essentials of Forensic Medicine and Toxicology by KS Narayan Reddy 29/e

36. Ans. a. 1st molar (Refer discussion)

Ref: The Essentials of Forensic Medicine and Toxicology by KS Narayan Reddy 29/e

37. Ans. c. Muscarine (Refer previous discussion)

Ref: The Essentials of Forensic Medicine and Toxicology by KS Narayan Reddy 29/e

38. Ans. c. High Court (Refer previous discussion)

Ref: The Essentials of Forensic Medicine and Toxicology by KS Narayan Reddy 24/e

39. Ans. d. Cruciate shaped wound (Refer previous discussion)

Ref: The Essentials of Forensic Medicine and Toxicology by KS Narayan Reddy 29/e p195

40. Ans. a. Mongols *Ref: The Essentials of Forensic Medicine and Toxicology by KS Narayan Reddy 29/e 54*

Type of Skull	Cephalic index	Race
Dolicocephalic (long-headed)	70 to 75	Pure Aryans, Aborigines and Negroes
Mesaticephalic (medium-headed)	75 to 80	Europeans and Chinese.
Brachycephalic (short-headed)	80 to 85	Mongolian

41. Ans. a. 304 A *Ref: The Essentials of Forensic Medicine and Toxicology by KS Narayan Reddy 29/e 34*

Sec 300 IPC	Definition of culpable homicide amounting to murder.
Sec 304-A IPC	Death caused by rash and negligent act–2 years.
Sec 320 IPC	Grievous hurt–definition
Sec 375 IPC	Rape–definition

42. Ans. a. 15 years (Refer previous discussion)

Ref: The Essentials of Forensic Medicine and Toxicology by KS Narayan Reddy 29/e p359

43. Ans. a. Cross examination (Refer previous discussion)

Ref: The Essentials of Forensic Medicine and Toxicology by KS Narayan Reddy 29/e

44. Ans. b. Phenol (Refer previous discussion)

Ref: The Essentials of Forensic Medicine and Toxicology by KS Narayan Reddy 29/e p478

45. Ans. c. Fetal death (Refer previous discussion)

Ref: The Essentials of Forensic Medicine and Toxicology by KS Narayan Reddy 29/e

Ultrasound features of intauterine fetal death

- Absent fetal heart beat
- Occasional findings
  - Overlapping of skull bones (Spalding sign)
  - Soft tissue edema: skin > 5 mm
- Uncommon findings
  - Thrombus in fetal heart
  - Gas shadow in fetal heart (Robert's sign).

46. Ans. d. Tympanic membrane

Ref: The Essentials of Forensic Medicine and Toxicology by KS Narayan Reddy 29/e

Primary blast injury

- Damage to **internal organs without visible external signs** of injury that occurs as a direct result of the **pressure wave** contacting the body
  - Most commonly involve air-filled organs and air-fluid interfaces
  - **Middle ear-most sensitive** tympanic membrane rupture
  - **Lungs: Blast lung**
  - **Gastrointestinal tract:** Abdominal hemorrhage and perforation (lower small intestine or cecum).

Secondary blast injury

- Damage to the **body with visible external signs of injury** that occurs as a result of contact with **objects** that are propelled by the blast wave.

Tertiary blast injury

- Blast wave **displacing the body** and the body contacting some object in the environment.

47. Ans. a. No specific violation of law needs to be proved (Refer previous discussion)

Ref: The Essentials of Forensic Medicine and Toxicology by KS Narayan Reddy 29/e p34

48. Ans. a. Yellow oleander poisoning (Refer previous discussion)

Ref: The Essentials of Forensic Medicine and Toxicology by KS Narayan Reddy 29/e

49. Ans. d. Forced alkaline dieresis

Ref: The Essentials of Forensic Medicine and Toxicology by KS Narayan Reddy 29/e

Treatment of methanol poisoning:

- Gastric lavage: 5% Sodium bicarb
- Ethyl Alcohol 50% 1ml/kg IV every 2 hours for 5 days. (Maintain blood alcohol level of 100–150 mg%)
- Hemodialysis is the treatment of choice.
- Fomepizole
- Folic acid: 50–75 mg/ 4 hours increases elimination of formic acid.
- Dextrose, Vitamin B1
- Maintain serum electrolyte to optimum level.

QUESTIONS 2015

1. **Blue-green postmortem staining is due to:**
   a. Hydrogen sulfide poisoning
   b. Sodium nitrite poisoning
   c. Cyanide poisoning
   d. Carbon monoxide poisoning
2. **Palatoprint is obtained from which part of hard palate:**
   a. Anterior part
   b. Middle part
   c. Posterior part
   d. Any of the above
3. **A person fired a bullet but it did not go off and when the second time he fired, two bullets came out. This kind of bullet is known as:**
   a. Ricochet bullet
   b. Dum-dum bullet
   c. Tandem bullet
   d. Tracer bullet
4. **In fingerprint study, minimum number of similarities required is:**
   a. 12
   b. 8
   c. 28
   d. 24
5. **In Gustafson method of age estimation from dentition, the most reliable criteria is:**
   a. Root transparency
   b. Secondary dentin
   c. Attrition
   d. Cementum apposition
6. **Exhumation order is given by:**
   a. Chief judicial magistrate
   b. Executive magistrate
   c. Investigating officer
   d. Second-class magistrate
7. **Deadborn after birth, all are seen except:**
   a. Maceration
   b. Adipocere
   c. Rigormortis
   d. Mummification
8. **Which is a character of male skull compared to female skull:**
   a. Prominance of frontal part
   b. Square-shaped orbits
   c. Less prominent glabella
   d. Smoothly curved frontonasal angulation

ANSWERS AND EXPLANATIONS

1. **Ans. a. Hydrogen sulfide poisoning**

Ref: The Essentials of Forensic Medicine and Toxicology; KSN Reddy, 27/e p139

Color of postmortem lividity (hypostasis)

- Normal–Bluish pink which later turns into bluish purple
- Hydrogen sulfide–Bluish green
- Carbon monoxide–Bright cherry red
- Cyanide–Pink
- Phosphorus–Dark brown
- Nitrates–Reddish brown
- Chlorates–Chocolate brown
- Aniline–Deep blue
- Opiates–Black

2. **Ans. a. Anterior part**

Ref: Bansode Shriram C, Kulkarni Meena M; Importance of palatal rugae in individual identification; Journal of forensic and dental sciences; Year: 2009 | Volume: 1/Issue Number: 2/p77-81

- Rugae are anatomical folds or wrinkles, the irregular fibrous connective tissue located on the anterior third of the palate, behind the incisive papilla. They are also called 'plica palatine'.
- In the anterior part of the palate, these structural details like the rugae are individual-specific and permanent.
- The palatoprints can be used in the same way as fingerprints.

3. Ans. c. Tandem bullet

Ref: The Essentials of Forensic Medicine and Toxicology; KSN Reddy, 27/e p200

Peculiar effects of bullet

Yawning bullet	Bullet traveling in an irregular fashion instead of traveling nose-on
Tumbling bullet	Bullet that rotates end-on-end during the motion
Tandem bullet	Bullet remains in the barrel and during subsequent firing, two bullets one behind the other are projected out and they may hit the body from the same or different wounds
External Recocheting	The bullet before striking the target strikes some intervening object first and then after recocheting and rebounding from these hits the object.
Internal Recocheting	Bullet hitting the cranial cavity
Souvenir bullet	Bullet lying in the body part since long. Chronic lead poisoning is possible
Frangible bullet	Fragment upon impact often to the point of disintegration
Kennedy phenomenon	Surgical alteration of bullet injury
Bullet embolism	Bullet enters large vessel

4. Ans. a. *Ref: Review of Forensic medicine and Toxicology, Gautum Biswas; 2/e p73*

DACTYLOGRAPHY (fingerprint system; dermatoglyphics; Galton system):

- This system was first used in India in 1858, by Sir William Herschel.
- Sir Francis Galton systematized this method in 1892.
- Fingerprint Bureau was first established in Kolkata.
- Classification:
  - Loops (about 67 percent), (2) Whorls (about 25 percent), (3) Arches (about 6 to 7 percent) (4) Composite form (about 1 to 2 percent).
- The final identification of any fingerprint is made by comparison of many details of characteristics which occur throughout the ridge areas and by the sequence in which these characteristics occur, **but not by comparing the patterns.**
- **In practice, 10 to 12 points of fine comparison are accepted as proof of identity.**
- The patterns are not inherited and paternity cannot be proved through fingerprint patterns.
- The fingerprint patterns are distinctive and permanent in individuals.
- The pattern is different even in identical twins.

5. Ans. a. Root transparency

Ref: The Essentials of Forensic Medicine and Toxicology; KSN Reddy, 27/e p63

After 21 years, age can be determined by examining few characteristic features in the teeth. Gustafson's method uses the following:

1. Attrition
2. Periodontitis
3. Secondary Dentin
4. Root Resorption
5. Cementum Apposition
6. Transparency of Root (most reliable criteria): It is the method used for the deceased.

Anterior teeth are more reliable than posterior teeth.

- Mixed Dentition: (6–12 years)
- Mixed Dentition occurs from Eruption of First Permanent Teeth (First Molar) to the Last Canine.
- Remember that the total number of teeth increase only when the Permanent Molars erupt. It is because all other permanent teeth erupt by 'pushing' out a milk teeth.
- The number of teeth increases from 6 months to 2 years and at two years, it is 20 (5 × 4).
- At the sixth year, the number increases from 20 to 24, because the first molar erupts and no tooth falls (Remember that there are 4 first molars–Upper Right, Upper Left, Lower Right, Lower Left)
- From 7 to 12 years, the number remains 24 because as and when a tooth erupts, it displaces another and the number remains constant.

- There is an addition of more from the age of 12 to 14 when the second Molar erupts and the total number becomes 28.
- Then the number remains constant till 17 and again 4 more are added from 17 to 25 and the number is 32.

6. **Ans. b. Executive magistrate**

Ref: The Essentials of Forensic Medicine and Toxicology; KSN Reddy, 27/e p118

- Exhumation is the digging out of an already buried body from the grave.
- There is no time limit for exhumation in India.
- **Authorisation:** The body is exhumed only when there is a written order from the Executive Magistrate.

Magistrate inquest (S 176 Cr PC)
• Conducted by Collector, Tahsildar, Deputy Commissioner, Revenue divisional officer • Death in police custody and while under police interrogation • Death due to police firing • Death in prisons, reformatories, Borstal school • Death in psychiatric hospitals • Dowry deaths • Exhumation

7. **Ans. b. Adipocere**

Ref: The Essentials of Forensic Medicine and Toxicology; KSN Reddy, 27/e p282

Signs of dead born: (any of the following signs)

1. Rigor mortis at delivery.
2. Maceration:
   - Aseptic autolysis, and is the usual change.
   - This occurs when the dead child remains in the uterus for about three or four days surrounded with liquor amnii but the exclusion of air.
   - The earliest sign of maceration is skin slippage, which can be seen in 12 hours after the death of the child in utero.
   - Gas in great vessels (aorta in 12 hours) of fetus indicates fetal death.
   - Collapse of the vertebral column occurs.
   - It has a sweetish, disagreeable odor.

Spalding's Sign:

- Loss of alignment and overriding of the bones of the cranial vault occurs due to shrinkage of the cerebrum after death of the fetus.
- In the early stage, there is only loss of alignment without overriding.

3. **Mummification:** When the fetus dies from deficient supply of blood, when liquor amni is scanty, and when no air enters uterus.

8. **Ans. b. Square-shaped orbit**

Ref: The Essentials of Forensic Medicine and Toxicology; KSN Reddy, 27/e p56

Difference between male and female skull

Features	Male	Female
Frontal eminence	Sloping, less prominent	Vertical, less prominent
Parietal eminence	Less pronounced	More pronounced
Occipital protuberance	Prominent	Less prominent or absent
Glabella	More prominent	Less prominent and smooth
Supraorbital ridges	More prominent	Less prominent or absent
Frontonasal junction	Distinct angulation	Smooth curved
Orbits	Square-shaped, placed relatively low on face, margins are rounded	Rounded, higher on face, margins are sharp
Cheek bones	Heavy, broad and laterally arched	Light, small and compressed

Contd...

Contd...

Features	Male	Female
Zygomatic arch	More prominent	Less prominent
Mastoid process	Large and rounded	Small and pointed
Foramen magnum	Large	Small
Palate	Large, broad and 'U'-shaped	Small and parabola in shape

Differences of Pelvis

Features	Male	Female
General body	Heavy, rough and deep funnel-shaped	Light, smooth and flat bowl-shaped
Preauricular sulcus (Attachment of anterior sacroiliac ligament)	Not frequent, narrow and shallow	More frequent, broad and deep
Acetabulum	Large, 52 cm in diameter and directed laterally	Small, 46 cm in diameter and directed anterolaterally
Obturator foramen	Oval and large	Triangular and small
Greater sciatic notch (Diagnostic)	Narrow, deep and 'V'-shaped. The angle fits into index finger and middle finger	Wide, shallow and 'U' or 'L'-shaped. Fits into the thumb and index finger
Ischial tuberosity	Inverted	Everted and widely separated
Subpubic angle	'V'-shaped and angle is 70 to 75	'U'-shaped and angle is 90 to 100
Pelvic cavity	Heart-shaped and conical	Oval, spacious, broad and rounded
Sacroiliac articulation	Large and extends 2.5 to 3 segments	Small and extends 2 to 2.5 segments
Sacrum	Tall and narrow. Uniformly curved and body of 1st vertebra larger	Short and wide. Upper half almost straight and lower half curves forward. 1st V is small

Differences between male and female mandible

Features	Male	Female
General	Large and thick	Small and thin
Chin	Square-shaoped	Rounded
Height	Taller	Smaller
Condyles	Large	Small
Ramus	Broad	Small
Angle of body and ramus	Less obtuse and everted	More obtuse and inverted

Chapter

5 Microbiology

J Suria Kumar

HISTORY

Antony Van Leeuwen Hoeck

- Founder of Microscope
- Little animalcules

Louis Pasteur

- Father of Microbiology
- Proposed theory of fermentation
- Sterilization methods – Pasteurization, Autoclave, Steam sterilizer and Hot air oven (PASH)
- Preparation of vaccines for – Chicken Cholera, Anthrax, Rabies, (CAR)
- Disproved spontaneous generation theory (Abiogenesis theory)

Joseph Lister

- Father of Modern Antiseptic surgery
- Used Carbolic acid as an antiseptic agent.

Robert Koch

- Father of Medical Microbiology/Father of Bacteriology
- Koch Phenomenon – Demonstration of allergy in TB
- Discovery of Bacillus anthracis, Vibrio cholera, Mycobacterium tuberculosis (CAT – Cholera, Anthrax, Tuberculosis)
- Smears and staining by Aniline dye, Abbe condenser
- Solid culture media concept by using gelatin and then agar-agar
- **Proposed Koch's Postulates** (4+1)
  - The organism must be present in the lesions in every case of the infectious disease.
  - It should be possible to isolate the organism in pure culture from the lesions of the infectious disease
  - The same lesion must result when the isolated organism is inoculated into a suitable healthy host.
  - The same organism must be isolated again from the lesion of the host.
  - Specific antibody to the organism should be demonstrable in the serum of the host suffering from the lesion. (Fifth one added later).
- M. leprae, B. burgdorferi, T. pallidum, Ricketssiae, Chlamydia and Viruses – not obeying Koch postulates

Paul Ehrlich

- First person described Acid-Fast stain
- Ehrlich phenomenon and Genus Ehrlichia

- Proposed side chain theory for Ab production
- Toxin and antitoxin standardization

Other Important contributors

Name	Discovery
Ruska	Electron Microscope
Karry B Mullis	Polymerase Chain Reaction (PCR)
Hansen	Mycobacterium leprae
Alexander Ogston	Staphylococcus
Neisser	Neisseria gonorrhoeae
Kleb and Loeffler	Corynebacterium diphtheria
Nicolaier	Clostridium tetani
Frankel	Streptococcus pneumoniae
Schauddin and Hoffmann	Treponema pallidum
Roux and Yersin	Yersinia pestis
Bordet and Gengou	Bordetella pertussis
Priesz and Nocard	Corynebacterium pseudotuberculosis
Battey	Mycobacterium intracellulare
Hoffmann	Corynebacterium pseudodiphtheriticum
Whitmore	Burkholderia pseudomallei
Johne	Mycobacterium paratuberculosis
Frisch	Klebsiella rhinoscleromatis
Pfeiffer	Haemophilus infuenzae
Koch–Week	Haemophilus aegypticus
Friedlander	Klebsiella pneumoniae
Abel	Klebsiella Ozeana
Prowazekii	Rickettsia prowazekii
Goodpasture	Cultivation of Viruses in Egg
Edward Jenner	Method of vaccination – small pox
Metchnikoff	Phagocytosis
Wright	Opsonisation
Domagk	Scientific chemotherapy – prontosil
Alexander Flemming	Penicillin
Ferdinand Cohn	Bacterial Endospores

Characteristics	Eukaryote	Prokaryote
Nucleus, nucleolus, Nuclear membrane, Ribo Nucleo-protein	Present	Absent
Cell division	Mitosis, Meiosis	Binary fission
Chromosome	Many, liner, Diploid DNA	One, Circular, Diploid DNA
Cell wall	Sterols (also Mycoplasma)	NAM/NAG
Membrane bond Organelles-Mitochondria, ER, Golgi bodies	Present	Absent
Respiration	Via Mitochondria	Via Mesosome
Cytoskeleton	Present	Absent
Ribosome	80s (60S + 40S)	70s (50S + 30S)
Pinocytosis	Present	Absent

Morphology and Physiology of Bacteria

- Kingdom Protista
  - Prokaryotes: E.g Bacteria and blue green algae
  - Eukaryotes: Fungi, algae (other than blue green) and protozoa

Microscopy

Resolution power	
Human eye	0.2 mm (millimeter)
Light microscope	0.2 μm (micrometer)
EM	0.2 nm (nanometer)

Types of microscopy

	Phase Contrast Microscope	Fluorescence microscope	Dark Field Microscopy	Electron microscope
Principle	Converts slight differences in refractive index and cell density into easily detectable variations in light intensity	Fluorescent compounds, when excited by incident light of one wavelength, emit light of a longer wavelength and thus a different color when exposed to UV rays.	Light scatteres by the object enters the objective and reach the eye.	Electron beam is used instead of ligt and Electromagnets are used instead of lenses
Requirements	Devices transforming the subtle changes in light waves passing through the specimen into differences in light intensity.	Auramine O, Acridine orange, and Fluorescent Isothiocyanate.	High intensity light source Condenser with special Circular stopper	Vaccuam Negative stain-Heavy metal salt coating – lead citrate and uranium acetate, Phosphotungstic acid
Applications	Intracellular structures – bacterial spores, granules, and organelles,	Cyclospora (Auto fluorescence) Acridine orange dyes (QBC) – malarial parasites, Auramine phenol – M. tuberculosis	Live thin organisms – spirocheates and Flagella	Tiny organisms – Viruses TEM and SEM – Internal and External

Staining Methods

Demonstrates Size, Shape and arrangement with structural details of the bacteria by coloring the agent.

Gram's Stain

- Hans Christian Grams (1884)
- Grouping bacteria into two: Gram positive and Gram negative
- GPB–**violet**- they have a relatively thick amorphous cell wall.
- Gram–negative bacteria take counter stain, appearing **Pink**.
- Classification of bacteria based on Gram staining:

		Gram reaction	
		Positive	Negative
Morphology	Cocci	Staphylococcus, Streptococcus Pneumococcus	Meningococcus, Gonococci, Veillonella, Moraxella
	Bacilli	Corynebacterium Clostridium Bacillus Listeria Actinomycetes/Nocardia, Mycobacteria etc	Enterobacteriaceae, Vibrio, Pseudomonas Hemophilus Bordetella Brucella etc

Differences between Gram positive and Gram negative bacterial cell wall

Characters	Gram positive cell wall	Gram negative cell wall
Cell wall	Thick 15–25 nm	Thin 10–15 nm
Lipid content	2–5%	15–20%
Teichoic acid	Present	Absent
Sporulation	Some species	Absent
Lipopolysaccharide in outer membrane (endotoxin)	Absent	Present
Aromatic amino acid	Absent	Present
Variety of amino acid	Few	Several
Lysozyme	Sensitive	Resistant

- Neisseria contains a shorter version of LPS called lipo-oligosaccharide (LOS).
- **Acid-fast stain**
  - First discoverd by Paul Ehrlich
  - Ziehl-Neelsen (ZN) staining method.
  - Acid-fast bacilli (AFB) – bright red in stained smears
  - Modifications of Ziehl-Neelsen staining and applications

Conc. H_2SO_4	Organism/Structure
25%	M. tuberculosis
5%	M. leprae
1%	Nocardia, Coccdian parasites, Eggs of T. saginata, Sperm head
0.5%	Spores and Rhodococcus

  - Kinyoun's Method – Cold AFB Staining
- **Negative staining**
  - India ink/Nigrosin,
  - In negative staining, the background is stained, while the structures to be demonstrated is not stained
  - Demonstration of Capsule and Spirocheates
- **Impregnation methods**
  - To visualize too thin bacteria by impregnating Siver on the bacteria,
  - Treponema pallidum, Leptospira, Borellia
  - Demonstration of flagella.
  - Eg: Fontana staining, Levediti staining
- **Albert's stain/Neisser's stain/Ponder's stain**
  - Staining the volutin granules (metachromatic granules) of Corynebacterium diphtheriae.

Bacterial Cell Structures and Functions

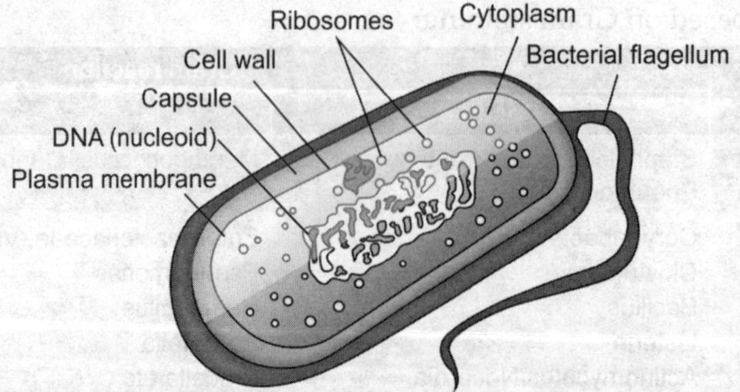

Fig. 5.1: Structure of a bacterial cell

Cell wall

- Rigidity and Shape
- Prevents from osmotic lysis
- Shape, Structure and act as barrier

Cell membrane – lacking sterols like cholesterol (except in mycoplasma)

Cytoplasm – Ribosomes- site of protein synthesis

- Mesosomes- principal sites of respiratory enzymes in the bacteria
- Intracytoplasmic inclusions – Storage of nutrients/energy

Nucleus

- Single super coiled circular DNA
- Feulgen stain
- Plasmids – Extra-chromosomal DNA – carry antibiotic resistance genes and production of toxins or enzymes.

Glycocalyx (Slime layer)

- A loose network of polysaccharide fibrils that surrounds cell walls.
- Biofilm formation and adherence of bacteria to surfaces Synthesized by surface enzymes.
- Contains prominent antigenic sites.

Capsule

- Invasiveness of bacteria by escaping from phagocytosis.
  Demonstration of capsule by Negative staining, Quellung reaction and M'Faydean capsule stain

Composition of capsules of various bacteria

Organism	Capsular component
Pneumococcus	Polysaccharide
Meningococcus	Polysaccharide
H. influenza	Polysaccharide
Bacillus anthracis	Polypeptide (d–glutamate)
Streptococcus pyogenes	Hyaluronic acid

Capsule and Slime layer – both are present in Streptococcus salivarius

Atypical forms of bacteria

- Cell wall deficient forms (L Forms) – Mycoplasma (Stable L forms), Spheroplast (G –ve), protoplast (G +ve).
- L – Lister Institute.
- Pleomorphic bacteria – Proteus, Yersinia pestis, Bacteroides and Hemophilus
- Involution forms

Surface appendages

Flagella

- Thread-like appendages made up of flagellin embedded in the cell envelope.
- Organ of locomotion

Flagellar arrangement	Example
Monotrichous (single polar flagellum)	Vibrio cholerae
Lophotrichous (multiple polar flagella)	Campylobacter jejuni
Peritrichous (distributed all over the surface)	Salmonella, Escherichia
Amphitrichous (single flagellum at both the ends)	Alcaligenes faecalis
Atrichous (No flagella)	Klebsiella pneumoniae
Endoflagella/Axial Filaments	Spirocheates

Demonstration of flagella by

- Flagellar stain – Tannic acid staining (Leifson method)
- Silver impregnation technique
- Dark ground, Phase contrast and Electron microscope
- By demonstration of motility – Craige tube, hanging drop, semisolid Motility Medium,
- Antiflagellar serum – Motility inhibition

Various types of motility in bacteria

Type of Motility	Organism
Cork screw, Rotatory and Flexion Extension	Spirocheates
Darting	Vibrio, Aeromonas and Plesiomonas, Campylobacter, Spirillum
Gliding	Mycoplasma
Tumbling	Listeria
Stately	Clostridium
Swarming	Proteus
Spinning	Fusarium gyrans
Twitching	Bartonella quintana
Gliding	Mycoplasma

Fimbriae or pilli

- Organ of adhesion and Antigenic
- Pillins – structural proteins
- Agglutination of sheep RBC
- Inhibited by mannose-four types (Type I – Mannose Sensitive)
- Sex pilli helps in conjugation
- Form surface pellicle in liquid culture

Bacterial Spores

- Endospores
- Not reproductive structures
- Withstand boiling and many disinfectants
- High dipicolic acid content/calcium dipicolinate
- Present in Aerobic Bacillus spp and anaerobic Clostridium.

Bayer's junction – found in Gram-negative bacteria.

- Region of the wall where the inner leaflet of the outer membrane is contiguous with the outer leaflet of the cell membrane.

Characteristic	Viruses	Bacteria	Fungi	Protozoa and Helminths
Cells	No	Yes	Yes	Yes
Approximate diameter (microns)	0.02–0.2	1–5	3–10 (yeasts)	15–25 (trophozoites)
Nucleic acid	Either DNA or RNA	Both DNA and RNA	Both DNA and RNA	Both DNA and RNA
Type of nucleus	None	Prokaryotic	Eukaryotic	Eukaryotic
Ribosomes	Absent	70S	80S	80S
Mitochondria	Absent	Absent	Present	Present
Nature of outer surface	Protein capsid and lipoprotein envelope	Rigid wall containing peptidoglycan	Rigid wall containing chitin	Flexible membrane
Motility	None	Some	None	Most
Method of replication	Not binary fission	Binary fission	Budding or mitosis	Mitosis

Growth and Nutrition of bacteria

- Generation time – The average time required for cell numbers to double under optimum condition.

Generation time	Example
20 minutes	Escherichia coli
20 hours	Mycobacterium tuberculosis
14 days	Mycobacterium leprae

Classification based on Temperature requirement

Psychrophiles	Grow within a temperature range of 0–20°C.
Mesophiles	Grow within a temperature range 25°C and 40°C, Most pathogenic bacteria are Mesophiles.
Thermophiles	Grow at a high temperature range of 55°C – 80°C Eg. Thermus aquaticus, Bacillus stereothermophilus

Bacterial Growth Curve

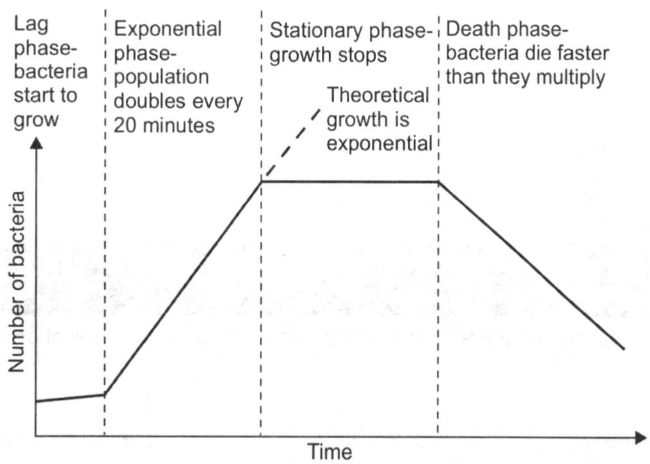

Fig. 5.2: Bacterial growth curve

Lag phase	Increase in size, No change in number, metabolite-depleted cells adapt to new environment
Log phase	Increase in numbers, Uniform staining, Biochemically active, more susceptible to antibiotics
Stationary phase	Exhausting essential nutrients, Accumulation of toxic products, Sporulation, Gram variability, Production of Exotoxins, antibiotics and Storage granules, No change in numbers
Decline phase	Cells may die due to toxic products, Involution form, Decrease in cell numbers

Bacterial growth is assessed in three ways:

- Viable cell counts, optical density and Metabolic products

Growth requirements pH Requirements

- Ideal pH for pathogenic bacteria lies between pH 7.2 – pH 7.6
- Bacteria grow in acidic pH – Lactobacilli – below pH 4
- Bacteria grow in alkaline pH – Vibrio cholerae – 8.2–8.8

Classification based on Oxygen Requirement

Obligate aerobes	Grow only in the presence of oxygen, contain enzymes catalase, Peroxidase and superoxide dismutase which protects them from the toxic effects of Nascent Oxygen E.g Vibrio, Pseudomonas
Facultative anaerobes	Aerobes, but can also grow in the absence of oxygen, E.g. Escherichia coli.
Micro aerophilic	Grow in the presence of low oxygen tension (5% -10%) e.g. Leptospira, Campylobacter
Aerotolerent	Anaerobes, but withstand exposure to oxygen E.g, Cl.perfringens
Obligate anaerobes	Grow only in the absence of oxygen. e.g. Clostridia
Capnophilic	Require higher amounts of carbon dioxide growth E.g Neisseria, H. influenzae, B. abortus

Light

- Phototrophs – Deriving energy from sunlight
- Chemotrophs – Deriving energy from chemical sources
- Organotrophs – Requires organic sources of hydrogen donor
- Most pathogens belongs to Chemo – Organotrophs

Toxins

Toxins may aid in invasiveness, damage cells, inhibit cellular processes, or trigger immune response and damage.

Structural Toxins

Endotoxins (Lipopolysaccharide)

- LPS is part of the Gram-negative outer membrane.
- Toxic portion is lipid A: generally released by death of cell.
- Exception: N. meningitides, which over-produces outer membrane fragments.

Exotoxins

- Protein toxins, secreted by bacterial cells
- A-B component protein toxins
- **B** component **B**inds to specific cell receptors to facilitate the internalization of A.
- **A** component is the **A**ctive (toxic) component

Cytolysins: lyse cells by damaging membrane.

Comparison of properties of exotoxins and endotoxins

Property	Exotoxin	Endotoxin
Source	Certain species of gram-positive and gram-negative bacteria	Cell wall of gram-negative bacteria and Listeria
Secreted from cell	Yes	No
Chemistry	Polypeptide	Lipopolysaccharide
Location of genes	Plasmid or bacteriophage	Bacterial chromosome
Toxicity	High (fatal dose on the order of 1 g)	Low (fatal dose on the order of hundreds of micrograms)
Clinical effects	Various effects	Fever, shock
Mode of action	Various modes	Includes TNF and interleukin-1
Antigenicity	Induces high-titer antibodies called antitoxins	Poorly antigenic
Vaccines	Toxoids used as vaccines	No toxoids formed and no vaccine available
Heat stability	Destroyed rapidly at 60°C (except staphylococcal enterotoxin)	Stable at 100°C for 1 hour
Typical diseases	Tetanus, botulism, diphtheria	Meningococcemia, sepsis by GNB

Sterilization and Disinfection

Sterilization

- Killing or removal of all microorganisms, including bacterial spores.

Disinfection

- Process that destroys or removes all pathogenic organisms or organisms capable of giving rise to infection.
- No destruction of bacterial endospores.
- Used only on inanimate objects because, in the concentrations required to be effective, they can be toxic to human and other animal tissue.

Germicide/microbicide

- Agent that kills pathogenic microorganisms, used on inanimate materials or on living tissue, but it cannot kill spores.

Antisepsis

- Practice that prevents the entry and multiplication of pathogenic agents into living tissues

Classification of sterilization

- Physical methods
- Chemical methods

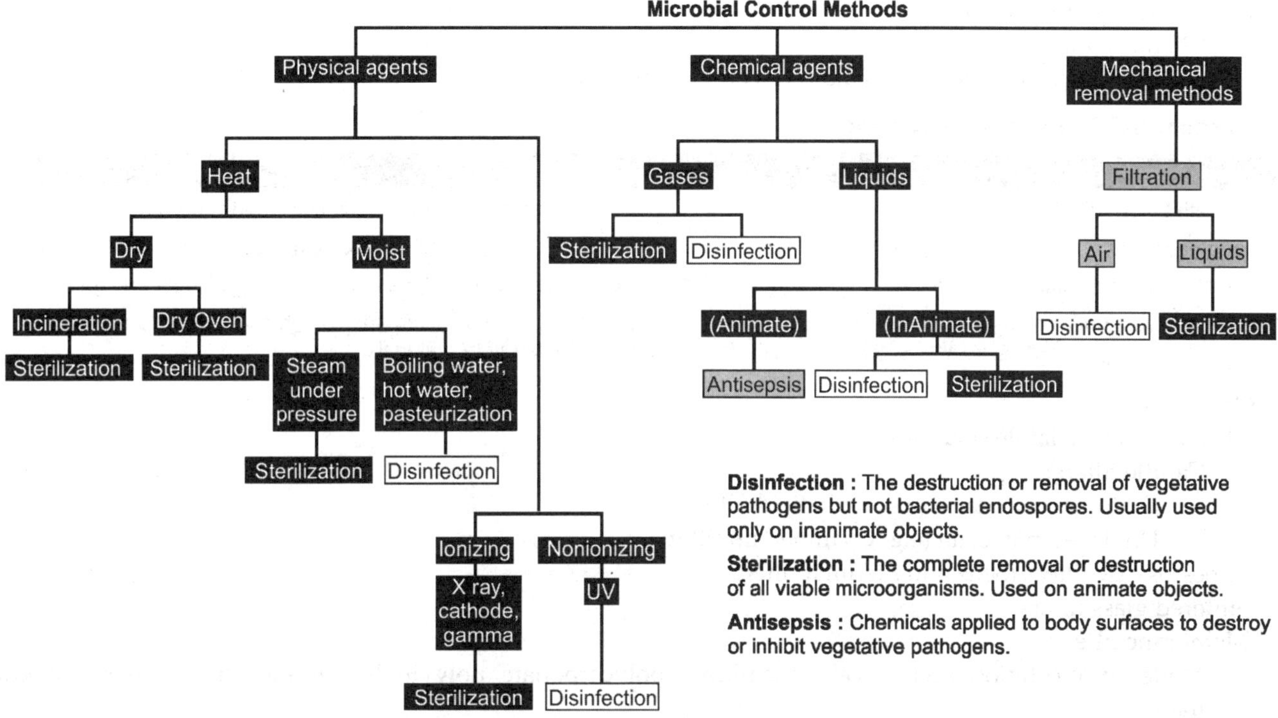

Fig. 5.3: Sterilization and disinfection-physical methods

Physical methods of sterilization

- Sunlight.
- Heat – Flaming, Red Heat, Dry heat, Moist heat, Incineration
- Filtration.
- Radiation.
- Sound (sonic) waves.

Sunlight – Sterilization of water in tanks, rivers and lakes.

Dry Heat – Protein denaturation, Oxidative damage and the toxic effect of increased level of electrolytes.

- Flaming, Incineration and Hot air oven
- Hot air oven – 160°C for 1 hour
- Materials sterilized: Glass ware, forceps, liquid paraffin, grease, fat, glycerol, dust powder
- Quality Control: Non toxigenic strain of Clostridium tetani, Browne tube

Moist heat – Coagulation and denaturation of protein

- Sterilization at a temperature below 100°C
  - Pasteurization: Milk
    - Holder method: 63°C – 30 minutes and cooling to 13°C
    - Flash method: 72°C – 15–20 minutes

- Vaccine bath: 60°C for 1 hour
- Inspissation: 80°C – 85°C, 30 minutes for 3 consecutive days
- Sterilization at a temperature of 100 °C
  - Boiling: 10–30 minutes
  - Koch's or Arnold's steam sterilizer: 90 miutes
  - Tyndallization: 20 minutes for 3 consecutive days, intermittent sterilization
- Sterilization at a temperature above 100°C
  - Autoclaves – 121°C for 15 min (15 lb/inch^2)
  - Control – B. stearothermophillus and Browns tube

Sterilization controls: Determine the efficacy of sterilization Thermocouples,

- Chemical indicators
- Bacteriological spores (e.g. Bacillus stereothermophilus).

Types and uses of moist heat sterilization

Method	Uses
Water bath below 100°C	For sterilization of serum, body fluids and vaccines
Water bath at 100°C	For sterilization of glass, metal and rubber items
Arnold steamer: steaming at 100°C	For sterilization of culture media containing sugar and gelatin
Autoclave: steam under pressure	For sterilization of culture media and other operation theatre as well as laboratory materials

Filtration

- Ideal for thermo labile solutions
  - Candle filters:
    - Diatomaceous earth (e.g. Berkefield filters)
    - Unglazed porcelain (e.g. Chamberlain filters)
- Asbestos disc filters (Seitz and Sterimat filters)
- Sintered glass filters
- Membrane filters:
  - Made up of cellulose acetate, cellulose nitrate, polycarbonate, polyvinylidene fluoride, or other synthetic materials.
  - Average pore diameter – 0.22µ
- Air filters – HEPA
- Syringe filters

Radiation

Types	Uses
Ionizing radiation: Cobalt 60, X-rays, gamma rays, Cosmic rays **(Cold Sterilization)**	Antibiotics, hormones, sutures, disposable items such as syringes, infusion sets and catheters etc.
Non-ionizing radiation: Infrared and Ultraviolet	Disinfection of clear surfaces in OTs, laminar flow hoods

Sound (sonic) waves

- High-frequency soundwaves disrupt cells.

Disinfection

Types of disinfectants

Group	Example
Phenolic compounds	Phenol
Diphenyl compounds	Hexachlorophene and Chlorheximide
Halogens	Fluorine, Bromine, Chlorine, and Iodine

Contd...

Contd...

Group	Example
Alcohols	Ethyl alcohol and Isopropyl alcohol
Aldehydes	Formaldehyde and Glutaraldehyde
Gaseous agents	Ethylene oxide, formaldehyde gas and BPL
Surface active agents	Detergents, wetting agents and emulsifiers.
Oxidizing agents	Halogens, hydrogen peroxide, $KMnO_4$
Acridine dyes	Acriflavine, euflavine, proflavine and aminacrine
Aniline dyes	Gentian violent, crystal violet and malachite green

Spaulding's Classification of disinfectant based on efficacy

Equipment	Example	Level of sterilization/disinfection
Critical	Contact with Sterile Body tissues. Cardiac catheters, Endoscopes enter into sterile body cavities	Sterilization
Semi Critical	Contact with Nonintact skin and Mucous membranes. USG Probe, Colonoscope, Laryngoscope	High level Disinfection (HLD) 2% Cidex, 35% H2O2
Non Critical	Contact with intact skin. Stethoscope, BP cuff	Intermediate level 70% alcohols, hypochlorites

- Prions: Hypochlorite for 1 hour or NaOH for 1 hour.

Testing of disinfectants

- Phenol coefficient test – Rideal walker and Chick Martin test (Best),
- Capacity (Kelsey-Sykes) test,
- In-use (Kelsey and Maurer) test.

Sporicidal agents (EFGH)

- Ethylene oxide, Formaldehyde, Glutaraldehyde, Hypochlorite, H_2O_2
- O-Phthalic acid, Peracetic acid
- Autoclave, Hot air oven, Plasma sterilization

Biological Sterilization Indicator

Hot air oven	Cl. tetani non toxigenic strain, B.subtilis, B.atrophaeus
Autoclave	B.stearothermophillus (Geobacillus stearothermophilus)
Filtration	Pseudomonas diminuta, Serratia
Ionizing radiation	Bacillus pumilus
Ethylne oxide	B.globigi
LTSF	B.stearothermophillus (Geobacillus stearothermophilus)

Various methods of sterilization for various materials

Material	Method of sterilization
Milk	Pasteurization
Inoculating loop	Red Heat
Glasswares – Paraffin, glass syringe, flask, slide, oil, grease, fat, glycerol	Hot air oven
Clinical thermometer	Isopropyl alcohol
Culture Media	Autoclave
OT, entryway, ward, lab fumigation	Formaldehyde, UV
Cystoscope, bronchoscope, endoscope	Glutaraldehyde (cidex)

Contd...

Contd...

Material	Method of sterilization
Heart lung machine, respirators and dental equipment.	Ethylene oxide
Toxins, Vaccine, sera, antibiotic, sugar	Filtration
Sharp instrument	5% Cresol, Hot Air Oven
Disposable syringes	Gamma radiation
Plastic syringe, cadgut, swab, catheter	Ionizing radiation
Culture media, all instrument except sharp and glass, all suture except catgut	Autoclave
Culture media containing egg or serum	Inspissation
Skin	Tincture iodine, 70% ethanol
Aprons	Autoclave
Animal carcases, soiled dressings	Incineration

Various concentrations of Commonly used disinfectants

Disinfectant	Concentration
Ethyl alcohol	70%
Isoprophyl alcohol	70%
Glutaraldehyde	2%
Lysol	2.5%
Savlon (Chlorhexidine and cetrimide)	2%, 5%
Dettol (Chloroxylenol)	4%
Bleaching powder (Calcium hypochlorite)	14 gm in 1 litre of water
Sodium hypochlorite	1%, 0.1% & 5%
Betadine (Iodophore)	2%
Hydrogen Peroxide	3 % (Wound debridement) 35% (Sterilizing H_2O_2)

CULTURE METHODS AND MEDIA

Culture Methods

- **Streak culture**
  - Useful method for obtaining discrete colonies and pure cultures.
- **Lawn culture**
  - Useful for carrying out antibiotic sensitivity testing by disc diffusion method (Kirby-Bauer Method)
  - For bacteriophage typing
  - Producing large amount of bacterial growth required for preparation of bacterial antigens and vaccines
- **Pour-plate culture**
  - Used to quantitate bacteria in urine cultures
  - To estimate viable bacterial count in a suspension.
  - Miles – Misra method
- **Stroke culture**
  - Provides pure growth of bacteria for carrying out diagnostic tests.
- **Stab culture**
  - Used for maintaining stock cultures.
  - For demonstration of oxygen requirement of the bacteria

- **Liquid culture**
  - Used for blood culture and for sterility tests, where, the concentration of bacteria is small.
  - It does not provide a pure culture of the bacteria
- **Aerobic culture**
  - Aerobic bacteria
  - Inoculated culture plates are incubated in at 37°C for overnight
- **Anaerobic culture methods**
  - Obligate anaerobes
  - Robertson cooked meat broth (RCM), Thioglycolate broth and neomycin blood agar.
  - Environment is free of oxygen, followed by incubation at 35°C for at least 48 hours.
  - McIntosh-Fildes anaerobic jar, Gas pack system and Anaerobic glove box

Culture Media

- **Basic Ingredients**
  - Agar or Agar-agar-long chain polysaccharide, it has no nutritive value and biochemically inert.
  - Peptone
  - Meat extract
- **Simple/basal media**
  - Peptone water – Peptone + NaCl
  - Nutrient broth – Peptone + meat extract + NaCl
  - Nutrient agar – Nutrient broth + 2% agar
- **Complex media** – Added ingredients for growth or bringing out certain property
- **Defined media** – Exact quantity of each chemical is known
- **Enriched media** contains – blood, serum, egg
  - E.g. Blood agar, Chocolate agar, Loeffler's serum slope, LJ medium
- **Enrichment broth (liquid media)** – Selectively allows certain organism to grow and inhibit others
  - E.g. Tetrathionate (S.typhi), APW – Vibrio, Selenite F-Shigella
- **Selective media (solid media)** – Selectively allows certain organism to grow and inhibit others
  - Crystal violet blood agar – Streptococcus
  - Wilson blair bismuth sulfite medium – Salmonella typhi
  - Thiosulphate Citrate Bilesalt Sucrose agar (TCBS) – Vibrio
- **Transport media** – **Maintains** viability of desired pathogenic bacteria without multiplication.

Streptococcus pyogenes	Pike's media
Neisseria gonorrheal	Stuart (charcoal swab), Amies medium
Vibrio cholerae	VR, Autoclaved sea water, Carry Blair
Shigella	Sach's Buffered glycerol saline
Bordetella	Modified Stuart's (with casmino acid), Mischulow's charcoal agar and Dacron or calcium alginate swab used

- **Differential media**
  - Mac Conkey agar
  - Cystein Lysine Electrolyte Deficient agar (CLED)

Growth Requirements	
Arginine	E.coli
Glutathione	Gonococci
Cholesterol	Mycoplasma
Aryl sulphate, amide	Atypical mycobacteria
Glycerol	Mycobacterium tuberculosis

Contd...

Contd...

Growth Requirements	
Sulfonamides	Rikettsia
Tryptophan	Salmonella typhi
L-cysteine	Listeria monocytogens
Sodium chloride	Vibrio parahaemolyticus
Factor x and v	H. influenzae

Bacterial Genetics

Bacteria have one copy of their DNA – haploid genome

Structure of DNA

- Proposed by Waston and Crick
- Key basic component of gene
- Consists of large number of genes
- DNA – sugar is D-2-deoxyribose.
- Gene is a segment of DNA that carries codons specifying for a particular polypeptide.
- Double helix structure, with a sugar-phosphate backbone containing purines (adenine and guanine) and pyrimidine pyrimidines (thymine and cytosine) bases.
- The two complementary strands are held together by hydrogen bonds.

Structure of RNA

- RNA – the sugar is D-ribose
- Single stranded
- The RNA contains the nitrogenous base uracil instead of thymine that is present in DNA.
- On the basis of structure and function, the RNA can be differentiated into three types:
  - Messenger RNA (mRNA), ribosomal RNA (rRNA) and transfer RNA (tRNA).

Mutations

- A mutation is a change in the base sequence of DNA that usually results in insertion of a different amino acid into a protein and the appearance of an altered phenotype.
- Silent mutation: without phenotypic expression
- Caused by a change in base sequence of DNA due to:
  - Addition
  - Deletion
  - Replacement/Substitution of one or more base in the nucleotide sequence of DNA.
  - Duplication
  - Inversion
- Point Mutation: Change in single nucleotide
- Multisite Mutation: Change in large number of basepairs
- Mutation types:
  - Base substitution (missense mutation and nonsense mutation),
  - Frame shift mutation and
  - Mutations due to transposons or insertion sequences.
- Mutation causing agents (Mutagens)
  - Viruses (mutator bacteriophage),
  - Chemicals- nitrous acid, alkylating agents, benzpyrine and base analogues
  - Radiation (X-ray and ultraviolet light).

- Mutations in the bacteria causes a lot of change in various properties of mutant bacteria
  - Drug susceptibility
  - Antigenic structure
  - Virulence

Plasmids

- Extra chromosomal DNA substances.
- Circular and double stranded DNA molecules that encode traits that are not essential for bacterial viability.
- Plasmids are of different types:
  - F factor (Fertility),
  - R factors (Resistance)
  - Col factor (Colicin)
- Plasmids confer new properties to recipient bacteria
  - Resistance to one or several antibiotics,
  - Production of toxins,
  - Synthesis of cell surface structures required for adherence or colonization
- Plasmids integrated with host chromosome is known as episomes.

Methods of Transfer of DNA between bacterial cells

- Transformation
- Transduction
- Conjugation

Transformation – process of the transfer of DNA itself from bacterium to another.

- When purified DNA is injected into the nucleus of a bacterial cell the process is called as transfection.
- Griffith's Test

Transduction – transfer of a portion of the DNA from one bacterium to another mediated by a bacteriophage.

- Bacteriophages encode diphtheria toxin, botulin toxin, cholera toxin and erythrogenic toxin.
- Transduction is of two types: generalized and specialized.
- Lysogenic Conversion

Conjugation – Discovered by Lederberg and Tatum

- Process of transfer of DNA from the donor bacterium to the recipient bacterium.
  - Occurs between two closely related species
  - It occurs mostly in Gram negative bacteria
  - Donor ability of the bacteria is determined by specific conjugative plasmids called fertility (F+) plasmids or sex plasmids.
  - Pilus is one of the most important proteins that form the sex pilus or conjugation tube.
    - The sex pilus produces a bridge between conjugating cells in Gram negative bacteria.
    - The transfer of plasmids during conjugation is responsible for the spread of multiple drug resistance among bacteria.

Transfer of DNA within bacterial cells

- Occurs by transposons, which are mobile DNA of 2000–20000bp.
- They can transfer DNA from one site of the bacterial chromosome to another site or to a plasmid – transposition.
- They are also called as jumping genes.
- The transposons codes for drug resistance enzymes, toxins or a variety of metabolic enzymes.
- This is responsible for antigenic changes seen in Neisseria gonorrhoae, Borrelia reccurentis and Trypanosoma.

Recombination

- After the DNA is transferred from one donor bacterium to the recipient, it combines with the chromosome of the bacterium by a process called recombination.
- Recombination is of two types: homologous and non-homologous.

Genetic engineering and molecular methods

Genetic engineering techniques – isolate virtually any gene with a biochemically recognizable property.

Steps

- Preparation of DNA fragments with restriction enzymes
- Physical separation of differently sized DNA fragments
- Enzymes for dicing, splicing, and reversing nucleic acids
  - Restriction endonucleases used for clipping the polynucleotide strands of DNA – restriction fragments.
  - Restriction endonucleases – EcoRI and HindIII
  - Ligase is an enzyme necessary to seal the sticky ends together by rejoining the phosphate-sugar bonds of DNA
- Methods used to size, synthesize, and sequence DNA
  - Hybridization of DNA to RNA – Northern blots.
  - Hybridization of DNA to DNA – Southern blots.
  - Antibodies are used to detect cloned genes by binding to their protein products by the Western blot.

Molecular diagnosis

- **DNA Sequencing**
  - Reveals gene structure.
  - Methods used- Maxam-Gilbert technique and Sanger technique
- **Nucleic acid probes**
  - These are DNA and RNA segments labeled with radioisotopes or enzymes which hybridize to complementary nucleic acids with high degree of specificity.
  - DNA probes – only detect DNA in specimens but without any amplification
  - DNA probes are available for identification of culture isolates and for direct detection of microbes in clinical specimens.

Application of DNA Probes

- Direct detection of microbes (e.g. M. tuberculosis, S. pyogenes, C. albicans) in clinical specimens.
- Diagnosis of uncultivable bacteria (e.g. Chlamydia, rickettsia, etc.) .
- Strain identification for epidemiological typing.
- Identification of virulence factors of microbial agents.
- Identification of toxins (e.g. diphtheria toxin)
- **Polymerase chain reaction – PCR**
  - Requires:
    - Taq Polymerase-withstand the high temperature
    - Primers
    - Nucleotides, Mg
  - Steps:
    - DNA extraction from micro-organism
    - Amplification of extracted DNA – 3 steps
      - Denaturation (95°C),
      - Primer annealing (55°C),
      - Extension (72°C)
  - Gel electrophoresis of amplified product
- PCR – amplified methods
- Real-time PCR – Recent development.

Gene therapy

- Technique for replacing a faulty gene with a normal one in individuals with fatal or extremely debilitating genetic diseases.

- There are two strategies:
  - Ex vivo therapy
  - In vivo therapy.

IMMUNOLOGY

Infection and Immunity

Infection

Based on relationship to host organisms may be classified as

- Saprophytes
  - Parasites – Commensals and Pathogens
- Types of Infection
  - Primary
  - Re-infection
  - Secondary infection
  - Focal infection
  - Nosocomial infection
  - Iatrogenic infection
  - Latent infection
- Sources of Infection
- Humans
  - Case
  - Carrier
    - Healthy carrier
    - Convalescent carrier
    - Contact carrier
    - Paradoxical carrier
- Animals
  - Reservoir host
  - Amplifier host
  - Insects – Mechanical vectors and Biological vectors
- Soil and Water
- Food
- Methods of transmission
  - Direct contact
  - Inhalation
  - Ingestion
  - Inoculation
  - Insects
  - Congenital
  - Iatrogenic and laboratory associated infection
- Factors Predisposing to Microbial Pathogenicity
- Pathogenicity
- Virulence
  - Attenuation – reduction in virulence
  - Exaltation – enhancement of Virulence
- Adhesion
  - Glycocalyx
  - Adherence proteins

- Lipoteichoic acids
- Fimbriae

- Invasiveness – ability to spread to host tissue after establishing infection
  - Hyaluronidase
  - Collagenase
  - Streptokinase
  - Hemolysins
  - Leukocidins
- Toxigenicity – Endo and Exo toxins

Immunity

- Refers to resistance exhibited by host towards to injury caused by microorganism or its products

Innate immunity	Acquired immunity
Resistance to infection that an individual possess from birth by its genetic or constitutional makeup.	Resistance to infection that an individual acquires during his life
Species or Racial or Individual specific	Active or passive and artificial or natural
Occurs in Minutes	Occurs in days
Diversity limited	Against wide range of infection
Non specific	Specific
No memory	Memory Present
Phagocyte (monocyte, macrophage, neutrophils, dendritic cell), NK cells Alternate complement pathway, Acute phase protein (CRP, MBP, serum amyloid protein), Inflammation, fever, Skin and mucosal barrier	T cell, B cell, Classical complement

Active immunity	Passive immunity
Produced actively by host immune system	Received passively
Induced by infection or immunogen	Induced by transferred antibody
Long lasting	Short
Lag period present	No Lag period
Memory present	No Memory
Booster doses-useful	Subsequent doses-Less affective
Negative phase may occur	No Negative phase
In Immunodeficiency- not useful	useful

Local Immunity

- Produced at mucosal surfaces – GIT or respiratory mucosa
- Provided by IgA antibody
- Induced by infection or by live vaccination

Adaptive Immunity

- Passive transfer of Immunologically Competent T cells
- Tried in Treatment for Lepromatous leprosy
- Transfer factor

Herd immunity

- Overall immunity of a community to a pathogen
- If herd immunity is good – chance of epidemic is less

- Eradication of a communicable disease – depends on good Herd immunity
- Provided by mass vaccination by live vaccination to all individual at same time.

Concomitant Immunity (Infection Immunity)

Immunity persists till the infection persists. E.g Malaria, Syphilis

Antigen, Antibody and Antigen antibody reaction, Complement

Antigen

- Antigen – has to component
  - Immunogenicity
  - Immunological reactivity (antigenicity) with antibody
- Hapten – No Immunogenicity but retain antigenicity
  - Simple hapten – Univalent, non precipitating with its antibody, only blocks the site on antibody
  - Complex hapten – Polyvalent, precipitating with its antibody.
  - Hapten becomes immunogenic by combing with carrier molecule.
- Epitope: Antigenic determinant
- Paratope: Antigen binding site of an antibody
  - T cell recognize linear/sequential epitope
  - B cell recognize conformational epitope

Antigenicity depends on:

- Size – Larger size, more antigenic
- Chemical – Protein > carbohydrate > lipid > Nucleic acids
- Susceptibility to Tissue enzyme – (latex and amino acid are non-antigenic)
- Foreignness (More foreignness – More antigenic)
- Route of entry
- Genetic constituent
- Specificity
  - Tissue specific
  - Iso specific – Human RBC
  - Auto specific – HLA, self antigens
  - Organ specific

Heterophile specificity

Paul Bunnel	EBV with sheep RBC
Weil felix	Proteus OX2,OX19,OX K with Ricketssia alkali stable polysaccharide
Cold Agglutination test	Mycoplasma with human O+ve RBC at 4°C
Streptococcus MG	Mycoplasma
Forssman antigen	Lipid-CHO complex, present all except rabbit. So anti-Forssman anibody can be prepared in rabit
Non treponemal test for syphilis	VDRL and RPR (Flocculation test) – Treponemal antibody detected by using Cardiolipin antigen prepared from beef heart
Autoimmunoconsequences	Acute rheumatic fever and glomerulonephritis (Streptococcal antigens and human tissue)

T Independent Ag	T dependent Ag
Simple – LPS, capsule, flagella	Chemically Complex
Dose dependent Immunogenicity	Immunogenic over wide range of dose
Limited antibody response-IgM and IgG3	All antibody can be raised
No memory	Memory present
No macrophage processing	Macrophage processing step is needed
Slowly metabolized	Rapidly metabolized

Antibody

- Papain digestion produces:
  - 2 Fab portion – antigen binding site
  - 1 Fc portion – biological function like complement attachment site, adherence to monocyte
- 2 Heavy and 2 Light chain
- Heavy chain – μ, γ, α, E, δ
- Light chain – kappa/lambda
- Hinge region – rich in cysteine, prolin

Properties of Human Immunoglobulins

Property	IgG	IgA	IgM	IgD	IgE
Percentage of total immunoglobulin in serum (approx)	75	15	9	0.2	0.004
Serum concentration (mg/dL) (approx)	1000	200	120	3	0.05
Sedimentation coefficient	7S	7S or 11S	19S	7S	8S
Molecular weight (x1000)	150	170 or 400	900	180	190
Structure	Monomer	Monomer or dimer	Monomer or pentamer	Monomer	Monomer
H chain symbol					E
Complement fixation	+	–	+	–	–
Transplacental passage	+	–	–	–	–
Mediation of allergic responses	–	–	–	–	+
Found in secretions	–	+	–	–	–
Opsonization	+	–	–	–	–
Antigen receptor on B cell	–	–	+	?	–
Polymeric form contains J chain	–	+	+	–	–

- Serum concentration – GAMDE

  IgM Antibody Examples: O Antibody in typhoid, Reaginic Antibody in syphilis, Antibody of ABO Grouping, Rh system (IgG), Reaginic Ab in syphilis

Immunoglobulin Specificity

- Idiotype – Based on antigenic determinant in paratope
- Isotype – Difference between Ig of different classes and subclasses
- Allotype – Difference between immunoglobulin of same classes between different individual in same species.

Ig	Major Functions
IgG	Types- IgG1>2>3>4, Main antibody in the secondary response. Opsonizes bacteria, making them easier to phagocytize. Precipitation,Fixes complement, which enhances bacterial killing. Neutralizes bacterial toxins and viruses. Crosses the placenta. Appear late, indicates past/chronic infection, Secreted in placenta, breast. IgG4 – No complement activity, IgG2 – Not crossing placenta, IgG3 – Maximum in classical pathway activation.
IgA	Secretory IgA prevents attachment of bacteria and viruses to mucous membranes. Does not fix classical complement. 2nd most abundant, Types – IgA1-monomer, minor IgA2 – Surafce/mucosal IgA – Dimer joined by J chain and secretory piece (from epithelium) Responsible for – Alternate Compliment, Mucosal/local immunity
IgM	Produced in the primary response to an antigen. 1st to appear following infection, indicates recent infection.1st to appear in intrauterine life also (20 weeks), Fixes complement. Agglutination, Haemolysis, Opsonization, Classical complement. Does not cross the placenta. Antigen receptor on the surface of B cells. High Molecular Weight, J Chain
IgD	Uncertain. Found on the surface of many B cells as well as in serum. Surface Ig
IgE	Mediates immediate hypersensitivity (type 1) by causing release of mediators from mast cells and basophils upon exposure to antigen (allergen). Defends against worm infections by causing release of enzymes from eosinophils. Does not fix complement. Main host defence against helminth infections. Homocytotropic, Reaginic antibody

Abnormal Immunoglobulins

- Bence Jones Protein
- Coagulates at 50°C, redissolve at 70°C, Elevated in Multiple myeloma
- Light chain of immunoglobulin i.e. Kappa or lambda (but never both in same patient)
- Unchecked proliferation of single clone of plasma chain
- Waldenstrom Macroglobulinemia (IgM)
- Heavy chain disease – Fc part of heavy chain
- Cryoglobulinemia – Precipitate at low temp, dissolve at room temp
- Seen with – HCV, myeloma, SLE, autoimmune disease

Antigen Antibody Reaction

Precipitation

- Definition: Soluble Antigen reacts with Antibody and forms insoluble precipitate floccules
- Ring tests: Ascoli thermo precipitation test, Lancefield grouping
- Flocculation tests: VDRL, RPR, Kahn test, standardization of toxin
- Immuno-diffusion: Elek gel precipitation (C. diphtheriae), Eiken (E.coli)
- CIEP – αFP, Antigen of Cryptococcus and Meningococcus
- Rocket electrophoresis
- Prozone Phenomenon: Antibody Excess (Marrack's lattice hypothesis)

Single diffusion in one dimension	Oudin procedure
Single diffusion in two dimension	Radial immunodiffusion
Double diffusion in one dimension	Oakley-Fulthrope procedure
Double diffusion in two dimension	Ouchterlony procedure

Agglutination

- Definition – Insoluble (Particulate) Antigen reacts with Antibody, forms visible clumps

Widal test	Enteric fever
Standard agglutination test (SAT)	Brucella
Microscopic agglutination test (MAT)	Leptospira
Direct Agglutination Test (DAT)	Leishmania
Weil-Felix test	Rickettsia
Paul Bunucl	EBV
Coombs test	Incomplete (IgG) Antibody

- Passive agglutination test (PHA)
- Soluble antigen is coated on carrier particle like RBC, latex
  - So that a precipitation reaction can be converted to an agglutination reaction and hence better visualized.
  - E.g. – TPHA(syphilis), Rose Waaler test (Rheumatoid arthritis)
- RPHA (Reverse Passive Hemagglutination test)
  - Antibody is coated on a surface of carrier particle like RBC to detect antigens, E.g. – HBsAg

CFT

- Syphilis – Wasserman, TPI
- Sabin – Feldman test – Toxoplasma
- CFT for viral diseases

Western blot

- PAGE (Polyacrylamide gel electrophoresis): Electrophoretically mobilize and separate the antigen fragments
- Nitrocellulose membrane (NCM) blotting: Antigenic fragments are blotted on NCM
- Enzyme immunoassay: to detect theAntigens/antibodies in serum of the patient

STRUCTURE OF IMMUNE SYSTEM AND IMMUNE RESPONSE

Lymphoid System – Lymphoid Organ + Lymphoid Cells

Lymphoid Organ

- Central/Primary – Thymus and bursa of Fabricius (birds)/Bone Marrow (human)
- Peripheral/Secondary – Spleen, Lymph Node, MALT (GIT and Resp), Liver

Lymphoid Cells

- T and B Cells, NK Cell, Macrophage/dendritic cell

Thymus

- 3rd and 4th pharyngeal pouch cortex – T lymphocytes, nurse cell, medulla – epithelial cells, lymphocytes, Hassal's corpuscle
- Progenitor T cells passed through thymus – 1% released out, rest destroyed (self-reacting T cells)
- T cells are educated – Acquire Thymus Ag – T dependent T cells
- Defect in thymus – CMI
- Runt disease – nude mice and DiGeorge syndrome

Bursa of Fabricius and Bone marrow

- Bursa of Fabricius – Birds and Bone marrow(BM) – humans
- All lymphocytes originates in BM, B cell proliferates in BM

Lymphocytes

- Short lived lymphocyte – life span 2 week, effector cells
- Long lived lymphocyte – life span 2–3 years, memory cells
- Markers:
  - CD 10, 19, 22, 23 – B cell markers
  - CD 3, 4, 7, 8 – T cell markers

T Kymphocyte

- Blast transformation occurs by
  - Anti CD3, phytohemagglutinin (PHA) and concavalin
- Formation starts from Yolk Sac – fetal liver – BM – Thymus In Thymus:
- CD7 +ve Pro T cell enter thymus, Pre T cell (CD2 and CD3)
- Immature T cell – CD1, 4, 8 and T cell receptor
- TCR – α β or γ δ
- TCR $\gamma\delta$ – IEL and intracellular organism like MTB

CD4 T cells – MHC II restriction site (60%)

- TH1 – secrete IL2 and IFN γ
  - IFN γ – Activate macrophage, B cell (IgG2b)
  - IL2 – T cell growth factor, DTH Tcell, NK cell γ LAK cell
- TH2 – secrete IL4, 5, 6, 10
  - IL4 – Inhibit Th1, Chemo attractant, class switch IgE and IgG
  - IL5 – class switch IgA, Chemo attractant to eosinophil

CD 8 expressing cells – MHC I restriction site (30%)

- T cytotoxic cells (Tc cells) – cause cytotoxic lysis of target cells
- T suppressor cells (Ts cells) – suppress immune response
- IL12 – promote Th1

B Lymphocytes

- 10–20% of total lymphocyte
- Also act as APC – mediated by surface IgM receptors
- CD40 of B cell attach to CD40L of T cell – leads to B cell maturation
- Possess Fc Receptor
- CD21 – EBV receptor, CD2 – measles receptor
- Microvilli present on surface
- Blast transformation occurs by:
  - Endotoxin, Anti Ig, EBV and Super Antigen

Macrophages

- Derived from the bone marrow
- Has role in phagocytosis, secretion of cytokines and antigen presentation
- Killing of cells by Phagocytosis and phagolysosome fusion and lysosomal degranulation.
- Also by generating oxygen free radical

Peripheral blood	Monocytes
Brain	Microglia
Bone	Osteoclasts
Any solid tissue	Histiocyte
Liver	Kupfer cells,
Kidney	Mesangial cells,
Lung	Alveolar macrophage
Inflammation site	Multinucleated cell and epitheliod cell

Dendritic Cell

- Act as APC during primary immune response
- BM derived (separate lineage)
- Transport the presented Antigen to lymph node
- Possess MHCII > MHC I and B7
- No phagocytic activity
- Types:
  - Myeloid
  - Lymphoid
  - Interstitial
  - Langerhans
  - Follicular:
    - Special type of dendritic cell
    - Doesn't possess any MHCII and No antigen presentation combine with antigen–antibody complexes
    - Fc receptors found on the surfaces
    - Act on memory B cell

NK Cell

- Natural killer cell/Null cell/large granular lymphocytes (LGL)/lymphokine activated cell (LAC)
- Constitutes 5–10% of total lymphocyte
- Nonspecifically kills viruses without any prior sensitization (No Memory cells)
- NK cell – LAK transformation is induced by IL2
- Possess indented nuclei and several granules
- NK cells are Not MHC restricted
- Possess CD16 and CD 56 markers

- Used in treatment of – renal cell carcinoma
- Mediates ADCC –Antibody dependent cytotoxicity
  - CD16 (FcR like) recognized Fc portion of antibody bound to a target cell
  - Then, NK cell release perforins and granazyme which lyses the target cells
  - Cytotoxicity to virus infected cells and malignant cells, parasitic infection

HLA/MHC

- Transplantation antigen – determining histocompatibility
- HLA I, II, III
- Play a central role in antigen recognition
- MHC-short arm of chromosome 6 in humans
- Highly polymorphic – 24 alleles – HLA A, 50-HLA B
- Alleles – co-dominantly expressed
- Class I MHC genes – glycoprotein-all nucleated cells
  - Present peptide antigen to Tc cells (CD8 T Cells)
  - Processing of virus infected cells and tumour cells
- Class II MHC genes – glycoprotein on all antigen presenting cells
  - Present peptide antigen to Th cells (CD4 T Cells)
  - Regulates immune response
  - Plays a central role in initiation of the immune response to transplantation antigens
- Class III MHC genes–genes coding C2, C4, properdin, factor B, C3 convertase, TNF, HSP

Class I MHC	Class II MHC
• Present in all nucleated cells • Present the Ag to the CD8 cells • Function – Graft rejection, Cell mediated cytolysis, Hormone receptor • Heavy α chain – 3 globular domain • α1 – α2 Groove: Ag peptide binding groove • α3 – CD8 Binding groove • β2 microglobulin	• Present in APC(macrophage) • Present the Ag to the CD4 cells • Function – GVH and MLR • Heterodimer • α chain – globular domain- α1, α2 • β chain – β1, β2 • α1 – β1 Groove: Ag peptide binding groove • β2 – CD4 Binding groove

Immune Response

- Humoral
- Cell mediated
  - Primary Immune response
  - Secondary Immune response

Immune response curve

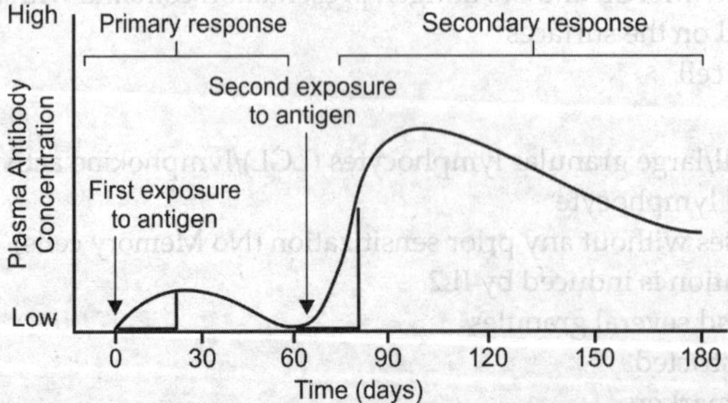

Fig. 5.4: Immune response curve

Hypersensitivity Reaction (Acid)

Mediator	Type	Reaction
Antibody (IgE)	I (immediate, **A**naphylactic)	IgE antibody is induced by allergen and binds to mast cells and basophils. When exposed to the allergen again, the allergen cross-links the bound IgE, which induces degranulation and release of mediators, e.g., histamine. Atopy – Asthma, allergic rhinitis (hay fever), food allergies, atopic eczema, Anaphylaxis, Theobald smith phenomena, Schultz Dale phenomena, Prausnitz Kustner reaction, Casoni test. Passive cutaneous anaphylaxis
Antibody (IgG)	II (**C**ytotoxic)	Antigens on a cell surface combine with antibody; this leads to complement-mediated lysis, e.g., transfusion, erythroblastosis fetalis Autoimmune haemolytic anaemia. C3a, C5a-Goodpasteur syndrome, Pemphigus vulgaris, Bullous pemphigous, rheumatic fever, vasculitis
Antibody (IgG)	III (**I**mmune complex)	Antigen–antibody immune complexes are deposited in tissues, complement is activated, and polymorphonuclear cells are attracted to the site. They release lysosomal enzymes, causing tissue damage. Arthus reaction, serum sickness, Hypersensitivity Pneumonitis(farmer's lung), PSGN, Subacute bacterial endocarditis, Microbial antigen – Strep. pyogenes, M.leprae, Treponema, Plasmodium, Trypanosome, HBV, HCV, EBV, Dengue, SLE, Rh A, PAN, Schick test, Hyperacute graft rejection
Cell Mediated	IV (**d**elayed)	Helper T lymphocytes sensitized by an antigen release lymphokines upon second contact with the same antigen. The lymphokines induce inflammation and activate macrophages, which, in turn, release various mediators. Manotoux/Heaf, Leprosy type I, contact dermatitis and Frie test

Immunodeficiency: Deficiency in

- B cells (antibody), (2) T cells, (3) complement, and (4) phagocytes.
- Congenital or Acquired

Important congenital immunodeficiencies			
Deficient Component and Name of Disease	**Specific Deficiency**	**Molecular Defect**	**Clinical Features**
B cell			
X-linked (Bruton's)	Absence of B cells; very low Ig levels	Mutant tyrosine kinase	Recurrent bacterial infections, especially of respiratory tract, caused by pyogenic bacteria such as pneumococci
Selective IgA	Very low IgA levels	Failure of heavy-chain gene switching	Recurrent infections, especially of the sinuses and lung, caused by pyogenic bacteria
T cell			
Thymic aplasia (DiGeorge's)	Absence of T cells	Defective development of pharyngeal pouches; not a genetic disease	Viral, fungal, and protozoal infections; tetani
Chronic mucocutaneous Candidiasis	Deficient T-cell response to Candida	Unknown	Skin and mucous membrane infections with Candida
Combined B and T cell			
Severe combined immunodeficiency (SCID)	Deficiency of both B-cell and T-cell function	Either defective IL-2 receptor, defective recombinases, defective kinases, absence of class II MHC proteins, or ADA or PNP deficiency	Bacterial, viral, fungal, and protozoal infections
Complement			
Hereditary angioedema	Deficiency of C1 protease inhibitor	Too much C3a, C4a, and C5a generated	Edema, especially laryngeal edema

Contd...

Contd...

Important congenital immunodeficiencies			
Deficient Component and Name of Disease	**Specific Deficiency**	**Molecular Defect**	**Clinical Features**
C6,7,8	Insufficient C6,7,8	Unknown	Neisseria infections
Phagocytes			
Chronic granulomatous disease	Defective bactericidal activity because no oxidative burst	Deficient NADPH oxidase activity	Pyogenic infections, especially with Sta. aureus and Aspergillus

Tumor Immunology

- **TSTA** – Tumor specific tumor antigen
  - Chemical induced – tumor specific
  - Virus induced – virus specific
- **TATA** – tumor associated tumor antigen
  - Also present normally, but elevated in malignancy
  - Alfa feto protein, Carcino embryonic Ag
  - Prostate specific Ag, CA 125, Beta HCG
  - Immunomodulator like
    - Monoclonal Ab – against tumor antigen
    - Tumor vaccine
    - Corynebacterium parvum, BCG, Thalidomide, Levamisole

Transplantation Immunology

Rejection response

- Direct pathway – recipient T cells recognize intact donor APC containing MHC molecules
- Indirect pathway – Recipient APC s process the donor-MHC antigen before presenting it to recipient T cells.
- Primary graft rejection-first set response-12 to 14 days
- Second set rejection – immunological memory, skin-faster rejection – in 5–6 days
- Mechanisms of rejection
  - Sensitization phase and effectors phase

GVH (Graft Versus Host Reaction)

- Occurs when Graft mounts an immune response against host tissue.
- GVHR
  - Graft contains immunocompetent cells
  - Recipient has transplant ag that is absent in graft
  - Recipient has not rejected graft
  - Recipient cannot respond immunologically
- Embryos or neonates, adults in immunosuppression
- Runt disease, Skin, liver and GI tract – main target organs of GVHD.

Prevention of transplant rejection

- ABO typing, HLA – typing by Serology (Microcytotoxicity, Mixed leukocyte reaction) and Molecular methods-PCR – RFLP.

SYSTEMIC BACTERIOLOGY

Gram Positive Cocci

Two types:
- Catalase positive – Staphylococcus, Micrococcus
- Catalase negative – Streptococcus, Pneumococci, Enterococcus

Staphylococcus

- Sir Alexander Ogston (1880): Establish the etiology and named as Staphylococci. Isolate non-virulent Staphylococci from skin surfaces.

Coagulase positive (tube and slide)	Coagulase negative
Staphylococcus aureus	S. epidermidis
Staph schleferi	S. saprophyticus
Staph hyicus and Intermedius (animal)	S. hemolyticus
Staph lugdunensis: slide coagulase +ve and tube coagulase –ve	

Antigenic structure and Virulence factors

Cell wall associated structures	Activity
Capsular polysaccharide	Inhibits opsonisation and Phagocytosis
Peptidoglycan	Confers cell rigidity and induces inflammatory response
Teichoic acid	Helps in adhesion to mucosal surfaces and prevent opsonisation
Clumping factor/Bound coagulase	Responsible for slide coagulase reaction
Protein A	Antiphagocytic, anti-complement, chemotactic Binds to Fc of IgG leaving Fab free to bind to Ag – Co agglutination
Extracellular factors	**Activity**
α hemolysin	Inactivated at 700C reactivated paradoxically at 100°C Lyses rabbit > sheep and human red blood cells Leucocidal, Cytotoxic, dermonecrotic, lethal
β Hemolysin	Sphingomyelinase, Lyses sheep RBC, but not human or rabbit RBC, Exhibits hot-cold phenomenon
γ Hemolysin	Bicomponent proteins, Lyses rabbit sheep and human red blood cells
δ Hemolysin	Detergent likc, Lyses rabbit, sheep and human red blood cells
Leucocidins/Panton valentine toxin	Two components F and S Damage PMN and macrophages
Synergohymenotropic toxin	Bicomponent toxin – γ and Leucocidins – Community acquired MRSA
Epidermolytic toxin (Exfoliative toxin)	Mainly belong to phage group II 2 Types: A: heat stable, chromosomal gene B: heat labile, Plasmid controlled Scalded skin syndrome Severe – Ritters disease (newborn), TEN (adult) Mild – Pemphigus neonatorum, bullous impetigo
Enterotoxins	Produced by 50% of clinical isolates Cause food poisoning IP: 1–6 hours due to preformed toxin Vomiting due to Vagus Nerve and vomiting centre stimulation Heat stable (not destroyed after heating food) Multiple antigenic type (A–E, G–I, K–M) (MCtype A)

Contd...

Contd...

Toxic shock syndrome toxin	Most strains belong to phage group I Enterotoxins F/pyrogenic exotoxinC (MC) > B,C Use of vaginal tampon Anti TSST1 Ab is protective Rash, desquamation and Multiorgan failure T/T – Clindamycin (reduces toxin synthesis)
Extracellular enzymes	**Activity**
Coagulase Enzyme	Enzyme is secreted into the surrounding Requires coagulase reacting factor (CRF) present in plasma for action Responsible for tube coagulase test
Others – Staphylokinase (fibrinolysin), Hyaluronidase, Deoxyribonuclease, Lipase, Protease	

Superantigens

- Act on Vβ of TCR (T-cell receptor)
- Don't require antigen presentation by macrophage, directly stimulate non specific T cells
- Leads to massive release of cytokines and polyclonal B cell activation
  Example: Staph – TSST, Exfoliative toxin, Enterotoxins, SPE.

Free coagulase	Bound coagulase/(clumping factor)
Enzyme secreted into medium Act with CRF (Coagulase reacting factor) 8 types identified (MC Type A) Heat labile Tube Coagulase test	Constituent of cell wall Independent of CRF Only one type Heat stable Slide Coagulase test

Staphylococcus aureus: Characteristic features:

Coagulase +ve Heat stable thermonuclease DNAse Phosphatase (also S.epidermidis) Golden yellow pigmentation	Hemolysis Ferment mannitol Black colony on Pot tellurite agar Gelatin liquefy Protein A

Medium

- 5% sheep blood agar – shows pin head shaped colony with narrow zone of β haemolysis
- MacConkey agar – minute pink colonies – means Lactose fermenting
- Selective medium
  - Milk salt agar (8–10% NaCl)
  - Mannitol salt agar- with 7.5% NaCl + 1% Mannitol
  - Ludlam's lithium chloride and tellurite media
- Media for pigment – Milk agar, Glycerol monoacetate agar, Tween agar, incubation at 22°C – 25°C
- Golden yellow pigmentation (due to beta carotene) – Non diffusible
- Nutrient agar slope – Oil paint appearence

Staphylococcus are differentiated from Micrococcus by

Properties	Staphylococcus aureus	Micrococcus
Hugh Leifson's oxidative fermentative test	Fermentative	Oxidative
Furazolidone	Sensitive	Resistant
Bacitracin (0.04IU disc)	Resistant	Sensitive

S. aureus is the MC agent for

- Skin and soft tissue infection
- Botryomycosis

- Tropical pyomyositis – S. aureus, (acute bacterial myositis – GrA Streptococcus)
- Osteomyelitis, septic arthritis, postoperative parotitis, Paronychia

Points to Remember

- MC method for typing of S.aureus – Phage typing (pattern method)
- Drug resistance in S.aureus transferred by – Transduction (MC) > conjugation
- MC site of colonization – Skin
- MC cause of Native valve endocarditis – MC: S.aureus
- MC cause of Early prosthetic valve endocarditis (<12m) – S.epidermidis and late prosthetic valve endocarditis (>12m) – Str Viridans
- Endocarditis in IV drug users – Rt sided-MC: S.aureus, Lt sided – MC: Enterococcus > S.aureus
- MC organism in late onset nosocomial pneumonia – Staph.aureus
- MC organism in SSI (surgical cite infection) – Staph. aureus

Coagulase Negative Staphylococcus (CONS) normal flora of skin

- *S. epidermidis* (MC CONS) – produce polysaccharide glycocalyx (slime) (Biofilm production) – Escape from phagocytosis
- Endocarditis with insertion of valvular prosthesis and Ventricular shunt infections leading to bacteremias.
- *S. saprophyticus* – causes UTI in young sexually active female. novobiocin resistant
- S.haemolyticus – mot common strain in resistance (MRSA +ve, VRSA +ve)
- Resistance by Staphyococci:
  - Penicillin resistance (Penicillin, Oxacillin, Methicillin)
  - Glycopeptide resistance (Vancomycin)

Mechanism of Resistance

- Production of β-lactamase (penicillinase)
- Change in the bacterial surface receptors
- Tolerence to Penicillin

MRSA: Methicillin Resistant Staphyloccoccus Aureus

- Definition – Methicillin MIC 8 μg/ml or more, Oxacillin MIC 4 μg/ml or more
- Resistance is chromosomally mediated (mec A gene)
  - Due to altered PBP 2a (MC) > hyper production of β lactamase
  - Treatment: Vancomycin is DOC
  - Others – Teichoplanin, linezolid, streptogramin, cipro/levofloxacin, cotrimoxazole, clindamycin, mupirocine, minocycline
  - Newer: Aptomycin, Ceftobiprole, Tigecycline, Oritavancin

Treatment

Penicillin sensitive strains	Penicillin G
Penicillin allergic patients	Cefazolin
TSST infection	Clindamycin
Food poisoning	No antibiotic (caused by preformed toxin)
MRSA	Vancomycin
MRSA carriers	Mupirocin
VRSA	Quinopristin, Dalfopristin, Linezolid

Streptococcus

- Gram positive cocci arranged in chains (due to division in single plane)
- Catalase Negative/Nonsporing

- Fresh isolates form capsule which is made up of Hyaluronic acid. It protects the organism from phagocytosis.

Cultural characteristics:

- Virulent stains produce matt colonies (finely granular)
- Avirulent strains produce glossy colonies
- Capsulated strains produce mucoid colonies.

Capsule:

- Gr A, C: Hyaluronic acid capsule
- Gr B,D: Polysaccharide capsule
- Sensitivity to Bacitracin is employed as a convenient for differentiating Strep. pyogens from other haemolytic stains. (Maxtred observation)
- Longest chain is formed by Strap.salivarius (non pathogenic)

Selective media: crystal violet – Blood agar and PNF medium (Polymyxin Neomycin Fusidic acid)

Strep. Pyogenes (Group A)

- Structural components of *Strept pyogenes* and Human tissue with which it cross reacts and produces damage (molecular mimicry)
- Capsular hyaluronic acid – Synovial fluid
- Cell wall protein M – Myocardium
- Cell wall carbohydrate – Cardiac valves
- Cytoplasmic membrane – Vascular intima
- Peptidoglycan – Skin antigens

Virulence factor	Activity
Antigens in the cell wall	
Lipoteichoic acid	Mediates adherence to fibronectin receptors on epithelial cells
M protein	Mediates adherence to epithelial cells, inhibits phagocytosis
Capsule	
Hyaluronic acid capsule	Inhibits phagocytosis
Enzymes and Toxins	
Erythrogenic toxin (SPE)	3 types (SPE A, B and C). Type A and C bacteriophage coded, B toxin chromosomal Mediated. Act as a Superantigen. Dick test – (ID injection) – detect susceptible individuals Schultz Charlton reaction (blanching of rash after injection of antibodies) – diagnosis of scarlet fever
Streptolysin O	Produced by group A, C and G streptococci. Oxygen labile, Serum stable Also Pneumolysin, tetanolysin, perfringolysin Acts by binding to cholesterol in the cell membrane and producing hole in it. It is strongly antigenic and rise of ASO > 200 Todd units, indicates recent streptococcal infection
Streptolysin S	Oxygen stable, Serum soluble Hemolysis on the surface of an aerobic blood agar plate. Not antigenic.
Streptokinase	Fibrinolysin (activate plasminogen) Rapid spread of infection by preventing the formation of fibrin barrier. This property is also used therapeutically in treatment of coronary thrombosis.

Contd...

Contd...

Virulence factor	Activity
Deoxyribonuclease	Streptodornase (4 types- A, B, C, D) Anti-DNAase B > 300–350μ is useful for the retrospective diagnosis of skin infections (pyoderma) where ASO is usually low Liquefy thick pus. Applied therapeutically in empyema (Streptodornase & streptokinase)
Hyaluronidase	M type 4 and 22 (non-capsulated)
Serum opacity factor	Lipoproteinase enzyme

Pathogenicity

- Mucoid colonies are virulent because of polysaccharide capsule will impart virulence and protect the organism from l phagocytosis.
- Hair like pili (fimbria) project through the capsule. The pili consist partly of M protein and are covered with lipoteichoic acid which is responsible for the attachment of Streptococci to the epithelial cells.
- Pharyngitis/sore throat – MC infection.
- Complication – otitis media, quinsy, Ludwig's angina, meningitis, pneumonia
- Scarlet fever and TSS (pyrogenic toxin (or) Dick toxin
- Impetigo – Seen in young individual. (School sore)
- Erysipelas – Seen in elder. Affects superficial lymphatics.
- Puerperal sepsis

Nonsuppurative sequelae

- ARF (Acute rheumatic fever)
- Acute glomerulonephritis – can occur either after skin or throat infection. Produced by gp A also group C may be involved; Most cases of AGN occur about one week after group A type 12 infections.
- Erythema nodosum, Reactive arthritis and Guttate psoriasis

	Acute rheumatic fever	Acute glomerulonephritis
Site	Throat	Skin > Throat
Prior sensitization	Essential	Not
Serotype	Any	Pyodermal – 49, 53–55, 59–61, Pharyngitis – 1, 12
Immune response	Marked	Moderate
Complement level	Unaltered	Low
Genetic susceptibility	Present	No
Repeated attack	Common	No
Penicillin prophylaxis	Indicated	No
Course	Progressive	Spontaneous resolution
Prognosis	Variable	Good

- Reinfection is common due to multiplicity of M protein.

Streptozyme test

- Passive haemagglutinin test
- Sensitive and specific screening test for Streptococcal infection
- Positive test shows suggestive of Streptococcal infection of skin (or) throat.

Treatment

Pharyngitis and Impetigo	Benzathine penicillin G
Erysipelas/cellulitis	Mild to moderate: Procaine penicillin Severe: penicillin G
Necrotizing fasciitis/myositis	Surgical debriment (most important) penicillin G along with Clindamycin
Pneumonia/Empyema	Draining of pus with penicillin G
Streptococcal toxic shock syndrome	penicillin G, Clindamycin, IV-Immunoglobulin
Note: Penicillin allergic patient Erythromycin is the drug of choice	

Group B Streptococci

S. Agalactiae Causes

- Early onset and late onset neonatal meningitis (MC)
- Early onset – first 5 days, usually due to ascending infection in utero > colonization during birth
- Late onset: after 1 week, acquires infection from hospital personnel and colonization during birth
- Most commonly due to capsular strain type III.
  Presumptive identification
- CAMP +ve (arrow head haemolysis with Staphylococcus)
- Hippurate hydrolysis test +ve pigment production
- Penicillin is the DOC. Vancomycin is DOC if penicillin allergy.

Group C Streptococci

- Human pathogen is Strep. equisimilis
- Beta haemolytic colonies
- Part of the normal flora of throat.
- Ferment trehalose and ribose (Str. pyogenes ferment only trehalose not ribose)
- It produces streptolysin O and streptokinase (Strep. equisimilis is the source of streptokinase used for thrombolytic therapy)
- DOC is Penicillin G

Group F Streptococci

- Minute streptococci
- Human pathogen is Str. MG
- Cause primary atypical pneumonia.
- Cold agglutinin is diagnostic

Group D Streptococci

- Differentiated from other *Streptococci* by ability to grow in presence of 40% bile and hydrolyze esculin. They can be further divided into Enterococci and Non-enterococci
  Enterococci – Important Characteristic
- Growth in presence of **6.5% NaCI, 40% bile, at pH 9.6 and at 45°C** (Heat resistance), 0.1% methylene blue milk.
- Most strains are **resistant to penicillin**, aminoglycoside and sulfonamides.
- Combination therapy with penicillin and aminoglycoside is effective.
- Disease – UTI, endocarditis, intra-abdominal infection, meningitis
- Most commonly associated with human disease *Enterococcus fecalis* and *Enterococcus faecium*
- Penicillin resistance: Production of β-lactamase (Enterococcus faecalis)
- Altered penicillin binding protein(Enterococcus faecium)
- Enterococcal resistance: Van A, Van B and Van C gene

Nonenterococcus – S. bovis and S. equinus

- Penicillin sensitive, inhibited by 6.5% NaCI, 40% bile, at pH 9.6 and at 45°C
- Non-hemolytic
- Cause UTI, Endocarditis in the patient with neoplasm of GIT i.e., Carcinoma or polyp. (Indirect evidence of carcinoma in early stages)

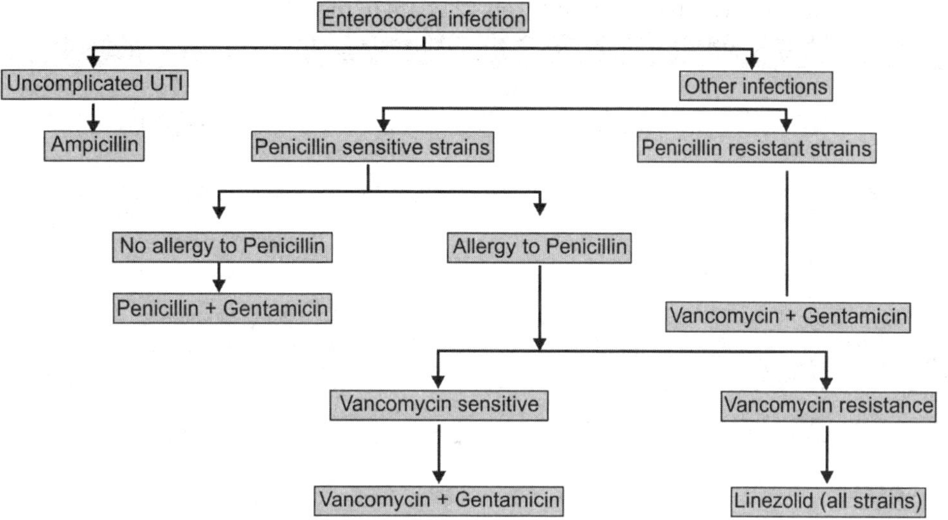

Viridans streptococci

- **S. salivarius, S. sanguis, S. mitis, S. mutans**
- α hemolytic, mouth commensals, usually sensitive to penicillin
- Nonpathogenic strains
- Produce endocarditis in person with preexisting cardiac lesion.
- *S.mutans* – dental caries, *S sanguis(MC)* – endocarditis
- Viridians streptococcal bacteremias occur frequently in neutropenic patients, particularly after bone marrow transplantation or high dose chemotherapy for cancer.
- Treatment: Bacteremia in neutropenic patients – Vancomycin
- Dental caries-Penicillin

S. pneumoniae

- α hemolytic colonies but under anaerobic condition – β hemolytic
- Gram positive/Capsulated
- Diplococcic (flame shaped/lanceolate shaped)

Antigenic structure

- Capsular Ag – 90 types (type 3 most virulent), SSS (specific soluble substances), typing by Quellung reaction
- Carbohydrate Ag – CRP precipitates with this Ag.
- Pneumolysin (thiol activated toxin, exerts a variety of effects on ciliary cells and PMN's and also activates the classical complement pathway)
- Autolysin – amidase – cleaves Peptidoglycan layer – leads to draughtsman shape colony and bile solubility
- IgA_1 Protease
- Anticapsular antibody provides the best specific protection

Pathogenicity

- Commensal in nasopharynx – 5%(adult), 20%(children) – in throat
- Pneumonia – In adults – type 1–8 (most virulent type-3), In Children – 6, 14, 19, 23

- Meningitis
- Others – otitis media, sinusitis, peritonitis etc.
- Penicillin resistance-due to altered PBP 2b(chromosomal)
- **Vaccine:** 1. Polysaccharide vaccine (23 valent) – Not useful for <2 years as T cell independent, Indication- splenectomy, sickle cell patient, DM, chronic heart/lung/renal/liver disease.
- *Conjugated vaccine* (7 valent) – can be given children <2 years (6 months to 3 years)

Character	S. Pneumoniae	S. Viridians
Morphology	Lanceolate/flame	Round
Arrangement	Diplo/Pairs	Long chains
Bile solubility	+	–
Capsule (Quellung test)	+	–
Inulin fermentation	+	–
Optochin sensitivity	S	R
Colony in BA	Draughtsman	Dome
Liquid medium turbidity	Uniform	Granular
Animal pathogenicity	+	–
Virulence	+	–

Gram Negative Cocci

- N meningitidis,
- N. gonorrhoeae,
- Moraxella,
- Veillonella

Neisseria

Gram Negative cocci (diplococci), Catalase and oxidase +ve

N. meningitidis	N. gonorrhoeae
Capsulated	Non-capsulated
Lens shaped (Diplococci with adjacent sides flattened)	Kidney shaped
Ferments Glucose and Maltose	Glucose only
Rarely have plasmids	Usually possess plasmid and more drug resistant
Extra or intracellular	Mostly intracelular
Strict aerobes	Growth can occur anaerobically

N. meningitides (Meningococcus)

Antigenic Determinants and Virulence Factors

- Capsular polysaccharide: inhibits phagocytosis, are of 13 serogroups
- Most meningococcal disease: A B, C, Y, 29E and W 135
- Group A – epidemics, C – sporadic, B-both
- Serogroup further classified based on OMP (outer membrane protein)
- Endotoxin and LOS (Lipooligosaccharide): produce generalized Shwartzman reaction and Water House–Friderichsen Syndrome
- IgA 1 protease: IgA1 protease cleaves subclass IgA 1 and inactivates it.
- Pili: allow to adhere and antiphagocytic

Pathogenicity

- MC source – human carriers
- Nasopharyngeal carrier- children mainly – 5–10% (inter epidemic), 20–90% (during epidemic)
- MC Route – hematogenous > olfactory Nerve > conjunctiva
- Deficiency of terminal complement components (C5–C9) → increase risk of meningococcal infection
- Outbreak in Hajji pilgrims in 1990 – due to group A, W135
- High prevalence – sub-Saharan belt of Africa
- Seasonal variation – MC in winter spring

Clinical feature

- Fulminant meningococcemia – septic shock, DIC, rashes and Water House – Friderichsen Syndrome (DIC induced micro thrombi, hemorrhage, B/L adrenal hemorrhage)
- Meningitis- common in 3–5 year age

Diagnosis

- Culture media – Chocolate agar, Muller Hilton agar, Thayer martin media – 35c at 5–10% CO2
- Sample – CSF, Blood and nasopharyngeal swab (for carriers)
- LDH and neuraminidase in CSF
- Antibody – retrospective evidence only

Treatment

- Cefotaxime and ceftriaxone is DOC
- Rifampicin or ciprofloxacin for carriers and prophylaxis

Vaccine

- Polyvalent vaccine containing – A, C, Y, W-135 immunity lasts for 3 years
- No vaccine for GpB: capsule is poorly immunogenic and sialic acid residue in capsule cross react with human brain tissue (fatal autoimmune consequences)
- Not useful – below 3 years (capsule is poorly immunogenic < 3 years as it is T independent Ag), C/I-pregnancy.

N. gonorrhea

- Obligate human parasite
- Many women are asymptomatic and may act as a reservoir of infection
- Highly transmissible by sexual contact and Vertical transmission to neonates may occur during passage through an infected birth canal
- Genotypic (PFGE, AFLP) typing may be undertaken to differentiate between strains of gonococci, e.g. in child abuse cases.
- Based on Pilli divided to – 4 types (T_1–T_4)
- T_1 T_2: Numerous pili P^+ P^{++}, and are virulent
- T_3 and T_4 – Non pillated or P^-, avirulent, forms smooth suspension
- Auxotyping is done
- IP – 2–8 days

Antigenic Structure (Virulence)

Organism related

- Pilli – important role in attachment, Antiphagocytic
- Outer membrane protein – protein I, II, and III
- Protein I – Serves as a basis for serotyping
- Protein II – associated with adherence, present in opaque colony (opacity associated OMP)
- IgA 1 protease – also present in Meningococcus, Pneumococci, H. influenzae

- Lipooligosaccharide: Toxicity is due to endotoxic effect.
- Transferrin binding protein (TBP 1 and 2)
- Lactoferrin binding protein
- Porin
- Resists Phagocytosis
- Re-infections occur, because protective immunity does not develop

Host factors

- Terminal complement deficiency
- Activation of phospholipasec and sphingomyelinase.

Clinical feature

Gonorrhoea in males

- Male – MC is urethritis (doesn't involve testes)
- MC of septic arthritis in adult (MC knee joint)
- Disseminated gonococcal infections (DGI) commonly manifest as arthritis, tenosynovitis, or pustules in the skin. MC associated with Porin A1 and AHU auxotype
- MC seen in people with Blood group B urethral stricture and sterility
- Gastrointestinal: proctitis (asymptomatic in many);
- Occular: hyper-acute conjunctivitis, periorbital cellulitis;

Gonorrhoea in females

- MC of PID worldwide (India MC is MTB)
- Cervicitis (adult vagina is resistant to Gonococcus, so Less severity)
- Salpingitis and Sterility/ectopic pregnancy due to scarring of tubes
- Vagina not infected (stratified squamous epithelium) in adolescent females.
- Complication – water can perineum, Fitz Hugh Curtis syndrome (perihepatitis), metastatic complications (Endocarditis, arthritis, nephritis)

Gonorrhoea in pregnant women: Fetal loss, abortion, premature delivery

Gonorrhoea in neonates: Babies born to infected mother – Ophthalmia neonatorum

Gonorrhoea in children: vulvovaginitis

Selective media

- Thayer Martin (VCN) and Modified Thayer Martin (VCNT)
- Modified New York city medium
- Chocolate agar
- Chaco Nair Medium

Transport media – charcoal impregnated swabs/medium (stuart/Amies media)

- For longer holding period – CO_2 generating system (JEMBEC system or Gono Gaspak system)
- Sample – Urethral discharge, endocervical swab (high vaginal swab not recommended) and rectal swab
- Urethral discharge demonstrating intracellular diplococci – for males 90% sensitive but for females it is only 50–60% Sensitivity, due to presence of normal flora confounding interpretation.
- So, Endocervical culture is recommended – 90% Sensitive
- Serology – CFT – Poor sensitivity and false positives

Treatment – DOC – Cefotaxime and ceftriaxone

- Penicillin allergic patients: Quinolones can be given
- Patient allergic to Cephalosporin and Quinolones: Spectinomycin (Doc)
- Mostly resistant to Penicillin due to Penicillinase production
- NG has got remarkable capacity to alter its antigenic structure.
- Ophthalmia neonatorum – 1% slver nitrate eye drops (Crede's Method)

Gram Positive Bacilli

- Spore forming – Bacillus, Clostridium
- Nonspore forming – Corynebacterium, Listeria, Erysipelothrix, Mycobacterium,
- Nonsporing anaerobe – Actinomycetes, Propionobacterium, Bifidobacterium, Lactobacillus
- Bacillus – aerobe and Clostridium – Anaerobe

Corynebacterium

- C. diphtheriae – Kleb-Loeffler bacillus
- Club shaped, Chinese letter and cuneiform arrangement
- Possess metachromatic granules (Inorganic polyphosphates) – Babe Earnst or polar body
- Special stain – Albert, Ponder, Neisser stain

On the basis of morphology on tellurite medium C. diphtheriae has four biotypes

McLeod classification	Gravis	Intermedius	Mitis
Colonies on PTA	Daisy head	Frogs eggs colony	Poached egg
Starch Fermentation	+ve	–ve	–ve
Toxigenic strains	100%	95–99%	80–85%
Occurrence	Epidemic	Epidemic	Endemic
Complication	Paralytic and Hemorrhagic	Hemorrhagic	Obstructive
Hemolysis	Variable	Nonhemolytic	Hemolytic
Morphology	Short, no granules	Long barred, poor granules	Long curved, prominent granules

All 3 types are nitrate +ve, Belfanti (fourth biotypes) – Nitrate –ve variant of Mitis

Culture

- Loffler's serum slope (Enriched medium):
  - Earliest growth (6–8 hours)
  - Granules best developed
  - Water of condensation can be used for animal pathogenicity
- Selective medium
  - Potassium tellurite (0.04%) – black colonies in 2 days due to tellurite reduction.
  - Tinsdales, Hoyles medium, McLeod's medium

  Clinical diphtheria – 3 species
- C. diphtheriae (with four biotypes), C. ulcerans and C. pseudotuberculosis – all produce Diphtheria toxin and black colony on PTA
- C. diphtheriae – urease negative but C. ulcerans and C. pseudotuberculosis – urease positive

Diphtheria toxin (DT)

- Bacilli is noninvasive but DT released locally and absorbed in circulation and produce systemic manifestation So diphtheria is toxemia but not bacteremia – organism cannot be demonstrated in blood
- Skin/local lesions – by non toxigenic strain strains, so vaccine has no role
- Toxin A fragments → A inhibit elongation factor → inhibits protein synthesis, Fragment B – for transportation of fragment A inside cell
- Depends on iron concentration (0.14 mg per/μl optimum), 0.5 mg per/μl will inhibit toxin production
- DT is coded by β phage (tox phage)
- Park William 8 strain of C. diphtheriae is used as a source of toxin for diphtheria toxoid (DPT vaccine)
- Toxigenicity or Virulence test of C. diphtheria
- In vivo tests – Subcutaneous test and Intradermal, Guinea pig or rabbit used, mice is resistant to diphtheria
- In vitro tests – Elek gel precipitation test, PCR detecting Tox gene, ELISA/ICT detecting toxin
- Immunization does not prevent nasopharyngeal carriage.

Schick test

- Susceptibility test before starting immunization (now obsolete)

Pathogenicity

- Natural infection only in man.
- Pseudo membrane formation on tonsil, posterior pharyngeal wall.
- Source – carriers (Nasal carries are particularly dangerous – shed large no. of bacilli)
- Faucial diphtheria – (MC), bull neck – cervical lymphadenopathy
- Malignant diphtheria- severe toxemia in faucial type
- Laryngeal – dangerous, mandates tracheostomy
- 1st muscle involved – palatopharynges
- Cutaneous diphtheria: caused by non-toxigenic strains, punched out ulcers
- Ciliary but not papillary paralysis occurs – So blurred vision with intact light reflex
- Neurological complication- occurs in 1st/2nd week
- Systemic – myocarditis, peripheral neuropathy
- Cardiac damage is permanent but Nerve recovery usually occurs
- Invasive infection – very rare, factors- pre-existing cardiac anomaly, IV drug abuser, cirrhosis.
- C. diphtheria does not need to be toxigenic to establish localized infection.

  Diagnosis – Usually clinical, not to wait for lab confirmation
- Gram staining of throat swab and culture followed by toxigenicity testing

Treatment

- C. diphtheriae sensitive to penicillin, Erythromycin, Rifampicin; but antibiotics do not neutralize circulating toxin. So, antibiotics + antitoxin given
- Erythromycin active for treatment of carriers

Prevention

- Vaccine- active immunization by toxoid – to prevent diphtheria, but can't prevent carrier stage

  DPT – DT, TT and pertussis (whole cell or acellular component)
- Diphtheria toxoid – 2 types. Fluid toxoid(formalinized) and
- Adsorbed toxoid- more immunogenic (aluminum phosphate > hydroxide)
- Both whole cell killed B.pertussis and acelluar pertussis component increases potency of DT(adjuvant)
- Whole cell killed B.pertussis is encephalogenic and short lasting immunity while acelluar pertussis component (DTaP) is devoid of neurological complication.
- Quadruple vaccine – (DPT+ Hib) – DT and TT increases immunogenicity of Hib.

Non Diphtheria Corynebacterium

- Those which cause infection in immunocompetent individual
- C. ulcerans – cause bovine mastitis, mimic respiratory diphtheria, transmitted by cow milk
- C. pseudotuberculosis (Preisz-Nocard bacilli) – affect sheep and horse, granulomatous lymphadenitis
- C. minutissimum (causes erythrasma)-lipophilic Corynebacteria, grown in media containing 20% fetal calf serum, fluorescence on UV light (corel red colour)

Those which cause opportunistic infections

- C. jeikeium (multidrug resistant): opportunistic pathogen in immunocompromised responding to vancomycin
- C.tenuis- trichomycosisaxillaris (pigmented nodules around axillary and pubic hair shafts)

C.parvum – immunomodulator

Diphtheroids:

- Commensal corynebacteria normally present in the skin and mucous membrane resembles C. diphtheria morphologically.
- C. xerosis and C. hofmannii are Diphtheroids differentiated by biochemical test and toxigenicity testing.

	C. Diphtheria	Diphtheroids
Morphology	Weakly Gram positive Metachromatic granules Pleomorphism present Chinese letter pattern	Strongly Gram positive Less or absent Little Pleomorphism No specific arrangement
Culture	Grows on enriched media	Grows on ordinary media
Biochemical reaction	Glucose – fermented	Glucose and sucrose – fermented
Toxigenicity	Toxic	Non-toxic

Bacillus

- Aerobic gram positive spore forming bacilli (heat resistant spores)
- Most common contaminants in bacteriological culture media.
- All are motile (peritrichous flagella) except – B.anthracis
- *B. anthracis* – highly pathogenic, non motile, zoonotic disease

B.anthracis

- Kochs postulates based on *B. anthracis*
- First bacterial attenuated vaccine (Louis pasteur)
- First pathogenic bacteria seen under microscope (Pollender)
- First communicable disease transmitted by infected blood (Davaine)
- First to be isolated in pure culture (Robert Koch)
- Used as a biological warfare (2001 outbreak)

Presumptive diagnosis

- Selective medium – PLET media(Polymyxin, Lysozyme, Ethylene Diamine Tetra Acetic Acid, Thallous Acetate)
- In culture: arranged long chains, end of bacilli are swollen and truncated (**bamboo sticks** appearance)
- Agar plate culture shows opaque, raised, greyish white colonies (**Frosted glass** appearance)
- Microscopy: edge of the agar plate seen under low power (10X) objective demonstrate log, interlacing chains of bacilli resembling locks of matted hair. (**Medusa head** appearance)
- In gelatin stab: **Inverted fir tree** appearance
- Solid media with penicillin – **String of pearl** appearance
- **MC fadyean** reaction – polypeptide capsule seen when stained with polychrome methylene blue
- Immunofluorescence microscopy – to confirm diagnosis
- Spores found in soil or in culture and never in animal body/Tissues

Virulence factor

- **Anthrax toxin** – 3 fraction
  - Edema factor – ↑cAMP
  - Protective factor-binding (Ab is protective)
  - Lethal factor
- Alum precipitated toxoid vaccine (containing protective antigen)
- Capsule-polyglutamate-plasmid mediated, live attenuated spore vaccine (Sterne, Mazucchi), polypeptide capsule is pathognomonic for bacillus
- Anthrax: It is a zoonotic disease (cattle and sheep)
- Man acquires infection through:
- Cutaneous type – by small cuts or skin abrasion, use of shaving razors used for animal, insect bite. Spontaneous resolution.
- Pulmonary type – by spore inhalation, Intestinal type – by ingestion of meat

Types of anthrax

- Cutaneous anthrax (Hide porter's disease) – MC (95%), but usually self-limiting – Dock worker, butcher, abattoir, farmer
- Malignant pustule (black eschar surrounded by non-pitting edema)
- Pulmonary anthrax – Woolsorter's disease (inhalation of spores) – hemorrhagic mediastinitis, causes mediastinal widening in X ray, fatal
- Intestinal anthrax – fatal, following eating carcasses of animal dying of anthrax
- All 3 form can lead to – hemorrhagic meningitis and septicemia (less in cutaneous type)
- Agent of Bioterrorism → recently used by Afghanistan (spores enclosed in paper were mailed)
- Ascoli thermo precipitin test – to demonstrate anthrax Ag

Bacillus cereus

- Motile, lacks capsule, causes food poisoning
- Can also cause opportunistic infections like endocarditis, bacteremia, LRTI, meningitis
- Presence of B. cereus at least $>10^5$/gm of stool – considered diagnostic.
- Selective media – MYPA (Mannitol, Egg Yolk, Phenol Red, Polymyxin Agar)

Diagnosis

- Gram stain: Gram positive bacilli with capsule
- India Ink: clear hallow around bacteria represents capsule
- Giemsa stained smears: red capsule around purple bacilli
- Direct Fluorescent antibody test: capsule demonstration
- M'Fadyean reaction: polychrome methylene blue stain
- Animal inoculation: intraperitoneal inoculation in mice or guinea pig
- Antibody detection: ELISA, Indirect Hemagglutination test
- Antigen detection test: Ascoli's thermo precipitation test

B. cereus	Diarrheal type	Emetic type
IP	8–16 hours	1–5 hours (preformed toxin)
Food	Cooked meat/vegetable	Rice (Chinese fried rice)
Toxin	Resemble heat labile toxin of E.coli	Resemble heat stable toxin of E.coli
Mechanism	Entertoxin cause fluid accumulation	Emetic toxin production
Clinical feature	Diarrhea, fever, rarely nausea	Vomiting, abdominal cramps
Serotype	2, 6, 8, 9,10, 12	1, 3, 5

Clostridium

- Gram Positive, spore forming, Anaerobes.
- All motile except – Cl.tetani type VI and Cl perfringes
- Spore – Spherical and terminal – **Drum Stick shaped – Cl tetani**
- Oval and terminal – **tennis racket shaped – Cl. tertium**
- Noncapsulated (except Cl.perfringes)
- Motility – stately motile
- Found normally in feces – Cl.perfringes, Cl. Difficle
- Invasive strains produce toxemia – Cl.perfringes, Cl tetan.
- Noninvasive strain: C.botulinum

Cl. perfringes

- Non motile, Spores oval, subterminal
- Toxigenic and invasive
- 4 LethalToxins – α, β, ε, i : 5 types (A–E)

- Target Haemolysis in blood agar
- Litmus Milk reaction (+)
- Naegler reaction (+) d/t q toxin – opalescence on egg yolk media – lecithinase – inhibited by antisera.
- Spores are not produced in tissue.

Infections

Gas gangrene

- Established causes – Cl. Perfringes type–A, Cl.novyi, Cl.septicum
- No PMN in spite of extensive tissue damage
- IP short for Cl. Perfringes, Pain and crepitus-characteristic
- Gram staining – **GPB without spore** – Cl. Perfringes
- Citron body and boat shaped GPB – Cl.septicum
- GPB with oval sub terminal spore – Cl.novyi
- Surgery, DOC – Penicillin+clindamycin and hyperbaric O_2

Food Poison – Type A – Enterotoxin (Similar to cholera and EPEC)

Necrotizing enteritis (Pigbel – Fire bowels) due to β toxin of type C

Cl. tetanus

- Motile, swarming

Two toxins:

- Tetanospasmin – Blocks release of inhibitory transmitter glycine and GABA: spastic paralysis and Tetanolysin

Tetanus

- 1st symptom – ↑masseter tone (trismus/lock jaw) then descending tetanus
- Hands feet are spared
- Mentation unimpaired, brisk deep tendon reflex
- Shorter IP leads to graver the prognosis
- Noninfectious – no person to person spread
- Diagnosis is always clinical, microscopy is unreliable

Prevention

- TT– 2 doses at 1–2 m interval followed by 2 boosters after 1 year and 6 year
- Others – DPT, HTIG, Combined immunization

Clostridium botulinum

- Botulinum toxin: Most toxic known to human (MLD = 1 μg)
- BT – Blocks release of acetylcholine – flaccid paralysis
- 8 types (A–G), A, B and E: Human disease
- All except C2 are-neurotoxin, C2-enterotoxin
- Type C, D–bacteriophage coded

Types

- Food-borne botulism: Preformed toxin of Canned food
- Symptoms – Diplopia, dysphasia, dysarthria, **constipation**, symmetric descending paralysis, decreased Deep tendon reflexes
- Wound botulism
- Infant botulism (spore ingestion) – Floppy Child syndrome
- Ingestion of spores, toxin released inside, source-honey

Cl. difficile

- Pseudo membranous Colitis after antibiotics like Clindamycin, Ampicillin
- Rx – Metronidazole > Vancomycin

- Toxins: A (Enterotoxin) and B (Cytotoxin)
- Both glucosylate the GTP binding protein
- Toxin Can be demonstrated on Hep2 or ELISA

Listeria Monocytogenes

- L. monocytogens, L. ivanovii
- Gram positive coccobacilli
- Aerobe/Microaerophillic
- Tumbling motility/somersault motility with peritrichous flagella
- Beta hemolytic – Listeriolysin (Histolysin)
- CAMP test positive (Block hemolysis), catalase positive
- Motile at 25°C and Non motile at 37°C,
- Grow at 4°C (Cold enrichment)
- Move from cell to cell by means of **actin rockets**—filaments of actin polymerize and propel the bacteria through the membrane of one human cell and into another.
- Umbrella pattern turbidity in semisolid medium.
- Granulamatosis infantiseptica
- Meningitis and Meningoencephalitis in infants and elderly
- Conjunctivitis, Endocarditis and Abscess
- Treatment of invasive disease consists of trimethoprim-sulfamethoxazole, Combinations, such as ampicillin and gentamicin or ampicillin and trimethoprim-sulfamethoxazole can also be used. Listeria gastroenteritis typically does not require treatment.

Erysipelothrix

- Gram +ve bacilli, Non-motile, Non-sporing, long filaments and α hemolysis
- E.rhusiopatathiae produces H_2S
- 2 species: E.rhusiopatathiae and E.tonsillarum
  - Pathogenesis: causes erysipeloid skin lesion, Occupational hazard of fish handler and veterinary surgeons
  - E.rhusiopatathiae causes red disease.

Actinomycetes

- A. israeli
- Gram positive, anaerobic and Non-Acid fast filamentous bacteria
- Endogenous infection
- Cervicofacial – MC
- Thoracic
- Abdominal
- Pelvic
- Punch actinomycosis
- Lumpy Jaw in cattles
- Indurated swelling – Yellow sulphur granules – Sun Ray appearance
- Spidery molar tooth colonies, Fluffy ball appearance in liquid medium
- **Treatment:** Penicillin, Clindamycin, Metronidazole, Surgical removal

Nocardia

- Nocardia asteroids and Nocardia brasiliensis
- Discovered by Edmund Nocard
- Gram positive, aerobic and Acid fast filamentous bacteria

- Sabroud's dextrose agar, Nutrient agar – pigment production
- Paraffin bait technique – isolation from culture
- **Disease:** Nocardiosis – Pulmonary (HIV – Pneumonia)
- Cutaneous forms – Mycetoma
- **Diagnosis:** Specimen: Pus, sputum, granules
- Microscopy – Grams and Acid fast staining
- **Treatment:** Amikacin, Cefotaxime

Mycobacterium

Mycobacterium – Name was derived from their branching filamentous form, mould like pellicle in liquid media and cell wall contains mycolic acid.

M tuberculosis complex – include 4 species

- *M. tuberculosis*
- *M. bovis* (bovine tubercle bacillus)
- *M. africanum* (intermediate between M tuberculosis & M bovis)
- *M. microti* (vole tubercle bacillus)
- Generation time 14 – 15 hours
- Incubation – 6-8 week
- Acid fastness – due to presence of mycolic acid in cell wall
- Phage types in M.tuberculosis: Four types: A, B, C, I
  - Type A: worldwide distribution
  - Type I (intermediate between A and B): prevalence in india
- Type 33D: can lyse M.tuberculosis, M.bovis, M.africanum but not BCG.

M tuberculosis	M bovis
Shape – Curved, long, beaded, less uniformly stained	Straight, short, stout, uniformly stained
Rough, tough, buff colony	White, smooth, moist colony
Eugonic growth	Dysgonic growth
Glycerol enhances growth	Glycerol inhibits growth
Tween 80 hydrolysis – variable	Tween 80 hydrolysis – negative
Niacin and nitrate +ve, Neutral red (+)	Niacin, Nitrate, NR (-)
Pathogenic to G. pig, but Not to rabbit	Pathogenic to both
Obligate aerobe	Microaerophilic
Not susceptible	Susceptible to TCH (thiophen 2-carboxylic acid hydrazine)
Both are equally pathogenic to human	

Pathogenicity

- Escapes from macrophages by inhibiting acidification and Fusion of the phagolysozome and HSN IV.
- Virulence factor-lipoarabinomannan, HSP, Sulphalipids. **Not Cord factor**

Clinical Feature

Pulmonary TB

- Primary TB – Ghon focus: subpleural focus in lower lobe of lungs
- Ghon focus + hilar lymphadenopathy = **Primary complex**
- Ghon focus + Fibrosis and calcification = **Ranke complex**
- Simons focus = Post primary/secondary tuberculosis: upper lobe focus in adults, LN rare, necrosis, cavitations and hematogenous spread
- Assman focus = Infraclavicular lesion

Extrapulmonary TB

- MC site LN (cervical) > pleural TB,
- Skeletal TB, MC Site is spine (Pott's spine)
- TB meningitis (Tuberculoma)
- Gastrointestinal TB, MC site caecum, ileum
- TB pericarditis, MC cause of chronic constrictive pericarditis
- Scrofuloderma – skin lesion due to breakdown of underlying TB foci
- Lupus vulgaris – MC TB skin lesion, Female, face and neck, **apple jelly nodule**,
- Genitourinary tuberculosis: Sterile pyuria, sterility

Lab Diagnosis

Microscopy

(a) AFB smear

- Ziehl Neelsen staining – detection limit 10^4 bacilli/ml of sputum
- RNTCP recommended – 25% Con.Sulphuric acid as a decoloriser.
- Used for monitoring, assessing the severity
- Two sputum samples are collected – early morning and spot

(b) Fluorescent staining – Auramine/rhodamine – Used for rapid screening

Culture

- Detection limit 10 to 100 viable organism
- Digestion and Decontamination procedures for sputum
  - Petroff's method (4%Na OH)
  - N-acetyl-Lcysteine (NALC)
  - Oxalic acid

Solid Media

- Egg Based – Lowenstein Jensen , Petragnani, Dorset
- Blood Based Media – e.g. Tarshis
- Potato based media – Pawlosky medium
- Serum based media – Loffler's serum slope
- Agar Based Media: Middle brook 7H11 and 7H10

Liquid media – Middle brook 7H9, Dubos, Proskauer, Sula, Sauton

Used for drug susceptibility, Ag and vaccine preparation

Antimicrobial Sensitivity methods:

- Resistance ratio method
- Absolute concentration method
- Proportion method – RNTCP recommended

Automated culture method – detects growth faster

- BATEC – Radiometric detection of 14 CO_2 using 14 C labeled substrates (palmitic acid) – radioactive substance used
- BacT/ALERT – colorimetric detection of pH change by liberating CO_2 by Mtb
- ESP – detection of change in pressure by production of CO_2 by Mtb
- MGIT – Mycobacteria Growth Indicator Tube: Fluorescent based
- Septicheck system: (Biphasic) – Contain 3 solid media (modified LJ, middle brook 7H11 and chocolate agar)

Molecular methods: RT PCR – GeneXpert and Line Probe Assay

Rapid methods: SEROLOGY IS BANNED BY WHO (from September 2011)

PCR : detecting IS6110 gene

Diagnosis of Latent TB

Tuberculin test

- Mantoux – 0.1 ml PPD (5TU) given ID–
- Induration: >15 mm – always +ve, 10–14 mm – +ve/BCG/NTM, 6–9 mm – BCG/NTM, < 5 mm – always-ve
- Heaf test (multiple puncture), Tine test – disposable prong with dries PPD
- Indicator of
  - Active infection in infants
  - Prevalence of infection
  - Past exposure in adult

False Positive	BCG vaccination, atypical Mycobacterial infection
False Negative	Immunocompromised, Miliary TB, measles, Severe malnutrition,

- Repeated test at different site: false negative/equivocal reaction may turn Positive
- Uses:
  - To diagnose active TB infection
  - To select the population for BCG vaccination
  - Used as an indication for successful BCG vaccination
  - To measure the prevalence of infection in community

Vaccine

- BCG: Bacilli Calmette Guerin
- Live attenuated vaccine
- Route: Intradermal Left deltoid)
- 0–80% efficacy, immunity last for 10–15 years
- BCG strain: M bovis attenuated in glycerol bile potato medium
- Indication – newborn soon after birth, no need after 2 years
- C/I – infect with active HIV, AFB +ve mother, Generalized eczema skin lesions over the inoculum site)
- Benefits: 1. protect from TB
  - 2.50–80% protection from Leprosy and Leukemia
- Adverse effects:
  - Local: abscess, ulcer, keloid
  - Regional: lymphadenitis
  - Systemic: fever, otitis media, erythema nodosum
- Recombinant vaccines and DNA vaccines – under trial

Drug Resistance

- INH – KatG, Inh A, ahpC
- R – rpoB gene (RNA polymerase B)
- Z – Pnc A (Pyrazinamidase)
- E – emb A, B, C (Arabinosyl transferase)
- S – rpSL – ribosomal protein subunit 12
- MRDTB: Resistance to Rif + INH
- XDRTB: MDRTB + Quinolone + one among the second line injectables (amikacin/capreomycin/kanamycin)

Neonatal TB

- Before delivery: If mother chest X-ray and sputum AFB +ve: mother given ATT (HRE)
- After delivery: If mother chest X-ray and sputum AFB +ve then, mother to be given ATT (HRE) + baby (INH for 9–12 m) + screening of household contacts
- Separation from mother or withhold of breastfeeding is not advised.

NTM/MOTT/ Atypical Mycobacteria

NTM differentiated from MTB complex by:

- Resistance to both paranitrobenzoic acid and TCH
- Opportunistic pathogens in humans
- Aryl sufatase and Amidase test +ve, NNN test – negative
- Non pathogenic for guinea pig but pathogenic for mouse
- Resistant to ATT drugs
- Strong Catalase +ve
- Grow at 25°C and 44°C
- NTM strains should be incubated at 25°C, 37°C and 44°C.

Atypical (environmental) Mycobacteria

Runyon group	Nature	Species
I Photo chromogen	Pigmentation only in light	M kansasii, M marinum, M simiae
II Scoto chromogen	Pigmentations only in light and dark	M. scrofulaceum, M szulgai, S.gordonae
III Non-chromogen	No Pigmentation	MAC, M xenopi M. ulcerans
IV Rapid growers	Grows within a week	M chelonei, M fortuitum

Diseases Caused by Atypical Mycobacterium

Pulmonary infection like TB	*M kansasii, MAC, M simiae*
Swimming pool granuloma	*M marinum*
Chronic ulcers	*M marinum*
Buruli ulcer	*M. ulcerans*
Johne's Disease	*M. paratuberculosis*
Disseminated disease	*M avium intracellulare (MAC)*
Posttrauma abscess	*M chelonei, M fortuitum*
Lymphadenopathy	*M avium intracellulare, M. scrofulaceum*

- Tween 80 hydrolysis: *M kansasii, M marinum*

Mycobacterium Leprae

- Non-cultivable on artificial medium, generation time: 14 days
- Grows well in cooler part of body (skin, testes, peripheral nerve, anterior eye)
- 5% H_2SO_4 Acid Fast
- Intracellulare – as parallel cigar bundles of bacilli bound with lipid like glia (globi) present inside foamy macrophage (Virchow's or lepra cell)
- Bacteriological index – total no of leprae bacilli
- Morphological index – The % of solid uniformly stained live bacilli in tissues
- MI is more meaningful for assessing the progress of patients on chemotherapy

Epidemiology

- Transmission- nasal secretion
- IP – 2–5 year
- Not highly communicable, intimate and prolong contact necessary
- Most affected area – Southeast Asia and Brazil – In India (MC-Bihar > Orissa > UP)

Animal model

- Foot pad of mouse: Shepard model
- Nine banded armadillo is highly susceptible to leprosy, due to low body temperature.
- Other – Korean chipmunk, Indian pangolin, Slender loris, European hedgehog

Antigenic structure

- LAM – B (Lipoarabinomannan B) is highly immunogenic and used in serodiagnosis of leprosy.
- PGL – 1 (phenolic glycolipid 1)

Classification

- Ridley Jopling classification: TT, BT, BB, BL, LL
- Madrid classification: LL, TT, borderline/dimorphous, indeterminate
- Indian classification – Madrid + pure neuritic type

Lepromatous	Tuberculoid
AFB + ++ multibacillary	+/–
Skin lesion many, poorly marginated, multiple infiltrative nodules, Leonine facies	Few, sharply demarcated, symmetric
Nerve lesion-late	Early anesthetic skin lesion
Lepromin test Negative	Lepromin test Positive
Antibodies +++	Antibodies-
CMI low	Normal
Biological false positive in VDRL test	Not causing BFP in VDRL
Involve any organ – except CNS and lungs, also warm area of skin (axilla, groin, scalp)	MC nerve involved – Ulnar > post auricular, Medial popliteal Nerve is never involved
Type II lepra reaction Positive	Type II lepra reaction Negative
Granuloma formation: Absent	Granuloma formation: common
Bad prognosis	Good prognosis

Lepra Reaction Type I

- Hypersensitivity reaction Type IV,
- Associated with borderline
- If occurs before treatment – downgrading reaction occurs towards LL
- If occurs after treatment – upgrading reaction occurs towards TT
- MC feature – edema
- MC nerve – Ulnar N
- DOC – glucocorticoid > clofazemine, thalidomide

Type II Lepra Reaction

- Hypersensitivity reaction Type III,
- Associated with BL, LL
- Usually follows sulfonamide therapy, but may precede t/t
- MC – crop of painful erythematous papule
- Central cytokine involves – TNFα
- DOC – thalidomide, glucocorticoid, clofazemine and antipyretics

Type III – Lucio phenomenon – HSNIII, associated with diffuse LL, both thalidomide, glucocorticoid not affective

- Mycobacterium lepramurium – rat leprosy-grows on Ogawa's egg yolk medium

Anti-Leprosy Vaccines

- BCG
- Armadillo-derived killed *M leprae*
- BCG and Killed *M leprae*
- ICRC bacillus (Indian Cancer Research Center)

Lepromin reaction: 0.1 ml Lepromin given intradermal

- Early/Fernandez – 2–3 days – Induration like tuberculin (DTH) – indicates Inf. in past (not useful)
- Late/Mitsuda – 3–4 weeks: nodule, necrosis, ulcer

- Measure of CMI induced by injected Lepromin (doesn't say about the past exposure)
- Applications: 1. classifcation of leprosy lesions, 2. Assess prognosis, 3. Assess resistance to leprosy in individuals

Lab diagnosis

- Sample- minimum 4 skin (slit skin)+ ear lobule+ nasal mucosa – grading of smear is done based on MI.
- Acid fast staining with 5% sulfuric acid
- Mouse food pad inoculation
- Ab to PGL1

Treatment

- Paucibacillary – (I, TT, BT) – Rifampicin(monthly) + dapsone daily – for 6 months
- Multibacillary – (BB, BL, LL) – Rifampicin(monthly) + dapsone daily + clofazemine daily – till 2 years or smear –ve
- Single lesion – (ROM) – rifampicin + ofloxacin + minocycline – single dose

Bordetella

Bordet and Gengou bacillus

- B. pertussis
- B. parapertussis
- B. bronchiseptica (motile with peritrichous flagella)
- B. avium (motile with peritrichous flagella)

B. pertussis

- Gram negative coccobacilli
- Bipolar metachromatic granules
- Thumbprint appearance – smears
- Obligate aerobe
- Culture: Bordet Gengou – glycerol – potato extract defibrinated Blood Agar – bisected pearls or mercury drop colonies, Aluminum paint appearance
- Regan Lowe medium (transport medium), Lacey DFP medium
- Phase variation – I to IV, I – virulent (encapsulated), IV – Avirulent

Virulence factors

Pertussis toxin	Lymphocytosis
Agglutinogen	K ag and fimbriae, attachment
Filamentous hemagglutinin	Fusion of bacteria
Heat labile toxin,	Vasoconstriction and Inflammatory reaction
Tracheal Cytotoxin	Destruction of ciliated respiratory epithelium
Adenylate cyclase	Inhibition of chemotaxis, Phagocytosis, ↑cAMP
LPS	
Pertactin (OMP)	

Pathogenesis

- Source of infection – patient in early stage
- IP – 1–2 weeks
- No healthy carrier
- Secondary Attack rate of more than 90%
- Pertussis (100 day cough) – 3 stages
- Catarrhal – 1–2 weeks – cough fever, malaise, highly infectious, +ve culture and smear

- Paroxysmal – 2–4 weeks – whooping cough, vomiting, usually culture and smear negative
- Convalescent stage – decrease in the severity of the disease
- Piracy of adhesion due to PT and FHA
- **Specimen** – Cough plate method, West's post nasal swab, per nasal swab
- Whooping cough – other organisms – Mycoplasma, Adenovirus.
- **DOC** – Erythromycin
- Maternal antibody confer no immunity against pertussis
- **Vaccine** – DPT/DTaP

Brucella

- Bruce bacillus
- Mediterranean fever, Malta fever, Undulant fever, Brucellosis
- B. melitensis – Goat, (MCC: Undulant fever) (Most pathogenic)
- B. abortus: Cattle
- B. suis : Pig
- B. canis : Dog
- B. ovis : Sheep
- B. neotome : Rat
- Gram Negative coccobacilli, Obligate Aerobe (B. abortus – capnophilic)
- Bipolar staining
- Intracellular organisms affecting RES
- Transmitted by ingestion – Raw milk intake & contact with animal excreta
- IP: 10–30 days
- Antigens: M and A, M more in melitensis, A more in abortus
- Reference phage is Tbilisi phage

Diagnosis

- Culture: Blood (Castaneda method). and Bone Marrow culture is ideal
  - Growth improved by Erythritol
  - Catalase +ve, Ox +ve, Urease+ve
  - Strauss reaction seen in Male guinea pigs
- *Serology* – Standard Agglutination Test (SAT) for IgM detected using B. abortus Ag – Acute brucellosis
  - False Negative due to blocking Ab and prozone phenomenon. (removed by prior heating/Dilution with 4%Nacl/coomb test)
  - Blocking/Non agglutinable antibodies: IgG, IgA
  - False Positive: Cross reacting Ab in Yesinia. Cholera, Tularemia (removed by agglutination absorption test)
  - CFT and ELISA – for chronic infection
- Animals: Rose Bengal Card test, Milk Ring Test, Whey agglutination test
- Brucellin Skin test: past exposure to brucella.
- **Management:** Doxycycline and Rifampicin or streptomycin with tetracycline
  - Neuro and CVS brucellosis: Doxycycline, Rifampicin and Cotrimoxazole.
  - No human vaccine available,

Hemophilus

- Blood loving bacteria
- Gram negative coccobacillus, Pleomorphic
- Require accessory growth factors V (NAD) and X (Hemin)
- Killed by cold temperature (Refrigeration)

- First member – H. aegypticus by Robert Koch
  - H. influenzae (Pfeiffer's bacillus)
  - H. ducreyi, H. Parainfluenzae
  - H. aphrophilus, H. Paraaphrophilus

H. influenzae

- Capsulated, Exclusive human pathogen
- First organism complete genome is mapped
- Requires factor X and V
- Oxidase and Catalase positive
- Sheep blood agar – Satellitism (Due to Factor V)
- Chocolate agar, Levinthal's medium (iridescent colonies), Filde's agar
- 8 biotypes, Meningitis caused by Biotype I
- Capsular polysaccharide antigen – six types
- Meningitis by serotype B (Poly Ribitol Phosphate – PRP)
- Protective in nature
- Pilli – attachment, OMP – Invasion, IgA Protease
- Meningitis, Pneumonia, laryngoepiglottitis, otitis media
- Specimen: CSF, Blood
- Microscopy – Gram staining, Quellung Reaction,
- ELISA, CIEP, Latex agglutination, Coagglutination
- Cefotaxime, ceftazidime
- Hib – PRP vaccine, Effective children more than 2 years.

H. aegypticus

- Koch – Week's bacillus
- Pink eye
- Brazilian purpuric fever

H. ducreyi

- Soft sore – chancroid – Painful Lymph nodes
- School of Fish and Rail road appearance
- Bipolar staining
- Chocolate agar with 1% isovitalex, Vancomycin.

ENTEROBACTERIACEAE

Family Characteristics

Gram –ve bacilli	Non fastidious	Oxidase negative
Catalase +ve	Reduce Nitrate to Nitrite	Aerobic or facultative anaerobe
Mostly Motile	Glucose fermenters	

Classification: based on Lactose fermentation (pink colony on MacConkey)

Lactose fermenter – Escherichia, Klebsiella

Non Lactose fermenter – Shigella, Salmonella, Proteus, Yesinia

Late Lactose fermenter – Shigella sonnei

Escherichia Coli

- Motile by Peritrichous flagella, Fimbriated, some strains capsulated
- Hemolytic on blood agar

- Biochemical reactions: IMViC: ++– (indole +ve, methyl red +ve, VP –ve, citrate-ve)
- Antigenic structure
  - Somatic Ag O: Heat stable, LPS, 175 serotypes
  - Flagellar antigen H: heat labile, 75 types
  - Capsular Ag K: attachment, 103 types
  - Fimbrial Ag: F
- Normal colon commensal strains: early O groups (1, 2, 3, 4 etc);
- Enteropathogenic strains, "later" O groups (26, 55, 86, 111 etc.)

Virulence Factors

Surface antigens

- "O" antigen (LPS): endotoxic; inhibits phagocytosis
- K antigen; protects from phagocytosis
- Fimbriae: Mannose resistant in uropathogenic E.coli
- CFA (I–IV) colonizing factor antigens in ETEC
- "P" Fimbriae in uropathogenic E.coli

Toxins

- Hemolysin
- Enterotoxins – LT,ST,VT

LT (heat labile)	ST (heat stable)	VT
Resembles cholera toxin in structure- A,B5 A-↑ cAMP, B-binds GM1 ganglioside	↑ cGMP	Inhibit ribosome and protein synthesis
Plasmid coded	Plasmid coded	Phage coded
Ligated rabbit ileal loop test (18 hours) Adult rabbit skin test Steroid production in Y1 mouse adrenal cell culture Elongation in Chinese hamster ovary cells Latex Agglutination, ELISA, DNA probe-differentiate ST and LT	Ligated rabbit ileal loop test (6 hours) Intra gastric in infant mouse	Shiga like toxin or verocytotoxin Identical to Shiga toxin, but not neutralized by shiga antitoxin Cytotoxic to Vero cells

Clinical infections

- **UTI:** MC cause of UTI – E.coli
- "Early" O groups 1, 2, 4, 6, 7, 18, 75
- Cystitis and lower UTI – mostly due to ascending infection, lack K Ag
- Pyelonephritis and upper UTI- mostly due to descending infection, possess K antigen
- Virulence factor and Hemolysin, P fimbriae, mannose resistant fimbriae
- Kass' concept of "significant Bacteriuria – $>10^5$/ml of urine"

Diarrhea

EPEC

- Diarrhea in infants and children, sporadic diarrhea in adults
- Nontoxigenic, noninvasive
- Adhere to intestinal mucosa and disrupt brush border–attaching effacing lesions

ETEC

- Acute watery diarrhea in infants and adults: traveler's diarrhea
- Pathogenesis: LT, ST (plasmid mediated), Fimbrial proteins (Colonization Factor Ag), noninvasive
- Diagnosis – Typing, Demonstration of toxins

EIEC

- Dysentery like disease in all ages
- Pathogenesis: Epithelial cell invasion by virulence marker Ag(VMA)
- Called atypical E coli (lactose Nonfermenter), resembles Shigella flexneri
- Diagnosis – HeLa and Hep2 cell invasion assay, Sereny's test

EHEC (VTEC)

- O157 : H7 and bloody diarrhea in all ages
- Pathogenesis- VT1 and or VT2, Capillary microangiopathy, Causes HUS and HC
- Diagnosis: β-glucuronidase negative, do not ferment sorbitol and rhamonose)
- VT1 and VT2 probes, Demonstration of VT1 and VT2 in Vero cell lines

EAEC

- Persistent diarrhea especially in developing countries
- Most are "O" un-type able but "H" type able
- Aggregated in a "Stacked Brick" formation on Hep2 cell lines
- EAST 1 (enter aggregative heat stable Enterotoxins)

DAEC

- Diffusely adherent to epithelial cells

Treatment

- UTI – fluoroquinolones
- Diarrhea – fluid and electrolyte balance, No antibiotics

Klebsiella

- Capsulated, LF, Nonmotile, produce mucoid colonies,
- *K. pneumoniae* – Urease +ve – causes pneumonia, UTI, abdominal, wound and surgical site infection,
- Friedlander Pneumonia: Multiple abscess formation with severe bronchopneumonia and Chronic destructive lesions
- *K.ozaenae,* – causes ozaenae (foul smelling nasal discharge)
- *K.rhinoscleromatis* – causes rhinoscleroma

Proteus

- Pleomorphic
- Motile, NLF, **PPA+ve** (phenyl alanine deaminase +ve), urease+ve, H_2S+ve, fishy/seminal smell
- Swarming on blood agar
- Organism which swarm – Proteus, Clostridium tetani, V parahemolyticus, V alginolyticus, Serratia
- Diene's phenomenon – to know the relatedness between different strains of Proteus
- Forms struvite stone in bladder in alkaline urine
- Nonmotile strains of Proteus (Basis of Weil Felix) –OX 19, OX2: Pr vulgaris), OX K (Pr mirabalis)

Shigella

- Nonmotile, NLF, causes dysentery
- 4 Species – Sh. Dysenteriae, Sh. Flexneri, Sh. Boydii, Sh. sonnei
- All are Catalase +ve except – Sh. Dysenteriae type 1
- All are Mannitol fermenting except – Sh. Dysenteriae
- All are anerogenic except – Sh. Flexneri biotypes – New castle, Manchester
- All are lactose nonfermenter except – Sh. sonnei (late lactose fermenter)

- Ornithine decarboxylase+ve, ONPG+ve – Sh. Sonnei
- Most hardier – Sh. sonnei
- MC in world – Sh. sonnei
- MC in India – Sh. flexneri
- Serotyping – Sh. dysenteriae – 10, Sh. flexneri – 6+2, Sh. Boydii-18 Serotypes, Sh. Sonnei-1
- Colicin typing done for – Sh. Sonnei
- Sh. Dysenteriae; Ty 1 – Shiga bacillus: causes HUS, forms Shiga toxin
- Ty 2 – Schmitzi – indole +ve
- Ty 3–7 – Large and Sachs group

Pathogenicity

- Endotoxin – LPS – Diarrhea, ulcers
- Exotoxin – by Sh. Dys type – I
- Neurotoxin
- Enterotoxin – ShET 1 and 2
- Cytotoxin – acts on Vero cell lines: VT
- Invasive – VMA: virulence marker antigen
- Infective dose – 10 organisms: Salmonella and Vibrio – 10^6 10^8
- Complications: Reactive Arthritis, Toxic Neuritis, Intussusception, HUS, TPP

Diagnosis

- Specimen – mucus flakes of stool
- Transport media – Sach's buffered glycerol saline
- Selective media – DCA, XLD, SS, HE Agar
- Enrichment Broth – G.N broth, Selenite F broth
- Treatment : Ampicillin, Cotrimoxazole, ceftriaxone

Salmonella

- Motile by means of Peritrichous flagella- except *S. gallinarum pullorum*
- *Enteric fever* – S. Typhi, S Paratyphi A, B, C
- DNA hybridization study – 7 group: all pathogenic-gr1
- Kaufmann White Scheme – 2399 serotypes-based on – O, H, Vi Ag

H antigen

- Heat and alcohol labile. Formaldehyde stable, More immunogenic, appears late
- Reacts to H Ab – forms large loosed fluffy clumps
- Exist in two alternative phases – monophasic are S.Typhi , S. Paratyphi A

O Antigen

- Heat stable formaldehyde labile polysaccharide
- Less immunogenic, appears early, goes early
- Reacts to O Ab – forms granular chalky clumps

Vi Antigen

- Surface polysaccharide covering O Ag
- Heat labile when present it renders the bacterium inagglutinable by O antiserum
- Possessed by S Typhi and S. Paratyphi C, Citrobacter
- Poorly immunogenic, but protective
- Absence of Vi Ab – poor prognosis
- Persistence in coalescent stage – carier state
- Epidemiological typing of S.Typhi – by Vi specific bacteriophage

Lab diagnosis

- Enrichment media – Tetrathionate broth, Selenite F broth, GN broth
- Selective media – DCA, XLD, SS, HE Agar
- Need tryptophan as growth factor

Biochemical reaction

- H_2S +ve except strains of *S. paratyphi A*
- Citrate + except *S. Typhi, S. paratyphi A*
- Non Lactose Fermenting colonies on Macconkey agar
- Gas +ve except S.Typhi
- Indole, Urease –ve

Enteric fever

- Step ladder-fever, rose spots, coated tongue
- Culture – blood, faeces, urine, bone marrow, rose spots etc
- Demonstration of circulating Ag
- Demonstration of Antibodies in serum

Weekwise diagnosis of choice:

- 1st week – Gold standard – Duodenal content culture > BM culture>blood culture (best – combination of all 3)
- Blood culture sensitivity – 90% in 1st week, 75% in 2nd weeks, 60% in 3rd weeks
- Clot culture – higher sensitive than blood culture
- End of 1st week – widal
- 2nd and 3rd week – stool and urine culture
- Stool culture – +ve in both case/carrier, +ve even if after antibiotic start

Detection of Antibodies: Widal

- Antibodies – appear by end of 1st week, peaks 3rd week then falls
- 4 fold rise – highly significant between 1st and 3rd week
- Titre of 1 : 100 of O agglutinins : significant, 1 : 200 of H agglutinins – significant
- H agglutinins appears late and disappears late
- Rise in O indicate recent infection
- Anamnestic reaction – false +ve in unrelated infection
- Patients treated with chloramphenicol: false negative

Carriers

- Chronic carrier – >1 year, 3% in India,
- Mainly in biliary tract, gall bladder and rarely urinary tract
- Fecal carriers MC, but Urine carriers – more dangerous than fecal carriers
- Detected by – Vi agglutinins: 1 : 10 or fecal/urine culture

Treatment

- Ciprofloxacin, ceftriaxone, alternate: Azithromycin
- MDR S.Typhi – R/Ampicillin, cotrimoxazole, chloramphenicol
- DOC for MDRS – quinolone
- Nalidixic acid resistant S Typhi – DOC-higher or longer doses of cipro/ofloxacin

Nontyphoidal Salmonella

- Salmonella septicemia – typically caused by *S. cholerasuis*
- Salmonella gastroenteritis
- Zoonotic food poisoning
  - Food like meat, egg, milk
  - S. Typhimurium, commonest species: 30–40%
  - Others are S. Enteritidis, S Dublin, S. Newport, S. Heidelberg

Vaccine

- Parental – (a) killed WC 2 doses 6 weeks apart (b) TAB vaccine booster at 3 years, (c) purified Vi
- Oral –Ty 21a: Gal E mutant – 3 doses on alternate days

Vibrio

- All are halophilic except V.cholerae, mimicus
- Gram negative curved rods: comma shaped
- Single polar flagella: darting motility – Also by Campylobacter
- Oxidase positive, Non/late lactose fermenter but sucrose +ve
- Indole +ve and Nitrate +ve: cholera red reaction
- String test +ve with Sodium deoxycholate

Culture media

Transport media	Venkatraman Ramakrishnan (VR) medium Cary blair medium, Autoclaved sea water
Enrichment media	APW (alkaline peptone water) Monsurs taurocholate tellurite peptone water
Selective media	Bile salt agar (BSA) Monsurs gelatin taurocholate trypticase tellurite agar (GTTA) Thiosulphate citrate bile sucrose (TCBS) – yellow (V cholera), green (V parahemolyticus)

Vibrio cholerae
- 01 { Classical, El Tor } { Ogawa, Inaba, Hikojima }
- 02-0138 and 0140-0206 } Non-01 non-0139
- 0139 Bengal

- 1st – 6th pandemics- started in Indian subcontinent and due to classical Vibrio
- 7th pandemic – started in Indonesia, due to Eltor, less severe illness and more carriers
- Eltor is much hardier/resistant than classical, but produce less severe cholera, more carrier than cases
- MC Serotype – Ogawa > Inaba > hikojima: agglutinated by both antisera.

O139 Vibrio

- Bengal strains – 1st in 1992 from Chennai
- Capsulated, might be invasive
- Arise from Eltor by horizontal transfer
- Clinically and epidemiologically indistinguishable from O1
- Not neutralized by O1 antisera
- Currently – both O1 Eltor and O139 coexist.
- Classical Vibrio still reported from Bangladesh.

Biotypes of V. choleral O1	Classical strain	El Tor
Hemolysis	–	+
Chick erythrocyte agglutination	–	+
Polymyxin B (50u)	+	–
Group IV phage susceptibility	+	–
Eltor Phage V susceptibility	–	+
VP	–	+
CAMP	–	+

Cholera

- Occurs only in man: rice water stools
- Maintained in sea water in inter epidemics
- Acid labile, so require high infective dose of 106/ml
- TCP – toxin co-regulatory pilus – adhesion
- Cholera Toxin: CT – resembles heat labile toxin of E. coli: LT.
- CT – A unit – ADP ribosylation of G protein →↑ Adenyl cyclase →↑ cAMP, B unit – binds to ganglioside receptors
- LPS – has no role in pathogenesis

Treatment

- DOC in adult – Doxycycline: if resistant, then Quinolones
- DOC in children – cotrimoxazole
- DOC in pregnancy – Furazolidone
- DOC for chemoprophylaxis – Tetracycline
  - **Halophilic Vibrio** – High NaCl tolerance *V. parahemolyticus (7%), V. alginolyticus (10%), V. vulnificus (8%)*
- Causes food poisoning (sea fish), green colony on TCBS (sucrose –ve)
  - ***V. parahemolyticus*** – Shows kanagawa phenomenon on wagatsuma agar
- Capsulated, bipolar staining, Peritrichous flagella
  - ***V. vulnificus***- lactose fermentative
  - **Vaccines** – Killed whole organism and Oral Vaccine – Killed and Live

Yesinia pestis

- Gram negative
- Bipolar staining – Safety pin appearance – Wayson's/methylene blue stain/Giemsa stain
- Pleomorphic no growth at 22°C
- Optimum temp: 27°C but capsule grows best at 37°C
- Stalactite growth in broth
- Production of pigmented colonies on medium containing haemin
- **Antigenic structure**
  - F1envelope Ag – inhibits phagocytosis
  - V and W proteins – inhibits phagocytosis
  - Pesticin, fibrinolysin, coagulase
  - Plague Toxin – Endotoxin and murine toxin:both exo and endotoxin activity
  - Ability to synthesize purine

Plague

- Zoonotic in rodents
- **Urban plague:** Man and rodents, Bubonic septicemic, Pneumonic plague
- Wild or Sylvatic plague – Wild rodents squirrels
- Transmitted by Rat flea: *Xenospsylla cheopsis in North India and X. astia in south India*
- India – outbreak in 1994 in Beed-Latur district (Maharashtra), then in 2002 (Simla)
- IP – Bubonic and septicemic (2–7 days), Pneumonic (1–3 days)
- Mode – Bubonic – flea bite > contact with rodent,
- Pneumonic-Man-Man by Inhalational
- Highly infectious and fatal is Pneumonic plague

Lab diagnosis

- Smear from bubo-bipolar staining-methylene blue staining
- Fluorescent Ab staining

- Culture-blood and bubo aspirate
- Ab to F1 Ag – >128
- Treatment – Streptomycin: DOC
- Vaccine-Killed (Haffkine institute, Mumbai) – immunity lasts for 6 months and Live attenuated

Yersiniosis

- Yesinia infection other than Y. pestis
- *Y. pseudotuberculosis and Y. enterocolitica*
- Both motile at 25°C, not at 37°C
- Cold enrichment done for culture

Y. pseudotuberculosis

- Zoonosis
- grows at 22°C, urease +ve
- Mesenteric lymphadenitis, resembling appendicitis, Erythema nodosum

Y. enterocolitica

- Causes acute enterocolitis, terminal ileitis and lymphadenitis.
- Reactive arthritis in HLA B27 pts.

Pasteurella multocida

- Zoonotic, wound infection, flu like

Francisella tularensis

- Tularemia: a disease of rodents, originally described Tulare country, California
- Mode of transmission – Direct contact with rodents > Tick bite > Inhalation and Ingestion
- Capsulated, intracellular, Fastidious, filamentous, filterable and divide by budding and binary fission
- Francis blood dextrose cysteine agar
- Local ulceration with lymphadenitis, Typhoid like fever

Pseudomonas aeruginosa

MC nosocomial pathogen because

- Ubiquitous water and soil organism
- Wide temp range 5°C to 42°C
- Produces biofilm – glycocalyx
- Resistant to disinfectant, antiseptics and multidrug resistance due to R-plasmids

Virulence factor

- Exotoxin A – NADase like, inhibiting protein synthesis
- Exotoxin S – Ribosylation of GTP binding protein
- Others – Capsule/slime layer, Exotoxin S, U, Y, protease, elastase, Hemolysin, Endotoxin

Distinguishing Characteristics

- Oxidase – positive, non-fermenting
- Motile with polar flagella
- Pigments: Pyocyanin (blue–green) by P. aeruginosa and Fluorescein (greenish yellow) – by all spp
- Pigmentation is Produced in King's media
- Selective media – cetrimide agar
- Grape – like fruity odor
- Slime layer – alginate
- Non-lactose fermenting colonies on MacConkey

Infections

- Burn patients infection
- Malignant otitis media, Shanghai fever
- Cellulitis: blue – green pus
- Neutropenic patients – causes Pneumonia and septicemia
- Chronic Granulomatous Disease (CGD)
- Ecthyma gangrenosum
- UTI in Catheterized patients
- Cystic fibrosis – by high slime producing strains (alginate)

AntiPseudomonal drugs

Penicillin – Piperacillin, Mezlocillin, Ticarcillin Cephalosporin – Ceftazidime, cefoperazone, cefipime Carbapenems – imipenem, meropenem Monobactam – Aztreonam	Aminoglycoside – Tobra, Genta, Amikacin Quinolone – Cipro, Levofloxacin Other – PolymyxinB, Colistin

Burkholderia

- GNB, NF, OX +ve, Resistant to polymyxinB,
- Bipolar stained
- Zoonotic, agent of bioterrorism,
- Occupational spread, t/t– ceftazidime/Carbapenems

B. pseudomallei

- Causative agent of *melidiosis* – Glanders like disease
- Motile
- Zoonotic – rodents
- Humans – Pulmonary infections like TB, lymphadenopathy

Burkholderia mallei

- Non-motile
- Zoonotic – horse
- Mallein test – like tuberculin test
- Causes: Glanders, nodules in Respiratory system and Farcy-skin with prominent lymphatics underneath
- Strauss reaction – intraperitoneal injection in male guinea pig causes – testicular swelling

HACEK group of organisms

- Fastidious slow growing bacteria, normal or oral cavity, causes endocarditis
  - **H**aemophillus species – parainfluenzae, aprophilus, paraaprophilus
  - **A**ctinobacillus actinomycetemcomitans.
  - **C**ardiobacterium hominis,
  - **E**ikenella corrodens – corrodes on blood agar
  - **K**ingella kingae

Campylobacter Jejuni

- Kampylos – Curved/Spiral GN, Gullwing shaped
- Unsheathed single polar flagellum
- Darting motility
- Microaerophilic – 5% O_2, 85% N_2, 10% CO_2
- Thermophilic – 42°C
- Mode-ingestion of contaminated food-raw milk

- Mechanism of diarrhea – Heat labile Enterotoxin: LT resembling CT + Invasion like Shigella + Cytotoxin
- Culture – Transport: Cary Blair medium
- Selective medium: Skirrow's, Campy BAP, Butzler, charcoal based media, Blaser's and Preston medium

Helicobacter Pylori

- H. pylori, H. cinaedi, Curved rod, motile unipolar tuft of lophotrichous flagella
- Microaerophilic and abundant production of urease
- MC in childhood, low socioeconomic status, crowding

Disease

- Acute gastritis: Antrum MC
- Peptic ulcer disease – 80% duodenal ulcer and 60% gastric ulcer
- Chronic atrophic gastritis, autoimmune gastritis
- Adenocarcinoma of stomach and esophagus and MALTomas
- Group I carcinogen (More potent carcinogen)
- Virulence – Cytotoxin associated gene (cag), Vacuolated cytotoxin gene (vag), urease
- H. cinaedi – MC in HIV positive homosexuals, Isolated from rectal swabs

Diagnosis

Invasive

- Warthin starry silver staining
- Culture – Skirrow's Campylobacter medium and Chocolate agar
- Biopsy urease test (at least 3 biopsy) – most sensitive, quick, simple
- PCR

Noninvasive

- Urea breath test – Follow up, Negative after treatment
- Serology: ELISA, Ag detection in stool

Treatment

- OCM, OCA, OBTM regimens

Legionella

- Pleomorphic Poorly Gram negative bacilli
- Silver impregnation staining
- Buffred Charcoal Yeast Extract Medium (BCYE medium)
  - Cut glass apperance
  - Fastidious requiring iron and cysteine
- **Reservoir** – Aerosols from A/C
  - Transmission – Inhalation of Aerosols from contaminated A/C
  - No human to human transmission
  - Risk Factors – Smokers, alcohol, Immunosuppression, hairy cell leukemia
- **Pathogenesis**
  - Facultative intracellular pathogen and Endotoxin, Coiling phagocytosis
- **Legionnaires' disease** (Atypical/walking Pneumonia) – CAP, Diarrhea, encephalitis, MC extra pulmonary site – heart (myocarditis and pericarditis)
- Numerous PMN, but no organism in sputum
- **Pontiac Fever** – Non fatal flu like symptoms

- **Diagnosis**: DFA (Direct Fluorescent Antibody) on biopsy
  - Fourfold increase in antibody
  - MC – L. pneumophila serogroup – **SG1**
- L. micdadei – Acid-fast (**Pittsburgh pneumonia agent**)
- Latex agglutination test
- Treatment – Ciprofloxaxin, Tetracycline

Treponema pallidum

- Spiral shaped Organism
- Medically Import Spirochetes
  - Treponema
  - Leptospira
  - Borrelia
- Discovered by Fritz Schaudinn and Erich Hoffmann
  - *Treponema pallidum* – Syphilis
  - *Treponema pertenue* – Yaws
  - *Treponema carateum* – Pinta
- Motile and Presence of endoflagella (axial filaments)
- Not cultivable in Artificial media
- Pathogenic – Nicholas strain – Rabbit testicular passage
- Nonpathogenic – Reiter strain – Smith – Nogutchi's Medium
- Solely Human pathogen and No reservoirs

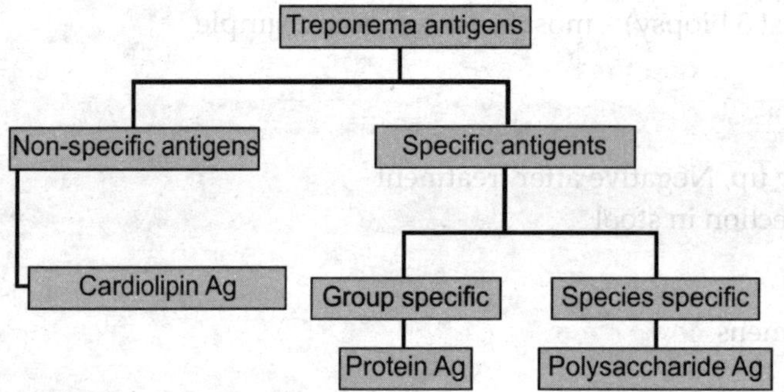

- Nospecific Virulence factors
- Inflammatory response to immune complexes
- Uses Host Fibrinectin for latency

Clinical features

Primary syphilis	Secondary syphilis	Tertiary syphilis
IP: 10 to 90 days Painless, Indurated Hard chancre (Huntarian chancre) Involvement of local lymph nodes Resolves spontaneously: 3–6 weeks Lesion contains organisms	2 to 8 weeks after primary syphilis Lymphadenopathy and maculopapular rash Condyloma latum Spirochetes are Abundant in lesions Lesions resolve but disease continues in one third of patients	5 to 20 years after primary syphilis Multisystem organ involvement CNS – Neurosyphilis Chronic meningitis – degenerative changes Psychosis, GPI Tabes dorsalis Cardiovascular syphilis – Aortitis leads to aneurysm Gummas – Destructive, localized granulomas Bone, skin etc

- Latent syphilis
  - No lesions, Early latency and Late latency
  - Serology is the only method for diagnosis

- Congenital syphilis
  - Bone and teeth deformities
  - Saddle nose
  - Saber shins
  - Clutton's joints
  - Hutchinson's teeth
  - Mulberry molars

Laboratory diagnosis

- Microscopy – Specimens
  - Exudate from lesion, Lymph node aspirate and Biopsy
  - Dark field microscopy
  - Staining – Fontana – Fluids and LevidiT – Tissues

Nonspecific tests Standard tests of syphilis (STS)	Specific tests	
	Pathogenic	Nonpathogenic
VDRL, RPR, Khan, Wasserman Toluidine red unheated serum test (TRUST)	FTA-Ads, TPA (K) TPHA, EIA (E) TPI (L)	RPCFT

K – killed, L – live, E – Extract

Reagin antibody tests: VDRL – Lecithin and RPR – Cardiolipin

- Ideal Monitoring tool
- Nonspecific and more Biological false positive
- PCR

Interpretation of Syphilis Serological tests

Non-treponemal tests (RPR/VDRL)	Treponemal tests (TPHA/FTA-ADS)	Possible explanation
Positive	Positive	Syphilis – Recent or previous Yaws or pinta
Positive	Negative	No syphilis, False positive
Negative	Positive	Exposure to Syphilis, Non Treponemal infections
Negative	Negative	No syphilis or incubation period

Penicillin is DOC, Allergic to penicillin Doxycycline

Leptospira

- Leptospira – obligate aerobes
  - *L. interrogans* – parasitic strains – >23 serogroup and >230 serovars
  - *L. biflexa* – free living saprophytic strains
- Zoonotic (rat)
- Transmission- direct contact with animal(occupational)
- India- MC in TN, Andaman, Kerala
- Clinical Stage- Anicteric (90%), Icteric – (10%) – Weil's disease (hepatorenal syndrome).
- Both type can be divided into – septicemic (1st week) or immune stage (meningitis, uveitis, rash) – after 2nd week

Diagnosis

- Septicemic stage (blood/csf), immune stage (urine)
- Microscopy – dark field- detection limit 10^4/ml, phase contrast, silver impregnation
- **Culture** – EMJH, Fletcher, Korthoff Medium
- Incubation at 28–30C for 13 weeks, tedious, Sunless than serology
- **Serology** – Genus specific – CFT, ELISA, Microscopic aggl test (MAT) – gold standard (Sero group and serovar specific)

Borrelia

Relapsing fever

- B. recurrentis – Epidemic or louse borne relapsing fever – Exclusively human
- B. duttoni, B. hermesii – Endemic or tick borne relapsing fever – Rodents
- Antigenic variation leads to relapse

Lab diagnosis

- Microscopic examination – Blood – wet film under dark ground or phase contrast microscope
- Giemsa and Leishman stain
- Animal inoculation mice – intra peritoneal infection
- ELISA, PCR
- OXK may be positive

Lyme's disease

- B. burgdorferi – Tick borne
- Erythema chronicum migrans, dissemination, persistent infection

Lab diagnosis

- Isolation from skin lesions or blood – modified Kelley's medium
- Microscopic detection – Dark ground, phase contrasts, Immunofluorescence, silver staining
- Antigen in urine

Borrelia vincentii

- Commensal of mouth
- Vincent's angina – ulcerative gingivostomatitis (predisposing conditions such as malnutrition, viral infection)
- Often associated with fusiform bacillus (Fusobacterium fusiformis)

Chlamydia

- Gram Negative, Obligate intracellular bacilli.
- Lack Peptidoglycan and Ability to produce ATP – Energy parasite
- Possess RNA and DNA.
- Multiply in the host cell cytoplasm – formation of inclusion bodies
- Elementary body – Extracellular – infectious, RNA = DNA
- Reticulate body – Intracellular – replicative, RNA > DNA

Agent	Character	Serotype	Disease
C. trachomatis	Compact inclusions with glycogen matrix Natural parasite of human Leave the host cell with a scar	Biovar TRIC – A, B, Ba, C	Trachoma
		Biovar TRIC – D-K	Inclusion conjunctivitis infant pneumonia Genital chlamydiasis
		Biovar LGV – L1, L2, L3	LGV
Chlamydaphila psittaci	Natural parasite of birds Leave host cell by lysis	Many	Psittacosis (Pneumonia) Inhalational route
Chlamydaphila pneumoniae TWAR agent	Exclusively human pathogen	One serotype	Atypical pneumonia atherosclerosis, asthma, sarcoidosis

- Generation time 24–48 hours and division by binary fission

Antigen

- Genus specific: LPS : CFT
- Species specific: Envelope Ag
- Serovar specific: Major OMP

Diagnosis

- **Specimen:** infected ocular and genital specimens
- **Microscopy:** Stain by Casteneda, Macchiavello, Giminez, Lugol's Iodine (only for C.trachomatis), IF using monoclonal About both inclusion and elementary body
- **Culture:** Mice (infective by only C.psittaci and LGV), Yolk sac, McCoy Cells and HeLa, Hep2 for *C.pneumoniae*
- **Serology:** MicroIF, CFT, ELISA
- **PCR**

Treatment

- C. trachomatis – Azithromycin
- C. psittaci – Tetracycline
- C. pneumoniae – Erythromycin and Tetracycline

C.trachomatis

- MC cause of STD worldwide
- MC cause of ophthalmic neonatorum, NGU, epididymitis
- NGU complications – Reiter syndrome (conjunctivitis/urethritis/polyarthritis)
- Fitz Hugh Curtis syndrome – perihepatitis
- Inclusion conjunctivitis – neonate (inclusion blenorrhea), adult (swimming pool conjunctivitis)

Trachoma

- Chronic conjunctivitis – follicular hypertrophy, papillary hyperplasia, pannus, cicatrization
- Inclusion body seen only in established trachoma I–IV

LGV

- MC by L2 > L1, L3
- LGV serovars are more inversive than others
- MC LN involved – pararectal and intrapelvic nodes
- Pain less ulcer + painful LN
- Esthiomone (elephantiasis of vulva) rectal stricture, hemorrhagic proctitis
- Skin test: Frie's test

Inclusion body

Psittacosis	Levinthal Colle Lille body
LGV	Miyagawa corpuscle
Trachoma	Halbersteater Prowazeki body

Nongonococcal Urethritis: NGU

- Chlamydia trachomatis
- Mycoplasma genitalium and hominis
- Ureoplasma urealyticum
- Trichomonas vaginalis
- Candida albicans
- Herpes virus
- Cytomegaloviru

Mycoplasma

- Mycoplasma and Ureaplasma
- Mycoplasma pneumoniae
- Very small, filterable, Flagella, pili–absent but some strains show gliding mobility
- No cell wall – Highly Pleomorphic, Coccoid and filaments, L forms
- Need cholesterol as a growth factor
- Gliding motility with fimbriae
- Dienes or Giemsa stain, Poorly Gram Negative
- Mycoplasma pneumoniae: Primary Atypical Pneumonia (PAP)/Walking pneumonia
- Ureoplasma urealyticum: NGU, non chlamydial urethritis, epididymitis, Vaginitis and cervicitis
- Culture medium: PPLO broth (bovine heart infusion broth, 20% horse serum, 10% fresh yeast extract) – Fried Egg colony

Lab Diagnosis

- **Sample** – Throat swab, Respiratory secretions, Sputum, BAL
- Culture – PPLO broth, Tetrazolium reduction test
- Serological tests – **Detection of antigen**
  - Immunofluorescence
  - HAI
  - PCR

Detection of antibody

- Cold agglutinins
- Streptococcus MG test
- CFT (Complement Fixation Test)
- ELISA for IgM, IgG and IgA

DOC: Erythromycin

Rickettsiaceae

- Obligate intracellular pathogen transmitted by arthropod
- Not cultivable in cell free media – except Bartonella
- Most severe – Rocky mountain spotted fever
- Mild – R pox, Eschar Seen in Scrub typhus
- Boutonneuse fever, Vesicular/vericelliform rash – Rickettsial pox
- Transovarial transmission occurs only in tick – i.e. Rocky Mountain spotted fever, Indian tick typhus

Group	Species	Disease	Vector
Typhus group	R. prowazekii	Epidemic typhus and Brill Zinsser	Louse
	R. typhi	Endemic typhus	Flea
Spotted fever group	R. rickettsii	Rocky mountain spotted fever	Tick
	R. conori	Indian tick typhus	Tick
	R. akari	Rickettsial pox	Mite (gamasid)
Scrub typhus	O. tsutsugumashi	Scrub typhus	Mite (trombiculid)

Lab diagnosis

- Isolation – in lab animals, hens egg and cell cultures
- Direct detection of the organisms and their antigens – giminez, Machiavello and Giemsa stain

Neil Mooser Reaction

- Male guinea pig intraperitoneal inoculation
- Rocky mountain spotted fever – scrotal necrosis
- Epidemic typhus – only fever, but negative tunica reaction
- R.typhi/conori/akari – fever and positive tunica reaction (testicular inflammation)

Serology - Weil Felix reaction

- Cross reacting alkali stable polysaccharide Ag in nonmotile strains of P.vulgaris (OX2, X19) and P. mirabilis (OXK)
- False +ve if proteus infection present
- Rise in titre more meaningful

Weil Felix	OX2	OX19	OXK
Epidemic typhus	+	++++	–
Endemic Typhus	+	++++	–
RMS Fever	+ to ++++	++++	–
Scrub typhus	–	–	+++

Scrub typhus

- Mite and chigger borne
- Affect rats in deserts, rain forest
- Eschar at site, rash lymphadenopathy, high OXK titre in Weil Felix test.

Coxiella Burnetii

- It survives holders method of pasteurization of milk
- Transmitted without arthropod (respiratory mode)
- No skin rash in Q fever.
- Zoonotic (wild animal)
- Produces interstitial pneumonia, shows latency

Ehrlichia

- Multiply with in membrane bound vacuoles in phagocytes (morula)
- *E sennetsu* – illness resembling Glandular fever; (lymphoid hyperplasia and atypical lymphocytosis)
- *E. chaffeensis* – Infects monocytes and produce febrile illness. Transmitted by ticks
- *E.* phagocytophila – infects granulocytes, Transmitted by ticks

Bartonella

- Involve RBC
- *B. bacilliformis* – Oroya fever, verruga peruana, Carrion's disease
- *B. quintana* – trench fever, louse borne
- *B. hensalae* – cat scratch diseases, Lymphadenopathy, Bacillary angiomatosis

Rat Bite Fever

- Streptobacillary moniliformis and Spirillum minus

Streptobacillary moniliformis:

- Gram negative, highly Pleomorphic bacillus
- String of bead appearance, nonmotile, fastidious
- Rat bite fever
- Haverhill fever – Erythema arthriticum epidemicum
- Lab diagnosis – Grow on culture media containing blood serum or ascitic fluid
- L forms – fried egg appearance

Spirillum minus – motile, causes Sudoku fever and non cultivable.

Gardnerella vaginalis

- Bacterial vaginosis,
- Gram variable – Gram Negative coccobacilli
- Other organisms implicated in BV – *Mycoplasma, Mobilincus, Prevotella,* Peptostreptococcus.
- BV is characterized by thin profuse vaginal discharge, pH > 4.5, fishy odor and Clue cells
- Nugent scoring used for diagnosis

VIROLOGY

General Properties of Virus

Virus Vs Bacteria:

Property	Virus	Bacteria
Nucleic acid	DNA or RNA	Both
Binary fission	No	Yes
Cellular organelle	Absent	Present
Cellular organization	No	Present
Location	Intracellular	Intra/Extra cellular
Resistant to	Antibiotics (exception- Rifampicin to Pox virus)	Sensitive
Culture in artificial media	No	Can be grown (except Rickettsia Chlamydia)
Ribosome	Absent	Present

Size of viruses

- Size – determines by
  - Ultrafiltration in gradcol membrane of graded porosity
  - Ultracentrifugation
  - Electron microscopy
- Largest – Pox virus (300 nm) – Possess elementary body (Lateral body)
- Smallest – Parvo virus (20 nm)

Shape of viruses

- Structure – consists of nucleocapsid (Nucleic acid and protein layer capsid)
- Capsid is made up capsomere units
- Most of the viruses are roughly spherical except:
  - Rabies – Bullet
  - Pox virus – Brick
  - Ebola virus – Filamentous
  - Tobaco mosaic virus – Rod
  - Space vehicle – Adenovirus

Nucleic acid

- Made up either DNA or RNA
- DNA viruses – Herpes, HBV, Adeno, Papova, Parvo and Pox (HHAPPP)
- RNA viruses
- All the RNA viruses are single stranded except Reoviruses (double stranded RNA)
- All the DNA viruses are double stranded except Parvoviruses (single stranded RNA)

Symmetry

- Icosahedral – All DNA viruses except Pox virus and most of the RNA viruses
- Helical – Few RNA viruses (Bunya, Myxo, Rhabdo, Filoviridae)
- Pox – complex symmetry

Envelop

Enveloped Virus

- Made up lipoprotein subunits called peplomere
- Lipid part is host cell membrane derived and protein part is virus derived,
- Envelop provides chemical, physical and biological properties to the cell.
- Ether sensitive, heat labile, pleomorphic

Non-Enveloped virus:

- Ether resistant, heat stable and non-pleomorphic
- DNA-Parvo, Adeno, Papova **(PAP)**
- RNA-Picorna, Astrovirus, Calcivirus, Reovirus **(PARC)**

Segmented RNA (BORA)

- Bunya (4 segments)
- Orthomyxovirus (8 segments)
- Rota (10 segments)
- Arena (2 segments)

Positive sense virus

- Picorna virus
- Toga virus
- Calci virus
- Corona virus
- Filovirus

Replication

- **Adsorption**
  - Most specific step requires respective receptors
  - If bypassed then any virus can attack any cell.
- **Penetration**
- **Uncoating**
- **Biosynthesis**
- DNA Viruses – Replicates in nucleus (except-Pox)
- RNA Virus – Replicates in Cytoplasm (except Myxo and Retro virus)
- Viral protein is synthesized only in cytoplasm
- Positive sense RNA virus:
  - Viral RNA itself acts as mRNA
  - Infectious and translated directly to protein
- Negative Sense RNA virus:
  - Have polarity opposite to mRNA
  - Noninfectious and possess their own RNA polymerase for transcription to form mRNA.
  - E.g. Myxo, Rabies
- Retroviruses
  - Viral reverse transcriptase converts viral ssRNA to dsDNA
  - Then dsDNA integrates with host DNA.
- Maturation
- Assembly
- Release
  - Bacteriophage – by host cell lysis
  - Animal virus – usually without lysis (Myxo – by budding)
  - Exception – Picorna- by host cell lysis

Viral Cultivation

Animal inoculation

- Coxsackievirus – Infant suckling Mice – Cox A-flaccid paralysis, Cox B-spastic paralysis
- Arbovirus

Egg inoculation

- Chorioamniotic membrane – Produce pocks. E.g. Vaccinia, Variola, HSV
- Yolk sac – Arbovirus, chlamydia, Rickettsia
- Amniotic membrane – Influenza culture
- Allantoic cavity – vaccine preparation for Influenza, Yellow(17D), Rabies (Flury)

Tissue culture

- **Organ culture** – tracheal ring (Corona virus)
- **Explant culture** – adenoid (Adeno virus)

Cell line:

- **Primary cell line** – Undergo limited division (5–10), diploid karyosome
  E.g. Rhesus kidney cell line, Human amniotic cell line, chick embryo fibroblast
- **Secondary cell line** – Undergo moderate cell division(10–50), diploid karyosome, E.g. Human fibroblast used for CMV
- **Continuous cell line** – Tumour cell lines, indefinite divisions, haploid karyosome. Not suitable for vaccines, E.g.- HeLa, Hep2, BHK
- **Cytopathic effect**
  - Crenation of cells and degeneration of entire cell sheet: Enterovirus
  - Syncytium formation: Measles virus, RSV, Parainfluenza, HIV
  - Large granular clumps like grapes: Adenovirus
  - Cytoplasmic vacuolation – SV40
  - Diffuse roundening of cells – Herpes
  - Large lysis: Polio virus

Inclusion Bodies

Intracytoplasmic

- Negri body – Rabies
- Guarnieri body – Vaccinia,
- Paschen body – Variola
- Bollinger body – Fowl pox
- Molluscum body – Molluscum contagiosum virus

Intranuclear

- Cowdry A (HAY) – Herpes (Lipschultz body), Yellow fever (Torres body)
- Cowdry B (BAP) – Adeno, Polio
- Both – Measles, CMV

Viral Interference

- When two viruses infect a cell, one inhibits the multiplication of the other virus, seen in Rubella and Polio

Viral Hemagglutination

- Myxovirus, Rabies, Arbo, Pox
- Elution (Neuraminidase) – only in Myxovirus (except RSV and Measles)
- Hemadsorption – RBC adsorbed onto virus infected cell surface
- Mumps, Influenza, Parainfluenza

Transfer Through Placenta

- Coxsackie B
- Hepatitis B, C
- Parvo B19
- HIV
- Measles, Mumps
- Cytomegalovirus and Herpes
- Rubella

Viral Vaccine

Inactivated Vaccine

- Salk polio – formalinized MKD
- Influenza
- Japanese B – (Nakayama) formalinized mouse brain
- Hepatitis B (subunit –HBsAg cloned in yeast)
- Rabies – BPL, Semple and non neural (PVC, PCEC, HDC)

Live Vaccine

- Sabin Polio – Avirulent MKD
- Influenza – egg
- Japanese B – (14–14–2)
- MMR
- Yellow (17D) – chick embryo
- Smallpox
- Oka Strain – Varicella
- Towne and AD – CMV
- Jerryl Lynn – Mumps
- Edmonston – Zagreb – Measles
- RA 27/3 – Rubella

Herpes

HSV 1 and 2 – Features

- HSV 1: lesion around mouth,
- HSV 2: lesion around genital infection,
- Transmission – HSV1 – contact droplet inhalation, HSV2 – sexual mode
- HSV 2 larger pocks in Chick embryo
- HSV 2 replicates well Chick embryo fibroblast
- HSV 2 more temperature sensitive
- HSV 2- more neurovirulent
- HSV 2 more drug resistance
- Antigen detection and PCR also can differentiate.

Characters	Alpha	Beta	Gamma
Replicative cycle	Fast (12–18 hours)	Slow (>24 hours)	Slow
Host range	Wide	Narrow	Narrow
Latency	Sensory ganglia	Salivary gland	Lymphoid tissue.
Cytopathology	Rapid, Cytolytic	Slow, Cytomegaly	Lympho-proliferative
Virus	HSV 1, 2, VZV	CMV, HHV 6, 7	EBV, HHV 8
Latency	Neuron	CMV-Secretory glands, kidney, organs and tissues HHV 6, 7-Lymphoid tissue	Lymphoid tissue

Clinical Feature

Mucosal

- MC site – buccal mucosa
- Most frequent primary lesion – gingivostomatitis, pharyngitis
- Most frequent recurrent lesion – herpes labialis
- MC cause of ulcerative stomatitis – HSV
- Secondary bacterial infection is common with—Streptococcus, Pneumococcus

CNS

- MC sporadic acute viral encephalitis
- Molaret meningitis (Aseptic meningitis)
- MC site – temporal lobe
- Most imp diagnosis – brain biopsy
- Transverse myeltis, GBS

Cutaneous

- MC site – Face
- Herpetic whitlow – seen in doctor, nurse
- Erythema multiforme – MC cause – HSV

Ophthalmic

- Acute keratoconjunctivitis
- Dendritic ulcer – Topical acyclovir, IFN

Genital

- HSV II MC than HSV I

Diagnosis

- TZANCK smear of keratinocyte
- Toluidine blue staining of base of vesicle reveals multinucleated giant cell with faceted nuclei & homogenously stained ground glass appearance.
- Type A intranuclear inclusion body in Giemsa stain
- Isolation – CAM, primary human kidney cell line

Varicella Zoster

- MC site – Spinal cord-D3 to L2 (chickenpox) or Trigeminal N-Ophthalmic branch (Zoster)
- Contact with either chickenpox or zoster patient leads to only chickenpox but not zoster.
- One attack gives lifelong immunity
- Source-infected individuals
- Portal of entry-respiratory tract or conjunctiva
- Incubation period – 2 weeks
- Infectious during initial stage – 2 days before and 5 days after the onset of rash.
- Rash- usually start in trunk, rapid evolution, appears in crops, centripetal distribution
- Chicken pox is a disease of childhood
- When occur in adult, it is more severe with bullous and hemorrhagic rash
- Complication:
  - Varicella pneumonia
  - Myocarditis, nephritis, encephalitis, cerebellar ataxia
  - Reye's syndrome – fatty liver after salicylate
- Vaccine – Oka strain (live attenuated) and VZIG

- Treatment- acyclovir, Steroid is contraindicated.
- Zoster:
  - Reactivation of latent virus
  - Trigeminal N (Ophthalmic branch)
  - Segmented and unilateral.
  - Affect Geniculate ganglia – **Ramsay Hunt syndrome** characterized by
  - Tetrad – Facial Nerve palsy + vesicle on tympanic membrane, External auditory meatus and tongue

Chickenpox in pregnancy:

- For mother – high risk for pneumonia
- 1st half of pregnancy – asymptomatic
- Fetal varicella syndrome – skin lesion, limb hypoplasia, choriodoretinitis and CNS defects
- Infection near delivery – congenital/neonatal Varicella
- If mother gets infection >1 week before delivery – then baby is mostly asymptomatic due to maternal antibody

CMV

- Largest member of Herpes virus family
- Enlargement of the virus infected cell
- Intranuclear and cytoplasmic inclusion body – owl's eye
- Spread slowly and requires close contact
- Route – via secretions, sexual, Blood transfusion
- Exhibit strict host specificity

Congenital – Cytomegalic inclusion disease

- Hepatosplenomegaly
- Microcephaly,
- Mental retardation
- 3Cs – chorioretinitis, cerebral calcification, convulsion
- Infants are highly infectious
- Transmit the virus in urine for 3–5 year

Acquired

- Mononucleosis like syndrome:
  - Occurs in adult (following Blood Transfusion/Post kidney transplant)
  - Atypical lymphocytosis seen
  - Paul Bunnel test is negative
- Post kidney transplant infection

Lab diagnosis

- Specimen – urine, saliva, cervix secretion, semen
- Culture – human fibroblast cell line,
- Growth occurs in 2–3 weeks, can be improved by shell vial technique
- IgM or fourfold rise of IgG
- pp65 antigenemia
- DNA PCR
- Transplacental CMV infection:
  - At Birth – IgG antibody +ve, IgM just appearing
  - At 1month – IgG antibody +ve, IgM peak
- Post natal CMV infection:
  - Birth – IgG antibody +ve, IgM –ve
  - 1 month – IgG antibody +ve, IgM just appearing
  - 3 month – IgG+, IgM peak

Treatment

- Gancyclovir, Foscarnet, Valgancyclovir, Cidofovir,

EBV

- Attach to CD21/CR2 receptor on B cell
- But atypical lymphocytosis occurs with T cell
- B cell become immortalized, polyclonally activated leading to hypergammaglobulinemia
- Not highly contagious, Spread slowly
- Intimate oral contact required
- Source – Saliva (Kissing disease)
- Commonly found in hyperendemic malaria areas
- Disease:
  - Hodgkin lymphoma and Burkitt's lymphoma
  - Nasopharyngeal Ca– Risk factor – genetic, salted shell fish (nitrosamine), herbal snuff. Chinese males
  - Duncan syndrome – X linked lymphoproliferative disorder
  - Infectious Mononucleosis

Infectious Mononucleosis

- Glandular fever
- Seen in nonimmune young adults following primary infection with EBV
- Incubation period 4–8weeks
- Characterized by:
  - Atypical T cell,
  - Lymphadenopathy
  - Hepatosplenomegaly and Rash
- Heterophile Antibody to sheep RBC – Paul Bunnel test
- Confirmed by monospot test/differential absorption test

HHV 6

- Sixth disease
- Exanthem subitum, Roseola infantum

HHV 8

- Kaposi sarcoma,
- Primary effusion lymphoma

Other DNA Viruses

Smallpox

- Variola – largest virus, possess ds DNA,
- Brick shaped,
- Only DNA virus which replicates in cytoplasm
- Smallpox-Eradicated from world – 1980
- Still can be a potential agent of bioterrorism
- Paschen body (Variola), Guarneri body (Vaccinia)
- Vaccinia pocks on CAM – larger necrotic and hemorrhagic than Variola
- Ceiling temperature- Vaccinia: 41°C, Variola: 38°C
- Live vaccine using Vaccinia virus
- Vaccinia but not Variola can produce plaques on chick embryo

Smallpox Eradication is successful because

- Exclusively human pathogen, no reservoir
- Source – patient only, No carriers
- Highly affective Live vaccine-
  - Prepared from Vaccinia
  - Freeze dried vaccine (more stability) and multiple puncture technique

Molluscum contageosum

- Seen in children and young adult
- Pearly white wart like nodule on skin composed of eosinophilic inclusion bodies.
- Human are the only host.
- Cannot be grown in egg or tissue culture and animal.
- Sexually transmitted.

Adenovirus

- DNA, non enveloped, space vehicle shaped.
- Ideal vector for recombinant technology
- Manifestation:
  - Hemorrahgic cystis – Adenovirus type 11 and 21
  - Infant diarrhoea – Adeno 40, 41
  - STD – Adenovirus type 37
  - Epidemic conjunctivitis – Adenovirus type 8, 19, 37 (shipyard eye)
  - Swimming pool conjunctivitis – Adenovirus type 3, 7, 14
  - Pharyngitis and Pneumonia – Adenovirus type 3 and 7
- Adeno-associated virus – defective virus – requires Adenovirus for multiplication

Parvovirus

- Smallest, ss DNA, Parvo B 19.
- **5th** disease
- Causes **Erythema infectiosum** – characterized by rash, arthralgia, lymphadenopathy
- **Slapped cheek** appearance – rash 1st on cheek
- Causes **aplastic crisis** in sickle cell anemia patients
- Pregnancy – causes nonimmune fetal hydrops
- Transmission- respiratory route/blood

Papovavirus

Human Papillomavirus:

- Ca cervix
  - Low risk – type 6, 11 – CIN
  - High risk – type 16, 18, 31, 33 – Ca Cx
  - Risk factor – early sex, multiple sex, multiparous, OCP
- Condyloma acuminata/genital wart – by Type 6, 11
- Common wart/verruca vulgaris – by Type 1, 2, 3, 4
- Epidermodysplasia verrucoplasia
- Vaccine
  - Prophylactic – using HPV 16/18 late structural protein L1
  - Therapeutic – using HPV 16/18 Early non structural protein E6/E7

Other Papova viruses:

- JC virus – Hodgkin disease and PML (progressive multifocal leukoencephalopathy)
- BK virus- renal infection

- Polyoma virus
- Simian Vacuolating virus

Myxo Virus

Orthomyxo

- Influenza A, B, C
- Segmented RNA, unstable
- Both hemagglutinin (HA) and Neuraminidase (NA) spikes present,
- Hemagglutination is reversible (Elution)

Influenza

- Influenza – A, B, C
- Antigenic Shift – Results in Pandemic – MC seen in Type A
- Antigenic drift – Results in Epidemic – MC seen in A,B
- HA Ag – H1 to H15 – Protective
- NA antigen – N1 to N9, less protective
- MC manifestation – URTI
- MC complication:
  - Bacterial pneumonia > viral pneumonia
  - Reye's syndrome – with **Type B** (following aspirin)

Diagnosis

- Egg inoculation – Amniotic cavity – by A, B, C Allanotic cavity by only A
- Hemagglutination with Fowl and Guinea pig RBC
- Type A – agglutinates with Guinea pig, B-both, C – agglutinates with fowl RBC at 4°C
- Ag detection from nasopharyngeal cells by Immunfluroscence
- Four fold rise of Antibody by – Hemagglutination inhibition test (HAI)
- Vaccine – Killed, Live, Recombinant

Avian Flu

- H5N1
- Seen from 2003 onwards
- Only bird to human transmission seen, but no human-human transmission seen
- Highly virulent (as PB1F2 targets host mitochondria, induces apoptosis)

H1N1 2009 Flu

- April 2009
- Pandemic – Including India
- Recombination of 4 strain – (1 Human + 2 Swine + 1 Avian)
- Swine influenza strain causing pandemics so far
- H1N1 classical (1918), H1N2, H3, N2, currently 2009 H1N1 recombinant strain
- Human to human transmission seen
- Less virulent (as it lacks PB1F2 gene)
- Diagnosis – by RT PCR detecting HA and NA genes
- Treatment – NA Inhibitor – Oseltamivir (Tamiflu), Zanamivir
- Resistant to Amantadine
- Vaccine
  - Injectable killed – HA protein
  - Live nasal spray – HA protein

Paramyxo

- Parainfluenza, Measles, Mumps, RSV, Metapnemuovirus, New castle virus
- HA spike present in – Parainfluenza, Mumps, Measles
- NA spike present in – Parainfluenza, Mumps
- Single RNA, stable
- Inclusion body – intracytoplasmic (only for measles it is both intracytoplasmic and intranuclear)

Mumps

- MC cause of Parotitis (Nonsuppurative enlargement)
- Complications
  - Epididymo – Orchitis (U/L > B/L) – seen in 1/3rd of post pubertal male patients
  - Aseptic meningitis
  - Pancreatitis
  - Diabetes – Mumps, Rubella, Coxsackie B4
- Resolve except deafness
- Secondary attack – 85%
- Human – only host,
- Source – only patients, no carriers
- MC seen in Children
- Once infected, gives lifelong immunity
- Transmission – Droplet, saliva, Direct contact, Fomite borne, urine
- Saliva is infectious from –1 to +2 week of parotitis
- Specimen – urine, saliva, CSF
- Lab diagnosis:
  - Isolation – Egg, MKC,
  - IgM Antibody by ELISA
  - CFT using S Antigen
  - Antibody to S antigen (internal Ag) appear early, goes early – indicates acute infection
  - Antibody to V antigen (surface Ag) appear late, goes late
- Vaccine – Jeryl Lynn strain (at 9 months) and MMR. The vaccine confers 95% protection for a period of 12 years.

Measles

- Rubeola
- MC childhood rash
- Source – cases only, no subclinical/carrier stage
- Highest secondary attack rate – 90%
- Period of communicability – 4 days before and 5 days after the appearence of rash
- Incubation Period – 10 days
- Koplik's spot – pathognomic, appear before rash
- Rash – appear at 4th day fades after 4 day, MC site is face and neck
- Diagnosis:
  - Antigen detection by Immunofluorescence (also +ve before rash)
  - Warthin finkeldey giant cell
  - Isolation from nose, throat, conjunctiva and blood – Amniotic route and Primary Human/Monkey Kidney cell lines.
- Complication
  - Diarrhea
  - Pneumonia
  - Otitis media

- Encephalitis,
- **SSPE** – (subacute sclerosing panencephalitis) – high titer antibody in CSF is diagnostic
- Suppressed delayed hypersensitivity (false –ve Mantoux test and worsening of TB)

- Recovery from measles leads to – recovery from asthma
- Vaccine
  - Prepared – chick embryo or human diploid cell line
  - Age – given at 9 months (maternal antibody disappears)
  - Can be given at 6 months if measles outbreak seen (2nd dose to be given at 9 month)
  - Type – Live attenuated- Edmonston-Zagreb strain or combined (MMR, MR, MMRV)
  - Side effect – toxic shock syndrome (contamination of vial), mild measles like illness
  - Vaccination to contacts – given within 3 days is effective (IP of vaccine strain is 7 days and wild strain is 10 days)
  - Immunoglobulin – can also be given 3 days (in this case live vaccine is given after 8–12 weeks).

Respiratory Syncytial Virus

- No H and N
- MC cause of post natal bronchilitis in children
- Also causes pneumonia and otitis media
- Age – **6 weeks – 6 months**, new borne are protected due to maternal antibody
- RSV – MC precipitating factor for Acute asthma
- Rhino – MC precipitating factor for Ac exacerbation of chronic asthma
- Reinfection – milder illness
- Causes epidemics in winter (temperate) and rainy (tropics)
- Culture – giant cell and Syncytial formation

Parainfluenza Virus

- Parainfluenza type 1 and 2 – causes **Croup** (acute laryngotracheobronchiolitis)
- Parainfluenza type 3 – LRTI
- Type 3 – more Endemic and affects <1 years, causes shipping fever in cattle
- Type 1 and 2 – affect preschool children

Rubella

- German measles,
- Belongs to family Togaviridae, Not a Myxovirus
- Identified by interference with Echovirus
- Source – cases
- One week before and after the appearance of the rash
- IP–2–3 weeks
- Transmission – droplet, contact, sexual
- Rash on day 1 (face), Lymphadenopathy
- **Forchheimer spots** seen
- Congenital Rubella
  - 1st trimester – risk is maximum, after 5th month – risk negligible
  - Classical Congenital Rubella syndrome – Triad – cataract, deafness, PDA
  - Expanded Congenital Rubella syndrome – myocarditis, hepatosplenomegaly, bone lesion
- **Vaccination – RA 27/3 live attenuated**
  - Prepared from Human diploid cell line
  - Given after 1 year,

Picornaviridae

Include two major groups of human pathogens:

- Enteroviruses – Polio and Coxsackie
- Rhinoviruses

Poliovirus

- 3 subtypes
  - Type 1 – MC wild type
  - Type 2
  - Type 3 – MC cause of vaccine associated paralysis
- CFT detects
  - C Ag (coreless),
  - D Ag (dense Ag, type specific)
- Risk factors
  - Following tonsillectomy,
  - Pregnancy
  - IM injection
  - Muscular activity,
  - Coxsackie A,
  - Genetic predisposition
- Pathogenesis
  - Mode of transmission – Faeco oral > Inhalation > conjunctiva
  - Spread – hematogenous spread, direct neural spread-Following Tonsillectomy
  - Site of action – Anterior horn of spinal cord
  - Earliest change in neuron **– Nissl body** degeneration
  - Pathological changes always more extensive than distribution of paralysis
- Clinical types
  - In apparent infection – 90–95%,
  - Abortive infection – 5–10%
  - Aseptic meningitis (nonparalytic) – 0.1%
  - Paralytic (<0.1%) – Ascending flaccid paralysis

Lab diagnosis:

- Blood, throat swab, CSF, feces (till 6 weeks)
- Isolation – Monkey kidney tissue culture followed by Neutralization test.
- Neutralizing Antibody – comes early, stay long
- CFT Antibody – Anti C – comes early, goes early, Anti D – comes late, goes late
- OPV – Type1-1L, 2-2L, 3-3L TCID50, MgCl2, pH<7

Polio vaccine	Salk (Injectable)	Sabin (Oral)
Preparation	Formalin killed preparation of all 3 types in MKC	Each dose contains • Type 1–10 lakh, Type 2–2 lakh • Type 3–3 lakh of TCID50, • Stabilized in MgCl2, pH<7
Safety	Relatively more safer	Safer except in immunocompromised pt
Efficiency	80–90% by full course	90–100% by 1 or 2 doses Efficacy decreases by • Interference by other enteroviruses • Frequent diarrheal disease • Breastfeeding
Economy	Relatively expensive	Economical

Contd...

Contd...

Polio vaccine	Salk (Injectable)	Sabin (Oral)
Duration of protection	Need booster doses periodically	Long lasting
In epidemics	Cannot be used	Can be used
Herd immunity	Not provided	Provided
Local mucosal immunity	Not provided	Provided (IgA antibody)

Coxsackie virus

Group A Coxsackie virus	Group B Coxsackie virus
Suckling mouse inoculation Flaccid paralysis Generalized myositis	**Suckling mouse inoculation** Spastic paralysis Focal myositis Necrosis of brown fat Pancreatitis, hepatitis, myocarditis, encephalitis
Herpangina (vesicular Pharyngitis) Hand-foot-and-mouth disease (Also by Enterovirus-71) Acute hemorrhagic conjunctivitis (Cox-A24 and Enterovirus 70) Pneumonitis of infants Diarrhea URTI, Fever with rash	Pleurodynia (epidemic myalgia)/Bornholm disease – B1, B5 Myocarditis, pericarditis Diabetes mellitus – B4 Pneumonia
	Both Cox A and B Aseptic meningitis (MC–A7), encephalitis, cold, hepatitis

Rabies virus

- Bullet shaped, –ve sense RNA virus
- Reservoir
  - Urban Rabies – Dog 99%, cat
  - Wild life Rabies – Fox, Jackal, Wolf
- Source – Saliva of Rabid animal
- Mode of transmission – Bite(MC), Lick on abrasion, corneal transplant, air borne
- Speed of Rabies progress in axons: 12–24 mm/day, In sensory nerve 200–400 mm/day
- Earliest symptom – Neuritic pain at bite site
- Sensory N → UMN → sympathetic → mental system
- Incubation period – 1–3 month,
- IP is shorter in children and upper limb bite (than lower limb bite)
- Mechanism-Neural apoptosis, ↓Acetyl choline

Street virus	Fixed virus
Freshly isolated,	After serial passage
Produce Negri body	Doesn't Produce Negri body
Affect salivary gland	Doesn't affect salivary gland
Incubation Period-1–12 week	IP-5–6 days, Used for vaccine

Furious Rabies	Dumb Rabies
80% of all cases	20% of all cases
Hydrophobia,	No hydrophobia
No-fever, Fasciculation, Percussion edema	Fever, Fasciculation, Percussion edema present
Paralytic, Proximal muscle	Paralytic, Proximal muscle
Seen in unvaccinated individuals	Associated with partial vaccine course

Antemortem diagnosis

- Direct Fluorescent Antibody test
  - corneal impression smear (30% Sn, in late stage),
  - hair follicle of nape of neck
- Antibody in CSF – RFFIT and IFA
- RNA detection by RT-PCR

Postmortem diagnosis

- Negri body
  - Pathognomic, Hippocampus
  - Absent in 20% cases
  - Seller's technique – methylene blue and basic fuchsin
- Mouse – intrathecal inoculation,
- Isolation
- DFA on brain smear.

Vaccine

- Neural
  - Semple, BPL, Infant brain
  - Poor immunogenic, encephalogenic
- Non neural
  - Purified chick embryo cell (PCEC)
  - Purified vero cell (PVC)
  - Human diploid cell (HDC)
- Pre Exposure – 3 doses-at day 0, 7, 28
- Post exposure – 6 doses, at day 0, 3, 7, 14, 28 and 90 days

Arboviruses

Arboviruses Common in India

- Hemorrhagic – Dengue, Chikungunya, KFD
- Encephalitis – Japanese B, Westnile, Sindbis
- Rare – Ganjam, Vellore, Chandipura, Bhanja
- Yellow fever NOT found in India

Animal Reservoirs

- In many cases, the actual reservoir is not known.
- Birds: Japanese encephalitis, St Louis encephalitis, EEE, WEE
- Pigs: Japanese encephalitis (Amplifier host)
- Monkeys: Yellow Fever
- Rodents: VEE, Russian Spring-Summer encephalitis

Clinical Features

- Fever and rash with athralgia – non-specific.
- Encephalitis – e.g. EEE, WEE, St Louis encephalitis, Japanese encephalitis.
- Hemorrhagic fever – e.g. yellow fever, dengue, Crimean-Congo hemorrhagic fever, Chikungunya, Hanta
- Hemorrhagic fever with shock – Dengue

Lab Diagnosis

- Serology
  - HAI Antibody, CFT antibody, neutralizing antibody
  - ELISA – MAC ELISA (IgM), IgG ELISA

- Indicators:
  - IgM detection
  - Seroconversion of IgG,
  - Four fold rise in titer of IgG of paired sera
- Isolation – Suckling mice brain, Mosquito inoculation
- Culture-mosquito cell lines: C3/36 cell line
- Detection of antigen – NS1 Antigen (ELISA and ICT)
- Detection of RNA (RT–PCR)

Japanese Encephalitis

- 1st seen in Japan as "Summer encephalitis" epidemics
- Called 'B' – to distinguish from encephalitis A (encephalitis lethargica/von economo disease)
- Affect from Korea to India and Malayasia
- Vector: C. tritaeniorhynchus, C. vishnui – India
- India – Vellore, TN-AP-KA border, now world wide
- Reservoir: Ardeid (wading) birds
- Amplifying hosts – Pigs, bats
- Incidental hosts-Horses, humans, others
- The most common cause of epidemic encephalitis.
- Seasonal variation
  - Temperate area (June – September) and
  - Subtropical areas (March – October)
- Live attenuated vaccine (14–14–2)
- Inactivated vaccine (Nakayama strain)

Dengue

- DEN 4 serotypes – 1, 2, 3, 4 – Type 3 MC
- Vector – Aedes aegypti mosquito
- Mixed infection: Antibody dependent enhancement
- Clinical features
  - Dengue fever: Biphasic, Saddle back, Break bone fever Maculopapular rash
  - Dengue Hemorrhagic Fever
  - Dengue Shock Syndrome (DSS)

Chikungunya

- Fever, rash, arthralgia (name derived-doubled up due to joint pain)
- Differ from Dengue
  - Hemorrhagic manifestations rare,
  - Chikungunya outbreaks are shorter
- Vector – Aedes aegypticus
- 1964 outbreak – Africa, India (Vellore, Pondicherry, Chennai)
- 1973–2005 – No outbreaks
- Re-emerged in 2005 – Hyderabad, Karnataka, Maharashtra
- Reason of re-emergence
  - New vector – Aedes albopictus
  - Viral factor – E1 glycoprotein mutation of virus,
  - More rural involvement

Yellow fever virus

- Endemic- West Africa and Central South America.
- Reservoir

  - Forest – Monkey and forest mosquito
  - Urban – cases urban mosquito
- 2 major forms:
  - Wild YF – cycle involving primates and forest mosquitoes.
  - Urban YF is – cycle involving human to human by Aedes aegypti mosquito.
- **Don't Exist in India** – because
  - Aedes aegypticus is present in East costal area in India (where as YF is endemic in West Africa)
  - Strict vigilance and Quarantine for the travelers
  - Cross reacting Dengue antibody provides protection
  - But YF immunization doesn't protect from Dengue
- Incubation period – **3–6 days**
- Clinical feature – Hemorrhages, Fever, Platelet dysfunction, Relative bradycardia, Jaundice
- Liver – midzonal necrosis, Councilman bodies
- **Torres** bodies (intranuclear inclusion body)
- Darkar vaccine – mouse brain vaccine, risk of encephalitis
- 17D Live attenuated vaccine
  - Prepared in India (CRI, Kasuli)
  - Chick embryo, no risk of encephalitis
  - Single dose given s.c
  - 95% effective within 10 days of inoculation
  - Reimmunization required every 10 years for travelers
  - Cholera and YF vaccine shouldn't be given together
  - Measures in airport
    - Unprotected travelers – 6 days quarantine
    - Aedes aegypti index <1 400 mt surrounding airport

Kyasanur Forest Disease

- Hemorrhagic fever
- Tick borne
- Seen in Kyasanur Forest in Shimoga District, Karnataka

Incubation Period

- Dengue—5–6 days,
- Chikungunya—5–6 days,
- Japanese B—5-15 days,
- Yellow Fever—3–6 days,
- KFD—4–8 days

Hemorrhagic virus (Non Arthropod borne)

Hantavirus:

- HF with renal syndrome –
- Rodent borne (MC route – inhalation from rodent excreta)
- Hanta pulmonary syndrome – by Sin Nombre virus

Others – Marbug, Ebola, Lassa

Hepatitis Viruses

Viral causes of hepatitis

- Hepatitis A, B, C, D, E, G
- Yellow fever virus, Cytomegalovirus, Epstein bar virus, Herpes simplex virus

- Rubella virus, Entero virus

	HAV	HBC	HCV	HDV	HEV
Common name	Infectious	Serum	Non A non B Post transfusion	Delta agent	Non A non B Enteric transmitted
Family	Entero 72	Hepadna	Flavi	Viroid like	Calci
Onset	Abrupt	Insidious	Insidious	Abrupt	Abrupt
Age	Children	Any	Adult	Any	Young adult
Route	Feaco-oral	Blood, sexual, vertical	Blood, sexual, vertical	Blood, sexual	Feaco-oral
I.P (days)	15–50	50–150	15–150	15–50	15–50
Mortality	<0.5%	1–2%	0.5–1%	High	Usually 1–2% and Pregnancy 20–40%
Chronic carrier	No	Yes	Yes	Yes	No
Oncogenic	Nil	Present (neonate)	Present	Nil	Nil
Associated other feature	Secondary attack rate 10–20%	HCC, cirrhosis, Autoimmune disorder like AGN, arthritis, PAN	HCC, cirrhosis, Autoimmune- AGN, arthritis, cryo-globulinemia	HCC, cirrhosis, fulminant hepatitis	Secondary attack rate 1–2%
Not seen in western countries					

Laboratory diagnosis of Hepatitis

HAV	HBV	HCV	HDV	HEV
HAV – IgM – HAV – RNA	HBsAg – Acute, chronic, carrier HBeAg – active infection Anti HBc – IgM – Acute, window period IgG – chronic infection Only Anti HBs – vaccination HBV DNA – active infection, viral load (monitoring infection) Anti HBe – epidemiological marker	Antibody by 3rd generation ELISA using NS5 Antigen HCV RNA Genotyping – 7 sub types	HBsAg Anti HBc IgM – Coinfection IgG – Superinfection HDV Ag HDV RNA Anti HD IgM	Anti HBE Antibody EM of stool HEV RNA

HBV

- HBV – ds DNA virus (double strand is incomplete)
- DNA polymerase has double action – DNA dependent DNA polymerase + Reverse transcriptase activity
- Has 3 form-spherical, tubular, Dane particle (complete)
- > 1/3rd of world population are infected with HBV
- Pathogenesis- immune mediated
- Hepatocyte carrying viral antigen subjected to Antibody dependent NK cell/CD8 T cell cytotoxicity
- In absence of affective immune system-leads to carrier state (infants)
- Animal model – chimpanzee
- HBV doesn't grow in conventional cell line

HBV Gene

- S gene (HBsAg)
- Core gene – HBcAg
- Pre core – HBeAg
- P gene – DNA polymerase
- X gene – Regulatory gene

Mutants

- Precore mutant – unable to form HBeAg, medeterrian
- Escape mutant – unable to form HBsAg-ve (S gene mutation)
  - Seen in infant borne to HBeAg +ve mother
  - Seen in Liver transplant recepient receiving combined HBV Vaccine + Immunoglobulin

HBV Carrier

- >6 months
- India ranks 2nd (China 1st)
- Populations can be divided into
  - Low endemicity – carrier rate – <2% (North India)
  - Intermediate – 2–8% – India
  - High endemicity – >8% (south India)
- **Super carriers** – High HBsAg, HBeAg, HBV DNA, DNA Polymerase
- **Simple carrier** – Low HBsAg, No HBeAg
- **Carrier rate**: Following infection
  - 5–10% of adult becomes carrier
  - 50% of children becomes carrier
  - 90% of neonate becomes carrier

Transmission

- Blood (MC route in developing) – highly infectious than HIV
- Vertical
  - During delivery
  - In-utero
  - Breastfeeding
  - HBeAg +ve mother – high risk
- Sexual (MC route in developed country)
- Direct skin contact with open skin lesion
- High risk occupation-paramedical workers, sex workers
- Though HBV can survive in Mosquito, but no transmission seen.
- Age- Developed country (Young adults), Developing country (younger age)
- No seasonal variation

Disease	HAV IgM	HAV IgG	HBsAg	HBe AG/HBV DNA	ANTI–HBc IgM	ANTI –HBc IgG	ANTI –HBs
Acute hepatitis A virus (HAV)	+	+/–					
Previous HAV	–	+					
Acute hepatitis B virus (HBV)			+	+	–/+	–	–
"Window"*			–	–	+	–	–
Chronic HBV healthy carrier			+	–	–	+	–
Chronic HBV infective carrier			+	+		+	
Previous HBV			–	–	–	+	+
Vaccinated			–	–	–	–	+

*The window period of HBV disease occurs after infection has been resolved but before anti-HBs can be detected.

Vaccine

- HBsAg subunit—prepared by using candida as a vector
- Three dose—0, 1, 5 months
- Booster after 5 years if Anti HBS <10 IU/ml
- Non responder—5–10%
- Neonate born to HBV mother—**HBIG + Vaccine** (with in 12 hours)
- Newer—containing whole HBsAg (i.e. Pre S1 + Pre S2 + S)

HCV

- Belongs to Flaviviridae
- ssRNA, enveloped
- 50–80% of patients develops–chronic infection
- Carrier rate—1–20%
- Affect only human
- MC cause of post transfusion hepatitis
- Mode of transmission—BT, IV drug abuser, sexual, vertical
- Antigenic diversity—6 genotype
- Hence, affective vaccination is difficult
- 3rd generation ELISA detecting antibody against NS5 Ag
- RNA PCR

HGV

- Flavivirus
- Also known as GB virus
- SsRNA
- Mode of transmission – BT, sexual, vertical
- Associated with – Acute, chronic, fulminant hepatitis

HIV

Discovered in 1983 (USA), In India – 1986 (Chennai)

Antigen:

- Envelope antigens (gp 160)
  - Spike antigen – gp 120 (principal antigen)
  - Transmembrane pedicle protein (gp 41)
- Shell antigen
  - Nucleocapsid protein-p18
  - Core antigen
  - Principal core antigen-p24
  - Other core antigens-p15, p55
- Polymerase antigens
  - p31, p51, p66

Types of HIV

- HIV– I and HIV–2
- HIV–1—divided into 3 groups—M (major), O (outlier), N (new)
- M group–10 subtypes or clades (A to J)
- After J, the sub clades are named as CRF. (Circulating recombinant forms)
- 90% HIV cases in AP, TN, Karnataka, Maharashtra, Nagaland and Manipur (High burden states)

Mode of transmission

Type of exposure (risk %)
Sexual (0.1–1%)
Blood transfusion (>90%)
Tissue or donation of organ (50–90%)
Injection and injuries (0.3%)
Mother to baby (30%)
High viral load found in – blood, genital secretion, CSF

- **Receptors**—binds to gp120 of HIV
  - All cells expressing CD4 molecules like T helper cells (T tropic strains),
  - Macrophages (M tropic strains)
  - Dendritic cells and
  - Glial cells
- **Co-Receptors**—binds to gp – 41 of HIV
  - CXCR4 (X4) – T tropic strains
  - CCR5 (R5) – M tropic strains

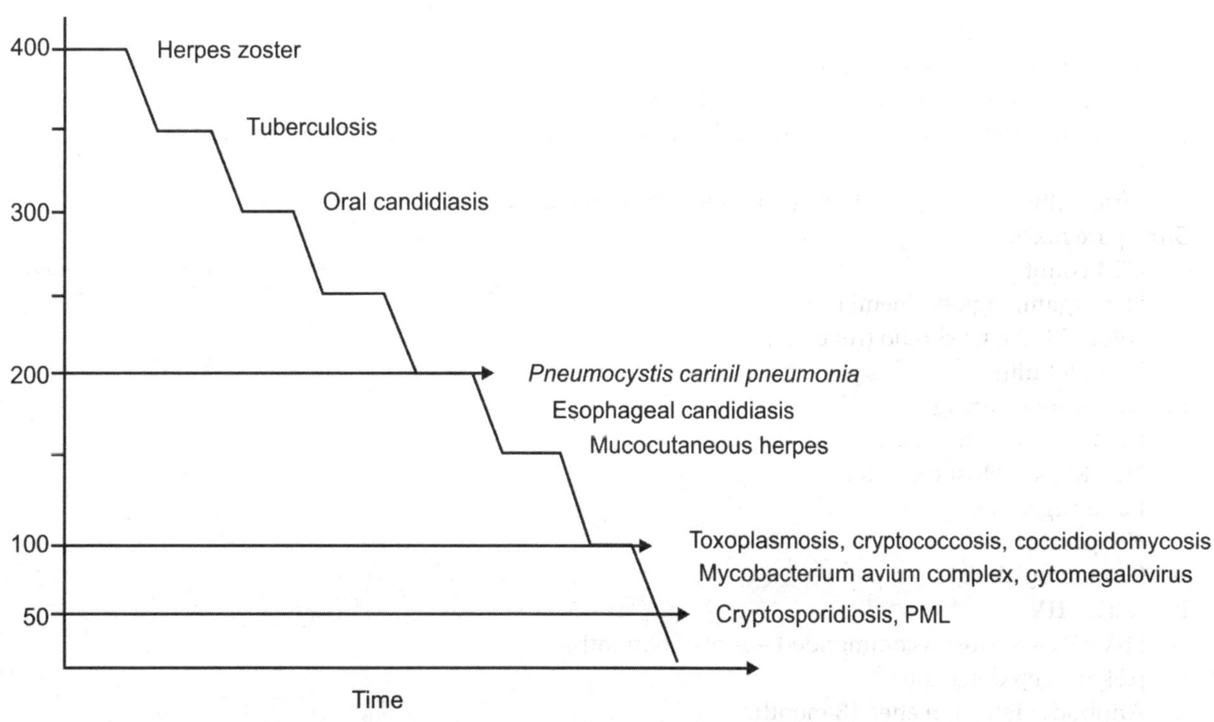

Fig. 5.5: Opportunistic infections in relation with CD4 count

HIV-related infections most frequently encountered in India				
Bacterial	**Viral**	**Fungal**	**Parasitic**	**Other illnesses**
Tuberculosis	Herpes simplex virus infection	Candidiasis	Cryptosporidiosis	AIDS dementia complex
Bacterial respiratory infections	Oral hairy leukoplakia	Cryptococcosis	Microsporidiosis	Invasive cervical cancer

Contd...

Contd...

	Varicella zoster virus disease	Pneumocystis jiroveci pneumonia	Isosporiasis	Non-hodgking lymphoma
Salmonella infection	Cytomegalovirus disease	Penicilliosis	Giardiasisww Stongyloides	
	Human papillomavirus infections		Toxoplasmosis	

*Rare infections include those due to Bartonella henselae, Rhodococcus equil, atypical mycobacterioses and human herpesvirus (HH5)-8 infections

Lab Diagnosis of HIV

- **Screening**—Rapid
  ELISA
  - 1st generation ELISA—crude preparation of HIV antigen is used
  - 2nd generation ELISA—recombinant Ag
  - 3rd generation ELISA—synthetic oligopeptide
  - 4th generation ELISA—Combination of recombinant. And synthetic Peptide and detect both HIV antgen (p24) and Antibody
- **Confirmatory**
  - Antibody detection:
    - Western blot-uses whole virus lysates
    - Immunofluorescence assay
    - Radioimmunoprecipitation assay (RIPA)
    - Line immunoassay (LIA)—recombinant/synthetic Antigen used—More specific
  - HIV RNA
  - Viral culture—Co-cultivation with un infected PBMC + IL2
- **Surrogate markers**
  - CD4 count
  - Hypergammaglobulinemia
  - Altered CD4: CD8 ratio (reversal)
  - Beta globulin
- **Prognosis/monitoring**
  - CD4 T cell count—most commonly used
  - HIV RNA—Most consistent
  - P24 antigen detection
  - Neopterin
  - β2 macroglobulin
- **Pediatric HIV**
  - HIV DNA—Most recommended—Age of 6 months
  - p24 antigen detection
  - Antibody detection after 18 months
- **Diagnosis in window period**
  - Initial time when the antibody detection methods are negative
  - p24 antigen detection (30% sensitive)
  - HIV RNA—best
- Guidelines for post exposure prophylaxis (PEP)
  - Body fluid considered at risk—blood, genital secretion, CSF and other body fluid
  - Body fluid not considered at risk—tear, sweat, saliva, feces
  - PEP should be started within 2 hours.

Guidelines for post exposure prophylaxis: PEP		
Exposure code	**HIV status code**	**Regimen**
1	1	Not required
1	2	Basic
2	1	Basic
2	2	Expanded
3	½	Expanded

Exposure code:
- EC1—Mild exposure – mucous membrane/non-intact skin with small volumes
- EC2—**Moderate exposure:** mucous membrane/non intact skin with large volumes **OR** percutaneous superficial exposure with solid needle
- EC3—**Severe exposure:** percutaneous with large volume by hollow needle, deep puncture

HIV status code:
- SC 1. HIV +ve, asymptomatic, CD count high, low viral load
- SC 2. HIV +ve, symptomatic, CD count low high viral load

Basic regimen—Zidovudine + Lamivudine for 4 weeks
Expanded regimen—Basic + Indinavir for 4 weeks

Causes of Viral Gastroenteritis

- Rotavirus
- Enteric adenovirus, type 40, 41
- Calcivirus:
  - e.g. Norwalk,
  - Outbreaks associated with uncooked **shellfish** in older children
  - Calci–means 32 cup shaped depression on virus surface
- Astroviruses
- Coronavirus
- H1N1

SLOW VIRUS DISEASES

- Definition: group of viruses which cause slow, progressive, neurodegenerative disease of CNS with long incubation period and high mortality rate.
  - Scrapie (sheep)
  - Bovine spongiform encephalopathy
  - Sporadic Creutzfeldt-Jakob disease (humans)
  - Variant Creutzfeldt-Jakob disease (humans)
- Character:
  - Very long Incubation periods ranging from months to years
  - Predilection to CNS
  - Slow growth rate and Genetic predisposition

Group A	Group B	
Visna – Demyelinating disease of sheep Maedi – hemorrhagic pneumonia of sheep,	Kuru – tremor, due to cannabalism Gerstmann-Straussler-Scheinker (GSS) syndrome, Creutzfeldt-Jakob disease Fatal familial insomnia Scrapie (sheep) Mink encephalopathy, Bovine spongiform encephalopathy (BSE)—Mad Cow Disease	Subacute sclerosing panencephalitis–measles Progressive multifocal leucoencephalopathy PML—(JC virus)

GENERAL PARASITOLOGY

Human parasites are divided as:
- Protozoa
- Helminths

Subkingdom Protozoa is further divided into four Phylum:
- Sarcomastigophora—Consists of Amoebae and Flagellates
- Apicomplexa—Coccidian parasites and Piroplasmida
- Ciliophora—Balantidium
- Microspora—Microsporida

Subkingdom Helminths or Metazoa in further divided into two phylum:
- Nemathelminths—consists of Class Nematoda
- Platyhelminths—consists of Class Cestoda and Trematoda

Amoeba

Parasitic Amoeba (alimentary canal)	Free living Amoeba
Entamoeba histolytica Entamoeba coli Entamoeba dispar Endolimax, Iodamoeba	Naegleria fowleri Acanthamoeba spp. Balamuthia spp.

Flagellates

Intestinal and Genital	Blood
Giardia lamblia Trichomonas	Trypanosoma Leishmania

Coccidian Parasites	Piroplasmida
Isospora Microsporidium Toxoplasma gondii Sarcocystis Cyclospora Cryptosporidium parvum	Plasmodium Babesia

Protozoan Parasites that infects humans by oral route

Parasite	Infective form
Entamoeba histolytica	Mature quadrinucleate cyst
Giardia lamblia	Mature cyst
Balantidium coli	Mature binucleate cyst
Cryptosporidium parvum	Thick-walled oocyst
Cyclospora	Oocyst
Isospora belli	Mature oocyst with 2 sporocyst
Toxoplasma gondii	Oocyst, Tissue cyst, Tachyzoite
Sarcocystis hominis	Sarcocyst

Nematodes that infect humans by oral route

Parasite	Infective form
Ascaris lumbricoides	Egg
Capillaria philippinensis	Larva
Dracunculus medinensis	Third stage larva (in Cyclops)

Contd...

Contd...

Parasite	Infective form
Enterobius vermicularis	Egg
Trichenella spiralis	Encysted larva
Trichuris trichiura	Egg
Trichostrongylus spp.	Larva
Angiostrongylus spp.	Larva

Parasites transmitted by

Sexual route	Transplacental	Blood transfusion	Conjunctiva	Skin
G. lamblia E. vermicularis T. vaginalis	Plasmodium T. gondii T. cruzi	Babesia L.donovani Plasmodium T. gondii T. cruzi	Acanthamoeba T. cruzi	A. duodenale N. americanus S. stercoralis Acanthamoeba Schistosoma

Parasites transmitted by bite or contamination of wound by infective forms of Arthropod vectors

Parasite	Arthropod
Plasmodium spp	Anopheline mosquito
Trypanosoma cruzi	Reduvid bug
Trypanosoma brucei	Tsetse fly
Leishmania donovani	Sandfly
Brugia malayi	Mosquito
Loa loa	Deer fly
Wucheriria bancrofti	Mosquito
Onchocerca volvulus	Black fly
Mansonella spp.	Culicoides spp. mosquitoes

INTESTINAL AMOEBAE, FREE-LIVING AMOEBA AND BALANTIDIUM COLI

Intestinal Amoebae

Habitat—Trophozoites of Entamoeba histolytica live mucosa and sub mucosa of Large intestine of man.

Morphology Three Stages

- Trophozoites—Feeding stage of the parasite, which is actively motile in freshly passed dysenteric stool, contains **phagocytosed RBCs.**
- Pre-cystic stage—It secrets highly refractile cyst wall around it and becomes cyst.
- Cystic stage—Mature cyst contain 4 nuclei and its cytoplasm contains 1–4 chromatoid bodies and glycogen mass.

Life Cycle

- Definitive host—Man
- Infective form—Mature quadrinucleate cyst
- Mode of infection—food or water contaminated with cyst
- Mode of transmission—**faeco-oral route** and Sexual transmission (20–30% in homosexuals)
- Reservoir of infection—Asymptomatic carriers

Culture Media

- Boeck and Drbohlav's Media
- Locke's egg serum/egg albumin
- Nelson's Medium
- Craig's Medium
- Monoxenic Medium—Cultivating *E. histolytica* with Trypanosoma cruzi
- Diamond Axenic Medium

Virulence Factors

Cysteine proteinase/enterotoxin/Cytotoxin—assists organism in digesting the extracellular matrix and invading tissues.

Host Factors Influencing Course of Infection

Stress, Malnutrition, Alcoholism, Corticosteroid therapy and immunodeficiency

Clinical Syndromes

Incubation period—4 days to a year

- **Asymptomatic infection—most frequent**
- **Symptomatic infections:**
  - Uncomplicated intestinal infection—diarrhea, cramps and flatulence
  - Acute amoebic dysentery
  - Chronic amoebic dysentery
  - Amoeboma—localised tumor-like lesion results from chronic ulceration
  - Hepatic amoebiasis
- **Metastatic infections:**
  - Pulmonary amoebiasis
  - Cerebral amoebiasis
  - Splenic abscess
  - Cutaneous amoebiasis
- **Entamoeba coli, E.dispar,** E. hartmanni, E. polecki, Iodamoeba butschlii and Endolimax nana-nonpathogenic intestinal amoebae.

Free-living Amoebae

	Naegleria fowleri	Acanthamoeba
Disease	Primary amoebic meningo-encephalitis	Granulomatous amoebic Meningo-encephalitis Ulcerative keratitis
Portal of entry	Nose	Upper respiratory tract
Predisposing factor	Swimming in contaminated water	Immunodeficiency
Clinical course	Acute	Subacute-Chronic
Pathology	Acute Suppurative changes	Granulomatous inflammation
Tissue form	Trophozoites	Cyst and trophozoites
Culture	Frequently positive	Negative
Trophozoites	Single pseudopodium	Thorn like Pseudopodium
Flagellate form	Present	Absent
Leukocytes in CSF	Neutrophils	Lymphocytes

Ciliate Parasites

- **Balantidium coli**—only ciliate parasite of humans.
- Inhabiting the large intestine, cecum, and terminal ileum, feeding on bacteria.
- The parasite may also invade the intestinal mucosa causing ulceration.
- Morphology—Trophozoites and cysts.
- Extra intestinal spread to the liver, lungs, and urogenital tract is rarely observed.
- Infection occurs by ingestion of cysts in contaminated food or drink.
- Pigs represent the source of infection for humans.
- Symptoms of the disease—**balantidiasis**—may range from mild colitis and diarrhea to clinical manifestations resembling severe dysentery.

FLAGELLATES

Giardia Lamblia

Habitat

Mucosa of duodenum and upper ileum of man.

Morphology two forms:

- **Trophozoites**—Tear-drop shaped/racket shaped/piriform shaped
  - It has 2 nuclei, 4 pairs of flagella, 2 Axostyles, 2 parabasal body and Ventral sucking disk
- **Cyst**—Mature cyst consists of 4 nuclei and cysts are passed in faeces.

Life cycle

- Infective stage—Cyst
- Route of infection—Faeco-oral route
- Trophozoite has **falling—leaf like motility**

Susceptibility to infection

- Children
- Immunocompromised individual
- Individuals with Achlorhydria and Hypochlorhydria (Gastric acidity weakens the cyst wall and excystation is completed in duodenum)

Pathogenesis

- It causes abnormalities of villous structure and causes malabsorption (lipids and lipid soluble vitamins)

Clinical Disease

- Symptomatic children—watery diarrhea or chronic diarrhea with malabsorption
- Older patients—epigastric pain, flatulence, low grade fever, diarrhea with foul smelling stool.
- **Traveller's diarrhea**
- Gall bladder infection—biliary colic and jaundice

Lab diagnosis

- Samples collected—stool sample and duodenal contents
- Microscopy—iodine and Saline wet mount—demonstrates either trophozoites or cyst
- **String test/Entero test**—bile stained mucus is collected for examination of trophozoites.
- Serology—antigen or antibody detection by ELISA and Immuno-fluorescent method

Treatment—Metranidazole/Tinidazole

Trichomonas Vaginalis

Habitat

- Urethra, vagina and prostate

Morphology

- Only trophozoite form, which is pear- shaped consists of 5 flagellas. No cystic stage.

Life cycle

- Mode of transmission—Sexual route
- Reservoir of infection—woman
- Infective stage—Trophozoites

Clinical disease

- **Incubation period—4-28 days**
- In women—Asymptomatic or vaginitis and UTI
- In men—Asymptomatic or Urethritis, Prostatitis and Cystitis

Lab diagnosis

- Sample collected—Vaginal, and urethral discharges, Prostatic secretions or Urine sediment
- Microscopy (wet mount)—Actively motile **(Jerky motility)** trophozoites observed
- Staining—Geimsa and papanicolaou stain used
- Culture—More sensitive (93%)
- Serology—Indirect haemagglutination, gel diffusion
- Gene probes—DNA probes used
- PCR

Treatment

Drug of choice—Metronidazole

- **Haemoflagellates**
  Lie in the blood or tissues of man, who serves as definitive hosts.
- **Trypanosoma spp.**
- **Leishmania spp.**
  Major blood and tissue-dwelling flagellates of humans

Trypanosomes infecting man

Parasite	Vector	Morphological forms	Disease
T. brucei subspecies T. brucei gambiense T. brucei rhodesiense T. brucei brucei	Tsetse fly	Trypomastigotes and Epimastigotes	African trypanosomiasis
Trypanosoma cruzi	Triatomid bug	Amastigotes and Trypomastigotes	South American trypanosomiasis (Chagas' disease)

Comparison of West African and East African Trypanosomiasis

Point of comparison	West African (gambiense)	East African (rhodesiense)
Organism	T. b. gambiense	T. b. rhodesiense
Vectors	Tsetse flies (palpalis group)	Tsetse flies (morsitans group)
Primary reservoir	Humans	Antelope and cattle
Human illness	Chronic (late CNS disease)	Acute (early CNS disease)
Duration of illness	Months to years	<9 months

Contd...

Contd...

Point of comparison	West African (gambiense)	East African (rhodesiense)
Lymphadenopathy	Prominent	Minimal
Parasitemia	Low	High
Diagnosis by rodent inoculation	No	Yes
Epidemiology	Rural populations	Workers in wild areas, rural populations, tourists in game parks

Trypanosoma Cruzi

Clinical spectrum of disease

Acute stage of infection:

- Incubation period 1–2 weeks
- Chagoma—Dusky-red swelling at site of entry of T. cruzi
- Conjunctival swelling, unilateral swelling of lids (Romana's sign)
- Generalized lymphadenopathy, enlargement of liver and spleen

Chronic stage of infection:

- **Heart**—thinning of the ventricular walls, biventricular enlargement, apical aneurysms, atrophy of myocardial cells and conduction-system involvement.
- GIT—varying degrees of dilatation **(mega disease)** of esophagus and colon

Laboratory Diagnosis

Acute Chagas' disease—requires the detection of parasites.

- Microscopic examination of fresh anticoagulated blood or of the buffy coat—demonstrates motile organisms.
- Giemsa-stained thin and thick blood smears.
- Microhematocrit tubes containing acridine orange—QBC examination useful.
- PCR or hemoculture in special media—when repeated attempts to visualize the organisms are unsuccessful.
- Hemoculture—takes several weeks to give positive results.
- Serologic testing **plays no role** in diagnosing acute Chagas' disease.

Chronic Chagas' disease

- Detection of specific antibodies that bind to T. cruzi antigens.
- Demonstration of the parasite is **not** of primary importance.
- **The radioimmune precipitation assay (Chagas' RIPA)** is a highly **sensitive and specific** confirmatory method for detecting antibodies to T. cruzi
- The use of PCR assays to detect T. cruzi DNA in chronically infected persons has been studied extensively.

Treatment—Nifurtimox and benznidazole- drugs used

Trypanosoma Brucei

Also called—African sleeping sickness

Pathogenesis and clinical course

- Trypanosomal chancre—appears a week or so after the bite of an infected tsetse fly.
- A systemic febrile illness occurs when parasites disseminated through the lymphatics and bloodstream.
- **Stage I disease:**
  - Without central nervous system (CNS) involvement with widespread lymphadenopathy, splenomegaly and myocarditis
  - Enlargement of posterior cervical lymphnodes or **Winterbottom's sign**
- **Stage II diseas:**
  - **Iinvolves invasion of the CNS,** with protean neurologic manifestations with abnormalities in the CSF.
  - A picture of progressive indifference and daytime somnolence develops (hence the designation "sleeping sickness")

Laboratory Diagnosis

- A definitive diagnosis—detection of the parasite.
- Microscopy—Chancre fluid/lymph node aspirate/CSF—wet mount- demonstrates highly motile Giemsa-stained thin and thick films of serial blood samples useful.
- QBC examination—Mcrohematocrit tubes containing acridine orange.

Treatment

	Clinical Stage	
Causative Organism	**I Normal CSF)**	**II Abnormal CSF)**
T. brucei gambiense (West African)	Pentamidine Alternative: Suramin	Eflornithine Alternative: Melarsoprol
T. brucei rhodesiense (East African)	Suramin	Melarsoprol

Leishmania

Leishmania spp. causing human disease:

Species/sub spp.	Disease	Geographical distribution
Leishmania donovani L.donovani donovani L.donovani infantum L.donovani chagasi	Visceral Leishmaniasis of old and new world	Midddle east, Africa, Indian subcontinent
Leishmania tropica Leishmania major Leishmania aethiopica	Cutaneous Leishmaniasis old world	Midddle east, Ethiopia, India
Leishmania braziliensis complex Leishmania mexicana complex	Cutaneous and mucocutaneous Leishmaniasis new world	Mexico, Central and South America

Morphological forms—amastigote (reticuloendothelial system of man)—promastigote (sandfly vector)—infective form

Laboratory diagnosis

- Microscopy—stained peripheral blood smear examination
- Lymphnode aspirate/bone marrow aspiration—smear and culture
- Blood culture—NNN medium
- Tissue culture
- Serological tests—Napier's aldehyde test and chopra's antimony test
- Leishmanin (Montenegro) skin test

Treatment—Pentavalent antimonials (sodium stibogluconate) and amphotericin B

Plasmodium species and babesia

- Malaria is caused by a parasite called **Plasmodium,** which is transmitted via the bites of infected anopheline mosquitoes. In the human body, the parasites multiply in the liver, and then infect red blood cells.

Plasmodium spp. causing malaria as follows:

Life Cycle

- Man—Intermediate host.
- Mosquito—Definitive host
- Sporozoites are infective forms
- Present in the salivary gland of female anopheles mosquito
- After bite of infected mosquito sporozoites are introduced into blood circulation.

Characteristics of plasmodium species infecting humans

Characteristic	P. falciparum	P. vivax	P. ovale	P. malariae
Duration of intrahepatic phase (days)	5.5	8	9	15
Duration of erythrocytic cycle (hours)	48	48	48	72
Red cell preference	Younger cells (but can invade cells of all ages)	Reticulocytes and cells up to 2 weeks old	Reticulocytes	Older cells
Morphology	Usually only ring forms, banana-shaped gametocytes	Irregularly shaped large rings and trophozoites; enlarged erythrocytes; Schüffner's dots	Infected erythrocytes, enlarged and oval with tufted ends; Schüffner's dots	Band or rectangular forms of trophozoites common
Pigment color	Black	Yellow-brown	Dark brown	Brown-black
Ability to cause relapses	No	Yes	Yes	No
Disease	Malignant tertian malaria	Beningn tertian malaria	Ovale tertian malaria	Quartan malaria

Clinical features of malaria

- Fever
- Sweating
- Anemia
- Splenomegaly
- Irritability
- Coma, retinal hemorrhages
- Algid malaria (a shock like syndrome)
- Respiratory distress syndrome

Complications

- Cerebral malaria
- Back water fever
- Malarial hyperpyrexia
- Gastrointestinal disorders
- Algid malaria
- Recrudescence—**P. falciparum** infection
- Relapse—**P. vivax** infection
- Nephrotic syndrome—**P. malariae** infection

Laboratory diagnosis

- Microscopy—for demonstration of parasites and for speciation
- Stained peripheral blood smear examination (thick and thin smears)—**Gold standard** method
- Quantitative Buffy Coat examination—Rapid method for detection of parasites
  The QBC method is the simplest and most sensitive method for diagnosing the following diseases:
  - Malaria
  - Babesiosis
  - Trypanosomiasis
  - Filariasis (elephantiasis, Loa-Loa)
  - Relapsing fever (borreliosis)
- Antigen Detection (pLDH and HRP-2 Ag detection)—Immunochromatographic tests—Rapid and simple
- Serology—antibodies against malaria parasites detected by indirect immunofluorescence (IFA) or enzyme-linked immunosorbent assay (ELISA).
- Molecular Diagnosis—Parasite nucleic acids are detected using polymerase chain reaction (PCR).
- P. knowlesi is known as quotidian malaria

Treatment

Choroquine—drug of choice in all forms of susceptible in all forms of acute malaria
Radical cure—primaquin
Other alternatives

- Quinine plus Doxycycline or Tetracycline
- Quinine plus Clindamycin

Newer alternatives

- Mefloquine
- Halofantril.

Babesia

- Intra erythrocytic protozoa
- Tick borne malaria like illness in animal
- Zoonotic—opportunistic to human
- Species:
  - B. microti,
  - B. bovis

Species	B. microti	B. bovis/divergens
Distribution	North America	Europe
Host	Rodent	Cattle
Immunity of host	Spleen is usually normal	Seen in spleenectomised and immunocompromised patient
Clinical feature	Asymptomatic/mild fever	Severe, but no cerebral involvement
Clinical Course	Self limiting	Severe, fulminant

COCCIDIAN PARASITES

Toxoplasma Gondii

- It is a coccidian protozoan—worldwide distribution
- Infects a wide range of animals and birds but does not appear to cause disease in them. The normal final hosts are strictly the **cat** and in which the oocyst-producing **sexual stage** of toxoplasma can develop.
- Morphological forms:
  - **Oocyst**—each oocyst has 2 sporocysts and each sporocyst containing 4 sporozoites.
  - **Tachyzoites**—rapidly multiplying crescentic cells, which initiate the **acute stage** of disease.
  - **Bradyzoites**—Tachyzoites penetrate nerve cells, especially of the brain and eye, where they multiply slowly (as bradyzoites) to form **quiescent tissue cysts**, initiating the **chronic stage** of disease.

Clinical forms

- Most human infections are **asymptomatic.**
- **Fulminating fatal infections** may develop in patients with **AIDS**, presumably by alteration of a chronic infection to an acute one.
- In immunosuppressed individuals—results in retinitis or chorioretinitis, encephalitis, pneumonitis,
- **Congenital infection** develops only when nonimmune mothers are infected during pregnancy (first time), is usually of great severity.
  - **Prenatal toxoplasmosis is a major cause of blindness and other congenital defects.**
  - Congenital infection leads to stillbirths, chorioretinitis, intracerebral calcifications, psychomotor disturbances, and hydrocephaly or microcephaly.
- Postnatal toxoplasmosis is less severe.

Culture

- T gondii may be cultured only in the presence of **living cells, in cell culture or eggs**.
- Optimal growth is at about 37–39°C in living cells.

Pathogenesis

- The tachyzoite directly destroys cells of the reticuloendothelial system.
- Humans are relatively resistant, but a low-grade lymph node infection resembling infectious mononucleosis may occur.

Laboratory Diagnosis

- Serology—**Sabin-Feldman dye test**—depends upon the appearance of antibodies (in **2–3 weeks),** that will render the membrane of laboratory-cultured living T gondii impermeable to alkaline **methylene blue**.
- **Treatment**
  - Acute infections—combination of **pyrimethamine** and **sulfadiazine** or trisulfapyrimidines.
  - Alternatives—spiramycin, **clindamycin, trimethoprim-sulfamethoxazole**,
  - In pregnancy—spiramycin is recommended.

Other Coccidian parasites

- Cryptosporidium parvum
- Cyclospora cayetanensis
- Isospora belli
- Sarcocystis hominis, S.suihominis and S.lindermanii
- Blastocystis hominis
- Microsporidia

Comparison of coccidian parasites causing diarrhea in immunocompromised host

Property	Cryptosporidium	Cyclospora	Isospora
Size	4–6 μ size	8–10 μ	10–20 μ
Shape	Round	Round	Oval
Cyst contains	4 sporozoites	2 sporoblast, each having 2 sporozoites	2 sporoblast, each having 4 sporozoites
Acid fast	Uniformly acid fast,	Variable acid fast	Uniformly acid fast,
Autofluoroscence	No, but can be stained with fluorescent dye	Autofluoroscence ++	Autofluoroscence +/–
Treatment	Trimethoprim-sulfamethoxazole (co-trimoxazole)	Trimethoprim-sulfamethoxazole (co-trimoxazole)	Spiramycin, Nitazoxanide

Microsporidium

- Characterized by a unicellular spore containing a coiled spring-like tubular polar filament through which the sporoplasm is forcibly discharged into a host cell.
- A modified trichrome -blue stain may detect microsporidia in urine, stool, and nasopharyngeal specimens.
- Transmission is chiefly by ingestion of spores in food or water.
- Transplacental transmission is common.
- Nonpathogenic in immunologically intact persons but a continuing threat to the immunocompromised.
- They often occur along with cryptosporidium in AIDS patients.

Cestodes

According to Habitat

- **Pseudophylladian cestodes**
  - Diphyllobothrium latum/fish tape worm

- **Cyclophylladean cestodes adult worm in humans**
  - Taenia saginata/beef tapeworm
  - Taenia solium/pork tape worm
  - Hymenolepis nana/dwarf tape worm
  - Hymenolepis diminuta/Rat tape worm
  - Dipylidium caninum/ Double-pored dog tape worm

Cestodes that infect humans by oral route

Parasite	Infective form
Diphyllobothrium latum	Pleurocercoid larva
Echinococcus granulosus	Egg
Echinococcus multilocularis	Egg
Hymenolepis nana	Egg
Hymenolepis diminuta	Cystecercoid larva
Multiceps spp.	Egg
Spirometra	Procercoid and Pleurocercoid larva
Taenia saginata	Cysticercus bovis
Taenia solium	Cysticercus cellulosae or Egg

- Cestodes, or tapeworms, are segmented worms
- Habitat- adults reside in the GIT & larvae can be found in any organ.

Intestinal cestodes—humans are definitive host

- Taenia saginata and T. solium
- Diphyllobothrium,
- Hymenolepis,
- Dipylidium caninum.

Tissue cestodes (larval-stage)—humans are intermediate host

- Echinococcus granulosus
- Sparganum
- Multiceps spp.

Taenia solium—human may be either the definitive or the intermediate host.

Taenia saginata and T. solium

Characters	Taenia saginata	Taenia solium
Length	5–10 metres	2–3 metres
Scolex	Large and quadrate	Small and globular
Neck	Short	Long
Proglottid	1000–2000	Less than 1000
Larva	Cysticercus bovis	Cysticercus cellulosae

- Both taenia saginata and T. solium causes intestinal taeniasis.
- T. solium in addition causes cysticercosis in humans, when they act as intermediate hosts. (consumption of egg)

Characters	Intestinal taeniasis	Cysticercosis
Infective stage	Cysticercus cellulosae	Taenia solium egg
Clinical symptoms	Intestinal symptoms only	Depending on the location of the cyst
Diagnosis	Demonstration of eggs in the faeces	Demonstration of larvae in tissues.

Man acquires cysticercosis by:

- Ingestion of food and water contaminated with eggs
- **Auto infection** through anus-hand-mouth transfer of eggs.
- Reverse peristalsis of eggs throwing back the eggs to duodenum where they hatch and cause tissue infection.

Cysticercosis

- Potentially dangerous systemic disease.
- Most commonly found in subcutaneous and intermuscular tissues followed by the **eye and then the brain.**

Neurocysticercosis

- Most serious form of cysticercosis.
- Two types:
  - Parenchymal
  - Extra-parenchymal
- Convulsions, intracranial hypertension and psychiatric disturbances are the three important manifestations.

Echinococcus

Character	Echinococcus granulosus	Echinococcus multilocularis	Echinococcus vogeli	Echinococcus oligarthus
Length	2–7 mm	1.2–3.7 mm	3.9–5.6 mm	1.9–2.9 mm
Proglottid	3–4	4–5	3	3
Larva	Unilocular	Multilocular	Polycystic multilocular	Polycystic multilocular
Host Definitive: Intermediate:	 Dog Man, sheep, cow	 Fox Man, rodents	 Dog Man, rodents	 Cat Man, rodents

- **Echinococcus granulosus—hydatid tape worm or dog tape worm.**
- Hydatid cyst is the larval stage.
- Causes cystic echinococcosis or hydatid disease in man and other herbivorous animals.

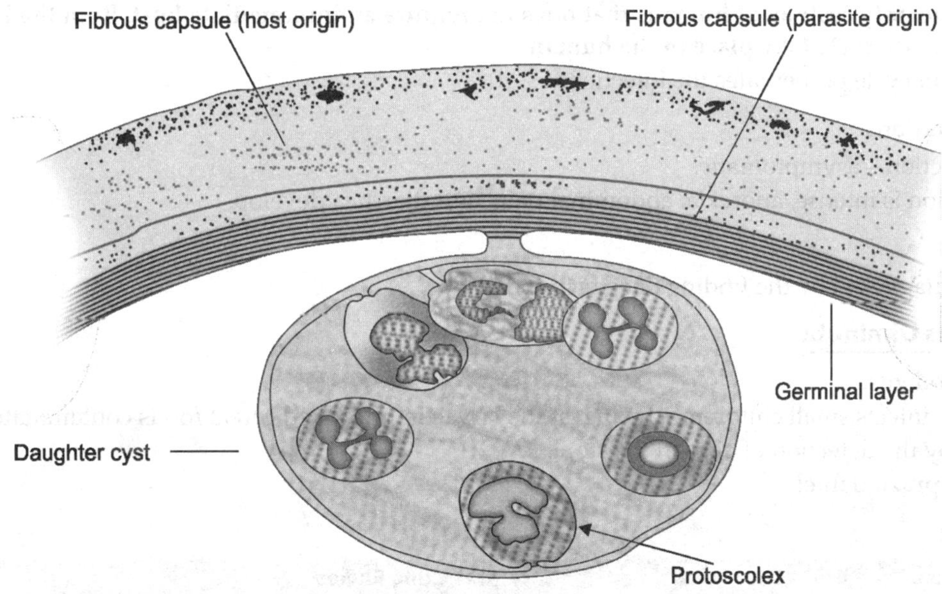

Fig. 5.6: Hydatid cyst wall

Life cycle

- Definitive host—dog and wild carnivores
- Intermediate hosts—man and other herbivorous animals.
- Man is an accidental host.
- Eggs—infective stage of the parasite.

Clinical features

- Hepatomegaly with or without palpable abdominal mass.
- Bone—rapid erosion leading to fractures.
- Other sites—tumor like condition or an abscess.

Parasitic Diagnosis

- Hydatid fluid microscopy – on wet mount examination protoscolices appear as colourless white **structures.**
- **Acid fast staining of centrifuged deposit—acid fast scolices and protoscolices seen.**
- **Casoni's skin test—immediate hypersensitivity reaction.**
- IHA, CIEP, ELISA and western blot used for the detection of antibodies.
- Detection of antigen:
  - In serum by ELISA, CIEP, latex agglutination test etc.
  - Recently, in urine by CoA or CIEP.
- Imaging methods like USG, MRI and X-ray are of immense importance to show the size and condition and to pinpoint the exact location of the cysts.

Treatment

- Surgery is the mainstay of this condition.
- Albendazole and mebendazole are the only antihelminthics useful in cystic echinococcosis.
- Percutaneous Aspiration Injection Reaspiration (PAIR) of the cyst is the latest alternative to surgery.

Hymenolepis nana-dwarf tapeworm

- Infection—fecal/oral contamination
- Common among institutionalized children.
- **H. nana is the only cestode of humans that does not require an intermediate host. Both the larval and adult phases of the life cycle take place in the human.**
- **Autoinfection** cycle perpetuates the infection.

Clinical Manifestations

- H. nana infection—asymptomatic.
- When infection is intense, anorexia, abdominal pain, and diarrhea develop.

Diagnosis

- Infection is diagnosed by the finding of eggs in the stool.

Hymenolepiasis Diminuta

- Cestode of rodents
- Occasionally infects small children, who ingest the larvae in uncooked cereal foods contaminated by **fleas**
- Diagnosed by the detection of eggs in the stool.
- Treatment—praziquantel

Class Trematoda

• **Intestinal Flukes** – Fasciolopsis buski – Heterophyes heterphyes – Gastrodiscoides hominis – Metagonimus Yokogawai	• **Lung Flukes** – Paragonimus westermani
• **Liver Flukes** – Fasciola hepatica – Fasciola gigantica – Clonorchis sinensis – Opisthorchis viverrini – Opisthorchis felineus	• **Blood Flukes** – Schistosoma haematobium – Schistosoma mansoni – Schistosoma japonicum

Parasite	Infective form
Clonorchis sinensis	Metacercaria
Fasciola hepatica	
Fasciola gigantica	
Fasciolopsis buski	
Opisthorchis viverrini	
Opisthorchis felineus	
Paragonimus westermani	
Metagonimus yokagawai	
Heterophyes heterophyes	
Gastrodiscoides hominis	
Schistosoma	Cercaria

Scientific and common name	Epidemiology	Disease-Producing from and its location in host	How infection occurs	Major disease manifestations, diagnostic stage and specimen of choke
Fasciolopsis buski (large intestinal fluke)	Far east	Adults live in small intestine	Ingestion of encysted matacercariae on raw vegetation	Edema, eosinophilia, diarrhea, malabsorption, and even death in heavy infection; diagnosis: eggs in feces
Fasciola hepatica (sheep liver fluke) (zoonosis)	Worldwide (in sheep-raising and cattle-raising areas), humans (accidental host), sheep (natural host)	Adults live in bile ducts	Ingestion of encysted metacercariae on raw vegetation	Traumatic tissue damage and irriation to the liver and bile ducts, jaundice and eosinophilia can occur; diagnosis: eggs in feces
Clonorchis sinensis (Oriental or Chinese liver fluke)	Far east	Adults live in bile ducts	Ingestion of encysted metacercariae in uncooked fish	Chronic fibrotic disease resembling tuberculosis (cough with blood-tinged sputum); diagnosis: eggs in sputum or feces
Heterophyes heterophyes; Metagonimus yokogawai (the heterophyids)	Far east	Adults live in small intestine	Ingestion of encysted metacercariae in uncooked fish	No intestinal symptoms unless very heavy infection; diagnosis: eggs in feces
Schistosoma mansoni (Manson's blood fluke, bilharziasis, swamp fever)	Africa, middle east, and south America	Adult in venules of the colon (eggs trapped in liver and other tissues)	Fork-tailed cercariae burrow into the capilary bed of feet, legs, or arms	Granuloma formation around eggs (i.e., in liver, intestine, and bladder), toxic and allergic reactions: nephrotic syndrome; diagnosis: eggs in feces and rectal biopsy, rarely in urine
Schistosoma japnicum (Oriental blood fluke)	Far east	As for Schistosoma mansoni	As for Schistosoma mansoni	As for Schistosoma mansoni, but symptoms are more severe because of greater egg production; diagnosis: eggs in feces and rectal biopsy, rarely in urine

Contd...

Contd...

Scientific and common name	Epidemiology	Disease-Producing from and its location in host	How infection occurs	Major disease manifestations, diagnostic stage and specimen of choke
Schistosoma haematobium (bladder fluke)	Africa, middle east, and Portugal	Adults in venules of bladder and rectum, eggs caught in tissues	As for Schistosoma mansoni	Bladder colic with blood and pus, nephrotic syndrome, symptomatic symptoms are mild, pulmonary involvement from eggs in lugs, has been associated with cancer of the bladder; diagnosis: eggs urine, rarely in feces
Swimmer's itch (zoonosis)	Worldwide	Cercariae of schistosomes that usually parasitize mammals and birds enter human skin	Fork-tailed cercariae burrow into skin of human in water	Allergic dermal response to repeated penetration, schistosomules do not develop to adults

Class Nematoda

- **Intestinal Nematodes**

Small Intestine
Ascaris lumbricoides/common round worm
Ancylostoma duodenale/hookworm
Necator americanus/American hookworm
Strongyloides stercoralis
Trichinella spiralis
Large Intestine
Enterobius vermicularis/seat worm/Pin worm
Trichuris trichuira/whip worm

Tissue or Somatic Nematode

Lymphatic system Wuchereria bancrofti Brugia malayi	**Mesentery** Mansonella perstans Mansonella ozzardi
Conjunctiva Loa loa	**Lungs** Strongyloides stercoralis
Subcutaneous tissues Dracunculus medinensis/Guinea worm Loa loa/African eye worm Onchocerca volvulus	

General characteristics:

- Unsegmented, elongated and cylindrical
- Separate sexes
- Buccal capsule present
- GIT is complete
- Body cavity is present
- Size: Smallest <5 mm—trichinella spiralis, strongyloides stercoralis
  - Largest > 1 metre—dracanculus medinensis
- Body is covered with a tough cuticle.

According to egg/larva producing capacity

Name	Birth to	Example
Viviparous	Larva	D. medinensis W. bancrofti B. malayi T. spiralis
Oviparous	Laying eggs	A. lumbricoides T. trichiuria A. duodenale N. americanus E. vermicularis
Ovo-viviparous	Egg containing larva which immediately hatchout	S.stercoralis

Mode of infection

Mode	Forms	Examples
Ingestion	Eggs contaminated food Growing embryo in intermediate host Encysted embryo in flesh	A. lumbricoides, E. vermicularis T. trichiura D. medinensis T. spiralis
Penetration through skin	Filariform larva	A. duodenale N. americanus S. stercoralis
Bite	Blood sucking insects	Filarioideae
Inhalation	Dust containing eggs	A. lumbricoides E. vermicularis

Human Intestinal Parasitic Nematodes

Parasitic Nematode					
Feature	Ascaris lumbricoides (Roundworm)	Necator americanus Ancylostoma duodenale (Hookworm)	Strongyloides stercoralis	Trichuris trichiura (Whipworm)	Enterobius vermicularis (Pinworm)
Infective stage	Egg	Filariform larva	Filariform larva	Egg	Egg
Route of infection	Oral	Percutaneous	Percutaneous or autoinfection	Oral	Oral
Gastrointestinal location of worms	Jejunal lumen	Jejunal mucosa	Small-bowel mucosa	Cecum, colonic mucosa	Cecum, appendix
Pulmonary passage of larvae	Yes	Yes	Yes	No	No
Principal symptoms	Rarely gastrointestinal or biliary obstruction	Iron-deficiency anemia in heavy infection	Gastrointestinal symptoms; malabsorption or sepsis in hyperinfection	Gastrointestinal symptoms, anemia	Perianal pruritus
Diagnostic stage	Eggs in stool	Eggs in fresh stool, larvae in old stool	Larvae in stool or duodenal aspirate; sputum in hyperinfection	Eggs in stool	Eggs from perianal skin on cellulose acetate tape
Treatment	Mebendazole Albendazole	Mebenda zole	Ivermectin Albendazole	Mebendazole Albendazole	Mebendazole

Trichuris trichiura—(whip worm)

- **Eggs:**
  - **Brown, bile stained egg**
  - Barrel shaped with a mucus plug at each pole.
  - contains an unsegmented ovum
  - Floats in saturated solution of common salt.
  - Embryonated egg is infectious

Pathogenesis and clinical disease—trichuriasis.

- Acute appendicitis—when the worm inhabits in appendix.
- C/o abdominal pain, mucus diarrhoea, blood streaked stool and loss of weight.
- Prolapse of rectum in massive trichuriasis.

Laboratory diagnosis:

- Stool examination- characteristic egg.
- Adult worm occasionally found in stool.

Treatment-thiabendazole and mebendazole.

Ascaris Lumbricoides

- Largest intestinal nematode parasite of humans—40 cm in length.
  Clinical Features
  - Nonproductive cough
  - Burning substernal discomfort
  - Dyspnea
  - Blood-tinged sputum are less common
- Chest X-ray—evidence of **eosinophilic pneumonitis—Löffler's syndrome**
- In heavy infections—pain and small-bowel obstruction, perforation, intussusception, or volvulus, biliary colic, cholecystitis, cholangitis, pancreatitis, intrahepatic abscesses.
- In highly endemic areas, intestinal and biliary ascariasis can mimic **acute appendicitis and gallstones** as causes of surgical acute abdomen.

Laboratory Findings

Hookworm—A. duodenale and N. americanus

- Infective larvae may provoke pruritic maculopapular dermatitis **(ground itch")** at the site of skin penetration as well as serpiginous tracks of subcutaneous migration in previously sensitized hosts
- Chronic hookworm infection leads—iron deficiency.
- **Hypochromic microcytic anemia, occasionally with eosinophilia or hypoalbuminemia, is characteristic of hookworm disease.**

Laboratory diagnosis

Treatment—albendazole, mebendazole

Strongyloides Stercoralis

- Dwarf thread worm—Smallest pathogenic nematode causing human infection

Clinical spectrum

- Acute strongyloidosis—presents as acute watery or mucoid diarrhoea
- Chronic strongyloidosis—diffuse abdominal pain, nausea, vomiting, diarrhoea
- Hyper-infection syndrome—corticosteroides, tacrolimus, chemotherapeutic agents, radiation therapy etc.

Laboratory diagnosis

- Specimens to be collected:
  - Stool
  - Duodenal aspirate
  - Sputum
  - Urine, etc.
- Larval demonstration in stool-low sensitivity ~ 20%.
- For isolation of larvae:
  - Baermann method
  - Harada Mori filter paper method—not very sensitive.
  - Agar plate method—96% sensitive but laborious and time consuming.
- Skin test
- Serology—IgG ELISA – about 85–95% sensitivity.

Treatment

- Ivermectin is drug of choice or thiabendazole and albendazole.

TISSUE NEMATODE

Filarial Worms

Characteristics of the filaria

Organism	Periodicity	Vector	Location of Adult	Microfilarial Location	Sheath
Wuchereria bancrofti	Nocturnal Subperiodic	Culex Anopheles Aedes	Lymphatic tissue Lymphatic tissue	Blood	+
Brugia malayi	Nocturnal Subperiodic	Mansonia, Anopheles Coquillettidia, Mansonia	Lymphatic tissue Lymphatic tissue	Blood	+
B. timori	Nocturnal	Anopheles	Lymphatic tissue	Blood	+
Loa loa	Diurnal	Chrysops (deerflies)	Subcutaneous tissue	Blood	+
Onchocerca volvulus	None	Simulium (blackflies)	Subcutaneous tissue	Skin, eye	–
Mansonella ozzardi	None	Culicoides (midges)	Undetermined site	Blood	–
M. perstans	None	Culicoides (midges)	Body cavities, mesentery, perirenal tissue	Blood	–
M. streptocerca	None	Culicoides (midges)	Subcutaneous tissue	Skin	-

Parasites associated with malignancy

Parasites	Malignancy
Schistosoma haematobium	Squamous cell carcinoma of urinary bladder
Clonorchis sinensis	Cholangiocarcinoma of liver, bile duct and Adenocarcinoma of pancreas
Opisthorchis viverrini	Cholangiocarcinoma of bile duct

Parasites causing anemia

Parasite	Type of anemia
Ancylostoma duodenale	Iron deficiency
Necator americanus	Iron deficiency
Babesia	Hemolytic
Plasmodium spp.	Autoimmune hemolytic
Trichuris trichiura	Iron deficiency
Leishmania donovani	Autoimmune hemolytic
Diphyllobothrium latum	Vit. B12 Deficiency/Megaloblastic

Parasites causing auto-infection

- Strongyloides stercoralis
- Taenia solium
- Hymenolepis nana
- Enterobius vermicularis
- Capillaria philippinensis
- Cryptosporidium parvum

Acid fast parasites

- Egg of taenia saginata
- Oocyst of isospora belle
- Oocyst of cyclospora
- Oocyst of cryptosporidium parvum

Non-bile stained eggs

- Hook worm
- Enterobius vermicularis
- Hymenolepis nana

MYCOLOGY

General properties

Eukaryotic	Nonmotile
DNA and RNA	Devoid of chlorophyll
Sexual and asexual reproduction	Cell wall—Chitin, Mannan and Polysaccharides
Cytoplasmic membrane Ergosterol	Nuclei + nuclear membrane and nucleolus
Uni and Multicellular	Yeast, Molds, Hyphae, Mycelium
Vegetative and Aerial mycelium	Fungal culture media—Sabouraud's dextrose agar (SDA)—pH 5.6

Classification

- **Systemic classification/taxonomical classification**

Class	Hyphae	Spores	Type
Zygomycetes	Nonseptate	Sporangiospores Zygospores	Asexual Asexual
Ascomycetes	Septate	Ascospores	Sexual
Basidiomycetes	Septate	Basidiospores	Sexual
Deuteromycetes	Septate	Lack of sexual state	

- **Morphological classification**

Yeast	Round/Oval Unicellular	Budding	Cryptococcus Rhodotorula
Yeast Like	Pseudohyphae	Budding	Candida Blastoscizomyces Trichosporon
Molds	Hyphae	Sexual and Asexual Spores	Dermatophytes, Aspergillus, Penicillium and Zygomycetes
Dimorphic	Yeast – 37°C Mold – 25°C		Penicillium marneffii Histoplasma capsulatum Coccidioidomycosis Para coccidioidomycosis Blastomyces Sporothrix schenckii Candida albicans (not thermally)

Reproduction of fungi

Sexual spores	Zygospores, Ascospores, and Basidiospores
Asexual spores **Aerial spores** **Vegetative spores**	Arthrospores, Blastospores, and Chlamydospores Microconidia, Macroconidia Sporangiospores, and Conidiospores,

Clinical Classification

Type	Anatomic Location	Disease
Superficial	Hair shaft, Dead layer of skin	Pityriasis versicolor, Tinea nigra
Cutaneous	Epidermis, hair and Nails	Dermatophytes
Subcutaneous	Dermis and Sub cutis	Chromoblastomycosis, Phaeohyphomycosis, Sporotrichosis Rhinosporidiosis Mycetoma agents
Systemic	Internal organs	Coccidioidomycosis, Paracoccidioidomycosis, Histoplasmosis, Blastomycosis and Cryptococcosis.
Opportunistic	Internal organs	Aspergillosis, Zygomycosis, Pneumocystitis Jiroveci Penicillium marneffei Cryptococcus neoformans

Superficial Mycosis

Fungi	Disease Caused	Characteristics	Lab diagnosis
Malassezia furfur (Pityrosporum orbicularae).	Pityriasis versicolor Rich area of sebaceous glands. Starum corneum hot and humid weather.	Lipophilic—SDA overlaid with olive oil—creamy colonies	KOH preparation Spaghetti and meat balls appearance LPCB—bottle shaped cells
Exophiala/Hortaea wernickii	Tinea nigra Well demarcated brown-back macular lesions, commonly seen on palms and soles.	Phaeoid/dematiaceous fungi Yeast-like growth on SDA	KOH mount of skin scrapping-Darkly pigmented yeast like cells and Septate branched hyphae
Piedraia hortae	Black piedra Superficial infections of the hair.	ASci—parasitic phase SDA Culture—chlamydospores	KOH mount of the hair nodule-club shaped asci with ascospores
Trichosporon beigelli Yeast-like fungi	White piedra hair of scalp, moustache and beard	Mycelium rapidly fragments to arthroconidia	KOH mount of hair–Intertwined hyphae/arthro/blastoconidia

Cutaneous Mycosis

- MC superficial mycosis—Dermatophytosis/tinea/ring worm infection
- Dermatophytes—Molds infecting superficial keratinized tissues like skin, hair, and nail.

Human pathogenic Dermatophytes classified into 3 genera and 42 species

- Trichophyton : Hair, Skin and Nail : 24 Species
- Epidermophyton : Skin and nail : 16 Species
- Microsporum : Hair and Skin : 2 Species

Classification based on habitat and host preferences

Groups	Character	Example
Anthropophilic	Adapted to live on human host. Human to human transmission	Trichophyton rubrum, Microsporum audouinii, Epidermophyton floccosum
Zoophilic	Adapted to live on animal host. Animal to human transmission	Trichophyton verrucosum, Microsporum canis.
Geophilic	Saprophytic, found in soil and dead organic substances. Occasional infections to humans	Microsporum gypseum, Trichophyton ajelloi.

Dermatophytid/id reaction:

- Belongs to telomorphic genera arthroderma (sexual state)

Morphology:

- In lesions: Hyphae and arthrospores seen.
- In culture: Septate hyphae with asexual spores (Micro and Macroconidia)

Microscopically differentiated based on Macro and Microconidia

Dermatophyte	Trichophyton	Microsporum	Epidermophyton
Macroconidia	Rare, thin walled, smooth, Single	Numerous, thick walled, rough Exept M. audouinii	Numerous, smooth walled
Microconidia	Abundant	Rare	Absent

Clinical syndromes—classified based on the site affected.

Clinical Types	Causative Dermatophytes
Tinea capitis (scalp hair)	Trichophyton spp and Microsporum spp.
Favus (scalp hair)	T. schoenleinii, rarely T. violaceum, M. gypseum
Kerion (scalp hair)	T. verrucosum, T. mentagrophytes
Tinea corporis (body skin)	T. rubrum and any other Dermatophytes
Tinea barbae (Beard)	T. rubrum, T. mentagrophytes and T. verrucosum
Tinea imbricate (concentric lesions of skin)	T. concentricum
Tinea unguium (nail plate)	T. rubrum, T. mentagrophytes and E. floccosum
Tinea pedis (Athlete foot)	T. rubrum, T. mentagrophytes and E. floccosum
Tinea cruris (jock itch)	E. floccosum, T. rubrum, and T. mentagrophytes
Tinea manuum (palm infection)	T. rubrum, T. mentagrophytes and E. floccosum
Endothrix hair infection—Arthrospores found inside the infected hair shaft.	T. Tonsurans, T. violaceum, T. schoenleinii (TVS)
Ectothrix hair infection—Arthrospores form sheath around the infected hair shaft	T. Mentagrophytes, M. audouinii, M. canis (MAC)

Lab diagnosis

- Specimens—infected hair, nail clippings and skin scrapings.
- 10% KOH mount preparation—branched septate hyphae.

- Wood's lamp examination (UV light)—infected hair appears bright green fluorescent, mainly for hair infection by microsporum spp.
- Fungal culture—SDA with antibiotics chloromphenicol and cycloheximide. Growth appears in 10 days to 3 weeks.

Hair perforation test		
Positive	T.mentagrophytes (urease positive)	Microsporum canis
Negative	T.rubrum, (urease negative)	Microsporum equinum

- Drug of choice—oral griseofulvin.

Subcutaneous Mycosis

- lesions in subcutaneous tissues and overlying skin with or without extension to bone and muscle.
- Causative agents are low pathogenic potential introduced into the body by trivial trauma.

Causative agents of subcutaneous mycosis

Disease	Etiological agents
Mycetoma	Fungi (eumycotic) and bactertia (actinomycotic)
Chromoblastomycosis	Fonsecaea spp, phialophora spp, cladophialophora spp.
Phaeohyphomycosis	Exophiala spp., bipolaris, wangiella spp.
Sporotrichosis	Sporothrix schenckii
Rhinosporidiosis	Rhinosporidium seeberi

Mycetoma

- Chronic granulamatous disease—feet and hands
- Common in tropical and subtropical countries.
- Gill from Madurai
- Tumefactions, draining sinuses and discharging granules (Triad)
- Actinomycetoma accounts nearly 65% of mycetomas and eumycetoma accounts about 35%.
- *Actinomadura madurae* is the major causative agent.
- Lab diagnosis—demonstration of the fungi or fungal elements in granules, pus and biopsy tissue by microscopy.

Chromoblastomycosis

- Slowly progressing granulomatous infection, caused group of phaeoid fungi.
- Development of warty nodules and cauliflower like lesions at the site of infection.
- Lab diagnosis—H and E staining—demonstration of small clusters of round and dark brown, thick walled cells—sclerotic bodies in tissues is characteristic.
- In PAS staining—sclerotic bodies/copper penny bodies are red in colour

Rhinosporidiosis

- Chronic granulomatous disease, characterized by development of red, friable polyps in the nose, conjunctiva or eye.
- Causative agent *Rhinosporidium seeberi.*
- *R. seeberi* cannot be cultured in cell-free artificial media.
- Lab diagnosis—demonstration of *R. seeberi* in tissue sections stained with H and E stains. Hyperplastic surface epithelium and stroma embedded with sporangia containing hundreds of Sporangiospores.

Sporotrichosis

- *S. schenckii*—dimorphic fungi.
- Infection is introduced in skin by trauma (thorn prick injury)

- Rose Gardener's disease'.
- Draining lymphatic system involvement is characteristic.
- Lab diagnosis—demonstration of asteroid bodies in pus of abscesses by microscopy and isolation of fungi in culture.
- Lacto phenol blue (LPCB) wet mount of the colony shows cigar-shaped yest like cells.
- Drug of choice of cutaneous sporotrichosis—itraconazole, KI
- Drug of choice for extracutaneous sporotrichosis—IV amphotericin B.

Opportunistic Mycosis

- These fungi usually cause infections in persons with impaired host defense.
- They do not cause disease in most of the immunocompetent hosts.

Disease	Causative fungus
Candidiasis	Candida albicans, Candida tropicalis, C.krusei etc
Meningitis	Cryptococcus neoformans
Aspergillosis	Aspergillus flavus, Aspergillus niger and A. fumigatus
Zygomycosis	Mucor, Rhizopus and Absidia spp.
Penicilliosis	Penicillium marneffei
Pneumocystis Jiroveci Pneumonia	Pneumocystis jiroveci

Zygomycetes

- Mucormycosis/phycomycosis
- *Mucor, Rhizopus* and *Absidia*.
- Invasive fungal infection in immunocompromised patients.
- *Rhizopus* species are the MC causative agents of zygomycosis in humans
- Angioinvasion leading to ischemia, necrosis, and infarction More prone to patients with acidosis secondary to renal insufficiency, diarrhea, and aspirin intake.
- Rhinocerebral zygomycosis—common in patients with DM
- KOH mount—broad, irregularly set Aseptate hyphae with right-angled branches
- Culture on SDA—is dense and hairy growth
- Surgical removal of necrotic, infected tissues and DOC—Amphotericin B

Pneumocystis Jiroveci

- Previously known as Pneumocystis carinii,
- Most common opportunistic infection in HIV-infected patients.
- Three Morphologic stages:
  - The trophozoite or tropic form
  - Sporozoite—precystic form, and
  - Cyst which contains several intracystic bodies (spores).
- Transmission of infection occurs by inhalation.
- Defects in both cellular immunity and humoral immunity allow development of the disease.
- P. jiroveci causes Pneumonia, in HIV patients with their CD4 cells count below 200/µl and patients with primary immune deficiencies
- Chest radiographs—show diffuse bilateral infiltrates extending from the perihilar region.
- Induced sputum and bronchoalveolar lavage (BAL) is ideal sample sensitivity more than 90%.
- Open lung biopsy has 100% sensitivity and specificity.
- HPE by Wright, Cresyl violet, and Giemsa stain—detect both the trophozoite and cyst forms, but not the cyst wall.
- Methenamine silver, Gram—Weigert, and Toluidine blue stain—Cyst wall.

- Direct immunofluorescence using monoclonal antibodies is more sensitive
- Does not respond to treatment with antifungal agents.
- Combination of trimethoprim and sulfamethoxazole is the drug of choice.
- Pentamidine and atovaquone are alternative drugs.
- Chemoprophylaxis with septran in HIV positive patients

Penicillium Marneffei

- Dimorphic fungi causing penicilliosis
- Colony—obverse—greenish yellow with red center and brick red pigment on the reverse side,
- Characteristic virulence is proliferation inside macrophages
- Cervical lymphadenitis resembling tuberculosis in immunocompetent hosts.
- Disseminated infection only in immunocompromised hosts—HIV patients.
- Allergic diseases and mycotoxicoses and Infects only man and bamboo rat.
- Specimens—skin and mucosal scrapings, sputum, stool, blood, urine, lymph node, bone marrow, lung and liver biopsy specimens.
- Stains—H and E, PAS, Wright's, and calcofluor white stain.
- Immunohistochemical assay using monoclonal antibody is used in tissues
- Antigen detection in serum and urine.—LAT
- IV Amphotericin B for 2 weeks followed by oral itraconazole for 10 weeks.

Aspergillosis

- *Aspergillus fumigatus* and *aspergillus niger, aspergillus flavus* and *aspergillus terreus.*
- Walls of the hyphae are septate and parallel, but in *mucor* and *rhizopus* walls are aseptate and more irregular.
- The conidia form radiating chains
- Rapid grower in SDA, produces colonies within 1–2 days with velvety surface.
- Causes invasive infections in immunocompromised host.
- Angioinvasion, leading to infarction, hemorrhage, and necrosis of lung tissues.
- Produces toxic metabolites that inhibit phagocytosis, facilitating dissemination of the infection.
- Do not form normal flora of humans.
- Allergic bronchopulmonary aspergillosis (Hypersensitivity reaction), Chronic necrotizing pulmonary aspergillosis, aspergilloma, invasive aspergillosis.
- Mycotoxicosis
- KOH preparation—septate hyphae with characteristic dichotomous branching at an angle of 45°, on SDA different *Aspergillus* species produce colonies of various colors—*A. fumigatus*—Green, *A. A. flavus—yellow, A. niger—Black* colonies.
- Estimation of serum galactomannan, a major constituent of *aspergillus* cell wall is useful in diagnosis of invasive aspergillosis.
- Amphotericin B is used for treatment of invasive aspergillosis.

Candidiasis

- Most common fungal pathogen affecting humans.
- These are true opportunistic pathogens that take advantage of the host compromised immune status.
- *C. albicans* is ovoid or spherical yeast with a single bud.
- It forms the part of the normal flora of the mucus membrane of the gastrointestinal, genitourinary, respiratory tract.
- It produces pseudohyphae in the cultures and in tissues.
- *Candida* grows readily on SDA and on bacteriological culture media.
- *C. albicans* produces creamy white, smooth colonies with a yeasty odor.
- Alteration in CMI may cause extensive superficial candidiasis.

- The humoral antibodies appear to play minimal role in protection against the disease.
- **Cutaneous candidiasis:** *Candida* species in immunocompetent host can cause infection of any warm and moist parts of the body exposed to environment. It causes infection of the nail, rectum, and other skin folds.
- **Mucocutaneous candidiasis:** Mucocutaneous candidiasis (oral thrush, perianal disease, etc.) is the most common manifestation of candidiasis. *Candida* species can cause severe oropharyngeal and esophageal candidiasis in HIV patients.
- **Chronic mucocutaneous candidiasis:** Chronic, treatment-resistant, superficial *Candida* infection of the skin, nails, and oropharynx.
- **Systemic candidiasis:** These include endocarditis, gastrointestinal tract candidiasis, respiratory tract candidiasis, genitourinary candidiasis, and hepatosplenic candidiasis. Systemic candidiasis may be candidemia and disseminated candidiasis.
- **Disseminated candidiasis:** Patients with severe neutropenia is the most important predisposing condition for life-threatening infection caused by Candida.
- Specimens—These include exudates or tissues for microscopy obtained from skin or nails.
- Demonstration of Gram-positive, oval, budding yeast with pseudohyphae
- Demonstration of pseudohyphae indicates colonization and tissue invasion
- On SDA—typical creamy white, smooth colonies with yeasty odour.
- Germ tube test (Reynold-Braude phenomenon)—rapid method for identification of C. albicans and Candida dubliniensis.
- Chlamydospore production on cornmeal agar at 20°C is positive by C. albicans and *Candida dubliniensis*.
- CHROM agar allows for the presumptive identification of several Candida species by showing different colors of the colonies depending on the Candida species.

Nonculture Candida detection tests:

- Candida mannan assay,
- Candida heat-labile-antigen assay,
- D-arabinitol assay,
- D-inositol assay, and
- 1, 3-beta-D-glucan assay.
- **Serological tests** are not that useful in diagnosis of patients with candidiasis because antibodies against Candida appear in sera of patients as well as in that of normal persons.
- **Skin test** with Candida antigen—delayed-hypersensitivity test (an indicator of functions of the CMI).
- Antifungal agents like azoles (fluconazole, triazole ketoconazole), nystatin, and amphotericin B.
- C. glabrata and Candida krusei are less susceptible/resistant to amphotericin B and other azoles (ketoconazole, fluconazole, etc).

Cryptococcus neoformans

- Cryptococcus neoformans/European Blastomycosis,
- Acute to chronic disease caused by an encapsulated yeast, *C. neoformans.*
- Cryptococcosis is the most common life-threatening fungal disease in HIV.
- There are 3 varieties and 4 serotypes (A, B, C & D) based on antigenic specificity of the capsular polysaccharide-
  - *C. neoformans* var grubi (serotype A)
  - *C. neoformans* var gattii (serotype B/C)—causes disease in immunocompetent patients and respond slowly to treatment
  - *C. neoformans* var *neoformans* (serotype D) causes disease in immunocompromised patients, e.g., AIDS.
- It is a true yeast with an oval and spherical budding yeast cell.
- Polysaccharide capsule composed of mannose, xylose, and glucuronic acid.
- It is gram-positive budding yeast cell.

- On SDA medium—smooth, convex, mucoid, cream-colored colonies at 20–37°C.
- Teleomorphic/sexual state is *Filobasidiella neoformans*.
- CMI is mediated by natural killer cells and T lymphocytes kills *Cryptococci.*
- Causes serious infections in patients with impaired CMI.
- Transmitted by inhalation.
- Cryptococcal polysaccharide capsule has antiphagocytic properties.
- Pulmonary cryptococcosis in immunocompetent
- CNS cryptococcosis—Subacute or chronic meningitis and meningoencephalitis
- Disseminated nonpulmonary non-CNS cryptococcosis—occurs most commonly in patients with AIDS and other immunosuppressed conditions.
- Specimen—CSF, sputum, pus, and brain biopsy tissue.
- Demonstration of the yeast by smear and isolation in culture is diagnostic.
- Methenamine silver stain or Periodic acid-Schiff stains used for demonstration of the capsule in tissue specimen.
- In India ink preparation of CSF, capsule (clear halo around the yeast cell) can be demonstrated in 25–50% of patients with cryptococcal meningitis.
- *C. neoformans* also produces melanin (black colonies), when incubated on Bird-seed agar/Niger seed agar
- Latex agglutination test (LAT) used to detect cryptococcal polysaccharide antigen in the serum or CSF for diagnosis of meningitis.
- Amphotericin B is the drug of choice.
- Hepatitis is an adverse effect of ketoconazole
- Woods light—Microsporum and T. schoenleinii—green, Pitiriasis rosea—Yellow
- Mycotoxins—Aflatoxin—Aspergillus flavus—hepatotoxicity
- LSD—Mental disorders
- Mycetism—GI disease caused by fungi itself

Systemic Mycosis

- Systemic mycosis is caused by fungi of soil, which are inherently virulent and cause disease in healthy humans.
- Infection is by inhalation of the spores of the fungi and lung is the primary target organ.

Causative agent	Dimorphism	Morphology	Disease	Laboratory diagnosis
Coccidioides immitis	Present	Spherule in tissues, which is resistance to host defenses	Coccidioido mycosis Valley fever or Desert rheumatism	Demonstration of spherules containing endospores by H and E or PAS stain. Culture
Paracoccidioides brasiliensis	Present	Multiple budding yeast cells—Mickey Mouse head or Pilot wheel appearance	Para coccidioidomycosis South American Blastomycosis	Microscopy Culture—SDA
Histoplasma capsulatum	Present	Thin, branching, acroco hyphae with tuberculate acroconidia and micoconidia	Darling' s diasese, RES Pulmonary histoplasmosis	Wright/giemsa stain, L A test
Blastomyces dermatitidis	Present	septate hyphae forming conidiophores bearing piriform conidia and broad based budding yeast cells	North American Blastomycosis Pneumonia	Culture—SDA ELISA

- H. dubosii-African histoplasmosis

QUESTIONS

1. Which of the following is not a feature of exotoxin? (2014)

a. High antigenicity
b. Neutralised by antibodies
c. Heat stable'
d. Protein in nature

2. Mechanism of development of resistance to penicillin in Streptococcus pneumonia is: (2014)

a. Production of Beta lactamase
b. Mutations in the penicillin binding proteins on the bacterial surface
c. Changes in the membrane permeability to penicillin
d. Production of an alternative penicillin binding protein

3. A New agent was developed to increase the recognition of foreign antigens by Antigen presenting cells. True regarding the physiological aspects of APCs (2014)

a. Antigen is presented via MHC–I complexes
b. APCs are required before a response to viruses are generated
c. Direct antibody stimulation still requires APC's
d. Antigen processed by APC are recognized by CD 4+ T Cells

4. True regarding thymus is: (2014)

a. Mature thymocytes express CD 4 and CD 8
b. Thymocytes whose T Cell receptor bind with high affinity to self-antigens and MHC Complexes are Clonally deleted
c. Mature thymocytes express surface IgM and IgD
d. CD 4 and CD 8 double positive cells are eliminated by a process of negative selection

5. A 16-year-old male patient presents with headache, fever and neck stiffness for the past 24 hours. similar history was present one year back. CSF analysis shows WBC's–400 ml, with 90% neutrophils. Gram staining shows gram negative diplococcic. The immune system affected in this condition is: (2014)

a. B lymphocytes
b. T lymphocytes
c. Immunoglobulins
d. Complement system

6. All the following are true about Staphylococcus aureus except: (2014)

a. Coagulase positive
b. Catalase negative
c. DNAse positive
d. Indole negative

7. There was a sudden outbreak of MRSA infection in a general ward. The best method for reducing the MRSA outbreak in the ward and to reduce the transmission is: (2014)

a. Encourage regular hand wash
b. Clean the walls and floors with chlorhexidine
c. Screen the ward staff using nasal swabs and exclude those with positive culture for MRSA
d. Close the ward for 1 month

8. A 37-year-old person, poorly controlled case of type-I DM presents with painful, red, swollen middle finger with redness extending to metacarpophalangeal joint. A diagnosis of cellulitis is made and treated with antibiotics. What is the organism causing this condition? (2014)

a. Pseudomonas aeruginosa
b. Klebsiella Pneumoniae
c. MRSA
d. Streptococcus pyogenes

9. 19 years old male patient comes to the emergency department with complaints of urethral discharge, 1 week after having unprotected sex. Gram staining reveals numerous neutrophils, some gram negative intracellular diplococci. He was treated with ceftriaxone 250 mg i.m 5 days later he returns with the same complaints. What is the diagnosis? (2014)

a. Chlamydia trachomatis
b. Penicillin resistant Neisseria gonorrhea
c. Reinfection with Neisseria gonorrhea
d. Ureaplasma urealyticum

10. A strain of E.coli isolated from urine is resistant to third generation cephalosporins. The mechanism of development of resistance is: (2014)

a. Extended spectrum Beta-Lactamases
b. Decreased permeability
c. Active effux of Beta-Lactam agents
d. Alteration of PBP's

11. Infection that can be acquired in laboratories except: (2014)

a. Brucellosis
b. Tuberculosis
c. Pertussis
d. Melioidosis.

12. A child present culosis. Steroids are not indicated in: (2014)
a. Tuberculoma
b. Endobronchial tuberculosis
c. Pleural effusion
d. Progressive primary pulmonary disease

13. Agent used in interferon gamma release assay for diagnosing latent tuberculosis is: (2014)
a. MPT 64
b. Mycolic acid
c. Lipoarabinomannan
d. ESAT-6

14. 45 years old female patient presents with duodenal ulcer. The most sensitive test for the detection of H. Pylori is: (2014)
a. Urea breath test
b. Serology
c. Biopsy and culture
d. Stool antigen test

15. Channel activated by cholera toxin: (2014)
a. Adenylate cyclase
b. Guanyl cyclase
c. ABC transport channel
d. Iron transport channel

16. A 25 years old male presents with 2 months history of loose stools and weight loss. Laboratory diagnostic tests are positive for HIV. Presence of which of the following disease is most likely in diagnosing HIV/AIDS: (2014)
a. Lyme disease
b. Glandular fever
c. Oropharyngeal candidiasis
d. Pulmonary TB

17. Parotid enlargement in a HIV infected child is characterized in which stage of AIDS, according to WHO? (2014)
a. Stage 1
b. Stage 2
c. Stage 3
d. Stage 4

18. Indication for varicella immunoglobulin is: (2014)
a. A pregnant woman non-immune to Varicella Zoster, exposed to a child with chickenpox 12 days ago
b. A pregnant woman non-immune to Varicella Zoster, exposed to mother with shingles
c. A pregnant woman with no history of chickenpox develops shingles
d. Pregnant woman previously treated with varicella immunoglobulin 10 days ago, but reexposed to a case of chickenpox.

19. Negri bodies are pathological inclusions seen in some pathological conditions. They are seen in all the following areas except: (2014)
a. Pyramidal neurons of hippocampus
b. Subcortical white matter
c. Basal ganglia
d. Purkinje cells of cerebellum

20. Modality not employed in the diagnosis of respiratory viruses in laboratory: (2014)
a. ELISA
b. Immunofluorescence
c. Single Radial Hemolysis
d. Hemagglutination

21. Morphological appearance of Pneumocystis jiroveci infection of lung is best characterized by: (2014)
a. Hemorrhagic and necrotizing pneumonia
b. ARDS with wide spread hyaline membrane formation
c. Interstitial pneumonitis with foamy intra alveolar exudates
d. Broncho pulmonary abscess formation

22. Which infection cannot spread in laboratory?
a. TB (2014)
b. Brucellosis
c. Meliodosis
d. Pertusis

23. False about Staphylococcus aureus is: (2014)
a. Coagulase positive
b. Catalase positive
c. Oxidase positive
d. DNAse positive

24. Craigie tube is used to differentiate between:
a. Virulent and avirulent strains (2014)
b. Rough and smooth strains
c. Motile and non-motile strains
d. Capsulated and non-capsulated strains

25. Espundia is a condition seen in: (2014)
a. Endemic syphilis
b. Malaria
c. Lympho Granuloma Venereum
d. Mucocutaneous leishmaniasis

26. Best disinfectant for endoscopes is:
a. Hypochlorite (2014)
b. Formaldehyde
c. Glutaraldehyde
d. Chlorhexidine

27. Immunoglobulin that activates the alternate complement pathway is (2014)
a. Ig A
b. Ig G
c. Ig M
d. Ig E

28. Transfer of genetic material in between bacteria through pili termed as: (2014)
a. Transduction
b. Conjugation
c. Transformation
d. Transfection

29. Percentage of total lymphocytes formed by null cells: (2014)
a. 0–1%
b. 2–3%
c. 5–10%
d. 10–15%

30. All these are the properties of exotoxin except:
a. Heat stable (2014)
b. Highly antigenic
c. Neutralized by antibodies
d. Protein in nature

31. Salmonella species are characterized by all except: (2014)
a. Acid and gas production from fermenting glucose
b. Citrate synthesis
c. H2S production
d. Indole negative

32. Which of the following bacterium is non-motile?
a. Klebsiella spp. (2014)
b. Citrobacter spp.
c. Escherichia spp.
d. Salmonella spp.

33. HIV infects which of the following cells? (2014)
a. NK cells
b. T-helper cells
c. T suppressor cells
d. Plasma cells

34. All are true about Koch's postulates except: (2014)
a. Disease should be susceptible to broad spectrum antibiotics
b. Organism causing lesion can be isolated from lesion
c. Organism can be cultured in artificial media
d. Organism causes similar lesion if inoculated in other person

35. All are live vaccines except: (2013)
a. BCG
b. Salk vaccine
c. Measles
d. Mumps

36. All are motile except: (2013)
a. Klebsiella
b. E.coli
c. Salmonella
d. Citrobacter

37. Immunoglobulins are seen as surface antigens on:
a. Neutrophils
b. Monocytes
c. NK Cells
d. B cells

38. Ig secreted in secondary immune response is:
a. Ig G (2013)
b. Ig M
c. Ig A
d. Ig E

39. Cytomegalovirus false statement:
a. Ds DNA
b. Uncommon in immunocompetent
c. Retinitis is uncommon if CD more than 200
d. Virus is eliminated by foscarnet

40. Mycobacteria exclusively affecting skin: (2013)
a. Mycobacterium marinum
b. Mycobacterium fortuitum
c. Mycobacterium xenopi
d. Mycobacterium chelonei

41. All are true about culture media except: (2013)
a. Best medium for anaerobes is chocolate agar
b. LJ medium is used for tubercle bacilli
c. Blood agar supports fastidious organisms
d. Loeffler's serum slope is used for Corynebacterium diphtheria

42. MHC II is present in: (2013)
a. Langerhans cell
b. Dendritic cell
c. T cell
d. NK cell

43. False regarding NK cells (2013)
a. NK cell activity is augmented by interferons
b. Initial response in viral infection
c. Active against tumour cells
d. MCH restricted

44. True about Northern blot technique: (2013)
a. Detects DNA
b. Detects RNA

c. Detects proteins
d. Detects post translational modifications in proteins

45. True statement regarding MRSA is: (2013)
a. Ceftriaxone is preferred for treatment of superficial MRSA infections
b. MRSA isolates produce β-lactamase
c. The mecA gene of MRSA encodes for penicillin-binding protein 2a (PBP2a), which has high affinity for β-lactam antibiotics
d. Pulsed gel field electrophoresis is used for typing

46. Aerogenic shigella: (2013)
a. Shigella flexneri Type 6
b. Shigela dysenteriae Type 1
c. Shigella sonnei
d. Shigella boydii type 4

47. Pathogenic and non-pathogenic Cryptococcus can be differentiated by all except: (2013)
a. Growth at 37°
b. Ability to hydrolyse urea
c. Colour reactions on canavanine-glycine-bromthymol blue
d. Melanin production

48. All are used for Gram staining except: (2013)
a. Carbol fuchsin
b. Alcian blue
c. Methyl violet
d. Sarfanine

49. Which of the following is a photochromogen?
a. Mycobacterium kansasii (2012)
b. Mycobacterium fortuitum
c. Mycobacterium gordonae
d. Mycobacterium xenopi

50. Mycobacterium simiae belongs to which of the following? (2012)
a. Scotochromogen
b. Photo chromogen
c. Nonphotochromogen
d. Rapid grower

51. Periportal fibrosis is caused by: (2012)
a. S. hemotobium
b. S. japanicum
c. S. manosni
d. S. intercalatum

52. Russel bodies and Mickulicz cells: (2012)
a. Rhinosporidiosis
b. Rhinoscleromatosis
c. Atrophic rhinitis
d. Mucormycosis

53. Miyagawa granulocorpusles bodies are seen in:
a. Lymphogranuloma venereum (LGV) **(2012)**
b. Chylamydia pneumonia
c. Mycoplasma
d. Chlamydia transhomatosis

54. Guarneri bodies are found in: (2012)
a. Smallpox
b. Herpes virus
c. Adenovirus
d. Coxsackie virus

55. Which one of the following is a dimorphic fungus? (2012)
a. Histoplasma capsulatum
b. Candida albicans
c. Aspergillus fumigates
d. Pneumocystis carinii

56. Thayer martin is selective medium for: (2012)
a. Neisseria gonorroheae
b. Streptococcus pyogenes
c. Streptococcus agalactiae
d. Streptococcus pneumonia

57. Malignant pustulosis is observed in: (2012)
a. Anthrax
b. Actinomycotic mycetoma
c. Plague
d. Cutaneous mycormycosis

58. Zoonotic infection in an agricultural labourer can be caused by all except: (2012)
a. Tetanus b. Q fever
c. Leptospirosis d. Plague

59. Which of the following is false regarding sporotrihosis: (2012)
a. It spreads by lymphatics
b. Caused by S. schenkii
c. Medilar bodies
d. Potassium iodide is drug of choice

60. Primary amoebic encephalitis caused by: (2012)
a. Naegleria fowleri
b. Acanthameba spp.
c. Entamoeba hartmanni
d. Balmuthia mandrillaris

61. Griffith's experiment on pneumococci using mouse was: (2012)
a. Lysogenic phage conversion
b. Translation
c. Transformation
d. Conjugation

62. Staphylococcal capsule is made up of: (2012)
a. Hyaluronic acid
b. Polysaccharide
c. Polypeptide
d. Poly-D-glutamic acid

63. Virulence marker antigen VMA used in the diagnosis of: (2012)
a. Mycobacterium tuberculosis
b. Atypical mycobacterium
c. Pneumococcus
d. Enteroinvasive E. coli (EIEC)

64. Most common zoonotic disease transmitted from animal to human: (2012)
a. Brucellosis
b. Rabies
c. Leptospirosis
d. Anthrax

65. Causative organism of Weil disease is: (2012)
a. Leptospira interrogans
b. Leptospira biflexa
c. Leptospira wolbachii
d. Leptospira inadai

66. Which of the following is not actively involved in cell mediated immunity? (2012)
a. NK cell
b. Cytotoxic T cell
c. Helper cell
d. B cell

67. Which specimen shouldn't be refrigerated before primary inoculation? (2011)
a. CSF
b. Urine
c. Sputum
d. Pus

68. Multidrug resistance through plasmids is transferred by: (2011)
a. Transduction
b. Transfection
c. Conjugation
d. Recombination

69. Swarming motility is shown by: (2011)
a. Proteus
b. Cholera
c. Shigella
d. Salmonella

70. False positive test against treponemal antigen is seen in: (2011)
a. HIV
b. Infectious mononucleosis
c. Lyme's disease
d. SLE

71. Coxsackie A virus causes all except: (2011)
a. Aseptic meningitis
b. Herpangina
c. Hand, foot and mouth disease
d. Bornholm's disease

72. The most efficient antigen presenting cell present in the skin is: (2011)
a. Dendritic cell
b. Macrophages
c. Langerhan's cell
d. Kupffer cells

73. Normal percentage of CD4 cells at birth is: (2011)
a. 45% of T cells
b. 45% of T cells
c. 65% of T cells
d. 80% of T Cells

74. Which of the following is a dimorphic fungus? (2011)
a. Rhizopus
b. Sporothrix schenckii
c. Tinea versicolor
d. Microsporum

75. Which is Eaton agent? (2011)
a. Mycoplasma
b. H.influenzal
c. Klebsiella
d. Chlamydia

76. VDRL is most sensitive in the diagnosis of which stage of syphilis? (2011)
a. Primary
b. Secondary
c. Tertiary
d. Reactivation

77. Which agent is effective in killing spores? (2011)
a. Alcohol
b. Phenol
c. Chlorine
d. Formaldehyde

78. Gas gangrene is caused by? (2010)
a. Clostridium botulium
b. Clostridium perfingens
c. Clostridium difficile
d. Clostridium tetani

79. Non motile clostridia is: (2010)
a. Clostridium tetanomorphum
b. Clostridium histolyticum
c. Clostridium septicum
d. Clostridium pefringens

80. False regarding brucellosis is: (2010)
a. Transmitted my milk ingestion
b. Cephalosporins is the drug of choice
c. Causes gastroenteritis
d. Causes spinal spondylosis

81. Other name of Cachetin is: (2010)
a. TNF-alpha
b. IL-2
c. IL-12
d. IFN- gamma

82. Which of these is sporicidal? (2010)
a. Alcohol
b. Phenol
c. Chlorine
d. Glutaraldehyde

83. Toxic shock syndrome caused by Staphylococcus is due to: (2010)
a. Hemolysins
b. Super antigens
c. Coagulase
d. Hyaluronidase

84. Which is the largest pathogenic bacillus? (2010)
a. Bacillus cereus
b. Bacillus subtilis
c. Bacillus megaterium
d. Bacillius anthracis

85. Ritter's disease is caused by: (2010)
a. Pseudomonas aeruginosa
b. Pneumococcus
c. Bacillus anthracis
d. Staphylococcus aureus

86. Basophilic inclusion bodies seen in: (2010)
a. Polio virus
b. Adenovirus
c. Measles virus
d. Herpes virus

87. The cyclic trend seen with influenza is due to
a. Antigenic drift (2010)
b. Antigenic shift
c. Endemicity
d. Virulence

88. Quadrivalent HPV vaccine protects against: (2010)
a. HPV 6, 11, 16, 18
b. HPV 6, 11, 31, 32
c. HPV 16, 18, 31, 35
d. HPV 11, 16, 30, 33

89. Thick walled fungal resting spores formed by condensation of hyphal elements is: (2010)
a. Basidiospore
b. Arthrospore
c. Chlamydospores
d. Blastospore

90. Which of the following cell has both T lymphocyte and B lymphocyte function: (2009)
a. Plasma Cell
b. T-lymphoblast Cell
c. B-lymphoblast cell
d. NK cell

91. Gram negative antigen is injected in a rabbit intradermally followed by a second intravenous injection 24 hours later. It developed a hemorrhagic and necrotic lesion at the site of the first injection. What is this reaction? (2009)
a. Schwartzman reaction
b. Schultz-dale phenomenon
c. P-K-reaction
d. Arthus reaction

92. Which of the following is an oncogenic retrovirus?
a. HTLV-1 (2009)
b. HPV
c. EBV
d. HBV

93. The disease called "lumpy jaw" is produced by:
a. Actinomyces israelii (2009)
b. Streptomyces
c. Nocardia asteroids
d. Rhizopus nigricans

94. Which of the following statement is true about bacterioides? (2009)
a. It is gram positive bacilli
b. It is strictly aerobic
c. It may cause peritonitis
d. Presence in stool culture indicates need for treatment

95. Most common cause of traveller's diarrhea is:
a. EHEC (2009)
b. ETEC
c. EPEC
d. EIEC

96. All mycobacteria produces pigment except:
a. M. kansasii (2009)
b. M. simiae
c. M. avium
d. M. scrofulaceum

97. Northern blot is used for identification of: (2008)
a. RNA
b. DNA
c. Protein
d. Antibodies

98. Nongranular fungal disease is: (2008)
a. Cryptococcosis
b. Blastomycosis
c. Candidiasis
d. Paracoccidoidomycosis

99. Phage typing is useful in classification of all except: (2008)
a. Staphylococcus
b. Streptococcus
c. Cholera
d. Salmonella

100. Pinta is caused by: (2008)
a. T pertenue
b. T pallidum
c. T carateum
d. Borrelia burgdorferi

101. Maximum exposure to HIV is seen in: (2008)
a. Intrapartum period
b. Breastfeeding
c. 1st Trimester
d. 3rd Trimester

102. Bacterial adherence to epithelium is mediated through: (2008)
a. Sex pili
b. Fimbriae
c. Flagella
d. Mesosomes

103. All the following organisms lack capsule except: (2008)
a. Histoplasma capsulatum
b. Cryptococcus neoformans
c. Candida albicans
d. Coccidioides immitis

104. Ova with terminal spines is feature of: (2008)
a. Schistosoma japonicum
b. Schistosoma mansoni
c. Schistosoma haematobium
d. Schistosoma mekongi

105. The Tzanck test, which aids in the diagnosis of herpes simplex infection, is a search for: (2008)
a. Intracytoplasmic inclusion bodies
b. Koilocytic cells
c. Virus shedding from pustular lesions
d. Multinucleated giant cells

106. A bone marrow transplant recipient becomes febrile and hypoxic and chest films demonstrate diffuse interstitial pneumonia. What is the most likely causative agent? (2008)
a. BK virus
b. Cytomegalovirus
c. Herpes simplex virus
d. Paramyxovirus

107. Chlamydia trachomatis is associated with the following except: (2008)
a. Endemic trachoma
b. Inclusion conjunctivitis
c. Lymphogranuloma venereum
d. Community acquire pneumonia

108. Rectal prolapsed is associated with: (2008)
a. Trichuris trichiura
b. Strongyloides sterocoralis
c. Necator americanus
d. Trichinella spiralis

109.Serum sickness is due to which type of hypersensitivity? (2007)
a. Type I
b. Type II
c. Type III
d. Type IV

110. Most common site of infection with Cryptococcus neoformans is: (2007)
a. Lung
b. Meninges
c. Skin
d. Bone

111. All are true about streptococcal infections except:
a. Throat infection more common in age group of 5–15 years (2007)
b. Skin infection more common in age <3 years
c. 15–20% colonization of mucosal surfaces
d. Scarlet fever more common <3 years

112. Which of the following activates the classical complement pathway? (2007)
a. Immune complex
b. Lipopolysaccharide
c. Exotoxin
d. Zymosan

113. Which leukotriene is the adhesion factor for the neutrophil on the cell surface to attach endothelium? (2007)
a. B4
b. C4
c. D4
d. E4

114. Oil and Grease are sterilized by: (2007)
a. Hot air oven
b. Autoclaving
c. Filtration
d. Irradiation

115. Which of the following is not true of Steptococcus pneumonia? (2007)
a. Bile insoluble
b. Bleaching on chocolate agar
c. Causes meningitis
d. Possesses capsule

116. Coxsackie A virus causes all except: (2007)
a. Aseptic meningitis

b. Herpangina
c. Hand foot and mouth disease
d. Bornholm's disease

117. Motile clostridia is: **(2007)**
a. Clostridium tetanomorphum
b. Clostridium histolyticum
c. Clostridium septicum
d. Clostridium perfringens

118. Warthin finkeldy cells are found in: **(2006)**
a. Measles
b. Mumps
c. Molluscum contagiosum
d. Herpes simplex infection

119. SARS is due to: **(2006)**
a. Hantavirus
b. Orthomyxovirus
c. Coronavirus
d. Respiratory syncytial virus

120. Prozone phenomenon is due to: **(2006)**
a. Antigen excess
b. Antibody excess
c. Excessive immune complex
d. Acute phase reactants

121. Which of the following is not a coccidian parasite? **(2006)**
a. Isospora
b. Toxoplasma
c. Blastomyces
d. Cyclospora

122. Which of the following is catalase positive?
a. Staph epidermidis **(2006)**
b. Enterococcus
c. Streptococcus
d. Pneumococcus

123. Toxoplasma infection in first trimester causes:
a. Achorioretinitis **(2006)**
b. Cardiac defets
c. Neural tube defects
d. Hearing defects

124. Hyperinfective syndrome is seen in: **(2006)**
a. Enterobius
b. Strongyloidosis
c. Ascariasis
d. Trichuriasis

125. Which parasite is not found in muscle? **(2006)**
a. Trichuris
b. Toxoplasma
c. Trichinella
d. Sarcocystis

126. The Entamoeba species that is morphologically identical to E. histolytica is: **(2006)**
a. E. coli
b. E. dispar
c. E. hartmanni
d. E. gingivalis

127. A liquid medium which selective favours the growth of pathogenic bacteria and inhibits the commensal bacteria is known as: **(2006)**
a. Enriched medium
b. Selective medium
c. Enrichment medium
d. Differential medium

128. A liquid medium which selective favours the growth of pathogenic bacteria and inhibits the commensal bacteria is known as: **(2006)**
a. Enriched medium
b. Selective medium
c. Enrichment medium
d. Differential medium

129. Vector for Visceral leishmaniasis in India is
a. Phlebotomus orientalis **(2006)**
b. Phlebotomus major
c. Phleobotomus argentipes
d. Lutzomyia longipalpis

130. Which of the following is not the function of complements? **(2006)**
a. Cell lysis
b. Antiviral action
c. Promotes phagocytosis
d. Toxin neutralization

131. Definitive host for echonococcus granulosus is:
a. Man **(2006)**
b. Dog
c. Cattle
d. Pig

132. True about mesosomes are all except: **(2006)**
a. Site of bacterial respiration
b. They are invagination of plasma membrane
c. They coordinate nuclear division
d. They are more prominent in Gram negative bacteria

133. All are true about plasmid except: **(2006)**
a. Cannot replicate
b. Vectors for gene transfer
c. Circular DNA molecules found in bacteria
d. Are also present in yeasts

134. Plasmid DNA-Chromosomal DNA combines to form: **(2006)**
a. Mesosome
b. Ribosome
c. Transposon
d. Episome

135. All mycobacteria produces pigment except:
a. M. kansasii
b. M. simiae
c. M. avium
d. M. scrofulaceum

136. Most common cause of traveler's diarrhea is:
a. EHEC
b. ETEC
c. EPEC
d. EIEC

137. False regarding active immunity is:
a. Induced by infection or immunogens
b. Effective only after lag period
c. No negative phase
d. Booster effect on subsequent dose

ANSWERS AND EXPLANATIONS

1. Ans. c. Heat stable *Ref: Ananthanarayan and Paniker: Textbook of Microbiology, 9/e p75, (2013).*

- Exotoxins are proteins, highly antigenic, toxoidable, neutralized by antibodies and heat labile. Endotoxins are extremely heat stable.

2. Ans. b. Mutations in the penicillin binding proteins on the bacterial surface.
Ref: Ananthanarayan and Paniker: Textbook of Microbiology, 9/e p225, (2013).

- Streptococcus pneumoniae become resistance to penicillin is due to mutation or gene transfer.
- The mode of resistance is not the production of beta lactamases
- It is due to alteration of the penicillin binding protein on the bacterial cell surface.

3. Ans. d. Antigen processed by APC are recognized by CD 4+ T Cells
Ref: Ananthanarayan and Paniker: Textbook of Microbiology, 9/e p138, (2013).

- Activation of both the humoral and cell mediated immune responses require cytokines produced by T_H cells.
- T helper cells can recognize only the antigens that are displayed together with Class II MHC molecules on the surface of Antigen presenting cells (APCs).

4. Ans. d. CD 4 and CD 8 double positive cells are eliminated by a process of negative selection
Ref: Kuby Immunology, 7/e p48, (2013).

- Thymus is the site where a large diversity of T cells is produced and so they can recognize and act against a myriad number of antigen—MHCs (major histocompatibility complexes).
- Thymocytes express neither CD4 nor CD8, markers associated with mature T cells. They are therefore called double negative (DN) cells. DN cells first travel to the region under the thymic capsule, a region referred to as the subcapsular cortex, where they proliferate and begin to generate their T-cell receptors.
- Thymocytes that successfully express TCRs begin to express both CD4 and CD8, becoming double positive (DP) cells, and populate the cortex, the site where most (85% or more) immature T cells are found.
- The thymus induces the death of those T cells that cannot recognize antigen–MHCs.
- It also induces death of those T cells that react with self-antigen MHC and pose a danger of causing autoimmune disease.
- **Negative selection** is the induction of death in lymphocytes bearing receptors that react too strongly with self-antigens.

5. Ans. d. Complement system
Ref: Ananthanarayan and Paniker: Textbook of Microbiology, 9/e p126, (2013).

- The deficiency of terminal complements (C5–C9) leads to recurrent meningococcal infections and toxoplasma infections.

6. Ans. b. Catalase negative
Ref: Ananthanarayan and Paniker: Textbook of Microbiology, 9/e p200, (2013).

- Staphylococcus aureus is MR, VP, Catalase and Coagulase positive and Indole negative.
- Catalase is the test used to differentiate Staphylococcus from Streptococcus.

7. Ans. a. Encourage regular hand wash

Ref: Ananthanarayan and Paniker: Textbook of Microbiology, 9/e p204 (2013).

Hand hygiene is the oldest, simplest, cost effective and most effective method to reduce the transmission of MRSA infection in health care settings.

Guideline for isolation precautions: Preventing transmission of infectious agents in healthcare settings, CDC, 2007

8. Ans. d. Streptococcus pyogenes *Ref: Ananthanarayan and Paniker: Textbook of Microbiology, 9/e p679, (2013).*

- Cellulitis is not a skin infection as such, but it can develop by extension from skin or wound infections. It usually manifests as an acute inflammation of subcutaneous connective tissue with swelling and pain and often with marked constitutional signs and symptoms.
- Most common cause for cellulitis is Streptococcus pyogenes.

9. Ans. c. Reinfection with Neisseria gonorrhea *Ref: Harrison's Infectious diseases, 1/e p467, (2010).*

- Acquiring high levels of antibody to outer membrane protein, Rmp (reduction modifiable protein, formerly called protein III), may be especially likely to become reinfected with N. gonorrhea because Rmp antibodies block the effect of bactericidal antibodies to porin and LOS.
- Rmp shows little, if any, inter strain antigenic variation; therefore, Rmp antibodies potentially may block antibody-mediated killing of all gonococci.
- True failure of treatment with a recommended regimen is rare and should prompt an evaluation for reinfection or consideration of an alternative diagnosis.

10. Ans. a. Extended spectrum beta lactamases *Ref: & Sherries Medical Microbiology, 6/e p426 (2014).*

- Extendedspectrum β-lactamases (ESBLs) because their range includes multiple cephalosporins.
- The laboratory detection of ESBLs is complex, as is their naming scheme (CTX-M, TEM, OXA, SHV, etc).
- From a clinical perspective, they are significant because treatment with any generation of cephalosporin may lead to clinical failure.
- Carbapenems are the drug class of choice for treating infections caused by ESBL-producing organisms.

11. Ans. c. Pertussis *Ref: Mackie and McCartney, Practical Medical Microbiology, 14/e p38–39, 418*

- Tularemia, Plague, Psittacosis, coccidioidomycosis, Tuberculosis, Brucellosis, Meliodosis, Anthrax are the common laboratory acquired infections

12. Ans. d. Progressive primary pulmonary disease

Ref: Ananthanarayan and Paniker: Textbook of Microbiology, 9/e p351, (2013).

- Steroids may reduce host resistance, thus favoring the conversion of asymptomatic infection into disease and it is contraindicated in children with progressive primary pulmonary disease.
- It may leads to disseminated Tuberculosis.

13. Ans. d. ESAT-6 *Ref: Sherries Medical Microbiology, 6/e p500, (2014).*

- Mycobacteria do not produce classic exotoxins or endotoxins although a protein called early secreted antigenic target (ESAT-6) causes cytolysis and is associated with virulence.
- Current vaccine strategies are focused on boosting the immunogenicity of either BCG or new recombinant strains with new virulence-associated antigens such as ESAT-6.
- Sometimes the results of the tuberculin skin test are equivocal, particularly in persons who have been vaccinated with BCG or who live in areas where NTM mycobacteria are highly prevalent in the environment.
- In an effort to improve diagnostic accuracy, whole-blood gamma-interferon release assays (IGRAs) have been commercially developed. These assays are based on the host's immune responses to specific M. tuberculosis antigens ESAT-6 and CFP-10 (culture fitrate protein-10), which are absent from most NTM mycobacteria and BCG. These tests detect interferon gamma that is released by sensitized CD4 T cells in response to these antigens.

14. Ans. c. Biopsy and Culture

Ref: Ananthanarayan and Paniker: Textbook of Microbiology, 9/e p401 (2013) & Sherries Medical Microbiology, 6/e p570 (2014).

- Culture of biopsy specimen is the more sensitive method for the diagnosis of H.pylori infection.
- Urea breath test is a rapid method with reliable sensitivity

15. Ans. a. Adenylate cyclase *Ref: Ananthanarayan and Paniker: Textbook of Microbiology, 9/e p308, (2013).*

- The A1 fragment of the cholera toxin causes prolonged activation of cellular adenylate cyclase and accumulation of cAMP leads to outpouring large quantities of water and electrolytes in to small intestinal lumen.

16. Ans. c. Oropharyngeal candidiasis *Ref: Sherries Medical Microbiology, 6/e p325 (2014).*

- Oropharyngeal candidiasis is an AIDS defining illness. It commonly occurs in Immunocompromised individuals.

17. Ans. b. Stage 2 *Ref: HIV and AIDS: Basic Elements and Priorities by S. Karthikeyan, Springer publications (2007)*

- As per WHO clinical staging, parotid enlargement in children falls on Stage 2.

18. Ans. b. A pregnant woman non-immune to Varicella Zoster, exposed to mother with shingles
Ref: Harrison's Infectious diseases, 1/e p745, (2010).

- γ-Globulin of high varicella-zoster virus antibody titer (varicella-zoster immune globulin) can be used to prevent the development of the illness in patients exposed to varicella who are at high risk of developing severe disease.
- It has no therapeutic value after varicella has started.
- It should be administered within 72–96 hours after exposure.

Recommendations for Vzig Administration

Exposure criteria

1. **Exposure to person with chickenpox or zoster**
   a. Household: residence in the same household
   b. Playmate: face-to-face indoor play
   c. Hospital
   Varicella: same 2 to 4-bed room or adjacent beds in large ward, face-o-face contact with infectious staff member or patient, visit by a person deemed contagious
   Zoster: intimate contact (e.g., touching or hugging) with a Person deemed contagious
   d. Newborn infant: onset of varicella in the mother ≤5 days before delivery or ≤48 hours after delivery; VZIG not indicated if the mother has zoster.
2. Patient should receive VZIG as soon as possible but not >96 hours after exposure

Candidates (Provided they have significant exposure) include

1. Immunocompromised susceptible children without a history of varicella or varicella immunization
2. Susceptible pregnant women
3. Newborn infants whose mother had onset of chickenpox within 5 days before or within 48 hour after delivery
4. Hospitalized premature infant (≥28 weeks of gestation) whose mother lacks a reliable history of chickenpox or serologic evidence of protection against varicella
5. Hospitalized premature infant (<28 weeks of gestation or ≤1000-g birth weight), regardless of maternal history of varicella or varicella-zoster virus serologic status

19. Ans. b. Subcortical white matter
Ref: Ananthanarayan and Paniker: Textbook of Microbiology, 9/e p534, (2013).

- Pathognomonic lesion of rabies is the Negri body, an eosinophilic cytoplasmic inclusion distributed throughout the brain, particularly in the hippocampus, pyramidal neurons, cerebral cortex, Purkinje cells of cerebellum and dorsal spinal ganglia.

20. Ans. a, b, c, d. *Ref: Ananthanarayan and Paniker: Textbook of Microbiology, 9/e p500, (2013).*

- Respiratory viruses are best diagnosed by Immunofluorescence, Ag detection by ELISA, Hemagglutination and radial immunodiffusion.
- Single radial hemolysis test used for quantitation of complement-fixing antibodies to non-hemagglutinating viruses.

21. Ans. c. Interstitial pneumonitis with foamy intra-alveolar exudates
Ref: Ananthanarayan and Paniker: Textbook of Microbiology, 9/e p614, (2013).

- Histologically, PCP is characterized by alveoli filed with desquamated alveolar cells, monocytes, organisms, and fluid, producing a distinctive foamy, honeycombed appearance.

22. Ans. d. Pertusis *Ref: Mackie and McCartney, Practical Medcial Microbiology, 14/e p38–39, 418*

- Tularemia, Plague, Psittacosis, coccidioidomycosis, Tuberculosis, Brucellosis, Meliodosis, Anthrax are the common laboratory acquired infections

23. Ans. c. Oxidase positive *Ref: Ananthanarayan and Paniker: Textbook of Microbiology, 9/e p206, (2013).*

- Staphylococcus is oxidase negative where micrococcus is oxidase positive (modified)

24. Ans. c. Motile and non-motile strains

Ref: Ananthanarayan and Paniker: Textbook of Microbiology, 9/e p47, (2013).

- Separation of motile and non motile can be effected by using Craigie's tube.
- In Craigie's tube method a wide tube containing semisolid agar (0.2%) is used.
- A short, narrow tube, open at both ends, is placed into the agar of the tube in such a way that the upper end of the tube projects well above the agar.
- The bacterial strain is inoculated into the inner tube, and after 8–16 hours of incubation, subcultures made from top of the agar outside the central tube yield a population of motile cells.

25. Ans. d. Mucocutaneous leishmaniasis *Ref: Paniker 's Textbook of Medical Parasitology, 7/e p62, (2013).*

- New world mucocutaneous and cutaneous leishmanisis (espundia) are caused by L. brazilensis and L. mexicana. Vector is sandy of genus Lutzomyra
- Mucocutaneous involvement leads to nodules inside the nose, perforation of the nasal septum, and enlargement of the nose and lips (espundia)

26. Ans. c. Glutaraldehyde *Ref: Ananthanarayan and Paniker: Textbook of Microbiology, 9/e p34, (2013).*

- 2% buffered solution of glutaraldehyde is an effective disinfectant.
- Used to disinfect hospital and laboratory equipments.
- Glutaraldehyde usually disinfects objects within time frame of 10 minutes but may require as long as 12 hours to destroy all spores.
- Glutaraldehyde is especially effective against tubercle bacilli, fungi, and viruses.
- It can be used for cleaning cystoscopes and bronchoscopes, corrugated rubber anesthetic tubes and face masks, plastic endotracheal tubes, metal instruments, and polythene tubing.

27. Ans. a. IgA *Ref: Ananthanarayan and Paniker: Textbook of Microbiology, 9/e p122, (2013).*

- Alternate complement pathway is activated by microbial endotoxins, IgA, IgD, cobra venom and nephritic factor.
- Classical pathway is activated by Ag-Ab reaction and involved antibodies are IgM and IgG.

28. Ans. b. Conjugation *Ref: Ananthanarayan and Paniker: Textbook of Microbiology, 9/e p60, (2013).*

- The genetic information can be transferred from one bacterium to another.
- There are three general methods for genetic exchange in bacteria:
- Transformation: Direct uptake of naked DNA
- Transduction: Mediated by a bacteriophage
- Conjugation: Direct contact through pilli

29. Ans. c. 5–10% *Ref: Ananthanarayan and Paniker: Textbook of Microbiology, 9/e p137, (2013).*

30. Ans. a. heat stable *Ref: Ananthanarayan and Paniker: Textbook of Microbiology, 9/e p75, (2013).*

- Refer the table in the text which shows the difference between exo and endo toxins

31. Ans. b. Citrate synthesis *Ref: Ananthanarayan and Paniker: Textbook of Microbiology, 9/e p291, (2013).*

- Salmonellae ferment glucose, mannitol, and maltose, forming acid and gas. S. Typhi is an exception, which does not ferment the sugars.
- They do not ferment lactose, sucrose, or salicin and do not produce indole.
- Most salmonellae except S. Paratyphi A, S. Choleraesuis, and some other species produce H2S.
- They are MR positive and VP negative and citrate positive
- Salmonellae are catalase positive and oxidase negative.

32. Ans. a. Klebsiella spp. *Ref: Ananthanarayan and Paniker: Textbook of Microbiology, 9/e p280, (2013).*

- Klebsiella is devoid of flagella and not motile.
- Escherichia coli, Salmonella typhi and Citrobacter motile with peritrichous flagella

33. Ans. b. T-helper cells *Ref: Ananthanarayan and Paniker: Textbook of Microbiology, 9/e p574, (2013).*

- HIV is having tropism over CD4 (T helper) cells due to the presence of CCR5(R5) and CXCR4 (X4) receptors on the surface of the cell.
- HIV also infects the following cells in a lesser extent

34. Ans. a. Disease should be susceptible to broad spectrum antibiotics

Ref: Ananthanarayan and Paniker: Textbook of Microbiology, 9/e p4, (2013) and Mandell, Douglas, and Bennett's: Principles and Practice of Infectious Diseases, 8/e p38, (2015).

Molecular Koch's postulates are originally described by Dr. Falkow .

- "The phenotype or property under investigation should be associated with pathogenic members of a genus or pathogenic strains of a species." Additionally, the gene in question should be found in all pathogenic strains of the genus or species but be absent from nonpathogenic strains.
- "Specific inactivation of the gene(s) associated with the suspected virulence trait should lead to a measurable loss in pathogenicity or virulence." Virulence of the microorganism with the inactivated gene must be less than that of the unaltered microorganism in an appropriate animal model.
- "Reversion or allelic replacement of the mutated gene should lead to restoration of pathogenicity." In other words, reintroduction of the gene into the microbe should restore virulence in the animal model.
- "The gene, which causes virulence, must be expressed during infection."
- "Immunity must be protective."

35. Ans. b. Salk vaccine *Ref: Ananthanarayan and Paniker: Textbook of Microbiology, 9/e p83, (2013).*

- Live attenuated vaccines
  - Bacille Calmette–Guérin (BCG)
  - Smallpox vaccine
  - Oral polio vaccine (OPV – Salk))
  - Mumps, measles, and rubella (MMR) vaccine
  - Yellow fever vaccine
- Live vaccines are usually contraindicated for use in immunocompromised patients
- Killed Inactivated Vaccines
  - Typhoid
  - Cholera
  - Pertussis
  - Pneumococcal
  - Rabies,
  - Hepatitis B (Sub unit)
  - Influenza vaccines

36. Ans. a. Klebsiella *Ref: Ananthanarayan and Paniker: Textbook of Microbiology, 9/e p276, (2013).*

- E.coli, Salmonella and Proteus are motile with peritrichous flagella.
- Klebsiella is devoid of flagella and non-motile

37. Ans. d. B cells *Ref: Ananthanarayan and Paniker: Textbook of Microbiology, 9/e p136, (2013).*

- Each immunologically competent B cell possesses receptor for either IgM or IgD that can combine with one antigen or closely related antigens.
- After binding of the antigen, the B cell is activated to proliferate and form a clone of cells. Selected B cells are transformed to plasma cells that secrete antibodies specific for the antigen
- B cells possess surface IgM, which acts as a receptor for antigen.
- Some B cells may also carry on their surface IgD as receptor for the antigen.
- There are many other molecules expressed on the surface of the B cells, which serve different functions. Eg.Ia protein and CR1

38. Ans. a. Ig G *Ref: Ananthanarayan and Paniker: Textbook of Microbiology, 9/e p97, (2013).*

- In response to infection, IgG antibodies appear late after appearance of IgM antibodies, but persists for a longer period. IgM – Primary immune response and IgG secondary Immune response
- Protection against the microorganisms present in the blood and tissues.

- Distributed equally in the intra- and extravascular compartments.
- It is the only immunoglobulin that crosses the placenta; hence, it confers natural passive immunity to the newborns. (IgG2 subtype – no placental transfer)
- Takes part in precipitation, complement fixation, and neutralization of toxins and viruses.

39. Ans. b. Uncommon in immunocompetent

Ref: Ananthanarayan and Paniker: Textbook of Microbiology, 9/e p473, (2013), and Sherries Medical Microbiology, 6/e p262, (2014).

- Human cytomegalovirus (CMV) is a β-herpesvirus named for the cytopathic effct it produces in cell culture.
- In addition to nuclear inclusions ("owl's eye cells"), CMV produces perinuclear cytoplasmic inclusions and enlargement of the cell (cytomegaly)
- High infection rates in early childhood and early adulthood
- Present in urine, saliva, semen, and cervical secretions
- Serious disease of fetus may develop with primary maternal infection
- CMV lung, visceral, and eye infections in Immunocompromised patients
- **Congenital infection**—Virus culture or viral DNA assay positive at birth or within 1 to 2 weeks (to distinguish from natally or perinatally infected infants, who will not begin to excrete virus until 3 to 4 weeks after delivery).
- **Perinatal infection**—Culture-negative specimens at birth but positive specimens at 4 weeks or more after birth suggest natal or early postnatal acquisition.
- Seronegative infants may acquire CMV from exogenous sources, such as from blood transfusion.
- **Immunocompromised patients**—Demonstration of virus by viral antigen or DNA in blood documents viremia.
- Demonstration of inclusions or viral antigen in diseased tissue (eg, lung, esophagus, or colon) establishes the presence of CMV infection, but does not provide proof that CMV is the cause of disease unless other pathogens are excluded.

40. Ans. a. Mycobacterium marinum *Ref: Ananthanarayan and Paniker: Textbook of Microbiology, 9/e p358, (2013).*

- Mycobacterium kansasii: Pulmonary disease
- Mycobacterium marinum: Swimming pool granuloma
- Mycobacterium simiae: Pulmonary disease (rare)
- Mycobacterium scrofulaceum: Lymphadenopathy
- Mycobacterium xenopi: Chronic pulmonary disease
- Mycobacterium avium complex: Pulmonary disease, lymphadenopathy,and disseminated disease
- Mycobacterium ulcerans: Buruli ulcer
- Mycobacterium fortuitum: Post-trauma chronic abscesses

41. Ans. Best medium for anaerobes is chocolate agar

Ref: Ananthanarayan and Paniker: Textbook of Microbiology, 9/e p47, (2013).

- The commonly used media for anaerobic culture are
  - Robertson cooked meat broth,
  - Thioglycollate broth,
  - Willis and Hobbs' media,
  - Neomycin blood agar.
- Blood agar and chocolate agar are enriched media

42. Ans. b. Dendritic cell *Ref: Ananthanarayan and Paniker: Textbook of Microbiology, 9/e p138, (2013).*

- Dendritic cells are very important for presentation of the antigen to T cells during primary immune response.
- They are bone marrow-derived cells that express class II MHC proteins and present antigen to CD4+ T cells.
- They have little or no phagocytic activity.
- They also serve as professional APCs, although macrophages and B cells are the major APCs

43. Ans. d. MHC restricted *Ref: Ananthanarayan and Paniker: Textbook of Microbiology, 9/e (2013), p137*

- Natural killer (NK) cells are morphologically described as large granular lymphocytes (LGL).
- They are named as natural killer cells due to their ability to kill certain virally infected cells and tumor cells without prior sensitization.
- Their activities are not enhanced by exposure and are not specific for any virus.
- NK cells comprise approximately 5–10% of peripheral lymphocytes and are found in spleen and peripheral blood.
- Kill virus-infected cells and tumor cells.
- Nonspecific killing of virus-infected cells and tumor cells.
- Killing is independent of antigen presentation by MHC proteins.
- Mechanism of killing is by perforins and granzymes, which cause apoptosis of target cell
- Killing is activated by failure of a cell to present antigen with class I MHC or by reduction of class I MHC proteins on the cell surface

44. Ans. b. Detects RNA *Ref: Ananthanarayan and Paniker: Textbook of Microbiology, 9/ e p65, (2013).*

- Southern blot is a method used for detection of a specific DNA sequence in DNA samples. Southern blotting combines transfer of electrophoresis-separated DNA fragments to a filter membrane and subsequent fragment detection by probe hybridization. The method is named after its inventor, the British biologist **Edwin Southern.**
- Northern blotting, the name was extrapolated from Southern blotting. The northern blot is a technique used to study gene expression by detection of RNA (or isolated mRNA) in a sample.
- Identification of a specific protein in a complex mixture of proteins can be done by a technique known as **western blotting**. Western blotting (also called **immunoblotting** because an antibody is used to specifically detect its antigen) was introduced by Towbin, et al. in 1979 and is now a routine technique for protein analysis.

45. Ans. d. Pulsed gel field electrophoresis is used for typing

Ref: Ananthanarayan and Paniker: Textbook of Microbiology, 9/e p204, (2013), and Sherries Medical Microbiology, 6/e p443, (2014).

- Alterations in the β-lactam target, the peptidoglycan transpeptidases (oftn called penicillinbinding proteins, or PBPs), are the basis for resistance to methicillin.
- These MRSA strains are also resistant to the other penicillinase-resistant penicillins such as oxacillin.
- The most common mechanism is the acquisition of a gene (mecA) coding for a new transpeptidase, which has reduced affinity for β-lactam antibiotics, but is still able to carry out its enzymatic function of cross-linking peptidoglycan.

46. Ans. a. Shigella flexneri Type 6 *Ref: Ananthanarayan and Paniker: Textbook of Microbiology, 9/e p286, (2013).*

47. Ans. c. Colour reactions on canavanine-glycine-bromthymol blue

Ref: Ananthanarayan and Paniker: Textbook of Microbiology, 9/e p613, (2013).

- Properties of pathogenic C. neoformans:
  - It grows at 37°C (98.6°F),
  - Assimilates inositol
  - Produces urease
  - Produces melanin in bird seed/niger seed agar (blackish—brown colonies)
  - Does not produce mycelia on cornmeal agar.

48. Ans. b. Alcian blue *Ref: Ananthanarayan and Paniker: Textbook of Microbiology, 9/e p13 (2013).*

- Gram stain was devised by Hans Christian Gram, a Danish microbiologist, in 1884,
- The Gram staining method essentially consists of four steps:
  - Primary staining with basic dyes, such as methyl violet, crystal violet, etc.
  - Application of mordant in the form of dilute solution of iodine.
  - Decolorization with ethanol, acetone, or aniline.
  - Counterstaining with acidic dyes, such as carbol fuchsin, safranine, or neutral red.
- Gram positive—purple/violet color, gram negative—pink color

49. Ans. a. M kansasii *Ref: Ananthanarayan and Paniker: Textbook of Microbiology, 9/e p359, (2013).*

- Examples for photochromogens are M. kansasii, Mycobacterium marinum, and Mycobacterium simiae.

50. Ans. b. Photo chromogen

Ref: Ananthanarayan and Paniker: Textbook of Microbiology, 9/e p359, (2013).

- As per the Runyon's classification, M.simiae belongs to Photochromogen.

51. Ans. c. S mansoni *Ref: Paniker's Textbook of Medical Parasitology, 7/e p146, (2013).*

- The eggs of S. manosni deposited in the gut wall cause inflammatory reactions leading to microabscesses, granulomas, hyperplasia, and eventual fibrosis.
- Egg granulomas are found in the distal part of the colon and rectum.
- Ectopic lesions include hepatosplenomegaly and periportal firosis, portal hypertension, as some of the eggs are carried through portal circulation into liver.
- Portal hypertension may cause gastrointestinal hemorrhage.

52. Ans. b. Rhinoscleromatosis *Ref: Ananthanarayan and Paniker: Textbook of Microbiology, 9/e p281, (2013).*

- Rhinoscleroma is a chronic granulomatous bacterial disease of the nose that can sometimes infect the upper respiratory tract.
- It most commonly affects the nasal cavity—the nose is involved in 95–100 per cent of cases—however, it can also affect the nasopharynx, larynx, trachea, and bronchi.
- Slightly more in females than males are affected and patients are usually 10 to 30 years of age.
- It is caused by Klebsiella rhinoscleromatis—subspecies of Klebsiella pneumoniae—a gram-negative, encapsulated, nonmotile, rod-shaped bacillus (diplobacillus), member of the Enterobacteriaceae family.
- It is sometimes referred to as the "Frisch bacillus".
- Russell bodies, and pseudoepitheliomatous hyperplasia, and groups of large vacuolated histiocytes containing Klebsiella rhinoscleromatis (Mikulicz cells) are Pathognomic.

53. Ans. a. LGV *Ref: Ananthanarayan and Paniker: Textbook of Microbiology, 9/e p421, (2013).*

Psittacosis	Levinthal-Cole-Lille (LCL) inclusion bodies
LGV	Miyagawa corpuscle
Trachoma	Halberstaedter Prowazek (HP) body

54. Ans. a. Smallpox *Ref: Ananthanarayan and Paniker: Textbook of Microbiology, 9/e p444, (2013).*

Inclusion bodies

Intracytoplasmic:

- Negri body—Rabies
- Guarnier body—vaccinia (small pox—vaccine starin),
- Paschen body—variola (small pox—pathogenic strain),
- Bollinger body—fowl pox
- Molluscum body—molluscum contagiosum virus

Intranuclear:

- Cowdry A (HAY)—herpes (lipschultz body), Yellow fever (torres body)
- Cowdry B (BAP)—adeno, polio
- Both—measles, CMV

55. Ans. a. Histoplasma capsulatum *Ref: Ananthanarayan and Paniker: Textbook of Microbiology, 9/e p590, (2013).*

- Dimorphic fungi are hyphal/mycelial forms in the soil and in the cultures at 22–25°C and yeasts or other structures in human tissue and in the culture at 37°C
- Examples include Coccidioides immitis, Paracoccidioides braziliensis, Histoplasma capsulatum, Blastomyces dermatitidis, and Sporothrix schenckii

56. Ans. a. Neisseria gonorrhoeae *Ref: Ananthanarayan and Paniker: Textbook of Microbiology, 9/e p231, (2013).*

- Selective media used for isolation of gonococci
- Thayer Martin medium (chocolate agar medium containing antibiotics, such as colistin, nystatin, and vancomycin)
- Modified New York City medium (a translucent medium containing vancomycin, colistin, trimethoprim, and either nystatin or amphotericin B)

57. Ans. a. Anthrax *Ref: Ananthanarayan and Paniker: Textbook of Microbiology, 9/e p247, (2013).*

- In cutaneous anthrax, the skin in the surrounding areas may become edematous and necrotic, but not purulent is called eschar, which is black colored and the lesion is called "malignant pustule" due to its characteristic appearance;

58. Ans. a. Tetanus

Disease	Pathogen	Animals involved	Mode of transmission
Haemorrhagic fevers–ebola virus disease	Ebolavirus	Chimpanzees, gorillas, fruit bats, monkeys, forest antelope and porcupines	Through body fluids, organs
Rabies	Rabies virus	Commonly—dogs, bats, monkeys, and cats	Through saliva by biting, or through scratches from an infected animal.
Anthrax	Bacillus anthracis	Commonly—grazing herbivores such as cattle, sheep, goats, camels, horses, and pigs	By ingestion, inhalation or skin contact of spores
Influenza	Influenza virus	Horses, pigs, domestic and wild birds, wild aquatic mammals such as seals and whales, minks and farmed carnivores.	Droplets transmitted through air
Leptospirosis	Leptospira interrogans	Rats, mice, dogs,	Direct or indirect contact with urine of infected animals
Bovine spongiform encephalopathy (BSE)	Prions	Cattle	Through eating meat or bone meal of made from infected animals.
Brucellosis	Brucella	Cattle, Goats	Infected milk or meat
Foodborne illnesses, commonly diarrheal diseases	Campylobacter, Escheria coli, Salmonella Shigella species	Animals domesticated for food production (Cattle, poultry)	Food made from infected animals
Haemorrhagic fevers–Marburg viral haemorrhagic fever, Lassa fever, Crimean-Congo haemorrhagic fever (CCHF)	Varies—Commonly Viruses	Varies (sometimes unknown), Commonly—camels, hares, hedgehogs, cattle, sheep, goats, horses and swine	Infection usually occurs through direct contact with infected animals
Bovine Tuberculosis	Mycobacterium bovis	Infected cattle, deer, llamas, pigs, domestic cats, wild carnivores (foxes, coyotes) and omnivores (possums, mustelids and rodents)	Milk, exhaled air, sputum, urine, faeces and pus from infected animals
Cysticercosis and Taeniasis	Taenia solium	Commonly—pigs	Eating water or food contaminated with the tapeworm eggs (Cysticercosis) or raw or undercooked pork meat contaminated with cysticerci (taeniasis), the larval form of the tapeworm
Echinococcosis	Echinococcus granulosus	Dogs, foxes, wolves, sheep, and rodents	Eating organs contaminated with the cysts of the worm
African sleeping sickness (Rhodesian/zoonotic)	Trypanosoma brucei rhodesiense	Range of wild animals and domestic livestock	Transmitted by the bite of the tsetse fly

59. Ans. c. Medlar bodies *Ref: Ananthanarayan and Paniker: Textbook of Microbiology, 9/e p601, (2013).*
- Sporotrichiosis shows asteroid bodies.
- Medlar bodies/copper penny bodies are the characteristic feature of chromoblastomycosis

60. Ans. a. Naegleria fowleri *Ref: Paniker's Textbook of Medical Parasitology, 7/e p148, (2013).*
- Naegleria Fowleri is the only species of genus Naegleria, which infects man. N. fowleri causes the disease primary amoebic meningoencephalitis (PAM), a brain infection that leads to destruction of brain tissue.
- Granulomatous amoebic encephalitis (GAE) and chronic amoebic keratitis (CAK)—caused by Acanthamoeba.

61. Ans. c. Transformation *Ref: Ananthanarayan and Paniker: Textbook of Microbiology, 9/e p59, (2013).*
- Griffith's experiment on mice demonstrated that neither of the mice died when injected separately with a live, noncapsulated Pneumococcus (nonvirulent) and heat-killed, capsulated Pneumococcus (nonvirulent), but the mice died when they were injected with a mixture of both these strains.
- From the dead mice, he could isolate live, capsulated pneumococci, which were virulent.
- He demonstrated that some factor in heat-killed, capsulated pneumococci had transferred the material for capsule synthesis in the noncapsulated strains of the bacteria, making them virulent

62. Ans. b. Polysaccharide *Ref: Sherries Medical Microbiology, 6/e p433, (2014).*
- The cell wall of S. aureus consists of a typical Gram-positive peptidoglycan interspersed with considerable amounts of teichoic acid.
- The peptidoglycan of the cell wall is commonly overlaid with polysaccharide and surface proteins. Although thin polysaccharide capsules are frequently present, their signifiance in human infections is unknown

63. Ans. d. Enteroinvasive E. coli (EIEC)
Ref: Ananthanarayan and Paniker: Textbook of Microbiology, 9/e p279, (2013).
- The EIEC strains have the ability to invade and destroy the colonic epithelium, producing a disease characterized initially by watery diarrhea.
- This ability of E. coli to invade cells is determined by a large plasmid, which codes for outer membrane antigens called the "virulence marker antigens" (VMA).
- The bacteria lyse the phagocytes and multiply in the cell cytoplasm.
- This process of epithelial cell destruction with inflammatory infiltration leads to the development of ulcers in intestine.

64. Ans. a. Brucellosis *Ref: Jawetz, Melnick, and Adelberg's Medical Microbiology, Twenty-Sixth Edition. Page No 271*

65. Ans. a. L interrogans *Ref: Ananthanarayan and Paniker: Textbook of Microbiology, 9/e p381, (2013).*
- Approximately 10% of the patients develop icteric manifestations of the leptospirosis, otherwise known as Weil's disease.
- The disease is characterized by the development of jaundice and it shows two distinct phases of septicemic and immune.

66. Ans. d. B cell
Ref: Ananthanarayan and Paniker: Textbook of Microbiology, 9/e p152, (2013).
- Cell-mediated immunity (CMI) is a specific type of acquired immune response mediated by sensitized T cells (T—helper, T—Cytotoxic, Natural Killer cells).
- This form of immunity is transferred from donor to recipient with intact lymphocytes; hence it is called cell-mediated immune reaction.

67. Ans. a. CSF *Ref: Ananthanarayan and Paniker: Textbook of Microbiology, 9/e p329, (2013).*
- H. influenzae is very sensitive to low temperatures, the CSF specimen should never be refrigerated in a suspected case of bacterial meningitis.

68. Ans. c. Cojugation *Ref: Ananthanarayan and Paniker: Textbook of Microbiology, 9/e p62, (2013).*
- The R factor—Resistance factors are extrachromosomal plasmids.
- They are circular with double-stranded DNA.
- R factors occur in two sizes: large plasmids (mol. wt. 60 million) and small plasmids (mol. wt. 10 million).
- The large plasmids are conjugative "R" factors, which contain extra DNA to code for the conjugation process.

- The small plasmids contain only the "r" genes and are not conjugative.
- R factor consists of two components: the resistance transfer factor (RTF) and resistant determinant (r).
- The RTF is responsible for conjugational transfer, while each r determinant carries resistance for one of the several antibiotics

69. Ans. a. Proteus *Ref: Ananthanarayan and Paniker: Textbook of Microbiology, 9/e p282, (2013).*

- P. mirabilis and P. vulgaris typically spread or swarm on surface of the medium.
- Organisms spread on the surface of the plate in successive waves to form a thin filmy layer in concentric circles. This is known as swarming
- E.g
- Proteus
- Cl. Tetani
- V. alginolyticus

70. Ans. c. Lyme's disease *Ref: Ananthanarayan and Paniker: Textbook of Microbiology, 9/e p376, (2013).*

- In lyme disease, VDRL is non reactive but FTA-Abs is positive.
- All the other choices are examples of false positive against treponemal antibodies.

71. Ans. d. Bornholm's disease

Ref: Ananthanarayan and Paniker: Textbook of Microbiology, 9/e p492, (2013), and Sherries Medical Microbiology, 6/e p213, (2014).

- Bornholm's disease (Epidemic Pleurodynia), Myocarditis, Pericarditis, Juvenile diabetes, orchitis and Post viral fatigue syndrome are caused by Group B Coxsackie virus.
- Incubation period: 2–10 days

72. Ans. c. Langerhan's cell *Ref: Ananthanarayan and Paniker: Textbook of Microbiology, 9/e p138, (2013).*

- Langerhan's cells in the skin possess the features of Macrophages and dendritic cells. They process and present the antigen that reach the dermis

73. Ans. d. 80% of T cells

Ref: Lymphocyte subsets in healthy children from birth through 18 years of age: the Pediatric AIDS Clinical Trials Group P 1009 study.J Allergy Clin Immunol. 2003 Nov; 112(5): 973–80

74. Ans. b. Sporothrix schenckii *Ref: Ananthanarayan and Paniker: Textbook of Microbiology, 9/e p590, (2013).*

- Example for Dimorphic fungi are
  - Thermally dimorphic: Histoplasma, Blastomyces. Coccidiodes, Paracoccidioides, Sporothrix, Penicillium marneffei
  - Non thermally dimorphic: Candida albicans

75. Ans. a. Mycoplasma *Ref: Ananthanarayan and Paniker: Textbook of Microbiology, 9/e p388, (2013).*

- First M. pneumoniae was considered as a virus rather than a bacterium, when Eaton and colleagues cultured the causative agent of human primary atypical pneumonia (PAP) or "walking pneumonia".
- The terms 'walking pneumonia' and 'atypical pneumonia' were coined to describe the unresponsiveness of pneumonia inducing mycoplasma infections to antibiotics like penicillin.
- Eaton's agent could be grown in chicken embryos and passed through a filter that excluded normal bacteria. Eaton suggested the possibility that the disease was caused by a mycoplasma.

76. Ans. b. Secondary *Ref: Ananthanarayan and Paniker: Textbook of Microbiology, 9/e p375, (2013).*

Stage	VDRL	FTA-ABS	TPHA
Primary	70–80	85–100	65–85
Secondary	100	100	100
Late	60–70	95–100	95–100

77. Ans. d. Formaldehyde *Ref: Ananthanarayan and Paniker: Textbook of Microbiology, 9/e p37 (2013),*

- Chlorine, Phenol and Alcohol are Intermittent level disinfectants which kills the all microbial pathogens, Mycobacterium, Non enveloped Viruses except spores.
- Formaldehyde, Glutaraldehyde and Hydrogen peroxide are high level disinfectants which kills spores.

78. Ans. b. Clostridium perifringens *Ref: Ananthanarayan and Paniker: Textbook of Microbiology, 9/e p257, (2013).*

- Gas gangrene causative agents
  - Clostridium perfringens
  - Clostridium novyi
  - Clostridium sordelli
  - Clostridium septicum

79. Ans. d. Clostridium perfringens *Ref: Ananthanarayan and Paniker: Textbook of Microbiology, 9/e (2013), p252*

- All the clostridia are motile with peritrichous flagella except Clostridium perfringens and Clostridium tetani type VI.

80. Ans. b. Cephalosporins is the drug of choice

Ref: Ananthanarayan and Paniker: Textbook of Microbiology, 9/e p344, (2013).

- Drug of choice for Brucellosis is Doxycycline

81. Ans. a. TNF-alpha *Ref: Ananthanarayan and Paniker: Textbook of Microbiology, 9/e p155, (2013).*

- Tumor necrosis factor (TNF-α) is produced by activated macrophages in response to microbes, especially the lipopolysaccharide of Gram-negative bacteria.
- It is an important mediator of acute inflammation.
- Cachetin is a protein that is released by activated macrophages as an immune system defense and, when the defense is overwhelmed, is a cause of cachexia or toxic shock

82. Ans. d. Glutaraldehyde *Ref: Ananthanarayan and Paniker: Textbook of Microbiology, 9/e p37, (2013)*

- Chlorine, Phenol and Alcohol are Intermittent level disinfectants which kills the all microbial pathogens, Mycobacterium, non enveloped Viruses except spores.
- Formaldehyde, glutaraldehyde and hydrogen peroxide are high level disinfectants which kills spores.

83. Ans. b. Super antigens *Ref: Ananthanarayan and Paniker: Textbook of Microbiology, 9/e p202, (2013).*

- Staphylococcal toxic shock syndrome (STSS) is caused by TSST.
- The toxin is a superantigen, which causes STSS by stimulating the release of large amounts of interleukins IL-1 and IL-2 in the body.
- The STSS is an acute and potentially life-threatening condition similar to gram-negative sepsis and septic shock. STSS is a multisystem disease characterized by fever, hypotension, myalgia, vomiting, diarrhea, mucosal hyperemia, and an erythematous rash followed by desquamation of the skin, particularly on palms and soles.
- This condition was first documented among the menstruating women who used highly absorbent vaginal tampons; the vaginal swab from these women showed a heavy growth of S. aureus.

84. Ans. d. Bacillius anthracis *Ref: Ananthanarayan and Paniker: Textbook of Microbiology, 9/e p245, (2013).*

- It is a very large bacillus measuring 31–1.6 μm in width and 3–10 μm in length.

85. Ans. d. Staphylococcus aureus *Ref: Ananthanarayan and Paniker: Textbook of Microbiology, 9/e p203, (2013).*

- Staphylococcal scalded skin syndrome (SSSS) is caused by the exfoliative toxin, exfoliatin.
- The condition is seen commonly in infants and children. It is associated with extensive exfoliation of the skin, in which outer layer of the epidermis is separated from the underlying tissue and is characterized by the appearance of extensive bullae.
- These bullae when ruptured may leave behind scalded, red, tender skin. The lesion typically starts periorificially or in skin folds. It usually resolves within 10 day's time.
- Pemphigus neonatorum and bullous impetigo are the milder forms, whereas Ritter's disease in the newborn and toxic epidermal necrolysis (TEN) in the older persons are the severe forms of the SSSS

86. Ans. b. Adenovirus *Ref: Ananthanarayan and Paniker: Textbook of Microbiology, 9/e p444, (2013).*

Viral inclusion bodies:

- Intracytoplasmic:
  - Henderson-peterson bodies in molluscum contagiosum
  - Negri bodies in rabies
  - Guarnieri bodies (B type inclusion bodies) in small pox

- Intranuclear:
  - Acidophilic
    - Cowdry Type A
      - ◊ Varicella zoster virus
      - ◊ Herpes simplex virus
      - ◊ Yellow fever virus (Torres bodies)
    - Cowdry Type B
      - ◊ Polio
  - Basophilic
    - Cowdry Type B
      - ◊ Adenovirus
      - ◊ Cytomegalovirus—Owl eye
- Intranuclear and Intracytoplasmic:
  - Measles

87. Ans. a. Antigenic drift *Ref: Ananthanarayan and Paniker: Textbook of Microbiology, 9/e p499, (2013).*

- The gradual, sequential, regular antigenic change in influenza virus is known as antigenic drift.
- This occurs due to minor antigenic changes in the HA or NA occurring at frequent intervals.
- This is caused even by a single mutation affecting HA glycoprotein.
- The antigenic drift is characterized by changes in certain epitopes in the HA, while others are being conserved.
- Reason for Cyclic trend in influenza

88. Ans. a. HPV6, 11, 16, 18 *Ref: Sherries Medical Microbiology, 6/e p339, (2014).*

- Two recombinant virus-like particle vaccines comprising viral capsid L polypeptide namely bivalent vaccine, Cervarix (HPV 16 and 18), and quadrivalent vaccine, Gardasil (HPV types 6, 11, 16, and 18) are licensed in the United States.
- Both vaccines are subunit recombinant vaccines that are noninfectious and elicit neutralizing antibodies that provide protection against commonly prevalent HPV that cause cervical cancers and genital warts.
- HPV vaccine is indicated for girls at the start of sexual activity.
- The vaccine can be administered to girls aged 9 to 12 years and to adolescent girls and women aged 13 to 26 years who have not completed or started the vaccine.
- Gardasil can be given to adolescent boys and men aged 13 to 26 years to prevent genital warts.
- Cervarix and Gardasil are given intramuscularly as a three-dose series over a 6-month period.
- Vaccinated females should continue Pap smear and HPV screening, because other HPV genotypes than those included in the vaccine can cause cervical cancer.

89. Ans. c. Chlamydospores *Ref: Ananthanarayan and Paniker: Textbook of Microbiology, 9/e p613, (2013).*

- Arthrospores are formed by fragmentations of the ends of hyphae, resulting in rectangular thick-walled spores. They are the infective stage of C. immitis.
- Chlamydospores arise by rounding and thickening of hyphal segments. They are round and thick walled. The terminal chlamydospores help in the identification of C. albicans.
- Blastospores are formed by budding process from parent cells, such as yeast. Some yeasts, such as C. albicans can form multiple buds that do not detach from the parent yeast, thus producing elongated structures called pseudohyphae.

90. Ans. b. T-lymphoblast cell *Ref: Ananthanarayan and Paniker: Textbook of Microbiology, 9/e p130, (2013).*

- A lymphoblast is a different form of a naive lymphocyte that occurs when the lymphocyte is activated by an antigen (from antigen-presenting cells) and increased in volume by nucleus and cytoplasm growth as well as new mRNA and protein synthesis.
- The lymphoblast then starts dividing and making clones of its original naive cells. Finally the dividing cells differentiate into effector cells, known as Plasma Cells (for B cells), Cytotoxic T cells, and Helper T cells.
- Lymphoblasts are immature cells which typically differentiate to form mature lymphocytes.
- Normally lymphoblasts are found in the bone marrow
- B lymphoblast will perform only B cell function while T Lymphoblast will perform primarily T cell function along with B cell function.

91. Ans. a. Schwartzman reaction *Ref: Ananthanarayan and Paniker: Textbook of Microbiology, 9/e p165, (2013)*

- A rabbit injected intradermally with a small quantity of lipopolysaccharide (endotoxin) followed by a second intravenous injection 24 hours later will develop a hemorrhagic and necrotic lesion at the site of the first injection.
- This reaction has no immunologic basis.
- This phenomenon is otherwise named as **Sanarelli phenomenon**

92. Ans. a. HTLV-1 *Ref: Ananthanarayan and Paniker: Textbook of Microbiology, 9/e p566, (2013).*

- HPV, EBV and HBV are oncogenic DNA viruses.
- Example for Oncogenic retroviruses
  - Mouse mammary tumor virus
  - Human T-lymphotropic virus (HTLV-1, HTLV-2, HTLV-5),
  - Rous sarcoma virus (chickens)
  - Human immunodeficiency virus (HIV-1, HIV-2), Visna virus (sheep), Caprine arthritis/ encephalitis virus (goats)

93. Ans. a. Actinomyces israelii *Ref: Ananthanarayan and Paniker: Textbook of Microbiology, 9/e p391, (2013).*

- Bollinger found a mould like organism in a lumpy jaw lesion in cattle.
- Ray like appearance—Actinomyces (Actinomyces—ray fungus)
- Anaerobic and non acid fast
- Fluffy ball appearance in liquid culture.

94. Ans. c. It may cause peritonitis *Ref: Ananthanarayan and Paniker: Textbook of Microbiology, 9/e p269, (2013).*

- Bacterioides are gram negative cocobacilli
- They possess polysaccharide capsule and produces enterotoxin.
- Source is from intestine (normal flora)
- Causes abdominal abscess and peritonitis (Opportunistic pathogen)

95. Ans. b. ETEC *Ref: Ananthanarayan and Paniker: Textbook of Microbiology, 9/e p279, (2013).*

- Entero toxigenic Escherichia coli is the causative agent of Traveler's diarrhea. Serotypes 6, 8, 15, 25, 27, 167 are involved.
- Labile toxin (LT) and Stable toxin (ST), CFA (I-IV) are the virulent factors.
- Watery diarrhea without fever and inflammation.

96. Ans. c. M. avium

Ref: Ananthanarayan and Paniker: Textbook of Microbiology, 9/e p359, (2013) and Sherries Medical Microbiology, 6/e p492, (2014).

- As per the Runyon's classification of Atypical mycobacteria, M. avium, M. intracellulare, M. ulcerens and M. xenopi are classified under non photo chromogens.
- M. kansasii and M. simiae belongs to photochromogens and M. scrofulaceum belongs to scotochromogens.

97. Ans. a. RNA *Ref: Ananthanarayan and Paniker: Textbook of Microbiology, 9/e p65, (2013).*

- Refer explanation of Q. no10, 2013

98. Ans. c. Candidiasis *Ref: Ananthanarayan and Paniker: Textbook of Microbiology, 9/e p605–615, (2013).*

- Blastomycosis caused by Blastomyces dermatitidis.
- Paracoccidoidomycosis caused by Paracoccidiodes immitis.
- Cryptococcosis caused by Cryptococcus neoformans.
- All the three fungi infections manifest as suppurative and granulomatous lesions.
- Candidiasis is usually a non granular infection, but hyper keratic granulomatous lesions occur in chronic mucocutaneous candidiasis as a result of immunodeficiency disorders like T cell disorders with or without endocrinopathy.

99. Ans. b. Streptococcus *Ref: Ananthanarayan and Paniker: Textbook of Microbiology, 9/e p456–460, (2013).*

- Phage typing has been the mainstay of strain discrimination and is widely used in epidemiological studies
- Staphylococcus aureus phage typing is carried out by pattern method, where a set of 23 standard typing phages of S. aureus is used to type staphylococcal isolates and distinguish them from one another by their patterns of susceptibility to lysis.

- Other organisms typed by Phage typing method are Proteus, S.typhi, (Nicolle's complementary phage typing), Vibrio cholerae, H. influenzae. Brucella abortus (Tblisi (Tb)–reference phage) and Bacillus anthracis.

100. Ans. c. T carateum *Ref: Ananthanarayan and Paniker: Textbook of Microbiology, 9/e p370, (2013).*

- T. pallidum consists of
  - T. pallidum subspp. pallidum causing venereal syphilis,
  - T. pallidum subspp. endemicum causing endemic syphilis or bejel,
  - T. pallidum subspp. pertenue causing yaws,
  - T. pallidum subspp carateum causes pinta.
  - Pinta, Bejel and Yaws are non-venereal in nature.

101. Ans. a. Intrapartum period *Ref: Ananthanarayan and Paniker: Textbook of Microbiology, 9/e p583, (2013).*

- The risk of vertical transmission is greatly increased during intra partum period due to an increase in duration of contact with the maternal blood and cervical vaginal secretions.

102. Ans: b. Fimbriae *Ref: Ananthanarayan and Paniker: Textbook of Microbiology, 9/e p74, (2013).*

- Bacterial adherence to the cell surface is mediated by specialized molecules. The various molecules that mediate adherence to the cell surface are called adhesins.
- These adhesins allow the bacteria to adhere to the surface of human cell, thereby promoting their ability to cause disease.
- Microorganism that lacks this mechanism are nonpathogenic.
- Bacterial adhesins can be divided into two major groups: pili (fimbriae) and nonpilus adhesins (afimbrial adhesins).

103. Ans. b. Cryptococcus neoformans

Ref: Ananthanarayan and Paniker: Textbook of Microbiology, 9/e p605–615 (2013).

- Histoplasma capsulatum, Candida albicans and Coccidiodes immitis lacks capsule.
- Cryptococcus neoformans possesses polysaccharide capsule which helps to evade the immune response.
- Capsule is demonstrated by negative staining technique. (India ink and Nigrosin)

104. Ans. c. Schistosoma haematobium *Ref: Paniker's Textbook of Medical Parasitology, 7/e p148, (2013).*

- Ova with terminal spine—S. hematobium
- Ova with lateral spine—S. mansoni
- Ova with knob—S. japonicum
- Ova with diminutive spine on the lateral axis-a. Schistosoma mekongi

105. Ans. d. Multinucleated giant cells *Ref: Ananthanarayan and Paniker: Textbook of Microbiology, 9/e p470, (2013).*

- Tzanck smear is useful for the cytological identification of viruses in the scraping obtained from the base of the vesicular lesion.
- In this procedure, the vesicular lesion is aseptically ruptured, and the base of the lesion is scrapped with a sterile scalpel.
- The scraping from the base of the lesion is smeared on a glass slide, air dried, fixed, and usually stained with 1% aqueous solution of toluidine blue' for 15 seconds.
- Demonstration of typical multi nucleated giant cells with faceted nuclei and homogenously stained ground glass chromatin or cowdry type A intranuclear inclusion bodies by giemsa or Wright stain is diagnostic of HSV infection.
- This method shows variable sensitivity of 40–80% for diagnosis of HSV.

106. Ans. b. Cytomegalovirus *Ref: Harrison's Infectious diseases 1/e p753, (2010).*

- In liver transplants, CMV induces a variety of syndromes, including fever and leukopenia, hepatitis, pneumonitis, esophagitis, gastritis, colitis, and retinitis.
- CMV disease may be an independent risk factor for both graft loss and death.
- The period of maximal risk is between 1 and 4 months after transplantation, although retinitis may be a later complication.
- The transplanted organ is particularly vulnerable as a target for CMV infection; thus there is a tendency for CMV hepatitis to follow liver transplantation and for CMV pneumonitis to follow lung transplantation.
- CMV pneumonia occurs in 15–20% of bone marrow transplant recipients; the case-fatality rate is 84–88%, although the risk of severe disease may be reduced by prophylaxis or preemptive therapy with antiviral drugs.

- The risk is greatest 5–13 weeks after transplantation, and identified risk factors include certain types of immunosuppressive therapy, acute graft-versus-host disease, older age, viremia, and pretransplantation seropositivity.

107. Ans. d. Community acquired pneumonia

Ref: Ananthanarayan and Paniker: Textbook of Microbiology, 9/e p419, (2013).

- Chlamydia trachomatis causes endemic trachoma, inclusion conjunctivitis and lymphogranuloma venereum.
- About one-third to one-half of all cases of interstitial pneumonia in infantsdue to C. trochomatis.
- Develops in a child between 6 weeks and 6 months of age and has a gradual onset.
- The child is usually afebrile, but develops difficulty in feeding, a characteristic staccato (pertussis-like) cough, and shortness of breath.
- This disease is rarely fatal, but may be associated with decreased pulmonary function later in life.

108. Ans. a. Trichuris trichiura

Ref: Paniker's Textbook of Medical Parasitology, 7/e p173, (2013) and Sherries Medical Microbiology, 6/e p852, (2014).

- Trichuris trichiura (whip worm)—Man is the definitive host.
- Habitats in Large intestine.
- There is no pulmonary passage in the life cycle.
- It causes "**Dysentery syndrome**" with bloody diarrhea that mimics infection with bacterial pathogens such as shigella.
- Heavy worm burdens may cause tenesmus, the sensation that one needs to defecate continuously, and this may lead to **prolapse of the rectum through the anus**, particularly when the host is straining at defecation or during childbirth.

109. Ans. c. Type III

Ref: Ananthanarayan and Paniker: Textbook of Microbiology, 9/e p166, (2013) and Sherries Medical Microbiology, 6/e p41, (2014).

- Serum sickness is the systemic form of Type III hypersensitivity.
- It was described by Von Pirquet and Schick
- Occurs 7–12 days after injecting the high concentration of foreign serum (e.g Diphtheria toxin)
- Fever, Myalgia, Lymphadenopathy, Glomerulonephritis, Splenomegaly and urticarial rashes are the manifestations.
- Pathogenesis—formation of immune complexes.
- Single dose may serve both as sensitizing and shocking dose. This the unique feature of serum sickness.

110. Ans. b. Meninges

Ref: Ananthanarayan and Paniker: Textbook of Microbiology, 9/e p613, (2013) and Sherries Medical Microbiology, 6/e p746 (2014).

- The primary disease caused by Cryptococci is a chronic meningitis. The onset is slow, even insidious, with low-grade fever and headache progressing to altered mental state and seizures.
- In the cerebrospinal fluid (CSF) and in tissues, the inflammatory response is often remarkably muted.
- Most patients have some obvious form of immune compromise, although some show no demonstrable immune defect.
- Associated with soil and bird droppings and inhalation of Yeasts or basidiospores.
- Antiphagocytic capsule is prime factor and Melanin provides oxidative protection in macrophage.
- Cryptococcus gattii is more likely to produce pulmonary infection and less likely to invade the CNS.
- In the CNS, C. gattii may cause localized lesions as opposed to the diffuse meningoencephalitis typical of C. neoformans.

111. Ans. d. Scarlet fever more common <3 years

Ref: Ananthanarayan and Paniker: Textbook of Microbiology, 9/e p211, (2013) and Harrison's Infectious diseases 1/e p182, (2010).

- The group A Streptococcus (S pyogenes) is the cause of "strep throat," which can lead to scarlet fever, rheumatic fever, and rheumatic heart disease; the ability of some strains to cause catastrophic deep tissue infections led British tabloids to apply the gory label "flesh-eating bacteria."

- Scarlet fever is most common in children aged 2–10 years; usually follows group A streptococcal pharyngitis.
- Strawberry tongue/sand pepper appearance.
- Group A streptococcal pharyngitis is primarily a disease of children 5–15 years of age; it is uncommon among children <3 years old, as is rheumatic fever.

112. Ans. a. Immune complex

Ref: Ananthanarayan and Paniker: Textbook of Microbiology, 9/e p121, (2013) and Sherries Medical Microbiology, 6/e p27, (2014).

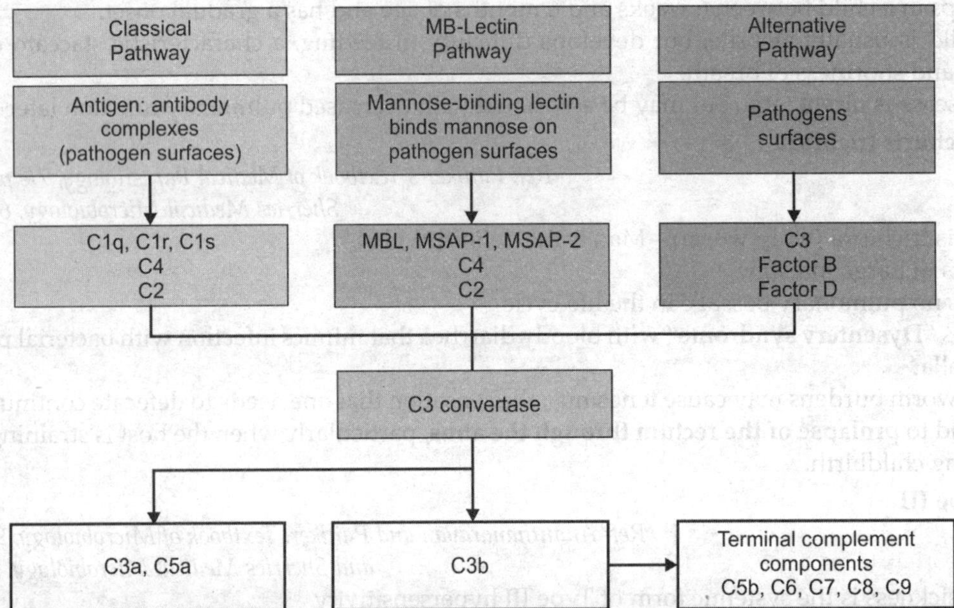

- Complement activation involves a series of enzymatic reactions that culminate in the formation of C3 convertase, which cleaves complement component C3 into C3b and C3a. The production of the C3 convertase is where the three pathways converge.
- C3a is a peptide mediator of local inflammation. C3b binds covalently to the bacterial cell membrane and opsonizes the bacteria, enabling phagocytes to internalize them.
- C5a and C5b are generated by the cleavage of C5 by a C5 convertase. In addition, C5a is a powerful peptide mediator of inflammation.
- C5b promotes the terminal components complement to assemble into a membrane-attack complex

113. Ans. a. B4

Ref: Ananthanarayan and Paniker: Textbook of Microbiology, 9/e p164, (2013) and Kuby Immunology, 7/e p458 (2013).

- Leucotrienes are derived by Lipooxygenase pathway from arachidonic acid.
- Leukotriene C4, D4, E4 and F4 are often called cysteinyl leukotrienes due to the presence of the amino acid cysteine in their structure. The cysteinyl leukotrienes make up the slow-reacting substance of anaphylaxis (SRS-A).
- Leukotriene B4 is synthesized in vivo from Leukotriene A4 by the enzyme LTA4 hydrolase. Its primary function is to recruit neutrophils to areas of tissue damage, though it also helps promote the production of inflammatory cytokines by various immune cells.

114. Ans. a. Hot air oven *Ref: Ananthanarayan and Paniker: Textbook of Microbiology, 9/e p30, (2013).*

- Powder, Oil, Grease, Glasswares, liquid paraffin, metal sharps and swabs are sterilized by hot air oven.
- The holding temperature for Oil and grease is 150°C for one hour.
- For Ophthalmic cutting instruments, the holding temperature is 150°C for two hours.

115. Ans. a. Bile insoluble *Ref: Ananthanarayan and Paniker: Textbook of Microbiology, 9/e p222, (2013).*

- Inulin fermentation, Bile solubility, Optochin sensitivity, Quellung reaction and Lanceolate shape are the classical characteristics of streptococcus pneumoniae.

116. Ans. d. Bornholm's disease

Ref: Ananthanarayan and Paniker: Textbook of Microbiology, 9/e p492, (2013) and Sherries Medical Microbiology, 6/e p213, (2014).

- Bornholm's disease (Epidemic Pleurodynia), Myocarditis, Pericarditis, Juvenile diabetes, orchitis and Post viral fatigue syndrome are caused by Group B Coxsackie virus.
- Incubation period: 2–10 days

117. Ans. d. Clostridium perfringens *Ref: Ananthanarayan and Paniker: Textbook of Microbiology, 9/e p252, (2013).*

- All the clostridia are motile with peritrichous flagella except Clostridium perfringens and Clostridium tetani type VI.

118. Ans. a. Measles

Ref: Ananthanarayan and Paniker: Textbook of Microbiology, 9/e p512, (2013) and Sherries Medical Microbiology, 6/e p190, (2014).

- In measles, the lymphoid tissues show hyperplastic changes, and large multinucleated reticuloendothelial giant cells are called as Warthin finkeldy cells

119. Ans. c. Coronavirus

Ref: Ananthanarayan and Paniker: Textbook of Microbiology, 9/e p559, (2013) and Sherries Medical Microbiology, 6/e p182 (2014).

- SARS is caused by a novel, new coronavirus
- Risk of transmission from an infected to an uninfected person is greatest around day 10 of illness
- Coronaviruses were so named for the crown-like appearance of their virions on electron microscopy. These viruses are the second most important cause of the common cold; rhinoviruses being the first cause.
- Severe acute respiratory syndrome (SARS)-associated coronavirus (SARS-CoV) is a newly described coronavirus in 2002.
- The virus causes an atypical pneumonia called SARS, a serious and potentially life-threatening viral infection of humans
- Recently, a new coronavirus (Novel Coronavirus 2012, now called MERS coronavirus) was isolated from a patient in the Middle East that caused a fatal respiratory disease leading to renal failure.
- This virus is similar to SARS, but still different than SARS and other human coronaviruses.

120. Ans. b. Antibody excess *Ref: Ananthanarayan and Paniker: Textbook of Microbiology, 9/e p105, (2013).*

- In an agglutination or precipitation reaction, the zone of relatively high antibody concentrations within which no reaction occurs.
- As the antibody concentration is lowered below the prozone, the reaction occurs. This phenomenon may be due simply to antibody excess or it may be due to blocking antibody or to nonspecific inhibitors in serum.
- This is also called **as Hook's effect**

121. Ans. c. Blastomyces *Ref: Paniker's Textbook of Medical Parasitology, 7/e p87 (2013).*

- Cryptosporidium and Microsporidium are other examples for coccidian parasites.

122. Ans. a. Staph epidermidis

Ref: Ananthanarayan and Paniker: Textbook of Microbiology, 9/e p52 (2013) and Sherries Medical Microbiology, 6/e p83 (2014).

- Catalase is an enzyme that catalyzes the reduction of toxic hydrogen peroxide to oxygen and water
- When a colony is placed in hydrogen peroxide, liberation of oxygen as gas bubbles can be seen.
- This test is particularly useful in differentiation of Staphylococci (positive) from streptococci (negative), but also has taxonomic application to Gram-negative bacteria.
  - Staphylococci (important not confuse it with streptococci)
  - Pseudomonas aeruginosa
  - Aspergillus fumigatus
  - Candida

- Enterobacteriaceae (specially Klebsiella and Serratia both of which can cause pneumonia and U)
- Neisseria (Gonorrhea and Meningitidis)
- Vibrio
- Nocardia
- Campylobacter and Helicobacter
- Gardnerella vaginalis
- Mycobacterium Tuberculosis also produce a heat sensitive catalase (active only in body temperature) so it become catalase negative at 68.0 "F
- **None of the anaerobes**

123. Ans. a. Chorioretinitis *Ref: Paniker's Textbook of Medical Parasitology, 7/e p90 (2013).*

- This occurs when the mother gets primary toxoplasma infection, whether clinical or asymptomatic, during the pregnancy.
- The risk of fetal infection rises with progress of gestation; from 25%, when the mother acquires primary infection in first trimester to 65% in the third trimester. Conversely, the severity of fetal damage is highest, when infection is transmitted in early pregnancy.
- Mothers with chronic or latent Toxoplasma infection, acquired earlier, do not ordinarily infect their babies. But in some women with latent or chronic infection, the tissue cyst may be reactivated during pregnancy and liberate trophozoites, which may infect the fetus in utero
- The manifestations of congenital toxoplasmosis include chorioretinitis, cerebral calcifications, convulsions, strabismus, deafness, blindness, mental retardation, microcephaly, and hydrocephalus.

124. Ans. b. Strongyloidosis *Ref: Paniker's Textbook of Medical Parasitology, 7/e p180, (2013)*

- Largest nematode known to cause human infection: Ascaris lumbricoides.
- Smallest Nematode known to cause human infection: Strongyloides stercoralis.
- In debilitated individuals and particularly in those with cellular immune defects, extensive internal reinfection takes place, leading to an enormous number of adult worms in the intestines and lungs and larvae in various tissues and organs. This is known as **hyperinfection Syndrome**.
- Severe malnutrition, lepromatous leprosy, lymphoreticular malignancies, acquired immunodeficiency syndrome (AIDS), immunosuppressive drugs, and other situations, in which cellmediated immunity is defective, predispose to this condition.
- Hyperinfection is an important hazard of steroid therapy and other instances of prolonged immunosuppression as in transplant patients.
- During hyperinfection, the filariform larvae may enter into arterial circulation and lodge in various organs e.g. heart, lungs, brain, kidney, pancreas, liver, and lymphnodes. Manifestations depend on the sites affected.
- Brain abscess, meningitis, and peritonitis are major fatal complications.
- It has been reported that circulating Strongyloides larvae may carry intestinal bacteria, causing septicemia

125. Ans. a. Trichuris *Ref: Paniker's Textbook of Medical Parasitology, 7/e p173, (2013) and Sherries Medical Microbiology, 6/e p852, (2014).*

- Trichuris trichiura (whip worm) has no tissue migratory phase.
- It causes **"Dysentery syndrome"** with bloody diarrhea that mimics infection with bacterial pathogens such as Shigella.
- Heavy worm burdens may cause tenesmus, the sensation that one needs to defecate continuously, and this may lead to prolapse of the rectum through the anus, particularly when the host is straining at defecation or during childbirth.
- Toxoplasma and Trichinella—man is the dead end host.
- Toxoplasma—brady cyst, Trichenella—larvae in Striated muscle

126. Ans. b. e. dispar

Ref: Paniker's Textbook of Medical Parasitology, 7/e p18, (2013) and Sherries Medical Microbiology, 6/e p813, (2014).

- It has been proposed that pathogenic and nonpathogenic strains though morphologically identical may represent 2 distinct species—the pathogenic strains being E. histolytica, and the nonpathogenic strains reclassifid as E. dispar.
- Trophozoites of E. dispar contain bacteria, but no RBCs

	E. histolytica	E. dispar
Ingested RBC	+	–
Zymodeme pattern	II, VI, VII, XI	I, III
Concavalin A Agglutination	+	–
Animal pathogenicity	+	–

128. Ans. c. Enrichment medium *Ref: Ananthanarayan and Paniker: Textbook of Microbiology, 9/e p42 (2013).*

- Liquid media contain substances that inhibit the growth of all but a few bacteria but at the same time facilitate growth of certain bacteria.
- E.g Selenite F broth, Tetrathionate broth and Alkaline peptone water

129. Ans. c. Phlebotomus argentipes

Ref: Paniker 's Textbook of Medical Parasitology, 7/e p52, (2013).

Vector species responsible for transmission of Leishmania donovani	
Country	*Phlebotomus species*
India	P. argentipes
China, Bangladesh	P. chineses P. sergenti
Sudan and Africa	P. pemicious P. orientalls (Sudan) P. longicupis P. sergenti
Mediterrean Countries	P. pemicious P. papatasii P. majaor P. tobbi
Middle East and Russia	P. perfulievi P. papatasii
Central Asia	P. papatasii
South America	P. longipalpis P. intermudias P. lutzi

130. Ans. d. Toxin neutralization

Ref: Ananthanarayan and Paniker: Textbook of Microbiology, 9/e p125, (2013).

- The following are the functions of complement.
- Phagocytosis
- Hypersensitivity reaction II and III
- Chemotaxis
- Autoimmune disease (SLE)
- Endotoxic shock
- Cytolysis
- Immune adherence
- Antiviral activity

131. Ans. b. Dog

Ref: Paniker's Textbook of Medical Parasitology, 7/e p127, (2013). Sherries Medical Microbiology, 6/e p892, (2014).

- The larva of Echinococcus granulosus (dog tapeworm) causes unilocular hydatid cyst disease. Multilocular hydatid disease is caused by E. multilocularis,
- E. granulosus is one of the smallest tapeworm
- Dogs are the most important definitive hosts.

- The intermediate hosts are usually sheep. Humans are almost always dead-end intermediate hosts.
- Prevention of human disease involves not feeding the entrails of slaughtered sheep to dogs.
- Pig is the definitive host for B.coli and intermediate host for T. solium.
- Cattle are intermediate host for t. saginata.

132. Ans. d. They are more prominent in Gram negative bacteria

Ref: Ananthanarayan and Paniker: Textbook of Microbiology, 9/e p18, (2013).

- Mesosomes are vesicular convoluted or multilaminated structures formed as invagination of the plasma membrane into the cytoplasm.
- They are analogous to the mitochondria of eukaryotic cell and are the principal sites of respiratory enzymes in bacteria.
- Two types: Septal and lateral are.
- The septal mesosome attached to the bacterial DNA and coordinates nuclear and cytoplasmic divisions during binary fission.
- Mesosomes are otherwise named as chondroids.
- They are more prominent in Gram Positive cells.

133. Ans. a. Cannot replicate

Ref: Ananthanarayan and Paniker: Textbook of Microbiology, 9/e p55, (2013).

- A plasmid is a small DNA molecule within a cell that is physically separated from a chromosomal DNA and can replicate independently.
- They are most commonly found in bacteria as small, circular, double-stranded DNA molecules.
- Involved in toxin production, virulence, Drug resistance and vector for genetic engineering.

134. Ans. d. Episome

Ref: Ananthanarayan and Paniker: Textbook of Microbiology, 9/e p55, (2013) and Sherries Medical Microbiology, 6/e p378, (2014).

- Integrated form of plasmid DNA with chromosomal DNA is episome.
- A DNA segment containing insertion sequences able to mediate movement between plasmids and chromosome; may also contain one or more recognizable genes is transposon.
- Transposons are otherwise called as Jumping genes.

135. Ans. C. M. avium

Ref: Ananthanarayan and Paniker: Textbook of Microbiology, 9/e p359, (2013) and Sherries Medical Microbiology, 6/e p492, (2014).

- As per the Runyon's classification of Atypical mycobacteria, M. avium, M. intracellulare, M. ulcerens and M.xenopi are classified under non photo chromogens.
- M. kansasii and M.simiae belongs to photochromogens and M. scrofulaceum belongs to scotochromogens.

136. Ans. B. ETEC

Ref: Ananthanarayan and Paniker: Textbook of Microbiology, 9/e p279(2013).

- Entero toxigenic Escherichia coli is the causative agent of Traveler's diarrhea. Serotypes 6, 8, 15, 25, 27, 167 are involved.
- Labile toxin (LT) and Stable toxin (ST), CFA (I-IV) are the virulent factors.
- Watery diarrhea without fever and inflammation.
- Causative agents for Traveler's diarrhea.

E. coli, enterotoxigenic	20–75%
E. coli, enteroaggregative	0–20%
E. coli, enteroinvasive	0–6%
Shigella spp	2–30%
Salmonella spp	0–33%
Campylobacter jejuni	3–17%
Vibrio parahemolyticus	0–31%
Aeromonas hydrophila	0–30%
Giardia lamblia	less than 20%

Entamoeba histolytica	0–5%
Cryptosporidium sp	less than 20%
Rotavirus	0–36%
Norwalk virus	0–10%

137. Ans. c. No negative phase *Ref: Ananthanarayan and Paniker: Textbook of Microbiology, 9/e p81, (2013) and Kuby Immunology, 7/e p8, (2013).*

- Clinical/subclinical infection leads to active natural immunity and Vaccination leads to active artificial immunity.
- Memory and Negative phase are the characteristic features of active immunity.
- During development of active immunity, there is a **Negative phase** where the level of measurable immunity is lower than it was before the antigenic stimulus.

QUESTIONS 2015

1. Best method for prevention of MRSA infection in health care settings is
a. Vaccines
b. Handwashing
c. Routine screening
d. Use of Higher antibiotics

2. Pick the true statement regarding Plasmids:
a. Non self replicatives
b. Acts as messenger RNA
c. Involved in transformation
d. Involved in conjugational transfer between strains

3. EHEC strain associated with HUS is:
a. O157 : H7
b. O7 : H157
c. O37 : H14
d. O157 : H9

4. Gas gangrene and Tetanus caused by which group of bacteria:
a. Campylobacter
b. Clostridium
c. Citrobacter
d. Cardiobacterium

5. The following is RNA virus
a. Hepatitis B virus
b. Polyoma virus
c. Herpes virus
d. HIV–1

6. All the following statements are true regarding endotoxins except:
a. Neutralized by specific antibodies
b. Heat stable
c. Somatic antigen
d. Poorly antigenic

7. Specific test to diagnose H.pylori infection is:
a. Urea breath test
b. Culture
c. Barium Meal
d. Animal inoculation

8. Heart lung machine is best sterilized by:
a. Ethylene oxide
b. Cidex
c. Isoprophyl alcohol
d. Formaldehyde

9. Protein degrading enzyme secreted by:
a. Gonococci
b. Pneumococci
c. Staph.aureus
d. Enterococci

10. Role of bacterial capsule is:
a. Support
b. Transport
c. Anti phagocytic
d. Adhesion

ANSWERS AND EXPLANATIONS

1. Ans. b. Handwashing *Ref: Ananthanarayan and Paniker: Textbook of Microbiology, 9/e p204, (2013).*

- Handwashing is the oldest, simplest and most effective method for prevention of MRSA out break in health care settings.

2. Ans. d. Involved in Conjugational transfer between strains

Ref: Ananthanarayan and Paniker: Textbook of Microbiology, 9/e p60, (2013).

- Plasmids are self replicative extrachromosomal elements frequently transferred by conjugation

3. Ans. a. O157 : H7

Ref: Ananthanarayan and Paniker: Textbook of Microbiology, 9/e p279, (2013).

- HUS is caused by Entero Hemorrhagic E coli strain O157 : H7. Its also caused by O26 : H1

4. Ans. b. Clostridium *Ref: Ananthanarayan and Paniker: Textbook of Microbiology, 9/e p251, (2013).*

- Gasgangrene is caused by Clostridium welchii and Tetanus is caused by Clostridium tetani.

5. Ans. d. HIV–1 *Ref: Ananthanarayan and Paniker: Textbook of Microbiology, 9/e p429, (2013).*

- Herpes, Hepatitis B, Pox, Adeno, Parvo and papova are DNA viruses.

6. Ans. a. Neutralized by specific antibodies

Ref: Ananthanarayan and Paniker: Textbook of Microbiology, 9/e p75, (2013).

- Only exotoxins are neutralized by specific antibodies not endotoxins.

7. Ans. b. Culture *Ref: Ananthanarayan and Paniker: Textbook of Microbiology, 9/e (2013), p400.*

- Culture is the gold standard test and urea breath test is the rapid test to diagnose H. pylori infection.

8. Ans. a. Ethylene oxide *Ref: Ananthanarayan and Paniker: Textbook of Microbiology, 9/e p35, (2013).*

- As per Spaulding's classification, critical equipments like Heart lung machines are best sterilized by ETO

9. Ans. a. Gonococci *Ref: Ananthanarayan and Paniker: Textbook of Microbiology, 9/e p231, (2013).*

- Gonococci and Meningococci produced IgA1 protease that spilts and inactivates IgA

10. Ans. c. Antiphagocytic *Ref: Ananthanarayan and Paniker: Textbook of Microbiology, 9/e p18, (2013).*

- The main role of bacterial capsule is to escape from phagocytosis

Chapter

6 Pathology

Marquess Raj

CELL INJURY AND CELLULAR ADAPTATION

Cell injury–Reversible vs irreversible cell injury

Reversible cell injury	Irreversible cell injury
• Cellular swelling • Loss of microvilli • Formation of cytoplasmic blebs • ER swelling • Ribosomal detachment • Myelin figures • Clumping of nuclear chromatin	• Flocculent, amorphous mitochondrial densities • Swelling and disruption of lysosomes • Plasma membrane damage • Pyknosis • Karyolysis • Karyorrhexis

Necrosis

- Two pathological processes take place in necrosis
  - Enzymatic digestion of the cell.
  - Denaturation of proteins
- **Morphology**
  - Increased eosinophilia attributable in part to loss of the normal basophilia imparted by the RNA in the cytoplasm
  - Dead cells may ultimately be replaced by large, whorled phospholipids masses called myelin figures
  - Calcifiation of such fatty acid residues results in the generation of calcium soaps.
  - Nuclear changes
    - Karyolysis, the basophilia of the chromomatin may fade
    - Pyknosis, nuclear shrinkage and increased basophilia
    - Karyorrhexis, nucleus undergoes fragmentation.

Types of necrosis

Type of necrosis	Pathology	Examples
Coagulative necrosis	Loss of nucleus with cellular outline being preserved associated with ischemia	Solid organs -Heart, kidney, liver
Liquefactive necrosis	Enzymatic destruction of cells with abscess formation	Soft organ-Brain
Caseous necrosis	Cheese like appearance of necrotic material	Tuberculosis
Fat necrosis	Action of lipases on fatty tissue	Breast, omentum, pancreas
Fibrinoid necrosis	Complexes of antigen and antibodies are deposited in vessel wall with leakage of fibrinogen out of vessels	Malignant hypertension, Wegener's granulomatosis, Ashoff bodies in rheumatic heart disease, PAN
Gangrenous necrosis	Necrosis of tissue with superadded putrefaction	Dry gangrene similar to coagulative necrosis Wet gangrene similar to liquefactive necrosis

Apoptosis

- Specialized form of ***programed cell death.***

Morphology

- Cell shrinks in size and has dense eosinophilic cytoplasm
- Nuclear chromatin condensation followed by fragmentation
- Formation of cytoplasmic membrane blebs
- Breakdown of the cell into fragments (apoptotic bodies)
- Phagocytosis of apoptotic bodies by adjacent cells or macrophages
- **Lack of an inflammatory response**

Stimulus for Apoptosis

- Cell injury and DNA damage
- Lack of hormones, cytokines, or growth factors
- Duct obstruction.
- Receptor-ligand signals
  - Fas binding to the Fas ligand
  - TNF binding to TNFR1
- Apoptosis is regulated by genes

Apoptosis inhibitor–bcl-2	Apoptosis stimulator–p–53
Prevents release of cytochrome C from mitochondria Binds to pro Apaf-1	Elevated by DNA injury and arrests the cell cycle If DNA repair is impossible, p-53 stimulates apoptosis

Execution of apoptosis

- Mediated by cascade of caspases
- Release of cytochrome C from mitochondria

Examples of apoptosis

Physiological apoptosis	Pathological apoptosis
• Embryogenesis and development	• Viral diseases: viral hepatitis (Councilman bodies).
• Hormone dependent apoptosis (menstruation)	• Graft vs host disease
• Thymus: selective death of lymphocytes	• Cystic fibrosis: duct obstruction and pancreatic atrophy

Cellular Adaptation

- Cellular adaptation is the result of a persistent stress or injury
- Adaptive responses are potentially reversible once the stress has been removed
- Some forms of adaptation may precede or progress to malignancy. eg: Metaplasia.

Atrophy

Decrease in cell size.

- **Causes of atrophy**
  - Decreased workload/disuse
  - Decreased blood supply → Ischemia (MC cause atherosclerosis)
  - Decreased nerve supply
  - Lack of hormonal stimulation
  - Malnutrition
  - Aging
- **Microscopy:** Small shrunken cells with lipofuscin granules
- EM: Decreased intracellular components and autophagosomes

Hypertrophy

- An *increase in cell size and functional ability* due to increased synthesis of intracellular components or in simple terms 'increase in mass.'
- Causes of hypertrophy

Increased mechanical demand	Increased endocrine stimulation
Physiologic: skeletal muscle with exercise Pathologic: cardiac muscle in HT	Puberty Gravid uterus Lactating breast

Hyperplasia

- An increase in the ***number of cells***

Physiological hyperplasia	Pathological hyperplasia
Female breast at puberty and during pregnancy Pregnant uterus (hyperplasia + hypertrophy)	Endometrial hyperplasia Benign prostatic hyperplasia

Metaplasia

- A reversible change of one cell type to another,usually in response to chronic irritation
- For example, one bronchial epithelium in response to tobacco smoking
- Two intestinal metaplasia in Barret's esophagus.

Dysplasia

- An abnormal proliferation of cells that is characterized by changes in cell size, shape, and loss of cellular organization
- Dysplasia is not cancer but may progress to cancer (preneoplastic lesion)
- Full thickness dysplasia or dysplasia involving entire thickness of the epithelium but not breaching the basement membrane is carcinoma in situ
- **Dysplasia is reversible**
- Examples: cervical dysplasia, actinic keratosis, and oral leukoplakia.

Other cellular alterations during injury

- Intracellular accumulations

Intracellular accumulations	Pathogenesis	Examples
Lipids	↑ Fatty acid synthesis ↑ Esterification of Fatty acids into triglycerides ↓ Fatty acid oxidation ↓ Apoprotein synthesis	• Triglycerides (e.g., fatty change in liver cells) • Cholesterol (e.g., atherosclerosis, xanthomas) • Complex lipids (e.g., sphingolipid accumulations) • Fatty change in heart–tigered effect or thrush breast appearance
Proteins	Excessive protein turnover or loss	• Nephrotic syndrome–Protein accumulates in PCT in proteinuria as reabsorption droplets • Multiple myeloma–Russel bodies intracytoplasmic accumulation of Ig in plasma cells
Exogenous pigments	Anthracotic pigmentation of the lung is secondary to the inhalation of carbon dust Tattoos	
Endogenous pigments	Lippofuscin	• Wear and tear pigment • Perinuclear yellow–brown pigment • Indigestable material within lysosomes • Common in liver and heart

Contd...

Contd...

Intracellular accumulations	Pathogenesis	Examples
	Melanin	• Black-brown pigment • Found in melanocytes and substantia nigra
	Hemosiderin	• Golden yellow-brown granular pigment • Found in areas of hemarrhage or bruises • Prussian blue stain demonstrates hemosiderin

- Hyaline changes
  - Nonspecific term used to describe any intra or extra cellular alteration that has a pink homogenous glassy appearance on H & E stain

Intracellular hyaline	Extracellular hyaline
• Renal proximal tubule protein reabsorption droplets • Russell bodies–seen in multiple myeloma Alcoholic hyaline or Mallory body	• Hyaline arteriosclerosis seen in DM • Amyloid • Hyaline membrane disease of the newborn

Giant Cells

Types of giant cell	Examples
Langhans giant cell	TB and Sarcoidosis
FB giant cell	TB, Leprosy, Brucellosis, Syphilis Aschoff's cells in rheumatic heart disease
Viral giant cell	Warthin-Finkedley–measles Adenovirus Herpes virus HIV
Resorptive giant cell	Osteoclasts Syncitiotrophoblast cells
Tumor giant cell	RS cell in Hodgkins disease

Inflammation

Acute Inflammation: Starts immediately following cell injury and lasts for a few minutes or one or two days. That is (24–48 hrs).

Features of acute inflammation:

1. Vascular changes

Alteration in vessel caliber and flow	• Initial transient vasoconstriction of arterioles. (lasts few seconds) • Persistent vasodilation • Slowing of circulation–Stasis of RBC's
Changes in vascular permeability	• Increased capillary blood pressure • Increased vascular permeability to proteins • Exudation of protein rich fluid resulting in edema

CELLULAR EVENTS: MARGINATION ADHESION CHEMOTAXIS PHAGOCYTOSIS

Neutrophilic Granules

Primary (azurophilic) granules	Smaller specific/secondary granules
• Acid hydrolases • BPI (Bacterial permeability increasing protein) • Cationic proteins • Cathepsin G • Defensins	• Alkaline phosphatase • Phospholipase A2 • Collagenase • Leukocyte alkaline phosphatase • Lysozyme

Contd...

Contd...

Primary (azurophilic) granules	Smaller specific/secondary granules
• Elastase • Phospholipase A2 • Lysozyme	• Lactoferrin • Vitamin B12 binding proteins

Genetic Defects of Leukocyte Function

Defects of adhesion: Leukocyte adhesion defects (LAD)	• LFA-1 and Mac-1 subunit defects lead to impaired adhesion (LAD-1) • Absence of sialyl-Lewis X, and defect in E-and P-selectin sugar epitopes (LAD-2)
Defects of chemotaxis/phagocytosis	• Microtubule assembly defect leads to impaired locomotion and lysosomal degranulation (Chediak-Higashi Syndrome) • Components of Chediak Higashi: Autosomal recessive disorder • Oculocutaneous albinism • Susceptible to pyogenic infections • Anemia • Bleeding tendency • Neutrophils and their precursors and monocytes demonstrate large granules (peroxidase +)
Defects of microbicidal activity: Chronic granulomatous disease (CGD)	• Deficiency of NADPH oxidase that generates superoxide, therefore no oxygen-dependent killing mechanism (CGD) • Diagnosis: CGD is detected by NBT (nitroblue tetrazolium test)

Acquired Defects of Leukocyte Function

Defects of Chemotaxis	Thermal injury, DM, Malignancy, Sepsis, Immuno deficiency
Defects of Adhesion	Hemodialysis, DM
Defects of Phagocytosis and Microbicidal activity	Leukemia, Anemia, Sepsis, DM, Neonates and Malnutrition

Chemical mediators of inflammation

- Plasma Proteases
  - Kinin system–Bradykinin, Substance P, Kallikrin
  - Complement system. For example C3a, C5a–Anaphylatoxins
  - Coagulation system. For example FDP's.
- Arachidonic acid (AA) metabolites
  - Via cyclooxygenase pathway–Prostaglandins, thromboxane
  - Via lipoxygenase pathway–leukotrienes
  - **Note:** AA is derived from essential fatty acid linoleic acid
  - Corticosteroids inhibit Phosholipase A2
  - Aspirin inhibits cyclooxygenase.
- Lysosomal constituents
- Oxygen derived free radicals
- PAF (platelet activating factor)
- Cytokines
- Growth factors
- Vasoactive amines. For example histamine, serotonin
- Chemokines (4 classes).
  - C × C–alpha. For example IL18.
  - CC-beta. For example MCP, Eotaxin.
  - C-gamma. For example specific for lymphocytes.
  - C × 3C–For example Fractaline.

Complement

- 20 complement proteins present and are numbered from C1 to C9
- Heat labile factors–Alexine or Complement

Difference between classical and alternate pathway

Features	Classical pathway	Alternate pathway
Activators	Ig M > Ig G4> Ig G1> Ig G2	Ig A1, Ig A2, Ig D, Ig G4
C3 convertase	C4b2b	C3bBb
C5 convertase	C4b2b3b	C3bBb3b
Factors	Decreased C1, C2, C3, C4 with Normal factor B	Decreased factor B and C3 with Normal C1, C2, C4

Complement pathway

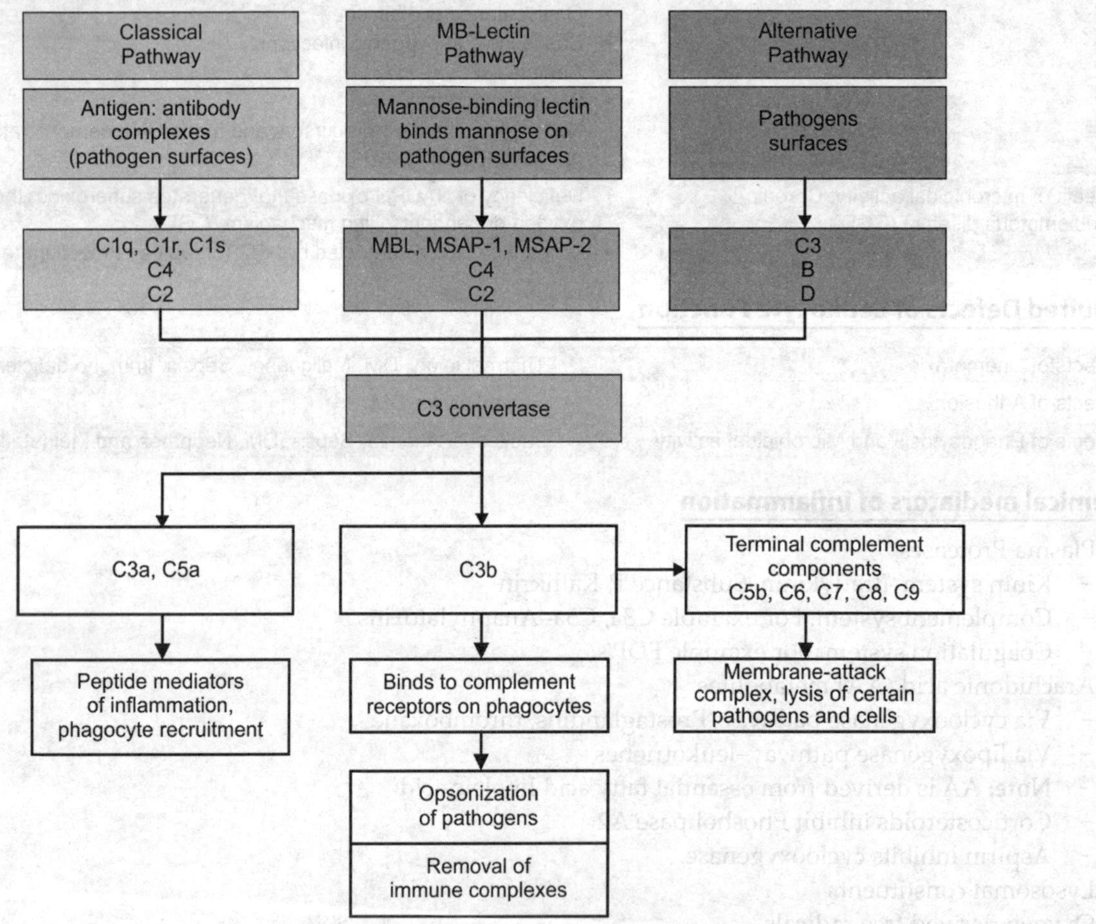

Functions of complement

Anaphylotoxins–C3a, C5a	Opsonization–C3b
Chemotaxis–C5a	Membrane attack complex–C5 to C9

Regulation of complement

Decay accelerating factor increases C3 convertase dissociation	Factor I proteolytically cleave C3b
CD 59 inhibits formation of Membrane attack complex	Factor H, Factor I, CD 46–prevent excessive alternate pathway activation

Complement synthesis

Site of synthesis	Complement involved
Liver	C3, C6, C9
GIT	C1
Macrophage	C2, C4
Spleen	C5, C8

Complement system disorders

Complement deficiency	Diseases associated
C1 esterase inhibitor	Hereditary angioneurotic edema
Early complements of classical pathway (C1, C2, C4)	Collagen vascular disorders, pyogenic infections
C3 and its regulatory protein	Severe recurrent pyogenic infections
C5–C9	Meningococcal and Toxoplasma infections
D, I	Pyogenic infections
Properdin	Neisseria infections
H	Hemolytic uremic syndrome
Decay accelerating factor	Paroxysmal nocturnal hemoglobinuria

Morphologic Types of acute inflammation:

- **Suppurative or purulent:** Exudate is rich in neutrophils. For example lung abscess.
- **Cattarhal inflammation:** Characterised by copius mucus discharge. For example allergic rhinitis.
- **Fibrinous:** Exudate is high in plasma proteins especially fibrin; seen in membrane-line body cavities. For example pericarditis. pleuritis.
- **Serous:** High fluid, low protein and cell content. For example burn blister.

Note neutrophils all the time are not present in all cases of acute inflammation-Exceptions:
- In viral and rickettsial infections, lymphocytes are the principal inflammatory cell
- In classic allergy and some parasitic infections, eosinophils dominate throughout
- In typhoid fever, the predominant cells are always the macrophages
- In most forms of acute dermatitis, lymphocytes are most abundant
- In clostridial gas gangrene neutrophils are not present

Chronic Inflammation

- **Definition:** An inflammatory response of prolonged duration (weeks or longer)
- **Associated events:** Development of specific humoral and cell-mediated immune response within 7–10 days of exposure

Cellular Elements

- **T-lymphocytes**: Following activation by antigen, produce lymphokines that attract blood monocytes to leave blood vessels go into tissue; activate macrophages
- **Plasma cells**: Synthesize specific antibodies against specific antigens
- **Macrophages**: Phagocytosis; produce chemokines that influence B-and T-cell function.

Causes of Chronic Inflammation

- Persistent infections by low toxicity organisms of which evoke delayed hypersensitivity—TB, leprosy, fungi
- Prolonged exposure to toxins or a nondegradable antigen—silicosis, atherosclerosis, alcoholism
- Autoimmunity: A self-perpetuating immune reaction is evoked by autoantigens with production of autoantibodies.

Histologic Types of CI

- **Granulomatous**
  - Infectious. For example (TB, schistosomiasis, syphilis, catscratch disease, deep fungal infections, leprosy, LGV)
  - Non-infectious/idiopathic. For example (sarcoidiosis, beryliosis, crohn disease)
  - Immune granulomas. For example (Wegeners granulomatosis)
  - Nonimmune granulomas.
- **Nongranulomatous or diffuse**
  - Chronic nonviral infections: Ineffective T-cell response is evoked while microorganisms survive and multiply within macrophages (lepromatous leprosy)
  - Chronic viral infections: Production of killer T-lymphocytes or cytotoxic antibodies that act with complement
  - Chronic chemical intoxication: Necrotic cells are targets of immune response.

Repair: Proliferation of cells and tissues to replace lost structures,usually accompanied by collagen deposition.

Classification of cells and tissues

Labile cells	Quiescent/stable cells	Permanent cells
• Surface epithelium of skin, oral cavity, vagina, cervix. • Lining mucosa of all excretory ducts of glands. • Epithelium of GIT, uterus, urinary tract. • Cells of bone marrow, hematopoietic cells.	• Low level of replication • Undergo rapid division in response to stimuli • Parenchymal cells of liver kidney and pancreas • Mesenchymal cells- fibroblasts, smooth muscle, vascular endothelial cells, lymphocytes and leukocytes, osteocytes	• Skeletal and cardiac muscle cell and nerve cells.

Wound healing

Healing by primary intention	Healing by secondary intention
• In wounds with opposed edges like surgical incisions. • Limited amount of injury. • Scab formation. • Re-epithelization through mitosis of basal cells. • Minimal granulation tissue formed • Fibrous union	• In wounds with separated edges or extensive loss of cells and tissue • Large tissue defect to be filled • Inadequate regeneration • Abundant granulation tissue formed • Wound contraction is prominent cells involved–myofibroblasts

Types of Collagen

- **Type I:** Major collagen of bone, skin, tendon and mature scars
- **Type II:** Major collagen of cartilage
- **Type III:** Abundant in blood vessels, uterus and GIT; first collagen deposited in wound healing
- **Type IV:** Found onlyin basement membranes
- **Types V and VI**: Found in most tissues
- **Types VII**: Dermoepidermal junction.

HEMODYNAMIC DISORDERS

Types of edema

- Localized edema

Edema of venous obstruction	Ascites	Pulmonary edema
• Lower limb venous obstruction (thrombosis) → impaired venous outflow	• Special type of localized edema.	• Most often caused by increased pulmonary venous pressure secondary to left heart failure.

Contd...

Contd...

Edema of venous obstruction	Ascites	Pulmonary edema
→ increase local hydrostatic pressure → edema	• Accumulated fluid can be transudate or exudates	• In infection (pneumonia), pulmonary edema is caused by increased permeability of pulmonary capillaries. • Pulmonary edema may occur in generalized edema caused by hypoalbuminemia of end stage liver disease

- Generalized edema
  - Cardiac failure
  - Renal failure
  - Starvation

Transudate vs Exudate

Features	Transudate edema fluid	Exudate edema fluid
Causes	CCF, Constrictive pericarditis	Malignant neoplasms, Infection, Lymphatic obstruction
Appearance	Clear	Turbid
Specific gravity	<1.015	>1.015
Protein content	<1.5 g/dL	>3 g/dL
Cells	None	Neutrophils
Fibrinogen	Absent	Present Clots spontaneously

Hyperemia and Congestion

Features	Hyperemia	Congestion
Process	Active–arteriolar dilatation	Passive–impaired venous outflow
Edema	Absent	Present
Color of tissue	Red	Bluish red
Seen in	Inflammation	Right heart failure, Portal venous obstruction in cirrhosis

Chronic Venous Congestion

- **Pathological changes** of chronic venous congestion: In long-standing congestion:
  - Stasis of poorly oxygenated blood → chronic hypoxia → parenchymal cell death.
  - Capillary rupture at the sites of chronic congestion → hemorrhage and **accumulation of hemosiderin-laden macrophages**

CPC–Lungs

- Chronic passive congestion of the lungs is typically secondary to left heart failure.
- It is accompanied by extravasation of RBCs into the alveolar spaces → these RBCs are taken up by macrophages.
- These hemosiderin laden macrophages are known as 'heart failure cells'
- Macrophages also enter the interstitial spaces, where they stimulate fibroblasts to produces collagen àfibrosis.
- Grossly the organ is fibrotic and brown in Color due to the fibrosis, called brown induration.

CPC–Liver

- Seen in right heart failure, obstruction of IVC.
- The area around the central vein is least oxygenated (Zone 3). Area around the portal tract is best oxygenated (Zone 1)

- Hypoxic injury affects the area around the central vein–centrilobular necrosis.
- Alternate areas of centrilobular necrosis and viable liver resembles a nutmeg on gross called 'nutmeg liver.

CPC–Spleen

- In congestive splenomegaly the spleen becomes fibrotic due to repeated infarcts accumulates hemosiderin, microscopically seen are 'Gamna-Gandy nodules' or Siderofibrotic nodule.

Thrombosis Introduction

- Thrombosis is a pathological process characterized by intravascular clotting in a living person
- Three factors influence thrombus formation (VIRCHOW'S TRIAD).
  - Endothelial (vessel wall) injury (most important)
  - Stasis and turbulence of blood flow
  - Blood hypercoagulibility.

Thrombosis–Pathogenesis

- Damaged endothelial cells produce or release procoagulant substances (e.g., thromboplasmin, von Willebrand factor), whereas the production of anticoagulant substances (e.g., nitric oxide, thrombodulin) is reduced.
- Loss of endothelial cells exposes the underlying basement membrane or collagen in the wall of the blood vessels, allowing bindings of platelets to these structures (mediated by vWF) → formation of platelet aggregates and initiates the formation of thrombi.

Emboli

- Emboli are particulate, fluid, or gaseous material carried by the blood stream from the site of their origin to other parts of the body. For example fat emboli, tumor emboli, etc.

Emboli–Pulmonary Emboli

- Pulmonary embolism is most often caused by venous thromboemboli originating in the veins of the lower extremities
- May present in several forms:
  - Occlusion of the main pulmonary artery or its main branches → sudden death.
    - Saddle embolus.
  - Occlusion of the branches of the pulmonary artery will cause infraction of the lung parenchyma
  - Nonocclusive emboli in branches of the pulmonary artery do not produce ischemia and may be clinically unrecognized. Overtime, these thrombi become organized → narrows the lumen of pulmonary artery branches → pulmonary hypertension.

Infarction

- **Definitions:**
  - Infarct: Area if ischemic necrosis.
  - Infarction: The process that leads to ischemic infract.
  - Causes: Infarction results from sudden reduction of blood supply to an area. Infarcts can be classified pathologically as:
  - Arterial–caused by obstruction of an artery.
  - Venous–caused by obstruction of venous outflow.
  - Hypotensive–caused by hypoperfusion of tissues by arterial blood that typically occurs in shock and is related to hypotension.

- Types of infarct

Red infarct (Hemorrhagic infarct)	Pale infarct (White infarct)
• Seen in venous occlusion	• Seen in arterial occlusion
• Area of infarct–Dual blood supply	• Area of infarct–Single blood supply
• Brain, Gut, Liver, Ovary, Testis	• Heart, Kidney, Spleen

General Sequence of Tissue Change Infarction:

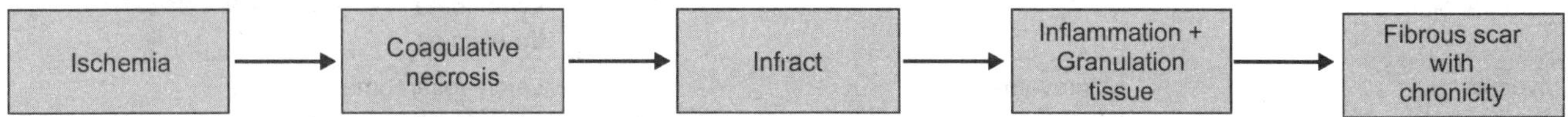

Shock

- Definitions: Shock is a condition caused by hypoperfusion of tissue with blood.
- It may be classified as:
  - Cardiogeneic, due to heart failure (myocardial pump failure)
  - Hypovolemic, due to fluid, blood or plasma loss
  - Distributive (hypotensive) due to peripheral vasodilatation
  - Common to all types of shock is a circulatory collapse and tissue hypoxia or anoxia → multiple organ failure.

Type of shock	Causes	Principal mechanisms
Cardiogeneic	Myocardial infarction Ventricular rupture Arrhythmia Cardiac temponade Pulmonary embolism	Failure of myocardial pump owing to intrinsic myocardial damage. Extrinsic pressure, or obstruction to outflow
Hypovolemic	Hemorrhage Fluid loss, e.g., vomiting, diarrhea, burn, or trauma	Inadequate blood or plasma volume
Distributive (hypotensive)	Sepsis (septic shock), caused by bacterial toxins Anaphylaxis (anaphylactic shock) Neurogenic stimuli (severe pain, spinal cord or brain injury)	Loss of peripheral vascular tone and pooling of blood in peripheral circulation

NEOPLASIA

Neoplasm	Hamartoma	Choristoma
An abnormal mass of tissue, the growth of which exceeds and is uncoordinated with that of normal tissues and persists in the same excessive manner even after cessation of the stimulus which evoked the change	Disorganized but benign-appearing masses composed of cells indigenous to the particular site. For examples bronchial hamartoma	Normal rest of tissue in an abnormal site For examples pancreatic tissue in stomach

Tissue of origin	Benign	Malignant
	Composed of one parenchymal cell type	
Mesenchymal origin	Fibroma Lipoma Sarcoma Osteoma	Fibrosarcoma Liposarcoma Chondrosarcoma Osteogenic sarcoma

Contd...

Contd...

Tissue of origin	Benign	Malignant
Endothelium	Hemangioma Lymphangioma Meningioma	Angiosarcoma Lymphangiosarcoma Synovial sarcoma
		Mesothelioma Invasive meningioma
Hematopoietic cells		Lymphoma Leukemia
Myocyte	Leiomyoma Rhabdomyoma	Leiomyosarcoma Rhabdomyosarcoma
Epithelium	Adenoma Papilloma Cystadenoma Bronchial adenoma Renal tubular adenoma Liver cell adenoma Transitional cell papilloma Hydatiform mole	Squamous cell carcinoma Basal cell carcinoma Adenocarcinoma Papillary carcinoma Cystadenocarcinoma Bronchogenic carcinoma Renal cell carcinoma Hepatocellular carcinoma Transitional cell carcinoma Choriocarcinoma Seminoma Embryonal carcinoma
Melanocyte	Nevus	Malignant melanoma
Composed of more than one neoplastic cell type–Mixed tumors, derived from one germ cell layer		
Salivary gland	Pleomorphic adenoma	Malignant mixed salivary gland tumor
Renal angle		Wilms tumor
Composed of more than one neoplastic cell type, derived from more than one germ cell layer		
Totipotential cells in gonads or in embryonic rests	Mature teratoma Dermoid cyst	Immature teratoma Teratocarcinoma

Differences between Benign and Malignant Tumors

Characteristic	Benign	Malignant
Differentiation and anaplasia	Well differentiated Tissue of origin is identifiable	Lack of differentiation
Pleomorphism (Tumor cells vary in size and shape)	None	Present
Rate of growth	Progressive and slow	Erratic and Slow to rapid
Mitoses	Rare and normal	Numerous and abnormal mitotic forms seen
Local invasion	Absent	Present
Metastasis	Absent	Present
Capsule	Present	Absent
Nuclear—cytoplasmic ratio.	Normal (1:4 to 1:6)	High N:C ratio

Pathways of Spread of Cancers

Lymphatic spread	Hematogenous spread	Seeding of body cavities and surfaces
Carcinomas	Sarcomas	Occurs when a malignant neoplasm penetrates into a natural cavity like peritoneal cavity,pleural cavity and Subarachnoid space

Contd...

Contd...

Lymphatic spread	Hematogenous spread	Seeding of body cavities and surfaces
Involvement follows anatomical routes of drainage	Veins are involved more commonly as arterial walls are thicker to penetrate	Transplantation via mechanical manipulation (e.g., surgical incision, needle tracts) may occur but is relatively rare
Cancers of the inner quadrants of the breast metastasise along the nodes along the internal mammary artery	Osteogenic sarcoma RCC HCC Follicular carcinoma of the thyroid Choriocarcinoma	Mucus secreting ovarian carcinomas fill the peritoneum Forming a gelatinous neoplastic mass called–pseudomyxoma pertonei

Grading and Staging

Tumor grading	Tumor staging
• Degree of differentiation • Histologic estimate of the malignancy of a tumor • Number of mitosis. Grading • Grade 1–Well–differentiated • Grade 2–Moderately–differentiated • Grade 3–Poorly–differentiated • Grade 4–Undifferentiated	• Clinical estimate of the size andextent of tumor spread TNM staging system criteria • T: Size of the primary tumor • N: Extent of regional lymph node spread • M: Presence of metastatic disease • In general, staging is a better predictor of prognosis than tumor grade

Chemical Carcinogenesis

Carcinogenesis is a multistep process involving a sequence of initiation (mutation) followed by promotion (proliferation)

Initiators	• Direct—acting chemical carcinogens. These are mutagens that cause cancer directly by modifying DNA. • Indirect—acting chemical carcinogens (procarcinogens). These require metabolic conversion to form active carcinogens
Promoters	• Cause cellular proliferation of mutated (initiated) cells • Proliferation of a mutated cellmaylead to accumulation of additional mutations

Chemical	Tumor
Polycyclic hydrocarbons	Squamous cell carcinoma of lung, oropharynx, cervix, larynx Transitional cell carcinoma bladder Pancreatic adenocarcinoma
Arsenic	Basal cell carcinoma, CA Lung, Epidermal hyperplasia
Benzene	Acute myelogenous leukemia
Chromium, Radon, Uranium	CA Lung
Beta naphthylamine, Aniline dyes	CA Urinary bladder
Nitrosamines	CA Esophagus, CA Stomach
Azodyes, Aflatoxins, OCPs, Thorotrast, Alcohol	Hepatoblastoma
Vinyl chloride, Thorotrast, Arsenic	Angiosarcoma of liver
Immunosuppressants	Non Hodgkins Lymphoma
Alkylating agent	Acute myelogenous leukemia, CA Bladder
Saccharin	CA Bladder
Estrogens	CA Breast, CA Endometrium, CA Liver
Diethyl stilbestrol	Clear cell carcinoma vagina
Phenacetin	Transitional cell carcinoma of renal pelvis and bladder

Microbial Carcinogenesis

Microbial agent	Malignancy associated
EBV	Burkitt's lymphoma, Primary CNS large B-cell lymphoma, CA Nasopharynx
HTLV–1	Adult T-cell leukemia/lymphoma
HTLV–2	Hairy cell leukemia, Chronic T-cell lymphoproliferative disorder
HTLV–3	AIDS
HPV–1, 4	Benign squamous papilloma
HPV–2, 7	Butcher's warts
HPV–6, 11	Condyloma acuminate
HPV–16, 31	CIN, Squamous cell carcinoma cervix/anal canal/penis
HPV–18	Adenocarcinoma cervix
HHV–8	Kaposi's sarcoma, Primary effusion lymphoma
HIV	Diffuse large B-cell lymphoma, Burkitt's lymphoma
HCV	Lymphoplasmacytic lymphoma
H.pylori	MALToma
Boca virus	CA Urinary bladder
Clonorchis sinensis, Opisthorchis viverni	Cholangiocarcinoma
Chronic bacterial infection	CA in draining sinuses
Gonococci, Chlamydia	CA Ovary, Cervix and Anal canal
Schistosomiasis	CA Bladder, Liver and Rectum

Radiational Carcinogenesis

Type of radiation	Tumor associated
Ionizing radiation	Leukemia, CA Thyroid and Breast
Ultraviolet radiation	Melanoma, BCC and SCC, Carcinoma in xeroderma pigmentosum

Carcinogenesis

- Carcinogenesis is a multistep process
- Development of all human cancers requires the accumulation of multiple genetic changes
  - Inherited germ line mutations
  - Acquired mutations
- A tumor is derived from a monoclonal expansion of a mutated cell
- Most important mutations involve
  - Growth promoting genes (protooncogenes)
  - Growth inhibiting tumor suppressor genes
  - The genes regulating apoptosis

Activation of growth promoting oncogenes	Inactivation of tumor suppressor genes
• Proto oncogenes are normal cellular genes involved with growth and cellular differentiation • Oncogenes are derived from proto oncogenes by either – A change in the gene sequence, resulting in a new gene product (oncoprotein) – Loss of gene regulation resulting in over expression of the normal gene product • Mechanisms of oncogene activation – Point mutations – Chromosomal translocations	• Definition-Tumor suppressor genes encode proteins that regulate and suppress cell proliferation by inhibiting progression of the cell through the cell cycle • Mechanisms of action – p53 prevents a cell with damaged DNA from entering S-phase – Rb prevents the cell from entering S-phase until the appropriate growth signals are present • Knudson's 'two hit hypothesis': both genes must be inactivated for oncogenesis

Contd...

Contd...

– Gene amplification – Insertional mutagenesis • Activated oncogenes lack regulatory control unregulated cellular proliferation	• Mode of action of inherited germ-line mutations – First hit: inherited germ-line mutation – Second hit: acquired somatic mutation • Examples of inherited germ-line mutations – Familial retinoblastoma – Li-Fraumeni syndrome

Apoptosis regulators

Antiapoptotic molecules	Proapoptotic molecules
Bcl–2 Bcl–XL Mcl–1	Bad Bim Bid Puma P53 Noxa

- Molecular pathogenesis of cancer
  - Self-sufficiency in growth signals
  - Insensitivity to growth inhibitory signals
  - Evasion of apoptosis
  - Limitless replicative potential
  - Development of sustained angiogenesis
  - Ability to invade and metastasize
  - Genomic instability.

Diagnosis of cancer

Microscopic examination of tissue	• Complete excision • Biopsy • Fine needle aspiration • Cytologic smears (Pap smear)
Immunohistochemistry	• Maybe helpful in confirming the tissue of origin of metastatic or poorly differentiated tumors • Monoclonal antibodies which are specific for a cellularcomponent . All of the serum tumor markers (listed below) – Thyroglobulin: thyroid cancers – S100:melanoma and neural tumors – Actin: smooth and skeletalmuscle – CD markers: lymphomas/leukemias
Ancillary tests	• Electron microscopy • Flow cytometry • Cytogenetics • PCR/DNA probes

IMMUNITY

Types of immunity

Innate immunity	Adaptive immunity
Present from birth	Acquired in nature
First line of defense	Second line of defense
No prior exposure to antigen	Prior exposure to antigen–present
Nonspecific	Specific
No immunological memory	Immunological memory present

Components of immunity

Innate immunity	Adaptive immunity
Epithelial barriers Phagocytes, NK cells, Dendritic cell Plasma proteins	Cell mediated immunity Humoral immunity

Types of immunity

Features	Active immunity	Passive immunity
Production	Actively by host immune system	Received passively
Induction	Infection/Immunogen	Transfer of readymade antibody
Duration	Long lasting	Short lived
Lag phase	Present	Absent
Immunological memory	Present	Absent
Booster doses	Useful	Less effective
Negative phase	Present	Absent
Immunodeficiency diseases	Not useful	Useful

Cells of immune system

Bone marrow (B-cells)	Thymus (T-cells)	Null cells	Dendritic cells
	• CD 8+ T-cell • CD 4+ T-cell	• K cell • NK cell (LGL cell)–LAK cells (IL–2) and NK/T cell (CD–3)	• Interdigitating dendritic cell • Mature dendritic cell • Follicular dendritic cell

Location of lymphocytes

Lymphoid organs	T-lymphocytes	B-lymphocytes
Lymph node	Paracortical areas	Cortical areas
Spleen	Periarteriolar sheaths	White pulp
Other peripheral organs		MALT of tonsils and Peyer's patches of GIT

Types of Lymphocytes

Features	B-cell	T-cell
Origin	Bone marrow	Bone marrow
Maturation	Bone marrow	Thymus
Peripheral smear finding	15–25%	65–85%
Ag receptors	Membrane bound Ig	T-cell receptors
CD markers	CD–19, 20, 21, 22, 23	CD–1, 2, 3, 4, 7, 8
Rosettes	EAC rosette, EBV receptors	SRBC rosette, Measles receptor
Thymus specific antigens	Absent	Present
Surface Ig	Present	Absent
Receptor for Fc fragment of Ig G	Present	Absent
Surface microvilli	Present	Absent
Blast transformation	Occurs by anti Ig; Mediated by endotoxin, S. aureus (cowan I strain) and EBV	Occurs by anti CD 3; Mediated by Phytohemagglutinin and Concavalin mediated
Tolerance	Negative selection–immature B-cells in bone marrow	Positive selection–mature T-cells in thymic cortex Negative selection–self reactive T-cells in cortex, cortico medullary junction and medulla of thymus

Classification of T-cells

Types of T-cells	Surface markers	Target cells	Functions
Helper/Inducer T-cell	CD 4+ T-cells	MHC class II	Growth of T-cells and Macrophages
Suppressor T-cell	CD 8+ T-cells	MHC class I	Down regulate immune response
Cytotoxic/Cytolytic/Killer T-cell	CD 8+ T-cells	MHC class I	Kill and lyse target cells carrying foreign antigen
Memory cell	CD 4+ T-cells and CD 8+ T-cells	MHC class I	Provide memory and anamnestic response

Types of CD 4+ Helper cells

TH 1 cell	TH 2 cell	TH 17 cell
IL–2, INF–γ ↓ • Activation of macrophage • Delayed hypersensitivity • Defense against intracellular microbes	IL–4, IL–5 ↓ • Production of Ig E • Defense against helminthic parasites	IL–17 ↓ • Recruitment of neutrophils and monocytes • Defense against fungi and extracellular bacteria

Classes of HLA molecules

Class I gene	Class II gene	Class III gene
Comprised of HLA–A, B, C, E, F, G loci	Comprised of HLA–D locus	
Codes for MHC–I molecule	Codes for MHC–II molecule	Codes for complement proteins C2 and C4, TNF–α and TNF–β, Heat shock proteins, Properidin and 21–hydroxylase enzyme
Present on all nucleated cells and platetlets	Present on B cells, Macrophages, Dendritic cell, Endothelial cells, Fibroblasts	
Detected by alloantisera	Detected by mixed lymphocyte reaction	
Present antigen to CD 8+ T-cell	Present antigen to CD 4+ T-cell	
Required for virus infected cells, cancer cells and graft rejection	Required for graft versus host response	Involved in autoimmune disorders

HLA and Disease Association

HLA class	Disease association
HLA–Class I	
B–27	Spondyloarthropathies Ankylosing spondylitis Reiter's syndrome Acute anterior uveitis Reactive arthritis Psoriatic arthritis
B–8	Graves' disease Myasthenia gravis
B–51	Behcet's disease
B–47	Congenital adrenal hyperplasia
CW–6	Psoriasis vulgaris
HLA–Class II	

Contd...

Contd...

HLA class	Disease association
DR–2	Japanese SLE Multiple sclerosis Narcolepsy Goodpasture's syndrome
DR–3	Graves' disease Myasthenia gravis Type I DM Dermatitis herpetiformis Chronic active hepatitis Sjogren's syndrome
DR–4	Type I DM Pemphigus vulgaris Rheumatoid arthritis
DR–5	Juvenile arthritis
DR–8	Type I DM
DQ–1	Pemphigus vulgaris
DQ–2, 8	Gluten sensitive enteropathy
DQ–7	Bullous pemphigoid
DQ–8	Type I DM

Hypersensitivity Reactions

Hypersensitivity reaction	Mechanism	Effects	Examples
Type I (Immediate or reaginic HSN)	• Ab-IgE (cytotropic) • Cells-IgE B cell, mast cells, basophils, eosinophil • Pivoted role- by T H2 cell • Most important vasoactive amine: Histamine • Slow reacting substance of anaphylaxis (SRS-A) = leukotrienes (LT B_4, C_4, D_4, E_4)	Systemic acute anaphylaxis	• Penicillin allergy • Bee sting • Insect bites • Anaphylactic shock
		Local anaphylaxis (Atopy)	• Urticaria • Angioedema • Hay fever • Some forms of asthma; eczema • Casoni's test • Theobald smith phenomenon • Schultz dale phenomenon • Prausnitz kustner (PK) reaction
Type II (Cytotoxic or cytolytic) HSN	• Ab: IgG or IgM • Lysis or phagocytosis by opsonization • Most commonly involves blood cells	Complement dependent	• Transfusion reactions • Erythroblastosis fetalis • AI hemolytic anemia • Pemphigus syndrome • Bullous pemphigoid • Perinicious anemia • Thrombotic phenomenon • Acute rheumatic fever
	• Ab-usually IgG sometimes IgE	Type VI HSN =	• Phagocytosis of tumor cells or parasite

Contd...

Contd...

Hypersensitivity reaction	Mechanism	Effects	Examples
	• Cell lysis without phagocytosis by monocytes, neutrophil, eosinophils and NK cells	Antibody dependent cell mediated cytotoxicity (ADCC)	
	• Antireceptor antibody • Stimulation • Inhibition	Type V HSN = Antibody mediated cellular dysfunction	• Thyrotoxicosis/grave's disease • Myasthenia gravis
Type III (Immune complex) HSN	• Ab- IgG or IgM • Ag-Ab complex activate complement→ attack neutrophil → release of lysosomal enzymes	Local immune complex disease (arthus reaction)	• PAN • Farmer's lung • Hypersensitivity pneumonitis • Arthus reaction
		Systemic immune complex (serum sickness)	• SLE • Certain forms of acute glomerulonephritis • Rheumatoid arthritis • Hyperacute graft rejection • Infective endocarditis • Henoch-Schonlein purpura • Schick test • Type 2 lepra reaction (ENL)
Type IV (Cell mediated) HSN	• Ab- No antibody • Initiated by specifically sensitized T-lymphocytes	Delayed type by CD_4 T H1 cells	• Tuberculin test • Lepromin test • Type I DM • Fairley's (Schistosomiasis) test • Frie's (LGV) test • Granulomatous inflammation • Contact dermatitis • Defence against intracellular pathogen • Type I lepra reaction
		Cell mediated cytotoxicity by CD-8 T-cells	• Graft rejection • Resistance to virus infection • Tumor immunity

Transplant Rejection

Types of rejection	Pathways	Antigen presenting cells	Effects
T-cell mediated rejection	Direct pathway (Acute graft rejection)	CD 4 and CD 8 T-cells of host	Graft tissue damage by perforin granzyme and Fas–Fas ligand pathways
	Indirect pathway (Chronic graft rejection)	CD 4 T-cells	
Antibody mediated rejection (B-cell)	Hyperacute rejection		Preformed antidonor antibodies
	Acute rejection		Inflammation, Complement mediated cytotoxicity, ADCC

Hypersensitivity of Rejection Reaction

Rejection reaction	Type of hypersensitivity reaction	Target site in transplantation
Hyperacute	Type II–Cytotoxic Type III–Immune complex	Small blood vessels in donor tissues
Acute	Type II–Cytotoxic	Parenchymal cells

Contd...

Contd...

Rejection reaction	Type of hypersensitivity reaction	Target site in transplantation
	Type III–Immune complex	Small blood vessels
Chronic	Type III–Immune complex Type IV–Cell mediated	Small blood vessels

Acquired immuno deficiency syndrome

Strains of HIV

HIV–1	Macrophage–tropic (R5 virus) strain	CCR5 receptor	Infects monocytes/macrophages and T-cells
HIV–2	T-cell–tropic (X4 virus) strain	CXCR4 receptor	Infects activated T-cell lines

Major Antigens of HIV

HIV antigens	Subtypes
Envelope antigens	Spike antigen–gp 120 Transmembrane pedicle protein–gp 41
Shell antigen	Nucleocapsid protein–p 18
Core antigen	p 24, p 15, p 55
Polymerase antigen	p 31, p 51, p 66

Stages of HIV Infection

Stages of HIV infection	Inference
Acute HIV infection	Asymptomatic
Seroconversion	Transient illness–fever, malaise, myalgia, arthralgia, pharyngitis, maculopapular rash
Persistent generalized lymphadenopathy	Nodes > 1 cm diameter at 2 extra inguinal sites, persisting for 3 months or longer
AIDS–related complex	Prodromal AIDS symptoms (fever, night sweats, diarrhea, weight loss) and MINOR opportunistic infections
Acquired immune deficiency syndrome	HIV infected individual with CD 4+ T cell count < 200/mL

Laboratory Diagnosis of AIDS

Test	Significance
HIV ELISA	Screening test for HIV infection Sensitivity >99.9%
Western blot	Confirmatory test for HIV infection Specificity >99.99%
CBC	Anemia, neutropenia, thrombocytopenia
Absolute CD4 lymphocyte count	Widely used predictor of HIV progression. Risk of progression to an AIDS, opportunistic infection or malignancy is high with CD4<200 cells/micro litre
CD4 lymphocyte percentage	Risk of progression to an AIDS, opportunistic infection or malignancy is high with <14%
HIV viral load test	Measure the amount of replicating virus
β_2 microglobulin	Cell surface protein indicative of macrophage–monocyte stimulation . Levels >3.5 mg/dl
p 24 antigen	Indicates active HIV replication captured during window period
HIV RNA by PCR	PCR amplification of cDNA generated from viral RNA
HIV RNA by bDNA	Measurement of levels of particles associated HIV RNA in a nuclei acid capture assay employing signal amplification
HIV RNA by NASBA	Isothermic nuclei acid amplification with internal controls

Opportunistic infection in relation with CD 4+ cells

CD 4+ cells < 50	CD 4+ cells–50 to 200	CD 4+ cells–200 to 500
Disseminated MAC Histoplasmosis CMV retinitis CNS lymphoma	Pneumocystis carinii Toxoplasmosis Crytococcosis Cryptosporidiosis Coccidioidomycosis	Tuberculosis Herpes simplex Herpes zoster Vaginal candidiasis Hairy leukoplakia Kaposi's sarcoma

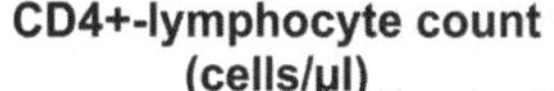

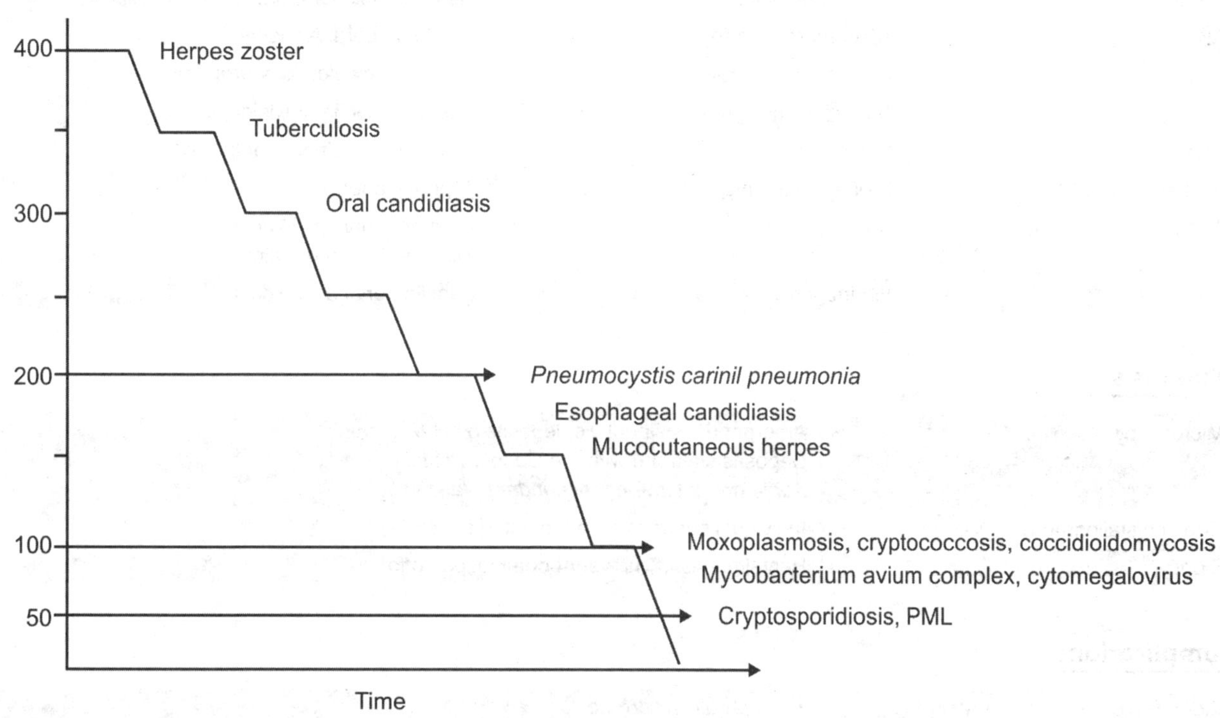

Fig. 6.1: Association between opportunistic infections and CD4^{+} -Lymphocyte Count

Opportunistic Bacterial Infection in AIDS Individuals

M.tuberculosis	Atypical mycobacterial infections	Salmonellosis
Nocardiosis	Campylobacter	Legionellosis

Opportunistic Viral Infection in AIDS Individuals

Cytomegalo virus	Herpes simplex virus	Varicella zoster virus	Japanese encephalitis

Opportunistic Parasitic Infection in AIDS Individuals

Toxoplasma gondii	E.histolytica	Cyclospora cayetanensis
Cryptosporidium parvum	Giardia lamblia	Leishmania
Isospora belli	Naegleria fowleri	Strongyloides stercoralis
Microsporidium	Acanthamoeba culbertsoni	

Opportunistic Fungal Infection in AIDS Individuals

Candida albicans	Mucor	Aspergillosis	Cryptococcosis
Histoplasma capsulatum	Coccidioides immitis	Blastomyces dermatidis	

Amyloidosis

Amyloid protein	Precursor	Disease
AL	Ig light chain	Multiple myeloma
AA	SAA	Secondary or reactive amyloidosis
$A\beta_2$ m	β_2 microglobulin	Hemodialysis associated amyloidosis
Aβ	Aβ precursor protein	Senile cerebral Alzheimer's
ATTR	Mutant Transthyretin	Familial amyloidotic neuropathy
	Normal Transthyretin	Systemic senile amyloidosis
ACal	Calcitonin	Medullary carcinoma of thyroid
AIAPP	Islet amyloid polypeptide	Type II diabetes
AANF	ANP	Isolated atrial amyloidosis Misfolded prion protein
Aα	Fibrinogen	Familial renal amyloidosis

Diagnosis

Microscopy	Amorphous eosinophilic deposits on H & E stain Deposits stain red with the *Congored stain* *Apple green birefringenceunder polarized light*
X-ray crystallography	Individual subunits form β pleated sheets
Biopsy	Rectalmucosa,Gingiva, Abdominal pad offat

Complications

Kidney	• Nephroticsyndrome • Progressive renal failure
Heart	• Restrictive cardiomyopathy • Low voltage EKG • Cardiac arrhythmias and CHF
Liver and Spleen	• Hepatosplenomegaly
GI tract	• Tongue enlargement • Malabsorption

GENETICS

Genetic disorders are broadly classified as

- Monogenic disorders or single gene disorder or Mendelian disorder
- Multifactorial disorders (previously called polygenic disorders)

Mendelian disorders

Definition: Mendelian disorders are characterized by single gene mutations.

Mutation

A. Point mutation

Silent mutation	Hemoglobin	6th position of β chain
	Hb Milwaukee	Glutamate
	Hb Bristol	Aspartate
	Hb Sydney	Alanine
Missense mutation	Acceptable mutation	Hb–hikari (β chain)
	Partially acceptable mutation	Hb–S (β chain)
	Unacceptable mutation	Hb–M Boston (α chain)
Nonsense mutation	Coding codon → Stop codon	β-thalassemia
	Stop codon → Coding codon	α-thalassemia

B. Frame shift mutation
- Cystic fibrosis–Deletion of phenylalanine at 508th position in CFTR gene

C. Trinucleotide repeat sequence

Coding region	Noncoding region
Huntington's chorea	Myotonic dystrophy Fragile X-syndrome

D. Splice site mutation–Myotonic dystrophy, β-thalassemia

IMPORTANT PRINCIPLES THAT CAN CHARACTERIZE SINGLE-GENE DISEASES

Mechanism	Description	Example
Variable expression	Most genetic diseases vary in the degree of phenotypic expression: some individuals may be severely affected, whereas others are more mildly affected	Neurofibromatosis
Incomplete penetrance	A disease-causing mutation is said to have incomplete penetrance when some individuals who have the disease genotype do not display the disease phenotype	Hereditary hemochromatosis
Delayed age of onset	Many individuals who carry a disease-causing mutation do not manifest the phenotype untillater in life. This can complicate the interpretation of a pedigree	Huntington's disease
Pleiotrophy	Pleiotropy exists when a single disease-causing mutation affects multiple organ systems.	Marfan syndrome
Locus heterogeneity	Locus heterogeneity exists when the same disease phenotype can be caused by mutations in different loci	Osteogenesis imperfecta

General Characteristics of Autosomal Dominant and Recessive Diseases

Features	Autosomal Recessive	Autosomal Dominant
Onset	Early uniform onset (infancy/childhood)	Variable onset (may be delayed into adulthood)
Penetrance	Complete penetrance	Incomplete penetrance with variable expression
Mutation	Usually an enzyme protein	Usually a structural protein orreceptor
Requires	Mutation of both alleles	Mutation of one allele

Autosomal Recessive Disorders

System	Disorder
Nervous	Neurogenic muscular atrophies Friedreich ataxia Spinal muscular atrophy
Metabolic	Cystic fibrosis Phenylketonuria Galactosemia Homocystinuria Lysosomal storage disorder α_1-Antitrypsin deficiency Wilson disease Hemochromatosis Glycogen storage diseases
Hematopoietic	Sickle cell anemia Thalassemias
Endocrine	Congenital adrenal hyperplasia
Skeletal	Ehlers Danlos syndrome (some variants) Alkaptonuria

Autosomal Dominant disorders

System	Disorder
Nervous	Huntington disease Neurofibromatosis Myotonic dystrophy Tuberous sclerosis
Urinary	Polycystic kidney disease
Gastrointestinal	Familial polyposis coli
Hematopoietic	Hereditary spherocytosis von Willebrand disease
Skeletal	Marfan syndrome Ehlers Danlos syndrome (some variants) Osteogenesis imperfecta Achondroplasia
Metabolic	Familial hypercholesterolemia Acute intermittent porphyria

X-Linked Recessive disorders

System	Disease
Musculoskeletal	Duchenne muscular dystrophy Menkes disease Pelizaeus–Merzbacher disease
Hematopoietic	Hemophilia A and B Chronic granulomatous disease G6PD deficiency
Immune	Agammaglobulinemia Wiskott-Aldrich syndrome
Metabolic	Diabetes insipidus Lesch-Nyhan syndrome
Nervous	Fragile X syndrome

X-Linked Autosomal disorders

- Vitamin D resistant rickets.
- Incontinentia pigmenti.
- Oro facial digital syndrome

MitochondrialInheritance

- Males and females affected
- Only females transmit the disease
  - For example Leber Hereditary Optic Neuropathy.

Two Important Concepts of Single Gene Disorders

Anticipation	Genomic imprinting
• Pattern of inheritance in which individuals in the most recent generations of a pedigree develop a disease at an earlier age or with greater severity than do those in earlier generations • Characteristic of trinucleotide repeat disorders • For example, Myotonic Dystrophy, Fragile X Syndrome	• Genetic phenomenon by which certain genes are expressed in a parent-of-origin-specific manner. • Inheritance process independent of the classical Mendelian inheritance. • For example, When the allele inherited from the father is mutated-Prader-Willi Syndrome and When the allele inherited from the mother is mutated- Angelman Syndrome

Multifactorial Disorders

Disorders arising from the combined actions of environmental influences and 2 or more mutant genes having additive effects.

Examples:

- Cleft lip and cleft palate
- Congenital heart disease
- Coronary heart disease
- Hypertension
- Gout
- Diabetes mellitus
- Pyloric stenosis

Glycogen Storage Disorders

Glycogen storage disorder		Enzyme defect
I	von Gierke's disease	Glucose 6 phosphatase
II	Pompe's disease	Acid maltase
III	Forbe's or Cori's disease	Debranching enzyme
IV	Anderson's disease	Branching enzyme
V	McArdle's disease	Muscle phosphorylase
VI	Her's disease	Liver phosphorylase
VII	Tauri's disease	Phosphofructo kinase–1
VIII		Liver phosphorylase kinase
IX		Liver and Muscle phosphorylase kinase
X		c-AMP dependent protein kinase
XI	Fanconi–Bickel	Glucose transporter–2

Mucopolysaccharidoses

Mucopolysaccharidoses	Enzyme defect
Hurler syndrome (MPS–1)	L-Iduronidase
Hunter syndrome (MPS–2)	Iduronate sulfatase

DISORDERS OF RED BLOOD CELLS AND COAGULATION

Anemia

- Decrease in the oxygen carrying capacity of blood.
- Reduction in the concentration of hemoglobin in the peripheral blood below the normal for the age and sex of the patient.

Classification of Anemia

Mechanism	Specific examples
Nutritional deficiencies	
Deficiencies affecting DNA synthesis	B12 and folate deficiencies
Deficiencies affecting hemoglobin synthesis	Iron deficiency anemia
Erythropoietin deficiency	Renal failure, anemia of chronic disease
Immune-mediated injury of progenitors	Aplastic anemia, pure red cell aplasia
Inflammation-mediated iron sequestration	Anemia of chronic disease
Primary hematopoietic neoplasms	Acute leukemia, myelodysplasia, myeloproliferative disorders
Space-occupying marrow lesions	Metastatic neoplasms, granulomatous disease
Infections of red cell progenitors	Parvovirus B19 infection
Unknown mechanisms	Endocrine disorders, hepatocellular liver disease
Decreased Red Cell Production	
Inherited genetic defects	
Defects leading to stem cell depletion	Fanconi anemia, telomerase defects
Defects affecting erythroblast maturation	Thalassemia syndromes

Blood loss

Acute blood loss	Trauma
Chronic blood loss	Gastrointestinal tract lesions, gynecologic disturbances

Increased red cell destruction (hemolysis)

Inherited genetic defects	
Red cell membrane disorders	Hereditary spherocytosis, hereditary elliptocytosis
Enzyme deficiencies	
Hexose monophosphate shunt enzyme deficiencies	G6PD deficiency, glutathione synthetase deficiency
Glycolytic enzyme deficiencies	Pyruvate kinase deficiency, hexokinase deficiency
Hemoglobin abnormalities	
Deficient globin synthesis	Thalassemia syndromes
Structurally abnormal globins (hemoglobinopathies)	Sickle cell disease, unstable hemoglobins
Acquired and genetic defects	
Deficiency of phosphatidylinositol-linked glycoproteins	Paroxysmal nocturnal hemoglobinuria
Antibody-mediated destruction	Hemolytic disease of the newborn (Rh disease), transfusion reactions, drug-induced, autoimmune disord
Mechanical trauma	

Microangiopathic hemolytic anemias	Hemolytic uremic syndrome, disseminated intravascular coagulation, thrombotic thrombocytopenia purpura
Cardiac traumatic hemolysis	Defective cardiac valves
Repetitive physical trauma	Bongo drumming, marathon running, karate chopping
Infections of red cells	Malaria, babesiosis
Toxic or chemical injury	Clostridial sepsis, snake venom, lead poisoning
Membrane lipid abnormalities	Abetalipoproteinemia, severe hepatocellular liver disease
Sequestration	Hypersplenism

Anemia's Due to Nutritional Deficiency

The 2 most common nutrients associated with anemia are

1. Iron deficiency–Microcytic hypochromic anemia.
2. B12 deficiency or folate deficiency–Marocytic anemia → with increasing severity Megaloblastic anemia.

Iron Deficiency Anemia

Normal forms of iron (Fe) and iron metabolism

- Functional iron is found in hemoglobin, myoglobin, and enzymes (catalase and cytochromes)
- Ferritin is the physiological storage form (plasma **ferritin:** total body Fe)
- Hemosiderin: degraded ferritin + lysosomal debris (Prussian blue positive)
- Iron is transported by transferrin
  - Transferrin levels: Total iron-binding capacity (TIBC) (normal = 300 mg/dl)
  - Normal % saturation = 1/3 saturation (as normal serum iron is 100 mg/dl)
- Sequence of events during iron deficiency

Decreased storage iron	Decreased serum ferritin Decreased BM iron (detected by Prussian blue stain)
Decreased circulating iron	↓ serum iron ↑ TIBC ↓ % saturation
Formation of microcytic/hypochromic anemia	Decreased MCV

Macrocytic Anemias

- **Megaloblastic anemias:**
  - Basic cause is impaired DNA synthesis (delayed mitoses) while **RNA is not impaired**
  - This produces a **nuclear-cytoplasmic asynchrony** that affects all rapidly proliferating cell lines, including cells of bone marrow, GI tract, etc.
  - Smear findings

RBCs	WBCs	Platelets
Macro-ovalocytes Autohemolysis in BM	Giant metamyelocytes in bone marrow. Hypersegmented neutrophils (>5 lobes)	No changes

- **Megaloblastic anemia due to vitamin B12 deficiency**
- Causes of B12 deficiency
  - Dietary deficiency (takes years to develop)
  - Decreased absorption, which may be caused by any of the following:
    - Decreased IF associated with gastrectomy or pernicious anemia
    - Pancreatic insufficiency (pancreatic proteases normally breakdown B12-R complexes in duodenum)
    - Intestinal malabsorption due to parasites (fish tapeworm, a.k.a. Diphyllobothrium latum), bacteria (blind-loop syndrome), or Crohn disease of ileum

- Lab tests
  - Low serum B12 level and increased serum homocysteine
  - Increased methylmalonic acid in urine
  - Schilling test
    - Pernicious anemia: abnormal with correction by IF
- **Megaloblastic anemia due to folate deficiency:**
- Causes include
  - Dietary deficiency (takes only month to develop)
  - Seen in chronic alcoholics and elderly.
  - Decreased absorption
  - Increased requirement for folate
    - Pregnancy
    - Infancy
- Decreased utilization: folate antagonists used in chemotherapy
  - Lab tests
    - Low serum folate levels and increased serum homocysteine

Note: Neurologic symptoms do not occur with folate deficiency.

RBC indices in different disorders

Anemia	MCV	MCH	MCHC
Macrocytic	↑	↑	Normal
Microcytic	↓	Normal	Normal
Microcytic hypochromic	↓	↓	↓
Normocytic normochromic	Normal	Normal	Normal

Anemia of Chronic Disease (AOCD)

- Characterized by iron being trapped in bone marrow macrophages
- Lab findings: increased serum ferritin with decreased TIBC
- Chronic inflammatory disorders may be associated with **increased IL-1**, which causes increased lactoferrin, which, in turn, traps iron in bone marrow macrophages.

Comparison of anemias

Parameters	Iron deficiency anemia	Anemia of chronic disease	Thalassemia minor	Sideroblastic anemia
Serum. Iron	↓	↓	Normal	↑
TIBC	↑	↓	Normal	↓
% saturation	↓	↓	Normal	↑
Serum. Ferritin	↓	↑	Normal	↑

APLASTIC ANEMIA

Causes of Aplastic Anemia

Acquired	Constitutional
• Idiopathic • Drugs and Chemicals • Ionising radiation • Infections: Viral hepatitis, CMV, Parvovirus B19 EBV • PNH, GVHD, Pregnancy	• Fanconi anemia • Dyskeratosis congenita • Schwachman Diamond syndrome

Hemolytic Anemia

- Hemolytic anemia is due to hemolysis, i.e. the abnormal breakdown of red blood cells
- Hemolytic anemia has the following features
  - A shortened red cell life span, i.e. premature destruction of red cells
  - **Elevated erythropoietin level** and increased erythropoiesis in the marrow and other sites
  - **Increased** reticulocyte count
  - Accumulation of the **products of hemoglobin** catabolism.

Difference between Extravascular and Intravascular Hemolysis

Extravascualr hemolysis	Intravascular hemolysis
• Hereditary spherocytosis • Thalassemia • Sickle cell anemia • Autoimmune hemolytic anemia • Drug induced immune hemolytic anemia • G-6-PD deficiency	• Paroxysmal nocturnal hemoglobinuria • G-6-PDdeficiency • Clostridial toxin • Falciparum malaria • Mechanical injury to red cells – Defective cardiac valves – Thrombin in microcirculation • Sickle cell anemia (minor)

Parameters	Extravascular hemolysis	Intravascular hemolysis
Site	RE cell organs- spleen, BM	In circulating blood
S. Methalbumin	Negative	Positive
Plasma hemoglobin	Negative	Positive
S. Ferritin	Normal or ↑	↓
S. bilirubin (unconjugated)	↑↑	↑
S. LDH	↑	↑↑
Urine hemoglobin	Negative	Positive
Urine Hemosiderin	Negative	Positive
Tissue iron in spleen, liver	↑	↓

Hereditary Spherocytosis

Definition: Autosomal dominant disorder that is due to a defect involving spectrin (Most commonly) in RBC membrane, which causes a decrease in the RBC surface membrane (spherocytosis).

Structural defect in Hereditary Spherocytosis

Membrane cytoskeleton that lies closely opposed to the internal surface of the plasma membrane is responsible for elasticity and maintenance of RBC shape.

Membrane skeleton consists:

- Spectrin-The chief protein component.
- Ankyrin and band 4.2 (paladin)-Binds spectrin to band 3
- Band 3-A transmembrane ion transport protein.
- Band 4.1-Binds spectrin to glycophorin A, a transmembrane protein.
  - Ankyrin → Most common
  - Band 3 → second most common
- Spherocytes are not flexible and are removed in spleen by macrophages (i.e., extravascular hemolysis), which causes
  - Splenomegaly with a mild to moderate hemolytic anemia
  - Chronic hemolysis produces increased bilirubin and an increased risk for jaundice and pigment gallstones

- Increased risk for acute red-cell aplasia due to parvovirus B19 infection
- Lab tests
  - **Osmotic fragility test**
  - Normal MCH with increased MCHC
- Splenectomy–corrects the condition.

Glucose-6-Phosphate dehydrogenase (G6PD) deficiency:

- Pathogenesis:
  - Deficiency of glucose-6-phosphate dehydrogenase (G6PD) results in decreased levels of the antioxidant glutathione (GSH)
  - RBCs are sensitive to injury by oxidant stresses leading to hemolysis
- G6PD is the rate-limiting enzyme in the hexose mono phosphate shunt
  - G6PD normally produces NADPH, which keeps glutathione reduced
  - Glutathione protects by breaking down hydrogen peroxide.
- **X-linked inheritance**
  - Hemolysis is secondary to acute oxidative stress, such as oxidative drugs (primaquine, sulfonamides, anti-TB drugs), and more typically by viral or bacterial infections
- Oxidation of hemoglobin forms Heinz bodies
  - Heinz bodies cannot be seen with normal peripheral blood stains (Wright-Giemsa)
  - Need supravital stains (methylene blue and crystal violet) to see Heinz bodies
  - Heinz bodies are 'eaten' by splenic macrophages (extravascular hemolysis), which may form bite cells.

Sickle Cell Anemia

Genetics: Abnormality: single nucleotide change in codon causes valine (neutral) to replace normal glutamic acid (acidic) at the 6th position of the β-globin chain.

- Heterozygous (AS): trait
  - About 8% of African Americans are heterozygous for hemoglobin S. Patients with sickle trait have fewer symptoms than those with sickle disease
  - Have resistance to Plasmodium falciparum infection (malaria)
- Homozygous (SS): disease (sickle cell anemia)

Factors affecting formation of irreversibly sickled red blood cells

- Increased concentration (dehydration) makes symptoms worse; decreased concentration (with thalassemia) makes symptoms better
- Decreased pH decreases oxygen affinity and makes symptoms worse
- Increased hemoglobin F makes symptoms better (rationale for therapy with hydroxyurea, which increased blood hemoglobin F levels)
- Presence of hemoglobin C (SC: Double-heterozygote individual) makes symptoms better

Increased RBC destruction causes a severe hemolytic anemia

- Erythroid hyperplasia in the bone marrow
- Increased bilirubin leads to jaundice and gallstone (pigment) formation

Capillary thrombi result from sickle cells blocking small vessels and may cause

- Vaso-occlusive (painful) crisis
- Hand-foot syndrome (swelling) in children
- Autosplenectomy, which is seen in older children and adults
  - Howell-Jolly bodies will appear in peripheral blood after autosplenectomy
  - Results in increased incidence of infections (encapsulated organisms)
- Increased incidence of Salmonella osteomyelitis (leg pain)
- Leg ulcers.
- Risk of aplastic crisis (especially with parvovirus B19 infection)
- Emergencies: Priapism and acute chest syndrome.

Pathophysiology

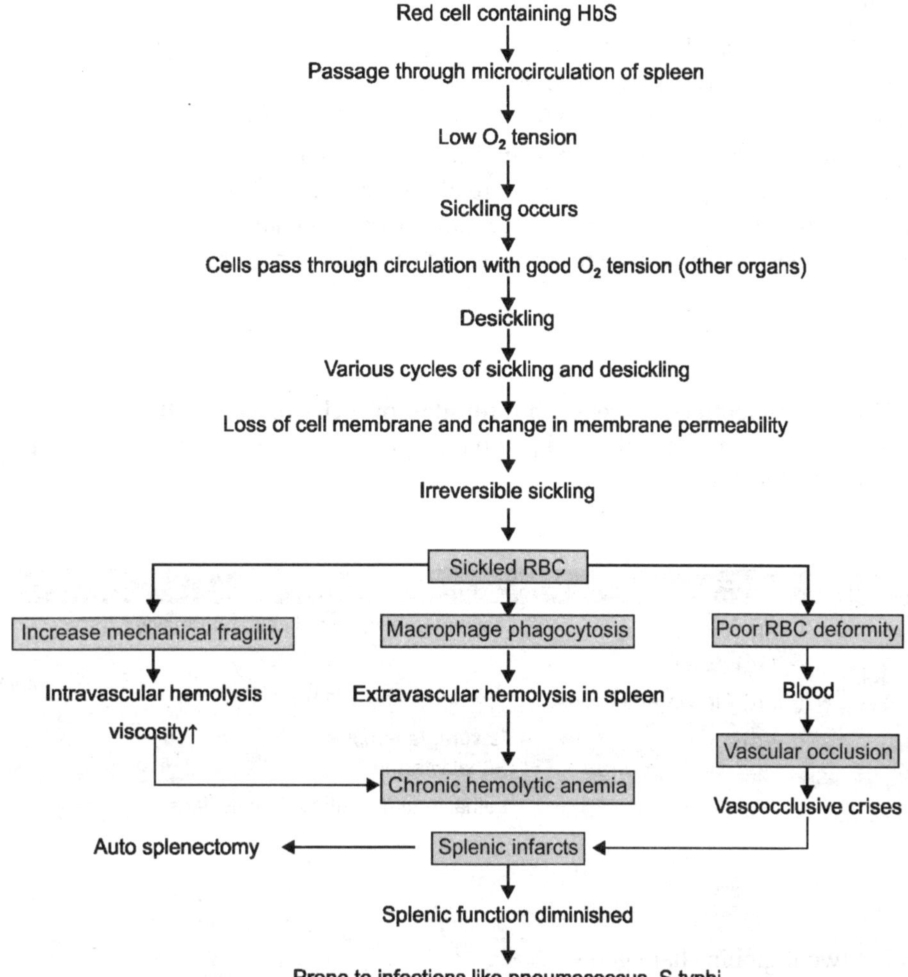

Lab Tests for Hemoglobin S

- Sickling test (metabisulfite test, which can not tell sickle cell disease from sickle cell trait)
- Hemoglobin electrophoresis
- HPLC
- Prenatal diagnosis: genetic testing (by Chorionic Villous Sampling)

Therapy includes hydroxyurea (increases hemoglobin F)

Note: Irreversible sickle cells are responsible for hemolytic anemia. Reversible sickle cells are responsible for vasoocclusive symptoms.

Hemoglobin C Disease

- Abnormality: Single nucleotide change in a codon causes lysine (basic) to replace normal glutamic acid (acidic) at the beta 6 position.
- Signs: Mild normochromic-normocytic anemia, splenomegaly, target cells, and rod-shaped crystals in RBCs (the latter being characteristic)

Thalassemia Syndromes

Normal and abnormal hemoglobins

HbA (α2 β2)–Normal Adult hemoglobin (95%).

HbA2 (α2 δ2)–Adult hemoglobin (5%). Elevated in β thalassemia trait >8%

HbF (α2 γ2)–Fetal hemoglobin (2%) consitutes > 90% of Hb in β-Thal minor.

Thalassemias are quantitative, not qualitative, abnormalities of hemoglobin

- α-Thalassemia has decreased α-globin chains with relative excess β chains
- β-Thalassemia has decreased β-globin chains with relative excess α chains.

Thalassemia provides a protective advantage to carriers, such as against malaria.

α-Thalassemia

Genetics

- There are a total of four α-globin chain genes **(but number of α chains is TWO)**
- Chains are normally expressed prenatally and postnatally; therefore, there is prenatal and postnatal disease
- α-Thalassemia is due to gene deletions

Clinical Disease States

Clinical syndromes	Genotype	Clinical features	Molecular genetics
Silent carrier	(- α/αα)	Asymptomatic; no red cell abnormality	Mainly gene deletion
α-thalassemia trait	(- -/αα)-Asians (-α/-α)-African-Americans	Asymptomatic, like β-thal minor	
Hb H disease	(- -/-α)	Severe; resembles β-thal intermedia	
Hydrops fetalis	(- -/- -)	Lethal in utero without transfusions	

β-Thalassemia

Genetics

- There are a total of two β-globin chain genes
- They are expressed postnatally only (therefore only postnatal disease and not prenatal).
- **Mechanism:** Mainly due to point mutations, which form either some β-chains (β^+) or none (β°)

Type	Peripheral smear	Bone marrow findings
Thalassemia major (Cooley anemia) (β^+/β^+ or β^0/β^0) Allelic homogenicity	Severe anemia, anisocytosis, microcytic hypochromic red cells, target cells, nucleated cells, basophilic stippling, Howel jolly bodies MCH, MCV, MCHC reduced HbF increased	Hypercellular with erythroid hyperplasia, reversal of normal M:E ratio, pink inclusions in normoblast
Thalassemia intermedia	Anemia	Hypercellular
Thalassemia minor or trait (β°/β or β°/β) Allelic heterogenicity	Microcytic hypochromic cells with basophilic stippling target cells MCH, MCV, MCHC reduced HbF mildly increased HbA2 drastically increased	Hypercellular with erythroid hyperplasia

NESTROF test–Naked Eye Single Test Red cell Osmotic Fragility–screening test

Qualitative estimation of HbH–Apt test

Quantitative estimation of HbH–Kleihauer test

Autoimmune Hemolytic Anemia (AIHA)

Features	Warm antibody type	Cold antibody type
Immunoglobulin	Ig G > Ig A	Ig M
Causes	Idiopathic SLE, RA B-cell neoplasm Methyldopa, Penicillin	Idiopathic Mycoplasma, IM Lymphoid neoplasm Paroxysmal cold hemoglobinuria
Mechanism	Extravascular hemolysis	Extravascular hemolysis in cold agglutinin Intravascular hemolysis in cold hemolysin
Complement activity	Ab not fix the complement but active at 37 °C	Ab react at 4–6 °C, dissociate at 30 °C or above

Paroxysmal Nocturnal Hemoglobinuria (PNH)

- **Abnormality:** Decreased glycosyl phosphatidyl inositol (GPI)-linked proteins, deficient in three GPI-linked proteins that regulate complement activity.
  - Membrane inhibitor of reactive lysis (MIRL), or **CD59** [Q]; **(MOST IMPORTANT)**
  - C8 binding protein
  - Decay–accelerating factor (DAF), or CD55;
    - The function of DAF is to inhibit the activation of the complement cascade by breaking down C3 convertase
    - Deficiency of DAF results in increased complement activity
    - All cells in blood have increased sensitivity to the lytic actions of complement
- Symptoms are episodes (paroxysms) of hemolysis at night.
- Acidosis in vivo, which occurs during sleep (breathing slowly retains CO_2) and exercise (lactic acidosis), causes activation of complement
- PNH is a clonal **stem cell disorder** that therefore affects all cell lines
- Pancytopenia in peripheral blood: Anemia, leukopenia, thrombocytopenia
- **Complications:** increased risk for aplastic anemia, leukemia, and venous thrombosis
- Lab tests for PNH
  - Sucrose in vitro (sucrose lysis test)
  - Acidosis in vitro (Ham's test)
  - Flow cytometry

Inclusions to be Included In Your Mind

- **Basophilic stippling** results from cytoplasmic remnants of RNA indicate reticulocytosis seen in lead poisoning and megaloblastic anemia.
- **Howell-Jolly bodies** are remnants of nuclear chromatin-severe anemias or patients after splenectomy.
- **Pappenheimer bodies** are composed of iron found in the peripheral blood following splenectomy.
- **Ring sideroblasts** have iron trapped abnormally in mitochondria, forming a ring around nucleus in sideroblastic anemia.
- **Heinz bodies** result from denatured hemoglobin seen with G6PD deficiency.

Hemostasis and Bleeding Disorders

- **Hemostasis:**
  - Sequence of events leading to the cessation of bleeding by the formation of a stable fibrin-platelet homeostatic plug
  - Homeostasis involves interactions between the vascular wall, platelets, and the coagulation system

PRIMARY HEMOSTASIS

- Endothelial cell injury exposes the extracellular matrix.
- Platelets adhere to the vWF
- Platelet activation leading to shape change, contraction and secretion.
- Platelet aggregation

Platelet Adhesion

- Subendothelial collagen exposed
- Activation of platelet membrane receptor, glycoprotein Ib/IX
- Adhesion is mediated by vWF protein

Platelet Granules

α granules	δ granules
• P selectin • Fibrinogen • Fibronectin • Factor V and VIII • Platelet factor 4 • PDGF • TGF–β	• ADP • ATP • Ionized calcium • Histamine • Serotonin • Epinephrine

Congenital Abnormalities of Platelet Function

Functional Platelet Disorders

Inherited	Acquired
Disorders of adhesion	
Bernard Soullier syndrome von Willebrand disease	Uremia Acquired vWF
Disorders of aggregation	
Glanzmann thrombasthenia Afibrinogenemia	FDP inhibition Dysproteinemia Drugs–Ticlopidine, Gp IIb/IIIa inhibitors
Disorders of granule release	
Oculocutaneous albinism Chediak Higashi syndrome Grey platelet syndrome	Cardiopulmonary bypass Myeloproliferative disorders NSAIDs

Glanzmann thrombasthenia (GT): Platelet aggregation refers to platelets binding to other platelets.

- Patients with GT have a deficiency of GpIIb-IIIa and defective platelet
- Aggregation. Abnormality of platelet aggregation (aggregation defects or primary wave defects) is Glanzmann thrombasthenia (GT)
- These patients have a normal prothrombin time (PT) and
- Normal partial thromboplastin time (PTT).

Bernard-Soulier syndrome (BSS): Bernard–Soulier–second M.C inherited bleeding disorder.

- Platelet adhesion refers to platelets binding to subendothelial collagen via von Willebrand's factor.
- (vWF) serves as a molecular bridge between the receptor Gp Ib/IX or CD 42 on
- platelets to collagen.
- A deficiency of Gp Ib/IX or CD 42 is seen in Bernard-Soulier syndrome, which has clinical signs similar to von Willebrand's disease.

SECONDARY HEMOSTASIS

Fibrin Clot Formation

- Activation of coagulation cascade
- Generation of thrombin
- Formation of a fibrin clot

Coagulation

- Contact activation-Intrinsic system
- Tissue factor activation–Extrinsic
- Common path- amplification
- Fibrin formation
- Fibrin lysis.

Coagulation Cascade

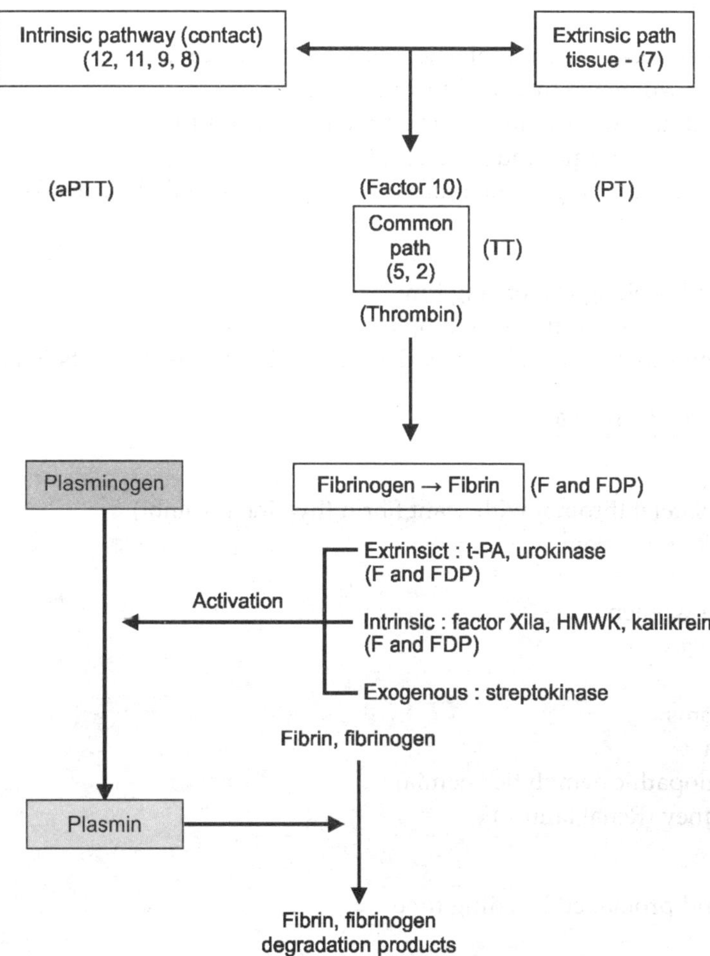

Common Platelet Disorders

Thrombocytopenia	Qualitative defect
• Decreased production • Aplastic anemia • Tumor	• von Willebrand disease • Bernard-Soulier Synd Autosomal recessive Deficiency of platelet GpIb/IX Defective platelet adhesion

Contd...

Contd...

Thrombocytopenia	Qualitative defect
• Increased destruction • ITP • TTP • DIC • Hypersplenism	• Glanzmann Thrombasthenia Autosomal recessive Deficiency of Gp IIb-IIIa Defective platelet aggregation

Immune Thrombocytopenic Purpura

Etiology

- *Antiplatelet antibodies against platelet antigens such as Gp IIb-IIIa and Gp Ib-IX*
- Platelets are destroyed peripherally in the spleen by macrophages, which have Fc receptors that bind IgG-coated platelets.

Forms of ITP

- Acute ITP: Seen in children following a viral infection. Self-limited disorder
- Chronic ITP: Usually seen in women in their childbearing years
  - May be the first manifestation of systemic lupus erythematosus (SLE)
  - Petechiae, ecchymoses, menorrhagia, and nose bleeds.
  - Splenomegaly is not present and if present alternative diagnosis should be considered.

Lab Diagnosis

- Decreased platelet count and prolonged bleeding time.
- Normal prothrombin time (PT) and partial thromboplastin time (PTT).
- Peripheral blood smear shows thrombocytopenia with enlarged immature platelets (megathrombocytes)

Thrombotic Thrombocytopenic Purpura

Pathology

- Widespread formation of platelet thrombi with scant fibrin (hyaline thrombi)
- No activation of the coagulation system
- Clinical findings
  - Most often affects adult women.
  - *Pentad of characteristic signs.*
    - Pyrexia
    - Neurologic symptoms
    - Thrombocytopenia
    - Anemia (Microangiopathic hemolytic anemia)
    - Dysfunction of Kidney (Renal failure)

Lab Diagnosis

- Decreased platelet count and prolonged bleeding time
- Normal PT and PTT
- Peripheral blood smear shows thrombocytopenia and schistocytes, and reticulocytosis

Hemolytic Uremic Syndrome (HUS)

- Occurs most commonly in children
- Follows a gastroenteritis with bloody diarrhea
- Organism: Verotoxin-producing *E. coli O157:H7*
- Similar clinical pentad

Coagulation

- Coagulation factors
  - The majority of the clotting factors are produced by the liver
  - Are proenzymes that must be converted to the active form
  - Some conversions occur on a phospholipid surface
  - Some conversions require calcium
- Intrinsic coagulation pathway is activated by the contact factors
  - Contact with subendothelial collagen
  - High molecular weight kininogen (HMWK)
  - Kallikrein
- Extrinsic coagulation pathway is activated by the release *of tissue factor*
- Laboratory tests for coagulation
  - *Prothrombin time (PT)*
    - *Tests the extrinsic and common coagulation pathways* VII, X, *V, prothrombin, fibrinogen*
  - *Partial thromboplastin time (PTT)*
    - *Tests the intrinsic and common coagulation pathways. XII, XI, IX,VIII, X, V, prothrombin, fibrinogen*
  - *Thrombin time (TT) tests for adequate fibrinogen levels*
  - *Fibrin degradationproducts (FDP) tests the fibrinolytic system (increased with DIC)*

Hemophilia A (classic hemophilia)

- Deficiency *of factor VIII*
- X-linked recessive
- Clinical features
  - Predominately affects males
  - Symptoms are variable dependent *on the degree of deficiency*
  - Spontaneous hemorrhages into joints (hemarthrosis)
  - Easy bruising and hematoma formation after minor trauma
  - Severe prolonged bleeding after surgery or lacerations
  - No petechiae *or ecchymoses*
- Lab findings
  - Normal platelet count and bleeding time
  - Normal PT and *prolonged PTT*

Hemophilia B (Christmas Disease)

- Deficiency of *factor IX*
- X-linked recessive
- Clinically identical to hemophilia A

Acquired Coagulopathies

- Vitamin K deficiency: Decreased synthesis *of factors II,VII, IX,X, and protein C and S*
- Liver disease: Decreased synthesis *of virtually all clotting factors*

von Willebrand Disease

- **Definition:** Inherited bleeding disorder characterized by either a deficiency *or* qualitative defect in von Willebrand factor. Three types;
  - Type 1–AD, reduced quantity of circulating vWF
  - Type 2–AD,qualitative defects in vWF
  - Type 3–AR, quantitative deficiency.
- vWF is normally produced by endothelial cells and megakaryocytes

- Clinical features
  - Spontaneous bleeding from mucous membranes
  - Prolonged bleeding from wounds
  - Menorrhagia in young females
  - Bleeding into joints is uncommon
- Lab findings:
  - Normal platelet count and a prolonged bleeding time
  - Normal PT with often a prolonged PTT
  - Abnormal platelet response to ristocetin (adhesion defect) is an important diagnostic test
  - Treatment: Treat mild cases (type I) with desmopressin (an antidiuretic hormone [ADH] analog), which releases vWF from Weibel Palade bodies of endothelial cells

Disseminated Intravascular Coagulation (DIC)

- DIC is always secondary to another disorder
- Causes
  - Obstetric complications (placental tissue factor activates clotting)
  - AML M3 (cytoplasmic granules in neoplastic promyelocytes activate clotting)
  - Adenocarcinomas (mucin activates clotting)
  - Gram negative sepsis (tumor necrosis factor [TNF] activates clotting)
  - Micro organisms (especially meningococci and rickettsiae)
- Pathology
  - Results in widespread microthrombi
  - Consumption of platelets and clotting factors causes hemorrhages
- Lab diagnosis
  - Platelet count is decreased
  - Prolonged PTIPTT
  - Decreased fibrinogen
  - Elevated fibrin split products (D-dimers)
- Treatment: Treat the underlying disorder

DISORDERS OF WHITE BLOOD CELLS

- Hemopoietic stem cells are CD34 and c-Kit positive. (c-Kit-CD 117)

Lymphopoiesis

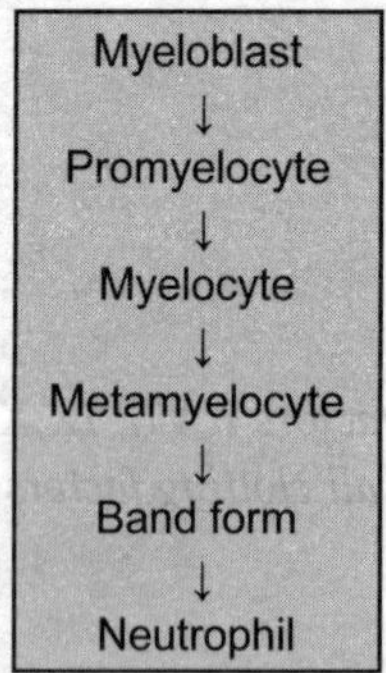

- Child under age 10 years: 10% fat to 90% cells
  Normal adult marrow, the ratio of fat to hematopoietic element is → **1:1**
- Normal Myeloid to Erythroid ratio → **3:1**

Agranulocytosis

- Significant reduction in the neutrophils → susceptible for bacterial and fungal infection

- Pathogenesis
  - Inadequate/ineffective granulopoiesis.
  - Accelerated removal of neutrophils from blood.
- **MC** cause of Agranulocytosis → **DRUG TOXICITY**
- Severe infection when the neutrophil count goes <500/ mm^3
- Some severe infections → many immature granulocytes like promyelocytes. myelocytes and metamyelocytes may appear in the blood simulates myeloid Leukemia, known as

LEUKEMOID REACTION

- Presence of immature granulocytes in PS is also termed shift to 'LEFT'
- This can pose diagnostic difficulty as leukemoid reaction can mimic CML
- In CML also there are increasedimmature granulocytes in the PS.

Differences between Leukemoid Reaction and CML

Feature	Leukemoid reaction	CML
Nature of disease	Reactive	Myeloproliferative disorder
TLC	10–50 × 10^9/L	100–500 × 10^9/L
Toxic granules in neutrophils	Positive	Negative
Basophilia	Negative	Positive
Eosinophilia	Negative	Positive
LAP score	↑↑ (150–350)	↓↓ (0–40)
pH chromosome	Negative	Positive

Reactive Proliferations of White Blood Cells

Leukocytosis

Neutrophilia	Eosinophilia
• Increased bone marrow production–acute inflammation association with pyogenic infection • Increased release from bone marrow storage pool–corticosteroid, stress or endotoxin • Increased bands ("left shift") in peripheral blood is characteristic • Reactive changes – Dohle bodies–aggregates of rough endoplasmic reticulum – Toxic granulations (prominent granules in neutrophils) – Cytoplasmic vacuoles in neutrophils – Increased LAP (whereas it is decreased in CML)	• Allergies and asthma • Parasites • Certain cancers (adenocarcinoma) • Drugs

Monocytosis	Lymphocytosis
Certain chronic diseases–IBD, Collagen vascular diseases,TB and some infections	Acute (viral) diseases Chronic inflammatory processes

Acute Leukemias

- Peripheral blood has decreased mature forms and increased immature forms called blasts, which have immature chromatin with nucleoli
- Bone marrow has increased immature cells (blasts); the diagnostic criteria is
- **20% blasts** in the bone marrow
  - Acute symptoms are secondary to marrow failure, which can produce marrow suppression (causing anemia and fatigue), → WBCs (permitting infections and fever), and → platelets (inducing bleeding).

Who Classification of Acute Myeloid Leukemia

Class	Prognosis	Fab subtype	Morphology/comments
AML with genetic aberration			
AML with t(8;21)(q22;q22); CBFα/ETO fusion gene	Favorable	M2	Full range of myelocytic maturation; Auer rods easily found; Abnormal cytoplasmic granules
AML with inv(16)(p13;q22); CBFβ/MYH11 fusion gene	Favorable	M4eo	Myelocytic and monocytic differentiation; Abnormal eosinophilic precursors with abnormal basophilic granules
AML with t(15;17)(q22;11-12); RARα/PML fusion gene	Intermediate	M3	Numerous Auer rods, often in bundles called 'faggots'; Primary granules usually very prominent (M3 subtype); High incidence of DIC
AML with t(11q23;v); diverse MLL fusion genes	Poor	M4, M5	Usually some degree of monocytic differentiation
AML with normal cytogenetics and mutated NPM	Favorable	Variable	Detected by immunohistochemical staining for NPM
AML with MDS like features			
With prior MDS	Poor	Variable	Diagnosis based on clinical history
AML with multilineage dysplasia	Poor	Variable	Maturing cells with dysplastic features typical of MDS
AML with MDS-like cytogenetic aberrations	Poor	Variable	Associated with 5q-, 7q-, 20q aberrations
AML therapy related			
	Very poor	Variable	If following alkylator therapy or radiation therapy, 2- to 8-year latency period, MDS-like cytogenetic aberrations; if following topoisomerase II inhibitor (e.g., etoposide) therapy, 1- to 3-year latency, translocations involving MLL (11q23)
AML–NOS			
AML, minimally differentiated	Intermediate	M0	Negative for myeloperoxidase; Myeloid antigens detected on blasts by flow cytometry
AML without maturation	Intermediate	M1	>3% of blasts positive for myeloperoxidase
AML with myelocytic maturation	Intermediate	M2	Full range of myelocytic maturation
AML with promyelocytic maturation	Intermediate	M3	Promyelocytic leukemia.
AML with myelomonocytic maturation	Intermediate	M4	Myelocytic and monocytic differentiation
AML with monocytic maturation	Intermediate	M5a,	In M5a subtype, nonspecific esterase-positive monoblasts and pro-monocytes predominate in marrow and blood
		M5b	M5b subtype, mature monocytes predominate in the blood
AML with erythroid maturation	Intermediate	M6a	>50% dysplastic maturing erythroid precursors and >20% myeloblasts
		M6b	>80% erythroid precursors without myeloblasts
AML with megakaryocytic maturation	Intermediate	M7	Blasts of megakaryocytic lineage predominate; detected with antibodies against megakaryocyte-specific markers (GPIIb/IIIa or vWF); Associated with marrow fibrosis; MC AML in Down syndrome

Myeloblasts

- Myeloblasts may have intracytoplasmic rods (stain red) called Auer rods
- Auer rods are abnormal lysosomes (primary granules) that are pathognomonic of myeloblasts and not found in ALL
- Auer rods also stain positive with myeloperoxidase (MPO) or Sudan-black B stain
- Auer rods are most commonly found in M3 AML
- The tissue form of AML is called granulocytic sarcoma (chloroma).

Cytochemical stain	Specificity
Myeloperoxidase	Granules of Neutrophils (primary and secondary), eosinophilsandmonocytes, Auer rods
Sudan black B	Granules of Neutrophils (primary and secondary), eosinophil andmonocytes, Auer rods
Naphthol AS-D chloroacetate esterase ('specific' esterase)	Granules of neutrophils and mast cells; Auer rods are usually negative except in AML associated with t(15;17) and t(8;21)
a-naphthyl acetate esterase ('non-specific' esterase)	Monocytes and macrophages, megakaryocytes and platelets, most T-lymphocytes and some T-lymphoblasts (focal)
a-naphthyl butyrate esterase ('non-specific' esterase)	Monocytes and macrophages, variable staining of T-lymphocytes
Periodic acid–Schiff	Neutrophil lineage, leukaemic promyelocytes (diffuse cytoplasmic), eosinophil cytoplasm but not granules, basophil cytoplasm, Erythroblasts, megakaryocytesand platelets (diffuse plus granules), some T- and B-lymphocytes, many leukaemic blast cells (blocks, B more than T)
Acid phosphatase	Neutrophils, most T-lymphocytes, T-lymphoblasts (polar), variable staining of eosinophils, monocytes and platelets, strong staining of macrophages, plasma cells and megakaryocytes and some leukemic megakaryoblasts
Toluidine blue	Basophil and mast cell granules
Perls' stain	Hemosiderin in erythroblasts, macrophages and, occasionally, plasma cells

Prognostic Factors in AML

Good prognosis	Bad prognosis
Age < 40 years M2, M3, M4 forms of AML Blast cell with Auer rod TLC < 25 x 109/L t(15;17), t(8;21), inv 16 Rapid response to therapy Leukemia without preceding MDS	Age < 2 years or > 55 years M0, M6, M7 forms of AML Complex karyotypes TLC > 100 x 109/L Deletions 5q, 7q Delayed response to therapy AML with preceding MDS

Acute Lymphoblastic Leukemia

FAB classification of ALL

L 1 ALL	L 2 ALL	L 3 ALL
Best prognosis	Worst prognosis	Very worst prognosis
Small homogeneous blast Scanty cytoplasm Indistinct nucleoli	Large heterogeneous blast Abundant cytoplasm Intended nuclei	Large homogeneous blast Abundant cytoplasm Cytoplasmic vacuolation

Immunological Classification of ALL

Features	B-cell lineage (More common)	T-cell lineage (Less common)
Immunophenotyping	Immunoglobulins, CD 19 and CD 20	CD 1, CD 2, CD 5, CD 7, CD 3, CD 4, CD 8
Associated disease pattern	Pancytopenia	Mediastinal mass, lymphadenopathy, splenomegaly
Genetics	Loss of function mutation in PAX 5, E2A and EBF or balanced t(12;21) affecting Tel and AML 1 genes	Gain of function mutation in NOTCH 1 gene

Prognostic factors in ALL

Good prognosis	Bad prognosis
Age 2–10 years	Age <1 or >10 years
Female sex	Male sex
L1 cell	L2 or L3 cell
Peripheral blast count <1,00,000	Peripheral blast count >1,00,000
Pre B-cell phenotype	Pre T-cell phenotype
Absence of mediastinal mass	Presence of mediastinal mass
Hyperdiploidy or t (12;21)	Pseudodiploidy or t (9;22) or t (8;14) or t (4;11)
Trisomy 4, 7 and 10	

LYMPHOID NEOPLASMS

Who Classification of Lymphoid Neoplasm

Precursor B-cell neoplasm	Peripheral B-cell neoplasm
• Precursor B lymphoblastic leukemia	• Chronic lymphocytic leukemia • B-cell prolymphocytic leukemia • Lymphoplasmacytic lymphoma • Splenic and nodal marginal zone lymphoma • Extra nodal marginal zone lymphoma • Mantle cell lymphoma • Follicular lymphoma • Marginal zone lymphoma • Hairy cell leukemia • Plasma cell myeloma • Diffuse large B-cell lymphoma • Burkitt lymphoma

Precursor T-cell neoplasm	Peripheral T-cell neoplasm
• Precursor T-lymphoblastic leukemia	• Angioimmunoblastic T-cell lymphoma • Large granular lymphocytic leukemia • T-cell prolymphocytic leukemia • Peripheral T-cell lymphoma
	• Anaplastic large cell lymphoma • Mycosis fungoides • Enteropathy associated T-cell lymphoma • Panniculitis like T-cell lymphoma • Hepatosplenic T-cell lymphoma • Adult T-cell lymphoma • NK/T-cell lymphoma • NK cell leukemia

Hodgkins lymphoma	
Classic subtypes	**Nonclassical subtype**
• Nodular sclerosis • Mixed cellularity • Lymphocyte rich • Lymphocyte depletion	• Lymphocyte predominant

Laboratory Investigations of Leukemias and Lymphomas

Leukemia/Lymphoma	Serum findings	Bone marrow	Biochemical findings
Acute lymphoblastic leukemia	↑ WBC count; Pancytopenia with few or no blast; Blasts–PAS +++	Hypercellular with blasts 20% of amrrow cells	↑serum uric acid; ↑serum phosphates; ↑serum LDH; Hypocalcemia
Acute myelogenous leukemia	↑ WBC count; Anemia, Neutropenia, Thrombocytopenia; Balsts–MPO, NSE or Sudan black +++	Hypercellular with blasts 20% of amrrow cells	↑serum uric acid; ↑serum phosphates; Hypocalcemia; ↑serum muraminidase (M4, M5 AML); ↑ FDP (M3 AML)
Myelodysplastic syndrome	Giant platelets; Macrocytes; Poikilocytes; Monocytosis	Pseudo Pelger Huet cells; Ringed sideroblasts; Pawn ball megakaryocytes; Dohle bodies	
Chronic myelogenous leukemia	Thrombocytosis; ↑↑ leucocytosis; Immature white cells; Eosinophilia; Basophilia	Hypercellular with decreased erythroid precursors; Abnormal megakaryocytes; Pseudo gaucher cells	↓LAP score; ↑serum uric acid; ↑serum LDH; ↑ Vitamin B12; ↑ serum ALP
Chronic lymphocytic leukemia	Low hemoglobin; ↑ TLC with lymphocytosis; Smudge cell; Basket cell; Parachute cell	Hypercellular with blasts 30% of amrrow cells	↓ level of surface immunoglobin heavy and light chains; CD 19 ++ CD 20 ++ CD 23 ++ CD 5 ++

Leukemoid Reaction

- Absence of lymphadenopathy, hepatosplenomegaly, hemorrhage
- Presence of immature cells/blasts to < 5%
- Presence of increased LAP score
- Presence of toxic granulations and Dohle bodies

Cytogenetics of Non Hodgkins Lymphomas

Type of neoplasm	Cytogenetics	Immunophenotyping
Follicular lymphoma	t (14;18) Increased expression of bcl-2	bcl-2 protein, surface Ig, CD 19⁺, CD 20⁺, CD 10⁺ (CALLA) and CD 5⁺
Mantle cell lymphoma	t (11;14) Increased expression of cyclin D1	Cyclin D1, surface Ig, CD 5⁺ CD 23⁺
Burkitt's lymphoma	t (8;14) Increased expression of c-MYC	Bcl-6 protein, surface Ig, CD 19⁺, CD 20⁺, CD 10⁺ (CALLA)
Marginal zone lymphoma	t (11;18)	CD 20⁺, CD 10⁺, CD 5⁺
Hairy cell leukemia	? TNF α	Surface Ig,, CD 19⁺, CD 20⁺, CD 11c⁺, CD 25⁺ and CD 103⁺; TRAP positivity

Laboratory Investigations of Non Hodgkins Lymphomas

Type of neoplasm	Lymph node biopsy	Blood findings	Bone marrow
Follicular lymphoma	Centerocytes ++ Centeroblasts ++	Lymphocytosis	Para trabecular lymphoid aggregates
Mantle cell lymphoma	Centerocytes ++ Centeroblasts –	Lymphocytosis	Para trabecular lymphoid aggregates
Burkitt's lymphoma	Presence of high mitotic index of lymphoid cells		
Hairy cell leukemia	Hairy cells	Pancytopenia; Atypical lymphoid cells; Hairy cells	Dry tap; Honey comb appearance; Fried egg appearance

Working Formulation Classification of NHL

Low grade NHL	Intermediate grade NHL	High grade NHL
• Small lymphocytic NHL • Follicular small cleaved NHL • Follicular mixed small cleaved and large cell NHL	• Follicular large cell NHL • Diffuse small cleaved NHL • Diffuse large cell NHL • Diffuse mixed small cleaved and large cell NHL	• Burkitt's lymphoma • Immunoblastic lymphoma • Lymphoblastic lymphoma

Hodgkins Lymphoma

Features	Hodgkins lymphoma	Non hodgkins lymphoma
Localization	Single group of LN	Multiple peripheral LN
Spread	Contiguous	Non contiguous
Nodal involvement	Mesenteric nodes, Walderyer ring, Extranodal involvement uncommon	Mesenteric nodes, Walderyer ring, Extranodal involvement common

WHO classification of Hodgkin's lymphoma

Nodular sclerosis	Mixed cellularity	Lymphocyte rich	Lymphocyte depleted	Lymphocyte predominant
Most common type of HL	Most common type of HL in India		Associated with HIV	
M = F	M > F	M > F	M > F	M > F
Reed Sternberg cell variant in lacunar cell (clear space surrounding cell)	Has eosinophils and plasma cells and Reed Sternberg cell in maximum numbers	Mononuclear and Reed Sternberg cell in low numbers	Reed Sternberg cell– pleomorphic, mummified AND necrobiotic	LH cells (pop corn cells) with absence of B-cell
Cells are CD 15^+ and CD 30^+	Cells are CD 15^+ and CD 30^+	Cells are CD 15^+ CD 30^+ and CD 20^-	Cells are CD 15^+ and CD 30^+	Cells are CD 15^-, CD 30^-, CD 20^+, $BCL6^+$ and EMA^+
No association with EBV	Associated with EBV	Associated with EBV	Associated with EBV	No association with EBV
Excellent prognosis	Very good prognosis	Good to excellent prognosis	Poor prognosis	Excellent prognosis
Adolescent and young adult	Biphasic incidence	Old age group	Old age group	Young males

Mycosis Fungoides (MF) and Sezary Syndrome (SS)

- MF is a malignant T-cell disorder (post-thymic CD4 cells) but has a better prognosis than ATLL
- Clinical: Generalized pruritic erythematous rash (no hypercalcemia)

- Sequence of skin changes (stages): Inflammatory eczematous → plaque stage → tumor nodule stage
- Micro reveals atypical PAS-positive lymphs in epidermis (epidermotropism); aggregates of these cells are called **Pautrier microabscesses**
- **Cerebriform Sezary cells** in peripheral blood: Sezary syndrome (which is also associated with a generalized exfoliative skin rash)

WHO Criteria for Diagnosis of Polycythemia Vera

Major criteria	Minor criteria
• Hemoglobin >18.5 mg/dL in men or >16.5 mg/dL in women or evidence of increased red cell volume • Presence of JAK2 mutation	• Hypercellular bone marrow biopsy with panmyelosis with prominent erythroid, granulocytic and megakaryocytic hyperplasia • Low serum erythropoietin levels • Endogenous erythroid colony formation in vitro

Criteria for Multiple Myeloma

Major criteria	Minor criteria
• Plasmacytomas in tissue biopsy • Marrow plasmacytosis with > 30% plasma cells • M spikes in serum electrophoresis • > 3.5 g/dl for Ig G and > 2 g/dl for Ig A or 1 g/dl of κ or λ light chain excretion on urine electrophoresis in absence of amyloidosis	• Lytic bone lesions • Marrow plasmacytosis 10–30% • Monoclonal globulin spikes present in lower level

Leucocyte Alkaline Phosphatase Scoring

High LAP score	• Infection • Inflammatory disorder • Growth factor therapy • Pregnancy • OCP • Stress • Myeloproliferative disorders except CML • Drugs–Lithium, Corticosteroid, Estrogen
Abnormally high LAP score	• Polycythemia vera • Myelofibrosis
Decreased LAP score	• Chronic phase of CML • Paroxysmal nocturnal hemoglobinuria

Immunophenotyping and Flow Cytometry

Leukemias/Lymphomas	Enzymes positivity	CD positivity	CD negativity
AML	MPO + Sudan black + Chloroacetate esterase +		
AML–Monocytic	NSE +	13, 33, 34	
AML–Erythroleukemia	Glycophorin A +		
AML–M7		41, 61	
ALL	PAS +		
CLL	Surface Ig ++	5, 9, 23	FMC 7
Hairy cell leukemia	TRAP + FMC 7 +	19, 20, 25, 103	5, 23
Mantle cell lymphoma	Surface Ig ++	5, 19, 20	23

Contd...

Contd...

Leukemias/Lymphomas	Enzymes positivity	CD positivity	CD negativity
Follicular lymphoma	Surface Ig ++	10, 19, 20, 22	5
Diffuse large B-cell lymphoma		20, 45	3, 5
Anaplastic large cell lymphoma	EMA + ALK +	3, 30	15, 20
Precursor B-cell ALL	Tdt ++	10, 19	
Early Pre B-cell ALL	Tdt ++ Cytoplasmic Ig M heavy chain	10, 19	
Burkitt's lymphoma	Surface Ig ++	10, 19, 20	
Granulocytic sarcoma	MPO + Lysozyme ++		
Hodgkin's lymphoma (Classical)		15, 30	
HL (Lymphocytic predominance type)		20, 45	15, 30

CARDIOVASCULAR AND RESPIRATORY PATHOLOGY

Blood vessels

Arteriosclerosis

Hyaline arteriosclerosis	Hyperplastic arteriosclerosis
Benign nephrosclerosis Diabetes mellitus Hypertension	Malignant hhypertension Monckeberg sclerosis

Aneurysms

- Localized abnormal dilation of a blood vessel or the heart.

True aneurysm	Pseudaneurysm
When aneurysm involves intact thinned out arterial wall or heart	Defect in vascular wall leading to an extravascular hematoma that freely communicates with the intravascular space

Pathology

- Intrinsic abnormality in vessel wall connective tissue. For example, Marfans syndrome
- Weakening of vessel wall by loss of connective tissue. For example, Systemic hypertension → narrowing of the vasa vasorum, which causes outer medial ischemia.
- Most common cause of aneurysms of abdominal aorta–Atherosclerosis
- Most common site of atherosclerotic aneurysm–below renal artery bifurcation
- Most common predisposing factor in aneurysms of ascending aorta–Hypertension
- Most common part of aorta affected in Tertiary syphilis or Leutic aneurysms–Thoracic aorta

Aortic Dissections–De Bakey's Classification

Proximal lesions or Type A or Debakey 1 and 2	Distal lesions or Type B or Debakey 3
Involve both the ascending and descending aorta or just the ascending aorta	Distal to subclavian artery

Other Aneurysms

- **Rasmussen's aneurysm:** Involves bronchial arteies, seen in TB → can cause massive hemoptysis when ruptures.
- **Berry aneurysm:** Most common cause of subarachnoid hemorrhage.

- **Charcot-Bouchard aneurysm:** Aneurysms involving cortical vessels seen in hypertension.
- **Mycotic aneurysm:** Misnomer caused due to bacteria, e.g. following Salmonellagastroenteritis.

Vasculitis

Classification of Vasculitis is by Chapel Hill Nomenclature

Type of vasculitis	Example	Significance
Large vessel vasculitis–Aorta and large branches	Giant cell (Temporal) arteritis Takayasu arteritis.	• Both are characterized by granulomatous inflammation • GCA is associated with polymyalgia rheumatica • Elevated ESR. • Seen in individuals > 50 years.
Medium vessel vasculitis–Main visceral arteries and their branches	Polyarteritis nodosa (PAN)	• PAN–necrotizing inflammation. • Invoves renal arteries,spares the pulmonary circulation
	Kawasaki disease (KD)	• Kawasaki disease also called muco-cutaneous lymph node syndrome. • Coronary arteries are involved with aneurysm formation and or thrombosis
Small vessel vasculitis-Arterioles,venules,capillaries	Wegeners granulomatosis (WG)	• Granulomatous inflammation involving respiratory tract and kidney. • Associated with PR3 ANCA
	Churg-Strauss syndrome	• Involves the pespiratory tract,associated with eosinophilia and asthma. • Associated with MPO-ANCA's
	Microscopic polyangiitis	• Few immune deposits • Pulmonary cappilaritis is common. • Associated with MPO-ANCA's

Kaposi Sarcoma(KS)

Pathogenesis

- Vascular tumor
- Lesions are characterized by the **proliferation of spindle cells**
- Regardless of the subtype 95% KS lesions are infected with **Human Herpes virus 8(HHV-8) or KS associated herpcsvirus (KSHV)**
- Rare in paediatric AIDS
- Incidence is more when AIDS is acquired by sexual route

Chronic, classic or European KS	Lymphadenopathic/ African/Endemic KS	Transplant associated KS	AIDS associated KS
• Not associated with HIV • ↑ risk in homosexuals • Asymptomatic and remain localized to the skin and subcutaneous tissue but persistent	• Localized or generalized LN • Extremely aggressive • Sparse skin lesions • Associated with HIV	• Months to years after transplant recipients on high dose immuno-suppression • Aggressive • Skin lesions absent	• Male homosexuals • With the use of HAART incidence come down to <1% • No site predilections • Gut involvement and dissemination occur early

Natural History of Atherosclerosis

Type	Gross	Microscopy
Clinically silent		
Type I	Fatty dot	Isolated macrophage; foam cell
Type II	Fatty streak (Earliest sign of atherosclerosis)	Intracellular lipid accumulation

Contd...

Contd...

Type	Gross	Microscopy
Type III	Intermediate lesion	Type II change + small extracellular lipid pool
Clinically silent or overt		
Type IV	Atheroma	Type II + core of extracellular lipids
Type V	Fibro atheroma	Lipid core + Fibrotic core
Type VI	Complicated lesion	Surface defect, hemorrhage and thrombus

Histopathology of Atheroma

Atherosclerosis–deposition of atheroma/fibrofatty plaque consisting of raised focal lesion. Plaque is present in the intima, has a lipid core and a covering of fibrous cap

- Fibrous cap–smooth muscle cells, macrophages, foam cells
- Shoulder area–cellular area around cap having macrophages, smooth muscle cells and T-lymphocytes
- Necrotic core–debris of dead cells, foam cells, cholesterol clefts.

Myocardial Response

Feature	Time
Cessation of aerobic respiration or onset of ATP depletion	Within seconds
Loss of contractility	<2 mins
ATP reduced to 50% of normal	10 mins
ATP reduced to 10% of normal	40 mins
Irreversible cell injury	20–40 mins
Microvascular injury	>1 hour

Myocardial Infarction

- Definition: Localized area of cardiac muscle necrosis due to ischemia
- Distribution of coronary artery thrombosis
  - Left anterior descending (LAD) = 45%
  - Right coronary artery (RCA) = 35%
  - Left circumflex coronary artery (LCA) = 15%
- Transmural infraction
  - Most common
  - Ischemic necrosis of > 50% of myocardial wall
- Subendocardial infraction ischemic necrosis of < 50% of myocardial wall.

Serum Markers used to Diagnose Myocardial Infarction

	Elevated by	Peak	Returns to normal by
CK–MB	4–8 hrs	18 hrs	2–3 days
Troponin I and T	3–6 hrs	16 hrs	7–10 days
LDH	24 hrs	3–6 days	8–14 days

Morphology of Myocardial Infarction

Time	Gross	Light microscopy
Reversible injury		
0–30 min	None	None
Irreversible injury		
20 mins to 4 hr	None	Waviness of fibres at border

Contd...

Contd...

Time	Gross	Light microscopy
4–12 hr	Occasional dark mottling	Beginning of coagulative necrosis, edema and hemorrhage
12–2 4 hr	Dark mottling	Ongoing coagulative necrosis, marginal contraction band necrosis, beginning of neutrophilic infiltration
1–3 days	Mottling with yellow tan infarct in center	Coagulative necrosis, interstitial neutrophilic infiltrate
3–7 days	Hyperemic borders, central yellow tan softening	Beginning of disintegration with dying neutrophils, early phagocytosis by macrophages
7–10 days	Maximum yellow tan and soft depressed red-tan margin	Early formation of fibrovascular granulation tissue at margins
10–14 days	Red gray depressed infarct borders	Well established granulation tissue and collagen deposition
2–8 weeks	Gray white scar progressive from border towards infarct core	Collagen deposition, ↓ cellularity
>2 months	Scarring complete	Dense collagenous scar

Rheumatic fever	Marantic endocarditis	Libman sack's endocarditis	Infective endocarditis
Small, warty Firm Friable	Small, warty Friable	Medium sized Flat, Verrucous Irregular	Large Bulky Irregular
Along lines of closure	Along lines of closure	On surface of cusps In pocket of valves	Vegetations on valve cusps
Sterile	Sterile	Sterile	Non sterile (Bacteria)
Embolization uncommon	Embolization common	Embolization uncommon	Embolization very common
In rheumatic heart disease	In M3 AML, pancreatic cancer, deep vein thrombosis, trousseau syndrome	In SLE	In infective endocarditis

Right Heart Failure

Etiology	• Left sided heart failure • Pulmonary or tricuspid valve disease • Cor pulmonale
Gross appearance	• RVH and dilation
Complications	• Chronic passive congestion of the liver → Nutmeg liver • Cardiac cirrhosis (only with long-standing congestion) • Lungs–Brown induration on gross. • Intra-alveolar hemosiderin-laden macropages("heart failure cells") on microscopy

Valvular Heart Disease

Valvular heart diseases	Significance
Degenerative calcific aortic valve stenosis	• Most common valvular abnormality • Definition: Age-related dystrophic calcification, degeneration, and stenosis of the aortic valve • Common in congenital bicuspid aortic valves • Results in concentric left ventricular hypertrophy and CHF • Increased risk of sudden death
Mitral valve prolapsed	• Associated with Marfan"s syndrome • Asymptomatic with a mid-systolic click on auscultation • Gross: Enlarged, floppy mitral valve leaflets that prolapse into the atrium or 'Hooding.' • Microscopy: Myxomatous degeneration

Contd...

Contd...

	• Complications – Infections endocarditis and septic emboli – Rupture of chordate tendineae and mitral insufficiency – Sudden death (rare)
Acute rheumatic heart disease	• Myocarditis–Aschoff body: Area of fibrinoid necrosis and surrounded by macrophages, lymphocytes, and plasma cells • Fibrinous pericarditis called 'bread and butter' pericarditis. • Endocarditis: Involves mitral and aortic valves • Fibrin vegetations along the lines of the closure • MacCallum Plaques: Left Atrial endocardial thickening • Complications – Mitral stenosis and CHF – Infectious endocarditis.

Rheumatic Valvular Heart Disease/Acute Rheumatic Fever

- Rheumatic fever is a systematic inflammatory disease, triggered by a pharyngeal infection with Group A B hemolytic streptococci
- Mechanism: Molecular mimicry-in genetically susceptible individuals, the infections results inproduction of antibodies that cross-react with cardiac antigens.
- Clinical findings
  - Symptoms occurs 2–3 weeks after a pharyngeal infection
  - Lab findings: Elevated antistreptolysin O
  - Modified Jones criteria

Major	Minor
Migratory polyarthritis Pancarditis Subcutaneous nodules Skin rash (erythema marginatum) Sydenham's chorea	Fever Arthralgias Elevated acute phase reactants
Diagnosis requires: two major or one major and two minor	

Cardiomyopathy

Dilated cardiomyopathy	• Most common form of cardiomyopathy • Definition: Cardiac enlargement with dilation of all four chambers resulting in progressive congestive heart failure • Etiology – Idiopathic (majority of cases) – Alcohol
	– Drug related–adriamycin(doxorubicin) and cocacine – Viral myocarditis–Coxsackievirus B andenteroviruses – Parasitic infections-chagas disease – Pregnancy related • Echocardiogram: Decreased ejection fraction • Presentation: Progressive CHF • Complications: Mural thrombi and cardiac arrhythmia • Prognosis: Poor; 5 year survival = 25% • Treatment: Heart transplantation
Hypertrophic cardiomyopathy	• Synonyms: Asymmetrical septal hypertrophy, idiopathic hypertrophic subaortic stenosis (IHSS) • Etiology – Hereditary: Autosomal dominant disorder (>50% of cases) – Idiopathic

Contd...

Contd...

	• Common cause of sudden cardiac death in young athletes • Gross – Asymmetrical cardiac hypertrophy – The ventricular outflow tract is often obstructed by the septal hypertrophy • Microscopy: Cardiac myofiber hypertrophy and disarray
Restrictive cardiomyopathy	• Definition: Uncommon form of cardiomyopathy caused by diseases that produce restriction of cardiac filling during diastole • Etiology – Amyloidosis – Sarcoidosis – Endomyocardial fibroelastosis – Loeffler's endomyocarditis.

Cardiac Tumor

Cardiac myxoma	Cardiac rhabdomyoma
• Benign tumor usually arising within the left atrium near the fossa ovalis. • Most common benign tumor in adults.. • Microscopyy: Stellate-shaped cells or spider cells within a myxoid background • Complications-Tumor emboli and Ball-valve obstruction of the valves	• Benign tumor usually arising within the myocardium • Most common benign tumor in children • Associated with tuberous sclerosis

Most common primary malignant tumor in adults is angiosarcoma
Most common cardiac tumor is metastasis.

RESPIRATORY SYSTEM

Obstructive Versus Restrictive Lung Disease

Obstructive Airway Disease	Restrictive Lung Disease
• Increased resistance to air flow secondary to obstruction of airways • FEVI/FVC ratio is decreased	• Decreased lung volume and capacity • Decreased TLC and VC
Asthma Chronic bronchitis Emphysema Bronchiectasis	Chest wall disorders Obesity, kyphoscoliosis, polio, Pulmonary effusion Interstitial/infiltrative diseases ARDS Pneumoconiosis Idiopathic Pulmonary fibrosis

Chronic Obstructive Pulmonary Disease (COPD)

Chronic Bronchitis

- Clinical diagnosis: Persistent cough and copious sputum production for at least 3 months in 2 consecutive years
- Highly associated with smoking (90%)
- Microscopy
  - Hypertrophy of bronchial mucous glands (Reid index)
  - Increased number of goblet cells
  - Hyper secretion of mucus
  - Bronchial squamous metaplasia and dysplasia (smokers)
- Complications
  - Increased risk for recurrent infections

- Pulmonary HTN leading to right heart failure (cor pulmonale)
- Lung cancer

Emphysema

- Definition: Destruction of alveolar septa distal to terminal bronchioleresulting in enlarged air spaces and a loss of elastic recoil, without fibrosis
- Etiology
  - Protease/antiprotease imbalance
  - Proteases (including elastase) are produced by neutrophils and macrophages, which are stimulated by smoke and pollution.
  - Antiproteases include α-1 antitrypsin, α-1 macroglobulin, and secretory leukoprotease inhibitor

Manifestations Related to Area of Involvement

• Centriacinar (Centrilobular)	• Panacinar (Panlobular)
• Proximal respiratory bronchioles involved, distal alveoli spared • Most common type (95%) • Associated with smoking • Distribution: Worst in apical segments of upper lobes	• Entire acinus involved • α-1 Antitrypsin deficiency • Distribution: Entire lung; worse in bases of lower lobes

Gross

- Overinflated, enlarged lungs
- Enlarged, grossly visible air spaces
- Formation of apical blebs and bullae (centriacinar type)

Asthma

- Definition: Hyperreactive airways, resulting in episodic bronchospasm when triggered by certain stimuli
- Extrinsic (type I hypersensitivity reaction)
  - Allergic (atopic)
    - Most common type
    - Childhood and young adults; (+) family history
    - Allergens: pollen, dust, food, molds, animal dander, etc.
  - Occupational exposure: fumes, gases, and chemicals
- Intrinsic (unknown mechanism)
  - Respiratory infections (usually viral)
  - Stress
  - Exercise
  - Cold temperatures
  - Drug induced (aspirin)
- Asthmatic attacks characterized by wheezing, severe dyspnea, coughing.
- Status asthmaticus: Potentially fatal unrelenting attack
- Sputum cytology
  - Curschmann's spirals: Twisted mucous plugs admixed with sloughed epithelium
  - Eosinophils (elevated IL 5 levels)
  - Charcot–leyden crystals: eosinophil membrane protein
- Microscopy
  - Mucous plugs
  - Hypertrophy of mucous glands with goblet cell hyperplasia
  - Inflammation (especially with eosinophils)
  - Edema
  - Hypertrophy of bronchial wall smooth muscle

Bronchiectasis

- Definition: Abnormal permanent airway dilatation with chronic necrotizing inflammation
- Cough, fever, purulent sputum, dyspnea
- Causes
  - Bronchial obstruction: foreign body, mucous, tumor, etc.
  - Necrotizing pneumonias
  - Cystic fibrosis
  - Kartagener's syndrome
    - Autosomal recessive
    - Immotile cilia due to defect of dynein arms
    - Bronchiectasis, sinusitis, situs inversus and sterility.
- Gross: Dilated bronchi and bronchioles extending out to the pleura
- Complications: Abscess, septic emboli, cor pulmonale, amyloidosis

Respiratory Distress Syndromes

- **Adult respiratory distress syndrome (ARDS)**
  - Synonyms: Diffuse alveolar damage (DAD), shock lung
  - Definition: Diffuse damage of alveolar epithelium and capillaries, resulting in progressive respiratory failure that is unresponsive to oxygen treatment
  - Causes: Shock, sepsis, trauma, gastric aspiration, radiation, oxygen toxicity, drugs, pulmonary infections, and many others)
  - Microscopy
    - Interstitial and intra-alveolar edema
    - Interstitial inflammation
    - Loss of type I pneumocytes
    - Hyaline membrane formation
- **Respiratory distress syndrome of the newborn**
  - Synonym: Hyaline membrane disease of newborn (HMD).
  - Associated with
    - Prematurity (gestational age of < 28 weeks has a 60% incidence)
    - Maternal diabetes
    - Multiple births
    - C-section delivery
  - Defect: Deficiency of surfactant
  - Lab findings: Lecithin: Sphingomyelin ratio <2
  - Microscopy: Atelectasis and hyaline membrane formation
  - Treatment: Surfactant replacement and oxygen
  - Prognosis: Overall mortality ~ 30%
  - Complication of oxygen treatment in newborns
    - Bronchopulmonary dysplasia
    - Retrolental fibroplasia (retinopathy of prematurity).

Bronchogenic Carcinoma

Histological variants of lung cancer

Squamous cell carcinoma	Adenocarcinoma	Small or oat cell carcinoma	Large cell carcinoma
	Overall most common type of cancer MC in non smokers and females	Most malignant form of lung carcinoma; Associated with smoking Commoner in smokers	

Contd...

Contd...

Squamous cell carcinoma	Adenocarcinoma	Small or oat cell carcinoma	Large cell carcinoma
Central location	Peripheral location	Central location	Peripheral location
p 53 mutation	K–RAS mutation	Expression of Bcl–2 gene	
Presence of keratin pearls	Presence of glandular pattern; Positive for mucin and thyroid transcription factor (TTF-1)	Salt and pepper pattern; Azzopardi effect (Basophilic staining of vascular walls); Presence of neurosecretory granules, chromogranin, synaptophysin and leu–7	Cells–large nuclei, prominent nucleoli, moderate amount of cytoplasm
Hypercalcemia due to PTHrP		SIADH and Cushing syndrome	Gynecomastia

Bronchial Carcinoids

- Younger age group; age < 40
- Gross: Polypoid intrabronchial mass–'collar button leison'
- Microscopy: Small, round, uniform cells growing in nests (organoid pattern)
- EM: Cytoplasmic dense core neurosecretory granules.

Metastatic Carcinoma to the Lung

- Most common malignant neoplasm in the lung
- Gross: Multiple, bilateral, scattered nodules
- Common primary sites: Breast, stomach, pancreas, colon

GASTROINTESTINAL TRACT AND HEPATOBILIARY PATHOLOGY

Liver

Unconjugated vs Conjugated Bilirubinemia

Unconjugated (indirect) bilirubinemia	Conjugated (direct) bilirubinemia
• Increased RBC turnover (haemolytic anemias) • Physiologic (newborn babies) • Hereditary (Gilbert and Crigler–najjar syndromes)	• Biliary tract obstruction • Biliary tract disease (PSC and PBC) • Hereditary (Dubin–Johnson and Rotor's syndromes) • Liver disease (cirrhosis and hepatitis)

Biliary Cirrhosis

Features	Secondary biliary cirrhosis	Primary biliary cirrhosis	Primary sclerosing cholangitis
Causes	Extrahepatic bile duct obstruction, Biliary atresia, Gallstones, Strictures, Cystic fibrosis, Choledochal cysts and Pancreatic head carcinoma	Possibly autoimmune	Possibly autoimmune
Clinical features	No sex predilection Pruritis, jaundice, dark urine, light stools hepatosplenomegaly	Female to male 6:1 Signs and symptoms similar to secondary biliary cirrhosis Xanthomas and xanthelasmas	Female to male 1:2 Same as secondary biliary cirrhosis
Lab diagnosis	Conjugated hyperbilirubinemia ↑ ALP, bile acids, cholesterol	Antimitochondrial antibodies +ve Elevated conjugated bilirubin Elevated ALP and 5'–nucleotidase	Elevated serum IgM Hypergammaglobulinemia

Contd...

Contd...

Features	Secondary biliary cirrhosis	Primary biliary cirrhosis	Primary sclerosing cholangitis
Microscopy	Bile stasis in bile ducts Bile duct proliferation	Florid duct lesion Dense lymphocytic infiltration in portal tracts with non caseating granulomatous inflammation	Periductal portal tract fibrosis(onion skin fibrosis) Segmental destruction of portal tracts Cholangigram: Beaded appearance Complications: Biliary cirrhosis and cholangiocarcinoma.

Cirrhosis

- Definition: End–stage liver disease characterized by disruption of the liver architecture by bands of fibrosis that divide the liver into nodules of regenerating liver parenchyma
- Aetiology-Alcohol, Viral hepatitis, Biliary tract disease, Hemochromatosis, Cryptogenic/idiopathic, Wilson's disease, α-1-antitrypsin deficiency
- Gross
  - Micronodular: Nodules < 3 mm
  - Macronodular: Nodules > 3 mm
  - Mixed micronodular and macronodular
  - At the end stage, most disease result in a mixed pattern, and the etiology may not be distinguished based on the appearance.
- Mechanism: Fibrosis is produced by the Ito cell (hepatic stellate cell)
- Consequences

Portal hypertension	Decreased detoxification	Decreased synthesis
Ascites Splenomegaly/hypersplenism Esophageal varices Hemorrhoids Caput medusae	Hepatic encephalopathy Spider angiomata Palmar erythema Gynecomastia	Hypoalbuminemia Decreased clotting factors

Viral Hepatitis

Common virus name	Hepatitis A (HAV)	Hepatitis B (HBV)	Hepatitis C (HCV)	Hepatitis D (HDV)	Hepatitis E (HEV)
Common disease name	'infectious'	'serum'	'posttransfusion' or 'non-A, non-B'	'delta'	'enteric'
Virus	Picorna virus naked capsid RNA	Hepadna virus enveloped DNA	Flavivirus Qenveloped RNA	Defective enveloped circular–RNA	Calici virus naked capsid RNA
Transmission	Fecal–oral	Parenteral, sexual	Parenteral, sexual	Parenteral, sexual	Fecal–oral
Onset	Abrupt (varies)	Insidious(varies)	Insidious (varies)	Abrupt (varies)	Abrupt (varies)
Severity	Mild	Occasionally severe	Usually subclinical	Co–infection with HBV occasionally severe; super–infection with HBV often severe	Normal patients: mild; pregnant patients: severe
Mortality	<0.5%	1–2%	0.5–1%	High to very high	Normal patients: 1-2%; pregnant patients: 20%
Chronicity or carrier state	No	Yes	Yes (high)	Yes	No

Contd...

Contd...

Common virus name	Hepatitis A (HAV)	Hepatitis B (HBV)	Hepatitis C (HCV)	Hepatitis D (HDV)	Hepatitis E (HEV)
Clinical disease	Acute hepatitis	Acute hepatitis Chronic hepatitis Cirrhosis Hepatocellular carcinoma (HCC)	Acute hepatitis Chronic hepatitis Cirrhosis HCC, HCC	Acute hepatitis Chronic hepatitis Cirrhosis	Acute hepatitis
Laboratory diagnosis	Symptoms and anti–HAV IgM	Symptoms and serum levels of HBsAg, HBeAg, and anti–HBc IgM	Symptoms and anti–HCV ELISA	Anti–HDV ELISA	

Hepatitis B Terminology and Markers

Abbreviation	Name and description
HBV	Hepatitis B virus, a hepadnavirus (enveloped, partially double–stranded DNA virus); Dane particle = infections HBV
HBsAg	Antigen found on surface of HBV; also found on spheres and filaments in patient's blood: positive during acute disease; continued presence indicates carrier state
HBsAb	Antibody to HBsAg; provides immunity to hepatitis B
HBcAg	Antigen associated with core of HBV
HBcAb	Antibody to HBcAg; positive during window phase; IgM HBcAb is an indicator of recent disease
HBeAg	A second, different antigenic determinant on the HBV core; important indicator of transmissibility
HBeAb	Antibody to e antigen; indicates low transmissibility
Delta agent	Small RNA virus with HBsAg envelope; defective virus that replicates only in HBV–infected cells

Hepatitis A Serology

Acute or recent infection	Anti–HAV IgM
Prior infection or immunization	Anti–HAV IgG

Hepatitis B Serology

Clinical scenario	HBsAg HBeAg* HBV–DNA	HBcAb IgM	HBcAb IgG	HBsAb IgG
Acute infection	+	+	–	–
Window period	–	+	–	–
Prior infection	–	–	+	+
Immunization	–	–	–	+
Chronic infection	+	–	+	–

Amebic Liver Abscess

- Organism: Entamoeba histolytica
- Gross: Necrotic abscess filled with brown paste like material ('Anchovy paste')

Alcoholic Liver Disease

Fatty change (steatosis)	Alcoholic hepatitis
• Reversible with abstinence • Gross: enlarged, yellow, greasy liver • Microscopy – Centrilobular macrovesicular steatosis(reversible) – Eventual fibrosis around the central vein(irreversible)	• Microscopy – Hepatocyte swelling (Ballooning) and necrosis – Mallory bodies (Cytokeratin intermediate filaments) – Neutrophils – Fatty change – Eventual fibrosis around the central vein

Alcoholic cirrhosis
• Develops in 15% of alcoholics • Micronodular cirrhosis • Most common disease requiring liver transplantation in adults

Metabolic Liver Disease

- Wilson's disease (hepatolenticular degeneration)
  - Definition: Genetic disorder of copper metabolism resulting in accumulation of toxic levels of copper in various organs
  - Genetics: Autosomal recessive (chromosome 13) and WD gene (ATP7B) codes for a hepatocyte canalicular copper–transporting ATPase
  - Mechanism: Decreased biliary excretion of copper
  - Presents in childhood or adolescence with liver disease
  - Distribution of disease
    - Liver: Fatty change, chronic hepatitis, and micronodular cirrhosis
    - Cornea: Kayser–Fleischer rings (copper deposition in Descemet's membrane)
    - Brain: Neurological and psychiatric manifestations, movement disorder.
- Diagnosis
  - **Decreased** serum ceruloplasmin levels
  - Increased tissue copper levels (liver biopsy)
  - Increased urinary copper excretion.
- Hemochromatosis
  - Definition: Increased levels of iron, leading to tissue injury
  - Causes
    - Hereditary (primary)
    - Recessive disorder (HLA–H gene on chromosome 6p); Mechanism: Increased small–intestine absorption of iron
    - Secondary (example: transfusions for chronic anemias).
  - Epidemiology-Males: females = 5:1
  - Distribution of disease
    - Liver: Micronodular cirrhosis and HCC (200 times the normal risk ratio)
    - Pancreas: Dabetes mellitus
    - Skin: Hyperpigmentation ("bronzing")
    - Heart: Congestive heart failure and cardiac arrhythmias
    - Gonads: Hypogonadism.
  - Diagnosis
    - Markedly elevated serum iron and ferritin
    - Prussian blue stain and increased tissue iron levels (liver biopsy).
- α-1-antitrypsin deficiency
  - Definition: Autosomal recessive disorder characterized by production of defective α-1-antitrypsin (α1-AT), which accumulates in hepatocyte's and caused liver damage and low serum levels of α1-AT
  - Genetics
    - α1-AT is produced by the Pi gene (chromosome 14)
    - More than 75 gene variants described
    - PiM: the normal, most common form (90%)
    - Most other variants also produce normal α1-AT levels
    - PiS deficiency variants: mildly reduced levels
    - PiZ deficiency variant: markedly reduced levels
    - Homozygous PiZZ have severe reduction (15% of normal) in enzyme levels

- Distribution of disease
  - Liver: Micronodular cirrhosis and an increased risk of HCC
  - Lungs: Panacinar emphysema
- Microscopy: PAS positive, eosinophilic cytoplasmic globules within hepatocyte's.

Hemodynamic Liver Disease

Budd–Chiari syndrome (hepatic vein thrombosis)

- Definition: Occlusion of the hepatic vein by a thrombus, often resulting in death
- Aetiology
  - Polycythemia Vera
  - Pregnancy
  - Oral contraceptives
  - Paroxysmal nocturnal hemoglobinuria
  - Hepatocellular carcinoma
  - Idiopathic
- Microscopy: Centrilobular congestion and necrosis

Chronic passive congestion of the liver

- Definition: "backup of blood" into the liver, usually due to right–sided heart failure
- Nutmeg appearance, ie, pattern of alternating dark (congested central areas) and light (portal tract areas) liver parenchyma
- Microscopy: Centrilobular necrosis congestion
- Complications-Centrilobular necrosis: Ischemic necrosis of centrilobular hepatocytes and Long–standing congestion → centrilobular fibrosis → cardiac cirrhosis

Benign Liver Tumors

Hemangioma	Hepatic adenoma
• Most common primary tumor of the liver	• Seen in young women • Related to oral contraceptive use

Malignant Liver Tumors

Hepatocellular carcinoma	Cholangiocarcinoma
• Most common primary malignant tumor of the liver • Etiology: Cirrhosis, hepatitis B and C virus, alcohol, aflatoxin B1, α1-AT def. • HCC invades vascular channels (hepatic vein). • Tumor marker: α-fetoprotein(AFP) • Fibrolamellar variant: younger age, fibrous bands, and better prognosis	• Uncommon (<10%) • Risk factors – Thorotrast – Clonorchis sinensis (liver fluke)

Angiosarcoma	Metastasis to liver
• Rare, malignant vascular neoplasm • Chemical carcinogens: vinyl chloride, thorotrast, and arsenic	• Most common tumor found within the liver • Common primary sites: colon, breast, and lung

PANCREATIC PATHOLOGY

Acute Hemorrhagic Pancreatitis

- Etiology

Gall stones	Alcohol	Hypercalcemia
Shock	Infections, Drugs	Hyperlipidemia
Trauma	Scorpion stings	Hyperthermia

- Mechanism: Pancreatic acinar cell injury results in activation of pancreatic enzymes and enzymatic destruction of the pancreatic parenchyma.
- Lab findings: Elevation of serum amylase and lipase
- Gross
  - Focal pancreatic hemorrhage and liquefaction
  - Chalky, white–yellow fat necrosis of adjacent adipose tissue
- Microscopy
  - Liquefactive necrosis of pancreatic parenchyma
  - Acute inflammation
  - Enzymatic fat necrosis
  - Necrosis of blood vessels causes hemorrhage.
- Complications
  - May develop acute respiratory distress syndrome (ARDS) or disseminated intravascular coagulation (DIC)
  - Pseudocyst
  - Pancreatic calcification
- Prognosis: Severe cases have a 30% mortality rate.

Chronic Pancreatitis

- Middle–age male alcoholics
- Definition: Chronic inflammation, atrophy, and fibrosis of the pancreas secondary to repeated bouts of pancreatitis
- Gross: firm, white, fibrotic pancreas
- Microscopy
  - Extensive fibrosis and parenchymal atrophy
  - Chronic inflammation
- Clinical features
  - Abdominal pain
  - Pancreatic insufficiency and malabsorption
- Complications
  - Pancreatic calcification
  - Pseudocyst
  - Diabetes (late complication)

Pancreatic Tumors

Gastrinoma (G-cell tumor)	Glucagonoma (α-cell tumor)
• Tumor produces gastrin • Zollinger–Ellison syndrome	• Tumor produces glucagon • Hyperglycemia (diabetes), anemia, and skin rash
– Elevated serum gastrin – Gastric hyperacidity – Intractable peptic ulcers • May arise outside the pancreas • Associated with MEN I	

Somatostatinoma (δ-cell tumor)	VIPoma
• Tumor produces somatostatin • Somatostatin inhibit – Insulin secretion → diabetes – Gastrin secretion → hypochlorhydria – Cholecystokinin secretion → gallstones and steatorrhea	• Tumor produces vasoactive intestinal peptide (VIP) • WDHA syndrome: watery diarrhea, hypokalemia, and achlorhydria

Pancreatic Carcinoma

- Most common between ages 60 and 80
- Risk factors: smoking
- Clinical presentation
  - Vague signs and symptoms until late in the course
  - Abdominal pain
  - Migratory thrombophlebitis or Trosseau syndrome
  - Obstructive jaundice
- Site: Pancreatic head (60%), body (15%), and tail (5%)
- Microscopy
  - Adenocarcinoma arising from the duct epithelium
  - Tumor desmoplasia and perineural invasion are common.
- Tumor markers: CEA and CA19-9
- Treatment: Surgical excision (whipple procedure)
- Prognosis: very poor; 1–year survival ~ 10%.

GASTROINTESTINAL TRACT PATHOLOGY

Esophagus

- Barrett's esophagus
  - Definition: Metaplasia of the squamous esophageal mucosa to a more protective columnar type because of chronic exposure to gastric secretions.
  - Cause: Gastroesophageal reflux disease (GERD)
  - Gross: Irregular gastroesophageal (GE) junction with tongues of red granular mucosa extending up into the esophagus
  - Increased risk of dysplasia and esophageal adenocarcinoma
- Esophageal carcinoma

Squamous cell carcinoma (SCC) of the esophagus	Adenocarcinoma of the esophagus
• Epidemiology – SCC is the most common type – Males > females; age usually > 50 – African Americans > Caucasians • Risk factors – Heavy smoking and alcohol use – Achalasia – Plummer–Vinson syndrome – Tylosis – Prior lye ingestion	• Arises in the distal esophagus • Associated with Barrett's esophagus and dysplasia • Prognosis: poor

Stomach

Hypertrophic Gastropathy

Menetrier's disease	Zollinger–Ellison syndrome
• Middle–aged men • Gross: Enlarged rugal folds in the body fundus • Microscopy: Massive foveolar hyperplasia with replacement of the parietal and chief cells • Decreased acid production • Protein losing enteropathy • Increased risk of gastric cancer	– Pancreatic gastrinoma producing gastrin – Gross: Enlarged rugal folds – Increased acid secretion – Presentation: multiple intractable peptic ulcers

Chronic Gastritis

Definition: Chronic inflammation of the gastric mucosa resulting in eventual atrophy (chronic atrophic gastritis)

	Fundic type (type A)	Antral type (type B)
Features	• Autoimmune atrophic gastritis • Involves the body and the fundus • Auto antibodies to parietal cells and/or intrinsic factor • Loss of parietal cells • Decreased acid secretion • Increased serum gastrin (G-cell hyperplasia) • Pernicious anemia: Megaloblastic anemia due to lack of intrinsic factor and B12 malabsorption	• Helicobacter pylori-Curved, gram–negative rods • Urease producing • Risk of infection increases with age • Associated with chronic gastritis (type B) • Associated with duodenal and gastric peptic ulcers • Associated with gastric carcinoma
Gross pathology	Loss of rugal folds in the body and fundus	
Histopathology	• Mucosal atrophy with loss of glands and parietal cells • Chronic lymphoplasmacytic inflammation • Intestinal metaplasia	• H. pylori organisms are visible in the mucous layer of the surface epithelium • Foci of acute inflammation • Chronic inflammation with lymphoid follicles • Intestinal metaplasia
Increased risk of	Gastric carcinoma	Gastric carcinoma

Chronic Peptic Ulcer (Benign Ulcer)

Peptic ulcer

- Definition: Ulcers of the distal stomach and proximal duodenum caused by gastric secretions (hydrochloric acid and pepsin) and impaired mucosal defenses
- Etiology
  - Chronic NSAID and aspirin use
  - Steroids
  - Smoking
  - H. pylori infection
- Complications
  - Hemorrhage
  - Iron deficiency anemia
  - Penetration into adjacent organs
  - Perforation (X-ray shows: free air under the diaphragm)
  - Pyloric obstruction

Duodenal peptic ulcer	Gastric peptic ulcer
• More common than gastric ulcers • Associations	• Associated with H. pylori (75%) • Location: lesser curvature of the antrum
– H. pylori (~100%) – Increased gastric acid secretion – Increased rate of gastric emptying – Blood group O – Multiple endocrine neoplasia (MEN) type I and Zollinger Ellison syndromes • Classic presentation: Burning epigastric pain 1–3 hours after eating, which is relieved by food	• Gross – Small (<3 cm), solitary ulcers – Round or oval shape – Sharply demarcated, "punched-out" ulcers – Overhanging margins – Radiating mucosal folds • Classic presentation: Burning epigastric pain, which worsens with eating

Gastric Carcinoma (Malignant Ulcer)

- Risk factors

Smoked fish and meat	Pickled vegetables	Nitrosamines
Benzopyrene	H. pylori infection	Chronic atropic gastritis
Smoking	Blood group A	Bacterial overgrowth in stomach
Prior subtotal gastrectomy	Menetrier's disease	

- Location: Lesser curvature of the antrum
- Gross
  - Large (> 3 cm), irregular ulcer
  - Heaped–up margins and a necrotic ulcer base
  - May also occur as a flat or polypoid mass
- Lauren's classification

Intestinal type	Diffuse type
• Gland–forming adenocarcinoma	• Diffuse infiltration of stomach by poorly differentiated tumor cells

- Signet-ring cells: Nucleus is displaced to the periphery by intracellular mucin
- Linitis plastica: Thickened "leather bottle"–like stomach
- Metastasis
  - Virchow's (sentinel) node: left supraclavicular lymph node
  - Krukenberg's tumor: spread to the ovary

Small and Large Intestine

Malabsorption Syndromes

- Celiac sprue
  - Synonyms: Gluten–sensitive enteropathy, nontropical sprue
  - Definition: Hypersensitivity to gluten (and gliadin), resulting in loss of small bowel villi and malabsorption
  - Genetic predisposition: HLA–B8, DR3, and DQ
  - Microscopy
    - Loss of villi
    - Increased intraepithelial lymphocytes
    - Increased plasma cells in the lamina propria
- Associated with dermatitis herpetiformis
- Whipple's disease
  - Definition: Rare infectious disease involving many organs, including small intestines, joints, lung, heart, liver, spleen, and CNS.
  - Males; age 30–50
  - Organism: Trophermyma whippleii
  - Microscopy: Small bowel lamina propria is filled with macrophages stuffed with PAS–positive, rod–shaped bacilli.

Crohn's Disease Versus Ulcerative Colitis

Feature	Crohn's disease	Ulcerative colitis
Most common site	Terminal ileum	Rectum
Distribution	Mouth to anus	Rectum → Colon "back–wash" ileitis
Spread	Discontinuous/skip	Continuous
Gross features	• Focal aphthous ulcers with intervening normal mucosa • Linear fissures • Cobblestone • Thickened bowel wall • "Creeping fat"	• Extensive ulceration • Pseudopolyps
Microscpic features	Noncaseating granulomas	Crypt abscesses
Inflammation	Transmural	Limited to mucosa and submucosa

Contd...

Contd...

Feature	Crohn's disease	Ulcerative colitis
Complications	• Strictures • "String sing" on barium studies • Obstruction • Abscesses • Fistulas • Sinus tracts	• Toxic megacolon
Genetic association		HLA–B27
Extraintestinal manifestations	Uncommon	Common (ie, arthritis, spondylitis, primary sclerosing cholangitis, erythema nodosum, pyoderma gangrenosum)
Cancer risk	Slight 1–3%	5–25%

Colonic Adenocarcinoma

- Risk factors
  - Low–fiber diet
  - Diet low in fruits and vegetables
  - High red meat and animal fat consumption
  - Adenomatous polyps
  - Hereditary polyposis syndromes
  - Lynch syndrome
  - Ulcerative colitis
- Genetics–mutations of APC gene, K-ras oncogene, DCC gene, P53 gene

	Right-sided cancer	Left-sided cancer
Gross	Polypoid mass	Circumferential growth producing a "napkin-ring" configuration
Barium studies	Polypoid mass	"Apple core" lesion
Presentation	Bleeding • Occult blood in stool • Iron deficiency anemia	Change in bowel habits • Constipation or diarrhea • Reduced caliber stools • Obstruction

Staging: Modified Dukes (Aster–Collar) staging system

Carcinoid Tumors

- Neuroendocrine tumor often producing serotonin
- Locations: Appendix (most common) and terminal ileum
- Metastasis to the liver may result in carcinoid heart disease.
- Carcinoid syndrome-Diarrhea, Cutaneous flushing, Bronchospasm and wheezing, Fibrosis
- Diagnosis: Urinary 5–HIAA (5- hydroxyindoleacetic Acid)

RENAL PATHOLOGY

Types of Renal Stones

Stones	Formation	Shape	Lucency
Struvite/Triple stone	Alkaline urine	Coffin lid shaped	Radiopaque
Calcium oxalate stone	Acidic urine	Needle/Square envelope shaped	Radiopaque
Cystine stone	Acidic urine	Hexagonal	Radiopaque
Uric acid stone	Acidic urine	Diamond/Barrel shaped	Radiolucent

Urinary Casts

Urinary casts	Significance
Hyaline casts	Concentrated urine, Febrile disease, After heavy exercise
RBC casts	Glomerular injury
WBC casts	Interstitial nephritis, Pyelonephritis
Broad granular casts	Chronic renal failure
Pigmented muddy brown granular casts	Tubular necrosis
Lipid cast	Nephritic syndrome, Renal lupus

Collagen Mutated Diseases

Genetic mutation in chain	Disease
Gene encoding α5 chain of collagen type IV	Alport syndrome
Gene encoding α4 chain of collagen type IV	Benign familial hematuria/Thin membrane disease
Gene encoding α3 chain of collagen type IV	Good pasture syndrome

Cystic Disease of Kidney

Autosomal recessive polycystic kidney disease	Autosomal dominant polycystic kidney disease
• Synonym: Childhood polycystic kidney disease • Bilaterally enlarged kidneys • Multiple small cysts in the cortex and medulla • The cysts are oriented in a radial fashion with their long axis at right angles to the capsule • Associations: May also have multiple hepatic cysts and congenital hepatic fibrosis	• Synonym: Adult polycystic kidney disease • Incidence: Affects 1 in 1000 people • Genetics – Autosomal dominant inheritance – Mutation of PKD1 gene on chromosome 16 – The PKD1 gene produces a transmembrane protein called polycystin 1 – Other mutations involve PKD2 and PKD3 genes • Presents with renal insufficiency, hematuria, and hypertension • Abdominal masses and flank pain • Liver cysts • Berry aneurysms of the circle of Willis • Mitral valve prolapse • Colonic diverticula

Glomerular Diseases

Clinical Syndromes in Glomerular Disease

Nephritic syndrome	Nephrotic syndrome
Hematuria (RBC casts) Hypertension Azotemia Oliguria Proteinuria (< 3.5 g/day)	Sever proteinuria (>3.5 g/day) Hypoalbuminemia (<3 g/dl) Generalized edema Hyperlipidemia Lipiduria

Types of Glomerular Nephritis

Disease	Light microscopy	Fluorescence	Electron microscopy
Post streptococcal GN	Proliferation of endothelail and mesangial cells	Ig G, Ig M, C3 deposits in mesangium	
RPGN–I		Linear GBM deposits of Ig G and C3	
RPGN–II		Lumpy bumpy granular pattern of staining	
RPGN–III		No Ig or Complement deposits in GBM	

Contd...

Contd...

Membranous glomerulopathy	Diffuse capillary wall thickening	Granular Ig G, C3	Subepithelial deposits
Minimal change disease	Lipid deposit in tubules	Negative	Loss of foot process of podocytes
Focal segmental glomerulosclerosis	Focal and segmental sclerosis and hyalinosis	Focal–Ig M and C3	Loss of foot process of podocytes, Epithelial denudation
Membranoproliferative glomerulonephritis	Mesangial proliferation, BM thickening and splitting	Ig G + C3 and C1q + C4	Subendothelial deposits
Ig A nephropathy	Mesangial widening and proliferation	Mesangial deposition of Ig A, C3 and properdin	
Alport syndrome	Presence of foam cells in interstitial cells		Irregular foci of thickening and thinning in GBM with splitting and lamination of lamina densa (BASKET WEAVE appearance)
Good pasture syndrome	Focal necrosis, Intra-alveolar hemorrhage, Type II pneumocyte hypertrophy		Linear deposits of Ig along alveolar septa and GBM

Glomerular Deposits

Subepithelial	Acute glomerulonephritis Membranous GN Heymann GN RPGN (some cases) MPGN type 1
Subendothelial	MPGN type 1 SLE Acute GN
Basement membrane	MPGN type 2 Membranous glomerulopathy
Mesangial	Ig A nephropathy HSP Anti GBM diseases like RPGN and good pasture syndrome

Diseases of the Tubules and Interstitium

- **Acute tubular necrosis (ATN)**
  Acute renal failure associated with reversible injury to the tubular epithelium
  - Clinical features
    - ATN is the most common cause of acute renal failure.
    - Oliguria and elevation of blood urea nitrogen (BUN) and creatinine
    - Metabolic acidosis and hyperkalemia
    - Urinalysis shows dirty brown granular casts and epithelial casts

Ischemic ATN	Nephrotoxic ATN
• Most common cause of ATN • Is due to decreased blood flow caused by serve hemorrhage, severe renal vasoconstriction, hypotension, dehydration, or shock	• Drugs (eg, Polymyxin, methicillin, gentamicin, sulfonamides) • Radiographic contrast agents • Heavy metals (eg, mercury, lead, gold) • Organic solvents (eg, carbon tetrachloride, chloroform, methylalcohol) • Ethylene glycol (antifreeze) • Mushroom poisoning • Phenol • Pesticides • Myoglobin

- **Acute pyelonephritis**
  Bacterial infection involving the renal pelvis, tubules, and interstitium
- Pathogenesis
  – Ascending infection is the most common route
  – Organisms
    - Gram-negative enteric bacilli
    - Escherichia coli, proteus, klebsiella, nitrobacterium
  – Predisposing factors: Urinary obstruction, vesicoureteral refluxpregnancy, urethral instrumentation, diabetes mellitus, benign prostatic hypertrophy, and other renal pathology
- **Diabetic nephropathy**

Renal artery atherosclerosis	Hyaline arteriolosclerosis of afferent and efferent arterioles
Diffuse glomerulosclerosis • Nephritic syndrome • Increased mesangial matrix and mesangial proliferation • Thickened basement membrane	Nodular glomerulosclerosis (Kimmelstiel–Wilson disease) • Nephrotic syndrome. • Nodular PAS (+) deposits of mesangial matrix • Thickened basement membranes
Pyelonephritis and necrotizing papillitis	Renal failure

Tumors of the Kidney

- Benign tumors of the kidney
  – Angiomyolipomas
    - Hamartomas composed of fat, smooth muscle, and blood vessels.
    - Common in patients with tuberous sclerosis
- Renal cell carcinoma (RCC)-Hypernephroma
  – Incidence
    - Males > female
    - They are most common from ages 50–70
  – Risk factors
    - Cigarette smoking
    - Chronic analgesic use
    - Asbestos exposure
    - Chronic renal failure and acquired cystic disease
    - Von Hippel–Lindau disease
  – Gross
    - Large solitary yellow mass found most commonly in the upper pole
    - Areas of necrosis and hemorrhage are commonly present
    - The tumor often invades the renal vein and may extend into the vena cava and heart
  – Microscopy
    - Clear cell carcinoma
      1. Most common type
      2. Polygonal cells with clear cytoplasm
  – Papillary carcinoma
  – Chromophobe carcinoma
    Sarcomatoid RCC (poor prognosis)
  – Clinical features
    - "Classic" triad (10%): hematuria, palpable mass, and flank pain
    - Paraneoplastic syndromes from ectopic hormone production
      1. Polycythemia (erythropoietin production)
      2. Hypertension (rennin production)
      3. Cushing's syndrome (corticosteroid synthesis)

4. Hypercalcemia (PTH–like hormone)
5. Feminization or masculinization (gonadotropin release)
- May cause amyloidosis, a leukemoid reaction, or eosinophilia

- **Wilms tumor (nephroblastoma)**
  - Peak age: 2–5 years
  - Risk factors
    - WAGR syndrome–Wilms tumor, aniridia, genital anomalies, and mental retardation
    - Beckwith–Wiedemann syndrome
    - Denys Drash syndrome
  - Tumor suppressor genes
    - WT-1 (11P13)
    - WT-2 (11P15)
  - Presents as a large abdominal mass
  - Gross: Large solitary tan mass
  - Microscopy
    - Metanephric blastema
    - Epithelial elements (immature glomeruli and tubules)
    - Stroma.

Genital System and Miscellaneous

Male Genital System

Condyloma acuminatum	Squamous cell carcinoma
• Warty, cauliflower-like growth • Human papilloma virus (HPV) serotypes 6 and 11	• Increased risk in uncircumcised males • Human papilloma virus (HPV) serotypes 16 and 18 • Premalignant leisons: Bowen's disease, bowenoid papulosis, Erythroplasia of Queyrat

Germ Cell Tumors

Seminomas versus nonseminomatous Germ cell tumors

Seminomas	Nonseminomatous germ cell tumors
Seminoma	Embryonal, yolk sac, choriocarcinoma, teratoma
Radiosensitive	Not radiosensitive
Chemosensitive	Chemosensitive
Late metastasis	Early metastases to retroperitoneal lymph nodes
Excellent prognosis	More aggressive

- **Germ cell tumors**

Seminoma	Most common germ cell tumors in adults age 15-35 Tumor marker: Placental alkaline phoshatase (PLAP) positive AFP negative Extremely radiosensitive Prognosis: Excellent; early stage 95% cure Variant: Spermatocytic seminoma—older males, excellent prognosis
Embryonal carcinoma	Age 20s-40s Tumor markers: nonspecific, may have alpha–fetoprotein (AFP) and/or beta human chorionic gonadotropin(Beta-hCG) More aggressive then seminoma
Choriocarcinoma	Highly malignant with widespread metastasis Hemotogenous spread to lungs and liver–Cannon ball metastasis

Contd...

Contd...

Endodermal sinus tumor	Most common germ cell tumor in children Microscopy: Schiller-Duval bodies Tumor markers: Alpha–fetoprotein (AFP)
Teratoma	Majority (99%) are malignant. Gross: Often cystic masses that may contain cartilage and bone Microscopy: Contains ectoderm, endoderm, and mesodermal tissue in a haphazard arrangement Immature elements and malignant transformation are often seen
Mixed germ cell tumors	As many as 60% of germ cell tumors are mixed and contain more then one component. Teratocarcinoma : Teratoma+ embryonal carcinoma.

- Sex cord stromal tumors
  - Leydig cell tumors –Reinke crystalloids seen.

Prostate

Benign hypertrophy of prostate	CA prostate
• Enlarged prostate with well-demarcated nodules in the transition and periurethral zones • Prostate specific antigen (PSG) may be elevated but is usually <10 ng/ml	• Commonly arises in the posterior aspect of the peripheral zone • Presentation – Often clinically silent – May present with lower back pain secondary to metastasis to vertebral column through Bateson's paravertebral plexus • Gleason grading system is used • Metastasis – Commonly goes to the obturator and pelvic lymph nodes – Osteoblastic bone metastasis to the lumbar spine • Alkaline phosphatase elevated with metastasis

Female Genital System and Breast

Vulva

Condyloma cuminatum	Cervical carcinoma
• Verrucous, wart like lesions. • May occur on the vulva, perineum, vagina, and cervix. • Associated with human papilloma virus (HPV) serotypes 6 and 11	• Peak incidence in the 40s • Most common malignant tumor of the female genital tract in india • Risk factors – Early age of first intercourse – Multiple sexual partners – Multiple pregnancies – Oral contraceptive use – Smoking – STDs – Immunosuppresion • HPV – High-risk types 16, 18, 31, and 33 – Viral oncogenes E6 (binds to p53) and E7 (binds to Rb)

Uterus

Endometriosis

- Definition: Presence of endometrial glands and stroma outside the uterus
- Most commonly affects women of reproductive age
- Common sites-Ovary, Ovarian and uterine ligaments, Pouch of douglas, Serosa of bowel and bladder, Peritoneal cavity

- Gross
  - Red–brown serosal nodules ("powder burns")
  - Endometrioma: ovarian "chocolate" cyst
- Clinical presentation
  - Chronic pelvic pain
  - Dysmenorrhea and dyspareunia
  - Rectal pain and constipation
  - Infertility

Endometrial carcinoma
- Epidemiology-Most commonly affects post menopausal females
- Risk factors
  - Early menarche and late menopause
  - Obesity
  - Chronic anovulation
  - Estrogen–producing therapy (ERT) and tamoxifen
  - Estrogen replacement therapy (complex atypical hyperplasia)
  - Lynch syndrome: Colon, endometrial, and ovarian cancers
- Most common type: Endometroid adenocarcinoma

Ovary

Polycystic ovarian disease (Stein-Leventhal syndrome)

Clinical presentation	Laboratory findings
• Young females of reproductive age • Oligomenorrhea or secondary amenorrhea • Obesity • Hirsutism • Infertility	• Elevated luteinizing hormone (LH) • Low follicle stimulating hormone (FSH) • Elevated testosterone

Epithelial ovarian tumors
- Arise from the ovarian surface epithelium
- Most common form of ovarian tumor
- Cystadenoma-Most common benign ovarian tumor and Microscopy: Simple serous or mucinous lining
- Borderline tumors (tumors of low malignant potential)
- Cystadenocarcinoma
  - Most common malignant ovarian tumor
  - Microscopy: Stratified serous or mucinous lining with tufting, Papillary structures with psammoma bodies, Stromal invasion
- Hereditary risk factors-BRCA-1: Breast and ovarian cancer, Lynch syndrome
- Tumor marker: CA 125
- Commonly spread by seeding the peritoneal cavity–'Pseudomyxoma peritonei'

Ovarian germ cell tumors
- Teratoma (dermoid cyst)
  - Vast majority (>95%) are benign
  - Commonly occur in the early reproductive years
  - Elements from all three germ cell layers are present
    - Ectoderm: skin, hair, adnexa, and neural tissue
    - Mesoderm: bone and cartilage
    - Endoderm: thyroid and bronchial tissue
  - Struma ovarii: preponderance of thyroid tissue
  - Immature teratoma: histological immature tissue.

- Dysgerminoma
  - Malignant germ cell tumor
  - Common in young adults–female counterpart of seminoma
  - Risk factors: Turner's syndrome and pseudohermaphrodites
  - Radiosensitive
  - Good prognosis
- Yolk sac tumor (endodermal sinus tumor) –"Schiller Duval bodies."
- Choriocarcinoma.

Ovarian Sex Cord-Stromal Tumors

Ovarian fibroma	• Most common stromal tumor • Meigs' syndrome: fibroma + ascites + pleural effusion
Granulosa cell tumor	• Potentially malignant • Estrogen producing tumor–hormonally active • Clinical presentation – Perpubertal → precocious puberty – Reproductive age → irregular menses – Postmenopausal → vaginal bleeding • Microscopy – Polygonal tumor cells with grooves–coffee bean appearance. – Formations of follicle-like structure (Call-Exner bodies) • Complications: endometrial hyperplasia and cancer
Sertoli–Leidig cell tumor	• Androgen producing tumor • Clinical presentation: virilization • Complications: risk of female pseudohermaphrodite

Metastatic tumors to the ovary-Breast cancer, Colon cancer, Endometrial cancer and Gastric "signet-ring-cell" cancer (Krukenberg's tumor)

Gestational trophoblastic disease

Hydatidiform mole (molar pregnancy)

Properties **of a partial mole versus those of a complete mole**

Features	Partial mole	Complete mole
Ploidy	Triploid	Diploid
Number of chromosomes	69	46 (all paternal)
β-HCG	Elevated (+)	Elevated(+++)
Chorionic villi	Some are hydropic	All are hydropic
Trophoblast proliferation	Focal	Marked
Fetal tissue	Present	Absent
Invasion mode	10%	10%
Choriocarcinoma	Rare	2%

Invasion moles: a mole that invades the myometrium of the uterine wall.

Choriocarcinoma

- Malignant germ cell tumor derived from the trophoblast
- Gross: Necrotic and hemorrhagic mass
- Microscpy: Proliferation of cytotrophoblasts, intermediate trophoblasts, and syncytiotrophoblasts
- Hematogenous spread to lungs, brain, liver, etc
- Responsive to chemotherapy.

ADDENDUM-IMPORTANT DISEASES THAT COULD BE ASKED AS MCQ's

Endocrine System

Hashimoto's thyroiditis

- Definition: Chronic autoimmune disease characterized by immune destruction of the thyroid gland and hypothyroidism
- Microscopy
  - Lymphocytic inflammation with germinal centres
  - Epithelial "Hürthle cell" changes
- May be associated with other autoimmune disease (SLE, RA, SS [Sjögren's syndrome], etc)
- Complication: Increased risk of non-Hodgkin's lymphoma (NHL) B-cell lymphoma

Thyroid Neoplasia

Papillary carcinoma	Follicular carcinoma
• Epidemiology – Account for 80% of malignant thyroid tumors – Females > males; age 20–50 – Risk factor: radiation exposure • Microscopy – The tumor typically exhibits a papillary pattern – Occasional psammoma bodies – Clear "Orphan Annie eye" nuclei – Nuclear grooves – Intranuclear cytoplasmic inclusions • Lymphatic spread to cervical nodes is common • Prognosis: excellent Q; 20-year survival = 90%	• Accounts for 15% of malignant thyroid tumors • Females > males: age 40–60 • Hematogenous metastasis to the bones or lungs is common

Medullary carcinoma	Anaplastic carcinoma
• Accounts for 5% of malignant thyroid tumors • Arises from C cells (parafollicular cells) and secrets calcitonin • Microscopy: nests of cells in an amyloid stroma • Minority (25%) are associated with MEN II and MEN III syndromes	• Presentation – Females>males; age>60 – Firm, rapidly enlarging, bulky mass • Prognosis: very aggressive and rapidly fatal

Histological Variants of Thyroid Carcinoma

Type of carcinoma	Cytogenetics
Follicular CA	Mutation of H-RAS, N-RAS, K-RAS PAX8-PPARγ1 fusiont(2;3)(q13;p25)
Papillary CA	Mutation of BRAF Mutation of RAS Rearrangement of tyrosine kinase receptor RET or NTRK-1RET/PTC rearrangements
Medullary CA	Mutation of RET gene
Anaplastic CA	Mutation of p53

Pheochromocytoma

- Definition: Tumor of the adrenal medulla, which produces catecholamines
- Microscopy: Characteristic "Zellballen" or cell nests
- "Rule of 10's"
  - 10% occur in children
  - 10% are bilateral
  - 10% occur outside the adrenal gland

- 10% are malignant
- 10% are familial (MEN II and III)

- Diagnosis: Elevated urinary vanillylmandelic acid (VMA)

Multiple Endocrine Neoplasia

	MEN–1	MEN–II A	MEN–II B
Pituitary	Adenoma ++		
Parathyroid	Hyperplasia ++ Adenoma ++	Hyperplasia ++	
Pancreatic islets	Hyperplasia ++ Adenoma ++ Carcinoma ++		
Adrenal	Cortical hyperplasia	Pheochromocytoma ++	Pheochromocytoma ++
Thyroid		C–cell hyperplasia ++ Medullary carcinoma ++	C–cell hyperplasia ++ Medullary carcinoma ++
Endocrine changes			Mucocutaneous ganglioneuromas, Marfanoid habitus
Mutant gene loci	MEN 1	RET	RET

QUESTIONS

1. A Patient have acquired syndrome associated with defective breakdown and disposal of intracellular fatty acids. Which intra cellular organelle is concerned with this mechanism? (2014)
a. Mitochondria
b. Peroxisomes
c. Lysosomes
d. Smooth endoplasmic reticulum

2. Flipped pattern of LDH seen in: (2012)
a. Muscular dystrophy
b. Acute Myocardial infarction
c. Lymphoma
d. Hemolytic anemia

3. Patient presented within chest pain to emergency room and dies within 12 hours of arrival. After 5 days, autopsy shows necrosis in Myocardium. What is the type of necrosis? (2012)
a. Coagulative
b. Fibrinoid
c. Caseous
d. liquefactive

4. Touton giant cells are seen in: (2012)
a. Xanthoma
b. Sarcoidosis
c. Tuberculosis
d. Foreign body granuloma

5. Metastatic calcification of the gastrointestinal tract commonly affects the mucosa of: (2012)
a. Stomach
b. Esophagus
c. Ileum
d. Rectum

6. All are true regarding apoptosis except: (2013)
a. Associated with inflammation
b. Phagocytosis of breakdown products
b. Programmed cell death
d. Cell shrinkage

7. Caspases are associated with: (2013)
a. Apoptosis
b. Cell injury
c. Necrosis
d. Inflammation

8. Apoptosis is initiated by (2014)
a. Caspases
b. DNA
c. Antibodies
d. MAP kinase

9. Metaplasia occurs in all of the following except: (2012)
a. Stem cells
b. Squamous cells
c. Columnar cells
d. Transitional cells

10. Stellate granuloma is seen in: (2012)
a. Cat's scratch disease
b. Syphilis
c. Lymphogranuloma venereum
d. Actinomycosis

11. **One of the following is not a characteristic of apoptosis: (2006)**
   a. Cell shrinkage
   b. Chromatin condensation
   c. Bleb formation
   d. Karyolysis and karyorhexxis
12. **Rubor is inflammation due to: (2011)**
   a. Decreased tissue oncotic pressure
   b. Decreased oncotic pressure in arterioles
   c. Constriction of the capillaries
   d. Dilatation of the arterioles
13. **Mediator of acute inflammation not derived from cell is: (2014)**
   a. Histamine
   b. Leukotrienes
   c. Kinins
   d. Cytokines
14. **Which among the following does not secrete Interleukin 1 alpha: (2009)**
   a. Lymphocyte
   b. Fibroblast
   c. Macrophage
   d. Endothelium
15. **Which of the following is a multilineage stimulator? (2007)**
   a. IL 1 b. IL 2
   c. IL 3 d. Stem cell factor
16. **The macrophage to epitheliod conversion in Mycobacterium tuberculosis infection is mediated by: (2011)**
   a. TNF alpha
   b. IFN-g
   c. IL-4
   d. TGF-Beta
17. **Regarding DIC all the following features are correct except: (2007)**
   a. Increased fibrin degradation products
   b. Decreased platelets
   c. Increased fibrinogen levels
   d. Prolonged Thrombin time (TT)
18. **Most accurate statement regarding DIC is:(2014)**
   a. Removal of the underlying cause leads to complete resolution
   b. Associated with increased serum fibrinogen levels
   c. Normal clotting parameters exclude DIC
   d. DIC is associated with increased levels of D-dimer
19. **A 50 years old male patient develops cardiogenic shock following acute myocardial infarction. The urine output decreases in next few days. Urea levels–90 mg/dl, creatinine–4.5 mg/dl. Urine analysis reveals no glycosuria or proteinuria, traces of blood present and numerous hyaline casts is present. Later he develops polyuria and the urea and creatinine levels fall. The pathological findings coinciding with the above situation is: (2014)**
   a. Patchy tubular necrosis
   b. Glomerular crescents
   c. Mesangial immune complex deposition
   d. Hyperplastic arteriosclerosis
20. **Marker of Melanoma: (2014)**
   a. S 100 b. Ck 20
   c. MTLF d. Vimentin
21. **Which of the following marker is used to diagnose rhabdomyosarcoma: (2014)**
   a. Desmin
   b. Synaptophysin
   c. Myeloperoxidase
   d. Cytokeratin
22. **True statement regarding follicular cell carcinoma of thyroid: (2014)**
   a. Hematogenous spread
   b. Commonly multifocal
   c. Readily diagnosed by FNAC
   d. Most common carcinoma of thyroid
23. **All are true regarding medullary carcinoma of thyroid except (2014)**
   a. It arises from C cells
   b. Secrete high levels of calcitonin
   c. It is dependent on TSH
   d. Most cases are familial
24. **Most cases of paraneoplastic syndrome are associated with which type of lung carcinoma? (2013)**
   a. Small cell Ca
   b. Bronchogenic Ca
   c. Bronchoalveolar Ca
   d. Adeno Ca
25. **Which of the following conditions is not associated with malignany? (2013)**
   a. Down syndrome
   b. NF I
   c. Turner syndrome
   d. Deletion of chromosome 13
26. **Para neoplastic syndrome in which antibodies are absent is? (2013)**
   a. Lamber-eaton syndrome
   b. Necrotizing myelopthy
   c. Limbic encephalopathy
   d. Stiff person syndrome

27. C Myc on chromosome 8 is seen in: (2013)
a. Burkitt's lymphoma
b. Follicular lymphoma
c. Mantle cell lymphoma
d. Body cavity lymphoma

28. HPV- tumorogenesis is mediated by: (2013)
a. Cyclin A inactivation
b. p16 inactivation
c. p21 inactivation
d. Cyclin E inactivation

29. Immumohistochemical marker of lung adeno carcinoma is: (2013)
a. Thyroid transcription factor
b. Fibrillary protein
c. Chromogranin
d. Synaptophysin

30. Xeroderma pigmentosum is caused due to defect in: (2012)
a. Base pair
b. Nucleotide excision repair
c. Mismatch repair
d. Translocation

31. Which of the following is not a chromosome breakage disorder? (2012)
a. Bloom syndrome
b. Fanconi anemia
c. Ataxia telangiectasia
d. Duchenne muscular dystrophy

32. This type of Kaposi sarcoma was predominantly found is South African children: (2012)
a. Classical type
b. Lymphadenopathic type
c. AIDS related type
d. Transplant associated type

33. Migratory thrombophlebitis is seen in all except: (2012)
a. Ca pancreas
b. Ca prostrate
c. Ca lung
d. Ca breast

34. Small cell Ca lung, DNA of the necrotic cells get deposited on vessels (2012)
a. Psammoma body
b. Azzopardy effect
c. Button collar lesion
d. Necrotic diathesis

35. In which of the following malignancies histological Grade is a good prognostic indicator? (2011)
a. Soft tissue sarcoma
b. Renal cell ca
c. Malignant Melanoma
d. ALL

36. True about familial polyposis colon cancer syndrome: (2011)
a. Autosomal recessive transmission
b. Associated with fibroma and osteomas
c. Associated with brain tumors
d. 100% chance of colon carcinomas

37. True statement regarding Bloom syndrome is:
a. Raised Ig M (2010)
b. Absent Ig A
c. Decreased Ig M
d. Raised Ig E

38. Superior sulcus tumor of the lungs characteristically present with: (2010)
a. Horner's syndrome
b. Breathlessness
c. Hemoptysis
d. Pancosast tumor

39. Oral hairy leukoplakia related to: (2010)
a. EBV
b. Candidiasis
c. Mycormycosis
d. Human papilloma virus

40. Medullary thyroid carcinoma occurs due to the mutation of: (2010)
a. RET
b. P53 gene
c. RASH-RAS, K-RAS, N-RAS
d. BRCA-1

41. Askin tumor: (2010)
a. Primitive neuroectodermal tumor in chest
b. Cholangiocarcinoma arising from bifurcation of bile duct
c. Lung adenocarcinoma involving apical region
d. Enterochromaffin cell tumor

42. Which is not a small round cell tumor? (2009)
a. Osteosarcoma?
b. Ewing's sarcoma
c. Neuroblastoma
d. Wilm's tumor

43. All are oncogenic viruses except: (2008)
a. Hepatitis C
b. Ebstein Barr virus
c. Human Metapneumovirus
d. Papilloma virus

44. Superior sulcus tumor of the lungs characteristically present with: (2008)
a. Horner's syndrome
b. Breathlessness
c. Hemoptysis
d. Pancoast tumor

45. EBV causes all except: (2008)
a. Kaposi sarcoma
b. Nasopharyngeal Ca
c. Burkitt lymphoma
d. Infectious mononucleosis

46. Which is false regarding von meyenberg complex? (2007)
a. Bile duct microhamartomas
b. Dilated bile ducts
c. Free of pigmented material
d. Premalignant

47. c-myc on chromosome 8 is seen in: (2007)
a. Burkitt's lymphoma
b. Follicular lymphoma
c. Mantle cell lymphoma
d. Body cavity lymphoma

48. Klatskin tumor: (2007)
a. Primitive neuroectodermal tumor in chest
b. Cholangiocarcinoma arising from bifurcation of bile duct
c. Lung adenocarcinoma involving apical region
d. Enterochromaffin cell tumor

49. All are true regarding oral hairy leukoplakia except: (2010)
a. It is premalignant
b. Associated with EBV infection
c. Seen in HIV infected patients
d. Hyperkeratosis on HPE

50. Juvenile papillomatosis is cause by: (2011)
a. HPV
b. EBV
c. CMV
d. Hierpes virus

51. Osteoblastic metastases is seen in: (2014)
a. Lung Ca
b. Prostate Ca
c. Breast Ca
d. Hepatocellular Ca

52. EBV causes all except: (2010)
a. Kaposi sarcoma
b. Nasopharyngeal Ca
c. Burkitt lymphoma
d. Infectious mononucleosis

53. Atypical lymphocytes in infectious mononucleosis are made up of: (2012)
a. CD4⁺ T-cells
b. CD 8⁺ T-cels
c. Plasma cells
d. NK cells

54. Allograft rejection is an example of with type of hypersensitivity reaction: (2014)
a. Immediate hypersensitivity
b. Delayed hypersensitivity
c. Swartzmans reaction
d. GVHD

55. In Alzheimer's disease, plaque is made up of: (2014)
a. Tau protein
b. Beta amyloid
c. Huntington
d. Alpha synnuclein

56. Goodpasture syndrome has antibodies against: (2013)
a. Collagen 1
b. G-y or x-y of collagen
c. Collagen 4
d. Collagen 2

57. Mucus plugs containing epithelial cell aggregations arranged as Whorls of shed epithelium in the airway muscle plugs seen in bronchial asthma is known as: (2013)
a. Charcot leyden crystals
b. Curshmann spirals
c. ?
d. ?

58. Type 2 lepra reaction is an example of which type of hypersensitivity reaction: (2013)
a. Type 1 hypersensitivity reaction
b. Type 2 hypersensitivity reaction
c. Type 3 hypersensitivity reaction
d. Type 4 hypersensitivity reaction

59. Amyloidosis deposition most commonly occurs in: (2012)
a. Renal vessels
b. Knee joints
c. Skin
d. Cornea

60. Immune complex deposition is the basic underlying pathology in which type of hypersensitivity reaction: (2012)
a. Type 1 b. Type 2
c. Type 3 d. Type 4

61. Immune complex mediated hypersensitivity is classified as: (2010)
a. Type 1 Hypersensitivity reaction
b. Type 2 Hypersensitivity reaction
c. Type 3 hypersensitivity reaction
d. Type 4 hypersensitivity reaction

62. Amyloid deposits are seen in which thyroid malignancy: (2010)
a. Medullary Ca
b. Papillary Ca
c. Anaplastic Ca
d. Follicular Ca

63. SS-A (Ro) and SS-B (LA) antibodies found in sjogren syndrome are targeted against: (2009)
a. DNA topoisomerase 1
b. Histones
c. Ribonucleoproteins
d. Native DNA

64. Biopsy of parotid gland in Sjogren's shows: (2010)
a. Lymphocytes
b. Neutrophils
c. Eosinophils
d. Basophils

65. A New agent was developed to increase the recognition of foreign antigens by Antigen presenting cells. True regarding the physiological aspects of APC's: (2014)
a. Antigen is presented via MHC-I complexes
b. APC's are required before a response to viruses are generated
c. Direct antibody stimulation still requires APC's
d. Antigen processed by APC are recognized by CD 4+ T-Cells

66. True regarding thymus is: (2014)
a. Mature thymocytes express CD 4 and CD 8
b. Thymocytes whose T Cell receptor bind with high affinity to self-antigens and MHC Complexes are Clonally deleted
c. Mature thymocytes express surface IgM and IgD
d. CD 4 and CD 8 double positive cells are eliminated by a process of negative selection

67. True statement regarding autosomal dominant disorder: (2014)
a. Present early in life
b. Complete penetrance common
c. New germ cell mutations in old fathers
d. ??

68. Defect in xeroderma pigmentosum: (2011)
a. Mismatch repair
b. Base excision repair
c. Nucleotide excision repair
d. Double strand break repair

69. All the following disorders are inherited except: (2011)
a. Protein S deficiency
b. Antiphospholipid antibody syndrome
c. Protein C deficiency
d. Factor V Leiden mutation

70. Which of the following conditions exhibit allelic heterogenicity: (2010)
a. Beta thalassemia
b. Sickle cell disease
c. HOCM
d. Duchenne muscular dystrophy

71. All are true regarding Klinefelter's syndrome except: (2008)
a. Small Testes
b. Webbing of neck
c. Gynecomastia
d. Increased FSH levels

72. The term 'sequence' in genetics means: (2007)
a. Order of nucleotides
b. Order of aminoacids in tRNA
c. ?
d. ?

73. CGG repeat sequence is found in:
a. Fragile X syndrome
b. Huntingtons chorea
c. Dentatorubropallidolusyian atrophy
d. Machado Joseph disease

74. Juene's syndrome is inherited as: (2006)
a. AR b. AD
c. XR d. XD

75. Zebra bodies seen in: (2008)
a. Niemann-Pick's disease
b. Taysach's disease
c. Pompe's disease
d. Krabbe's disease

76. A 17 year old pregnant woman has scattered small, raised lesions on trunk and axillary freckles. The mode of inheritance of this condition: (2014)
a. Autosomal dominant
b. Autosomal recessive
c. X-linked dominant
d. X-linked recessive

77. The following condition is not a single gene disorder: (2014)
a. Arrhythmogenic right ventricular cardiomyopathy
b. Hypertrophic cardiomyopathy
c. Dilated cardiomyopathy
d. Mitral valve prolapse

78. CDE marker of stem cell is: (2008)
a. CD 34 b. CD 1
c. CD 19 d. CD 21

79. Most severe form of hereditary spheroytosis is caused by the mutation of: (2014)
a. Ankyrin
b. Alpha spectrin
c. Beta spectrin
d. Band 3

80. **Surface protein not present in Red blood cell membrane is: (2013)**
   a. Nebulin
   b. Ankyrin
   c. Spectrin
   d. Glycophorin
81. **Which of the following infections can be transmitted during blood transfusion: (2013)**
   a. Dengue
   b. CMV
   c. Hepatitis G
   d. Parvovirus
82. **Maximum storage time for Platelets is: (2013)**
   a. 5 days 20-24 deg Celsius
   b. 5 days 1 to 7 deg Celsius
   c. 5 days 25-28 deg Celsius
   d. 57days 26-28 deg Celsius
83. **All are platelet aggregators except: (2013)**
   a. ADP
   b. Thromboxane
   c. Steroids
   d. PGD2
84. **Best indicator of hemolysis in peripheral smear is: (2012)**
   a. Target cells
   b. Acanthocytes
   c. schistocytes
   d. basophilic stippling
85. **Which of the following conditions is due to membrane receptor defect: (2011)**
   a. Beta thalassemia
   b. Familial hypercholesterolemia
   c. HSP
   d. Sickle cell disease
86. **Sequestration crisis of sickle cell anemia is characterized by all except: (2011)**
   a. Severe abdominal pain
   b. Reduced reticulocyte count
   c. Sudden hypovolemia
   d. Increased splenomegaly
87. **Osmotic fragility of RBCs are increased in:**
   a. Hereditary Spherocytosis (2011)
   b. Sickle cell anemia
   c. Thalessemia
   d. PNH
88. **Which of the following is not a feature of anemia of chronic disease: (2009)**
   a. Increased TIBC
   b. Increased serum iron
   c. Increased serum serum ferritin
   d. Increased bone marrow iron
89. **Paroxysmal nocturnal hemoglobinuria occurs due to defective: (2006)**
   a. CD 55 b. CD 21
   c. CD 45 d. CD 34
90. **42 years old female presents with tiredness. There was no H/O smoking, drug abuse or alcohol comsumption. Hb 7.8 g/L, MCV–72 fL., WBC–7.6 × 109/μL, platelet count 3, 50, 000/μL. Serum ferritin levels–8 μg/L (15-300 μg/L). She was started on oral iron therapy and her Hb condition during review was 80 g/L. The cause for failure of treatment is: (2014)**
   a. Acquired sideroblastic anemia
   b. Inadequate iron dosage
   c. Poor compliance to oral iron
   d. Folate deficiency
91. **True regarding abnormal hemoglobins are:**
   a. HBS is caused by single base mutation (2014)
   b. In thalassemia, persistence of HbF indicates bad prognosis
   c. Alpha thalassemia is due to deficiency of Beta chain production
   d. Genes for alpha and beta chains are present in the same chromosome
92. **Severe herditary spherocytosis is seen due to the defect of the following protein (2014)**
   a. Spectrin
   b. Ankyrin
   c. Band 3
   d. Band 4.2
93. **A 29 years old female with 30 weeks of pregnancy is receiving subcutaneous low molecular weight heparin for pulmonary embolism. Now she is developing bruises. BP in left lateral position is 125/75 mm Hg. Next immediate step is:**
   a. Platelet count (2014)
   b. Factor X-a levels
   c. APTT
   d. Serum albumin levels
94. **Even after screening of blood before transfusion, post transfusion hepatitis is common because: (2014)**
   a. Most cases of post transfusion hepatitis are caused by hepatitis C virus
   b. Most hepatitis B carriers do not have detectable HbS antigen in serum
   c. Available tests are not sensitive to detect HbS antigen
   d. Most cases of post transfusion hepatitis are caused by CMV

95. A 55 year old presents with bleeding gums. He is an alcoholic, has petechia. The vitamin deficiency associated with this condition is: (2014)
a. Vitamin B1
b. Vitamin B12
c. Vitamin C
d. Vitamin E

96. Which virus is implicated in Burkitts lymphoma: (2014)
a. EBV
b. HTLV
c. HPV
d. HHV8

97. Bad prognostic indicators in childhood leukemia are all except: (2014)
a. Infancy
b. T(9,22) translocation
c. Slow response to initial therapy
d. Hyperdiploidy

98. LAP score is decreased in: (2013)
a. CML
b. Polycythemia
c. Pregnancy
d. Bacterial infection

99. Chronic myeloproliferative disorder includes all except: (2010)
a. CML
b. Polycythemia vera
c. Essential thromboytosis
d. Erthyroleukemia

100. Auers rods are: (2010)
a. Condensation of granules within cytoplasm
b. Aggregated ribosomes
c. Aggregated globin chains
d. Lysosymal granules > condensation of granules within cytoplasm

101. All transretinoic acid (ATRA) is used in the treatment of: (2010)
a. APML
b. CML
c. ALL
d. CLL

102. Which of the following subtypes of Hodgkin's lymphoma is not associated with Ebstein Barr virus infection? (2009)
a. Lymphocyte rich
b. Mixed cellularity
c. Lymphocyte depletion
d. Nodular sclerosis

103. Translocation of t(8:14) is characteristic of: (2009)
a. Burkitt's lymphoma
b. Hairy cell leukemia
c. Mantle cell lymphoma
d. Follicular lymphoma

104. Burkitt's lymphoma is associated with: (2008)
a. T (8,14)
b. T (9,22)
c. T (154,17)
d. Deletion of 5 chromosome

105. Lymphocyte predominance subtype of Hodgkin's disease is characterized by: (2006)
a. CD15
b. CD30
c. CD20
d. EBV

106. To assess prognosis and effect of treatment in a case of AML, which of the following is used? (2006)
a. Cytogenetics
b. Flow cytometry
c. FAB classiciation
d. Leukocyte count

107. Morphological appearance of Pneumocystis jiroveci infection of lung is best characterized by: (2014)
a. Hemorrhagic and necrotizing pneumonia
b. ARDS with wide spread hyaline membrance formation
c. Interstital pneumonitis with foamy intra-alveolar exudates
d. Broncho pulmonary abscess formation

108. Carcinoid tumors of lung arises from: (2014)
a. Type-II pneumocytes
b. Kulchitsky (K) cells
c. Mucus (goblet) cells
d. Clara cells

109. Small deposits of neuroendocrine cell hyperplasia in scarred lungs are known as:
a. Teratoma
b. Tumorlet
c. Carcinoid
d. Hamartoma

110. In takayasu arteritis, most common artery involved is: (2014)
a. Common carotid artery
b. Subclavian artery
c. Renal artery
d. Inferior mesenteric artery

111. True regarding aortic aneurysm are all except:
a. Sacccular aneurysm involves whole circumference (2013)
b. True aneurysm involves all 3 layers
c. Atherosclerosis is the commonest cause
d. False aneurysm is not covered by all 3 layers

112. Macullums patch is usually seen in: (2013)
a. Left atrium
b. Left ventricle
c. Right atrium
d. Right ventricle

113. All the following are features of benign hypertension except: (2013)
a. Fibrinoid necrosis
b. Hyalinising and medial hyperplasia
c. Intimal hyperplasia
d. Nephrosclerosis

114. Reid index is useful in the diagnosis of: (2012)
a. Chronic bronchitis
b. Bronchial asthma
c. Bronchiectasis
d. Emphysema

115. Russel bodies and Mikulicz cells seen with following condition: (2012)
a. Rhinosporidiosis
b. Rhinoscleromatosis
c. Atrophic rhinitis
d. Mucormycosis

116. "Aschoff bodies" are seen in: (2011)
a. Rheumatoid arthritis
b. Rheumatic fever
c. Bacterial endocarditis
d. Marantic endocarditis

117. True statement regarding bronchial carcinoid is:
a. Highly radiosensitive (2011)
b. High chances of Metastasis
c. Carcinoid syndrome does not manifest
d. Terminal bronchioles are the commonest site

118. Lepidic cells are seen in: (2010)
a. Lepromatous Leprosy
b. Rhabdomyoma
c. Glioblastoma
d. Cardiac myxomas

119. Earliest lesion seen in atherosclerosis is: (2010)
a. Fatty streaks
b. Intimal thickening
c. Fibrinoid necrosis
d. Plaque

120. Which cell does not take part in atherogenesis?
a. Neutrophil (2010)
b. Platelet
c. Monocyte
d. Smooth muscle

121. Aschoff nodules are characteristically seen in:
a. Rheumatic carditis (2008)
b. Infective endocarditis
c. Viral Myocarditis
d. Libamn-Sacks endocarditis

122. Infective endarteritis is characteristically seen in:
a. PDA (2008)
b. VSD
c. TOF
d. Tricuspid atresia

123. Pulmonary surfactant is synthesized by: (2007)
a. Type I pneumocytes
b. Type II pneumocytes
c. Clara cells
d. Endothelium

124. Which of the following virus has been found to play a role in the genesis of atherosclerosis?
a. CMV (2007)
b. HIV
c. EBV
d. Coxsackie B

125. All the following cause dilated cardiomyopathy *except*: (2007)
a. Alcoholism
b. Hemochromatosis
c. Fredreich ataxia
d. Sarcoidosis

126. A 45-year-old man with cirrhosis due to α1-antitrypsin deficiency receives a liver transplant. He is at an increase risk of developing which of the following types of emphysema? (2007)
a. Centriacinar
b. Paraseptal
c. Panacinar
d. Compensatory

127. Which of the following is a characteristic feature of malignant hypertension? (2007)
a. Fibrinoid necrosis
b. Hyalinising and medial hyperplasia
c. Intimal hyperplasia
d. Nephrosclerosis

128. Most common site for peripheral aneurysm is:
a. Popliteal (2006)
b. Profunda femoral
c. Femoral
d. External iliac

129. Regarding cause of fatty liver, true statement about pathogenesis is: (2012)
a. Decrease beta oxidation of fat
b. Decreased triglycerides
c. Decreased fatty acid mobilization
d. Increased catabolism

130. Which is not a pathologic feature H. pylori chronic gastritis? (2014)
a. Eosinophilic infiltrates
b. Intraepithelial neurtrophil deposits
c. Intestinal gland formation in stomach
d. Subepithelial plasma cell deposits

131. Most common benign tumor of oesophagus is:
a. Lipoma (2014)
b. Leiomyoma
c. Hamartoma
d. Hemangioma

132. Classical liver lobule is present around: (2012)
a. Portal vein b. Hepatic artery
c. Central vein d. Bile duct

133. Regarding Fibrolamellar Carcinoma of liver: All of the following are true except: (2012)
a. Equal incidence in males and females
b. Constitute 5% of hepatocellular carcinoma
c. Prognosis is bad
d. Common in young males and female adults

134. Primary sclerosing cholangitis associated with which of the following condition? (2011)
a. Adenoca pancreas
b. Adenoca GB
c. Cholangiocarcinoma
d. HCC

135. True regarding Hepatocellular carcinoma (HCC) is: (2010)
a. NASH is a risk factor
b. OCPs are implicated
c. Focal Nodular Hyperplasia is premalignant
d. Chromosomal abnormalities are seen

136. Type of anemia seen in H. pylori infection:
a. Microcytic anemia (2010)
b. Megaloblastic anemia
c. Normocyic anemia
d. Aplastic anemia

137. Most common site of Ca stomach? (2010)
a. Lesser curvature
b. Greater curvature
c. Antrum
d. Fundus

138. Which statement best describes the tears seen in Mallory-Weiss syndrome? (2009)
a. Longtitudinal tears in lower 1/3 esophagus
b. Circumferential tears in lower 1/3 esophagus
c. Longtitudinal tears in middle 1/3 esophagus
d. Circumferential tears in middle1/3 esophagus

139. Most common site of gastric cancer is: (2008)
a. Lesser curvature of stomach
b. Greater curvature of stomach
c. Fundus
d. Antrum

140. Histological scoring of chronic hepatitis does not include: (2007)
a. Periportal inflammation
b. Portal fibrosis
c. Bridging necrosis
d. Cholestasis

141. Antimitochondrial antibodies are seen in:
a. Primary biliary cirrhosis (2006)
b. Autoimmune hepatitis
c. Sclerosing cholangitis
d. Secondary biliary cirrhosis

142. Small intestinal tuberculous ulcer is characteristically: (2006)
a. Transverse ulcer
b. Longitudinal ulcer
c. Multiple oval ulcers
d. Serpiginous ulcers

143. All the following are features of acute pancreatitis except: (2014)
a. Increased amylase
b. Hypocalcemia
c. Hypoglycemia
d. Leukoctosis

144. 45 years old female patient presents with duodenal ulcer. The most sensitive test for the detection of H. Pylori is: (2014)
a. Urea breath test
b. Serology
c. Biopsy and culture
d. Stool antigen test

145. Mutation of STK II/LKB I gene results in:
a. Peutz Jegher's syndrome (2014)
b. Cowden syndrome
c. Familial adenomatous polyposis
d. Hereditary nonpolyposis colorectal cancer

146. True regarding gamma glutamyl transferase:
a. Synthesized only in liver (2014)
b. Levels are increased in fatty liver
c. Better indicator of infectious hepatitis than for cholestasis
d. Isolated increase of GGT in patients with prostatic carcinoma indicated hepatic metastasis

147. Which of the following does not a cause of CRF?
a. Membranous glomerluonephritis (2013)
b. FSGN
c. PSGN
d. Membranoproliferative

148. Which of the following features in histologpathology increases the chances of contralateral kidney involvement in Wilm's tumor? (2013)
a. Nephrogenic rests
b. Degree of mitosis
c. Pleomorphic cells
d. Cellular atypia

149. Cerebellar hemangioblastoma and retinal tumors are seen in: (2012)
a. von Hippel Lindau syndrome
b. Neurofibromatosis type 1
c. Tuberous sclerosis
d. Neurofibromatosis type 2

150. Wilm's tumor chromosome is: (2012)
a. 13q
b. 13p14
c. 11p13
d. 17

151. Mesangial cell contraction is brought about by which of the following chemical mediator? (2012)
a. Histamine
b. Bradykinin
c. Nitric oxide
d. PAF

152. Glomerular capillary permeability, which substance is least lost in urine: (2012)
a. Albumin
b. Hemoglobin
c. Myoglobin
d. Inulin

153. IgA nephropathy over expresses: (2012)
a. CD 51
b. CD 61
c. CD 71
d. CD 81

154. Kimmesteil Wilson lesion is: (2011)
a. Hyaline arteriosclerosis
b. Nodular glomerulosclerosis
c. Renal Amyloid deposits
d. Renal Glycogen deposits

155. RPGN is characterized by: (2011)
a. Crescent formation
b. Splitting of basement membrance
c. Neutrophil infiltration of interstitium
d. Glomerulosclerosis

156. Ig A deposition in glomeruli is seen in: (2010)
a. SLE nephritis
b. PSGN
c. MPGN
d. HSP nephritis

157. Subendothelial deposits in glomerulus are characteristically seen in: (2008)
a. Lupus nephritis
b. IgA nephropathy
c. Post infectious nephritis
d. Goodpasture disease

158. Pauci-immune glomerulonephritis is seen in (2008)
a. Post-transplantation in Alport's syndrome
b. Microscopic polyangitis
c. Henoch-Scholein purpura
d. Lupus Nephritis

159. Wire loop lesion seen in lupus nephritis is due to: (2006)
a. Capillary wall thickening
b. Basement membrane thickening
c. Subepithelial deposits
d. Sclerosis of mesangium

160. True in a child with post streptococcal glomerulonephritis is: (2014)
a. Mircroscopic heamaturia decreases within 4 weeks
b. Serum triglyceride levels increases
c. Severe renal dysfunction is an indication for biopsy
d. Serum C3 levels are normal

161. Which of the following lesion is characteristic of diabetic nephropathy? (2008)
a. Hyaline arteriosclerosis
b. Nodular glomerulosclerosis
c. Renal Amyloid deposits
d. Fibrinoid necrosis

162. Negri bodies are not found in which part of CNS? (2014)
a. Basal ganglia
b. Hippocampus
c. Purkinje nucleus
d. White matter

163. Histological feature of lobular carcinoma of breast is: (2011)
a. Single file pattern
b. Pleomorphic cells in sheets
c. Cribriform pattern
d. Pseudo palisade arrangement

164. Extramammary Paget's disease MC seen in: (2011)
a. Vulva
b. Vagina
c. Penis
d. Axial

165. An adolescent boy presents with endocrinopathy, fibrous dysplasia of bone and hyperpigmentation. The probable diagnosis is: (2011)
a. Alagille syndrome
b. MacCune Albright syndrome
c. MEN type 1
d. NEM type 2

166. True statement regarding Meningioma is: (2011)
a. More common in Men
b. 50% are malignant
c. 95% cure rate following Radiotherapy
d. Arise from arachnoid layer

167. 'Pseudopalisading' arrangement of malignant cells is characteristic of: (2009)
a. Glioblastoma
b. Ependymoma
c. Oligodendroglioma
d. Medulloblastoma

168. Brown tumor is seen with: (2008)
a. Hyperparathyroidism
b. Hypoparathyroidism
c. Hypothyroidism
d. Hyperthyroidism

169. All are true regarding Paget's disease *except*:
a. Increased osteolytic activity (2008)
b. Increased osteoblastic activity
c. Occurs in young women
d. Increased chances of malignancy

170. Cerebellar hemangioblastoma and retinal tumors are seen in: (2007)
a. von Hippel Lindau syndrome
b. Neurofibromatosis type 1
c. Tuberous sclerosis
d. Neurofibromatosis type 2

171. Most common tumor of pineal gland is: (2007)
a. Hemangioma
b. Germinoma
c. Teratoma
d. Embryonal Carcinoma

172. Impaired glucose tolerance is seen in deficiency of: (2014)
a. Selenium b. Chromium
c. Manganese d. Molybdenum

173. 50 years old male presents with polyuria, polydipsia and weight loss for 3 months. Presence of one of the following in this patient is diagnostic of Diabetes mellitus: (2014)
a. Urine dipstick test 3+ glucose
b. Fasting plasma glucose 135 mgs/dl
c. Fasting plasma glucose 117 mgs/dl
d. Two-hour plasma glucose 180 mgs during an oral glucose tolerance test

174. The reinke crystalloid is seen in______ (2014)
a. Yolk sac tumor
b. Teratoma
c. Gonadoblastoma
d. Leydig cell tumor

175. Lewy bodies in parkinson disease have: (2014)
a. Alpha synuclein
b. Beta synuclein
c. Barkin
d. Alpha synuclein and barkin

176. A 16 year old male patient presents with head ache, fever and neck stiffness for the past 24 hr. similar history was present one year back. CSF analysis shows WBC's-400 ml, with 90% neutrophils. Gram staining shows gram megative diplococcic. The immune system affected in this condition is: (2014)
a. B-lymphocytes
b. T-lymphocytes
c. Immunoglobulins
d. Complement system

ANSWERS AND EXPLANATIONS

1. Ans. c. Lysosomes *Ref: Robbins, SA Vol 1/e p62, 149*

Acid hydrolases secreted by lysosomes are responsible for the catabolism of abnormal macromolecules derived from turnover of intracellular orgasnelles (autophagy) or macromolecules obtained from outside the cells (heterophagy).

Several classes of disorders fall under–Lysosomal storage disorders.

- Glycogenosis–Eg. Type 2 Pompe's disease.
- Sphingolipidoses–Eg. Tay Sach's disease.
- Sulfatidoses–Eg. Niemann Pick disease Types A and B.
- Mucopolysaccharidoses–Eg. Hurler syndrome.

2. **Ans. b. Acute Myocardial infarction**

Ref: Henry's: Clinical Diagnosis and Management by Laboratory Methods, 21/e p246

"Flipped" LDH pattern is seen in MI (LDH1 greater than LDH2). Usually LDH-2 is the predominant form in the serum. A LDH-1 level higher than the LDH-2 level (a "flipped pattern") suggests myocardial infarction (damage to heart tissues releases heart LDH, which is rich in LDH-1, into the bloodstream).

Other uses of LDH in Lab Medicine.

- LDH is an indicator of hemolysis–Diagnosis of hemolytic anemia.
- LDH is often measured in HIV patients as a nonspecific marker for pneumonia due to Pneumocystis jiroveci (PCP).
- Differentiation of exudates and transudate. The usual criterion is that a ratio of fluid LDH versus upper limit of normal serum LDH of more than 0.6 or $\frac{2}{3}$ indicates an exudate
- Elevated LDH is often the first clinical sign of dysgerminoma (female counterpart of seminoma).

3. **Ans. a. Coagulative** *Ref: Coagulative nercrosis Patterns of Necrosis Robbins, SA Chapter 1 vol 1/e p43*

Coagulative necrosis is the type of necrosis expected in myocardium following infarction. In coagulative necrosis the basic architecture of the cells is preserved but the nuclear changes observed in necrosis (karyolysis, karyorrhexis and pyknosis) are can be appreciated.

Definition: A localized area of coagulative necrosis is an infarct.

4. **Ans. a. Xanthoma** *Ref: Dermatology: 2-Volume Set. St. Louis: Mosby. p14, 15*

Touton giant cells are seen in xanthoma. Touton giant cells are a type of multinucleated giant cell seen in lesions with high lipid content such as

- Fat necrosis,
- Xanthoma
- Xanthogranulomas and
- Dermatofibroma

5. **Ans. a. Stomach** *Ref: Robbins: SA vol 2/e p52*

Stomach is the most common site for metaplastic calcification in the GIT. Metastatic calcification is almost always associated with disordered calcium homeostasis. Inadvertently hypercalcemia is present in Metastatic calcification.

Pathologic forms of calcification

Dystrophic calcification	Metastatic calcification
Seen in dead tissue Serum calcium levels–normal/or raised Seen at the sites of necrosis	Seen in living tissue Serum calcium levels–raised Seen in lungs, kidneys, stomach, systemic artery and pulmonary veins
Examples • Rheumatic heart disease • Atheromatous plaque • TB lymph node • Meningioma • Mesothelioma • Papillary CA of thyroid, ovary and salivary gland • Prolactinoma, Glucagonoma	Examples • Hyperparathyroidism • Renal failure • Vitamin D intoxication • Sarcoidosis • Milk alkali syndrome • Multiple myeloma • Metastatic bone tumors

6. **Ans. a. Associated with inflammation** *Ref: Robbins, SA vol 1/e p52*

Absence of inflammation is the hallmark of apoptosis .

Important points

- Programmed cell death
- **No inflammatory reaction.**[Q]

Morphological features

- Cell shrinkage
- Chromatin condensation
- Cytoplasmic blebs and apoptotic bodies eg; Councilman body in viral hepatitis
- Phagocytosis of apoptotic cells by macrophages

Proapoptotic proteins	Antiapoptotic proteins
• Bak • Bax • Bim • Caspases • Bcl-2	• Bcl-2 • Bcl-x • Apaf-1 • AIF

7. Ans. a. Apoptosis *Ref: Robbins: SA Vol 1/e p56*

Apaf–1 activates caspases and induces apoptosis.

Proapoptotic genes	Antiapoptotic genes
Bax, Bid, Bak, Bim, Bad	Bcl-2, Bcl-xL or Mcl-1

8. Ans. a. Caspases *Ref: Robbins: SA Vol 1/e p52*

Programed cell death is apoptosis

9. Ans. a. Stem cells *Ref: Robbins: SA Vol 1/e p61*

Metaplasia is a reversible change in which one differentiated cell type (epithelial and mesenchymal) is replaced by another cell type. Metaplasia is a response to chronic inflammation. For example, Barrets metaplasia–Squamous epithelium in the lower esophagus is replaced by intestinal type epithelium.

Stem cells do not undergo metaplasia. Examples of stem cells are given below. Stem cells reside is specialized locations called 'niches.'

Name of the cell	Location	Function
Oval cells	Canals of Herring of liver	Forming hepatocytes and biliary cells
Satellite cells	Basal lamina of myotubule	Differentiate into myocyte after injury
Limbus cells	Canals of Schlemm	Stem cells for cornea
Ito cells	Subendothelial space of Disse	Stores vitamin A and source of collagen for cirrhotic liver
Paneth cells	Bottom of crypts	Host defense against microbes

10. Ans. a. Cat's scratch disease *Ref: Robbins: SA Vol 1 Table 3-8/e p98*

Stellate granulomas are noted in cat scratch disease.

Granuloma is a lieson seen on microscopy in certain forms of chronic inflasmmation where the antigen inciting the inflammation is easily nondegradable or hardy.

Infectious granulomatous disease. Examples	Non-Infectious granulomatous disease. Examples
Tuberculosis	Sacrcoidiosis
Cat-scratch disease	Crohns disease
Schistosomiasis	Berylliosis

11. Ans. d. Karyolysis and karyorhexxis *Ref: Robbins: SA Vol 1/e p53*

The following have been described under morphological features noted in apoptosis;

- Cell shrinkage
- Chromatin condensation
- Formation of cytoplasmic blebs and apoptotic bodies
- Phagocytosis of the apoptotic bodies by macrophages.

Karyolysyis and karyorhexxis are more specific for necrosis.

Note –The latest edition of Robbins describes 2 new terms 'Necroptosis and pyroptosis',

- Necroptosis is caspase independent and triggered by viral proteins or ligation of TNFR1
- Pyroptosis is caspase dependent.

12. Ans. d. Dilatation of the arterioles *Ref: Robbins: Pathologic Basic of Disease, SA /e p73*

Dilatation of the arterioles. Vasodilation is the earliest manifestations of acute inflammation[q]. It is brought about by the action of several mediators notably histamine on vascular smooth muscle in the arterioles. The result is increased blood flow,which is the cause of erthema (redness or rubor).

The cardinal signs of inflammation are dolor, calor, rubor, tumor and loss of function. The first 4 signs all ending with 'or' were described by Celsus. Loss of function was described by Rudolph Virchow–The father of pathology.

13. Ans. c. Kinins *Ref: Table 3-4 Robbins: Pathologic Basic of Disease, SA /e p83*

Kinins are derived from plasma given below is the list of inflammatory mediators, their source and actions.

Mediator	Source	Action
Histamine	Mast cells, basophils, platelets	Vasodilation, Increased Vascular permeability, endothelial activation
Prostaglandins	Mast cells, Leukocytes	Vasodialtion, pain, fever
Leukotrienes	Mast cells, Leukocytes	Increased Vascular permeability, chemotaxis, leukocyte adhesion and activation
Cytokines (TNF, IL1, IL6)	Mast cells, endothelial cells, macrophages	endothelial activation
Chemokines	Leukocytes, Mast cells	chemotaxis, leukocyte activation
PAF	Leukocytes, Mast cells	Vasodilation, Increased Vascular permeability, leukocyte adhesion, degranulation and oxidative burst
Complement	Plasma (produced in liver)	leukocyte chemotaxis and activation, Vasodilation
KInins	Plasma (produced in liver)	Increased Vascular permeability, smooth muscle contraction, Vasodilation, pain

14. Ans. a. Lymphocyte *Ref: Table 3.6 Robbins: Pathologic Basic of Disease, SA e p86*

- TNF derived from–Macrophages, mast cells and T-lymphocytes.
- IL1 derived from–Macrophages, endothelial cells and epithelial cells.
- BothTNF and IL-1 are produced by macrophages and dendritic cells.
  - TNF is produced by lymphocytes but there is no mention of IL 1 in the literature.

15. Ans. c. IL 3 *Ref: Internet sources*

16. Ans. b. IFN-g *Ref: Robbins Pathologic Basic of Disease, SA e p210*

The activated macrophages in type 4 hypersensitivity are called epitheloid cells.

Type 4 hypersensitivity is synonymous with delayed type hypersensitivity or granulomatous inflammation.

Granulomatous reaction features;

- Strong CD 4 + T helper 1 lymphocyte activation (TH1)activation.
- High IFN g levels-IFN g is the mediator which converts TH1 into epitheloid cells (Refer to fig. 6-20/ e p210 SA edition–Really worth it !).
- Usually TH1 cells predominate in granulomatous reaction. Schistosomiasis is an exception-TH2 cells contribute to the lesions.

17. Ans. c. Increased fibrinogen levels *Ref: Robbins Pathologic Basic of Disease, Vol 1 SA /e p663*

- DIC is characterized by formation of fibrin thrombi which occlude the microcirculation.
- As fibrin thrombi are formed the levels of fibrinogen decrease.

18. Ans. a. Removal of the underlying cause leads to complete resolution

Robbins Pathologic Basic of Disease, p663 vol 1 SA edition Let us do a stepwise elimination process. As discussed in the previous question option B is out.

The following points are from Guidelines for the diagnosis and management of disseminated intravascular coagulation–British journal of hematology. Vol 145 Issue 1.

- There is no single laboratory test that can establish or rule out the diagnosis of DIC.
- The PT or aPTT is prolonged in about 50–60% of cases of DIC at some point during the course of illness.
- Fibrinogen levels can be normal in as many as 57% of patients. So ↓ fibrinogen is not the rule in all cases of DIC.
- In fact the most common abnormal parameter in 98% of DIC cases is thrombocytopenia.
- FDP and D-Dimer can be elevated in any case of thromboembolism Eg. Pulmonary embolism and are not DIC specific.

The above points when considered eliminate options C and D. What remains is option A, which is rather classical medical teaching." In DIC treat the underlying cause."

19. Ans. a. Patchy tubular necrosis *Ref: Robbins Pathologic Basic of Disease, p927 Vol 2 SA edition*

One of the sequelae of cardiogenic shock is fall in cardiac output and consequent renal hypoperfusion.

Renal hypoperfusion

↓

Renal ischemia

Acute tubular necrosis or acute tubular injury(ATI).

ATI most commonly affect the PCT and is patchy.

2 conditions can cause ATI.

- Shock or loss of blood supply (Most common cause)
- Toxins.

Quick revision of the other options:

- Glomerular crescents are seen in RPGN (Rapidly progressive glomeruloneplritis)
- Mesangial immune complex deposition = Antigen antibody complex deposition. Eg. SLE, PAN, PSGN.
- Hyperplastic arteriosclerosis is a feature of malignant hypertension.

20. Ans. a. S 100 *Ref: Rook's Textbook of Dermatology and Robbins Pathologic Basis of Disease, 8/e p1171-5*

21. Ans. a. Desmin *Ref: Robbins Pathologic Basis of Disease, 8/e p265*

22. Ans. a. Hematogenous spread *Ref: Robbins Pathologic Basis of Disease, SA edition, vol 2/e p1097*

Follicular carcinoma–Thyroid

- Frequent in areas with dietary iodine deficiency.
- More common in women 3:1.
- Mostly unifocal.
- Distiction between follicular carcinoma and adenoma cannot be made on basis of FNAC. For distinction extensive tissue sampling is required.
- The most common malignant neoplasm of thyroid is papillary carcinoma.

23. Ans. c. It is dependent on TSH *Ref: Robbins Pathologic Basis of Disease, SA e p1099*

Medullary carcinoma–Thyroid

- Neuroendocrine neoplasm originating from the parafollicular cells or C cells of the thyroid.
- 70% of medullary carcinomas arise sporadically while the rest are part of MEN 2A and MEN 2B.
- Activation of RET protooncogene plays an important role in both development of familial and sporadic medullary cancer.
- Multicentricity and bilaterality is common in medullary cancer.
- Amyloid deposits can be seen.

Considering the options given,We can choose either between C or D–TSH has not been described aside medullary Ca in the literature and is more incorrect compared to option D.

24. Ans. c. Bronchoalveolar Ca *Ref: Robbins Pathologic Basis of Disease, SA Vol 1/e p331*

Paraneoplastic syndrome–Hormones liberated by malignant tumor cause symptoms unrelated to anatomical location of the tumor.

- Most common paraneoplastic syndrome–Cushing syndrome.
- Amongst cancers of the lung small cell carcinoma of the lung is known to cause many paraneoplastic syndromes including SIADH and Cushing syndrome.

Please refer to table 7-11 in pg.331 vol 1 SA edition.

25. Ans. c. Turner syndrome *Ref: Robbins Pathologic Basis of Disease, SA Vol 1/e p279*

Down syndrome is associated with increased risk of malignancy as there is defective DNA repair in Downs

Defective DNA repair syndromes:

- Ataxia–telangectasia.
- Bloom syndrome.
- Fanconi anemia.
- Xeroderma pigmentosum.
- Li-Fraumeni syndrome results from germline mutations in p53 gene.

Both NF 1 and NF 2 are associated with malignancy. Features of both NF 1 and NF 2 are given below.
Neurofibromatosis type 1–Features:
- **Gliomas** of the optic nerve.
- Pigmented nodules of the iris- Lisch nodules.
- Cutaneous hyperpigmented macules–'cafe au lait' spots.

Neurofibromatosis type 2–features:
- Bilateral 8th nerve schwannomas.
- Gliomas.
- Meningiomas.
- Ependymoma of the spinal cord.
- Deletion of chromosome 13 is implicated in retinoblastoma.

By elimination the most appropriate option is C.
Turner syndrome is associated with lymphangioma as lymphangioma is a benign tumor.

26. Ans. b. Necrotizing myelopthy

Ref: Robbins Pathologic Basis of Disease, 8/e p:
Harrison's Online. Chapter 101. Paraneplastic Neurologic Syndromes.

There are no autoantibodies involved in the pathogenesis of necrotizing myelopathy.
- Lamber-eaton syndrome–Antibodies that block Ach release by blocking presynaptic calcium channel. Most commonly associated with small cell Ca. Lung
- Limbic encephalopathy-The main antibodies within this group are those against voltage-gated potassium channels (VGKC) and anti-N-methyl-D-aspartate receptors (NMDAR)
- Stiff person syndrome- GAD(Glutamic acid decarboxylase) antibodies.

27. Ans. b. Follicular lymphoma *Ref: Robbins Pathologic Basis of Disease, SA, Vol 1/e p288*

The myc proto-oncogene is expressed in all cells. It is mutated in a number of human cancers.
- MYC translocation–Burkitt's lymphoma.
- N-MYC amplification–Neuroblastoma.
- L-MYC amplification–Small cell carcinoma lung.

28. Ans. c. p21 inactivation *Ref: Robbins Pathologic Basis of Disease, SA, Vol 1/e p327*

2 viral genes E6 andn E7 are implicated in the carcinogenesis of cervical cancer.
E6 degrades p53. E7 inactivates cell cycle regulators p21 and p27.

29. Ans. a. Thyroid transcription factor *Ref: Robbins Pathologic Basis of Disease, SA, Vol 2/e p714*

Thyroid transcription factor (TTF) is a tumor marker used for the Dx of adenoCa Lung. Tumor markers in lung Ca are classified as non-small cell (NSCLC) and small cell lung cancer (SCLC).

Markers in NSCLC	Markers in SCLC
• CEA • TPA • TTF • CYFRA 21-1 • Ferritin • CA19-9 • CA50 • CA242 • H-K-N-ras mutations and p53 mutation	• BN/GRP • CK-BB • NCAM • IL-2R • IGF-I • Transferrin • ANP • mAb (cluster 5), Le-y and c-N-L-myc mutation

30. Ans. b. Nucleotide excision repair *Ref: Robbins and Cotran Pathologic Basis of Disease, SA, Vol 2/e p314*

Xeroderma pigmentosum is an inherited autosomal recessive syndrome of defective DNA repair.
- Individuals with Xeroderma pigmentosum run high-risk of developing cancers of the skin following exposure to UV rays
- This is due to accumulation of pyrmidine dimers
- Normally such pyrmidine dimers are repaired by nucleotide excision repair system
- Nucleotide excision repair system is defective in Xeroderma pigmentosum.

31. Ans. d. Duchenne muscular dystrophy *Ref: Robbins and Cotran Pathologic Basis of Disease, SA, Vol 2/e p314*

Chromosome breakage disorders are characterized by defective DNA repair and are inherited in an autosomal recessive pattern.

For example, bloom syndrome

- Downs syndrome
- Ataxia telangectasia
- Fanconi anemia.

32. Ans. b. Lymphadenopathic type

Ref: Chapter 11. Blood vessels; p518; Robins and Cotran Pathologic Basic of Disease: SA, Vol 2/e

Features of KS

- Vascular tumor
- Lesions are characterized by the proliferation of spindle cells
- Regardless of the subtype 95% KS lesions are infected with Human Herpes virus 8(HHV-8) or KS associated herpesvirus(KSHV)
- Rare in paediatric AIDS
- Incidence is more when AIDS is acquired by sexual route

Chronic, classic or European KS	Lymphadenopathic/ African/Endemic KS	Transplant associated KS	AIDS associated KS
• Not associated with HIV • ↑ risk in homosexuals • Asymptomatic and remain localized to the skin and subcutaneous tissue but persistent	• Localized or generalized LN • Extremely aggressive • Sparse skin lesions • Associated with HIV	• Months to years after transplant recipients on high dose immunosuppression • Aggressive • Skin lesions absent	• Male homosexuals • With the use of HAART incidence come down to <1% • No site predilections • Gut involvement and dissemination occur early

33. Ans. d. Ca breast *Ref: Chapter 7. Neoplasia; table 7-11; Robbins Pathologic Basis of Disease, SA, Vol 1/e p331*

Migratory thrombophlebitis or Trosseau syndrome is described in Ca. Pancreas. It is not described in Ca. Breast.

Mondors thrombophlebitis occurs post mastectomy in Ca. breast.

34. Ans. b. Azzopardy effect *Ref: Sternberg's Diagnostic surgical pathology. Vol 1/e p1140*

Azzopardi effect is seen in small cell carcinoma of lung. The Azzopardi effect is encrustation of blood vessels with nuclear basophilic material which represents nuclear material.

35. Ans. a. Soft tissue sarcoma *Ref: Robbins Pathologic Basic of Disease, 8/e*

- Stage is a good prognostic indicator for carcinomas.
- Grade is a good prognostic indicator for sarcomas.

36. Ans. d. 100% chance of colon carcinomas *Ref: Robbins Pathologic Basic of Disease, SA, Vol 2/e p*

Colorectal adenocarcinoma develops in 100% of untreated FAP patients before the age of 30 and always before the age of 50.

Classic FAP syndrome	Gardner syndrome
• Typically 500–2500 colonic adenomas • Minimum of 100 for diagnosis Q • Also have polyps in stomach and SI • Cancer prevention measures include early detection and prophylactic colectomy in siblings Q and first degree relatives at risk	• Intestinal polyps Q • Multiple osteoma Qs (mandible, skull, long bones) • Epidermal cysts, Fibromatosis Q • Retroperitoneal fibrosis Q, Desmoid tumor • Risk of duodenal, thyroid and Ampullary ca Q • Congenital hypertrophy of retinal pigment epithelium Q
Attenuated FAP syndrome • Fewer polyps • Risk of cancer 50%	**Turcot syndrome** • Colonic polyps Q • CNS tumors Q (APC mutation–medulloblastomas; HNPCC mutations–glioblastomas)

37. Ans. c. Decreased Ig M *Ref: Robbins Pathologic Basic of Disease, 8/e p314*

Decreased Ig M is a feature of Bloom syndrome.

38. Ans. d. Pancosast tumor *Ref: Robbins Pathologic Basic of Disease, SA/e p719*

Pancoast tumor is synonymous with superior pulmonary sulcus tumor. These tumors tend to invade the cervical sympathetic plexus and cause the symptoms associated with Horner's syndrome.

39. Ans. a. EBV *Ref: Robbins Pathologic Basic of Disease, SA. Vol 2/e p730*

Oral hairy leukoplakia-EBV

Hairy leukoplakia is a distinctive lesion on the lateral border of the tongue that is usually seen in immunocompromised patients and is caused by EBV.

40. Ans. a. RET *Ref: Robbins Pathologic Basic of Disease, SA, Vol 2/e p1095*

Familial medullary carcinomas occur in MEN 2 and are associated with germline RET mutations.

- However chromosomal rearrangrements involving RET, such as the RET/PTC translocations are seen in papillary Ca. Thyroid and not in medullary carcinoma.

41. Ans. a. Primitive neuroectodermal tumor in chest

Ref: Benbrahim Z et al. Askin's tumor: a case report and literature review. World j Surg Oncol. 2013; 11:10

Askin tumor

- Rare tumor
- Primitive neuroectodermal tumor of the thoracopulmonary region
- Presenting in childhood
- In adults is rare
- CD99 + just like Ewings and Synovial sarcoma.

42. Ans. d. Wilm's tumor *Ref: Robbins Pathologic Basic of Disease, SA, Vol 1/e p481*

WIlm's tumor is a tripahsic tumor composed of epithelial, blastemal and stromal elements.

Small round cell tumors are listed below

- Lymphoma
- Neuroblastoma
- Ewings sarcoma
- Rhabdomyosarcoma
- PNET

Wilm's tumor is a triphasic tumor composed of epithelial, stromal and blastemal elements.

43. Ans. c. Human Metapneumovirus

Option 'C' is the answer by exclusion. There is sufficient evidence in Robbins that options A, B and D cause cancer. Metapneumovirus is the second most common cause (after the *respiratory syncytial virus*) of lower respiratory infection in young children.

44. Ans. d. Pancoast tumor *Ref: Robbins Pathologic Basic of Disease, SA/e p719*

45. Ans. a. Kaposi sarcoma *Ref: Robbins Pathologic Basic of Disease, SA/e p869*

46. Ans. a. Bile duct microhamartomas *Ref: Robbins Pathologic Basic of Disease, SA/e p86*

Von meyeburg complex is a biliary hamartoma and not a malignancy.

47. Ans. a. Burkitt's lymphoma *Ref: Robbins Pathologic Basic of Disease, SA /e p597*

All forms of Burkitt lymphoma are highly associated with translocations of the MYC gene on chromosome 8 that lead to increased MYC protein levels.

48. Ans. b. Cholangiocarcinoma arising from bifurcation of bile duct

Ref: Robbins Pathologic Basic of Disease,SA, Vol 2/e p824

Klatskin tumor-Cholangiocarcinoma arising from bifurcation of bile duct.

- Klatskin tumor–Extra hepatic perihilar tumor.
- Located at junction of right and left hepatic ducts.
- 50–60% of all cholangiocarcinomas are perihilar.

49. Ans. a. It is premalignant *Ref: Robbins Pathologic Basic of Disease, SA, Vol 2/e p731*

Oral hairy leukoplakia–Hairy leukoplakia is a distinctive oral lesion on the later border of the tongue that is usually seen in immunocompromised patients and is caused by EBV.

- Associated with HIV.
- Microscopy shows hyperparakeratosis and acanthosis.

- Characteristic cells seen are–balloon cells.
- Leukoplakia is precancerous lesion but not oral hairy leukoplakia.

50. Ans. a. HPV *Ref: Robbins Pathologic Basic of Disease, SA, Vol 2/e p739*

Papillomas are benign neoplasms caused by HPV types 6 and11.

51. Ans. b. Prostate Ca *Ref: Robbins Pathologic Basis of Disease, SA, Vol 2/e p986,1207*

Mets to bone can be either blastic, lytic or mixed. Osteblastic metastases are characteristic of prostatic carcinoma. Osteolytic mets seen in: Ca Kidney, lung, melanoma, Cancers of GIT.

52. Ans. a. Kaposi sarcoma *Ref: Robbins Pathologic Basic of Disease, SA, Vol 1/e p518*

Kaposi sarcoma (KS) is a vascular neoplasm caused by human herpes virus 8 (HHV8).
The other 3 options are caused by EBV.

53. Ans. b. CD 8⁺ T-cells *Ref: Robbins Pathologic Basic of Disease, SA, Vol 1/e p361*

Please refer to this line from Robbins, The ATL's seen in the blood, characteristic of EBV infection are mainly EBV specific CD8+ cytotoxic T-cells,but also include CD16+ NK cells.

EBV–stimulates a B-cell response but the atypical lymphocytes seen in the blood are not B lymphocytes but CD8 T helper cells predominantly.

54. Ans. b. Delayed hypersensitivity *Ref: Robbins Pathologic Basis of Disease, SA, Vol 1/e p231*

Important points in transplant pathology.

The main reason for rejection of the donor tissue by the recipient are differences in HLA alleles.

The best tissue donor (for say kidney or heart) is always an identical twin.

- Hyperacute rejection (happens on operation table)–Mediated by complement and pre-existing antibodies.
- Acute rejection (happens in days)–Mediated by formed antibodies and T cells.
- Chronic rejection (takes months to years)–Mediated by T-cells.

55. Ans. b. Beta amyloid *Ref: Robbins Pathologic Basis of Disease, SA, Vol 1/e p257*

(A β) constitutes the core of cerebral plaques found in Alzheimer disease,as well as senile cerebral amyloidiosis where amyloid is deposited in the walls of the blood vessels.

56. Ans. c. Collagen 4 *Ref: Robbins Pathologic Basis of Disease, SA, Vol 1/e p206*

Table 6-3. Goodpasture syndrome is characterized by antibodies against basement membrane of glomeruli and alveoli.

57. Ans. c. ? *Ref: Robbins Pathologic Basis of Disease, SA, Vol 1/e p682*

The answer is sometimes in the question itself! Curschmann spirals represent mucus plugs extruded from subepithelial mucus gland ducts or bronchioles. Charcot leyden crystals are derived from a eosinophil protein called galectin-10.

58. Ans. C. Type 3 hypersensitivity reaction *Ref: Robbins Pathologic Basis of Disease, SA, Vol 1/e p207*

Lepra reaction–2 Types.

- Type 1 lepra reaction–Type 4 hypersensitivity
- Type 2 lepra reaction–Type 3 hypersensitivity.

59. Ans. a. Renal vessels *Ref: Robbins Pathologic Basis of Disease, SA, Vol 1/e p261*

- Kidney is the most common organ involved in amyloidosis.
- Most common site in kidney where amyloid gets deposited is the glomerulus.
- Amyloid also gets deposited in BM (basement membrane) causing 'thickened' BM. of the options provide A is the best choice.

60. Ans. c. Type 3 *Ref: Robbins Pathologic Basis of Disease, SA, Vol 1/e p207*

Type 3 hypersensitivity is synonymous with immune complex-mediated hypersensitivity.

- Localized immune complex deposition is called 'arthus reaction.'

61. Ans. c. Type 3 hypersensitivity reaction *Ref: Question above.*

62. Ans. a. Medullary Ca *Ref: Robbins Pathologic Basis of Disease, SA, Vol 1/e p259*

- Amyloid deposition is associated with medullary carcinoma of thyroid. The amyloid protein deposited is calcitonin (A cal).

63. Ans. c. Ribonucleoproteins *Ref: Robbins Pathologic Basis of Disease, SA, Vol 1/e p226*

90% of patients with sjogrens syndrome have antibodies directed against 2 RNA antigens SS-A(Ro) and SS-B(La).

64. Ans. a. Lymphocytes *Ref: Robbins Pathologic Basis of Disease, SA, Vol 1/e p227*

The earliest histological feature is perivascular and periductal lymphocytic infiltration of both the major and minor salivary glands.

Diseases with chronic inflammation which can eventually transform into a B-cell lymphoma.

- Sjogrens syndrome.
- Hashimotos thyroiditis.

65. Ans. d. Antigen processed by APC are recognized by CD 4+ T-Cells

Ref: Robbins Pathologic Basis of Disease, SA, Vol 1/e p191

Points relevant to APC's (Antigen presenting cells)

- The most important cell involved in presenting antigens to T-cells are dendritic cells.
- Production of antibodies does not require that the antigen is presented to B-lymphocytes. Nevertheless abs are generated by this mechanism too.
- A response to viruses and tumor cells is generated by NK cells first,hence option C is wrong.
- Antigen is presented via MHC-2 complexes this in turn generates a CD 4 T-lymphocytic response. Thus of all options provided D is the best.

66. Ans. b. Thymocytes whose T-Cell receptor bind with high affinity to self-antigens and MHC Complexes are Clonally deleted

Fundamentals of Immunology-Paul. Mature thymocytes can either express CD 4 or CD 8 but nor both. So it is clear that there is no possibility of double positivity of CD 4 and CD 8.

- B-cell precursors express IgM and IgD.
- The true statement is therefore thymocytes whose T-Cell receptor bind with high affinity to self-antigens and MHC Complexes are Clonally deleted.

67. Ans. c. New germ cell mutations in old fathers *Ref: Robbins Pathologic Basis of Disease, SA edition Vol 1 p140*

Features of AD disorders

- Both males and females are affected.
- Siblings have 50% chance of inheriting the disease if any one of the parents are affected.
- Incomplete penetrance and variable expressivity.

68. Ans. c. Nucleotide excision repair *Ref: Robbins Pathologic Basic of Disease, SA edition, Vol 1 p314*

- Xeroderma pigmentosa-disorder of DNA repair.
- In individuals with the disease exposure to UV rays cause pyrimidine dimers to accumulate preventing normal DNA replication.
- Several proteins are involved in 'DNA excision repair'.
- Mutation in any one can give rise to XP.

69. Ans. b. Antiphospholipid antibody syndrome *Ref: Robbins Pathologic Basic of Disease, SA edition Vol 1 p124*

Antiphospholipid antibody syndrome

- APLA is always acquired whether primay or secondary.
- Primary APLA–Absence of AI cause/Idiopathic.
- Secondary APLA–AI disease like SLE, drugs, Postimmunsuppression

70. Ans. a. Beta thalassemia *Ref: Robbins Pathologic Basic of Disease, SA edition Vol 1 p638*

Allelic heterogenecity is a phenomenon in genetics where in which mutations at the same locus by whatever mechanism cause a similar phenotype.

For example, Beta thalassemia can be caused by several different mutations in the beta globin gene.

71. Ans. b. Webbing of neck *Ref: Robbins Pathologic Basic of Disease, SA edition Vol 1 p164*

- Webbing of neck is a feature of Turners syndrome.
- Both Klinefelter and Turner syndrome involve sex chromosome mutations.

Klinefelter syndrome

- Karyotype: 47 XXY
- Caused by meiotic nondisjunction
- Common cause of male hypogonadism

- Lab diagnosis
  - Elevated FSH and LH
  - Low levels of testosterone
- Clinical findings
  - Testicular atrophy
  - Infertility due to azoospermia
  - Eunuchoid body habitus
  - High-pitched voice
  - Female distribution of hair
  - Gynecomastia.

72. Ans. a. Order of nucleotides *Ref: Robbins Pathologic Basic of Disease, SA edition Vol 1 p168 and Internet Sources Order of nucleotides within DNA is a sequence*

73. Ans. a. Fragile X syndrome *Ref: Robbins Pathologic Basic of Disease, SA edition vol 1 p168, Table 5-8.*

CGG repeat is found in Fragile X syndrome.

74. Ans. a. AR *Ref: Internet sources.*

75. Ans. a. Niemann-Pick's disease *Ref: Robbins Pathologic Basic of Disease, SA edition Vol 1 p153*

- Niemann-Pick's disease–inherited deficiency of spingomyelinase
- Concentric lamellelated myelin figures called 'Zebra bodies' which represent spingomyelin accumulation are seen on electron microscopy.

76. Ans. a. Autosomal dominant *Ref: Robbins Pathologic Basic of Disease, SA edition Vol 2 p1249*

The clinical features described ar compatible with Neurofibromatosis type 1. Not sure why they have described pregnancy in the question

Other lesions seen with NF 1 are:

- Lisch nodules–Iris hamartomas
- Optic nerve gliomas
- Cafe au lait spots.

77. Ans. ??

This is an unfair question. After extensive searching I have concluded all of the options provided are single gene disorders. In almost any question paper there will be controversial questions. Instead of brooding over questions such as these it is advised that students skip suck junk.

A single gene disorder is one which is inherited in a classic mendelian pattern of inheritance.

- Arrhythmogenic right ventricular cardiomyopathy–AD
- Hypertrophic cardiomyopathy–AD
- Dilated cardiomyopathy–AD in >50% cases
- Mitral valve prolapse–Mostly AD but AR inheritance also is described.

78. Ans. a. CD 34 *Ref: Robbins Pathologic Basic of Disease, SA edition, p590, Table 13-5*

Given below is not copy/paste of the table in Robbins–I have tabulated important makers used in flow cytometry for cancer diagnosis.

Antigen designation	Normal cellular distribution
CD 1	Thymocytes and Langerhans cells
CD 4	Helper T-cells
CD 8	Cytotoxic T-cells
CD 10	Pre B-cells and germinal center B-cells
CD 19	Pre B-cells and mature B-cells but not plasma cells
CD 20	EBV receptor, Mature B-cells and follicular dendritic cells
CD 64	Mature myeloid cells
CD 16	NK cells and granulocytes
CD 56	NK cells and granulocytes
CD 14	Monocytes
CD 34	Pluripotent stem cell
CD 45	LCA–Leucocyte common antigen present on all leukocytes

79. Ans. b. Alpha spectrin *Ref: Nelson and Robbins Pathologic Basis of Disease, SA edition, p632*

Hereditary spherocytosis: Salient points

- Normal lifespan of RBC–120 days in HS it is reduced by 10–20 days
- Not a fatal disorder–Splenectomy corrects the disease.
- Autosomal dominant disorder.
- Structural defect in Hereditary spherocytosis.
  - Ankyrin→ Most common
  - Band 3 → second most common

Lab tests

- Osmotic fragility test–Obsolete test–importance only in entrance exams.
- Normal MCH with increased MCHC

80. Ans. a. Nebulin *Ref: Robbins Pathologic Basis of Disease, SA edition, p632*

Nebulin has not been described as a cytoskeletal protein, in fact nebulin is a protein related to muscle (refer Ganong).

81. Ans. a, b, c and d

Ref: Dacie and Lewis, Practical hematology. Robbins Pathologic Basis of Disease, SA edition and Harrison's principles of internal medicine, 18/e, chapter 113, transfusion biology and therapy.

Microorganisms transmissable by transfusion-All options provided are transmissible through transfusion.

Viruses	Prions	Bacteria	Parasites
• Hepatitis viruses–A (rare), Band C • Hepatitis G–Blood borne pathogen. Hence can be transmitted through blood. (Rare) • HIV 1 and 2 • Human parvovirus B19. • CMV • EBV • HTLV 1 and 2 • Dengue (rare)	Creutzfeldt Jacob disease (CJD and variants)	• Treponema pallidum • Brucellosis • Bacterial contamination	• Malaria • Trypanasoma • Toxoplasma • Babesia • Leishmania

82. Ans. a. 5 days 20–24 deg Celsius *Ref: Dacie and Lewis, Practical hematology*

Platelets are stored in a platelet agitator @ 20–24 deg Celsius for 5 days

83. Ans. d. PGD2 *Ref: Robbins Pathologic Basis of Disease, SA edition, p84, Table 3–5*

- There should absolutely be no doubt that ADP and TXA2 are platelet aggregators.
- PGD2 is a vasodilator and its role in platelet aggregation is not described.

84. Ans. c. Schistocytes *Ref: Robbins Pathologic Basic of Disease SA edition p663–665*

- The best indicator of hemolysis on PS are schistocytes.
- Schistocytes are seen when RBC's are broken in the microcirculation when they try to negotiate through microthrombi for example, DIC, HUS or when they are mechanically broken by mechanical valves etc.

85. Ans. b. Familial hypercholesterolemia *Ref: Robbins Pathologic Basic of Disease, SA edition, p147*

- Hereditary hypercholesterolemia is a receptor disease that is consequence of a mutation in the gene encoding the receptor for LDL.
- Options Aand D are not receptor defects.
- Hemolysis can be seen in OptionA, C and D.
- Interestingly patients with inherited red cell membrane receptor defects have abnormal lipid profiles.

86. Ans. b. Reduced reticulocyte count *Ref: Robbins Pathologic Basic of Disease, SA edition, p638*

- Several crises can occur in SSA.
- Sequestration crisis–Occurs in children with intact spleens.
- Massive entrapment of sickle cells in the spleen leads to splenic enlargement, hypovolemia and shock.
- Reticulocyte increase is expected in hemolytic crisis and not in sequestration crisis where immature RBC's come out of the marrow to compensate for the hemolysis.

- Option A–Abdominal pain can be attributed to splenomegaly.
- Of all the options B is most inappropriate.

87. Ans. a. Hereditary Spherocytosis *Ref: Robbins Pathologic Basis of Disease, SA edition, p632*
Hereditary Spherocytosis–OFT is increased

88. Ans. a. Increased TIBC *Ref: Robbins Pathologic Basic of Disease, SA edition, p652*

- Increased TIBC is never a feature of anemia of chronic disease.
- Serum Iron can be normal early during course of the disease but eventually increases.

Iron studies–Table (Indispensible for any entrance not just JIPMER)

	Iron deficiency	AOCD	Thal. Minor	Sideroblastic
Serum. Iron	↓	↓	Normal	↑
TIBC	↑	↓	Normal	↓
% saturation	↓	↓	Normal	↑
Serum. Ferritin	↓	↑	Normal	↑

89. Ans. a. CD 55 *Ref: Robbins Pathologic Basic of Disease, SA edition, p643*
Lab tests for PNH

- Sucrose in vitro (sucrose lysis test): obsolete
- Acidosis in vitro (Ham's test): obsolete
- Flow cytometry is considered to be the 'Gold standard' for diagnosis of PNH now.
- Flow can detect small molecules CD 16 and Cd 66b for granulocytes.
- CD 55 and CD 59 for red cells and platelets.
- Flow cytometry is more sensitive than Ham's test.

90. Ans. a. Acquired sideroblastic anemia
The clinical history given correlates with classic microcytic hypochromic anemia or IDA.

- Acquired sideroblastic anemia is an iron overload condition and therefore either serum iron or serum ferritin should be elevated, so option A is out
- Folate deficiency causes megalobalstic anemia and has no role in the pathogenesis od IDA
- Most commonly it is failure to comply to iron therapy rather than inadequate iron dosage (unless a quack prescribes iron) that results in no improvement in Hb
- Please excuse no references for this!

91. Ans. a. HBS is caused by single base mutation *Ref: Robbins Pathologic Basic of Disease, SA edition, p635*
The option C for starters makes no sense and is eliminated. So is option D as the genes for alpha and beta chains are not present in the same chromosome.

- Consider option B-The predominant Hb in β Thalassemia major is Hb F and it carries a bad prognosis.
- In fact β Thalassemia major is the only thalassemia where Hb F is significantly increased.
- Remember that the dominant Hb in β Thalassemia minor is adult Hb($\alpha 2\beta 2$).
- Option B does not specify α or β thalassemia and is 'Vague'
- Option A is true as "Sickle cell anemia is caused by a point mutation in the 6th codon of beta globin chain ehich leads to replacement of a glutamate residue with a valine residue."

92. Ans. a. Spectrin *Ref: Robbins Pathologic Basis of Disease, SA edition, p632*

93. Ans. c. APTT
The clinical history describes a patient developing bruises following LMWH therapy.

- Basically the question is intended to test logical approach to bleeding disorders.
- The first step that should be done in assessment of bleeding disorder is determining the type of bleed, ie. whether petechia/purpura or echymosis /bruise.
- The first investigation if the patient has petechia/purpura would be a platelet count.
- Here the patient has a larger bleed a bruise, so some abnormality with clotting exists (coagulation factors) and the investigation of choice would be an APTT.
- Also bear in mind that heparin therapy used to be monitored by CT now APTT has replaced CT.
- BT is a good investigation to pin point if there is an abnormality with platelets.

94. Ans. b. Most hepatitis B carriers do not have detectable HbS antigen in serum

Ref: Essentials of hematology, Kawthalkar.

Transfusion associated hepatitis B

- Most common infection transmitted through transfusion is Hep B. followed by Hep C.
- Donor blood is usually screened for HBsAg, anti-HBc, anti-HCV.
- Most hepatitis B carriers do not have detectable HbS antigen in serum(prevalence is 1.5-4% in India) and that is the reason infected blood still reaches the patients.
- HBV DNA amplification by polymerase chain reaction should be ideally done on all donor units to eliminate the possibility of infected blood being transfused.

95. Ans. c. Vitamin C *Ref: Robbins Pathologic Basis of Disease, SA edition, p443*

The clinical history describes a chronic alcoholic with bleeding gums. Though thiamine deficiency is seen in alcoholics it has nothing to do with gum bleeds and petechiae. This is a good old case of scurvy.

96. Ans. a. EBV *Ref: Robbins, SA edition vol 1 p597*

Burkitt lymphoma is caused by EBV.

Types

- African(endemic); Sporadic; In HIV patients

Morphology:

- High mitotic index
- Starry sky pattern[Q]
- The neoplastic cells in Burkitt lymphoma have a similar morphology to blasts of ALL-L3
- These blasts posses vacuoles which are positive for Oil red O and Sudan black (fat stains)[Q].

Cytogenetics

- Translocation (8;14)[Q]
- Express IgM, CD19, CD20, CD10, BCL6
- All endemic tumors are infected with EBV

Clinical features

Endemic: Mass involving mandible and can involve kidneys, ovaries and adrenal glands

- Sporadic: Abdominal mass involving ileocaecum and peritoneum
- Rapidly progressive and can involve CNS
- Chemotherapy is the treatment of choice.

97. Ans. b. T(9,22) translocation *Ref: Harissons: Textbook of internal medicine, 19/e*

The most common leukemia in childhood is ALL.

Time and time again such questions have been repeated. Please memorize the prognosis criteria for both ALL and AML.

Prognostic factors in ALL

Good prognosis	Bad prognosis
• Age 2–10 years • Female sex • L1 cell • Peripheral blast count <1,00,000 • Pre B-cell phenotype • Absence of mediastinal mass • Hyperdiploidy or t(12;21) • Trisomy 4, 7 and 10	• Age <1 or >10 years • Male sex • L2 or L3 cell • Peripheral blast count >1,00,000 • Pre T-cell phenotype • Presence of mediastinal mass • Pseudodiploidy or t(9;22) or t(8;14) or t(4;11)

98. Ans. a. CML *Ref: Kawthalkar: Essentials of Hematology*

LAP or leukocyte alkaline phoshatase is increased in inflammatory condition such as bacterial infection, burns, pregnancy.

Leukocyte alkaline phosphatase (LAP) is found within white blood cells. White blood cell levels of LAP can help in the diagnosis of certain conditions.

- Higher levels are seen in polycythemia vera (PV), essential thrombocytosis (ET), primary myelofibrosis (PM), and theleukemoid reaction.

- Lower levels are found in CML in the chronic phase (During accelerated phase and blast crisis LAP levels increase) and PNH.

99. Ans. d. Erthyroleukemia *Ref: Robbins,SA edition Vol 1 p613, 616*

Erthyroleukemia is AML (M6) in the FAB classification

Important points are tabulated below

Class	Fab subtype	Morphology	Comments
AML, minimally differentiated	M0	Negative for myeloperoxidase; myeloid antigens detected on blasts by flow cytometry	
AML without maturation	M1	>3% of blasts positive for myeloperoxidase	Few Auer rods
AML with myelocytic maturation	M2	Full range of myelocytic maturation	Many Auer rods,t(8:21),good prognosis.Chloromas +
AML with promyelocytic maturation	M3	Promyelocytic leukemia	t(15:17), associated with DIC, Many Auer rods, responds to ATRA
AML with myelomonocytic maturation	M4	Myelocytic and monocytic differentiation	Nonspecific esterase-positive monoblasts
AML with monocytic maturation	M5	In M5 subtype, and promonocytes predominate in marrow and blood	Organomeggaly, lymphadeno pathy, gum hypertrophy associated. NSE +,older patients.
AML with erythroid maturation	M6a, M6b	Erythroid/myeloid subtype (M6a) defined by >50% dysplastic maturing erythroid precursors and >20% myeloblasts; pure erythroid subtype (M6b) defined by >80% erythroid precursors without myeloblasts	Erythroblasts are PAS +
AML with megakaryocytic maturation	M7	Blasts of megakaryocytic lineage predominate	Detected with antibodies against megakaryocyte-specific markers (GPIIb/IIIa or vWF). Often associated with marrow fibrosis. Most common AML in Down syndrome

100. Ans. a. Condensation of granules within cytoplasm

Ref: Robbins Pathologic Basic of Disease, SA edition, Vol 1 p613

- Auer rods–Needle like condensation of azurophilic granules.
- Maximum number of Auer rods are seen in acute promyelocytic leukemia or AML t(15:17).
- Dot like condensation of granules called 'phi granules' can also be seen in AML t(15:17).

101. Ans. a. APL *Ref: Robbins Pathologic Basic of Disease,SA edition, Vol 1 p614*

- ATRA is used in the treatment of APML, i.e. acute promyelocytic leukemia.
- Currently AMPL has the best prognosis.

102. Ans. d. Nodular sclerosis *Ref: Robbins, SA edition, Vol 1 p609, Table 13-8*

Reed **Hodgkin Lymphoma** Associated with BCL 2 translocation.

- Distinguished from other lymphomas by the presence of Reed Stenberg's cells in the background of non-neoplastic inflammatory cells

Nodular sclerosis RS cells: CD15+ CD30+ **EBV-** CD45-	Frequent ***lacunar cells***, occasional diagnostic R-S cells Background rich in T-cells, eosinophils, macrophages and plasma cells	Most common type (70%) more common in females **Excellent** prognosis
Mixed cellularity RS cells: CD15+ CD30+ 70% EBV +	Frequent mononuclear and **diagnostic R-S cells**, background rich in T-cells, macrophages, eosinophils and plasma cells	M>F, Biphasic incidence, Young adults and >50 Good prognosis

Lymphocyte rich RS cells: CD15+ CD30+ CD45- 40% EBV +	Frequent mononuclear and R-S cells, background rich in T-cells	Uncommon Good prognosis
Lymphocyte depletion RS cells: CD15+ CD30+ Most EBV +	Reticular variant: frequent R-S cell with paucity of background reactive cells	**Common in HIV** infected individuals and in developing countries
Lymphocyte predominance RS cells: CD15- CD30- CD20+ BCL6+ EBV-	Frequent ***L and H (popcorn) cell*** in a background of follicular dendritic cells and reactive B-cells	Young males with cervical or axillary lymphadenopathy Excellent prognosis

- Both HL and NHL present with painless enlargement of neck nodes.
- Cyclical high grade fever (Pel-Epstein fever).
- **Note:** CD15+ CD30+ positivity is seen in RS cells of all types except lymphocyte predominant type.

103. Ans. a. Burkitt's lymphoma *Ref: Robbins, Vol 1, 9/e p597*

t(8:14) is seen in Burkitt's lymphoma[Q]. The hallmark of follicular lymphoma is t(14:18)[Q].

104. Ans. a. T(8,14) *Ref: Robbins, Vol 1 9/e p597*

105. Ans. c. CD20 *Ref: Robbins, Vol 1 9/e p609*

106. Ans. a. Cytogenetics *Ref: Robbins, Vol 1 9/e p614*

Cytogeneti lies at the heart of prognostication of AML.

Risk Group Cytogenetic Abnormality.

- Low risk- inv(16), t(16;16), t(8;21), t(15;17)
- Intermediate Risk-Normal cytogenetics, +8, t(9;11); other chromosomal abnormalities

Poor Risk- 5, 5q-, -7, 7q-, 11q23 other than t(9;11), inv(3), t(3;3), t(6;9),

107. Ans. c. Interstital pneumonitis with foamy intra-alveolar exudates *Ref: Robbins, Vol 1 9/e p253*

Sternberg's surgical pathology.

- Alveolar spaces filled with pink, foamy amorphous material composed of proliferating fungi and cell debris
- Fungi are 4–6 microns, cup/boat shaped cysts
- Hyaline membranes and granulomatous response also can be seen with P. jiroveci pneumonia but of all the options provided 'C' is the best.

108. Ans. b. Kulchitsky (K) cells *Ref: Robbins, Vol 2 9/e p719*

Carcinoid tumor arises from neuroendocrine cells. Specialised neuroendocrine cells called "Kulchitsky cells", occurring in the epithelia lining the lumen of the digestive tract and the respiratory tract that release serotonin.

109. Ans. b. Tumorlet *Ref: Robbins, Vol 2 9/e p719*

Tumorlets–small, inconsequential, hyperplastic nests of neuroendocrine cells seen in areas of scarring and chronic inflammation.

110. Ans. b. Subclavian artery *Ref: Robbins, Vol 1, 9/e p508*

Takayasus Arteritis

- Granulomatous inflammation of the aorta and its major branches.
- Also known as pulseless disease–absent pulses in upper extremities.
- Characteristically involves the aortic arch.
- Though the carotid artery can also be involved, subclavian occlusion is commoner.

111. Ans. b. True aneurysm involves all 3 layers *Ref: Robbins, Vol 1, 9/e p501*

Saccular aneurysm does notinvolve all the 3 layers.

- Most common cause of aneurysms of abdominal aorta–Atherosclerosis.
- Most common site of atherosclerotic aneurysm–below renal artery bifurcation.
- Most common predisposing factor in aneurysms of ascending aorta–Hypertension.
- Most common part of aorta affected in Tertiary syphilis or Leutic aneurysms–Thoracic aorta.
- Mycotic aneurysms–Aneurysm ocuuring as a result of bacterial infection. The term 'mycotic' is a misnomer.
- In fact, Staphylococcus and Salmonella spp. are the two most commonly cultured organisms in mycotic aneurysms.

112. Ans. a. Left atrium *Ref: Robbins, Vol 1, 9/e p557, 558*

Leisons seen in RHD.

- Aschoff body :Area of fibrinoid necrosis and surrounded by macrophages, lymphocytes, and plasma cells
- Fibrinous pericarditis called 'bread and butter' pericarditis.
- Endocarditis:Involves mitral and aortic valves
- Fibrin vegetations along the lines of the closure
- MacCallum Plaques: Left Atrial endocardial thickening

113. Ans. a. Fibrinoid necrosis *Ref: Robbins, SA edition Vol 1 p490*

- Fibrinoid necrosis is a feature of malignant hypertension.
- With elevated blood pressure in malignant hypertension the following changes occur;
- Increase in smooth-muscle cells in a laminar configuration, which leads to total and subtotal occlusion of the vessels.
- The renal vessels demonstrate a concentric obliteration of arterioles (Onion skin fibrosis).
- These changes are part of hyperplastic arteriolosclerosis.
- The changes described in options B, C and D are seen in benign nephrosclerosis.

114. Ans. a. Chronic bronchitis *Ref: Robbins, Vol 2, 9/e p679*

Reid index is the increased ratio of thickness of the mucus gland layer to the thickness of the wall between the epithelium and cartilage. Normal Ried index is 0.4. The following microscopic features are observed in chronic bronchitis;

- Hypertrophy[Q] of bronchial mucous glands.
- Increased number of goblet cells[Q]
- Hyper secretion of mucus[Q]
- Thus increased Reid index is observed in chronic bronchitis.

115. Ans. b. Rhinoscleromatosis

Ref: Chapter 30 Histopathology Practical; pathology Review: by Dr. Sinhasan SP, PARAS Publications, 1/e

Rhinoscleromatosis–Miculicz cells and Russel bodies.

116. Ans. b. Rheumatic fever *Ref: Robbins, Vol 1, 9/e p557, 558*

117. Ans. c. Carcinoid syndrome does not manifest *Ref: Robbins, Vol 2, 9/e p*

Bronchial carcinoids

- Younger age group; age < 40
- Gross: polypoid intrabronchial mass–'collar button leison'
- Microscopy: small, round, uniform cells growing in nests (organoid pattern)
- EM: cytoplasmic dense core neurosecretory granules
- 10% of tumors cause carcinoid syndrome. But robbins states that these tumors have hardly secretory activity and metastasize only rarely.

118. Ans. d. Cardiac myxomas *Ref: Robbins, Vol 1, 9/e p576*

Cardiac myxoma

- Benign tumor usually arising within the left atrium near the fossa ovalis.
- Most common benign tumor in adults..
- Microscopyy: Stellate-shaped cells or spider cells within a myxoid background
- Complications-Tumor emboli and Ball-valve" obstruction of the valves.

119. Ans. a. Fatty streaks *Ref: Robbins, Vol 2 9/e p496*

The earliest change seen in atherosclerosis is a fatty streak. Even the blood vessels of infants can have fatty streaks.

120. Ans. a. Neutrophil *Ref: Robbins, Vol 2, 9/e p496*

Atherosclerosis is a chronic disease. Neutrophils are not involved in the pathogenesis of atherosclerosis.

121. Ans. a. Rheumatic carditis *Ref: Robbins, Vol 1, 9/e p557, 558*

122. Ans. a. PDA *Ref: Robbins Pathologic Basic of Disease, SA edition p535*

123. Ans. b. Type II pneumocytes *Ref: Robbins Pathologic Basic of Disease, SA edition p670*

124. Ans. a. CMV *Ref: Robbins Pathologic Basic of Disease, SA edition p496*

Herpes virus, CMV and Chlamydophilia pneumonia have been linked to atherosclerosis.

125. Ans. c. Fredreich ataxia *Ref: Robbins Pathologic Basic of Disease, SA edition p565*

DCM-Causes

- Idiopathic (majority of cases)
- Alcohol
- Drug related–driamycin (doxorubicin) and cocacine
- Viral myocarditis–Coxsackievirus B and enteroviruses
- Parasitic infections–chagas disease
- Pregnancy related.

126. Ans. c. Panacinar *Ref: Robbins Pathologic Basic of Disease, Vol 1, SA edition p675*

127. Ans. a. Fibrinoid necrosis *Ref: Robbins Pathologic Basic of Disease, Vol 1, SA edition p490*

128. Ans. a. Popliteal *Ref: Robbins Pathologic Basic of Disease, Vol 1, SA edition p501*

129. Ans. a. Decrease beta oxidation of fat *Ref: Robbins. SA ed Vol. 2 chapter 18 p844*

Mechanisms underlying fatty liver are:

- Decreased mitochondrial fatty acid β oxidation.
- Increassed endogenous fatty acid synthesis or enhanced delivery/mobilisation of fatty acids from periphery to liver.
- NADH ® Increase in free fatty acids(↑Tg's).
- In alcoholic fatty liver direct hepatotoxicity to alcohol also contributes to fatty liver.
- There is decreased catabolism of fatty acids. NADH when elevated inhibits FFA catabolism.

130. Ans. a. Eosinophilic infiltrates *Ref: Robbins, Vol 2, 9/e p*

Leisons seen with H. Pylori gastritis.

- Follicular gastritis and plasma cells in the lamina propria.
- Active inflammation if neutrophils present in glandular of surface epithelial layer.
- Intestinal metaplasia.
- Organism is a curved and spirochete like present along the mucus layer.

131. Ans. b. Leiomyoma *Ref: Robbins,Vol 2, 9/e p758*

- The most common beingn tumor of esophagus is leiomyoma.
- High incidence and multiple tumors are seen in MEN 1.

132. Ans. c. Central vein *Ref: Robbins, Vol 2, 9/e p822*

From a metabolic perspective the liver is composed of hexagonal units called lobules. The central structure in the hepatic lobule is the central vein. Necrosis around the cental vein is thereby termed centrilobular. The area around the central vein corresponds to Zone 3–least oxygenated zone.

133. Ans. c. Prognosis is bad *Ref: Robbins, Vol 2, 9/e p873*

Fibrolamellar carcinoma

- Young males and females (20–40 yrs)
- Not associated with cirrhosis or HBV
- Better prognosis
- Presents with large, hard scirrhous tumor with fibrous bands coursing through it
- Encapsulated
- Alpha fetoprotein not elevated.

134. Ans. c. Cholangiocarcinoma *Ref: Robbins, Vol 2, 9/e p860*

- Primary sclerosing cholangitis is an autoimmune condition characterized by progressive inflammatory and sclerosing destruction of intra and extrahepatic bile ducts.
- Biliary intraepithelial neoplasia can occur in cases of PSC and eventually cholangiocarcinoma can develop.

135. Ans. a. NASH is a risk factor *Ref: Robbins, Vol 2, 9/e p870*

- Chronic liver disease is the greatest risk factor for development of HCC.
- OCP's are implicated in Hepatocellular adenoma.
- NAFLD is a precursor lesion implicated in HCC.

136. Ans. a. Microcytic anemia *Ref: Robbins, Vol 2, 9/e p763*

- H.pylori infection most often presents as a predominantly antral gastritis. This is in contrast to autoimmune gastritis which spares the antrum.
- H.pylori gastritis–Microcytic hypochromic anemia.
- Autoimmune gastritis → Vitamin B12 deficiency → Megaloblastic anemia.

137. Ans. c. Antrum *Ref: Robbins, Vol 2, 9/e p772*

Gastric adenocarcinoma

- Most common malignancy of the stomach.
- Most common site–Antrum.
- Lesser curvature is involved more than the greater curvature.
- Though lesser curvature is given amongst the options provided. The best option is 'C'.

138. Ans. a. Longitudinal tears in lower 1/3 esophagus *Ref: Robbins, Vol 2, 9/e p754*

- Mallory Weiss tears are described as roughly linear lacerations which are longitudinally oriented ranging from few millimeters to several centimeters.
- MW tears occur in the distal third of esophagus usually crossing the GE junction.

139. Ans. d. Antrum *Ref: Robbins, Vol 2, 9/e p772*

140. Ans. d. Cholestasis *Ref: Robbins, Vol 2, 9/e p837*

Cholestasis is described as a feature of acute hepatitis and not chronic hepatitis.

Changes seen in chronic hepatitis

- Chronic persistent hepatitis: Inflammation confined to portal tracts
- Fatty change. especially marked with hepatitis C.
- Chronic active hepatitis: Inflammation spills into the parenchyma, causing an interface hepatitis[Q] (piecemeal necrosis of limiting plate).
- Necrosis may extend from one portal tract to another–bridging necrosis[Q].
- Hepatitis B often has "ground glass" hepatocytes (cytoplasmic HBsAg[Q])
- Fibrosis around portal tracts or periportal fibrosis[Q]. Periportal fibrosis is indicative of irreversible injury[Q].
- Cirrhosis,

141. Ans. a. Primary biliary cirrhosis *Ref: Robbins, Vol 2, 9/e p858*

AMA are seen in PBC.

142. Ans. a. Transverse ulcer *Ref: Robbins, Vol 1, 9/e p374*

- The intestinal ulcers seen in TB are classically transverse ulcers.
- The ulcers in seen in typhoid are longitudinal, caused due to ulceration of the Peyer's patches.

143. Ans. c. Hypoglycemia *Ref: Robbins, Vol 2, 9/e p887*

- There is no doubt that elevated serum amylase and lipase are noted with acute pancreatitis.
- The first enzyme to rise is serum amylase (24 hrs) followed by lipase (72 hrs).
- Hypocalcemia is also described in reliable texts and hypocalcemia is attributed to the increased formation of calcium soaps (dystrophic calcification).
- Glycosuria occurs in 10% of the cases. Hypoglycemia has not been described in reliable texts like Robbins, Merck Manual, Wallachs' etc. Thus though theroritically hypoglycemia can occur because of insulin release from an inflamed gland it is not the option to be selected in exam!

144. Ans. c. Biopsy and Culture *Ref: Robbins, Vol 2, 9/e p887*

RUT (rapid urease test), seology and stool antigen detection have more than 90% sensitivity in the detection of H.pylori. However 100% sensitivity is expected with biopsy and culture, demonstrating the organism with special stains like Giemnase (not giemsa), Warthin Starry, etc.

145. Ans. b. Cowden syndrome *Ref: Robbins, Vol 2, 9/e p806*

Syndrome	Mean age at presentation	Mutated genes	GI lesions	Extra GI manifestations
Juvenile polyposis	< 5	SMAD, BMPR1A TGF-β	Risk of gastric, SI, colonicand pancreatic adenoCA	Congenital malformations, digital clubbing

Contd...

Contd...

Syndrome	Mean age at presentation	Mutated genes	GI lesions	Extra GI manifestations
Peutz-Jeghers polyps	10–15	STK 11, AMP kinase related pathway.	Arborizing polyps; Small intestine > Colon > Stomach; Colonic Adeno Ca	Risk of Ca pancreas, breast, lung, ovary; pigmented macules
Cowden syndrome	<15	PTEN (Chr 10), PI3K/ AKT	Multiple hamartomas involving organs derived from all the 3 germinal layers	Facial trichilemmomas[Q] Acral keratoses; Oral papilloma Risk of breast and thyroid cancers
Cronkhite-Canada syndrome	>50	Non hereditary, unknown cause	Hamartomatous polyps throughout the GI	Ectodermal anomalies like nail atrophy, skin pigmentation and alopecia
Tuberous sclerosis		TSC1, TSC2	Hamartomatous polyps	Mental retardation, epilepsy, Renal angiomyolipoma.
Familial adenomatous polyposis (FAP) syndrome	10–15	APC mutation	Multiple adenomas	Congenital retinal pigment epithelium hypertrophy
Turcot syndrome	10–15	APC mutation	Colonic polyps	CNS tumors (medulloblastomas; glioblastomas)

146. Ans. b. Levels are increased in fatty liver *Ref: Interpretation of diagnostic tests, Wallach 8/e p51, 52*

- GGT is a membrane bound enzyme in decreasing order of abundance in liver, proximal renal tubules, brain, prostate and pancreas.
- GGT generally parallels changes in serum ALP, LAP and 5 nucleotidase.
- Not very sensitive in hepatitis but last enzyme to return to normal in acute hepatitis.
- Elevated in fatty liver parallels AST and ALT.
- GGT is elevated in the absence of liver metastasis especially melanoma, carcinoma of the breast and lung. Highest levels in RCC.

147. Ans. c. PSGN *Ref: Robbins, SA edition Vol 2 p909*

Complete recovery in > 95% of cases in children is the rule in PSGN.

Acute post–streptococcal glomerulonephritis (PSGN)

- Most common cause of nephritic syndrome in children[Q].
- Occurs 2-4 weeks after a streptococcal infection of the throat or skin.
- Organism: β–hemolytic group A streptococci[Q]
- May be caused by other bacteria, viruses, and parasites and systemic diseases (SLE[Q] and polyarteritis nodosa [PAN[Q]])
- Laboratory studies
  - Elevated antistreptolysin[Q] (ASO) titers
  - Low serum complement[Q]
- Light microscopy
  - Hypercellular glomeruli with neutrophils and monocytes.
  - Red cell casts in the renal tubules (nephritic syndrome).[Q]
- Immunofluorescence: Granular deposits of IgG, IgM, and C3 throughout the glomerulus[Q]
- Electron microscopy: Subepithelial (humps[Q]) immune complex deposits.

148. Ans. a. Nephrogenic rests *Ref: Robbins, SA edition Vol 1, p452*

Wilms Tumor

- Accounts for 85% of all pediatric tumor.
- Presentation before 10 years of age.
- Nephrogenic rests are considered as precursor lesions from which nephroblastoma can develop.

149. Ans. a. von Hippel Lindau syndrome *Ref: Robbins, SA edition Vol 2, p1317*

Von-Hippel Lindau disease
- Autosomal dominant
- Gene located on chromosome 3p
- Hemangioblastomas of the CNS and cysts involving the pancreas, liver and kidneys are seen.
- Patients have a predisposition to developing RCC.
- Hemangioblastomas are seen in the CNS and retina.

150. Ans. c. 11p13 *Ref: Robbins, SA edition, Vol 1 p452*

Wilms tumor (nephroblastoma)
- Peak age: 2–5 years
- Risk factors
  - WAGR syndrome–Wilms tumor, aniridia, genital anomalies, and mental retardation
  - Beckwith–Wiedemann syndrome
  - Denys Drash syndrome
- Tumor suppressor genes

1. WT-1 (11P13)
2. WT-2 (11P15)

- Presents as a large abdominal mass
- Microscopy–Triphasic tumor
  - Metanephric blastema
  - Epithelial elements (immature glomeruli and tubules)
  - Stroma.

151. Ans. d. PAF *Ref: Internet sources*

Mesangial cell contaction induced by endothelin is mediated by release of PAF.

152. Ans. a. Albumin *Ref: Robbins, SA edition, Vol 2 p900*

- The permeability characteristics of the glomerular filtration barrier allow discrimination among various protein molecules, depending on their size (the larger the less permeable) and charge (the more cationic, the more permeable).
- This is important in the virtual exclusion of albumin from the filtrate as albumin is an anionic molecule.

153. Ans. c. CD 71 *Ref: http://www.ncbi.nlm.nih.gov/pubmed/14691748*

154. Ans. b. Nodular glomerulosclerosis *Ref: Robbins, SA edition, Vol 2 p939*

Nodular glomerulosclerosis seen in DM is also called Kimmelstiel–Wilson disease^{Q} or 'Christmas ball 'disease.

Diabetic nephropathy manifestations
- Renal artery atherosclerosis^{Q}.
- Hyaline arteriolosclerosis of afferent and efferent arteriole ^{Q} s.
- Diffuse glomerulosclerosis

1. Nephritic syndrome ^{Q}.
2. Increased mesangial matrix and mesangial proliferation ^{Q}.
3. Thickened basement membrane ^{Q}

- Nodular glomerulosclerosis (Kimmelstiel–Wilson disease ^{Q})
  - Nephrotic syndrome.
  - Nodular PAS (+) deposits of mesangial matrix ^{Q}.
  - Thickened basement membranes ^{Q}.
- Pyelonephritis and necrotizing papillitis ^{Q}.
- Renal failure ^{Q}.

155. a. Crescent formation *Ref: Robbins, SA edition Vol 2 p939*

IgA nephropathy (Berger's disease) presents with recurrent gross hematuria ^{Q} in children and young adults following a respiratory infection ^{Q} often.
- Hematuria is a feature of nephritic syndrome. Please refer table above.
- The rest of the options provided present as nephritic syndrome.
- Associated with celiac sprue and Henoch–Schonlein purpura Q

156. Ans. d. HSP nephritis *Ref: Robbins, SA edition Vol 2, p939*

Rapidly progressive glomerulonephritis (RPGN)

- Synonym: Crescentic glomerulonephritis
- Clinical feature: Rapid progression to severe renal failure in weeks or months

Rapidly progressive (crescentic) glomerulonephtitis-Classification

Type I RPGN (anti-GBM antibody)	Type II RPGN (immune complex)	Type III RPGN (pauci-immune)
• Idiopathic Q • Good pasture syndrome Q	• Post infectious Q • SLE Q • IgA Q nephropathy • HSP Q	• Antineutrophil Cytoplasmic antibodies Q • Wegener granulomatosis Q • PAN Q

- Light microscopy
  - Hypercellular glomeruli
  - Crescent formation in bowman's space
  - Crescents are composed of proliferating parietal epithelial cells Q, monocytes and macrophages.
- Immunofluorescence
  - Variable
  - May show granular or linear deposits of immunoglobulin and complement
- Electron microscopy
  - Variable
  - May or may not have electron–dense deposits
  - GBM disruption and discontinuity is commonly seen
- Prognosis: Poor with rapid progression to acute renal failure and endstage renal disease

157. Ans. a. Lupus nephritis *Ref: Robbins, Vol 1, 9/e p224*

Subendothelial immune complex deposits may create a circumferential thickening of the capillary wallforming 'wire loop' structures on microscopy.

158. Ans. b. Microscopic polyangitis *Ref: Robbins, Vol 2, 9/e p940*

- Pauci-immune is a general term used to refer any form of vasculitis that is associated with minimal evidence of hypersensitivity upon immunofluorescence and a lack of anti-GBM antibody.
- Pauci-immune glomerulonephritis is seen in Churg-Strauss syndrome and microscopic polyangitis.

159. Ans. a. Capillary wall thickening *Ref: Robbins, Vol 1, 9/e p224*

160. Ans. c. Severe renal dysfunction is an indication for biopsy *Ref: Robbins, SA edition, Vol 2, p909*

- Though most children with PSGN recover completely some may progress to CRF.
- Renal biopsy is an indication in cases where recovery does not occur
- Low complement levels are noted in PSGN especially C3 levels.
- C2 and C4 may be low to start with but eventually return to normal.
- Hematuria may take months to recover in PSGN, sometimes may take 3 months.
- Hyperlipidemia/hypertriglyceridemia is a feature of nephrotic syndrome and not PSGN.

161. Ans. b. Nodular glomerulosclerosis *Ref: Robbins, SA edition Vol 2 p939*

Nodular glomerulosclerosis seen in DM is also called Kimmelstiel–Wilson is characteristic of DM. Though hyaline arteriolosclerosis of afferent and efferent arterioles can be seen in DM, nodular glomerulosclerosis is more specific.

162. Ans. d. White matter *Ref: Robbins, SA edition Vol 2, p1277*

Negri bodies are described in all the options provided.

- Negri bodies are round or oval inclusions within the cytoplasm of nerve cells of animals infected with rabies. They are most frequently seen in pyramidal cells of Ammon's horn in Hippocampus and Purkinje cells of the cerebellum.
- They are also seen in the cells of the medulla (brain stem) and various other ganglia including basal ganglia. Negri bodies are also seen in the neurons of salivary glands and tongue.

163. Ans. a. Single file pattern *Ref: Robbins, SA edition Vol 2, p1065*

- The characteristic histologic feature of lobular carcinoma of the breast is "Indian file pattern".
- This refers to the battle formation of red Indians in a single row.

164. Ans. a. Vulva *Ref: Robbins, SA edition Vol 2, p999*

- Extramammary Pagets disease presents as erythematous patches on the skin of genital organs.
- Vulva is the most common site to be invovlved in extra mammary pagets disease.
- Malignant cells are positive for Alcian blue, PAS, mucicarmine and cytokeratin 7.

165. Ans. b. MacCune Albright syndrome *Ref: Robbins, SA edition Vol 2, p1206*

MacCune Albright syndrome

- Mono-ostotic or polyostotic fibrous dysplasia[Q].
- Café au lait spots[Q].
- Precocious puberty due to endocrinopathy.

166. Ans. d. Arise from arachnoid layer *Ref: Robbins, SA edition Vol 2 p1314*

Meningioma arises from the arachnoid cap cells also known as meningothelial cells.

167. Ans. a. Glioblastoma *Ref: Robbins, SA edition Vol 2 p1308*

Pseudopalisading necrosis is a feature of GBM (glioblastoma multiforme).

168. Ans. a. Hyperparathyroidism *Ref: Robbins, SA edition Vol 2. p1191*

Three leisons have been described in the bone in hyperparathyroidism:

- Osteopoeosis.
- Brown tumors–Bone loss predisposes to microfracutes and secondary hemorrhages that elicit an influx of macrophages and an ingrowth of reparative fibrous tissue, creating a mass of reactive tissue, known as brown tumor.
- Osteitis fibrosa cystica.

169. Ans. c. Occurs in young women *Ref: Robbins, SA edition Vol 2, p1191*

- Both osteolytic and osteoblastic activity occur in Pagets disease.
- Individuals with Pagets disease are at risk of developing benign lesions like giant cell tumor, giant cell reparative granuloma and extraosseous masses of hematopoietic tissue.
- Osteosarcoma and fibrosarcoma are 2 dreaded complications of Pagets disease.
- Pagets disease occurs in individuals more than 50 years of age and is more common in males.

170. Ans. a. von Hippel Lindau syndrome *Ref: Robbins, SA edition Vol 2 p1191*

von Hippel Lindau disease–Associated lesions

- Pheochromocytoma
- Paraganglioma
- Renal cell carcinoma
- Hemangioblastoma
- Pancreaticendocrine neoplasm.

171. Ans. a. Hemangioma *Ref: Robbins, SA edition Vol 2, p1191*

The most common tumor of pineal gland is germinoma.

172. Ans. b. Chromium

Glucose intolerance can occur with chromium deficiency in patients who are on long term total parenteral nutrition.

173. Ans. b. Fasting plasma glucose 135 mgs/dl *Ref: Chapter 13, Interpretation of Diagnostic Tests–Wallach, p702*

The following are the criteria for diagnosis of DM in nonpregnant adults.

- Random plasma glucose >200 mg/dl when there are classical symptoms.
- Fasting blood glucose >126 mg/dl.
- 2 hour plasma glucose > 200 mg/dl after 75 G glucose load.
- Any of the above must be confirmed the subsequent day.

Of the options provided B seems to the best.

174. Ans. a. Yolk sac tumor *Ref: Robbins, SA edition Vol 2, p977*

- Call-Exner bodies = Granulosatheca cell tumor

- Reinke crystalloids = Hilus cell tumor (pure leydig cell tumor)
- Schiller Duval bodies = Endodermal sinus tumor
- A. Robbins, Vol 2, 9/e p1294

175. Ans. a. Alpha synuclein *Ref: Robbins, Vol 2 9/e p1294*

These are single or multiple, cytoplasmic, eosinophilic, round to elongated inclusions that often have a dense core surrounded by a pale halo. Ultrastructurally, Lewy bodies are composed of fine filaments, densely packed in the core but loose at the rim; these filaments are composed of α-synuclein.

176. Ans. d. Omplement system *Ref: Robbins, Vol 1 9/e p89*

The clinical history describes apatient with Niesseia meningitis and the individual described has a complement deficiency and hence he is not able to form a bactericidal MAC against Niesseria.

High yield points that can be asked as MCQ's

Guide to special stain

To demonstrate	Method	Result
Acid fast bacilli	Ziehl Neelson	AFB-bright red; other tissue pale blue
Amebae	Heidenhain's iron hematoxylin	Amebae-black
Amyloid	Congo red Crystal violet	Amyloid-pale pink Nuclei-blue Amyloid magenta
Argentaffin	Masson fontana (also melanin)	Argentaffin-black Background-pink
Bacteria	Brown and Brenn	Grm +ve blue Gram –ve red Background-yellow
Bile	Stein's	Bile emerald green
Calcium	von Kossa Alizarin Red	Calcium-black Calcium-orange red
Connective tissue	Masson trichrome	Muscle-red Collagen-blue or green Nuclei black
Elastic tissue	Vehoeff's van Gieson's	Elastic tissue-Blac Muscle-yellow Collagen red
DNA	Feulgen	DNA-red Background-green
Fat	Frozen section Oil red 0, Sudan black, Sudan 3.	Fat-orange red Nuclei-blue
Fibrin	Mallory's phosphotungstic acid Hemotoxylin	Fibrin-blue Nuclei-blue Collagen-brownish red
Fungi	Gomori's Methenamine silver PAS	Fungi-black Background-green PAS +ve–red
Glycogen	Periodic acid Schiff-PAS	Rose to red
DNA and RNA	Methyl green–pyronin	DNA-green RNA-red
Hemosiderin	Perl's reaction	Hemosiderin-blue Background-pink
Mast cells	Toluidine blue (MCQ)	Mast cell granules violet to pink

Contd...

Contd...

To demonstrate	Method	Result
Mucin	Meyer's Muci-Carmine	Mucin-deep rose to red Nuclei-blue to black
Muscle	Masson trichrome	Muscle-red Collagen green or blue
Myelin sheath	Luxo fast blue	Myelin sheath-blue
Reticulin	Gordon and sweets	Reticulin fibre-black
Spirochetes	Levaditi	Spirochaetes-black Background-yellow
Astrocytes	Cajal's gold sublimate	Astrocytes and their processes-black
Basement membrane in kidney biopsies	John's silver methenamine	Basement membrane-black Background-light brown

Structures-AFB positivity

Mycobacterium tuberculosis	Oocyst of C.parvum	Sarcocystis
Mycobacterium leprae	Oocyst of Cyclospora	Sperm head
Atypical mycobacteria	Oocyst of Isospora	Hair shaft
Nocardia	Hydatid hooklet	Bacterial spores
Rhodococcus	Gordona	Tsukamurella
Legionella micdadei	T. solium egg	Schistosoma hematobium egg

Narrow spectrum fungal stains
- India ink–Cryptococcus
- Mucicarmine–Cryptococcus
- Fontana masson–Cryptococcus
- Congo red–Blastomyces.
- Wright–Histoplasma.

Patterns in histopathology

Pattern	Tumor
Cribriform	Adenoid cystic carcinoma
Biphasic	Synovial Sarcoma
Herring bone	Fibrosarcoma
Hobnail	Angiosarcoma
Indian file pattern	Lobular Ca. breast.
Storiform	Malignant fibrous histiocytoma and dermatofibrosarcoma protuberans.
Syncitial	Meningioma
Reticular	Yolk sac tumor
Trabecular	Oncocytoma

Some bodies and appearances
- Charcot Bouchard aneurysms–Hypertension
- Negri bodies–Rabies
- Hirano bodies–Alzheimer's disease
- Glomeruloid bodies–Glioblastoma multiforme
- Amphicytes–Ataxia telangiectasia
- Rosenthal fibers–Pilocytic astrocytoma, Alexander disease

- Lafora bodies–Myoclonic epilepsy
- Spinal muscular atrophy–Panfascicular atrophy
- Syphilis–Ghost vessels in cornea
- Flexner Wintersteiner rosettes (True rosettes)–Retinoblastoma and Neuroblastoma
- Homer Wright rosettes (False rosettes)–Ewing's sarcoma and Ependymoma

Picks disease	• Walnut brain • Knife edge appearance of brain
Mitochondrial myopathies	• Ragged red fibres • Parking lot inclusions
Dermatomyositis	• Grotton lesion • Lilac or heliotrope discoloration of upper eyelids • Perifascicular atrophy
Pelizalius Merzbacher disease	• Tigroid appearance of cerebral hemisphere

Serum tumor markers

- Intermediate filaments

Marker	Cell of origin	Tumors
Cytokeratin	Epithelial cells	Carcinomas
Vimentin	Mesenchymal cells	Sarcomas
Desmin	Smooth muscle/striated muscle	Leiomyosarcoma
Glial fibrillary protein	Glial cells	Glioma
S100	Neurons	Schwannoma Melanoma

- Enzymes

Enzyme	Cell of origin	Tumors
NSE (Neuron specific enolase)	Neurons	Neuroblastoma
Placental alkaline phosphatase	Seminiferous tubules	Seminoma
Prostatic acid phosphatase	Prostate	Prostate cancer

- Hormones

Hormones	Cell of origin	Tumors
Beta human chorionic gonadotropin (hCG)	Syncitiotrophoblasts	Choriocarcinoma
Calcitonin	"C" cells of the thyroid	Medullary carcinoma of the thyroid
Estrogen/Progesterone	Ovary, Breast	Ovarian tumors, Breast carcinomas

- Immunoglobulins

Immunoglobulins	Cell of origin	Tumors
Factor 8 Antigen	Endothelial cells	Angiosarcoma
Epithelial membrane antigen (EMA)	Arachnoid cap cells	Meningioma
PSA	Prostate	Prostate cancer
Carcinoembryonic antigen (CEA)	Oncofetal antigen secreted by embryonic cells	Carcinomas of the lung, pancreas, stomach, breast, and colon
CA-125	Oncofetal antigen secreted by embryonic cells	Ovarian cancer
CA19-9	Oncofetal antigen secreted by embryonic cells	Pancreatic cancer

QUESTIONS 2015

1. **Ring like enhancement with frontal lobe involvement with areas of necrosis:**
   a. Pilocytic astrocytoma
   b. Glioblastoma multiforme
   c. Meningioma
   d. Medulloblastoma
2. **First active cells in healing after tissue injury:**
   a. Mast cells
   b. Macrophages
   c. Lymphocytes
   d. Platelet
3. **Which are activated in apoptosis?**
   a. Caspases
   b. Oligonucleases
   c. Lipases
   d. Amylase
4. **Which of the following is a tumor supressor gene?**
   a. RAS b. Rb
   c. Myc d. Bcr
5. **Benzathine pencillins was infused to a child, after 2nd dose hypotension etc reactions develops. Which type of hypersensitivity?**
   a. Type 1
   b. Type 2
   c. Type 3
   d. Type 4
6. **A 50 years old lady with irregular overy massive ascites with palpable mass in right. Iliac fossa tumor marker?**
   A. CEA
   B. a-FP
   C. CA 19–9
   D. CA 125
7. **Polygenic inheritance seen in:**
   a. Huntington
   b. Penred syndrome
   c. Fragile X-syndrome
   d. Ankylosing spondylitis
8. **Incidence of which cancer increases in AIDS patient?**
   a. Squamous cell ca of esophagus
   b. Anaplastic ca of thyroid
   c. Basal cell Ca skin
   d. B-cell non-Hodgkin's lymphoma

ANSWERS AND EXPLANATIONS

1. **Ans. b. Glioblastoma multiforme** *Ref: Robbins Pathologic Basis of Disease, SA edition, Vol 2, p1308*
   Glioblastoma multiforme
   High grade CNS tumor (WHO–Grade 4)
   Primary: Tumor arises denovo.
   Secondary: Younger individuals.
   - Associated with genetic mutations
   - EGFR mutation in chromosome 7
   - IDH1 mutation
   - Del P 53.

   H/P–palisading necrosis
   - Glomeruloid bodies–represent vascular proliferation

   Ring like contrast enhancement is seen on imaging with GBM.
2. **Ans. c. Lymphocytes** *Ref: Robbins Pathologic Basis of Disease, SA edition, Vol 1, p101, Internet sources.*
   - Whenever there is tissue injury there is simultaneous injury to the vasculature present in the tissue as well.
   - The events of hemostasis and repair are closely intert wined.
   - Of the options provided platelet is the best answer, though macrophages have a central role in repair by clearing offending agents and dead tissue, providing growth factors for the proliferation of various cells, and secreting cytokines that stimulate fibroblast proliferation and connective tissue synthesis and deposition.
   - Lymphocytes are not required for the initiation of wound healing.

- The role of platelet rich fibrin in healing has been emphasized in recent times and in fact is being used in maxillofacial surgery.

3. Ans. c. Lipases *Ref: Robbins Pathologic Basis of Disease, SA edition, Vol 1, p55*

Activation of caspases is critical for apoptosis to be effected.

4. b. Rb *Ref: Robbins Pathologic Basis of Disease, SA edition, Vol 1, p291, Table7-7*

Tumor suppressor genes belong to the following classes:

- Inhibitors of mitogenic signaling pathways. For example, APC, NF1, NF2, PTEN.
- Inhibitors of cell cycle progression. For example, RB, CDKN2A.
- Inhibitors of pro growth programs of angiogenesis and metabolism. For example,VHL, STK11, SDHB, SDHD.
- Inhibitors of invasion and metastasis. For example, CDH 1
- Enablers of genomic stability. For example, TP53.
- DNA Repair factors. For example, BRCA1, BRCA2, MSH2, MLH1.
- Unknown mechanisms. For example, WT1, MEN1

5. Ans. a and b *Ref: Robbins Pathologic Basis of Disease, SA edition, Vol 1, p201,Table6-1*

Development of hypersensitivity on re-exposure to previously sensitized antigen is the classic mechanism in Type 1 hypersensitivity.

Type	Immune mechanisms	Histopathological leisons	Prototypical disorders
Type 1 hypersensitivity	Production of IgE antibody → immediate release of vasoactive amines and other mediators from mast cells → later recruitment of inflammatory cells.	Vascular dilatation,edema and smooth muscle contraction,mucus production, tissue injury and inflammation.	Anaphylaxis; allergies; bronchial asthma.
Type 2 hypersensitivity	Production of IgG,IgM → binds to antigen on target cell or tissue → phagocytosis or lysis of target cell by activated complement or Fc receptors; recruitment of leukocytes.	Phagocytosis and lysis of cells; inflammation;in some diseases functional derangements without cell or tissue injury (For example, Myasthenia gravis)	Autoimmune hemolytic anemia, Goodpasteur's syndrome.
Type 3 hypersensitivity	Deposition of antigen-antibody complexes → complement activation → recruitment of leukocytes by com	Inflammation,necrotising vasculitis (fibrinoid necrosis)	SLE,Serum sickness, Some forms of glomerulonephritis; Arthus reaction.
Type 4 hypersensitivity	Activated T lymphocytes → (1) release of cytokines (2)T cell mediated cytotoxicity	Perivascular cellular infiltrates; edema; granuloma formation; cell destruction	Contact dermatitis; multiple sclerosis; Type 1 DM, TB, Saecoidiosis.

6. Ans. d. CA 125 *Ref: Wallach's Interpretation of diagnostic tests 9/e p90*

CA stands for cancer antigen. Ca 125 is expressed on the surface of ovarian cancer cells and is used as a tumor marker in ovarian Ca diagnosis.

The history suggests a ovarian mass which is probably cancerous.

Cancer antigen	Derived from/nature	Uses
CA 15–3	Epithelial mucin	Marker for breast carcinoma Also increased in lung, ovarian, colorectal and liver Ca.
CA 19–9	Modified Lewis blood group antigen	Ca. pancreas (80%), hepatobiliary Ca (22-51%), gastric Ca (42%), Colon Ca (20%). Increased in cirrhosis, cholangitis, pancreatitis and hepatitis.
CA 27.29	Monoclonal ab to glycoprotein Muc 1	Increased in colon,gastric, hepatic, pancreatic, ovarian and pancreatic Ca. Benign conditions–Breast, liver, kidney and ovarian disorders.

Contd...

Contd...

Cancer antigen	Derived from/nature	Uses
CA 125	Glycoprotein present of the surface of ovarian cancer cells	Fallopian tube tumors (100%), nonmucinous epithelial ovarian cancer (85%), cervical adenocarcinoma (83%), Endometrial Ca (50%),Trophoblastic tumors (45%), NHL (20%), Cirrhosis (66%)

7. Ans. d. Ankylosing spondylitis *Ref: Robbins Pathologic Basis of Disease, SA edition, Vol 2, p1213*

- Polygenic inheritance refers to inheritance of a phenotypic characteristic that is attributable to 2 or more genes and can be measured quantitatively.
- Approximately 90% of patients with ankylosing spondylitis are HLA B 27 positive.
- Associations have been found with IL 23 receptor gene also.
- Huntington disease is a autosomal dominant disease.
- Penred syndrome is inherited in an autosomal recessive pattern.
- Fragile X syndrome as the name suggests is X linked.

8. Ans. d. *Ref: Robbins Pathologic Basis of Disease, SA edition, Vol 1, p254*

- Lymphomas occur with a markedly increased rate in individuals with AIDS.
- Roughly 5% of individuals present with lymphoma.
- Unchecked B cell proliferation ultimately culminates in NHL.
- Other cancers like carcinoma of the cervix, anal cancer, and Kaposi sarcoma are associated with HIV.
- Lymphocyte depletion variant of Hodgkins lymphoma is associated with HIV.

Chapter

7 Pharmacology

Ravindra

GENERAL PHARMACOLOGY

Essential Drugs

Essential drugs are drugs which are safe, economical, effective, and satisfy the priority health needs of the population.

- In India 4th Edition Essential Drug List (EDL) was released in July 2013. It has Essential Drugs, Surgical Products and Sutures List.
- The WHO Model List of Essential Medicines was first published in 1977. Since then it is updated after every 2 years. The 18th edition for adults was released in April 2013.
- WHO Model List of Essential Medicines for Children is a separate list for children up to 12 years has been released in 2007. The 4th edition for children was released in April 2013.

Orphan Drugs

Used for diagnosis, treatment or prevention of rare disease or condition. Examples are:

- Sodium nitrite
- Fomepizole
- Liposomal Amphotericin – B
- Rifabutin
- Succimer
- Digoxin antibody – Digibind
- Liothyronine (T3).

Prodrug is an inactive chemical precursor that is converted to the active drug by biologic processes inside the body.

Prodrug	Active form
Levodopa	Dopamine
Enalapril	Enalaprilat
α-Methyldopa	α-Methylnorepinephrine
Dipivefrine	Epinephrine
Sulindac	Sulfide metabolite
Proguanil	Cycloguanil
Prednisone	Prednisolone
Bacampicillin	Ampicilin
Sulfasalzine	5-aminosalicylic acid
Cyclophosphamide	Aldophosphamide, phosphoramide mustard, acrolein
Fluorouracil	Fluorouridine monophosphate
Mercaptopurine	Methylmercaptopurine ribonucleotide
Acyclovir	Acyclovir triphosphate

Transport

Energy	Type	Property	Example
Energy not required	Passive diffusion	Lipid soluble drugs	Acidic drugs and basic drugs
	Filtration	Through membrane pores	Glomerular filtration of drugs
	Facilitated diffusion	Translocation via transporters	GLUT4 transporter
Energy required	Active transport	ATP required	ABC, OCT, OAT, SGLT

Therapeutic Drug Monitoring

- The measurement of plasma concentration of drug and adjusting its dose.
- Done for drugs having narrow therapeutic index and whose response cannot be measured.
- For example, Phenytoin, phenobarbitone, carbamazepine, tacrolimus, cyclosporine, lithium, etc.

Low Therapeutic Range Drugs

- Lithium
- Theophylline
- Amino glycosides
- Digoxin
- Lignocaine
- Anticonvulsants, e.g. Phenytoin.

	Nonionized drug	Ionized drug
Lipid solubility	Yes	No
Placenta, cornea, and BBB	Cross	Poorly cross
Absorption from stomach and intestine	Rapid	Slow
Vd	Higher	Lower
Dialysis	Not effective	Effective

Acidic vs Basic Drugs

	Acidic drugs	Basic drugs
Binds to	Albumin	Alpha 1 Acid Glycoprotein
Variation	So decrease in albumin increases the free level of acidic drugs. For example, Liver failure, Nephrotic syndrome	So increase in the Alpha – 1 Acid Glyco protein level, decreases the free level basic drugs. For example, Cancer, Arthritis
Absorption	In acidic pH (Stomach) Because acidic drugs will be lipid soluble in acidic pH	In basic pH (Intestine) Because basic drugs will be lipid soluble in basic pH
Excretion	In basic pH Because acidic drugs will be lipid insoluble in basic pH So in barbiturate toxicity alkalinize the urine	In acidic pH Because basic drugs will be lipid insoluble in acidic pH So in quinine toxicity acidify the urine
Examples	Phenytoin, Salicylates, Phenylbutazone, Warfarin	Propranolol Quinidine, Lignocaine, Imipramine

Parameter	Numerator	Denominator	Unit
Volume of Distribution(Vd)	Drug administered IV	Plasma concentration	ml
Clearance (Cl)	Rate of elimination of a drug	Plasma concentration	ml/min
Rate of Elimation (Re)	Amount of drug eliminated	Time taken	mg/min

Contd...

Contd...

Parameter	Numerator	Denominator	Unit
Half-life (t1/2)	0.693 × Vd	Clearance	min
Therapeutic Index (TI)	Median Lethal Dose (LD50)	Median Effective Dose (ED50)	—
Bioavailability	Area under curve for IV route	Area under curve for oral	%
Relative Bioavailability	Area under curve of A ×100%	Area under curve of B	%
Loading Dose	Vd × Target plasma Concentration	—	mg
Maintenance Dose	Cl × Target plasma Concentration	—	mg

Bioavailability: The fraction of drug that reaches the systemic circulation in an unchanged form. Bioavailability depends on rate and extent of drug absorption, presystemic (hepatic) metabolism and elimination. It is calculated by comparing the area under curve (AUC) for IV route and AUC of oral route. Either the plasma concentration or urinary concentration of the drug can be used.

Most important for drugs with high first pass metabolism and narrow therapeutic index

- Intravenous/Intra-arterial: 100%
- Intramuscular and Subcutaneous: 75 to 100%
- Oral and inhalational: 5 to 100%
- Per rectal: 35 to 100%
- Transdermal: 70 to 100%.

Kinetics of Elimination

First order kinetic	Zero order kinetic
Constant fraction of the drug is eliminated per unit time	Constant amount of the drug is eliminated per unit time
Directly proportional to plasma concentration	Independent of plasma concentration
Constant half-life and clearance	At higher plasma concentration half-life increases and clearance decreases
Most of the drugs follow first order kinetics	For example, Warfarin, Phenytoin, Alcohol, Salicylates, Tolbutamide, Theophylline

Metabolism of Drug

Metabolism maybe either

- Microsomal (present in smooth endoplasmic reticulum) e.g. All Phase I reaction and glucuronide conjugation
- Nonmicrosomal enzymes e.g. All Phase II reaction except glucuronide conjugation.

Atracurium a skeletal muscle relaxant **undergoes Hoffmann elimination** (Spontaneous degradation) and is safe in renal/liver failure patients.

Enzyme inhibitors	Enzyme inducers	Drugs undergoing acetylation are SHIP dance
• Ketoconazole • Isoniazid • Sodium valproate • Sulphonamides • Metronidazole • Omeprazole • Fluoroquinolone • Alcohol • Chloramphenicol • Cimetidine • Erythromycin	• Carbamazepine • Chloral hydrate • Griseofulvin • Rifampin • Alcohol • Phenobarbital • Phenytoin • Sulphonylureas	• Sulfonamides • Hydralazine • Isoniazid • Procainamide • Dapsone

Biotransformation

Phase I	Phase II	
• Oxidation • (Hydroxylation, Dealkylation, Deamination) • Reduction • Hydrolysis • Cyclization • Decyclization	• Microsomal	• Nonmicrosomal
	• Glucuronide conjugation	• Glutathione conjugation • Acetylation • Methylation • Sulfation

Drugs undergoing high first pass metabolism not given orally (remember **LIGHT**)

- Lignocaine
- Isoprenaline
- Hydrocortisone
- Testosterone.

Potency vs Efficiency

Potency	Efficiency
Amount of drug needed to produce a response	Maximum response that can be elicited by the drug
X-axis–More potent the drug towards right	Y-axis–Maximum height maximum efficacious
Antagonist acts by decreasing the potency of drug	Noncompetitive antagonist acts by decreasing the efficiency
Potency refers to EC50 (or) ED50	Efficacy

Competitive antagonism	Noncompetitive antagonism
Parallel, Right shift of the DRC	Nonparallel, Right shift of the DRC
Maximum response remains the same	Maximum response is much reduced
Reversible by addition of agonist	Irreversible and Unsurmountable by addition of agonist
For example, Ach and Atropine at muscarinic receptors	For example, Phenoxybenzamine at alpha receptors

Adverse Reactions

Classification of Adverse Reaction

Type A	Augmented reactions	Hypoglycemia with Insulin
Type B	Bizarre reactions	Anaphylaxis – Penicillin allergy
Type C	Chronic reactions	Diclofenac – Analgesic Nephropathy
Type D	Delayed reactions	Teratogenesis, Carcinogenesis
Type E	End of use reactions	Adrenocortical insufficiency due to sudden withdrawal of corticosteroids
Type F	Failure of therapy	

Pregnancy Risk Category

A	No risk
B	Human study are lacking but animal studies shows no teratogenicity
C	Both human and animal studies are lacking but potential benefit warrants its use
D	Evidence of risk is proved. Potential benefit are high
X	Definitely risk, definitely contraindicated

Safer Drugs in Pregnancy

Anticoagulation	Heparin
Antimalarial	chloroquine
Antithyroid	Prophythiouracil
Antihypertensive	Hydrolazine/methyl dopa → CCB → Cardio selective B blocker → Prazocin/clonidine
Muscle relaxant	δ-tubocurarin
HIV	Zidovudine/Nevirapine
Toxoplasmosis	Spiramycin
Anticonvulsant	Phenobarbital
Eclampsia	Magnesium sulfate
UTI	Nitrofurantoin, Ampicillin, Cephalosporins
ATT	Rifampicin + Isoniazid

Clinical Trial

Phase	Unit of study	Purpose
Preclinical trials		
Phase 0	Animals	Pretesting in animals
Clinical trials		
Phase 1	Healthy human volunteers	Establishment of safety and nontoxicity
Phase 2	Patients	Establishment of effectiveness
Phase 3	Patients	Comparison between older/existing drugs
Phase 4	Patients	Assessment of long-term side effects

Phase 1 – Maximum tolerable dose of drug given.

Phase 3 – Randomized control trial and new drug launched in market after phase 3.

Phase 4 – Longest phase of trial and postmarketing surveillance done.

Pharmacovigilance Programme of India (PvPI)

- The Central Drugs Standard Control Organisation (CDSCO), New Delhi, under MOHFW, Government of India has initiated a pharmacovigilance programme of India in July, 2010.
- The National Coordinating Center is located in Indian Pharmacopoeia Commission (IPC), Ghaziabad, (UP).
- The vision of PvPI is to promote patient safety by monitoring drug safety and to reduce the risk associated with use of drugs.
- WHO Headquarters for Pharmacovigilance is in Uppsala Monitoring Centre, (UMC), in Sweden.

AUTONOMIC NERVOUS SYSTEM AND AUTACOIDS

ANS Neurotransmitters

<table>
<tr><th></th><th>Preganglionic</th><th colspan="2">Postganglionic</th></tr>
<tr><td rowspan="4">Sympathetic system</td><td rowspan="4">Ach</td><td colspan="2">NA</td></tr>
<tr><td>Renal and mesenteric vasculature</td><td>Dopamine</td></tr>
<tr><td>Sweat glands</td><td>Ach</td></tr>
<tr><td>Adrenal medulla</td><td>Adrenaline</td></tr>
<tr><td>Parasympathetic system</td><td>Ach</td><td colspan="2">Ach</td></tr>
</table>

Actions of sympathetic system	Systems	Actions of parasympathetic system
Increases heart rate and conduction	Heart	Decreases heart rate and conduction
Bronchodilatation	Bronchus	Bronchoconstriction
Decreases movements	GIT	Stimulates movements
Decreases urine outflow	Bladder	Stimulates urine outflow
Mydriasis	Pupil	Miosis
Decreases secretions (except sweating)	Glands	Stimulates secretions

Cholinergic Receptors

Nicotinic receptor		Muscarinic receptors				
N_N	N_M	M1	M2	M3	M4	M5
Ganglia, Adrenal medulla	Neuromuscular junction	Gastric ganglia, CNS	Heart	Eye, GIT, Bladder, Bronchus, Glands, CNS	CNS	CNS

Parasympathomimetic Drugs

Parasympathomimetic drugs		Drugs	
Direct acting parasympathomimetics		Acetyl choline, Pilocarpine, Bethanechol, Methacholine, Carbachol	
Indirectly acting parasympathomimetics	Reversible	Lipid soluble	Physostigmine, Tacrine, Donepezil, Rivastigmine, Gallantamine
		Water soluble	Neostigmine, Pyridostigmine, Edrophonium
	Irreversible	Organophosphates	Malathion, Parathion, DFP, Chlorpyrifos, Ecothiophate, Tabun, Sarin, Soman
		Carbamates	Carbaryl, Propoxur, Aldicarb

Antiglaucoma Drugs

Glaucoma drugs		Drugs	
Drugs decrease aqueous secretion	β blockers	Cardioselective	Betaxolol, Levobetaxolol
		Noncardioselective	Timolol, Levobunolol, Cartelol
	α2 agonist	Brimonidine, Apraclonidine	
	CA inhibitors	Acetazolamide, Dorzolamide, Brinzolamide	
Drugs increase aqueous outflow	Increases trabecular outflow	Miotics	Pilocarpine, Physostigmine
		α2 agonist	Dipivefrin
	Increases uveoscleral outflow	Latanoprost, Bimatoprost	

Cholinergic Drugs

- Maximum nicotinic effect is seen with carbachol
- Brinzolamide and acetazolamide are contra indicated in pt with allergy to sulphonamide
- Atropine does not inhibits bile secretion
- Antimuscarinic agent is contraindicated in glaucoma and BPH
- Atropine is useful in the treatment of poisoning with amanita inocybe and not preferred in amanita muscaria
- Atropine can be used both in OP and carbamate poisoning but Pralidoximes are CI in carbamate poisoning
- Pralidoxime acts by reactivating cholinesterase enzyme
- Ganglion blockers: Trimethaphan used to produce controlled hypotension and Mecamylamine has been tried for smoking cessation.

- Other drugs for smoking cessation Vareniciline- nicotinic agonist, Nicotine patch, Bupriopion Amfebutamine, Clonidine, Rimonabant (banned due to risk of suicidal tendency), Topiramate, Nortyptaline.

Anticholinergics

Natural alkaloids	Semi-synthetic derivatives	Synthetic compounds		
		Mydriatics	**Antisecretary – antispasmodic**	**Antiparkinsonian**
Atropine Hyoscine Nonselective antagonists	Homatropine Ipratropium Bromide Tiotropium bromide	Cyclopentolate, Tropicamide	Quaternary compounds: Propantheline, Oxyphenonium, Clidinium, Isopropamide, Glycopyrrolade. Tertiary amines: Dicyclomine, Oxybutynin, Flavoxate, Pirenzepine, Telenzepine	Trihexiphenidyl, Procylidine, Biperidin, Benztropine,

	Cholinergic actions	Anticholinergic actions	Drugs
M1	Gastric glands → HCl secretion	Prevents peptic ulcer disease	Pirenzepine telenzepine
M2	• Decrease HR –ve chronotropic • Decrease conduction –ve dromotropic	Tachycardia	Atropine → used in AV block Digitalis induced bradycardia
M3	**S** Salivation Sweating	Dry mouth Hyperthermia	Atropine preanesthetic
	L Lacrimation	Dry eyes	
	U Urination	Urinary retention	Dicyclomine, flavoxate and oxybutynin, tolterodine used in urinary incontinence
	D Defecation **G** GE movt increased	Constipation	Hyoscine, dicyclomine, propantheline, oxyphenonium and clidinium are useful as antispasmodic agents Darifenacin is used for irritable bowel syndrome
	E Emesis	Antiemetic	Glycopyrrolate and atropine as preanesthetic
	A Accommodation of eye Ach – miosis	Passive mydriasis	Atropine (longest), homatropine, cyclopentolate and tropicamide (shortest) used for RE assessment and fundoscopy
	BC Bronchoconstriction	Bronchodialatation	Ipratropium and tiotropium used in COPD and bronchial asthma
	D Dilatation of Blood vessels **E** Erection of Penis	Hypertension	
M1 to M5	CNS	Atropine cause delirium Hyoscine is CNS depressant Many tricyclic antidepressants has anticholinergic properties	Scopolamine (t.d patch) prevents motion sickness Hyoscine (truth serum) used as lie detector Central anticholinergic agents are used in prevention of drug induced Parkinsonism e.g. trihexiphenidyl (benzhexol), benztropine and biperidin

Adrenergic Receptors

α-Actions	β-Actions
Rise in BP (by vasoconstriction)-alpha 1	Fall in BP (by vasodilatation)-beta 2
Cardiac arrhythmia at higher doses	Increase the rate and force of contraction-beta 1
No effect on bronchioles	Bronchodilatation-beta 2

Contd...

Contd...

α-Actions	β-Actions
Intestinal relaxation, sphincter contraction	Intestinal relaxation
Bladder-trigone contraction	Detrusor relaxation
Uterine contraction, piloerection	Uterine relaxation-beta 2
Splenic capsule contraction	Splenic capsule relaxation
Inhibition of insulin secretion-alpha 2	Augmentation of insulin secretion

Actions

- Adrenaline – Strong α1, α2, β1, β2 and weak β3 activity
- Noradrenaline – Strong α1, α2, β1 and no β2 activity
- Isoprenaline – Strong β1, β2 and β3 activity.

Dopamine

Dose of dopamine	Receptor	Action
Low (< 2 μg/kg/min)	D1	Dilates renal and mesenteric blood vessels
Moderate (2–10 μg/kg/min)	β1	Inotropic > chronotropic
High (> 10 μg/kg/min)	A	Vasoconstriction

Dobutamine

- Derivative of DA, acts on both α and β adrenergic receptors but not a D1 or D2 receptor.
- It increases force of cardiac contraction and output, without significant change in heart rate, peripheral resistance and BP.

Adrenergic Agonist

- The rate limiting step in the synthesis of catecholamine is hydroxylation of tyrosine.
- Uptake I inhibited by cocaine, imipramine and doxipine.
- Activation of prejunctional alpha 2 receptors on sympathetic nerve endings is associated with decrease in cAMP formation GI type of GPCR.
- Overuse of certain decongestants that are indirectly acting sympathomimetic can lead to a diminished response. Tachyphylaxis in such cases is most probably due to reduced stores of available neurotransmitter.
- β1 Selective agonist is Dobutamine.
- Midodrine is an Alpha 1 receptor agonist used in the management of postural hypotension.
- Clonidine is a ∝2 selective antagonist.
- Therapeutic window phenomena is seen in TCA, clonidine and glipizide.
- Dale's vasomotor phenomenon is because of stimulation of β2 receptor. Adrenaline acts on ∝1, ∝2, β1 and β2.
- Adr is predominantly vasopressor agent, acting through ∝1 receptor. But if alpha blocker is given first, pressure effect of Adr is blocked, and produces only fall in BP, due to β2 mediated vasodilatation.
- Phenyl propanolamine is a sympathomimetic drug which has been associated with hemorrhagic stroke.

Anorectic Agent Used in Obesity

	Sympathomimetic	Serotoninergic	Hormonal	Newer drugs
Action	On appetite center	Satiety center		
Drugs	Phentermine PPA Diethyl proplon Mazindol	Fenfluramine Dexfenfluramine	Thyroxine	Orlistat Olestra Leptin Sibutramine

Erectile Dysfunction

Drugs causing erectile dysfunction	Treatment of erectile dysfunction
• Anti HT – β blocker, clonidine, alpha methyldopa, thiazide • Antipsychotic – phenothiazine • Antidepressant – SSRI, MAO inhibitors • Anxiolytic – BZD • Miscellaneous – Metaclopropamide, Opioid, Nicotine	• Oral- sildenalfil, yohimbine, phentolamine, apomorphine, trazadone, L-argininie • Intracavernosal injection – alprostadil, papaverine, phentolamine • Transcutaneous – GTN, papaverine, minoxidil, alprostadil cream, gel, paste • Herbal – Ginseng, kava, gincobiloba

Directly acting sympathomimetics	
Catecholamines	**Noncatecholamines**
Endogenous catecholamines: Dopamine noradrenaline adrenaline **Exogenous catecholamines:** Isoprenaline, fenoldopam dobutamine, dopexamine	**α1 agonists:** • Oxymetazoline and Xylometazoline: Nasal decongestants. • Methoxamine and Mephentermine: Increase BP • Phenylephrine used as mydriatic (no cycloplegia). **α2 agonists:** • Clonidine and α methyldopa: Rx of hypertension • Apraclonidine and brimonidine: Topically for Rx of glaucoma • Tizanidine: muscle relaxant • Dexmeditomidine is used for preanesthetic medication. **β1 agonists: prenaltrenol** **β2 agonists:** • Used in bronchial asthma and uterine relaxants (Formoterol, Isoxsuprine Ritodrine, Salbutamol Salmeterol, Terbutaline)

Indirectly acting sympathomimetics	Mixed action sympathomimetics
• Noradrenaline reuptake inhibitor: Cocaine and TCA • Tyramine → cheese reaction (in patients on MAO inhibitors) • Methylphenidate (Amphetamine) DOC for attention deficit hyperkinetic disorder (ADHD). • Modafinil: Used in narcolepsy and obstructive sleep apnea	• Ephedrine and pseudoephedrine: nasal decongestants • Indirect action: Enhance the release of NA • Direct action: activates adrenergic receptors • Ephedrine is vasopressor of choice in pregnancy.

∝1 selective agonist	∝1 selective antagonist	∝2 selective agonist	∝2 selective antagonist	Nonselective μ blockers	
Phenylephrine	Prazocin	Clonidine	Yohimbine	Phenoxybenzamine	• Ergotamine
Methoxamine	Terazosin	Apraclonidine	Idazoxan	Phentolamine	• Dihydroergotamine
Mephenteramine	Tamsulocin (∝1A subtype)	Guanafacine			• Tolazoline
Metaraminol		Guanabenz			• Chlorpromazine
Midodrine		Tizanidine			• Ergotoxin/Dihydro ergotoxine
		Brimonidine			• Ketanserin

Clonidine: Causes vasodialation	Uses	Adverse effects
• ∝2 agonist • ∝2 A subtype in brainstem • No dyslipidemia • No increase Rennin release	• HTN • Opioid withdrawal • Alcohol withdrawal • Nicotine withdrawal • Surgical and post OP Analgesia	• Rebound HTN • CNS depression • Sedation • Mental depression • Insomnia

Contd...

Contd...

Clonidine: Causes vasodialation	Uses	Adverse effects
	• To control diarrhea in diabetic neuropathy • Postmenopausal vasomotor • Symptoms • Pheochromocytoma	• Dry mouth, Nose, Eye • Constipation • Impotence • Salt/H_2O retention • Bradycardia

Prazocin: Causes vasodialation	Uses	Adverse effects
• Highly selective ∝1 blocker • No dyslipidemia • ∝1A subtype located in Prostate • ∝1B subtype located in blood vessels	• Improves carbohydrate metabolism • Symptomatic improvement in • BPH – ∝1A blockade • PVD – ∝1B blockade	• Postural hypotension – first dose effect – ∝1B blockade • Higher dose – impairment of ejaculation – not seen with Tamsulozin which blocks ∝1A subtype • Prolonged use develops tolerance

Directly acting	Agonist	Antagonist
Alpha 1	Phenylephrine	Prazosin
Alpha 2	Clonidine	Yohimbine

Yohimbine

- Activation of presynaptic receptors in PNS inhibits the release of NE.
- Activation of α2 receptors in CNS (postmedullary region) inhibits sympathetic nervous system. Yohimbine is a competitive antagonist for α2 receptors.
- It readily enters the CNS, where it acts to increase blood pressure and heart rate; it also enhances motor activity and produces tremors. α2 agonist clonidine has opposite action.
- Uses of Yohimbine: male sexual dysfunction, diabetic neuropathy and in the treatment of postural hypotension.

Idazoxan

- It acts as an antagonist for both α2 adrenergic receptor and imidazoline receptor.
- Idazoxan has been under investigation as an antidepressant, as an adjunctive treatment in schizophrenia (α2 receptor antagonism enhances therapeutic effects of antipsychotics).

Adrenergic Antagonist

- In an anginal patient with resting heart rate 60/mt, beta blocker of choice is Acebutalol
- Beta Blockers in HF: Metoprolol, Bisoprolol, and Carvedilol
- Antidote in case of β-blocker poisoning is Glucagon
- Glucagon acts via G protein coupled receptor – increase adenyl cyclase—cAMP
- Selective α1 A Blocker is – Tamsulosin
- Prazocin is the DOC for scorpion bite
- Postural hypotension is seen with Prazocin
- Rebound hypertension seen with clonidine.

Generation	β-blockers	
I	Nonselective	Propranolol, Timolol, Nadolol, Pindolol, Alprenolol, Oxprenolol
	With intrinsic sympathomimetic activity	Oxprenolol, Pindolol, Alprenolol
	Membrane stabilizing property	Propranolol, Pindolol

Contd...

Contd...

Generation	β-blockers	
II – Cardioselective	Selective β1 blockers	Nebivolol, Betaxolol, Bisoprolol, Acebutalol, Esmolol, Atenolol, Metoprolol, Celiprolol
	With intrinsic sympathomimetic activity	Celiprolol, Penbutalol, Acebutalol
	Membrane stabilizing property	Metoprolol, acebutolol
	Lipid insoluble β-blockers	Nadolol, Sotalol, Atenolol, Acebutolol, Betaxolol, Bisoprolol, Celiprolol
III – With additional vasodilator property	α-blockade	Labetalol, Carvedilol
	β2 agonism	Celiprolol, Carteolol
	Release of NO	Nebivolol
	Opening of K^+ channels	Tilisolol
	Inhibition of Ca^{2+} channels	Carvedilol, Bevantolol, Betaxolol

CARDIOVASCULAR SYSTEM, HEMATOLOGY AND EXCRETORY SYSTEM

Newer Drugs

Nesiritide	Human BNP analogue used in acute decompensated CHF
Omapatrilat/Sampatrilat	Vasopeptidase inhibitor used for the treatment of hypertension, myocardial infarction and congestive heart failure
Bosentan	Nonselective antagonist of endothelin receptor
Ambresentan	Selective ET-A receptor antagonist used in primary pul hypertension
Calcium sensitizer	Pimobendan,Levosibendan tried in heart failure
Icatibant	Bradykinin inhibitor

PD III Inhibitor

- Amrinone (Inamrinone)
- Milrinone
- Vesnarinone
- Enoximone
- Piroximone
- Fenoximone.

ACE Inhibitors

Drugs	Uses	ADR	Contraindications
Captopril Lisinopril Enalapril Quinapril Fosinopril Perindopril Ramipril Trandolapril Benazepril All ACE inhibitors are prodrug except captopril, lisinopril	Heart failure (all stages) Hypertension MI Diabetic nephropathy Scleroderma renal crisis	Cough Angioneurotic edema Fetopathic potential Hypotension Hyperkalemia and acute renal failure Dysgeusia Neutropenia; proteinurea	Pregnancy Bilateral renal artery stenosis Severe renal failure Hyperkalemia Pre-existing severe hypotension Severe aortic stenosis

Digoxin

Digoxin hemodynamic effect	Digoxin neurohormonal effect
• ↑Cardiac output • ↑LV ejection fraction • ↓LVEDP • ↑Exercise tolerance • ↑Natriuresis • ↓Neurohumoral activation	• ↓Plasma noradrenaline • ↓Peripheral nervous system activity • ↓RAAS activity • ↑Vagal tone • Normalizes arterial baroreceptors

Antiarrhythmic Drugs: Classification of Antiarrhythmic Drugs

Class of antiarrhythmic drugs		Drugs
Class I – Membrane stabilizing agents (Sodium channel blockers)	Moderately decrease dv/dt of 0 phase	Quinidine, Procainamide, Disopyramide
	Little decrease dv/dt of 0 phase	Lidocaine, Mexiletine
	Marked decrease dv/dt of 0 phase	Propafenone, Flecainide
Class II – Beta blockers		Propranolol, Sotalol, Esmolol
Class III – Agents widening AP (potassium channel blockers)		Amiodarone, Dronedarone, Dofetilide, Ibutilide
Class IV – Calcium channel blockers		Verapamil, Diltiazem
Class V		Digoxin, Adenosine, Magnesium, Atropine, Potassium

Uses of Antiarrhythmic Drugs

Flecainaide	Acute Rx of WPW syndrome
Ibutilide	Acute conversion of atrial fibrillation into sinus rhythm
Sotalol	Rx of atrial and ventricular tachyarrhythmias, AV re-entrant arrhythmias
Verapamil	Prophylaxis of PSVT
IV Adenosine	Rx of PSVT
Digoxin	Controls ventricular rate in atrial fibrillation and flutter
Magnesium	Rx of congenital and acquired long QT syndrome

DOC for Arrhythmias

Type of arrhythmias	DOC
Atrial flutter/Atrial fibrillation	Propranolol, Esmolol
PSVT	Adenosine
Ventricular tachycardia	Lignocaine, Magnesium
Ventricular fibrillation	Lignocaine, Bretylium
WPW syndrome	Flecainaide
Torsades de' pointes	Magnesium
Digitalis induced ventricular arrhythmias	Lignocaine, Phenytoin

Antihypertensive Drugs: Classification of antihypertensives

Class of antihypertensives		Drugs
Diuretics	Thiazides	Hydrochlorthiazide, Chlorthalidone, Bendroflumethiazide, Indapamide
	Loop diuretics	Furosemide, Torsemide, Bumetanide, Indacrinone
	Potassium sparing diuretics	Spironolactone, Epleronone, Amiloride, Triamterene

Contd...

Contd...

Class of antihypertensives		Drugs
Sympathoplegics	Central anticholinergics	Clonidine, α-methyldopa
	α2 agonists	Moxonidine, Rilmenidine
	Ganglion blockers	Hexamethonium, Trimethaphan, Mecamylamine
	Adrenergic neuron blockers	Reserpine, Guanethidine, Bretylium
	α blockers	Phenoxybenzamine, Phentolamine, Tolazoline
	β blockers	Nevibolol, Metoprolol, Esmolol, Atenolol, Acetutolol, Betaxolol, Bisoprolol, Celiprolol
	α + β blockers	Labetolol, Carvedilol
Vasodilators	Potassium channel openers	Hydralazine, Minoxidil, Diazoxide
	No releasers	Sodium nitroprusside, Hydralazine
	Dopamine agonist	Fenoldopam
	Calcium channel blockers	Verapamil, Diltiazem, Nifedipine, Nicardipine, Nimodipine, Nisoldipine, Niterndipine, Isradipine, Lacidipine, Felodipine, Amlodipine
Drugs decreasing the action of RAAS	Renin inhibitors	Aliskiren, Remikiren, Enalkiren
	ACE inhibitors	Captopril, Enalapril, Lisinopril, Ramipril, Perindopril, Trandopril, Fosinopril, Moexipril
	Angiotensin receptor blockers	Losartan, Valsartan, Irbesartan, Candesartan, Telmisartan, Eprosartan

Antihypertensive Choice in Various Clinical Situations

Clinical condition	Preferred antihypertensive drugs
Angina	β-blockers, CCB
BPH	α-blockers
Diabetes and hyperlipidemia	ACE inhibitors, ARB, CCB, α-blockers
Elderly and Isolated systolic hypertension	Diuretics, CCB
Low renin hypertension	Diuretics, CCB
High renin hypertension	ACE inhibitors, ARB, β-blockers
Asthma	Diuretics, CCB, ACE inhibitors, ARB
CHF	ACE inhibitors, Diuretics
Post MI	β-blockers, ACE inhibitors
PVD	CCB, α-blockers
Thyrotoxicosis	β-blockers
Pregnancy	β-blockers (Cardioselective, Labetalol), Methyldopa, Clonidine, Dihydropyridine, CCB, Hydralazine, Prazosin

Uses of Antihypertensive Drugs

Indapamide	Antihypertensive of choice for DM
Indacrinone	Gout
α-Methyldopa, Clonidine	Anti HT in pregnancy

Mecamylamine	Smoking cessation
Prazosin, Terazosin, Doxazosin	Anti HT of choice for patients with BPH
Alpha blockers	Safer in patients with DM, CAD, Gout
Carvedilol	Antioxidant, Antimitogen
Minoxidil	Alopecia in males
Riociguat (guanylate cyclase stimulator)	Chronic thromboembolic pulmonary HT
Aliskiren, Remikiren, Enalkiren	Oral treatment of chronic HTN

Drugs Employed in Hypertensive Emergencies

- Sodium nitropurusside
- Glyceryl trinitrate
- Diazoxide
- Hydralazine
- Esmolol
- Phentolamine
- Labetalol
- Indaramine
- Urapadil
- Furosemide.

Malignant Hypertension

Immediate onset	Late onset
• Diazoxide • Sodium nitropurusside • Trimethaphan	• Enalapril • Hydralazine • Labetalol • Methyldopa

Antianginal Drugs: Classification of Antianginal Drugs

Class of antianginal drugs	Drugs
Nitrates	Glycerotrinitrate, Isosorbide dinitrate
Calcium channel blockers	Verapamil, Diltiazem
Beta blockers	Propranolol, Metoprolol, Atenolol
Potassium channel openers	Nicorandil
pFOX inhibitors	Trimetazidine, Ranolazine
Sodium channel blockers	Ranolazine, Ivabradine

Nitric Oxide Donors

- Sodium nitroprusside
- Organic nitrates
- Nitrities
- Fenoldopam – selective α1 agonist useful in HT emergency
- Propofol
- Nebivolol
- Nipradilol.

Nitrates

- Preload reduction
- Decreased O_2 consumption
- Reduction in end diastolic size and pressure
- Better ventricular emptying
- Increased subendocardial perfusion during diastole.

Adverse effects	Uses
• Reduction of preload and afterload • Slight decrease in tpr • Hypotension • Reflex tachycardia • Thrombing headache • Flushing, palpitation and fainting • Methemoglobinemia • Rashes – pentaerthrytal tetranitrate • Tolerance – decrease SH radicals • Dependence • Monday morning headache	• Angina pectoris • CHF and LVF • MI • Billiary colic • Esophageal spasm • Cyanide poisoning

Calcium Channel Blockers

- Least Effect on AV Conduction – Nifedipine
- Highest oral bioavialability – Amlopdipine
- Longest elimination half-life – Amlodipine
- Highest plasma protein binding – Felodipine
- Least plasma protein binding – Diltiazem
- Antiplatelet – Nifedipine
- Cerebral Hemorrhage – Nimodipine

Potassium Channel Openers

Drugs	Uses of potassium channel openers
• Minoxidil • Diazoxide • Nicorandil • Pinacidil • Cromakalim	• Hypertension • Angina • CCF • Alopecia • Peripheral vascular disease • Bronchial Asthma • Antihypoglycemic • Premature labor • Erectile impotence • Urinary incontinence

Hypolipidemic Drugs

Classes of hypolipidemic drugs	Drugs
HMG CoA reductase inhibitors	Lovastatin, Simvastatin, Atorvastatin, Rosuvastatin, Pravastatin, Pitavastatin
Bile acid sequestrant	Cholestyramine, Colestipol, Colesevelam
Lipoprotein lipase activators	Clofibrate, Gemfibrozil, Bezafibrate, Fenofibrate
Lipolysis and TGL synthesis inhibitor	Nicotinic acid
Sterol absorption inhibitor	Ezetimibe, Avasimibe
Miscellaneous drugs	Probucol, Gugulipid, Torcetrapib, Anacetrapib, Lomitapide

Drugs	Mechanism of action	Effect of lipids (%)
HMG CoA reductase inhibitors	Decreased cholesterol synthesis by inhibition of rate limiting HMG-CoA reductase	LDL ↓ 20–55 HDL ↑ 5–15 TGL ↓ 10–35
Bile acids Sequestrant	Decreased bile acid absorption, increased hepatic conversion of cholesterol to bile acids, increased LDL receptors on hepatocytes	LDL ↓ 15–30 HDL ↑ 3–5 TGL not affected
Fibric acid derivatives (Gemfibrozil, bezafibrate, fenofibrate)	Increase activity of lipoprotein lipase, decreased release of fatty acids from adipose tissue	LDL ↓ 5–20 HDL ↑ 10–20 TGL ↓ 20–50
Nicotinic acid	Decreased production of VLDL, decreased lipolysis in adipocytes	LDL ↓ 15–25 HDL ↑ 20–35 TGL ↓ 20–50

Diurteics

Diuretics	Site of action	Mechanism of action
Loop diuretics	Thick ascending limb of loop of henle	Inhibition of $Na^+/k^+/cl^-$ co-transport in luminal membrane
Thiazides	Early DT	Inhibition of Na^+/cl^- co-transport
Amiloride	Late DT/CT	Inhibition of luminal membrane Na^+ channel and has Na^+ K^+ exchange
Spironolactone	Late DT/CT	ADH antagonist
Osmotic	PT, descending limb of loop of henle, CT	Passive water reabsorbtion is reduced
CA enzyme inhibitor	PT, also DT	Increases excretion of HCO_3, Na, KCl and water

Diuretic Points

Diuretics	Clinical significance
Frusemide	To treat LVF and Pulmonary edema
Ethacrynic Acid	Highly ototoxic
Bumetanide	Most potent
Mersalyl	Kidney damage
Thiazides	Used to treat kidney stones
Metalozone	Useful even in severe renal failure
Indacrinone	Used in gouty arthritis

Diuretic	Body pH
CA inhibitor	Metabolic acidosis
LOOP	Metabolic alkalosis
Thiazide	Metabolic alkalosis
K^+ Sparing	Metabolic acidosis

Adverse Effects of Diuretics

Frusemide ADR	Thiazides ADR	Spironolactone ADR
Hypokalemia Dehydration Hyponatremia GI upset	Hypokalemia Hyperuricemia Mg depletion Hyperglycemia	Hirsuitism Gynaecomastia hyperkalemia

Contd...

Contd...

Frusemide ADR	Thiazides ADR	Spironolactone ADR
Hearing Loss (ethacrynic acid) Allergy (Sulfonamides) Caution (pregnancy)	Hyperlipidemia Hypercalcemia Impotence	

- **Only diuretic that does not require access to the tubular lumen to induce a diuretic effect is** Spironolactone
- **Canrenone is the active form of** Spironolactone
- **Eplerenone is a** selective aldosterone antagonist.

Antidiuretic

	V1	V2	V3
Location	Vascular smooth muscle/platelet/ hepatocyte	CT (kidney) Vascular endothelium	Anterior pituitary
Functions	Vasoconstriction Vascular smooth muscle contraction Platelet aggregation glycogenolysis	Antidiuretic Increase release of factor VIII, von Willebrand factor vasodilatation	Release of ACTH
Mechanism of action	GqCPR → PLC/IP3-DAG-Ca^{++}	GsCPR → cAMP	GqCPR → PLC/IP3-DAG-Ca^{++}
Agonist and USE	Arginine vasopressin **Terlipressin** Bleeding esophageal varices	Desmopressin Central DI Type I van Willebrand's disease Primary nocturnal enuresis	Arginine vasopressin

Thrombolytic, Anticoagulants and Antiplatelets

Fibrinolytic agents	Antagonists of fibrinolytics
• Streptokinase, Urokinase, Anistreplase • Alteplase, Reteplase, Tenecteplase from r-DNA technology	• EACA • Tranexamic acid • Aprotinin

Inhibition of Synthesis of Clotting Factor by Warfarin

- First factor VII (plasma t ½ 6 hours)
- Next factor IX (t ½ 24 hours)
- Factor X (t½ 40 hours)
- Prothrombin (t ½ 60 hours).

Warfarin

- Monitored by PT and INR.
- No alteration in bleeding time.

Potentiation of Warfarin Action

Enzyme inhibitors	Displacing warfarin from protein binding site	Excretion of Vit K	Reducing Vit K absorption
Metronidazole Chloramphenicol Disulfiram Erythromycin Cimetidine Allopurinol Amiodarone Celecoxib	Co-trimoxazole Indomethacin Phenytoin Phenobarbitone Phenylbutazone Ethacrynic acid	Liquid paraffin	Broad spectrum antibiotics

Inhibition of Warfarin Action

Enzyme inducers	Inhibiting warfarin absorption	Increased synthesis of clotting factor
Barbiturates Rifampicin Griseofulvin carbamazepine	Cholestyramine Sucralfate	Estrogen OCP

Warfarin side effects	Treatment of warfarin poisoning
Alopecia Bleeding Oral (GI intolerance) Dermatitis Teratogenicity	Fresh frozen plasma Inj Vit K 1 IV infusion phytonadione Monitor INR (International Normalized Ratio)

Heparin

- Strongest organic acid
- Monitor aPTT
- Activate Antithrombin III – inhibits both IIa and Xa.

Side Effects

- A-alopecia
- B-bleeding
- O-osteoporosis
- U-urticaria
- T-thrombocytopenia
- Sec hyperaldosteronism – hyperkalemia.

Anticoagulants

Oral anticoagulants		Parenteral anticoagulants	
Vit K inhibitors	Warfarin, Dicumarol, Acenocoumarin, Phenindione	Direct thrombin inhibitors	Hirudin, Lepirudin, Bivalirudin, Argatroban, Melagatran
Factor Xa inhibitor	Rivaroxaban, Apixaban	Indirect thrombin inhibitors	Unfractionated heparin
Direct thrombin inhibitor	Ximelagatran, Dabigatran		LMW heparin – Enoxaparin, Dalteparin, Tinzaparin
			Fondaparinux, Idraparinux

GP-IIb/IIIa receptor blockers	Abciximab monoclonal antibody	Tirofiban nonpeptide	Eptifibatide peptide
Mechanism of action	Steric hindrance and Conformational changes	Mimics native protein sequence in receptor	
Biologic half-life (h)	12–24	4–8	
Reversible with platelet infusions	Yes	No	
Speed of reversibility	Slow (>48 h)	Fast (2 h)	
FDA-approved labelling	PCI	Unstable angina	PCI, Unstable angina

- Antiplatelet drugs – prolongs bleeding time
- Anticoagulant – prolongs clotting time
- Heparin (intrinsic pathway) – prolongs aPTT
- Warfarin (extrinsic pathway) – prolongs PT.

ENDOCRINOLOGY

Mechanism of Action of Hormones

Nuclear receptors		T3, T4, Estrogen, Progesterone, Testosterone	
Cytoplasmic receptors		Glucocorticoids, Mineralocorticoids	
Membrane receptors	Tyrosine kinase	Insulin, GH, Prolactin	
	GPCRs	K^+ channel opening	Somatostatin
		IP3/DAG/Ca^{2+}	Vasopressin, Oxytocin, TRH, GnRH
		Decrease cAMP	Prolactin inhibiting hormone
		Increase cAMP	V2 receptors of vasopressin

Receptors for Hormones

Membrane Receptors

Seven transmembrane GPCRs (Serpentine receptors)	Tyrosine kinase receptors (Insulin, IGF-1)
Cytokine receptors (Growth hormone, Prolactin)	Serine kinase receptors (Activin, TGF-β)

Nuclear Receptors

AF–1	DBD	Hinge	LBD	AF–2
Amino terminus	Central domain	Hinge portion	Carboxy terminus	
Activates transcription	Binds to hormone response elements	Permits flexibility	Binds ligand	Interacts with coactivators and facilitates transactivation

Examples – Glucocorticoids, Mineralocorticoids, Androgen, Estrogen, Progestin, Thyroid hormones, Vitamin D.

G Proteins Coupled Receptors

Small G proteins		Large heterotrimeric G proteins
Rab family	Regulation of vesicle traffic	3 subunits – α, β, γ
Rho/Rac family	Interaction between cytoskeleton and cell membrane	α unit bound to GDP and it separates from βγ subunit. The intrinsic GTPase activity of α subunit converts GTP to GDP and leads to reassociation of α with βγ subunit
Ras family	Growth regulation	5 families – G_s, G_i, G_t, G_q, G_{13}

Effector pathways of GPCRs

- Adenyl cyclase: c-AMP pathway (via G_s, G_i)
- Phospholipase C: IP_3-DAG pathway (via G_q)
- Channel regulation.

Three major families of G-proteins

G_s β – adrenergic receptor ACTH receptor FSH receptor	Couples to adenylate cyclase • Stimulates AC activity • Increases cAMP • Activates protein kinase A
G_i α_2 – adrenergic receptor M2 muscarinic receptor	Couples to adenylate cyclase • Inhibits AC activity • Decreases cAMP • Inhibits protein kinase A

G_q α_1 – adrenergic receptor M1, M3 muscarinic receptors Angiotensin receptor	Couples to phospholipase C • Increases IP_3 – DAG • Increases intracellular Ca^{2+} • Activates protein kinase C

Pituitary Hormones

Anterior: Gonadotrophins, Growth hormone, Prolactin, TSH, ACTH.
Posterior: Oxytocin, Vasopressin.

Gonadotrophin Releasing Hormone

	GnRH agonist	GnRH antagonist
Drugs	Leuprolide, Goserelin, Busorelin, Naferelin, Desorelin, Histrelin, Tritprelin	Ganirelix, Cetrorelix, Abarelix
Action	For Induction of ovulation To treat Delayed Puberty Cryptorchidism	To treat DUB, Endometriosis, Fibroid Carcinoma Prostate Contraception Premenstural syndrome

Growth Hormones (GH) and Growth Hormone Releasing Hormone (GHRH)

- Recombinant growth hormones (**somatrem and somatropin**): Pituitary dwarfism and AIDS related wasting
- **IGF-1 (MECASERMIN):** Useful for GH resistant dwarfism
- Pegvisomant is a GH receptor antagonist indicated for the treatment of acromegaly.

Somatostatin: Octreotide (somatostatin analogue) others are sandostatin, vapreotide, seglitide, lanreotide

- Used in acromegaly, islet cell tumors, bleeding due to esophageal varices, secretory diarrhea, thyrotrope adenoma – increased TSH.

Prolactin

- Prolactin release is inhibited by Dopamine.

Drugs causing decrease prolactin level – Dopamine agonist	Drugs causing increase prolactin level – Dopamine antagonist
Dopamine, Bromocriptine, Apomorphine, Pergolide, Piribedil, Ropinirole, Pramipexole	Cholrpromazine, Haloperidol, Metochlopromide, Reserpine, Methyldopa

Bromocriptine is a dopamine agonist used in treatment of hyperprolactinemia, acromegaly, parkinsonism.

Treatment of Diabetes Mellitus

- Type I DM (IDDM) is treated only by insulin.
- In type II DM (NIDDM), orally active drugs and or insulin is tried.

Insulin preparations

Rapid acting	Insulin lispro Insulin aspart Insulin glulisine
Short acting	Soluble insulin Semi lente
Intermediate acting	Lente insulin Neutral protamine hagedorn's
Long acting	Ultra lente Insulin glargine Insulin detemir

Oral Hypoglycemic Agents

Enhance insulin secretion

Sulfonylureas (K-ATP channel blockers)	I – Tolbutamide	Safer in elderly and those prone to hypoglycemia, Controls postprandial hyperglycemia
	II – Glibenclamide, Glipizide, Gliclazide, Glimepride	Potent drugs with lower incidence of hypoglycemic attacks
Meglitinide analogues	Repaglinide, Nateglinide	Stimulates insulin secretion and limits postprandial hypoglycemia
GLP-1 receptor agonists	Exenatide, Liraglutide	Lowers postprandial hypoglycemia, fasting blood glucose, HbA1c and body weight Produces anorectic effect
DPP-4 inhibitors	Sitagliptin, Vidagliptin, Saxagliptin, Alogliptin, Linagliptin	Boosts postprandial insulin release, decreases glucagon secretion, lowers meal time and fasting blood glucose

Overcome insulin resistance

Biguanide (AMP-K activator)	Metformin	Suppresses hepatic gluconeogenesis, enhances insulin mediated glucose uptake in skeletal muscle and fat, promotes peripheral glucose utilization
Thiazolidinediones (PPARγ activator)	Pioglitazone, Rosiglitazone, Troglitazone	Suppresses hepatic gluconeogenesis, activator of genes regulating fatty acid metabolism and lipogenesis in adipose tissue, lowers HbA1c and insulin levels

Miscellaneous drugs

α-glucosidase inhibitors	Acarbose, Voglibose, Miglitol	Reduces postprandial glycemia, lowers HbA1C levels
Amylin analogue	Pramlintide	Delay gastric emptying, retard glucose absorption and promotes satiety
Dopamine D2 receptor agonist	Bromocriptine	Suppresses glycemic peak, reduce body weight
SGLT-2 inhibitor	Dapagliflozin, Canagliflozin	Produces round the clock glucosuria, lowers blood glucose levels

Adrenal Cortex: Divided into Three Regions

- Zona Glomerulosa — Secretes aldosterone
- Zona Fasciculata — Secretes glucocorticoids
- Zona Reticularis — Secretes sex steroids.

Steroids and Their Peculiarities

Features	Steroid
Maximum glucocorticoid activity	Dexamethasone, Betamethasone
Maximum mineralocorticoid activity	Aldosterone
Glucocorticoid with maximum mineralocorticoid activity	Hydrocortisone
Least potent glucocorticoid	Cortisone
Most potent glucocorticoid	Betamethasone
Selective mineralocorticoid action (with no glucocorticoid activity)	DOCA
Selective mineralocorticoid action (with no mineralocorticoid activity)	Methylprednisolone, Triamcinolone, paramethasone, dexamethasone, Betamethasone

Corticosteroids Side Effects

Cushing habitus	Cataract	Glaucoma	Skin lesions
Osteoporosis	Suppression of HPO axis	Infection	Purple striae
Retarded growth	Peptic ulcer	Delayed wound healing	

Glucocorticoid Synthesis Inhibitors

Glucocorticoid synthesis inhibitors	Mechanism of action	Use
Metyrapone	Inhibits 11 β hydroxylase	Cushing syndrome (Safe in pregnancy)
Aminoglutethimide	Inhibits cholesterol side chain cleavage; Inhibits aromatase	CA breast
Mitotane	Atrophy of zona fasciculata and reticularis	Medical adrenalectomy
Trilostane	Inhibits 3 β hydroxysteroid dehydrogenase; Inhibits aromatase	
Ketoconazole	Inhibits 3 β hydroxysteroid dehydrogenase and 17 α hydroxylase	Cushing syndrome

Corticosteroid Receptor Antagonist

- Mifepristone
- Spironolactone
- Epleronone
- Drospirenone.

Thyroxine Synthesis

Steps in the Synthesis of Thyroid Hormone

- Iodide trapping (Na^+/I^- symporter)
- Oxidation of iodide (peroxidase)
- Iodide organification (iodine+3 tyrosine = mit, iodine + 3, 5 tyrosine = dit)
- Coupling of mit or dit — t4, t3
- Endocytosis of thyroglobulin (t4, t3, mit, dit) from colloid into follicular cell
- Proteolysis of thyroglobulin
- Thyroid hormone secretion (t4, t3)
- Deiodination (mit and dit within follicular cell, t4–t3 in peripheral circulation.

Classification of Anti thyroid drugs

Classes of antithyroid drugs	Drugs
Inhibitors of $Na^+ - I^-$ symporter	Thiocyanate, Fluborate, Perchlorate, Pertechtenate, Nitrates
Thyroid peroxidase inhibitors	Propylthiouracil, Carbimazole, Methimazole
Inhibitors of thyroid hormone release	Na I, KI, Lugol's iodine
Drugs causing thyroid gland destruction	Iodine – 131
Drugs inhibiting peripheral conversion of T4 to T3	Propranolol, Propylthiouracil, Amiodarone
Adjuvant antithyroid drugs	Beta blockers, Diltiazem, IV methylprednisolone

Sex Steroids

Androgens

Actions of Testosterone

- Feedback inhibition of LH secretion from pituitary
- Internal genitalia development in male fetus

- **Spermatogenesis** in testes
- Hematopoisis – Stimulation **of erythropoiesis.**

Danazol

Indications – Endometriosis, Benign Fibrocystic Disease, Hereditary Angio Neurotic edema, DUB, Precocious Puberty, Fibroid.

Antiandrogens

- Steroid synthesis inhibitors: Ketoconazole.
- 5-α reductase inhibitors: Finasteride.
- Androgen receptor inhibitors: Cyproterone, Flutamide, bicalutamide.

Estrogens

Selective estrogen receptor modulators (SERMs)

- **Clomiphene, tamoxifen, doloxifene, toremifene, fulvestrant, raloxifene and ormeloxifene** are SERMs
- Tamoxifen, doloxifene and toremifene: Breast carcinoma
- Fulvestrant (SERD) used in **tamoxifen resistant breast cancer**
- Raloxifene, **lasofoxafene** is used for osteoporosis
- Centchroman (ormeloxifene, Saheli) treatment of DUB.

Aromatase Inhibitors

I generation		Aminoglutethamide
II generation	Steroidal (Suicidal)	Formestane, Exemestane
	Nonsteroidal (Reversible inhibitor)	Letrozole, Anastrozole, Fadrozole, Vorozole

- These are useful for the treatment of tamoxifen resistant breast carcinoma.

Progestins

- Medroxyprogesterone acetate (IM, Oral)
- Megestrol acetate (Oral)
- Dyhydrogesterone (Oral)
- Hydroxyprogesterone caproate (IM) (long acting injection)
- Newer compound – Nomegesterol acetate (Oral).

Selective progesterone receptor modulator Asoprisnil, ulipristal.

Side Effects of Progestins

- Endometrial carcinoma
- Stroke
- Thromboembolism
- Rectal/colorectal carcinoma
- Ovarian cancer
- Gall bladder and liver disease
- Dementia
- Breast carcinoma.

Drugs for Osteoporosis

Antiresorptive agents	Bone forming agents	Both actions
• Bisphosphonates • Estrogen and SERM • Calcium Salts • Vitamine D and Analogs • Calcitonin • Thiazide diuretics	• Fluoride • Androgen and Anabolic Steroid • Parathormone	• Strontium ranelate

Biphosphonates

MOA: Inhibit bone resorption by suppressing the activity of osteoclasts (inhibition of farnesyl pyrophosphate synthesis) and secondarily bone formation

I generation	II generation	III generation
• Medronate • Clodronate • Etidronate	• Alendronate • Pamidronate • Ibadronate	• Risedronate • Zoledronate

Uses of Bisphonates

- Paget's disease
- Hypercalcemia
- Osteoporosis

ADR: esophageal and gastric irritation (common), renal failure, osteonecrosis of the jaw, subtrochanteric (femur) fractures.

Vitamin D and Analogs

Vitamin D2	**Ergocalciferol**
Vitamin D3	**Cholecalciferol**
25 OH Vitamin D3	**Calciferol**
1,25 (OH)2 Vit D3	**Calcitriol**

Therapeutic Uses of Vit D

- Nutritional rickets
- Metabolic rickets and osteomalacia
- Hypoparathyroidism
- Osteoporosis
- Fanconi syndrome
- Psoriasis.

Vitamin D Disorders

Vit D dependent rickets-Type I	Vit D dependent rickets-Type II	Vitamin D resistant rickets
• Autosomal recessive • Defective conversion of 25OHD-calcitriol (1α hydroxylase defect) • Treatment is Vit D	• Autosomal recessive • Defective receptor Vit-D (mutation) • Treatment is parenteral Ca^{2+}	• X-linked dominent • Hypophosphatemic rickets • Renal tubular defect in reabsorbtion of phosphate • Treatment is high dose OV Vit D along with inorganic phosphate

CENTRAL NERVOUS SYSTEM

Antidepressants

TCAs and selective serotonin reuptake inhibitors (SSRI): Selective blockade of serotonin transporter (SERT) and norepinephrine transporter (NET)

- Fluoxetine
- Fluoxamine
- Paroxetine
- Sertraline
- Citalopram.

Newer Antidepressents

- SNRI (serotonin and noradrenaline reuptake inhibitor) – Venlafaxine
- NDRI (noradrenaline dopamine reuptake inhibitor) – Bupropion
- NARI (noradrenaline reuptake inhibitor) – Reboxetine
- NASSA (noradrenergic and specific serotoninergic antidepressants) – Mirtazepine
- SARI (serotonin antagonist and reuptake inhibitor) – Trazadone, Nefazodone
- NSRE (noradrenaline serotonin reuptake enhancer) – Tianeptin
- RIMA (reversible inhibitor of MAO - A) – Meclobemide, Broforamine

Antidepressant with

Sedative effect	Amitriptaline, Doxepine, Trazadone
Stimulant effect	SSRI, Bupriopion
Antipsychotic effect	Amoxepine
No anticholinergic effect	SSRI, Desimpramine, Trazadone
No cardiac activity	Lofepramine, Mianserine
No weight gain	SSRI except paroxitine
Depression with sexual problem	Use – Trazadone, Bupriopion, Mirtazapine Avoid – SSRI
Used to control panic disorders	Paroxetine, Fluoxetine
OCD	Fluvoxamine, Clomipramine, Citalopram
Phobia	Paroxetine, Moclobemide
Post-traumatic stress disorders	Paroxetine with alprazolam
Used for treating bulimia nervosa	Fluvoxamine and Fluoxetine
Used to treat nicotine dependence and smoking cessation	Bupropion

Lithium

Mood stabilizing drugs	Lithium – uses	Lithium – adverse effects
Lithium carbonate Carbamazepine Sodium valproate Olanzapine Resperidone Clonidine Verapamil Nimodipine	• Acute manic episode • Prophylaxis in bipolar depression • Recurrent neuropsychiatric illness • Cluster headache • Cancer chemotherapy induced leukopenia and agranulocytosis • Inappropriate ADH secretion syndrome	Nausea, vomiting, mild diarrhea Thirst, polyuria Fine tremor CNS toxicity, Renal DI Thyroid dysfunction CI – Pregnancy, sick sinus syndrome

Antipsychotics

Typical antipsychotics block D2 receptors. EPS is seen as ADR.

Atypical antipsychotic does not block D2 receptors. EPS is not seen as ADR.

Classifications

Phenothiazines	Butyrophenones	Thioxanthenes	Atypical antipsychotic agents
Chlorpromazine Triflupromazine Thioridazone Trifluoperazine Fluphenazine	Haloperidol Trifluperidol Droperidol Penfluridol	Thiothixene Flupenthixol Other hetrocyclic: Pimozide Loxapine Reserpine	Clozapine Quetiapine Olanzapine Risperidone Sertindole Ziprasidone Aripiprazole

Clozapine

- 5 HT2/ALPHA antagonist
- Suppress Positive/Negayive Symptoms of Schizhophrenia, Potent Anticholinergic
- Useful for Resistant Schizophrenia
- Adverse effects – Agranulocytosis – 1%, Seizure, Weight gain, Sedation++, Myocarditis.

Antiparkinsonian Drugs

Drugs affecting brain dopaminergic system	
Dopamine precursor	Levodopa
Peripheral decarboxylase inhibitors	Carbidopa, Benserazide
Dopaminergic agonists	Bromocriptine, Ropinirole, Pramipexole
MAO-B inhibitor	Selegiline, Rasagiline
COMT inhibitor	Entacapone, Tolcapone
Glutamate antagonist (Antiviral)	Amantadine
Drugs affecting brain cholinergic system	
Central anticholinergics	Trihexyphenidyl, Procyclidine, Biperiden
Antihistaminic	Orphenadrine, Promethazine

Antiepileptic Drugs

Classification of antiepilectics

Barbiturate	Phenobarbitone
Deoxybarbiturate	Primidone
Hydantoin	Phenytoin, Fosphenytoin
Iminostilbene	Carbamazepine, Oxycarbazepine
Succinimide	Ethosuximide
Aliphatic carboxylic acid	Valproic acid
Benzodiazepines	Clonazepam, Diazepam, Lorazepam, Clobazam
Phenyl Triazine	Lamotrigine
Cyclic GABA analogues	Gabapentin, Pregabalin
Newer drugs	Topiramate, Zonisamide, Levetiracetam, Vigabatrin, Tiagabine, Lacosamide

MOA of Antiepileptics

MOA of antiepileptic	Drugs
Inhibition of use dependent Na^+ channels	Phenytoin, Carbamazepine, Valproate, Topiramate, Lamotrigine, Lacosamide
Inhibition of inhibitory neurotransmission	Barbiturates, Benzodiazepines, Ganaxolone, Gabapentin, Vigabatrin, Tiagabine
Decrease in excitatory neurotransmission	Glutamate, Aspartate, Felbamate, Topiramate
Inhibition of Ca^{2+} channels	Ethosuximide, Valproate, Lamotrigine

Phenytoin Toxicity

Acute toxicity	Chronic toxicity
• Cardiac arrhythmias • Nystagmus • Ataxia • Diplopia • Vertigo	• Hyperglycemia • Hirsutism,acne • Hypertrophy of gums • Hypersensitivity – rashes, SLE • Hydantoin syndrome

DOC for Various Seizures

Types of seizures	Drug of choice
Absence seizures	Valproate
GTCS	Valproate
Myoclonic seizures	Valproate
Atonic seizures	Valproate
Tonic seizures	Valproate
Clonic seizures	Valproate
Partial seizures	Carbamazepine
Infantile spasms	ACTH
Infantile spasm with tuberous sclerosis	Vigabatrin
Febrile seizures	PR Diazepam
Status epilepticus	IV Lorazepam
Status in eclampsia	Magnesium sulfate

Opioids

Actions ascribed to different types of opioid receptor

μ (Mu)	κ (Kappa)	δ (Delta)
Analgesia Respiratory depression Sedation Euphoria Miosis Muscular rigidity Reduced GI motility Physical dependence (morphine type)	Analgesia Respiratory depression (low ceiling) Dysphoria Miosis (low ceiling) Sedation Reduced GI motility Physical dependence (nalorphine type)	Analgesia Respiratory depression Affecting behavior Reinforcing actions Reducing GI motility Proconvulsant

Classification of Opioids

Natural opium alkaloids	Morphine, Codeine
Semisynthetic opioids	Diacetylmorphine, Pholcodeine, Ethylmorphine
Synthetic opioids	Pethidine, Fentanyl, Methadone, Tramadol, Dextropropoxyphene

Opioid Agonist and Antagonist

Mixed opioid	Agonist	Antagonist
Buprenorphin	μ	κ, δ
Nalbupine, Pentazocin, Dezocine	κ	μ
Butorphanol	κ	

Uses of Opioid Antagonist

Naloxone	Rx of acute opioid poisoning
Nalmefene	Maintenance drug for opioid poisoning Prevent relapse after de-addiction Prevent alcohol craving in chronic alcoholics
Naloxone	Neonatal resuscitation

Opioid De-addiction

Short duration	Long duration/maintenance	Relapse prevention
• Beta blockers/Clonidine	• Methadone	• Naltrexone

Uses of Opioids

IV morphine	Myocardial infarction, Acute pulmonary edema
Codeine, Pholcodeine, Dextromethorphan, Noscapine	Cough suppressants
Loperamide, Diphenoxylate	Noninfective diarrhea
Morphine	Preanesthetic medication
Pethidine	Reduces shivering after anesthesia (α2 receptor action)
Methadone	Neuropathic/Cancer pain
Methadone	Opioid abuse and Opioid rotation treatment

Migraine

Drug therapy of Migraine

Severity	Drug therapy
Mild	Simple analgesics/NSAIDs (antiemetic)
Moderate	NSAIDs combinations/triptans/ergot alkaloids (antiemetic)
Severe	Triptans/ergot alkaloids (antiemetic) + Prophylaxis

Classification of Antimigraine Drugs

Simple analgesics	Paracetamol, Aspirin
Nonsteroidal anti-inflammatory drugs	Ibuprofen, Naproxen, Diclofenac, Mephenamic acid, Indomethacin
Antiemetics	Metoclopramide, Domperidone, Prochlorperazine
Ergot alkaloids	Ergotamine, Dihydroergotamine
Selective 5-HT agonists	Sumatriptan, Rizatriptan

Prophylaxis of Migraine

β-blocker	Propranolol, Metoprolol, Atenolol, Timolol
Tricyclic antidepressants	Amitriptyline
Calcium channel blockers	Verapamil, Flunarizine
Anticonvulsants	Valproic acid, Gabapentin, Topiramate
5-HT antagonist	Methysergide, Cyproheptadine

Sedative/Hypnotics

Barbiturates	Long acting	Phenobarbitone
	Short acting	Butobarbitone, Pentobarbitone
	Ultra short acting	Thiopentone, Methohexitone
Benzodiazepines	Hypnotic	Diazepam, Flurazepam, Nitrazepam, Flunitrazepam, Temazepam, Triazolam, Quazepam, Midazolam
	Anticonvulsant	Diazepam, Clonazepam, Clobazem, Lorazepam
	Antianxiety	Diazepam, Oxazepam, Lorazepam, Alprazolam, Chlordiazepoxide
	Muscle relaxant	Diazepam
Newer hypnotics		Zopiclone, Zolpidem, Zaleplon
Other drugs		Chloral hydrate, Glutethimide, Meprobamate, Ramelton, Tasimelton

Gout

Acute gout	Chronic gout	
NSAIDs Colchicine's Corticosteroids	Uricosuric	Synthesis inhibitors
	Probenicid Sulfinpyrazone Benzbromarone Rasburicase Pegloticase	Allopurinol Febuxostat

Rheumatoid Arthritis

Disease modifying Antirheumatoid drug

TNF – α blocking agent	Etanercept, Adalimumab, Infliximab, Golimumab, Certolizumab
Antimetabolite	Methotrexate
Sulfonamides	Sulfasalazine, Sulfapyridine
Immunosuppressant	Leflunomide, Azathioprine, Mycophenolate mofetil, Cyclosporine, Cyclophosphamide, Abatacept (Co-stimulation inhibitor), Tocilizumab (MAB against IL – 6), Tofacitinib
Antimalarial	Chloroquine, Hydroxychloroquine
Old drugs	Gold, d-penicillamine

Rx of Neurodegenerative Diseases

Alzhemer's Disease	Anticholinesterases (Donepezil, rivastigmine and galantamine), Tacrine more hepatotoxic Memantine: NMDA antagonist that slows down the progression
Huntingtion's Chorea	D2 blockers like chlorpromazine, haloperidol as well as Olanzapine. Tetrabenazine (dopamine deplete) and reserpine

Amyotrophic Lateral Slerosis (ALS)	Riluzole (NMDA antagonist)
Multiple Sclerosis	Frequency of relapse can be decreased by: beta-interferon or glatiramer Spasticity can be decreased by: baclofen or tizanidine Monoclonal antibody: natalizumab (A.E: progressive multifocal leuco encephalopathy) Fingolimod: sphingosine-1 phosphate receptor modulator-used in relapsing forms of MS Dalfampridine: oral K channel blocker, improves walking in patients with MS
WILSON'S Disease	D-Penicillamine, Trientine, Zinc sulfate

RESPIRATORY SYSTEM AND GASTROINTESTINAL TRACT

Drugs for Peptic Ulcer

Peptic ulcer drugs

Antacids	Systemic antacid	Sodium bicarbonate
	Nonsystemic antacid	Aluminium hydroxide, Magnesium trisilicate, Megaldrate, Magnesium hydroxide
	Antifoaming agent	Simethicone
Drugs decreasing acid secretion	Proton pump inhibitors	Omeprazole, Pantoprazole, Esomeprazole, Lansoprazole, Rabeprazole
	H2 blockers	Cimetidine, Ranitidine, Famotidine, Roxatidine, Nizatidine, Loxatidine
	Anticholinergics	Propantheline, Oxyphenonium, Pirenzipine, Telenzipine
Drugs increasing protective factor	PGE 1 analogue	Misoprostol
	PGE 2 analogues	Enprostil, Rioprostil
Ulceroprotectives		Sucralfate, Colloidal bismuth subcitrate, Rebamipide and Ecabet
Anti H.pylori drugs	Triple regimen (2 weeks)	Lansoprazole + Amoxicillin + Clarithromycin
	Quadruple regimen (2 weeks)	Lansoprazole + Amoxicillin + Clarithromycin + Bismuth subcitrate
Ulcer healing drug		Carbenoloxone

Misoprostol (PGE 1 analogue) is the most specific drug for Rx and prevention of NSAID induced peptic ulcer (DOC is PPI).

Antihelicobacter Pylori Drugs

- Metronidazole/tinidazole
- Amoxicillin
- Clarithromycin
- Tetracycline
- Colloidal bismuth subcitrate
- Omeprazole/Lansoprazole.

Rx of Inflammatory Bowel Disease

- **Aminosalicylates 5ASA**
- **Glucocorticoids**
- **Purine analogs** Azathioprine and 6-MP
- **Methotrexate**
- **Anti TNFa therapy:** Infliximab, adalimumab and certolizumab
- **Natalizumab:** targeted against α-4 subunit of integrins.

Antiemetic Drugs

- **Drugs for motion sickness: Hyoscine**
- **Cinnarizine** used Rx of vertigo
- **Doxylamine (antihistamic) with pyridoxine (Vit B6):** Safest antiemetic drug in pregnancy
- **Chemotherapy and radiotherapy induced vomiting:** 5HT3 blockers like ondansetron DOC
- **Aprepitant (substance P antagonist)**: Selective NK-1 receptor antagonist
- **Dronabinol (a cannabinoid).**

Antitussives

Expectorants	Antitussives
Potassium iodide acts directly (by irritating bronchial glands) and indirectly (by gastric irritation) to increase bronchial secretion Mucolytic: Bromhexine and Ambroxol	Cough suppressants, Only for dry (nonproductive) cough Antitussives include codeine, pholocodeline, noscapine, and dextromethorphan

Drugs for Bronchial Asthma

Mechanism of action		Drugs
Bronchodilators	β_2 sympathomimetics	Salbutamol, Terbutaline, Bambuterol, Salmeterol, Formoterol, Ephedrine
	Methylxanthine	Theophylline, Aminophylline, Choline theophyllinate, Doxophylline
	Anticholinergics	Ipratropium bromide, Tiotropium bromide
Leukotriene antagonist		Montelukast, Zafirlukast
Mast cell stabilizers		Sodium cromoglycate, Ketotifen
Corticosteroids	Systemic	Hydrocortisone, Prednisolone
	Inhalational	Beclomethasone, Budesonide, Fluticasone, Flunisolide, Ciclesonide
Anti IgE antibody		Omalizumab

Rx of acute attack of bronchial asthma (bronchodilators)

Sympathomimetics	Parasympatholytics	Methyl xanthenes
• Fastest acting drugs by inhalational route • Adrenaline, isoprenaline and ephedrine • Selective β2 agonists (Salbutamol (albuterol), pirbuterol and terbutaline) for acute attack asthma • Not suitable for prophylaxis because of shorter duration of action • Salmeterol, bambuterol and formoterol are long acting β2 selective agonist	• More effective for COPD than bronchial asthma • Ipratropium and tiotropium are anticholinergic drugs (selective M3 antagonists) that can be used by inhalational route • Bronchodilators of choice in patients of bronchial asthma on β blocker therapy	• Caffeine, aminophylline, theophylline and theobromine • Inhibits phosphodiesterase

ANTIMICROBIAL AGENTS

Classification of Antibiotics According to Its Mechanism of Action

Mechanism of action	Drugs
Inhibition of cell wall synthesis	Penicillin, Cephalosporins, Vancomycin, Cycloserine, Bacitracin, Fosfomycin
Leakage from cell membrane	Polymyxin B, Colistin, Bacitracin, Nystatin, Amphotericin B, Hamycin
Inhibit protein synthesis	Tetracycline, Clindamycin, Chloramphenicol, Linezolid, Erythromycin

Contd...

Contd...

Mechanism of action	Drugs
mRNA code misreading	Aminoglycosides
Inhibition of DNA gyrase	Quinolones
Interfere DNA function	Rifampicin, Metronidazole
Interferes DNA synthesis	Acyclovir, Zidovudine
Interaction with intermediary metabolism	Sulfonamides, Sulfones, PAS, Trimethoprim, Pyrimethamine, Ethambutol

Protein Synthesis Inhibitors

Event	Antibiotic(s) and Binding Site(s)	Mechanism(s)
• Formation of initiation complex	Aminoglycosides (30S)	Interfere with initiation codon functions—block association of 50S ribosomal subunit with mRNA-30S (static); misreading of code incorporation of wrong AA (-cidal)
• Amino-acid incorporation	Tetracyclines (30S)	Block the attachment of aminoacyl tRNA to acceptor site (-static)
• Formation of peptide bond	Chloramphenicol (50S)	Inhibit the activity of peptidyltransferase (-static)
• Translocation	Macrolides and clindamycin (50S)	Inhibit translocation of peptidyl-tRNA from acceptor to donor site *(-static)*

Post Antibiotic Effect

Aminoglycoside, Quinolone, Rifampicin, Carbapenem, Azithro and Clarithromycin

Antibiotic Use in Pregnancy

Maternal ADR

- **Tetracycline** – Fulminant hepatic failure for mother
- **Erythromycin estolate** – Cholestatic jaundice for mother.

Fetal ADR

- Supha and Cotrimoxazole – Kernicterus
- Tetracycline – Teeth and Bone Problem
- Aminoglycoside – Ototoxicity
- Quinolones – Arthropathy
- Clarithromycin – Teratogenic
- Chloramphenicol – Grey Baby Syndrome.

Important Mechanisms of Drug Resistance

Groups	Mechanism of resistance
Beta lactams	Inactivating enzyme (beta lactamase)
Tetracyclines	Efflux pump (decreased concentration in the cell)
Chloramphenicol	Inactivating enzyme (acetyl transferase)
Fluoroquinolones	Altered DNA gyrase with reduced affinity
Sulfonamides	For large amount of PABA, Decreased activity of folate synthase
Aminoglycosides	Inactivating enzyme
Macrolides	Decreased permeability or efflux pumps

Antipseudomonal Drugs

Beta lactam antibiotics	Carboxypenicillins	Carbenicillin, Ticarcillin
	Ureidopenicillin	Piperacillin, Azlocillin, Mezlocillin
	Monobactams	Aztreonam
	Cephalosporins	Ceftazidime, Cefperazone, Moxalactam, Cefepime, Cefpirome
	Carbapenems	Imipenem, Doripenem, Meropenem
Fluoroquinolones	Ciprofloxacin, Pefloxacin	
Polypeptide antibiotics	Colistin, Polymixin B	
Aminoglycosides		

Beta-Lactam Antibiotics Penicillins

- **Cephalosporins**
- **Monobactams, e.g. aztreonam**
- **Carbapenems, e.g. imipenem**
- **Beta lactamase inhibitors, e.g. clavulanic acid, sulbatum, tazabactum**

Penicillins

Based on the susceptibility to penicillinase and spectrum of action, penicillins are classified as:

- **Narrow spectrum penicillinase susceptible** penicillin G and penicillin V
- **Narrow spectrum penicillinase resistant** methicillin, nafcillin, oxacillin, cloxacillin
- **Wide spectrum penicillinase susceptible:**
  1. **Aminopenicillins** – Amoxicillin, ampicillin, bacampicillin
  2. **Carboxypenicillins** – Carbenicillin, ticarcillin
  3. **Ureidopenicillins** – Piperacillin, azlocillin, mezlocillin
  4. **Amidinopenicillin** – Gram negative except pseudomonas-Mecillinam

MOA: They bind to penicillin binding proteins (PBPs) on bacterial membrane and inhibit transpeptidase enzyme preventing the cross linking of peptidoglycan chains.

Cephalosporins

These are β-lactam antibiotics having 7-amino cephalosporanic acid nucleus.

First generation		Second generation		Third generation		Fourth generation	
Oral	Parenteral	Oral	Parenteral	Oral	Parenteral	Parenteral	Fifth generation
Cephalexin Cefadroxil Cephradine Cephaloridine	Cephalothin Cefazolin	Cefaclor Cefuroxime axetil	Cefuroxime Cefotetan Cefoxitin	Cefixime Cefopodoxime proxetil Cefdinir Ceftibuten	Cefotaxime Ceftizoxime Ceftriaxone Ceftazidime Cefoperazone Moxalactam	Cefepime Cefpirome	Ceftobiprole – parenteral Ceftraroline-IV
USES of 5th generation cephalosporin – MRSA, community acquired pneumonia.							

Sulfonamides Classification

Absorbed rapidly, excreted rapidly	Absorbed poorly, locally acting in the bowl	Topically used	Long acting
Short acting – sulfadiazine, sulfisoxazole **Medium acting** – sulfamethaxazole	Sulfasalazine	Silversulfadiazine mafenide sulfacetamide	sulfadoxine

Aminoglycosides

Site of action	Drugs	
Systemic aminoglycosides	Streptomycin Gentamycin Kanamycin Tobramycin	Amikacin Sisomicin Netilmicin
Oral aminoglycosides	Neomycin	Framycetin
Newer aminoglycosides	Paromomycin Ribostamycin Arbekacin Bekanamycin Dibekacin	Spectinomycin Hygromycin B Isepamicin Astromicin Verdamicin

Uses of Aminoglycosides

Aminoglycosides	Uses
Gentamicin, Tobramicin, Amikacin	Against gram negative organism
Streptomycin	Treatment of TB, Plague, Tularemia
Amikacin	Second line anti TB drug and for MDR TB
Neomycin, Framycetin	Used for topical bacterial infections
Neomycin	Gut sterilization in hepatic encephalopathy
Spectinomycin	Single dose treatment for penicillinase producing Neisseria gonorrhea

Side Effects of Aminoglycosides

Hearing loss	Vestibular dysfunction
Amikacin, Kanamycin, Neomycin	Streptomycin, Gentamicin

	Maximum	Minimum
Nephrotoxicity	Neomycin > Gentamicin	Streptomycin
Ototoxicity	Amikacin (Auditory), Streptomycin (Vestibular)	Netilmicin
Neuromuscular blockade	Neomycin > Streptomycin	Tobramycin

Classification of Tetracyclines

Group – I	Tetracycline, Chlortetracycline, Oxytetracycline
Group – II	Demeclocycline, Lymecycline
Group – III	Doxycycline, Minocycline

Uses of Tetracyclines

Tetracycline analogues	Uses
Tetracycline	LGV, Granuloma inguinale, Chlamydial pneumonia, Cholera, Brucellosis, Plague prophylaxis, H.pylori
Doxycycline	Relapsing fever, Lyme's disease, Rickettsial and Chlamydial infections, Malaria prophylaxis, Amebiasis
Minocycline	Meningococcal carrier state, Leprosy (ROM regime)
Demeclocycline	SIADH

Classification of Fluoroquinolones

Generation of fluoroquinolones	Drugs
First	Norfloxacin, Lomefloxacin
Second	Ciprofloxacin, Ofloxacin
Third	Levofloxacin, Gatifloxacin, Pefloxacin, Sparfloxacin
Fourth	Moxifloxacin, Fleroxacin, Garenoxacin, Gemifloxacin, Trovafloxacin

Uses of fluoroquinolones	Uses
Ciprofloxacin	Antipseudomonal fluoroquinolone, Prophylaxis of neutropenic patients
Ciprofloxacin	Prophylaxis of anthrax and meningococcal meningitis
Sparfloxacin	Against gram positive organisms
Levofloxacin, Gatifloxacin, Gemifloxacin, Moxifloxacin	Respiratory fluoroquinolones
Moxifloxacin, Trovafloxacin	Against gram positive and gram negative organisms and anerobes

Urinary Antiseptics

Favorable urinary pH for AMA

Acidic	Alkaline	pH immaterial
Nitrofurantoin Methenamine Tetracycline Methicillin Cloxacillin	Cotrimoxazole Aminoglycosides Cephalosporines Fluroquinolone	Chloramphenicol Ampicillin Colistin

Epsilometer test is done to detect antibiotic susceptibility.

Macrolides

Classification of Macrolides

Macrolides	Uses
Erythromycin	Chancroid, Corynebacterium, Campylobacter infections, Legionella infections, Atypical pneumonia, Whooping cough
Azithromycin and Roxithromycin	H.influenza and Neisseria infections Urogenital infections Chlamydia, MAC, Toxoplasma
Clarithromycin	Rx and prophylaxis of MAC Peptic ulcer by H.pylori
Spiramycin	Toxoplasmosis in pregnancy
Tacrolimus	Immunomodulator

Other Protein Synthesis Inhibitors

Protein synthesis inhibitors	Uses
Glycylcyclines – Tigecycline	Serious complicated skin and intra-abdominal infections Against MRSA, VRSA, Streptococci, Enterococci, Anerobes, Legionella
Ketolides – Telithromycin	Same as Macrolides
Lincosamides – Clindamycin, Lincomycin	Against anerobes like Bacteriodes and Propionbacterium DOC for Group A Streptococcal infection along with penicillin Pneumocystis jiroveci, Toxoplasma gondii

Contd...

Contd...

Protein synthesis inhibitors	Uses
Streptogramins – Quinpristinn and Dalfopristine	DOC for Penicillin resistant pneumococci, MRSA, VRSA and Methicillin resistant Enterococcus fecalis
Oxazolidinones – Linezolid	Against MRSA, VRSA and VRE
Pleuromutilins – Retapamulin	Topical treatment of MSSA
Lipopeptide – Daptomycin	Treatment of organisms resistant to linezolid and streptogramins, MRSA, VRSA, Penicillin resistant pneumococci

Antitubercualr Drugs

First line drugs	Second line drugs	
	Old drugs	Newer drugs
Isoniazid (H) Rifampin (R) Pyrazinamide (Z) Ethambutol (E) Streptomycin (S)	Thiacetazone, Para-aminosalicylic acid PAS, Ethionamide, Cycloserine Kanamycin, Amikacin, Capreomycin	Ciprofloxacin, Ofloxacin Clarithromycin, Azithromycin Rifabutin, Sparfloxacin

Important Features of Different Antitubercular Drugs

Drug	Mechanisms of action and resistance	Adverse effects
Isoniazid	Inhibit mycolic acid synthesis High level resistance – deletion in Cat K gene (codes for Catalase)	Hepatitis, Peripheral neuritis, Hemolysis in G6PD deficiency, SLE in slow acetylators
Rifampin	Inhibits DNA dependent RNA polymerase Resistance due to mutation in repo B gene	Proteinuria, Hepatitis, Flu-like syndrome, Red orange urine, Thrombocytopenia
Ethambutol	Inhibits synthesis of arabinogalactan (cell wall component)	Dose dependent retro bulbar neuritis, ↓visual acuity and Red – green blindness
Pyrazinamide	Action similar to that of INH Resistance due to mutation in the gene which encodes for enzyme generation in the active metabolite	Polyarthralgia, myalgia, Hepatitis and Rash Hyperuricemia, phototoxicity, ↑porphyrin synthesis
Streptomycin	Protein synthesis inhibitor	Deafness, Vestibular dysfunction and Nephrotoxicity

MAC – Treatment: REC regimen (Rifabutin + Ethambutol + Clarithromcin or Azithromycin)

RNTCP Guidelines: Treatment Categories: DOTS

New (former categories I and III)	Previously treated (former category II)
New sputum smear-positive, New sputum smear-negative, New extrapulmonary tuberculosis, others	Sputum smear-positive relapse, Sputum smear-positive failure, Sputum smear-positive treatment after default, Sputum smear-negative or who have Extra-pulmonary disease who can have recurrence
$2H_3R_3Z_3E_3 + 4H_3R_3$	$2H_3R_3Z_3E_3S_3 + 1H_3R_3Z_3E_3 + 5H_3R_3E_3$
2 months Intensive phase + 4 months continuation phase Four drugs at Thrice-weekly Schedule for 2 months Intensive phase and Two drugs at Thrice-Weekly Schedule for remaining 4 months continuation phase	3 months Intensive phase + 5 months continuation phase Five drugs at Thrice-weekly Schedule for initial 2 months followed by Four drugs for next 1 month Intensive phase Three drugs at Thrice-weekly Schedule for remaining 5 months continuation phase

H: Isoniazid (300 mg),
R: Rifampicin (450 mg),

Z: Pyrazinamide (1500 mg),
E: Ethambutol (1200 mg),
S: Streptomycin (750 mg).

Note:

- Patients who weigh > 60 kg will receive additional Rifampicin 150 mg.
- Patients who > 50 years old receive Streptomycin 500 mg.
- Patients who weigh < 30 kg receive drugs as per body weight.
  - **DOTS is for TB and DOTS-Plus is for MDR-TB.**

MDR-TB: DOTS-Plus

Multi-drug-resistant tuberculosis (MDR-TB) is defined as TB which is resistant to at least isoniazid (INH) and rifampicin (RMP).

Grouping Drugs

Group	Class	Drugs
1	First-line oral anti-TB agents	Isoniazid (H); Rifampicin (R); Ethambutol (E); Pyrazinamide (Z)
2	Injectable anti-TB agents	Streptomycin (S); Kanamycin (Km); Amikacin (Am); Capreomycin (Cm); Viomycin (Vm).
3	Fluoroquinolones	Ciprofloxacin (Cfx); Ofloxacin (Ofx); Levofloxacin (Lvx); Moxifloxacin (Mfx); Gatifloxacin (Gfx)
4	Oral second-line anti-TB agents	Ethionamide (Eto); Prothionamide (Pto); Cycloserine (Cs); Terizadone (Trd); Para-aminosalicylic acid (PAS)
5	Agents with unclear efficacy (not recommended by WHO for routine use in MDR-TB patients)	Clofazimine (Cfz); Linezolid (Lzd); Amoxicillin/Clavulanate (Amx/Clv); Thioacetazone (Thz); Imipenem/Cilastatin (Ipm/Cln); High-dose isoniazid (high-dose H); Clarithromycin (Clr)

RNTCP CATEGORY IV REGIMEN for Treatment of MDR TB:

6 (9) Km Ofx (Lvx) Eto Cs Z E/18 Ofx (Lvx) Eto Cs E

Antileprosy Drugs

Multibacillary leprosy – 12 months	Paucibacillary leprosy – 6 months
Rifampicin – 600 mg once monthly supervised Dapsone – 100 mg OD Clofazimine – 300 mg once monthly supervised and 50 mg OD	Rifampicin – 600 mg once monthly supervised Dapsone – 100 mg OD
	ROM regimen – Rifampicin + Ofloxacin + Minocycline single dose therapy

Antiretroviral Agents

CLASS	Drugs	Special points
Nucleoside reverse transcriptase inhibitors (NRTI)	Zidovudine Didanosine Lamivudine Stavudine Abacavir Zalcitabine Emtricitabine Apricitabine	• All NRTIs are excreted by the kidney(require dosage adjustment in RF) except ABACAVIR which is metabolized by alcohol dehydrogenase. • All NRTIs including tenofovir may cause lactic acisosis, hepatomegaly, steatosis by inhibiting mammalian mitochondrial DNA polymerase • Abacavir is a Nucleoside Reverse Transcriptase Inhibitors (NRTI's). Hypersensitivity reaction is due to HLA B 5701 allele

Nucleotide RTI	Tenofovir	Not require bioactivation by kinases
Non-nucleoside reverse transcriptase inhibitors (NNRTI)	Efavirenz Nevirapine Delavirdine Etravirine Rilpivirine	Rashes/headache/nausea, Fatigue, Hepatitis Neuropsychiatric manifestation
Protease Inhibitors (PI)	Amprenavir Fosamprenavir Indinavir Saquinavir Ritonavir Tipranavir Lopiniavir Atazanavir Nelfinavir Darunavir	• All PI agents, except fosamprenavir, carry the risk of hyperlipidemia, fat maldistribution (buffalo hump), hyperglycemia, and insulin resistance • The concurrent use of saquinavir and ritonavir is contraindicated because of QT prolongation • Ritonavir a potent CYP3A4 inhibitor used to 'boost' the levels of other PI agents, thus acting as a 'pharmacokinetic enhancer'
Integrase Inhibitor	Raltigranavir Elvitegranavir	Metabolized by glucuronidation (not cytochrome P450)
Fusion Inhibitors	Enfuvirtide Maraviroc	Binds to Gp 41 sub unit of HIV envelope Maraviroc is CCR-5 inhibitor

Prior to the initiation of Abacavir – Test for the presence of HLA-B5701 allele is recommended.

Drugs Safer in Pregnancy

Zidovudine, Lamivudine, Nevirapine, Lopinavir, Ritonavir.

Antiherpes Drugs

Acyclovir: Herpes simplex virus (HSV-1 and 2) and varicella zoster virus (VZV).

- It is a guanosine analogue activated by a virus specific kinase acyclovir monophosphate and then by host kinase to form acyclovir triphosphate.
- **Valacyclovir** has a long half life and gets converted to acyclovir by hepatic metabolism.
- **Famciclovir** is a prodrug of penciclovir.

Ganciclovir: CMV and HSV and acts by inhibiting DNA polymerase.

- **Ganciclovir is the drug of choice for CMV infections including retinitis.**
- Dose limiting ADR is **myelosuppression.**

Cidofovir: HSV, CMV, adenovirus and papilloma virus.

- Dose limiting toxicity is nephrotoxicity.

Foscarnet: CMV infections

It does not require phosphorylation for activity.

ADR: Nephrotoxicity, hypocalcemia and CNS problems.

Other Drugs for HSV: Vidarabine, idoxuridine, trifluridine, fomivirsen and docosanol.

- **Fomivirsen** is the first antisense oligonucleotide and is active against CMV retinitis by intravitreal route
- It can cause iritis, vitreitis and changes in intraocular pressure
- **Idoxuridine** is used only topically for keratoconjunctivitis by HSV
- **Docosanol** is a long chain saturated alcohol that can be used topically for herpes labialis.

ANTI-INFLUENZA DRUGS

Amantadine and rimantadine: Prevent uncoating of influenza A virus (not influenza B).

- Amantadine can cause adverse effects like livedo reticularis and ankle edema.
- Amantadine is also used in parkinsonism.
- Rimantadine is longer acting than amantadine.

Oseltamivir and zanamavir: Neuraminidase inhibitors preventing the virion release by causing clumping of mature virions of both influenza A and influenza B (Bird flu)

- Oseltamivir (TAMIFLU) is an oral prodrug (ADR: nausea and vomiting)
- Zanamavir is administered intranasally (ADR: bronchospasm).

Other Antivirals

- **Palivizumab:** Human monoclonal antibody for RSV
- **Imiquimod:** HPV
- **Rhinovirus/Enterovirus:** Pleconaril

Drugs in clinical trials:

- **Maribavir:** DNA synthesis inhibitor – CMV
- **Peramivir:** (Neuraminidase inhibitor) – influenza

Antifungal Agents

According to the mechanism of action the antifungal agents can be classified as

- **Drug altering membrane permeability**
  - Azoles: Inhibit 14 – sterol demethylase, prevent ergosterol synthesis, and lead to the accumulation of 14 – methylsterols.
    - Triazoles, e.g. Fluconazole, itraconazole, voriconazole
    - Imidazoles, e.g. Ketoconazole, miconazole, clotrimazole
  - Allylamines: Naftifine and terbinafine, inhibit squalene epoxidase and prevent ergosterol synthesis.
  - Polyenes, e.g. Amphotericin B, nystatin, hamycin. They bind to ergosterol in fungal cell membranes and increase membrane permeability.
- **Drug blocking nucleic acid synthesis,** e.g. Flucytosine
- **Drugs disrupting microtubule function,** e.g. Griseofulvin
- **Drugs inhibiting cell wall synthesis,** e.g. Caspofungin, nikkomycin. These are echinocandins, which inhibit the formation of glucans in the fungal cell wall.

Antimalarial Drugs

Primary tissue schizonticides (Causal prophylaxis)		Proguanil, Primaquine, Pyrimethamine
Erythrocytic schizonticides (Acute attacks and Suppressive prophylaxis)	Fast acting	Chloroquine, Mepacrine, Quinine, Mefloquine, Halofantrine, Atovaquone, Artemisinin derivatives
	Slow acting	Proguanil, Pyrimethamine, Sulfonamides, Tetracyclines
Exoerythrocytic schizonticides (Radical cure)		Primaquine
Sporonticides/Gametocides (Prevent malarial transmission)	P.vivax	Chloroquine, Mepacrine, Quinine
	P.vivax and P.falciparum	Proguanil, Primaquine, Pyrimethamine, Artemisinin

Remember the Uses of Chloroquine as 'My Girl's RED LIP'

- M = Malaria
- G = Giardiasis
- R = Rhematoid arthritis
- E = Extraintestinal amebiasis
- D = DLE
- L = Lepra reaction
- I = Infectious mononucleosis
- P = Photogenic reactions.

Classification on Antiamebic Drugs

Class of antiamebic drugs	Drugs
Tissue amebicides	Chloroquine
Luminal and Tissue amebicides	Nitroimidazoles (Metronidazole, Tinidazole, Secnidazole, Ornidazole), Emetine, Dehydroemetine
Luminal amebicides	Diloxanide furoate, Paromomycin, Iodoquinol, Quiniodochlor, Tetracyclines

Classification of antihelminthic Drugs

Antihelminthic drugs	Drugs
Drugs inhibiting polymerization of beta tubulin	Albendazole, Mebendazole, Thiabendazole, Triclabendazole
Drugs causing spastic paralysis (NN receptor agonist)	Pyrantel palmoate, Levamisole
Drugs causing flaccid paralysis (GABA agonist)	Piperazine, Ivermectin
Drugs altering microfilarial membrane and increasing phagocytosis	Diethyl carbazine
Drugs causing uncoupling of oxidative phosphorylation	Bithionol, Niclosamide
Drugs causing influx of calcium	Praziquantel

Antihelminthic	Mechanism of action	Parasites susceptible
Mebendazole	Inhibits polymerization of β-tubulin of susceptible worms → live worms expelled	Round worm, Hook worm, Whip worm, Pin worm, Trichinella spiralis
Pyrantel palmate	Inhibits cholinesterase in worms → persistent depolarization → spastic paralysis → live worms expelled	Ascaris, Enterobius, Ancylostoma, Strongyloides
Piperazine	Hyperpolarization of muscle by GABA agonistic action → flaccid paralysis → live worms expelled	Ascaris, Enterobius
Ivermectin	Potentiates glutamated gated Cl- channel and increases GABA transmission in worms → hyperpolarization and paralysis of worms → dead worms expelled	Pediculosis, Scabies, Onchocerca, Strongyloides, Ascaris, Cutaneous larva migrans
Praziquantel	Increased muscular contraction and spastic paralysis of worms → dead worms expelled	Trematode, Cestodes
Levamisole and tetramisole	Ganglionic stimulation → tonic paralysis → live worms expelled	Ascaris, Ancylostoma, Strongyloides
Diethyl carbamazepine	Hyperpolarization of muscles → live worms expelled	Microfilaria of bancrofti, malayi, loa loa, Onchocerca
Niclosamide	Inhibits oxidative phosphorylation in mitochondria	Cestodes

CHEMOTHERAPY AND IMMUNOSUPPRESSANTS

Antineoplastic drugs: Divided on the basis of stage of cell cycle at which they act into two groups – cell cycle specific (CCS) and cell cycle non-specific (CCNS)

Phase	CCS drugs	CCNS drugs (AAAAAAM)
G1	Etoposide	Platinum compounds Alkylating agents, Anthracyclines, Actinomycin D, cAmptothecins Mitomycin-C
S	Antimetabolites	
G2	Bleomycin, Etoposide	
M	Vinca alkaloids, Taxanes (MTV)	

Classification of Anticancer Drugs

Alkylating agents	Nitrogen mustards	Mechlorethamine, cyclophosphamide, ifosfamide, melphalan,
	Ethyleimines	Thio-TEPA, hexamethylmelamine (altreatmine)
	Alkyl sulfonates	Busulphan
	Nitroso ureas	Carmustine, lomustine, streptozocin
	Triaines	Procarbazine, temozolomide
Platinum compounds	Cisplatin, carboplatin, oxaliplatin	
Antimetabolites	Pyrimidine analogs	5-FU, cytarabine, gemcitabine
	Purine analogs	6-MP, 6-thiogunanine, pentostatin, cladribine
	Folic acid analogs	Methotrexate, vinblastine, vinorelbine
Natural productus	Vinca alkaloids	Vincristine, vinblastine, vinorelbine
	Taxanes	Paclitaxel, docetaxel
	Epipodophylotoxins	Etoposide, teniposide
	Camptothecins	Topotecan, irinotecan
	Antitumor antibiotics	Anthracyclines (d aunorubicin, doxorubicin, epirubicin, darubicin, mitoxantrone), bleomycin, dactinomycin, mitomycin-C
	Enzymes	I-Asparaginase
Hormones and related agents	Corticosteroids	Prednisolone, prednisone
	Antiestrogens	SERMs and Aromatase inhibitors E.g.: Tamoxifen, Aminoglutethimide, formestane, exemestane, anastrozole, vorozole, letrozole, etc.
	Progestins	Medroxyprogesterone acetate
	Estrogen	Diethylstilbestrol, ehineyl estradiol
	Androgens	Testosterone
	Antiandrogens	Flutamide
	GnRH analogs	Leuprolide, goserelin, nafareline, busureline, histerelin
	GnRH antagonists	Cetorelix, ganirelix, abarelix
Miscellaneous agents	Arsenic compounds	As_2O_3
	Adenosine deaminase inhibitor	Pentostatin
	Tyrosine kinase inhibitors	Imatinib, geftinib, erlotinib
	Retinoids	Isotretinoin

Inhibiting DNA or RNA synthes: Cell Cycle Specific (S-phase)

Folic acid	Purine	Pyramidine
Methotrexate Pemetrexed	Thioguanine Mercaptopurine Fludarabine Pentostatin Cladribine	Cytarabine Flurouracil Floxuridine Gemcitabine Capecitabine

Distinctive toxicities of antimetabolites	
6-MP and 6TG	Hepatotoxicity
5-FU	Hand and foot syndrome, neurotoxicity
Capecitabine	Hand and foot syndrome
Cytarabine	Cerebellar ataxia
Fludarabine	Arthralgia
Gemcitabine	Diarrhea

Anticancer Antibiotics

- Actinomycin D (Dactinomycin)
- Daunorubicin
- Mitomycin
- Bleomycin
- Doxorubicin
- Mitoxantrone
- Mithramycin → Plicamycin

All anticancer drugs acts by intercalating between DNA strands and Interfere with its template function.

Alkylating Agents

- Busulfan
- Carmustine (Nitrosoureas), Lomustine, Semustine
- Chlorambucil
- Cyclophosphamide
- Melphalan, Dacarbazine, Mechlorethaminle, Ifosfamide
- Thiotepa
- Cell cycle nonspecific, secondary neoplasia are common.

Most leukemogenic alkylating agent – Melphalan

- Only alkylating agent which act by inhibiting RNA and protein synthesis (rest mainly affect DNA) – Decarbazine.

Distinctive toxicities of alkylating agents	
Cyclophosphamide	Alopecia, hemorrhagic cystitis
Ifosfamide	Hemorrhagic cystitis
Busulphan	Pulmonary fibrosis, hyperpigmentation. Adrenal insufficiency
Cisplatin	Emesis, Nephrotoxicity, ototoxicity, peripheral sensory neuropathy
Procarbazine	Secondary leukemias, disulfiram like reactions

Protectants

- Granulocyte Colony stimulating factors (CSF) – Filgrastim.
- (GM-CSF) Sargramostim in chemo-therapy induced neutropenia
- Acrolein conjugator Mesna in hemorrhagic cystitis
- Iron chelator: Dexrazoxane (doxorubicin induced cardiomyopathy)
- Thrombopoietic growth factors Oprelvekin (interleukin-11, IL-11)
- Reversal of resistance – verapamil.

Immunosuppressants Drugs

- Glucocorticoids-prednisolone, methyl prednisolone
- Cyclosporin, Tacrolimus, Sirolimus.

Cytotoxic Drugs

Purine Analogues

- Azathioprine
- Mycophenolate.

Pyramidine Analogues

- Leflunamide
- Folate analogue

- Methotrexate
- Cyclophosphamide.

Immunosuppressants – Antibodies

- Lymphocyte Immunoglobulin (LIG, ATG)
- Rh(D) immunoglobulin

Monoclonal antibodies:

- Daclizumab – IL2 inhibitor
- Basiliximab
- Infliximab
- OKT3, muromonab (CD3 T-cell)

THALIDOMIDE used for multiple myeloma, type 2 lepra reaction.

Monoclonal Antibodies

Name	MOA	Indications	Toxicity
Rituximab	Anti CD20	B-cell lymphoma CLL	• Infusion related (fever, urticaria, hypotension) • Late onset neutropenia
Alemtuzumab	Anti CD52	B-cell CLL T-cell lymphoma	• Infusion related • T-cell depletion with infection
Daclizumab	Anti CD25a IL2	T-cell mycosis fungodies	• Fever, Arthralgia • Asthma, Hypotension
Gemtuzumab	Anti CD33	AML, Myelodysplasias	• Infusion related • Bone marrow suppression • Hepatic toxicity
Trastuzumab	Anti HER2/neu (ErbB-2)	• Breast cancer	• Cardiomyopathy • Infusion related
Cetuximab	Anti EGFR	• Nonsmall cell lung cancer	• Skin rash (in 75% patients) • Colorectal cancer • Infusion related • Breast cancer, Pancreatic cancer
Bevacizumab	Anti VEGF	• Colorectal cancer	• Hypertension • pulmonary hemorrhage • GIT perforation • Proteinuria • Congestive heart failure
Omalizumab	Anti IgE	Bronchial asthma (in chronic asthma as a rescue medication and in status asthmatics	• Injection site reactions (stinging, brushing, induration)

Infliximab	Anti TNFa	Rheumatoid arthritis Crohn's disease	Infusion related Upper respiratory tract infections Urinary infections
Adalimumab	Anti TNFa	Rheumatoid arthritis	
Etanercept (not a monoclonal Ab)	Anti TNFa	Rheumatoid arthritis	
Efalizumab	Anti LFA-1 CD11	Organ transplantation Psoriasis	LFA-1, lymphocyte function associated antigen 1.

Basiliximab	Il-2	Immunosuppressant
Palivizumab	Fusion protein	RSV
Alefacept	LFA-3	Plaque psoriasis
Natalizumab	Integerin- alpha 4	Multiple sclerosis
Donesumab	RANL L	Osteoporosis

Ofatumumab	CD20	SLE
Belimumab	BLyS	SLE
Epratuzumab	CD22	SLE
Ocrelizumab	CD20	SLE
Donesumab	Rank ligand	Osteoporosis
Taclizumab	IL-6R	SLE

Gene therapy: refers to the introduction of functional genetic material into target cell to replace or supplement defective genes, or to modify target cells so as achieve therapeutic goals.

Approaches in gene therapy	Applications of gene therapy
• Gene modification • Gene insertion • Gene transfer • Gene deletion	• Cystic fibrosis, severe combined immune deficiency • Growth hormone deficiency, Familial hypercholesterolemia • Lesch-Nyhan syndrome, Parkinsonism, Alzheimer's • Gaucher's disease, Multiple sclerosis, DMD, Cancer, HIV

Neoplasm	Chemotherapeutic agent of choice	Neoplasm	Chemotherapeutic agent of choice
Multiple myeloma	Melphalan		
Carcinoma pancreas	Gemcitabine	Hairy cell leukemia and CLL	Cladiribin
Choriocarcinoma	Methotrexate	Carcinoma prostate	Flutamide
Brain tumors	Nitroso urease	CML	Imatinib
Esophagus	Cisplatin	Wegener's granulomatosis	Cyclophosphamide

NEWER DRUGS: FDA APPROVED NEWER DRUGS 2012–14

Name		MOA	Use
GIT	Linaclotide	Guanylyl Cyclase Agonist	Constipation associated IBS
	Crofelemer	CFTR and CaCC channel inhibitors	Diarrhea in AIDS
CVS	Vedolizumab	Blocks integrin α4β7 (LPAM-1, lymphocyte Peyer's patch adhesion molecule 1)	Ulcerative colitis and Crohn's disease
	Apixaban	Xa inhibitor	Stroke and systemic embolism (atrial fibrillation)
	Peginesatide acetate	Synthetic, pegylated erythropoiesis-stimulating agent	Anemia due to chronic kidney disease
	Avanafil	PDE5 inhibitor	Erectile dysfunction
	Vorapaxar	Thrombin receptor (protease-activated receptor, PAR-1) antagonist	Thrombotic cardiovascular events in patients with a history of myocardial infarction or peripheral arterial disease
NS	Florbetapir f-18	Radioactive diagnostic agent	Estimates β-amyloid plaques in Alzheimer's disease
	Taliglucerase alfa	r- β-gluco cerebrosidase	Gaucher's disease
	Mirabegron	Adrenergic Agonist	Overactive bladder
	Perampanel	i-AMPA Glutamate Receptor Antagonist	Partial – Onset seizures
	Dimethyl fumarate	GSH depletion and increase in HO-1 (anti-inflammatory stress protein)	Relapsing multiple sclerosis
	Tasimelteon	Selective agonist for the melatonin receptors MT1 and MT2 in the suprachiasmatic nucleus	Non-24-hour sleep–wake disorder
	Droxidopa	Synthetic amino acid prodrug for norepinephrine and epinephrine capable of crossing BBB	Neurogenic orthostatic hypotension

Contd...

Contd...

	Name	MOA	Use
RS	Aclidinium bromide	Antimuscarinic agent	COPD
	Bedaquiline (diarylquinoline)	Subunit c mycobacterial ATP synthase inhibitor	Pulmonary multidrug-resistant tuberculosis
	Ivacaftor	Potentiate CFTR	Cystic fibrosis with mutation in CFTR gene
	Lucinactant	Pulmonary surfactant	Respiratory distress syndrome
Chemotherapy	Cobicistat; elvitegravir; Emtricitabine; tenofovir	CyP450 Inhibitor; HIV-1 Integrase Inhibitor; NRTI; Nucliotide RTI	HIV-1 Infection
	Raxibacumab	mAb to Bacillus anthracis toxin	Anthrax
	Miltefosine	Inhibitor of Akt [protein kinase B (PKB)]	Leishmania donovani, L braziliensis, L guyanensisor, L panamensis infection
	Efinaconazole	A triazole antifungal inhibiting 14α-demethylase	Onychomycosis of the toe nails due to Trichophyton rubrum or Trichophyton mentagrophyte
	Dalbavancin	Lipoglycopeptide antibiotic inhibiting peptido-glycan synthesis in cellwall	ABSSSI (acute bacterial skin and skin structure infections) caused by designated Susceptible Gram-positive microorganisms
	Tedizolid	Inhibition of protein synthesis by binding to the 50S subunit of the bacterial ribosome	
Endocrine	Pasireotide	Somatostatin analogue	Cushing's disease
	Lorcaserin	5-HT 2C receptor agonist	Obesity
	Teduglutide,	GLP2 analogue	Short bowel syndrome
	Albiglutide	Glucagon-like peptide-1 agonist (GLP-1 agonist). DPP 4-resistant GLP 1 dimer fused to human albumin.	Type 2 diabetes
	Canagliflozin, Dapagliflozin	Sodium-glucose transport protein subtype 2 (SGLT2) inhibitor	Type 2 diabetes
	Lomitapide	Microsomal triglyceride transfer protein inhibitor	Homozygous familial hypercholesterolemia
	Alogliptin	Dipeptidyl peptidase 4 inhibitor	Type 2 diabetes
	Mipomersen	Antisense oligonucleotide	Homozygous familial hypercholesterolemia
	Ospemifene	Selective estrogen receptor modulator (SERM)	Dyspareunia – pain during sexual intercourse in woman
Others	Ingenol Mebutate	Apoptosis (unknown)	Actinic keratosis
	Tofacitinib	JAK inhibitor	Rheumatoid arthritis
	Tafluprost	PG- F receptor agonist	Open-angle glaucoma
	Ocriplasmin	r-Human Plasmin	Vitreo macular Adhesion
	Elosulfase Alfa	Synthetic N-acetylgalactosamine-6-sulfatase	Mucopolysaccharidosis type IVA (Morquio syndrome)
	Metreleptin	Synthetic analog of the hormone leptin	Leptin deficiency in patients with congenital or acquired generalized lipodystrophy
	Apremilast	Phosphodiesterase 4 (PDE4) inhibitor	Psoriatic arthritis
	Siltuximab	Monoclonal antibody that binds to interleukin-6	Multicentric Castleman's disease

Contd...

Contd...

	Name	MOA	Use
Oncology	Radium Ra-^{223} dichloride	Radioactivity	Castration-resistant prostate cancer
	Glucarpidase	r-bacterial enzyme degrades methotrexate	Methotrexate toxicity
	Choline C-11	Radiolabelled choline analogue	Diagnosis of recurrent Prostate Cancer
	Enzalutamide	Androgen rec. inhibitor	Metastatic castration-resistant prostate cancer
	Teriflunomide	Dihydroorotate dehydrogenase inhibitor	Relapsing forms of multiple sclerosis
	Regorafenib	Multikinase inhibitor (RET, VEGFR1, –2, –3, KIT)	Metastatic colorectal cancer
	Omacetaxine	Inhibits initiation of protein translation	CML
	Ponatinib	Multikinase inhibitor (BCR–ABL, KIT, RET, FLT3)	CML
	Bosutinib	Bcr–Abl inhibitor	Ph+ CML
	Axitinib	VEGF 1, 2, 3 inhibitor	Renal cell carcinoma
	Vismodegib	Smoothened receptor (SMO) Hedgehog pathway inhibitor	Basal cell carcinoma
	Ado-Trastuzumab Emtansine	mAB trastuzumab linked to the cytotoxic agent mertansine	HER2 +ve metastatic breast cancer
	Pertuzumab	mAb to HER2	HER2 +ve breast cancer
	Dabrafenib Mesylate	B-Raf inhibitor	Metastatic melanoma
	Trametinib	MEK inhibitor	Metastatic melanoma
	Pomalidomide	Thalidomide analog Upregulates IFN gamma, IL-2 and IL-10 and Down regulates IL-6	Multiple myeloma
	Carfilzomib	20s Proteasome Inhibitor	Multiple myeloma
	Cabozantinib	Multikinase inhibitor (RET, MET, VEGF, KIT, FLT3)	Medullary thyroid cancer
	Ziv-Aflibercept	r-Fusion Protein binding VEGFA, VEGFB and PIGF	Colorectal cancer
	Ramucirumab	Vascular endothelial growth factor receptor 2 (VEGFR2) antagonist	Gastric cancer
	Ceritinib	(Anaplastic lymphoma kinase) ALK inhibitor	Anaplastic lymphoma kinase (ALK)-positive metastatic non-small-cell lung cance

Other Newer Drugs

DMOAD

- Diacerin (IL-1 antagonist)
- Licofelone (combined COX-LOX inhibitor)

Cardiovascular Drugs

Name	MOA	Indications	Toxicity
Nesiritide	Recombinant from of BNP (Brain natriuretic peptide)–Natriuretric–Diuretic–Vasodilator	Refractory CHF	Hypotension
Omapartrilat	Vasopeptidase inhibitor Inhibits ACE and NEP → BNP ANP AT II	Congestive heart failure	Hypotension
Ibutilide/ Dofetilide	Selective K channel blocker (inward rectifying K chennal blocker)	Atrial fibrillation	Torsades de pointes

Hypolipidemic Drugs

Name	MOA	Indications	Toxicity
Ezetimibe	Decreased cholestrol absorption • Compensatory increase in cholesterol synthesis in liver so, always combined with a statin (synergistic effect)	Primary hypercholesterolemia	None reported
Torcetrapib (CETP inhibitor)	CETP mediates Transfer of TG from LDL to HDL • Transfer of cholesterol from HDL to LDL So, toretrapib increase HDL by inhibiting its degradation in liver because TG loaded HDL, is destroyed by liver	Hypercholesterolemia	None reported

Antiretroviral Drugs

Name	MOA	Indications	Toxicity
Enfuvirtide	Fusion Inhibitor	HIV positive adults (only in treatment experienced)	Injection site reaction
Emtricitabine	• Nucleoside reverse transcripatase inhibitor • Same as lamivudine but 10 times more potent	HIV infection	Nonspecific

Antiemetic Drugs

Name	MOA	Indications
Dronabinol	Stimulates CB, cannabinoid receptor on neurons in and around vomiting centre Also stimulates appetite	Cancer chemotherphy induced vomiting aids with anorexia (to stimulate appetite)
Aprepitant	• Antagonist of NK, subtype of tachykinin receptor	Cancer chemotherapy induced vomiting (delayed phase)

Antihepatitis Drugs

Name	MOA	Indications	Toxicity
Adefovir	Inhibits HBV DNA polymerase	Chronic HBV infection Lamivudine resistant NBV Infection	Nephrotoxicity
Lamivudine	• Inhibits HBV DNA polymerase • Inhibits HIV reverse transcriptase	Chronic HCV infection	
Ribavirin	Inhibits viral replication	Chronic HCV infection (given with infection	Rash, wheezing, conjunctival irritation
Interferon	• Protein synthesis inhibitor	Chronic HBV infection Chronic HCV infection HIV associated kaposi sarcoma condylomata accuminata	Acute influenza like syndrome

Tyrosine Kinase Inhibitor

Name	MOA	Indications	Toxicity
Imatinib mesylate	Inhibitor of ABL, PDGFR, KIT	CML CMML, HES GIST	Nausea, Vomiting, Muscle cramps
Geftinib	Inhibits EGFR type	Non-small-cell-lung cancer (ERB BI or HERI)	Diarrhea Acne Pruritis
Erlotinib	Inhibits EGFR type	Non-small-cell-lung cancer	Diarrhea Interstitial lung disease

QUESTIONS

1. **Mechanism of action of azoles:** (2014)
   a. Inhibition ergosterol synthesis
   b. Squalene epoxidase inhibitor
   c. Mitotic inhibitor
   d. Micropore formation
2. **Fusion inhibitor approved for use in HIV is:**
   a. Enfuvirtide (2014)
   b. Efaviranez
   c. Empricitabine
   d. Atazaravir
3. **Which antiplatelet agent is a prodrug?**
   a. Aspirin (2014)
   b. Ticlopidine
   c. Prasugrel
   d. Ticagrelor
4. **Which of the following drug has least value in heart failure?** (2014)
   a. Antiplatelet agents
   b. Beta blockers
   c. Diuretics
   d. ACE inhibitors
5. **Which statin is given to an 8 years old child with heterozygous familial hypercholesterolemia?**
   a. Simvastatin (2014)
   b. Pravastatin
   c. Atorvastatin
   d. Lovastatin
6. **True regarding loading dose are all except:**
   a. Achieves target levels fast (2014)
   b. Rapid activation of receptors
   c. Depends on volume of distribution
   d. Proportional to the half life of the drug
7. **Which is not a pleiotropic effect of statins?**
   a. Reduce LDL cholesterol (2014)
   b. Improve endothelial stability
   c. Anti-inflammatory/antioxidant
   d. Reduce plaque rupture
8. **Antiarrhythmic drug causing hypothyroidism is:**
   a. Lidocaine (2014)
   b. Propanolol
   c. Aminodarone
   d. Procainamide
9. **Only thiazide used in renal failure when GFR is less than 30–40 ml/min:** (2014)
   a. Chlorthiazide
   b. Chlorthialidone
   c. Metolazone
   d. Methylclothiazide
10. **Which of the following drug causes capillary leak syndrome?** (2014)
    a. GM CSF
    b. GCSF
    c. Filgristin
    d. Peg filgrastim
11. **Heparin injection releases which of the following:**
    a. Lipoprotein lipase (2014)
    b. Nitric oxide
    c. cGMP
    d. Hormone sensitive lipase
12. **Heparin induced thrombocytopenia is reversed by:** (2006)
    a. Warfarin
    b. Enoxaparin
    c. Danaparoid
    d. Ardeparin
13. **Lenalidomide coadministration with which another drug increases the risk of thrombosis?**
    a. Alcohol (2014)
    b. Barbiturate
    c. Glucocorticoids
    d. Antibiotics
14. **Pregnant woman is on valproate for juvenile myoclonic epilepsy. Alternative monotherapy of choice:** (2014)
    a. Carbamazepine
    b. Phenytoin
    c. Leviteracitam
    d. Lacasomide
15. **Which of the following drug causes aseptic meningitis?** (2014)
    a. Intrathecal dexamethasone
    b. Cisplatin
    c. Intrathecal methotrexate
    d. Doxorubicin
16. **Administration of disulfiram in an alcoholic can cause all these side effects except:** (2014)
    a. Flushing
    b. Headache
    c. Hypertension
    d. Nausea
17. **Which beta blocker has membrane stabilizing property?** (2014)
    a. Metoprolol
    b. Atenolol
    c. Propranolol
    d. Esmolol

18. Which of the following drugs does not penetrate blood brain barrier and cause central effects? (2014)
a. Glycopyrrolate
b. Hyoscine hydrobromide
c. Hyoscine butylbromide
d. Atropine

19. Which beta blocker has antioxidant property? (2014)
a. Celiprolol
b. Carvedilol
c. Betaxolol
d. Propanolol

20. False regarding Cytochrome P450 is: (2013)
a. Found only in bone marrow
b. CYP3A4 is the most common isoform
c. Participate in Phase 1 Xenobiotic reactions
d. They are present in Smooth Endoplasmic reticulum within cells

21. Drug used in the treatment of overactive bladder causing xerostomia is: (2013)
a. Serfanacin
b. Oxybutynin
c. Trospium
d. Solefenacin

22. Drug used in narcoanalysis is: (2013)
a. Cocaine
b. Pethidine
c. Atropine
d. Scopolamine

23. True about beta blockers all except: (2013)
a. Postural hypotension
b. Bradycardia
c. Glucagon used for toxicity
d. Lipid soluble drug (cause bad dreams)

24. Glucagon hydrochloride is used in poisoning of: (2013)
a. Beta blocker
b. Calcium channel blocker
c. Tricyclic antidepressants
d. SSRI

25. Ethanol is used in Ethylene glycol poisoning. What is the mechanism of action? (2013)
a. Competitive inhibiton of alchohol dehydrogenase
b. Competitive inhibition of aldehyde dehydrogenase
c. Competitive inhibition NADPH oxidase
d. Non-competitive inhibition of aldehyde dehydrogenase

26. False regarding cocaine is: (2013)
a. Cause tachycardia and hypertension
b. Half life is 3 hours
c. Not suppress the stress of surgery
d. It is very short acting

27. Which of the following drugs is not used for the treatment of anaerobic infections? (2009)
a. Penicillin
b. Clindamycin
c. Chloramphenicol
d. Gentamicin

28. Proton pump inhibitor used along which of the following antiplatelet drug can decrease its antiplatelet activity? (2013)
a. Clopidogrel
b. Aspirin
c. Ticlodipine
d. Thrombospondin

29. Drug used in both type of diabetes is: (2013)
a. Exanitide
b. Pioglitasone
c. Alpha glucosidase inhibitors
d. Pramlintide

30. Which of the following impairs GI motility? (2013)
a. Erythromycin
b. Verapamil
c. Botulinum
d. Nitroglycerine

31. All are true regarding Mechanism of action except: (2013)
a. Chloramphenicol – Protein synthesis
b. Tetracycline – Cell wall synthesis
c. Metronidazole – DNA
d. Penicillin – Cell wall synthesis

32. Drug used in neoadjuvant chemotherapy in Ca esophagus is: (2013)
a. 5FU+Cisplatin
b. Cisplatin
c. Adriamycin
d. Mitomycin

33. All are true regarding phase II biotransformation reaction except: (2013)
a. Converts drug to lipid soluble
b. Introduces covalent bonds
c. Attachment of polar compounds
d. Produces large molecular weight product

34. Highly plasma protein bound opioid among the following is: (2012)
a. Pethidine
b. Fentanyl
c. Sufentanyl
d. Meperidine

35. Which is not side effect of aminodarone? (2012)
a. Pulmonary fibrosis
b. Torsades de pointes
c. Atrial fibrillation
d. Bradycardia

36. Which of the following is a direct rennin inhibitor? (2012)
a. Aliskiren
b. Losartan
c. Perindopril
d. Vernakalant

37. Which of the following antibiotic is a glycopeptides? (2012)
a. Clindamycin
b. Vancomycin
c. Azithromycin
d. Linezolid

38. Which should not be given in liver failure?
a. Acetazolamide (2012)
b. Frusemide
c. Eplerenone
d. Spironolactone

39. Anticraving drug used in alcohol dependence:
a. Naltrexone (2012)
b. Methadone
c. Vareniciline
d. Rimonabant

40. Antiepileptic drug of choice in child treated with ketogenic diet? (2012)
a. Carbamazipine
b. Phentoin
c. Valproate
d. Lamotrigine

41. Phenobarbitone in mother causes all in baby except: (2012)
a. Hypoglycemia
b. Ataxia
c. Neonatal drowsiness
d. Vitamin K deficiency

42. Entry of new drug into the market:
a. Phase 1 (2012)
b. Phase 2
c. Phase 3
d. Phase 4

43. Seizures are caused by all except: (2012)
a. Cyclosporine
b. Olanzapine
c. Tramodol
d. Propofol

44. Which drug can be administered through all routes? (2012)
a. Fentanyl
b. Paracetamol
c. Penicillin G
d. Azithromycin

45. All are true: (2012)
a. Famciclovir is the prodrug of penciclovir
b. Penciclovir does not cause chain termination
c. Penciclovir triphosphate has lower affinity for the viral DNA polymerase than acyclovir triphosphate
d. Incidence of mammary adenocardinoma increased in female rats

46. Diarrhea is a side effect of: (2012)
a. Amitryptiline
b. Metformin
c. Atropine
d. Codeine

47. Which of the following is a calcium sensitizing agent? (2012)
a. Levosimendan
b. Cinacalcet
c. Alendronate
d. Teriparatide

48. Mesalamine is used in: (2012)
a. Ulcerative colitis
b. Diabetes
c. Erectile dysfunction
d. Tinea corporis

49. All are true about Buspirone except:
a. Not a benzodiapezine (2012)
b. Is a antianxiety drug
c. Used as sedative hypnotic
d. Used as antidepressant

50. Drug bound to alpha 1 acid glycoprotein are all except: (2012)
a. Lignocaine
b. Tolbutamide
c. Quinidine
d. Propranolol

51. A patient is on propanolol. Adverse effects of beta blocker are all except: (2012)
a. Seizures
b. Rebound tachycardia
c. Hypotension
d. Poor response to hypoglycemia

52. Which drug acts by inhibiting protein synthesis?
a. Ciprofloxacin (2012)
b. Penicillin
c. Erythromycin
d. Nalidixic acid

53. **Which of the following drug causes interstitial nephritis? (2012)**
 a. Methicillin
 b. Cloxacillin
 c. Amoxycillin
 d. Pipercillin

54. **Linezolid belongs to which class of Drugs? (2011)**
 a. Macrolide
 b. Aminoglycoside
 c. Oxazolidinones
 d. Streptogamins

55. **Which of the following antibiotics has a Nonspecific MAO Inhibitor activity? (2011)**
 a. Tazobactum
 b. Ampicillin
 c. Spectinomycin
 d. Linezolid

56. **Which antipsychotic has maximum hypotensive side effect: (2011)**
 a. Flufenazine
 b. Trifluoperazine
 c. Thioridazine
 d. Haloperidol

57. **Drug most active against for Bacteriodes fragilis is? (2011)**
 a. Cefipime
 b. Ceftazidime
 c. Cefoxitin
 d. Cefotetan

58. **Which of the following is a Phase 1 reaction in xenobiotics? (2011)**
 a. Hydroxylation
 b. Methylation
 c. Conjugation
 d. Acetylation

59. **Intranasal calcitonin used for: (2011)**
 a. Postmenopausal osteoporosis
 b. Paget's disease
 c. Secondary hypoparathyroidism
 d. Hypercalcemia

60. **Which group of drugs potentiates the action of neuromuscular blockers? (2011)**
 a. Aminoglycosides
 b. Cephalosporins
 c. Ampicillin
 d. Penicillin

61. **Clonidine acts on: (2011)**
 a. Vasomotor center
 b. Sympathetic nerve
 c. Autonomic ganglia
 d. Vascular smooth muscle

62. **Which alpha 2 agonist is used to relieve spasticity in amyotrophic lateral sclerosis? (2011)**
 a. Clonidine
 b. Brimonidine
 c. Apraclonidine
 d. Tizanidine

63. **All of the following drugs produce active metabolites except: (2011)**
 a. Propranolol
 b. Procainamide
 c. Diazepam
 d. Fexofenadine

64. **Vasopressin inhibited by: (2011)**
 a. Alcohol
 b. Carbamazepine
 c. Clofibrate
 d. Chlorpropamide

65. **Which of the following is least protein bound? (2011)**
 a. Morphine
 b. Sufentanyl
 c. Meperidine
 d. Fentanyl

66. **Proton pump inhibitors for peptic ulcer disease should be taken: (2011)**
 a. Before breakfast
 b. After breakfast
 c. Before dinner
 d. After dinner

67. **Which of the following antidiabetic medications does not cause weight gain? (2011)**
 a. Rosiglitazone
 b. Glibenclamide
 c. GLP-1 analagues
 d. Metformin

68. **All the following can occur with tetracycline therapy during pregnancy except: (2011)**
 a. Teeth discoloration
 b. Gingival hyperplasia
 c. Raised ICT
 d. Reduced bone growth

69. **Imatinib mesylate is used in the treatment of: (2011)**
 a. GIST
 b. Seminoma
 c. Malt
 d. Zollinger Ellison syndrome

70. **Antihelminthic contraindicated in seizure disorder is: (2011)**
 a. DEC
 b. Albendazole
 c. Piperazine
 d. Pyrantel pamoate

71. **Which of the following is not true regarding morphine? (2010)**
   a. Causes cerebral vasodilation
   b. Inhibits urinary voiding reflex
   c. Causes direct stimulation of chemoreceptor trigger muscle tone in high doses
   d. Reduces muscle tone in high doses

72. **Methotrexate is an example for which of the following class drugs? (2010)**
   a. Altibiotic
   b. Alkylating agent
   c. Biologic response modifier
   d. Folic acid analogue

73. **Which is not true regarding disulfiram? (2010)**
   a. It is irreversibly inhibits aldehyde dehydrogenase
   b. It has several active metabolites
   c. It can be given to a patient who has abstained from alcohol for atleast 6 hours
   d. Sensitization to alcohol can last as long as 14 days after last intake of disulfiram

74. **All the following drugs inhibit cytochrome P-450 except: (2010)**
   a. Alcohol
   b. Cyclophosphamide
   c. Isoniazid
   d. Disulfiram

75. **All are true regarding mifepristone except: (2010)**
   a. It is a pure antagonist
   b. Ineffective against mineralocorticoids
   c. No antiestrogenic side effects
   d. Antiandrogenic action

76. **Grey color and yellow fluorescence in infant teeth is caused by: (2010)**
   a. Phenytoin
   b. Porphyria
   c. Tetracycline
   d. Barbiturate

77. **Which of the following is a selective COX-2 inhibitor? (2010)**
   a. Diflunisal
   b. Piroxicam
   c. Sulindac
   d. Parecoxib

78. **Which of the following is not a uricosuric drug? (2010)**
   a. Probenecid
   b. Benzbromarone
   c. Sulfinpyrazone
   d. Febuxostat

79. **Dyslipedimia is least commonly seen with: (2010)**
   a. Amprenavir
   b. Atazanavir
   c. Saquinavir
   d. Nelfinavir

80. **Drug not acting on cell wall is: (2010)**
   a. Dactinomycin
   b. Cycloserine
   c. Amoxicillin
   d. Bacitracin

81. **Which of the following is an example of a phase 1 xenobiotic reaction? (2010)**
   a. Acetylation
   b. Hydroxylation
   c. Methylation
   d. Glucuronidation

82. **Sucralfate does not interfere with the absorption of: (2010)**
   a. Phenoxy methyl penicillin
   b. Ciprofloxacin
   c. Phenytoin
   d. Digoxin

83. **Which of the following is not seen with thiazide diuretics? (2010)**
   a. Hypokalemia
   b. Hypercalcemia
   c. Hyperuricemia
   d. Metabolic acidosis

84. **Ivermectin is indicated in all of the following except: (2010)**
   a. Ascaris
   b. Filariasis
   c. Malaria
   d. Oncocerciasis

85. **Maximum bicarbonate loss occurs with: (2010)**
   a. Acetazolamide
   b. Furosemide
   c. Thiazide
   d. Spirinolactone

86. **A drug which is an alpha agonist and orally used prodrug for autonomic insufficiency and postural hypotension is: (2010)**
   a. Metamphetamine
   b. Midodrine
   c. Phenylephrine
   d. Metaraminol

87. **Drug contraindicated in severe hypertriglyceridemia is: (2010)**
   a. Fibrates
   b. Simvastatin
   c. Niacin
   d. Cholestyramine

88. Which of the following best depicts the mechanism of action of thiazolidinediones?
a. Improving insulin sensitivity (2010)
b. Modifying receptors of beta cells
c. Increasing insulin secretion
d. Increasing number of GLIT-4

89. All the following are beta-blockers except:
a. Esmolol (2009)
b. Sotalol
c. Celiprolol
d. Formoterol

90. True statement regarding bromocriptine is: **(2009)**
a. It acts as agonist to dopamine receptors
b. It can be used in active peptic ulceration
c. It does not cause postural hypotension
d. It has possible neuroprotective effect

91. Which of the following is contraindicated in early pregnancy? (2009)
a. Heparin
b. Phenytoin
c. Chloroquine
d. Penicillin

92. Insulin sensitivity increases with following treatment except: (2009)
a. Metformin
b. Acarbose
c. Exercise
d. Fasting

93. All the following are anticonvulsants except:
a. Lamotrigine (2009)
b. Methylphenidate
c. Vigabatrin
d. Topiramate

94. Side effect of valvular heart disease is seen with:
a. Pergolide (2009)
b. Methylphenidate
c. Amphetamine
d. Pramipexole

95. Side effect of acute pancreatitis is due to following anti-HIV drugs: (2009)
a. Lamivudine
b. Zidovudine
c. Didanosine
d. Zalcitabine

96. Short acting antihistamine is: (2009)
a. Cetirizine
b. Promethazine
c. Hydroxyzine
d. Acrivastine

97. Sumatriptan is contraindicated in: (2009)
a. Asthma
b. DM
c. Sepsis
d. Peripheral vascular disease

98. The following macrolides are used for toxoplasmosis except: (2009)
a. Erythromycin
b. Clarithromycin
c. Azithromycin
d. Spiramycin

99. Following are third generation cephalosporins except: (2009)
a. Cefuroxime
b. Ceftriaxone
c. Ceftazidime
d. Cefotaxime

100. The mechanism of action of cephalosporin is: **(2009)**
a. Interferes with cell wall synthesis
b. Inhibition of DNA gyrase
c. Inhibition of protein synthesis
d. Inhibition of DNA polymerase

101. Autoinduction of biotrasformation and action as a hormone is seen in: (2009)
a. Carbamazepine
b. Cimetidine
c. Corticosteroid
d. Thyroxine

102. Selective decrease in IgA is seen with administration of: (2009)
a. Phenytoin
b. Diazepam
c. Clonazepam
d. Phenobarbitone

103. Which of the following is prothrombotic?
a. Thrombomodulin (2009)
b. PGI2
c. Heparin
d. ADP

104. Which of the following is not an analeptic agent?
a. Doxapram (2009)
b. Nikethamide
c. Doxacurium
d. Propylbutamide

105. The neurotransmitter secreted by postganglionic sympathetic fibers innervating sweat glands is:
a. Norepinephrine (2009)
b. Epinephrine
c. Acetylcholine
d. Dopamine

106. Which of the following drugs is used to treat chlamydia infection in pregnancy? (2009)
a. Doxycyclin
b. Erythromycin
c. Meropenem
d. Tetracycline

107. Troglitazone is the drug used in the treatment of: (2009)
a. Petit mal epilepsy
b. Type 2 diabetes mellitus
c. Hyperlipidemia
d. Osteoporosis

108. Which of the following is not an alpha-2 stimulant? (2009)
a. Guanabenz
b. Guanadrel
c. Clonidine
d. Alpha methyl dopa

109. 99% of degradation of 131I occurs in: (2009)
a. 26 days
b. 36 days
c. 46 days
d. 56 days

110. Niacin toxicity causes all except: (2009)
a. Hepatitis
b. Diabetes
c. Hypertriglyceridemia
d. Macular edema

111. Which of the following has the highest affinity for 5HT3 receptors? (2008)
a. Dolasetron
b. Granisetron
c. Ondansetron
d. Palonosetron

112. Which of the following drugs is found to be effective in both epilepsy and migraine? (2008)
a. Valproate
b. Lamotrigine
c. Vigabatrin
d. Flunarizine

113. Which of the following is not an example an NNRTI? (2008)
a. Efavirenz
b. Etravirine
c. Emtricitabine
d. Delavirdine

114. Heparin treatment is monitored by: (2008)
a. APTT
b. PT
c. CT
d. BT

115. Which of the following group of drugs is used in the treatment of Kala Azar? (2008)
a. Spiramycin
b. Sodium stibogluconate
c. Praziquantel
d. Niclosamide

116. Antihelicobacter pylori drugs include all of the following except: (2008)
a. Amoxicillin
b. Clarithromycin
c. Metronidazole
d. Sucralfate

117. Which of the following proton pump inhibitors is known to inhibit CYP2C19? (2008)
a. Pantoprazole
b. Omeprazole
c. Rabeprazole
d. Dexlansoprazole

118. ACE inhibitors are contraindicated in all the following except: (2008)
a. Bilateral renal artery stenosis
b. Elderly hypertensive
c. Diabetic microalbuminuria
d. Severe renal failure

119. Which of the following is a cardiotoxic anticancer drug? (2008)
a. Bleomycin
b. Doxorubicin
c. 5FU
d. Dactinomycin

120. The neurotransmitter secreted by postganglionic sympathetic fibers innervating sweat glands is: (2008)
a. Norepinephrine
b. Epinephrine
c. Acetyl choline
d. Dopamine

121. Opioid induced respiratory depression can be reversed with: (2008)
a. Naloxone
b. Theophylline
c. Artificial ventilation
d. Doxapram

122. Which group of drugs potentiates the action of Neuromuscular blockers? (2008)
a. Aminoglyosides
b. Cephalosporins
c. Ampicillin
d. Penicillin

123. Antihelminthic contraindicated in seizure disorder is: (2008)
a. DEC
b. Albendazole
c. Piperazine
d. Pyrantel pamoate

124. Which of the following is the most beta-1 selective antagonist? (2007)
a. Acebutolol
b. Atenolol
c. Metoprolol
d. Bisoprolol

125. Calcium channel blocker which is usually used in subarachnoid hemorrhage is: (2007)
a. Nimodipine
b. Diltiazem
c. Verapamil
d. Flunarizine

126. Drug induced cirrhosis is not seen with:
a. Methotrexate (2007)
b. Phenobarbitone
c. Valproic acid
d. Amiadraone

127. Which of the following is not used in the prophylaxis of febrile seizures? (2007)
a. Sodium valproate
b. Carbamazepine
c. Phenobarbitone
d. Diazepam

128. Which of the following drugs will not cause hypothyroidism? (2007)
a. Ethambutol
b. Lithium
c. Amiodarone
d. Pyraxinamide

129. Atropine is added with diphenoxylate to:
a. Increase effects (2007)
b. Decrease side effects
c. Decrease abuse potential
d. Enhance absorption

130. Monitoring of drug levels is not required with:
a. Lithium (2007)
b. L-Dopa
c. Digoxin
d. Phenytoin

131. Carbamazepine toxicity is precipitated by:
a. Erythromycin (2007)
b. Vitamin K
c. Theophyllin
d. Phenytoin

132. The drug of choice for management of infantile spasm is: (2007)
a. Phenytoin
b. Valproate
c. ACTH
d. Diazepam

133. All are true about buspirone except:
a. Not a benzodiazepine (2007)
b. Is an antianxiety drug
c. Used as sedative hypnotic
d. Used as antidepressant

134. Which is a characteristic adverse effect of chronic amiodarone therapy? (2007)
a. Corneal deposition
b. Cataract
c. Glaucoma
d. Retinal pigmentation

135. Drug of choice for treatment of gastrointestinal stromal tumors is: (2007)
a. Rituximab
b. Imatinib mesylate
c. Anagrelide
d. Denileukin difititox

136. All are true about Phase II trials except:
a. Safety and efficacy (2006)
b. Done in healthy human volunteers
c. Therapeutic exploratory trial
d. Positive evidence in Phase I is a prerequisite

137. All are true about Nefopam except:
a. Non-opioid (2006)
b. Decreases PG synthesis
c. Causes seizures
d. Prevents shivering

138. Bromocriptine inhibits: (2006)
a. Prolactin
b. Vasopressin
c. Imipramine
d. Levodopa

139. All of the following are useful against MRSA except: (2006)
a. Vancomycin
b. Linezolid
c. Retapamulin
d. Streptogramin

140. Dexmedetomidine is a new drug used in:
a. General anesthesia (2006)
b. Treatment of VRSA
c. Hypertension
d. Multiple sclerosis

141. NMDA antagonist used in Alzheimer's disease is: (2006)
a. Memantine
b. Rivgastigmine
c. Donepezil
d. Galantamine

142. Which one of the following is not an NMDA receptor? (2006)
a. Kappa
b. Kainite
c. AMPA
d. Glutamate

143. Which drug is used to suppress lactation? (2006)
a. Bromocriptine
b. Metoclopramide
c. Domperidone
d. Prolactin

144. Rate of elimination of drug is: (2006)
a. Clearance
b. T1/2
c. Biotransformation
d. Bioavailability

145. Ondansetron is not useful for: (2006)
a. Chemotherapy – induced nausea and vomiting
b. Postoperative and postradiation emesis
c. Reduce carving in alcoholism
d. Chemotherapy induced hypercuriemia

146. Longest acting triptan: (2006)
a. Rizatriptan
b. Zolmitriptan
c. Naratriptan
d. Frovatriptan

147. Least sedative antihistaminic is: (2006)
a. Cetrizine
b. Hydroxyzine
c. Chlorpheniramine
d. Carbinoxamine

148. Drug of choice for treating extended spectrum beta lactamase (ESBL) organism is: (2006)
a. Aztreonam
b. Imipenem
c. Cefipime
d. Ceftazidime

149. Aztreonam differs from imipenam in: (2006)
a. Not active against enterobacteriaceae
b. Aztreonam is effective against ESBL whereas imipenam is not
c. In penicillin allergy, aztreonam tolerated but not imipenam
d. Aztreonam does not penetrate CSF in contrast to imipenam

ANSWERS AND EXPLANATIONS

1. **Ans. a. Inhibition ergosterol synthesis** *Ref: KD Tripathi's Essentials of Medical Pharmacology 7/e*

According to the mechanism of action the antifungal agents can be classified as:

A. Drug altering membrane permeability
- Azoles: inhibit 14-sterol demethylase, prevent ergosterol synthesis, and lead to the accumulation of 14-methylsterols.
- Triazoles, e.g. Fluconazole, itraconazole, voriconazole
- Imidazoles, e.g. Ketoconazole, miconazole, clotrimazole
- Allylamines: Naftifine and terbinafine, inhibit squalene epoxidase and prevent ergosterol synthesis.
- Polyenes, e.g. Amphotericin B, nystatin, hamycin. They bind to ergosterol in fungal cell membranes and increase membrane permeability.

B. Drug blocking nucleic acid synthesis, e.g. Flucytosine
C. Drugs disrupting microtubule function, e.g. Griseofulvin
D. Drugs inhibiting cell wall synthesis, e.g. Caspofungin, nikkomycin. These are echinocandins, which inhibit the formation of glucans in the fungal cell wall.

2 **Ans. a. Enfuvirtide** *Ref: Goodman and Gilman's The Pharmacological Basis of Therapeutics 12/e*

Entry inhibitors are enfuvirtide and maraviroc
Integrase inhibitor are raltegravir and elvitegravir
Enfuvirtide is a peptide that blocks the interaction between the N36 and C34 sequences of the gp41 glycoprotein by binding to a hydrophobic groove in the N36 coil. This prevents formation of a six-helix bundle critical for membrane fusion and viral entry into the host cell.

3. **Ans. b. Ticlopidine and c. prasugrel** *Ref: Goodman and Gilman's The Pharmacological Basis of Therapeutics, 12/e*
P2Y12 antagonists are thienopyridines and Non-thienopyridines acting on P2Y12 receptor on platelets and causing inhibition of ADP-induced platelet aggregation.
Thienopyridines irreversibly inhibit P2Y12, a major ADP receptor on the platelet surface include ticlopidine, clopidogrel and prasugrel. All three drugs are prodrugs.
Non-thienopyridines reversibly inhibit P2Y12 and these include Cangrelor (IV), Ticagrelor (oral) and Elinogrel.
4. **Ans. a. Antiplatelet agents** *Ref: Goodman and Gilman's The Pharmacological Basis of Therapeutics 12/e; Ref: Katzung (2012) Basic and clinical pharmacology 12/e.*

Drug groups used in heart failure:

Chronic heart failure	Acute heart failure
• Diuretics • Aldosterone receptor antagonists • Angiotensin – converting enzyme inhibitors • Angiotensin receptor blockers • Beta blockers • Cardiac glycosides • Vasodilators	• Diuretics • Vasodilators • Bipyridines • Beta agonists • Natriuretic peptide – nesiritide

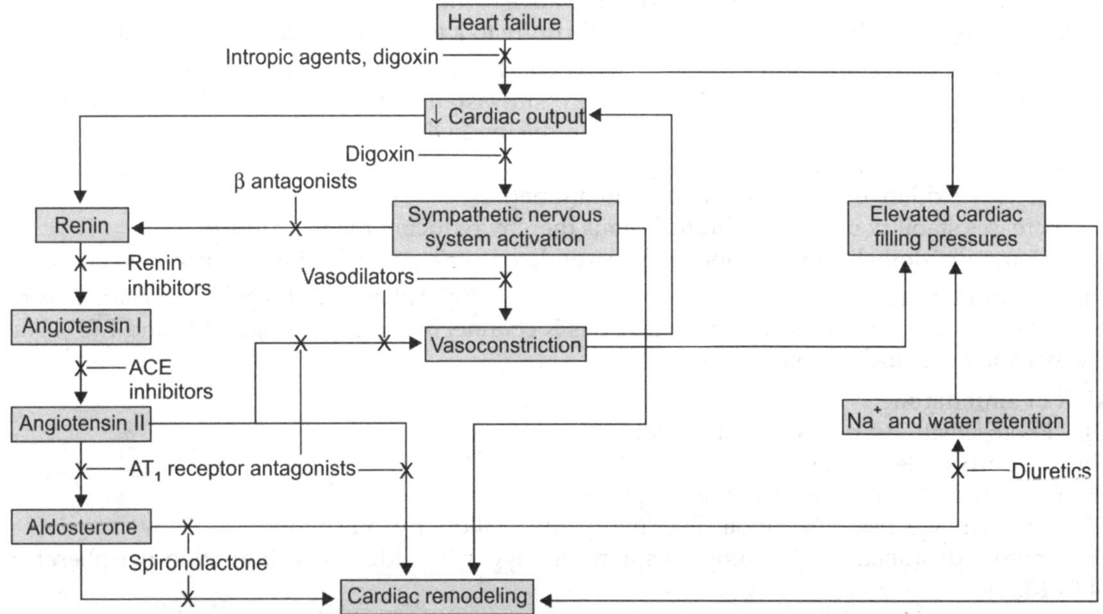

Classification and treatment of chronic heart failure

ACC/AHA stage	NYHA class	Description	Management
A	Prefailure	No symptoms but risk factors present	Treat obesity, hypertension, diabetes, hyperlipidemia, etc.
B	I	Symptoms with severe exercise	ACEI/ARB, β blocker, diuretic
C	Class II	Symptoms with marked exercise	Add aldosterone antagonist, digoxin; CRT (cardiac resynchronization therapy), hydralazine/nitrate
	Class III	Symptoms with mild exercise	
D	IV	Severe symptoms at rest	Transplant, LVAD (left ventricular assist device)

Management of Acute Heart Failure

Intravenous treatment is the rule in acute heart failure.

- Diuretics – furosemide is the most commonly used (venodilation property).
- Dopamine or Dobutamine – positive inotropic drugs – most useful in severe hypotension.

- Levosimendan
- Vasodilators – nitroprusside, nitroglycerine, and nesiritide (Vd act by reduction in afterload)
- Conivaptan a V1a and V2 receptor antagonist used for hyponatremia in acute heart failure due to increased vasopressin activity.

5. **Ans. b. Pravastatin** *Ref: Goodman and Gillman's Pharmacological Basis of Therapeutics 12/e*
'HMG-CoA Reductase inhibitors are useful alone or with resins, niacin, or ezetimibe in reducing levels of LDL. The choice of statins should be based on efficacy (reduction of LDL-C) and cost. Three drugs (lovastatin, simvastatin, and pravastatin) have been used safely in clinical trials involving thousands of subjects for 5 or more years. Some statins have been approved for use in children with heterozygous familial hypercholesterolemia. Atorvastatin, lovastatin, and simvastatin are indicated for children more than 11 years. Pravastatin is approved for children more than 8 years.'

6. **Ans. d. Proportional to the half-life of the drug** *Ref: Katzung (2012) Basic and Clinical Pharmacology 12/e*
Loading dose
The *loading dose* is one or a series of doses that maybe given at the onset of therapy with the aim of achieving the target concentration rapidly due to rapid activation of receptors.
Loading dose = Volume of distribution × target plasma concentration
A loading dose maybe desirable if the time required to attain steady state by the administration of drug at a constant rate (4 elimination t1/2 values) is long relative to the temporal demands of the condition being treated. Disadvantage if sensitive individual exposed abruptly to a toxic concentration of a drug.

7. **Ans. a. Reduce LDL cholesterol** *Ref: Goodman and Gillman's Pharmacological Basis of Therapeutics 12/e*
Lovastatin, atorvastatin, fluvastatin, pravastatin, simvastatin, rosuvastatin and pitavastatin are HMG-CoA reductase inhibitors. They are most effective in reducing LDL.
Pleiotropic effects of statins are:
   - Decrease oxidative stress and vascular inflammation
   - Increases stability of atherosclerotic lesions thereby reducing plaque rupture
   - Enhances endothelial production of the vasodilator nitric oxide, leading to improved endothelial function.

8. **Ans. c. Amiodarone** *Ref: Katzung (2012) Basic and clinical pharmacology 12/e*
Amiodarone – Class III antiarrhythmic drug has K channel blocker (prolongs APD and ERP), Na channel, Ca channel and beta blocking properties.

   ADR of amiodarone:
   Plz – Photosensitivity, pigmentation of skin
   Check – Corneal deposition
   PFT Pulmonary fibrosis. Peripheral neuropathy
   LFT Liver damage, pseudoalcoholic liver injury and Mallory hyaline bodies
   TFT Thyroid dysfunction – hypothyroidsm, rarely hyperthyroidism and inhibition peripheral conversion of T4 to T3.
   The drug available for the treatment of resisitant cases of atrial fibrilation is Amiodarone

9. **Ans. c. Metolazone** *Ref: Goodman and Gillman's Pharmacological Basis of Therapeutics 12/e*
Thiazide diuretics inhibit the Na^+– Cl^- symporter in PCT.
'Thiazide diuretics are used for the treatment of edema associated with heart (congestive heart failure), liver (hepatic cirrhosis), and renal (nephrotic syndrome, chronic renal failure, and acute glomerulonephritis) disease.
Most thiazide diuretics are ineffective when the GFR is < 30–40 mL/min, except of metolazone and Indapamide

10. **Ans. a. GM CSF** *Ref: Katzung (2012), Basic and Clinical Pharmacology 12/e*

11. **Ans. a. Lipoprotein lipase** *Ref: Goodman and Gillman The Pharmacological Basis of Therapeutics 12/e*
'Heparin 'clears' lipemic plasma *in vivo* by causing the release of lipoprotein lipase into the circulation. Lipoprotein lipase hydrolyzes triglycerides to glycerol and free fatty acids.
The clearing of lipemic plasma may occur at concentrations of heparin below those necessary to produce an anticoagulant effect. Rebound hyperlipemia may occur after heparin administration is stopped.
High doses of heparin can interfere with platelet aggregation and thereby prolong the bleeding time. In contrast, LMWHs and fondaparinux have little effect on platelets.'

12. Ans. c. Danaparoid *Ref: Goodman and Gilman's The Pharmacological Basis of Therapeutics 12/e*

Heparin – induced thrombocytopenia (HIT) is the development of thrombocytopenia due to the administration of UFH for a minimum of 7 days

Heparin – induced thrombocytopenia and thrombosis (HITT): HIT predisposing to thrombosis is called HITT.
Incidence: 1–4% of individuals treated with UFH.

Etiology: In HIT, the immune system forms antibodies against platelet factor 4 (PF4). The IgG antibodies form a complex with heparin and PF4 in the bloodstream. The tail of the antibody then binds to the FcγIIa receptor, a protein on the surface of the platelet. This results in platelet activation and the formation of platelet microparticles, which initiate the formation of blood clots; the platelet count falls as a result, leading to thrombocytopenia.

Treatment: Patients who develop HIT are treated by discontinuance of heparin and administration of a direct thrombin inhibitor.

13. Ans. c. Glucocorticoids *Ref: Goodman and Gillman's The Pharmacological Basis of Therapeutics 12/e*

Lenalidomide is a immunomodulatory derivatives of thalidomide (IMiD) was used in the treatment of the myelodysplastic syndrome with the chromosome 5q31 deletion, relapsed or refractory multiple myeloma. 'Thromboembolic events occur with increased frequency in patients receiving thalidomide or lenalidomide, but particularly in combination with glucocorticoids and with anthracyclines. Anticoagulation reduces this risk and seems indicated in patients presenting with risk factors for clotting, but anticoagulant prophylaxis has not been evaluated prospectively.'

14. Ans. c. Leviteracitam *Ref: Goodman and Gillman's, The Pharmacological Basis of Therapeutics 12/e*

Seizure type	Features	Antiseizure drugs
Myoclonic seizure	A brief (perhaps a second), shock like contraction of muscles that maybe restricted to part of one extremity or maybe generalized.	Valproate, clonazepam levetiracetam

'The most common generalized epilepsy is referred to as juvenile myoclonic epilepsy, accounting for ~10% of all epileptic syndromes.'

15. Ans. c. Intrathecal methotrexate *Ref: Katzung (2012), Basic and Clinical Pharmacology 12/e*

16. Ans. c. Hypertension *Ref: Goodman and Gillman's The Pharmacological Basis of Therapeutics 12/e*

When ethyl alcohol enters the body, oxidation of acetaldehyde is inhibited by disulfiram (aldehyde dehydrogenase inhibitor). When ethanol is consumed in the presence of disulfiram, acetaldehyde accumulates and causes an unpleasant reaction of facial flushing, nausea, vomiting, dizziness, and headache.

Remember: Alcohol dehydrogenase is inhibited by fomepizole and aldehyde dehydrogenase is inhibited by disulfiram.

17. Ans. c. Propranolol *Ref: Goodman and Gillman's, The Pharmacological Basis of Therapeutics 12/e*

Beta blockers with membrane stabilizing activity or local anesthetic activity, similar to lidocaine, that is independent of beta blockade. Such drugs include propranolol, acebutolol, and carvedilol.

Pindolol, metoprolol, betaxolol, and labetalol have slight membrane-stabilizing effects.

18. Ans. a. Glycopyrrolate *Ref: KD Tripathi, Essentials of Medical Pharmacology 7/e*

Glycopyrrolate is a quaternary amine, lipid insoluble polar compound does not penetrate blood brain barrier, a competitive antagonist at M3 receptors. It reduces smooth muscle and secretory activity of gut. So used in irritable bowel syndrome and diarrhea.

19. Ans. b. Carvedilol *Ref: Goodman and Gilman's The Pharmacological Basis of Therapeutics 12/e*

Carvedilol blocks beta 1, beta 2, and alpha 1 receptors.

It has antioxidant (decrease the biosynthesis of ROS and oxygen radicals.) and anti-inflammatory effects: may contribute to cardio protective effects.

It has membrane – stabilizing activity

It lacks intrinsic sympathomimetic activity.

It produces vasodilation.

It protects cell membranes from lipid peroxidation.

It prevents low density lipoprotein (LDL) oxidation.

It also inhibits ROS-mediated loss of myocardial contractility, stress-induced hypertrophy, apoptosis, and the accumulation and activation of neutrophils.

At high doses, carvedilol exerts Ca^{2+} channel-blocking activity.

It does not increase receptor density and is not associated with high levels of inverse agonist activity.

The drug is FDA-approved for use in hypertension, congestive heart failure, and left ventricular dysfunction following MI.

20. Ans. a. Found only in bone marrow *Ref: Goodman and Gilman's The Pharmacological Basis of Therapeutics 12/e*

Let me explain about each options

Option a:

Microsomal enzymes (mono oxygenases, cytochrome p450 and glucoronyl transferase) maybe induced or inhibited by other drugs.

CYP3A4 carries out biotransformation of largest number of drugs.

21. Ans. b. Oxybutynin *Ref: Katzung Basic and Clinical Pharmacology 12/e p122*

M3 receptors predominate than M2 receptors in the human urinary bladder. M3 receptor blockers provide relief of overactive bladder like Oxybutynin, Trospium, Darifenacin, Solifenacin, Tolterodine, Fesoterodine and Propiverine.

An alternative treatment for urinary incontinence refractory to antimuscarinic drugs is intrabladder injection of botulinum toxin A which acts by interfering with the co-release of ATP with neuronal acetylcholine. Imipramine, a TCA drug with strong anti-muscarinic actions, has long been used to reduce incontinence in institutionalized elderly patients.

22. Ans. d. Scopolamine *Ref: KD Tripathi, Essentials of Medical Pharmacology 7/e*

Drugs used in Narcoanalysis are muscarinic receptor antagonist – scopolamine, benzodiazepines such as midazolam, flunitrazepam, barbiturates including sodium thiopental (Sodium Pentothal) and amobarbital (sodium amytal).

23. Ans. a. Postural hypotension *Ref: Goodman and Gilman's The Pharmacological Basis of Therapeutics 12/e*

Clinical pharmacology of the beta receptor blocking drugs:

- Hypertension
- Ischemic heart disease
- Cardiac arrhythmias
- Heart failure
- Obstructive cardiomyopathy
- Dissecting aortic aneurysm
- Glaucoma
- Migraine headache
- Tremors
- Anxiety
- Bleeding from esophageal varices
- Hyperthyroidism

ADR of beta blockers: BBC DRIVe

- Bradycardia
  - Bronchoconstriction
  - Claudication
  - Dyslipidemia – Lipids
- Reduced sensitivity to hypoglycemia
  - Negative Inotropic action
  - Vivid dreams and nightmares

24. Ans. a. Beta blocker *Ref: Katzung (2012), Basic and Clinical Pharmacology 12/e p1033*

- Stimulation of the glucagon Gs protein coupled receptor results in activation of adenylate cyclase and increased levels of intracellular cAMP.
- Heart is stimulated (rate and force), without access to β receptor.

25. Ans. a. Competitie inhibition of alcohol dehydrogenase

Ref: Katzung (2012), Basic and Clinical Pharmacology 12/e p398

Ethylene glycol is first metabolized to glycolaldehyde by the enzyme alcohol dehydrogenase, then to glycolate, glyoxylate, and oxalate. Glycolate and oxalate are responsible for the metabolic acidosis and renal damage. Fomepizole and ethanol are competitive inhibitors of methanol to alcohol dehydrogenase. They competes with methanol for the active site. As ethanol is added, less methanol can bind to alcohol dehydrogenase's active sites. Formaldehyde is produced at a slower rate.

Treatment of Ethylene glycol poisoning: Early IV fomepizole is initiated immediately at a dose of 15 mg/kg; repeat every 12 hours, and continued until the patient's serum ethylene glycol concentration drops below a toxic threshold (20–30 mg/dL). Intravenous ethanol is an alternative to fomepizole in ethylene glycol poisoning. Ethanol loading dose is calculated so as to give a blood level of at least 100 mg/dL (42 g/70 kg in adults). Hemodialysis effectively removes ethylene glycol and its toxic metabolites and is recommended for patients with a serum ethylene glycol concentration above 50 mg/dL, significant metabolic acidosis, and significant renal impairment.

Antidotes	Poisoning
Theophylline	Adenosine
Succimer, Dimercaptosuccinic acid (DMSA)	Lead
Pyridoxine	Isoniazid
Prussian blue	Thallium
Protamine sulfate	Heparin
Pralidoxime chloride (2-PAM)	Organophosphate insecticides
Phytomenadione (Vitamin K) and FFP	Warfarin
Physostigmine sulfate	Anticholinergic
Octreotide	Oral hypoglycemic agents
Naloxone hydrochloride	Opioid
N-acetylcysteine	Paracetamol (acetaminophen)
Methylene blue	Methemoglobinemia
Leucovorin	Methotrexate and trimethoprim
Glucagon	Beta blocker, calcium channel blocker
Flumazenil	Benzodiazepine
Ethanol or fomepizole	Ethylene glycol and methanol
Digoxin Immune Fab antibody (Digibind and Digifab)	Digoxin
Deferoxamine mesylate	Iron
amyl nitrite, sodium nitrite, or thiosulfate	Cyanide
Calcium gluconate	Hydrofluoric acid
Calcium chloride	Calcium channel blockers
Beta blocker	Theophylline
Atropine	Organophosphate and carbamate insecticides

26. Ans. b. Half-life is 3 hours *Ref: Goodman and Gilman's The Pharmacological Basis of Therapeutics 12/e*

Cocaine: First ocular LA, Mydriasis, corneal sloughing, only LA causing vasoconstriction and increases blood pressure (act as sympathomimetic due to inhibition of noradrenaline reuptake), rise in BP, only ester not metabolized by esterase. It is metabolized in liver.

Cocaine never be given by intravenous route or with adrenaline.

27. Ans. d. Gentamicin *Ref: Katzung (2012), Basic and Clinical Pharmacology 12/e p813-816*

Anerobic infections

Effective: Metronidazole, Clindamycin, Chloramphenicol, Cefamycin, Penicillin, Sulbactam + beta–lactam

Not effective: Aminoglycosides, Aztreonam, Fluroquinolones except 4th generation, Cotrimoxazole.

28. Ans. a. Clopidogrel *Ref: Goodman and Gilman's The Pharmacological Basis of Therapeutics 12/e*

Most importantly CYP2C19 is involved in the metabolic activation of clopidogrel. Clopidogrel-treated patients with the loss-of-function CYP2C19*2 allele exhibit reduced platelet inhibition compared with those with the wild-type CYP2C19*1 allele and experience a higher rate of cardiovascular events. Concomitant administration of proton pump inhibitors, which are inhibitors of CYP2C19, with clopidogrel, produces a small reduction in the inhibitory effects of clopidogrel on ADP-induced platelet aggregation.

29. Ans. d. Pramlintide *Ref: Goodman and Gilman's The Pharmacological Basis of Therapeutics 12/e*

Pramlintide, a synthetic analog of amylin,

- It is an injectable (s/c) antihyperglycemic agent that modulates postprandial glucose levels.
- It is approved for preprandial use in persons with type 1 and type 2 diabetes.
- It is administered in addition to insulin in those who are unable to achieve their target postprandial blood sugar levels.
- Pramlintide suppresses glucagon release, delays gastric emptying, and has CNS mediated anorectic effects.
- It is rapidly absorbed after subcutaneous administration; levels peak within 20 minutes, and the duration of action is less than 150 minutes.
- Pramlintide is renally metabolized and excreted.

The major adverse effects of pramlintide are hypoglycemia and gastrointestinal symptoms, including nausea, vomiting, and anorexia.

30. Ans. a. Erythromycin *Ref: Goodman and Gilman's The Pharmacological Basis of Therapeutics 12/e*

Motilin a peptide hormone found in the GI M cells and in some enterochromaffin cells of the upper small bowel, is a potent contractile agent of the upper GI tract. The effects of motilin can be mimicked by erythromycin. This property is shared to varying extents by other macrolide antibiotics, including oleandomycin, azithromycin, and clarithromycin. The best established use of erythromycin as a prokinetic agent is in patients with diabetic gastroparesis, where it can improve gastric emptying in the short-term. Erythromycin – stimulated gastric contractions can be intense and result in 'dumping' of relatively undigested food into the small bowel. Currently, mitemcinal (GM-611), a macrolide nonantibiotic and motilin receptor agonist, shows promise for the treatment of gastroparesis.

31. Ans. b. Tetracycline – cell wall synthesis

Ref: Katzung (2012), Basic and Clinical Pharmacology 12/e p818

Tetracyclines are broad-spectrum bacteriostatic antibiotics that inhibit protein synthesis. They bind reversibly to the 30S subunit of the bacterial ribosome, blocking the binding of aminoacyl-tRNA to the acceptor site on the mRNA-ribosome complex. This prevents addition of amino acids to the growing peptide. Tetracyclines are active against many gram-positive and gram-negative bacteria, including certain anerobes, rickettsiae, chlamydiae, and mycoplasmas.

32. Ans. a. 5FU+Cisplatin *Ref: Goodman and Gilman's The Pharmacological Basis of Therapeutics 12/e*

- Week 1, 5, 8, and 11
- Inj. 5FU 750 mg/m2 D1–D4 continuous IV Infusion
- Inj. Cisplatin 75 mg/m2 D1
- Followed by RT 50 Gy

33. Ans. a. Converts drug to lipid soluble

Ref: Goodman and Gilman's The Pharmacological Basis of Therapeutics 12/e

Biotransformation Reaction are two types:

Phase I: Nonsynthetic (drugs maybe activated, unchanged or most often inactivated)

A polar group is either introduced or unmasked, so the drug molecule becomes more water-soluble and can be excreted. Reactions in general produce a more water-soluble and less active metabolites. The majority of metabolites are generated by a common hydroxylating enzyme cytochrome P450.

Phase II: Synthetic/Conjugation (drug or Phase I metabolite enter Phase II reaction, conjugated drug usually inactivated)

These reactions involve covalent attachment of small polar endogenous molecule such as glucuronic acid, sulfate, or glycine to form water-soluble compounds. The final compounds have a larger molecular weight.

Phase I/Nonsynthetic reactions:
- Oxidation
- Reduction
- Hydrolysis
- Cyclization
- Decyclization.

Nonsynthetic reaction					
Oxidation		Reduction	Hydrolysis	Cyclization	Decyclization
cyp450 dependent	Cyp450 independent	Chloralhydrate	Procaine	Proguanil	Barbiturate
Propranolol	Chlorpromazine	Chloramphenicol	Lignocaine		Phenytoin
Phenytoin	Desimipramine	Halothane	Pethidine		
Warfarin	Propylthiouracil		Procainamide		
Pentabarbitol	Ethanol				

Phase II Reactions (synthetic reaction) needs energy:
- Glucuronidation
- Sulfate conjugation
- Acetylation
- Glycine conjugation
- Methylation
- Transulfuration
- Glutathione conjugation
- Mercapturic acid synthesis.

Glucuronide	Acetylation (SHIP)	Methylation	Sulfate	Glycine	Glutathione	Nucleotide synthesis
Chloramphenicol Aspirin Phenacetin Morphine Metronidazole	sulfonamide Hydralazine INH Procainamide	Adrenaline Histamine Nicotinic acid	Chloramphenicol Adrenal steroids Sex steroids	Salicylates	Paracetamol Ethacrynic acid	Anticancer purine and pyramidine necleotides

Mnemonics:
- All reaction starting with 'De' are Phase I reaction
- Dealkylation, Desulfuration, Decyclization, Deamination, Dechlorination
- All reaction starting with 'G' are Phase II reaction
- Glucorinide conjugation, Glycine conjugation, Glutathione conjugation.

34. Ans. c. Sufentanyl *Ref: Katzung (2012), Basic and Clinical Pharmacology 12/e*

Pethidine or Meperidine is 60–80% bound to plasma proteins, primarily albumin and α_1-acid glycoprotein. 85% of fentanyl is bound to proteins and 90% of Sufentanil is protein bound.

35. Ans. c. Atrial fibrillation *Ref: Goodman and Gilman's The Pharmacological Basis of Therapeutics 12/e p834-837*

6 Ps of Amiodarone:
- Prolongs action potential duration (Torsades de pointes)
- Pulmonary alveolitis and fibrosis
- Peripheral conversion of T4 to T3 is inhibited
- Photosensitivity
- Pigmentation of skin
- Peripheral neuropathy.

Amiodarone side-effects + Toxicity are a 'BITCH'

Bradycardia/**B**lue man
- **I**nterstitial Lung Disease
- **T**hyroid (hyper and hypo)

- Corneal (occular)/Cutaneous (skin)
- Hepatic/Hypotension when IV (due to solvents)

36. Ans. a. Aliskrein *Ref: Goodman and Gilman's The Pharmacological Basis of Therapeutics 12/e p779*

Aliskiren binds the active site of renin to block conversion of angiotensinogen to AngI, thus reducing the consequent production of AngII.

Aliskiren is an effective antihypertensive agent that is well tolerated in monotherapy and combination therapy. It has cardioprotective and renoprotective effects in combination therapy; however, long-term advantages still need to be establizhed.

Adverse Events

Mild gastrointestinal symptoms such as diarrhea observed at high doses, abdominal pain, dyspepsia, and gastroesophageal reflux; headache; nasopharyngitis; dizziness; fatigue; upper-respiratory tract infection; back pain; angiodema; and cough (cough is much less common than with ACE inhibitors). Like other RAS inhibitors, aliskiren is not recommended in pregnancy.

37. Ans. b. Vancomycin *Ref: Goodman and Gilman's The Pharmacological Basis of Therapeutics 12/e p539-1542*

Glycopeptides vancomycin produced by *Streptococcus orientalis* and Teicoplanin produced by *Actinoplanes teichomyetius.* Other lipoglycopeptides are telavancin, oritavancin, and dalbavancin.

Vancomycin: Cell wall synthesis inhibition, inhibit tansglycosylase. Not absorbed orally. Given IV. Has wide distribution and excreted through GF.

ADR – Dose dependent nerve deafness and nephrotoxicity. Histamine release by vancomycin when given rapid IV causes skin allergy, hypotension and red man syndrome.

USES – MRSA, Strep. Viridans endocarditis, E. faecalis causing endocarditis (along with AGs) and Corynebacterium infections.

Orally used for pseudomembranous enterocolitis.

38. Ans. a. Acetazolamide *Ref: Katzung (2012), Basic and Clinical Pharmacology 12/e p256-258*

Carbonic anhydrase inhibitor–induced alkalinization of the urine decreases urinary excretion of NH^{4+} (by converting it to rapidly reabsorbed NH^{3}) and may contribute to the development of hyperammonemia and hepatic encephalopathy in patients with cirrhosis.

Drugs CI in liver disease

- Erythromycin estolate – Acute hepatic failure
- Acetazolamide – hepatic encephalopathy
- Tetracycline
- Pyrazinamide
- Pefloxacin.

Dose reduction in liver failure

- INH
- RIF
- Chloamphenicol
- Clindamycin

39. Ans. a. Naltrexone *Ref: Katzung (2012), Basic and Clinical Pharmacology 12/e p396*

Effects of blood alcohol levels in the absence of tolerance

Blood level, g/dL	Usual effect
0.02	Decreased inhibitions, a slight feeling of intoxication
0.08	Decrease in complex cognitive functions and motor performance
0.20	Obvious slurred speech, motor incoordination, irritability, and poor judgment
0.30	Light coma and depressed vital signs
0.40	Death

Management of alcohol withdrawal syndrome is by long-acting benzodiazepines, chlordiazepoxide and diazepam. Three drugs—disulfiram, naltrexone, and acamprosate—have FDA approval for adjunctive treatment of alcohol dependence. Other drug is clonidine.

40. Ans. c. Valproate *Ref: Goodman and Gilman's The Pharmacological Basis of Therapeutics 12/e*

The **ketogenic diet** is believed to be effective in glucose transporter protein 1 (GLUT-1) deficiency, pyruvate dehydrogenase deficiency, myoclonic-astatic epilepsy, tuberous sclerosis complex, Rett syndrome, severe myoclonic epilepsy of infancy (Dravet syndrome), and infantile spasms.

41. Ans. a. Hypoglycemia *Ref: Goodman and Gilman's The Pharmacological Basis of Therapeutics 12/e*

Antiepileptic drugs and congenital malformations:
- Phenytoin – cleft palate
- Valproic acid – spina bifida
- Topimarate – teratogenicity in aminal testing.

Epilepsy in Pregnancy

Mother: Phenobarbitone, folic acid 5 mg/day – throughout pregnancy and Phytonadione (III trimester)
Child: Examine for congenital abnormality. Give Inj. Vit K
Eclampsia with fits: IV Magnesium sulfate

42. Ans. d. Phase 4 *Ref: Goodman and Gilman's The Pharmacological Basis of Therapeutics 12/e*

Phase		Done in	
0	Micro dosing (IND is submitted before starting)	3–10 subjects	Done in healthy volunteers to obtain preliminary pharmacokinetic data Dose: 1/100th of proposed therapeutic dose to a maximum of 100 μg and for protein products, the maximum limit is 30 nanomoles
I	Human pharmacology and safety (IND is submitted before starting)	15–50 subjects	First in human study Done in healthy volunteers or volunteer patients (Anticancer/anti retro viral drug) • To evaluate pharmacokinetics (ADME) • To determine dose limiting toxicity (DLT) • To identify maximum tolerated dose (MTD) and biologically active dose Safety and tolerance data
II	Therapeutic exploration and dose raging	50–300 patients	First in patient/disease study Efficacy, safety and dose ranging May involve comparison with placebo Surrogate end points (biomarkers used) Fast track approval of drugs
III	Therapeutic confirmation and comparison (NDA is submitted after finishing)	250–1000 + patients	Randomized controlled trials Bioequivalent studies Multicentre trials Confirms efficacy
IV	Therapeutic use (postlicensing studies, Postmarketing Surveillance)	2000–10000+ patients	Approved drug used in treatment Surveillance for long-term safety and efficacy Postmarketing studies, pharmacoeconomic studies pharmacoepidemiology studies Pharmacovigilance Drug utilization studies Drug interactions Newer indications can be identified

43. Ans. b. Olanzapine *Ref: Goodman and Gilman's The Pharmacological Basis of Therapeutics 12/e*

Drugs and other substances that can cause seizures
Alkylating agents (e.g., busulfan, chlorambucil) **Antimalarials** (chloroquine, mefloquine) **Antimicrobials/antivirals** Beta lactam and related compounds Quinolones

Contd...

Contd...

Drugs and other substances that can cause seizures
Acyclovir
Isoniazid
Ganciclovir
Anesthetics and analgesics
Meperidine
Tramadol
Local anesthetics
Dietary supplements
Ephedra (ma huang)
Gingko
Immunomodulatory drugs
Cyclosporine
OKT3 (monoclonal antibodies to T-cells)
Tacrolimus
Interferons
Psychotropics
Antidepressants
Antipsychotics
Lithium
Radiographic contrast agents
Theophylline
Sedative-hypnotic drug withdrawal
Alcohol
Barbiturates (short-acting)
Benzodiazepines (short-acting)
Drugs of abuse
Amphetamine
Cocaine
Phencyclidine
Methylphenidate
Flumazenil in benzodiazepine-dependent patients.

44. Ans. a. Fentanyl *Ref: Katzung (2012), Basic and Clinical Pharmacology 12/e p542*

Fentanyl

- Parenteral: 50 mcg/mL for injection
- Fentanyl Transdermal System: 12.5, 25, 50, 75, 100 mcg/h delivery
- Fentanyl Buccal: 100, 200, 400, 600, 800 mcg oral lozenge
- Fentanyl Lollypop: 200, 400, 600, 800, 1200, 1600 mcg lozenge on a stick
- Patient Controlled Transdermal Iontophoretic Fentanyl System: 40 mcg per dose for delivery.

45. Ans. a. Famiciclovir is the prodrug of penciclovir

Ref: Katzung (2012), Basic and Clinical Pharmacology 12/e p848-849

Famciclovir is well absorbed orally (BA of 75%) and is converted rapidly to penciclovir (Oral BA is 5%).

46. Ans. b. Metformin *Ref: Goodman and Gilman's The Pharmacological Basis of Therapeutics 12/e*

'The most common side effects of metformin are gastrointestinal. Approximately 10–25% of patients starting this medication report nausea, indigestion, abdominal cramps or bloating, diarrhea, or some combination of these. Metformin has direct effects on GI function including glucose and bile salt absorption. Use of metformin is associated with 20–30% lower blood levels of Vitamin B12 probably due to malabsorption, but neurological or hematological consequences of this have not been reported. Most GI adverse effects of metformin abate over time with continued use of the drug, and can be minimized by starting at low doses and gradually titrating to a target dose over several weeks, and by having patients take it with 'meals.'

47. Ans. a. Levosimendan *Ref: Katzung (2012), Basic and Clinical Pharmacology 12/e p218*

Levosimendan is a calcium sensitizer – it increases the sensitivity of the heart to calcium, thus increasing cardiac contractility without a rise in intracellular calcium also appears to inhibit phosphodiesterase and to cause some vasodilation in addition to its inotropic effects. Some clinical trials suggest that this drug maybe useful in patients with heart failure, and the drug has been approved in some countries

48. Ans. a. Ulcerative colitis *Ref: Katzung 12/e p1101*

'5-ASA absorbed from the small intestine and does not reach its distal part. To overcome the rapid absorption of 5-ASA from the proximal small intestine, drugs have been designed to deliver 5-ASA to various distal segments of the small bowel or the colon. These include sulfasalazine, olsalazine, balsalazide, and various forms of mesalamine. 5-ASA drugs induce and maintain remission in ulcerative colitis and are considered to be the first-line agents for treatment of mild to moderate active ulcerative colitis. Their efficacy in Crohn's disease is not proven.'

Disease severity	Therapy	Responsiveness to therapy
Severe	Surgery natalizumab cyclosporine TNF antagonists intravenous corticosteroids	Refractory
Moderate	TNF antagonists oral corticosteroids methotrexate azathioprine/6-mercaptopurine	
Mild	Budesonide (ileitis) topical corticosteroids (proctitis) antibiotics 5-aminosalicylates	Responsive

Therapeutic pyramid approach to inflammatory bowel diseases. Treatment choice is predicated on both the severity of the illness and the responsiveness to therapy. Agents at the bottom of the pyramid are less efficacious but carry a lower risk of serious adverse effects.

49. Ans. c. Used as sedative hypnotic *Ref: Katzung (2012), Basic and Clinical Pharmacology 12/e p376, 284*

Buspirone, a 5-HT 1A partial agonist, is an effective non-benzodiazepine anxiolytic. Buspirone relieves anxiety without causing marked sedative, hypnotic, or euphoric effects. The drug is used in generalized anxiety states but is less effective in panic disorders.

Newer Antianxiety Drugs

Zolpidem, Zolpicone, Zaleplon acts on w1 type of benzodiazepine receptor

Buspirone and Ipsapirone are 5-HT 1A partial agonist

50. Ans. b. Tolbutamide *Ref: Goodman and Gilman's The Pharmacological Basis of Therapeutics 12/e*

	Acidic drugs	Basic drugs
Binds to	Albumin	Alpha-1 acid glycoprotein
Variation	So decrease in albumin increases the free level of acidic drugs. e.g. Liver failure, Nephrotic syndrome	So increase in the Alpha-1 acid glycoprotein level, decreases the free level of basic drugs. e.g. Cancer, Arthritis
Examples	Phenytoin, Salicylates, Phenylbutazone, Warfarin, Tolbutamide	Propranolol Quinidine, Lignocaine, Imipramine

51. Ans. b. Rebound tachycardia *Ref: Goodman and Gilman's The Pharmacological Basis of Therapeutics 12/e*

Beta-blockers: side effects 'BBC DIVeR':
- Bradycardia
- Bronchoconstriction
- Claudication
- DysLipidemia
- Negative Inotropic action
- Vivid dreams and nightmares
- Reduced sensitivity to hypoglycemia

52. Ans. c. Erythromycin a macrolide antibiotic
Ref: Goodman and Gilman's The Pharmacological Basis of Therapeutics 12/e

Event	Antibiotic(s) and binding site(s)	Mechanism(s)
Formation of initiation complex	Aminoglycosides (30S)	Interfere with initiation codon functions—block association of 50S ribosomal subunit with mRNA-30S (static); misreading of code incorporation of wrong AA (-cidal)
Amino-acid incorporation	Tetracyclines (30S)	Block the attachment of aminoacyl tRNA to acceptor site (-static)
Formation of peptide bond	Chloramphenicol (50S)	Inhibit the activity of peptidyltransferase (-static)
Translocation	Macrolides and clindamycin (50S)	Inhibit translocation of peptidyl-tRNA from acceptor to donor site *(-static)*

53. Ans. a. Methicillin *Ref: Katzung (2012), Basic and Clinical Pharmacology 12/e p796*

In patients with renal failure, penicillin in high doses can cause seizures. Nafcillin is associated with neutropenia; oxacillin can cause hepatitis; and methicillin causes interstitial nephritis (and is no longer used for this reason).

54. Ans. c. Oxazolidinones *Ref: Goodman and Gilman's The Pharmacological Basis of Therapeutics 12/e p1537*

Linezolid: First of oxazolidinones

Acts by inhibiting Protein synthesis by binding with 23s fraction of 50s, Primarily Bacteriostatic except St. pneumococci (CIDAL), Resistant cases of Gr+ve aerobe/anerobe/MRSA, Infection by vancomycin resistant E. fecium (VRSA, VRE) and other MDR organisms, NO ACTION AGAINST Gr (–) ve

ADR-Thrombocytopenia, neutropenia, MAO inhibitory property.

55. Ans. d. Linezolid *Ref: Goodman and Gilman's The Pharmacological Basis of Therapeutics, 12/e p1537-8*

Linezolid is a oxazolidinones acts by inhibiting protein synthesis by binding with 23s fraction of 50s, Primarily Bacteriostatic except St. pneumococci (CIDAL), Resistant cases of Gr+ve aerobe/anerobe/MRSA, Infection by vancomycin resistant E. fecium (VRSA, VRE) and other MDR organisms, NO ACTION AGAINST Gr (-) ve

ADR: Thrombocytopenia, neutropenia, MAO inhibitory property.

56. Ans. c. Thioridazine *Ref: Goodman and Gilman's The Pharmacological Basis of Therapeutics 12/e*

ADRs of Thioridazine:

Prolong QT interval, degenerative retinopathies, anticholinergic side effects, orthostatic hypotension and cardiotoxicity, Hyperprolactinemia, weight gain, extrapyramidal side effects: tardive dyskinesia and neuroleptic malignant syndrome. Blood dyscrasias such as agranulocytosis, leukopenia and neutropenia.

57. Ans. d. Cefotetan *Ref: Basic and clinical Pharmacology by Katzung 12/e p806*

Cefotetan and cefoxitin IV, has activity versus bacteroides fragilisallows for use in abdominal/pelvic infections

Cefepime Intravenous, fourth-generation drug, broad activity with improved stability to chromosomal β lactamase

58. Ans. a. Hydroxylation *Ref: Goodman and Gilman's The Pharmacological Basis of Therapeutics 12/e*

Explained in previous questions regarding biotransformation

59. Ans. a. Postmenopausal osteoporosis *Ref: Goodman and Gilman's The Pharmacological Basis of Therapeutics 12/e*

Diagnostic Uses of Calcitonin

Calcitonin is a sensitive and specific marker for the presence of medullary thyroid carcinoma (MTC) that can be hereditary (25%) or sporadic (75%) and is present in all patients with the multiple endocrine neoplasia type 2 (MEN2) syndromes.

Therapeutic Uses of Calcitonin

Calcitonin lowers plasma Ca^{2+} and phosphate concentrations in patients with hypercalcemia, Paget's disease, and in some patients with osteoporosis.

Salmon calcitonin is approved for clinical use and is available as a **nasal spray**, once-daily treatment of **postmenopausal osteoporosis**.

Side effects of calcitonin: Nausea, hand swelling, urticaria, and rarely, intestinal cramping.

60. **Ans. a. Aminoglycosides** *Ref: Goodman and Gilman's The Pharmacological Basis of Therapeutics 12/e*

Aminoglycosides in the order of decreasing potency for neuromuscular blockade are neomycin, kanamycin, amikacin, gentamicin, and tobramycin. Susceptibility to neuromuscular blockade by aminoglycosides is more with anesthesia, neuromuscular blockers and in patients with myasthenia gravis.

MOA: AGs inhibit prejunctional release of Ach.

Treatment: Intravenous calcium salt and AchE Inhibitors (e.g., edrophonium and neostigmine).

61. **Ans. a. Vasomotor center** *Ref: Katzung Section III Cardiovascular-Renal Drugs. Figure 11–3, p172*

Sites of action of the major classes of antihypertensive drugs.

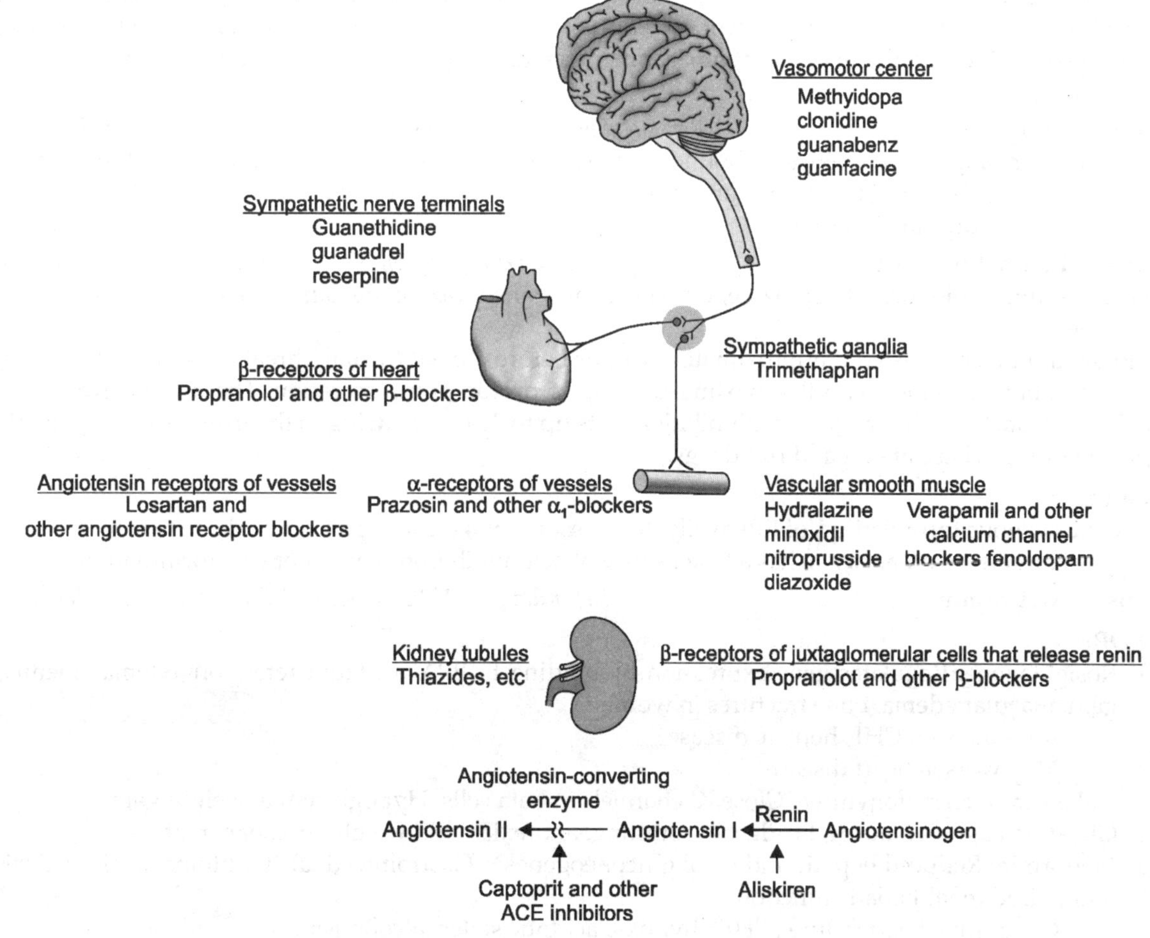

62. **Ans. d. Tizanidine** *Ref: Goodman and Gilman's The Pharmacological Basis of Therapeutics 12/e p626*

ALS is a progressive degenerative disease of spinal motor neurons leading to weakness and eventually paralysis often fatal within 2–3 years of onset. No treatment arrests the underlying pathologic process in ALS. The drug riluzole (reduce excitotoxicity by diminishing glutamate release) has modest effect.

To reduce spasticity: Tizanidine a congener of clonidine ($\alpha 2$ adrenoceptor agonist) and Baclofen, a $GABA_B$ receptor agonist are tried.

63. Ans. d. Fexofenadine *Ref: Goodman and Gilman's The Pharmacological Basis of Therapeutics 12/e*

List of active drugs producing active metabolites

Active drug	Active metabolite
Phenacetin	Paracetamol
Phenylbutazone	Oxyphenbutazone
Primidone	Phenobarbitone
Codeine	Morphine
Diazepam	Oxazepam
Digitoxin	Digoxin
Spironolactone	Canrenone
Procainamide	Acetylprocainamide
Propranolol	Hydroxypropranolo

64. Ans. a. Alcohol *Ref: Goodman and Gilman's The Pharmacological Basis of Therapeutics 12/e*

Alcohol reduces the calcium-dependent secretion of vasopressin by blocking voltage-gated calcium channels. Chlorpropamide, Clofibrate and Carbamazepine: Increases the action of ADH on the kidney and are useful in central DI.

65. Ans. a. Morphine *Ref: Goodman and Gilman's The Pharmacological Basis of Therapeutics 12/e*

Pethidine or Meperidine is 60–80% bound to plasma proteins, primarily albumin and α1-acid glycoprotein. 85% of fentanyl is bound to proteins and 90% of sufentanil is protein bound.

While PB for morphine is 30–40%.

66. Ans. a. Before breakfast *Ref: Katzung (2012), Basic and Clinical Pharmacology 12/e p1087*

Proton pump inhibitors: Omeprazole, esomeprazole, lansoprazole, dexlansoprazole, rabeprazole and pantoprazole.

PPI should be administered approximately 1 hour before a meal (usually breakfast), so that the peak serum concentration coincides with the maximal activity of proton pump secretion. The drugs have a short serum half-life of about 1.5 hours, but acid inhibition lasts up to 24 hours owing to the irreversible inactivation of the proton pump. These are hit and run drugs.

Points:

The intravenous formulations of PPI available are esomeprazole and pantoprazole.

Immediate-release omeprazole has a faster onset of acid inhibition than other oral formulations.

67. Ans. d. Metformin *Ref: Katzung (2012), Basic and Clinical Pharmacology 12/e p764-5*

ADRs:

a. Rosiglitazone: Regulates gene expression by binding to PPAR-γ. Fluid retention, edema, anemia, weight gain, macular edema, bone fractures in women
   - Cannot use if CHF, hepatic disease
   - May worsen heart disease

b. Glibenclamide: sulfonylurea, Close K^+ channels in beta cells. Hypoglycemia, weight gain

c. GLP-1 analagues: Nausea, headache, vomiting, anorexia, mild weight loss, pancreatitis

d. Metformin: Reduced hepatic and renal gluconeogenesis. Gastrointestinal symptoms, lactic acidosis, CI use if impaired renal/hepatic function
   - Congestive heart failure (CHF), hypoxic/acidotic states, alcoholism.

All the 4 drugs are used in Type 2 diabetes. Metformin can cause weight loss more than GLP1 analogues so tried in obesity and metabolic syndrome.

68. Ans. b. Gingival hyperplasia *Ref: Katzung (2012), Basic and Clinical Pharmacology 12/e p812*

Toxicity of tetracycline:

- These are contra-indicated in pregnancy due to the risk of fetal tooth enamel dysplasia and irregularities in the fetal bone growth and also they may cause fulminate hepatic failure to the mother.
- Treatment of young children with tetracycline may cause dentition abnormalities.

- **Teeth/bone-Midpregnancy-5 months:** Decidious teeth affected, brown discoloration, more susceptible to caries
- **Baby (3 month 6 years):** Affect crown of permenant dentition, suppression of bony growth
- **Outdated tetracycline use may lead to fanconi's syndrome (a type of renal tubular acidosis) due to Epitetracycline Anhydrotetracycline, Epianhydrotetracycline metabolites**
- Tetracycline may exacerbate pre-existing renal dysfunction although these are not directly nephrotoxic
- **Demeclocycline (maximum) and doxycycline can result in photosensitivity**
- Antianabolic effect
- Increased intra cranial pressure (pseudotumor cerebral)
- DI- demeclocycline
- Vestibular toxicity- minocycline
- Hypersensitivity/super infection

69. Ans. a. GIST *Ref: Goodman and Gilman's The Pharmacological Basis of Therapeutics 12/e*

- **Inhibitors of the BCR-ABL Kinase: Imatinib, Dasatinib, and Nilotinib**
- **USES of Imatinib:** Chronic myelogenous leukemia (CML), GIT stromal cell tumor
- **ADR-** Nausea, vomiting, edema, muscle cramps, elevation of transaminases, neutropenia, Thrombocytopenia
- **Dasatinib** is approved for patients with CML resistant to imatinib in and for pH^+ ALL who are resistant to prior therapies
- **Nilotinib** is approved for patients with CML resistant to prior imatinib therapy
- **Epidermal Growth Factor Receptor (EGFR) Inhibitors**: Gefitinib, Erlotinib
- These drugs inhibit this EGFR linked TK pathway by binding to tyrosine kinase-ATP binding site
- **USES:** Metastatic nonsmall cell lung cancer and other solid tumors
- **ADR:** Diarrhea, acneiform skin rash, anorexia
- The EGFR tyrosine kinase inhibitors erlotinib and gefitinib bind to the kinase domain and block the enzymatic function of EGFR.
- The monoclonal antibodies cetuximab and panitumumab bind specifically to the extracellular domain of EGFR.

70. Ans. c. Piperazine *Ref: Katzung (2012), Basic and Clinical Pharmacology 12/e p943*

Piperazine causes paralysis of ascaris by blocking acetylcholine at the myoneural junction; unable to maintain their position in the host, live worms are expelled by normal peristalsis.

Occasional mild adverse effects include nausea, vomiting, diarrhea, abdominal pain, dizziness, and headache. Neurotoxicity and allergic reactions are rare. CI: Pregnancy, impaired renal or hepatic function, or to those with a history of epilepsy or chronic neurologic disease.

71. Ans. d. Reduces muscle tone in high doses *Ref: Katzung (2012), Basic and Clinical Pharmacology 12/e p551*

An intensification of tone in the large trunk muscles called truncal rigidity reduces thoracic compliance and thus interferes with ventilation. The effect is more with lipid-soluble opioids (eg, fentanyl, sufentanil, alfentanil, remifentanil). Truncal rigidity can be prevented by concomitant use of neuromuscular blocking agents.

72. Ans. d. Folic acid analogue *Ref: Katzung (2012), Basic and clinical pharmacology 12/e p959*

Methotrexate (MTX) is a folic acid analogue that binds to the active catalytic site of dihydrofolate reductase (DHFR) resulting in inhibition of tetrahydrofolate (THF) synthesis. The biologic effects of MTX can be reversed by administration of the reduced folate leucovorin (5-formyltetrahydrofolate).

Uses: Breast cancer, head, and neck cancer, osteogenic sarcoma, primary central nervous system lymphoma, non-Hodgkin's lymphoma, bladder cancer, choriocarcinoma.

73. Ans. c. It can be given to a patient who has abstained from alcohol for atleast 6 hours

Ref: Goodman and Gilman's The Pharmacological Basis of Therapeutics 12/e

The drug never should be administered until for the patient who has abstained from alcohol for at least 12 hours. In the initial phase of treatment, the daily dose should be taken in the morning, the time when the resolve not to drink maybe strongest. Sensitization to alcohol may last as long as 14 days after the last ingestion of disulfiram because of the slow rate of restoration of ALDH. Disulfiram and/or its metabolites can inhibit many enzymes with sulphydryl groups and inhibits hepatic CYPs.

74. Ans. b. Cyclophosphamide *Ref: Goodman and Gilman's The Pharmacological Basis of Therapeutics 12/e*

KISS Me On FACE	Enzyme inhibitors	C GRAPPS	Enzyme inducers
K	Ketoconazole	C	Carbamezapine
I	Isoniazid	G	Chloral hydrate
S	Sodium valproate	R	Griseofulvin
S	Sulfonamides	A	Rifampin
Me	Metronidazole	P	Alcohol
On	Omeprazole	P	Phenobarbital
F	Fluoroquinolone	S	Phenytoin
A	Alcohol		Sulfonylureas
C	Chloramphenicol,		
E	Cemitidine		
	Erythromycin		

75. Ans. a. It is a pure antagonist *Ref: Goodman and Gilman's The Pharmacological Basis of Therapeutics 12/e*

76. Ans. c. Tetracyclines *Ref: Goodman and Gilman's The Pharmacological Basis of Therapeutics 12/e*

Toxicity of tetracycline is explained in previous questions

77. Ans. d. Parecoxib *Ref: Goodman and Gilman's The Pharmacological Basis of Therapeutics 12/e*

Selective COX-2 inhibitors: celecoxib, rofecoxib, valdecoxib and its prodrug parecoxib, etoricoxib, and lumiracoxib. The relative degree of selectivity for COX-2 inhibition is lumiracoxib = etoricoxib > valdecoxib = rofecoxib ≫ Celecoxib. Celecoxib currently is the only COX-2 inhibitor licensed for use in U.S.

Parecoxib is the only COX-2–selective NSAID administered by injection and useful analgesic for the peri-operative period when patients are unable to take oral medication

78. Ans. d. Febuxostat *Ref: Goodman and Gilman's The Pharmacological Basis of Therapeutics 12/e p997-8*

Gout can be treated by:

- Drugs that relieve inflammation and pain (NSAIDs, colchicine, glucocorticoids)
- Drugs that prevent inflammatory responses to crystals (colchicine and NSAIDs)
- Drugs that act by inhibition of urate formation (allopurinol, febuxostat) or to augment urate excretion (probenecid)

Uricosuric drugs are probenecid, sulfinpyrazone, benzbromarone and losartan compete with urate for the transporter.

Febuxostat is a nonpurine inhibitor of xanthine oxidase approved for hyperuric patients with gout attacks, but not recommended for treatment of asymptomatic hyperuricemia.

HINT: Febu**xostat: xo = xanthine oxidase, stat = static or inhibitor**

79. Ans. b. Atazanavir *Ref: Goodman and Gilman's The Pharmacological Basis of Therapeutics 12/e*

Patients treated with atazanavir had significantly lower fasting triglyceride and cholesterol concentrations than patients treated with nelfinavir, lopinavir, or efavirenz (suggesting a reduced propensity to cause these side effects). Atazanavir is not known to cause glucose intolerance.

Anti HIV drug classification:

Nucleoside Reverse Transcriptase Inhibitors	Non-nucleoside Reverse Transcriptase Inhibitors	Protease Inhibitors
Zidovudine	Nevirapine	Saquinavir
Didanosine	Efavirenz	Indinavir
Stavudine	Delavirdine	Ritonavir
Zalcitabine	Etravirine	Nelfinavir
Lamivudine	**Entry Inhibitors**	Amprenavir
Abacavir	Enfuvirtide	Lopinavir
Emtricitabine	Maraviroc	Atazanavir
Nucleotide Reverse Transcriptase Inhibitors	**Integrase Inhibitor**	Fosamprenavir
Tenofovir disoproxil	Raltegravir	Tipranavir
		Darunavir

80. Ans. (a) Dactinomycin *Ref: Goodman and Gilman's The Pharmacological Basis of Therapeutics 12/e*

Cell wall synthesis inhibitors

Drugs	MOA
Cycloserine	Alanine racemase and alanine ligase
Vancomycin	Transglycosylase
Bacitracin (polypeptide)	Dephosphorylation of bactoprenol
Beta lactums	Transpeptidase
Fosfomycin	Enolpyruvate transferase

81. Ans. b. Hydroxylation *Ref: Goodman and Gilman's The Pharmacological Basis of Therapeutics 12/e*

82. Ans. a. Phenoxy methyl penicillin *Ref: Goodman and Gilman's The Pharmacological Basis of Therapeutics 12/e*

Explained in previous questions regarding biotransformation.

83. Ans. d. Metabolic acidosis *Ref: Goodman and Gilman's The Pharmacological Basis of Therapeutics 12/e*

Diuretics	Route of access	Site of action	Mechanism of action
Loop diuretics	Organic acid secretory system	Thick ascending limb of loop of henle	Inhibition of $Na^+/k^+/cl^-$ co-transport in luminal membrane
Thiazides	-do-	Early DT	Inhibition of Na^+/cl^- co-transport
Amiloride	Organic base secretory system	Late DT/CT	Inhibition of luminal membrane Na^+ channel and has Na^+ K^+ exchange
Spironolactone	Through peritubular circulation	-do-	ADH antagonist
Osmotic	Glomerular filtration	PT, descending limb of loop of henle, CT	Passive water reabsorbtion is reduced
CA enzyme inhibitor	Secreted through PT	PT, also DT	Increases excretion of HCO_3, Na, Kcl and water

Drug Toxicity

Loop diuretics	**Thiazides**	**Spirinolactone**
Hypokalemia	**Hypokalemia**	Drowsiness
Dehydration	**Hyperuricemia**	Confusion
Dilution Hyponatremia	Mg depletition	Mental upset
GI upset	Hyper Glycemia	Hirsutism
Hearing Loss (Ethacrynic acid)	Hyper Llpidemia	Gynecomastia
Allergy (Sulfonamides)	**Hyper Calciemia**	Impotence
Caution (pregnancy)	Torsade de Pointes (Hypokalemia)	Menstrual irregularity

84. Ans. c. Malaria *Ref: Goodman and Gilman's The Pharmacological Basis of Therapeutics 12/e*

Ivermectin: GABA agonist, Does not cross BBB

DOC: Onchocerciasis: Ochocerca volvulus and strongyloidosis

Alternative uses: Filariasis, Cutaneous larva migrans, Ascaris lumbricoides (roundworm)

Orally: Scabies, pediculosis. Single dose 0.2 mg/kg, River blindness control programme – WHO

ADR: Mazzotti reaction, avoid in children of less than 5 years old.

85. Ans. a. Acetazolamide *Ref: Goodman and Gilman's The Pharmacological Basis of Therapeutics 12/e*

Diuretic	Urine NaCl	Urine HCO_3	Urine K^+	Body Cl^-	Body pH
CA inhibitor (Acetazolamide)	+	+++	+	+	Acidosis
Loop	++++	–	+	–	Alkalosis
Thiazide	++	+/–	+	–	Alkalosis
K^+ Sparing	+	–	–	–/+	Acidosis

86. Ans. b. Midodrine

Ref: Goodman and Gilman's The Pharmacological Basis of Therapeutics, 12/e; Midodrine is an alpha-1 agonist and orally used prodrug used for autonomic insufficiency and postural hypotension. ADRs include: Hypertension, Reflex bradycardia, Dry mouth, sedation, rebound hypertension upon abrupt withdrawal.

Other alpha-1 agonists are Methoxamine, Phenylephrine, Mephentermine, Metaraminol.

87. Ans. d. Cholestyramine *Ref: Goodman and Gilman's The Pharmacological Basis of Therapeutics 12/e*

Bile Acid-Binding Resins: Colestipol, cholestyramine, and colesevelamare useful only for isolated increases in LDL. The resin-induced increase in bile-acid production is accompanied by an increase in hepatic triglyceride synthesis, which is of consequence in patients with significant hypertriglyceridemia (baseline triglyceride level > 250 mg/dL).

Cholestyramine

Bind bile acid in the intestine interrupting their enterohepatic circulation
Fecal excretion of bile salts and CH is increased
Increases the activity of hepatic HMG CoA reductase-poor long term efficacy
Reduction of plasma LDL-CH

- Level of VLDL and TG are not altered or maybe increased
- HDL levels are affected little
- They are suitable only when LDL-CH are raised and TGs are normal i.e type IIa
- Also useful in relieving itching of obstructive jaundice and bile salt mediated diarrhea

ADR: GI complication, decreased absorption of Vit K, digitalis, warfarin, thiazide, pravastatin, fluvastatin

88. Ans. a. Improve insulin sensitivity *Ref: Goodman and Gilman's The Pharmacological Basis of Therapeutics 12/e*

Thiazolidinediones are ligands for the peroxisome proliferation activating receptor (PPAR) receptors, involved in the regulation of genes related to glucose and lipid metabolism. Pioglitazone and rosiglitazone are insulin sensitizers and increase insulin-mediated glucose uptake by 30–50% in patients with type 2 diabetes.

89. Ans. d. Formoterol *Ref: Goodman and Gilman's The Pharmacological Basis of Therapeutics 12/e*

Non-selective

A. Without intrinsic sympathomimetic: Propranolol, sotalol, Timolol, Nadolol
B. With intrinsic sympathomimetic: Pindolol, Oxprenolol, Alprenolol, Carteolol
C. With additional alpha blocking: Labetalol, carvedelol, Dilevalol

Cardioselective: Metoprolol, atenolol, acebutalol, bisoprolol, esmolol, betaxolol, celiprolol

Selective (beta 2): Butoxamine.

90. Ans. a. It acts as agonist to dopamine receptors *Ref: Katzung (2012), Basic and Clinical Pharmacology 12/e p489*

Bromocriptine

Synthetic ergot derivative, potent dopamine agonist
Agonist at D2, partial agonist antagonist at D1 and weak α blocking property

Actions of bromocriptine

- Decreasing prolactin release
- Increasing GH release in normal individual but decrease the same from pituitary tumours causing acromegaly
- Antiparkinsonism action
- Stimulatig CTZ
- Hypotension – (alpha blocking and central suppression of postural reflex)
- Decreased GI motility.

Uses

- Hyperprolactinemia
- Acromegaly
- Parkinsonism
- Hepatic coma
- Suppression of lactation and breast engorgement.

Side effects

Early: Nausea, vomiting, postural hypotension

Late: Behavior alteration, mental confusion, psychosis, abnormal movements.

91 **Ans. b. Phenytoin** *Ref: Goodman and Gilman's The Pharmacological Basis of Therapeutics 12/e*

Safer Drugs In Pregnancy

Anticoagulation	Heparin
Antimalarial	Chloroquine
Antithyroid	Prophythiouracil
Antihypertensive	Hydrolazine/methyl dopa → CCB → Cardio slective B blocker → Prazocin/clonidine
Muscle relaxant	d-tubocurarine
HIV	Zidovudine/Nevirapine
Toxoplasmosis	Spiramycin
Anticonvulsant	Pheno barbital
Eclampsia	Magnesium sulphate
UTI	Nitro furantoin, Ampicillin, Cephalosporins
ATT	Rifampicin + Isoniazide

92. **Ans. d. Fasting** *Ref: Goodman and Gilman's The Pharmacological Basis of Therapeutics 12/e*

93. **Ans. b. Methylphenidate** *Ref: Goodman and Gilman's The Pharmacological Basis of Therapeutics 12/e*
Amphetamine an Indirect-Acting Sympathomimetics acts by release of norepinephrine and, to some extent, dopamine. Amphetamine like compounds are Methamphetamine (attention deficit hyperactivity disorder), Phenmetrazineis (anorexiant) and Modafinil (narcolepsy).

Classification of Antiepileptic drugs

- **Prolongation of sodium channel inactivation:** Phenytoin and phosphenytoin, carbamazepine and Oxcarbazepine, Lamotrigine, Zonisamide, Topiramate, Valproate
- **Inhibition of T-Type Calcium Current:** Ethosuximide, Trimethadione, Valproate
- **Facilitation of GABA Mediated Action:** Benzodiazepine, Barbiturate, Gabapentin, Tiagabine, Vigabatrin, Ganaxolone, valproate
- **Inhibition of Exitatory Neurotransmission:** Felbamate, Topiramate, Remacemide, Lamotrigine.

94. **Ans. a. Pergolide** *Ref: Goodman and Gilman's The Pharmacological Basis of Therapeutics 12/e*
Pergolide, an ergot derivative, directly stimulates both D1 and D2 receptors was used for Parkinsonism. Its use has been associated with the development of valvular heart disease.

95. **Ans. c. Didanosine** *Ref: Goodman and Gilman's The Pharmacological Basis of Therapeutics 12/e*
ADR of didanosine include peripheral neuropathy and pancreatitis, as consequence of mitochondrial toxicity. Combining didanosine with stavudine, increases the risk and severity of both toxicities. Acute pancreatitis is a rare but potentially fatal complication of didanosine.

96. **Ans. b. Promethazine** *Ref: Goodman and Gilman's The Pharmacological Basis of Therapeutics 12/e*

97. **Ans. d. Peripheral vascular disease** *Ref: Goodman and Gilman's The Pharmacological Basis of Therapeutics 12/e*
5-HT 1D/1B agonists (triptans, eg, sumatriptan) are used for migraine headache.
ADRs of triptans are altered sensations (tingling, warmth, etc), dizziness, muscle weakness, neck pain, Chest discomfort and for parenteral sumatriptan, injection site reactions.
Naratriptan and eletriptan are CI in severe hepatic or renal impairment or peripheral vascular syndromes; frovatriptan in patients with peripheral vascular disease; Zolmitriptan in patients with Wolff-Parkinson-White syndrome.

98. Ans. a. Erythromycin *Ref: Katzung (2012), Basic and Clinical Pharmacology 12/e p813-814*

Toxoplasmosis: TOC-Pyrimethamine, in combination with sulfadiazine, Alternative is clindamycin.

Macrolides are used for toxoplasmosis are Clarithromycin, Azithromycin and Spiramycin

Tetracycline and erythromycin are alternative therapies for the treatment of intestinal amebiasis.

99. Ans. a. Cefuroxime *Ref: Goodman and Gilman's The Pharmacological Basis of Therapeutics 12/e*

First generation		Second generation		Third generation		Fourth G.	Fifth G.
Oral	Parenteral	Oral	Parenteral	Oral	Parenteral	Parenteral	
Cephalexin Cefadroxil Cephradine Cephaloridine	Cephalothin Cefazolin	Cefaclor Cefuroxime Axetil	Cefuroxime Cefotetan Cefoxitin	Cefixime Cefopodoxime Proxetil Cefdinir Ceftibuten	Cefotaxime Ceftizoxime Ceftriaxone Ceftazidime Cefoperazone Moxalactam	Cefepime Cefpirome	Ceftobiprole – parenteral Ceftraroline-IV

100. Ans. a. Interferes with cell wall synthesis

Ref: Goodman and Gilman's The Pharmacological Basis of Therapeutics 12/e

Cephalosporins are β-lactam antibiotics having 7-amino cephalosporanic acid nucleus. They inhibit synthesis of the bacterial peptidoglycan cell wall (transpeptidase inhibitor).

101. Ans. d. Thyroxine *Ref: Katzung (2012), Basic and Clinical Pharmacology 12/e p684-685*

102. Ans. a. Phenytoin *Ref: Goodman and Gilman's The Pharmacological Basis of Therapeutics 12/e p593*

103. Ans. d. ADP *Ref: Rang and Dale Pharmacology Textbook 8/e*

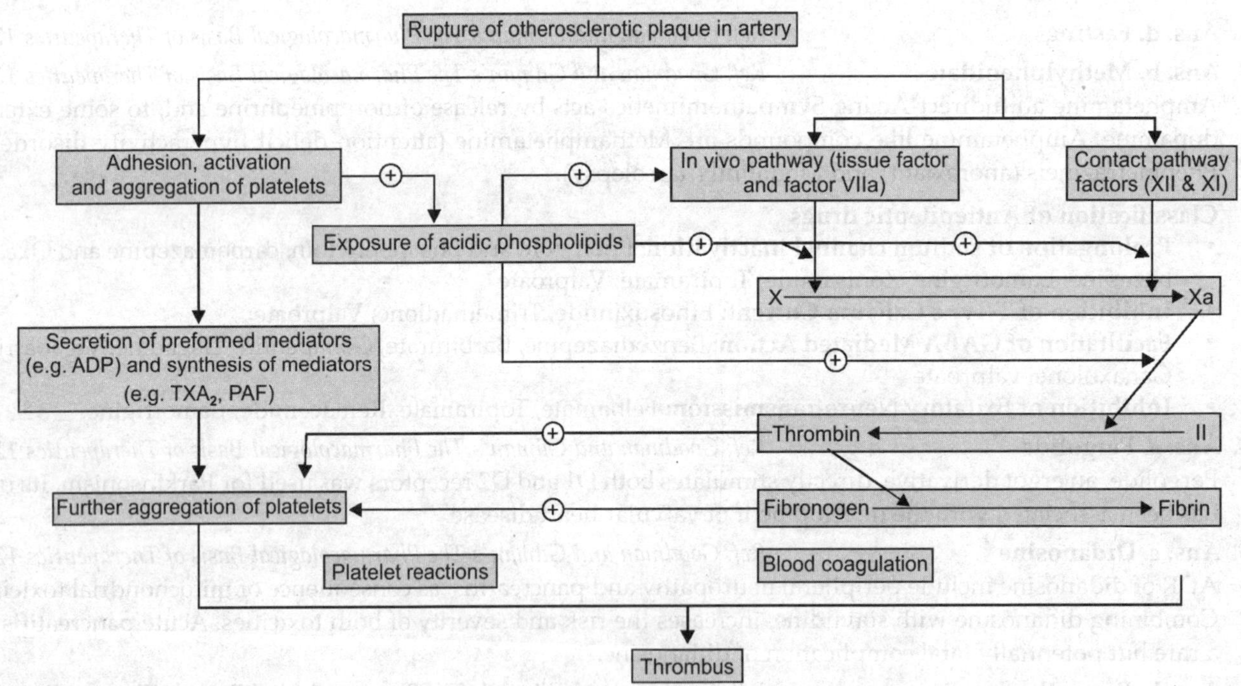

104. Ans. c. Doxacurium *Ref: Goodman and Gilman's The Pharmacological Basis of Therapeutics 12/e*

Classification of Sk M Relaxants

- **NM Blockers** (Non-depolarizing/competitive blockers)

These drugs decrease the transmission of impulse across NMJ either by inhibiting nicotinic NM receptor or by consistently depolarizing the muscle end plate.

- **Nondepolarizing:**
  - **Long acting: (> 35′):** d-Tubocurarine, Gallamine, Pancuronium, Doxacurium. Pipecuronium
  - **Intermediate acting: 20–35′:** Vecuronium, Atracurium, Rocuronium, Rapacuronium
  - **Short acting: 10–20′:** Mivacurium

- **Depolarizing blockers:** Succinyl choline, Decamethonium
  - **Centrally acting drugs:** Diazepam, clonazepam, Baclofen, Tizanidine, Carisoprodol, Chlorzoxazone, Methocarbamol
  - **Directly acting:** Dantrolene
  - **Miscellaneous:** Quinine, botulinum toxin A, B

105. Ans. c. Acetylcholine *Ref: Katzung (2012), Basic and Clinical Pharmacology 12/e*

Four Basic Kinds of Cholinergic Nerves

1. All preganglionic nerves in the ANS, both sympathetic and parasympathetic
2. Postganglionic nerves of the PSNS and a few SNS nerves
3. Motor nerves on skeletal muscles
4. Cholinergic nerves within the CNS.

106. Ans. b. Erythromycin *Ref: Katzung*

Chlamydia	First choice	Alternative
C trachomatis	Tetracycline, azithromycin	Clindamycin, ofloxacin
C pneumonia	Tetracycline, erythromycin	Clarithromycin, azithromycin
C psittaci	Tetracycline	Chloramphenicol

Erythromycin is used to treat Chlamydia infection in pregnancy

107. Ans. b. Type 2 diabetes mellitus *Ref: Goodman and Gilman's The Pharmacological Basis of Therapeutics, 12/e p1261-62*

Thiazolidinediones have benefit in the prevention of type 2 diabetes by reducing insulin resistance

Thiazolidinediones	Pioglitazone	Rosiglitazone
MOA	Regulates gene expression by binding to PPAR-γ and PPAR-α	Regulates gene expression by binding to PPAR-γ
Pk	Oral • Long-acting (> 24 h)	
ADR	Fluid retention, edema, anemia, weight gain, macular edema, bone fractures in women	
CI	CHF, hepatic disease	

Because of the hepatotoxicity observed with **troglitazone**, a discontinued drug, the FDA continues to require monitoring of liver function tests before initiation of Tzd therapy and periodically afterward.

108. Ans. b. Guanadrel *Ref: Goodman and Gilman's The Pharmacological Basis of Therapeutics 12/e*

Alpha-2 agonists: Clonidine, Apraclonidine, Guanfacine, Guanabenz, Brimonidine, Alphamethyldopa

MOA: Decrease sympathetic outflow from brain to periphery resulting in decrease PVR and blood pressure. Decrease nerve-evoked release of sympathetic transmitters and decrease production of aqueous humor

Uses: Adjunctive therapy in shock, hypertension, to reduce sympathetic response to withdrawal from narcotics, alcohol, and tobacco. Glaucoma

Remarks: Apraclonidine and brimonidine used topically for glaucoma and ocular hypertension

Methyldopa is converted in CNS to alpha-methyl NE, an effective alpha$_2$ agonist.

109. Ans. d. 56 days *Ref: Goodman and Gilman's The Pharmacological Basis of Therapeutics 12/e*

Iodine 131 is a radioisotope with a half-life of 8 days.

Around 7 half-life is required for a drug to degrade by 99%.

So 7 x 8 = 56 days is the answer

110. Ans. c. Hypertriglyceridemia *Ref: Goodman and Gilman's The Pharmacological Basis of Therapeutics 12/e*

Antihyperlipidemic drugs are

- HMG-CoA reductase inhibitors—the statins
- Bile acid–binding resins
- Nicotinic acid (*niacin*)
- Fibric acid derivatives
- The cholesterol absorption inhibitor *ezetimibe*

NIACIN:
MOA: Decreases catabolism of apo AI, reduces VLDL secretion from liver
Niacin is used to increase HDL, decrease lipoprotein (a) [Lp(a)], LDL, and triglycerides
ADR: Gastric irritation, flushing, low incidence of hepatic toxicity, may reduce glucose tolerance.
Rarer reversible side effects include toxic amblyopia and toxic maculopathy.

111. Ans. d. Palonosetron *Ref: Goodman and Gilman's The Pharmacological Basis of Therapeutics 12/e*

The 5-HT_1, 5-HT_2, and 5-$HT_{4–7}$ receptor families are members of GPCRs and the 5-HT_3 receptor is a ligand-gated ion channel that gates Na^+ and K^+.

Seratonin receptor	Action	Drug examples	Clinical disorder
5-HT_{1A}	Partial agonist	Buspirone, ipsaperone	Anxiety, depression
5-$HT_{1B/1D}$	Agonist	Sumatriptan	Migraine
5-$HT_{2A/2C}$	Antagonist	Methysergide, risperidone, ketanserin	Migraine, depression, schizophrenia
5-HT_3	Antagonist	Ondansetron	Chemotherapy-induced emesis
5-HT_4	Agonist	Cisapride	GI disorders
SERT (5-HT transporter)	Inhibitor	Fluoxetine, sertraline	Depression, obsessive-compulsive disorder, panic disorder, social phobia, post-traumatic stress disorder

5-HT3 Antagonists in Chemotherapy-Induced Nausea/Emesis

Drug	Receptor interactions	$T_{1/2}$
Ondansetron	5-HT_3 antagonist and weak 5-HT_4 antagonist	3.9 h
Granisetron	5-HT_3 antagonist	9–11.6 h
Dolasetron	5-HT_3 antagonist	7–9 h
Palonosetron	5-HT_3 antagonist; **highest affinity** for 5-HT_3 receptor in this class	40 h

112. Ans. a. Valproate *Ref: Goodman and Gilman's The Pharmacological Basis of Therapeutics 12/e*

Prophylaxis
- Beta Blockers: Propranolol except BB with ISA
- 5-HT_2 Receptor Blockers: Pizotifen, Cyproheptadine, Methysergide
- Ca^{++} Channel Blocker: Verapamil, Flunarizine
- Tricyclic Antidepressants: Amitryptyline
- Anticonvulsants: Valproic acid, gabapentin, topiramate
- Clonidine, CRRP antagonist.

Acute Attack
- Simple analgesics+Antiemetics
- Dopamine antagonists, Ergotamine (5-HT_1 Partial Agonist),
- Triptans (5-HT_1 b/1D Agonist): Sumatriptan, Zolmitriptan, Naratriptan, Rizatriptan, Eletriptan, Almotriptan, Frovatriptan
- Note: Frovatriptan is the longest acting and rizatriptan is the fastest acting congener.
- ADR: Coronary vasospasm so CI in ischemic heart disease, hypertension, epilepsy, hepatic or renal impairement and pregnancy

113. Ans. c. Emtricitabine *Ref: Goodman and Gilman's The Pharmacological Basis of Therapeutics 12/e*

Classification of Antiretro viral drugs explained in previous questions

114. Ans. a. aPTT *Ref: Goodman and Gilman's The Pharmacological Basis of Therapeutics 12/e*
- Antiplatelet drugs – prolongs bleeding time
- Anticoagulant – prolongs clotting time
- Heparin (intrinsic pathway) – prolongs aPTT
- Warfarin (extrinsic pathway) – prolongs PT
- Thrombin time is prolonged in afibrogenemia and dysfibrogenemia.

115. Ans. b. Sodium stibogluconate *Ref: Goodman and Gilman's The Pharmacological Basis of Therapeutics 12/e*

Leishmaniasis

- Cutaneous leishmaniasis caused by – Leishmania tropica
- Mucocutaneous leishmaniasis caused by – Leishmania braziliensis
- Visceral leishmaniasis caused by – Leishmania donovani (Kala-Azar)

Treatment of Kala Azar

- **Sodium stibogluconate:** Primary treatment for all forms of disease, given parenterally, cardiotoxic (QT prolongation)
- **Other drugs:** Meglumine antimoniate, Amphotericin B, Pentamidine, miltefosine and sitamaquine, paromomycin, ketaconazole, mepacrine, INF γ and Allopurinol
- **Cutaneous leishmaniasis:** Primary: Sodium stibogluconate
- Other drugs: Meglumine antimoniate or Amphotericin B or Pentamidine or Fluconazole or metroidazole
- **Mucocutaneous leishmaniasis:** Liposomal Amphotericin B

116. Ans. d. Sucralfate *Ref: Goodman and Gilman's The Pharmacological Basis of Therapeutics 12/e*

Antihelicobacter pylori drugs are proton pump inhibitor + amoxicillin + clarithromycin or Bismuth + metronidazole + tetracycline + proton pump inhibitor.

117. Ans. b. Omeprazole *Ref: Goodman and Gilman's The Pharmacological Basis of Therapeutics 12/e*

For cyp2c19: Omeprazole, lansoprazole and Clopidogrel

118. Ans. c. Diabetic microalbuminuria *Ref: Goodman and Gilman's The Pharmacological Basis of Therapeutics 12/e*

ACE Inhibitors suited for:	**Contra indicated:**
• High renin cases/those on low salt diet	• Bilateral renal atrery stenosis
• Physically/intellectually and sexually active pts	• Pregnancy
• Diabetic specially with nephropathy	• Hyperkalemia
• Coexisting angina, post MI	**Caution in:**
• LVD/CHF	• Pt. on high dose diuretic therapy
• LVH	• Pre-existing dry cough
• Gout/PVD/dyslipidemia	

119. Ans. b. Doxorubicin *Ref: Goodman and Gilman's The Pharmacological Basis of Therapeutics 12/e*

Cardiomyopathy is the most important long-term toxicity of doxorubicin. An acute form is characterized by abnormal electrocardiographic changes, including ST- and T-wave alterations and arrhythmias. Chronic, cumulative dose-related toxicity (usually total doses of > 550 mg/m^2) progress to congestive heart failure.

120. Ans. c. Acetyl choline *Ref: Goodman and Gilman's The Pharmacological Basis of Therapeutics 12/e*

- Main NT of postganglionic sympathetic nervous system is Noradrenaline
- Dopamine in mesenteric and renal vasculature
- Adrenaline in adrenal medulla
- Acetyl choline in sweat glands

121. Ans. a. Naloxone *Ref: Goodman and Gilman's The Pharmacological Basis of Therapeutics 12/e*

Pure Antagonist of Opioid receptor:

- Naloxone
- Naltrexone
- Nalmefene

Naltrexone:

- Chemically related to naloxone, More potent, Orally active, Long acting 1–2 days
- Suitable in post addicts, But produces hepato toxicity

Naloxone:

- Competitive antagonist of all receptors
- Low dose: mu receptor; high dose: kappa and delta
- Blocks all actions except sedation
- Suppress dysphoria and psychomimmetic effects

- Ppt. Morphine withdrawal in dependents
- Blocks endogenous opioids
- Blocks placebo, acupuncture and stress – analgesia
- Antagonizes resp. depression by N_2O and diazepam
- Only parenteral administration
- T ½ 1 hour in adult 3 hours in children

Uses of Naloxone: Morphine poisoning, Neonatal asphyxia, to reverse respiratory depression, intraspinal opioid analgesia, diagnosis of opioid dependence, reverses alcohol intoxication, elevate BP in shock.

122. Ans. a. Aminoglycosides *Ref: Goodman and Gilman's The Pharmacological Basis of Therapeutics 12/e*

Explained previously

123. Ans. c. Piperazine *Ref: Goodman and Gilman's The Pharmacological Basis of Therapeutics 12/e*

Piperazine: Mild adverse effects include nausea, vomiting, diarrhea, abdominal pain, dizziness, and headache. Neurotoxicity and allergic reactions are rare. Piperazine compounds should not be given to women during pregnancy, to patients with impaired renal or hepatic function, or to those with a history of epilepsy or chronic neurologic disease.

124. Ans. d. Bisoprolol *Ref: Goodman and Gilman's The Pharmacological Basis of Therapeutics 12/e*

Beta-1 selective antagonists are

- Acebutolol
- Atenolol
- Bisoprolol – highly **cardioselective**
- Betaxolol
- Esmolol
- Metoprolol
- Celiprolol
- Nebivolol – **most cardioselective**

125. Ans. a. Nimodipine *Ref: KD Tripathi, Essentials of Medical Pharmacology 7/e*

Calcium channel blockers – dihydropyridines (DHP) – nifedipine, amlodipine, felodipine, isradipine, nicardipine, nisoldipine, nimodipine, and clevidipine

Nimodipine is a short-acting DHP, due to its high lipid solubility it penetrates blood-brain barrier very efficiently. It selectively relaxes cerebral vasculature and approved for prevention and treatment of neurological deficit due to cerebral vasospasm following subarachnoid hemorrhage or ruptured congenital intracranial aneurysms. Side effects are headache, flushing, dizziness, palpitation and nausea.

Nifedipine, diltiazem, amlodipine, and felodipine appear to provide symptomatic relief in Raynaud's disease.

HINT: Nifedipine, nicardipine, nisoldipine, nimodipine... confusion in using for SAH because all starts from *ni.* Remember *mood* is related to CNS. So answer is Nimodipine.

126. Ans. b. Phenobarbitone *Ref: Goodman and Gilman's The Pharmacological Basis of Therapeutics 12/e*

127. Ans. b. Carbamezapine *Ref: Goodman and Gilman's The Pharmacological Basis of Therapeutics 12/e*

For children at high-risk of developing recurrent febrile seizures, rectally administered diazepam at the time of fever may prevent recurrent seizures and avoid side effects of chronic phenobarbitone and valproate therapy.

128. Ans. a. Ethambutol *Ref: Katzung (2012), Basic and Clinical Pharmacology 12/e p243-516*

Hypothyroidism: Lithium, iodides, sulfonamides, amiodarone, phenylbutazone, carbimazole, acetazolamide, phenytoin, pyrazinamide (0.2%).

129. Ans. c. Decrease abuse potential *Ref: Katzung (2012), Basic and Clinical Pharmacology 12/e p1095*

Loperamide and diphenoxylate are not used for opioid analgesia but for the treatment of diarrhea. As antidiarrheal drugs, they are used in combination with atropine. The atropine is added in a concentration too low to have a significant antidiarrheal effect but is presumed to further reduce the likelihood of abuse.

130. Ans. b. L-Dopa *Ref: Goodman and Gilman's The Pharmacological Basis of Therapeutics 12/e*

Indications for therapeutic drug monitoring include:

- There is relationship between plasma drug concentration and the pharmacological effect.
- Knowledge of the drug level influences management.

- Narrow therapeutic window.
- Patient compliance problems.
- The drug dose cannot be optimised by clinical observation alone.

Examples of drugs analyzed by therapeutic drug monitoring:

- Aminoglycosides (gentamicin)
- Antiepileptics (carbamazepine, phenytoin and valproic acid, phenobarbitone)
- Lithium
- Antipsychotics (clozapine)
- Digoxin
- Tacrolimus, Cyclosporine.

131. Ans. a. Erythromycin *Ref: Goodman and Gilman's The Pharmacological Basis of Therapeutics 12/e*

Erythromycin metabolites inhibit cytochrome P450 enzymes and thus, increase the serum concentrations of numerous drugs, including theophylline, carbamazepine, warfarin, cyclosporine, and methyl prednisolone. Erythromycin increases serum concentrations of oral digoxin by increasing its bioavailability.

Carbamazepine is itself an enzyme inducer, so the increased metabolic capacity of the hepatic enzymes may cause a reduction in steady-state carbamazepine concentrations and an increased rate of metabolism of other drugs, e.g. primidone, phenytoin, ethosuximide, valproic acid, and clonazepam.

132. Ans. c. ACTH *Ref: Goodman and Gilman's The Pharmacological Basis of Therapeutics 12/e*

Epileptic spasms, infantile spasms, juvenile spasms, West syndrome or West's syndrome is a rare epileptic disorder. West syndrome in modern usage is the triad of infantile spasms, a pathognomonic EEG pattern (called hypsarrhythmia), and developmental regression.

Etiology: A malfunction in the regulation of the GABA transmission process and hyperproduction of the Corticotropin-releasing hormone (CRH).

Treatment:

Prednisone, ACTH, Vigabatrin

Other drugs pyridoxine therapy, topiramate, lamotrigine, levetiracetam and zonisamide.

NOTE: The ketogenic diet has been shown to be effective in treating infantile spasm.

133. Ans. c. Used as sedative hypnotic *Ref: Goodman and Gilman's The Pharmacological Basis of Therapeutics 12/e*

Explained in previous questions

134. Ans. a. Corneal deposition *Ref: Goodman and Gilman's The Pharmacological Basis of Therapeutics 12/e*

Explained in previous questions

135. Ans. b. Imatinib mesylate *Ref: Goodman and Gilman's The Pharmacological Basis of Therapeutics 12/e*

Gastrointestinal stromal tumors (GISTs) are the most common mesenchymal neoplasms of the gastrointestinal tract. Most occur in the stomach and gastric GISTs have a lower malignant potential than tumors found elsewhere in the GI tract. GISTs arise in the smooth muscle pacemaker interstitial cell of Cajal. Mutations in the KIT gene (CD117) (85%), PDGFRA gene (10%), or BRAF kinase (rare).

Imatinib is an inhibitor of the tyrosine kinase domain of the Bcr-Abl oncoprotein and prevents phosphorylation of the kinase substrate by ATP. It also inhibits receptor tyrosine kinases for platelet-derived growth factor receptor (PDGFR), stem cell factor, and c-kit.

Imatinib is approved for use as first-line therapy in chronic phase CML, in blast crisis, and as second-line therapy for chronic phase CML that has progressed on prior interferon-alfa therapy.

Imatinib is also effective in of gastrointestinal stromal tumors expressing the c-kit tyrosine kinase.

ADR of Imatinib: Fluid retention with ankle and periorbital edema, diarrhea, myalgias, congestive heart failure.

Sunitinib inhibits multiple RTKs (PDGFR-α and PDGFR-β, VEGF-R1, VEGF-R2, VEGF-R3, and c-kit). It is approved for the treatment of advanced renal cell cancer and for the treatment of gastrointestinal stromal tumors (GIST) after disease progression on or with intolerance to imatinib.

ADR: Skin rash, fatigue and asthenia, bleeding complications, cardiac toxicity leading to congestive heart failure.

Regorafenib was FDA approved in 2013 for advanced GISTs that cannot be surgically removed and that no longer respond to imatinib and sunitinib. Regorafenib shows antiangiogenic activity due to its dual targeted VEGFR2-TIE2 tyrosine kinase inhibition.
ADR: Weakness or fatigue, loss of appetite, hand-foot syndrome (palmar-plantar erythrodysesthesia), diarrhea, mouth sores (mucousitis), weight loss, infection, high blood pressure, and changes in voice (dysphonia).

136. Ans. b. Done in healthy human volunteers
Ref: Goodman and Gilman's The Pharmacological Basis of Therapeutics 12/e

Explained in previous questions.

137. Ans. b. Decreases PG synthesis *Ref: Goodman and Gilman's The Pharmacological Basis of Therapeutics 12/e*

Nefopam is a centrally-acting but nonopioid analgesic drug used for the relief of moderate to severe pain as an alternative to opioid, in the prevention of shivering, to combat severe hiccups.
It is contraindicated in people with epilepsy and with MAO inhibitors.
Action: voltage-gated sodium channel blocker and inhibition of serotonin, dopamine and noradrenaline reuptake.

138. Ans. a. Prolactin *Ref: Goodman and Gilman's The Pharmacological Basis of Therapeutics 12/e*

Explained in previous questions.

139. Ans. c. Retapamulin *Ref: Goodman and Gilman's The Pharmacological Basis of Therapeutics 12/e*

For MRSA (Methicillin-resistant *Staphylococcus aureus*)

Glycopeptide antibiotics: Vancomycin and teicoplanin are used.

For VISA (Vancomycin intermediate-resistant *Staphylococcus aureus*)

Linezolid, quinupristin/dalfopristin, daptomycin, ceftaroline, and tigecycline are used to treat infections that do not respond to glycopeptides

140. Ans. a. General anesthesia *Ref: Katzung (2012), Basic and Clinical Pharmacology 12/e*

141. Ans. a. Memantine *Ref: Goodman and Gilman's The Pharmacological Basis of Therapeutics 12/e*

Types of Alzheimer's disease:

1. Late onset: Genes involved:
   - Epsilon 4 (ε4) allele at the apolipoprotein E (ApoE) locus (chromosome 19).
   - The ApoE gene encodes a protein responsible for lipid transport.
   - ApoE ε4 allele carriers lower overall age at onset for Alzheimer disease.
2. Familial (< 1%). Genes involved:
   - Amyloid precursor protein (chromosome 21)
   - Presenilin 1 (chromosome 14)
   - Presenilin 2 (chromosome 1).

Treatment:

	Donepezil	Rivastigmine	Galantamine	Tacrine[a]	Memantine
Inhibition[b]	AChE	AChE, BuChE	AChE	AChE, BuChE	NMDA
Mechanism of inhibition	Noncompetitive	Noncompetitive	Competitive	Noncompetitive	Noncompetitive
Typical maintenance dose	10 mg once daily	9.5 mg/24h (transdermal) 3-6 mg twice daily (oral)	8–12 mg twice daily 16–24 mg/day (XR)	20 mg, four times daily	5–10 mg twice daily
FDA-approved indications	Mild-severe AD	Mild-moderate AD,	Mild-moderate AD	Mild-moderate AD	Moderate-severe AD
Adverse effects	Nausea, vomiting, loss of appetite, weight loss, diarrhea, dizziness, muscle cramps, insomnia, vivid dreams, etc.			And hepatotoxicity	Constipation, dizziness, headache

[a]Tacrine is not used because of hepatotoxicity
[b]AChE: Acetylcholinesterase, BuChE: Butyrylcholinesterase, NMDA: N-methyl-D-aspartate

142. Ans. a. Kappa *Ref: Katzung (2012), Basic and Clinical Pharmacology 12/e p367*

Primary excitatory neurotransmitter in the CNS is glutamate.

Glutamate receptors can be divided into two groups

1. Ionotropic glutamate receptors (iGluRs) form the ion channel pore.
2. Metabotropic glutamate receptors (mGluRs) that involves G proteins.

Type	Name	Agonist(s)	Antagonists
Ionotropic (iGluRs)	NMDA receptor	NMDA	Felbamate Memantine
	Kainate receptor	Kainate	Topiramate
	AMPA receptor	AMPA	Topiramate, phenobarbital and lamotrigine
Metabotropic	mGluR	Under research	

143. Ans. a. Bromocriptine *Ref: Katzung (2012), 12/e Basic and clinical pharmacology*

For lactation suppression: Diethylstilbestrol, bromocriptine, cabergoline are used (off label)

Prolactin causes lactation. Dopamine suppress prolactin, so dopamine antagonists like metaclopramide and domperidone has hyperprolactinemia as side effect.

Dopamine agonist (Decrease Prolactin)

- Dopamine
- Bromocriptine
- Apomorphine
- Pergolide
- Piribedil
- Ropinirole
- Pramipexle
- **Increased prolactin SECRETION-**
- **Dopamine antagonist**
- Cholrpromazine
- Haloperidol
- Metochlopromide
- **Dopamine depleters**
- Reserpine
- Methyldopa.

144. Ans. a. Clearance *Ref: Katzung (2012) Basic and Clinical Pharmacology 12/e p38*

- **Rate of elimination of drug is** the amount of drug eliminated (in units of weight like grams) per unit time.
- Total body clearance is the rate of elimination of a drug divided by its plasma concentration.
- Rate of elimination is directly proportional to plasma concentration in **FIRST ORDER KINETIC**
- Rate of elimination is independent of plasma concentration **ZERO ORDER KINETIC**

Clearance (C_L) = Rate of elimination of a drug/Plasma concentration

Rate of elimination = Amount of drug eliminated/Time taken

145. Ans. d. Chemotherapy induced hyperuricemia *Ref: Katzung (2012) Basic and Clinical Pharmacology 12/e p1099*

146. Ans. d. Frovatriptan *Ref: Katzung (2012) Basic and Clinical Pharmacology 12/e p286*

Explained

147. Ans. a. Cetrizine *Ref: Katzung (2012) Basic and clinical pharmacology 12/e*

148. Ans: Imipinem *Ref: Katzung (2012) Basic and Clinical Pharmacology 12/e p800-802*

Extended-spectrum β-lactamases (ESBLs), hydrolyze both cephalosporins and penicillins. Carbapenems are highly resistant to hydrolysis by penicillinases and cephalosporinases, but they are hydrolyzed by metallo-β-lactamase and carbapenemases.

149. Ans. c. In penicillin allergey aztreonam tolerated but not imipenam

Ref: Katzung (2012) Basic and Clinical Pharmacology 12/e p800-802

Carbapenams are Doripenem, ertapenem, imipenem and meropenem

Monobactam is Aztreonam

Aztreonam: Spectrum of activity is limited to aerobic gram-negative rods (including P aeruginosa). Unlike other β-lactam antibiotics, they have no activity against gram-positive bacteria or anerobes. If a patient develops severe hypersensitivity reaction to a penicillin, all other beta lactam antibiotic are contraindicated except aztreonam (cross sensitivity is not present) to treat serious infections such as pneumonia, meningitis, and sepsis caused by susceptible gram-negative pathogens.

Carbapenam: Spectrum of activity against many gram-negative rods, including P aeruginosa, gram-positive organisms, and anerobes. Imipenem is inactivated by dehydropeptidases in renal tubules, resulting in low urinary concentrations. So, it is administered together with an inhibitor of renal dehydropeptidase, cilastatin. Doripenem, ertapenem and meropenem do not require inhibitor of renal dehydropeptidase.

Carbapenems are used in treatment of infections caused by extended-spectrum β-lactamase-producing gram-negative bacteria. ADRs are nausea, vomiting, diarrhea, skin rashes, and reactions at the infusion sites. Excessive levels of imipenem in patients with renal failure may lead to seizures. Patients allergic to penicillins may be allergic to carbapenems.

QUESTIONS 2015

1. Cotrimoxazole can be given with:
a. Warfarin
b. Metronidazole
c. Glibenclamide
d. Phenytoin

2. What is not a radiosensitizer?
a. Hydroxyurea
b. Mitomycin
c. Gemcitabine
d. Cyclophosphamide

3. All are true regarding vancomycin toxicity except:
a. No toxicity with oral medication
b. Irreversible ototoxicity
c. Dose dependent nephrotoxicity
d. Red neck syndrome

4. Complications of cyclosporine therapy are all except:
a. Bone marrow toxicity
b. Hyperkalemia
c. Hirsuitism
d. Nephrotoxicity

5. Patient on morphine for c/c pain. What is the effect of addition of partial agonist?
a. More sedation
b. Reduction in analgesia
c. Respiratory depression
d. Constipation

6. Cisplatin toxicity are all except:
a. Neurotoxicity
b. Ototoxicity
c. Nephrotoxicity
d. Myelosuppression

7. Which of the following can cause dangerous hyperkalemia?
a. Frusemide and propranolol
b. Amiloride and hydrochlorothiazide
c. Lisinopril and amiloride
d. Losartan and hydrochlorothiazide

8. Hepatitis with cholestatic jaundice occurs most frequently as an adverse reaction to the following preparation of erythromycin:
a. Erythromycin base
b. Erythromycin stearate
c. Erythromycin estolate
d. Erythromycin ethyl succinate

9. Bisphosphonates act by:
a. Apoptosis of osteoclasts
b. Inhibiting farnesyl pyrophosphate synthase
c. Bone resorption
d. Both a and b

10. In paracetamol overdose concerning acute liver failure, which is NOT TRUE
a. Albumin is good index for liver failure
b. N-acetyl cysteine is beneficial in acute paracetamol poisoning
c. Administration of GSH is not effective
d. Toxic metabolite is N-acetylbenzoiminoquinone

11. The following statements are true of oral anticoagulants except:
a. They interfere with an early step in the synthesis of clotting factors

b. Irrespective of the dose administered, their anticoagulant effect has a latency of onset of 1–3 days
c. Their dose is adjusted by repeated measurement of prothrombin time
d. They are contraindicated during pregnancy

12. Which beta blocker has antioxidant property?
a. Celiprolol
b. Carvedilol
c. Betaxolol
d. Propranolol

ANSWERS AND EXPLANATIONS

1. Ans. b. Metronidazole *Ref: Goodman and Gilman's The Pharmacological Basis of Therapeutics 12/e*

GG: The most important interactions of the sulfonamides involve those with the oral anticoagulants, the sulfonylurea hypoglycemic agents, and the hydantoin anticonvulsants. In each case, sulfonamides can potentiate the effects of the other drug by mechanisms that appear to involve primarily inhibition of metabolism and, possibly, displacement from albumin. Dosage adjustment may be necessary when a sulfonamide is given concurrently.

Metronidazole should be used with caution in patients with active disease of the CNS because of its potential neurotoxicity. The drug also may precipitate CNS signs of lithium toxicity in patients receiving high doses of lithium. Plasma levels of metronidazole can be elevated by drugs such as cimetidine that inhibit hepatic microsomal metabolism. Moreover, metronidazole can prolong the prothrombin time of patients receiving therapy with coumadin anticoagulants. The dosage of metronidazole should be reduced in patients with severe hepatic disease.

2. Ans. d. Cyclophosphamide *Ref: Goodman and Gilman's The Pharmacological Basis of Therapeutics 12/e*

HU is a potent radiosensitizer as a consequence of its inhibition of RNR (Flanagan et al., 2007) and has been incorporated into several treatment regimens with concurrent irradiation (i.e., cervical carcinoma, primary brain tumors, head and neck cancer, non-small cell lung cancer).

Gemcitabine is a very potent radiosensitizer, likely the result of its inhibition of RNR, depletion of dATP, and inhibition of DNA repair (Flanagan et al., 2007) and should not be used with radiotherapy except in closely monitored clinical trials.

Mitomycin is a potent radiosensitizer, teratogen, and carcinogen in rodents.

3. Ans. a. No toxicity with oral medication *Ref: Katzung (2012), Basic and Clinical Pharmacology 12/e*

Vancomycin at the site of injection causes phlebitis and infusion-related flushing caused by release of histamine called 'red man' or 'red neck' syndrome. Chills and fever may occur. Nephrotoxicity is uncommon with current preparations. Administration with another ototoxic or nephrotoxic drug, such as an aminoglycoside, increases the risk of these toxicities. Ototoxicity can be minimized by maintaining peak serum concentrations below 60 mcg/mL

4. Ans. a. Bone marrow toxicity *Ref: Katzung (2012), Basic and Clinical Pharmacology 12/e*

Toxicities include nephrotoxicity, hypertension, hyperglycemia, liver dysfunction, hyperkalemia, altered mental status, seizures, and hirsutism. However, cyclosporine causes very little bone marrow toxicity. While an increased incidence of lymphoma and other cancers (Kaposi's sarcoma, skin cancer) have been observed in transplant recipients receiving cyclosporine (because the drug induces TGF-β, which promotes tumor invasion and metastasis)

5. Ans. b. Reduction in analgesia *Ref: Katzung (2012), Basic and Clinical Pharmacology 12/e*

Partial agonist to patients receiving pure agonist drugs can reduce analgesic effect.

Generic name	Mu	Delta	Kappa	Receptor effects
Pentazocine	Partial agonist		Agonist	–
Nalbuphine	Antagonist		Agonist	Ceiling to the respiratory depressant effect
Buprenorphine	Partial agonist/ Antagonist	Antagonist	Antagonist	In opioid dependence. No analgesia and respiratory depression diversion for illicit intravenous abuse

Contd...

Contd...

Generic name	Mu	Delta	Kappa	Receptor effects
Suboxone	Antagonist			
Butorphanol	Partial agonist		Agonist	–

6. **Ans. d. Myelosuppression** *Ref: Katzung (2012), Basic and Clinical Pharmacology 12/e*
Platinum analogs are Carboplatin, Cisplatin and Oxaliplatin
MOA: They kill tumor cells in all stages of the cell cycle and bind DNA through the formation of intrastrand and interstrand cross-links, thereby leading to inhibition of DNA synthesis and function. The primary binding site is the N7 position of guanine, but covalent interaction with the N3 position of adenine and O6 position of cytosine can also occur.
Uses: non-small cell and small cell lung cancer, esophageal and gastric cancer, cholangiocarcinoma, head and neck cancer, and genitourinary cancers, particularly testicular, ovarian, and bladder cancer.
ADR of cisplatin: Nephrotoxicity, peripheral sensory neuropathy, ototoxicity, nerve dysfunction.
Myelosuppression is exhibited more by Carboplatin and Oxaliplatin.

7. **Ans. c. Lisinopril and amiloride** *Ref: Katzung (2012), Basic and Clinical Pharmacology 12/e*
Potassium-sparing diuretics (Amiloride, Eplerenone, spironolactone, triamterene) shows additive hyperkalemic effect with ACE inhibitors, Angiotensin II receptor blockers, Potassium-sparing diuretics and Potassium supplements. This is especially a problem in presence of renal impairment.

8. **Ans. c. Erythromycin estolate** *Ref: Katzung (2012), Basic and Clinical Pharmacology 12/e*
Erythromycins, particularly the estolate, can produce acute cholestatic hepatitis (fever, jaundice, impaired liver function), probably as a hypersensitivity reaction. Most patients recover from this, but hepatitis recurs if the drug is readministered. Other allergic reactions include fever, esinophilia, and rashes.

9. **Ans. d. Both a and b** *Ref: Goodman and Gilman's The Pharmacological Basis of Therapeutics 12/e*
Bisphosphonates include etidronate, pamidronate, alendronate, risedronate, tiludronate, ibandronate, and zoledronate.
MOA: Bisphosphonates accumulate to a high concentration only in bones as Bisphosphonate molecules preferentially 'stick' to calcium and bind to it. Bisphosphonates, when attached to bone tissue, are 'ingested' by osteoclasts and kill it.
Non-N-containing bisphosphonates like Etidronate and Tiludronate competes with adenosine triphosphate (ATP) in the osteoclast initiating its apoptosis, leading to an overall decrease in the breakdown of bone.
Nitrogenous bisphosphonates like Pamidronate, Alendronate, Ibandronate, Risedronate and Zoledronate inhibit farnesyl pyrophosphate synthase, an enzyme in the mevalonate pathway (HMG-CoA reductase pathway) that appears to be critical for osteoclast survival.

10. **Ans. a. Albumin is good index for liver failure**
Ref: Goodman and Gilman's The Pharmacological Basis of Therapeutics 12/e
Serum albumin has a half-life of approximately 20 days and is therefore a poor marker of acute hepatic failure
When acetaminophen intake far exceeds therapeutic doses, the glucuronidation and sulfation pathways are saturated, and the P450-dependent becomes important.
N-acetyl cysteine replenishes hepatic glutathione which in turn binds the toxic metabolite N-acetylbenzoimi-noquinone of paracetamol.
Administration of GSH is not effective because it does not cross cell membranes readily.
Liver transplantation may be required for patients with fulminant hepatic failure.

11. **Ans. a. They interfere with an early step in the synthesis of clotting factors**
Ref: Katzung (2012), Basic and Clinical Pharmacology 12/e
Oral anticoagulant interfere with an late steps in the synthesis of clotting factors (Factors 2, 7, 9, 10)
Classification:
Indirect Thrombin Inhibitors: Unfractionated heparin (UFH), low-molecular-weight heparin (LMWH), and the synthetic penta-saccharide fondaparinux
Parenteral Direct Thrombin Inhibitors: Hirudin, Bivalirudin, Argatroban and Melagatran.
Oral Direct Thrombin Inhibitors: Dabigatran etexilate mesylate

Oral Direct Factor Xa Inhibitors: Rivaroxaban and apixaban
Warfarin and Other Coumarin Anticoagulants.

12. Ans. b. Carvedilol

Ref: Goodman and Gilman's The Pharmacological Basis of Therapeutics 12/e

Carvedilol blocks $beta_1$, $beta_2$, and $alpha_1$ receptors.
It has antioxidant (decrease the biosynthesis of ROS and oxygen radicals.) and anti-inflammatory effects: may contribute to cardio protective effects
It has membrane-stabilizing activity
It lacks intrinsic sympathomimetic activity.
Carvedilol produces vasodilatation.
Carvedilol protect cell membranes from lipid peroxidation.
It prevents low density lipoprotein (LDL) oxidation.
Carvedilol also inhibits ROS-mediated loss of myocardial contractility, stress-induced hypertrophy, apoptosis, and the accumulation and activation of neutrophils.
At high doses, carvedilol exerts Ca^{2+} channel-blocking activity.
Carvedilol does not increase receptor density and is not associated with high levels of inverse agonist activity .
The drug is FDA-approved for use in hypertension, congestive heart failure, and left ventricular dysfunction following MI.

Chapter 8 Preventive Social Medicine

A Balaji

Henry Siegerist, the medical historian has stated that every system of medicine was developed as one of the aspects of culture.

Primitive medicine

Supernatural theory of disease.

The primitive man attributed disease and all human suffering to the wrath of gods, the invasion of body by evil spirits.

Indian system of medicine

AYUSH: Ayurveda, Unani, Sidha, Homeopathy

Ayurveda

- Implies the 'knowledge of life'.
- The tridosha theory of disease is practiced in ayurveda.
- The celebrated Ayurvedic medicine authorities were Atreya, Charaka, Susruta, and Vaghbhatt.
- Atreya is acknowledged as the first great Indian physician and teacher.
- Susruta: The father of Indian surgery.

Changing concepts in public health—Four distinct phases

1. Disease control phase (1880–1920)
   - Public health was largely a matter of sanitary legislation and sanitary reforms aimed at the control of man's physical environment.
2. Health promotional phase (1920–1960)
   - C.E.A. Winslow defined public health as the science and art of preventing disease, prolonging life and promoting health through organized community effort.
   - The evolution of health centers is an important contribution of history of public health. The second great movement was Community Development Programme to promote village development through community participation.
3. Social engineering phase (1960–1980)
   - Social and behavioral aspects of disease and health were given a new priority.
4. Health for all phase (1981–2000)
   - Attainment of a level of health that will permit all people 'to lead a socially and economically productive life'.

CONCEPT OF HEALTH AND DISEASE

Definition of health	Concept of well-being
• The widely accepted definition of health given by World Health Organization is 'Health is defined as a state of complete physical, mental and social well-being and not merely an absence of disease or infirmity'.	• Objective components: Standard of living, level of living • Subjective components: Quality of life **Standard of living** It refers to the usual scale of our expenditure, the goods we consume and the services we enjoy. It depends on income, occupation, standards of housing, educational, recreational and other services utilized

Contd...

Contd...

Definition of health	Concept of well-being
Quality of life Defined by WHO as 'the condition of life resulting from the combination of the effects of complete range of factors (environment, education, other services, etc.) **Physical Quality of Life Index:** PQLI It consolidates three indicators, viz. 1. Infant mortality, 2. Life expectancy at age one, and 3. Literacy. PQLI has not taken per capita GNP into consideration. The scale of 0 to 100, where 0 represents an absolutely defined worst performance and 100 represents an absolutely defined best performance.	**Human development index** Defined as composite index of combining three indicators 1. Longevity (life expectancy at birth), 2. Knowledge (adult literacy rate and mean years of schooling) and 3. Income (real GDP per capita in purchasing power parity in US dollars) HDI value ranges between 0 to 1, • 0.8 and above means high human development category, • 0.5 to 0.799 medium human development category and • < 0.5 low human development category. • India comes in the medium human development category, ranking at number 136.

QALY: Quality Adjusted Life Years

- It is measure of disease burden including both the quality and quantity of life lived (year of life lived with perfect health)
- Number of years of life added by intervention
- Use for assessing the value for money of a medical intervention

DFLE: Disability Free Life Expectancy

- Also called as active life expectancy
- Average number of years an individual is expected to live free of disability if current pattern of mortality and disability continue to apply

DALY

- The **Disability: Adjusted Life Year (DALY)** is a measure of overall disease burden, expressed as the number of years lost due to ill-health, disability or early death
- DALYs are calculated by taking the sum of these two components
- In a formula:

DALY = YLL + YLD.

- The DALY relies on an acceptance that the most appropriate measure of the effects of chronic illness is time, both time lost due to premature death and time spent disabled by disease
- One DALY, therefore, is equal to one year of healthy life lost

Indicators of health	Importance
Health care delivery indicators	It reflects the equity of distribution of health resources Examples, doctor population ratio, population bed ratio, population per health subcenter
Health policy indicators	Single most indicator of political commitment is allocation of adequate resources Examples, proportion GNP spent on health services
Socioeconomic indicators	Do not directly measure health But important for interpretation of indicators health care Examples, rate of population increase, per capita GNP, level of unemployment, dependency ratio, percapita calore availability, etc.
Indicators for provision of health care	Availability, accessibility, utilization, quality of care
Health status indicator	Low birth weight, nutritional status, IMR, life expectancy at birth, maternal mortality rate, disease specific mortality, prevalence of disability

Concept of Disease: WHO has defined health but not disease
Disease literally mean without ease, the opposite of ease
Disease is a physiological/psychological dysfunction
Illness is a subjective state of the person who feels aware of not being well
Sickness is a state of social dysfunction
Concepts of Prevention:
Primordial Prevention
Prevention of emergence of risk factors

Contd...

Contd...

Primary Prevention
Action taken prior to the onset of disease
- Health Promotion
  - Health education
  - Environmental Modification
  - Nutritional interventions
  - Life-style and behavioral change
- Specific Protection
  - Immunization
  - Specific nutrients
  - Chemoprophylaxis
  - Protection from carcinogens
  - Protection against accidents

Secondary Prevention
- Action taken to prevent the progress of disease
- Early diagnosis and treatment

Tertiary Prevention
Action taken to prevent or reduce the impairment and disability

Disability limitation

Disease	→	Impairment	→	Disability	→	Handicap
(Accident)		(loss of foot)		(cannot walk)		(Unemployed)

Rehabilitation
- Medical: Restoration of function
- Vocational: To earn livelihood
- Social: Restoration of family
- Psychological: Restoration of personal dignity

PRINCIPLES OF EPIDEMIOLOGY AND EPIDEMIOLOGICAL METHODS

Introduction

Epidemiology is derived from the word epidemic which is a very old world word dating back to the 3rd century. **Epi = among; demos = people; logos = study.**

In 1927, W.H. Frost became the first professor of epidemiology in US.

Later Major Greenwood became the first professor of epidemiology and medical statistics in the University of London.

- Epidemiology has been defined by John M. Last in 1988 as 'The study of the distribution and determinants of health related states or events in specified populations, and the application of this study to the control of health problems'.

Tools of measurement
- Rate
- Ratio
- Proportion

Rate
A rate measures the occurrence of some particular event in a population during a given period of time
Nothing but a statement of the risk of developing a condition
A rate comprises the following elements numerator, denominator, time specification and a multiplier

$$\text{Death rate} = \frac{\text{Number of deaths in one year} \times 100}{\text{Mid year population}}$$

Ratio
- It measures a relation in size between two random quantities
- Simply ratio is the result of dividing one quantity by another
- Numerator is not a component of denominator in ratio

Contd...

Contd...

- Expressed as x:y or x/y

$$\text{Sex ratio} = \frac{\text{Total Number of females in a population}}{\text{Total Number of males in the same population}}$$

Proportion

- It is a ratio which indicates the relation in magnitude of a part of the whole
- Numerator is always included in the denominator
- Usually expressed in percentage

$$= \frac{\text{Total number of children with malnutrition at a certain time} \times 100}{\text{Total number of children in the village at the same time}}$$

Observational studies: This type of study allow nature to take its own course; the investigator just observes but does not intervene.

Descriptive study is limited to a description of the occurrence of a disease in a population.

Analytical study: Analyses the relationship between health status and other variables.

Ecological studies

- In an ecological study, the units of study are populations or groups of people rather than individuals
- These studies are conducted by comparing populations in different countries at the same time
  Example: Comparison of air pollution level and mortality rate at the same time in different countries.

Cross sectional study or prevalence study

- Single examination of a cross section of population at one point in time
  Example: prevalence of skin diseases among school children.

Experimental or interventional studies

- Intervention or experimentation involves attempting to change a variable in one or more groups of people
  Example: testing a new treatment on a selected group of patients.

Randomized controlled trials or clinical trials

- Study population is randomly allocated into groups called treatment and control groups, and the results are assessed by comparing the outcome in the two groups.
  Example: testing an antihypertensive drug among hypertensives. Those who undergo therapy are treatment groups and those who do not undergo therapy are control groups
- Usually conducted among patients attending tertiary care institutions/hospitals/dispensaries, etc.

Field trials

- Field trials, in contrast to clinical trials, involve people who are disease free but presumed to be at risk
- Data collection done at the field.

Community intervention trials

- In this form of study the treatment groups are communities rather than individuals
- This is particularly appropriate for diseases easily influenced by the intervention directed at group behavior
  Example: cardiovascular disease

Case series study

- Number of patients with a specific disease are described but are not compared with those of a reference population

Steps in descriptive epidemiology	Basic steps in case control study	Basic steps in a cohort study
1. Defining the population to be studied 2. Defining the disease under the study	• Selection of cases and controls • Selection of cases • Selection of controls	• Selection of study subjects • Obtaining data on exposure • Selection of comparison groups

Contd...

Contd...

Steps in descriptive epidemiology	Basic steps in case control study	Basic steps in a Cohort study
3. Describing the disease by – Time – Place – Person 4. Measurement of disease 5. Comparing with known indices 6. Formulation of an etiological hypothesis	• Matching • Measurement of exposure • Analysis • Estimation of exposure rates • Estimation of risk	• Follow-up • Analysis

Short-term fluctuation: (TYPES OF EPIDEMICS)

The best known short term fluctuation is the occurrence of epidemic.

Three major types of epidemics

1. Common source epidemics
   - Single exposure or point source epidemic
   - Continuous or multiple exposure epidemics
2. Propagated epidemics
3. Slow (modern) epidemic.

Common source, single exposure epidemic

- Known as point source epidemics, Example: Food poisoning

Features:

- The exposure to the disease agent is brief and simultaneous
- All cases occur within one incubation period
- Curve has only one peak, no secondary waves
- Clustering of cases within a narrow interval of time
- Not always due to exposure to an infectious agent.

Common source, multiple exposure epidemics

- The exposure from the same source may be prolonged, continuous, repeated not necessarily at the same time, Example: a commercial sex worker may be a common source in gonorrhea outbreak, since she will infect her clients over a period of time
- Epidemics: beyond the range of one incubation period
- No evidence of secondary cases from the infected persons

Propagated epidemics

- Most often of infectious origin
- Results from person to person transmission of an infectious agent
- The curve shows a gradual rise and tails off over a longer period of time
- Periodic fluctuations

Seasonal trend

- Well known examples are measles, varicella, malaria

Cyclical trend

- Influenza pandemics known to occur at 7–10 years intervals

Long term or secular trends

- Implies consistent tendency of a disease to change in a particular direction or a definite movement in one direction, Examples: coronary heart disease, diabetes

ANALYTICAL EPIDEMIOLOGY

The objective is to test the hypothesis.

Two types

1. Case control studies
2. Cohort studies

Case Control Studies

- Called retrospective studies
- First common approach to test causal hypothesis.

- Three distinct features of case control studies

a. Both exposure and outcome have occurred before start of the study
b. The study proceeds backwards from effect to cause
c. It uses a control or comparison group to support or refute an inference.

Steps in case control studies

- Selection of cases and controls.
- Selection of cases.
- Definition of cases.
- Sources of cases.
- Selection of controls
  - Controls must be free from the disease
  - Must be similar to the cases as possible.
- Selection of cases and controls is crucial to the interpretation of the results of the case control studies.
- Failure to select comparable controls can introduce bias which is called selection bias.
- Matching: Is defined as the process by which we select controls in such a way that they are similar to cases.
- Confounding factor: Defined as one which is associated both with exposure and disease, and is unequally distributed in study and control groups.
- Measurement of exposure
  - Information about exposure should be obtained in the same manner both for cases and controls
  - Obtained by interviews, questionnaires, or by studying past records of cases, employment records
- Analysis
  - Exposure rates among cases and controls to suspected factor
  - Estimation of disease risk associated with exposure (odds ratio)

	Cases (lung cancer)	Controls (without lung cancer)
Smokers	a	B
Nonsmokers	c	d
Totals	a + c	b + d

Exposure rates among cases = a/a + c × 100

Exposure rats among controls = b/b + d × 100

Estimation of risk (odds ratio) = ad/bc

Bias in case control studies

Bias is any systematic error in the determination of the association between the exposure and the disease.

Types of bias in case control study

- Confounding bias
- Memory or recall bias
- Selection bias
- Berkesonian bias
- Interviewer's bias.

Nested case control study: Case control study done in a cohort study
- A nested case control study draws its cases and controls from a cohort population that has been followed for a period of time
- It utilizes the exposure data originally collected before the onset of disease, thus reducing the risk of recall bias
- It includes cases and controls drawn from the same cohort, thus decreasing the chances of selection bias.

Cohort Study (Prospective study, longitudinal study, incidence study, forward looking study, follow up study)

- Features of a cohort study
- Population are identified prior to the development of the study
- The study groups are followed for a period of time
- The study proceeds from cause to effect
- Cohort is defined as a group of people who share a common characteristic.

Types of cohort studies

- Prospective study
- Retrospective study
- Combination of both prospective and retrospective study.

Prospective study

- The outcome has not yet occurred at the time of investigation begins.

Retrospective cohort study or historical cohort study or non concurrent cohort study

- Outcomes have all occurred before the start of investigation
- The investigator goes back in time, to select his study groups from existing records and traces them forward through time, usually up to the present time.

Combination of both retrospective and prospective cohort studies

- The study population is identified from past records, and is assessed till date and followed up in future for further assessment of outcome.

Analysis in cohort study

Incidence rates of disease among exposed and nonexposed

Estimation of risk

Cigarette smoking	Developed lung cancer	Did not develop lung cancer	Total
Yes	a	b	a+b
No	c	d	c+d

Incidence rates among exposed (smokers) = a/a + b × 1000

Incidence rates among nonexposed (nonsmokers) = c/c + d × 1000

Estimation of risk

$$\text{Relative risk (risk ratio)} = \frac{\text{Incidence rates disease among nonexposed}}{\text{Incidence rates of disease among exposed}}$$

- Direct measure of strength of association
- RR of 1 indicates no association
- RR > 1 suggests positive association between the exposure and the outcome.

Attributable risk:

$$\frac{\text{Incidence of disease rate among exposed} - \text{Incidence of disease rate among non-exposed}}{\text{Incidence of disease rate among exposed}} \times 100$$

AR means to what extent the disease under study can be attributed to the exposure

Population attributable risk

$$\frac{\text{Incidence of disease in the total population} - \text{Incidence of disease among nonexposed}}{\text{Incidence among the total population}} \times 100$$

Provides an estimate of amount by which the disease could be reduced in that population if the factor under study could be controlled or eliminated.

Case control study	Cohort study
Proceeds from effect to cause	Proceeds from cause to effect
Starts with the disease	Starts with the people exposed to risk factor
Involves few number of subjects	Involves large number of subjects
Yields relatively quick results	Long follow up period, involving delayed results
Suitable for study of rare diseases	Suitable for study of rare exposures
Yields only estimate of RR (odds ratio)	Yields incidence rates, RR and AR
Inexpensive	Expensive

Randomized Controlled Trials

- Randomization: Statistical procedure by which the participants are allocated into groups usually called study and control groups to receive or not to receive an experimental or therapeutic procedure
- Randomization is an attempt to eliminate bias and allow for comparability
- By randomization we can eliminate selection bias
- Randomization is done only after the participant has entered the study.

Bias in RCT

Subjective bias: Participants may subjectively feel better or report improvement if they knew they were receiving a new form of treatment.

Observer bias: The observer measuring the outcome of a trial may be influenced if he knows beforehand the particular procedure or therapy to which the patient has been subjected

Bias in evaluation: The investigator may subconsciously give a favorable report of the outcome of the trial.

Blinding

- Single blind trial: Participant is not aware
- Double blind trial: Neither the doctor nor the participant is aware
- Triple blind trial: The participant, observer, person who is analyzing the data are all blind.
- Ideally triple blinding should be used
- But most frequently used one is double blinding.

Concurrent Parallel Study Designs

- Comparisons are made between two randomly assigned groups, one group exposed to specific treatment, and the other group not exposed.
- Patient remain in the study group or the control group for the duration of investigation

Crossover Type of Study Designs

- With this type of study design, each patient serves as his own control
- As before, the patients are randomly assigned to a study group and control group
- The study group receives the treatment and the control group does not
- Then the two groups are observed over time
- Then the treatment is withdrawn for a period of time till the elimination of the medication from the body
- Then the groups who received treatment are changed into the control group and the control groups are given the treatment this time.

Advantages

- All patients can be assured that sometime during the course of the study, they will receive the new therapy.

Disadvantages

- Not suitable if the drug of interest cures the disease
- Not suitable if the drug is effective during a certain stage of disease
- If the disease changes radically during the period of treatment.

Association and Causation

- Association may be defined as the concurrence of two variables more often than expected by chance.
- In other words, events are said to be associated when they occur more frequently together.
- Association does not imply a causal relationship.
- The terms association and relationship are often used interchangeably.

Causation

- A cause of a disease is an event or condition which plays an important role in producing the disease
- A single causal factor on its own is often neither necessary or sufficient for producing the disease, e.g. smoking is a factor in causing stroke
- The concept of cause embodied in the germ theory of disease is generally referred to as a one to one relationship between causal agent and disease.

Multifactorial causation

- The concept by Pattenkofer of Munich during 19th century was an early proponent of multifactorial causation.
- Then scientists came to know after several years during emergence of non-communicable diseases that single causation theory was over simplification and that there are other factors in the etiology of diseases.
- The doctrine of one to one relationship between cause and disease has been shown to be untenable not only for noncommunicable diseases but also for microbial diseases, e.g. tuberculosis, leprosy.

Web of causation

- This model of disease causation was suggested by MacMohan and Pugh.
- This model is ideally suited in the study of chronic diseases, where the diseases caused not only due to the individual presence of causal factors but due to complex interrelationship between these factors.

Association can be grouped under three headings

1. Spurious association
2. Indirect association
3. Direct association.

ADDITIONAL CRITERIA FOR JUDGING CAUSALITY

- In the absence of evidence to incriminate a cause certain additional criteria have been evolved for deciding when an association may be considered a causal association.
- Bradford Hill and others have pointed out that the likelihood of a causal relationship is increased by the presence of the following criteria.
- Temporal association: Cause precedes the disease
- Strength of association: RR
- Specificity of the association: Specific to the system affected
- Consistency of association: Repeated observation
- Biological plausibility: Site of involvement
- Coherence of association: Concurrent occurrence.

INFECTIOUS DISEASE EPIDEMIOLOGY

Nosocomial Infection

An infection acquired by a patient during the stay in the hospital, either from the hospital staff, or from other patients. It includes infection acquired in the hospital but appearing after discharge. Example infection of surgical wounds

Opportunistic Infection

Infection by an organism that takes the opportunity provided by a defect in host defense to infect the host and hence cause the disease. Example: H. simplex, M. tuberculosis.

Latrogenic infection (Physician induced)

Any infection introduced during the hospital procedures or therapeutic regimen by the physician professional activity or from other health professionals. Example: Urinary infection following catheterization, hepatitis B infection following injection or blood transfusion.

Contamination: The presence of an infectious agent on a body surface, or in clothes beddings, dressings, or other inanimate articles or substances including milk, water and food.

Pollution: Implies the presence of offensive, but not necessarily an infectious matter in the environment. Example: Air pollution.

Infestation: The lodgment, development and reproduction of arthropods on the surface of the body or in the clothing. Example: Head louse, body lice infestation.

Host: A person or animal, birds and arthropods, that affords subsistence or lodgment to an infectious agent under natural conditions.

Obligate host or compulsory host: Obligate host means the only host status available for a particular disease. Example: Man in measles, typhoid and poliomyelitis.

Definitive host or primary host or final host: Host in which the parasite attains maturity or passes its sexual stage are primary or definitive hosts. Example: Mosquito in malaria (sporogony sexual cycle), man in Filariasis.

Intermediate or secondary host or alternate host: Those in which the parasite is in a larval stage or asexual state are secondary or intermediate host. Example: Man in malaria (schizogony asexual cycle), mosquito in Filariasis

Transport host or mechanical carrier: It is a carrier in which the organism remains alive but does not undergo multiplication or development. Example: Housefly

Infectious disease: A clinically manifest disease of man or animals resulting from an infection.

Contagious disease: A disease that is transmitted through contact. Example: Scabies, trachoma.

Epidemic: The unusual occurrence of a disease in a community clearly in excess of 'expected occurrence'.

Endemic: It refers to the constant presence of a disease or infectious agent within a given geographic area or population group, without importation from outside.

Hyperendemic: The disease is constantly presently at a high incidence and or prevalence rate and affects all age groups equally.

Holoendemic: A high level of infection beginning early in life and affecting most of the child population than adults. Example: Malaria

Sporadic: Means scattered about. The cases occur irregularly, haphazardly from time to time and generally infrequently.
The cases are few and separated widely in space and time. Example: Polio, tetanus.

Pandemic: An epidemic usually affecting a large proportion of the population, occurring over a wide geographic area such as a section of nation, the entire nation, entire continent or the world.
Example: Influenza pandemics.

Exotic: Diseases which are imported into a country in which they do not otherwise occur. Example: Rabies in UK.

Zoonoses: An infection or infectious disease transmissible under natural conditions from vertebrate animals to man. Example: Rabies, plague

Anthropozoonoses: Infections transmitted to man from vertebrate animals.
Example: Rabies, plague

Zooanthroponoses: Infections transmitted from man to vertebrate animals.
Example: Human tuberculosis in cattle

Amphixenoses: Infections maintained in both man and lower vertebrate animals that may be transmitted in either direction.
Example: T.cruzi, S.japonicum

Direct zoonoses: Infections which transmitted from an infected vertebrate host to a susceptible vertebrate host by direct contact, by contact with fomite, or by mechanical vector.
The agent does not undergo any propogative or developmental changes.
Example: Rabies, brucellosis

Cyclozoonoses: Infections which require more than one vertebrate host species, but no invertebrate host, in order to complete the developmental cycle of the agent.
Example: Human taeniasis, echinococcosis

Metazoonoses: Infections which are transmitted biologically by invertebrate vectors in which the agent multiplies or develops, or both, and there is always an extrinsic incubation period before transmission to another vertebrate host.
Example: Arbovirus infections, plague

Saprozoonoses: Have both a vertebrate host and a non-animal developmental site or reservoir. Non-animal sites may include soil, plants, etc.
Example: Larva migrants, Mycoses

Epizootic: An outbreak of disease in an animal population.
Example: Swine flu (influenza), Q fever.

Epornithic: An outbreak of disease in bird population.
Example: Bird flu (influenza).

Enzootic: An endemic occurring in animals.
Example: Anthrax, bovine tuberculosis.

Source: The source of infection is defined as 'the person, animal, object or substance from which an infectious agent passes or is disseminated to the host.

Reservoir

- Any person, animal, arthropod, plant, soil, or substance in which an infectious agent lives and multiplies, on which it depends primarily for survival.
- In short, the reservoir is the natural habitat in which the organism metabolizes and replicates. Example: Hookworm infection, the reservoir is man, but the source of infection is the soil contaminated with infectious larvae.

Carrier

- An infected person or animal that harbors a specific infectious agent in the absence of discernible clinical disease and serves as a potential source of infection for others.
- It may be either due to inadequate treatment or immune response resulting in a carrier state.
- Less infectious than cases
- Epidemiologically more dangerous than cases
- Carriers may be classified
  - By type: Incubatory, convalescent, healthy
  - By duration: Temporary, chronic
  - Portal of exit: Urinary, intestinal, respiratory, others
  - Pseudo carriers: Carriers of avirulent organisms, epidemiologically not important.

Incubation period: Time interval between invasion by an infectious agent and appearance of the first sign or symptom of the disease in question.

Median incubation period: Defined as the time required for 50% of the cases to occur following exposure.

Latent period: This term is used in noninfectious diseases as the equivalent of incubation period in infectious diseases. This is defined as the period from disease initiation to disease detection

Importance of incubation period

- Tracing the source of infection
- Period of surveillance (or quarantine)
- Immunizations
- Identification of type of epidemic
- Prognosis

Primary case
Refers to the first case of a communicable disease introduced into the population unit being studied
Secondary case
Cases which develop from contact with primary case
Serial interval
The gap in time between the onset of primary case and the secondary case is called serial interval
Generation time
The interval of time between receipt of infection by a host and maximal infectivity of that host.
Generation time roughly equal to the incubation period.
Communicable period
The time during which an infectious agent may be transferred directly or indirectly from an infected person to another person.
An important measure of communicability is secondary attack rate.

Isolation	Quarantine
Isolation of the infected person	Restriction of freedom of the healthy contacts
Isolated for the period of communicability	Restricted for the longest incubation period of the disease
Types Standard Strict High security Protective	Types Absolute Modified–exclusion of child from school Segregation–removal of susceptible child to home of immune person

HERD IMMUNITY

It is the level of resistance of a community to a particular disease.
Elements contributing to herd immunity:

- Occurrence of clinical and subclinical infection in the herd
- Immunization of the herd
- Herd structure
  - In polio and diphtheria herd immunity due to immunization programmes help in elimination of the disease
  - In case of small pox it is not the herd immunity but elimination of source of infection was crucial in eradication
  - In case of tetanus herd immunity cannot protect the individual
  - It is never possible nor necessary to attain 100% herd immunity.

Cold Chain

- System of storage and transport of vaccines at low temperature from the manufacturer to the actual vaccination site.
- Vaccine failure will occur if not properly stored and transported.

Compartment in which it is stored	Vaccines
Freezer compartment	Polio and measles
Stored in cold part but never allowed to freeze	Typhoid, DPT, TT, DT, BCG and diluents

Most vaccines except polio can be stored up to 5 weeks at PHC between 4 to 8 degree C.

Cold Chain Equipment

WIC: Walk In Cold Room	Located at regional level, meant to store vaccine up to 3 months and serve 4–5 districts
Deep freezers (300L) Ice lined Refrigerators(300/240L) capacity	Supplied to all districts, DF: Used for preparing ice packs (polio, measles)
Small DF and ILR (140L)	Provided to PHCs, urban family planning centers
Vaccine carriers or cold boxes	To shift the vaccines to the peripheral level
Vaccine carriers	To carry small quantities of vaccines (16 to 20 vials), 4 fully frozen ice packs are used for lining the sides
Day carriers	Quantity of carrying 6–8 vials, two fully frozen ice packs are kept inside

SCREENING OF DISEASE

- Defined as 'the search for unrecognized disease or defect by means of rapidly applied tests, examinations or other procedures in apparently healthy individuals'.
- Screening differs from periodic health examinations in the following respects
- Capable of wide applications
- Relatively inexpensive
- Requires little physician time. In fact the physician is not required to administer the test, but only to interpret.

Screening test	Diagnostic test
Done on apparently healthy individuals	Done on those who are sick
Test result are final	Not final but modified in view of sum of all evidence
Less accurate	More accurate
Less expensive	More expensive
Not a basis of treatment	Used as a basis of treatment

Lead Time

- Time lag between disease onset and the usual time of diagnosis.
- In this period, there are usually a number of critical points which determine both severity of the disease and the success of any treatment in reversing.
- Screening of the disease done before the disease reaches this usual time of diagnosis.

Uses of Screening

- Case detection
- Prescriptive screening
- Presumptive identification of unrecognized disease, which does not arise from a patient's request
  - Example: Neonatal screening
- People are screened for their own benefit
- Control of disease
- Prospective screening
- People are examined for the benefit of others
  - Example: Screening of immigrants for infectious diseases
- Reduce the spread of infectious disease
- Research purposes

- Screening may be performed for research purposes
  - Example: Many chronic diseases whose natural history is not fully known
- Educational opportunities
- Creating public awareness and for educating health professionals
  - Example: Screening for diabetes.

Criteria for Screening

Disease

- Disease should be an important public health problem
- There should be recognizable latent or asymptomatic stage
- Test that can detect the disease prior to the onset of signs and symptoms
- Facilities should be available for confirmation of test
- Evidence that early detection and treatment reduces morbidity and mortality.

Screening test

- Acceptability: Painful, discomforting or embarrassing are not likely to be acceptable to the population
- Repeatability: (Reliability, Precision, Reproducibility). Test must give consistent results when repeated more than once on the same or material, under the same conditions.
- Validity (accuracy), refers to what extent the test accurately measures what it has to measure. Two components, sensitivity, specificity. The word sensitivity was introduced by Yerushalmy in 1940s. Sensitivity is defined as the ability of a test to identify correctly all those who have the disease, which is true positive. Specificity is defined as the ability of a test to identify correctly those who do not have the disease, that is, true negative.
- Predictive value of a positive test: Indicates the probability that a patient with a positive test result has the disease. The predictive value of a positive result falls as disease prevalence declines.
- Yield: Is the amount of previously unrecognized disease that is diagnosed as a result of the screening effort.
- Screening test must satisfy the criteria of not only acceptability, repeatability and validity but also yield, simplicity, safety, rapidity, and cost.

Evaluation of a screening test

Screening test results	Diseased	Not diseased	Total
Positive	a	B	a + b
Negative	c	D	c + d
Total	a + c	b + d	a + b + c + d

Sensitivity = a/(a + c) × 100 Specificity = d/(b + d) × 100 Predictive value of positive test = a/(a + b) × 100 Predictive value of negative test = d/(c + d) × 100 Percentage of false negatives = c/(a + c) × 100 Percentage of false positives = b/(b + d) × 100 Prevalence of the disease = (a + c)/(a + b + c + d) × 100	• TP is directly related to sensitivity • TN is directly related to specificity • FP is inversely related to specificity • FN is inversely related to sensitivity • PPV is directly related to prevalence of disease • NPV is inversely related to prevalence of disease
Predictive value of a positive test (PPV) • Indicates the probability that a patient with a positive test result has the disease. NPV (predictive value of a negative test) • Probability that a person with a negative test does not have the disease Bayer's theorem $PPV = \frac{(\text{Sensitivity} \times \text{prevalence})}{(\text{Sensitivity} \times \text{Prevalence}) + (1-\text{specificity})(1-\text{prevalence})} \times 100$ $NPV = \frac{\text{Specificity} \times (1-\text{prevalence})}{(\text{Specificity} \times (1-\text{prevalence}) + (1-\text{sensitivity}) \times \text{prevalence}} \times 100$	• **If the population has more false positives** • PPV will be low • Prevalence of the disease is low • **If the population has more false negatives** • Negative predictive value of the test is low

EPIDEMIOLOGY OF COMMUNICABLE DISEASES, NONCOMMUNICABLE DISEASES

Chickenpox–Varicella

- Caused by Varicella-zoster virus
- Characterized by vesicular rash with fever
- Chickenpox and herpes zoster are now regarded as different host responses to the same etiological agent
- Agent HHV: 3 virus, primary infection causes chickenpox
- Source of infection: Usually a case of chickenpox
- Period of communicability: Ranges from 1 to 2 days before the onset of rash and 4 to 5 days there after
- SAR 90%, MC affects Children less than 10 years of age and one attack gives durable immunity. Portal of entry of the virus is through the respiratory tract.
- Incubation period: Usually 14 to 16 days.

C/F Rashes are symmetrical, first appear on the trunk and then comes on the face, arms and legs. Centripetal. Mucosal surfaces are generally involved. Rashes are pleomorphic,(different stages of rashes seen at one time), fever rises whenever the crops of rashes appear.

- Vesicles filled with clear fluid: Dew drops appearance on the skin.
- Mortality less than 1% and there is no specific treatment for the disease.
- A live attenuated OKA strain vaccine developed in Japan has been use in field trials.

Measles (Rubeola–Red spots)

- Caused by RNA paramyxovirus, there is only one serotype. The only source of infection is a case of measles. Carriers are not known to occur. The period of communicability is approximately 4 days before and 5 days after the appearance of rash. Infection confers lifelong immunity.
- MC age group: Six months and 3 years in developing countries and usually over 5 years in developed countries. The mortality rate is 400 times more in malnourished children.
- Incubation period: Ten days from exposure to onset of fever, and 14 days to appearance of rash.

C/F–Prodromal phase: Begins 10 days after infection and lasts until day 14. A day or two before the appearance of rash Koplik's spots appear on the buccal mucosa opposite to first and second upper molar teeth. Koplik's spots are small, bluish white spots on a red base, smaller than a size of head of a pin. Their presence is pathognomonic of measles.

- The next phase is eruptive phase which is characterized by typical, dusky red macular and maculopapular rash which begins behind the ears. The rash fades in the same order of appearance leaving a brownish discoloration which may persist for 2 months or more.
- The most common complications are–measles associated diarrhea, pneumonia, and otitis media. The more serious complications are neurological complications which include febrile convulsions, encephalitis, and SSPE.
- SSPE: Subacute sclerosing pan encephalitis rare complication–7/million cases of natural measles. This is characterized by progressive mental deterioration leading to paralysis, probably due to persistence of virus in the brain.
- Encephalitis: 1/1000 cases of measles.

Control measures

- Isolation for 7 days after the onset of rash
- Immunization of contacts within 2 days of exposure (If vaccine is contraindicated: IG should be given within 3 to 4 days of exposure).

Eradication of measles

- Achieving an immunization coverage rate of 96% and the cumulation of immunity gap be prevented

WHO measles elimination strategy

Catch-up: One time nationwide vaccination campaign targeting usually all children aged 9 months to 14 years regardless of measles disease or vaccination status.

Keep-up: Routine vaccination coverage of 95% of each successive birth cohort.

Follow-up: Subsequent nationwide vaccination campaign every 2 to 4 years targeting all children born after catch up campaign.

Influenza

- Caused by influenza virus: 3 types A, B and C. No cross immunity between them.
- It has two distinct antigens: Hemaglutinin and neuraminidase. H–antigen initiates the infection and N antigen is responsible for the release of the virus from the infected cell.
- Sudden complete or major change: In the antigenic components **antigenic shift:** Results from genetic recombination of human with animal or avian virus. Antigenic shift causes major epidemic or pandemic. When the antigenic change is gradual over a period of time it is called a **drift:** Results from point mutation. Influenza C–antigenically stable.
- Hemaglutinin antibody: Resists initiation of infection which neutralizes the virus. Neuraminidase antibody: Decreases the severity of disease and decreased ability to transmit virus to contacts.
- Incubation period: 18 to 72 hours.

Influenza Vaccines

- Killed vaccine–Chick embryo vaccine: Protection lasts for 3 to 6 months. 0.5 ml, Sc.
- Live attenuated vaccines: Nose drops, which stimulates both local and systemic immunity.
- Newer vaccines
- Split virus vaccine: Subvirion vaccine, low antigenicity, several doses required, recommended for children.
- Neuraminidase specific vaccine: Subunit vaccine containing only N antigen
- Recombinant vaccine
- Anti viral drugs
- Amantadine and Rimantadine: Block penetration of Influenza virus in the host cell and prevent virus replication.
- Dosage: 100 mg twice a day for 3 to 5 days. These drugs are not effective against B, C serotypes.

Control of ARI

Count the breaths

Fast breathing:

- 60 per min or more in a child less than 2 months of age
- 50 per min or more in a child aged 2 months to 12 months
- 40 per min or more in a child aged 12 months up to 5 years

Very severe pneumonia: Not able to drink, convulsions, abnormally sleepy or difficult to wake, stridor in a calm child or severe malnutrition

Severe pneumonia: Nasal flaring, chest indrawing

Pneumonia: No chest indrawing bu only fast breathing

No Pneumonia: No chest indrawing or no fast breathing

Treatment

Pneumonia: Cotrimaxazole–5 days

Severe pneumonia: Benzyl penicillin or Ampicillin or Chloramphenicol

Very severe pneumonia: Chloramphenicol IM–DOC or the alternate is IM injections of cloxacillin and gentamycin

Diphtheria

- Cause by Cornybacterium diphtheriae.
- The bacteria produces powerful exotoxin which is responsible for the formation of a greyish or yellowish membrane (false membrane), with well: Defined edges and the membrane cannot be wiped away.
- Three types Gravis, Mitis, Intermedius: Gravis infection tend to be more severe.
- Carriers are common sources of infection: Ration ranges from 95 carriers to 5 clinical cases. Immunization does not prevent the carrier state.
- The nasal carriers are more dangerous as the source of infection because of more frequent shedding of the agent.

- A case or carrier is considered as noncommunicable when at least 2 cultures properly obtained from nose and throat 24 hours apart are negative for diphtheria bacilli. It affects the age group of 1 to 5.
- Incubation period: 2 to 6 days.
- Patient with severe disease may have marked edema of submandibular area and the anterior portion of the neck along with lymphadenopathy giving: **Bull necked appearance**.
- Cutaneous diphtheria: Often appears as a secondary infection of a previous skin abrasion or infection.
- All cases, suspected cases and carriers: Isolated for 14 days or until proved fee infection
- DOC: Carriers 10 day course of oral erythromycin.

Whooping Cough–Hundred Day Cough

- Caused by B. pertusis and parapertusis.
- No subclinical cases or chronic carrier state. The infective period extends from a week after the exposure to about 3 weeks after the onset of the paraoxysmal stage. SAR 90% in unimmunized individuals.
- Age: Infants and preschool children. Incidence and mortality are more among female than male children. Incubation period: 7 to 14 days.
- C/F–Catarrhal stage: Lasting about 10 days and paraoxysmal stage: 2 to 4 weeks and convalescent stage: 1 to 2 weeks.
- Cases: Erythromycin is probably the drug of choice course given for 10 days.
- Contacts: 10 days course of ampicillin or erythromycin.

Meningococcal Meningitis

- Caused by N. meningitides, the fatality of untreated case 80% and with early diagnosis and treatment the fatality can be reduced to 10%.
- Group A and C cause for major epidemics. This is a delicate organism, dies rapidly on exposure to heat and cold. Carriers are the most important source of infection. Cases rapidly lose their infectiousness within 24 hours of specific treatment.
- Incubation period: 3 to 4 days
- Cases–DOC: Penicillin. Carriers Rifampicin 600 mg BD for two days or Sulfadiazine: 1g BD for two days. Vaccines–group A, C, Y and W 135 available.

Tuberculosis

Prevalence of infection:

- It is the percentage of individuals who show a positive reaction to the standard tuberculin test.

Incidence of infection (Annual infection rate):

- It is the percentage of population under study who will be newly infected by Myco. Tuberculosis among the noninfected of the preceding survey during the course of one year.
- Also known as 'tuberculin conversion' index, this parameter is considered one of the best indicators for evaluating the tuberculosis problem and its trend.

Prevalence of disease or case rate:

- It is the percentage of individuals whose sputum is positive for tubercle bacilli on microscopic examination.
- Best available practical index to estimate the number of infection cases or 'case load 'in a community.

Incidence of new cases:

- It is the percentage of new tuberculosis cases (confirmed by bacteriological examination). It would reveal the trend if the problem in the community.

Prevalence of 'suspect' cases:

- This is bases on X-ray examination of chest. No epidemiological significance can be attached to this index.

Prevalence of drug-resistant cases:

- It is the prevalence of patient excreting tubercle bacilli resistant to anti-tuberculosis drugs. Index is directly related to chemotherapy.

Tuberculin Test

- The tuberculin test was discovered by Von Pirquet in 1907.
- A positive reaction to the test is generally accepted as evidence of past or present infection by M. tuberculosis.
- The tuberculin test is the only means of estimating the prevalence of infection in a population.

Mantoux Test

- The Mantoux test is carried out by injecting intradermally on the flex or surface of the forearm 1 TU of PPD in 0.1 ml. The result of the test is read after 72 hours (3rd day).
- Induration alone is measured (horizontal transverse diameter of induration in millimeters. Reactions exceeding 10 mm are considered 'positive'. Those less than 6 mm are considered' negative'. Those between 6 and 9 mm are considered 'doubtful'.
- Those showing 20 mm or more induration have greater chances of developing tuberculosis than those showing 10 mm induration.
- Those with less than 5 mm induration have more risk of developing tuberculosis than those with 6–9 mm induration (reaction of 10 mm or more to 1 TU PPD) indicates that the person is infected with M. tuberculosis; it does not prove that the person is suffering from the disease.
- A positive reaction is significant in younger age groups. If a child below 2 years is found to be tuberculin positive, it is an indirect evidence of an active tuberculosis lesion in the body even if it is not manifest.

BCG

- Two to three weeks after a correct intradermal injection of a potent vaccine, a papule develops at the site of vaccination. In size and reaches a diameter of about 4 to 8 mm in about 5 weeks.
- It then subsides or breaks into a shallow ulcer, rarely open, but usually seen covered with a crust. Healing occurs spontaneously within 6 to 12 weeks leaving a permanent, tiny round scar, typically 4–8 mm in diameter. This is a normal reaction.

DOTS-Plus

- The goal of DOTS-Plus is to prevent further development and spread of MDR-TB

A case of tuberculosis • Diagnosed with at least one sputum specimen positive for AFB **OR** • Culture positive for M. TB **OR** • RNTCP endorsed rapid diagnostic molecular test positive for TB **OR** • Diagnosed clinically without microbiological confirmation and initiated on ATT	• **Smear positive:** At least one initial sputum smears positive for AFB in a well functioning EQA system • **Smear negative:** At least two negative smears, but tuberculosis suggestive symptoms and X-ray abnormalities or Positive culture
• **Return after default:** • A patient who returns sputum smear positive, after having left treatment for at least two months.	• **Cured** • **Initially smear positive patient who completed treatment and had negative smear result on at least two occasions. (one at treatment completion)**

Category I (RED BOX)	Category II (BLUE BOX)
New Cases • New sputum positive • New sputum negative • New extra pulmonary • New others • 2 (HRZE) 3 + 4 (HR) • Test sputum at 2 months, 4 months and 6 months • If positive at 2 months continue IP for one more month and then complete the treatment in 7 months	Previously Treated • Sputum smear positive relapse • Sputum smear positive failure • Sputum smear positive treatment after default • Others • 2 $(HRZES)_3$ + 1 $(HRZE)_3$ + 5 $(HRE)_3$ • Test sputum at 3 months, 5 months and 6 months and completion of treatment. • If positive at 3 months continue IP for one more month and test sputum at 4 months (if positive–send it to culture and sensitivity as it might by MDR TB)

INTESTINAL INFECTIONS

Poliomyelitis

Poliomyelitis is primarily an infection of the human alimentary tract but the virus may infect the central nervous system in a very small percentage (about 1 percent).

Poliomyelitis eradication: Epidemiological basis

- Poliomyelitis is eradicable because man is the only host.
- A long-term carrier state is not known to occur.
- Oral polio vaccine, which is easy to administer and relatively cheap.
- Live vaccine virus, by multiplying in the intestine can interrupt the transmission of the wild polioviruses.

Agent

- The causative agent is the poliovirus which has three serotypes 1, 2 and 3. Most outbreaks of paralytic polio are due to type-1 virus.
- Reservoir of infection: Most infection are subclinical. It is estimated that for every clinical case, there may be 1000 subclinical cases in children and 75 in adults. No chronic carriers.

Period of Communicability

The cases are most infectious 7 to 10 days before and after onset of symptoms.

a. Age: The most vulnerable age is between 6 months and 3 years.
b. Sex: Ratio of 3 males to one female.
c. Risk factors: Provocative or risk factors have been found to precipitate an attack of paralytic. Fatigue, trauma, intramuscular injections, operative procedures such as tonsillectomy undertaken especially during epidemics of polio and administration of immunizing agents particularly alum-containing DPT.

Clinical Spectrum

- Inapparent (subclinical) infection: 91 to 96%
- Abortive polio or minor illness: 4 to 8%
- Nonparalytic polio: 1%
- Paralytic polio: Occurs in less than one percent. The predominant sign is asymmetrical flaccid paralysis
- Tripod sign may be present, i.e. the child finds difficulty in sitting and sits by supporting hands at the back and by partially flexing the hips and knees
- Descending, proximal muscle groups are more involved as compared to distal ones. No sensory loss.

OPV

The advantages of OPV are:

- Since given orally, it is easy to administer and does not require the use of highly trained personnel.
- Induces both humoral and intestinal immunity.
- Antibody is quickly produced in a large proportion of vaccines, even a single dose elicits (except in topical countries) substantial immunity.
- The vaccine excretes the virus and so infects others who are also immunized thereby.
- Useful in controlling epidemics, and
- Relatively inexpensive.

Strategies for Polio Eradication in India

- Conduct Pulse Polio Immunization days every year for 3–4 years or until poliomyelitis is eradicated.
- Sustain high levels of routine immunization coverage.
- Monitor OPV coverage at district level and below.
- Improve surveillance capable of detecting all cases of AFP due to polio and nonpolio etiology.
- Ensure rapid case investigation, including the collection of stool samples for virus isolation.

- Arrange follow-up of all cases of AFP at 60 days to check for residual paralysis.
- Conduct outbreak control for cases confirmed or suspected to be poliomyelitis to stop transmission.

Mopping Up

The strategy of 'mopping up' involves door-to-door immunization in high risk districts, where wild poliovirus is known or suspected to be still circulating.

VIRAL HEPATITIS

Hepatitis A

- Hepatitis A (formerly known as 'infections' hepatitis or epidemic jaundice) is an acute infectious disease causes by hepatitis A virus.

Epidemiological Determinants

Agent factors

- **Agent:** Enterovirus (type 72) of the Picornaviridae family.
- **Reservoir of infection:** The human cases are the only reservoir of infection. There is no evidence of a chronic carrier state.
- **Period of infectivity:** The risk of transmitting HAV is greatest form 2 weeks before to 1 week after the onset of jaundice.
- **Infective material:** Mainly man's feces.

Modes of transmission

- **Fecal-oral route:** Water-borne transmission food-bone.
- **Sexual transmission:** Occur mainly among homosexual men because of oral-anal contact.

Incubation period: 15 to 45 days

Prevention and containment

- Control of reservoir: The use of 0.5 percent sodium hypochlorite has been strongly recommended as an effective disinfectant.
- Control of susceptible population: Globulin to induce passive immunity. It is recommended for 1. Susceptible persons travelling to highly endemic areas. 2. Close personal contacts of patients with HAV, and 3. For the control of outbreaks in institutions.

Hepatits B

- Hepatitis B (formerly known as 'serum' hepatitis) transmitted usually by the parenteral route. Long incubation period (6 weeks to 6 months).
- In approximately of cases, HBV infection fails to resolve and the affected individuals then become persistent carriers 5 to 15 percent of the virus
  - Epidemiological determinants:
  - Agent factors:
    - **Agent:** Discovered by Blumberg. HBV is a complex, 42 nm, double-shelled DNA virus, originally known as the **'Dane particle'**. The purified 22 mm particles are used in the preparation of hepatitis B vaccine.
    - **Reservoir of infection:** Man is the only reservoir of infection which can be spread either from **carriers** or from **cases.** The risk of an adult becoming a carrier following acute infection is 5 to 10 percent; in infants, it may exceed 50 percent.
    - **Infective material:** Contaminated blood is the main source of infection.
  - Host factors:
    - Age: Mortality from fulminant hepatitis B is approximately 70 percent.

Humoral and Cellular Responses

- HBsAg (23): The appearance of HBsAg is the first evidence of infection, appearing before biochemical evidence of liver disease.
- Anti-HBs (23): Disappearance of HBsAg and the appearance of anti-HBs signals recovery from HBV infection, noninfectivity and immunity.
- Anti-HBc (23): IgM anti-HBc appears shortly. After HBsAg is detected. (HBcAg alone does not appear in serum). Its presence in the setting of acute hepatitis indicates a diagnosis of acute hepatitis B.
- HBeAg (23): HBeAg indicates viral replication and infectivity. Persistence of HBeAg in serum beyond 3 months indicates an increased likelihood of chronic hepatitis B.
- HBV DNA (23): The presence of HBV DNA in serum generally parallels the parallels the HBeAg, although HBV DNA is a more sensitive and precise marker of viral replication and infectivity.

Mode of transmission:

- Parenteral route
- Perinatal transmission
- Sexual transmission: particularly male homosexuals.

Incubation period

- The median incubation period is said to be lower than 100 days.

PREVENTION AND CONTAINMENT

Hepatitis B Vaccine

- RDNA-Yeast Derived Vaccine: The recombinant DNA vaccine elaborated from cultures of yeast cloned with HBsAg s-gene. The dose for adult is 10–20 micrograms initially (depending on the formulation) and again at 1 and 6 months.
- Hepatitis B Immunoglobulin (HBIG)
- Immediate protection, (a) Surgeons, nurses or laboratory workers. (b) Newborn infants of carrier mothers, and (c) Sexual contacts of acute hepatitis B patients. The HBIG should be given as soon as possible after an accidental inoculation (ideally within 6 hours and preferably not later than 48 hours. At the same time the victim's blood is drawn for HBsAg testing. If the test is negative, vaccination should be started immediately and a full course given. If the test is positive for surface antibody, no further action is needed.
- The recommended dose is 0.05 to 0.07 ml/kg of body weight (33); two doses should be given 30 days apart.

Passive-Active Immunization

- Combined procedure is ideal both for prophylaxis of persons accidentally exposed to blood known to contain hepatitis B virus, and for prevention of the carrier state in the newborn babies of carrier mothers.
- HBIG (0.05–.0.07 ml/kg) should be given as soon as possible and within 24 hours, if possible.
- Hepatitis B virus vaccine 1.0 ml (20 mcg/1.0 ml) should be given intramuscularly within 7 days of exposure, and second and third doses should be given one and six months, respectively, after the first dose.

Hepatits C

- In India HCV antibodies have been found in 2 percent of voluntary blood donors.
- The hepatitis C virus is a single-stranded RNA virus with properties similar to those of flavivirus.
- The virus is mainly transmitted through transfusion of contaminated blood or blood products.
- Up 50% of cases are related to intravenous drug users who share needles.
- The incubation period averages 6–7 weeks. High rate of (more than 50%) chronic hepatitis, which may lead to cirrhosis of liver or liver cancer. More likely to d so in men than in women. Interferon is the only drug that has been found effective in the treatment of HCV infection.

Hepatits E

- The infection caused by the hepatitis E virus (HEV) which was discovered in 1990, is essentially a waterborne disease. Formerly termed enteric ally transmitted hepatitis non-A, non-B RNA virus Water or food supplies, contaminated by feces, in which the virus is excreted have been implicated in major outbreaks incubation period of 2–9 weeks, a self-limiting acute viral hepatitis appears, lasting for a period if several weeks, which us followed by recovery.
- No case of chronic disease has reported. Mainly young adults aged 14–40 years.
- HEV has a propensity to induce a fulminating form of acute disease (the mortality ranges between 0.5% to 4%), particularly in pregnant women. A mortality that may reach about 80% of such cases.
- Diagnosis is made by the level of anti-HEV antibodies in the serum. No confirmatory assay is currently available.
- No specific treatment for hepatitis E. Recovery from hepatitis E is always complete. No vaccine or specific immunoglobulin prophylaxis is available.

Nomenclature and definitions of hepatitis viruses, antigens and antibodies

- Hepatitis A: Infectious hepatitis, picornavirus, Hepatovirus, lifetime persistence
- Hepatitis B: Serum hepatitis, hepadnavirus, Soluble antigen, HBV replication, with high titers if HBV in serum and with infectivity of serum
- Indicators past infection with immunity to HBV, from HBIG, or immune responsefrom HBV vaccine
- Presence in serum of HBsAg carrier suggests lower titer of HBV
- Indicators recent infection with HBV
- Hepatitis C: Post-transfusion hepatitis. Flavivrus Hepacivirus
- Hepatitis D: Delta hepatitis, causes infection only in presence of HBV
- Hepatitis E: Enterically transmitted hepatitis virus. Fecal-oral or waterborne transmission Calicivirus
- Hepatitis G: Flavivirus.

Enteric Fever

Typhoid fever is the result of systemic infection mainly by S.typhi found only, in man. The term 'enteric fever' includes both typhoid and paratyphoid fevers.

Agents Factors

- Agent: S.typhi is the major cause of enteric fever. S. Para A and S. para B are relatively infrequently (7). S.typhi has three main antigens–O, H and VI
- The antibody to the somatic antigen (O) is usually higher in the patient with the disease, and the antibody to the flagellar antigen (H) is usually higher in immunized individuals.

Host Factors

- Highest incidence of this disease occurs in the 5–19 years of age group.
- More cases are reported among males than females, probably as a result of increased exposure to infection.
- Carrier rate is more in females.

Incubation Period

- Usually 10–14 days. But it may be as short as 3 days or as long as three weeks depending upon the dose of the bacilli ingested.

Modes of Transmission

- Typhoid fever is transmitted via the fecal–oral route or urine–oral routes.

Reservoir of Infection: Man

Carriers: In most chronic carriers, the organisms persist in the gall bladder and in the biliary tact. A chronic carrier state may be expected to develop in 2 to 5 percent of cases.

Clinical Features

- The fever ascends in a step ladder fashion. There may be marked constipation, especially in early stage or 'pea soup' diarrhea. There is a marked abdominal distension.
- There is a leucopenia and blood.
- The rash (rose spots) commonly appears during the second week of disease.
- Complications occur in about 30 percent of untreated cases.

Investigations

Widal test–AB detection–blood test, Blood culture, Urine culture, Stool culture.

Widal Test

- Measures agglutinating antibody levels of O and H antigen
- Test usually performed in acute serum before giving one dose of antibiotic
- Gives high false positive and false negative
- False positive: cross reacting with other paratyphi antigens
- False negative: 30% because of prior antibiotic therapy
- Usually O antibodies appear on day 6 to 8 and H antibodies on day 10 to 12 after the onset of disease.

Control and Prevention

Control of reservoir, Control of sanitation and immunization

Control of Reservoir

Carriers

- Identification: The VI antibodies are present in about 80 percent of chronic carriers.
- Treatment: The carrier should be given an intensive course of ampicillin (4–6 g a day) together with Probenecid (2 g/day) for 6 weeks.
- Surgery: Cholecystectomy with concomitant ampicillin therapy has been regarded as the most successful approach to the treatment of carriers. Cure rate may be as high as 80 percent.

Control of Cases

- Early diagnosis
- Notification
- Isolation: Treated in the hospital if the infection is severe
- Treatment: Fluoroquinolones are the DOC
- Disinfection of urine and feces–5% cresol for 2 hours
- Follow-up: After 2 to 3 months for S.typhi and after 12 months for detection of carrier state.

Immunization

- Antityphoid vaccines
- VI polysaccharide vaccine: subunit vaccine single dose SC or IM
- Efficacy is 72% for 1 to 2 years
- Typhoral vaccine: Live attenuated vaccine
- Enteric coated capsule
- One capsule is administered on days 1, 3, 5 days one hour before meal
- Protection lasts for at least for 3 years and booster required after 3 years.

Yellow Fever

Arboviruses

- Arthropod borne viral diseases: Viruses which are maintained in nature principally or through biological transmission between susceptible vertebrate arthropods by hematogogous arthropods

- Group A: (Alpha viruses) Sindbis, Chikunkunya viruses
- Group B: (Flaviviruses) Dengue, KFD, JE, West Nile
- Yellow fever: Agent Flavivirus—(Group B Arbovirus)
- Reservoir: Monkey in forest, man in urban area
- Vector: Aedes aegypti, Immunity: After one attack lifelong immunity
- International certificate of vaccination: Validity of certificate begins 10 days after date of vaccination and extends up to 10 years
- Control of Yellow fever
- Vaccination 17 D vaccine: Live attenuated vaccine and administered subcutaneously
- Mosquito control measures.

Japanese Encephalitis

- Caused by group B arbovirus (flavivirus)
- Transmitted by culex tritaeniorhynchus–most important vector
- Man is the incidental dead end host
- Pigs are amplifiers of the virus
- Incubation period: 5 to 15 days
- Case fatality rate: 20 to 40%
- The average period between the onset of illness and death is about 9 days
- Mouse brain vaccine: Nayakama or beijing strain
- Cell culture vaccine: Beijing p3 strain
- Cell culture live attenuated vaccine: SA-14-14-2–currently used in UIP in UP, Assam, West Bengal, and Karnataka.

Kyasanur Forest Disease

- Transmitted by ticks, first recognized in shimoga district of Karnataka, it was called as monkey disease, later named after the locality Kyasanur forest.
- Gropup B viruses, rats and squirrels are main reservoirs of infection
- Monkeys are amplifying hosts
- Cattles are required for maintenance of ticks population
- Man is an incidental dead end host
- Transmitted mainly by hemophysalis spinegera and turtura
- No evidence of man to man transmission
- Incubation period: 3 to 8 days
- Case fatality rate: 5 to 10%.

Tetanus

- DPT: 6, 10, 14 weeks as DPT, followed by 18 months–1st booster and then second booster at 5–6 years–DT, then third booster–at 10 years TT alone
- Adults: TT–two doses with a gap of 4 to 6 weeks and then first booster after one year, then second booster may not be required after 5 years in developing countries
- Prevention after injury
- Wounds less than 6 hours old, clean, non penetrating and with negligible tissue damage.

TT given according to the immunity status or previous immunization status

- A: Has had a complete course of toxoid or a booster within past 5 years–nothing more required
- B: Has had a complete course of toxoid or a booster more than 5 years–less than 10 years–toxoid 1 dose
- C: More than 10 years–toxoid 1 dose
- D: Has not had a complete course of toxoid or immunity status not known–tetanus toxoid complete course
- A: Nothing required

- B: Toxoid 1 dose
- C: Toxoid 1 dose and human TET Ig
- D: Toxoid complete course and human TET Ig

Leprosy

Indian classification

- Indeterminate type: 1 or 2 vague hypopigmented macules and definite sensory impairment. Lesions bacteriologically negative.
- Tuberculoid: 1 or 2 well defined lesions, flat or raised, hypopigmented or erythematous and are anesthetic. Bacteriologically negative
- Borderline: 4 or more lesions, well or ill defined, bacteriological positivity variable
- Lepromatous: Diffuse infiltration or numerous flat or raised, poorly defined, shiny, smooth symmetrically distributed bacteriologically positive lesions
- Pure neuritic type: Nerve involvement but no skin involvement. Bacteriologically –ve.

Early reaction of Fernandez:	Late reaction of Mitsuda:
• Delayed hypersensitivity to soluble constituents of leprosy bacilli • Inflammatory response develops within 24–48 hours and disappears after 3–4 days • If the diameter of the red area is > 10 mm at the end of 48 hours it is considered positive • Indicates whether a person is previously sensitized or not to lepra bacilli • Corresponds Mantoux reaction in TB	• Becomes apparent after 7 days and reaches maximum in 3 or 4 weeks • The test is read on 21 days • A nodule more than 5mm diameter at the site of inoculation is considered positive • Indicates CMI • BCG vaccine converts lepromin negative to positive

Reversal reaction	Relapse
Occurs **during chemotherapy** or within 6 months of stopping treatment	Only **when chemotherapy has been stopped** after an interval of > 6 months
Abrupt and sudden	Slow and insidious
Existing lesions become edematous erythematous and tender	May show erythema and infiltration but **no tenderness**
Several **new lesions appear**	Minimal new lesions
Lesions may ulcerate	No ulceration
Multiple nerve involvement	Single nerve involvement
Rapid response to steroid treatment	No response

Rabies

- Rabies caused by Lyssavirus type 1
- Water is the most effective natural barrier to rabies
- A 'Rabies-free' area is defined as one in which no case if indigenously acquired rabies has occurred in human or any animal species of 2 years
- Reservoirs is the domestic dogs in urban rabies
- Rabies in man is the dead end infection
- Transmission by animal bites, licks on abraded skin or mucosa, aerosols, person to person by bite, corneal and organ transplantation
- Incubation period 3–8 weeks.

Rickettsial Zoonoses

Diseases	Agent	Vectors	Mammalian reservoirs
Typhus group			
Epidemic typhus	R. prowazekki	Louse	Humans
Murine typhus	R. typhi	Flea	Rodents
Scrub typhus	R. tsutsugamushi	Mite	Rodents

Contd...

Contd...

Diseases	Agent	Vectors	Mammalian reservoirs
Spotted fever group			
Indian tick typhus	R. conorri	Tick	Rodents
Rocky mountain fever	R. rickettsii	Tick	Rodents, dogs
Ricketssial pox	R. akari	Mite	Mice
Others			
Q fever	C. burnetii	Nil	Cattle, sheep and goats
Trench fever	Rochalimea quintana	Louse	Humans

DEMOGRAPHY AND FAMILY PLANNING

Scientific Study of Human Population

Demographic Cycle

- High stationary: High BR and DR, cancel each other
- Early expanding: DR begins to decline, BR–unchanged
- Late expanding: DR Declines still further, and BR tends to fall
- Low stationary: Low BR and Low DR, Austria–zero GR, UK, Denmark, Belgium
- Declining: BR lower than DR, Germany and Hungary.

If the GR < than 0.5 slow growth, 0.5–1 moderate growth, 1–1.5 rapid growth, .5 to 2 very rapid growth, > 2 Explosive growth.

Some demographic data likely to be asked in exams

Global	India
• TFR: 2.5 • GR: 1.2 • CBR: 20 • CDR: 8	• TFR: 2.68 • GR: 1.54–21st edition Park–2008 data • But Census web site gives 1.64–2011 • CBR: 22.8 • CDR: 7.4 • Percentage of population more than 60–7.2% • 901 per 1000 males • Total dependency ratio: 61.1% • Young age dependency: 53.1% • Old age dependency: 8.02% • Density of population: 345 per sq km • Population: 2011–1210.2 millions • Life expectancy males: 63.9 and females: 66.9

Eligible Couple

- Currently married couple wherein the wife is in the reproductive age, which is generally assumed to lie between the ages of 15 to 45
- Couples need of family planning services.

Target Couples

- Couple who have had 2–3 living children and family planning was largely directed to such couples.

Couple Protection Rate

- Indicator of prevalence of contraceptive practice in the community
- Percent of eligible couples effectively protected against childbirth by one or the other approved methods of family planning (sterilization, IUD, condom, oral pills).

General Fertility Rate

- Number of live births per 1000 women in reproductive age group (15 to 44 or 49)
- Better measure of fertility than crude birth rate because the denominator is restricted to the number of women in the child bearing age group rather than whole population.

Family Size

- Approximate magnitude of completed family size is given by TFR which means average number of children a woman would have during her reproductive years, bearing children at the same rates as the woman now in each age group.

Gross Reproductive Rate

- Average number of girls that would be born to a woman if she experiences the current fertility pattern throughout her reproductive span **assuming no mortality.**

NRR-Net Reproductive Rate

- Defined as the number of daughters a newborn girl will bear during her lifetime assuming age specific fertility and mortality rates.
- NRR of 1 is equivalent to attaining approximately the 2 child norm. NRR = 1 can be achieved only if at least 60% of eligible couples are effectively practising family planning.

Barrier Methods

Condom

- Prevents semen from being deposited in vagina
- Failure rate–3 to 14 per 100 women years
- Failure–Incorrect use

Advantages: Easily available, safe and inexpensive, easy to use, no side effects, do not require any medical supervision, light compact and disposable, provides protection against not only pregnancy and also against STD.

Disadvantages: Slip off, tear, interfere with sex sensation.

Female Condom

- Pouch made up of polyurethane which lines the vagina
- High cost and acceptability is the problem
- 5 to 21 per 100 women years of typical users.

Diaphragm (Dutch Cap)

- Made of synthetic rubber
- Failure rate–6–12 per 100 women years
- Inserted before sexual intercourse and must remain in place for not less than 6 hours after the intercourse.

Vaginal Sponge

- Trade name TODAY, Nonoxynol 9
- Small polyurethane foam sponge
- Failure rate–20 to 40 per 100 women years.

Intrauterine devices

- Nonmedicated or inert IUDs: First generation IUDs
  - Made of polyethylene, loops, spirals, coils, rings
  - Lippes loop: Double S shaped, impregnated with barium sulfate
  - Attached with thread at the end to find out the presence

- Exists four sizes A ,B, C, D: The latter being the largest
- Larger the size greater its antifertility effect
- Copper IUDs: Second generation
- Hormone IUDs: Third generation.

Copper IUDs

- Cu–7: 2 to 3%
- Cu–T: 200–4 years, 3%
- Newer
  - T Cu–220 C
  - T Cu–380 A or Ag–12 years, 0.5 to 0.8%
  - Nova T: 5 years
- Multiload–ML: Cu–250
- ML: Cu–375
- The numbers included in the names of the devices refer to the surface area of the copper on the device
- Effectiveness of the Cu devices is directly related to the amount of copper surface area.

Hormonal IUDs

- Most widely used–progestasert–38 mg of progesterone which releases 65 mcg daily. 1.3 to 1.6%–failure rate
- LNG–20 (Mirena)–Levonorgestrel, releases 20 mcg daily, effective for 10 years, failure rate 0.2%. Less number of ectopics.

Mechanism of action of IUDs

- Foreign body reaction (cellular and biochemical changes): Impair the viability of ovum
- Reduce the chance of fertilization rather than implantation
- Hormone releasing IUDs: Increase the viscosity of the cervical mucus.

Contraindication

Absolute: Suspected pregnancy, vaginal bleeding of undiagnosed etiology, cancer of Cx, vagina, previous ectopic pregnancy

Relative contraindication

- Menorrhagia, anemia, history of PID, purulent cervial discharge, congenital anomalies, unmotivated females.
- Timing of insertion: During menstruation or within 10 days of menstruation

Side Effects

- Bleeding (MC), pain, PID, uterine perforation, ectopic pregnancy, expulsion.

Hormonal Contraceptives

Oral

- Combined pill: 0.3 mg of Norgesterel, 0.03 mg of ethinyl estradiol
- Progesterone only pill: Render cervical mucus viscous
- Post coital pill: IUD inserion within 72 hours, 50 mcg of estrogen 2 tablets immediately followed by 2 tablets 12 hours later
- Once a month pill: Quinestrol long acting estrogen given with short acting progestogen
- Male pill: Gossypol Oligospermia and Azoospermia.

Depot Formulations

- Injectables: DMPA, IM,150 mg, every 3 months NET-EN–IM, 200 mg, 60 days–Both INJ given at 5th day of menstruation, deep IM, injection site should not be massaged

- Injectables: Combined (P and O) Cyclofem, cycloprovera, mesigyna, given at once monthly intervals
- Subcutaneous implants: Norplant, 35 mg, levonorgestrel, effective for 5 years
- Vaginal rings: Containing levonorgestrel, hormone is absorbed through vaginal mucosa, ring is worn in vagina.

Side Effects

- Cardiovascular: MI, cerebral thrombosis, veinous thrombosis
- Carcinogenesis: Increasing incidence of Cx cancer
- Metabolic effects: Rise in BP, blood clotting, altered lipid metabolism, accelerate atherogenesis
- Liver disorders: Hepatic adenoma, cholestatic jaundice
- Ectopic pregnancies: POP
- Weight gain, breast tenderness, headche and migraine.

Beneficial Effects

Give protection against–benign breast diseases, ovarian cyst, Fe-df anemia, PID, ectopic, ovarian cancer.

MATERNAL AND CHILD HEALTH

Antenatal Care

Antenatal Visits

- Ideally the mother should attend the AN clinic once a month during first 7 months, twice a month the next month, and thereafter, once a week, if everything is normal. (more than 10 visits)
- If not a minimum of 4th visits covering the entire period of pregnancy, 1st visit within 12 weeks, 2nd visit between 14–26 weeks, 3rd visit 28 to 34 weeks and 4th visit 36 weeks and term.
- **The central purpose of antenatal care is to identify 'high-risk' mothers as early as possible.**

High-risk mothers	At risk infants
• Elderly primi (30 years and above) • Short statured primi (140 cm and below) • Malpresentations, viz breech, transverse lie, etc. • Antepartum hemorrhage, threatened abortion • Preeclampsia, eclampsia • Anemia • Twins, hydramnios • Previous still birth, IUD, Manual removal of placenta • Elderly grandmultipara • Prolonged pregnancy (14 days after EDD) • H/O previous caesarean or instrumental delivery • Pregnancy associated with general disease, like CVD, DM etc.	• Birth weight less than 2.5 kg • Twins • Birth order 5 and more • Artificial feeding • Weight below 70% of the expected weight • Failure to gain weight during three successive months • Children with PEM, diarrhea • Working mother/one parent

Home visiting by the female health worker is the back bone of all MCH services.

Warning Signals During Pregnancy

- Swelling of the feet
- Fits
- Headache
- Blurring of vision
- Bleeding or discharge per vagina.

Neonatal Care

- The first week of life is the most crucial period in the life of an infant.
- In India, 61.3% of all infant deaths occur within the first month of life. Of these, more than half may die during the first week of birth.
- The risk of death is greatest during **the first 24 to 48 hours** after birth.

MEASURING THE BABY

Birth Weight

- Should be taken preferably **within the first hour** of life, before significant post natal weight loss has occurred
- The child is weighed to the **nearest 100 g** according to the standard method for weight measurement
- **Length (height)**
- Should be recorded **within first 3 days** using infantometer
- Length is taken to the **nearest 0.1 cm.**

Low Birth Weight

Defined as a birth weight of less than 2.5 kg (up to and including 2.499 kg)

- **Preterm**–Babies born before the end of 37 weeks (less than 259 days)
- **Term**–Babies born between 37 completed weeks to less than 42 weeks (259 days to 293 days)
- **Post-term**–Babies born at 42 completed weeks or any time thereafter (294 days and over)
- **Small for date babies (SFD)**–These may be born at term or pre term. **They weigh less than the 10th percentile for the gestational age.** These babies are clearly the result of **retarded intrauterine fetal growth.**
- **In most parts of India, the mean birth weight is between 2.7 and 2.9 kg.**

GROWTH CHART

- The growth or road to health chart **first designed by David Morley**
- WHO growth chart prototype has 2 reference curves. The upper reference curve represents the 50th percentile for boys and the lower reference curve the 3rd percentile for girls. Thus, the chart can be used for both sexes.

The Growth Chart used in India has Four Reference Curves

- The topmost curve corresponds to 80% of the median, the lower lines represent 70%, 60% and 50% of that standard.
- If a child's weight is between 80% to 70% it indicates first degree or mild malnutrition, 70% to 60% indicates second degree or moderate malnutrition, 70% to 60% indicates third degree or severe malnutrition.
- The growth charts being used in **ICDS in India contains 3 reference lines,** representing 80%, 60% and 50% of the reference standards.

Uses of Growth Chart

- Growth monitoring, diagnostic tool, planning and policy making, educational tool, tool for action, evaluation of effectiveness of control measures and tool for teaching.

School Health Services

- School health committee (1961) recommends that 10 acres of land be provided for high schools and 5 acres for primary schools with additional one acre of land per 100 students.
- Exterior walls should have a minimum thickness of 10 inches and should be heat resistant.
- No class rooms should accommodate more than 40 students.
- Per capita space for students in a class room should not be less than 10 sq ft.
- Desks should be of minus type.
- Combined door and window area should be at least 25% of the floor space.
- One urinal for 60 students and one latrine for 100 students.

Breastfeeding

- Under normal conditions, Indian mothers secrete 450 to 600 ml of milk daily
- The energy value of human milk is 70 kcals/100 ml
- Breastfeeding week–August 1 to 7.

Components of Breast Milk

Protein

- In general cows milk contains 3 times more protein content than human milk–33g/l and 11g/l respectively but lact-albumin is twice the amount seen in human milk.
- Human milk contains more cystine, essential for the prematures.
- It is rich in taurine.
- Human milk protein are almost completely digested and absorbed, whereas cows milk protein is excreted by the infant undigested producing whitish curdy stool.
- IgG, lysozyme, which are non-nutritive, but antiinfective.
- Human milk is virtually a living fluid.

Fats

- Human milk is similar to the cows milk as far as fat content is concerned.
- But it differ in two ways.
- Essential polyunsaturated fatty acids, especially linoleic acid and alpha-linoleic acid are higher in human milk.
- The fats of human milk are easy to digest and absorb for the infant.
- Unabsorbed fatty acids of cows milk interfere with calcium absorption.

Carbohydrates

- Carbohydrate content is more in human milk compared to breast milk (H–70g/l, C–50g/l).
- Human milk contains more lactose.
- Useful for growing brain.
- Lactose helps in growing of beneficial bacteria (lactobacillus) in the intestine which inhibits the growth of harmful bacteria.
- Lactobacillus help to keep the intestinal contents acidic.

Vitamins and Minerals

- Vitamin D is present in the human milk in the water soluble form. (H-50 IU, C-25IU).
- Human milk contains more Vitamin A and Vitamin C than cows milk (Vit C-60 mg/l).
- Iron is seen in small quantity but has a very high level of bioavailability.
- Coefficient of intake of the iron in breast milk may be as high as 70%, but only 30% in cows milk.

MCH Indicators

Maternal Mortality Rate

- Maternal mortality rate measures the risk of women dying from puerperal causes and is calculated by

$$\frac{\text{Total number of female deaths due to complications of pregnancy, childbirth or within 42 days of delivery from puerperal causes in an area during a given year}}{\text{Total number of life births in the same area and year}} \times 1000$$

Ideally the denominator should include all deliveries and abortions.

Late Maternal Death

The death of a woman from direct or indirect obstetric causes more than 42 days but less than one year after termination of pregnancy.

Pregnancy Related Death

Death of a woman while pregnant or within 42 days of termination of pregnancy, irrespective of the cause of death.

Causes of Maternal Deaths

Direct obstetric causes

Those resulting from obstetric complications of the pregnant state (pregnancy, labor and puerperium), from interventions, omissions, incorrect treatment, or from a chain of events resulting from any of the above

Indirect obstetric causes

Those resulting from previous existing disease or disease that developed during pregnancy and which was not due to direct obstetric causes, but which was aggravated by physiological effects of pregnancy.

Mortality in Infancy and Childhood

Fetal Death

Death after the 20th or 28th week of gestation (the definition of length of gestation varies between countries).

Stillbirth Rate

$$SR = \frac{\text{Fetal deaths weighing over 1000 g at birth}}{\text{Total live + stillbirths weighing over 1000 g at birth}} \times 1000$$

Death of a fetus weighing 1000 g (this is equivalent to 28 weeks of gestation).
WHO has recommended the term stillbirth be applied to a fetus born dead, and weighing over 500 g–birth weight most frequently associated with a gestation period of 22 weeks.
But for international comparison, suggested 1000 g or with a gestation of 28 weeks.

Perinatal Mortality Rate

- Perinatal period defined as period lasting from the 28th week of gestation to the seventh day after birth
- Baby weighing 1000 g or gestation period of 28 weeks or body length (crown to heel) of at least 35 cm should be used.
- But the preferred criterion is birth weight.

$$PMR = \frac{\text{Late fetal deaths (28 weeks gestation and more)} + \text{Early neonatal deaths (first week) in one year}}{\text{Total live births in the same year}} \times 1000$$

WHO Expert Committee Definition

$$PMR = \frac{\text{Late fetal and early neonatal deaths weighing over 1000 g at birth}}{\text{Total live births weighing over 1000 g at birth}} \times 1000$$

Importance of Perinatal Mortality Rate

With the decline of infant mortality rate to low levels in developed countries, PMR has assumed greater significance as a yardstick of obstetric and pediatric care.

Two types of death rates are included in still births (late fetal deaths and early neonatal deaths) because the factors responsible for these two types of deaths are often similar.

- A proportion of deaths which occur after birth are incorrectly registered as stillbirths, thereby inflating the stillbirth rate and lowering the neonatal death rate.
- The perinatal mortality rate, being a combination of stillbirths and early neonatal deaths, is not influenced by this error.
- The value of perinatal mortality rate is that it gives a good indication of the extent of pregnancy wastage as well as the quality of the MCH care.
- It reflects the results of maternity care clearly than the neonatal death rate as previously thought.

Neonatal Mortality Rate

$$\text{PMR} = \frac{\text{Number of deaths of children under 28 days of age in a year}}{\text{Total live births in the same year}} \times 1000$$

- Neonatal mortality rate is directly related to the birth weight and gestational age.
- NMR is a measure of intensity with which endogenous factors affect life.
- Most common cause of NMR is prematurity (28%) followed by infection (26%) and then birth asphyxia (23%), congenital anomalies (8%), neonatal tetanus (7%), diarrheal diseases (3%), and other causes (7%).
- Neonatal mortality rate is greater in boys throughout the world, because boys are biologically more fragile than girls.

Postneonatal Mortality Rate

$$\frac{\text{Number of deaths of children between 28 days and one year of age in a given year}}{\text{Total live births in the same year}} \times 1000$$

- Postneonatal mortality rate is dominated by the exogenous factors (environmental and social)
- In developed countries the main cause of PNMR is congenital anomalies
- Diarrhea and respiratory infections are the main causes of death in India.

Infant Mortality Rate

$$\frac{\text{Number of deaths of children less than 1 year of age in a year}}{\text{Number of live births in the same year}} \times 1000$$

- Most important indicator of the health status of a community but also of the level of living of people in general and effectiveness of MCH services in particular.
- In general IMR reflects the socioeconomic development of a country.

Under 5 Mortality Rate

It measures the probability of dying between birth and exactly 5 years of age.

$$\frac{\text{Number of deaths of children less than 5 years of age in a year}}{\text{Number of live births in the same year}} \times 1000$$

Next to the neonatal causes (37%), acute respiratory infections constitute 19% of cause of death.

NUTRITION AND HEALTH

Nutritive Value of Foods

Cereals

Rice

- Rice belongs to cereal group which constitute the bulk of the daily diet.
- Energy provided by 100 g of rice is 345 Kcal.
- The protein content of rice varies from 6–9 percent.
- Good source of B group of vitamins especially thiamine.
- The milling process deprives the rice grain of its valuable nutritive elements (thiamine, riboflavin)
- Cereal proteins are deficient in lysine but rice is an exception.
- Rice proteins are richer in lysine. So it is called better quality protein cereal.
- Parboiling preserves the nutritive quality of rice.

Wheat

- Next to rice Wheat is the most important cereal.
- The protein content of wheat varies from 9 to 16%, the limiting amino acids are lysine and threonine.

- Whole grain wheat flour is richer source of Vitamin B than refined white flour.
- Maida or white flour which represents 70% extraction of wheat is poorer from the nutrition stand point.

Maize (Corn or Bhutta)

- Maize ranks next to rice and wheat in human consumption.
- The yellow variety of maize contains significant amount of carotenoid pigments.
- Maize is fairly rich in fat.
- The proteins of maize are deficient in tryptophan and lysine and they contain excess of leucine.
- Excess of leucine interferes in the conversion of tryptophan into niacin and thus aggravates the pellagrogenic action of maize.
- Maize is also used in the manufacture of breakfast foods such as cornflakes.

Jowar

- Jowar is also known as Kaffir corn or Milo
- It is a major crop grown in India next only to wheat and rice
- The protein content of jowar varies from 9 to 14% and the proteins are limiting in lysine and threonine
- Certain varieties of jowar have a high leucine content and consumption of these varieties is associated with pellagra.

Ragi

- Cheapest among millets.
- Nutritive value–protein–7.3%, fat–1.3%, carbohydrates–72%, calcium–344 gm/100 gm of ragi.
- Popular millet in Andhra Pradesh and Karnataka
- Ragi flour is cooked and eaten as porridge.

Pulses (Legumes)

- Pulses comprise a variety of grams, also known as dals
- Pulses contain 20 to 25% of proteins, which is double that found in wheat and three times that found in rice. Hence they are called 'Poor man's meat'
- Pulse proteins contain more protein than eggs, fish or flesh
- In regard to quality pulse proteins are inferior to animal proteins
- Pulse proteins are poorer in methionine and to a lesser extent in cystein but rich in lysine
- Pulses are rich in minerals and B group vitamins
- Germinating pulses contain higher concentration of Vitamin B and Vitamin C.
- Presence of high amounts of certain sugars known as oligosaccharides is known to be associated with flatulence.

Soybean

- Richest source of proteins among pulses.
- Limiting amino acid is methionine
- Cooked and eaten as dal and also in other forms like mixing it with atta for chapattis, soybean milk in baby foods, etc.
- Nutritive Value–432 kcal/100 g
  - 43.2 g/100 g
  - 19.5 g/100 g.

Egg

- Egg contains all the nutrients except carbohydrate and vitamin C
- An egg weighing 60 grams contains 6 g of protein, 6 g of fat, 30 mg of calcium and 1.5 mg of iron and supplies 70 Kcal of energy
- Egg proteins contain all the nine essential amino acids needed by the body in right proportions
- Except for Vitamin C egg contains all the fat soluble vitamins.

- Boiled egg is nutritionally superior than raw egg because boiling destroys avidin a substance which prevents the body from obtaining biotin (B complex Vitamin)
- The cholesterol content of egg is 250 mg/egg
- Net protein utilization which combines in a single value the biological value and digestibility coefficient, is 100 for egg.

Milk

- Best and most complete of all foods
- Good source of proteins, fats, sugars, vitamins and minerals
- The chief protein of milk is casein
- The other important proteins are lactalbumin and lactoglobulin
- Milk proteins contain all essential amino acids
- The fat content of milk varies from 3.4% to 8.8%
- Milk fat is a good source of retinol and vitamin D
- The carbohydrate in milk is lactose or milk sugar
- Milk is rich in calcium and contains almost all minerals, but it is a poor source of iron.

Constituent	Breast milk	Cow's milk
Proteins	**11**	**33**
• Casein	4	28
• Soluble proteins	7	5
Lipids	35	35
Carbohydrates	**70**	**50**
• Lactose	62	50
• Nitrogenous oligosaccharides	8	0
Minerals	2	8
• Ca	0.33	1
• P	0.15	1
• Fe	**0.4–1.5 mg**	**0.3–0.5 mg**
Vitamins		
• C	60 mg	20 mg
• D	50 IU	25 IU
Energy	640–720 Kcal	650 Kcal

COMMUNITY NUTRITION PROGRAMMES

- Vitamin A prophylaxis programme
- Nutritional anemia control programme
- National goitre control programme
- National IDD control programme
- Special nutrition programme
- Balwadi nutrition programme
- ICDS programme
- Midday meal programme (School lunch programme)

Xerophthalmia (Dry eye)

- Refers to all the ocular manifestations of Vitamin a deficiency
- MC among 1 to 3 years age group
- Prevention and control
- Short term action

- Administration of large doses of vitamin A orally in recommended doses to vulnerable groups–1 lac IU to children of less than one year, followed 2 lac IU every six months till 5 years of age
- Medium term action
  - Promote regular and adequate intake of Vitamin A
  - By fortification of certain foods–Dalda (vanaspathi)
- Long term action
  - Persuading people especially mothers to consume generally dark green leafy vegetables, other Vitamin A rich foods
  - Improvement in environmental conditions
- Immunization against infectious diseases.

Vitamin A

- Halibut liver oil is the richest source of vitamin A (900000 mcg/g)
- Beta carotene has the highest vitamin A activity
- First clinical sign of vitamin A deficiency is conjunctival xerosis
- Xerophthalmia is most common in 1–3 years.

Short term action: Vitamin A prophylaxis

Age	Oral dose of Retinol palmitate	Time
< 12 months	100000 IU	Once every 4–6 months
> 12 months	200000 IU	Once every 4–6 months
New born	50000 IU	At birth
Women of child bearing age	300000 IU	Within one month of giving birth
Pregnant and lactating women	5000 IU or 20000 IU	Everyday Everyweek

Medium Term Action

- Food fortification.

Long term action

- Consumption of dark green leafy vegetables generously
- Promotion of breastfeeding
- Improvements of environmental health such as ensuring safe and adequate water supply and construction and maintenance of sanitary latrines to safeguard against diarrhea
- Immunization against infectious diseases such as measles
- Prompt treatment of diarrhea and associated infections
- Health education.

Folate

- Folic acid deficiency produces megaloblastic anemia, glossitis, cheilosis and GI disturbances such as diarrhea, distension and flatulence
- Severe folate deficiency may even cause infertility or sterility
- Folate requirements
- Healthy adults–100 mcg
- Children–100 mcg
- Pregnancy–400 mcg
- Lactation–150 mcg.

Vitamin B_{12} Requirement

Adults	1 mcg/day
Pregnancy and lactation	1.5 mcg/day
Infants and children	0.2 mcg/day

Vitamin D

Age group	Daily requirement of vitamin D
Adults	2.5 mcg or 100 IU
Infants and children	5.0 mcg or 200 IU
Pregnancy and lactation	10 mcg or 400 IU

CONTROL OF IDD

Iodized Salt

- Most widely used public health measure
- Level of iodization is fixed at 30 ppm at the production point and 15 ppm at consumer level
- Most economical, convenient and effective means.

Iodized Oil

- IM injection of iodized oil (poppy seed oil), dosage 1 ml
- 1 ml will provide protection for about 4 years
- But more expensive
- Difficulty–reaching every person in the community
- Oral administration of iodine as iodized oil or sodium iodate tablets
- Technically simpler
- More costly than intramuscular injections
- Manpower training–Health workers
- Mass communication–Creating awareness
- Monitoring and surveillance through network of labs–iodine in water, iodine in salt for quality control.

MIDDAY MEAL PROGRAMME

- School lunch programme–1961
- Objective is to attract the children for admission to schools and retain them so that literacy status of children improves.

Principles

- Meal should be a supplement and not a substitute
- Should supply at least on third of total energy requirement and half of the protein requirement
- Cost should be low
- Cooked with the locally available foods
- Reorientation of food habits
- Incorporation of nutrition education
- Improving school attendance
- Improve the educational performance.

INTEGRATED CHILD DEVELOPMENT SERVICES

- To improve the nutritional and health status of the children in the age group of 0 to 6 years
- To lay the foundations for proper psychological and social development of the child
- To reduce the morbidity, mortality, malnutrition and school drop out
- To enhance the capability of the mother and nutritional needs of the child through proper nutrition and health education.

Beneficiaries

- Pregnant women
- Nursing mothers
- Other women of 15 to 45 years
- Children less than 3 years
- Children in the age group 3 to 6 years
- Adolescent girls 11–18 years.

Population Norms Under ICDS

- Rural/Urban projects
  - 1 for AWC for 400–800 population
  - 2 for AWC for 800–1600 population
  - 3 for AWC for 1600–2400 population
  - ONE AWC for multiples of 800 population
  - ONE MINI AWC 150–400 population
- For Tribal/hilly/riverine/desert–and other difficult areas
- 1 AWC for 300–800 population
- 1 MINI AWC for 150–300 population

Community development block in rural areas
Tribal development block in tribal areas and group of slums in urban areas
Rural/Urban project–per 1,00,000 population (100 villages)
Tribal project–35,000 population (50 villages)

Pregnant Women

- Health check-up–An check-up, iron and folic acid tablets are provided
- Immunization against tetanus
- Supplementary nutrition–Women of low income group, to get 600 calories and 18 to 20 grams of protein
- Nutrition and health education.

Children Under 3 Years

- Supplementary nutrition–500 calories and 12–15 grams of proteins
- Immunization—Against 6 vaccine preventable diseases
- Health check-up—Growth monitoring, watch over miles stones, treatment of diseases like diarrhea, dysentry, ari, etc. deworming, prophylaxis against Vitamin A deficiency, maintenance of health cards and records
- Referral services—Referral of serious cases at the right time.

Children of 3 to 6 Years

- Supplementary nutrition
- Immunization
- Health check-up
- Referral services
- Non-formal education–Non-formal preschool education is imparted, to develop desirable attitude and behaviour through organized play and creative activity.

Adolescent Girls 11 to 18 Years

- Supplementary nutrition–500 calories and 20 to 25 grams of protein
- Nutrition and health education
- Malnurished children
- 800 calories and 20 to 25 grams of proteins.

• Kishori Shakti Yojana–implemented using ICDS infrastructure, target–11 to 18 year old adolescent girls, Addresses towards self development, nutrition and health status, literacy skills, vocational skills. • Nutrition programme for adolescent girls–focus on undernourished adolescent girls–11 to 19 years – 11 to 15 years–less than 30 kg and 15 to 19 years–less than 35 kg are covered under the scheme – 6 kg of food grain is provided to each beneficiary	• Rajiv Gandhi Scheme for Empowerment of adolescent girls–(SABLA scheme)–Pilot basis • The SABLA scheme aims at empowering Adolescent Girls of 11–18 years by improving their nutritional and health status, up gradation of home skills, life skills and vocational skills. • The girls will be equipped with information on health and family welfare, hygiene and guidance on existing public services. • SABLA would be a 100% Centrally Sponsored scheme for all inputs except nutrition component which will be on 50:50 shared basis between Central and State Government.

Nutritional Anemia in India

- Iron deficiency anemia is a major form of nutritional anemia
- The incidence varies 60 to 70% among women and young children
- The second common nutritional anemia is folate deficiency anemia
- It affects 25 to 50% of pregnant women in India.

Causes of Nutritional Anemia

- Inadequate intake
- Poor bioavailability of dietary iron
- Excessive losses of iron from the body
- Infections like malaria
- Infestations like hookworm.

Control and Prevention

- Iron and folic acid supplementation
- Iron fortification
- Others strategies–Health education and control of infections
- Daily supplementation of iron and folic acid
  - To pregnant women
  - Lactating mothers
  - Children 12 years

Eligibility criteria–Hb, between 10 and 12 g/dl

Pregnant and lactating mothers

- One tablet of iron and folic acid containing 100 mg of elemental iron (300 mg of ferrous sulphate) daily, 0.5 mg (500 mcg) of folic acid daily, 2 to 3 months (100 days).

Children

- One tablet of iron and folic acid containing 20 mg of elemental iron (60 mg of ferrous sulphate), 0.1 mg (100 mcg) of folic acid.

Iron fortification

- Ferric orthophosphate or ferrous sulphate with sodium bisulphate to fortify with salt
- All segments of population may get benefited.

Calorie, protein and iron requirement

RDA Energy	RDA Protein
• Pregnant women–+300,	• +15 g
• Lactation 0–6 months–+550, • 6 to 12 months–+400	• +25 g • +18 g

FOOD TOXICANTS

Aflatoxins–Mycotoxins (storage fungus) produced by Aspergillus flavus, Aspergillus parasiticus

- These fungi infest food grains like–ground nut, maize, wheat, rice, etc.
- Aflatoxins–B1 and G1–hepatotoxins
- More prevalent in Rajasthan and Gujarat.

Ergot–This is due to field fungus–claviceps fusiformis

- Severe vasoconstriction of capillaries resulting in peripheral gangrene, rarely fatal
- Easily removed by floating them in salt water.

Endemic ascites–Over all mortality–40%, causes ascites and jaundice, contamination of weed seeds of Crotalaria (Jhunjhunia plants)–contain pyrrolizidine alkaloids–hepatotoxins. Prevalent in Madhya Pradesh.

Epidemic dropsy–contamination of mustard oil with argemone oil

- Sangunarine is the toxic principle in argemone oil
- Interfers with oxidation of pyruvic acid which accumulates in the blood
- Sudden, non inflammatory swelling of legs, with diarrhea, dyspnea, cardiac failure
- Tests for the detection of argemone oil–nitric acid test, paper chromatography test (most sensitive test), detects argemone oil up to 0.0001%.

Nutritional Health Problem in India

Neurolathyrism

- Crippling disease of nervous system–gradually developing spastic paralysis of lower limbs–occurring in adults consuming the pulse lathyrus sativus (Khesari dal)–toxin is BOAA
- More prevalent in Madhya pradesh, Uttar pradesh, Bihar and Orissa
- Also reported in Maharashtra, West Bengal, Rajasthan, Assam, Gujarat
- Prevention–(removal of toxin)–steeping method, Parboiling, Genetic approach

Endemic Fluorosis–dental–1.5 to 3 mg/l, skeletal–3 to 6, MC in–Andhra Pradesh

ENVIRONMENT AND HEALTH

Sanitary Well

- A sanitary well is one which is properly located, well constructed and protected against contamination with a view to yield a supply of safe water
- Located 15 m away from the likely source of contamination
- Should be located in such a place that no user will have to carry water for more than 100 m (100 yards)
- The lining of the wall should be built of bricks or stones set in cement up to a depth of 6 m (20 feet)
- The lining should be carried 60–90 cm above the ground level
- Parapet wall up to a height of at least 70–75 cm above the ground
- Cement concrete platform round the well 1 m (3 feet) in all directions
- The top of the well should be covered by cement concrete with some gap for taking the water.

Contents	Rapid sand filter	Slow sand filter
Space	Occupies very little space	Requires larger area
Rate of filtration	5–15 cubicmeter/meter square/hour	0.1–0.4 cubic meter/meter square/hour
Effective size of the sand	0.4 to 0.7 mm	0.2 to 0.3 mm

Preliminary treatment	Chemical coagulation and sedimentation	Plain sedimentation
Washing	By backwashing	By scraping
Operation	Highly skilled	Less skilled
Removal of bacteria	98–99%	99.9–99.99%

Advantages of Sand Filters

Rapid sand filters	Slow sand filters
Can deal with raw water directly	Simple to construct and operate
No preliminary storage needed	Cost of construction is cheaper
Filtration is rapid 40 to 50 times that of slow sand filters and washing of the filters very easy	The physical, chemical and biological quality of water is very high

Principles of Chlorination

- Water to be chlorinated should be clear and free from turbidity
- Chlorine demand of the water should be estimated–Is the difference between the amount of chlorine added to the water and the amount of residual chlorine remaining at the end of a specific period of time (usually 60 minutes)
- This time is essential to kill bacteria and viruses
- The point at which the chlorine demand of the water is met is called the 'break-point'
- Recommended concentration of free chlorine is 0.5 mg/dl.

O-tolidine Test (OT test)

0.1 ml reagent is mixed with 1 ml of water–yellow colour appears within 10 seconds which shows free chlorine and the yellow colour that is produced after a lapse of 15 minutes is due to both combined and free chlorine.

Orthotolidine Arsenite Test

Modification of orthotolidine test to determine free and combined chlorine separately.

The errors caused by presence of interfering substances such as nitrites, iron and manganese all of which produce a yellow colour with o-tolidine, are overcome by the OTA test

Ozonation	Ultraviolet radiation
• Method of water disinfection on large scale • Relatively unstable gas • Powerful oxidizing agent • Eliminates undesirable odor, taste and color • Removes all chlorine from the water • Has strong virucidal effect • Dosage required for water treatment varies from 0.2 to 1.5 mg/l Disadvantages • No residual germicidal effect • Ozonation is usually employed in combination with chlorination	• This method of disinfection involves the exposure of a film of water up to about 120 mm thick, at a wavelength in the range of 200 to 295 nenometre Advantages • Exposure is for a short period • No foreign matter is introduced • No taste and odor produced • Over exposure does not result in any harmful effects Disadvantages • No residual effect • Lack of a rapid field test for assessing the treatment efficiency • Apparatus needed is expensive

Hardness of Water

- May be defined as soap destroying power of water
- Caused by mainly four dissolved compounds
  - Calcium bicarbonate,
  - Magnesium bicarbonate,
  - Calcium sulphate and
  - Magnesium sulphate

- Temporary hardness–Due to carbonates
- Permanent hardness–Due to non carbonate–like sulphates, chlorides, nitrites, etc
- Expressed in terms of milliequivalents per litre (mEq/l)
  - Soft water–less than 1 mEq/l (< 50 mg/l)
  - Moderately hard–1–3 mEq/l (50–150 mg/l)
  - Hard water–3–6 mEq/l (150–300 mg/l)
  - Very hard water–over (> 300 mg/l).

Monitoring of Air Pollution

The best indicators of air pollution are

- Sulfur dioxide,
- Smoke or soiling index,
- Suspended particles,
- Grit and dust measurement,
- Coefficient of haze and
- Air pollution index

Indices of Thermal Comfort

Air temperature, humidity, air movement, effective temperature, corrected effective temperature.

Corrected effective temperature

- Pleasant and cool–< 20 °C
- Cool and comfortable 20 to 25 °C
- Comfortable–25 to 27 °C
- Hot and uncomfortable–27 to 28 °C
- 28 + extremely hot
- 30 + intolerable hot.

Prevention and control of air pollution

- Containment–Prevention of escape of toxic substances in to ambient air
- Replacement–Replacing technological process causing air pollution
- Dilution–Establishment of green belts between industrial and residential areas is an attempt to dilution
- Legislation–Example Clean Air Act, to decrease the nuisance of air pollution, the Govt of India have enacted The Air (Prevention and Control of Pollution) Act in 1981.
- International action–International network of labs for monitoring and study of air pollution.

Light

Measurement of light

- Candela–brightness of source
- Lumen–Flow of light
- Lux–Amount of light reaching surface
- Lambert–Amount of light remitted by surface
- Day light factor–It is the ratio of instantaneous illumination indoors to illumination outdoors simultaneously multiplying by 100
- It is recommended that in living rooms, the day light factor should be at least 8% and in kitchens about 10%.
- Casual reading–100 lux, general office work–400 lux, watch making–2000–3000.

Noise

- Defined as unwanted sound
- The 20th century has been described as the century of noise
- Loudness is measured in Decibelss (dB)
- Normal conversation–60 to 65 dB, Whispering–20 to 30 dB
- A daily exposure up to 85 dB is about the limit people can tolerate without substantial damage to their hearing
- The frequency is denoted as Hertz (Hz)
- The human ear can hear frequencies from about 20 to 20000 Hz
- Auditory fatigue occurs at 90 dB
- Temporary hearing loss occurs in frequency range between 4000 to 6000 Hz
- Repeated or continuous exposure to noise around 100 decibels may result in a permanent hearing loss
- Exposure to noise above 160 dB may rupture the tympanic membrane and cause permanent loss of hearing
- SIL–Speech Interference Level 12 Db.

Housing standards

- Site–Elevated from surroundings, independent access to a street or road, away from breeding sources
- Set back–Open space all around the house
- Floor–Damp proof, height of the plinth should be 2 to 3 feet
- Walls–Should not absorb heat, 9 inch thick brick wall
- Roof–Should not be less than 10 feet (3 m)
- Rooms–At least 2 living rooms
- Floor area–100 square feet for occupancy by a single person
- Windows–At least one of them should open directly on to a open space, height of 3 feet from the ground
- Lighting–Day light factor should exceed 1%.

Medical Entomology

A study of the arthropods of medical importance is known as medical entomology which is an important branch of preventive medicine.

Transmission of arthropod borne diseases.

Three types of transmission

- Direct contact
- Directly transferred from man to man through close contact.

Example. Scabies, pediculosis.

- Mechanical transmission

The transmission of diarrhea, dysentry, typhoid, food poisoning, and trachoma by the housefly

- Biological transmission

When the disease agent multiplies or undergoes some developmental change with or without multiplication in the arthropod host it is called biological transmission

- Propagative

When the disease agent undergoes no cyclical change, but multiplies in the body of the vector (arthropod), transmission is said to be propagative

Example. Plague bacilli in rat fleas

- Cyclopropagative

The disease agent undergoes cyclical change and multiplies in the body of the arthropod

Example. Malarial parasite in anopheles mosquito

- Cyclodevelopmental

When the disease agent undergoes cyclical change but does not multiply in the body of the arthropod

Example. Filarial parasite in the Culex mosquito and Guinea worm embryo in Cyclops

Diseases transmitted

Mosquito • Malaria, Filaria, • Viral encephalitis (Japanes encephalitis) • Viral fevers (Dengue, West Nile) • Viral hemorrhagic fevers (Yellow fever, dengue hemorrhagic fever) Sandfly • Kala-azar • Oriental sore • Sandfly fever • Oraya fever **Mnemonic–SOOK** Tse tse fly–Sleeping sickness Rat flea • Bubonic plague • Endemic typhus • Chiggerosis • Hymenolepsis diminuta **Mnemonic–BEnTCH** Louse • Epidemic typhus • Relapsing fever • Trench fever • Pediculosis **Mnemonic–Evening rise of Temperature**	Hard tick • Tick typhus (T) • Viral encephalitis (v) • Tularemia (T) • Viral fever (v) • KFD–Kyasanur Forest Disease (K) • Tick paralysis (T) • Human babesiosis • Mnemonic–(TvTvKTv) Soft tick–Q fever and relapsing fever (QRST) Black fly–Onchocerciasis Reduvid bug–Chagas disease Trombiculid mite–Scrub typhus, Rickettsial pox Itch mite–Scabies

Characteristics	Anopheles	Culex	Aedes	Mansonia
Disease transmitted	Malaria	Bancroftian filariasis, JE, West Nile fever	Dengue and DHF, Chikungunya, Yellow fever, Rift valley fever	Malayan filariasis
Breeding habit	Clean water	Dirty polluted water	Artificial collections of water	Water bodies containing aquatic plants
Eggs	Laid singly,boat shaped with lateral floats	Laid in clusters/rafts	Laid singly,cigar shaped	Laid in star shaped clusters
Larvae	No siphon tube; rest parallel to undersurface of water	Siphon tube; rest perpendicular to undersurface of water	Siphon tube;rest in dark bottom corners	Siphon tube; rest attached to rootlets of plants
Pupae	Broad and short siphon tube	Long and narrow siphon tube	Long and narrow siphon tube	Long and narrow siphon tube
Adults	Inclined at an angle to surface Spotted wings	Hunch back rest	Stripes on body and legs	–
Flight range	3–5 km	11 km	100 m	–

Anopheles Mosquito

45 species of anopheles mosquitoes have been found in India

- Anopheles fluviatalis and An minimus found in foot hill regions
- An. Sundaicus and An. Stephensi found in coastal regions
- An. Culicifacies and An. Philippinensis in the plains

Transmits malaria and filaria (not in India)

- Male–Palpi are longer than proboscis, clubbed at the end, thick and bushy antenna seen
- Female–The palpi are smaller than the proboscis, not clubbed at the end, sparse antenna seen.

Culex Mosquito Adult

- Nuisance mosquitoes
- Culex fatigans is the important vector in India
- Breeds in dirty water collection (stagnant drains, cesspools, septic tanks, burrow pits)
- Strong winged mosquito can fly upto 11 km
- The peak biting time is at midnight
- During the day they rest indoors, on walls, underneath furniture, dark corners
- Transmits bancroftian filariasis, Japanese encephalitis, West Nile fever, viral arthritis.

Aedes Mosquito

- Striped or banded character of legs–Tiger mosquitoes
- First proved vector of a virus–Yellow fever
- Breeds in artificial water collection–Discarded tins, broken bottles, etc.
- Females are fearless biters and they bite during the day
- Do not fly over long distances usually less than 100 cms
- Under WHO international health regulations all international airports and seaports are kept free from all types of mosquitoes for a distance of 400 meters around the perimeter of ports
- Under the IHR–Aedes agypti index is defined as the ratio, expressed as percentage between the number of houses in the limited area on the premises of which actual breeding A. aegypti are found and the total number of houses examined in that area
- This index is kept at zero at all ports
- Transmits yellow fever(not in India), dengue, chikungunya, rift valley fever, filaria (not in India).

Mansonia Mosquito

- Big black or brown mosquitoes with speckling on their wings and legs
- Breed on certain aquatic plants especially pistia, water hyacinth
- The larvae and pupae are found attached to the rootlets of these plants by their siphon tubes.

Body Louse

- Belongs to phylum arthropoda, class insecta or hexapoda
- These are ectoparasites and are called as Pediculus humanus corporis
- The body is divided into head, thorax and abdomen
- The body is flattened dorsoventrally and the abdomen is elongated and consists of 9 segments
- Pair of antenna is seen which has five segments
- Maxillary palpi and proboscis are absent
- There are 3 pairs of legs on the ventral side of thorax which are strongly developed and adapted for maintaining firm hold on the host
- It transmits epidemic typhus, trench fever and louse borne relapsing fever.

Crab Louse

Pubic louse or Phthirus pubis

- Small and has square body
- Head impacted on the thorax
- 3 pairs of powerful legs
- Not proved to transmit any disease.

Sand Fly

- These are small insects, light or dark brown in colour
- Smaller than mosquitoes measuring 1.5 to 2.5 mm in length with their bodies and wings densely clothed with hair (hairy insect)

- Wings are upright and lanceolate shaped
- The legs are longer compared with the size of the body
- Diseases transmitted are Kala-azar, Sandfly fever, Oriental sore.

Rat Fleas

- Fleas are small bilaterally compressed, wingless insects with a hard chitinous exoskeleton and covered with backwardly directed strong bristles
- The body of the rat flea is divided into head, thorax and abdomen
- The head is conical in shape and is attached without a neck
- It has 3 pairs of legs attached to thorax
- The abdomen consists of 10 segments
- It transmits plague, endemic typhus or murine typhus, chiggerosis and Hymenolepsis diminuta.

Trombiculid Mites

- Trombiculidae is a family of mites called trombiculid mites (some common names are known as harvest mites, red bugs, and chiggers)
- Belongs to phylum Arthropoda and class Arachnida
- These are spider like arthropods and the body roughly a figure of 8 appearance
- The body not well demarcated into head, thorax and abdomen
- The adult male lives in soil and does not bite and it feeds on juices of certain vegetation
- It has 4 pairs of legs, the first pair is largest
- These are vectors of scrub typhus

Mite Larva

- This is very small, pale orange in color
- The larva has 3 pairs of legs
- It feeds on vertebrate host (rodent or man) and transmits scrub typhus
- The larval stage is the bitting stage and it is found as ectoparasite on field rodents
- The larval stage lasts for 1 to 3 weeks.

Itch Mite (Sarcoptes Scabei or Acarus Scabei)

- Female parasite burrows into epidermis and it breeds
- It is globular shaped or shaped like a tortoise
- Two pair of legs in front and two pair of legs behind
- Live for 2 months
- Control of itch mite
- 25% benzyl benzoate, HCH–0.5 to 1% strength of gamma HCH (lindane), tetmosol–5%, sulfur oinment–2.5% to 10%.

Hard Tick

- Belongs phylum arthropoda and class arachnida
- The body of tick is oval or oblong in outline and consists of one unit only, there being no differentiation into thorax and abdomen
- The body does not show segmentation and on the ventral side there are 4 pairs of well developed legs
- At the anterior end there is a movable head like structure, the capitulam
- Capitulam terminal, anterior in position and antenna are absent
- Dorsal surface of the body covered with a thin chitinous plate or shield called the scutum
- Hard tick transmits tick typhus, viral encephalitis, viral hemorrhagic fever, tularemia, tick paralysis and human babesiosis

Soft Tick

- Belongs phylum arthropoda and class arachnida
- The body of tick is oval or oblong in outline and consists of one unit only, there being no differentiation into thorax and abdomen
- The body does not show segmentation and on the ventral side there are 4 pairs of well developed legs
- Capitulam ventral in position or subterminal and antenna are absent
- Scutum completely absent
- Soft tick transmits Q fever, relapsing fever.

Cyclops (Water Flea)

- Belongs to phylum Arthropoda and Crustacea
- Commonly found in fresh water ponds, stepwells and brackish waters
- It is 1 mm in size white in color and can be just seen with naked eye
- The body is pear shaped semitransparent, a forked tail, 2 pairs of antenna, 5 pair of legs
- At the anterior portion of the Cephalothorax there are two pairs of segemented antenna
- Cyclops has a single median eye on the dorsal side of Cephalothorax
- Cyclops is the intermediate host of guinea worm disease and fish tape worm infestation.

Insecticides

Contact poisons				Stomach poisons
Natural	**Synthetic**			Paris green
Pyrethrum Rotenone Nicotine Mineral oils	Organo chlorine DDT, BHC Lindane, chlordane Dieldrin, aldrin	Organo phosphorous Abate, diazinon Chlorthion, malathion Fenthion, parathion Dichlorvos, chlorpyrifos	Carbamates Carbaryl Propoxur Dimetilan	Sodium fluoride Fumigants Hydrogen cyanide Sulfur dioxide Carbon disulfate

BIOSTATISTICS, HEALTH PLANNING, OCCUPATIONAL HEALTH AND GENETICS

The origin of the word statistics is from the word 'status' which means 'of the state'.

Definition

It is the science and art of **collection, compilation/classification, presentation/summarizing, analysis and interpretation** of numerical data concerned with biological events.

Biological events—example—births, deaths, diseases occurring among human beings.

Quantitative data

- Can be measured or counted

  Example—Age can be measured in months, years, days, height can be measured in centimeters or meters or feet

  Discrete—Can be counted–take only whole number values–number of visits, number of patients, etc.

  Continuous—Assume any value from 0 to infinity—age—continuous variable–although it can be measured in years, age can be measured in months, days, hours, minutes, seconds

  Weight and height are also continuous variables.

Qualitative data

- Do not have numerical values.

  Example–color of skin, color of hair, severity of disease, religion, sex

Nominal data–data divided into qualitative categories or groups, no order is seen. Examples–Male/Female, Black/White

Ordinal data–Data has meaningful order but no information about size of interval.

Students raking in class–1st, 2nd,3rd., Severity of illness–Mild, Moderate, Severe shows increasing severity. Like this meaningful order seen but no size difference.

Interval–Data has meaningful order and also meaningful interval. Example, Temperature in degree C or Fahrenheit. No meaningful ratio.

Ratio–Data has meaningful order and ratio also. Example, Pulse rate 120/m is twice as fast as pulse rate of 60/m.

Data Presentation

Graphical Presentation

- This is a **visual** presentation of data
- It makes data **interesting** and makes it understanding easy for illiterate persons
- It will give **meaningful impression** immediately

Bar Diagram

- Variables are depicted as bars of equal breadth
- Length of the bar is proportional to the frequency of variable
- The distance between bars is kept equal
- In **simple bar chart** a single variable is depicted.

Histogram

- It is an area diagram consisting of series of adjacent blocks (rectangles)
- Entire area covered by a rectangle represents the entire frequency and the area covered by the individual block represents the frequency of that particular variable
- X-axis represents class intervals
- Y-axis represents frequency
- Histogram can deal with the data with unequal class intervals.

Frequency Polygon

- If the midpoints of the bars are connected by a continuous line and the bars removed the resulting graph is called frequency polygon
- In frequency polygon, the two ends of the graph are allowed to touch x-axis.

Line Diagram

- Best form of graphical presentation is the line diagram
- Trend of events over a period of time can be noted
- It can also be used to compare proportionate change in two variables over a period of time
- The curve in line diagram–No need to touch x axis.

Scatter Diagram

- Used to show relationship between two quantitative variables
- Dependent variable depicted on y axis and independent variable depicted on x axis

Pictogram popular method of presenting data to illiterate people.

Measures of central tendency	**Measures of dispersion/variation**
Statistical averages Mean • Arithmetic average • Influenced by extreme values • Easy to calculate and understand • Most useful measure	**Range** • Simplest measure of dispersion • Difference between the highest and lowest values • Indicates only the extreme values and nothing about the dispersion

Median • Mid point of any observation • Not affected by extreme values Mode • Commonly occurring values • Easy to understand, not affected by the extreme values Skewness–It can be explained simply as follows. • If the mean minus median gives the answer with minus symbol then it is negatively skewed and vice versa. • Here 130 (Mean) –140 (Median) = –10 (negative skewed distribution) • If Mean = Median = Mode–then it is normal distribution	**Quartiles** • 25th and 75th percentiles • First locate the median. The first quartile is the 1st to 25th observation, second quartiles–25th to 75th, 75th to 100th observation–Third quartile – 25th to 75th–Interquartile range (Q3–Q1) **Standard deviation** • Measure of spread around the mean and should be used when the mean is employed as the measure of centre • Average deviation of the observations from the mean • Square root of the average of the squared deviations • Square root of sum of (x-m)2/N Variance–Square of SD • Coefficient of variation–ratio of SD and mean expressed as percentage

Normal Curve (De Moirre and Gauss)

Characteristics

- Bell shaped, bilaterally symmetrical infinitely large number of observations
- Area of the curve is 1
- Mean median and mode all coincide
- The distance of a value from the mean of the curve in units of standard deviation is called relative deviate or standard normal variate Z = x – m/SD.

Population

- In biostatistics the term population is used to denote the units under study
- Thus if we want to study all the individuals in a city, all individuals will form a population.

Sample

- Sample is the portion of the population selected by a process called sampling
- Instead of studying the entire population only a sample is studied.

Sampling Methods

When a large proportion of individuals or items or units have to be studied we take a sample.

Methods

- Simple random–Random numbers are assigned to the individuals. Each person has an equal chance of being drawn in the sample. Lottery method
- Systematic random–Every 5th or 10th unit or the person
- Stratified random–Done for unequally distributed groups in the population (religion)
- Divide the groups or strata then do the sampling proportionately.

Sampling Variation

- When the two samples of same size are drawn from a population their means show variation with reference to each other and with reference to the population mean
- This variation is called as sampling variation.

Depends on two factors

1. Variation in the universe (population)
2. Sample size–Lesser the sample size more will be the variation.

Test of Significance

When we select a sample for drawing inferences about the underlying population it is assumed that the sample is representative of the population to which it belongs

To check the above–We are doing test of significance

- SE of mean, SE of difference between two means, SE of proportion, SE of difference between two proportion
- Start with null hypothesis
- Find out the P value (probability)
- If the P value > 0.05–Not significant
- If the P value < 0.05–Significant.

Type 1 error

- False positive conclusion that the samples are different actually they are not
- This is called alpha error.

Type 2 error

- Drawing a false negative conclusion that there is no difference when actually there is a difference (missing the true difference), called as beta error.

Inference

- If the p value is small (smaller than the level of alpha P less than 5% or 0.05) it is statistically significant, i.e the probability of null hypothesis being true is small and hence it is rejected
- If it is more than level of alpha level P > 0.05 then the null hypothesis cannot be rejected.

Two independent variables
- Qualitative (nominal)–Chi square test
- Quantitative (continuous)–Student t test

Two related groups
- Qualitative (nominal)–McNemar's and Chi-square test
- Quantitative (continuous)–paired t test

More than 2 groups
- Qualitative–Chi square test
- Quantitative–ANOVA–F

Correlation

To find out the association between two variables

- Ranges from –1 to +1
- – 1–negative association
- + 1–positive association
- 0–no association.

Probability

- Relative frequency (chance) of occurrence of an event
- Probability value ranges from 0 to 1
- We use symbol p for probability of an event occurring. Symbol q for probability for the event not occurring
- The sum of p and q always equal to 1.

Laws of probability

- Addition law–The probability occurrence of any two (or more) mutually exclusive events is equal to sum of two individual probabilities
- Multiplication law of probability–The probability of simultaneous or successive occurrence of two or more independent events is equal to the product of their separate probabilities.

Hospital Waste Management

Categories

• Cat 1–Human anatomical waste • Cat 2–Animal waste • Cat 3–Microbiology and biotechnology waste • Cat–4 Waste sharps • Cat 5–Discarded medicines and cytotoxic drugs	• Cat 6–Solid waste (items contaminated with blood like cotton, dressings, casts, etc.) • Cat 7–Solid waste (tubings, catheters, IV sets) • Cat 8–Liquid waste • Cat 9–Incineration ash • Cat 10–Chemicals used in disinfection (insecticides, disinfectants)

Colored bags and disposal methods

Yellow bag–Cat 1, 2, 3, 6–Incineration/deep burial
Red bag–Cat 3, 6 and 7–Autoclaving/Chemical treatment/microwaving
Blue/White translucent–Cat 4 and 7–Autoclaving/microwaving/chemical treatment
Black–Cat 5, 9 and 10–Disposal in secured lanfill

HEALTH PLANNING IN INDIA

Health planning involves all steps taken to identify common health problems establishing priority to them and initiate integrated programmes.

Health planning in India is an integral part of national socioeconomic planning.

Bhore Committee, 1946

The Government of India in 1943 appointed the Health survey and Development Committee with Sir Joseph Bhore as Chairman, to survey the then existing position regarding the health conditions and health organization in the country and to make recommendations for the future development.

Recommendations

- Integration of preventive and curative services
- Short term–Primary health centers for 40,000 population
- Long term–Primary health units with 75 beds for each 10,000–20,000 population
- Formation of village health committee
- Provision social physicians
- Inter-sectoral approach to health services development
- There months training in preventive and social medicine to prepare social physicians.

Mudaliar Committee, 1962

Health Survey and Planning Committee.

The Mudaliar committee found that the quality of services provided by the primary health centers inadequate, and advised strengthening of the existing primary health centers before new centers were established.

Recommendations

- Strengthening of the district hospital with specialist services
- Appointing of regional deputy or assistant directors to supervise 2 or 3 district medical and health officers
- Each primary health center not to serve more than 40,000 population
- To improve the quality of health care provided by the primary health centers
- Constitution of all India health service on the pattern of Indian Administrative Service.

Chadha Committee, 1963

- This committee was appointed under chairmanship of Dr MS Chadha, the then Director General of Health Services, to advise about the necessary arrangements for the maintenance phase of National Malaria Eradication Programme.

- The committee suggested that the vigilance activity in the NMEP should be carried out by basic health workers (one per 10,000 population), who would function as multipurpose workers and would perform, in addition to malaria work, the duties of family planning and vital statistics data collection under supervision of family planning health assistants.

Mukherjee Committee, 1965

- The recommendations of the Chadha Committee, when implemented, were found to be impracticable because the basic health workers, with their multiple functions could do justice neither to malaria work nor to family planning work.
- The Mukherjee committee headed by the then Secretary of Health Shri Mukherjee, was appointed to review the performance in the area of family planning.
- The committee recommended separate staff for the family planning programme.
- The family planning assistants were to undertake family planning duties only.
- The basic health workers were to be utilized for purposes other than family planning.
- The committee also recommended to de-link the malaria activities from family planning so that the latter would received undivided attention of its staff.

Jungalwalla Committee, 1967

- This committee, known as the 'Committee on Integration of Health Services' was set up in 1964 under the chairmanship of Dr N Jungalwalla, the then Director of National Institute of Health Administration and Education (currently NIHFW).
- It was asked to look into various problems related to integration of health services, abolition of private practice by doctors in government services, and the service conditions of Doctors. The committee defined 'integrated health services' as:
  - A service with unified approach for all problems instead of a segmented approach for different problems
  - Medical care and public health programmes should be put under charge of a single administrator.

Recommendations

- Unified cadre, common seniority, recognition of extra qualifications, equal pay for equal work, special pay for special work, abolition of private practice by government doctors, and *improvement in their servicing conditions.*

Kartar Singh Committee, 1973

- This committee, headed by the Additional Secretary of Health and titled the 'Committee on multipurpose workers under Health and Family Planning' was constituted to form a framework for integration of health and medical services at peripheral and supervisory levels.

Its main recommendations were:

- Various categories of peripheral workers should be amalgamated into a single cadre of multipurpose workers (male and female).
- The erstwhile auxiliary nurse midwives were to be converted into MPW(F) and the basic health workers, malaria surveillance workers, etc. were to be converted to MPW(M).
- The work of 3–4 male and female MPWs was to be supervised by one health supervisor (male or female respectively).
- The present day lady health visitors to be designated as female health supervisors.
- One Primary Health Center should cover a population of 50,000.
- It should be divided into 16 subcenters (one for 3000 to 3500 population) each to be staffed by a male and a female health worker.

Shrivastav Committee, 1975

This committee was set up in 1974 as 'Group on Medical Education and Support Manpower' to determine steps needed to

- Reorient medical education in accordance with national needs and priorities
- Develop a curriculum for health assistants who were to function as a link between medical officers and MPWs.

It recommended immediate action for:

- Creation of bonds of paraprofessional and semiprofessional health workers from within the community itself.
- Establishment of three cadres of health workers namely–multipurpose health workers and health assistants between the community level workers and doctors at PHC.
- Development of a 'Refferal Services Complex'
- Establishment of a Medical and Health Education Commission for planning and implementing the reforms needed in health and medical education on the lines of University Grants Commission.
- Acceptance of the recommendations of the Shrivastava Committee in 1977 led to the launching of the Rural Health Scheme, wherein training of community health workers, reorientation training of multipurpose workers, and linking medical colleges to rural health was initiated.

Occupational Health

Factories Act

- The Factories Act dates as far back as 1881. The recent amendment being 1987.
- The act applies to the whole of India except the state of Jammu and Kashmir.
- A minimum of 500 Cu ft space for each worker has been prescribed.
- Appointment of Safety officers in every factory wherein 1000 or more workers are ordinarily employed.
- If 500 or more workers are employed–one Welfare Officer.
- The act specifies that wherein more than 250 workers–a canteen shall be provided.
- Should provide crèches–if more than 30 women workers are employed.
- The act prohibits employment of children below the age of 14 years and declares that age between 15 to 18 as adolescents.
- Adolescents should be duly certified by the Certifying surgeons.
- Adolescents employee are allowed to work only between 6 AM and 7 PM.
- Prescribes a maximum of 48 hours per week not exceeding 9 hours per day with ½ hour rest after 5 hours of continuous work.
- The total number of hours of work in a week including overtime shall not exceed 60 hours.

ESI Act–1948

- Extends to whole India excluding (mines, railways, defence establishments)
- Including small power using factories employing 10 to 19 persons and nonpower using factories wherein 20 or more persons are employed
- Shops
- Hotels and restaurants
- Cinemas and theatres
- Road and motor transport establishments
- Newspaper establishment
- Finance
- Employer contributes–4.75% of wages
- Employee contributes–1.75% of wages
- Employees with wages less than ₹ 50 per day are exempted from contribution
- Medical care–state government 1/8th and ESI corporation share 7/8th of total, medical care
- Medical benefit–OP, IP care
- Establishment having more than 1000 employees–1 full time dispensary with a IMO, 750–part time dispensary
- Sickness benefit–maximum period of 91 days continuously, 50% of average daily wages

- Extended sickness benefit is for a maximum period of 2 years
- Enhanced sickness benefit is payable to insured women for 14 days–for tubectomy and for 7 days in case of vasectomy in respect of male
- Amount equal to full wages
- Maternity benefit–12 weeks for pregnancy, 6 weeks for miscarriage. Benefit full wages
- Disablement benefit–70% as long as he is having temporary disability, permanent–pension
- Dependants benefit–death as a result of employment injury–70% of wages is given monthly to the dependents
- Funeral expense–₹ 5000
- Rehabilitation allowance.

OCCUPATIONAL DISEASES

- Byssinosis–inhalation of cotton fibre dust–textile workers.

Silicosis

- Among occupational diseases major cause of permanent disability and mortality, first reported in Kolar gold mines–karnataka–1947
- Caused by inhalation of dust containing free silica or silicon dioxide
- Silicotics are more prone to pulmonary tuberculosis
- X-ray–shows snow storm appearance
- Silicosis–notifiable disease under factories act and Mines Act–1952

Anthracosis

- Coal mine workers (simple pneumoconosis or PMF)
- Notifiable disease–Mines Act 1952, compensatable in the workmens compensation act, 1959

Bagassosis

- Inhalation of sugar cane dust, due to thermophilic actinomycete, (Thermoactinomyces sacchari).

Asbestosis

- Serpentine type or chrysolite type, amphibole type
- Amphibole type is more common–90%
- Peribronchial diffuse and basal in location, X-ray–ground glass appearance
- Silicosis–apical lobe is commonly involved.

Farmer's lung–inhalation of mouldy hay or grain dust (microspora faeni).

NATIONAL HEALTH PROGRAMMES

Malaria programme milestones • 1953–NMCP launched • 1958–NMEP launched	Ecotypes and control measures • Economic development project areas–Mass screening of incoming laborers, antilarval measures, **IRS/ITN/LLINs**
• 1977–MPO implemented • 1999–Renaming into NAMP • 2005–introduction of RDT • 2002–renaming NAMP into NVBDCP • 2009–introduction of LLINs • 2010–New drug policy 2010	• Urban malaria–chemical and biological larviciding, environmental measures, **ITNs and LLINs,** Focus IRS in areas where it is feasible, other personal protection procedures • Tribal malaria–associated with forest environment–**IRS/ITN/LLIN** and limited role for larval control

- The goals under the national strategies for malaria control
- At least 50% reduction in mortality due to malaria by the year 2010, as per National Health Policy–2002
- At least 80% of those suffering from malaria get correct, affordable and appropriate treatment
- Treatment should be given within 24 hours of reporting to the health system, by the year 2012
- At least 80% of those at high-risk of malaria get protected by effective preventive measures such as ITNs/LLINs or IRS by 2012

TREATMENT FAILURES IN MALARIA (DEFINITIONS)

Early treatment failure (ETF)	Late clinical failure (LCF)	Late parasitological failure (LPF)
Early treatment failure (ETF): Development of danger signs or severe malaria on Day 1, 2 or 3, in the presence of parasitemia; parasitemia on Day 2 higher than on Day 0, irrespective of axillary temperature; parasitemia on Day 3 with axillary temperature 37.5 °C; and parasitemia on Day 3, 25% of count on Day 0.	Late clinical failure (LCF): Development of danger signs or severe malaria in the presence of parasitemia on any day between Day 4 and Day 28 (Day 42) in patients who did not previously meet any of the criteria of early treatment failure; and presence of parasitemia on any day between Day 4 and Day 28 (Day 42) with axillary temperature 37.5 °C in patients who did not previously meet any of the criteria of early treatment failure.	Late parasitological failure (LPF): Presence of parasitemia on any day between Day 7 and Day 28 with axillary temperature < 37.5 °C in patients who did not previously meet any of the criteria of early treatment failure or late clinical failure. • Such cases of falciparum malaria should be given alternative ACT or quinine with Doxycycline. • Doxycycline is contraindicated in pregnacy, lactation and in children up to 8 years. Treatment failure with chloroquine in P. vivax malaria is rare in India.

Roll Back Malaria

- Global partnership founded in 1998 by the World Health Organization (WHO), the United Nations Development Program (UNDP), the UNICEF and the world bank.
- Its aim is to halve the world's malaria burden by 2010.
- Interim target
  - At least 60% of those suffering from malaria have prompt access to treatment within 24 hours of the onset of symptoms
  - At least 60% of those at risk of malaria, particularly pregnant women and children under five years of age benefit from insecticide treated bed nets and suffering
  - At least 60% of all pregnant women who are at risk of malaria, especially those in their first pregnancies, have access to chemoprophylaxis

Technical strategies of RBM

- Prompt access to effective treatment
- Promotion of insecticide treated bed nets and improved vector control
- Prevention and management of malaria in pregnancy
- Improving the prevention and response to malaria epidemics and malaria in complex emergencies
  - Encourage the research in new and better drugs, insecticides and malaria vaccines
  - Strengthening health system and capacity building
  - Encourage linkages to other programmes and involvement of private sector

API less than 1	API between 1 and 2	API between 2–5	API above 5
• Vector control by minor engineering procedures • Biological control by use of larvicides • Involving PRIs by sensitizing them in rural areas and municipal bodies in urban areas	• Vector control by source reduction and biological control • Active surveillance by ASHA /ANM/MPW	• Vector control by distribution of LLIN • Quality IRS for selective vector control	Areas with perennial transmission • 2 rounds of IRS with DDT and 3 rounds with malathion • Distribution of LLIN • Vector bionomics studies Areas with seasonal transmission • 1 round of IRS with DDT • Focal spray wherever and whenever needed • Distribution of LLIN

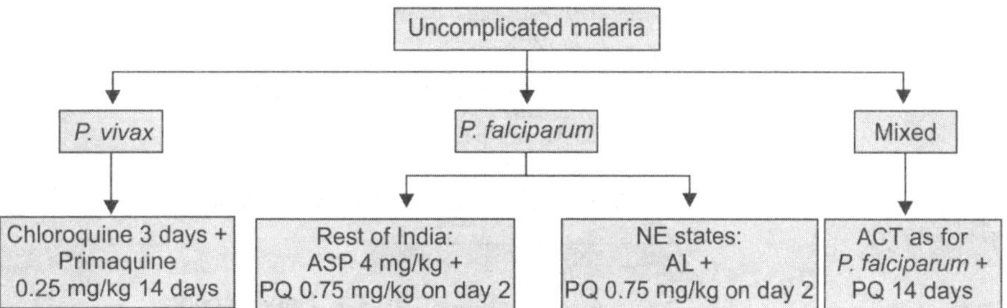

TUBERCULOSIS

Case definitions (Epidemiological definitions)

- Presumptive TB refers to a patient who presents with symptoms or signs suggestive of TB
- Bacteriologically confirmed TB case–A biological specimen is positive by smear microscopy, culture or WRD (WHO–RAPID DIAGNOSTIC)
- Clinically diagnosed TB case–One who does not fulfill criteria for bacteriological confirmation but has been diagnosed with active TB by a clinician or other medical practitioner who has decided to give the patient a full course of TB treatment
- **Mono resistance–resistance to one first line anti TB drug only**
- **Poly resistance–resistance to more than one first line anti TB drug (other than both isoniazid and rifampicin)**
- **Multi drug resistance–resistance to at least both isoniazid and rifampicin**
- Extensive Resistance to any fluorquinolone and at least one of three second line injectable drugs (capreomycin, kanamycin and amikacin)–in addition to multi drug resistance
- A pulmonary TB patient with bacteriologically confirmed TB at the beginning of treatment who was smear or culture negative in the last month of treatment and on at least one previous occasion–Cured
- A TB patient who completed treatment without evidence of failure but with no record to show that sputum smear or culture results were negative (test not done or results not available)–Treatment completed
- **A TB patient whose sputum smear or culture is positive at month 5 or later during treatment–Treatment failure**
- A TB patient who did not start treatment or whose treatment was interrupted for 2 consecutive months or more–**Lost to follow up**
- **The sum of cured and treatment completed–Treatment success**

HIV/AIDS programme

- 1986–first case of HIV was detected, National AIDS Committee was established under Ministry of Health
- 1992–NACP I–slow down the spread, National AIDS control board was constituted
- 1999–NACP II–focus on behavior change, state AIDS control societies established
- 2002–national AIDS control policy was adopted
- 2004–**antiretroviral treatment initiated**
- 2006–national policy on pediatric HIV formulated
- **Categories of districts**
  - Cat A–More than 1% ANC/PTCT prevalence in district at anytime in any of the sites in the last 3 years
  - Cat B–Less than 1% ANC/PTCT prevalence in all the sites during the last 3 years associated with more than 5% prevalence in any HRG
  - Cat C–Less than 1% in ANC prevalence in all sites during last 3 years with less than 5% in all STD clinic attendees or any HRG with known hot spots
  - Cat D–Less than 1% in ANC prevalence in all sites during last 3 years with less than 5% in all STD clinic attendees or any HRG or poor HIV data with no known hot spots

National blindness control programme

Diseases of focus globally

- Cataract
- Trachoma
- Onchocerclasis
- Childhood blindness
- Refractive Errors and Low Vision

The target diseases identified for Vision 2020 in India include:

- Cataract
- Childhood Blindness
- Refractive Errors and Low Vision
- Corneal Blindness
- Diabetic Retinopathy
- Glaucoma
- Trachoma (focal)

Contd...

Contd...

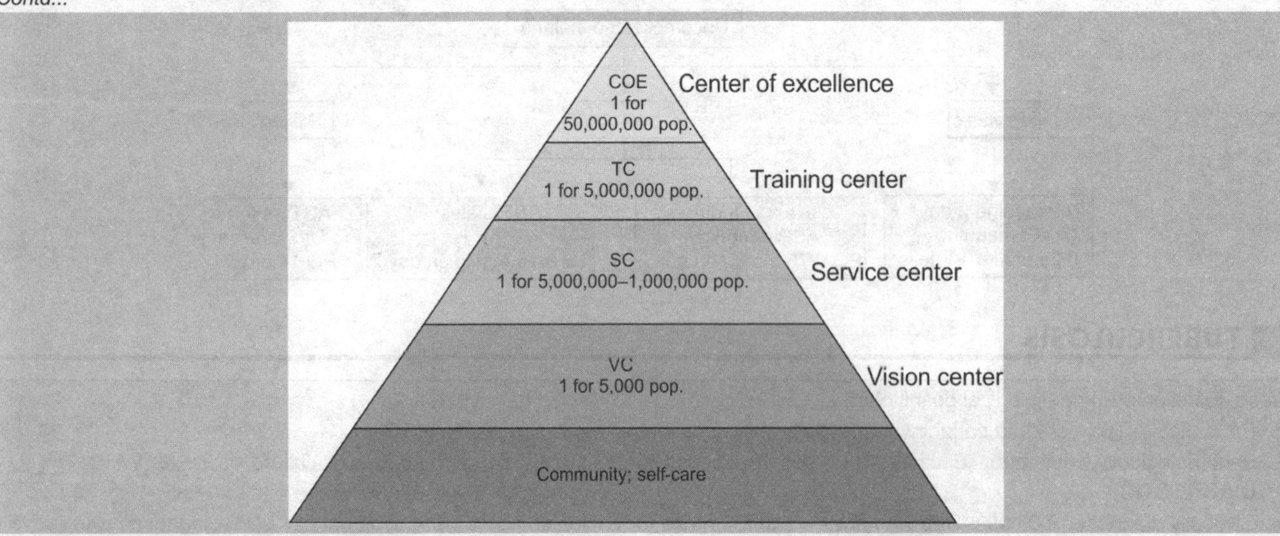

Miles stones–maternal and child health programmes

- 1992–CSSM programme
- 1997–RCH–I
- 2005–RCH–II
- 2005–NRHM
- 2013–RMNCH + A strategy
- 2013–National Health Mission
- 2014–India Newborn Action Plan (INAP)
- **SELECTION ASHA**
  - ASHA must be a resident of the village
  - The age group must be between 25 to 45 years
  - Formal education up to eighth class
  - The woman can be married/divorced/single
  - The general norm of selection will be one ASHA for 1000 population.

Facility based newborn care is divided into three levels

- MCH level I–PHC and sub-center level–for sick newborns → prompt referral
- MCH level II–Community health center (FRUs)–for sick newborns → (NBSU)–Newborn stabilization unit
- MCH level III–District hospital → Special Newborn care unit (SNCU)
- No MCH level IV is present as of now
- **NBCC–New born care corner–space within the delivery room in any health facility where immediate care is provided to all newborns at birth, which is mandatory for all health facilities at all levels.**

RBSK (Rashtriya Bal Swasthya Karyakram)

Launched to provide comprehensive health care and improve the quality of life of children through early detection of birth defects, diseases, deficiencies, and development delays including disability

RKSK (Rashtriya Kishor Swasthya Karyakram)

Launched to comprehensively address the health needs of adolescents in new dimensions like mental health, nutrition, substance misuse, injuries, and violence and noncommunicable diseases

- JSSK–Zero out of pocket expenditure for maternal and infant health services through free health care and referral transport entitlements.
- RBSK–Screening of children with birth defects, diseases, deficiencies, developmental delays.

NUHM

- 1 U–CHC per 2.5 lakh population (in patient facility–30 to 50 bedded)
- 1 U–PHC–per 50,000 population
- Mahila Arogya Samiti–per 50 to 100 households or 1000 to 2500 population
- 1 ANM per 10,000 population
- 1 community health volunteer (ASHA/USHA/LW)–200 to 500 households or 1000 or 2500 population

QUESTIONS

1. **Which is transmitted by Mansonia? (2014)**
   a. Bancroftian filariasis
   b. Japanese encephalitis
   c. Dengue
   d. Chickungunya

2. **Most abundant element in nature: (2014)**
   a. Fluorine
   b. Phosphorus
   c. Iodine
   d. Calcium

3. **Millennium development goal targets to reduce MMR in 2015 by: (2014)**
   a. 0.25
   b. 0.75
   c. 0.50
   d. 1.0
4. **Meta zoonosis is: (2014)**
   a. Plague
   b. Rabies
   c. Taenia
   d. Tapeworm
5. **All are live vaccines except: (2014)**
   a. BCG
   b. Yellow fever
   c. Salk vaccine
   d. Measles
6. **The color of bag used to dispose sharp wastes is: (2014)**
   a. Red
   b. Blue white translucent
   c. Yellow
   d. Black
7. **Preventing obesity is an example of which of the following types of prevention? (2014)**
   a. Primordial
   b. Primary
   c. Secondary
   d. Tertiary
8. **True statement regarding case control studies is: (2014)**
   a. Best to study rare diseases
   b. Moves from cause to effect
   c. Cost effective
   d. Large number of participants needed
9. **False statement regarding point source epidemic is: (2014)**
   a. Many secondary waves
   b. Cases occur in clusters
   c. All cases occur within one incubation period
   d. Rapid rise and fall
10. **Test of statistical significance are all except: (2014)**
    a. SD
    b. Standard error of mean
    c. Standard error proportion
    d. Chi-square test
11. **In NRHM, the ASHA workers are recruited from the same village. Which part of principles of primary health care is followed here? (2014)**
    a. Intersectorial coordination
    b. Equitable distribution
    c. Appropriate technology
    d. Community participation
12. **Iron requirement in lactating mother is: (2014)**
    a. 30 mg/day
    b. 34 mg/day
    c. 36 mg/day
    d. 38 mg/day
13. **For monitoring of food standards in international market, standard followed is: (2014)**
    a. Codex alimentarius
    b. AGMARK
    c. PFA (Prevention of Food adulteration Act)
    d. BIS
14. **Best assessment of protein quality is done through: (2014)**
    a. Net prostein utilization
    b. Protein biological value
    c. Digestibility coefficient
    d. Protein energy ratio
15. **Human developmental index includes all except: (2013)**
    a. Adult literacy
    b. Per capita income
    c. Life expectancy
    d. Infant mortality rate
16. **Measure of infectivity of a disease: (2013)**
    a. Incidence rate
    b. Prevalence rate
    c. Secondary attack rate
    d. Case fatality rate
17. **Recommended concentration of iodine in iodized salt at consumer level is: (2013)**
    a. 20 ppm
    b. 15 ppm
    c. 10 ppm
    d. 5 ppm
18. **Recommended residual chlorine level after 1 hour contact period is: (2013)**
    a. 0.5
    b. 1.0
    c. 1.5
    d. 2
19. **All are indicators of 'Physical Quality Life Index' except: (2013)**
    a. Real GDP per capita income
    b. Literacy
    c. Life expectancy at age one
    d. Infant mortality
20. **Ultra low volume fogging is done for: (2013)**
    a. DDT
    b. Malathion
    c. Pyrethroid
    d. Abate

21. Sampling is nonhomogenous group: **(2013)**
a. Simple random
b. Stratified random sampling
c. Clustered sampling
d. Systematic sampling

22. ESI sickness benefit scheme for confinement: **(2013)**
A. 60 days
B. 30 days
C. 15 days
D. 7 days

23. Target in RNTCP case detection for tuberculosis: **(2013)**
a. 70%
b. 95%
c. 85%
d. 90%

24. Cyclopropagative means: **(2013)**
a. Only development
b. Only multiplication
c. No development and no multiplication
d. Multiplication and development

25. Positive predictive value is: **(2013)**
a. a/a+c*100
b. d/b+d*100
c. a/a+b*100
d. d/c+d*100

26. Most cost effective intervention for NCD: **(2013)**
a. Primordial
b. Primary
c. Secondary
d. Specific protection

27. Criteria for incinerations of waste are all except: **(2013)**
a. Low heating volume
b. Percentage of combustible material greater than 60%
c. Percentage of noncombustible material less than 5%
d. Moisture content greater than 30%

28. The interval between the primary and the secondary case is called: **(2012)**
a. Serial interval
b. Generation time
c. Median incubation period
d. Latent period

29. The ability of a test to detect true negatives is: **(2012)**
a. Sensitivity
b. Specificity
c. PPV
d. NPV

30. Antibiotic in SAFE strategy is: **(2012)**
a. Azithromycin
b. Rifampicin
c. Penicillin
d. Tetracycline

31. Size of dust particles reaching alveoli: **(2012)**
a. < 5 microns
b. 5–10 microns
c. > 15 microns
d. 10–15 microns

32. Screening of coronary heart disease by: **(2012)**
a. LDH
b. Total serum cholesterol
c. LDL
d. HDL

33. Category 2 ATT in India: **(2012)**
a. Smear positive after 6 months therapy-default
b. Sputum positive
c. Seriously ill sputum negative
d. New smear positive extrapulmonary tb

34. Mosquito free airport perimeter: **(2012)**
a. 400 m
b. 100 m
c. 200 m
d. 500 m

35. Normal fluoride level in water: **(2012)**
a. 2.0 mg/l
b. 0.5 mg/l
c. 1.5 mg/l
d. 2.5 mg/l

36. ICDS programme under: **(2012)**
a. Ministry of H and FW
b. Ministry of Education
c. Ministry of Social Welfare
d. Ministry of GRD

37. During outbreak of an epidemic first thing to do: **(2012)**
a. Verification of diagnosis
b. Confirmation of the epidemic
c. Defining; the population at risk
d. Rapid searh for all cases

38. Subclinical infection is not seen in: **(2012)**
a. Measles
b. Mumps
c. Rubella
d. Japanse encephalitis

39. Which of the following is best in studying the decline in percentage of alcohol usage in men and women over several years? (2011)
a. Pie chart
b. Histogram
c. Frequency polygon
d. Line diagram

40. Point prevalence overestimates diseases with:
a. High incidence (2011)
b. Low incidence
c. Chronic course
d. High morality

41. A screening test for Ca breast has sensitivity of 90% and specificity of 90%. What is the chance that a patient with Ca breast remains undetected for two consecutive years? (2011)
a. 1/10
b. 2/10
c. 1/100
d. 2/100

42. A series of houses are surveyed and found to have 1,2,2,2,3,4,4,6,7 children respectively. Find the mean, median, and mode of the following:
a. 2,3,4, (2011)
b. 3,2,4
c. 2,3,2
d. 1,2,3

43. A study to evaluate the relationship between smoking and pregnancy was performed with history of smoking exposures taken during ANC visit and the child birth weight after delivery. This type of study is: (2011)
a. Case control
b. Prospective cohort
c. Cross-sectional
d. Clinical trial

44. Which of the following is not considered for selecting a screening test? (2011)
a. Disease burden
b. Physician's knowledge of the disease
c. Cost of the test
d. Treatment efficacy

45. A patient with cervical cancer is missed by a screening test and later diagnosed to have advanced disease. This time interval is called:
a. Lead time (2011)
b. Screening time
c. Serial interval
d. Generation time

46. Test used to study the ordinal data of two independent groups which are not distributed normally: (2011)
a. Student T-test
b. Paired T-test
c. Wilocoxon's signed rank test
d. Mann-Whitney U test

47. What is true about case fatality rate? (2010)
a. It is a ratio
b. It is not useful for acute disease
c. Related to virulence
d. Not useful in chronic diseases

48. Confounding factor can be eliminated by:
a. Matching (2010)
b. Correlation
c. Standardization
d. Randomization

49. Which is done even after control of disease?
a. Surveillance (2010)
b. Vaccination
c. Chemoprophylaxis
d. Prolonged treatment

50. Primary and secondary prevention of a disease is done for: (2010)
a. Control
b. Eradication
c. Elimination
d. Surveillance

51. A vaccine's efficacy is calculated to be 95%. It literally means: (2010)
a. 5 out of 100 children can get infection even after vaccination
b. 95% of children will not get the disease
c. 95% are no longer susceptible to infection following vaccination
d. 95% of the population is protected

52. Most sensitive parameter in monitoring iodine deficiency control programme is: (2010)
a. Goiter
b. Urine T3, T4
c. Growth retardation
d. Neonatal hypothyroidism

53. Which of the following is a killed vaccine?
a. Japanese encephalitis (2010)
b. Measles
c. BCG
d. Yellow fever

54. **Most common cause of death in the under five age group in developing countries is: (2010)**
    a. Malnutrition
    b. Respiratory diseases
    c. Diarrhea
    d. Road traffic accidents
55. **Which respiratory illness is more common in a paper mill worker? (2010)**
    a. Anthracosis
    b. Byssinosis
    c. Bagassosis
    d. Asbestosis
56. **RNTCP target level (2010)**
    a. 70% detection 85% cure
    b. 70% detection 85% cure
    c. 80% detection 75% cure
    d. 80% detection 75% cure
57. **The number of live births/no of females 15–45 in the population denotes: (2010)**
    a. General fertility rate
    b. Total fertility rate
    c. Gross reproduction rate
    d. Age specific fertility rate
58. **Following are louse-borne disease: (2009)**
    a. Endemic typhus
    b. KFD
    c. Lyme's disease
    d. Trench fever
59. **Point prevalence of a chronic disease is studied best by: (2009)**
    a. Case control study
    b. Cross-sectional study
    c. Historical cohort
    d. Cohort
60. **In Revised National TB Control Programme main-stay of diagnosis of pulmonary tuberculosis is: (2009)**
    a. Sputum AFB
    b. CXR
    c. Clinical examination
    d. PCR
61. **Yellow fever is not present in India because of absence of: (2009)**
    a. The virus
    b. The vector mosquito aedes
    c. Suitable atmospheric condition
    d. Susceptible individuals
62. **The approximate magnitude of completed family size from demographic point of view is given by: (2009)**
    a. TFR
    b. GFR
    c. NRR
    d. GRR
63. **According to WHO the minimum number of antenatal visits to prevent maternal mortality is: (2009)**
    a. 3
    b. 6
    c. 9
    d. 12
64. **What is the definition of blindness according to WHO? (2009)**
    a. Vision less than 3/60
    b. < 6/60
    c. < 6/18
    d. Only no light perception
65. **Which of the following is not a priority vaccine for the first years of life? (2009)**
    a. Hib
    b. Hepatitis B
    c. DPT
    d. BCG
66. **Which of the following rates is not only an indicator of mortality but also of the living standard of a community? (2009)**
    a. IMR
    b. PNMR
    c. MMR
    d. CDR
67. **Which of the following is a parametric test of significance? (2009)**
    a. U test
    b. T-test
    c. Chi-square test
    d. Kruskal-Wallis test
68. **Most common cause of blindness in India is: (2009)**
    a. Cataract
    b. Refractive error
    c. Glaucoma
    d. Diabetes
69. **Minimum educational requirement for ASHA: (2009)**
    a. Class eight or higher
    b. Class ten or higher
    c. Completed 10 + 2
    d. No educational qualification required

70. A patient with cervical cancer is missed by a screening test and later diagnosed to have advanced disease. This time interval is called:
a. Lead time (2009)
b. Screening time
c. Serial interval
d. Generation time

71. Sickness absenteeism is a useful index to assess:
a. Workers management relationship (2009)
b. Working environment
c. State of health of workers
d. Sincerity of the workers

72. When there is an extreme value, best indicator of average to be used is: (2008)
a. Median
b. Mean
c. Mode
d. Standard deviation

73. Pearl Index is: (2008)
a. Failure rate per 100 women years of exposure
b. Success rate per 100 women years of exposure
c. Failure rate per 1000 women years of exposure
d. Success rate per 1000 women years of exposure

74. The most important index of screening test for a patient: (2008)
a. Positive predictive value
b. Negative predictive value
c. Sensitivity
d. Specificity

75. Normal water fluoride level in mg/L: (2008)
a. 0.5–0.8
b. 1.5–2.0
c. 0.05–0.08
d. 5–8

76. A screening test for Ca breast has sensitivity of 90% and specificity of 90%. What is the chance that a patient with Ca breast remains undetected for two consecutive years? (2008)
a. 1/10
b. 2/10
c. 1/100
d. 2/100

77. Most common sources of lead to cause increased blood level is from: (2008)
a. Inhalation
b. Ingestion of food
c. Ingestion of water
d. Cutaneous

78. The term family size in demographic parlance means: (2008)
a. The total number of children women has borne at a point of time
b. The total number of children of couples
c. The total number of children by women borne in a female between 15–45 years
d. The total number of members in the family

79. Test used to study the ordinal data of two independent groups which are not distributed normally: (2008)
a. Student T test
b. Paired T test
c. Wilocoxon's signed rank test
d. Mann-Whitney U test

80. Which of the following is true about cohort study? (2008)
a. Incidence can be calculated
b. It is from effect to cause
c. It is inexpensive
d. Shorter time than case control

81. Which of the following disease is not included in international health regulations (2008)
a. Plague
b. Yellow fever
c. Cholera
d. Polio

82. The size of sand particle in slow sand filter is:
a. 0.1–0.2 mm (2008)
b. 2–0.3 mm
c. 0.3–0.4 mm
d. 0.4–0.5 mm

83. Which of the following is used to destroy algae in water? (2008)
a. Copper sulfate
b. Potassium permanganate
c. Hypochlorite
d. Bleaching powder

84. Validity of a screening test includes all except:
a. Sensitivity (2008)
b. Specificity
c. Repeatability
d. Accuracy

85. Vector of Japanese Encephalitis in South India is:
a. Culex tritaneorhyncus (2008)
b. Anopheles
c. Aedes
d. Mansonoides

86. All the following are examples of health promotion except: **(2007)**
a. Stop smoking
b. Installation of sanitary latrine
c. Chemoprophylaxis
d. Decreased salt intake

87. One of the following helps deliver of baby in the community: **(2007)**
a. Health worker female
b. Anganwadi worker
c. Health assistant female
d. Village health guide

88. Standard normal deviate is given by the formula:
a. $(x-\bar{x}/sd)$ **(2007)**
b. $(x-\bar{x})$ 2/sd
c. $(x-\bar{x})$ 2/sd
d. $(x+\bar{x})$/sd

89. Relative risk is assesses all of the following except:
a. Strength of association **(2007)**
b. Biological plausibility
c. Dose response
d. Temporality

90. Median incubation period means: **(2007)**
a. Time for 50% cases to occur
b. Time between primary case and secondary case
c. Time between onset of infection and period of maximum infectivity
d. Median of several incubation period

91. In census literacy rate is assessed by: **(2007)**
a. Attended literacy classes for one year
b. Ability to write signature
c. Ability to read and write
d. Attended schooling

92. Significance of difference between two proportions is best studied by: **(2007)**
a. 't' test
b. Chi-square test
c. ANOVA
d. Regression coefficient

93. All are true about normal response curve except:
a. Bell shaped **(2007)**
b. Total area of curve = 1
c. SD = 0
d. Mean, mode, median coincide

94. Minimum level of free chlorine in potable water is:
a. 1 mg **(2007)**
b. 0.5 mg
c. 0.2 mg
d. 0.7 mg

95. Annual blood smear examination rate in malaria survey is an indicator: **(2007)**
a. Disease rate
b. Infectivity rate
c. Operational efficiency
d. Carrier state

96. Chandler's endemic index is used in: **(2007)**
a. Dengue hemorrhagic fever
b. Malaria
c. Hookworm infestation
d. Cholera

97. PQLI does not include: **(2007)**
a. Infant mortality rate
b. Gross national product
c. Literacy rate
d. Life expectancy at 1 year of age

98. Culex mosquito transmits: **(2007)**
a. Yellow fever
b. Dengue fever
c. Tularemia
d. Japanese encephalitis

99. The extra calorie intake required for a lactating mother is: **(2007)**
a. 400 Kcal
b. 450 Kcal
c. 500 Kcal
d. 550 Kcal

100. Kuppuswamy's socioeconomic status classification includes all except: **(2007)**
a. Income
b. Occupations
c. Housing
d. Education

101. Net Reproductive Rate of 1 implies a Couple Protection Rate of: **(2007)**
a. 50
b. 60
c. 70
d. 80

102. A case of chickenpox should be isolated for a period of: **(2006)**
a. 6 days
b. 10 days
c. 12 days
d. 14 days

103. In RNTCP the most effective tool for case finding is:
a. Sputum examination **(2006)**
b. Radiology
c. Culture
d. Mantoux test

104. Most common cause of blindness in India is:
a. Cataract (2006)
b. Refractive error
c. Glaucoma
d. Diabetes

105. Indalone belong to following type of insecticide:
a. Stomach poison (2006)
b. Contact poison
c. Repellant
d. Block respiration

106. 'Confounding bias' in a case control study can be removed by: (2006)
a. Double blinding
b. By properly recalling events
c. Matching
d. By selecting representative population

107. A village has a total of 100 under five children. The coverage with measles vaccine in this age group is 60%. Following the occurrence of measles case in a child after a visit outside, 12 children developed measles. The secondary attack rate of measles is:
a. 12% (2006)
b. 33%
c. 30%
d. 15%

108. Who is ASHA? (2006)
a. Worker of a Non-Governmental Organization
b. Community level voluntary worker for health
c. Government health worker
d. Helper of Anganwadi

109. The limiting amino acid in Bengal gram is:
a. Methionine (2006)
b. Lysine
c. Leucine
d. Tryptophan

110. What is not true about Chi square test? (2006)
a. Nonparametric test
b. Continuous variables
c. Proportion
d. Compares more than 2 groups

111. All of the following are tests for milk pasteurization except: (2006)
a. Methylene blue
b. Phosphatase test
c. Standard plate count
d. Coliform count

112. All of the following are milk-borne diseases except: (2006)
a. Brucellosis
b. Pasturella
c. Streptococcal infections
d. Viral hepatitis

113. Maternal mortality rate the denominator is:
a. 1000 live births (2006)
b. 100 live births
c. 1000 total births
d. 100 total births

114. Regarding midday meal programme, true statement is: (2006)
a. ⅓ of calories and ½ of protein is supplemented
b. ½ of calories and ⅓ of protein is supplemented
c. ⅓ of calories and ⅓ of protein is supplemented
d. ½ calories and ½ of protein is supplemented

115. Amount of residual chlorine to be present after contact time should: (2006)
a. 0.5 mg/dl
b. 1 mg/dl
c. 1.5 mg/dl
d. 2 mg/dl

116. The minimum contact period after chlorination:
a. ½ hour (2006)
b. 1 hour
c. 2 hours
d. 3 hours

ANSWERS AND EXPLANATIONS

1. Ans. d. Chickungunya *Ref: Park's Textbook of Preventive and Social Medicine, 22/e p716*

- Anopheles transmits–Malaria and Filaria (but not in India)
- Culex transmits–**Bancroftian filariasis, JE**, West Nile fever, Viral arthritis
- Aedes transmits–Yellow fever, Dengue, **Chikungunya fever,** Rift valley fever, Filaria (not in India)
- Mansonoides transmits–Malayan (brugian) filariasis, **Chikungunya fever**

- Mansonia mosquito
- Big black or brown mosquitoes with speckling on their wings and legs

- Breed on certain aquatic plants especially pistia, water hyacinth
- The larvae and pupae are found attached to the rootlets of these plants by their siphon tubes

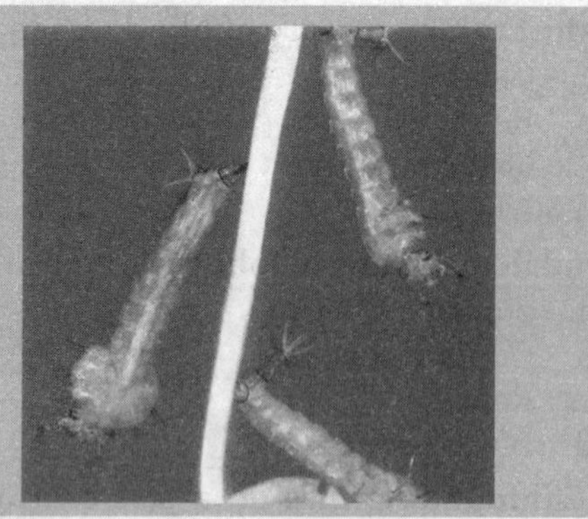

2. Ans. a. Fluorine *Ref: Park's Textbook of Preventive and Social Medicine, 22/e p579*

- Fluorine is the most abundant element in nature
- 96% of fluoride in the body is found in bone and teeth
- The major source of fluorine is drinking water
- Called as Double edged sword
- Recommended level of fluorides in drinking water in India is accepted as 0.5 to 0.8 mg/litre
- RDA for calcium is 600 mg for adults
- RDA for Iodine is 150 micrograms and during pregnancy the RDA is 250 mcg.

3. Ans. b. 0.75 *Ref: Park's Textbook of Preventive and Social Medicine, 22/e p835*

Millennium development goals (goal number)

- **Eradicate poverty and hunger–halve between 1990 and 2015, the proportion of people who suffer from hunger**
- **Achieve universal primary education**
- **Promote gender equality and empower woman**
- **Reduce child mortality–reduce by two thirds between 1990 and 2015, the under five mortality**
- **Improve maternal health–reduce by three quarters, between 1990 and 2015, the maternal mortality ratio**
- **Combat HIV and AIDS, Malaria and other diseases**
  - **Halted by 2015, and begun to reverse, the spread of HIV/AIDS**
  - **Have halted by 2015, and begun to reverse the incidence of malaria and major diseases**
- **Empower environment sustainability**
  - **Integrate the principles of sustainable development into country policies and programmes and reverse the loss of environmental resources**
- **Development a global partnership for development–provide access to affordable, essential drugs in developing countries**

Health related goals are (Goal number 1, 4, 5, 6, 7 and 8)

4. Ans. a. Plague *Ref: Park's Textbook of Preventive and Social Medicine, 22/e p251*

Meta-zoonoses are transmitted biologically by invertebrate vectors. In the invertebrate, the agent multiplies or develops, or both and there is always an extrinsic incubation (prepatent) period before transmission to another vertebrate host is possible. Examples, Arbovirus infections, Plague and Schistosomiasis.

• **Zoonoses**	• **Zooanthroponoses**	• **Direct zoonoses**	• **Cyclozoonoses**
• An infection or infectious disease transmissible under natural conditions from vertebrate animals to man. Example, rabies, plague • **Anthropozoonoses** • Infections transmitted to man from vertebrate animals. Example, rabies, plague	• Infections transmitted from man to vertebrate animals. Example, human tuberculosis in cattle • **Amphixenoses** • Infections maintained in both man and lower vertebrate animals that may be transmitted in either direction. Example, T. cruzi, S. japonicum	• Infections which transmitted from an infected vertebrate host to a susceptible vertebrate host by direct contact, by contact with fomite, or by mechanical vector. The agent does not undergo any propogative or developmental changes. Example, rabies, brucellosis	• Infections which require more than one vertebrate host species, but no invertebrate host, in order to complete the developmental cycle of the agent. Example, human teniasis, echinococcosis • **Saprozoonoses** • Have both a vertebrate host and a non animal developmental site or reservoir. Non animal sites may include soil, plants etc. Example, Larva migrants, Mycoses

5. Ans. c. Salk vaccine *Ref: Park's Textbook of Preventive and Social Medicine, 22/e p99*

Salk Vaccine–Killed vaccine–IPV–given subcutaneously or IM which induce circulating antibody, not useful in controlling epidemics.

• **Live vaccines**	• **Killed vaccines**
• BCG–intradermal–0.05 ml	• Typhoid
• Typhoid oral	• Cholera
• Oral polio–2 to 3 drops	• Pertusis
• Measles–Sc, 0.5 ml	• Plague
• Mumps	• Rabies
• Rubella	• Salk polio
• Yellow fever	• Influenza
• Influenza	• Hep B–Im
• Epi. Typhus	• JE
	• KFD

6. Ans (b) Blue white translucent *Ref: Park's Textbook of Preventive and Social Medicine, 22/e p739*

According to Park 22nd edition–The answer is 'b' choice–Sharp wastes (Category–4)–Category 4 and 7

Categories of biomedical waste management
- Cat 1–Human anatomical waste
- Cat 2–Animal waste
- Cat 3–Microbiology and biotechnology waste
- Cat–4 Waste sharps
- Cat 5–Discarded medicines and cytotoxic drugs
- Cat 6–Solid waste (items contaminated with blood like cotton, dressings, casts, etc.)
- Cat 7–Solid waste (tubings, catheters, iv sets)
- Cat 8–Liquid waste
- Cat 9–Incineration ash
- Cat 10–Chemicals used in disinfection (insecticides, disinfectants)

Color coding and disposal
- Yellow bag–Cat 1, 2, 3, 6–Incineration/deep burial
- Red bag–Cat 3,6 and 7–Autoclaving/Chemical treatment/microwaving
- Blue/White translucent–Cat 4 and 7–Autoclaving/microwaving/chemical treatment
- Black–Cat 5,9 and 10–Disposal in secured landfill

7. Ans. a. Primordial *Ref: Park's Textbook of Preventive and Social Medicine, 22/e p39, 40*

Preventing the development of risk factors falls under primordial prevention. (Action taken before the emergence of risk factors is called primordial prevention)

• Primordial–action taken prior to the emergence of risk factors	• Primordial and primary prevention
• Primary–action taken prior to the onset of disease	• Health promotion
• Secondary–action which halts the progress of the disease	• Specific protection
• Tertiary–measures taken to reduce or limit disabilities	• Secondary prevention
	• Early diagnosis and treatment
	• Tertiary prevention
	• Disability limitation
	• Rehabilitation

8. Ans. a. Best to study rare diseases *Ref: Park's Textbook of Preventive and Social Medicine, 22/e p71*

Case control studies proceed from effect to cause. Both exposure and outcome has already occurred before the initiation of the study. It is also called retrospective studies, which proceed backwards and involve very few number of subjects as compared to cohort studies which involve large number of study participants.

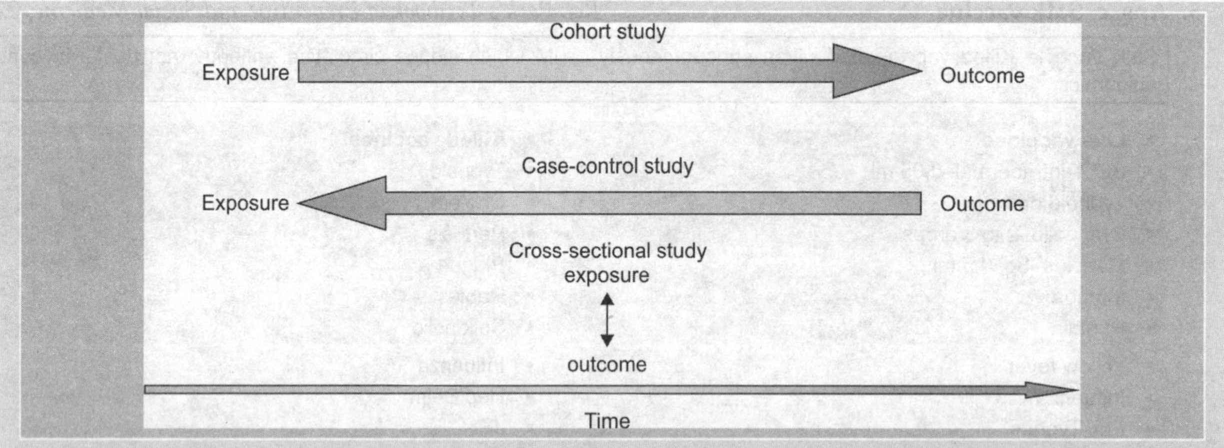

Case Control Study	Cohort Study
• Proceeds from effect to cause	• Proceeds from cause to effect
• Starts with the disease	• Starts with the people exposed to risk factor
• Involves few number of subjects	• Involves large number of subjects
• Yields relatively quick results	• Long follow up period, involving delayed results
• Suitable for study of rare diseases	• Suitable for study of rare exposures
• Yields only estimate of RR (odds ratio)	• Yields incidence rates, RR and AR
• Inexpensive	• Expensive

9. Ans. a. Many secondary waves *Ref: Park's Textbook of Preventive and Social Medicine, 22/e p62*

Point source epidemic is also called Common source single exposure–because the exposure is simultaneous, all the cases occur within one incubation period and the epidemic curve will have only one peak with no secondary curves or waves. Whereas slow rise and slow falls will be seen in propagated epidemics.

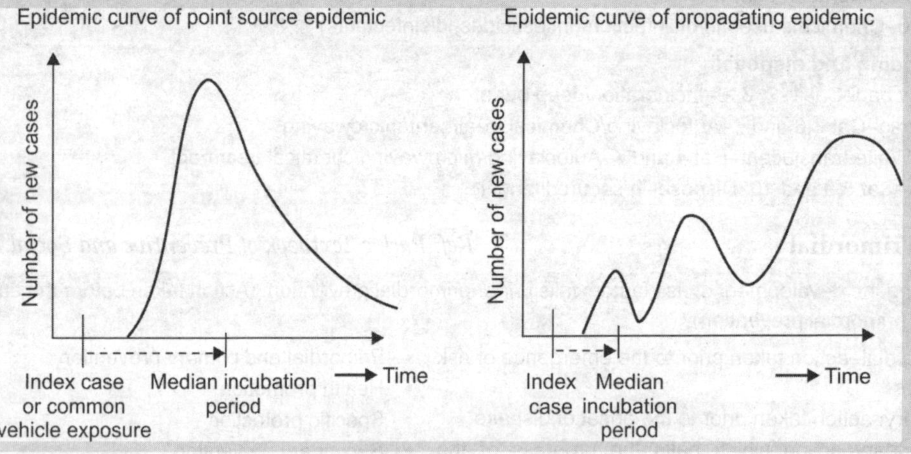

10. Ans. a. SD *Ref: Park's Textbook of Preventive and Social Medicine, 22/e p793*

1. Test of significance: These statistical tests done to assess the outcome of null hypothesis. These tests are done with standard error because it indicates how reliable an estimate of the mean is likely to be. Examples for tests of significance are parametric and nonparametric tests.
2. Parametric test of significance: Done for quantitative data–Example student *t*-test and ANOVA
3. Nonparametric test of significance: Done for qualitative data–Example–Chi-square test and McNemar's test
4. Standard deviation is nothing but the deviation from the mean in normal distribution and gives us the idea of the spread of the dispersion that the larger the SD the greater the dispersion of values about the mean.

11. Ans. d. Community participation *Ref: Park's Textbook of Preventive and Social Medicine, 22/e p20, 413, 833*

The concept of primary health care centers round people's participation in their own activities. The village health guide scheme in India is an example of community participation. Similarly ASHA scheme under NRHM, Anganwadi worker under ICDS scheme, Malaria Link volunteer scheme under NAMP, Training the Local Dais for clean delivery are all examples of community participation which is community responsibility.

12. Ans. a. 30 mg/day *Ref: Park's Textbook of Preventive and Social Medicine, 22/e p578, 590*

Page number 578.
Pregnant woman weighing 55 kg (Prepregnancy weight)–2.80 mg of iron should be absorbed for daily needs.
Lactating woman (0–6 months)–weighing 55 kg–1.65 mg of iron should be absorbed for daily needs.
Page number 590
Pregnant woman–35 mg/day is the iron requirement
Lactating woman–21 mg/day is the iron requirement
Because 30 mg/day is closer answer we can go for the choice–A

13. Ans. a. Codex Alimentarius *Ref: Park's Textbook of Preventive and Social Medicine, 22/e p612*

Food standards: Codex Alimentarius, PFA Standards, The Agmark Standards, Bureau of Standards.
Codex Alimentarius–principal organ of Joint FAO and WHO food standards programme formulates food standards for **international market**. The food standards in India are based standards of codex alimentarius.
PFA standards–the purpose of the PFA standards is to obtain a minimum level of quality of food stuffs.
ISI And AGMARK–Assurance and guarantee of good quality in accordance with the standards.

14. Ans. a. Net protein utilization *Ref: Park's Textbook of Preventive and Social Medicine, 22/e p588*

NPU–is the product of Biological value and digestibility coefficient. NPU is nothing but the amount of nitrogen retained in the body in relation to the total nitrogen intake. NPU is more complete expression of protein quality than amino acid score.
Amino acid score is amount of amino acid present in the test protein in relation to the reference protein.
The measure of protein quantity is protein energy ratio. (Energy from protein in relation to total energy in the diet).

15. Ans. d. Infant morality rate *Ref: Park's Textbook of Preventive and Social Medicine, 22/e p16*

- HDI–Defined as composite index of combining three indicators–longevity (life expectancy at birth), knowledge (adult literacy rate and mean years of schooling) and income (real GDP per capita in Purchasing power parity in US dollars).
- HDI value ranges between 0 to 1, 0.8 and above means high human development category, 0.5 to 0.799–medium human development categories and less than 0.5–low human development category.
- India comes in the medium (0.547) human development category, ranking at number 134.

- The dimensions used in HPI-1, for developing countries.
- A long and healthy life vulnerability to death at a relatively early age (probability at birth of not surviving to age 40.
- Knowledge–exclusion from the world of reading and communications.
- A decent standard of living–lack of access to overall economic provisioning (percentage of population not using an improved water source and the percentage of children under weight for age).
- **HPI is expressed as percentages.**
- HPI-2 includes the following dimensions, for developed countries.
- Probability at birth of not surviving to age 60.
- Exclusion from the world of reading and communications as measured by percentage of adults (16–65) lacking functional literacy skills.
- Percentage of people living below the income poverty line.
- **Social exclusion–as measured by the rate of long-term unemployment 12 months or more.**

16. Ans. c. Secondary attack rate *Ref: Park's Textbook of Preventive and Social Medicine, 22/e p58, 55, 96*

- Secondary attack rates

$$= \frac{\text{Number of exposed persons developing the disease within the range incubation period}}{\text{Total number of susceptible/exposed contacts}} \times 100$$

- The denominator consists of all persons who are exposed to the case
- Initially developed to measure the spread of infection in infectious diseases
- It is a measure of communicability

- Evaluating the effectiveness of control measures
- Secondary attack rate is limited to its application to infectious diseases in which the primary case is infective for only a short period of time measured in days (measles and chickenpox).

17. Ans: b. 15 ppm *Ref: Park's Textbook of Preventive and Social Medicine, 22/e p597*

- **Iodized salt**
- Most widely used public health measure
- Level of iodization is fixed at 30 ppm at the production point and 15 ppm at consumer level
- Most economical, convenient and effective means
- **Iodized oil**
- IM injection of iodized oil (poppy seed oil), dosage 1 ml
- 1 ml will provide protection for about 4 years
- But more expensive
- Difficulty–reaching every person in the community
- **Oral administration of iodine as iodized oil or sodium iodate tablets**
- Technically simpler
- More costly than intramuscular injections

18. Ans. a. 0.5 *Ref: Park's Textbook of Preventive and Social Medicine, 22/e p663; Suryakantha's Community medicine with recent advances 3/e p32*

Principles of chlorination
- Water to be chlorinated should be clear and free from turbidity
- **Chlorine demand** of the water should be estimated–is the difference between the amount of chlorine added to the water and the amount of residual chlorine remaining at the end of a specific period of time **(usually 60 minutes)**
- This time is essential to kill bacteria and viruses
- The point at which the chlorine demand of the water is met is called the **'break-point'**
- Recommended concentration of free chlorine is **0.5 mg/dl at the end of one hour**

19. Ans. a. Real GDP per capita income *Ref: Park's Textbook of Preventive and Social Medicine, 22/e p16*

• PQLI: Difficult to define, difficult to measure. It consolidates three indicators, viz. infant mortality, life expectancy at age one, and literacy. PQLI has not taken per capita GNP into consideration. • The scale of 0 to 100, where 0 represents an absolutely defined worst performance and 100 represents an absolutely defined best performance.	• Disability Indices • **Sullivan's index:** Expectation of life free of disability-computed by subtracting from the life expectancy the probable duration of bed disability and inability to perform major activities
Quality Adjusted Life Years • It is measure of disease burden including both the quality and quantity of life lived (year of life lived with perfect health) • Number of years of life added by intervention • Use for assessing the value for money of a medical intrevention	• **DFLE: Disability free life expectancy** • Also called active life expectancy • Average number of years an individual is expected to live free of disability if current pattern of mortality and disability continue to apply
• **HALE: Health Adjusted Life Expectancy** • HALE was previously called DALE: Disability Adjusted Life Expectancy • HALE is based on life expectancy at birth but includes an adjustment for time spent in poor health. • Equal number of years in full health that a newborn is expected to live based on current rates of ill health and mortality.	• **DALYs are calculated by taking the sum of these two components. In a formula:** – **DALY = YLL + YLD.** – **The DALY relies on an acceptance that the most appropriate measure of the effects of chronic illness is time, both time lost due to premature death and time spent disabled by disease.** – **One DALY, therefore, is equal to one year of healthy life lost.**

20. Ans. b. Malathion *Ref: Park's Textbook of Preventive and Social Medicine, 22/e p728-9*

Malathion–least of all organophosphorous, clear brown liquid, 100 to 200 mg/sq ft every 3 months, ULV–fogging–as Antiadult
Abate–(temephos)–extensively used in India as an antilarval–A. stephensi larva, 1 ppm, less effectve as adulticide
DDT–was discovered by German chemist Ziedler. But Paul Muller discovered the insecticidal properties of DDT. Active fraction is Para-para isomer. Can be used either as residual spray or space spary.
Synthetic pyrethroids are 10 times more effective than naturally occurring pyrethrins.

21. Ans. b. Stratified random sampling *Ref: Park's Textbook of Preventive and Social Medicine, 22/e p792*

Note: If there are nonhomogenous groups–the method of sampling adopted can be stratified random sampling method. Selecting randomly from inside each strata (nonhomogenous groups) is called stratified random sampling method.

Stratified random sampling method	**Cluster random sampling method**
• Principle – Classify population **into homogeneous subgroups (strata)** – Draw sample in each strata – Combine results of all strata • Advantage – More precise if variable associated with strata – All subgroups represented, allowing separate conclusions about each of them – Gives greater accuracy	• This method is used when units of population are natural groups or clusters such as villages, wards or blocks • Principle – Random sample of groups ('clusters') of units – In selected clusters, all units or proportion of units included • Advantages – Simple as no list of units required – Less travel/resources required

22. Ans. b. 30 days *Ref: Park's Textbook of Preventive and Social Medicine, 22/e p762*

Benefits to Employees

- Sickness benefit–maximum period of 91 days continuously, 50% of average daily wages
- Extended sickness benefit is for a maximum period of 2 years
- Enhanced sickness benefit is payable to insured women for 14 days–for tubectomy and for 7 days in case of vasectomy in respect of male. Amount equal to full wages
- Maternity benefit–12 weeks (84 days) for pregnancy, 6 weeks for miscarriage and for sickness arising out of confinement 30 days. Benefit full wages
- Disablement benefit–70%–as long as he is having temporary disability, permanent–pension
- Dependants benefit–death as a result of employment injury–70% of wages is given monthly to the dependents
- Funeral expense–₹ 5000

Benefits to Employers

Exemption from applicability of wokmen's compensation act, maternity benefit act, income tax act.

23. Ans. a. 70% *Ref: Park's Textbook of Preventive and Social Medicine, 22/e p394*

• NTP–1962 • Long-term objectives – One case infects less than one new person annually – The prevalence of infection in the age group below 14 years is brought down to less than 1% • Strategies – To detect maximum number of TB cases – To vaccinate the newborns and infants with BCG vaccine	RNTCP–1992, the salient features are to achieve • At least 85% cure rate of infectious cases through DOTS, • Case detection rate at 70% (through quality sputum microscopy) and involvement of NGOs. • Under RNTCP case finding is passive, that is patients presenting with suspicious of tuberculosis are screened through 3 sputum smear examination.

24. Ans. d. Multiplication and development *Ref: Park's Textbook of Preventive and Social Medicine, 22/e*

Transmission of arthropod borne diseases

Direct contact

- Directly transferred from man to man through close contact.
- Example. Scabies, pediculosis

Mechanical transmission

- The transmission of diarrhea, dysentry, typhoid, food poisoning, and trachoma by the housefly

Biological transmission

- When the disease agent multiplies or undergoes some developmental change with or without multiplication in the arthropod host it is called biological transmission
- **Propagative**
- When the disease agent undergoes no cyclical change, but multiplies in the body of the vector (arthropod), transmission is said to be propagative
- Example. Plague bacilli in rat fleas

- **Cyclopropagative**
- The disease agent undergoes cyclical change and multiplies in the body of the arthropod
- Example. Malarial parasite in anopheles mosquito
- **Cyclodevelopmental**
- When the disease agent undergoes cyclical change but does not multiply in the body of the arthropod
- Example. Filarial parasite in the Culex mosquito and Guinea worm embryo in cyclops

25. Ans. c. a/a+b*100 *Ref: Park's Textbook of Preventive and Social Medicine, 22/e p131*

- **Sensitivity** is defined as the ability of a test to identify correctly all those who have the disease, which is true positive.
- **Specificity** is defined as the ability of a test to identify correctly those who do not have the disease, that is, true negative.
- **Predictive value of** a positive test (PPV)
- Indicates the probability that a patient with a positive test result has the disease.
- NPV (predictive value of a negative test)
- Probability that a person with a negative test does not have the disease

Screening test results	Diseased	Non diseased	Total
Positive	a	b	a + b
Negative	c	d	c + d
Total	a + c	b + d	a + b + c + d

- Sensitivity = a/(a+c) * 100
- Specificity = d/(b+d) * 100
- Predictive value of positive test = a/(a+b) * 100
- Predictive value of negative test = d/(c+d) * 100

Positivity rate or prevalence of positivity = Total test positives/Total tested x 100
Negativity rate or prevalence of negativity = Total test negatives/Total tested x 100

26. Ans. b. Primary *Ref: Park's Textbook of Preventive and Social Medicine, 22/e p336*

The cost effective and low cost population wide interventions that can reduce the risk factors for NCDs are:
- Protecting people from tobacco smoking and banning smoking in public places
- Restricting access to retailed alcohol, enforcing bans on alcohol advertising and raising taxes on alcohol
- Enforcing drink–driving laws
- Restrictions on marketing of foods and beverages high in salt, fats and sugar
- Healthy nutrition environment in schools
- National physical activity guidelines (school based physical activity programmes)
- Protection against environmental or occupational risk factors for cancer.

All these above examples given in the Park's text book suggest it focuses on health promotion activities–which falls mostly under primary prevention. So the answer is more in favor of primary prevention than primordial prevention.

27. Ans. d. Moisture content greater than 30% *Ref: Park's Textbook of Preventive and Social Medicine, 22/e p735–736*

Incineration is a high temperature dry oxidation process, which reduces organic and combustible waste to inorganic incombustible matter and results in a very significant reduction of waste volume and weight.
The process is usually selected to treat wastes that cannot be recycled, reused or disposed off in a land fill site.
Incineration requires no pretreatment, provided that certain waste types are not included in the matter to be incinerated.
Characteristics of the waste suitable for incineration are:
- Low heating volume–above 2,000 Kcal/kg for single chamber incinerators and above 3500 Kcal/kg for pyrolytic double–chamber incinerators.
- Content of combustible matter above 60%
- Content of non combustible matter below 5%
- Content of non combustible fines below 20%
- Moisture content below 30%

Waste types not to be incinerated
- Pressurized gas containers
- Large amount of reactive chemical waste

- Silver salts and photographic or radiographic waste
- Halogenated plastics or PVC
- Waste with high mercury or cadmium content such as thermometers, used batteries and lead lined wooden panels
- Sealed ampoules or ampoules containing heavy metals.

Three kinds of incineration technology are of interest for treating health care waste.
- Double chamber pyrolytic incinerators which maybe especially designed to burn infectious health care waste
- Single chamber furnaces with static grate, which should be only when pyrolytic incinerators are not affordable
- Rotary kilns operating at high temperatures, capable of causing decomposition of genotoxic substances and heat–resistant chemicals.

28. Ans. a. Serial interval *Ref: Park 22/e p96*

Cases
- Index–the first case identified
- Primary–the case that brings the infection into a population
- Secondary–infected by a primary case
- Tertiary–infected by a secondary case.

Serial interval
- The gap in time between the onset of primary case and the secondary case is called serial interval.

Generation time
- The interval of time between receipt of infection by a host and maximal infectivity of that host
- Generation time roughly equal to the incubation period.

Some common definitions in infectious disease epidemiology

Infectivity (ability to infect) ***(number infected/number susceptible) x 100*** **Pathogenicity (ability to cause disease)** ***(number with clinical disease/number infected) x 100*** **Virulence (ability to cause death)** ***(number of deaths/ number with disease) x 100***	**Infection:** The entry, development or multiplication of an infectious agent in the body of man or animals. **Colonization:** The infectious agent just present in the tissue or organ of the human body or animals as normal flora. Colonization is nonpathogenic. Example, staphylococci in skin and nasopharynx
Subclinical or inapparent or covert or missed or abortive infection: The disease agent present in the host may multiply but does not manifest by signs and symptoms and the host contaminates the environment by continuously shedding the infectious agent. Example, poliovirus infection	**Latent infection:** In latent infection, the host does not shed the infectious agent which lies dormant within the host without producing signs and symptoms. Example, herpes simplex infection

Nosocomial infection: An infection acquired by a patient during the stay in the hospital, either from the hospital staff, or from other patients. It includes infection acquired in the hospital but appearing after discharge. Example, infection of surgical wounds
Opportunistic infection: Infection by an organism that takes the opportunity provided by a defect in host defense to infect the host and hence cause the disease. Example, H. simplex, M. tuberculosis. **Iatrogenic infection (physician induced):** Any infection introduced during the hospital procedures or therapeutic regimen by the physician professional activity or from other health professionals. Example, urinary infection following catheterization, hepatitis B infection following injection or blood transfusion.
Obligate host or compulsory host: Obligate host means the only host status available for a particular disease. Example, man in measles, typhoid and poliomyelitis. **Definitive host or primary host or final host:** Host in which the parasite attains maturity or passes its sexual stage are primary or definitive hosts. Example, mosquito in malaria (sporogony–sexual cycle), man in filariasis. **Intermediate or secondary host or alternate host:** Those in which the parasite is in a larval stage or asexual state are secondary or intermediate host. Example, Man in malaria (schizogony–asexual cycle), mosquito in filariasis.
Incubation period: Time interval between invasion by an infectious agent and appearance of the first sign or symptom of the disease in question. **Median incubation period:** Defined as the time required for 50% of the cases to occur following exposure. **Latent period:** This term is used in non infectious diseases as the equivalent of incubation period in infectious diseases. This is defined as the period from disease initiation to disease detection.

29. Ans. b. Specificity *Ref: Park 22/e p131*

Sensitivity is defined as the ability of a test to identify correctly all those who have the disease, which is **true positive.**
Specificity is defined as the ability of a test to identify correctly those who do not have the disease, that is, **true negative.**

30. Ans. a. Azithromycin *Ref:* http://www.who.int/blindness/causes/trachoma/en/

'SAFE'

International efforts to eliminate trachoma as a blinding disease will be based on the WHO-developed strategy–a combination of interventions known by the acronym 'SAFE' which stands for Surgery for trichiasis (inturned eyelashes), Antibiotics, Facial cleanliness and Environmental improvement.

These interventions will be community-targeted and will seek community involvement through the primary health care approach.

These decisions were taken at a meeting, convened by the WHO programme for the Prevention of Blindness and Deafness (PBD) and held at WHO's headquarters in Geneva from 25 to 26 November 1996. The meeting was attended by representatives of a number of international nongovernmental development organizations (INGDOs), the Edna McConnell Clark Foundation and the philanthropic section of Pfizer International Inc: The company that owns the patent of azithromycin, a new long-acting antibiotic which maybe used to fight trachoma. This drug is replacing tetracycline eye ointment, still used in many countries in trachoma treatment. Because of certain disadvantages, topical tetracycline has not been fully accepted in community-based programmes.

Azithromycin is already been used in those countries approaching the final elimination of trachoma as a blinding disease. The experience of Morocco, first country that used azithromycin in large-scale, nation wide elimination programme, has paved the way for the worldwide application of **azithromycin** as part of the SAFE strategy in the fight against the disease.

31. Ans. a. < 5 *Ref: Park 21/e p93, 94 and 751*

Droplet nuclei:

- These are type of particles implicated in the spread of airborne infection. They are tiny particles (1–10 Microns range) that represent the dried residue of droplets.
- They maybe formed by evaporation of droplets coughed or sneezed into the air, generated by automated devices (aerosols).
- Particles of 1 to 5 microns range are liable to be easily drawn into the alveoli of the lungs and maybe retained there.
- Particles of 10 mm or greater in diameter are filtered by nose.
- Those less 5 mm can penetrate deeply and reach alveoli.
- The droplet spread is usually, limited to a distance of 30–60 cm between the source and host.
- Pneumoconiosis: dusts with the size range 0.5 to 3 microns, is a health hazard producing, after a variable period of exposure, a lung disease known as Pneumoconiosis.
- The hazardous effects of dusts on the lungs depend upon a number of factors such as
  - Chemical composition
  - Fineness
  - Concentration of dust in the air
  - Period of exposure
  - Health status of the person exposed:

32. Ans. b. Total serum cholesterol: *Ref: Park 22/e p340*

Risk factors of CHD is multifactorial	
Nonmodifiable risk factors • Age • Sex • Family history • Genetic factors • Personality (?)	**Modifiable risk factors** • Cigarette smoking • High blood pressure • Elevated serum cholesterol • Diabetes • Obesity, sedentary habits, stress
Serum cholesterol • Elevated serum cholesterol is one of the factors which carried an increased risk of development of MI • High mean serum cholesterol (> 200 mg/dl)–have greater risk of developing CHD • LDL: Most directly associated with CHD	With newer techniques HDL and LDL have been further subdivided into sub-fractions. • Apolipoprotein A -1 (major HDL protein) • Apolipoprotein B–(major LDL protein) are better predictors of CHD than HDL cholesterol or LDL cholesterol respectively • Measurement of Apolipoproteins may replace lipoprotein cholesterol determinations in assessing the risk of CHD.

• VLDL: Associated with premature atherosclerosis (more strongly associated with peripheral vascular disease) • HDL: Protective against the development of CHD (> 40 mg.dl) • Cholesterol/HDL ratio: Ratio of less than 3.5 has been recommended as a clinical goal for CHD prevention.	• **For prediction of risk: LDL (among the choices is better)** • **But for overall screening for CHD–Total serum cholesterol–will be the first choice.**

33. Ans. a. Smear positive after 6 months therapy-default *Ref: Park text book 22/e p175*

Treatment categories and sputum examination schedule under RNTCP

Category–1 • New cases (red box) • Type of patients–New sputum smear-positive, new sputum smear negative, new extra-pulmonary, new others • Regimen–2(HRZE)$_3$ + 4 (HR)$_3$ • Test at 2 months • Smear Negative at 2 months–start CP, test sputum at 4 and 6 months • Positive at 2 months–continue IP for one more month and complete the treatment at 7 months Category–II • Previously treated (Blue box) • Type of patients: Sputum smear positive–relapse, failure, treatment after default • Regimen–2 (HRZES)$_3$ + 1 (HRZE)$_3$ + 5 (HRE)$_3$ • Test at 3 months • Smear Negative at 3 months–start continuation phase, test sputum again at 5 months, 6 months and again at completion of treatment	RNTCP will be using a **Standardized Treatment Regimen (Cat IV) for the treatment of MDR-TB cases (and** those with rifampicin resistance) under the programme. • Cat IV regimen comprises of 6 drugs–kanamycin, ofloxacin (levofloxacin), ethionamide, pyrazinamide, ethambutol, and cycloserine during 6-9 months of the Intensive Phase. – And 4 drugs–ofloxacin (levofloxacin), ethionamide, ethambutol, and cycloserine during the 18 months of the Continuation Phase. – *p-aminosalicylic acid (PAS) is included in the regimen as a substitute drug* if any bactericidal drug (K, Ofl, Z and Eto) or 2 bacteriostatic (E and Cs) drugs are not tolerated. – **RNTCP CATEGORY IV REGIMEN: 6 (9) Km Ofx (Lvx) Eto Cs Z E/18 Ofx (Lvx)Eto Cs E**	**Drug dosages and administration** • All drugs should be given in a single daily dosage under directly observed treatment (DOT) by a DOT Provider. • All patients will receive drugs under direct observation on 6 days of the week. On the 7th day (Sunday) the oral drugs will be administered unsupervised whereas injection kanamycin will be omitted. • If intolerance occurs to the drugs, ethionamide, cycloserine and PAS maybe split into two dosages and the morning dose administered under DOT. The evening dose will be self-administered. • The empty blister packs of the self-administered doses will be checked the next morning during DOT. • **Pyridoxine should be administered to all patients on an RNTCP Category IV regimen.**
• Positive at 3 months–continue IP for one more month, test sputum again at 4 months if sputum is positive send sputum for culture and sensitivity as it might be a case of MDR-TB		

Any patient treated with Category 1 who has a positive smear at 5 months of treatment should be considered a failure and started on category II treatment, afresh.

If category 1 patient sputum smear negative case fails to improve or if patient develops pulmonary signs and positive smear at the end of IP, it is considered treatment failure. Start Cat II treatment and confirm failure by culture and perform DST.

34. Ans. a. 400 m *Ref: Park 22/e p259*

- Under WHO international health regulations all international airports and seaports are kept free from all types of mosquitoes for a **distance of 400 meters around the perimeter of ports.**
- Under the IHR–Aedes agypti index is defined as the ratio, expressed as percentage between the number of houses in the limited area on the premises of which actual breeding A. aegypti are found and the total number of houses examined in that area.
- This index is kept at zero at all ports.

Anopheles	Culex	Aedes	Mansonia
The anopheles lays eggs singly and the eggs are boat shaped and posses lateral floats • 45 species of anopheles mosquitoes have been found in India	The Culex lays her eggs in small clusters or rafts, the eggs do not possess lateral floats • Nuisance mosquitoes • Culex fatigans is the important vector in India	The Aedes lays her eggs singly and the eggs are cigar shaped and do not possess lateral floats • Striped or banded character of legs–tiger mosquitoes • First proved vector of a virus–yellow fever	The Mansonoides lays her eggs in star shaped clusters attached to the under surface of certain aquatic plants, pista plants • Big black or brown mosquitoes with speckling on their wings and legs

Contd...

Contd...

Anopheles	Culex	Aedes	Mansonia
• Anopheles fluviatalis and An minimus found in foot hill regions • An. Sundaicus and An. Stephensi found in coastal regions • An. Culicifacies and An. Philippinensis in the plains • Transmits malaria and filaria (not in India)	• Breeds in dirty water collection (stagnant drains, cesspools, septic tanks, burrow pits) • Strong winged mosquito can fly up to 11 km • The peak biting time is at midnight • During the day they rest indoors, on walls, underneath furniture, dark corners • Transmits bancroftian filariasis, Japanese encephalitis, West Nile fever, Viral arthritis	• Breeds in artificial water collection–discarded tins, broken bottles etc., • Females are fearless biters and they bite during the day • Do not fly over long distances usually less than 100 m • Transmits yellow fever (not in India), Dengue, Chikungunya, rift valley fever, filaria (not in India)	• Breed on certain aquatic plants especially pistia, water hyacinth • The larvae and pupae are found attached to the rootlets of these plants by their siphon tubes • Mansonia transmits Malayan (Brugian) filariasis and Chikungunya fever
Anophelini (Larva) • Rest parallel to water surface • No siphon tube • Palmate hairs present on abdominal segments Culicine (Culex, Aedes, Mansonia)–Larva • Suspended with head downwards at an angle to water surface • Siphon tube present • No palmate hairs • **The larva of Mansonia mosquito attached to roots of the pista plants**		Culex/aedes	
Anophelini (Anopheles) • When at rest, inclined at angle to surface • Wings spotted • Palpi long in both sexes Culicini (Culex, Aedes, Mansonia) • When at rest, the body exhibits a hunch back • Wings are unspotted • Palpi are short in female		Anopheles	

35. Ans. b. 0.5 mg/l *Ref: Park, 22/e p579 and p671*

Fluorine
- Most abundant element in nature
- 96% of the fluorine in the body is found in bones and teeth
- Essential for normal mineralization of bones and formation of dental enamel
- Principal sources of fluorine: Drinking water and foods like sea fish, cheese, and tea are reported to be rich in fluorides
- It is a double edged sword (excess result in fluorosis and inadequate intake causes dental caries
- The recommended level of fluorides in drinking water in India is accepted as 0.5 to 0.8 mg/l
- The optimum level is accepted as 1 to 2 mg/l
- Mottling of teeth occurs at levels above 1.5 mg/l
- Lifetime daily intake of 3 to 6 mg/l or more is associated with skeletal fluorosis
- With the concentration of exceeding 10 mg/l causes crippling fluorosis.

Environment and health
- Fluoride accounts for about 0.3 g/kg of the earth's crust.
- Levels of daily exposure of fluoride depends on the geographic area
- Recommended maximum limit of concentration of fluoride in drinking water–1.5 mg/l.

36. Ans. c. Ministry of social welfare *Ref: Park 21/e p611*

- Initiated by Government of India
- Under ministry of social and women's welfare
- On behalf of national policy for children
- Started in 1975

Objectives
- To improve the nutritional and health status of the children in the age group of zero to six years
- To lay the foundations for proper psychological and social development of the child
- To reduce the morbidity, mortality, malnutrition, and school drop out
- To enhance the capability of the mother and nutritional needs of the child through proper nutrition and health education

Beneficiaries
- Pregnant women
- Nursing mothers
- Other women of 15 to 45 years
- Children less than three years
- Children in the age group three to six years
- Adolescent girls 11 to 18 years

Services provided under ICDS
- Supplementary nutrition:
  - 6 to 72 months–500 cal and 12 to 15 g of protein
  - Severely malnourished–800 cal and 20 to 25 g of proteins
  - Pregnant and nursing mothers–600 cal and 18 to 20 g of proteins
- Nutrition and health education
- Immunization
- Health check-up
- Non formal pre-school education

Population norms (revised)–2010
- Rural/urban projects
- **1 for AWC for 400–800 population**
- 2 for AWC for 800–1600 population
- 3 for AWC for 1600–2400 population
- one AWC for multiples of 800 population
- one mini AWC 150–400 population
- for tribal/hilly/riverine/desert–and other difficult areas
- 1 AWC for 300–800 population
- 1 mini AWC for 150–300 population

Administrative unit
- Community development block in rural areas
- Tribal development block in tribal areas and group of slums in urban areas
- Rural/urban project–per 1,00,000 population (100 villages)
- Tribal project–35,000 population (50 villages)

Community Nutrition Programmes

- **Vitamin A prophylaxis programme: Ministry of health and family welfare**
- **Nutritional anemia control programme: Ministry of health and family welfare**
- **National goitre control programme: Ministry of health and family welfare**
- **National IDD control programme: Ministry of health and family welfare**
- **Special nutrition programme: Ministry of health and family welfare**
- **Balwadi nutrition programme: Ministry of health and family welfare**
- **ICDS programme: Ministry of social welfare**
- **Mid day meal programme (school lunch programme): Ministry of education**

37. Ans. a. Verification of diagnosis *Ref: Park, 22/e p122–123*

Steps in investigation of epidemic
1. **Verification of diagnosis**
2. **Confirmation of the existence of the epidemic**
3. **Defining the population at risk**
4. **Rapid search for all cases**
5. **Data analysis**
6. **Formulation of hypothesis**
7. **Testing the hypothesis**
8. **Evaluation of ecological factors**

9. **Further investigation of population at risk**
10. **Writing the report**

Verification of diagnosis	Step–2
• **First step** • **Done as quickly as possible** • **Not necessary to examine all the cases to arrive at a diagnosis** • **A clinical examination of a sample of cases is more than sufficient followed by lab confirmation of diagnosis**	• **Confirmation of the existence of the epidemic** • **How ???????** – Compare the disease frequency with previous years

38. Ans. a. Measles

Ref: Park 22/e p138

Measles

- Caused by RNA paramyxovirus, there is only one serotype.
- **The only source of infection is a case of measles. Carriers and subclinical cases are not known to occur in measles.**
- The period of communicability is approximately 4 days before and 5 days after the appearance of rash. Infection confers life long immunity.
- MC age group–6 months and 3 years in developing countries and usually over 5 years in developed countries.
- The mortality rate is 400 times more in malnourished children.
- Incubation period–10 days from exposure to onset of fever, and 14 days to appearance of rash.
- **C/F**–Prodromal phase–begins 10 days after infection and lasts until day 14.
- A day or two before the appearance of rash Koplik's spots appear on the buccal mucosa opposite to first and second upper molar teeth.
- Koplik's spots are small, bluish white spots on a red base, smaller than a size of head of a pin. Their presence is pathognomonic of measles.
- The next phase is Eruptive phase which is characterized by typical, dusky red macular and acula-papular rash which begins behind the ears.
- The rash fades in the same order of appearance leaving a brownish discoloration which may persist for 2 months or more.
- The most common complications are measles associated diarrhea, pneumonia, and otitis media.
- The more serious complications are neurological complications which include febrile convulsions, encephalitis, and SSPE.
- SSPE–Subacute Sclerosing Pan Encephalitis–rare complication–1 in 3 lakh cases of natural measles. This is characterized by progressive mental deterioration leading to paralysis, probably due to persistence of virus in the brain.
- Encephalitis–1/1000 cases of measles.
- **Control measures**
  - Isolation for 7 days after the onset of rash
  - Immunization of contacts within 2 days of exposure (If vaccine is contraindicated–IG should be given within 3 to 4 days of exposure).
- **Eradication of measles**
  - Achieving an immunization coverage rate of 96% and the cumulation of immunity gap be prevented.
- **WHO measles elimination strategy**
  - **Catch-up:** One time nationwide vaccination campaign targeting usually all children aged 9 months to 14 years regardless of measles disease or vaccination status.
  - **Keep-up:** Routine vaccination coverage of 95% of each successive birth cohort.
  - **Follow-up:** Subsequent nationwide vaccination campaign every 2 to 4 years targeting all children born after catch up campaign.
  - **Measles vaccine:** Live attenuated vaccine, freeze dried product, contains sorbitol and hydrolyzed gelatin as stabilizers as well as neomycin but it does not contain thiomersal
  - **Reconstituted measles vaccine loses about 50% of its potency after 1 hour at 20 °C, it loses almost all potency after 1 hour at 37 °C and the vaccine is also sensitive to sunlight, hence it is kept in colored glass vials.**
  - After reconstitution, the vaccine must be stored in the dark at 2–8 °C and used within 4 hours.

Source of infection	Disease
Usually cases act as source of infection No carrier or subclinical cases	Measles, Chickenpox (latent infection is possible in chickenpox)
Large numbers of infections are subclinical (Both cases and subclinical infections)	Rubella
Both subclinical and clinical cases	Mumps
Both cases and carrier	Diphtheria
Both cases and carriers	Meningococcal meningitis

39. Ans. d. Line diagram *Ref: K Park, Parks Textbook of Preventive and Social Medicine 22/e p788*

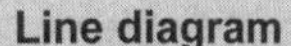

Line diagram
- Best form of graphical presentation is the line diagram
- Trend of events over a period of time can be noted
- It can also be used to compare proportionate change in two variables over a period of time
- The curve in line diagram–no need to touch x-axis

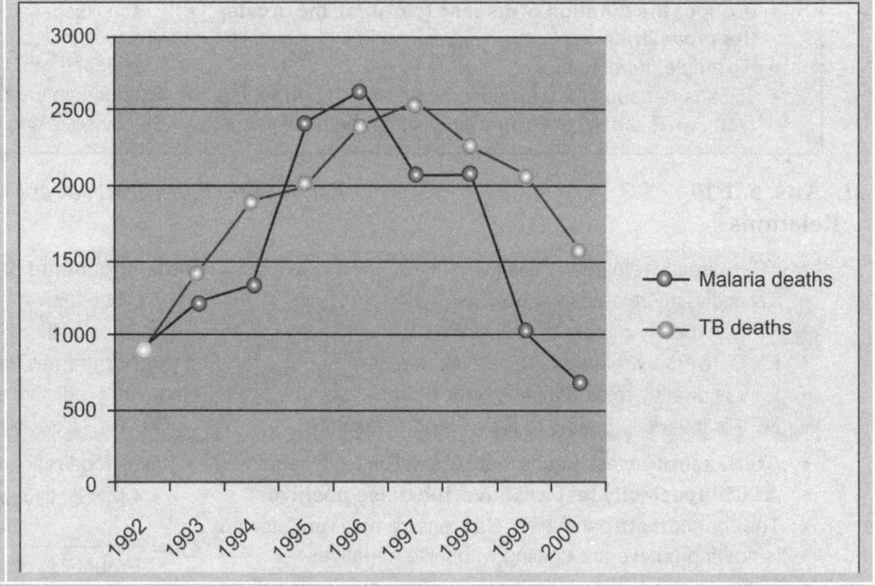

Type of data presentation methods

Quantitative data	Qualitative data
• Histogram • Frequency polygon • Frequency curve • Line diagram • Scatter diagram • Cumulative frequency diagram	• Bar diagram • Pie/sector diagram • Pictogram • Spot map

Histogram
- It is an area diagram consisting of series of adjacent blocks (rectangles).
- Entire area covered by a rectangle represents the entire frequency and the area covered by the individual block represents the frequency of that particular variable
- X-axis represents class intervals
- Y-axis represents frequency
- Histogram can deal with the data with unequal class intervals.

Frequency polygon

If the midpoints of the bars are connected by a continuous line and the bars removed the resulting graph is called frequency polygon in frequency polygon, the two ends of the graph are allowed to touch x-axis

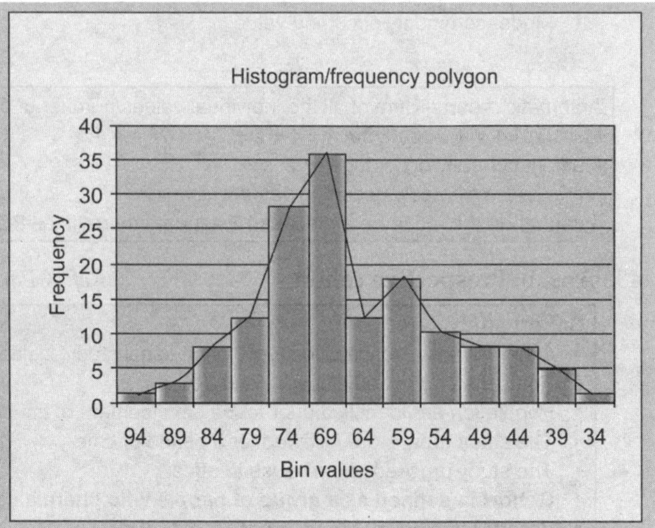

40. Ans. c. Chronic course *Ref: K Park, Parks Textbook of Preventive and Social Medicine 22/e p58*

Relation between incidence and prevalence
- Prevalence depends upon two factors, incidence and duration of illness.
- The relation between incidence and prevalence can be expressed as
- P = I × D

- P = incidence × mean duration

• **Longer the duration of disease (chronic), the greater its prevalence.** • Example, tuberculosis • This is because the new cases crop up throughput the year, while the old ones may persist for months or years.	• If the disease is acute and of short duration of illness either because of rapid recovery or death, the prevalence rate will below compared to incidence rate. • Example, influenza • Strictly speaking these events have no prevalence.

41. Ans. a. 1/10 *Ref: K Park, Parks Textbook of Preventive and Social Medicine 22/e p131*

Relations

• TP is directly related to sensitivity • TN is directly related to specificity • FP is inversely related to specificity • FN is inversely related to sensitivity • PPV is directly related to prevalence of disease • NPV is inversely related to prevalence of disease	**If the population has more false positives** PPV will be low Prevalence of the disease is low **If the population has more false negatives** Negative predictive value of the test is low
• A 90% sensitive test means that 10% will be false negatives • **A 90% specificity test will have 10% false positives** • The chance that a patient with Ca breast remains undetected is nothing but we are dealing with false negatives • Because the test is 90% sensitive the remaining will be 10% of false negatives which is 10/100 or 1/10.	• Likelihood ratio–ratio of probabilities $LR = \frac{\text{Probability of an individual with the disease having the test result}}{\text{Probability of an individual without the disease having the test result}}$

42. Ans. c. 2,3,2 *Ref: K Park, Parks Textbook of Preventive and Social Medicine 22/e p790*

Measures of central tendency/statistical averages
• Averages or centering constants–value in the distribution around which the other values are distributed
• Mean
  – Arithmetic mean–sum of frequencies/no of frequencies
• Median–middle value
• Mode–commonly occurring value
	Statistical averages
	• Mean–arithmetic average
	  – Influenced by extreme values
	  – Easy to calculate and understand
	  – Most useful measure
	• Median–mid point of any observation
	  – Not affected by extreme values
	• Mode–commonly occurring values
	  – Easy to understand, not affected by the extreme values

Arithmetic mean = Sum of all the individual values/number of observations
Mean = 1 + 2 + 2 + 2 + 3 + 4 + 4 + 6 + 7 = 31/7 = 4.42.
Median–centrally occurring value is 3.
Mode is–2 repeatedly occurring value which is 2.
4 cannot be the mode here, because 2 appears more times than number 4.

43. Ans. b. Prospective cohort *Ref: K Park, Parks Textbook of Preventive and Social Medicine 22/e p72*

Cohort study

- Other names–Prospective study, longitudinal study, incidence study, forward looking study, follow-up study
- **Features** of a cohort study
- Population are identified prior to the development of the study
- The study groups are followed for a period of time
- The study proceeds from cause to effect
- **Cohort is defined as a group of people who share a common characteristic**
- **Prospective study (concurrent)**
  - The outcome has not yet occurred at the time of investigation begins.
- **Retrospective cohort study or historical cohort study or non concurrent cohort study or**
  - Outcomes have all occurred before the start of investigation
  - The investigator goes back in time, to select his study groups from existing records and traces them forward through time, usually up to the present time.

- Combination of both retrospective and prospective cohort studies or ambidirectional
  - The study population is identified from past records, and is assessed till date and followed-up in future for further assessment of outcome.

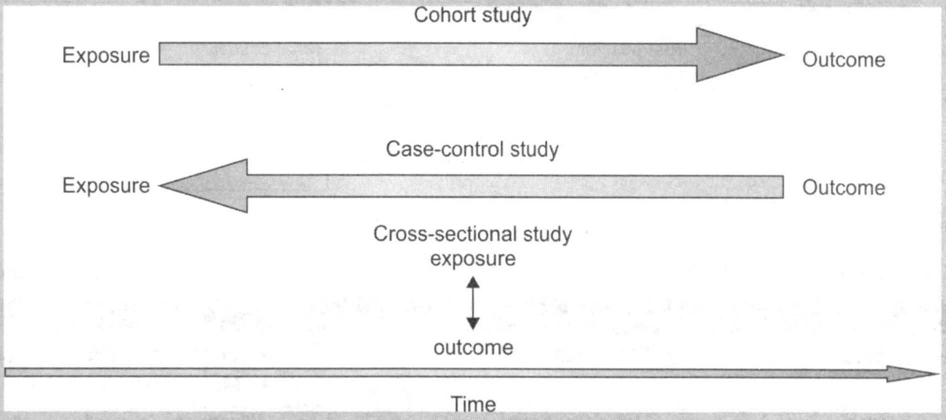

Cohort study

Exposure → Outcome

Case-control study

Exposure ← Outcome

Cross-sectional study
exposure
↕
outcome

Time

Exposure cohort study design

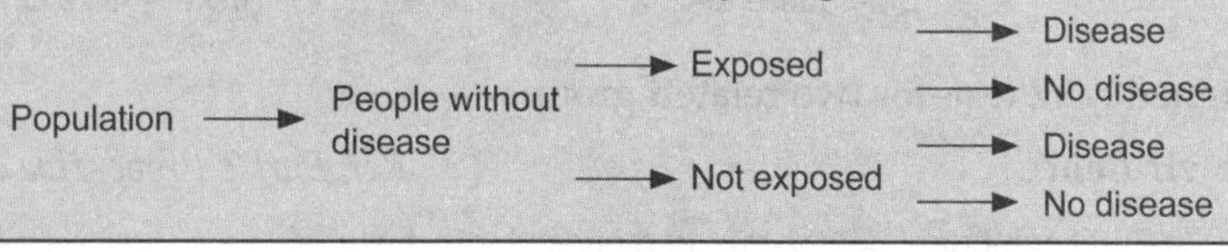

Population → People without disease → Exposed → Disease / No disease; → Not exposed → Disease / No disease

44. Ans. b. Physician's knowledge of the disease *Ref: Park, Text book of preventive and social medicine 22/e*

Before finalizing and performing the screening test to a large number of people to the community the test and the disease should fulfill certain criteria.

Criteria for the disease	Criteria for the disease
• Disease should be an important public health problem • There should be recognizable latent or asymptomatic stage • Test that can detect the disease prior to the onset of signs and symptoms • Facilities should be available for confirmation of test • Evidence that early detection and treatment reduces morbidity and mortality	• **Acceptability:** Painful, discomforting or embarrassing are not likely to be acceptable to the population. • **Repeatability:** (Reliability, precision, reproducibility). Test must give consistent results when repeated more than once on the same or material, under the same conditions. • **Validity (accuracy):** Refers to what extent the test accurately measures what it has to measure. • **Yield:** Is the amount of previously unrecognized disease that is diagnosed as a result of the screening effort. • Screening test must satisfy the criteria of not only acceptability, repeatability and validity but also yield, simplicity, safety, rapidity, cost.

Screening differs from periodic health examinations in the following respects
- Capable of wide applications
- Relatively inexpensive
- **Requires little physician time. In fact the physician is not required to administer the test, but only to interpret.**

45. Ans. a. Lead time *Ref: K Park, Parks Textbook of Preventive and Social Medicine. 22/e p127; Textbook of Public Health and Community Medicine. Armed Force Medical College, Pune 1/e p136, 224, 2009*

- **Time lag between disease onset and the usual time of diagnosis.**
- In this period, there are usually a number of critical points which determine both severity of the disease and the success of any treatment in reversing.
- Screening of the disease done before the disease reaches this usual time of diagnosis.

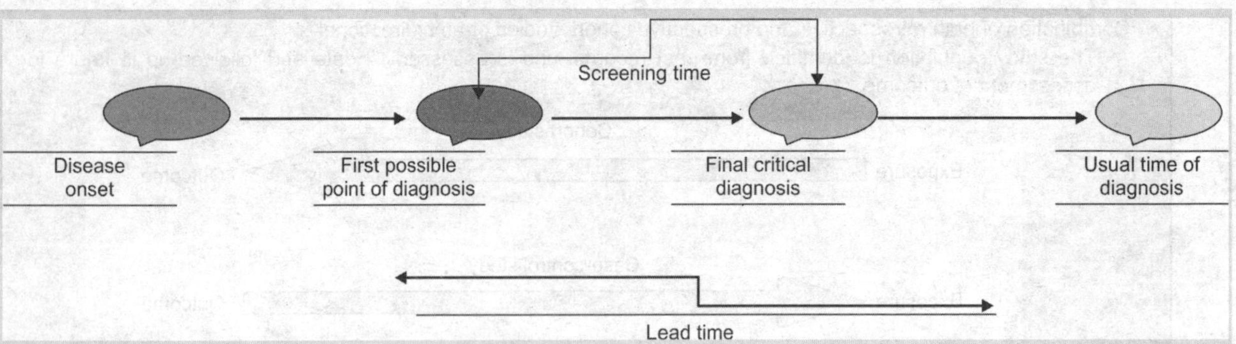

46. Ans. d. Mann-Whitney U test *Ref: Textbook of Community Medicine, AFMC, p275*

	Nominal data	Ordinal data
Two unrelated groups	Chi-square	• Wilcoxan's rank sum test • Mann-Whitney test
Two related groups	McNemar's test	Wilxcoxan's signed rank test
K unrelated groups	Chi-square test	Kruskal–Vallis One way Anova

Note: Wilcoxan's signed rank test–for two related groups.

47. Ans. c. Related to virulence *Ref: Park's Preventive and Social Medicine, 22/e p55*

- Case fatality rate = $\frac{\text{Total number of deaths due to a particular disease}}{\text{Total number of cases due to the same disease}} \times 100$

- Represents the killing power of disease
- Closely related to virulence
- Typically used in acute infectious diseases

- Case fatality rate is a measure of virulence
- Secondary attack rate is a measure of communicability
- Survival rate is a measure of prognosis.

Other measures of mortality

• Crude death rate $= \frac{\text{Number of deaths during a year}}{\text{Midyear population}} \times 100$ • Crude death rate have a major disadvantage, that is, they lack comparability for communities with populations that differ by age, sex, race, etc.	• Specific death rate • When analysis is planned to throw light on etiology, it is essential to use specific death rates. • Cause specific • Disease specific • Related specific groups
• Proportional mortality rate $= \frac{\text{Total number of deaths from the specific disease in a year}}{\text{Total deaths from all causes in that year}} \times 100$	• Survival rate $= \frac{\text{Total number of patients alive after 5 years}}{\text{Total number of patients diagnosed or treated}} \times 100$ • Method of describing prognosis • Used in cancer and chronic studies.

48. Ans. a. Matching *Ref: Park's Preventive and Social Medicine, 22/e p69*

Steps under case control study
1. Selection of cases and controls
2. Matching
3. Measurement of exposure

4. Analysis
5. Estimation of exposure rates and odds ratio (risk)

- **Matching**
- Is defined as the process by which we select controls in such a way that they are similar to cases
- **Confounding factor**
- Defined as one this is associated both with exposure and disease, and is unequally in study and control groups
- The crucial step which avoids this occurrence of confounding factor is matching.

49. Ans. a. Surveillance *Ref: Park's Preventive and Social Medicine, 22/e p118*

The **continuous scrutiny of the factors** that determine the occurrence and distribution of disease is termed as Surveillance. Types of surveillance: Active, Passive, and Sentinel surveillance.
Surveillance is the technical process done throughout the year irrespective of the incidence and prevalence of the disease. It will be regular process done even if the disease is under control.

- Surveillance goes beyond the passive reporting of cases
- It includes laboratory confirmation of presumptive diagnosis, finding out the source of infection, routes of transmission, identification of all cases and susceptible contacts; still others who are at risk in order finally to prevent the further spread of disease.

- Surveillance is systematic collection of morbidity and mortality data, the orderly consolidation of these data, special field investigation, and rapid dissemination of this information to those responsible for prevention and control
- Once control measures have been instituted, their effectiveness should be evaluated
- The ultimate objective of surveillance is prevention

• Monitoring	• Surveillance
– Continuous oversight of activities to ensure that they are proceeding according to plan. – It keeps track achievements, staff movements and utilization, supplies, and equipment and the money spent and immediate correction measures if anything goes wrong.	Continuous scrutiny of the factors that determine the occurrence of the disease The main objectives are – To provide information about new and changing trends – To provide the feedback – To provide the timely warning.

50. Ans. a. Control *Ref: Park's Preventive and Social Medicine, 22/e p37 and 38*

Disease control	Disease elimination	Disease eradication
Aims at reducing • Incidence of disease • Duration of disease • Risk of transmission • Effects of infection • Financial burden to the community • **Control activities may focus on primary prevention or secondary prevention, most control programmes combine two.** The concept of tertiary prevention is comparatively less relevant to control efforts. • In disease control, the disease agent is permitted to persist in the community at a level where it ceases to be a public health problem. • A state of equilibrium becomes established between the agent, host, and environment.	• Between control and eradication, an intermediate goal has been described, called 'regional elimination'. • The term elimination is used to describe interruption of transmission of disease. • Regional elimination is an important precursor of eradication.	• Eradication literally means to 'tear out by roots'. • Eradication of disease implies termination of all transmission of infection by extermination of the infectious agent. • As the name implies, eradication is an absolute process, and not a relative goal. • It is all or none phenomenon • It has been shown that once the morbidity of a disease reaches a very low level, a residual infection usually persists in the population leading to a state of equilibrium between the agent, host, and environment.

51. Ans. b. 95% of children will not get the disease *Ref: Park's Preventive and Social Medicine, 22/e http://www.who.int/influenza_vaccines_plan/resources/Session4_VEfficacy_VEffectiveness. PDF*

Vaccine efficacy	Vaccine effectiveness
Vaccine efficacy percentage reduction in disease incidence in a vaccinated group compared to an unvaccinated group under optimal conditions • Typically use objective outcomes e.g. lab-confirmed influenza • Designed to maximize internal validity (by randomization and allocation concealment) • Often at the expense of generalizability.	Where the balance rests depends upon understanding the **proportion of the disease burden that is vaccine preventable = Vaccine effectiveness** • At any vaccine cost, the greater the burden of disease and the greater the proportion that is vaccine preventable, the more **Cost effective** a program will be

Vaccine efficacy of different vaccines
- Chickenpox vaccine–95% (children)
- Measles vaccine–90%
- Rubella vaccine (RA 27/3)–95%
- Mumps vaccine–95%
- DPT (Pertusis component)–85%
- BCG vaccine–0 to 80%
- Viral Hepatitis A vaccine (Formaldehyde inactivated vaccine)–94%
- Viral Hepatitis B vaccine–95%
- OPV–85%

52. Ans. d. Neonatal hypothyroidism *Ref: Park's Preventive and Social Medicine, 22/e p579 and 596–597*

Control of IDD (IDD control programme)

Iodized salt
- Most widely used public health measure
- Level of iodization is fixed at 30 ppm at the production point and 15 ppm at consumer level
- Most economical, convenient and effective means
- **Iodized oil**
- IM injection of iodized oil (poppy seed oil), dosage 1 ml
- 1 ml will provide protection for about 4 years
- But more expensive
- Difficulty–reaching every person in the community
- Oral administration of iodine as iodized oil or sodium iodate tablets
- Technically simpler
- More costly than intramuscular injections
- Manpower training–health workers
- Mass communication–creating awareness
- Monitoring and surveillance through network of labs–iodine in water, iodine in salt for quality control
- Iodine is essential micronutrient
- Required for synthesis of the thyroid hormones
- The best sources of iodine are sea foods
- About 90% of iodine comes from the foods eaten, the reminder from drinking water
- The requirement of iodine for adults is placed at 150 micro grams.
- The recommendations of WHO of 250 mcg per day for iodine during pregnancy
- Epidemiological assessment of iodine deficiency (Indicators)
- Prevalence of Goiter
- Prevalence of cretinism
- Urinary iodine excretion
- Measurement of thyroid function
- Prevalence of neonatal hypothyroidism
- Neonatal hypothyroidism has been to be a sensitive indicator of environmental iodine deficiency
- Serum T4 levels–more sensitive indicator of thyroid insufficiency than T3

53. Ans. a. Japanese encephalitis *Ref: Park's Preventive and Social Medicine, 22/e; Ananthanarayan, Paniker CJ. Textbook of Microbiology. 8/e London: John Wiley and sons; 2009. p88, 451*

Immunizing agents
- Vaccines, Immunoglobulins and antisera
- Vaccine is an immunobiological substance designed to produce specific protection against a given disease.
- Prepared from–live modified organisms, inactivated or killed organisms, extracted cellular fractions, toxoids or combination of these.

Live vaccines	Live vaccines
• Prepared from live organisms which have been passed repeatedly in the lab in tissue culture or chick embryos and have lost their capacity to induce full blown disease but retain their immunogenicity • More potent	• Should not be administered to persons with immunodeficiency diseases • Pregnancy is the contraindication unless the risk of infection exceeds the risk of harm to the fetus of some live vaccines

• Multiply–antigenic dose is large • Have all major and minor antigenic components • Engage certain tissues of the body (e.g. intestinal mucosa–OPV) • Persistence of latent virus	• When two live vaccines are required they should be given at different sites or with an interval of at least 3 weeks • Live vaccines usually produce a durable immunity but not always as that of natural infection • Immunity is generally achieved with a single dose (exception OPV) • Properly stored to retain effectiveness
Inactivated or killed vaccines • Organisms killed by heat or chemicals • Usually safe and less allergic but less efficacious • Usually require two or three primary doses to produce durable immunity	**Toxoids** • The toxins produced by the organisms are detoxicated and used in the preparation of vaccines • The antibodies produced neutralize the toxic moiety produced during infection rather acting upon the organisms
• Usually booster doses are required • The only absolute contraindication is severe local or systemic reaction to a previous dose.	• Highly efficacious and safe immunizing agents.

Cellular fractions
- Vaccines prepared from cellular components of the bacteria or viruses
- For example, polysachharide antigen–from the capsule of pneumococcus
- Polypeptide–Hep B
- Efficacious and safe

Combinations
- More than one kind of immunizing agents are included in the vaccine
- Simple to administer
- Reduce costs
- Minimize the number of contacts of the patient with the health system
- DPT, DT, MMR
- Polyvalent vaccines–prepared from two or more strains of the same species (polio and influenza)

• **Normal human immunoglobulin**–antibody rich fraction obtained from donors • WHO definite standards–the Immunoglobulin preparation should contain at least 90% intact IgG, free from IgG aggregates, all IgG subclasses, low IgA concentration • Live vaccines should not normally given for 12 weeks after an injection Normal Human Ig and if a live vaccine has already given then NHIg should be given after 2 weeks	• **Specific immunoglobulins (hyper immunune)** • Contains at least 5 times the antibody potential preparations made from plasma of patients who have recently recovered from an infection–or are obtained from individuals who have been immunized against a specific infection • High antibody content and provide immediate protection • For example, Rabies Ig, Hep B, chickenpox prophylaxis • Administered IM • Peak blood levels are reached in 2 days after IM injections • Advantages: Freedom from Hep B, high Ab content, stable Ab content if properly stored • Allergic reactions are common–anaphylactic reactions.
• **Live vaccines** • BCG–intradermal–0.05 ml • Typhoid oral • Oral polio–2 to 3 drops • Measles–SC, 0.5 ml • Mumps • Rubella • Yellow fever • Influenza • Epi. Typhus.	• **Killed vaccines** • Typhoid • Cholera • Pertusis • Plague • Rabies • Salk polio • Influenza • Hep B–IM • JE • KFD.

54. Ans. b. Respiratory disease *Ref: Park's Preventive and Social Medicine, 22/e p530*

UNICEF defines this as the 'annual number of deaths of children age under 5 years expressed as a rate per 1000 live births'.
- UNICEF considers it as the single indicator of social development and well-being rather than GNP per capita.
- Under five mortality rate–reflects income, nutrition, health care and basic education.
- Child mortality rate = Number of under five deaths/Live births × 1000.

- MC common cause of under five mortality worldwide–Pneumonia (18%), preterm birth complication (14%), diarrhea (11%), intrapartum related complication (9%), malaria (7%), and neonatal sepsis, meningitis and tetanus (6%)
- Among the under five mortality (neonatal deaths causes constitute 40%)
- Current under five mortality rate in India–59/1000 (according 2010), worldwide under five mortality rate–57/1000 live births.

55. Ans. c. Bagassosis *Ref: Park's Preventive and Social Medicine, 22/e p751*

- **Byssinosis**–inhalation of cotton fibre dust–textile workers
- **Silicosis**–among occupational diseases major cause of permanent disability and mortality, first reported in Kolar gold mines–karnataka–1947
- Caused by inhalation of dust containing free silica or silicon dioxide
- Silicotics are more prone to pulmonary tuberculosis
- X-ray–shows snow storm appearance
- Silicosis–notifiable disease under Factories Act and Mines Act 1952
- **Anthracosis**–coal mine workers (simple pneumoconiosis or PMF)
- Notifiable disease–Mines Act 1952, compensatable in the Workmens Compensation Act, 1959
- **Bagassosis**–inhalation of sugar cane dust, due to thermophilic actinomycete, (Thermoactinomyces sacchari)–the sugar cane fiber which until recently went to waste is now utilitzed in the manufacture of **paper, cardboard and rayon**.
- **Bagasse control**–keeping the moisture content more than 20% and spraying 2% propionic acid
- **Asbestosis**–serpentine type or chrysolite type, amphibole type
- Amphibole type is more common–90%
- Peribronchial diffuse and basal in location, X-ray–ground glass appearance
- Mesothelioma, a rare form of cancer of the pleura and peritoneum, has been shown to have a strong association with the crocidolite variety of asbestos
- Silicosis–apical lobe is commonly involved
- **Farmer's lung**–inhalation of mouldy hay or grain dust (microspora faeni).

56. Ans. a. 70% detection 85% cure *Ref: Park's Preventive and Social Medicine, 22/e p394; and http://www.health.mp.gov.in/tb.htm (RNTCP document) 2012 revised*

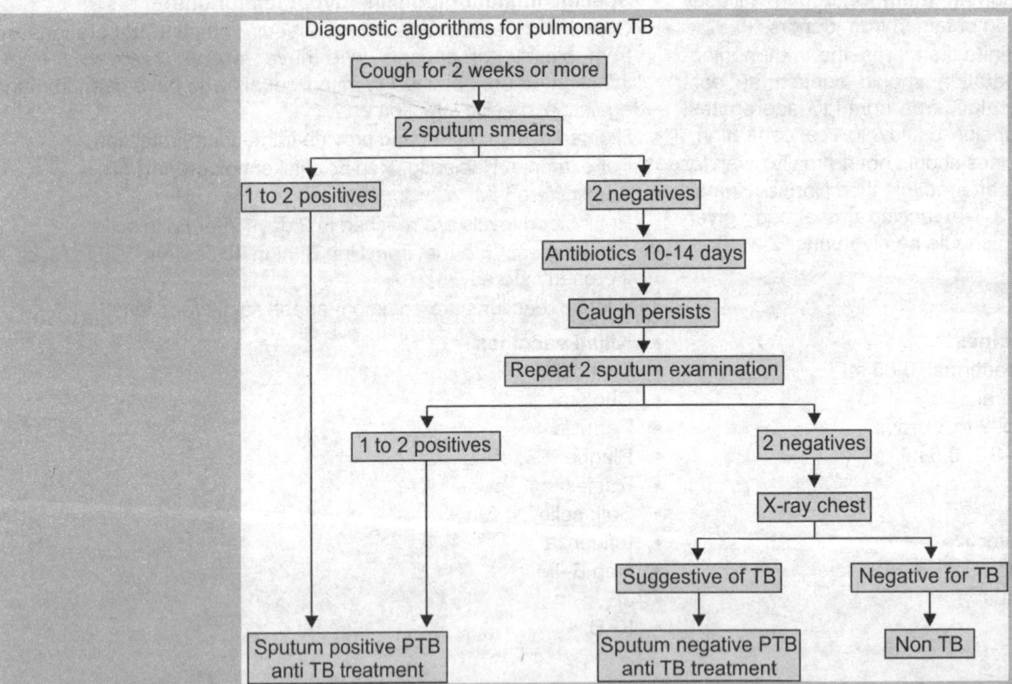

National Tuberculosis Programme–1962
- Long-term Objectives
  - One case infects less than one new person annually
  - The prevalence of infection in the age group below 14 years is brought down to less than 1%.

Organization
- State TB office–State TB officer
- State TB training and demonstration center–Director

- Strategies
  - To detect maximum number of TB cases
  - To vaccinate the newborns and infants with BCG vaccine.
- RNTCP–1992, the salient features are to achieve
  - At least 85% cure rate of infectious cases through DOTS,
  - Case detection rate at 70% (through quality sputum microscopy) and
  - Involvement of NGOs

- District TB centre–DTO
- Tuberculosis Unit–MOTC, STS, STLS (per 5 lakh population)
- Microscopy center (Per lakh population), treatment centers
- DOTS providers.

- Microscopy centers are established for every one lakh population and 1 TU for 5 lakh population
- Each DMC center has a skilled technician for diagnosis
- STLS–Senior TB Lab supervisor is appointed at TU and he will be in charge for every 5 microscopy centers to cross check all positive slides and 10% of negative slides

Lab network and External Quality Assessment (EQA)
- TU–STLS carries out onsite evaluation and blinded rechecking of the slides
- District TB Center–DTO–does blinded rechecking of the slides and maintaining good quality reagents and equipments.
- IRL–State level labs–Training to STLS and technicians, and undertakes onsite evaluation and panel testing of each DTC at least once a year.
- NRL–EQA of 8 to 11 states
- WHO supranational Lab–carry out anti TB drug sensitivity testing

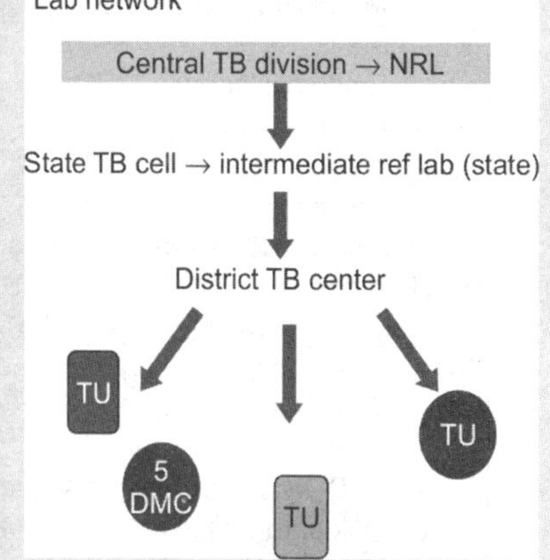

57. Ans. a. General fertility rate *Ref: Park's Preventive and Social Medicine, 22/e p450; and http://censusindia.go.in/vital_statistics/Vital-Rates/Vital-rates.aspx*

- **NRR (Net reproductive rate)** is defined as the number of daughters a newborn girl will bear during her lifetime assuming age specific fertility and mortality rates. NRR of 1 is equivalent to attaining approximately the 2 child norm. NRR = 1 can be achieved only if at least 60% of eligible couples are effectively practising family planning.
- **Family size:** Approximate magnitude of completed family size is given by TFR which means average number of children a woman would have during her reproductive years, bearing children at the same rates as the woman now in each age group.
- **Gross reproductive rate:** Average number of girls that would be born to a woman if she experiences the current fertility pattern throughout her reproductive span **assuming no mortality.**
- **General fertility rate**
- Number of live births per 1000 women in reproductive age group(**15 to 44 or 49**)
- Better measure of fertility than crude birth rate because the denominator is restricted to the number of women in the child bearing age group rather than whole population.
- **Age specific fertility rate:** 'Number of live births in a year to 1000 live women in any specified age group'.
- **Eligible couple:** Currently married couple wherein the wife is in the reproductive age, which is generally assumed to lie between the ages of 15 to 45
- Couples need of family planning services
- **Target couples:** Couple who have had two to three living children and family planning was largely directed to such couples
- **Couple protection rate:** Indicator of prevalence of contraceptive practice in the community
- Percent of eligible couples effectively protected against childbirth by one or the other approved methods of family planning (sterilization, IUD, Condom, oral pills).

58. Ans. d. Trench fever *Ref: K. Park Textbook of Preventive and Social Medicine, 22/e p755*

Diseases transmitted
- Mosquito
  - Malaria, Filaria,
  - Viral encephalitis (Japanes encephalitis)
  - Viral fevers (Dengue, West Nile)
  - Viral hemorrhagic fevers (Yellow fever, dengue hemorrhagic fever)
- Sandfly
  - Kala-azar
  - Oriental sore
  - Sandfly fever
  - Oraya fever

Mnemonic–SOOK
- Tse tse fly–Sleeping sickness
- Rat flea
  - Bubonic plague
  - Endemic typhus
  - Chiggerosis
  - Hymenolepsis diminuta

  Mnemonic–BEnTCH
- Louse
  - Epidemic typhus
  - Relapsing fever
  - Trench fever
  - Pediculosis

Mnemonic–Evening Rise of Temperature
- Hard tick
  - Tick typhus (T)
  - Viral encephalitis (v)
  - Tularemia (T)
  - Viral fever (v)
  - KFD–kyasanur forest disease (K)
  - Tick paralysis (T)
  - Human babesiosis

  Mnemonic–(TvTvKTv)
- **Soft tick**–Q fever and relapsing fever **(QRST)**
- Black fly–Onchocerciasis
- Reduvid bug–Chagas disease
- Trombiculid mite–Scrub typhus, Rickettsial pox
- Itch mite–Scabies

59. Ans. b. Cross-sectional study *Ref: K. Park Textbook of Preventive and Social Medicine, 22/e p67*

Cross-sectional study	Longitudinal study
• Simplest form of observational study • Based on single examination of a cross-section of population at one point in time • Also known as prevalence study • More useful for chronic than short lived diseases • Tells us about the distribution of disease in a population rather than its etiology • Time sequence which is required to establish concept of causativity • Distribution of events may suggest causal hypothesis which can be tested by analytical studies • Provides very little information about the natural history of disease or about the incidence of disease.	• Observations are repeated on the same population over a prolonged period of time by means of follow-up examinations • Useful to study the natural history of disease and its future outcome • Useful for identifying risk factors of disease • Useful for finding out the incidence rate or rate occurrence of new cases • But longitudinal studies are difficult to organize and more time consuming.

60. Ans. a. Sputum AFB *Ref: Textbook of Preventive and Social Medicine, 22/e p170 and 396*

Case finding tools in Tuberculosis

Sputum examination–method of choice for diagnosis under RNTCP, Under RNTCP–first priority is given to direct smear examination of sputum of patients.

Symptoms suggestive of tuberculosis
1. Persistent cough of about 3 or 4 weeks duration
2. Continuous fever
3. Chest pain
4. Hemoptysis.

Sputum examination

False positive	**False negative**
Because of red strain retained by scratches on the slide, accidental transfer of AFBs from a positive slide, or smear by environmental mycobacteria, presence of various particles that are acid fast. (e.g., food particles, precipitates, other microorganisms)	May arise due to inadequate sample, inappropriate sputum container, sputum stored too long, faulty sampling, faulty smear preparation, inadequate time spent, administrative errors like misidentification of patient, incorrect labeling or mistakes of documentation.

Radiography: Chest X-rays are useful for the diagnosis of smear negative pulmonary tuberculosis and TB in children. It is not routinely indicated in smear positive cases. It is useful in diagnosis pleural and pericardial effusion. It is essential in the diagnosis of military tuberculosis.

Sputum culture: Culture examination of sputum is only second in importance in a case finding programme. Culture of sputum is necessary for confirmation of failure and for evaluation of treatment outcomes in patients who received adapted treatment for drug resistant TB, and for extra-pulmonary tuberculosis cases.

Diagnostic algorithms for pulmonary TB

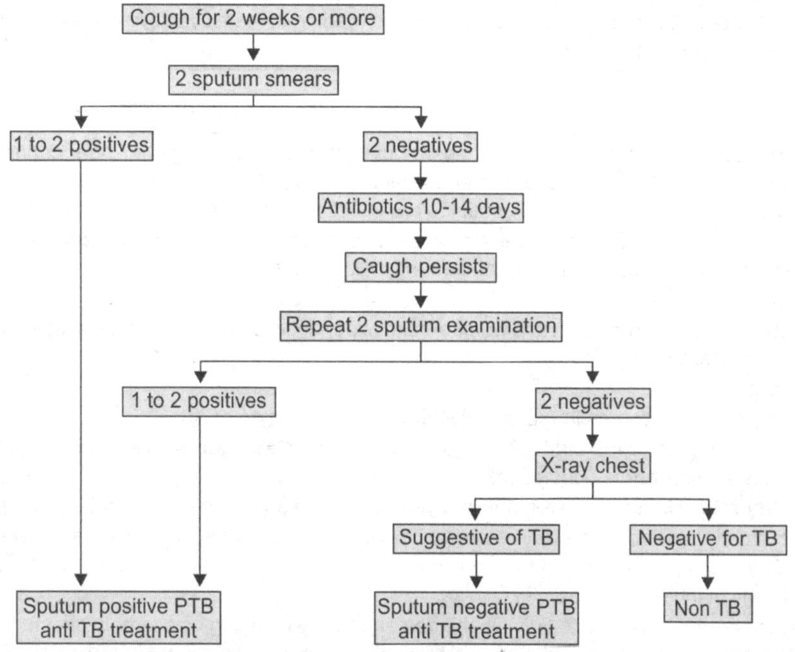

61. Ans. a. The virus *Ref: K. Park, Textbook of Preventive and Social Medicine, 22/e p257*

Yellow fever

- Arboviruses–Arthropod borne viral diseases–viruses which are maintained in nature principally or through biological transmission between susceptible vertebrate arthropods by hematophagous arthropods.
- Group A–(Alpha viruses) Sindbis, Chikungunya viruses
- Group B–(Flaviviruses) Dengue, KFD, JE, West Nile
- Yellow fever–Agent–Flavivirus–(Group B Arbovirus)
- Reservoir–Monkey in forest, Man in urban area
- Vector–Aedes aegypti, Immunity–After one attack lifelong immunity.

Modes of transmission

- Jungle cycle–transmission of yellow fever among monkeys–maintained by Aedes africanus and simpsoni
- Transmission from monkeys to man is accidental and is the result of penetration of man into the infected focus
- Urban cycle–person to person transmission by Aedes aegypti.

Clinical features

- Similar to other viral hemorrhagic fevers (dengue)
- Characterized by liver and renal involvement
- Fever, headache, jaundice, hemorrhagic manifestations–hemetemesis, malena, epistaxis)
- Albuminuria, anuria, shock, stupor and coma
- Death occurs between fifth and tenth day of illness.

Incubation period–3 to 6 days

- International certificate of vaccination–Validity of certificate begins 10 days after date of vaccination and extends up to 10 years.
- Yellow fever is an exotic disease (for India).

Control of Yellow fever

- In India there is no yellow fever
- Susceptible population is avãilable and Aedes is found in abundance but the yellow fever virus is absent
- The virus will enter into India in two ways
  - Through infected travellers
  - Through infected mosquitoes.
- Vaccination–17 D vaccine–Live attenuated vaccine and administered subcutaneously
- Mosquito control measures
- Travellers–all travellers including infants passing through endemic zones–posses vaccination certificate against yellow fever
  - If no such certificate is available–quarantine for a period of 6 days in a mosquito proof ward
  - Mosquitoes–airports and seaports are kept free from breeding of insect vectors at least 400 meters
  - Aedes aegypti index should be kept below one.

62. Ans. a. TFR *Ref: K. Park Textbook of Preventive and social medicine, 22/e p450*

NRR (Net reproductive rate) is defined as the number of daughters a newborn girl will bear during her lifetime assuming age specific fertility and mortality rates. NRR of one is equivalent to attaining approximately the two child norm. NRR is equal one can be achieved only if at least 60% of eligible couples are effectively practising family planning.

Family size–Approximate magnitude of completed family size is given by TFR which means average number of children a woman would have during her reproductive years, bearing children at the same rates as the woman now in each age group.

Gross reproductive rate

Average number of girls that would be born to a woman if she experiences the current fertility pattern throughout her reproductive span **assuming no mortality.**

General fertility rate

Number of live births per 1000 women in reproductive age group (**15 to 44 or 49**)

Better measure of fertility than crude birth rate because the denominator is restricted to the number of women in the child bearing age group rather than whole population.

Age specific fertility rate: 'Number of live births in a year to 1000 live women in any specified age group'.

Eligible couple–currently married couple wherein the wife is in the reproductive age, which is generally assumed to lie between the ages of 15 to 45

Couples need of family planning services

Target couples–couple who have had 2–3 living children and family planning was largely directed to such couples

Couple protection rate–indicator of prevalence of contraceptive practice in the community percent of eligible couples effectively protected against childbirth by one or the other approved methods of family planning (sterilization, IUD, Condom, oral pills)

Total dependency ratio = Children 0 to 14 years + more than 65 years of age divided by population between 15 to 64 years

Crude literacy rate = Number of literate persons/Total population × 100

Effective literacy rate = Number of literate persons aged 7 and above/Population aged 7 years and above × 100.

63. Ans. a. 3 *Ref: K. Park Textbook of Preventive and Social Medicine, 22/e p483*

Antenatal visits

- Ideally the mother should attend the antenatal clinic once a month during the first 7 months, twice a month during the next month, and thereafter once a week–if everything is normal.
- A minimum of 4 visits covering the entire period of pregnancy should be the target
- First visit–within 12 weeks, preferably as soon as the pregnancy is suspected
- Second visit–between 14 and 26 weeks
- Third visit–between 28 and 34 weeks
- Fourth visit–between 36 weeks and term
- It is advisable for the woman to visit medical officer at the PHC for an antenatal check-up during the period of 28–34 weeks. (third visit)
- Registration of pregnancy within 12 weeks is the primary responsibility of the ANM.

High-risk mothers
- Elderly primi (30 years and above)
- Short statured primi (140 cm and below)
- Malpresentations, viz breech, transverse lie, etc.
- Antepartum hemorrhage, threatened abortion
- Preeclampsia, eclampsia
- Anemia
- Twins, hydarmnios
- Previous stillbirth, IUD, Manual removal of placenta
- Elderly grandmulti
- Prolonged pregnancy (14 days after EDD)
- H/O previous cesarean or instrumental delivery
- Pregnancy associated with general disease, like CVD, DM, etc.

64. Ans. a. Vision less than 3/60 *Ref: K. Park Textbook of Preventive and Social Medicine, 22/e p371 and NPCB website*

Category	Worse than	Equal to or better than
Mild or no visual impairment 0		6/18
Moderate visual impairment 1		6/60
Severe visual impairment 2	6/60	3/60
Blindness 3	3/60	1/60
Blindness 4	1/60	Light perception
Blindness 5	No light perception	No light perception
Blindness 9	Undetermined or unspecified	Undetermined or unspecified

65. Ans. b. Hepatitis B *Ref: K. Park Textbook of Preventive and Social Medicine, 22/e*

66. Ans. a. IMR *Ref: K. Park Textbook of Preventive and Social Medicine, 22/e p16 and 525*

Concept of well-being
- Objective components–standard of living, level of living
- Subjective components–quality of life
- Standard of living–refers to the usual scale of our expenditure, the goods we consume and the services we enjoy. It depends on income, occupation, standards of housing, educational, recreational and other services utilized
- Level of living–consists of nine components: health, food consumption, education, occupation and working conditions, housing, social security, clothing, recreation and leisure and human rights. This is the parallel term used in United Nations documents
- Quality of life–defined by WHO as 'the condition of life resulting from the combination of the effects of complete range of factors (environment, education, other services, etc.)
- Physical Quality of Life Index (PQLI)–difficult to define, difficult to measure. It consolidates three indicators, viz. infant mortality, life expectancy at age one, and literacy. PQLI has not taken per capita GNP into consideration. The scale of 0 to 100, where 0 represents an absolutely defined worst performance and 100 represents an absolutely defined best performance.
- IMR is universally regarded not only as a most important indicator of the health status of a community but also of the level of living of people in general and effectiveness of MCH services in particular
- Infant mortality is given a separate treatment by demographers because
  - It is the largest single age–category of mortality
  - Causes of deaths at this age is specific and peculiar to this age
  - It is affected by quickly and directly by specific health program and hence may change more rapidly than the general death rate.

67. Ans. b. T-test *Ref: K. Park Textbook of Preventive and Social Medicine, 22/e*

	Parametric test	Nonparametric test
Based on	Normal distribution	Nonnormal distribution
Type of data	Quantitative data	Qualitative data
Compares	Means and SD	Percentages, proportions and fractions
Examples	Student t-test, Z-test, ANOVA	Chi-square test, McNemar's test, Fisher test

- **Two independent variables**
  1. Qualitative (nominal)–Chi-square test
  2. Quantitative (continuous)–Student t-test–unpaired t-test
- **Two related groups**
  1. Qualitative (nominal)–McNemar's and Chi-square test
  2. Quantitative (continuous)–paired t-test
- **More than 2 groups**
  1. Qualitative–Chi-square test
  2. Quantitative–ANOVA–F.

68. Ans. a. Cataract *Ref: K. Park Textbook of Preventive and Social Medicine, 22/e p371-2*

- In 2010, an estimated 285 million people worldwide were visually disabled, of whom nearly 39 million were blind, about 90% of them live in developing countries
- About 80% of blindness is preventable
- The most frequent causes of blindness in developed countries are accidents, glaucoma, diabetes, vascular diseases, cataract, and degeneration of ocular tissues and hereditary conditions
- In South East Asian Region, cataract is the single most common cause of blindness being responsible for 50 to 80% of all blindness
- Uncorrected refractive errors are being increasingly recognized as a cause of blindness and low vision in developing countries
- National survey on blindness (2007)
- Cataract–62.6%, refractive error–19.7%, glaucoma–5.8%.

69. Ans. a. Class eight or higher *Ref: K. Park Textbook of Preventive and Social Medicine, 22/e*

Selection ASHA
- ASHA must be a resident of the village
- The age group must be between 25 to 45 years
- Formal education up to eighth class
- The woman can be married/divorced/single
- The general norm of selection will be one ASHA for 1000 population.

National Urban Health Mission
- One UPHC: Per 50,000 population (Urban Primary Health Centre)
- Mahila Arogya Samiti: Per 50 to 100 households or 1000 to 2500 population
- One ANM per 10,000 population
- One community health volunteer (ASHA/USHA/LW): 200 to 500 households or 1000 or 2500 population

70. Ans. a. Lead time *Ref: K. Park Textbook of Preventive and Social Medicine, 22/e p127*

Lead time
Time lag between disease onset and the usual time of diagnosis.
In this period, there are usually a number of critical points which determine both severity of the disease and the success of any treatment in reversing.

Screening of the disease done before the disease reaches this usual time of diagnosis.

Screening test	Diagnostic test
Done on apparently healthy individuals	Done on those who are sick
Test result are final	Not final but modified in view of sum of all evidence
Less accurate	More accurate
Less expensive	More expensive
Not a basis of treatment.	Used as a basis of treatment.

71. Ans. c. State of health of workers *Ref: K. Park Textbook of Preventive and Social Medicine, 22/e p715*

Sickness absenteeism
- Sickness absence is an important health problem in industry.
- It may seriously impede production with serious cost repercussions, both direct as well as indirect.
- As the production techniques become more sophisticated, absenteeism tends to increase the adverse repercussions.
- Absenteeism is a useful index in industry to assess the state of health of workers, and their physical, mental and social well-being.
- **CAUSES**: The causes of sickness-absenteeism may not be entirely due to sickness:
  - **Economic causes:**
    - Studies have shown that if the worker is entitled to sick leave with pay, he tends to avail of this privilege by reporting sick. It is so well remarked that in industry the workers declare themselves fit or unfit for work, at their choice.
  - **Social causes:**
    - Certain social factors appear to influence sickness absenteeism in India.
    - These are the social and family obligations such as weddings, festivals, repair and maintenance of ancestral house and similar other causes.
    - Some of the workers who come from rural areas go back to their villages, for short or long periods, during sowing and harvest seasons.
  - **Medical causes:**
    - About 10% of the days lost were found to be due to occupational accidents. Respiratory and alimentary illnesses have also been found to be important causes.
  - **Non occupational cause:**
    - Certain nonoccupational causes such as nutritional disorders, alcoholism and drug addiction have also been found to be responsible for sickness-absenteeism.

- Prevention: The prevention/reduction of sickness absenteeism would result in better utilization of resources and maximizing the production.
- The method for reducing sickness absenteeism include:
  - Good factory management and practices
  - Adequate pre placement examination
  - Good human relations
  - Application of ergonomics.

72. Ans. a. Median *Ref: K. Park Textbook of Preventive and Social Medicine, 22/e p790*

Measures of central tendency
- Statistical averages
  - Mean–arithmetic average
    - Influenced by extreme values
    - Easy to calculate and understand
    - Most useful measure.
  - Median–midpoint of any observation
    - Not affected by extreme values.
  - Mode–commonly occurring values
    - Easy to understand, not affected by the extreme values.

Positive skew: The right tail is longer; the mass of the distribution is concentrated on the left It has relatively few high values.
- Example (observations): 1,2,3,4,100.

Negative skew: The left tail is longer; the mass of the distribution is concentrated on the right of the figure. It has relatively few low values. (observations): 1,1000,1001,1002,1003

- It can be explained simply as follows:
  - If the mean minus median gives the answer with minus symbol then it is negatively skewed and vice versa.
  - Here 130 (Mean)–140 (Median) = –10 (negative skewed distribution)
  - If Mean = Median = Mode–then it is normal distribution.

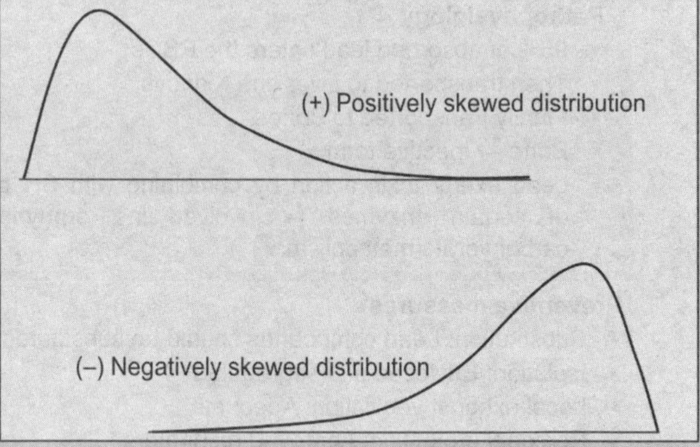

73. Ans. a. Failure rate per 100 women years of exposure
Ref: K. Park Textbook of Preventive and Social Medicine, 22/e p471

74. Ans. a. Positve predictive value *Ref: K. Park Textbook of Preventive and Social Medicine, 22/e p131*

75. Ans. a. 0.5–0.8 *Ref: K. Park Textbook of Preventive and Social Medicine, 22/e p579*

Fluorine
- Most abundant element in nature
- 96% of the fluorine in the body is found in bones and teeth.
- Essential for normal mineralization of bones and formation of dental enamel
- Principal sources of fluorine: Drinking water and foods like sea fish, cheese and tea are reported to be rich in fluorides.
- It is a double edged sword (excess result in fluorosis and inadequate intake causes dental caries.
- The recommended level of fluorides in drinking water in India is accepted as 0.5 to 0.8 mg/l
- The optimum level is accepted as 1 to 2 mg/l
- Mottling of teeth occurs at levels above 1.5 mg/l
- Lifetime daily intake of 3 to 6 mg/l or more is associated with skeletal fluorosis
- With the concentration of exceeding 10 mg/l causes crippling fluorosis
- Environment and health
- Fluoride accounts for about 0.3 g/kg of the earth's crust
- Levels of daily exposure of fluoride depends on the geographic area
- Recommended maximum limit of concentration of fluoride in drinking water–1.5 mg/l.

76. Ans. a. 1/10 *Ref: K. Park Textbook of Preventive and Social Medicine, 22/e p131*

77. Ans. a. Inhalation *Ref: K. Park Textbook of Preventive and Social Medicine, 22/e p752*

Lead poisoning

Lead	**Sources of lead**
• Widely used in variety of industries • Because of its properties • Low boiling point • Mixes with other metals easily to form alloys • Easily oxidized and corrosive • All lead compounds are toxic–lead arsenate, lead oxide, lead carbonate are the most dangerous • Lead sulfide–is least toxic.	• Industrial (occupational)–manufacture of storage batteries, glass manufacture, ship building, printing and potteries and rubber industries • Non-occupational–the greatest source of environment is Gasoline (exhausted from automobiles) • Drinking water, lead paints chewing or toys in case of children.
Modes of absorption • Inhalation–industrial exposure is mainly due to inhalation of fumes and dust of lead • Ingestion–Small quantities of lead trapped in the upper respiratory tract maybe ingested. May also be ingested in food/drinking water/contaminated hands • Skin–occurs only in organic compounds (Tetraethyl Lead) • Inorganic lead–not absorbed through skin. **Pathophysiology** • 95% of absorbed lead enters the RBCs • Then transported to Liver and Kidneys • Finally transported to Bones • Bone → Inactive form • Lead exerts toxic action by combining with SH groups of certain enzymes → involved in Porphyrin and carbohydrate metabolism.	**Clinical features** • Inorganic lead–abdominal colic, constipation, loss of appetite, blue line on gums, stippling of red cells, anemia, wrist drop and foot drop • Organic lead–CNS–insomnia, headache, mental confusion, delirium, etc. **Laboratory tests** • Coprophyrin in Urine (CPU)–useful screening test. (less than 150 microgram/Litre) • Aminolevulinic acid in Urine (ALAU)–exceeds 5 mg/L indicates clearly lead absorption • Lead in blood and urine: lead in urine > 0.8 mg/L indicates lead exposure and lead absorption • Blood lead level more than 70 microgram/100 ml • Basophilic stipling of RBC–sensitive parameter of the hematological response.

Preventive measures
- Substitution: Lead compounds should be substituted by less toxic metals
- Isolation: Enclosed and segregated
- Local exhaust ventilation: Adequate
- Personal protection: Approved respirators
- Good housekeeping: Floors, benches, machines–kept clean
- Working atmosphere: Kept below 2 mg/10 cu meters of air
- Periodic examination of workers: Laboratory investigations
- Personal hygiene: Handwashing before eating
- Health education: On risks of lead exposure and personal protection measures

Prevention of further absorption
- Chelating agents
- D-Penicillamine
- Ca-EDTA.

78. Ans. c. The total number of children by women borne in a female between 15–45 years

Ref: K. Park Textbook of Preventive and Social Medicine, 22/e p450

- **NRR (Net Reproductive Rate)** is defined as the number of daughters a newborn girl will bear during her lifetime assuming age specific fertility and mortality rates. NRR of 1 is equivalent to attaining approximately the 2 child norm. NRR = 1 can be achieved only if at least 60% of eligible couples are effectively practising family planning.
- **Family size:** Approximate magnitude of **completed family size** is given by TFR which means average number of children a woman would have during her reproductive years, bearing children at the same rates as the woman now in each age group.
- **Gross reproductive rate:** Average number of girls that would be born to a woman if she experiences the current fertility pattern throughout her reproductive span **assuming no mortality.**
- **General fertility rate:** Number of live births per 1000 women in reproductive age group **(15 to 44 or 49)**
- Better measure of fertility than crude birth rate because the denominator is restricted to the number of women in the child bearing age group rather than whole population
- **Age specific fertility rate:** 'number of live births in a year to 1000 live women in any specified age group'.

79. Ans. d. Mann-Whitney U test

Ref: Textbook of Community Medicine, AFMC, p257

	Parametric test	Nonparametric test
Based on	Normal distribution	Non-normal distribution
Type of data	Quantitative data	Qualitative data
Compares	Means and SD	Percentages, proportions and fractions
Examples	Student t-test, Z-test, ANOVA	Chi-square test, McNemar's test, Fisher test

	Nominal data	Ordinal data
Two unrelated groups	Chi-square	1. Wilcoxan's rank sum test 2. Mann-Whitney test
Two related groups	McNemar's test	Wilxcoxan-signed rank test
K unrelated groups	Chi-square test	Kruskal–Vallis One way ANOVA

80. Ans. a. Incidence can be calculated

Ref: K. Park Textbook of Preventive and Social Medicine, 22/e p72

Case control study	Cohort study
• Proceeds from effect to cause • Starts with the disease • Involves few number of subjects • Yields relatively quick results • Suitable for study of rare diseases • Yields only estimate of RR (odds ratio) • Inexpensive.	• Proceeds from cause to effect • Starts with the people exposed to risk factor • Involves large number of subjects • Long follow-up period, involving delayed results • Suitable for study of rare exposures • Yields incidence rates, RR and AR • Expensive.
Types of cohort study • Prospective study (concurrent) – The outcome has not yet occurred at the time of investigation begins. • Retrospective cohort study or historical cohort study or non-concurrent cohort study or	**Estimation of risk** $= \frac{\text{Incidence rates of disease among exposed relative risk (risk ratio)}}{\text{Incidence rates disease among nonexposed}}$ • Direct measure of strength of association
– Outcomes have all occurred before the start of investigation – The investigator goes back in time to select his study groups from existing records and traces them forward through time, usually up to the present time.	• RR of 1 indicates no association • RR > 1 suggests positive association between the exposure and the outcome

- Combination of both retrospective and prospective cohort studies or ambidirectional
  - The study population is identified from past records, and is assessed till date and followed-up in future for further assessment of outcome.

Attributable risk

$$= \frac{\text{Incidence of disease rate among exposed} - \text{Incidence of disease rate among nonexposed}}{\text{Incidence of disease rate among exposed}} \times 100$$

AR means to what extent the disease under study can be attributed to the exposure

- Population attributable risk

$$= \frac{\text{Incidence of disease in the total population} - \text{Incidence of disease among nonexposed}}{\text{Incidence of disease in the total population}} \times 100$$

- Provides an estimate of amount by which the disease could be reduced in that population if the factor under study could be controlled or eliminated.

81. Ans. d. Polio

Ref: K. Park Textbook of Preventive and Social Medicine, 22/e p112 and International; Health Regulation 2005, 2/e by WHO

82. Ans. b. 0.2–0.3 mm *Ref: K. Park Textbook of Preventive and Social Medicine, 22/e p662*

Slow sand filter

- **First used in 1804 in Scotland**
- Supernatant water above the sand bed whose depth varies from 1 to 1.5 meter
- Most important part of the filter is the sand bed
- The thickness of the sand bed is about 1.2 meter
- The effective diameter of the sand grains range between **0.2 to 0.3 mm**
- The sand bed presents some 15,000 sq meters of surface area
- Rate of filtration lies between 0.1 and 0.4 cubic meter/hr/square meter
- Venturimeter measures the sand bed resistance
- Cleaning is done by scraping.

Rapid sand filtration

First rapid sand filtration installed in 1884 in USA

Steps

1. Coagulation–treated with a chemical coagulant Alum
2. Rapid mixing
3. Flocculation
4. Sedimentation
5. Filtration

The effective size of sand particles 0.4–0.7 mm

The depth of the sand bed is usually about 1 meter

Cleaning is done by backwashing

Contents	Rapid sand filter	Slow sand filter
Space	Occupies very little space	Requires larger area
Rate of filtration	5–15 cubicmeter/meter square/hr	0.1–0.4 cubic meter/meter square/hr
Effective size of the sand	0.4 to 0.7 mm	0.2 to 0.3 mm
Preliminary treatment	Chemical coagulation and sedimentation	Plain sedimentation
Washing	By backwashing	By scraping
Operation	Highly skilled	Less skilled
Removal of bacteria	98–99%	99.9–99.99%

Advantages of sand filters

Rapid sand filters	Slow sand filters
Can deal with raw water directly	Simple to construct and operate
No preliminary storage needed	Cost of construction is cheaper
Filtration is rapid 40 to 50 times that of slow sand filters and washing of the filters very easy	The physical, chemical, and biological quality of water is very high

83. Ans. a. Copper sulfate *Ref: K. Park Textbook of Preventive and Social Medicine, 22/e p676 and http://www.cdc.gov/nceh/publications/books/housing/cha14.htm*

84. Ans. Repeatability *Ref: K. Park Textbook of Preventive and Social Medicine, 22/e p130*

- **Validity (accuracy)**, refers to what extent the test accurately measures what it has to measure.
- Two components of validity sensitivity, specificity. The word sensitivity was introduced by **Yerushalmy** in 1940s
- **Sensitivity** is defined as the ability of a test to identify correctly all those who have the disease, which is true positive.
- **Specificity** is defined as the ability of a test to identify correctly those who do not have the disease, that is, true negative.
- Sensitivity = a/(a+c) × 100
- Specificity = d/(b+d) × 100

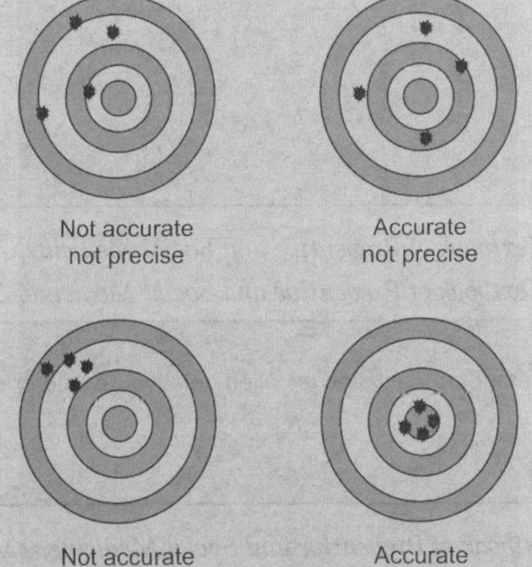

Repeatability. (Reliability, Precision, Reproducibility). Test must give consistent results when repeated more than once on the same or material, under the same conditions.

Repeatability is affected by

- Observer variation
- Intraobserver variation
  - Variations between repeated observations by the same observer on the same subject or material at the same time
  - Minimized by taking the **average of several** measurements at the same time
- Interobserver variation
  - Minimized by
    - Standardization of the procedure
    - Intensive training of the individuals
    - Making use of two or more observers for independent assessment
    - It is probable that these type of errors can never be eliminated
- Biological variation
  - Associated with many of the physiological variables like BP, Blood sugar, serum cholesterol, etc.
  - Changes in the parameters observed
  - Variations in the way the patient perceive their symptoms and answer
  - Regression to the mean
    - Tendency for values at the extremes of a distribution, either very high or low to regress towards the mean or average on repeat measurements.
- Errors relating to technical methods
  - Defective instruments
  - Erroneous calibration
  - Faulty reagents
  - Test itself might be inappropriate or unreliable.

85. Ans. a. Culex trilaeniorhynchus *Ref: Park's Textbook of Preventive and Social Medicine, 20/e p260–261*

- Caused by group B arbovirus (flavivirus)
- Transmitted by culex trilaeniorhynchus–most important vector
- Vectors–Culex trilaeniorhynchus, Culex vishnui, Culex gelidus
- Most important vectors in South India Culex trilaeniorhynchus and vishnui.
- Generally breed in irrigated rice fields, shallow ditches and pools.
- Rice fields are the most important breeding places
- These mosquitoes are primarily Zoophilic
- Man is the incidental dead end host
- Pigs are amplifiers of the virus
- Incubation period–5 to 15 days
- Case fatality rate–20 to 40%

- The average period between the onset of illness and death is about 9 days
- Mouse brain vaccine–Nayakama or Beijing strain
- Cell culture vaccine–Beijing p3 strain
- Cell culture–live attenuated vaccine–SA-14-14-2–currently used in UIP–in UP, Assam, West Bengal, and Karnataka.

86. Ans. c. Chemoprophylaxis *Ref: Textbook of Preventive and social medicine, K. park, 22/e p40-1*

Concepts of Prevention

- **Primordial Prevention**–Prevention of emergence of Risk Factors
- **Primary Prevention**–Action taken prior to the onset of disease
  a. **Health Promotion**
    i. Health education
    ii. Environmental Modification
    iii. Nutritional interventions
    iv. Lifestyle and behavioral change
  b. **Specific Protection**
    i. Immunization
    ii. Specific nutrients
    iii. Chemoprophylaxis
    iv. Protection from carcinogens
    v. Protection against accidents
- **Secondary Prevention**–action taken to prevent the progress of disease
  – Early diagnosis and treatment
- **Tertiary Prevention**–action taken to prevent or reduce the impairment and disability
  – Disability limitation
    Disease → Impairment → Disability → Handicap
    (accident) (loss of foot) (can not walk) (unemployed)
  – Rehabilitation
    - Medical–Restoration of function
    - Vocational–To earn livelihood
    - Social–Restoration of family
    - Psychological–Restoration of personal dignity.

87. Ans. a. Health worker female *Ref: K. Park Textbook of Preventive and Social Medicine, 22/e p849*

88. Ans. a. (x–x̄/sd) *Ref: K. Park Textbook of Preventive and Social Medicine, 22/e p792*

Relative deviate or standard normal deviate

The distance of a value (x) from the mean ($\bar{x}$) of the curve in units of standard deviation is called 'relative deviate or standard normal variate' and is usually denoted by Z

$$Z = \frac{(X - \overline{X})}{\sigma}$$

89. Ans. b. Biological plausibility *Ref: K. Park Textbook of Preventive and Social Medicine, 22/e p75,86*

- **Association** may be defined as the concurrence of two variables more often than expected by chance
- In other words, events are said to be associated when they occur more frequently together
- Association does not imply a causal relationship
- The terms association and relationship are often used interchangeably
- Multi-factorial causation
- The concept by Pattenkofer of Munich during 19th century was an early proponent of multi-factorial causation
- Then scientists came to know after several years during emergence of non-communicable diseases that single causation theory was over simplification and that there are other factors in the etiology of diseases

- **Causation**
- A cause of a disease is an event or condition which plays an important role in producing the disease
- A single causal factor on its own is often neither necessary or sufficient for producing the disease, e.g. smoking as factor in causing stroke
- The concept of cause embodied in the germ theory of disease is generally referred to as a **one to one** relationship between causal agent and disease
- Web of causation
- This model of disease causation was suggested by MacMohan and Pugh

- The doctrine of one to one relationship between cause and disease has been shown to be untenable not only for non-communicable diseases but also for microbial diseases, e.g. tuberculosis, leprosy.
- This model is ideally suited in the study of chronic diseases, where the diseases caused not only due to the individual presence of causal factors but due to complex interrelationship between these factors.

Bradford Hill and others have pointed out that the likelihood of a causal relationship is increased by the presence of the following criteria.
- Temporal association–cause precedes the disease
- Strength of association–RR (measured by relative risk)
- Specificity of the association–specific to the system affected
- Consistency of association–repeated observation
- Biological plausibility–site of involvement–This cannot be explained by the relative risk
- Coherence of association–concurrent occurrence.

90. Ans. a. Time for 50% cases to occur *Ref: K. Park Textbook of Preventive and Social Medicine, 22/e p62*

- **Incubation period:** Time interval between invasion by an infectious agent and appearance of the first sign or symptom of the disease in question
- **Median incubation period:** Defined as the time required for 50% of the cases to occur following exposure
- **Latent period:** This term is used in noninfectious diseases as the equivalent of incubation period in infectious diseases. This is defined as the period from disease initiation to disease detection.

91. Ans. c. Ability to read and write *Ref: K. Park Textbook of Preventive and Social Medicine, 22/e p447*

92. Ans. b. Chi-square test *Ref: K. Park Textbook of Preventive and Social Medicine, 22/e p755*

93. Ans. c. SD = 0 *Ref: K. Park Textbook of Preventive and Social Medicine, 211/e p788, Feb 2011*

- **Normal curve (De Moivre and Gauss)**
- **Other names–curve of error, gaussian curve**
- **Characteristics**
- Bell shaped, bilaterally symmetrical infinitely large number of observations
- Tail never touch the baseline
- Area of the curve is 1, SD is 1
- Mean median and mode all coincide
- The distance of a value from the mean of the curve in units of standard deviation is called relative deviate or standard normal variate Z = x – m/SD
- One SD on either side of mean covers 68% of values
- Two SD on either side of mean covers 95% of values
- Three SD on either side of mean covers 99% of values.

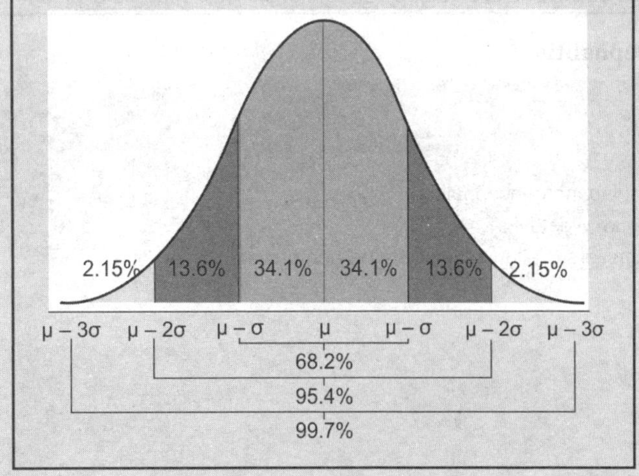

94. Ans. b. 0.5 mg *Ref: K. Park Textbook of Preventive and Social Medicine, 22/e p663; Community Medicine with Recent Advances, Suryakantha, 3/e p32*

Chlorination	Principles of chlorination
• Addition of chlorine in the form of chlorine gas, chloramine, perchloron, bleaching powder. • It is a supplement not a substitute for filtration. • Kills pathogenic bacteria but it has no effect on spores and certain viruses like, Polio, viral hepatitis • Apart from germicidal effect, it oxidizes iron, manganese, and H_2S, destroys taste producing organisms, it controls algae and slime organisms, and aids coagulation.	• Water to be chlorinated should be clear and free from turbidity • Chlorine demand of the water should be estimated–is the difference between the amount of chlorine added to the water and the amount of residual chlorine remaining at the end of a specific period of time (usually 60 minutes) • This time is essential to kill bacteria and viruses • The point at which the chlorine demand of the water is met is called the 'break-point' • Recommended concentration of free chlorine is 0.5 mg/dl.

95. Ans. c. Operational efficiency *Ref: K. Park Textbook of Preventive and Social Medicine, 20/e p227*

Malaria indices	
• Pre-eradication era • Spleen rate–percentage of children between 2 and 10 years of age showing enlargement of spleen (adults are excluded). Used for measuring the endemicity of malaria • Parasite rate–percentage of children between the ages 2 and 10 years showing malaria parasites in their films • Infant parasite rate–percentage of infants below the age of one year showing malaria parasites in their blood films. Most sensitive index of recent transmission of malaria.	• Annual parasite incidence–confirmed cases of malaria during one year/population under surveillance • ABER–number of slides examined/population under surveillance • At least 1% of population should be examined for blood smear for malaria monthly • This is index of operational efficiency.

96. Ans. c. Hookworm infestation *Ref: K. Park Textbook of Preventive and Social Medicine, 20/e p215*

97. Ans. b. Gross national product *Ref: K. Park Textbook of Preventive and Social Medicine, 22/e p16*

PQLI–difficult to define, difficult to measure. It consolidates three indicators, viz. infant mortality, life expectancy at age one, and literacy. PQLI has not taken per capita GNP into consideration.

The scale of 0 to 100, where 0 represents an absolutely defined worst performance and 100 represents an absolutely defined best performance.

Standard of living–refers to the usual scale of our expenditure, the goods we consume and the services we enjoy.

It depends on income, occupation, standards of housing, educational, recreational and other services utilized.

Level of living–consists of nine components: health, food consumption, education, occupation and working conditions, housing, social security, clothing, recreation and leisure and human rights. This is the parallel term used in United Nations documents.

98. Ans. d. Japanese encephalitis *Ref: Park 21/e*

Diseases transmitted

- Mosquito
  - Malaria, Filaria,
  - Viral encephalitis (Japanes encephalitis)
  - Viral fevers (Dengue, West Nile)
  - Viral hemorrhagic fevers (Yellow fever, dengue hemorrhagic fever)
- Sandfly
  - Kala-azar
  - Oriental sore
  - Sandfly fever
  - Oraya fever

  Mnemonic–SOOK
- Tse tse fly–Sleeping sickness

- Rat flea
  - Bubonic plague
  - Endemic typhus
  - Chiggerosis
  - Hymenolepsis diminuta

  Mnemonic–BEnTCH
- Louse
  - Epidemic typhus
  - Relapsing fever
  - Trench fever
  - Pediculosis

  Mnemonic–Evening Rise of TemPerature
- **Hard tick**
  - Tick typhus (T)
  - Viral encephalitis (v)
  - Tularemia (T)
  - Viral fever (v)
  - KFD–kyasanur forest disease (K)
  - Tick paralysis (T)
  - Human babesiosis

  Mnemonic: (TvTvKTv)
- **Soft tick:** Q fever and relapsing fever (QRST)
- Black fly: Onchocerciasis
- Reduvid bug: Chagas disease
- Trombiculid mite: Scrub typhus, Rickettsial pox
- Itch mite: Scabies

Anopheles mosquito	Culex mosquito adult	Aedes mosquito
• 45 species of anopheles mosquitoes have been found in India • Anopheles fluviatilis and An minimus found in foot hill regions • An. Sundaicus and An. Stephensi found in coastal regions • An. Culicifacies and An. Philippinensis in the plains • Transmits malaria and filaria (not in India) • Male: Palpi are longer than proboscis, clubbed at the end, Thick and bushy antenna seen • Female: The palpi are smaller than the proboscis, not clubbed at the end, Sparse antenna seen.	• Nuisance mosquitoes • Culex fatigans is the important vector in India • Breeds in dirty water collection (stagnant drains, cesspools, septic tanks, burrow pits) • Strong winged mosquito can fly up to 11 km • The peak biting time is at midnight • During the day they rest indoors, on walls, underneath furniture, dark corners • Transmits bancroftian filariasis, Japanese encephalitis, West Nile fever, Viral arthritis.	• Striped or banded character of legs–tiger mosquitoes • First proved vector of a virus–yellow fever • Breeds in artificial water collection–discarded tins, broken bottles, etc. • Females are fearless biters and they bite during the day • Do not fly over long distances usually less than 100 cms • Under WHO international health regulations all international airports and seaports are kept free from all types of mosquitoes for a distance of 400 meters around the perimeter of ports • Under the IHR–Aedes agypti index is defined as the ratio, expressed as percentage between the number of houses in the limited area on the premises of which actual breeding A. aegypti are found and the total number of houses examined in that area • This index is kept at zero at all ports • Transmits yellow fever (not in India), Dengue, Chikungunya, rift valley fever, filaria (not in India).

99. Ans. d. 550 Kcal *Ref: Park 21/e*

100. Ans. c. Housing *Ref: K Park Textbook of Preventive and Social Medicine, 21/e Feb 2011*

101. Ans. b. 60 *Ref: K Park Textbook of Preventive and Social Medicine, 21/e, p452, Feb 2011*

102. Ans. a. 6 days *Ref: Park 22/e p112*

Chickenpox–Varicella
- Caused by Varicella-zoster virus
- Characterized by vesicular rash with fever
- Chickenpox and herpes zoster are now regarded as different host responses to the same etiological agent
- Agent–HHV: 3 virus, primary infection causes chickenpox
- Source of infection: Usually a case of chickenpox
- Period of communicability: Ranges from 1 to 2 days before the onset of rash and 4 to 5 days there after
- SAR–90%, MC affects: Children less than 10 years of age and one attack gives durable immunity. Portal of entry of the virus is through the respiratory tract
- Incubation period: Usually 14 to 16 days
- C/F: Rashes are symmetrical, first appear on the trunk and then come on the face, arms and legs. Centripetal. Mucosal surfaces are generally involved. Rashes are pleomorphic,(different stages of rashes seen at one time), fever rises whenever the crops of rashes appear
- Vesicles filled with clear fluid: Dew drops appearance on the skin
- ISOLATION: 6 DAYS
- Mortality less than 1% and there is no specific treatment for the disease
- A live attenuated OKA strain vaccine developed in Japan has been use in field trials
- Live vaccine
- Children single dose because the seroconversion–95%
- 2 doses are required for >12 years–because the single dose vaccination gives only 78% seroconversion
- Postexposure within 3–5 days
- Duration of protection 10 years
- C/I
  - Immunocompromised individuals, including HIV-positive children and adults
  - Pregnant women
  - Persons allergic to neomycin

Salicylates should be avoided for 6 weeks (Reye's syndrome)

CNS	Pulmonary
• Cerebellar ataxia • Meningitis • Encephalitis • GB syndrome • Tranverse myelitis • Reye's syndrome.	• **Pneumonia (Varicella): Serious complication in adults** • ***Others*** – Myocarditis – Nephritis – Arthritis – Hepatitis – Bleeding diathesis.

103. Ans. a. Sputum examination *Ref: Park 22/e*

104. Ans. a. Cataract *Ref: Park p372*

Causes of blindness in India (2006–07) national survey on blindness

Cataract–62.6%, Refractive error–19.7%, Glaucoma–5.8%, Posterior segment pathology–4.7%, Corneal opacity–0.9%, posterior capsular opacification–0.9%
- In south East Asia region, cataract is the single most common cause of blindness being responsible for 50–80% of all blindness
- Uncorrected refractive errors are being increasingly recognized as a cause of blindness and low vision
- Leading cause of childhood blindness is Xeroppthalmia
- The most frequent cause of blindness in developed countries are accidents, glaucoma, diabetes, hypertension and cataract.

105. Ans. c. Repellant *Ref: Park 22/e p728*

Insecticides
- Insecticides: Contact poisons, stomach poisons, fumigants, repellants, synthetic pyrethroids
- Contact poisons: Natural and synthetic
- Natural: Pyrethrum, rotenone, derris, nicotine, mineral oils

- Stomach poisons: Paris green, Sodium fluoride
- Fumigants: HCN, methyl bromide, Sulfur dioxide, carbon disulfate
- Repellants: Metadiethyl toluamide, benzyl benzoate, indalone, dimethyl phthalate, ethyl hexanediol
- Synthetic pyrethroids: Resmethrin, Bioresmethrin, Pothrin
- Synthetic: Organochlorine, Organophosphorous, Carbamates
- Organochlorine: DDT, methoxychlor, HCH, Lindane, Chlordane, Dieldrin, Aldrin, kepone, mirex
- Organophosphorus: Chlorthion, malathion, parathion, dichlorvos, abate, methyl parathion, fenthion, diazinon, chlorpyrifos, Fenitrothion (OMS 43)
- Carbamates: Carbaryl, propoxur (OMS 33)
- Malathion: Least of all organophosphorus, clear brown liquid, 100 to 200 mg/sq ft every 3 months, ULV–fogging–as Anti adult
- Abate (temephos): Extensively used in India as an anti larval–A. stephensi larva, 1 ppm, less effectve as adulticide.

106. Ans. c. Matching *Ref: Park 22/e*

Bias in case control studies	Biases in RCT
• Bias is any systematic error in the determination of the association between the exposure and the disease	• **Subjective bias.** Participants may subjectively feel better or report improvement if they knew they were receiving a new form of treatment
• **Types of bias in case control study** – Confounding bias – Memory or recall bias – Selection bias – Berkesonian bias – Interviewer's bias. • **Confounding bias** • Defined as one which is associated both with exposure and disease, and is unequally in study and control groups, this can be avoided by MATCHING • **Memory or recall bias** • When cases and controls are asked questions about their past history, it may be more likely for the cases to recall the existence of certain events • **Selection bias** • May be difference in characteristics between cases and controls • **Berkesonian bias** • Different rates of admission to hospitals for people with different diseases • **Interviewers bias** • Bias also may occur when the interviewer knows the hypothesis and also knows who the cases are.	• **Observer bias:** The observer measuring the outcome of a trial may be influenced if he knows beforehand the particular procedure or therapy to which the patient has been subjected • **Bias in evaluation:** The investigator may be subconsciously giving a favorable report of the outcome of the trial • **Blinding avoids/reduces bias in RCT.** • **Single blind trial:** Participant is not aware • **Double blind trial:** Neither the doctor nor the participant is aware • **Triple blind trial:** The participant, observer, person who is analyzing the data are all blind • Ideally triple blinding should be used • But most frequently used one is double blinding • **Randomization:** Statistical procedure by which the participants are allocated into groups usually called study and control groups to receive or not to receive an experimental or therapeutic procedure • Randomization is an attempt to eliminate bias and allow for comparability • **By randomization we can eliminate selection bias.**

107. Ans. c. 30% *Ref: Park 22/e*

60% of the children are protected against the disease because they are vaccinated. They are not susceptible. Among the remaining 40 children, 1 (Primary case) child got infected with measles and then it was spread to 12 (secondary case) children. Primary case should be excluded from the numerator and the denominator. So finally s
SAR = 12/39 × 100 = 30.7%

Secondary attack rate = Number of exposed persons developing the disease within the range incubation period × 100 Total number of susceptible/exposed contacts • The denominator consists of all persons who are exposed to the case	• **Attack rate (case rate)** • An attack rate is an incidence rate (usually expressed as a percent), used only during epidemic. (when a population is exposed to risk for a limited period of time)

• Initially developed to measure the spread of infection in infectious diseases • It is a measure of communicability • Evaluating the effectiveness of control measures.	$\frac{\text{Number of new cases of a specified disease during a specified time interval}}{\text{Total population at risk during the same interval}} \times 100$
Limitations of secondary attack rate • Limited its application to infectious disease in which the primary case is infective for only a short period of time, measles • Sometimes difficult to identify susceptible population in all situations • Sometimes has a limited meaning when there are numerous subclinical cases	**Point prevalence** $\frac{\text{Number of all current cases (old and New) of a specified disease existing at a given point in time}}{\text{Estimated population at the same point in time}} \times 100$ • When the term prevalence rate alone is used, it is taken to mean point prevalence.

108. Ans. b. Community level voluntary worker for health *Ref: Park 22/e*

• Selection ASHA – ASHA must be a resident of the village – The age group must be between 25 to 45 years – Formal education up to eighth class – The woman can be married/divorced/single – The general norm of selection will be one ASHA for 1000 population.	NRHM–National rural health mission Launched in 2005 • **Provision of trained and supported Village Health Activist in underserved areas as per need (Accredited Social Health Activists, ASHA)** • Preparation of health action plans by Panchayats as mechanism for involving community in health • Strengthening SC/PHC/CHC by developing Indian Public Health Standards • Institutionalizing and substantially strengthening District level Management of Health (all districts) • Increase utilization of First Referral Units from less than 20% (2002) to more than 75% by 2010.
Roles and responsibilities of ASHA • Create awareness and provide information on nutrition, basic sanitation • Counsel the women–regarding birth preparedness, breastfeeding, immunization • Mobilize the community to utilize the services • Work with village health and sanitation committee of Gram Panchayat • Arrange escort/accompany preganant women • Provide primary medical care for minor ailments such as diarrhea, fevers and can be a DOTS provider • Depot holder for certain drugs (DRUG KIT) like ORS, Iron and folic acid, CQ, Disposable delivery kits, oral pills, etc. • Can provide newborn care and management of a range of common ailments (childhood illnesses) • Inform about births and deaths, unusual health problems in the community to PHC/Subcentre • Promote construction of household toilets	**Monitoring and evaluation of ASHA's work** **Process indicator** • Number of ASHA selected by due process • Number of ASHA's trained • Percentage of ASHA's attending the review meeting after one year **Impact indicators** • IMR • Child malnutrition rates • Number of cases of TB/Leprosy detected as compared to previous year **Outcome indicators** • Percentage of newborn who were weighed and families counseled • Percentage of children who received ORS • Percentage of deliveries with skilled assistance • Percentage of institutional deliveries • Percentage of JSY claims made to ASHA • Percentage of completely immunized in 12 to 23 months • Percentage of unmet of needs for contraception among BPL • Percentage of fever cases who received CQ within first week in a malaria endemic area.

109. Ans. a. Methionine *Ref: Park 22/e p564*

Pulses (legumes)	Cereals
• Pulses comprise a variety of grams, also known as dals • Pulses contain 20 to 25% of proteins, which is double that found in wheat and three times that found in rice. Hence they are called 'poor man's meat'	Rice • Rice belongs to cereal group which constitute the bulk of the daily diet • Energy provided by 100 g of rice is 345 kcal

- Pulse proteins contain more protein than eggs, fish or flesh
- In regard to quality pulse proteins are inferior to animal proteins
- **Pulse proteins are poorer in methionine and to a lesser extent in cystein but rich in lysine**
- Pulses are rich in minerals and B group vitamins
- Germinating pulses contain higher concentration of vit B and vit C
- Presence of high amounts of certain sugars known as oligosaccharides is known to be associated with flatulence

Soybean
- Richest source of proteins among pulses.
- **Limiting amino acid is methionine**
- Cooked and eaten as dal and also in other forms like mixing it with atta for chapattis, Soybean milk in baby foods, etc.
- Nutritive value–432 kcal/100 g
  43.2 g/100 g
  19.5 g/100 g

- The protein content of rice varies from 6–9 percent
- Good source of B group of vitamins especially thiamine
- The milling process deprives the rice grain of its valuable nutritive elements (thiamine, riboflavin)
- **Cereal proteins are deficient in lysine but rice is an exception**
- Rice proteins are richer in lysine. So it is called better quality protein cereal
- Parboiling preserves the nutritive quality of rice.

Wheat
- Next to rice wheat is the most important cereal
- The protein content of wheat varies from 9 to 16%, **the limiting amino acids are lysine and threonine**
- Whole grain wheat flour is richer source of vitamin B than refined white flour.
- Maida or white flour which represents 70% extraction of wheat is poorer from the nutrition stand point

Maize (corn or bhutta)
- Maize ranks next to rice and wheat in human consumption
- The yellow variety of maize contains significant amount of carotenoid pigments
- Maize is fairly rich in fat
- **The proteins of maize are deficient in tryptophan and lysine and they contain excess of leucine**
- Excess of leucine interferes in the conversion of tryptophan into niacin and thus aggravates the pellagrogenic action of maize
- Maize is also used in the manufacture of breakfast foods such as cornflakes.

110. Ans. b. Continuous variables

Ref: Park 22/e

	Parametric test	Nonparametric test
Based on	Normal distribution	Non-normal distribution
Type of data	Quantitative data (continuous variables)	Qualitative data
Compares	Means and SD	Percentages, proportions and fractions
Examples	Student t test, Z test, ANOVA	Chi-square test, McNemar's test, Fisher test

Two independent variables
1. Qualitative (nominal): Chi-square test
2. Quantitative (continuous): Student t-test–unpaired t-test

Two related groups
1. Qualitative (nominal): McNemar's and Chi-square test
2. Quantitative (continuous): Paired t-test

More than 2 groups
1. Qualitative: Chi-square test
2. Quantitative: ANOVA–F

111. Ans. a. Methylene blue

Ref: Park 22/e p608

Pasteurization of milk

Defined as the heating of milk to such temperatures and for such periods of time as are required to destroy any pathogens that may be present while causing minimal changes in the composition, flavor and nutritive value.

Methods of pasteurization
- **Holder method (Vat method)**

Tests of pasteurized milk
- **Phosphatase test**

This test is used to check the efficiency of pasteurization. This test based on the fact that raw milk contains an enzyme called phosphatase which is destroyed on heating at a temperature which corresponds closely with the standard time and temperature required for pasteurization. At 60 °C for 30 minutes phosphatase is completely destroyed.

In this process, milk is kept at 63–66 °C for at least 30 minutes, and then quickly cooled to 5 °C. This method is recommended for small and rural communities. In large cities, it is going out of use

- **HTST method**

Also known as 'High Temperature and Short Time' method. Milk is rapidly heated to a temperature of 72 °C, is held at that temperature for not less than 15 seconds, and is then rapidly cooled to 4 °C. This is now the most widely used method. Very large quantities of milk per hour can be pasteurized by this method

UHT method

Also known as 'Ultra High Temperature' method. Milk is rapidly heated usually in 2 stages (the second stage usually being under pressure) to 125 °C for a few seconds only. It is then rapidly cooled and bottled as quickly as possible.

- **Standard plate count**

The bacteriological quality of pasteurized milk is determined by the standard plate count. The limit is 30,000 bacterial counts per ml of pasteurized milk.

- **Coliform count**

Coliform organisms are usually completely destroyed by pasteurization, and therefore, their presence in pasteurized milk is an indication either of improper pasteurization or contamination after contamination.The standard is that coliforms be absent in even in 1 ml of milk.

112. Ans. b. Pasturella

Ref: Park 22/e p607

Milk is an efficient vehicle for a great variety of disease agents. The sources of infection or contamination of milk may be

- Diary animal
- Human handler
- The environment (contaminated vessels, polluted water, flies, dust, etc.).

Milkborne diseases

A joint FAO/WHO expert committee (1970) on Milk Hygiene classified milkborne diseases as under

1. Infections of animals that can be transmitted to man

Primary importance:

- Tuberculosis
- Brucellosis
- Streptococcal infections
- Staphylococcal enterotoxin poisoning
- Salmonelosis
- Q fever.

Less importance

- Cowpox
- Foot and mouth disease
- Anthrax
- Leptospirosis
- Tickborne encephalitis

2. Infections primary to man that can be transmitted through milk
   - Typhoid and Paratyphoid fevers
   - Shigellosis
   - Cholera
   - Enteropathogenic E. coli.

Nondiarrheal diseases

- Streptococcal infections
- Staphylococcal food poisoning
- Diphtheria
- Tuberculosis
- Enteroviruses
- Viral hepatitis.

113. Ans. a. 1000 live births

- The number of maternal deaths in a given period per 1,00,000 women of reproductive age group during the same period is **maternal mortality rate**
- Maternal mortality ratio measures the risk of women dying from puerperal causes and is calculated by

$$\frac{\text{Total number of female deaths due to complications of pregnancy, childbirth or within 42 days of delivery from puerperal causes in an area during a given year}}{\text{Total number of life births in the same area and year}} \times 1000$$

- Ideally the denominator should include all deliveries and abortions
- **Late maternal death:** The death of a woman from direct or indirect obstetric causes more than 42 days but less than one year after termination of pregnancy
- **Pregnancy related death:** Death of a woman while pregnant or within 42 days of termination of pregnancy, irrespective of the cause of death.

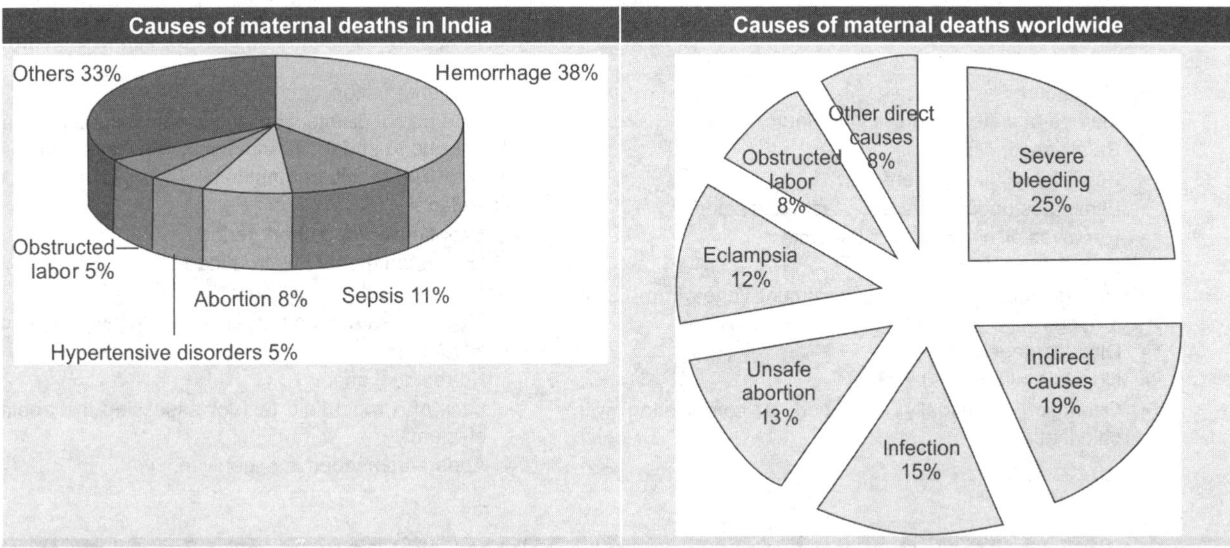

114. Ans. a. 1/3 of calories and ½ of protein supplemented *Ref: Park 22/e*

Midday meal programme
- School lunch programme
- Launched in 1961
- Objective is to attract the children for admission to schools and retain them
- So that literacy status of children improves
- Meal should be a supplement and not a substitute
- Should supply at least on third of total energy requirement and half of the protein requirement

Cost should be low
Cooked with the locally available foods
Re orientation of food habits
Incorporation of nutrition education
Improving school attendance
Improve the educational performance.

Midday Meal scheme: National Programme for Nutritional support to primary education
- Launched in 15th August 1995 revised in 2004
- Objective: Universalization of primary education by increasing enrollment, retention, and attendance and simultaneously impacting on nutrition
- 100% centrally sponsored scheme: 100 g per student per day with a minimum 300 calories and 8 to 12 grams of proteins to all children in Class I to IV
- Principles: Single dish meals, Cereal pulse ratio–3 : 1 to 5 : 1.

115. Ans. a. 0.5 mg/dl *Ref: Park's Textbook of Preventive and Social Medicine, 20/e p625 (Refer question number 15)*

116. Ans. b. 1 hour *Ref: Park's Textbook of Preventive and Social Medicine, 20/e p625*

Large scale disinfection
- Chlorination
- Ultraviolet radiation
- Ozonation

Chlorination	Principles of chlorination
• Addition of chlorine in the form of chlorine gas, chloramine, perchloron, bleaching powder • It is a supplement not a substitute for filtration • Kills pathogenic bacteria but it has no effect on spores and certain viruses like, Polio, viral hepatitis • Apart from germicidal effect, it oxidizes iron, manganese, and H_2S, Destroys taste producing organisms, it controls algae and slime organisms, and aids coagulation	• Water to be chlorinated should be clear and free from turbidity • Chlorine demand of the water should be estimated is the difference between the amount of chlorine added to the water and the amount of residual chlorine remaining at the end of a specific period of time (usually 60 minutes) • This time is essential to kill bacteria and viruses • The point at which the chlorine demand of the water is met is called the 'break-point' • Recommended concentration of free chlorine is 0.5 mg/dl.
• Ozonation • Method of water disinfection on large scale • Relatively unstable gas • Powerful oxidizing agent • Eliminates undesirable odor, taste and color • Removes all chlorine from the water • Has strong virucidal effect • Dosage required for water treatment varies from 0.2 to 1.5 mg/l • Disadvantages • No residual germicidal effect • Ozonation is usually employed in combination with chlorination.	• Ultraviolet radiation • This method of disinfection involves the exposure of a film of water up to about 120 mm thick, at a wavelength in the range of 200 to 295 nanometer • Advantages – Exposure is for a short period – No foreign matter is introduced – No taste and odor produced – Overexposure does not result in any harmful effects • Disadvantages – No residual effect – Lack of a rapid field test for assessing the treatment efficiency – Apparatus needed is expensive.

ONE LINER FOR PSM

1. Father of public health—John Snow
2. India's current HDI rank—136
3. MDG targets to be achieved by 2015
4. Father of multifactorial causation pattenkofer of munich and web of causation—MacMohan and Pugh
5. Spectrum of disease is also called as gradient of infection
6. The science of health and embraces all factors which contribute to healthful living
7. The Jakarta declaration on health promotion—July 1997
8. Ottawa charter incorporates five key action areas in health promotion
9. SMR is a measure of indirect standardization
10. SAR is a measure of communicability
11. Case fatality rate is a measure of virulence
12. Survival rate is a measures of prognosis
13. Index case is the case which comes to the notification
14. Emporitatrics: Study of health of travellers
15. Ergonomics: Study of healthy environment of employees
16. Eugenics: Modification of genes (genetic endowment)
17. Euthenics: Modification of environment (surroundings)
18. First step in investigation of epidemic is verification of diagnosis
19. Matching avoids confounding bias in case control study
20. Randomization avoids selection bias in RCT

21. Dropouts can be included for analysis in RCT
22. Best measure of stength of association is relative risk
23. Incubatory carriers: Mumps, measles, polio, pertusis, influenza, diphtheria, and hepatitis B
24. Convalescent carreir: Typhoid, cholera, dysentry (bacillary/amebic), diphtheria and whooping cough
25. Healthy carriers emerge from subclinical cases. Healthy carriers: Polio, cholera, meningococcal meningitis, salmonellosis and diphtheria
26. Diseases subject to international health regulations: Cholera, plague and yellow fever
27. Diseses under surveillance by who: Louseborne typhus fever, relapsing fever, paralytic polio, malaria, viral influenza–A, Sars, smallpox
28. Semmelweis: Demonstrated the value of handwashing with antiseptic solutions
29. Varicella pneumonia is the most common complication in neonates, adults and immunocompromised patients.
30. Period of communicability for measles is 4 days before and 4 days after the appearance of rash, but for chickenpox 1 to 2 days before and 4 to 5 days thereafter
31. No carrier state in measles (but some subclinical measles occur more often than previously thought)
32. The maximum infectivity for mumps is just before and at the onset of parotitis
33. Secondary attack rate of chickenpox 90%, SAR of mumps 86%, SAR of whooping cough 90%, SAR of measles 90%
34. In influenza antigenic shift: Due to genetic recombination whereas antigenic drift: Due to point mutation
35. Oseltamivir is the drug of choice for influenza
36. Drug of choice for treatment of diphtheria is penicillin or erythromycin
37. DOC for carriers for diphtheria is oral erythromycin, DOC for close contacts (non immunized)–penicillin or oral erythromycin
38. Meningococcal vaccine (men a) can be given for the less than 1 year of age
39. Meningococal conjugate vaccines are preferred over polysacharide vaccines due to their potential for herd protection
40. (Pneumococcal conjugate vaccine) PCV 7 now gradually removed from the marker. PCV 10 and PCV 13 are preservartive free and the vaccine must not be frozen
41. Extensive drug resistant tuberculosis: Resistance to any fluroquinolones and at least one of three second line injectable drugs (capreomycin, kanamycin, amikacin)
42. Prevalence of TB infection is measured by tuberculin positivity
43. Incidence of TB infection is measured by tuberculin conversion index (annual infection rate)
44. Incidence of tuberculosis case: Measured by sputum smear
45. Most common pathogen identified in children with acute diarrhea: Rotaviruses
46. Two live oral vaccines for rotavirus: Rotarix (monovalent) and rotateq (pentavalent)
47. Doxycycline is the drug of choice for chemoprophylaxis of cholera: 300 mg single dose
48. Annual parasitic incidence: Measure of malaria incidence in a community (> 2/1000 population means it belong to high-risk area
49. Aber: Should be at least 10%
50. Mosquitoes are allowed to feed on the patient and then dissected 2 weeks later—for detecting low density microfilaremia
51. Influence of cigarette smoking on coronary artery disease is considered to be synergistic with other risk factors
52. VLDL is strongly associated with peripheral vascular diseases
53. LDL is strongly associated with coronary heart disease, but recently apo lipoprotein a 1 (major HDL) and APO lipoprotein B (major LDL) are better predictors of CHD than LDL and HDL
54. Rules of halves is related to hypertension and rule of 100 is related to diabetes

55. Most common vector of JE is culex tritaeniorhynchus
56. Pigs are amplifying hosts in JE and monkeys are amplifying hosts in KFD
57. Quarantine period for yellow fever is 6 days
58. Case fatality rate of KFD–5 to 10%, CFR of JE–20 to 40%
59. Charles laveran: Discovered the malaria parasite, ronald ross: Discovered the malraia transmission by mosquitoes, grassi: Discovered the malaria is transmitted by anopheles mosquito
60. NRR of one can be achieved only when CPR exceeds 60%
61. Most common site occupational cancer is skin cancer, asbestosis: Crocidolite variety causes mesothelioma
62. Indicator of prevalence of contraceptive practice: Couple protection rate
63. Measure/indicator of contraceptive efficacy is pearl index
64. Major air pollutant (used as indicator of air pollution) is sulfur dioxide
65. Instrument used for measuring amount of bleaching powder for disinfection of well is Horrock's apparatus
66. Instrument used for measuring the residual chlorine: Chloroscope
67. Instrument used for measuring the air humidity: Sling psychometer, wind velocity is measured by anemometer, cooling power of air is measured by kata thermometer
68. Most common cause of maternal mortality rate is hemorrahge
69. Most common cause of neonatal mortality rate is prematurity
70. Most common cause of infant mortality rate is prematurity/low birth weight
71. Most common cause of postneonatal mortality is infections (respiratory infections followed by diarrhea)
72. Most common cause of under five mortality rate is neonatal casues (prematurity)
73. Minimum number of antenatal visits are four according to WHO, minimum number of postnatal visits–3
74. The limiting amino acid in wheat: Lysine and threonine
75. The limiting amino acid in maize: Lysing and tryptophan
76. The limiting amino acid in Soybeans: Methionine
77. The extracalories for pregnant mother + 350, first 6 months of lactation + 600 and second 6 months of lactation + 520
78. Age dependent indices for malnutrition: Height and weight
79. Age independent indices for malnutrition: Mid upper arm circumference and skin fold thickness
80. Weight for age and weight for height are both measures of acute malnutrition
81. Height for age is a measure of chronic malnutiriton
82. Toxic principle of neurolathyrism is BOAA, epidemic dropsy: Sangunarine, endemic ascites: Pyrrolizidine alkaloids
83. Acculturation is nothing but culture contact
84. Index of economic status of households called as wealth index
85. Hidden hunger: Micronutrient deficiency, Undernourishment: Chronic calorie deficiency (less than 1800 kcal/day)
86. Global hunger index includes proportion of undernourished population + children under weight + child mortality in percentage. For India the GHI–for the year 2014–17.8
87. Skewness is asymmetry and kurtosis is peakedness
88. Mean is affected by the presence of extreme values
89. Alpha error (type 1 error) is nothing but rejecting the null hypothesis when it is actually true
90. Sampling within the groups is called as stratified random sampling
91. Chi-square test is also called as test of goodness of fit
92. National antimalaria programme launched in the year 1999

93. National rural health mission launched in 2005, RNTCP–1992, RCH–1997, JSY–2005, RMNCH–A–2013, India newborn action plan launched in 2014, NMHP–1982, IDSP–2004, NFWP–1952
94. Planned end point of all activities objective
95. Ultimate desired state towards which objectives and resources are directed is called as goal
96. The benefits expressed in monetary terms to determine whether a given programme is economically sound is called cost benefit analysis
97. Longest path of the network is critical path method
98. Ayurveda medicine is based on three doshas whereas greek medicine based on four humors (phlegm, yellow bile, blood and black bile)
99. Walter Reed and his collegues demonstrated that yellow fever was transmitted by the aedes mosquito.
100. In the whole of north India, neural tube defects or spina bifida are the most common birth defects. In the rest of India, musculoskeletal disorders are most common such as club foot.

MILLENNIUM DEVELOPMENT GOALS (2000)

The Millennium Declaration adopted 8 development goals, 18 time-bound targets and 48 indicators to be achieved by 2015. Three of the 8 goals, 8 of the 18 targets and 18 of the 48 indicators are related to health

Baseline year 1990 and target year 2015

Goals

- Goal 1: Eradicate extreme poverty and hunger
- Goal 2: Universalize primary education
- Goal 3: Promote gender equality and empower women
- Goal 4: Reduce child mortality
- Goal 5: Improve maternal health
- Goal 6: Combat HIV/AIDS, malaria and other diseases
- Goal 7: Ensure environmental sustainability
- Goal 8: Global partnership for development

Programme	Year
STD control programme	1946
National family welfare programme	1952
National malaria control programme	1953
National filarial control programme	1955
National leprosy control programme	1955
National malaria eradication programme	1958
National tuberculosis programme National iodine control programme	1962
Minimum needs programme	1974
20 point programme	1975
National cancer control programme	1975-76
National programme for control of blindness	1976
Modified plan of operation	1977
National AIDS control programme	1987
CSSM programme	1992
Revised tuberculosis control programme	1992-93
Pulse polio immunization programme	1995
RCH programme RCH phase II	1997 2005

Contd...

Contd...

Programme	Year
Urban leprosy control programme	2005
National rural health mission Janani suraksha yojana	2005
National AIDS control programme phase III	2007

ACTS AND YEARS

Environment (protection) act	1986
Air (prevention and control of pollution) act	1981
Water (prevention and control of pollution) act	1974
The registration of births and deaths act	1969
The immoral traffic (prevention) act	1956
The consumer protection act	1986
The preconception and prenatal diagnostic techniques (prohibition of sex selection) act	1994
The workmen's compensation act	1923
The children act	1960
Juvenile justice act	1986
The child marriage restraint act	1978
Prevention of food adulteration act	1954
Dowry prohibition (amendment) act	1986
The epidemic diseases act	1897

QUESTIONS 2015

1. **SD+ or 1 (2) covers ______ % of ppl**
   a. 85
   b. 95
   c. 97
   d. 99
2. **True about observations 2, 1, 4, 2, 6:**
   a. Median is 3
   b. Mean is 3
   c. Median–5
   d. Mean–2
3. **Sensitivity is:**
   a. TP/TP + FN
   b. TP/TP + FP
   c. TP/TP + TN
   d. TN/TP + TN
4. **HDI INCLUDES all except:**
   a. Life expectancy at 1 year
   b. Life expectancy at birth
   c. Income
   d. Knowledge
5. **MTP Act introduced in the year:**
   a. 1971
   b. 1983
   c. 1967
   d. 1963
6. **MDG (Millennium development goal) 4 is related to:**
   a. Child mortality
   b. Maternal mortality
   c. Environment development
   d. Eradicate poverty
7. **First vaccine:**
   a. Jenner
   b. Ancient chinese physician
   c. John Snow
   d. Louis Pasteur

8. Double blind trial with placebo implies:
a. Study group does not know the drug
b. Clinician does not know the group
c. Investigator does not know the group
d. Participant does not know the group

9. Prospective study with drugs:
a. RCT
b. Case control study
c. Retrospective study
d. Nested case control study

10. Errors in significance test:
a. Type I corresponds to level of significance
b. Type II corresponds to level of significance
c. Type II is similar to power of study
d. Type I similar to power of study

11. Most repeated frequency in a distribution:
a. Mode
b. Median
c. Mean
d. Range

12. Prevalence:
a. Depends on both incidence and duration
b. Depends on only incidence of disease
c. Depends on only duration of disease
d. Depends on severity of disease

13. Incidence is:
a. New cases in a group for a defined period
b. Old cases in a group for a defined period
c. Old and new cases in a group for a defined period
d. Primary cases in a group for a defined period

14. Prevalence:
a. All current cases in populations
b. All new cases in populations
c. All old cases in population
d. All secondary cases in populations

ANSWERS AND EXPLANATIONS

1. Ans. b. 95 *Ref: Park 23/e p849*

According to Normal curve (normal distribution curve)
The following are the characteristics of the normal curve
- It is a bell shaped bilaterally symmetrical curve which has got infinite number of observations and hence both tails will not touch the X-axis
- Total area of the curve–1, SD = 1 (variance = 1) and Mean = median = mode
- Mean Plus or Minus 1 SD covers 68%, Mean plus or minus 2 SD covers 95%, Mean plus or minus 3 SD covers 99% of people in the normal curve.

2. Ans. a. Median is 3 *Ref: Park 23/e p847*

Answer–A (Mean–3), (Median–2) , (Mode–2)
Mean = Add all the values divide it by number = 15/5 = 3
- **Averages or centering constants: Value in the distribution around which the other values are distributed**
- Mean: Arithmetic average
  - Influenced by extreme values
  - Easy to calculate and understand
  - Most useful measure
- Median: Mid point of any observation
  - Not affected by extreme values
- Mode: Commonly occurring values
  - Easy to understand, not affected by the extreme values

3. Ans. a. TP/TP + FN *Ref: Park 23/e p139*

- Sensitivity = a (TP) / (a (TP) + c (FN)) × 100
- Specificity = d/(b + d) × 100
- Predictive value of positive test = a/(a + b) × 100
- Predictive value of negative test = d/(c + d) × 100
  - **Percentage of false negatives = c/(a + c) × 100**

- **Percentage of false positives = b/(b + d) × 100**
- **Prevalence of the disease = (a + c) / (a + b + c + d) × 100**
- **Accuracy = (a + d) / (a + b + c + d) × 100.**

4. Ans. a. Life expectancy at 1 year *Ref: Park 23/e p17*

- Defined as composite index of combining three indicators–longevity (life expectancy at birth), knowledge (adult literacy rate and mean years of schooling) and income (real GDP per capita in Purchasing power parity in US dollars)
- HDI value ranges between 0 to 1, 0.8 and above means high human development category, 0.5 to 0.799–medium human development category and less than 0.5 low human development category. India comes in the medium (0.547) human development category, ranking at number 136.

5. Ans. a. 1971 *Ref: Park 23/e p506*

MTP ACT–1971 LAYS THE DOWN

- The conditions under which a pregnancy can be terminated
- The person or persons who can perform such terminations
- The place where such terminations can be performed.

Conditions: Medical, eugenic, humanitarian, socioeconomic and failure of contraceptive devices

Persons:

- If the pregnancy does not exceed 12 weeks: Terminations can be performed by RMP having experience in OG.
- If it exceeds 12 weeks and 20 weeks the opinion of two RMP is necessary to terminate the pregnancy.

6. Ans. a. Child mortality *Ref: Park 23/e p28*

Millenium Development Goals

- Goal 1: Eradicate extreme poverty and hunger
- Goal 4: Reduce child mortality
- Goal 5: Improve maternal health
- Goal 6: Combat HIV/AIDS, malaria and other diseases
- Goal 7: Ensure environmnetal sustainability
- Goal 8: Develop global partnership for development

7. Ans. a. Jenner *Ref: http://www.ncbi.nlm.nih.gov/pmc/articles/PMC1200696/*

- Edward Jenner: Was an English physician and scientist who was the pioneer of smallpox vaccine, the world's first vaccine. He is often called father of immunology
- French bacteriologist: Louis Pasteur–demonstrated the presence of bacteria in air. He disproved the theory of spontaneous generation
- John Snow: Father of public health, did work on cholera epidemic
- Ancient Chinese physician: The Chinese were early pioneers of immunization, they practiced the variolation to prevent smallpox.

8. Ans. b. Clinician does not know the group *Ref: Park 23/e p83*

- **Single blind trial:** Participant is not aware
- **Double blind trial:** Neither the doctor nor the participant is aware
- **Triple blind trial:** The participant, observer, person who is analyzing the data are all blind
- Ideally triple blinding should be used
- But most frequently used one is double blinding.

9. Ans. a. RCT *Ref: Park 23/e p80-81*

- Experimental studies or intervention studies are similar in approach to cohort studies excepting that the conditions in which study is carried out are under the direct control of the investigator
- The aim of experimental studies: To provide scientific proof of etiological factors and to provide a method of measuring the effectiveness and efficiency of health services for the prevention and control and treatment of disease.

10. Ans. a. Type I corresponds to level of significance *Ref: Bhaskara Rao, Methods of Biostatistics, p81 and 82*

- Type I error is also called an "error of first kind" or Alpha error. The rejection of null hypothesis that is actually true.
- Statistical testing is based predominantly on error. In our studies of testing of null hypothesis we use an alpha error of 0.05 (5%) as the cut off for rejecting null hypothesis.
- This 5% (0.05) is the level of significance: Which is Type 1 error

11. Ans. a. Mode

Mean = Add all the values divide it by number = 15/5 = 3

- **Averages or centering constants: Value in the distribution around which the other values are distributed**
- Mean: Arithmetic average
  - Influenced by extreme values
  - Easy to calculate and understand
  - Most useful measure
- Median: Mid point of any observation
  - Not affected by extreme values
- Mode: Commonly occurring values
- Easy to understand, not affected by the extreme values.

12. Ans. a. Depends on both incidence and duration *Ref: Park 23/e p61*

• Prevalence depends upon two factors, **incidence and duration of illness**	• Longer the duration of disease (chronic), the greater its prevalence. • Example tuberculosis	• If the disease is acute and of short duration of illness either because of rapid recovery or death, the prevalence rate will below compared to incidence rate
• The relation between incidence and prevalence can be expressed as • P = I × D • P = Incidence and mean duration.	• This is because the new cases crop up throughput the year, while the old ones may persist for months or years.	• Example: Influenza • Strictly speaking these events have no prevalence.

13. Ans. a. New cases in a group for a defined period *Ref: Park 23/e p60*

Incidence rate is defined as 'the number of new cases occurring in a defined population during a specified period of time'

$$\text{Incidence} = \frac{\text{Total number of new cases of specific disease during a given time period}}{\text{Population at risk during that period}} \times 1000$$

14. Ans. a. All current cases in populations *Ref: Park 23/e p61*

- The term disease prevalence refers to all current cases (old and new) existing at a given point in time or over a period of time in a given population
- Although referred to as rate, prevalence rate is really a ratio
- Two types
  - Point prevalence
  - Period prevalence
- Defined as the number of all current cases (old and new) of a disease at one point of time, in relation to a defined population

$$\text{Number of all current cases (old and New) of a specified} = \frac{\text{Disease existing at a given point in time}}{\text{Estimated population at the same point in time}} \times 100$$

- When the term prevalence rate alone is used, it is taken to mean point prevalence:

Chapter

9

ENT

VJ Vikram

EAR

Anatomy

Pinna–yellow elastic cartilage.

Other yellow elastic cartilages are epiglottis, corniculate, cuneiform and tip of vocal part of arytenoid.

Eustachian Tube/Auditory Tube/Pharyngotympanic Tube

Three muscles

1. Tensor veli palatine (dilator tubae) opens tubal lumen
2. Levator veli palatine
3. Salpingopharyngeus
   - Tensor veli palatine: Mandibular branch of 5th nerve
   - Levator veli palatine and salpingopharyngeus—pharyngeal plexus
   - Infant ET is 18 mm at birth, forms 10° with the horizontal, at seven years becomes 45°
   - Adult ET 36 mm in length, makes 45° with the horizontal.

Tympanic Membarane

- Obliquely set so that posterosuperior part is more lateral than anteroinferior part 9–10 mm height, 8–9 mm width, 0.1 mm thick.
- A bright cone of light seen radiating from the tip of malleus to the periphery in the anteroinferior quadrant.

Macewen's triangle: The surgical landmark for mastoid antrum. Mastoid antrum is present at birth:

- **Mastoid tip**: It is absent at birth. Develops at 2 years.
- Korner's septum: Bony plate separating superficial Squamous from deep petrosal cells.
- **Physiology**: Sound wave reaches maximum frequency on basilar membrane and stimulates that segment.
- Higher frequencies are represented in the basal turns of cochlea and progressively lower ones towards apex.
- Inner ear fluids:
- Scala vestibule and scala tympani are filled with perilymph.
- Scala media is filled with endolymph.
- Endolymph: Fills membranous labyrinth, It is rich in K^+ ions, Secreted by stria vascularis of the crista
- Perilymph: Lies between bony and membraneous labyrinth, rich in Na^+ ion.

Otomycosis

- Aspergillus niger in subtropics and Candida albicans in tropics are the commonest.

Tuberculosis Otitis Media

Painless foul smelling ear discharge, severe conductive hearing loss which is out of proportion to symptoms.

O/E: Multiple perforations on TM is characteristic. Pale granulation tissue in middle ear and there Maybe facial palsy.

Malignant Otitis Externa

- Necrotizing otitis externa or skull base osteomyelitis
- Caused by Pseudomonas aeruginosa infection
- Presence of granulations at bony cartilaginous junction—Hall mark finding
- Most common nerve palsy—facial nerve.

Acute Suppurative Otitis Media

- Purulent inflammation of the mucoperiosteum of the middle ear cleft
- The most common organism: Streptococcus Pneumoniae followed by H. influenzae.

Clinical Stages

- Stage of congestion
- Stage of exudation
  - TM congestion, cart wheel appearance.
- Stage of suppuration
- Stage of resolution
  - A small central perforation in the pars tensa through which pulsatile discharge is seen (light house sign)
- **Stage of complications.**

Serous Otitis Media/Secretory Om/Mucoid Om/Glue Ear

- Nonpurulent sterile effusion accumulates in the middle ear cavity
- MCC of conductive deafness in children
- Persistent unilateral OME in adults rule out nasopharyngeal mass
- Symptoms: Hearing loss (< 40 dB)
- Otoscopy: TM dull and opaque with loss of light reflex, retracted, fluid level and air bubbles seen

Procedures to be known:

- Myringotomy: Incision over TM
- Myringoplasty: Repair of TM
- Ossiculoplasty: Reconstruction of ossicular chain
- Tympanoplasty: Repair of TM and ossicles.

Types of Tympanoplasty (Wullstein's Classification)

- Type I: Myringoplasty (TM perforation)
- Type II: TM perforation and erosion of malleus
- Type III: Myringostapedopexy/Columella tympanoplasty
  - Malleus and incus absent. Graft between oval stapes head (columella effect)
- Type IV: Only foot plate of stapes present. Graft between oval window and round window
  Foot plate exteriorized over which soundwaves act directly (baffle effect)
- Type V: Fenestration operation
- Type VI: Sono inversion.

Facial Nerve

Labyrinthine segment: Narrowest and shortest segment, first genu

Neuropraxia: Conduction block

- **Axonotemesis:** Injury to axons
- **Neurotemesis:** Injury to nerve.

Otosclerosis/Otospongiosis

- Disease of bony labyrinth where spongy bone replaces normal enchondral layer of bony otic capsule
- Most often the otosclerotic focus involves stapes leading to stapes fixation and conductive hearing loss.

Etiology

- Fistula ante fenestrum in front of oval window is the site of predilection in stapedial type
- Family history present, Autosomal dominant; Whites more affected than Negroes
- Females affected twice more than males. But in India males are more affected; Age 20–30 years
- Maybe initiated or made worse by pregnancy, menopause, after an accident or a major operation
- Van der Hoeve syndrome- triad of Osteogenesis imperfecta, Blue sclera and Otosclerosis.

Symptoms and Signs

Paracusis willisi-hears better in noisy surroundings

- **Schwartz sign**: Reddish hue seen on the promontory through TM, which indicates active focus
- In some cases a dip in the bone conduction curve appear at 2000 Hz which disappears after successful stapedectomy (**Carhart's notch**)
- **Bezold's triad-absolute negative Rinne's raised lower tone limit, prolonged bone conduction.**

Acoustic Neuroma/Vestibular Schwannoma/Neurilemmoma

- Tumors almost always arise from the Schwann cells of superior vestibular division of VIII nerve
- Cranial nerves: 5th nerve earliest to be involved
- **Hitzelberger's sign** (hypoesthesia of posterior meatal wall), loss of taste, decreased lacrimation are due to facial nerve involvement.

Glomus Tumor

Otoscopy

- Red reflex
- Rising sun appearance when the tumor arises from the floor of middle ear
- **Brown's sign** (pulsation sign) when ear canal pressure is increased, the tumor pulsates vigorously
- **Phelp's sign**: Destruction of bone between carotid canal and jugular foramen
- **Aquino sign**: Otoscopy shows blanching of tumor on compression of carotid reduces vascularity and arrests growth.

Meniere's Disease/Endolymphatic Hydrops

Three Cardinal symptoms

1. Episodic vertigo
2. Roaring tinnitus
3. Fluctuating hearing loss

Other Features

- Tullio phenomenon: Loud sounds produce vertigo
- Diplacusis: Tone of a particular frequency Maybe heard normal in one ear and higher pitch in the other ear
- Hennebert's Sign: False positive test fistula test also occurs in congenital syphilis

- Hennebert phenemenon: In perilymph fistula disequilibrium occurs in nose blowing
- **Lermoyez syndrome**: Variant of Meniere's disease in which hearing loss and tinnitus are relieved with episode of vertigo
- Drop attacks **(Tumarkin's otolithic crisis)** sudden drop attack without loss of bezold's Abscess: Pus breaks through the medial side of the **mastoid tip** and present as neck swelling.

Luc's abscess

- Meatal abscess when pus breaks through bony wall between antrum and osseous external meatus
  - **Citelli's abscess**: Pus tracks along the digastrics muscle and present as swelling in the digastic triangle
  - **Zygomatic abscess**: Presents at root of zygoma. Swelling in front and above pinna.

Gradenigo's Syndrome:

- Seen in petrositis (CSOM complications)
- Ear discharge
- Diplopia (CN VI paralysis)
- Retro orbital pain (CN V)

Melkerson's Syndrome:

- Facial paralysis
- Swelling of lips
- Fissured tongue.

Lateral/Sigmoid Sinus Thrombosis

- **Hectic Picket-fence type** of fever with rigors
- **Griesinger's sign**: Due to thrombosis of mastoid emissary vein, edema over posterior part of mastoid
- **Tobey-Ayer test:**
  - Compression of jugular vein on thrombosed side: no effect on CSF pressure
  - Compression of jugular vein on the normal side: rapid rise in CSF pressure
- **Crowe-Beck test:** Pressure on the jug vein on healthy side: engorgement of retinal and supraorbital veins.

NOSE

Maxillary and ethmoidal sinuses are present at birth. First radiological evidence of maxillary sinus is at 4–5 months after birth.

Little's Area

- Little's area: Situated in the anteroinferior part of nasal septum, just above the vestibule
- Common site of epistaxis in children.

Woodruff's Area

- Site of epistaxis in elderly
- Sphenopalatine artery anastomosis with posterior pharyngeal artery.

Nasal Cycle

Nasal mucosa undergoes rhythmic cyclical congestion and decongestion. When one nasal chamber is working total nasal respiration of both nasal chambers is carried by it every 21/2–4 hours.

Rhinoscleroma

- Chronic granulomatous disease caused by Klebsiella rhinoscleromatis or Frisch bacillus, a gram-negative coccobacillus
- Subdermal infiltration of the lower part of external nose and upper lip giving a wood feel
- Miculicz' cells (plasma cells) and Russel bodies (also seen in multiple myeloma).

Foreign Bodies in The Nose

- If a child presents with unilateral, foul smelling nasal discharge (sometimes blood stained), foreign body must be excluded
- Other important causes of unilateral blood stained nasal discharge
  - Rhinolith
  - Nasal diphtheria
  - Nasal myiasis.

Rhinophyma (Potato Tumor)

- Benign tumor due to hypertrophy of sebaceous glands of the tip of the nose

Kartagner's syndrome	Young syndrome	Churg-Strauss syndrome
• Bronchiectasis • Situs inversus • Ciliary dyskinesia	• Sinopulomonary disease • Azoospermia	• Asthma, Fever • Eosinophilia • Vasculitis, Granuloma

Maxillary Carcinoma

Ohngren's Classification

- An imaginary plane from medial canthus of eye to angle of mandible. Growth situated above this plane (suprastructural) have a poorer prognosis than those below it (infrastructural).

Lederman's Classification

- Uses two horizontal lines of sibileau. One passing through the floors of orbit and the other through the floors of maxillary antrum
- Suprastructure: Ethmoid, sphenoid and frontal sinuses and olfactory area of nose
- Mesostructure: Maxillary sinus and respiratory area of nose
- Infrastructure: Containing alveolar process.

Nasal Septal Perforation is Seen In

- Septal abscess/Septal myiasis
- Rhinolith or neglected foreign body
- TB, leprosy, lupus cause perforation of cartilaginous part
- Syphilis involves bony part
- Wegeners granulomatosis-total septal destruction
- Prolonged use of steroid sprays in nasal allergy
- Cocaine addicts
- Occupational-chromium plating, dichromate or soda ash manufacture, arsenic exposure.

Rhinolalia Clausa

- It is due to blockage of nasal cavity or nasopharynx
- Causes: Common cold, nasal allergy, nasal polyp, nasal mass, adenoids.

Rhinolalia Aperta

It is abnormal connection between the nasal cavity and oral cavity.

Causes: Velopharyngeal insufficiency, submucus palate, cleft palate, paralysis of soft palate, oroantral fistula.

Atrophic Rhinitis (Ozaena)

Mericiful anosmia: Patient unaware of foul smell due to anosmia.

CSF Rhinorrhea

- Discharge is clear, watery appears suddenly in a gush drops when bending forward (Tea pot sign) or straining
- Uncontrollable and cannot be sniffed back
- Not associated with sneezing, nasal congestion or lacrimation
- On collection in test tube it remains clear (Nasal discharge usually sediments)
- Glucose content > 30 mg/dl (Nasal discharge < 10 mg/dl)
- Beta 2 transferrin present (Absent in nasal discharge)
- In traumatic CSF leak. CSF and Blood are mixed **(Double ring sign or target sign).**

Oral Cavity/Pharynx/Larynx/Trachea

Action	Intrinsic muscle
Abductor of the Vocal Cords	Posterior Crico Arytenoid
Adductor of the Vocal Cords	Thyroarytenoids (external part); Interarytenoids (Transverse arytenoids) Lateral Cricoarytenoids
Tensor of Vocal Cord	Cricothyroid; Thyroid arytenoids (internal part) [VOCALIS]
Openers of laryngeal inlet	Thyroepiglottic (part of thyro arytenoid)
Closers of laryngeal inlet	Interarytenoids (oblique part); Interarytenoids (aryepiglottic part)

Nerve Supply

Motor	Sensory
All intrinsic muscles are supplied by Recurrent laryngeal nerve except for Cricothyroid which is supplied by External laryngeal nerve	Up to the level of Vocal Cords: Internal laryngeal N Below the level of Vocal Cords Recurrent laryngeal N

Laryngeal Cartilages

- Cricoids is the only cartilage forming complete ring
- VISOR angle: Angle between cricoids and thyroid cartilage
- Hyaline cartilage: Thyroid, cricoids and most of arytenoids
- Fibroelastic cartilage: Epiglottis, corniclate, cuneieform and tip of arytenoids.

Waldeyer's Ring

- A collection of subepithelial lymphoid tissue around the entrance to the pharynx

Inner ring	Outer ring
• Adenoids • Tubal tonsils • Lingual tonsils • Palatine tonsils	• Retropharyngeal node • Jugulodigastric node (tonsillar node) • Submandibular node • Submental node

- **Semon's law:** in all organic lesions abductor fibers are more susceptible and paralyzed earlier than the adductors
- **Wagner and Grossman hypothesis**: Cricothyroid receives innervations from SLN, keeps the vocal cord in paramedian position.

Thyroplasty

Isshiki's classification

Type	Procedure	Indication
I	Medialization of cord	Unilateral vocal cord paralysis Vocal fold atrophy Sulcus vocalis
II	Lateralization of cord	Spasmodic dysphonia Bilateral abductor paralysis
III	Shortening (Relax) of cord, To decrease pitch	To treat puberphonia; In those who have undergone gender transformation from female to male
IV	Lengthening (tighten) of cord, To increase pitch	To treat androphonia; converts male character of voice to female

Paterson Brown Kelly Syndorme/Plummer Vison Syndorme

- Females between 20–40 years
- Dysphagia
- Anemia
- Koilonychias, Glossitis and angular stomatitis
- **Bocca's sign**: Absence of laryngeal crepitation (postcricoids malignancy, perichondritis, foreign body cricopharynx).

Laryngomalacia

- Most common congenital anomaly of larynx
- Producing stridor
- Cry is normal
- Direct laryngoscopy shows elongated epiglottis (omega shaped) aryepiglottic folds and prominent arytenoids.

TB Larynx

- Affects posterior part more than the anterior part
- Almost always secondary to PT
- Most commonly affected part is the inter arytenoid fold
- Weakness of voice: earliest symptom
- Impairment of adduction: first sign
- Mamillated appearance: swelling in the interarytenoid region
- Mouse nibbled appearance: pseudoedema of glottis
- **Tripod sign**: in acute epiglottis, child sitting up and leaning forwards, unable to lie supine.

Surgical Anatomy of Larynx

Site	Subsite
Supraglottis	• Suprahyoid epiglottis (both lingual and laryngeal surfaces) • Infrahyoid epiglottis • Aryepiglottic folds (lateral aspect only) • Arytenoids • Ventricular bands (false cords)
Glottis	True vocal cords including anterior and posterior commissure
Subglottis	Up to the lower border of cricoids cartilage

Juvenile Nasopharyngeal Angiofiberoma

- Arises from posterior part of nasal cavity close to sphenoparietal foramen
- Commonly seen in males in second decade
- Profuse recurrent epistaxis is the most common symptom
- Broadening of nasal bridge, frog face deformity Maybe seen
- CT shows anterior bowing of posterior wall of maxillary sinus **(Antral sign or Holman-Miller sign).**

Laryngeal Carcinoma

- Etiology: Tobacco, Alcohol, Genetic, Asbestos, Mustard gas, previous radiation
- 90% are squamous cell carcinoma.

Supraglottic cancer	Glottis cancer	Subglottic cancer
• Early nodal metastasis to upper and middle jugular nodes • Bilateral nodes seen in epiglottic cancer • Hoarseness is a late symptom	• Most common type • Only local spread • No nodal metastases • Hoarseness is an early symptom (welcome cancer) hence detected early • Fixation of cord indicates spread to thyroarytenoid muscle (bad prognosis)	• Earliest symptom-stridor or laryngeal obstruction • Hoarseness is a late symptom • Nodal metastases to prelaryngeal, pretracheal and lower jugular nodes

Treatment of Glottis Carcinoma

Carcinoma in situ	• Best treated by transoral endoscopic CO_2 laser • If laser not available, stripping of vocal cords and tissues sent for biopsy • If biopsy shows invasive carcinoma give radiotherapy • If biopsy confirms only carcinoma in situ regular follow-up
T1 (limited to vocal cords)	• Radiotherapy is the treatment of choice
T1 (extension to anterior commissure or arytenoids)	• Radiotherapy is the best choice • If RT not available, frontolateral partial laryngectomy • If it fails total laryngectomy
T2 No (Supraglottic or subglottic involvement)	Cord mobile –radiotherapy → conservation laryngectomy → TL
	Cord mobility impairment → conservation laryngectomy → TL
T3 and T4 lesions	Total laryngectomy (TL)

Treatment of Subglottic Cancer

- T1 and T2 lesions: radiotherapy
- T3 and T4 lesions: total laryngectomy and postoperative radiation.

Treatment of Supraglottic Cancer

- T1 lesions: radiotherapy or CO_2 laser excision
- T2 lesions: supraglottic laryngectomy with or without neck dissection
- T3 and T4 lesions: total laryngectomy with neck dissection and postoperative RT.

Nasopharyngeal Carcinoma

- **Trotter's triad**: Conductive deafness (ET block], Ipsilateral temporoparietal neuralgia (involvement of CN V) and Palatal paralysis (CN X)
- **Jaccods's triad**: Ipsilateral ophthalmoplegia, amaurosis, ipsilateral neuralgia
- Enlargement of cervical lymph nodes: **Most common symptom** (60%) and most common region posterior cervical

- **Type:**
  - **Type I**: Squamous cell carcinoma
  - **Type II**: Nonkeratinizing carcinoma
  - **Type III**: Undifferentiated carcinoma.

Dysphagia Lusoria

- Aabnormal large vessel pressing on the esophagus and causing dysphagia
  - Right aortic arch
  - Double aortic arch
  - Abnormal right subclavian artery
  - Abnormal innominate artery
- Foreign body in Trachea lies in sagittal plane as it is a rigid structure—Seen better in lateral X-ray
- Foreign body in Esophagus lies in Coronal plane as it is not rigid—Seen better in Anteroposterior view.

QUESTIONS

1. A pregnant woman has deterioration of hearing loss. The tympanogram is likely to show: **(Repeat 2013)**
a. As type
b. Ad type
c. B type
d. C type

2. Sinuses present at birth are: **(Repeat 2012)**
a. Frontal and maxillary
b. Frontal and ethmoid
c. Maxillary and sphenoid
d. Maxillary and ethmoid

3. Average hearing at 500, 1000, 2000, Hz is 45 dB in the left ear. Percentage hearing loss in left ear is: **(2014)**
a. 0.45
b. 0.20
c. 0.30
d. 0.40

4. All are true regarding Adenotonsillectomy in children except: **(2014)**
a. Extracapsular hot tonsillectomy is done with cold knife
b. Grisel's syndrome is common in children
c. Sleep apnea is an indication
d. Cricothyroid region is high and anterior in children

5. BERA can be most accurate from which gestation? **(2014)**
a. 30 weeks
b. 32 weeks
c. 34 weeks
d. 28 weeks

6. In which TNM staging of glottis carcinoma, cancer limited to larynx with vocal cord fixation? **(2014)**
a. T1
b. T2
c. T3
d. T4

7. Not a component of Kiesselbach's plexus: **(Repeat 2011)**
a. Superior labial
b. Posterior ethmoidal
c. Sphenopalatine
d. Greater palatine

8. Mouth nibbled appearance of vocal cords is seen in: **(2013)**
a. Tb larynx
b. Syphilis
c. Achalasia cardia
d. Lupus

9. The frequency used in tympanometry is: **(2013)**
a. 256 Hz
b. 220 Hz
c. 222 Hz
d. 440 Hz

10 Mid tracheostomy is done at which of the following level? **(2013)**
a. 3–4 rings of tracheal cartilage
b. 5–6 rings
c. 1–2 rings
d. 2–3 rings

11. Osteomas common in which of the following sinus? **(2013)**
a. Frontal
b. Ethmoid
c. Maxillary
d. Sphenoid

12. Gutzman Pressure test: (2012)
- a. Laryngomalacia
- b. Puberphonia
- c. Laryngeal stenosis
- d. Subglottic hemangioma

13. Posterior ethmoidal sinus drain into: (2012)
- a. Sphenoethmoidal recess
- b. Superior meatus
- c. Inferior meatus
- d. Middle meatus

14. Which of the following does not form Waldeyer's ring? (2012)
- a. Palatine tonsils
- b. Adenoids
- c. Jugulodigastric node
- d. Lateral pharyngeal bands

15. Sound reaches maximum amplitude depending on its frequency at: (2012)
- a. Tympanic membrane
- b. Ear ossicles
- c. Semicircular canals
- d. Basilar membrane

16. True about tympanic membrane: (2012)
- a. Attached to oval window
- b. Forms an angle of 45 degree with external auditory canal
- c. Chorda tympani nerve passes through pars tensa
- d. Cone of light forms anterosuperior quadrant

17. Staging of glottic carcinoma of larynx with fixation of vocal cord is: (2012)
- a. T1
- b. T2
- c. T3
- d. T4

18. Endolymph is present in: (2012)
- a. Scala media
- b. Scala vestibule
- c. Scala tympani
- d. Cochlear aqueduct

19. Trotters triad includes all except: (2011)
- a. Diplopia
- b. Conductive deafness
- c. Ipsilateral temporoparietal neuralgia
- d. Palatal palsy

20. Macintosh curved blade laryngoscope is used in: (2011)
- a. Indirect laryngoscopy
- b. Direct laryngoscopy
- c. Video laryngoscopy
- d. Bronchoscopy

21. Which of the following arteries is not involved little's area anastomosis? (2011)
- a. Anterior ethmoid
- b. Sphenopalatine art
- c. Greater palatine artery
- d. Posterior ethmoid artery

22. Which of the following is not an objective hearing test? (2011)
- a. Impedance audiometry
- b. Otoacoustic emissions
- c. Brainstem evoked response
- d. Pure tone audiometry

23. Which of the following is false regarding Peritonsillar abcess? (2011)
- a. Usually presents with trimus
- b. The accumulation of pus is lateral to the superior constrictor muscle
- c. It does not involve the floor of mouth
- d. It causes bulge of the uvula/soft palate

24. Type of deafness seen in early stages of Meniere's disease: (2010)
- a. Low frequency conductive hearing loss
- b. Low frequency sensorineural hearing loss
- c. High frequency conductive hearing loss
- d. High frequency sensorineural hearing loss

25. Most common cause of acute otitis media in children: (2010)
- a. E coli
- b. H influenza
- c. Pneumococcus
- d. Staph aureus

26. Characteristic feature of TB otitis media: (Repeat) (2010)
- a. Multiple perforations in TM
- b. Mastoiditis
- c. Middle ear effusion
- d. Ear discharge

27. Most common site of fracture mandible: (2010)
- a. Ramus
- b. Angle of mandible
- c. Neck of the condyle
- d. Coronoid process

28. Perilymph communicates with subarachnoid space through: (2010)
- a. Ductus reunions
- b. Helicotrema
- c. Utriculosaccular duct
- d. Cochlear aqueduct

29. Level of tracheostomy is by which of the following anatomical landmark? (2013)
a. Cricoid cartilage
b. Isthmus of thyroid
c. 2nd tracheal ring
d. 3rd tracheal ring

30. Depolarization of cochlea due to: (2010)
a. Potassium influx
b. Potassium efflux
c. Sodium influx
d. Sodium efflux

31. Which among the following is not true about otosclerosis? (2009)
a. Hearing better in louder conditions
b. Eustachian tube is always abnormal
c. Tympanic membrane is normal
d. Bilateral progressive conductive deafness

32 For Grommet tube insertion in serous otitis media, the incision on tympanic membrane is made on: (2009)
a. Anteroinferior quardrant
b. Anterosuperior quadrant
c. Posterosuperior quadrant
d. Posteroinferior quadrant

33. Bezold's abscess is seen at: (2009)
a. Petrous tip
b. Mastoid tip
c. Digastric triangle
d. Subdurally

34. Which of the following is not a feature of Rhino–sporidiosis? (2009)
a. Bleeding polyp
b. Russell bodies are seen
c. Oral dapsone is useful in treatment
d. Bleeding is present

35. True statement about antrochoanal polyp is: (2009)
a. Often bilateral
b. Usually multiple
c. Arises from lateral wall
d. Recurrence is less common

36. A patient hears better in noise. Most likely diagnosis is: (2009)
a. Hyperacusis
b. Presbyacusis
c. Hypoacusis
d. Paracusis

37. Which of the following is not true about secretory otitis media? (2009)
a. Tympanic membrane is intact, retracted and lustreless
b. Hairline fluid level seen inside the tympanic cavity
c. Fistula test is positive
d. Politzerization affords relief

38. Mastoid tip develops by: (2008)
a. 1 year
b. 2 years
c. 3 years
d. 4 years

39. Advantage of flexible bronchoscopy is: (2008)
a. Can be done in awake patient
b. Can examine the subsegmental bronchi
c. Can be used in jaw and neck abnormalities
d. All the above

40. Deafness is seen with: (2008)
a. Essential hypertension
b. Congenital QT syndrome
c. Marfan syndrome
d. Turners syndrome

41. Acoustic neuroma commonly involves: (2008)
a. Superior vestibular nerve
b. Inferior vestibular nerve
c. Facial nerve
d. Cochlear nerve

42. All take part in anastomosis in little's area except: (2011)
a. Post ethmoid artery
b. Anterior ethmoid artery
c. Sphenopalatine artery
d. Greater palatine artery

43. Test for malingering of hearing loss: (2008)
a. Tympanometry
b. Lombard test
c. ABC test
d. Gringe test

44. Cottel's test is used to test the patency of the nares in: (2008)
a. Atrophic rhinitis
b. Rhinosporidiosis
c. Deviated nasal septum
d. Hypertrophied inferior turbinate

45. In a patient with hypertrophied adenoids the voice abnormality that is seen is: (2008)
a. Rhinolalia clausa
b. Rhinolalia aperta
c. Hot potato voice
d. Muffled voice

46. Abductor of the vocal cord is: (2008)
a. Lateral cricoarytenoid
b. Cricothyroid
c. Posterior cricoarytenoid
d. Interarytenoid

47. **Carhart's notch on otoscerosis is observed at:** (2013)
a. 1000 HZ
b. 2000 HZ
c. 3000 HZ
d. 4000 HZ

48. **One of the following abscesses occur in sterno-cleidomastoid sheath in relation to mastoid infection:** (2009)
a. Bezold's abscess
b. Meatal abscess
c. Luc's abscess
d. Citelli's abscess

49. **What is the symptom of a person with unilateral abductor paralysis?** (2007)
a. Dyspnea on excertion
b. Transient hoarseness
c. Husky voice
d. Inspiratory stridor

50. **Regarding acute vestibular neuronitis all are true except:** (2007)
a. Tinnitus and vertigo developing over 1–2 weeks
b. High frequency sensorineural hearing loss
c. Spontaneous nystagmus present
d. Usually follows an upper respiratory tract infection

51. **Most common complication of tracheostomy is:** (2007)
a. Pneumothorax
b. Surgical emphysema
c. Injury to large vessels
d. Injury to esophagus

52. **Which of the following is not seen in Meniere's disease?** (2007)
a. Vertigo
b. Tinnitus
c. Conductive hearing loss
d. Sensorineural hearing loss

53. **Which of the following ECG finding is associated with congenital deafness?** (2007)
a. Delta wave
b. Long QT
c. Short PR interval
d. T wave inversion

54. **All the following are features of Grandenigo's syndrome except:** (2007)
a. Flushing of skin over parotid
b. Retro orbit of pain
c. VI nerve palsy
d. Persistent ear discharge

55. **Barotraumatic otitis media is a result of:** (2007)
a. Rapid descent while in an aircraft
b. Rapid ascent while in an aircraft
c. Sudden acceleration while in a bus
d. Sudden deceleration while in a bus

56. **Laryngomalacia is characterized by:** (2007)
a. Usually present at about the age of 5 years
b. Biphasic stridor
c. Elongated epiglottis with thin aryepiglottic folds on laryngoscopy
d. Best treatment by epiglottectomy

57. **Bony septal perforation is seen in:** (2007)
a. Syphilis
b. Leprosy
c. TB
d. Lupus

58. **Modified Young's operation is done for:** (2007)
a. Atrophic rhinitis
b. Allergic rhinitis
c. Acute sinusitis
d. Chronic sinusitis

59. **Subjective interference is present in:** (2007)
a. Pure tone audiometry
b. Impedance
c. Otoacoustic emission
d. Brainstem evoked potential

60. **Most common presentation of nasopharyngeal carcinoma is:** (Repeat 2011)
a. Epistaxis
b. Cervical lymphadenopathy
c. Nasal obstruction
d. Hearing loss

61. **Otalgia referred pain is carried by all except:** (2007)
a. CNVII
b. CNVIII
c. CN X
d. C2 C3

62. **Rinne's positive means:** (2007)
a. Conductive hearing loss in ipsilateral ear
b. Conductive hearing loss in opposite ear
c. Normal hearing
d. AC < BC

63. **After Caldwell Luc operation, the person experiences loss of sensation over cheek, this is due to involvement of which nerve?** (2007)
a. Mandibular nerve
b. Vagus nerve
c. Maxillary nerve
d. Facial nerve

ANSWERS AND EXPLANATIONS

1. Ans. a. As type *Ref: Diseases of Ear, Nose and Throat by PL Dhingra, 5/e p98*

- History suggests worsening of hearing loss in pregnancy, which is characteristically seen in otosclerosis. The impedance audiometry in otosclerosis will show **As type of curve.**

Otosclerosis/Otospongiosis:

- Disease of **bony labyrinth** where **spongy bone replaces normal enchondral layer of bony otic capsule**
- Most often the otosclerotic focus **involves stapes** leading to stapes fixation and CHL.

Etiology

- **Fistula ante fenestrum**: In front of oval window is the most common site of predilection in stapedial type
- **Family history present**, Autosomal dominant; Whites more affected than Negroes
- **Females affected twice** more than males. But in India males are more affected; Age 20–30 years
- Maybe initiated or **made worse by pregnancy**, menopause, after an accident or a major operation
- **Van der Hoeve's syndrome: Triad of Osteogenesis imperfecta, Blue sclera and Otosclerosis.**

Symptoms and Signs

- Hearing loss: Painless progressive bilateral CHL
- **Paracusis willisi**: Hears better in noisy surroundings
- Tinnitus, Vertigo, Monotonuous soft speech
- TM: Normal and mobile
- **Schwartz sign**: Reddish hue seen on the promontory through TM, which indicates active focus
- TFTs: Negative Rinne, Weber lateralized to the ear with greater hearing loss
- In some cases a **dip in the bone conduction curve appear at 2000 Hz which disappears after successful stapedectomy (Carhart's notch)**
- **Bezold's triad: Absolute negative Rinne's raised lower tone limit, prolonged bone conduction.**

Treatment

- Medical: Sodium fluoride
- **Surgical: Stapedectomy (treatment of choice).** Replacement of stapes with Teflon or stainless steel or titanium piston.

Contraindications for stapedectomy

- Only hearing ear
- Associated Meniere's disease
- Young children
- Professional athletes, high construction workers, divers, frequent air travellers

Relative Contraindications: Otitis externa, TM perforation, Exostosis

Tympanograms

Has impedance part and acoustic reflex measurement to find middle ear status. Based on principle that when soundwaves stikes the tympanic membrane some energy is absorbed and some is reflected. We measure reflected sound and its variation with changes in EAC pressure plotted as tympanogram.

Delivers a tone of 220 Hz (Q)

Normal middle ear pressure: 0–150 mm H_2O

- Type A: Normal Tympanogram
- Type A_S: Otosclerosis, malleus fixation
- Type A_D: Ossicular Discontinuity/thin lax TM
- Type B: Middle ear fluid, Thick TM
- Type C: Retracted TM

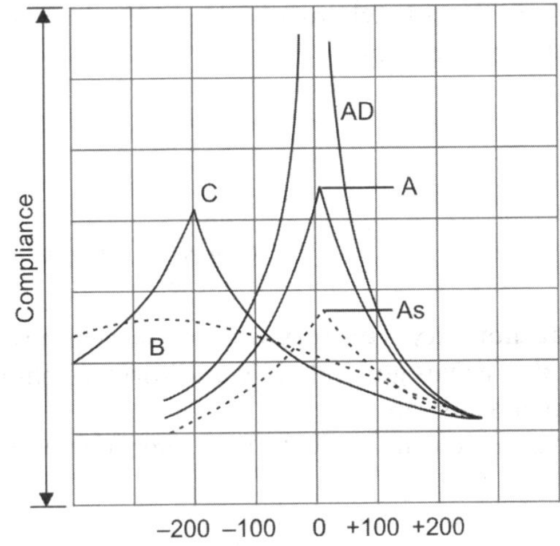

2. **Ans. d. Maxillary and ethmoid** *Ref: Diseases of Ear, Nose and Throat by PL Dhingra, 5/e p203*
   - **Maxillary** and **ethmoidal sinuses are present at birth. First radiological evidence of maxillary sinus is at 4–5 months after birth.**
   - **Ethmoidal sinus is pneumatized at birth** but maxillary sinus is not pneumatised until 4 years
   - **Earliest sinus to appear radiological–maxillary sinus at 4–5 months**
   - Spenoidal sinuses are present by 5 years of age, whereas the frontal sinuses begin to develop at 7–8 years and are not completely developed until adolescence.

	Status at birth	Growth	First radiologic evidence
Maxillary	Present at birth	Rapid growth from birth to 3 years and from 7–12 years. Adult size – 15 years	4–5 months after birth
Ethmoid	Present at birth Anterior group: 5 × 2 × 2 mm. Posterior group: 5 × 4 × 2 mm.	Reach adult size by 12 years	1 year
Frontal	Not present	Invades frontal bone at the age of 4 years. Size increases until teens	6 years
Sphenoid	Not Present	Reaches sella turcica by the age of 7 years, dorsum sellae by late teens and basis phenoid by adult age. Reaches full size between 15 years and adult age	4 years

3. **Ans. c. 0.30** *Ref: Diseases of Ear, Nose and Throat, by Mohan Bansal, p164*
   - Calculate the average of threshold of hearing speech frequencies of 500, 1000, 2000 Hz. Here it is 45 Db
   - Deduct from it 25 Db (as up to 25 dB loss is considered normal). 45–25 = 20.
   - Multiply it with 1.5 and its percentage is the percentage of hearing impairment of the ear. 20 × 1.5 = 30. Its percentage is 0.30.
   - To calculate the handicap percentage = [(Better ear % × 5) + worse ear %]/6
4. **Ans. a. Extracapsular hot tonsillectomy is done with cold knife**
   Ref: Textbook of Ear, Nose and Throat, by BS Tuli 2/e p480 and Dhingra p440
   - Extracapsular tonsillectomy: Complete tonsillectomy is done by dissection and snare method (cold knife) or electrocautery (hot tonsillectomy)
   - Intratonsillar tonsillectomy: Partial tonsillectomy in which capsule is preserved to reduce postoperative pain
   - Methods include microdebrider and by cold methods (cryosurgery, coblation, Harmonic scapel).

Grisel's syndrome
- It is nontraumatic atlantoaxial sublaxation results from inflammation in superior cervical region leading to stiffness of neck, spasm of sternocleidomastoid and deep cervical muscles

- The head is rotated away from the side where atlas has shifted forward
- Diagnosis confirmed with CT cervical spine
- Treatment
- Antibiotics.

Philadelphia Collar
Traction to reduce subluxation.

5. Ans. c. 34 weeks *Ref: Cloherty's Manual of Neonatal care, 6/e p646 and Dhingra 32*

BERA:
(Brainstem Evoked response audiometry/Auditory Brainstem response (ABR)
Measures electroencephalographic waves generated by auditory system in response to clicks
ABR is reliable after 34 weeks postnatal age
Preferred noninvasive screening method in NICU to find intergrity of auditory pathways through 8th nerve, pons and midbrain.
Measures hearing sensitivity in range of 1000–4000 Hz

- In normal persons 7 waves are produced in the first 10 ms
- I, III, V are most stable and used in measurements.
- Parameters studied are latency, interwave latency, amplitude.
- Anatomical site from where the waves arise
  - Wave I: Distal part of 8th Nerve
  - Wave II: Proximal part of 8th Nerve
  - Wave III: Cochlear nucleus
  - Wave IV: Superior Olivary complex
  - Wave V: Lateral colliculus
  - Waves VI and VII: Inferior Colliculus

Uses: Screening test in infants

- To determine threshold of hearing in children, uncooperative adults, malingers
- To diagnose retrocochlear pathology, e.g: Acoustic neuroma
- To diagnose brainstem pathology, e.g. Multiple sclerosis
- To monitor 8 th nerve intraoperatively in acoustic neuroma surgery.

6. Ans. c. T3 *Ref: Diseases of Ear, Nose and Throat by PL Dhingra, 5/e p328*

Glottis	
T_1	Tumor limited to vocal cord(s) (may involve anterior or posterior commissures) with normal mobility
T_1a	Tumor limited to one vocal cord
T_1b	Tumor involves both vocal cords
T_2	Tumor extends to supraglottis and/or subglottis, and/or with impaired vocal cord mobility
T_3	Tumor limited to the larynx with vocal cord fixation and/or invades paraglottic space and/or minor thyroid cartilage erosion
T_4a	Tumor invades through thyroid cartilage and/or invades tissues beyond the larynx (e.g. trachea, soft tissues of neck including deep extrinsic muscles of the tongue, strap muscles, thyroid, or esophagus)
T_1b	Tumor invades prevertebral space, encases carotid artery or invades mediastinal structures

7. Ans. b. Posterior ethmoidal *Ref: Diseases of Ear, Nose and Throat by PL Dhingra, 5/e p190*

Is situated in the Little's area in the anteroinferior part of nasal septum

- Four arteries anastamose here to form Kiesselbach's plexus
  a. Anterior ethmoidal artery
  b. Septal branch of sphenopalatine artery
  c. Septal branch of greater palatine artery
  d. Septal branch of superior labial artery

  This area is exposed to drying effect of inspiratory current and finger nail trauma
  Common site of epistaxis in children.

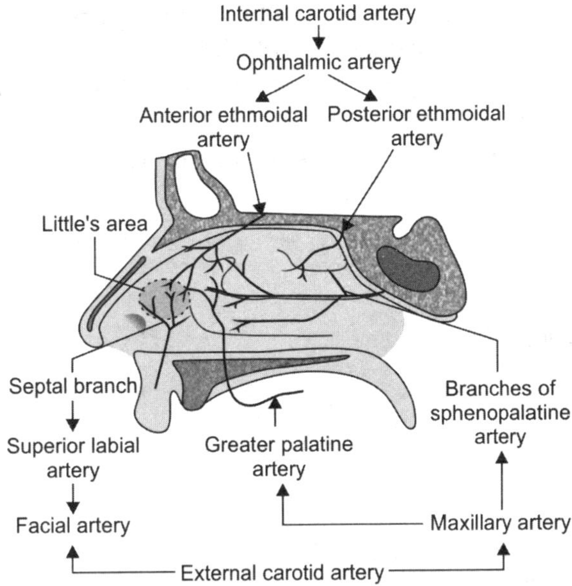

8. Ans. a. Tb larynx *Ref: Diseases of Ear, Nose and Throat by PL Dhingra, 5/e p312*

TB LARYNX

- Affects posterior part more than the anterior part
- Almost always secondary to PT
- Most commonly affected part is the arytenoids, interarytenoid fold.

C/F:z

- **Weakness of voice earliest symptom**
- **Pain radiating to ear due to ulceration**
- **Odynophagia.**

Examination Findings

- **Monocorditis**: Hyperemia of vocal cord with impairment of adduction-**first sign**
- Mamillated appearance: Swelling in the interarytenoid region
- Mouse nibbled appearance: Ulceration of vocal cord
- Ulceration and granulation over arytenoids and inter arytenoids
- Pseudoedema of epiglottis: Turban epiglottis
- Swelling of false vocal cord and aryepiglottic fold
- Diagnosis is by chest X-ray and sputum AFB examination
- Biopsy to rule out malignancy
- Treatment with ATT.

Lupus

- Affects anterior larynx
- Epiglottis is involved first
- Lupus of larynx is painless
- There is no pulmonary TB
- Treatment is with ATT.

Syphilis

- Present as smooth swelling which may ulcerate
- Occur in any part of larynx
  - Diagnosis is by biopsy and serology
  - Laryngeal stenosis is a frequent complication.

9. Ans b. 220 Hz *Ref: Diseases of Ear, Nose and Throat by PL Dhingra, 5/e p29*

Explanation: Refer Tympanometry part in question 1 of 2014

10. Ans. d. 2–3 rings *Ref: Diseases of Ear, Nose and Throat by PL Dhingra, 5/e p337*

Tracheostomy

- Tracheostomy is making an opening in the anterior wall of trachea and converting it into a stoma on the skin surface
- Indications are
  - Respiratory obstruction
  - Suction of retained secretions
  - Respiratory insufficiency
- Types are
  - Elective
  - Emergency
  - Based on the site.

High tracheostomy

- Opening Made above the isthmus of thyroid gland
- Through the 1st tracheal ring
- Done in malignancy of the larynx
- Increased risk of perichondritis and subglottic stenosis.

Mid tracheostomy

- Done through the 2nd and 3rd tracheal rings
- Most commonly done
- Isthmus has to be retracted or divided.

Low tracheostomy

- Done below the isthmus
- Through 4th and 5th tracheal rings
- Done when the airway is blocked at the upper tracheal level
- Risk of injuring the great vessels of neck.

11. Ans. a. Frontal sinus *Ref: Diseases of Ear, Nose and Throat by PL Dhingra, 5/e p219*

Sinus Osteomas

- Osteomas are most common in Frontal followed by ethmoid and then maxillary sinusitis
- Most are asymptomatic and detected incidentally on radiology of the sinuses
- May become symptomatic when they obstruct the sinus Ostia leading to sinusitis or mucocele formation
- May also cause pressure symptoms on the orbit, nose or cranium.

Incidence of Osteoma in Paranasal Sinus

- Frontal sinuses: 80%
- Ethmoid air cells: ~15%
- Maxillary sinuses: ~5%
- Sphenoid sinus: rare

Subtypes

Osteomas are, as the name suggests, osteogenic tumors composed of mature bone. **Three histological patterns are recognized.**

1. **Ivory osteoma**
   - Also known as eburnated osteoma
   - Most common
   - Dense bone lacking haversian system
2. **Mature osteoma**
   - Also known as osteoma spongiosum
   - Resembles 'normal' bone, including trabecular bone often with marrow

3. **Mixed osteoma**
   - Mixture of ivory and mature histology

They are associated with Gardener syndrome.

12. Ans. b. Puberphonia *Ref: Diseases of Ear, Nose and Throat by Mohan Bansal, 2013, p496*

- Puberphonia
- Failure of childhood high-pitched voice to low-pitched male voice after puberty in boys is called puberphonia.

Anatomy

Male and female larynx are identical until puberty, after which male larynx grows rapidly with lengthening of rima glottides which brings change in character of male voice (voice becomes lower pitch) while female larynx changes a little.

Treatment

- Speech therapy
- Gutzman's pressure test in which when thyroid prominence is pressed in a backward and downward direction it relaxes the outstretched cord and low tone is produced
- Type III thyroplasty (surgical shortening and relaxation of vocal cords).

13. Ans b. Superior meatus *Ref: Diseases of Ear, Nose and Throat by PL Dhingra, 5/e p149*

Openings in the meatus:

Inferior meatus	Nasolacrimal duct
Middle meatus	• Middle ethomidal air cells (forms a bulge- Bulla Ethmoidalis) • Frontal sinus opens into the infundibulum • Maxillary sinus and anterior ethmoidal sinus opens posterior to infundibulum
Superior meatus	Posterior ethmoidal sinus
Sphenoethmoidal recess	Sphenoid sinus

14. Ans: c. Jugulodigastric node *Ref: Diseases of Ear, Nose and Throat by PL Dhingra, 5/e p253*

Waldeyer's ring

A collection of subepithelial lymphoid tissue around the entrance to the pharynx:

- Adenoids
- Tubal tonsils in fossa of Rosenmuller
- Lingual tonsils
- Palatine tonsils
- Lateral pharyngeal bands
- Nodules in posterior pharyngeal wall

15. Ans. d. Basilar membrane *Ref: Diseases of Ear, Nose and Throat by PL Dhingra, 5/e p18*

Physiology: Soundwave reaches maximum frequency on basilar membrane and stimulates that segment. Higher frequencies are represented in the basal turns of cochlea and progressively lower ones towards apex.

16. Ans. b. Forms an angle of 45 degree with external auditory canal

Ref: Diseases of Ear, Nose and Throat by PL Dhingra, 5/e p4, Mohan Bansal p5

Tympanic Membarane

- Obliquely set so that posterosuperior part is more lateral than anteroinferior part 9–10 mm height, 8–9 mm width, 0.1 mm thick
- It forms an angle of 55 degree with deep EAC.

Pars tensa

- Forms most part of tympanic membrane
- Periphery thickened to form annulus tympanicus
- Central part is tented inwards at the level of tip of malleus and is called the umbo
- A bright cone of light seen radiating from the tip of malleus to the periphery in the anteroinferior quadrant.

Pars flaccid (Shrapnel's membrane)

- Situated above the lateral process of malleus between the notch of Rivinus and the malleolar folds
- The periphery is thickened to form annulus. It is not attached to oval window
- Chorda tympani runs on medial surface of tympanic membrane
- Cone of light forms in anteroinferior quadrant.

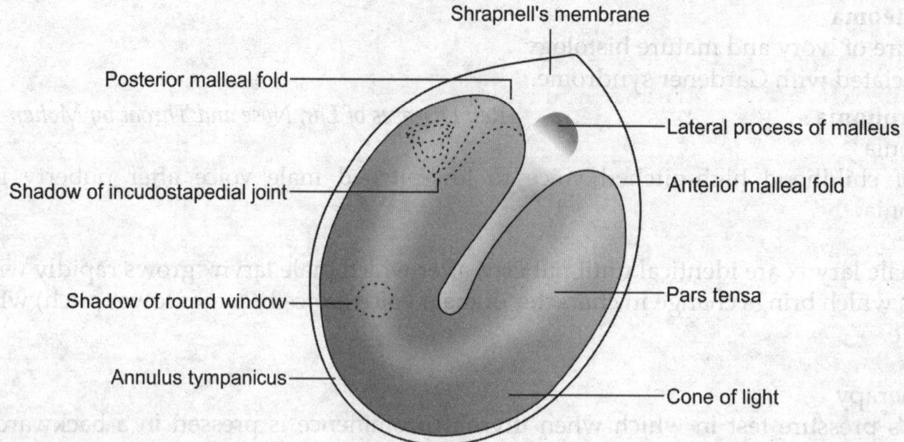

17. Ans: c. T3 *Ref: Diseases of Ear, Nose and Throat by PL Dhingra, 5/e p328*

Explanation: Refer question 6 of 2014

18. Ans. a. Scala media *Ref: Diseases of Ear, Nose and Throat by PL Dhingra, 5/e p12*

Inner ear fluids:

- Scala vestibule and scala tympani are filled with perilymph
- Scala media is filled with endolymph.

Endolymph:

- Fills membranous labyrinth
- It is rich in K^+ ions
- Composition is like intracellular fluid
- Secreted by stria vascularis of the crista and dark cells in utricle and ampullary end of the semicircular canals.

Perilymph:

- Lies between bony and membranous labyrinth
- Composition is like extracellular fluid
- Rich in Na^+ ions

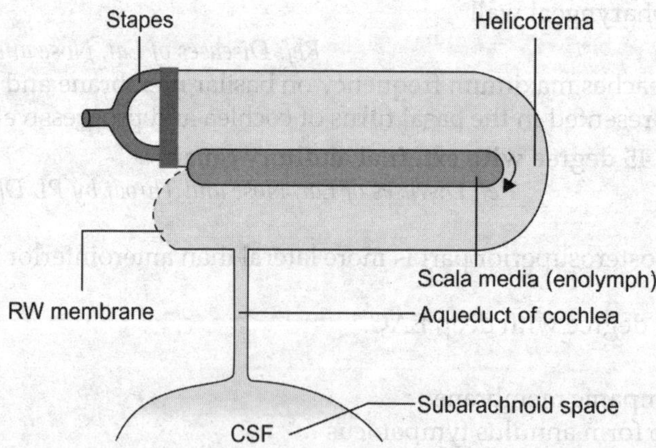

19. Ans. a. Diplopia *Ref: Diseases of Ear, Nose and Throat by PL Dhingra, 5/e p264*

Nasopharyngeal carcinoma

Etiology

- Genetic-prevalent among Chinese

- Virus-EBV
- Environmental: air pollution, tobacco smoking, opium smoking, nitrosamines from dry salted fish, smoke from burning incense and wood, vitamin C deficiency.

Clinical features

- Age: 5th to 7th decades; Males affected 3 times more
- Presence of unilateral SOM in an adult should rise the suspicion of nasopharyngeal growth
- Jugular foramen syndrome
- Horner's syndrome

Trotter's triad: Conductive deafness (ET block], Ipsilateral temporoparietal neuralgia (involvement of CN V) and Palatal paralysis (CN X)

Jaccods's triad: Ipsilateral ophthalmoplegia, amaurosis, ipsilateral neuralgia

Enlargement of cervical lymph nodes: **Most common symptom** (60%) and most common region posterior cervical.

Types:

- **Type I:** Squamous cell carcinoma
- **Type II:** nonkeratinizing carcinoma
- **Type III:** undifferentiated carcinoma

Diagnosis is with biopsy, CT scan, MRI

Treatment: Irradiation is the treatment of choice; Chemotherapy for stage III and IV cancers with Cisplatin +/- 5 FU.

20. Ans. b. Direct laryngoscopy *Ref: Otolaryngology by Scott–Brown. 7/e Diseases of Ear, Nose and Throat by PL Dhingra, Volume 1; 5/e p432, 434*

Mackintosh curved blade laryngoscope

- It is the most common blade used by anesthesist to intubate
- Indirect Laryngology is done using laryngeal mirrors and does not need any blade
- Video laryngoscopy is done using 70 degree or 45 degree endoscopes
- Bronchoscopy is done using bronchoscopes and may not need a blade for introducing them through the larynx.

Miller's straight blade is used for intubating neonates.

21. Ans. d. Posterior ethmoid artery

Explanation: Refer Question 1 of 2013

22. Ans d. Pure tone audiometry *Ref: Diseases of Ear, Nose and Throat by PL Dhingra, 5/e p27*

Pure tone audiogram.

- It is a **subjective** test depending on patients response to pure tones delivered by audiometer. **OAE, BERA are objective tests**
- Air conduction thresholds (AC) at 125, 250, 500, 1000, 2000, 4000, 8000 Hz and Bone conduction (BC) thresholds at 250, 500, 1000, 2000, 4000 Hz are measured.

Otoacoustic emissions

- OAEs are low intensity sounds produced by outer hair cells of a normal cochlea
- Do not disappear in 8th nerve damage as cochlear cells are normal

Use

- Screening test for hearing in neonates and uncooperative, mentally challenged after sedation as sedation does not affect OAE
- Distinguish cochlear from retrocochlear lesions
- Used to diagnose retrocochlear lesions especially auditory neuropathy

Types

a. Spontaneous OAE: Healthy persons with < 30 dB hearing loss

b. Evoked OAE: Elicited by sound stimulus
   i. Transient evoked OAE: Evoked by clicks
   ii. Distortion product OAE: Two tones are presented simultaneously to cochlea to produce distortion.

OAEs absent in:
- 50% normal individuals
- Cochlear lesions
- Middle ear disorder
- Hearing loss > 30 dB

(Brainstem Evoked response audiometry/Auditory Brainstem response (ABR)- refer question 5 of 2014.

23. Ans. b. The accumulation of pus is lateral to the superior constrictor muscle

Ref: Diseases of Ear, Nose and Throat by PL Dhingra, 5/e p278-279

Peritonsillar abscess
- In peritonsillar abscess the collection of pus is between the superior constrictor and the capsule of the tonsil.
- It is also called **Quinsy**
  - Common in adults
  - C/F: Fever, **odynophagia,** muffled or **hot potato voice**, halitosis, trismus.
  - O/E: Unilateral tonsillar enlargement with congestion, pushing uvula to opposite side, enlarged
- Tender jugulodigastric nodes.
  - Treatment is incision and drainage at most prominent point or at the junction of anterior pillar with the line drawn from base of uvula.

24. Ans. b. Low frequency sensorineural hearing loss

Ref: Diseases of Ear, Nose and Throat by PL Dhingra, 5/e p113

- Hearing loss in Meniere's disease is sensorineural type and is fluctuating.
- It is associated with episodic vertigo, tinnitus and sensation of fullness of ear.
- Early Meniere's has low frequency loss and the PTA curve is rising type.
- Later on the higher frequencies are affected and the PTA curve becomes flat and finally it becomes sloping type.

25. Ans. c. Pneumococcus *Ref: Diseases of Ear, Nose and Throat by PL Dhingra, 5/e p69*

Most common organisms ASOM in infants and children is:
- Streptococcus pneumonia: 30%
- Hemophilus influenza: 20%
- Moraxella catarrhalis: 12%
- Other organisms are like Streptococcus pyogenes, Staphylococcus aureus.

26. Ans. a. Multiple perforations in TM *Ref: Diseases of Ear, Nose and Throat by PL Dhingra, 5/e p83*

Tuberculosis Otitis Media
- Secondary to pulmonary TB
- Common in children, young adults
- Painless foul smelling ear discharge, severe conductive hearing loss which is out of proportion to symptoms
- O/E: Multiple perforations on TM is characteristic. Pale granulation tissue in middle ear and there Maybe facial palsy
- Investigations include culture of discharge, HPE of granulation tissue and chest X-ray to rule out pulmonary TB
- Treatment is ATT.

27. Ans. c. Neck of the condyle *Ref: Diseases of Ear, Nose and Throat by PL Dhingra, 5/e p199*

- Most common site of fracture mandible is the Condyle > Angle and Body > Symphysis
- Clinical features are that of pain and trismum
- O/e deviation of jaw to the opposite side, echymosis of the oral mucosa, malocclusion of teeth
- Treatment is with either open or closed reduction and fixation.

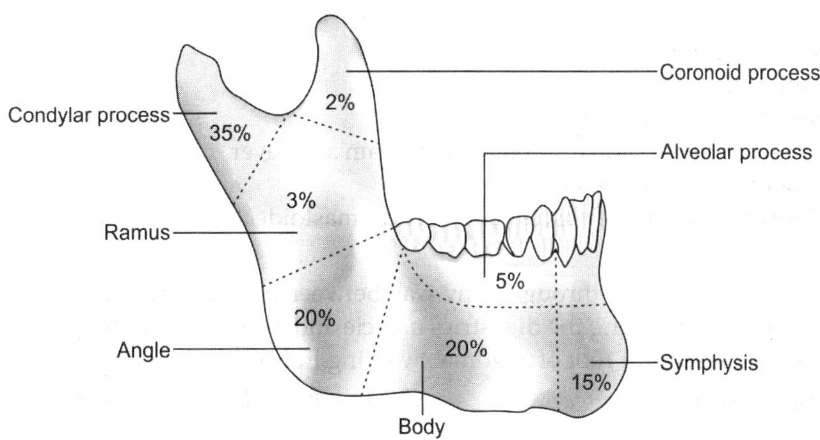

28. Ans. d. Cochlear aqueduct
Explanation: Question 7, 2012

29. Ans. b. Isthmus of thyroid *Ref: Diseases of Ear, Nose and Throat by PL Dhingra, 5/e p337*

Types of tracheostomy based on position

- High tracheostomy: Above the thyroid isthmus through the first tracheal ring
  - Increased risk of subglottic edema and stenosis
- Mid tracheostomy: At the level of thyroid isthmus, through the 2nd or 3rd tracheal ring
  - Isthmus is divided or retracted
  - Most commonly done
- Low tracheostomy: Below the isthmus
- Increased risk of injury to great vessels in the neck.

30. Ans. a. Potassium influx *Ref: Diseases of Ear, Nose and Throat by PL Dhingra, 5/e p13 and 19*

- There exists a potential difference approx (125 mv) between the K^+ rich endolymph (+ 80 mv) and the inner hair cells (–45 mv)
- When the ion channels of the hair cells open, K^+ is driven into the hair cells because of this potential difference and causes depolarization
- This mechanism helps to convert the mechanical energy of sound into electrical impulses
- This gradient and energy for transduction is provided by the Na^+/K^+ ATPase pump in stria vascularis.

31. Ans. b. Eustachian tube is always abnormal *Ref: Diseases of Ear, Nose and Throat by PL Dhingra, 5/e p98*

Eustachian tube is normal in otosclerosis. Refer question 1 of 2014

32. Ans. a. Anteroinferior quardrant *Ref: Diseases of Ear, Nose and Throat by PL Dhingra, 5/e p407*

- Myringotomy is a surgical procedure in which incision is made on the tympanic membrane to drain suppurative or nonsuppurative effusion of the middle ear or to provide aeration of middle ear in case of malfunctioning Eustachian tube.

Indications are:

- Asom with severe earache, incomplete resolution or with complications like mastoiditis.
- Secretory otitis media
- Aero-otitis media
- Atelectatic ear

Incision used are:

- Radial incision: Made in the anteroinferior quadrant in secretory otitis media
- Circumferential incision: Made in the posteroinferior quadrant in acute suppurative otitis media.

33. Ans. b. Mastoid tip *Ref: Diseases of Ear, Nose and Throat by PL Dhingra, 5/e p87*

Bezold's abscess: Follows acute coalescent mastoiditis

Pus breaks through the medial side of the **mastoid tip** and present as neck swelling

It may lie

i. Deep to sternocleidomastoid

ii. May reach parapharyngeal space

iii. Track along the carotid into mediastinum

There will be history of purulent otorrhea followed by pain and fever

O/E: Torticollis, tender swelling in the neck

Treatment–IV antibiotics, drainage of abscess and cortical mastoidectomy.

Luc's abscess

- Meatal abscess when pus breaks through bony wall between antrum and osseous external meatus
- **Citelli's abscess**: Pus tracks along the digastrics muscle and present as swelling in the digastric triangle
- **Zygomatic abscess**: Presents at root of zygoma. Swelling in front and above pinna.

34. Ans. b. Russell bodies are seen *Ref: Diseases of Ear, Nose and Throat by PL Dhingra, 5/e p172*

Rhinoscleroma

- Chronic granulomatous disease caused by Klebsiella rhinoscleromatis or Frisch bacillus, a gram-negative coccobacillus
- Subdermal infiltration of the lower part of eternal nose and upper lip giving a wood feel
- Miculicz' cells (plasma cells) and Russel bodies (also seen in multiple myeloma)
- Corin cells, morula cell, mott cells are also seen
- Gothic sign
- Potato nose, hebra nose, elephantiasis of nose
- Tapir nose (also in leishmaniasis)
- Treatment: streptomycin + tetracycline for 4–6 weeks.

35. Ans. d. Recurrence is less common *Ref: Diseases of Ear, Nose and Throat by PL Dhingra, 5/e p186-188*

Antrochoanal polyp	Ethmoidal polyp
Children	Adults
Infection	Allergy
Unilateral	Multiple, grape like clusters
Unilateral	Bilateral
Arise from maxillary sinus	Ethomidal sinus
Grows backwards to choana	Grows anteriorly
Recurrence uncommon- treatment Caldwell luc surgery	Common

36. Ans. d. Paracusis *Ref: Diseases of Ear, Nose and Throat by PL Dhingra, 5/e p98*

Paracusis willisii: Patient hears better in noisy environment.

- This is because people raise their voice in noise which will be near the patients hearing threshold
- Seen in otosclerosis.

Presbyacousis: Decreased hearing associated with aging.

37. Ans. c. Fistula test is positive *Ref: Diseases of Ear, Nose and Throat by PL Dhingra, 5/e p72-73, 47*

Serous otitis media/secretory om/mucoid om/glue ear

- Nonpurulent sterile effusion accumulates in the middle ear cavity
- MCC of conductive deafness in children
- Symptoms: Hearing loss (< 40 dB); Delayed and defective speech; Mild earache
- Otoscopy: TM dull and opaque with loss of light reflex, retracted, fluid level and air bubbles seen
- Hearing tests: TFTs and Audiometry show CHL
- Impedance Audiometry: Decreased compliance, flat curve, shift to negative side
- X-ray Mastoid: Clouding of air cells
- Treatment; Medical-Decongestant, Anti allergic, Antibiotics, Middle ear aeration (Valsalva maneuver)
- Surgical:

- Myringotomy and fluid aspiration: 2 incisions one in the anteroinferior and other anterosuperior quadrant of the TM to aspirate thick glue like secretions. (Beer can principle)
- **Grommet insertion**: Left in place till spontaneously extruded
- Tympanotomy (or) cortical mastoidectomy
- Treatment of the cause: Adenoidectomy, tonsillectomy.

Fistula Test

- The basis of this is to induce nystagmus by creating pressure changes in the external canal which are then transmitted to the labyrinth by using a Siegel's speculum or intermittenty pressure over the tragus.

Negative fistula test	Positive Fistula test
Normally the test is negative because pressure changes in the external canal cannot be transmitted to the labyrinth **False negative Fistula test** When cholesteatoma covers the site of fistula **False positive Fistula test** • Congenital syphilis (hyper mobile stapes footplate) • Meniere's disease (Hennebert's sign)	• Cholesteatoma (erosion of horizontal semicircular canal) • Fenestration operation (surgically created window in the Horizontal canal) • Post stapedectomy fistula (abnormal opening in the oval window) • Rupture of round window membrane

- Hennebert's phenomenon: Disequilibrium following nose blowing or lifting heavy objects
- Seen in perilymph fistula.

38. Ans. b. 2 years *Ref: Diseases of Ear, Nose and Throat by PL Dhingra, 5/e p441*

- Mastoid tip develops by 2 years of age
- Surgical importance: Since mastoid tip is not developed in less than 2 years, the facial nerve lies superficial and is at a risk of injury while making the postaural incision for mastoidectomy.
- Therefore the postaural incision should be made more slanting inferiorly to prevent damage to the facial nerve in children less than 2 years.

39. Ans. d. All the above *Ref: Diseases of Ear, Nose and Throat by PL Dhingra, 5/e p435*

- Flexible bronchoscopy is done using a flexible fiber optic bronchoscope
- It provides better illumination and magnification than the rigid bronchoscope
- Can be done under topical anesthesia in an awake patient and is especially useful for bedside examination of critically ill patients
- More useful adults and limited utility in children because of the problem in ventilation
- Can be used for taking biopsy, suctioning of secretions or mucus plugs and removing small foreign bodies.

40. Ans. b. Congenital QT syndrome *Ref: Diseases of Ear, Nose and Throat by PL Dhingra, 5/e p129*

Congenital deafness associated syndromes

Jervell and Lange–Nielsons syndrome

- Autosomal recessive
- Repeated syncopal attacks
- Congenital sensorineural hearing loss
- Prolonged QT in ECG.

Alports syndrome

Autosomal dominant or X linked

- Delayed on set of sensorineural hearing loss
- Hereditary progressive glomerulonephritis
- Corneal dystrophy.

Pendred syndrome

- Autosomal recessive
- Delayed onset of SNHL
- Retinitis pigmentosa
- Night blindness.

Treacher Collin syndrome and Aperts syndrome are associated with conductive hearing loss.

41. Ans. a. Superior vestibular nerve *Ref: Diseases of Ear, Nose and Throat by PL Dhingra, 5/e p124–126, BS Tuli p110*

Acoustic Neuroma/Vestibular Schwannoma/Neurilemmoma

- 80% of all CP angle tumors
- Benign encapsulated, extremely slow growing tumors
- Bilateral tumors seen in neurofibromatosis
- Tumors almost always arise from the Schwann cells of superior vestibular division of VIII nerve
- 40–60 years, no sex predilection
- Cochleovestibular symptoms: Earliest, progressive unilateral SNHL, tinnitus, difficulty in understanding speech out of proportion of pure tone hearing loss (characteristic of AN)
- Cranial nerves: 5th nerve earliest to be involved
- **Hitzelberger's sign** (hypoesthesia of posterior meatal wall), loss of taste, decreased lacrimation are due to facial nerve involvement
- Poor speech discrimination and Roll over phenomenon are seen
- Short Increment Sensitivity Index (SISI) shows a score of 0–20%
- Diminished or no response to calorie tests
- Gold standard for diagnosis: MRI with gadolinium enhancement
- Treatment: Surgical removal, cobalt - 60 gamma knife surgery

42. Ans. a. Post ethmoid artery *Ref: Diseases of Ear, Nose and Throat by PL Dhingra, 5/e p190*

Explanation: Refer Question 1 of 2013

43. Ans. b. Lombard test *Ref: Diseases of Ear, Nose and Throat by PL Dhingra, 5/e p42 (Repeat)*

- In Lombard's voice reflex test the patient is asked to read and slowly a masking noise is induced into his ear
- Normal patient will increase his vocal intensity in presence of background noise but a malingering patient will keep reading in the same internsity.

Other tests for malingering are:

a. Brainstem evoked response audiometry
b. Electrocochleography
c. Acoustic reflex threshold (not tympanometry)
d. Stenger test
e. Delayed auditory feedback test

ABC: Absolute bone conduction test—Patients bone conduction is compared with the examiners (assuming that the examiners hearing is normal).

44. Ans. c. Deviated nasal septum *Ref: Diseases of Ear, Nose and Throat by PL Dhingra, 5/e p164–165*

- In this test the cheek is pulled laterally and subjective improvement in the airway is assessed
- If there is relief in nasal obstruction then the test is positive and indicates an abnormality in the vestibular component of the nasal valve.

45. Ans. a. Rhinolalia clausa *Ref: Diseases of Ear, Nose and Throat by PL Dhingra, 5/e p334*

Rhinolalia clausa

- It is due to blockage of nasal cavity or nasopharynx
- Causes: Common cold, nasal allergy, nasal polyp, nasal mass, adenoids

Rhinolalia aperta

- It is due to failure of nasopharynx to cut off from oropharynx or abnormal connection between the nasal cavity and oral cavity.
- Causes: Velopharyngeal insufficiency, sub mucus palate, cleft palate, paralysis of soft palate, oroantral fistula.

46. Ans: c. Posterior cricoarytenoid *Ref: Diseases of Ear, Nose and Throat by PL Dhingra, 5/e p300*

Action	Intrinsic muscle
Abductor of the Vocal Cords	Posterior Cricoarytenoid
Adductor of the Vocal Cords	Thyroarytenoids (external part); Interarytenoids (Transverse arytenoids) Lateral Cricoarytenoids

Contd...

Contd...

Action	Intrinsic muscle
Tensor of Vocal Cord	Cricothyroid; Thyroidarytenoids (internal part) [VOCALIS]
Openers of laryngeal inlet	Thyroepiglottic (part of thyroarytenoid)
Closers of laryngeal inlet	Interarytenoids (oblique part); Interarytenoids (aryepiglottic part)

Nerve supply

Motor	Sensory
All intrinsic muscles are supplied by Recurrent laryngeal nerve except for Cricothyroid which is supplied by External laryngeal nerve	Up to the level of Vocal Cords: Internal laryngeal N Below the level of Vocal Cords Recurrent laryngeal N

Extrinsic Muscles of Larynx

Elevators		Depressors
Primary elevators (attached to thyroid cartilage)	Secondary elevators (attached to hyoid bone)	Sternohyoid
Stylopharyngeus	Mylohyoid	Sternothyroid
Salpingopharyngeus	Digastrics	Omohyoid
Palatopharyngeus	Stylohyoid	
Thyrohyoid	Geniohyoid	

47. Ans. b. 2000 HZ *Ref: Diseases of Ear, Nose and Throat by PL Dhingra, 5/e p97–100*

- Carhart's notch
- Carhart's notch is classically seen as a dip in bone conduction around 2 KHz in otosclerosis
- This notch will disappear after successful stapedotomy.

48. Ans. a. Bezold's abscess *Ref: Diseases of Ear, Nose and Throat by PL Dhingra, 5/e p87*

- **Bezold's abscess**: Follows acute coalescent mastoiditis
- Pus breaks through the medial side of the mastoid tip and present as neck swelling

It may lie

i. Deep to sternocleidomastoid

ii. May reach parapharyngeal space

iii. Track along the carotid into mediastinum.

There will be history of purulent otorrhea followed by pain and fever

O/E: Torticollis, tender swelling in the neck

Treatment–IV antibiotics, drainage of abscess and cortical matoidectomy.

Luc's abscess

- Meatal abscess when pus breaks through bony wall between antrum and osseous external meatus
  - **Citelli's abscess**: Pus tracks along the digastrics muscle and present as swelling in the digastric triangle
  - **Zygomatic abscess**: Presents at root of zygoma. Swelling in front and above pinna.

49. Ans. b. Transient hoarseness *Ref: Diseases of Ear, Nose and Throat by PL Dhingra, 5/e p318*

Recurrent laryngeal nerve (abductor) paralysis

- Ipsilateral paralysis of all muscles except cricothyroid
- Vocal cord does not move laterally during inspiration
- **Semon's law:** in all organic lesions abductor fibers are more susceptible and paralyzed earlier than the adductors
- **Wagner and Grossman hypothesis**: Cricothyroid receives innervations from SLN, keeps the vocal cord in paramedian position.

Unilateral RLN Paralysis

- One third patients asymptomatic
- Transient change in voice

- Voice gradually improves due to compensation by healthy cord which crosses midline to meet the paralyzed one
- No aspiration, airway obstruction, no treatment required.

Bilateral RLN Paralysis

- All intrinsic muscles paralyzed, vocal in median or paramedian position due to unopposed action of cricothyroid
- Airway obstruction: Dyspnea, stridor
- Voice is normal
- Treatment: Most cases require tracheostomy as emergency procedure
- Arytenoidectomy, Type II thyroplasty, Cordectomy are other procedures

Causes of recurrent laryngeal nerve paralysis

Right	Left	Both
Neck trauma Aneurysm of subclavian artery Carcinoma right lung apex Tuberculosis of cervical pleura	Trauma Bronchogenic cancer Ca thoracic esophagus Aortic aneurysm Mediastinal lymphadenopathy Enlarged left auricle Intrathoracic surgery	Thyroid surgery Thyroid carcinoma Ca cervical esophagus Cervical lymphadenopathy Idiopathic

50. Ans. b. High frequency sensorineural hearing loss

Ref: Diseases of Ear, Nose and Throat by PL Dhingra, 5/e p32

Vestibular neuronitis:

- Usually follows an upper respiratory tract infection
- Due to direct viral involvement on vestibular ganglion
- Characterized by sudden onset of severe vertigo which may last from few days to 2 weeks. Self-limiting.

There is **NO COCHLEAR** symptom

D/D for Pheripheral vertigo

- Meniere's disease
- BPPV
- Labyrinthitis
- Perilymph fistula.

51. Ans. b. Surgical emphysema

Ref: Diseases of Ear, Nose and Throat by PL Dhingra, 5/e p340, Mohan Bansal p513

- Out of the given options, surgical emphysema is the most common.
- Complications of tracheostomy
- Incidence of complications range from 5 to 40 %
- Most common complication occurring include hemorraghe (3.7 %), tube obstruction (2.7%), tube displacement (1.5%).
- Pneumothorax occurs due to injury to apical pleura.
- Complications can be divided into:
  - Immediate: Seen during surgery like hemorrhage, apnea, pneumothorax, injury to esophagus.
  - Intermediate: During first few hours or days like secondary bleeding, infection, tube block, tube displacement
  - Delayed: Seen in prolonged use of tube for weeks like laryngeal or tracheal stenosis, tracheoesophageal fistula and hemorrhage due to erosion of major vessel.

52. Ans. c. Conductive hearing loss *Ref: Diseases of Ear, Nose and Throat by PL Dhingra, 5/e p112*

- Disorder of endolymphatic system which is distended due to increased volume of endolymph
- Associated with allergy, hypothyroidism, Na and water retention
- Male predilection.

Cardinal symptoms

- Episodic vertigo: Attacks are in clusters and associated with nausea, vomiting, ataxia and nystagmus. There are periods of spontaneous remissions lasting for weeks, months or years.

- Roaring tinnitus: Low pitched
- Fluctuating hearing loss: Accompanies or precedes vertigo. Improves after attack, with each attack the hearing loss will add up and gradually the hearing will worsen.

53. Ans. b. Long QT *Ref: Diseases of Ear, Nose and Throat by PL Dhingra, 5/e p129*

Syndrome/Inheritance	Features	Onset/Type HL
Waardenberg's syndrome (AD)	White forelock Heterochromia iridis Vitiligo Dystopia cathorum	Congenital SNHL
Usher syndrome (AR)	Retinitis pigmentosa Night blindness	Delayed SNHL
Jervell and Lange-Neilson's syndrome (AR)	Repeated syncopal attacks Prolonged QT interval	Congenital SNHL
Alport syndrome (AD or X-linked)	Hereditary progressive GN Corneal dystrophy	Delayed Progressive SNHL
Treacher-Collins syndrome (mandibulofacial dysostosis) (AD)	Antimongoloid palpebral fissures Coloboma of lower lid Hypoplasia of mandible and malar bones Malformed pinna and meatal atresia Malformed malleus incus (stapes normal)	Congenital Conductive
Crouzon's syndrome (AD) (craniofacial dysostosis)	Frog eyes, Hypertelorism Parrot beak nose Mandibular prognathism Mental retardation	Congenital Conductive or mixed
Apert's syndrome (AD)	Syndactyly Features of Crouzon's syndrome	Congenital, Conductive (stapes fixation)
Klippel-Feil syndrome (AR)	Short neck Fused cervical vertebrae Spina bifida Atresia of ear canal	Congenital SNHL or mixed
Stickler's syndrome (AD)	Small jaw Cleft palate Myopia, Cataract Juvenile onset arthritis	Delayed Conductive or SNHL
Van der Hoeve's syndrome	Osteogenesis impertecta (H/O fractures) Blue sclera	Delayed CHL, SNHL or mixed
Pierre-Robin sequence	Micrognathia Glossoptosis Cleft plate	SNHL or conductive
Goldenhar's syndrome (facio-auriculo-vertebral dysplasia or oculo-auriculo –vertebral [OAV] syndrome)	Facial asymmetry Low set ears Atresia of ear canal Preauricular tags Cardiac abnormalities Hemivertebrae in cervical region Epibulbar dermoid Coloboma or upper lid	Mixed or conductive

54. Ans. a. Flushing of skin over parotid *Ref: Diseases of Ear, Nose and Throat by PL Dhingra, 5/e p89*

Gradenigo's syndrome:

- Seen in petrositis (CSOM complications)
- Ear discharge
- Diplopia (CN VI paralysis)
- Retro orbital pain (CN V)

- Diagnosis is by CT scan or MRI
- Treatment modified radical or radical mastoidectomy along with IV antibiotics.

55. Ans. a. Rapid descent while in an aircraft *Ref: Diseases of Ear, Nose and Throat by PL Dhingra, 5/e p74*

Barotrauma otitis media

Seen in rapid descent during flight, deep water diving leading to difference between atmospheric pressure and middle ear pressure > 90 mm Hg causing of locking of Eustachian tube.

- Locking occurs due to collapse of soft tissue into Eustachian tube.
- The negative middle ear pressure leads to transudation, hemorrhage and even rupture of TM and rupture of labyrinthine membrane with vertigo and sensorineural hearing loss.

C/F: Severe ear pain, hearing loss, tinnitus.

O/E: TM Maybe retracted, congested or ruptured. Middle ear may show bubbles or hemorrhagic effusion.

Treatment:Nasal decongestants, antihistamines and in severe cases myringotomy Maybe required.

56. Ans. c. Elongated epiglottis with thin aryepiglottic folds on laryngoscopy

Ref: Diseases of Ear, Nose and Throat by PL Dhingra, 5/e p314

Laryngomalacia

- Most common congenital anomaly of larynx
- Excessive flaccidity of supraglottis larynx which is sucked in during inspiration producing stridor
- Cry is normal
- Condition manifests at birth but usually disappears at 2 years
- Direct laryngoscopy shows elongated epiglottis (omega shaped) aryepiglottic folds and prominent arytenoids
- Treatment: Conservative, for severe cases tracheostomy.

57. Ans. a. Syphilis *Ref: Diseases of Ear, Nose and Throat by PL Dhingra, 5/e p166*

Septal perforation

Most common cause is trauma which can be due to surgery like SMR, cauterization for epistaxis, nose picking, pricked for ornaments wearing

Pathological perforation

- Septal abscess
- Nasal myiasis
- Rhinolith or neglected foreign body.

Perforation in cartilaginous part

- Lupus
- Tuberculosis
- Leprosy
  - Syphilis causes destruction of bony septum
  - Wegners disease causes total destruction of septum.

Drugs

- Prolonged use of steroid spray
- Cocaine addicts
- Workers in certain occupation, e.g. chromium plating, soda ash, arsenic compounds
  - Small perforations cause whistling sound
- Large perforation cause crusting and epistaxis
  - Treatment: Attempt to be made and find cause and treat it.
- Inactive small perforations closed by local flaps, silastic buttons
- Large perforation difficult to close
- Alkaline nasal douching.

58. Ans. a. Atrophic rhinitis *Ref: Diseases of Ear, Nose and Throat by PL Dhingra, 5/e p170*

Young's operation

- It is done as a treatment of atrophic rhinitis
- It involves closure of nasal cavity affected with atrophic rhinitis by creating mucocutaneous flaps
- They are opened after 6 months. In these cases mucosa may revert to normal and crusting reduced.

59. Ans. a. Puretone audiometry *Ref: Diseases of Ear, Nose and Throat by PL Dhingra, 5/e p27*

Explanation: Refer question 4 of 2011 and question 1 of 2014 for Tympanometry.

Pure tone audiogram

It is a **subjective** test depending on patient's response to pure tones delivered by audiometer.

60. Ans. b. Cervical lymphadenopathy *Ref: Diseases of Ear, Nose and Throat by PL Dhingra, 5/e p265*

Nasopharyngeal carcinoma

Etiology

- Genetic: Prevalent among Chinese
- Virus: EBV
- Environmental: Air pollution, tobacco smoking, opium smoking, nitrosamines from dry salted fish, smoke from burning incense and wood, vitamin C deficiency.

Clinical features

- Age: 5th to 7th decades; Males affected 3 times more
- Presence of unilateral SOM in an adult should rise the suspicion of nasopharyngeal growth
- Jugular foramen syndrome
- Horner's syndrome
- **Trotter's triad**: Conductive deafness (ET block], Ipsilateral temporoparietal neuralgia (involvement of CN V) and Palatal paralysis (CN X)
- **Jaccods's triad**: Ipsilateral ophthalmoplegia, amaurosis, ipsilateral neuralgia
- Enlargement of cervical lymph nodes: **Most common symptom** (60%) and most common region posterior cervical.

Types

I. Squamous cell carcinoma
II. Nonkeratinizing carcinoma
III Undifferentiated carcinoma

Diagnosis is with biopsy, CT scan, MRI

Treatment: Irradiation is the treatment of choice; Chemotherapy for stage III and IV cancers with Cisplatin +/– 5 FU.

61. Ans. b. CN VIII *Ref: Diseases of Ear, Nose and Throat by PL Dhingra, 5/e p143*

Nerve supply of external ear

Pinna	External auditory canal	Tympanic membrane
Greater auricular nerve (C2C3) Lesser occipital nerve (C2) Auriculotemporal nerve (mandibular branch of 5th nerve) Auricular branch of Vagus (Arnold's N) Facial nerve	Anterior wall and roof-auriculo temporal nerve Posterior wall and floor • **Arnolds nerve**	Anterior half of lateral surface-auriculotemporal Posterior half of lateral surface-Arnolds nerve Medial surface tympanic branch of 9th nerve **(Jacobson's N)**

These dermatomes are important for referred ear pain—Pain in ear due to distant lesions:

i. Via VN N: Auriculotemporal nerve
   a. Dental: Caries, apical abscess, impacted molar, malocculusion
   b. Oral cavity: Benign or malignant ulcerative lesions of oral cavity or tongue
   c. Temporomandibular joint disorders: Bruxism, osteoarthritis, recurrent dislocation, ill-fitting dentures
   d. Spenopalatine neuralgia.
ii. Via IX N: Jacobson nerve
   a. Oropharynx: Acute tonsillitis, Peritonsillar abscess, tonsillectomy. Benign and malignant ulcers of soft palate, tonsil and it's pillar.
   b. Base of tongue: Tuberculosis or malignancy
   c. Elongated styloid process.
iii. Via X N-Arnold's nerve
   a. Malignancy or ulcerative lesion of vallecula, epiglottis, larynx or laryngopharynx, esophagus.
iv. Via C2 and C3 N: Cervical spondylosis, cervical injury.

62. Ans. c. Normal hearing *Ref: Diseases of Ear, Nose and Throat by PL Dhingra, 5/e p26*

Rinne's test

- Positive: AC > BC normal
- Negative: BC > AC: Conductive hearing loss
- Reduced positive: Sensory neural hearing loss
- False negative: Unilateral profound deafness

63. Ans: c. Maxillary nerve *Ref: Diseases of Ear, Nose and Throat by PL Dhingra, 5/e p421*

Caldwell Luc Operation

- Caldwell Luc operation is a process of opening of maxillary antrum through canine fossa and nasoantral window is made through inferior meatus.

Indications:

- Chronic maxillary sinusitis
- Oroantral fistula
- Removal of foreign bodies
- Suspected neoplasm of antrum and biopsy
- Recurrent AC polyp
- # Maxilla or blow out # of orbit
- Approach to ethmoids
- Vidian neurectomy.

Contraindication: < 17 years

Complications:

- Postoperative bleeding
- Anesthesia of the cheek due to stretching of the infraorbital nerve (branch of maxillary nerve)
- Anesthesia of teeth
- Sublabial fistula
- Injury to nasolacrimal duct.

One liners:

- Meckel cave: On superior part of temporal bone houses Gasserian ganglion (V nerve)
- Bill's bar in internal acoustic meatus separates facial nerve from superior vestibular nerve
- Eward's law: States slow component of nystagmus is always flow of endolymph
- Most common site of injury to facial nerve in mastoid surgery is in second genu
- Pulsatile tinnitus is seen in glomus jugulare and arteriovenous shunts
- Sluders neuralgia is also called as anterior ethmoidal neuralgia
- Leprosy involves
- Syphilis bony septal perforation, tuberculosis affects cartilaginous framework
- Aspergillosis is the commonest fungal infection of nose and paranasal sinuses
- In children most common sinusitis is ethmoidal sinusitis
- Most common site of mucocele formation is frontal sinus
- Potts puffy tumor is subperiosteal abscess due to frontal sinusitis
- Ranula becomes plunging if it penetrates myelohyoid muscle
- Malignant change in erythroplakia is 17 times higher than in leukoplakia
- Killians dehiscence is a gap between oblique and transverse fibers of inferior constrictor
- Galen's anastomosis is between recurrent laryngeal nerve and internal laryngeal nerve
- Adenoids are clinically seen by 4 months and radiologically by 6 months
- Irwine moore's sign: Pressure on the anterior pillar results in expression of pus from tonsillar crypts
- Ludwigs angina is cellulitis of submandibular and sublingual space caused by periodontal disease
- Byrce's sign: Gurgling sound when swelling is presses in laryngocele
- Verrucous carcinoma are also called as Ackermann's tumor
- Most common LASER used in laryngotracheal lesion is CO_2 laser
- Sistrunk operation is treatment of choice for thyroglossal cyst.

QUESTIONS 2015

1. **Nerve supply of pyriform fossa:**
   a. Recurrent laryngeal nerve
   b. Internal laryngeal nerve
   c. External laryngeal nerve
2. **Definitive indication of tonsillectomy is:**
   a. 5 attacks in a year
   b. Recurrent glue ear
   c. Hypertrophy causing airway obstruction
   d. Streptococcal carrier
3. **Otalgia in tonsillitis is due to**
   a. Greater auricular
   b. Auricular branch of vagus
   c. Glossopharyngeal nerve
   d. Auriculotemporal nerve
4. **Most effective treatment of glue ear:**
   a. Decongestant nasal drops or spray
   b. Steroids
   c. Antibiotics
   d. Valsalva maneuver
5. **Cochlear implant stimulates:**
   a. Oval window
   b. Ganglion of auditory nerve
   c. Inner hair cells
   d. Outer hair cells

ANSWERS AND EXPLANATIONS

1. **Ans. b. Internal laryngeal nerve**

   ***Ref:** Diseases of Ear, Nose and Throat by PL Dhingra, 5/e p317*

   - Nerve supply of larynx
   - Motor: All muscles of larynx are supplied by the recurrent laryngeal nerve except the Cricothyroid which receives its innervations from external laryngeal nerve—a branch of superior laryngeal nerve
   - Sensory: Above the level of vocal cords and hypopharynx is supplied by internal branch of superior laryngeal nerve
   - Below the level of vocal cords by recurrent laryngeal nerve.

2. **Ans. c. Hypertrophy causing airway obstruction** *Ref: Diseases of Ear, Nose and Throat by PL Dhingra, 5/e p438*

   Tonsillectomy

   Absolute indications
   - Recurrent throat infection > 7 in 1 year or 5 per year for 2 years or 3 per year for 3 years
   - Peritonsillar abscess: 4–6 weeks after abscess is treated
   - Hypertrophy of tonsils causing airway obstruction, dysphagia, or interference with speech
   - Tonsillitis causing febrile seizures
   - Hypertrophy of tonsil causing sleep apnea, speech interference
   - Suspected malignancy.

   Relative indications
   - Diphtheria carriers, streptococcal carriers
   - Chronic tonsillitis.

   As a part of another operation
   - Palatopharyngoplasty for sleep apnea syndrome
   - Glossopharyngeal neurectomy
   - Removal of styloid process

   Contraindications
   - Acute infection of upper respiratory tract, even Acute tonsillitis
   - Children < 3 years
   - Submucous cleft palate
   - At the time of polio epidemic.

3. **Ans. c. Glossopharyngeal nerve** *Ref: Diseases of Ear, Nose and Throat by PL Dhingra, 5/e p143*

   Explanation: Refer question 5 of 2006

4. **Ans. a. Decongestant nasal drops or spray** *Ref: Diseases of Ear, Nose and Throat by PL Dhingra, 5/e p71*

   Explanation: Refer question 7 of 2009

5. **Ans. b. Ganglion of auditory nerve** *Ref: Diseases of Ear, Nose and Throat by PL Dhingra, 5/e p138*

   A cochlear implant works by electrical stimulation of auditory nerve where degeneration of hair cells has progressed to a point such that amplification provided by hearing aids is no longer effective.

Chapter

10 Ophthalmology

R Anjana

EMBRYOLOGY

Neural ectoderm	Surface ectoderm	Mesoderm
Epithelium of iris and ciliary body **Iris muscles (Sphincter and dilator pupillae)** Retina (all 10 layers) Optic nerve Melanocytes Secondary vitreous	Conjuctival and corneal epithelium Lacrimal and tarsal glands Lens Skin of lids and its derivatives (cilia)	Sclera Corneal stroma and endothelium Iris stroma Choroid Glial tissue of optic nerve Blood vessels Muscles of eye **(except iris muscles)** Trabecular meshwork Primary vitreous

- Pupillary reflex develops in the intra uterine life
- Fixation reflex between 2-4 months
- Fusional reflexes (stereopsis and accommodation) bet 4-6 months
- Macula develops by 2-4 months
- Cornea attains normal adult diameter by 2 years

ANATOMY

Extraocular Muscles: *Ref: Anatomy and physiology of eye, AK Khurana p291*

Origin: All recti muscle arise from annular tendon of Zinn at the apex of orbit

Insertion: Into the sclera after piercing tenon 's capsule

Muscles	Nerve Supply	Primary Action	Secondary Action
RECTI			
Superior rectus	Oculomotor nerve	***Elevation***	***Intorsion***
Inferior rectus	Oculomotor nerve	***Depression***	***extorsion***
Medial rectus	Oculomotor nerve	***Adduction***	
Lateral rectus	**Abducent nerve**	***abduction***	
Oblique			
Superior oblique	***Trochlear nerve***	***Intorsion***	***Depression***
Inferior oblique	***Oculomotor nerve***	***extorsion***	***Elevation***

Note: All superiors (superior oblique and superior rectus) are intortors. All inferiors are extortors

All **recti** are **ADDUCTORS**. All **obliques** are **ABDUCTORS.**

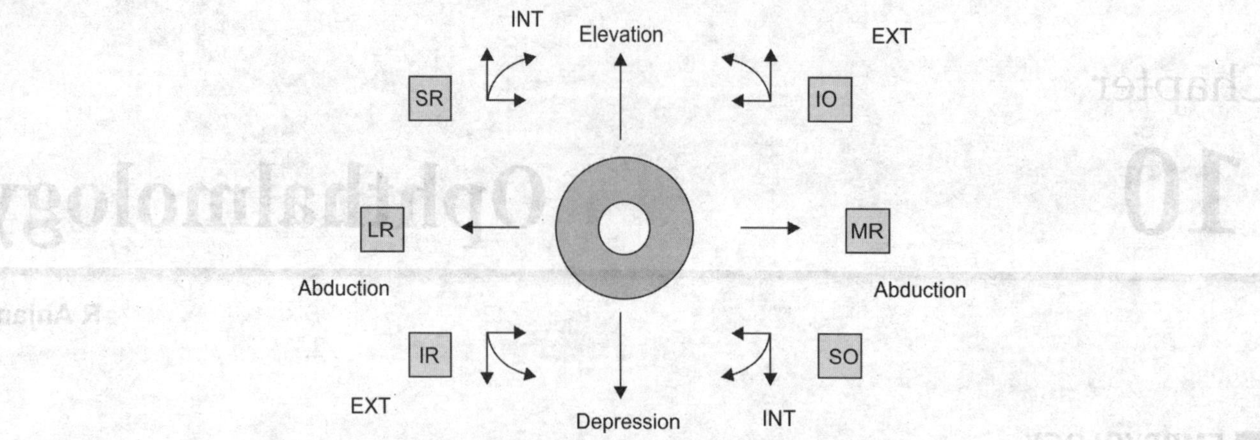

LONGEST MUSCLE: Superior Oblique; SHORTEST MUSCLE: inferior oblique

Only muscle **not arising from apex of orbit: INFERIOR OBLIQUE**

Refractive Indices of Various Structures of Eye: *Ref: Clinical optics by Andrew R Elkington p102*

Structure	Refractive index
Cornea	1. 376
Aqueous	1. 336
Lens 1. cortex 2. nucleus	 1. 386 1. 406
vitreous	1. 336

Highest REFRACTIVE INDEX: Lens (core/nucleus)

Highest refractive POWER: anterior surface of CORNEA

Total refractive power of eye: + 60 D

Ant surface of cornea + 48D

Posterior surface – 5D

Net refractive power of cornea + 43 (three fourth of total refractive power of eye which is 60D)

Layers of Cornea

From Anterior to posterior:

1. Epithelium
2. Bowmans membrane
3. Stroma
4. Dua's layer (latest 6th layer of cornea)
5. Descemet's membrane
6. Endothelium

Accomodation Reflex

Near reflex comprises of

- Accommodation: Ciliary muscle contracts and zonules relax: The anterior curvature of capsule increases (radius of curvature decreased from 10–6 mm)

- Convergence
- Miosis

Orbit

Volume of orbital cavity: 29ml ; volume of eye ball: 6 ml Ratio of volume of orbit: eyeball is 5: 1

Thinnest wall of orbit - medial wall (hence infections from ethmoid sinus can easily spread to orbit and cause orbital cellulitis)

Thickest wall – lateral wall

BLOWOUT FRACTURE: *Ref: Kanski's Clinical ophthalmology 7/e p873*

Fracture of floor (inferior) wall of orbit along with the bone covering infraorbital canal

Causes: sudden increase in intra orbital pressure by an impacting object > 5 cm (tennis ball, fist)

Types:

- *Pure blow out fracture:* Orbital rim or other facial bones not involved
- *Impure blow out fracture:* Involves other bones/rim

Features:

- Periorbital ecchymosis and edema
- Enophthalmos
- Restriction of Extraocular movement (elevation: due to entrapment of inferior rectus)
- Diplopia (d/t muscle muscle entrapment, hemorrhage, edema)
- Infra orbital anaesthesia (dlt involvement of infra orbital nerve)

Radiography (x ray orbit/ct): **TEAR DROP SIGN:** protrusion of orbital tissue into maxillary antrum

Management:

Conservative management: Antibiotics and anti inflammatory drugs

Surgical management (with bone graft, silicone plate) indicated in

- Fracture involving more than 1/3 rd of the globe
- Persisting diplopia
- Enophthalmos > 2 mm

Blow In Fracture: Sudden rise in pressure in maxillary antrum d/t facial trauma with elevation of bony fragments into orbit

Tumors Of Orbit

Most Common

- *MC Primary Orbital malignant tumor in children:* Embryonal sarcoma (aka Rhabdomyosarcoma)
- *MC Orbital tumor in childhood:* Capillary hemangioma

Embryonal Sarcoma (Rhabdomyosarcoma)

Derived from undifferentiated mesenchymal cells rest

Types:

- *Undifferentiated:* Consists of mass of loosely arranged cells
- *Differentiated:* Tumor cells have TADPOLE LTENNIS RACKET configuration with or without striations
- *Site:* MC in superonasal and retrobulbar regions
- *Treatment:* Radio/chemotherapy surgical excision for recurrent/radioresistant tumors.

Proptosis

Protrusion of eyeball out of the orbital cavity.

Types: 1. Axial 2. Eccentric

Axial	Eccentric
Due to lesions within muscle cone	Extraconal lesions
Examples: • Optic nerve glioma • Optic nerve sheath meningioma • Cavernous hemangioma	**Examples:** **Downward Displacement** Dermoid cyst Frontal mucocele Lacrimal gland tumors Thyroid orbitopathy **Upward Displacement** Lacrimal sac tumors Lymphoma Maxillary sinus tumor **Lateral Displacement** Ethmoid mucocele Lacrimal sac tumors Nasopharangeal tumors **Medial Displacement** Dermoid cyst Sphenoid wing meningioma

MC cause of proptosis in adults: both unilateral n bilateral: THYROID OPHTHAMOPATHY
In children: Unilateral: Orbital cellulitits
Bilateral: Metastasis from neuroblastoma (raccoon eyes)

Thyroid Ophthalmopathy: Eye Signs

- *Dalrypmle's sign:* Upper scleral show
- *Moebius sign:* Loss of convergence
- *Stellwag's sign:* Infrequent blinking and widening of palpebral fissure d/t lps involvement
- *Joffroy's sign:* Absence of wrinkling of forehead when asked to look upwards
- *von Graefe sign:* Lid lag sign
- *Jellinke s sign:* Increased pigmentation of eyelids

Gifford's test n naffziger's method: To diff proptosis from exophthalmos.

Lagophthalmos

Inadequate closure of eyelids can lead to exposure keratits

Causes

- **Facial nerve palsy:** Bells palsy, leprosy, sarcoidosis, csom, parotid tumors
- Proptosis and exophthalmous
- Cicatrical deformity of eyelid

Congenital dacrocystitis/congenital nasolacrimal duct obstruction:
Due to incomplete canalization of nasolacrimal duct most often the valve of hasner
Usually presents at 3rd week of life with watering and discharge.

Management

- < 1 year – lacrimal sac massage (Creigler's method)
- 1–4 years – probing, balloon catherterisation, silicone tube intubation
- > 4 years – dacrocyctorhinostomy (connection is established bet the lacrimal sac and middle meatus. can be done by external route or endonasally).
- *Dacrocystectomy:* Removal of lacrimal sac. Done in extremes of age, tumors of sac, TB of sac, fibrotic sac
- *Chalazion:* Chronic, noninfective, granulomatous inflammation of meibomian gland

- ***Hordeolum externum (stye):*** Acute suppurative inflammation of gland of Zeiss or moll
- ***Hordeolum internum:*** Suppurative inflammation of gland of meibomian gland.
- **Horners Syndrome (aka oculosympathetic paresis) due to involvement of sympathetic fibres:**

Classification

1. Central Horner's syndrome: lesions from hypothalamus to cilio-spinal centre of budge at c8-t2
2. Preganglionic Horner's syndrome: From c8 to t2 of spinal cord to the superior cervical ganglion
3. Postganglionic Horner's syndrome: Lesion in the course of postganglionic fibres.

Features

- Miosis due to paralysis of dilator pupillae
- Partial ptosis due to paralysis of muller's muscle of upper lid
- Enophthalmos
- *Heterochromia irides:* A feature of congenital Horner 's
- Anhydrosis: when the lesion is below superior cervical sympathetic ganglion
- *Cociane test:* When 4 % cocaine is instilled, normal pupils dilate but horner s donot dilate.

Preganglionic Horner's	Postganglionic Horner's
Anhydrosis of face and neck	Anhydrosis absent
Hydroxyamphetamine test: • When 10% Amphetamine instilled, pupils dilate	• Pupils do not dilate
Adrenaline/ phenylephrine test: • When adrenaline 1 in 100 or phenylephrine 10 % instilled, pupil dilate	• Dilation is more than normal/pre ganglionic horners because of denervation supersenstivity

Procedures and Instruments in Ophthal

Ophthalmoscopy: **Technique used to examine the retina (fundus)**

Direct Ophthalmoscopy (Uniocular)	Indirect Ophthalmoscopy (Binocular)
Condensing lens not used	**Condensing lens used**
Image: Erect, virtual	Real, inverted
Magnified up to 15 times	Magnified up to 5 times
Working distance as close to patient as possible	**Arms distance**
Brightness of illumination Less	**Brighter illumination used**
Periphery of retina not visualized (only posterior pole visualized ie 10°)	**Peripheries can be visualized (upto 37 °)**
Sclera indentation difficult	**Sclera indentation easily done**
Not useful in hazy media	**Useful in hazy media**
Steropsis absent	**Steropsis present (Depth perception)**

Tonometry: Technique used to measure intraocular pressure.

Types

- Indentation tonometry (e. g. Schiotz tonometer)
- Applanation tonometer (Goldmann's tonometer which is the GOLD STANDARD, macky marg, pneumatic, non contact tonometers)

Gonioscopy: Technique used to visualize angle of anterior chamber.

Types

- Direct (e. g. Koeppe's, barkan's)
- Indirect (e. g. Goldmann's, zeiss, posner and sussman)

Retinoscopy: Objective method of testing the refractive status by method of umphrey's

Types
- Mirror retinoscopy:
  - Single plane mirror
  - Pristley smith mirror combination of plane and concave mirror
- Self illuminated retinoscopy:
  - Spot retinoscope
  - Streak retinoscope.

Mydriatics, cycloplegics duration of action table

Drugs	Percentage	Duration of action
Atropine	1%	2 weeks
Homatropine	2%	2 days
Tropicamide	0. 5–1%	24 hours

- Drug which is only mydriatic not a cycloplegic: Phenylephrine
- Fastest acting: Tropicamide
- Pachymetry: To measure corneal thickness
- Keratometry: To measure corneal curvature
- Perimetry: To quantify visual fields
- Types
  - Kinetic perimetry (e. g. Bjerrum's screen)
  - Static perimetry (e. g. humphrey perimeter, octopus perimeter)
- Specular Microscopy: To visualize corneal endothelium

Lasers in Ophthalmology *(High yielding topic)*

Laser effect	Mechanism	Type of laser
Photocoagulation	Controlled burn	Argon laser Diode laser Krypton laser
Photovaporization		Argon laser Diode laser
Photodisruption	Optical break down to disrupt tissues by the formation of plasma	Nd yag laser
Photoablation	Ablation of corneal tissue without thermal damage	Excimer laser

Laser and uses

Lasers	Uses in ophthalmology
Nd yag laser (Neodymium Yttrium Aluminum Garnet)	Iridotomy (glaucoma angle closure) Capsulotomy (Posterior capsular opacification)
Argon laser	Laser ablation – trichiasis Trabeculoplasty (glaucoma open angle)
Holmium Yag laser	Endolaser Dacryocystorhinostomy
Excimer (excited Dimer)	Photo refractive keratectomy LASIK Laser assisted in situ keratomileusis Photo therapeutic keratoplasty- Superficial scars
HO: YAG (Holmium Yttrium Aluminum Garnet)	Laser thermal keratoplasty
Diode laser	Trabeculoplasty (glaucoma) Cyclo ablation (Absolute glaucoma)
Helium Neon Laser	Laser interferometry: To test the potential visual acuity in the presence of opacity in media

Errors of Refraction

	Myopia	Hypermetropia
Definition	Refractive state of eye where in the parallel rays of light coming from object at infinity are focused **in front of** the retina with accommodation at rest	Refractive state of eye where in the parallel rays of light coming from object at infinity are focused **behind** the retina with accommodation at rest
Types	• **Axial:** Due to increase in axial length of eye ball • **Curvatural:** Increase in corneal/lenticular curvature • **Index:** due to increase in refractive index (nuclear sclerosis) • **Positional:** Due to anteriorly placed lens	• **Axial:** Due to decrease in axial length of eye ball • **Curvatural:** Decrease in corneal/lenticular curvature • **Index:** Due to decrease in refractive index (nuclear sclerosis) • **Positional:** Due to posteriorly placed lens
Symptoms	Defective vision	Asthenopic symptoms due to excessive accommodation and defective vision
Correction: lenses used	Concave lens	Convex lens
Associated ocular findings	Prominent eyeball Deep anterior chamber **Fundus:** Large optic disk with temporal myopic crescent Degenerative changes and foster fuchs spots in macula	Size of eye ball may be small Anterior Chamber may be shallow Pseudopapillitis: Small Hyperemic disc sometimes with ill defined margins
Complications	Lattice degeneration Retinal detachment Posterior staphyloma	Recurrent styes, chalazion Accomdative convergent squint (by 2–3 years) Predisposition to develop primary narrow angle glaucoma

Pathological Myopia

Refractive error > – 6 D or axial length > 26 mm

Usually hereditary

Starts at 5 years of age and continue till 25 years of age

Ocular features

- Prominent eyes
- Anterior chamber deep
- Myopic chorioretinal degeneration
- Large pale disc with temporal crescent
- Foster Fuch's spots due to choroidal hemorrhages
- Lacquer cracks –linear breaks in bruchs membrane
- Posterior staphyloma

Astigmatism

Refractive state of eye where in the refraction varies in different meridian

Types: Regular and irregular astigmatism

Regular astigmatism:

1. **Simple *astigmatism:*** Wherein the rays are focused on the retina in one meridian and either in front (*simple myopic astigmatism*) or behind (*simple hypermetropic astigmatism*) the retina in the other meridian
   - ***Compound astigmatism:*** The rays of light in both the meridia are focused either in front or behind the retina and the condition is labelled as *compound myopic* or *compound hypermetropic astigmatism,* respectively

- *Mixed astigmatism* wherein the light rays in one meridian are focused in front and in other meridian behind the retina. Thus in one meridian eye is myopic and in another hypermetropic. Such patients have comparatively less symptoms as 'circle of least *diffusion*' is formed on the retina.

Optical treatment

- *Spectacles* with full correction of cylindrical power
- *Contact lenses.* Rigid contact lenses may correct up to 2-3 of regular astigmatism, while soft contact lenses can correct only little astigmatism. For higher degrees of astigmatism toric contact lenses are needed. In order to maintain the correct axis of toric lenses, ballasting or truncation is required.

2. **Surgical correction of astigmatism**

Irregular astigmatism: It is characterized by an irregular change of refractive power in different meridia.

Treatment

1. *Optical treatment* of irregular astigmatism consists of **contact lens** which replaces the anterior surface of the cornea for refraction.
2. *Phototherapeutic keratectomy* (PTK) performed with excimer laser may be helpful in patients with superficial corneal scar responsible for irregular astigmatism.

Refractive surgeries

Lasik

Laser in-situ keratomileusis (LASIK). In this technique first a flap of 130-160 micron thickness of anterior corneal tissue is raised. After creating a corneal flap midstromal tissue is ablated directly with an excimer laser beam, ultimately flattening the cornea this procedure is being considered the refractive surgery of choice for myopiaof up to – 12 D.

Patient selection criteria:

- Patients above 20 years of age,
- Stable refraction for at least 12 months.
- Absence of corneal pathology. Presence of ectasia or any other corneal pathology and a corneal thickness less than 450 mm is an absolute contraindication for LASIK.

Contact Lens

Types of contact lenses

- Hard lenses,
- Rigid gas permeable lenses, and
- Soft lenses.

- ***Hard lenses*** are manufactured from PMMA (polymethylmethacrylate). PMMA contact lenses are sparingly used in clinical practice because of poor patient acceptance.

  Disadvantages:
  - PMMA is practically impermeable to O_2 thus restricting the tolerance.
  - Being hard, it can cause corneal abrasions.
  - Being hydrophobic in nature, resists wetting but a stable tear film can be formed over it.
- ***Rigid gas permeable (RGP) lenses*** are made up of materials which are permeable to oxygen. Gas permeable lenses are commonly manufactured from copolymer of PMMA and silicone containing vinyl monomer.
- ***Soft lenses*** are made up of HEMA (hydroxymethymethacrylate), cover the entire cornea and extend 1–2 mm over the sclera

  Advantages: Being soft and oxygen permeable, they are most comfortable and so well tolerated.

  Disadvantages include problem of wettability, proteinaceous deposits, inferior optical quality, Giant papillary conjunctivitis, increased risk of keratitis.

Lens

Named cataracts

CATARACT	CONDITION ASSOCIATED
Sunflower cataract	Wilson s, chalcosis
Snowflake	True Diabetic cataract
Christmas tree	Myotonic dystrophy
Oil drop central opacities	Galactosemia
Shield cataract	Atopic dermatitis
Rossete (Early and late)	Traumatic cataract
Steroid induced	Posterior sub capsular (discoid)
Breadcrumb appearance Polychromatic lusture	Complicated cataract (Post subscapular cataract)
Anterior polar cataract	Alport syndrome

Reversible cataract: In diabates

Two types of cataract in diabetes:

- Senile cataract: Earlier onset
- True diabetic cataract or snow flake cataract. Common in type 1 diabetes.

Congenital cataract

Mc type: Punctuate or blue dot cataract

Mc type causing visual impairment: Lamellar or Zonular cataract.

Stages of Senile Ctatract:

Stages of maturation of cortical senile cataract:

- ***Stage of lamellar separation***
- ***Stage of incipient cataract.*** Two types
  - *Cuneiform senile cortical cataract:* Wedge-shaped opacities extending from equator towards centre.
  - Cupuliform cataract: Lies right in the pathway of the axial rays and thus causes an early loss of visual acuity.
- ***Immature senile cataract (ISC).*** lens may become swollen *'intumescent cataract'* Due to swollen lens anterior chamber becomes shallow (secondary angle closure glaucoma)
- ***Mature senile cataract (MSC).*** Lens becomes pearly white in color
- ***Hypermature senile cataract (HMSC).***
  - *Morgagnian hypermature cataract*: The whole cortex liquefies And the small brownish nucleus settles at the bottom.
  - *Sclerotic type hypermature cataract:* The cortex becomes disintegrated and the lens becomes shrunken. The anterior capsule is wrinkled and thickened.

Visual Loss in Cataract

- Painless and progressive loss of vision.
- Paitents with central opacities (Post. Subcapsular cataract) have early and more visual loss since the opacity lies on the nodal point of eye (Cataract causing highest visual morbidity)
- These patients see better when pupil is dilated due to dim light in the evening (day blindness).
- In patients with peripheral opacities (e. g. cuneiform cataract) visual loss is delayed and the vision is improved in bright light when pupil is contracted with poor vision at night (night blindness)
- In nuclear sclerosis, distant vision deteriorates due to progressive index myopia. Such patients may be able to read without presbyopic glasses. This improvement in near vision is referred to as 'second sight'.

Drug Induced Cataracts

1. Steroid (systemic)
2. Miotics (echothiophate, demecarium bromide, disopropyl fluorophosfate (DFP)
3. Amiodarone,
4. Chlorpromazine, busulphan,
5. Gold and allopurinol

After cataracts: Posterior capsular opacification.

Types

1. Elsching rings
2. Sommering pearls

Treatment: Yag capsulotomy

Cataract Surgeries

- Intracapsular cataract extraction (ICCE) The entire cataractous lens along with the intact capsule is removed. At present the only indications of ICCE is markedly **subluxated and dislocated lens.**
- Extracapsular cataract extraction (ECCE). In this technique, major portion of anterior capsule with nucleus and cortex are removed; leaving behind intact posterior capsule. Posterior chamber IOL is placed

Contraindications. The only absolute contraindication for ECCE is markedly subluxated or dislocated lens.

Major Advantage of ECCE over ICCE is that a Posterior chamber IOL can be implanted after ECCE, while it cannot be implanted after ICCE.

Types of extracapsular cataract extraction

The surgical techniques of ECCE are:

- Conventional extracapsular cataract extraction (ECCE),
- Manual small incision cataract surgery (SICS)
- Phacoemulsification

Calculation of IOL power (Biometry): The most common method of determining IOL power uses a regression formula called 'SRK (Sanders, Retzlaff and Kraff) formula'. The formula is P = A –2. 5L – 0. 9K

Where:

- P is the power of IOL,
- A is a constant which is specific for each lens type.
- L is the axial length of the eyeball in mm which is determined by A-scan ultrasonography.
- K is average corneal curvature, which is determined by keratometry

Lens Subluxation: Partially displaced lens with intact zonules in some regions

Etiology:

- Marfan's Syndrome (superotemporal)
- Homocystinuria (inferonasal)
- Weill marchesani syndrome
- Familial ectopia lentis

Glaucoma:

Defined as chronic progressive optic neuropathy characterized by optic disc changes, field changes with or without raised IOP

Classification

- ***Congenital and developmental glaucomas***
  - Primary congenital glaucoma (without associated anomalies).
  - Developmental glaucoma (with associated anomalies).

- ***Primary adult glaucomas***
  - Primary open angle glaucoma (POAG)
  - Primary angle closure glaucoma (PACG)
  - Primary mixed mechanism glaucoma.
- ***Secondary glaucomas***

PRIMARY DEVELOPMENTAL/CONGENITAL GLAUCOMA

When the disease manifests prior to age of 3 years, the eyeball enlarges and so the term'***buphthalmos***' (bull-like eyes) is used. Occurs due to trabeculodysgenesis.

Clinical features:

- TRIAD of photophobia, blepharospasm, lacrimation
- Corneal signs include its oedema, enlargement (diameter > 13 mm) and Descemet's breaks known as Haab's striae
- Lens becomes flat due to stretching of zonules and may even subluxate.
- Optic disc may show variable cupping and atrophy

Treatment:

- Goniotomy: Treatment of choice with clear cornea
- Goniopuncture
- Trabeculotomy
- Trabeculectomy + trabeculotomy

Primary Open Angle Glaucoma (POAG)

Characterised by slowly progressive raised intraocular pressure (> 21 mm Hg recorded on at least a few occasions) associated with characteristic optic disc cupping and visual fields with open angles in gonioscopy.

Clinical Features

Symptoms

- Usually asymptomatic
- *Frequent changes in presbyopic glasses*owing to accommodative failure due to constant pressure on the ciliary muscle.

Optic disk changes:

- Large, Vertically oval cupwith increased cup disc ratio (normal 0. 3-0. 4)
- Asymmetry of the cups. A difference of more than 0. 2 between two eyes is significant.
- Splinter haemorrhages present on or near the optic disk margin.
- Nasal shifting of retinal vessels which have the appearance of being broken off at the margin (Bayonetting sign)
- Lamellar dot sign the pores in the lamina cribrosa are slit-shaped and are visible up to the margin of the disk.
- Glaucomatous optic atrophy

Visual field defects:

- Paracentral scotoma (earliest clinically significant field defect)
- *Seidel's scotoma:* Paracental scotoma joins the blind spot to form a sickle shaped scotoma known as Seidel'sscotoma
- Arcuate or Bjerrum's scotoma
- Ring or double arcuate scotoma: When the two arcuate scotomas join together
- Roenne's central nasal step: When the two arcuate scotomas run in different arcs and meet to form a sharp right-angled defect at the horizontal meridian.

- Advanced glaucomatous field defects include retained central vision (tubular vision)

Treatment:

Medical management

- **Topical beta-blockers:** Which include Timolol maleate, Betaxolol (useful in asthmatics and cardiopulmonary disorders), Levobunolol, Carteolol
- Adrenergic drugs like epinephrine, dipivefrine, apraclonidine and Brimonidine (neuroprotective)
- Prostaglandin analogues: decreases the IOP by increasing the uveoscleral outflow of aqueous. egs Latanoprost, bimatoprost, travoprost
- **Carbonic anhydrase inhibitors:** Oral acetazolamide, Topical Dorzolamide

Other treatment options:

- Argon or diode laser trabeculoplasty
- Trabeculectomy

PRIMARY ANGLE CLOSURE GLAUCOMA

Rise in intraocular pressure occurs due to blockage of the aqueous humour outflow by closure of a narrower angle of the anterior chamber.

Predisposing risk factors

- Hypermetropic eyes with shallow anterior chamber.
- Eyes in which iris-lens diaphragm is placed anteriorly
- Plateau iris configuration.

Precipitating factors

- Dim illumination,
- Emotional stress,
- Use of mydriatics

Mechanism of rise in IOP

Mid dilatation of the pupil

↓

Increases the amount of apposition between iris and lens

↓

Resulting in relative pupil

↓

Iris pushed anteriorly (Iris bombe)

Raised IOP

↓

Long standing cases: Synechial angle closure (due to formation of peripheral anterior synechiae) and an attack of rise in IOP may last long

Stages

- Latent primary angle-closure glaucoma (primary angle-closure glaucoma suspect).
- Subacute (intermittent) primary angle-closure glaucoma.
- Acute primary angle-closure glaucoma
- Postcongestive angle-closure glaucoma

- Chronic primary angle-closure glaucoma
- Absolute glaucoma

Acute congestive Glaucoma

Symptoms

- Severe Pain with nausea, vomiting and prostrations
- Rapidly progressive impairment of vision, redness, photophobia and lacrimation
- Signs:
- Conjunctiva: circumcorneal congestion
- Cornea oedematous
- Anterior chamber is very shallow with aqueous flare or cells
- Angle of anterior chamber is completely closed as seen on gonioscopy
- Pupil is middilated, vertically oval and fixed. It is non-reactive to light
- IOP is markedly elevated

Management

Medical therapy

- Systemic hyperosmotic agent intravenous mannitol (1 gm/kg body weight) should be given
- initially to lower IOP.
- Acetazolamide (a carbonic anhydrase inhibitor)
- Pilocarpine eyedrops, Beta blocker eyedrop

Surgical treatment

- Peripheral iridectomy. It is indicated when peripheral anterior synechiae are formed in less than 50 percent of the angle of anterior chamber and as prophylaxis in the other eye.
  Laser iridotomy, a noninvasive procedure, is a good alternative to surgical iridectomy.
- Filtration surgery (like trabeculectomy): done in cases where IOP is not controlled with the best medical therapy following an attack of acute congestive glaucoma and also when peripheral anterior synechiae are formed in more than 50% of the angle of the anterior chamber.

Secondary glaucomas are named as follows:

- Lens-induced (phacogenic) glaucomas: which include
  - **Phacolytic glaucoma** (secondary open angle glaucoma) in leaky hypermature (morgagnian) cataract, in which trabecular meshwork is clogged by the lens proteins and macrophages which have phagocytosed the lens proteins.
  - **Phacomorphic glaucoma** (secondary angle-closure glaucoma) caused by: Intumescent lens, i.e. swollen cataractous lens pushing the iris forward causing acute angle closure attack. other causes include anterior subluxation or dislocation of the lens and spherophakia.
- Inflammatory glaucoma (glaucoma due to intraocular inflammation).
- Pigmentary glaucoma.
- Neovascular glaucoma (CRVO, Diabetic retinopathy)
- Glaucomas associated with irido-corneal endothelial syndromes.
- Pseudoexfoliative glaucoma.
- Glaucomas associated with intraocular haemorrhage.
- Steroid-induced glaucoma.
- Traumatic glaucoma.
- Glaucoma-in-aphakia.

Conj, Cornea, Sclera

Pterygium

- Pterygium is a wing-shaped fold of conjunctiva encroaching upon the cornea from either side within the interpalpebral fissure. The subconjunctival tissue undergoes **elastotic degeneration** and proliferates and encroaches the cornea. T
- Deposition of iron in corneal epithelium anterior to advancing head of pterygium ***-stocker's line.***

Parts

- *Head* (apical part present on the cornea),
- *Neck* (limbal part), and
- *Body* (scleral part) extending between limbus and the canthus.

Symptoms: usually asymptomatic. *Visual disturbances* due to corneal astigmatism induced due to fibrosis in the regressive stage or when it encroaches upon the pupillary area.

Treatment: Excision with amniotic membrane grafting or conjuctival autografting is treatment of choice

VERNAL KERATOCONJUNCTIVITIS (VKC) OR SPRING CATARRH

Recurrent, bilateral, interstitial, self-limiting, allergic inflammation of the conjunctiva due to hypersensitivity reaction to some exogenous allergen, such as grass pollens.

Clinical Features

Symptoms

- Burning and itching sensation
- Mild photophobia, lacrimation,
- Stringy (ropy) discharge, heaviness of lids.

Signs

- *Palpebral form:*
  - The typical lesion is characterized by the presence of hard, flat topped, papillae arranged in a ***'cobble-stone'* or *'pavement stone'***, fashion. In severe cases, papillaemay hypertrophy to produce cauliflower like excrescences of **'giant papillae'**. Conjunctival changes are associated with white ropy discharge.
- *Bulbar form.* It is characterized by:
  - dusky red triangular congestion of bulbar conjunctiva in palpebral area;
  - Gelatinous thickened accumulation of tissue around the limbus; and
  - Presence of discrete whitish raised dots along the limbus (Tranta's spots)
- *Mixed form.* It shows combined features of both
  - Palpebral and bulbar forms
  - ***Vernal keratopathy.***
  - Vernal keratopathy includes following 5 types of lesions:
    - *Punctate epithelial keratitis*
    - *Ulcerative vernal keratitis (shield ulcer)*
    - *Vernal corneal plaques*
    - *Subepithelial scarring* occurs in the form of a ring scar.
    - *Pseudogerontoxon* is characterized by a classical 'cupid's bow' outline.

Treatment

- *Topical antihistaminics* like olopatadine eyedrops
- *Mast cell stabilizers* such as sodium cromoglycate (2%) drops 4-5 times a day are quite effective in controlling VKC, especially atopic cases. It is mast cell stabilizer.

- *Topical steroids* like fluorometholone medrysone.
- *Topical cyclosporine* (1%) and tacrolimus eye ointment inunresponsive cases_

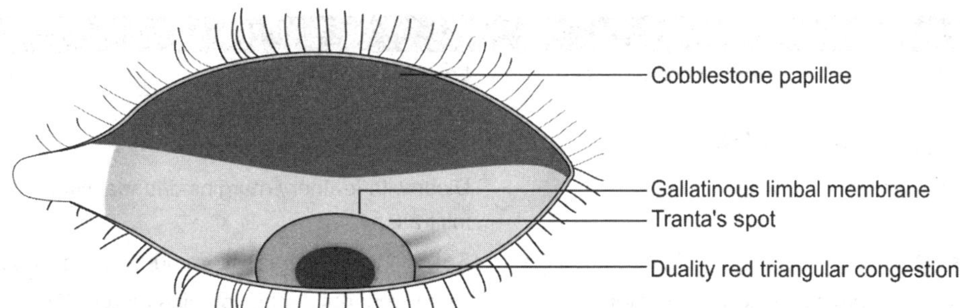

Fig. 10.1: Vernal keratoconjunctivitis

Trachoma

- Caused by Chlamydia trachomatis A, B, Ba, C
- Spread by 3Fs-Fingers, Fomites, Flies
- Forms epithelial inclusion bodies-Halberstader Prowazek Inclusion Bodies
- Conjuctiva-upper tarsal follicle which heals to form minute stellate scars
- Arlt's Line- fibrous band in the tarsal plate.
- Limbal follicles - Herbert follicles- Herbert Pits
- Cornea-Pannus- lymphocytic infiltration with vascularisation of cornea

Who Classification: (Fisto)

Stages	Features	Treatment
Follicles	> 5 follicles, > 0. 5 mm in upper tarsus	Needs treatment No scarring
Intense	> 50% palpebral blood vessels not seen	Urgent treatment Complications +
Scarring	Tarsal conj scarring with white fibrous bands	Inactive
Trichiasis	Atleast one trichiatic lash	Corrective surgery
Opacities	K opacity covering pupillary region	

Safe Strategy

S–Surgery for trichiasis and entropion
A–Antibiotics
F–Frequent face wash
E–Environmental sanitation

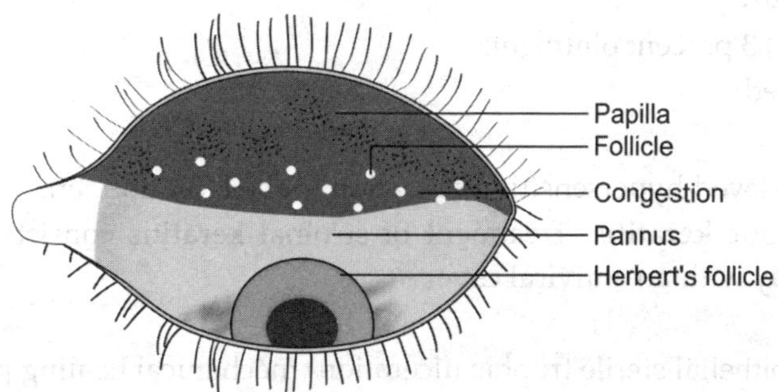

Fig. 10.2: Trachoma

Corneal ulcers:

Infective Keratitis

Differences between bacterial and fungal corneal ulcer:

Bacterial corneal ulcer	Fungal corneal ulcer
Very symptomatic: severe pain, photophobia and defective vision	Less symptomatic
Signs: lid edema, circumcorneal congestion	Signs more than symptoms
Well defined ulcer with stromal infiltration	Ulcer with feathery margins d/fungal filaments with stromal infiltration
Satellite lesions absent	Satellite lesions present, Immune ring may be seen
Hypopyon: sterile, mobile (due to polymorphs in anterior chamber)	Hypopyon: notsterile, contains fungal filament so immobile
Treatment: topical antibiotics like fluroquinolones (moxifloxin) started empirically and changed according to sensitivity of organisms	Treatment: topical antifungals like 5% natamycin, Voriconazole

Protozoal keratitis

Acanthamoeaba keratitis: Free living ameba

Etiology

- Contact lens wearers
- Bathing in swimming pools, open ponds

Features:

- Extremly painful due to perineural spread (radial keratoneuritis)
- Ring shaped ulcers
- Rapidly progressive

Treatment: Topical chlorhexidine 0. 3% drops, Propamidine eye drops, PHMB polyhexamethyl biguanide drops and Topical antibiotics for secondary bacterial infection

Recurrent ocular herpes

The virus which lies dormant in the trigeminal ganglion, periodically reactivates and causes recurrent infection.

- **Epithelial keratitis**
  - **Punctate epithelial keratitis**
  - **Dendritic ulcer** An irregular, zigzag linear branching shape knobbed at the ends. There is an associated marked diminution of corneal sensations.
  - **Geographical ulcer** due to use of steroids in dendritic ulcer.

Treatment of epithelial keratitis.

- Antiviral drugs (Aciclovir) 3 percent ointment:
  Steroids are contraindicated
  Stromal keratitis
  - **Disciform keratitis** delayed hypersensitivity reaction to the HSV antigen.
  - **Diffuse stromal necrotic keratitis**. Treatment of stromal keratitis consists of topical **steroid** eye drops instilled 4-5 times a day with an antiviral cover
- **Metaherpetic keratitis**
  Metaherpetic keratitis (Epithelial sterile trophic ulceration) mechanical healing problem

Treatment: lubricants (artificial tears), bandage soft contact lens and lid closure (tarsorrhaphy).

Herpes Zoster Ophthalmicus

Herpes zoster ophthalmicus is an acute infection of Gasserian ganglion of the fifth cranial nerve by the varicella-zoster virus

The **Hutchinson's rule**: Ocular involvement is frequent if the side or tip of nose presents vesicles (cutaneous involvement of **nasociliary nerve)**

Ocular lesions

- Conjunctivitis
- Zoster keratitis
  - Fine or coarse punctate epithelial keratitis
  - Microdendritic epithelial ulcers
  - Nummular keratitis
  - Disciform keratitis

  Neuroparalytic ulceration due to acute infection and Gasserian ganglion destruction.
  - Episcleritis and scleritis
  - Iridocyclitis with associated hypopyon and hyphaema (acute hemorrhagic uveitis).
- Acute retinal necrosis
- Anterior segment necrosis and phthisis bulbi.
- Secondary glaucoma. It may occur due to trabeculitis in early stages and synechial angle closure in late stages.

Interstitial Keratitis

Inflammation of the corneal stroma without primary involvement of the epithelium or endothelium.

Causes:

- Syphilis
- Tuberculosis
- Cogan's syndrome
- Malaria
- Leprosy
- Sarcoidosis

Syphilitic (luetic) interstitial keratitis

Pathogenesis

- Due to local antigen-antibody reaction
- Part of Hutchinson's triad, which includes: interstitial keratitis, Hutchinson's teeth and **vestibular deafness.**

Stages

- **Initial progressive stage: ground glass appaearnace of cornea** due to edema of endothelium and surrounding stroma
- ***Florid stage.*** Deep vascularization of cornea, consisting of radial bundle of brush-like vessels develops with hazy cornea- ***'Salmon patch appearance'***.
- ***Stage of regression.***

Treatment

- **Topical corticosteroid drops**
- ***Atropine eye ointment*** 1 percent 2-3 times a day.
- ***Keratoplasty*** is required in cases where dense corneal opacities are left.
- ***Systemic treatment*** Penicillin in high doses should be started to prevent development of further syphilitic lesions.

Deposition at various levels

Type of pigment	Disorders	Corneal location
Iron	Keratoconus – **Fleischer's ring** Old opacity – **Hudson stahlis line** Pterygium – **Stockers line** Filtering bleb- **Ferry s line** (trabeculectomy)	Epithelium Epithelium Epithelium Epithelium
Copper	Wilsons ds, chalcosis – **KF ring**	**Descemets membrane**
Melanin	Pigment dispersion syndrome – **krukenberg spindle**	endothelium

Keratoconus

Noninflammatory, ectatic condition of cornea in its axial part

Clinical features:

- Defective vision due to progressive myopia and **irregular astigmatism**
- **Fleischer's ring** at the base of cone (due to iron deposition in epithelium)
- Very fine, vertical, deep stromal striae **(Vogt lines)**
- On retinoscopy a **yawning reflex (scissor reflex)**
- On distant direct ophthalmoscopy-**oil droplet reflex**
- **Munson's sign:** localised bulging of lower lid when patient looks down

Complications: *Acute hydrops* due to rupture of Descemet's membrane- characterised by sudden development of corneal oedema associated with marked defective vision, pain, photophobia

Treatment

Falling vision may not be corrected by

- Glasses due to irregular astigmatism.
- Contact lenses (rigid gas permeable) usually improve the vision in early cases.
- In later stages penetrating keratoplasty may be required.

Sclera

Staphyloma: Staphyloma refers to a localised bulging of weak and thin outer tunic of the eyeball (cornea or sclera), lined by uveal tissue which shines through the thinned out fibrous coat.

Types

Types	Site	Causes
Anterior	Involving part or the whole of cornea, lined by iris	Sloughing corneal ulcer
Intercalary	Limbus and 2 mm from limbus, lined by ciliary body	Perforating injuries Marginal corneal ulcer Anterior scleritis Scleromalacia perforans Post surgical wound site Secondary glaucoma
Equatorial	2-8 mm from limbus, lined by chorois	Scleritis, pathological myopia, chronic uncontrolled glaucoma
Posterior	Posterior pole, lined by the choroid	Scleritis, pathological myopia, chronic uncontrolled glaucoma

Uveitis

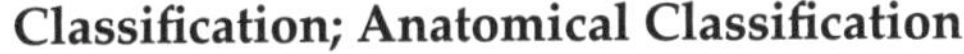

Classification; Anatomical Classification

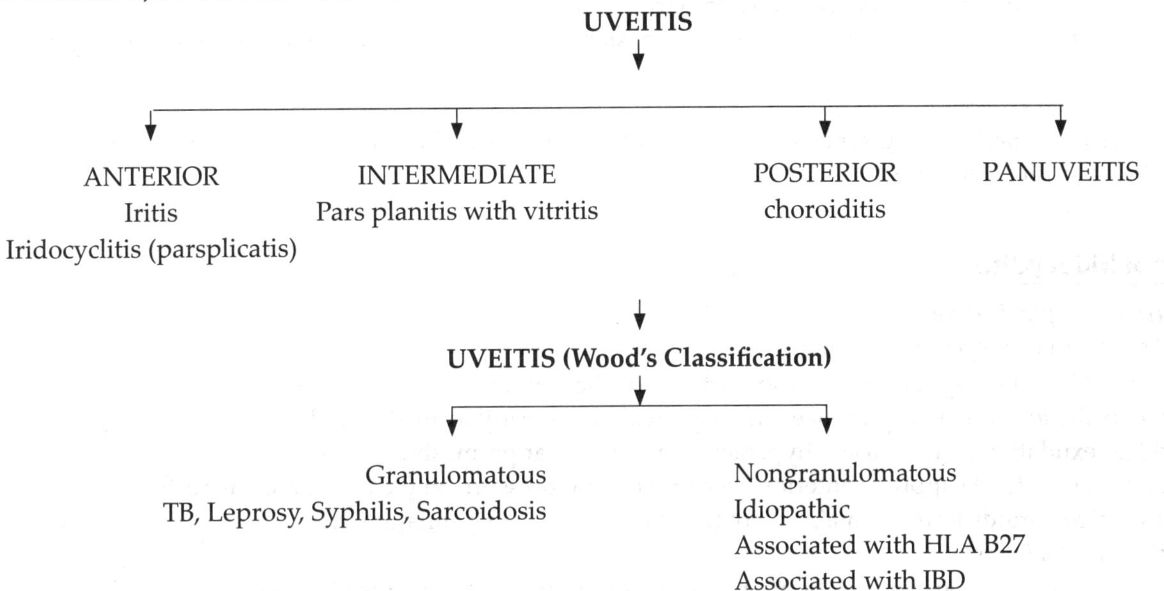

Etiological (Duke Elder's)

Classification

- Infective uveitis
- Allergic uveitis
- Toxic uveitis
- Traumatic uveitis
- Uveitis associated with non-infective systemicdiseases
- Idiopathic uveitis.

Anterior uveitis

Symptoms: ***Pain, Redness, Photophobia*** **and** ***Defective vision***

Signs

Circumcorneal congestion

Corneal signs

Keratic precipitates (KPs) are proteinaceous cellular deposits occurring at the back of cornea. types

- Mutton fat KPs:. in granulomatous uveitis
- Small and medium KPs (granular KPs)

Nongranulomatous uveitis and are composed of lymphocytes

Anterior chamber signs

- ***Aqueous cells***
- ***Aqueous flare.*** It is due to leakage of protein particles into the aqueous humour from damaged blood vessels demonstrated in slit lamp due to 'Brownian movements' or 'Tyndal phenomenon'.
- ***Hypopyon.*** sterile pus in the anterior chamber

- **Iris nodules:**
  - Koeppe's nodules at the papillary border
  - Busacca's nodules near the collarette and are large.

Posterior synechiae. These are adhesions between the posterior surface of iris and anterior capsule of crystalline lens. types:

- *Segmental posterior synechiae*
- *Annular posterior synechiae* (ring synechiae are 360° adhesions of pupillary margin to anterior capsule of lens leading to *'iris-bombe'* formation.
- *Total posterior synechiae*

Treatment of Iridocyclitis

- ***Mydriatic-cycloplegic drugs***

  Mode of action. In iridocyclitis, atropine
  - Pain relief by relieving spasm of iris sphincter and ciliary muscle
  - Prevents the formation of synechiae and may break the already formed synechiae .
  - Reduces exudation by decreasing hyperaemia and vascular permeability and
  - Increases the blood supply to anterior uvea byrelieving pressure on the anterior ciliary arteries.
- **Topical Corticosteroids** form the mainstay of treatment by reducing Inflammation.

  Sympathetic ophthalmitis:
  - Bilateral granulomatous panuveitis after penetrating trauma with prolapsed of uvea
  - After injury, it will take 4-8 weeks for sympathetic ophthalmitis to develop
  - Injured eye –exciting eye, normal eye –sympathizing eye
  - Causes –penetrating injuries dangerous site being iris and ciliary body
  - Pathogenesis: autoimmune reaction against uveal antigens
  - Earliest sign: **Retrolental flare** and cells
  - Keratic precipitates at back of cornea
  - Pathognomonic Feature: **Dalen fuch s nodule**: granulomas bet bruch s membrane and retinal pigment epithelium.

Treatment: Enucleation of exciting eye within 10 days of injury

Vogt- koyanagi -harada syndrome (VKH Syndrome): Uncommon multisystem autoimmune disorder characterized by chronic, bilateral, diffuse granulomatous uveitis associated with dermatological, neurological and auditory involvement.

Stages

- **Prodromal stage:**
  - Flu like symptoms with headache, nausea, meningism, dysacusia, tinnitus
- **Acute uveitic stage**:
  - Blurring of vision
  - B/L granulomatous anterior uveitis with variable degree of vitritis
  - Elevation of peripaplliary retinal choroid
  - Multiple serous retinal detachments and edema of optic nerve
- **Convalescent stage:**
  - Sunset glow fundus: depigmentation of choroid causing orange red discoloration
  - Siguira sign – perilimbal vitiligo
  - Alopecia, poliosis
- **Chronic recurrent stage**

Treatment: Topical/periocular/systemic steroids

Retina:

Anatomy

Innermost layer of eyeball

Both nervous tissue and blood vessels seen through naked eye

Consists of

- *Optic disk:* Size 1. 5mm
- *Macula:* consists of central depressed portion – fovea which is 2 disk diopter (3 mm) away from disk 1 mm below the horizontal meridian
- *Rods:* 120 million, more in mid periphery
- *Cones:* 6.5 million, more concentrated at fovea

Diabetic Retinopathy

Pathogenesis: It is a microangiopathy affecting retinal precapillary arterioles, capillaries and venules.

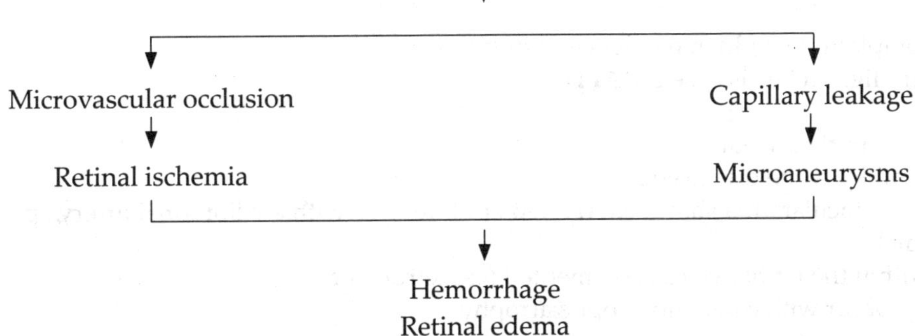

Classification

A. Nonprofilerative diabetic retinopathy

NPDR has been further classified as under:

- *Mild NPDR*
- *Moderate NPDR*
- *Severe NPDR.*
- *Very severe NPDR*

B. Profilerative diabetic retinopathy

The hallmark of PDR is the occurrence of neovascularization

- Neovascularization of Disc (NVD)
- Neovascularization elsewhere (NVE)

C. Diabetic Maculopathy

D. Advance diabetic eye disease (ADED)

These new vessels may proliferate in the plane of retina or spread into the vitreous as vascular fronds. Later on condensation of connective tissue around the new vessels results in formation of fibrovascular epiretinal membrane, vitreous detachment and vitreous hemorrhage.

Diabetic Papillopathy

Transient visual dysfunction associated with optic disk swelling.

Signs

- Defective vision 6/12
- Unilateral or bilateral disk swelling and hyperemia
- Disk surface telangiectasia.

CRAO

Central Retinal Artery Occlusion

Etiology

- Atherosclerosis-related thrombosis most common cause (75%) of CRAO.
- Emboli from the carotid artery and those of cardiac origin
- Retinal arteritis with obliteration (associated with giant cell arteritis) periarteritis (associated with polyarteritis nodosa, systemic lupus erythematosus, Wegner's granulomatosis and scleroderma)
- Tight encirclage in retinal detachment surgery.
- Thrombophilic disorders

Clinical features

Symptoms: Patient complains of sudden painless loss of vision.
Signs: Direct pupillary light reflex is absent **RAPD**
Fundus:

- Retinal arteries are markedly narrowed
- Retina becomes milky white due to edema
- Central part of the macular area shows **cherry-red spot**. In eyes with a cilioretinal artery, part of the macular will remain normal
- Blood column within the retinal veins is segmented (cattletrucking)
- Atrophic changes occur with consecutive optic atrophy.

Management

- *Immediate lowering of intraocular pressure* by intravenous mannitol and intermittent ocular massage. It may aid the arterial perfusion and also help in dislodging the embolus. Paracentesis of anterior chamber can be done
- *Vasodilators and inhalation of a mixture* of 5 percent carbon dioxide and 95 percent oxygen
- *Anticoagulants* may be helpful in some cases
- *Intravenous steroids* are indicated in patients with giant cell arteritis.

Cherry Red Spot

Causes

- Metabolic Storage Diseases:
  - Mucopolysaccharidosis
  - Hurler's disease
  - Tay-Sachs disease
  - MPS VII (Sly syndrome)
  - Farber's disease
  - GM1 gangliosidoses
  - Niemann Pick's disease
  - Sandhoff disease
  - Shprintzen-Goldberg syndrome
  - Lysosomal Storage Diseases

- Congenital Developmental Diseases: Leber's Congenital Amaurosis
- Hereditary/Familial:
  - Hallervorden Spatz disease
  - Krabbe disease
- Degenerative: Metachromatic leukodystrophy
- Vascular: Central retinal artery occlusion

AMAROUSIS FUGAX

Transient visual loss due to central retinal artery occlusion

Causes:
- CRAO
- Papilledema
- Migraine

CRVO

Central Retinal Vein Occlusion

Etiology
- Pressure on the vein by a sclerotic retinal artery (Due to hypertension, atherosclerosis)
- Hyperviscosity of blood as in polycythemia, multiple myeloma and macroglobulinemia
- Periphlebitis retinae
- Raised introcular pressure: common in patients with primary open-angle glaucoma
- Local causes are orbital cellulitis, facial erysipelas and cavernous sinus thrombosis
- Thrombogenic states like homocystinuria, factor v deficiency, antiphospholipid antibody syndrome, oral contraceptive pill usage.

Classification
- **Nonischemic CRVO:** Nonischemic CRVO (venous stasis retinopathy) is the most common clinical variety (75%).
- It is **Ischaemic CRVO:** Ischemic CRVO (Hemorrhagic retinopathy) refers to acute (sudden) complete occlusion of central retinal vein with neovascularisation at the disc (NVD) or in the periphery (NVE). *Macula* shows marked pigmentary changes and chronic cystoid oedema.

Nonischemic CRVO	Ischemic CRVO
VISION: moderate to severe loss	Severe loss
RAPD: absent	Present
• **Fundus**: Optic disc edema – mild to moderate • Mild tortuosity and venous dilatation • Dot n blot hemorrhages and flame shaped hemorrhages • Cotton wool spots absent • Macular edema may or may not be present	• Optic disk edema-severe • Venous changes –Marked • **Massive hemmorhages –TOMATO SPLASH FUNDUS** • Cotton wool spots • Macular edema

The most common cause of defective vision in crvo: MACULAR EDEMA

Complications. **Rubeosis iridis and neovascular glaucoma (NVG)** occur in more than 50 percent cases within 3 months (so also called **90 days glaucoma or 100th day**) A few cases develop vitreous hemorrhage and proliferative retinopathy.

Treatment. Panretinal photocoagulation (PRP) should be carried out when most of the intraretinal blood is absorbed, which usually takes about 3-4 months.

Macular edema: grid laser/intravitreal ANTI VEGF.

Retinal Detachment

Separation of neurosensory retina properfrom the pigment epithelium

Classification

- Rhegmatogenous or primary retinal detachment
- Tractional retinal detachment
- Exudative retinal detachment

Rhegmatogenous or primary retinal detachment

associated with a retinal break through which subretinal fluid (SRF) seeps and separates

Etiology

- Myopia
- Aphakia.
- Retinal degenerations:
  - Lattice degeneration (most common degeneration associated with rhegmatogenous RD)
  - Snail track degeneration.
  - White-with-pressure and white-without-or occult pressure.
  - Acquired retinoschisis.
- Trauma
- Senile posterior vitreous detachment (PVD).

Clinical features

symptoms. 3 fs

- **Flashes of light (photopsia)** due to irritation of retina by vitreous movements
- **Floaters:** Due to rapid vitreous degeneration
  Both of these symptoms are prodromal
- **Field defects with sudden painless loss of vision**

Signs

Marcus Gunn pupil (relative afferent papillary defect)

Fundus examination:

- Grey reflex
- In total detachment retina becomes funnel-shaped

Exudative or solid retinal detachment

It occurs due to the retina being pushed away by a neoplasm or accumulation of fluid beneath the retina following inflammatory or vascular lesions.

- *Systemic diseases*. These include: toxaemia of pregnancy, renal hypertension, blood dyscrasias and polyarteritis nodosa.
- *Ocular diseases.*
  - Inflammations such as Harada's disease, sympathetic ophthalmia, posterior scleritis, and orbital cellulitis;
  - Vascular diseases such as central serous retinopathy and exudative retinopathy of Coats
  - Neoplasms, e.g. malignant melanoma of choroid and retinoblastoma (exophytic type)
  - Sudden hypotony due to perforation of globe and intraocular operations.

Clinical features

- *Absence of* photopsia

Fundus:

- The exudative detachment is smooth and convex
- Shifting fluid characterized by changing position of the detached area with gravity is the hallmark of exudative retinal detachment.

Tractional Retinal Detachment

It occurs due to retina being mechanically pulled away from its bed by the contraction of fibrous tissue in the vitreous (vitreoretinal tractional bands).

Etiology

It is associated with the following conditions:

- Post-traumatic retraction of scar tissue especially following penetrating injury
- Proliferative diabetic retinopathy
- Retinopathy of prematurity
- Sickle cell retinopathy
- Proliferative retinopathy in Eales' disease.

Clinical features

- Tractional retinal detachment charcterised by presence of vitreoretinal bands with lesions of the causative disease.
- Shifting fluid is absent.

Retinal Vasculitis

Inflammation of the retinal vessels may be primary (Eales' disease) or secondary to uveitis.

Eales' disease: Idiopathic inflammation of the peripheral retinal veins characterised by recurrent vitreous hemorrhage.

Etiology. May be due to be hypersensitivity reaction to tubercular proteins.

Clinical features bilateral disease, typically affecting young adult males. Symptoms are sudden appearance of floater or painless loss of vision due to vitreous hemorrhage

Stages:

- Stage of inflammation: perivascular exudates and sheathing with superficial hemorrhages
- Stage of ischemia
- Stage of retinal neovascularization Bleeding from these vessels leads to recurrent vitreous hemorrhage.
- Stage of sequelae is characterized by development of complications such as proliferative vitreoretinopathy, tractional retinal detachment, rubeosis iridis and neovascular glaucoma.

Treatment of Eales' disease comprises:

- Medical treatment: oral corticosteroids and Anti TB therapy
- Laser photocoagulation for neovascularizion.
- Vitreoretinal surgery is required for nonresolving vitreous haemorrhage and tractional retinal detachment.

Retinal tamponade

Indications:

- To achieve retinal flattening by replacing vitreous
- To drain subretinal fluid
- To provide the internal tamponade of retinal breaks during the postoperative period

Types:

1. Expanding gases:

- Sulfur hexafluoride
- Perfluorethane
- Perfluoropropane

Indications: Superior Retinal breaks

Postoperative: Patients should have a particular head posture to prevent papillary block glaucoma and to give appropriate buoyancy effect

SILICON OIL: Low specific gravity

Acts as a tamponade, prevents migration of proliferative cells and VEGF into vitrius and provides hemostasis during surgery

Complications

- Emulsification (Inverse hypopyon)
- Cataract
- Glaucoma

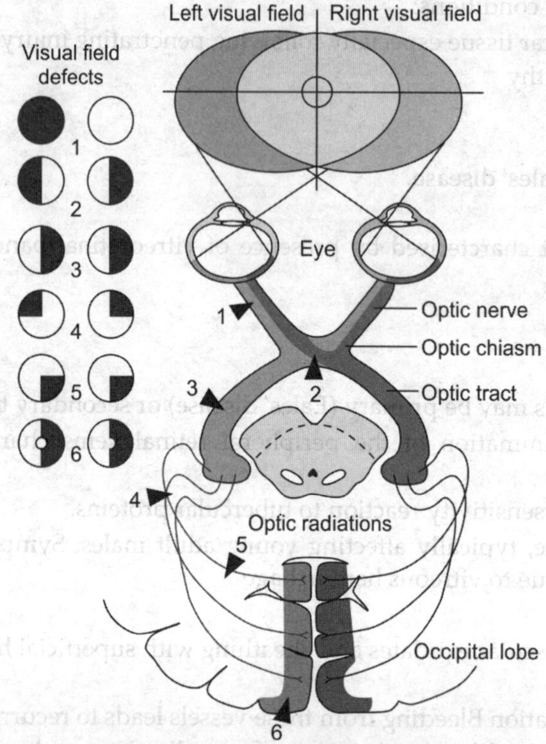

Fig. 10.3: Visual field defects

Sl. No.	Name	Site of Lesion
1	Monocular field defect	Optic nerve (same side)
2.	Bitemporal hemianopia	Lesions of optic chiasma (due to compression by pituitary tumors like pituitary adenoma, suprasellar tumors like craniopharyngioma, tb meningitis
3	Homonymous hemianopia (incongruous)	Optic tract (opposite side eg. Right homonymous hemianopia –left optic tract)
4	Superior homonymous quadrantopia	Temporal lobe
5	Inferior homonymous quadrantopia	Parietal lobe
6	Homonymous hemianopia, congruous, macular sparing	Occipital lobe (visual cortex)

Homonymous hemianopia with macular sparing: Mainly due to occlusion of posterior cerebral artery. Macular area of occipital cortex is supllied by branches from both middle cerebral and posterior cerebral artery, so there is macular sparing

Binasal hemianopia: Lesions which affect the lateral aspect of optic chiasma (By pressure from supraclinoid portion of sclerotic int. carotid arteries).

Postchiasmal lesions: Opposite field defect

Difference between papilledema and papillitis:

- Papilloedema is the swelling of optic nerve head due to raised intracranial pressure

- Papillitis ;inflammation of optic nerve head (optic neuritis)

	Papilledema	Papillitis
Vision	Normal (except in stage of optic atrophy where vision is grossly reduced)	Defective vision at presentation
Color vision	Usually normal	Affected (typically red green)
Rapd	Absent	Present
Disk swelling	Usually Bilateral	Usually unilateral
Nerve palsies	Sixth nerve palsy may be associated (false localizing sign)	Nil
Visual field defects	Enlarged blind spot	Central/Centrocecal Scotoma

Nystagmus:

Repetative, involuntary, to and fro movements of the eyeball.

Etiology:

- Physiological
- Pathological

Physiological nystagmus:

- Vestibular
- Optokinetic
- Eccentric gaze

Pathological nystagmus:

- Congenital
- Acquired: secondary to loss of vision

Due to toxins/metabolic:

- Alcohol
- Lithium
- Phenytoin
- Babituates
- Thiamine deficiency

Neurological

Lesions of midbrain, brainstem, vestibular apparatus

Squint

Definition: Visual axis of two eyes do not meet at the point of object of regard.

Classification

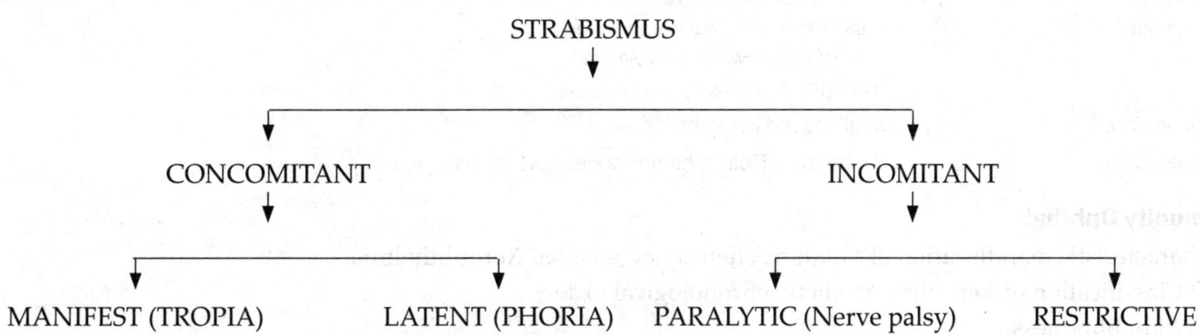

Esodeviation (Convergent Strabismus): Inward deviation:

Types

- Nonaccommodative
- Accommodative
- Partially accommodative

Exodeviation (Divergent strabismus): outward deviation:

Types

- Basic
- Convergence insufficiency
- Divergence excess

Miotics are used in accommodative squint in younger children less than 2 years who is unable to or refuses to use glasses

Drugs used: Pilocarpine ; anticholinesterase like di-isopropyl fluorophosphates, ecothiophate.

Drugs	Side Effects
Topical/Periocular steroids	Glaucoma (MC)
Systemic steroid	Cataract (MC)
Oxygen	**Retinopathy of prematurity**
Digitalis	**Disturbance of color vision** **Scotoma** **Photopsia**
Quinidine	**Optic neuritis**
Thiazides	**Xanthopsia (yallow vision)**
Amiodarone	**Corneal deposits (Vortex or Whorl keratopathy)**
Phenothiazines	**Oculogyric crisis**
Chloramphenicol	**Optic neuritis and atrophy**
Streptomycin	**Optic neuritis**
Chloroquine	**Macular changes** **Central scotoma** **Bull's eye maculopathy (pigmentary degeneration of retina)** **Chloroquine keratopathy** **Ocular palsy** **Ptosis** **ERG depression**
Iodochorhydroxyquin	Optic atrophy
Ethambutol	Optic neuritis and atrophy
Isoniazid	Optic neuritis and atrophy
Phenylbutazone	Retinal hemorrhages
Penicillamine	Ocular pemphigoid, Optic neuritis, Ocular myasthenia
Vitamin A	Papilledema, Retinal hemorrhages Loss of eyebrows and eyelashes Nystagmus, Diplopia
Vitamin D	Band shaped keratopathy
Salicylates	Nystagmus, Retinal hemorrhages cortical blindness

Community Ophthal

The characteristic manifestation of vitamin A deficiency is called Xerophthalmia.

WHO Classification of Xerophth-Almia (in chronological order)

XN—Night blindness

X1A—Conjuctival xerosis
X1B—Bitot's spots
X2—Corneal xerosis
X3A—Keratomalacia < 1/3rd corneal surface
X3B—Keratomalacia > 1/3rd corneal surface
XS—Corneal scar
XF—Xerophthalmic fundus

Night Blindness: Earliest manifestation; responds to vitamin A therapy.

Conjuctival xerosis: First appears in the temporal side in the interpalpebral area.

Bitot's Spot: In the xerotic areas, keratin and corynebacterium xerosis accumulate giving it a foamy or cheesy appearence.

Corneal Xerosis: Dry and lustreless cornea.

Keratomalacia: Colliquative necrosis (sterile corneal melting).

Scarring of the cornea.

Xerophthalmic fundus (Uyemura's fundus)

Treatment

Day	Oral	IM
Immediately, Day 1	2 lakh IU	1 lakh IU
Day 2	2 lakh IU	1 lakh IU
Within 1-4 weeks	2 lakh IU	1 lakh IU

Children between 6-11 months - half the above dose.
Children < 6 months - one-quarter of the above dose.

QUESTIONS

1. Gas used in retinal tamponade: (2014)
a. SF6 (sulfur hexafluoride)
b. Ethylene oxide
c. Nitrous oxide
d. CO_2

2. Vertically oval dilated pupil is seen in: (2014)
a. Neovascular glaucoma
b. Primary open angle glaucoma
c. Primary angle closure glaucoma
d. Acute congestive angle closure glaucoma

3. Vision not impaired in: (2014)
a. Berlin's edema
b. Optic neuritis
c. Papilledema
d. Uveitis

4. Which instrument is used to visualize the angle of anterior chamber? (2014)
a. Slit lamp examination
b. Keratometry
c. Gonioscopy
d. Indirect opthalmoscopy

5. Type of laser used in Laser iridotomy is: (2014)
a. CO_2 laser
b. Nd Yag laser
c. Excimer laser
d. KTP laser

6. Post-traumatic cataract: (2014)
a. Christmas tree
b. Rosette cataract
c. Sunflower cataract
d. Shield cataract

7. Which of the following is true regarding Horner's syndrome: (2014)
a. Constriction of pupil
b. Complete ptosis
c. Excessive sweating
d. Loss of accommodation

8. Not seen in vitreous hemorrhage: (2014)
a. Sudden vision loss
b. Floaters
c. Metamorphopsia
d. Absent fundus glow

9. Soft contact lenses are made-up of: (2014)
a. HEMA
b. Silicone
c. PMMA
d. Hydroxymethyl cellulose

10. All the following drugs cause retinal changes except: (2014)
a. Tamoifen
b. Amiadarone
c. Hydroxychloroquine
d. Vigabatrin

11. Extraocular muscle not supplied by oculomotor: (2014)
a. Superior oblique
b. Super rectus
c. Medial rectus
d. Inferior oblique

12. Which laser is used in LASIK? (2013)
a. Nd yag lesr
b. Excimer
c. CO2
d. Argon laser

13. Which gas is used for Retinal insufflations (Tamponade of lretina)? (2013)
a. SF6 sulfur hexafluoride
b. S3F8
c. S2F6
d. S4F10

14. Dalen fuch nodules are seen in: (2013)
a. TB
b. Sarcoidosis
c. Sympathetic ophthalmitis
d. Vogt-Koyanagi-Harada syndrome

15. False statement about retina is: (2013)
a. Only nerve tissue seen thru naked eye
b. Supplied by central retinal artery
c. Contain cones more than rods
d. Optic disk lateral to macula

16. Best response to goniotomy is seen with: (2013)
a. Congenital glaucoma
b. Primary angle closure glaucoma
c. Primary open angle glaucoma Adults
d. Primary open angle glaucoma Children

17. Posterior staphyloma is associated with: (2013)
a. Glaucoma
b. Uveoscleritis
c. Pathological myopia
d. All the above

18. Giant papillary conjunctivitis is associated with: (2013)
a. Hard Contact lens
b. Rigid gas permeable contact lens
c. Soft hydrophilic contact lens
d. INTACTS

19. Which of the following is a characteristic sign of diabetic retinopathy? (2013)
a. Increase in pericytes
b. Thinning of capillary basement membrane
c. Lipohyaline deposits Retinal pigment epithelium
d. Proliferation of endothelial cells

20. Posterior capsular opacification is a complication following: (2012)
a. PMMA hard contact lens
b. Intraocular lens
c. Rigid Gas permeable lens
d. Hydrophilic HEMA lens

21. All are true regarding Eale's disease except: (2012)
a. Sudden painless loss of vision
b. Bilateral involvement in 80% of cases
c. Young patients in 2nd and 3rd decade are affected
d. Inflammation of peripheral retinal arteries

22. Treatment of choice for congenital glaucoma: (2012)
a. Goniotomy
b. Trabaculoplasty
c. Conservative treatment
d. Laser iridectomy

23. The type of degeneration most common associated with retinal breaks is: (2012)
a. Paving stone degeneration
b. Lattice degeneration
c. Snow flake degeneration
d. Cystoids degeneration

24. Rubeosis iridis (Neovascularization) of iris is seen in: (2011)
a. Diabetic maculopathy
b. Hypertensive retinopathy
c. Primary open angle glaucoma
d. CRVO

25. Treatment of uveitis consists of: (2011)
a. Antibiotic and steroid
b. Steroid and Cycloplegic
c. Antibiotic and cyclopegic
d. Steroid and mydriatic

26. Pterygium causes visual disturbances due to: (2011)
a. Astigmatism
b. Myopia
c. Hypermetropia
d. Keratoconus

27. Amaurosis fugax caused by lesion/atherosclerosis in:
a. Internal carotid artery **(2011)**
b. MCA
c. ACA
d. Basilar artery

28. Photopsia are present in which of the following?
a. Retinal detachment **(2011)**
b. Open angle glaucoma
c. Uveitis
d. Central serous retinopathy

29. Blowout injury refers to what? (2011)
a. Fracture of orbit
b. Fracture of maxillary antrum
c. Fracture of nasal septum
d. Fracture of mandible

30. Bulls eye retinopathy is seen in toxicity of: (2011)
a. Quinine
b. Tobacco
c. Ethanol
d. Chloroquine

31. Salmon patch is seen in: (2011)
a. Interstitial keratitis
b. Disciform keratitis
c. Acne rosaea
d. Phlectenular keratitis

32. Visual field defect in a woman with pituitary adenoma compressing the optic chiasma: (2011)
a. Homonymous hemianopia
b. Bitemporal hemianopia
c. Binasal hemianopia
d. Quadrantanopia

33. The changes seen in accommodation during near reflex are all except: (2010)
a. Increase in curvature of lens
b. Contraction of ciliary muscle
c. Convergence of visual axis
d. Dilatation of the pupil

34. Most common malignant intraorbital tumor in childhood: (2010)
a. Malignant melanoma
b. Retinoblastoma
c. Rhabdomyosarcoma
d. Neuroblastoma

35. False about pathological myopia is: (2010)
a. Vitreous opacities
b. Retinal degeneration
c. Myopic crescents
d. Shallow ant chamber

36. Tractional retinal detachment is seen in: (2010)
a. Diabetic retinopathy
b. Hypertensive retinopathy
c. Pathological myopia
d. Malignant melanoma

37. Topical glucocorticoids in eyes causes: (2010)
a. Claucoma
b. Optic atrophy
c. Retinal detachment
d. Corneal ulcer

38. The characteristic feature of diabetic papillopathy:
a. Bulging optic disc with telengiectatic vessels
b. Multiple hemorrhagic spots **(2010)**
c. Optic disc pallor
d. Cupping of optic disc

39. Earliest manifestation of vitamin A deficiency is:
a. Conjunctival xerosis **(2009)**
b. Corneal xerosis
c. Bitot's spot
d. Night blindness

40. Sunflower cataract is seen in: (2009)
a. Blunt trauma
b. Diabetes
c. Chalcosis
d. Argyrosis

41. Steroid may be used in the treatment of which of the following type of herpes keratitis? (2009)
a. Superficial punctuate keratitis
b. Dendritic ulcer
c. Geographic ulcer
d. Disciform keratitis

42. Which of the following is the causes of blindness in partial retinal branch vein occlusion? (2009)
a. Cystoids macular edema
b. Macular hemorrhage
c. Vitreous hemorrhage
d. All the above

43. In a patient, highest visual morbidity is seen in:
a. Nuclear cataract **(2009)**
b. Intumescent cataract
c. Posterior subcapsular
d. Cuneiform cataract

44. For the treatment of a patient with after cataract which laser is used? (2009)
a. LASIK
b. Nd-YAG
c. Excimer
d. Argon

45. Reversible cataract is seen in which of following:
a. Galactosemia **(2009)**
b. Hypoparathyroidism
c. Diabetes mellitus
d. Trauma

46. Extorsion is a primary action of which of the following Extraocular muscle? (2009)
a. Medial rectus
b. Lateral rectus
c. Superior oblique
d. Inferior oblique

47. Gonioscopy is used to study: (2009)
a. Anterior chamber
b. Posterior chamber
c. Angel of anterior chamber
d. Retina

48. Anterior staphyloma is seen in: (2009)
a. Sloughing corneal ulcer
b. Scleritis
c. Glaucoma
d. Pathological myopia

49. Tear drop sign: (2008)
a. # floor of orbit
b. Retinoblastoma
c. Dry eyes
d. Congenital nasolacrimal duct obstruction

50. Papillary reflex begins at: (2008)
a. Intrauterine life
b. 3 months of age
c. 6 months of age
d. 4 months of age

51. Muscle of iris are derived from: (2008)
a. Neuroectoderm
b. Endoderm
c. Mesoderm
d. Mesencephalon

52. Hazy media can be examined with: (2008)
a. Indirect ophthalmoscopy
b. Direct ophthalmoscopy
c. Distant direct
d. Fluorescein angiography

53. Symblepharon is caused by: (2008)
a. Diphtheria
b. Gonococci
c. Chlamydia
d. Ophthalmia neonatorum

54. Iridectomy is a treatment option in: (2008)
a. Pigmentary glaucoma
b. Angle closure
c. Psuedoexfoliative glaucoma
d. Open glaucoma

55. Ring Scotoma is seen in: (2008)
a. Retinitis pigmentosa
b. End stage of glaucoma
c. CRAO with cilioretinal artery sparing
d. CRVO

56. To assess the refraction state of eye, the investigation done is: (2008)
a. USG-bscan
b. Retinoscopy
c. Binoculoscopy
d. Oprhalmoscopy

57. Cherry red spot in retina is a feature of: (2008)
a. Infantile Gaucher's disease
b. Niemann Pick disease
c. Fabry's disease
d. CRVO

58. Preganglionic and postganglionic Horner's syndrome are differentiated by application of:
a. Atropine **(2008)**
b. Pilocarpine
c. Timolol
d. Hydroxyl amphetamine

59. Axial proptosis is caused by: (2008)
a. Blowout fracture of the orbit
b. Maxillary tumor invading the orbit
c. Frontal mucocele
d. Optic glioma

60. Which of the following is used for treatment of myopia? (2008)
a. Nd YAG laser
b. Excimer laser
c. Argon laser
d. Hormium laser

61. Miotics are useful in which type of squint? (2007)
a. Accommodative squint
b. Paralytc squint
c. Divergent squint
d. Congenital squint

62. Extracapsular extraction of lens is not possible in:
a. Hypermature cataract **(2007)**
b. Immature cataract
c. Lens subluxation
d. Developmental cataract

63. KF ring in wilson's disease is seen at the level of:
a. Descemet's membrane **(2007)**
b. Epithelium
c. Endothelium
d. Stroma

64. Treatment of congenital dacryocystitis is: (2007)
a. Dacryocystectomy
b. Hydrostatic massage

c. Probing and syringing with antibiotics
d. Dacryocystorhinostomy

65. Cattle truck appearance on fundus examination is a feature of: **(2007)**
a. CRVO
b. Incomplete CRAO
c. Incomplete CRAO
d. Hypertensive retinopathy

66. Whorled keratopathy is seen with the use of:
a. Digoxin **(2007)**
b. Amiodarone
c. Ethambutol
d. Steroids

67. Herbert's pit is seen in: **(2007)**
a. Vernal conjunctivitis
b. Atopic conjunctivitis
c. Gonococcal conjunctivitis
d. Chlamydial conjunctivitis

68. Lagopathalmos is seen in: **(2007)**
a. Leprosy
b. Syphilis
c. Peripheral neuritis
d. HZV infection

69. Topical steroids is used in: **(2007)**
a. Interstitial keratitis
b. Bacterial keratitis
c. Fungal kertaitis
d. Herpetic dendritic keratitis

70. After injury, when does sympathetic ophthalmitis develop? **(2007)**
a. Immediately
b. After 1-2 weeks
c. After 4-8 weeks
d. After 1-2 years

71. Left homonymous hemianopia is due to lesion in:
a. Optic chiasma **(2006)**
b. Left optic radiation
c. Right optic radiation
d. Right optic tract

72. Giant papillary conjunctivitis is caused by: (2006)
a. Contact lens
b. Trichiasis
c. LASIK
d. SASEK

73. Most dangerous complication of trachoma is:
a. Ptosis **(2006)**
b. Pannus
c. Herbert pits
d. Follicles

74. Roving movement of eyeball in a 6-year-old child is due to: **(2006)**
a. Cerebellar dysfunction
b. Brainstem dysfunction
c. Congenital
d. All the above

75. Anterior staphyloma is seen in: **(2006)**
a. Sloughing corneal ulcer
b. Scleritis
c. Glaucoma
d. Pathological myopia

76. Treatment of irregular astigmatism: **(2006)**
a. Spectacles
b. Contact lens
c. Intra ocular contact lens
d. Tattooing

ANSWERS AND EXPLANATIONS

1. Ans. a. SF6 (Surfur hexafluoride)
Ref: Kanski Clincial Ophthalmology, 6/e p727-728; Modern Ophthalmology, 3/e, L. C. Dutta, p1753-1755

2. Ans. d. Acute congestive angle closure glaucoma *Ref: Bask's Essentials of Ophthalmology, 5/e*

3. Ans. c. Papilledema *Ref: Bask's Essentials of Ophthalmology, 5/e*

4. Ans. c. Gonioscopy *Ref: Bask's Essentials of Ophthalmology, 5/e*

5. Ans. b. Nd Yag laser *Ref: Multiple Sources: Basak, Kanski*

6. Ans. b. Rossette cataract *Ref: Multiple Sources, Kanski and Basak's Essential in Ophthalmology*

7. Ans. a. Constriction of pupil *Ref: Bask's Essentials of Ophthalmology, 5/e*

8. Ans. c. Metamorphopsia *Ref: Bask's Essentials of Ophthalmology, 5/e*

9. Ans. a. HEMA *Ref: Bask's Essentials of Ophthalmology, 5/e and Parson's Diseases of the Eye, 21/e p83*

10. Ans. b. Amiadarone *Ref: Bask's Essentials of Ophthalmology, 5/e Harrison's, Nelson's*

11. Ans. a. Superior oblique *Ref: Basak's Essentials of Opthalamology, 5/e*

12. Ans. b. Excimer laser
Ref: BASAK Essentials of Ophthalmology, 5/e p70; Kanski Clinical Ophthalmology 6/e p320-321

13. Ans. a. SF6 *Ref: Kanski Clincial Ophthalmology 6/e p727-728; Modern Ophthalmology 3/e, LC Dutta, p1753-1755*

14. Ans. c. Sympathetic ophthalmitis *Ref: Kanski Clincial Ophthalmology 6/e p465-467*

15. Ans. c and d *Ref: Anatomy and Physiology of eye; 2/e; AK Khurana; p140, 143*

16. Ans. a. Congenital glaucoma *Ref: Kanski Clincial Ophthalmology 6/e p417-419*

17. Ans. d. All the abvoe *Ref: Parson's Disease of the Eye 21/e p222-223*

18. Ans. c. Soft hydrophilic contact lens *Ref: Kanski Clincial Ophthalmology 6/e p218, 234*

19. Ans. d. Proliferation of endothelial cells *Ref: Kanski Clincial Ophthalmology 6/e p567*

20. Ans. b. Intraocular lens *Ref: Samar K Basak's Clinical Opthalmology*

21. Ans. d. Inflammation of peripheral retinal arteries *Ref: http://emedicine. medscape. com/article/Eales disease*

22. Ans. a. Goniotomy *Ref: Samar K Basak's Clinical Ophthalmoloy 2/e*

23. Ans. b. Lattice degeneration *Ref: Samar K Basak's Clinical Ophthalmoloy 2/e*

24. Ans. d. CRVO *Ref: Kanski Clinical Ophthalmology 7/e p553-554; Basak Essentials of Ophthalmology 5/e p310-312*

25. Ans. b. Steroid and cyclopegic
Ref: Basak Essentials of Ophthalmology 5/e p215; Kanski Clinical Ophthalmology 7/e p410-411

26. Ans. a. Astigmatism *Ref: Basak Essentials of Ophthalmology 5/e p153-156*

27. Ans. a. Internal carotid artery *Ref: Kanski: Clinical Ophthalmology; 7/e p563-564*

28. Ans. a. Retinal detachment
Ref: Basak Essentials of Ophthalmology 5/e p321; Kanski: Clinical Ophthalmology; 7/e p705

29. Ans. a. Fracture of orbit
Ref: Basak Essentials of Ophthalmology 5/e p421; Kanski: Clinical Ophthalmology; 7/e p873-874

30. Ans. d. Chloroquine *Ref: Clinical Ophthalmology; 7/e p864*

31. Ans. a. Interstitial Keratitis *Ref: Basak Essentials of Ophthalmology 5/e p185; Kanski: Clinical Ophthalmology; 7/e p572*

32. Ans. b. Bitemporal hemianopia *Ref: Kanski: Clinical Ophthalmology; 7/e*

33. Ans. d. Dilatation of the pupil *Ref: Kanski Clinical Ophthalmology 6/e p803; Parson's Diseases of the eye 22/e p58*

34. Ans. c. Rhabdomyosarcoma *Ref: Kanski Clinical Ophthalmology 6/e p200-201*

35. Ans. d. Shallow anterior chamber *Ref: Parson's Diseases of the Eye 22/e p73; Kanski Clinical Ophthalmology 6/e p654-655*

36. Ans. a. Diabetic retinopathy
Ref: Parson's Diseases of the Eye 22/e p323; Kanski Clinical Ophthalmology 6/e p654-655; Basak Disease of the Eye 5/e p324

37. Ans. a. Glaucoma *Ref: Parson's Diseases of the Eye p358; Kanski Clinical Ophthalmology 6/e p50*

38. Ans. a. Bulging optic disk with telengiectatic vessels *Ref: Kanski Clinical Ophthalmology 6/e p796*

39. Ans. d. Night blindness *Ref: Basak Disease of the Eye 5/e p474-476*

40. Ans. c. Chalcosis *Ref: Parson's Diseases of the Eye 22/e p258–259*

41. Ans. d. Disciform keratitis *Ref: Parson's Diseases of the Eye 22/e p202*

42. Ans. d. All the above *Ref: Kanski Clinical Ophthalmology 7/e p553-554; Basak Essential of Ophthalmology, 5/e p313*

43. Ans. c. Posterior subcapsular
Ref: Basak: Essential of Ophthalmology, 5/e p248; Parson's Diseases of the Eye 21/e p262

44. **Ans. b. Nd-YAG** *Ref: Parson's Diseases of the Eye 21/e p584*
45. **Ans. c. Diabetes mellitus** *Ref: Parson's Diseases of the Eye 21/e p263*
46. **Ans. d. Inferior oblique** *Ref: Kanski Clinical Ophthalmology 7/e p736-737*
47. **Ans. c. Angel of anterior chamber** *Ref: Kanski Clinical Ophthalmology 6/e p11*
48. **Ans. a. Sloughing corneal ulcer** *Ref: Parson's Diseases of the Eye 21/e p222-223*
49. **Ans. a. # floor of the orbit** *Basak: Essential of Ophthalmology, 5/e p421; Kanski Clinical Ophthalmology 7/e p873-874*
50. **Ans. a. Intrauterine life** *Ref: AK. Khurana comprehensive ophthalmology 5/e p11*
51. **Ans. a. Neuroectoderm** *Ref: Parson's Diseases of the Eye 21/e p5*
52. **Ref: A. Indirect ophthalmoscopy** *Basak: Essential of Ophthalmology, 5/e p87*
53. **Ans. a. Diphtheria** *Basak: Essential of Ophthalmology, 5/e p118-119*
54. **Ans. b. Angle closure** *Basak: Essential of Ophthalmology, 5/e p455*
55. **Ans. a. Retinitis pigmentosa** *Ref: Basak: Essential of Ophthalmology, 5/e p283*
56. **Ans. b. Retinoscopy** *Ref: Basak: Essential of Ophthalmology, 5/e p83, 529, 530, 532*
57. **Ans. b. Niemann Pick disease** *Ref: Kanski 7/e Clinical ophthalmology, p683-684*
58. **Ans. d. Hydroxy amphetamine** *Ref: Kanski 7/e Clinical ophthalmology, p812-814*
59. **Ans. d. Optic glioma**
    Ref: Basak Essentials of ophthalmology 5/e p361 and 371; Parson's Diseases of the eye 22/e p472
60. **Ans. b. Excimer laser**
    Ref: Kanski 7/e Clinical ophthalmology, p70; Kanski 7/e Clinical ophthalmology, p320-321
61. **Ans. a. Accommodative squint**
    Ref: J Whitwell, Proceeding of the Royal Society of Medicine 07/1958; 51 (6): 455-7.
62. **Ans. c. Lens subluxation**
    Ref: www. enjouranlofophthalmology. com/ejo18. htmly; Basak Essentials of Ophthalmology, 5/e p254, 260
63. **Ans. a. Descement's membrane** *Ref: Basak Essentials of ophthalmology 5/e p163*
64. **Ans. b. Hydrostatic massage**
    Ref: Basak Essentials of ophthalmology 5/e p387; Parson's diseases of the eye 22/e p464
65. **Ans. b. Incomplete CRAO** *Ref: Kanski 7/e Clinical ophthalmology, p563-564*
66. **Ans. b. Amiodarone** *Ref: Kanski 7/e Clinical ophthalmology, p862-863*
67. **Ans. d. Chlamydial conjunctivitis** *Ref: Parson's Diseases of the Eye; 21/e p172-175*
68. **Ans. a. Leprosy** *Ref: Parson's Diseases of the Eye; 21/e p 176; Basak Essentials of ophthalmology 5/e p117*
69. **Ans. a. Interstitial keratitis**
    Ref: Basak Essentials of ophthalmology 5/e p185; Kanski 7/e Clinical ophthalmology, p572
70. **Ans. c. 4-8 weeks** *Ref: Kanski 7/e Clinical ophthalmology, p465-467*
71. **Ans. d. Right optic tract** *Ref: Kanski's clinical Ophthalmology 6/e and Harrison's Online*
72. **Ans. a. Contact lens** *Ref: Kanski's clinical Ophthalmology 6/e p218, 234*
73. **Ans. b. Pannus: If trichiatic lash is the option, then that is the answer**
    Ref: Parson's Diseases of the Eye; 21/e p172-175
74. **Ans. d. All the above** *Ref: Parson's Diseases of the Eye; 21/e p494; Kanski's clinical Ophthalmology 6/e p830-833*
75. **Ans. a. Sloughing corneal ulcer** *Ref: Parson's Disease of the Eye 21/e p222-223*
76. **Ans: b. Contact lens** *Ref: Parson's Diseases of the Eye; 21/e p77; Basak Essentials of ophthalmology 5/e p77*

QUESTIONS 2015

1. Which of the muscle is not supplied by occulomotor nerve?
   a. Medial rectus
   b. Inferior rectus
   c. Lateral rectus
   d. Inferior oblique

2. Function of rod:
   a. Color vision
   b. Vision in dim light
   c. Vision in bright light

3. A patient with abdominal pain and painful red eye. Colonoscopy showing features of Chron's. Most probable diagnosis:
   a. Acute angle closure glaucoma
   b. Anterior uveitis

ANSWERS AND EXPLANATIONS

1. Ans. c. Lateral rectus
2. Ans. b. Vision in dim light (scotopic vision)
3. Ans. b. Anterior uveitis

Chapter

11 Medicine

Suthantira Kannan S

RESPIRATORY SYSTEM

Respiratory Failure

Type 1 respiratory failure (acute hypoxemic)	Type 2 respiratory failure
• Failure of oxygenation ($PO_2 < 60$) – PaO_2: Low – $PaCO_2$: Normal or Low – $P_{(A-a)}O_2$: Increased	• Defect in ventilation – PaO_2: Low – $PaCO_2$: **Increased** – $P_{(A-a)}O_2$: Normal
Causes: Due to alveolar flooding and failure of vasculature/shunts • Parenchymal diseases (V-Q mismatch) • Pneumonia • ARDS • Right to left shunt • Pulmonary edema • Embolism • Fibrosis	**Causes**: Due to hypoventilation, bronchospasm and reduced lung and chest wall compliance. • **Decreased CNS drive**: *For example:* CNS disorders-drug overdose, brainstem injury, sleep disordered breathing, hypothyroidism • **Weakness of respiratory muscles** *For example:* Myasthenia gravis, gullian-barre syndrome, amyotrophic lateral sclerosis, phrenic nerve injury myopathy and hypokalemia • **Kyphoscoliosis** • **Obstructive lung disease**

Type 3 respiratory failure (also called perioperative failure): due to lung atelactasis following GA.

Type 4 respiratory failure: due to hypoperfusion of respiratory muscles in shock

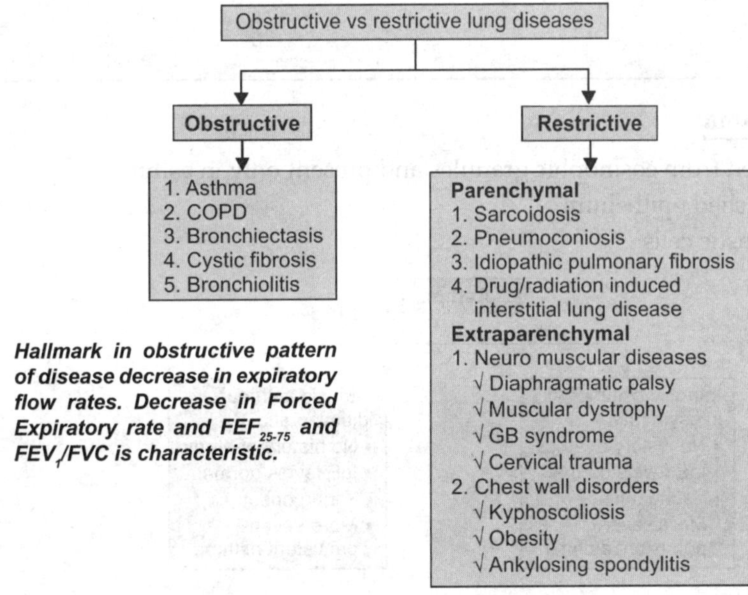

Spirometry	Obstructive	Restrictive
FEV1	Decreased (decreased out of proportion to FVC)	Decreased (decreased in proportion to FVC)
FVC	Decreased	Decreased
FEV1/FVC	Decreased	Normal or increased
FEF25-75	< 50% predicted	Decreased
TLC	Normal or elevated	Decreased
DLCO	Normal Decreased in emphysema	Decreased in parenchymal disease Normal in extraparenchymal disease

DLCO: Altered in disease affecting functional integrity of alveolar capillary membrane

Decreased	Increased
• Interstitial lung disease • Emphysema • Recurrent pulmonary embolism and primary pulmonary hypertension • Anemia	• Alveolar hemorrhage • Congestive cardiac failure • Asthma • Polycythemia

BRONCHIAL ASTHMA

- Chronic inflammatory disorder
- Airway hyperresponsiveness
- Airway epithelial shedding
- Subepithelial fibrosis and basement membrane thickening
- Hypertrophy and hyperplasia of smooth muscle
- Vascular congestion
- Microvascular leakage resulting in **airway edema** and plasma exudation
- **Mucus hypersecretion** leading to mucus plug that occlude airways
- Airway remodeling
- Autonomic neural control defect
- Mycoplasma and Chlamydia precipitate
- "hygiene hypothesis" is associated
- Vitamin D deficiency predispose

Microscopic Features of Asthma

Charcot leyden crystals: Derived from eosinophic granules and present only in asthma

Curshmann spirals: Whorls of shed epithelium

Creola bodies: Isolated metaplastic cells

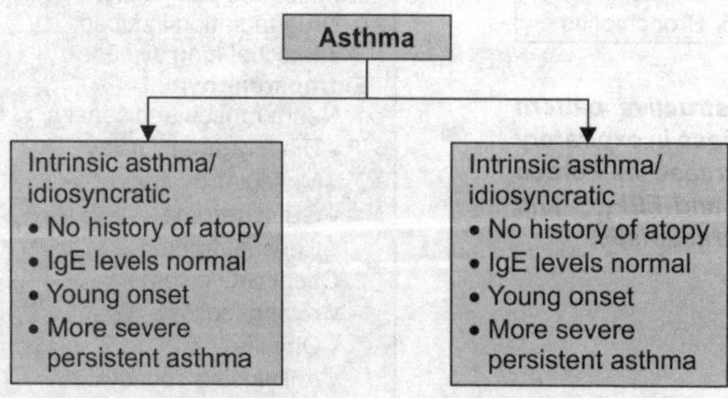

Lung Function Tests

- Reduced FEV_1, FEV_1/FVC ratio and PEF
- 15 minutes after an inhaled short beta acting agonist leads to reversibility of > 12% and 200 ml increase in FEV_1
- Exhaled nitric oxide- a recent noninvasive test to measure eosinophilic airway inflammation.

Treatment

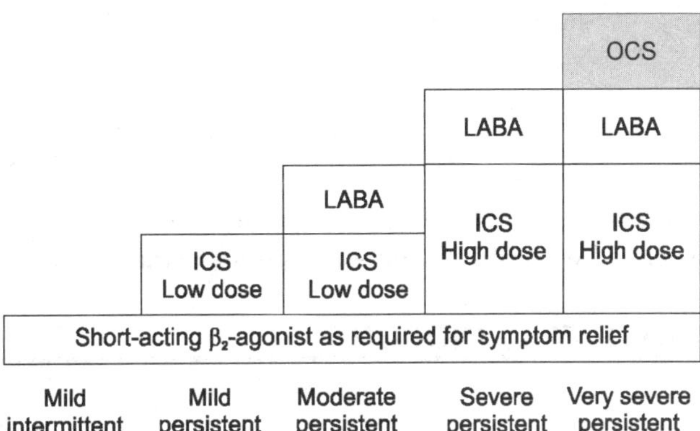

Main aim: Peak expiratory flow circadian variation < 20%

Factors associated with clearance of theophylline	
Increased Clearance: • Enzyme induction (rifampicin, phenobarbitone, ethanol) • Smoking (tobacco, marijuana) • High-protein, low-carbohydrate diet • Barbecued meat • Childhood	**Decreased Clearance:** • Enzyme inhibition (cimetidine, erythromycin, ciprofloxacin, allopurinol, zileuton, zafirlukast) • Congestive heart failure • Liver disease • Pneumonia • Viral infection and vaccination • High carbohydrate diet • Old age

HYPERSENSITIVITY PNEUMONITIS

Disease	Source	Antigen/Agent
Farmer's Lung	Mouldy hay, straw, grain dust	Micropolyspora faeni (the mophilic actinomycete)
Aspergillus fumigates		
Bird fancier's lung	Avian excreta, feathers	Avian serum proteins
Malt worker's lung	Maldy malting	Aspergillus clavatus
Byssinosis	Textile industries	Cotton, flax, hemp, dust
Bagassosis	Sugar cane dust (bagasse)	Thermoactinomyes sacchari
Humidifieror air conditioner lung-ventilation pneumonitis	Contaminated water in humidifier	Thermoactinomyes sacchari
Cheese washer's lung	Mouldy cheese	Penicilium casei
Maple bark stripper's lung	Bark from stored maple	Cryptostroma corticale
Cheese washer's lung	Moldy chees	Penicilium casei
Chemivle worker's lung	Polyurethane foam, varnishes, lacquer	Isocyanates
Compost lung	Compost	Aspergillus

Contd...

Contd...

Disease	Source	Antigen/Agent
Detergent worker's disease	Detergent	Bacillus subtilis enzymes (subtilisins)
Hot tub lung	Mold on ceiling, contaminated water	Cladosporium species
Mycobacterium avium complex		
Malt worker's lung	Moldy barley	A Fumigates or A. clavates
Miller's lung	Infested wheat flour	Sitophilus granarus (wheat weevil)
Sausage worker's lung	Dry sausage mold	Penicillum nalgiovense
Tabacco worker's lung	Mold on tobacco	Aspergillus nalgiovense
Tap water lung	Containminated tap water	Mycobacterium species

Smoking is associated with decreased incidence of hypersensitivity pneumonitis
Fibrosis is prominent in HP associated with BIRDS and emphysema is more common in farmer's lung.

ACUTE RESPIRATORY DISTRESS SYNDROME

Synonym for ARDS:

- Shock lung
- Blast lung
- Traumatic wet lung
- Congestive atelactasis
- Diffuse alveolar damage

Disorders associated with ARDS

Direct lung injury	Indirect lung injury	Miscellaneous causes
• Pneumonia • Aspiration of gastric contents • Pulmonary contusion • Near drowning • Toxic inhalation injury	• Sepsis • Severe trauma-bone#, head trauma, flail chest • Burns • Multiple transfusions • Drug overdose • Pancreatitis • Postcardiopulmonary bypass	• Renal failure • Liver failure • DIC • Eclampsia • Amniotic fluid emboli/air emboli • Hanging • High altitude

Definitions

Arterial $PO_2/FiO_2 < 200$ mm Hg is characteristic of ARDS, while a PaO_2/FiO_2 between 200 and 300 suggests acute lung injury

Phases

ARDS has three phases-exudative (first 7 days), proliferative (day 7 to day 21) and fibrotic.

Pathophysiology

- Due to damage to normally tight alveolar barrier, edema fluid rich in protein, accumulates in interstitial and alveolar spaces (noncardiogenic pulmonary edema)
- **The proteins aggregate in air spaces with cellular debris** and dysfunctional pulmonary surfactant to form hyaline membrane.
- It leads to decreased diffusion from alveolus to capillary but CO_2 being a water soluble gas diffuse from capillary to alveolus leading to **type 1 respiratory failure.**

Extra edge:

- **Left atrial pressure is normal in ARDS**
- **Left atrial pressure is elevated in cardiogenic pulmonary edema**

Diagnostic criteria

- Acute
- CXR: B/L infiltrates
- PCWP < 18 mmHg
- Total thoracic compliance < 30 ml/cm H_2O

Management

- Respiratory support: In early ARDS, CPAP with 40 to 60% oxygen
- Steroids protect those at risk of fat embolization
- Prognosis: overall mortality is 50 -75%

CARDIOVASCULAR SYSTEM

Heart Sounds

S1–First Heart Sound

Due to closure of AV Valves

2 components M1, T1

Separated by 20 msec.

SOFT S1	LOUD S1	VARIABLE S1	SPLITTING OF S1	REVERSE SPLITTING OF S1
MR TR RV/LV dysfunction Calcified MS/TS Prolonged PR interval obesity	MS TS High output states Short PR interval LA myxoma	AF Extrasystole Complete heart block	RBBB LV pacing LV ectopies Idioventricular rhythm of LV Ebsteins	LBBB RV pacing RV ectopies Idioventricular rhythm of RV Significant MS Severe LA myxoma

Loud S1 in MS is due to

- Thickened valves
- Wide opened valve during onset of systole
- Forceful closure of valve

Second Heart Sound S2

Due to the closure of semi lunar valves

A2 P2 separated by 30ms

During inspiration the split widens physiologically

SINGLE S2	
• TGA • TOF • TA • Severe AS	• Pulmonary Artesia • Severe PS • Aortic Artesia

WIDE SPLIT	
VARIABLE	FIXED
Early A2 • MR • VSD • Constrictive Pericarditis Late P2 • RBBB • LV ectopies • LV pacemakers • PS • PHT	• ASD (os type) • PAPVC • RV failure • Massive pulmonary embolism

REVERSE SPLITTING OF S_2 Mostly due to delayed closure of A_2 sometimes due to early P_2			
DELAYED A2	Electrical LBBB RV pacing RV ectopies	Mechanical LV outflow obstruction (AS, HOCM) SHT	Decreased impedance of systemic circuit Poststenotic dilatation PDA
EARLY P2	WPW synd type B		

S3–Third Heart Sound

- **Low pitched**
- Also known as proto diastolic sound or ventricular gallop
- Produced by initial passive filling of ventricles
- Occurs when

Increased filling of normal ventricle (physiological, high output state, ASD)
Normal filling of diseased ventricles (cardiomyopathy, cardiac failure)

CAUSES OF S_3	
Physiological	Pathological
• Children, young adults • Athletes • Pregnancy	• High output states • Congenital heart disease ASD, VSD, PDA • Regurgitant lesions AR, MR, TR • Cardiomyopathies • Constrictive pericarditis

RV S3

- ASD
- TR
  - LV S3 maybe physiological or pathological
  - RV S3 is always pathological

S4–Fourth Heart Sound

- **Low pitched**
- Also known as pre-systolic or atrial gallop
- Produced by rapid emptying of atrium into a non-compliant ventricle
- Causes of S4
  - HOCM
  - SHT, PHT
  - AS
  - CAD
- S4 is always pathologial

Pitches of Sounds

Low frequency	High frequency
• S3 • S4	• S1 • S2 • OS • Ejection click • Pericardial knock • Tumor plop • Prosthetic valve sounds

Diastolic sounds	Systolic sounds
Early • OS • Tumor plop • Pericardial knock • Opening-prosthetic valves Mid–S3 Late–S4	Early • Ejection click • Closing-prosthetic valves Mid to Late • Nonejection clicks

Events from A2

P2 Expiration → < 30 ms
P2 Inspiration → 40–50 ms
OS → 30–150 ms
Pericardial knock → 100–120 ms
S3 → 120–200 ms

Opening Snap

Produced by opening of AV valves
Due to sudden diastolic buckling of AV valve leaflets due to elevated atrial pressure

Causes

Apex	Tricuspid
• MS, MR	• TS, TR
• VSD	• ASD
• PDA	

A2–OS interval indicates the Left atrial pressure thereby the severity of MS. **As the severity increases A2-OS interval will become shorter**.

Mild MS → > 120 ms
Mod MS → 60–80 ms
Severe MS → 40–60 ms

In MS, OS is best heard between mitral and tricuspid area.

MURMURS

Systolic Murmurs			
Early systolic	**Mid (Ejection) systolic**	**Late systolic**	**Pan systolic**
• Small muscular VSD • Large VSD with PHT • Acute severe MR • Acute severe TR	• AS • PS • HOCM	• MVPS • TVPS • Papillary muscle dysfunction	• MR • TR • VSD

Diastolic murmurs		
Early diastolic	**Mid diastolic**	**Late diastolic**
• AR • PR • Graham steels murmur	• MS • TS • **Carry coombs**–acute Rh carditis • **Austin flint murmur** chronic AR • Acute severe AR • **Rytands murmur** of comp. block • High output states–flow MDM • VSD, PDA, MR, ASD, TR, TAPVC	• MS • TS • Atrial myxoma

Continuous murmur		
High pressure to low pressure shunt	**Normal flow through constricted vessel**	**Increased flow through normal vessel**
• PDA • Aorto pulmonary window • ALCAPA • Coronary AV fistula • ROSV • Lutembacher • AV fistula • Porto systemic shunt	• COA • Peripheral pulm artery stenosis • Carotid stenosis • Renal artery stenosis • Celiac, mesenteric artery stenosis	• Venous hum • Umbilical vein (cruveilheir) • Mammary soufflés • Uterine soufflés • Hepatoma • Nephroma • Thyrotoxicosis

To and Fro murmurs (Bi phasic murmurs)

Murmurs occuring through a single channel occupying mid systole and early diastole
Eg: AS with AR
PHT with PR

Systolico diastolic murmur

Murmurs occuring through different channels occupying systole and diastole
Eg: VSD with AR

Continuous murmur with diastolic accentuation

- RSOV
- Coronary AV fistula
- ALCAPA
- Pulm AV fistula
- Venous hum

Continuous murmur with cyanosis

- TAPVC
- Pulm AV fistula
- TOF] broncho
- TA] pulmonary
- Tricuspid atresia] collaterals

PULSE

- **Pulse pressure** = systolic–diastolic pressure
- Normal 30–60 mm Hg

Narrow PP (< 30 mm Hg)	(> 60) Wide PP
• CCF • AS • Cardiac tamponade • Dehydration	• AR • PDA • CHB • Hyperdynamic states

- **Mean arterial pressure** = diastolic + 1/3 PP
- Normal = 93 mm Hg
- **Normal pulse is called as CATACROTIC pulse**
  - Percussion wave → early systole
  - Anacrotic shoulder → jet of blood in aorta
  - Incisura → closure of aortic valve
  - Dicrotic wave → elastic recoil of aorta
  - Tidal wave → large systole

Pulse Character

Best assessed in carotid arteries

But characters of

- Pulses Bisferiens
- Pulses Alternans

Are best assessed in peripheral vessels like brachial and radial arteries

ANACROTIC PULSE	• Parvus et tardus • Slow rising, late peaking • Cause–severe AS
COLLAPSING PULSE	• Water Hammer pulse • Corrigan's pulse • Large volume • Rapid upstroke • Rapid down stroke • **Causes** – AR – PDA – AV fistula – ROSV
PULSES BISFERIENS	• 2 peaks **both in systole** • **Causes** – AS with AR, severe AR – HOCM, myocarditis
PULSES ALTERNANS	• Alternate small and large volume pulse • Due to cyclical changes in intracellular calcium and action potential • **Causes** – LV dysfunction – Following SVT
PULSES DICROTICUS	• Two peaks–one in systole, one in diastole • **Causes** (CCDDE) – LVF – Dehydration – Enteric fever – Cardiac tamponade – Dilated cardiomyopathy – Intra aortic balloon pumping

Contd...

Contd...

PULSES PARADOXUS	• Pulsus normalis aggregans • Inspiratory fall of systolic BP > 10 mm Hg • It is exaggeration of normal phenomenon • **Causes** – Cardiac tamponade – Constrictive pericarditis (1/3rd of pts) – COPD, Acute severe Asthma – Hypovolemic shock, massive pulmonary embolism
REVERSE PULSUS PARADOXUS	• Occurs in HOCM, IPPV, AV dissociation

CARDIAC FAILURE

- Massive pulmonary embolism is the MCC for acute corpulmonale
- Massive pulmonary embolism is the MCC for acute RV failure

Management of Heart Failure

- Diuretics
- ACE inhibitors
- Beta blockers
- Hydralazine/isosorbide
- Digoxin
- Spiranolactone

Drugs that prolong survival in CF

- ACE I
- ARB
- B blockers
- spironolactone

Inotropes

- Dobutamine–B1, B2 agonist
- Milrinone–PDE III inhibitor–inodilator
- Dopamine–B1, A 1, D1, D 2 agonist

Newer drugs

- Levosemendine
- Trimetazidine

Vasodilators

- NTG
- Nitroprusside
- Nesritide–recombinant BNP

Vasopressin antagonist

- Reduce body weight, edema
- Normalise serum sodium
- **Tolvaptan, conivaptan**

Interventions

- Intraaortic balloon pumping
- Lv assist devices
- Cardiac Tx

Device therapy

- Cardiac resynchornization
- Implantable cardiac defibrillators
- **Cardiac resynchornization**

Also called as biventricular pacing

Indications

- EF < 35%
- QRS > 120 ms
- NYHA III–IV

Can be combined with medical therapy

- **ICD**

Reduce the incidence of sudden cardiac death

Indications

- NYHA II–III
- EF < 35%

Can be combined with biventricular pacing

ECG

- P wave–atrial depolarization
- PR interval–conduction through atria to AV node
- PR segment–AV nodal delay
- QRS complex–ventricular depolarization
- T wave–ventricular repolarization
- QT interval–duration of ventricular electrical activity

U wave: **Repolarization of bundle branches and purkinje fibres**

Current of injury is-ST segment

Duration

- PR interval 120–200 ms
- QRS duration 100 ms
- QT interval 400–450 ms

AV BLOCKS		
First degree AV block Prolongation of PR interval > 200 ms	**Second degree AV block** Not all the P waves are followed by QRS complexes (not all the atrial impulses are conducted) **Atrial rate will be higher than ventricular rate**	**Third degree AV block** • Complete interruption of AV conduction • Ventricles takes a new pacemaker
		• AV dissociation • Slow ventricular rate – Junctional rhythm → 40–50 beats – Ventricular rhythm → 30–40 beats

Contd...

Contd...

AV BLOCKS			
	Type I second degree (Mobitz type I) Wenkebachs phenomenon PR interval gradually increases, finally a 'p' wave is not conducted.	**Type II (Mobitz type II)** Intermittent failure of 'p' wave to be conducted to the ventricles with normal preceding PR interval Type II has **poor prognosis** than type I Maybe associated with **abnormal QRS complexes** as it is distal his bundle block When associated with paroxysmal AV block (series of unconducted 'p') is an **indication for permanent pacemaker**.	

QT interval

- From the onset of Q wave to end of T wave
- Normal 400–450 ms
- Varies with RR interval
- Therefore it should be corrected
- QTc is corrected QT interval
- **BAZETT'S FORMULA**
- Corrected QT (QTC) = Bazett's Formula = QT Interval/√ (RR interval) RR Interval = 60/HR

QT PROLONGATION		QT SHORTENING
• **Hypocalcemia** • **Hypothermia** • **Hypokalemia** • **Hypomagnesimia** • **Hypothyroidism** • HOCM • MVP • Pulmonary embolism • MI • Myocarditis • CNS injury • Raised ICT	**Drugs** • Quinidine • Procaineamide • Disopyramide • Phenothiazines • TCA **Congenital** • Jervell –Lange- Nielsen synd • Romano–Ward synd	• Hypercalcemia • Hyperthermia • Digitalis • Vagal stimulation

Electrolyte Abnormalities in ECG

Hyperkalemia	**Flattening of P wave** **Prolongation of PR interval** **Widening of QRS complexes** ST segment shortening, disappearance QT shortening **Tall T wave**
Hypokalemia	**Disappearance of T** **Appearance of 'U' wave** First or second degree AV block
	ST segment depression **PR prolongation** **QT prolongation**
Hypercalcemia	Shortening of QT interval
Hypocalcemia	QT prolongation
Hypermagnesemia	Similar to Hyperkalemia
Hypomagnesemia	Similar to Hypokalemia

Arrythmias

Torsades de pointes

- Meaning–twisting of points
- Polymorphic VT
- Occurs in QT prolongation syndromes
- Delay in phase 3 of AP
- Rate 150–250
- Sudden death is common

Causes

Congenital

- Romano-ward syndrome
- Jervell Lange Neilson syndrome

Acquired

- Anti arrythmic drugs (I a, I c, III)
  - Quinidine, procainamide, disopyramide
- Encainide, flecainide
- Sotolol, Amiodarone

TCA

- Antibiotics–macrolides, azoles
- Terfinadine, cisapride, astimizole
- Metabolic
  - Hypokalemia
  - Hypocalcemia
  - Hypomagnesiemia

Treatment

- Congenital
  - Beta blockers
- Aquired
  - Atrial or ventricular overdrive pacing
  - Magnesium

Ventricular premature beats

Characteristics

- Premature discharge
- Bizarre QRS
- Secondary ST–T changes
- Constant coupling interval
- Compensatory pause complete
- Does not reset the rhythm
- Follows rule of Bigeminy

VT

- 3 or more VPDs occurring in series is called as ventricular tachycardia
- Characteristic feature include
  - AV dissociation
  - Capture beats
  - Fusion beats

Arrythmias Treatment

PSVT

- First choice–adenosine and verapamil
- Second choice–beta blockers

Av blocks

- Isoprenaline, atropine
- Permanent pacing for CHB and Mobitz II

Wolf Parkinsonwhite Syndrome

- Pre-excitation syndrome
- Aberrant pathway which connects atria and ventricle- **bundle of kent**
- More common in **males**
- Decreases with age
- May be associated with **Ebsteins, MVPs**

ECG
Normal P wave
Short PR interval
Slurred initial part of QRS
Slight widening of QRS
Secondary ST-T changes

Arrythmias in WPW syndrome

- AF
- Reciprocating SVT
- Treatment-radio frequency ablation
- SVT-vagal stimulation
  - Adenosine
  - Verapamil, diltiazem, beta blocker
- AF-DC version if life threatening
- procainamide
  - Ibutilide
- Cautious use of IV digoxin and IV verapamil as there is risk for VF

Digoxin Toxicity

Clinical features	Precipitated By ...	Treatment
• Anorexia, nausea, vomiting- earliest • Wt loss • **Yellow vision (Xanthopsia)** • Gynacomastia	• Advanced age • Renal insuffiency • Hypokalemia • Hypomagnesiemia	• Drug withdrawal • Potassium • Phenytoin • B blocker

Contd...

Contd...

Clinical features	Precipitated By ...	Treatment
• Delirium • Arrythmias – Non paroxysmal tachycardia with variable AV block – VPD, Bigeminy – VT – AV blocks • Digoxin converts atrial flutter in fibrillation	• Hyoxia • Hypercalcemia • Hypothyroidism • Drugs – Quinidine – Verapamil – Amioderone – propafenone	• Lignocaine • Pacemaker • Cardioversion • Digibind

Hemodialysis not useful

- Hemodialysis not useful **(K–BOD)**
- **K–Kerosine**
- **B–Barbiturates**
- **O–Oleander**
- **D–Digoxin**
- **Osborn waves** occurs in **hypothermia**

ISCHEMIC HEART DISEASE

Risk Factors

- Cigarette smoking
- Hypertension
- High LDL
- Low HDL
- DM
- Family H/O premature CAD
  - Males < 55 year
  - Females < 65 year
  - Age men >/45 year
  - Women >/65 year
- Infections-chlamydia

Life style risk factor

- Obesity (BMI > 30)
- Physical inactivity
- Atherogenic diet

Emerging Risk Factors

- Lipoprotein (a)
- Homocysteine
- High fibrinogen
- **HS CRP**

Metabolic Syndrome

- NCEP ATP III 2001 guidelines
  - 3 or more of

- Central obesity
  - WC men > 102 cm
  - Women > 88 cm
- Triglycerides >/150 mg%
- HDL < 40 mg% and < 50 mg% on medication
- BP > 130/85 mm Hg
- FBS > 100 mg%

- IDF criteria
  - W C Based on ethnicity
    - 90 cm–male
    - 80 cm–female
- For south Asians
- LDL/HDL is called as coronary risk ratio. It is a good predictor of coronary risk.

Classification of IHD

- Stable angina
- Acute coronary syndromes
  - Unstable angina
  - Myocardial infarction
    - STEMI
    - NSTEMI

Clinically ACS is divided into

- STEMI (red fibrin rich thrombi)
- NSTEMI/UA (white platelet rich thrombi)

Stable Angina

- Exertional angina pecotris
- Relieved in 5–10 min by rest or NG

UA

- Occurs at rest lasting for > 10 min
- Severe and new onset (4–6 wks)
- Crescendo pattern
- ECG showing ST depression and T inversion

NSTEMI

- UA + elevated bio marks

Investigations

ECG changes

- NSTEMI/UA–subendocardial ischemia
  - ST depression
- STEMI–ST elevation

STEMI

Hyper acute phase (< 30 min)	Acute Phase	Evolved phase (6 hrs)	Chronic phase (> 2 wk)
T wave become Tall	ST elevation	Q wave formation T–inversion	ST iso electric T upright Q persists/reduced/disappear

Localization

Location of MI	Leads to see in ECG
Inferior wall	II, III, aVF
Anterior wall	I, aVL, V1-v6
Lateral wall	I, aVL (high lateral), v5, v6
RVMI	v1-v2, rt sided leads (v4R)
Posterior wall	Only reciprocal changes in V1-v3 Associated with inferior or lateral infarct

Artery involvement

- LAD: **Anterior**, lateral, septal
- RCA: **Inferior** wall of LV, RV
- LCX: **Lateral**, post wall, inferior,

Prinzmetal variant angina:

- Seen in younger patients.
- Transient ST elevation with rest pain
- Multiple episodes of asymptomatic ST elevation (silent ischemia)
- Coronary angiography shows TRANSIENT CORONARY SPASM –diagnostic hallmark.
- Spasm most commonly seen in RCA
- CCBs and NITRATES are most effective.
- Aspirin increases the severity of attacks.

Bio Markers

Creatinine Phosphokinase	• Seen at 4–8 hrs • Peaks at 24 hrs • Normalization at 48–72 hrs • Limitation-less specific • CPK-MB/CPK ratio > 2.5 is highly suggestive of MI • CPK-MB also raised in – Myocarditis – Electrical cardioversion – Cardiac surgery
Troponin T	• Elevated even in small MI • Earlier rise than CPK • **DISADVANTAGES of Troponin-T** • Elevated for 7–10 days and therefore not useful in reinfarction during that time
MYOGLOBIN	**Earliest biomarker**

Nonspecific

- SGOT
- LDH
- Others
  - Polymorphonuclear leukocytosis
  - Increased ESR

Cardiac imaging

- 2D Echocardiogaphy
  - Wall motion abnormality

- RV infarct
- Ventricular aneurysm
- Pericardial effusion
- LV thrombus
- VSD, MR

- Radionuclide Imaging
  - Perfusion imaging with **thallium** 201 and Tc 99m stestamibi
  - Venticulography with Tc 99 m labelled RBCs
- In pts who are unable to walk pharmacological stress test is performed with IV
  - Dipyramidole
  - Adenosine
  - Dobutamine
- Information gained from stress test can be enhanced by radionuclide perfusion imaging with IV
  - Thallium 201
  - Tc 99 m sestamibi
  - PET scan using N-13 ammonia or rubidium
- Images taken at rest are compared with images
- taken immediately after exercise to detect the '**reversible Ischemia**'
- **Agatston score**-coronary calcium detected by imaging techniques.

Complications of MI

- **Pump Failure**
  - Primary cause of in hospital death

Classification (Killip)	
Class I	• No sign of pulmonary venous congestion
Class II	• Rales at lung bases • S3 gallop • Tachypnoea • Venous and hepatic congestion
Class III	• Severe heart failure and pulmonary edema
Class IV	• Shock, • Systolic BP < 90 mm Hg • Peripheral cyanosis • Mental confusion • Oliguria

- Prognosis–Mortality
- Class I: 0–5%
- Class II: 10–20 %
- Class III: 35–45 %
- Class IV: 85–95%

RV infarct

- One third of inferior wall infarct
- JVP increased
- Hypotension
- Lungs clear
- Kussmaul's sign +ve
- Hepatomegaly

Diagnosis

- RT sided leads v4R, ST elevation
- 2D echo
- RA catheterization shows features similar to constrictive pericarditis
  - Steep Y descent
  - Square root pattern

Arrhythmias Management

Prophylactic anti arrhythmic therapy is contraindicated
Routine use of beta blocker is indicated

VPD	No Treatment
Sustained VT	Amiadarone Procainamide Electroversion (nonsynchronized) Epinephrine/Amiadarone (if refractory to electrovertion)
AIVR	no treatment
Sinus tachycardia	beta blocker
AF/Afl	digoxin (In failure) beta blocker verapamil diltiazem synchronized/electroversion (refractory)
Acc. Junctional rhythm	RA/coronary sinus pacing
Sinus bradycardia	atropine, electrical pacing
Complete AV block	temporary pacing

- **Pericarditis**: Aspirin (650 mg qid)
- **Thrombo embolism**: Systemic anticoagulants

Mechanical complications

Ventricular septal rupture

- 3–7 days after reperfusion
- Chest pain, hypotension, SOB
- Harsh holosystolic murmur

Rupture of ventricular free wall

- 1–7 days of after reperfusion
- Present as tamponade
- Electromechanical dissociation

Papillary muscle rupture

- One day after MI
- Pulmonary edema, hypotension
- Present as acute MR

Management of ACS

- **UA/NSTEMI**
  - Bed rest
  - Oxygen

- **Anti-ischemic treatment**
  - Nitrates- SL/buccal spray 3 doses
  - IV nitrates
- **Beta blockers**
  - Oral beta blockers to target HR 50–60/min
  - IV beta blocker cautiously used for the risk of cardiogenic shock
- **Calcium channel blocker**
  - Diltiazem, verapamil for beta blockers nonresponding and intolerant

ACE I

Statins

Antithrombotic

- Aspirin
- Clopidogrel
- Prausgrel

IV antiplatelet agents

- Abciximab
- Epifibatide
- Tirofiban

Anticoagulants/anti thrombotic

- UFH
- Enoxapiridin-LMWH
- Fondaparinaux-indirect factor X a
- Bivalirudin–direct thrombin inhibitor
  - High risk → angiography after all medical management → PCI or CABG
  - Low risk → watchful waiting

Management of STEMI

- ECG changes indication for reperfusion
  - ST elevation > 2 mm in 2 contiguous precordial leads
  - ST elevation > 1 mm in 2 adjacent limb leads
  - New LBBB

PCI vs fibrinolysis

- GOAL
  - Door to needle time < 30 min
  - Door to balloon time < 90 min
- If EMS is available
  - EMS to balloon time < 90 min -PCI

PCI preferred when

- Diagnosis is in doubt
- **Cardiogenic shock** is present
- Bleeding risk is increased
- Symptom for 2–3 hrs (**Mature clot**)

Fibrinolysis

- Drugs
- SK

- Alteplase
- Tenectaplase
- Reteplase
- **Coronary angiography** should be performed after fibrinolytics
- Failure of perfusion–RESCUE PCI.

Dressler's Syndrome

- Occurs few weeks to few months after MI
- Due to autoimmunity to necrosed myocardial cells
- Persistent fever, pericarditis, pleuritis, joint pain, raised ESR
- Subside after few days
- Prolonged or severe symptoms are treated with high dose aspirin or even steroids

Pericardial Disease

Etiology

- Acute < 6 wks
- Sub acute 6 wks–6 months
- Chronic > 6 wks
  - **Idiopathic–most common**
  - Viral–coxsakie A, B, Echo, Mumps, Adeno
  - Pyogenic
  - Fungal–histo, coccido, candida, blasto
  - Others–syphilis, protozoal, parasites
  - MI
  - Uremia
  - Neoplasm
  - Myxoedema
  - Trauma
  - Radiation

Auto Immune

- Rheumatic
- Collagen vascular disorder
- Drugs–Hydralizine, Procainamide, Phenytoin,
  - INH, Minoxidil, Methysergide,
  - Anticoagulants
- Postcardiac injury–Dresslers syndrome (**fibrinous pericarditis**)

Blood in pericardium

- Neoplasm
- TB
- Acute Rheumatic fever
- Post cardiac injury
- Post MI
- Renal failure dialysis
- Dissecting aneurysm of aorta

Chest Pain

Presents only in acute pericarditis
Severe, retro sternal/left precardial, referred to neck, arm or left shoulder
Aggravated on lying supine and relieved by sitting up and leaning forward
May be accompanied by pleuritic chest pain

Pericardial Frictional Rub

- May have 3 components (**mid systolic, middiastolic, pre systolic**)
- High pitched, rasping, scratching or grating
- Left lower sternal boarder, end expiration, upright, leaning forwards
- Often inconstant

ECG Changes

Stage I

- Wide spread ST elevation, upward concavity in 2–3 limb leads and V2–V6
- Reciprocal changes only in V1 and aVR
- PR segment depression below TP segment–atrial involvement

Stage 2 (after few days)

- ST segment returns to normal

Stage 3

- T wave inverted

Stage 4 (weeks to months)

- T wave Returns to normal

Ewart's Sign

In pericardial effusion the base of the left lung may be compressed by the pericardial fluid–**patch of dullness and ego phony beneath the angle of scapula**

Diagnosis

- **Echo cardiography**: Sensitive, specific, noninvasive
- CT, MRI: Superior to ECHO in
- Loculated effusions
- Pericardial thickenings
- Pericardial masses

JUGULAR VENOUS PULSE

a → Right atrial contraction
x → Atrial relaxation
c → Tricuspid valve ascends during isovolumetric contraction phase
v → Venous filling of atrium
y → Tricuspid valve opens

Remember ...

- S1 precedes C wave
- S2 precedes Y descent

'a' WAVE	• **Absent** – Atrial fibrillation • **Prominent** – TS – PS – PHT
	• **Giant** – Regular → Junctional rhythm – Irregular → Complete heart block - Multiple ectopics
'X' DESCENT	• **Absent** – TR • **Prominent** – Cardiac tamponade – Constrictive pericarditis
'v' WAVE	• **Prominent** – TR
'y' DESCENT	• **Slow** – TS – RA myxoma • **Fast** – TR – Constrictive pericarditis • **Absent** – Cardiac tamponade

Remember in TR	Remember in cardiac tamponade	Remember in constrictive pericarditis
'x' descent → absent 'v' wave → prominent 'y' descent → prominent	X descent is prominent Y descent is absent	X descent is absent Y descent is prominent

Mnemonic PaY TaX-Pericarditis-Y descent; Tamponade-X descent

Kussmaul's Sign

Inspiratory increase in JVP

- Seen in
- Constrictive pericarditis
- Restrictive cardio myopathy
- RV infarct
- RV failure

Absent in cardiac tamponade

Friedreich's Sign

Rapid 'y' descent

Constrictive pericarditis

TR

CARDIAC TAMPONADE

Beck's Triad

- Hypotension
- Absent heart sounds

- JVP shows
  - Prominent 'x' descent
  - Absent 'y' descent

Kussmaul's sign absent

In cardiac tamponade ventricular filling is impeded throughout the diastole

Pulsus Paradoxus

Inspirational fall in systolic BP > 10 mm Hg

Mechanism in cardiac tamponade

Both ventricles are compressed by the tamponade and are not allowed to expand. Therefore increased venous return to the right ventricle causes bulging of the IVS into left ventricle thereby reducing the venous return to LV

ECG

- Decreased amplitude of QRS complexes
- Electrical alternans

ECHO

- Diagnostic
- Tricuspid and pulmonary valve flow velocities **increased** markedly during **inspiration**
- Pulmonary vein, mitral, aortic velocities **decreased** during **inspiration**
- **Diastolic collapse of RV free wall and RA**

Treatment

- Pericardiocentesis under echo or fluroscopic guidance
- MC approach–sub-xiphoid.

CONSTRICTIVE PERICARDITIS

Causes

Developing countries–TB

Developed Countries

- Viral/idiopathic pericarditis
- Trauma
- Cardiac injury
- Mechanical irradiation
- purulent infection
- Neoplasm
- RA, SLE
- CRF
- Histoplasma

Pericardium forms a **firm scar, calcified** encasing the heart and interferes with ventricular filling. **Ventricular filling is unimpeded during early diastole but reduced abruptly when the elastic limit of the pericardium is reached** (in cardiac tamponade ventricular filling is impeded throughout the diastole)

In both CT and CP

- Stroke volume reduces
- Ventricular end diastolic volume reduced
- Ventricular end diastolic pressure increased

In constrictive pericarditis

- 'x' descent absent in JVP
- 'y' descent prominent JVP
- Kussmauls sign positive
- **M shaped contour of atrial tracing** due to rapid 'x' and 'y' descent.
- **Square root sign in ventricular tracing** (also seen in restrictive cardio myopathy)
- Pulsus paradoxus positive in 1/3 of cases
- Acute LV failure andpulmonary edema are very uncommon
- RV failure features are predominant
- **Broad bent's sign**
  - Apical impulse is reduced and retracted in systole
- Heart sounds are diminished
- Pericardial knock is heard. High pitched, earlier than S3

Ascites is out of proportion to edema.it is called as **ascites precox**

ECHO–doppler

- During inspiration decreased flow to LV and increased flow to RV → leftward bulging of IVS
- Opposite during expiration

Restrictive cardiomyopathy differs from CP by

- Orthopnoea with LV failure
- Apex beat well defined
- LV hypertrophy
- Gallop sounds
- Bundle branch block
- Q wave in ECG
- Treatment-Pericardial resection

Constrictive pericarditis differs from RCMP by

- Absent LV failure (pulm edema)
- Less prominent apex beat
- Pericardial thickening
- Pericardial knock
- Low voltage QRS
- Diffuse flattening/T inversion
- ECHO → exaggerated resp variations
  - Equalization of diastolic pressure

NEPHROLOGY

Kidney

Clinical Syndrome

Nephrotic syndrome	Nephritic syndrome
Proteinuria > 3 g/day	Proteinuria 1–2 g/day
Massive edema	Hematuria
Hypoalbuminemia	RBC cast
Hypercholestrolemia	Pyuria
Microscopic hematuria	HT
	↓ GFR
	Fluid retention

Acute Nephritic Syndrome

- Hematuria
- Subnephrotic proteinuria
- Oliguria
- HT
- Renal failure–Azotemia

Nephrotic Syndrome

- Nephrotic proteinuria
- Hypo albuminemia
- Massive edema
- Hyperlipidemia

Loss	Effects
Albumin	Edema
AT III	Hypercoagulability
TBG	Hypothyroidism
Transferrin	Microcytic hypochromic anemia
Cholecalceferol binding protein	Hypocalcemia
Ceruloplasmin	Low copper levels

RPGN (ARF): Nephritic syndrome progressing to renal failure **within weeks**
CRF: Nephritic/Nephrotic syndrome progressing to renal failure **over years**

Pathological Syndromes

- Diffuse proliferative GN
- Mesangial GN
- Mesangioproliferative GN
- Membranous GN
- Minimal change GN
- Focal segmental glomerulo sclerosis
- Membrano proliferative GN
- Focal proliferative
- Cresentic nephritis

Pathologically GN is classified as

Proliferative	Sclerotic
• PSGN • MPGN • Lupus • Cryoglobulinemia • Endocarditis	• FSGS • MGN • Diabetic • Amyloidosis

Pathology vs Clinical

Nephritic syndrome	Nephrotic syndrome	RPGN
• Diffuse prolifertive • Membranoproliferative • Focal proliferative	• Minimal change • Membranous GN • FSGS	• Crescentic GN

Nephrotic syndrome

The **dyslipidemia pattern** in NS is

- ↑ TC
- ↑ LDL
- ↑ TG
- ↑ VLDL
- HDL–often decreased, but maybe variable.

Nephrotic Syndrome is a Hypercoagulable State Due to

- Low AT III
- High fibrinogen
- Low fibrinolysin
- Altered protein C and S
- Increased platelet aggregability

MCC of NS in
- Children: Minimal change disease (70–90%)
- Adult: Membranous nephropathy
- Systemic disease: DM

Usually the minimal change disease occurs as a primary disease.
But it can also be associated with

- Hodgkin's disease
- NSAID induced interstitial nephritis
- Allergies
- HIV

The microscopic features of MCD are

- Light microscopy–No abnormality
- IF microscopy–NO abnormality
- **Electron microscopy–fusion/effacement of foot processes**

The glomeruli appears normal, but the tubules (proximal) are often laden with lipids (due to increased hepatic production). So MCD is also called as **'Lipoid Nephrosis'** It is also called as **"Nil Lesion"**

Selective Proteinuria

The urine proteins in MCD is predominantly albumin. This is due to loss of anionic charge in the foot processess.

In children renal biopsy is needed only in

- **Steroid nonresponders.**
- **Steroid dependent**
  - 2 relapses while tapering
- **Steroid resistant**
  - No response to steroid in children
  - They may have FSGS on repeat biopsy
- **Frequent relapses**
  - 2 or more relapse in 6 months following tapering.

Response in Adult differs from Children

- The complete remission is less (80% vs 95%)
- Response is slow (8 weeks vs 24 wks)
- Relapses are less common
- Relapses are resistant to prednisolone

Postinfective GN/Post streptococcal GN

- It is an acute endocapillary proliferative GN
- The classic presentation is acute nephritic picture

Poststreptococcal GN

- Prototype for acute endocapillary proliferative GN (DPGN)
- Children 2–14 yrs
- Male > females
- Skin infections
  - M types 47, 49, 55, 57, 60, 2
  - GN: 2–6 weeks following skin infection
- Pharyngitis
  - M types 1, 2, 3, 4, 12, 25, 49
  - GN: 1–3 weeks following pharyngitis

Renal biopsy

- Diffuse proliferative
- **Humps**–subepithelial
- Subendothelial Ig G, Ig M, C_3, C_4, C_{3-9}

Hypo complimentemia

- ↓ C3, normal C4
- DPGN with subepithelial humps

Increased

- ASO
- Anti–DNA se
- Antihyaluronidase Ab

Prognosis

Good in children, worst in elderly

Hypocomplementemia

- PSGN
- MPGN
- Lupus
- Cryoglobulinemia
- Endocarditis
- In PSGN serum complement is transiently decreased
  - It returns to normal with in 6–8 weeks.

Normal complement

- **Anti-GBM disease**
  - Good-Pasteur syndrome
- **Pauci-immune glomerulonephritis**
  - Wegener's granulomatosis
  - Microscopic polyangitis

- **Immune complex mediated**
  - IgA nephropathy
  - Henoch-Schonlein purpura
  - Fibrillary glomerulonephritis

IgA nephropathy

- Commonest glomerulonephritis worldwide
- Also called as Berger's disease
- Affects children and young adults-males
- Recurrent painless haematuria
- Preceded by URI 1–2 days
- Resolves spontaneously but may have persistent proteinuria

IgA nephropathy–light microscopy

- Mesangioproliferative
- Focal proliferative
- Diffuse proliferative

IF–mesangial deposits of IgA (mainly IgA1)

PSGN	IgA nephropathy
Presents after 7–21 days of URI	2–4 days
C 3 level decreased	Normal
IgA level normal	Increased
Not recurrent	Recurrence
ASO titer increased	Normal

Causes of recurrent hematuria

- Alports syndrome
- IgA nephropathy
- Thin BM disease
  - Urolithiasis
  - Hypercalciuria

Membranous GN

Microscopy

- Light → Diffuse thickening of GBM
- Electron → Subepithelial deposits
- Immuno → IgG and C3 granular deposits

MCC of NS in Adults–30% of NS

- Membranous GN

Causes

Infections

- Hepatitis B
- Hepatitis C
- Schistosomiasis
- Malaria

Malignancy

- Solid tumors-breast, colon, lung, stomach, kidney, esophagus, neuroblastoma **Not with lymphoproliferative ca**

Rheumatological

- SLE
- RA
- Sjogrens

Drugs

- Gold
- Mercury
- Penicillamine
- NSAIDS
- probenecid

Renal Vein Thrombosis

MGN has highest reported incidence of Renal vein thrombosis, PE, DVT
Other causes are

- MPGN
- Amyloidosis
- Lupus nephritis

Clinical Features

- Flank pain
- Tenderness
- Hematuria
- Rapid decline in renal functions
- Proteinuria

Endothelial Damage

- Homocystinemia
- Endovascular intervention
- Surgery

Venous Stasis

- Dehydration
- Retroperitoneal fibrosis
- Abdominal neoplasm

Hyper Coagulable state

- APL Ab syndrome
- NS–MGN
- Protein C, S AT deficiency
- Factor V Leiden
- OCP
- Disseminated Malignancy

Rapidly Progressing GN

- GN which progress to renal failure rapidly within weeks.
- This clinical syndrome matches with the pathological finding of crescents in > 70% of the glomeruli.

Causes of RPGN

Type 1 (Anti-GBM antibody)	Type 2 (Immune complex)	Type 3 (pauci-immune)
• Idiopathic Anti-GBM • Goodpasteur syndrome	• Idiopathic • Acute PSGN • Lupus nephritis • HSP • IgA nephropathy • MPGN • Cryoglobulinemia • Postinfectious Glomerulonephritis	• Idiopathic • ANCA-small vessel vasculitis – Wegener's Glomerulnephritis – Microscopic polyangitis

Good pasture's syndrome

- Antibodies against α 3 chain of collagen IV
- Collagen IV is found in BM of kidney and alveoli
- Hematuria and hematemisis
- Anti GBM Ab positive
- RPGN

Light microscope

- DPGN
- Crescents

IF

- Linear deposits

MPGN

Biopsy

- Mesangial proliferation
- BM thickening
- Splitting of BM- **double contour/tram-track appearance**
- Electron microscopy
  - Type I: Subendothelial and mesangial deposits
  - Type II: Dense deposits in BM (dense deposit disease)

MPGN has high recurrence in transplant kidneys

- Splitting of BM-MPGN

GN in HIV are

- FSGS
- DPGN
- Mesangioproliferative GN
- MPGN
- Membranous GN

Most common and characteristic is FSGS

- The type of FSGS in HIV Associated Nephropathy is a **collapsing GN**
- Biopsy shows
  - Swelling of epithelial cells
  - Collapse of glomorular tuft

- TIN
- Cystic dilation of renal tubules

Clinical course is aggressive

Lupus Nephritis

- Lupus nephritis 30–50%
- Most serious manifestation
- **Nephrits and infections are most common cause of death in first decade of disease**
- Urine analysis is needed for all patients
- Renal biopsy useful for planning treatment

Classifiaction Lupus Nephritis

CLASS I	Minimal meangial LN
CLASS II	Mesangial proliferative LN
CLASS III	**Focal LN**, involving 50% of glomeruli • Subendothelial deposits A-Active–Proliferative C-Chronic–Sclerosing
CLASS IV	**Diffuse LN**, involving > 50% of glomeruli • Subendothelial deposits • WIRE LOOP lesions +
CLASS V	**Membranous LN** • Subepithelial deposits
CLASS VI	**Advanced sclerosed** • > 90% of glomeruli are sclerosed

LN-Treatment

- CLASS I, II, VI: Treatment not recommended
- CLASS III, IV: Aggressive immunosupression
  - High dose steroids + cyclophospamide/mycophenolate
- CLASS IV G with crescentic glomeruli–worst prognosis
  - High dose cyclophosphamide or mycophenolate
- CLASS V: Usually co exist with CLASS III/IV but may exist as isolated lesion
  - Alternate steroids + cyclophosphamide

LN RECURS in 10% of transplanted kidneys

- CLASS I: No treatment
- CLASS II: No treatment
- CLASS III: High dose steroids + CP/Myco
- CLASS IV: High dose steroids + CP/Myco
- CLASS V: Alternate day steroids + CPM
- CLASS VI: No treatment

Acute kidney injury

The most common cause of AKI-pre-renal.

Prerenal	• Hypovolemia • Decreased cardiac output • Decreased effective circulating volume
	– CCF – Liver failure • Impaired renal autoregulation – NSAIDS – ACE-I/ARB – Cyclosporine
Intrinsic	• **Glomerular**–acute GN • **Tubules and interstitium** – Ischemia – Sepsis/infection – Nephrotoxins
	Exogenous: Contrasts, Aminoglycosides, Cisplatin, Amphotericin-B **Endogenous**: Hemolysis, Rhabdomyolysis, Intratubular crystals, Myeloma
	• **Vascular**: Vasculitis, malignant HT, TTP-HUS
Postrenal	Bladder outlet obstruction

Exogenous	Endogenous
Contrasts	Hemolysis
Aminoglycosides	Rhabdomyolysis
Cisplatin	Intratubular crystals
Amphotericin-B	Myeloma

FeNa = U.Na/P.Na × P.Cr/U.Cr

- In pre-renal AKI < 1
- In intrinsic renal AKI > 1
- In pre renal/hypovolemia due to low tubular flow rate, there is increased recycling of urea. So the urea elevation is disproportionate to that of creatinine (i.e.)
- S.BUN/S.Cr > 20 in prerenal
  < 10 in renal

Indices	Prerenal	Renal
FeNa	< 1	1
U.Na	< 10	20
U.Cr/P.Cr	40	< 20
Urine osmolality	500	< 300
Sp.Gravity	> 1.020	1.010
P.BUN/P.Cr	20	< 10
Sediments	Hyaline cast	Muddy brown Granular cast

- **Hypocalcemia** is a feature of AKI of some specific causes like
  - Hemolysis
  - Rhabdomyolysis
  - Tumor lysis syndrome

Biochemical Findings of AKI

- Uremia
- Hyponatremia

- Hyperkalemia
- Hyperphosphatemia
- Hypocalcemia
- Acidosis
- Anemia and bleeding

Tumor Lysis Syndrome

The AKI in TLS is due to uric acid nephropathy.

Occurs in

- Burkitt's lymphoma
- ALL
- CLL
- Solid tumors (rare)

May occur spontaneously but usually after Rx (1- 5 days after)

Biochemical Findings

- Hyperuricemia
- Hyperkalemia
- Hyperphosphatemia
- Hypocalcemia
- ↑ LDH

Rx

- Allopurinol
- Rasburicase (recombinant urate oxidase)
- Alkalinization of urine
- Aggressive hydration

Noval Markers of Kidney Injury

- KIM–1 → kidney injury molecule–1
- NGAL → Neutrophil geratinaseassosiant
- B2 microglobulin
- α1 microglobulin
- Retinol binding protein
- Cystatin–C
- Micro albumin
- Clusterin
- IL–18
- Osteopontin

NKF K/DOQ1 guidelines classification

GFR ml/min/1.73	Stage
0 (risk factors)	0
1 (other evidence of damage)	≥ 90
2	60–90
3	30–59
4	15–29
5	< 15

The formulas for calculation of GFR

- Cockcroft–Gault formula
- MDRD formula

Cockcroft–Gault formula

$$Cr.Cl = \frac{(140-Age) \times (body\ weight) \times 0.85\ for\ women}{72 \times P.Cr}$$

The fluid and electrolyte imbalance in CKD includes

- Acidosis
- Hyponatremia
- Hyperkalemia
- Hypocalcemia
- Hyperphosphatemia

Hypokalemia

Is rare in CKD, may occur due to

- Marked reduction in dietary intake
- Diuretic excess
- GI loss
- Fanconi's syndrome
- RTA
- TIN

Neuromuscular Disorders in CKD

- Sleep disorders
- Fatigue, lethargy
- Asterixis
- Myopathy, irritability
- Peripheral neuropathy
- Restless leg syndrome
- Myoclonus
- Seizure
- Come
- Dialysis disequilibrium syndrome

Bone disease in CKD

High bone turnover	Low bone turnover
↑ PTH	↓ PTH
Osteitis fibrosa cystica	Adynamic bone disease
Brown's tumor	Osteomalacia
Rugger jersey spine	

Calciphylaxis (Uremic Arteriolopathy)

- Due to vascular occlusion by calcium deposition in arterioles.
- It is herald by livido reticularis
- It causes avascular necrosis in legs, thighs, abdomen, breasts, etc.

Rx of secondary hyperparathyroidism

Phosphate Binders

Calcium containing

- Calcium acetate
- Calcium carbonate

Disadvantages

- Causes Hypercalcemia
- Suppress PTH to such a extent to cause adynamic bone disease.

Noncalcium containing

- Sevalamer
- Lanthanum

Calcitriol analogues–Paricalcitol. Useful for PTH suppression without hypercalcemia

Indications for Dialysis

- Uremic symptoms
- Hyperkalemia
- Volume overload
- Acidosis
- Bleeding diathesis
- GFR < 10 ml/min/1.73 m^2
- Peripheral neuropathy
- Pericarditis

Renal Tubular Acidosis

- Type I: Distal (Selective)
- Type II: Proximal
- Tpe IV: Distal (Non Selective)

Type I	Type II RTA	Type IV
Inability of distal nephron to acidify urine (urine pH > 5.5)	Proximal tubular dysfunction	The most common form Characterized by **hyperkalemia**
Causes . Congenital Acquired–amphotericin B Ifosfomaide	Maybe inherited or acquired • **fanconi's synd** • Cystinosis • Tyrosinuria • Galactosemia	
Associated with hypokalemia, Hypocitrateuria, hypercalcuria-**nephrocalcinosis** Rickets, osteomalacia due to ca 2$^+$ loss	• Heriditary fructose intolerance • GSD type I • Lowe's syndrome • Acetozolamide • Topiramate	**Causes** Hyperaldosteronism Obstructive nephropathy Drugs-amiloride, spironolactone Renal transplant rejection

- Hypokalemia is common to both proximal (type II) and distal (type I) RTA.
- Hypercalciuria is a common feature between type I and II
- But in type I since the proximal tube function is intact it will lead to hypocitraturia.
- Hypercalciuria + Hypocitraturia promotes stone formation

NEUROLOGY

Headache

Migrane

Diagnostic criteria for migrane

Headache lasting for 4–72 hrs with

At least 2 of the following

- Unilateral pain
- Throbbing pain
- Aggravated on movements
- Moderate to severe

One of the following

- Nausea/vomiting
- Photophobia/phonophobia

More common in **females**

Two types

- Migrane with aura: Classical migrane
- Migrane without aura: Common migrane

Most common aura associated with migrane is **vision disturbance**

Focal neurological symptoms associated with migrane

- Parasthesia of face and hands
- Weakness
- Aphasia/dysphasia
- Mild confusion

Types of migrane

- **Ophthalmic migrane:** Partial 3rd and 4th N palsy
- **Retinal migrane**: Photophobia, mono-ocular altitudinal defects, loss of vision
- **Basilar migrane**: Vertigo, staggering, dysarthria
- **Hemiplegic migrane**: Autosomal dominant

Treatment-migrane

Drugs in acute attack

- NSAIDS, caffeine
- 5HT1 agonists–Triptans (selective)
- 5HT1 agonists–Ergot (nonselective)
- Dopamine antagonists (adjuncts)

Drugs for prophylaxis

- Pizotifen
- β blockers
- TCA
- Anticonvulsants–valproate, Gaba P, topiramate
- Methysergide
- Flunarazine
- Verapamil–no convincing evidence
- Nimodipine, Clonidine–No effect

Cluster Headache

- Occurs in clusters, which lasts for 6–12 weeks of daily headache
- Each Cluster is followed by a asymptomatic period of years
- More common in young males (5:1)
- Characterized by
  - Intense throbbing pain
  - Periorbital
  - Frequently nocturnal (> 50%)
  - Makes patient restless (migranept quiet)
  - Associated with vasomotor phenomenon–Nasal block, rhinorrhea, conjunctival congestion

SUNCT/SUNA

SUNCT

Shortlasting Unilateral Neuralgiform headache Conjunctival injection and Tearing

SUNA

- Shortlasting
- Unilateral
- Neuralgiform headache
- Autonomic features
  - Stabbing, sharp
  - Periorbital
  - Lasting for 5–240 seconds
  - 3–200 episodes/day
  - Associated with Conj congestion or autonomic symptoms.

Seizures

- Grand mal–Generalised tonic clonic
- Petit mal–absence

Classification of Seizure

Old Classification

- **Partial seizure**
  - Simple partial
  - Complex partial
  - Secondary generalization
- **Primary generalized seizure**
  - Absence
  - Tonic clonic
  - Tonic
  - Clonic
  - Atonic
  - Myoclonic
- **Unclassified**
  - Neonatal seizure
  - Infantile spasm

ILAE classification

- **Focal seizure**
  - Without dyscognitivesym
  - With dyscognitivesymp
  - Describe the generalized seizure
- **Generalized seizure**
  - Absense (typical, atypical)
  - Tonic clonic
  - Tonic
  - Clonic
  - Atonic
  - Myoclonic
- **Unclear**
  - Epileptic spasm

Absence Seizure

- Main seizure type in childhood 4–8 yrs
- Sudden brief lapses in consciousness without loss of postural control.
- Described as 'day dreaming'–by parents. 'poor school performance'–by teachers
- No post ictal confusion
- **Hyperventilation provokes**
- EEG–3 Hz spike wave pattern

Atypical Absence Seizure

- Longer duration
- More prominent motor signs
- EEG < 2.5 Hz frequency

3 Hz spike–wave pattern

Juvenile Myoclonic Epilepsy

- Older children and young adults
- Myoclonic jerks on awakening in morning
- Tonic clonic. Absence seizures can also occur
- Family H/O myoclonic jerks
- EEG 4–6 Hz spike pattern
- Rx–**sodium valproate**
- Occurs with **SSPE**

Drugs Used in Status Epilepticus

- Lorazepam/diazepam
- Phenytoin/fosphenytoin
- Phenobarbitone
- Midazolam, propofol, thiopentone
- Valproate instead of phenytoin in pts who are on valproate.

Treatment of Seizures

	Primary generalized, tonic, clonic, GTCS	Partial seizure	Absence seizure	Atypical absence, myoclonic, atonic
First line	Valproic acid lamotrigine	Carbamazepine phenytoin lamotrigine valproic acid	Ethosuximide	Valproic acid
Alternative	Phenytoin Carbamazepine Tropiramide Zonisamide Felbamate Primidone Phenobarbital	Topiramate Lenetiracetam Tiagabine Zonisamide Gabapentin Primidone Phenobarbital	Valproic acid lamotrigine clonazepam	Lamotrigine Topiramate Clonazepam

Special Cases:

- Infantile spasms: Vigabatrin;
- Febrile seizures: Diazepam (per rectal)
- Status epilepticus: Clonazepam (i.v.);
- Epilepsy in pregnancy: Phenobarbitone
- Seizures in eclampsia: Magnesium sulphate

Other MCQ oriented points from seizure

- Psychogenic nonepileptic convulsion is a new term for pseudoseizure
- Posttraumatic seizure occurs usually at 1–3 months after trauma.
- Pseudolymphoma is caused by phenytoin

Lennox Gastaut syndrome

Triad of

- Multiple seizure types
- Impaired cognitive functions
- < 3 Hz spike and wave

Rufinamide is the drug used in Lennox-Gestaut syndrome.

Mesial temporal lobe epilepsy syndrome (MTLE)

- Focal seizure with dyscognitive features
- Refractive to medical Rx
- Effective surgical management
- MRI shows hippocampal sclerosis

Intracranial bleed

CHRONIC SDH

- Common in elderly/clotting defects
- Injury will be trivial
- Headache, slow thinking, change in personality, seizure or mild hemiparesis is the usual presentation.
- DD–SOL brain, drug intoxication, stroke, and depression

Investigations

- CT with contrast-**hypernormal CT scan**

Rx

- Surgical evacuation with removal of the fibrous membrane.

Acute SDH

It is common in
- Elderly
- Alcoholics
- Boxers
- Patients on anticoagulants/clotting defects
- Trauma maybe minor or whiplash injury is enough

Presents as

- Lucid interval (1/3rd of cases). But is very characteristic of EDH
- Headache
- Slightly enlarged pupil
- Stupor, coma

Rx

- Burr drainage or
- Emergency craniotomy

SDH: Rupture of bridging veins
EDH: Rupture of middle meningeal artery
SDH: Lacunar shape/concave shape
EDH: Biconvex shaped/lenticular shape

Sub dural hematoma	Epi dural hematoma
• Lucid interval less characteristic • Injury minor • Usually not associated with skull bone # • Bleeding from veins • Imaging–lacunar shape	• Lucid interval more characteristic • Injury major • Usually associated with skull bone # • Bleeding from middle meningeal A • Lenticular shaped

Diffuse Axonal Injury

- Traumatic sheering force due to rapid acceleration or deceleration
- Rotational forces are more involved than linear forces
- Injury to the region where there is difference in density is more common. Eg: grey-white junction
- Presents as extended coma or vegetative state following trauma.

Features of base of skull fracture

- CSF leakage–rhinorrhea
- Pneumocephalus
- Cavernous carotid fistula
- Hemotymphanum
- Battle sign (echymosis over mastoid)
- Racoon sign (periorbital echymosis)

Subarachnoid Hemorrhage

- MCC for SAH–trauma
- MCC for non-traumatic SAH–rupture of Berry aneurysm
- III N palsy–posterior communicating artery aneurysm

- VI N palsy–cavernous sinus aneurysm
- II N palsy–ophthalmic artery aneurysm
- Retro orbital pain–MCA aneurysm
- Occipital/neck pain–PICA/AICA aneurysm

Points to remember

- III N palsy due to compression of aneurysm–early pupil involvement
- Due to DM neuropathy–late pupil involvement (Pupillary sparing)

85% of aneurysms–anterior circulation

15% of aneurysms–posterior circulation

3 common locations

- Terminal ICA
- MCA bifurcation
- Top of basilar artery

Risk of rupture is high in

- > 7 mm (< 10 mm 0.1% > 10 mm 1%)
- Top of basilar, origin of post communicating artery
- Previously ruptured aneurysm.

Headache and Neck Stiffness

- With fever–meningitis
- Without fever–SAH

Symptoms of SAH

- Headache-excruciating. 'worst headache of my life'
- Transient LOC
- Neck stiffness
- Nausea, vomiting
- Focal deficits (rare)

ICA, post communicating A–3rd N palsy

MCA bifurcation, anti communicating A– hemiparesis, aphasia, abulia

2 scoring system for SAH

- Hunt and Hess scale

Based on clinical presentation

- WFNS (world federation of neurological society) scale

Based on GCS and motor involvement

Causes for Late Neurological Deterioration in SAH

Vasospasm

MCC is vasospasm: It is due to the direct effect of clotted blood and breakdown products on arteries in subarachanoid space.

Presents as

- Appears 4–14 days after SAH

- Acute fluctuating focal deficits
- Decreased mental status.

Re-rupture

- First month 30%, peaks in 7 days

Hydrocephalus

- Progressive abulia, incontinence, gait difficulty

Hyponatremia

- Within 2 weeks after SAH
- Hypovolumic hyponatremia
- Mediated by ANP, BNP
- Cerebral salt wasting syndrome
- Spontaneous remission.

Stroke

UMN paralysis	LMN paralysis
Muscles affected in groups and not individually	Individual muscles maybe affected
Power decreased	Very much decreased
Atrophy slight	Marked atrophy up to 70%
Clasp knife Spasticity (hypertonia)	**Flaccidity (hypotonia)**
Superficial reflexes lost	Lost
Exaggerated tendon reflexes	**Hypotonia and loss of tendon reflexes**
Clonus maybe present	Absent
Babinski sign + (extensor plantar reflex)	**Babinski sign –ve**
Fasciculations absent	**Present**
Nerve conduction study normal	**Abnormal; denervation potential in EMG**

Lenticulostriate branch of MCA supplies

- Putamen, Globus pallidus
- Post limb of IC, Caudate nucleus.

Causes for ICH

- HT (MCC)
- Trauma
- Cerebral amyloid angiopathy

Risks

- Alcohol consumption
- Cocaine
- Methamphetamine
- Phenylpraopanolamine

Recombinant tissue plasminogen activator is used for IV thrombolysis in acute ischemic stroke.

Indications of tPA	C/I of tPA
• Clinical diagnosis of stroke • Onset ≤ 3 hrs • CT–no hemorrhage, no edema > 1/3 of MCA territory	• BP > 185/100 • Platelets < 1 lakh, HCT < 25% • Blood sugar < 50 or > 400 mg%
• Age ≥ 18 yrs • Consent	• Minor stroke • Rapidly improving • coma/stupor • Recent MI • GI bleed • Heparin with in 2 days, prolonged PTT, ↑ INR • Prior stroke 3 months, prior ICH • Major surgery–2 weeks

Administration

- Dose 0.9 mg/kg (max 90 mg)
- 10% as bolus, 90% over 1 hour
- If any decline in neurological status. Stop infusion, give cryoprecipitate, reimage

Time

- IV thrombolysis: 3 hrs
- Endovascular thrombolysis: 6 hrs
- Mechanical thrombolectomy: 8 hrs

Prourokinase-endovascular Thrombolysis

Platelet inhibition

Aspirin is the only drug that has been proved for acute management of stroke.

Abciximab should be avoided.

Hollenhorst Plaques-Retina show cholesterol crystals.

Stroke

- Ischemic–85%
- Hemorrhagic–15%

Ischemic

- Thrombolic–25%
- Embolic–75%

Remember these ...

Most common cause

- *Of stroke–embolic*
- *Of hemorrhage–intracerebral hemorrhage*
- *Of ICH–hypertension*
- *Of SAH–trauma*
- *Of spontaneous SAH–aneurysm rupture*
- *Site of ICH–putamen (basal ganglia)*

Lobar Function

Frontal	Temporal		Parietal		Occipital
Personality • Emotional control	**Dominant** • Auditory perception	**Nondominant** • Auditory perception	**Dominant** • Language • Calculation	**Nondominant** • Spatial orientation	• Visual processing
• Social behavior • Contralateral motor control • Language • Micturition • Language • Calculation • Spatial orientation • Constructional skills	• Language • Verbal memory • Smell • Balance	• Melody/pitch perception • Nonverbal memory • Smell • Balance		• Constructional skills	

Aphasia

- Categorical hemisphere–dominant hemisphere
- Representational hemisphere–nondominant hemisphere

Brocos area

- Inferior frontal gyrus of dominant lobe
- Area 44, 45

Wernicke's area

- Posterior temporal parietal region of dominant lobe
- Post part of area 22
- It includes angular gyrus and supra-marginal gyrus

Global: All modalities affected

Brocas: Only comprehension is spared

Sensory: Only fluency is spared

Conduction: Only repetition is affected

Transcortical: Repetition is spared in addition

	Comprehension	Fluency	Repetition	Naming, Reading, Writing
Global	—	—	—	—
Brocas	+	—	—	—
Wernicke's	—	+	—	—
Conduction	+	+	—	+
Transcortical motor	+	—	+	—

Other lesion in parietal lobe

- Supramarginalgyrus–gerstman'ssynd
- Angular gyrus–word blindness (dyslexia)

ACA territory

- Paralysis of leg–motor area
- Weakness of arm–corona radiata

- Bladder incontinence
  - Loss of social control- sup frontal gyrus
  - Loss of volitional control- paracentral lobule
- **Gagenhalten** paratonic rigidity–medial surface of frontal lobe
- Abulia–subcallosum
- Dyspraxia of left limb–corpus callosum

PCA involvement

- Anton's synd
- Balints synd
- cortical blindness
- dyslexia without dysgraphia
- Simultagnosia
- Prosagnosia
- Memory defect-Hippocampal lesion

ABCD-SPM

- Perforating branches (P2 synd)
  - Thalamic synd (Dejerine roussy)
    - Hemianaesthsia
    - Pain dysaesthesia
    - Choreathetosis
    - Intentional tremor

Thalamoperforate Synd

- Claudes synd–IL 3 N + cerebellar ataxia
- Webers synd–IL 3 N + CL hemiplegia
- Vertical gaze palsy–INC + RIMLF in midbrain
- Hemiballismus –subthalamic N

Lacunar infarct

- Lacunar infarct are due to lipohyalinosis of penetrating arteries, they manifest as
- **Pure motor hemiplegia-** internal capsule
- **Pure sensory**–ventral thalamus
- **Pure motor + dysarthria**–pons ventral
- **Clumsiness of hand-** pons ventral
- **Ataxia**–midbrain pons
- **Pseudobulbar palsy**–corticobulbar tract

Brainstem syndromes

Wallenberg syndrome–Lateral medullary syndrome

Structures involved ipsilateral	Symptoms
Descending tract of V nerve	Numbness, loss of Pain over face
Vestibular N	Vertigo, Nystagmus
Restiform body	Ataxia
Descending sympathetic tract	Horner's syndrome
IX and X nerve N	Dysphagia, hoarseness of voice
Nucleus tractussolitarius	Loss of taste
Cuneate and gracilius N	Numbness of arm, trunk and legs

Contralateral

- Decreased pain and temp over body- spinothalamic tract
- SPARED
  - 12th N
  - Pyramids
  - Medial leminiscus

Lateral medullary syndrome is due to occlusion of

- PICA
- Vertebral artery
- Lateral medullary arteries (partial synd)

Most common of these are vertebral artery occlusion (80% of cases)

Medial medullary syndrome

Is due to occlusion of vertebral arteries, lower basilar arteries or anterior spinal arteries.
The features are

Ipsilateral

- Paralysis and atrophy of tongue–Hypoglossal N

Contralateral

- Paralysis of body–Pyramids
- Loss of touch and vibration–Medial Leminiscus.

Features of Pontine Hemorrhage

- Acute onset
- Unconscious
- Pinpoint pupil–reacting to light
- Hyper pyrexia
- Quadreparesis
- Decerebrate rigidity

Brain Stem Syndromes

Midbrain

- Benedicts syndrome: IL 3rd N+CL hemiplegia+ CL tremor (Red nucleus)
- Weber's syndrome: IL 3rd+CL tremor
- Claudes syndrome: IL 3rd N+CL ataxia (cerebellar peduncle)

PONS

- Millard Gubler: IL 7th N
  - CL hemiplegia
- Fovilles: IL 6th N
  - IL 7th N
  - CL hemiplegia
- Mobius syndrome–congenital absence of 6th + 7th N nucleus. Teratogenic side effect of misoprostol.
- Melkerson Rosanthal syndrome–triad of
  - Facial edema
  - Fissured tongue
  - Facial palsy

Causes of B/L facial palsy

- GBS
- Leprosy
- Leukemia
- Lymes disease
- B/L Bells palsy
- Sarcoidosis

Mnemonic: GuLLLianBarrie Syndrome

CNS Infections

Normal CSF plasma glucose is 40–70 mg%. Varies according to blood sugar level. It is about 60% of plasma glucose i.e. CSF/S.glucose = 0.6

Normal Values of CSF

- Pressure: 90–180 cm of water
- Glucose: 40–70 mg%
- Protein: 15–45 mg%
- LDH < 20 U/L
- Chloride: 115–130 meq/L
- WBC: < 5 cells/ml
- DC: 40–80% lymphocytes
  - 15–45% monocytes
  - 0–6% polymorphs
- Epidemics are caused by meningococcus–B
- The tetravalent vaccination against meningococci contains only antigens of A, C, W-135, Y strain
- Most common organism causing meningitis is S.Pneumoniae
- 2nd most common–N.meningitis
- MCC in neonates–Group B streptococci
- E.coli

CSF in Pyogenic Meningitis

- Appearance–cloudy
- Pressure - > 180 cm water
- Proteins - > 45 mg%
- Glucose - < 40 mg%
- Chloride–decreased
- Cells–polymorphs
- Gram stain–positive for organisms

Complications

- Hydrocephalus
- Cranial N involvement
- Seizure
- Subdural effusion
- Subdural pyema
- Cerebral herniation
- Central D I

CT Appearance of TBM

- Exudates in basal cisterns–most characteristic
- Calcification of meninges
- Ventriculitis

CSF findings	TBM	Viral .M
Appearance	Slightly opaque	Clear
Pressure	Increased	Normal
Proteins	Increased	Moderate to N
Glucose	N or decreased	Normal
Chloride	Markedly decreased	Normal
Cells	Lymphocytes	lymphocytes

- Diffuse meningeal enhancement
- Enhancement in temporo frontal lobes
- Multiple hemorrhagic infarcts
- Hemorrhagic infarcts in B/L Thalamus

MRI Findings in Meningitis

- Pyogenic meningitis–diffuse meningeal enhancement with gadolinium contrast
- HSV meningitis–high signal intensity in temporal, orbito frontal region (in T2 weighed FLAIR imaging)
- VZV encephalitis–multi focal ischemic hemorrhagic infarction.
- Japanese Encephalitis–B/L thalamic Hemorrhagic infarct

Viral meningitis

- Enterovirus
  - Coxsakie
  - ECHO
  - Enterovirus(68–71)
- HSV 2
- Arthopode borne virus
- HIV

Viral encephalitis

- Herpes
  - HSV–1
  - VZV
  - EBV
- Arbovirus
  - La crosse
  - WNV
  - St Louis
- Neurocysticercosis MC parasite in CNC
- MC presentation–seizure
- MC site–Brain parenchyma

Rx

- Albendazole, Flubendazole and
- Praziquantal (not niclosamide)

Spinal Cord Diseases

Fasciculation are characteristic of LMN lesions. Active degeneration of anterior horn cells causes fasciculation.

- MND
- Syringomyelia
- Cervical spondylosis
- Primary muscular atrophy
- Recovery phase of poliomyelitis
- OPC poisoning

Fasciculations are absent in myopathies except

- Thyrotoxic myopathy
- Carcinomatous myopathy

Jaw Jerk

- Afferent–5th N
- Efferent–5th N
- Centre–Pons

Lesion should be above the level of Pons to cause a exaggerated jaw jerk

Spinal Shock Features

- Complete paralysis
- Flaccidity
- Loss of autonomic control
- **Flaccid sphincters**
- Paralytic ileus
- Urinary retention with overflow incontinence
- Absent genital reflexes

Duration–1–6 weeks

Syringomyelia Features

- Symmetric involvement
- 50% associated with Chiari type 1 malformation
- Dissociated sensory loss **at the level of lesion–**due to destruction of crossing fibres of spinothalamic tract
- Small muscle wasting - due to AHC destruction
- Fasciculation–due to AHC destruction
- UMN signs below the level of lesion–CST involvement
- Dissociated sensory loss **below the level of lesion–**spinothalamic tract involvement
- With Chiari malformations.shunting of hydrocephalus should be done first.

Brown Sequard syndrome

Due to hemi transaction of spinal cord

- LMN lesion at the level of lesion
- A zone of hyperesthesia at the level of lesion
- IL pyramidal tract
- IL posterior column
- CL spinothalamic tract

Motor Neuron Disease

- Primary lateral sclerosis–corticospinal tract only
- Progressive muscular dystrophy–anterior horn cells only
- Amyotrophic lateral sclerosis–AHC + CST
- Pseudobulbar palsy–UMN for cranial nerves
- Bulbar palsy–LMN for cranial nerves

Both AHC and CST involvement is a feature of ALS

Presentation of ALS

- Fasciculations
- Small muscle wasting of hands
- Hyper reflexia
- Spasticity of legs
- No sensory involvement

Features of Fredrich's Ataxia

- Loss of position and vibration–post column
- Ataxia - spinocerebellar
- Babinski +ve - CST
- Loss of tendon reflexes - dorsal root ganglia

Associated Features

- Cardiomyopathy
- DM
- Kyphoscoliosis, pescavus
- Optic atrophy
- Dementia

B 12 deficiency causes demyelination

So myelinated tracts are affected.

- Post column
- CST
- Peripheral nerves

TabesDorsalis

Structures Involved

- Dorsal root ganglia
- Posterior column
- Posterior root

Clinical Features

- Hypotonia
- Areflexia
- Bladder involvement
- Analgesia
- Joint insensitivity–Charcot joint
- Lightening pain
- Ataxia (pure sensory)
- Argyl Robertson pupil–neurosyphilis

Extrapyramidal Disorders

Parkinson's Disease - 4 cardinal features:

- **Parkinson's tremor**
  - Rest tremors
  - Absent during action
  - Slow frequency (4–7Hz)
  - Pill rolling tremors in some
- **Rigidity**
  - Lead pipe or cog wheel rigidity
- **Bradykinesia**
  - Mask like face, drooling of saliva, reduced blinking, reduced arm swing
  - Small and spidery hand writing (micrographia),
- **Postural instability**
  - **Postural reflexes lost**
  - Festinating gait (rapid small steps) difficulty in stopping suddenly and impaired balance on turning
- **Other Features**
  - Deep tendon reflexes normal
  - Babinski sign negative (plantor reflex - flexor)
  - Normal intelligence

Dementia

Treatable Causes

- Hypothyroidism
- Thiamine deficiency
- Vit B12 deficiency
- NPH
- SDH
- Chronic infection
- Brain tumors
- Drug intoxication
- Alcoholism
- Depression

Subcortical Dementia

- Pick's disease
- Progressive supranuclear palsy
- Parkinsonism
- Huntingtons
- AIDS dementia complex

Features	Subcortical	Cortical
Memory impairment	More severe	Less severe
Depression	More common	Less common
Extrapyramidal	More common	Less common

Pathology of Alzheimer's

- Medial temporal lobe–Entorhinal, perirhinal, hippocampus
- Lateral temporal

- Nucleus basalis of Meynert
- Lewy bodies are features of idiopathic Parkinson's disease

Risk factors	Protective
• Old age • Family H/O • Female • Low education • Aluminum • Mercury • Viruses • Down's syndrome	• Estrogen • NSAID

Etiopathogenesis of Alzheimer's

- Tau proteins
- Apolipoprotein E 4
- Preseneline 1 and 2
- Trisomy 21
  - Picks disease is a tau pathy

Contents of

- N.F tangles–hyper phosphorylated tau
- Senile plaques–β amyloid
- Lewy bodies–ubiquitin, α–synuclein

NPH is a triad of

- Gait ataxia
- Urinary incontinence
- Dementia

Features of progressive supra nuclear palsy (Steel Richardson syndrome)

- Frequent falls
- Hyper extended neck
- Vertical gaze palsy
- Axial rigidity
- Postural imbalance
- Dysarthria
- Mental changes–Dementia

Peripheral Neuropathy

- Proximal muscle weakness is a feature of myopathy
- Peripheral neuropathy causes distal muscle weakness

Peripheral Neuropathy

- **Wallarian degeneration–dying forward**
  - Proximal to distal
  - *For example*: Focal mononeuropathies (trauma)

- **Axonal degeneration–dying back**
  - Distal to proximal
  - *For example*: Metabolic causes
- Symmetrical degeneration–due to demyelination
  - *For example*: Immune, inflammatory mediators (GBS)

Examples for metabolic neuropathy

- Thiamine deficiency
- Pyridoxine deficiency
- Vit E
- Porphyria
- Arsenic
- Uremia
- Alcoholic
- Diabetic
- Amyloidosis

Motor	Sensory	Mixed
• ALS • Poliomyelitis • Lead • Dapsone • Porphyria • GBS • Eaton Lambert	• Cisplatin • Taxol • Pyridoxine • B12 deficiency • Paraneoplasm • Sjogrens	• DM • Uremia • Arsenic • Alcohol • OPC • Diptheria • AIDS • Leprosy

Factors reducing the possibility of GBS

- Asymmetric weakness
- Initial bladder/bowel symptom
- Severe symptoms at initiation of disease
- 50 mononuclear cells/cu.mm in CSF
- Well demarcated sensory level
- Others
  - Fever associated
  - Residual weakness

Hereditary Neuropathies

- Charcot-Marie-Tooth (CMT) disease is the most common type of hereditary neuropathy
- Four types. Most common is CMT 1.CMT 1-atrophy of muscles below knee-**inverted champagne bottle legs**.
- CMT3 is otherwise called as Dejerina ans Sottas.
- CMT4 is autosomal recessive.
- Hereditary neuropathy with liability to pressure palsy-HNPP (tomachulous neuropathy) is AD
- Present as recurrent episodes of focal entrapment neuropathy with attacks of numbness and weakness in peroneal, ulnar, radial, and median nerves (in descending order) or in brachial plexus distribution
- Tomaculae are sausage-shaped bodies that indicate segmental demyelination

Myasthenia Gravis

- Autoimmune destruction of Acetylcholine receptors (AChR) in post synaptic region
- Decreased number of AChRs

Antibodies

2 types of antibodies

- Anti AChR–antibodies
- Anti MUSK antibodies (muscle specific Kinase)

MUSK helps in arrangement of AChR

Anti MUSK ab positive patients have

- Prominent bulbar involvement
- Aggressive disease, respiratory paralysis
- Proximal muscle weakness

Anti MUSK is negative in MG limited to ocular muscles.

Clinical Features

- Women > men
- Increasing weakness on repeated use
- Distribution of weakness
  - Lids and ocular muscles (MC)
  - Facial muscles–snare
  - Tongue muscles–muschy speech
  - Palate, pharynx–dysphagia
- Tendon jerks are preserved

Diagnosis

- Antibodies (Anti AChRab, Anti MUSK ab)
  - **Sensitive and specific**
  - Positive in 85% of MG and 50 % of OMG
- Repetitive nerve stimulation test(RNT)–decremental response
- Single fibre EMG
- Endrophonium test (Tensilon test)
  - Reserved only for patients with negative antibodies and RNT

Associated abnormalities

- Thymic abnormalities–hyperplasia, Thymoma
- Thyroid abnormalities–Hashimoto's, Graves
- Autoimmune diseases–SLE, Rh.Arthritis

Treatment

- Pyridostigmine
- Thymectomy
- Immunosupressants–steroids, Azathioprine
- Plasmaperisis
- IVIg

Thymus and MG

Thymomas are associated with

- Hypogamaglobulinemia
- Pure red cell aplasia

- Graves disease
- Pernicious anemia
- Cushings, SIADH
- Polyglandular autoimmune syndrome II
- Connective tissue disorders

Muscle-like cells (myoid cells) which bear AChRs on their surface may be the autoantigen.

Thymic abnormalities are seen in 75% of MG

- 65 % hyperplasia
- 10% thymomas
- They present as superior mediastinal syndrome

Thymectomy

- Is indicated in all MG patients except
- < 15 yrs or > 55 yrs age
- isolated OMG patients
- Some cases show spontaneous remission following thymectomy

Drugs aggravating MG

- Antibiotics
  - Aminoglycosides
  - Quinolones
  - Macrolides
- Nondepolarising muscle relaxants
- Beta blockers
- Local anaesthetics and related drugs
  - Procaine
  - **Procainamide**
  - Lignocaine
- Quinine derivatives
  - Quinine
  - **Chloroquine**
  - Mefloquine
- Magnesium-**Decreases Ach release**
- Penicillamine **may cause MG**

MG vs LEMS

MG	LEMS
Postsynaptic defect	Presynaptic defect
Ab against AChR	Ab against P/Q type Ca channels
Ocular muscles are involved first	Proximal limb muscles involved first
DTR intact	DTR diminished
No autonomic changes	Autonomic changes
Decremental response to RNT	Incremental response to RNT
Pyridostigmine –DOC	3–4 Diaminopyrimidine (K Ch blocker)
Associated with Thymoma	Associated with small cell Ca lung

HEMATOLOGY

Sites of Hemopoiesis

- **Fetus**
- Ist trimester: Yolk sac
- IInd trimester: Spleen and liver
- IIIrd trimester: Mostly Bone Marrow

Adults

- Up to 20yrs: All bones
- After 20yrs: Flat bones
  - After 20 years red BM gets converted into yellow BM in long bones.

Normal Hematological Parameters

- **Hb:** 14–18 mg/dl
- **Serum iron:** 50–150 mcg/dl
- **Percentage saturation:** 30–50%
- **Serum Ferritin:** 50–200 mcg/L
- **TIBC:** 300–600 mcg/dl
- **HbA2:** 1.5–3.5 % of total Hb
- **HbF:** < 2% of total Hb

RBC indicies		Normal values
Mean corpuscular volume Indicates average size of the RBC (volume)	MCV = (hematocrit x 10)/ (red cell count x 10^6)	90 ± 8 femtolitres (fl)
Mean corpuscular hemoglobin	MCH = (hemoglobin x 10)/ (red cell count x 10^6)	30 ± 3 picograms (pg)
Mean corpuscular HB concentration	MCHC = hemoglobin x10)/ hematocrit, or MCH/MCV	33 ± 2%

The components of the CBC also help in the classification of anemia.

MCV	
Lower than normal **MCV (< 80)**	**Microcytosis**
High MCV values **(> 100)**	**Macrocytosis**
The **MCH and MCHC** reflect defects in hemoglobin synthesis (*hypochromia*)	

Blood smear also reveals variations in cell size (***anisocytosis***) and shape (***poikilocytosis***)
Red cell volume distribution width: The degree of anisocytosis usually correlates with increases in the RDW or the range of cell sizes. Normally 11–14%.

Morphological classification of anemia		
Microcytic hypochromic	**Normocytic normochromic**	**Macrocytic normochromic**
• Iron deficiency anemia • Thalassemia • Sideroblastic anemia • Lead toxicity • +/- anemia of chronic disease	• With high reticulocyte count • With low reticulocyte count (discussed later)	• Vit B12 deficiency • Folate deficiency • Thiamine deficiency

- **Basophilic stippling**: Diffuse fine or coarse blue dots in the red cell -representing RNA residue—especially common in lead poisoning
- **Howell-Jolly bodies**: Dense blue circular inclusions that represent nuclear remnants —their presence implies defective splenic function
- **Nuclei**: Red cells may be released or pushed out of the marrow prematurely before nuclear extrusion—often implies a myelophthisic process or a vigorous narrow response to anemia, usually hemolytic anemia
- **Parasites**: Red cell parasites include malaria and babesia
- **Polychromatophilia**: The red cell cytoplasm has a bluish hue, reflecting the persistence of ribosomes still actively making hemoglobin in a young red cell
- Vital stains are necessary to see precipitated hemoglobin called Heinz bodies.
- **Schistocytes are helmet**: Shaped cells that reflect microangiopathic hemolytic anemia or fragmentation on an artificial heart valve.
- **Echinocytes** are spiculated red cells with the spikes evenly spaced; they can represent an artifact of abnormal drying of the blood smear or reflect changes in stored blood. They also can be seen in **renal failure, Uremia** and malnutrition and are often reversible.
- **Acanthocytes** are spiculated red cells with the spikes irregularly distributed. This process tends to be irreversible and reflects underlying renal disease, abetalipoproteinemia, or splenectomy.
- **Hypersegmented neutrophils**: Hypersegmented neutrophils (multilobed polymorphonuclear leukocytes) are larger than normal neutrophils with five or more segmented nuclear lobes. They are commonly seen with folic acid or vitamin B12 deficiency.

IRON DEFICIENCY ANEMIA

Causes of IDA
• **Increased Demand for Iron** – Rapid growth in infancy or adolescence – Pregnancy – Erythropoietin therapy
• **Increased Iron Loss** – Chronic blood loss – Menses – Acute blood loss – Blood donation – Phlebotomy as treatment for polycythemia vera
• **Decreased Iron Intake or Absorption** – Inadequate diet – Malabsorption from disease (sprue, Crohn's disease) – Malabsorption from surgery (postgastrectomy) – Acute or chronic inflammation

Factors	Enhanced absorption	Reduced absorption
Dietary factors	• Increased heme iron • Increased animal food • Ferrous iron salts	• Decreased heme iron • Decreased animal food • Ferric iron salts
Luminal factors	• Acidic pH • Low molecular weight soluble chelates	• Alkaline pH (Pancreatic secretion) • Insoluble iron complexes
Systemic factors	• Iron deficiency • Increased erythropoiesis • Pregnancy • Hypoxia	• Iron overload • Decreased erythropoiesis • Inflammatory disorders

Stages of Iron Deficiency

	Normal	Negative iron balance	Iron–deficient erythropoiesis	Iron–deficient anemia
Marrow iron stores	1–3+	0–1+	0	0
Serum ferritin (gμ/L)	50–200	<20	<15	<15
TIBC (μg/dL)	300–360	>360	>380	>400
SI (μg/dL)	50–150	NL	<50	<30
Saturation (%)	30–50	NL	<20	<10
Marrow sideroblasts (%)	40–60	NL	<10	<10
RBC protoporphyrin (μg/dL)	30–50	NL	>100	>200
RBC morphology	NL	NL	NL	Microcytic/ hypochromic

Treatment

Oral Iron Preparations

Generic Name	Tablet (Iron content), mg	Elixir (Iron content), mg in 5 ml
Ferrous Sulfate	325 (65) 195 (39)	300 (60) 90 (18)
Extended release	525 (105)	
Ferrous fumarate	325 (107) 195 (39)	100 (35)
Ferrous gluconate	325 (39)	300 (35)
Polysaccharide iron	150 (150) 50 (50)	100 (100)

Typically, the reticulocyte count should begin to increase within **4–7 days after initiation of therapy and peak at 11/2 to 2 weeks.**

Intravenous Iron

It can be given to patients who are unable to tolerate oral iron; whose needs are relatively acute; or who need iron on an ongoing basis, usually due to persistent gastrointestinal blood loss also in patients with erythropoietin therapy in CRF.

Body weight (kg) × 2.3 × (15–patient's hemoglobin, g/dL) + 500 or 1000 mg (for stores)

- Test dose only for dextran compounds
- Very low incidence of anaphylaxis with newer preparations
- Ferric Carboxymaltose–hypophosphatemia.

Red Cell Transfusion

- Transfusion therapy is reserved for individuals who have symptoms of anemia, cardiovascular instability, continued and excessive blood loss from whatever source, and require immediate intervention.

HYPOPROLIFERATIVE ANEMIAS

It can be divided into four categories:

- Chronic inflammation,
- Renal disease,
- Endocrine and nutritional deficiencies (hypometabolic states), and
- Marrow damage

Anemia of Acute and Chronic Inflammation/Infection (the Anemia of Inflammation)

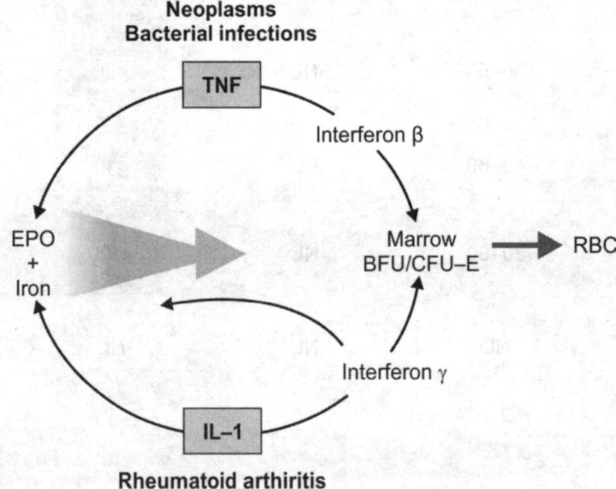

Suppression of erythropoiesis by inflammatory cytokines

- Through the release of tumor necrosis factor (TNF) and interferon (IFN-), neoplasms and bacterial infections suppress erythropoietin (EPO) production and the proliferation of erythroid progenitors [erythroid burst-forming units and erythroid colony-forming units (BFU/CFU-E)].
- The mediators in patients with vasculitis and rheumatoid arthritis include interleukin 1 (IL-1) and IFN-γ. (The red arrows indicate sites of inflammatory cytokine inhibitory effects)

Hepcidin

- Hepcidin, made by the liver, is increased in inflammation and acts to suppress iron absorption and iron release from storage sites.
- In iron deficiency, hepcidin levels are low and iron is much more efficiently absorbed
- Mutations in the genes encoding HFE, TfR2, hemojuvelin and **hepcidin** all lead to decreased hepcidin release and increased iron absorption, resulting in hemochromatosis.

Anemia of Chronic Renal Failure

- Normocytic normochromic, hypoproliferative.
- Anemia is primarily due to a failure to produce adequate amounts of erythropoietin and a reduced red cell survival.
- Normal serum iron, TIBC and ferritin levels.
- Level of anemia correlates with severity of renal failure.
- EPO therapy is the mainstay of treatment.
- Iron must be replenished in these patients to ensure an adequate response to EPO therapy.
- Dialysis has little effect.
- Peritoneal dialysis- improves anemia; hemodialysis- cause an associated iron deficiency anemia.

Endocrine Deficiency States

Testosterone and anabolic steroids augment erythropoiesis; castration and estrogen administration to males decrease erythropoiesis

Anemia in Liver Disease

- Smear may show **spur cells** and stomatocytes from the accumulation of excess cholesterol in the membrane from a deficiency of lecithin-cholesterol acyltransferase.
- **Red cell survival is shortened**, and the production of EPO is inadequate to compensate.
- In alcoholic liver disease, nutritional deficiencies are common and complicate the management.
- Folate deficiency from inadequate intake, as well as iron deficiency from blood loss and inadequate intake, can alter the red cell indices.

The two major forms of treatment of hypoproliferative anemias are transfusions and EPO.

Sideroblastic Anemia

- It is an uncommon form of anemia characterized by the presence of large number of sideroblasts in the bone marrow
- Here there is a defect in incorporating iron into the hemoglobin molecule within the erythrocyte.
- Sideroblasts are erythroid precursors with demonstrable **cytoplasmic iron.**
- Ring sideroblasts are erythroblasts in which there are minimum 5 siderotic granules covering **at least one third** of the circumference of the nucleus.
- Peripheral smear- **dimorphic** picture- mixture of microcytic hypochromic and macrocytic erythrocytes.

	Iron deficiency anemia	Thalassemia	Sideroblastic anemia	Anemia of chronic disease
Smear Microcytic (MCV < 80)	Microcytic hypochromic	Microcytic hypochromic	Microcytic hypochromic	NCNC > Microhypo
S. iron (50–150µg/dl)	Low (< 30)	Normal	Normal	↓(< 50)
TIBC (300–360 µg/dl)	High (> 360)	Normal	Normal	↓(< 300)
Percentage saturation (30–50%)	< 10 (↓)	N or ↑ (30–80)	N or ↑ (30–80)	↓(10–20)
Ferritin (50–200 µg/dl)	< 15 (↓)	↑(50–300)	↑(50–300)	Normal or ↑ (30–200)
Free erythrocyte porphyrin	↑	Normal	↑	↑
Hemoglobin pattern	Normal	Abnormal	Normal	Normal
RDW	↑	Normal	Normal	Normal

MEGALOBLASTIC ANEMIA

CAUSES
• Cobalamin deficiency • Folate deficiency • Therapy with antifolate drugs (e.g., methotrexate)
• Independent of either cobalamin or folate deficiency and refractory to cobalamin and folate therapy: – Some cases of acute myeloid leukemia, myelodysplasia – Therapy with drugs interfering with synthesis of DNA – Orotic aciduria (responds to uridine) – Thiamine-responsive megaloblastic anemia

- Most common cause of cobalamine deficiency is **malabsorption.**
- Most common cause of folate deficiency is either **decreased dietary intake** or **increased demand**.
- Body's stores of folate are low so deficiency arises suddenly.

Drugs causing megaloblastic anemia	
• **Anticonvulsant drugs** – Phenytoin – Primidone – Barbiturates	• **Purine antagonist** – 6-Mercaptopurine – 6-Thioguanine – Azathioprine
• **Folate antagonists** (inhibitors of Dihydrofolate reductase) – Methotrexate – Trimethoprim-sulfamethoxazole – Pyrimethamine – Cotrimaxazole – Pentamidine – Triamtrene	• **Pyrimidine antagonists** – 5-Fluorouracil – 6-Azauridine – Cytosine arabinose
• **Others** – Acyclovir – Zidovudine – Hydroxyurea – Procarbazine	• **N_2O** anesthesia– – Most common cause of **acute megaloblastic anemia**

Causes of thiamine deficiency
• Malabsorption • Dietary habits- polished rice • Alcoholic and food faddists, Chronic heart failure

Causes of cobalamine deficiency	
• Nutritional • Malabsorption • Gastric causes	• Vegans • Pernicious anemia • Congenital absence of intrinsic factor or functional abnormality • Total or partial gastrectomy
• Intestinal causes Intestinal stagnant loop syndrome:	• Jejunal diverticulosis, ileocolic fistula, anatomic blind loop, intestinal stricture, etc. • Ileal resection and Crohn's disease • Selective malabsorption with proteinuria • Tropical sprue • Transcobalamin II deficiency • Fish tapeworm

Pernicious Anemia

- Pernicious anemia (PA) may be defined as a severe lack of IF due to gastric atrophy.

Intestinal Stagnant Loop Syndrome

- Malabsorption of cobalamin occurs in a variety of intestinal lesions in which there is **colonization** of the upper small intestine by fecal organisms
  - ie. Malabsorption occurs secondary to bacterial overgrowth.

SCHILLING TEST: *(From Williams hematology)*
- Assays of Cobalamin Absorption and Intrinsic Factor.
- Test assays cobalamin absorption by measuring urinary radioactivity after an oral dose of radioactive cobalamin.

- After voiding, a fasting patient drinks 0.5 μCi (0.5–2.0 μg) of radioactive CnCbl in water.
- 24-hour urine collection is started.
- At 2 hours, 1 mg of unlabeled CnCbl is given intramuscularly (IM) to saturate the circulating cobalamin-binding proteins, after which the patient may eat.
- The amount of radioactivity in the 24-hour urine collection is measured.
- Normal subjects excrete at least 7 percent of the administered radioactivity in the first 24 hours.

- If excretion of radioactivity is low, the second part of the Schilling test is performed after a 5-day delay.
- The interval allows the unlabeled cobalamin given in the first part of the test to correct intestinal megaloblastosis.
- The procedure is the same except that 60 mg of active hog intrinsic factor is given orally with the radioactive cobalamin.
- If poor excretion in the first part resulted from intrinsic factor deficiency, excretion in the second part will be normal.

Intrinsic factor will not correct cobalamin malabsorption resulting from other causes.
Etiology for abnormal Schilling test may be deduced as follows..

Diagnosis	^{58}Co-Cbl	With IF	With Pancreatic enzyme	After 5 days of antibiotics
Pernicious anemia	Reduced	**Normal**	Reduced	Reduced
Chronic pancreatitis	Reduced	Reduced	**Normal**	Reduced
Bacterial overgrowth	Reduced	Reduced	Reduced	Normal
Ileal disease	Reduced	Reduced	Reduced	**Reduced**

Clinical Features

- Anemia
- Anorexia - marked, weight loss, diarrhea, or constipation.
- Jaundice (unconjugated), and reversible melanin skin hyperpigmentation
- Thrombocytopenia sometimes leads to bruising
- Oral manifestations:
  - **Macroglossia**
  - **Atrophic glossitis** - loss of papillae
  - Moeller's glossitis - Red patches or red lines on the ventrum
  - Angular chelitis
  - Sore tongue

General Tissue Effects of Cobalamin and Folate Deficiencies

Epithelial Surfaces of the mouth, stomach, and small intestine and the respiratory, urinary, and female genital tracts- macrocytosis
Neural Tube Defects: Anencephaly, meningomyelocele, encephalocele, and spina bifida
Cardiovascular Disease: Cerebrovascular, peripheral vascular, and coronary heart disease and with deep vein thrombosis.
Neurologic Manifestations: Bilateral peripheral neuropathy or degeneration (demyelination) of the posterior and pyramidal tracts.
Malignancy: Prophylactic folic acid in pregnancy- reduce the subsequent incidence of acute lymphoblastic leukemia.

Hematologic Findings- Peripheral Blood
Pancytopenia • Anemia- macrocytic with macro-ovulocytes • Hypersegmented neutrophils • Leukopenia due to a reduction in granulocytes and lymphocytes, but this is usually > 1.5 x 10^9/L Platelet count may be moderately reduced, rarely to < 40 x 10^9/L.
Bone marrow • Megaloblastic erythropoiesis • Giant and abnormally shaped metamyelocytes • Enlarged hyperpolyploid megakaryocytes

Treatment

Megaloblastic anemia (Vit B12/Folate deficiency)-establish which of the two deficiencies, folate or cobalamin

- If clearly established-Treat with appropriate vitamin
- No clearly established diagnosis-treat with both vitamin
- If only folic acid is administered in patient with vit B12 deficiency, worsening of neurological symptoms (cobalamine neuropathy) is seed despite an improvement in the hematological symptoms (anemia)

Prophylaxis - Folic acid, 400 g daily, should be given as a supplement before and throughout pregnancy.

HEMOLYTIC ANEMIAS

Intravascular hemolysis	Extravascular hemolysis
RBCs are degraded intravascularly	Degraded within the cells of reticuloendothelial system ie spleen/liver
Paroxysmal nocturnal hemoglobinuria • Erythrocyte fragmentation disorders • Transfusion reactions resulting from ABO isoantibodies • Paroxysmal cold hemoglobinuria • Acquired autoimmune hemolytic anemia (occasionally) **Associated with certain infections** • Blackwater fever in falciparum malaria • Clostridial sepsis **Caused by certain chemical agents** • Arsine poisoning • Snake and spider venoms • Acute drug reactions with glucose-6-phosphate dehydrogenase deficiency • Intravenous administration of distilled water **Thermal injury**	**Inherited disorder of hemoglobin or synthesis** • Thalassemia **Membrane structural defects** • Hereditary spherocytosis • Hereditary elliptocytosis syndromes • Acanthocytosis **Hereditary enzyme disorders** • Glucose-6-phosphate dehydrogenase deficiency • Pyruvate kinase deficiency **Acquired hemolytic anemias** • Autoimmune hemolytic anemia • Warm reacting (IgG) • Cold reacting (IgM) • Infectious agents • Malaria/IMN/Mycoplasma **Others** • Malignancy/DIC • TTP/HUS • Eclampsia/Preeclampsia
Plasma/serum • Bilirubin- ↑ unconjugated • Haptoglobin- absent • Plasma haemoglobin- ↑↑ • LDH- increased ↑↑	 • Bilirubin- ↑ unconjugated • Haptoglobin- ↓ • Plasma hemoglobin-N- ↑ • LDH- increased (variable)
Urine • Bilirubin- Absent • Hemosiderin- present • Hemoglobin–present in severe cases • Methemoglobinuria- immediately after iv hemolysis	 • Bilirubin- Absent • Hemosiderin- Absent • Hemoglobin–Absent

Contd...

Contd...

Intravascular hemolysis	Extravascular hemolysis
Hematologic • Routine blood film- polychromatophilia • Increased reticulocyte count • Erythroid hyperplasia	• Routine blood film- polychromatophilia • Increased reticulocyte count • Erythroid hyperplasia

Compensatory erythropoietic response of the bone marrow

Red cell destruction is a potent stimulus for erythropoiesis, which is mediated by erythropoietin (EPO) produced by the kidney

X- ray

- Expansion of marrow space- tubular bones/skull
- Bossing of skull

Compensated Hemolysis Versus HA

- In many cases the increased output of red cells from the bone marrow can fully balance an increased destruction of red cells
- Compensated hemolysis may become '**decompensated**'—i.e., anemia may suddenly appear—in certain circumstances, for instance pregnancy, folate deficiency, or renal failure, interfering with adequate EPO production
- Infection by parvovirus B19 can suppress erythropoiesis, which may cause a rather precipitous fall in hemoglobin; an occurrence sometimes referred to as **aplastic crisis**

Reticulocyte Count

Both intravascular and extravascular hemolysis are characterised by elevated retic count

Reticulocyte count	=	Percentage reticulocytes in RBC population
Corrected reticulocyte count	=	Percentage reticulocytes × (patient Hct/45)
Reticulocyte production index	=	Corrected reticulocyte count × Maturation time in peripheral blood in days (Normal values of all of above 0.5–1.5%)

Reticulocyte maturation time
1 day for Hct ≥40%;
1.5 days for Hct 30–40%;
2.0 days for Hct 20–30%;
2.5 days for Hct < 20%.

Reticulocyte count

Low /normal reticulocyte count (Reticulocyte production index <2.5)		
Hypoproliferative NCNC	Maturation defect Microcytic	Macrocytic
• Red cell aplasia • Fanconi's anemia • Marrow damage • Infiltration/fibrosis • Malignancy • Decreased stimulation • Chronic inflammation • Kidney disease	• Iron deficiency • Thalassemia • Lead toxicity • Sideroblastic anemia	• Vit B12 deficiency • Folate deficiency • Hypothyroidism • Drug toxicity • Refractory anemia(CDA)

High reticulocyte count (Reticulocyte production index > 2.5)
• Hemorrhage/hemolysis • Intravascular • Transfusion reactions • Snake bite • Thermal burns • PNH/PCH • Mechanical heart valves

HEREDITARY SPHEROCYTOSIS

- Classically the inheritance of HS is autosomal dominant (with the patients being heterozygous).

Gene	Protein produced	Disease(s) with certain mutation	Comments
SPTA1	α-spectrin	HS (recessive) HE (dominant)	Rare Mutations of this gene account for about **65% of HE**
SPTB	β-Spectrin	HS (dominant) HE (dominant)	Rare Mutations of this gene account for about **30% of HE**, including some severe forms
ANK1	Ankyrin	HS (dominant)	May account for **majority of HS**
SLC4A1	Band 3 (anion channel)	HS (dominant) Southeast asia ovalocytosis (dominant)	Mutations of this gene may account for about **25% of HS** Polymorphic mutation; clinically asymptomatic; protective against *Plasmodium falciparum*
Protein defects causing HS-Ankyrin > protein 3 > spectrin > Palladin			

Diagnosis

- In most cases, the diagnosis can be made on the basis of red cell morphology and of a test for osmotic fragility, a modified version of which is called the 'pink test'.
- HS is the only condition associated with high MCHC.

Osmotic fragility (OF) of red cells is defined as the ease with which the red cells are ruptured/hemolysed when exposed to hypotonic solution

↑Osmotic fragility (↓surface volume ratio)	Decreased OF (↑ Surface volume ratio)
• Hereditary spherocytosis • Autoimmune hemolytic anemia • Hereditary disease of newborn • Severe pyruvate kinase deficiency	• Thalassemia • Iron deficiency anemia • Sickle cell anemia • Post splenectomy • Reticulocytosis
(Conditions with spherocytes in blood)	(Conditions with target cells in the blood)

Treatment

Splenectomy has long been regarded as a prime, almost obligatory therapeutic measure in HS.

Current guidelines (not evidence-based) are as follows.

- Avoid splenectomy in mild cases.
- Delay splenectomy until at least 4 years of age, after the risk of severe sepsis has peaked.
- Antipneumococcal vaccination before splenectomy is imperative, whereas penicillin prophylaxis postsplenectomy is controversial.
- HS patients often may require cholecystectomy, in which case the practice has been to also carry out a splenectomy at the same time.

G-6PD deficiency

- G6PD gene is X-linked.
- Confers a relative resistance against *Plasmodium falciparum* malaria infection.
- G6PD deficiency is a prime example of an HA due to **interaction between an intracorpuscular cause and an extracorpuscular cause**, because in the majority of cases, hemolysis is triggered by an exogenous agent.
- The most typical feature is the presence of bizarre poikilocytes, with red cells that appear to have unevenly distributed hemoglobin ('hemighosts') and red cells that appear to have had parts of them bitten away ('**bite cells**' or 'blister cells').

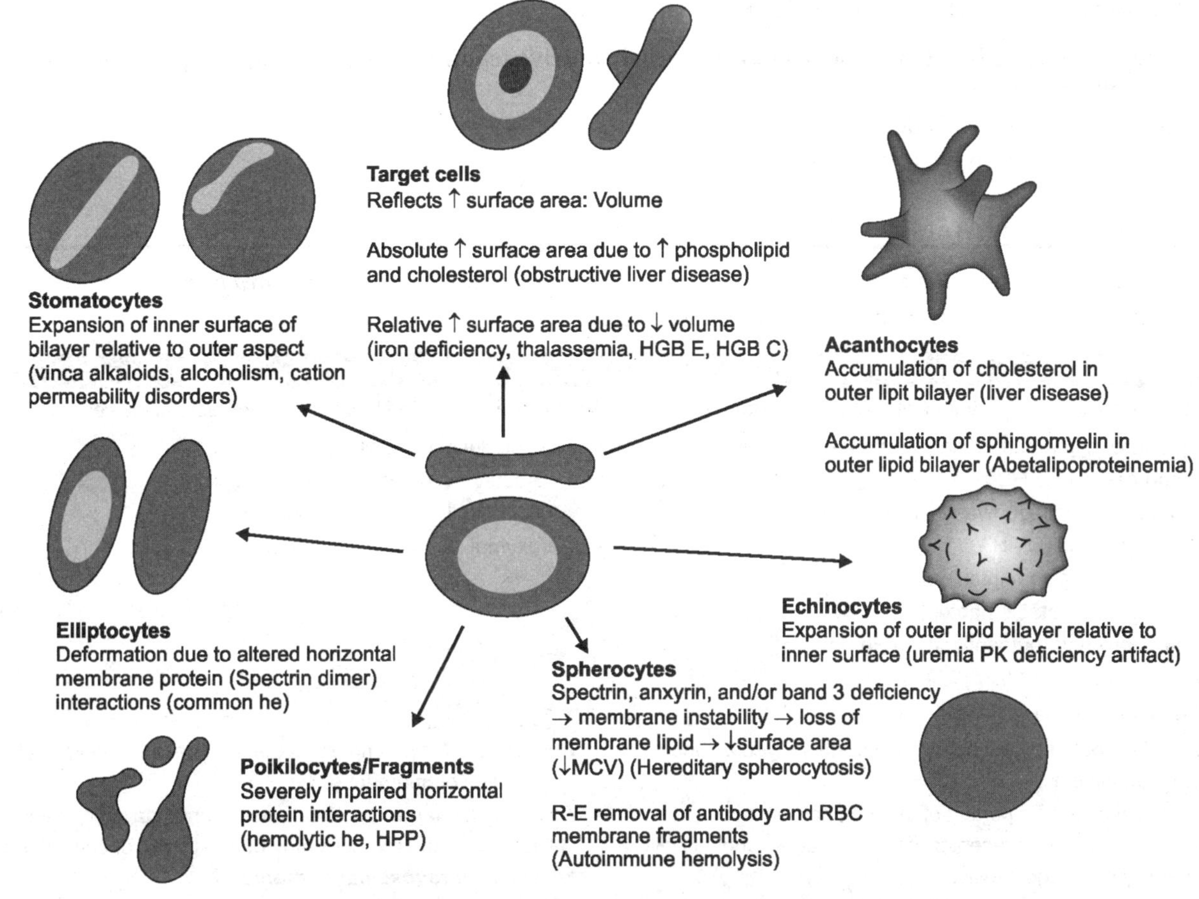

Diagrammatic representation of abnormal cells associated with alterations in the erythrocyte membrane

- Supravital staining with methyl violet that, if done promptly, reveals the presence of **Heinz bodies**, consisting of precipitates of **denatured hemoglobin** and regarded as a signature of oxidative damage to red cells.

Agent	Definitive risk	Possible risk	Doubtful risk
Antimalarials	Primaquine Dapsone/chlorproguanil	Chloroquine	Quinine
Sulphonamides/sulphones	Sulfamethoxazole Others Dapsone	Sulfasalazine	Sulfisoxazole
Antibacterials/Antibiotics	Cotrimoxazole Nalidixic acid Nitrofurantoin Niridazole	Ciprofloxacin Norfloxacin	Chloramphenicol *p*-Aminosalicylic acid
Antipyretic/analgesics	Acetanilide Phenazopyridine	Acetylsalicylic acid High dose > 3g/d	Acetylsalicylic acid < 3g/d Acetaminophen Phenacetin
Others	Naphthalene Methylene blue	Vitamin K analogues Ascorbic acid > 1 g Rasburicase	Doxorubicin Probenecid

Other Abnormalities of the Redox System:

Pyrimidine 5′-Nucleotidase (P5N) Deficiency: Highly distinctive feature- **basophilic stippling**- 3rd most common among red cell enzyme defects

- 1st most common- G-6PD deficiency
- 2nd most common- pyuvate kinase

AUTOIMMUNE HAEMOLYTIC ANEMIA

Except for countries where malaria is endemic, AIHA is the most common form of *acquired hemolytic anemia*
AIHA is caused by an autoantibody directed against a red cell antigen

Warm- antibody immunohemolytic anemia	Cold-antibody immunohemolytic anemia
Antibodies here bind with antigens at room temperature (37 °C)	Antibodies here bind with antigens at temperature lower than 37 °C
• Idiopathic autoimmune hemolytic anemia • Lymphomas- CLL/NHL • SLE and other collagen vascular diseases – Drug-induced (DI-IHA) – Penicillin (stable hapten) – Quinidine (unstable hapten) – α-methyldopa (autoantibody to Rh antigen) • Post viral infections • Other tumors (rare)	• Cold agglutinin disease – Acute: Mycoplasma infection, IMN – Chronic: Idiopathic, lymphoma • Paroxymal cold hemoglobinuria
• Red cell is coated by antibody, it will be destroyed by one or more mechanisms. • In most cases the Fc portion of the antibody will be recognized by the Fc receptor of macrophages, and this will trigger erythrophagocytosis. • Thus, destruction of red cells will take place wherever macrophages are abundant, i.e., in the spleen, liver, and bone marrow. • Spleen is the predominant site of red cell destruction. • Most of the phagocytosis-mediated red cell destruction takes place in the organs just mentioned, and it is therefore called ***extravascular hemolysis.***	• Antigen-antibody complex on the surface of red cells is able to activate complement (C). • As a result, a large amount of membrane attack complex will form, and the red cells may be destroyed directly; this is known as ***intravascular hemolysis***
• Positive direct and indirect Coomb's test at 37 °C for the presence of warm antibodies.	• Positive direct Coomb's test for detection of C3 on the red cell surface. • IgM responsible for coating antibodies are not found.

AIHA is diagnosed, a full screen for autoimmune disease is imperative.
In some cases, AIHA can be associated, on first presentation or subsequently, with autoimmune thrombocytopenia (**Evans's syndrome= AIHA+ Autoimmune thrombocytopenia**).

Treatment

- Severe acute AIHA can be a medical emergency.
- First line of treatmentof AIHA is **steroids**.
- Second line–long term **immunosupression** using low dose prednisolone.
- Chronic cases will benefit from splenectomy.
- Rituximab (anti-CD20), IV Ig are also used.
- In severe refractory cases, either auto- or allo-hematopoietic stem cell transplantation has been used, sometimes successfully.

Paroxysmal Cold Hemoglobinuria (PCH)

- PCH is a rather rare form of AIHA occurring mostly in children
- Triggered by a **viral** infection, usually self-limited, and characterized by the involvement of the so-called Donath-Landsteiner antibody.
- In vitro this antibody has unique serologic features: it has **anti-P specificity** and it binds to red cells only at a low temperature (optimally at 4 °C), but when the temperature is shifted to 37 °C, lysis of red cells takes place in the presence of complement.
- Consequently, in vivo there is intravascular hemolysis, resulting in hemoglobinuria.
- Active supportive treatment, including blood transfusion, is needed to control the anemia; subsequently, recovery is the rule.

Cold Agglutinin Disease (CAD)

- Chronic AIHA that usually affects the **elderly**.
- Antibody is usually IgM with an **anti-I specificity**.
- Antibody is produced by an expanded clone of B lymphocytes and its concentration in the plasma is high enough (monoclonal gammopathy)
- Since the antibody is IgM, CAD is related to **Waldenstrom macroglobulinemia** (WM)
- Mild forms- avoidance of exposure to cold
- More severe forms
  - Immunosuppressive/cytotoxic treatment with azathioprine or cyclophosphamide
  - Plasma exchange
  - Rituximab
- Blood transfusion is not easy because donar red cells are I- positive and are removed rapidly

HEMOGLOBINOPATHIES

- Structural hemoglobinopathies: Hemoglobins with altered amino acid sequences that result in **deranged function or altered physical or chemical properties**
  - Abnormal hemoglobin polymerization—HbS, hemoglobin sickling
  - Altered O_2 affinity
    - High affinity—polycythemia
    - Low affinity—cyanosis, pseudoanemia
  - Hemoglobins that oxidize readily
    - Unstable hemoglobins—hemolytic anemia, jaundice
    - M hemoglobins—methemoglobinemia, cyanosis
- **Thalassemias: Defective biosynthesis of globin chains**
  - Thalassemias
  - Thalassemias
  - δβ, ϒδβ, αβ Thalassemias
- **Thalassemic hemoglobin variants: Structurally abnormal Hb associated with co-inherited thalassemic phenotype**
  - HbE
  - Hb Constant Spring
  - Hb Lepore
- **Hereditary persistence of fetal hemoglobin:** Persistence of high levels of HbF into adult life
- **Acquired hemoglobinopathies**
  - Methemoglobin due to toxic exposures
  - Sulfhemoglobin due to toxic exposures
  - Carboxyhemoglobin
  - HbH in erythroleukemia
  - Elevated HbF in states of erythroid stress and bone marrow dysplasia

THALASSEMIA

The thalassemia syndromes are inherited disorders of α- or β-globin biosynthesis.

In β-thalassemia/Cooley's anemia,

Total or decreased synthesis of β chains resulting in marked decrease in HbA($\alpha2\beta2$)

- Compensatory increase of other chain

✱HbF (✱α2✱2. and ✱ HbA2 (✱α2δ2)

- Precipitation of excess unimpaired α chains
  - Excess α chains- destruction of RBCsà Anemia

Mutations in Thalassemia

- Most β-thalassemias are due to **point mutations**
- Most common site is intervening sequence-1 (IVS-1)/intron-1
- Most α-thalassemias are due to **gene deletions**

	Thalassemia Major	Thalassemia Intermedia	Thalassemia Minor
		GENERAL	
	Presents in early infancy	Present somewhere between the two extremes	Presents late Can lead a normal life except for mild persistent anemia
	Require repeated blood transfusion	Require occasional transfusions but are not dependent on blood transfusions for survival	Not dependent on blood transfusions
Life expectancy	20–28yrs	Normal	Normal
		HEMATOLOGICAL FINDINGS	
Hb	Hb- < 7 g/dl	Hb- 7–10 g/dl	Hb- > 10 g/dl
Microcytosis and hypochromia	+++	++	+
Basophilic stippling Ansiopoikilocytosis **Target cells**	++ +++ **+++**	+ ++ ++	+ ++ ++
Nucleated RBCs	+++	+/-	-
HbF HbA2	30–90% < 3.5%	20–100% < 3.5%	0–5% 3.5–8%
Bone marrow iron	++++	++	+/-
Iron overload	+	-	-
Treatment	Regular blood transfusions	Intermittent transfusions during exacerbation of anemia	No treatment

- Diagnosis is established by **Hb electrophoresis or HPLC**.
- Thal major- Splenectomy is required if the annual transfusion requirement (volume of RBCs per kilogram of body weight per year) increases by > **50%**.

Transfusional Hemosiderosis

Chronic blood transfusion can lead to blood borne infection, alloimmunization, febrile reactions, and lethal iron overload.

Iron-chelating agents

- Desferoxamine (Desferal) is for parenteral use
- Deferasirox is an oral iron-chelating agent

Skeletal Changes

Children develop characteristic '**chipmunk**' facies due to maxillary marrow hyperplasia and frontal bossing.

The skull is large and deformed by frontal and posterior bossing with the diploe increased in thickness to several times normal. The outer and inner tables are thin and the trabeculae are arranged in vertical striations, resulting in a '**hair-on-end/crew cut**' appearance. Most characteristic of thalassemia and sickle cell anemia. Also seen in other haemolytic anemias.

It's important to differentiate **iron deficiency (IDA) from thalassemia trait**

IDA	THALASSEMIA TRAIT
Microcytic hypochromic (MCV↓)	Microcytic hypochromic (MCV↓)
S.iron-↓	S.iron- Normal
Ferritin- ↓	Ferritin- ↑
Saturation- ↓	Saturation- ↑
TIBC- ↑	TIBC- Normal

Mentzer Index is based on the MCV and RBC count:

- MCV/RBC (10^6) > 14 (suggestive of iron deficiency)
- MCV/RBC (10^6) 12–14 (indeterminate)
- **MCV/RBC (10^6) < 12** (suggestive of **thalassemia trait** disorders)

Nestroft- Naked Eye Single Tube Red Cell Osmotic Fragility Test is used for screening thalassemia trait patients but is not diagnostic.

α-Thalassemias

Clinical syndrome	Genotype	Clinical features
Silent carrier	-/α α/α	Asymptomatic; no red cell abnormality
α-thalassemia trait	-/- α/α	Asymptomatic; like β-thalassemia minor
HbH disease	-/- -/α	Severe; resembles thalassemia intermedia
Hydrops fetalis	-/- -/-	Lethal in utero without transfusions

HbH Disease

- HbA production is only 25–30% normal.
- Fetuses accumulate some unpaired chains **(Hb Barts; ϒ-chain tetramers)** which has a very high oxygen affinity. It delivers almost no O_2 to fetal tissues.
- In adults, unpaired chains accumulate and are soluble enough to form β4 tetramers called HbH.
- HbH forms few **inclusions** in erythroblasts and precipitates in circulating RBC

Prevention

Antenatal diagnosis of thalassemia syndromes is now widely available.

DNA diagnosis is based on PCR amplification of fetal DNA, obtained by amniocentesis or chorionic villus biopsy followed by hybridization to allele specific oligonucleotides probes or direct DNA sequencing.

Hereditary Persistence of Fetal Hemoglobin

HPFH is characterized by continued synthesis of high levels of HbF in adult life. No deleterious effects are apparent, even when all of the hemoglobin produced is HbF.

SICKLE CELL ANEMIA

The sickle cell syndromes are caused by a mutation in the -globin gene that changes the sixth amino acid from glutamic acid to valine.

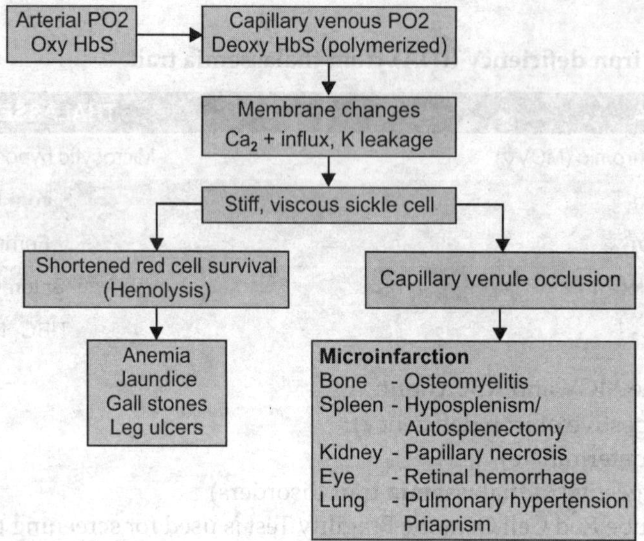

Factors Favoring Polymerization

- Hypoxia: 2, 3 diphosphoglycerate increases polymerization
- Acidosis (↓pH)
- High Hb concentration
- Combination of HbS with other Hemoglobins: Descending order of ability to co-polymerize are HbS, C, D, O, Arab, A, J, and F (least with F)

Painful Crisis

- Intermittent episodes of vaso-occlusion in connective and musculoskeletal structures produce ischemia manifested by acute pain and tenderness, fever, tachycardia, and anxiety.
- These recurrent episodes, called **painful crises**, are the most common clinical manifestation
- Management - vigorous hydration, thorough evaluation for underlying causes (such as infection), and aggressive analgesia (Morphine)

Hand-foot syndrome is caused by painful infarcts of the digits and dactylitis.

Hydroxyurea

- Mainstay of therapy for patients with severe symptoms.
- Hydroxyurea (10–30 mg/kg per day) increases fetal hemoglobin
- It also exert beneficial affects on RBC hydration, vascular wall adherence, and suppression of the granulocyte and reticulocyte counts

Antitumor drug **5-azacytidine** was the first agent found to elevate HbF- but never achieved widespread use because of concerns about acute toxicity and carcinogenesis.

Low doses of the related agent **5-deoxyazacytidine** (decitabine) can elevate HbF with more acceptable toxicity.

Bone marrow transplantation can provide definitive cures but is known to be effective and safe only in children

Representative abnormal hemoglobins with altered synthesis of function			
Designation	**Mutation**	**Population**	**Main clinical effects**[a]
Stickle or S	β6Glu→Val	African	Anemia, ischemic infarcts
C	β6Glu→Lys	African	Mild anemia; interacts with Hbs
E	β26Glu→Lys	Southeast Asian	Microcytuc anemia, splenimegly, thalassemic phenotype
Köln	β98Val→Met	Sporadic	Hemolytic anemia, Heinz bodies when splenectomized
Yakima	β99Asp→His	Sporadic	Polycythemia
Kansan	β102Asn→Lys	Sporadic	Mild anemia
M. Iwata	α87His→Tyr	Sporadic	Mrthemoglobinemia

PAROXYSMAL NOCTURNAL HEMOGLOBINURIA (PNH)

PNH is an acquired chronic HA characterized by persistent intravascular hemolysis subject to recurrent exacerbations. The molecular basis of the disease is due shortage of a unique glycolipid molecule GPI, through which proteins are anchored to surface.

Shortage of GPI is due in turn to a mutation in an X-linked gene, called PIG-A, required for an early step in GPI biosynthesis.

Triad makes PNH a truly unique clinical condition which includes

Hemolysis	• Because of increased activation of complement mediated destruction. • Hemoglobinemia, hemoglobinuria, hemosiderinuria, ↑LDH.
Pancytopenia	• Defective hematopoiesis due to defect at stem cell level. • ↓Granulocytes, Thrombocytopenia.
Venous thrombosis	• Complement activation stimulates platelet aggregation and hypercoagulability (Thrombosis despite thrombocytopenia). • Classic site–Hepatic vein- Budd Chiari syndrome. • Second common site - Cranial vein (Frank cerebral thrombosis- grave complication)

Leukocyte Alkaline Phosphate (LAP)

Low LAP	High LAP
• **PNH** • CML	• Polycythemia • Leukemoid reaction • Infection

Lab Findings

Anemia

- Mild to moderate to very severe; usually normomacrocytic, with unremarkable red cell morphology
- MCV is high, it is usually largely accounted for by reticulocytosis, which maybe quite marked (up to 20%)

Hemoglobinuria, the telltale sign of **intravascular hemolysis**.

Other features of IV hemolysis.

Bone Marrow

- Usually cellular, with marked to massive erythroid hyperplasia,
- At some stage of the disease, the marrow may become hypocellular or even frankly aplastic

Sucrose hemolysis test - unreliable

Acidified serum (Ham) test

The gold standard today is **flow cytometry**

- This can be carried out on granulocytes as well as on red cells.
- A bimodal distribution of cells, with a discrete population that is CD59-, CD55-, is diagnostic of PNH.

Major advance in treatment–**ECULIZUMAB**–monoclonal antibody against complement C5

PNH may progress to aplastic anemia

PNH-AA is treated with ATG or cyclosporine

APLASTIC ANEMIA, MYELODYSPLASIA, AND RELATED BONE MARROW FAILURE SYNDROMES

Hypoproliferative anemias are normochromic, normocytic, or macrocytic and are characterized by a low reticulocyte count

Bone marrow failure states include

- Aplastic anemia,
- Myelodysplastic syndrome (MDS),
- Pure red cell aplasia (PRCA), and
- Myelophthisis

More frequent in bone marrow failure is pancytopenia:

- Anemia
- Leukopenia
- Thrombocytopenia

Splenomegaly is characteristically **absent** in aplastic anemia

Differential diagnosis of pancytopenia		
Pancytopenia with hypocellular Bone marrow	Pancytopenia with cellular bone marrow	
	Primary bone marrow diseases	Secondary to systemic diseases
• Acquired aplastic anemia • Constitutional aplastic anemia (Fanconi's anemia, dyskeratosis congenita) • Some myelodysplasia • Rare aleukemic leukemia • Some acute lymphoid leukemia • Some lymphomas of bone marrow	• Myelodysplasia • Paroxysmal nocturnal hemoglobinuria • Myelofibrosis • Some aleukemic leukemia • Myelophthisis • Bone marrow lymphoma • Hairy cell leukemia	• Systemic lupus erythematosus • **Hypersplenism** • B12, folate deficiency • Overwhelming infection • Alcohol • Brucellosis • Sarcoidosis • Tuberculosis • Leishmaniasis

Hypocellular Bone Marrow ± Cytopenia
Q fever
Legionnaires' disease
Anorexia nervosa, starvation
Mycobacterium

Classification of aplastic anemia	
Acquired aplastic anemia	Inherited
• Radiation • Drugs and chemicals- idiosyncratic/regular effects • Viruses- – EBV (IMN) – Hepatitis (non A, non B, non C) – **Parvovirus B19 (transient aplastic crisis, PRCA)** – HIV-1 • Immune disorders – Eosinophilic fasciitis	• **Fanconi's anemia** • Dyskeratosis congenita • Shwachman-Diamond syndrome • Reticular dysgenesis • Amegakaryocytic thrombocytopenia

Contd...

Contd...

Classification of aplastic anemia	
Acquired aplastic anemia	**Inherited**
– Hyperimmunoglobulinemia – **Thymoma/thymic carcinoma** – Graft-versus-host disease in immunodeficiency • Paroxysmal nocturnal hemoglobinuria • Pregnancy • Idiopathic	• Familial aplastic anemias – Preleukemia (monosomy 7, etc.) – Nonhematologic syndrome (Down, Dubowitz, Seckel)

Classification of drugs most commonly implicated in causing aplastic anemia
Nonsteroidal analgesics – Phenylbutazone, indomethacin, ibuprofen, sulindac, diclofenac, piroxicam • Anticonvulsants – Hydantoins, carbamazepine, phenacemide • Antibiotics – Sulfonamides, chloramphenicol • Antiprotozoals – Quinacrine, chloroquine • Antithyroid drugs – Methimazole, propylthiouracil • Gold

Classification of aplastic anemia based on severity of pancytopenia
• **Severe aplastic anemia (SAA)** – Bone marrow cellularity < 25% – Two of three peripheral blood criteria: – Absolute neutrophil count < 500/mm³ – Platelet count < 20, 000/mm³ – Reticulocyte count < 60, 000/mm³ or < 1% corrected reticulocyte count
• **Very severe aplastic anemia (VSAA)** – Same as SAA with absolute neutrophil count < 200/mm³
• **Nonsevere (moderate) aplastic anemia** – Bone marrow cellularity < 25% – Peripheral blood cytopenias do not fulfill criteria for SAA

Bone marrow: Usually readily aspirated but dilute on smear, and the **fatty** biopsy specimen may be grossly pale on withdrawal; a **'dry tap' instead suggests fibrosis or myelophthisis**.

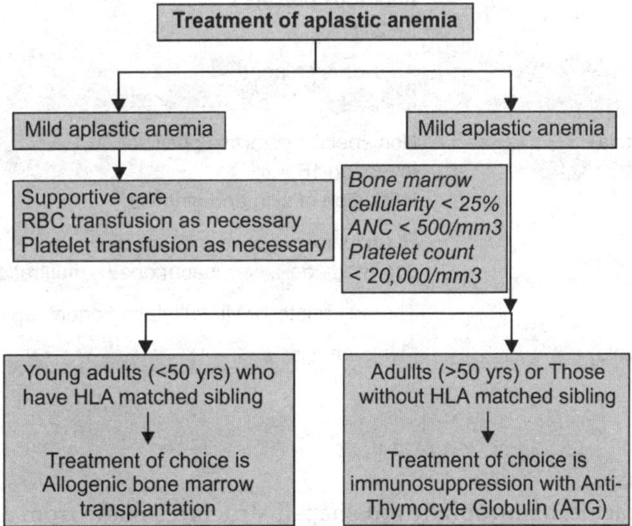

Aplastic anemia may be difficult to distinguish from the hypocellular variety of MDS:
MDS is favored by finding morphologic abnormalities, particularly of megakaryocytes and myeloid precursor cells, and typical cytogenetic abnormalities.

Characteristic	Myelodysplastic syndromes	Aplastic anemia
Cellularity	Usually increased or normal	Decreased
CD34	Normal to increased	Decreased
Erythropoiesis		
Megaloblatosis	Common	Common
Dyserythropoiesis	Common	Sometimes
Ringed sideroblasts	Common	Never
Myelopoiesis		
Increased blast	Common	Never
Megakaryocytes		
Dysplastic	Common	Never

[a]A Hypocellular bone marrow is found in up to 15% of cases of myelosysplastic syndromes.

Causes of microangiopathic HA

TTP HUS DIC	Hemangiomas March hemoglobinuria

ACUTE MYELOID LEUKEMIA

Classification

AML Type	Salient features
M0 (minimally differentiated AML)	Myeloperoxidase negative
M1 (AML without maturation)	Peroxidase positive Auer rods present
M2 (AML with maturation)	Auer rods present t(8;21)
M3 (acute promyelocytic leukemia)	Auer rods present t(15;27)
M4 (acute myelomonocytic leukemia)	Non specific esterase positive Inversion 16 Infiltration of skin and gingival
M5 (acute monocytic leukemia)	Peroxidase negative, nonspecific esterase positive Organomegaly, lymphadenopathy, infiltration of skin and gingiva
M6 (acute erythroleukemia)	Therapy related AML (alkylating agent, epipodophyllotoxin)
M7 (acute mega karyocytic leukemia)	Myelofibrosis

- M2-Commonest
- M7-Rarest
- M6-DiGuglielmo's disease

Auer rods are crystalline, refractile, azuurophilic rod shaped structures made from alignment of granules.

Seen	Absent in
Most frequently in AML-M3 (95–100%), AML-M2 (70%) May be seen in AML-M1, M4, M6 (30–50%) MDS with excess blasts in transformation	AML-M0 AML-M5a and AML-7

AML type	Chromosomal association
• M2	• t(8;21) (q22; qq22)- RUNX1/ETO fusion
• M3	• t(15;17)- RARA/PML fusion
• M5	• t(9;11)
• M4-Eo	• inv16–CBFB/MYH 11 fusion

Favourable prognostic features	Unfavorable prognostic features
Clinical factors	
< 45 yrs	< 2 years, > 60 yrs
De novo leukemia	Antecedent
TLC < 25, 000/mm^3	> 1, 00, 000/mm^3
No extramedullary disease	Extramedullary disease +
No CNS involvement	CNS involvement
Rapid cytoreduction	Delayed cytoreduction
Normal S.LDH	Elevated S.LDH
Morphology	
Auer rods +	Auer rods –
Eosinophils +	Eosinophils –
Megaloblastic erythroids -	Megaloblastic eryhroids+
Dysplastic megakaryocytes -	Dyplastic megs +
AML- M2, M3, M4	M0, M6, M7
Surface Markers	
CD34-, CD14-, CD13-	CD34+
HLA DR-	HLADR+
TdT-	TdT+
CD2+	CD7, CD56+, biphenotypic
MDR-1-	MDR–1+
Cytogenetics	
t(15;17), t(8;21), inv 16	–7, –5, del (7q), del (5q), 3q21, 3q26, complex karyotypes
Molecular prognostic markers	
NPM1, CEBPA mutation	WT1 mutation KIT mutation BAALC, ERG, MN1, EVI1 overexpression

APML

Present with bleeding tendencies and/or DIC Tretinoin- induces the differentiation of leukemic cells Aresenic trioxide- response in up to 85% of cases refractory to ATRA	Retinoic acid syndrome • Occurs within first 3 weeks treatment of retinoic acid • Fever, dyspnoea, chest pain, pulmonary infiltrates, pleural and pericardial effusions • Management- Glucocorticoids, Chemotherapy, supportive measures

Acute Lymphoid Leukemia

- Neoplasms of **immature pre-B and pre-T cells**
- 85% are pre-B cell tumors and present in childhood as leukemias
- Less common pre-T cell tumors present in adolescent males as lymphomas with thymomas
- **Most common tumors in childhood** (2nd most common–brain tumors)

B ALL

Pre-B cell ALL has been associated with poorer outcome compared to Early Pre-B ALL.
Most Early Pre B ALL are **CALLA positive**. It does not have independent prognostic significance.

Immunologic subtype	FAB subtype	Cytogenetic abnormalities
Pre-B ALL (75%)	L1, L2	t(9;22), t(4;11), t(1;19)
T-cell ALL (20%)	L1, L2	14q11 or 7q34
B-cell ALL	L3	t(8;14), t(8;22), t(2;8)

<table>
<tr><th></th><th>Precursor B-ALL</th><th>Common ALL</th><th>Pre B-ALL</th><th>Mature B-ALL</th></tr>
<tr><td>HLA-DR</td><td colspan="4" rowspan="4">Positive</td></tr>
<tr><td>cCD22</td></tr>
<tr><td>CD79a</td></tr>
<tr><td>CD19</td></tr>
<tr><td>TdT</td><td colspan="3">Positive</td><td>Negative</td></tr>
<tr><td>CD10</td><td>Negative</td><td colspan="2">Positive</td><td>Negative</td></tr>
<tr><td>cIgM</td><td colspan="2">Negative</td><td>Positive</td><td>Negative</td></tr>
<tr><td>sIg</td><td colspan="3">Negative</td><td>Positive</td></tr>
</table>

T-ALL

- Occurs in Older children and adults
- Male predilection
- Anterior mediastinal mass in half of the cases at presentation
- High WBC count > 1, 00, 000/mm^3
- Early testicular and CNS involvement

<table>
<tr><th></th><th>Pro-T-ALL</th><th>Pre-T-ALL</th><th>Cortical-T-ALL</th><th>Mature-T-ALL</th></tr>
<tr><td>TdT</td><td colspan="3">Positive</td><td>Negative</td></tr>
<tr><td>cCD3</td><td colspan="4">Positive</td></tr>
<tr><td>CD7</td><td colspan="4">Positive</td></tr>
<tr><td>CD2</td><td>Negative</td><td colspan="3">Positive</td></tr>
<tr><td>CD5</td><td>Negative</td><td colspan="3">Positive</td></tr>
<tr><td>CD4</td><td colspan="2">Negative</td><td rowspan="2">Positive for CD4 and CD8</td><td rowspan="2">Positive for CD4 or CD8</td></tr>
<tr><td>CD8</td><td colspan="2">Negative</td></tr>
<tr><td>CD1a</td><td colspan="2">Negative</td><td>Positive</td><td>Negative</td></tr>
<tr><td>sCD3</td><td colspan="3">Negative</td><td>Positive</td></tr>
</table>

Prognostic factors

Favorable	Unfavorable
Low WBC count	High WBC count
3–7 yrs	< 1, > 10 yrs
Female	Male
White	Black
Node, liver, spleen - Absent	Massive lymphadenopathy, hepatosplenomegaly
Testicular enlargement-absent	Testicular enlargement- present
No CNS involvement	CNS involvement- present
L1	L2
Early pre-B-cell	T-cell
Hyperdiploidy	Hypodiploidy
Trisomies 4, 10, 17; t(12;21) Tel aml	t(9;22), t(4;11), t(1;19)
Remission time- < 14 days	> 28 days
Minimal Residual Disease- < 10^{-4}	> 10^{-3}

Treatment of intracranial ALL

- Intrathecal chemotherapy (MTX, Cytarabine, Thiotepa) and cranial irradiation.

Why?

- Most children with ALL have subclinical CNS involvement at the time of diagnosis.
- Meninges act as a sanctuary site where leukemic cells are prevented from systemic chemotherapy because of blood brain barrier.
- So, CNS **prophylaxis** is routinely administered in both children and adults.

CNS relapse is very uncommon in AML.

ALL with eosinophilia

- Eosinophilia- reactive process
- t(5;14) rearrangement

Biphenotypic Leukemia

- Rare acute leukemias that express both myeloid and lymphoid associated antigens to degree that no single lineage can be assigned
- Scoring system- precisely defines this and distinguishes these cases from ALL with myeloid antigen expression or AML with lymphoid antigen expression

Points	B-Lineage	T-Lineage	Myeloid
2	CD 79 a, CD 22, Cyt IgM	CD 3 (m/cyt) Anti-TCR α/β Anti-TCR α/β	Anti-MPO (monoclonal) MPO cytochemistry
1	CD 19, CD10, CD20	CD 2, 5, 8, 10	CD117, CD 13, CD33, CD65s, Anti-MPO (polyclonal)
0.5	TdT, CD24	TdT, CD 7, CD1a	CD 14, CD15, CD64

> 2 points are required to assign a lineage.

CHRONIC MYELOPROLIFERATIVE DISORDERS

WHO Classification of chronic myeloproliferative disorders
Chronic myelogenous leukemia, bcr-abl–positive
Chronic neutrophilic leukemia
Chronic eosinophilic leukemia, not otherwise specified
Polycythemia vera
Primary myelofibrosis
Essential thrombocytosis
Mastocytosis
Myeloproliferative neoplasms, unclassifiable

CHRONIC MYELOID LEUKEMIA

The diagnosis of CML is established by identifying a clonal expansion of a hematopoietic stem cell possessing a reciprocal translocation between chromosomes 9 and 22.

This translocation results in the head-to-tail fusion of the breakpoint cluster region (***BCR***) **gene on chromosome** **22**q11 with the *ABL1* (named after the abelson murine leukemia virus) gene located on **chromosome 9**q34.

Clinical presentation

- Usually asymptomatic- discovered incidentally
- Non specific symptoms- fatigue, weight loss, malaise
- **Splenomegaly (massive)** - early satiety, left hypochondrial pain
- Uncommon presentations
- Granulocyte/platelet dysfunction- Infection, thrombosis and bleeding
- Leukostatic manifestations- CVA, MI, venous thrombosis, priaprism, visual disturbance

Peripheral smear

- Elevated WBC count
  - Both immature and mature forms in different stages of maturation
  - With the majority of cells being myelocytes, metamyelocytes, and band forms.
- Blasts < 5%
- Promyelocytes < 10%
- Eosinophilia (less common) and basophilia (often present)
- Thrombocytosis
- Patients are usually not anemic/mildly anemic

Bone marrow

- Hypercellular with left shifted myelopoiesis
- Myeloid erythroid ratio- increased
- Blasts < 5%

Deacreased LAP (Also in PNH)

- Indicates that although total number of granulocytes are increased, they are functionally impaired
- S.Vit B12 and Vit B12 binding proteins- increased

Cytogenetics

t(9;22)- bcr/abl fusion

Attachment of the *BCR* sequences to *ABL1* results in three critical functional changes:

- The Abl protein becomes constitutively active as a tyrosine kinase (TK) enzyme, activating downstream kinases that prevent apoptosis;

- The DNA-protein-binding activity of Abl is attenuated; and
- The binding of Abl to cytoskeletal actin microfilaments is enhanced.

Disease acceleration	Blast crisis
• Increasing degrees of anemia unaccounted for by bleeding or therapy • Cytogenetic clonal evolution or Blood or marrow blasts between 10 and 20%, blood or marrow basophils 20% or Platelet count < 100, 000/L	• Acute leukemia, with blood or marrow blasts 20% • Blast cells - myeloid, lymphoid, erythroid, or undifferentiated, based on morphologic, cytochemical, and immunologic features

- Disease progression: By acquisition of additional t(9;22), trisomy 8, or 17p (*TP*53 loss)
- Progressive de novo DNA methylation at the *BCR-ABL1* locus and hypomethylation of the *LINE-1* retrotransposon promoter herald blastic transformation
- Interleukin 1 may be involved in the progression of CML to the blastic phase.

Sokal index	Hansford system
Blast % Spleen size Platelet count Age Cytogenetic clonal evolution	Age Spleen size Blast% % of Eosinophil, basophil (Based on INF-α treated patients)

- Both Sokal and Hansford system are applicable to Imatinib treated patients
- Hansford system better than Sokal score for predicting survival time

Treatment

- Allogenic stem cell transplant- treatment of choice
- Imatinib mesylate (Gleevec)- functions through competitive inhibition at the ATP-binding site of the Abl kinase in the inactive conformation, which leads to inhibition of tyrosine phosphorylation of proteins involved in Bcr-Abl signal transduction
  - Given orally
  - Main side effects- fluid retention and myelosuppression
  - Not useful in blast crisis
- Dasatinib
  - Approved by the FDA for the treatment of all stages of CML with resistance or intolerance to prior therapy, including imatinib
- Nilotinib
  - Approved by the FDA for the treatment of chronic- and accelerated-phase CML with resistance or intolerance to prior therapy, including imatinib
  - Binds to the kinase domain in the inactive conformation
- IFN-α is FDA approved for CML but is only offered if all other options have failed

Remission	Criteria
Complete hematologic remission	WBC < 10, 000/L, normal morphology, hemoglobin and platelet counts, and disappearance of splenomegaly
Minimal cytogenetic remission	66–95% bone marrow metaphases with t(9;22)
Complete cytogenetic remission	No bone marrow metaphases with t(9;22)
Partial cytogenetic remission	1–35% bone marrow metaphases with t(9;22)
Minor cytogenetic remission	36–85% bone marrow metaphases with t(9;22)

Juvenile CML

- Skin rashes
- **Philadelphia chromosome absent**/BCR-ABL fusion negative

- Monocytosis
- HbF raised
- Poor prognosis

Causes of Erythrocytosis	
• **Relative Erythrocytosis** – Hemoconcentration secondary to dehydration, diuretics, ethanol abuse, androgens or tobacco abuse	
Absolute Erythrocytosis	
• **Hypoxia** – Carbon monoxide intoxication – High oxygen-affinity – Hemoglobin – High altitude – Pulmonary disease – Right to left cardiac or – Vascular shunts – Sleep apnea syndrome – Hepatopulmonary syndrome	• **Renal Disease** – Renal artery stenosis – Focal sclerosing or membranous glomerulonephritis – Postrenal transplantation – Renal cysts – Bartter's syndrome • **Drugs** – Androgens – Recombinant erythropoietin
• **Tumors associated with polycythemia vera** – Hypernephroma – Hepatoma – Adrenal adenoma – Pheochromocytoma • **Cerebellar hemangioblastoma** – Uterine fibromyoma – Meningioma	• **Familial (with normal hemoglobin function)** – Erythropoietin receptor mutation – VHL mutations (**Chuvash** polycythemia) – 2, 3-BPG mutation • **Polycythemia vera**

Polycythemia Vera

WHO criteria
Major criteria • Hb > 18.5 g/dl in men, > 16.5 g/dl in women or evidence of increased red cell volume • Presence of **JAK2 mutation**
Minor criteria • Hypercellular bone marrow biopsy with panmyelosis with prominent erythroid, granulocytic and megakaryocytic hyperplasia • Low serum erythropoietin level • Endogenous erythroid colony formation in vitro

Polycythemia Vera		
↑ Erythroid elements	**↑ Granulocyte elements**	**↑ Megakaryocytic elements**
Clinical features		
Erythrocytosis–polycythemia • Plethora/cyanosis • Neurological symptoms • Vertigo, tinnitus • Headache • Dizziness visual disturbances	Increased basophils Intense pruritis Peptic ulceration	↑ platelets (along with hyperviscosity) → Thrombosis and/or Platelet function abnormalities → Bleeding MC site- Upper GI from bleeding peptic ulcer
Lab features		
↑ RBC count, Hb, Hct ↑Blood viscosity ↓ESR	↑TLC ↑LAP Neutrophils–normal ↑Transcobalamine I and III ↑Vitamin B12 binding capacity	Increased platelet count Platelet function abnormalities Abnormal platelet aggregation studies

- **Spent phase:** Features of myelofibrosis develop
- Sometimes transform to AML

Myelofibrosis

Ineffective erythropoiesis → Leukoerythroblastic picture (immature leukocytes and nucleated RBCs in circulation)
Compensatory hematopoiesis → Enlarged spleen
Tear drop cells +, Dry tap on BMA
Abnormal large platelets (dysplastic megakaryoctes)

Causes of leucoerythroblastosis
Primary myelofibrosis
Secondary myelofibrosis • Infections – TB, fungal, HIV • Tumors – Metastatic carcinoma – Lymphomas, e.g. Hodgkins – Leukemias, e.g. CML, AML, Hairy cell – Plasma cell disorders- Multiple myeloma • Polycythemia vera • Lipid deposition – Gaucher's disease • Radiation therapy

Essential Thrombocytosis

- Diagnosis of exclusion
- Elevated platelet count is the hallmark (usually > 1000 X 10^9)
- WBC is only mildly elevated
- Haematocrit and RBC morphology- normal
- Philadelphia chromosome- absent
- LAP- normal or elevated

Cells and surface markers	
T-cells	CD1, CD3 (pan-T-cell marker), CD4, CD5, CD8
B-cells	CD10 (CALLA) CD19 (pan-B-cell marker), CD20, CD21, CD23, CD79a
Monocyte/Macrophage	CD11c, CD13, CD14, CD15, CD33, CD64
NK cell	CD16, CD56
Stem cell and progenitor cell	CD34
Activation marker	CD30
All leukocytes	CD45 (leukocyte common antigen, LCA)
Endothelium	CD31
Langerhans cell histiocytosis	CD1a
Tumor metastasis	CD44
Apoptosis	CD95
Plasma cell	CD38
Myelomonocytes	CD33
EBV receptor	CD21
Memory T-cell	CD 54RO

CLL

- Small lymphocytes mixed with larger cells called **prolymphocytes** which gather to form focal aggregates called **proliferation centers** which are pathognomic of CLL/SLL
- ***Smudge cells*** which are fragile CLL cells disrupted in the process of making slides
- Express CD19, CD20 and the ***specific markers CD23, CD5***

Clinical Features

- Usual age of presentation above 50
- Mostly asymptomatic
- Lymphocytosis is the hall mark of the disease
- Generalized lymphadenopathy, hepatosplenomegaly
- May transform in to prolymphocytic transformation or to a diffuse large B-cell lymphoma which is called **Ritcher syndrome**

Markers of poor prognosis in CLL (Wintrobes hematology)	
Routine	**Investigational**
• Advanced Rai or Binet stage • Male • "**Atypical**" morphology or CLL/PLL • Peripheral lymphocyte doubling time of < 12 months • $CD38^+$ • High β_2-microglobulin level • Diffuse marrow histology • High lactate dehydrogenase • Fludarabine resistance	• **Lack of IgV_H gene mutations** • Expression of ZAP-70 protein • Del 11q22–q23 (loss of ATM gene), del 17p13 (loss of p53), or trisomy 12 • Increased serum levels of CD23, tumor necrosis factor-α, and thymidine kinase

Multiple Myeloma

- Neoplastic proliferation of plasma cells
- The plasma cells proliferate from single clone of lymphocytes (monoclonal proliferation) and secrete homogenous Ig (monoclonal gammapathy)
- The monoclonal Ig present in blood is M component

Clinical Features

- Multiple punched out osteolytic lesions on X-rays is characteristic feature which present as pathological feature or bone pain. Vertebra are mostly involved
- Pancytopenia due to replacement of normal marrow elements by plasma cells
- Hypercalcemia
- Bence Jones light chain proteinuria which may lead to Renal failure and amyloidosis
- Frequent infections
- Cryoglobulinemia
- Hyperviscosity
- Abnormal coagulation

Lab Features

- Flame cells, Mott cells, Russel bodies (intracytoplasmic) and Dutcher bodies (intranuclear) in plasma cells
- Alkaline phosphatase level not increased

Diagnostic criteria
Monoclonal Gammopathy of Undetermined Significance (MGUS) • M protein in serum **< 30 g/L** • Bone marrow clonal plasma cells **< 10%**
• No evidence of other B cell proliferative disorders • No myeloma-related organ or tissue impairment (no end organ damage, including bone lesions)
Asymptomatic Myeloma (Smoldering Myeloma) • M protein in serum **≥ 30 g/L** *and/or* • Bone marrow clonal plasma cells **≥ 10%** • No myeloma-related organ or tissue impairment (no end organ damage, including bone lesions) or symptoms
Symptomatic Multiple Myeloma • M protein in serum and/or urine • Bone marrow (clonal) plasma cells or plasmacytoma • Myeloma-related organ or tissue impairment (end organ damage, including bone lesions)
Nonsecretory Myeloma • No M protein in serum and/or urine with immunofixation • Bone marrow clonal plasmacytosis ≥10% or plasmacytoma • Myeloma-related organ or tissue impairment (end organ damage, including bone lesions)
Solitary Plasmacytoma of Bone • No M protein in serum and/or urinec • Single area of bone destruction due to clonal plasma cells • Bone marrow not consistent with multiple myeloma • Normal skeletal survey (and MRI of spine and pelvis if done) • No related organ or tissue impairment (no end organ damage other than solitary bone lesion)

Treatment

- Alkylating agent **(melphalan)** + prednisolone
- For hyperviscosity syndrome: plasmapheresis
- For hypercalcemia: bisphosphonates, glucocorticoids.

Hairy Cell Leukemia

- Leukemic cells have fine hair like projections
- Express CD19, CD20, CD22, surface IgH which are B cell markers
- **CD11c, CD25, CD103 (diagnostic), CD116** are typical for hairy cell leukemia
- Tartrate resistant acid phosphatase positivity of cytoplasm.

Clinical Features

- Male to female–4:1
- **Massive splenomegaly** is the most common presentation
- 1/3rd patients present with **infections**
- **Pancytopenia**
- Hepatomegaly less common
- **Lymphadenopathy rare**
- Indolent course
- Bone marrow aspiration: cannot be aspirated easily **(dry tap).**

Treatment

- **Cladirabine** is the treatment of choice
- Others: **pentostatin, interferon-α, Rituximab (anti-CD20)**
- Splenectomy.

Mantle Cell Lymphoma

- Usually presents in 5th and 6th decade
- Painless lymphadenopathy, splenomegaly
- Multifocal mucosal involvement of the small bowel and colon produces **'lymphatoid polyposis'**
- Express **CD19, CD20, CD5 and Cyclin D1** (characteristic); CD23 –ve
- Most common translocation **(11;14)**
- Prognosis poor

Burkitt Lymphoma

Types → African (endemic); Sporadic; In HIV patients

Morphology

- High mitotic index
- Starry sky pattern

Cytogenetics

- Translocation **(8;14)**
- Express IgM, CD19, CD20, CD10, BCL6
- All endemic tumors are infected with **EBV**

Clinical Features

- Endemic: Mass involving mandible and can involve kidneys, ovaries and adrenal glands
- Sporadic: Abdominal mass involving ileocaecum and peritoneum
- Rapidly progressive and can involve CNS
- Chemotherapy is the treatment of choice
- Translocations
- t (8;14): Burkitt's Lymphoma, ALL (FAB type-3)
- t (15;17): Pro myelocytic leukemia (M3- AML)
- t (4;11): ALL
- t (11;14): CLL, Mantle cell lymphoma
- t (14;18) : B cell lymphoma

Hodgkin Lymphoma

Distinguished from other lymphomas by the presence of ***Reed Stenberg's cells*** in the background of non-neoplastic inflammatory cells

Nodular sclerosis R-S cells: CD15+ CD30+ EBV- CD45-	Frequent **lacunar cells**	**Most common** type (70%) more common in females Excellent prognosis
Mixed cellularity R-S cells: CD15+ CD30+ 70% EBV +	Frequent **mononuclear** and diagnostic R-S cells	M > F, **Biphasic** incidence, Young adults and > 50, commonest type in India Good prognosis
Lymphocyte rich R-S cells: CD15+ CD30+ CD45- 40% EBV +	Frequent mononuclear and R-S cells, background rich in T cells	Uncommon Good prognosis
Lymphocyte depletion R-S cells: CD15+ CD30+ Most EBV +	Reticular variant	Common in **HIV infected** individuals and in developing countries worst prognosis
Lymphocyte predominance R-S cells: CD15- CD30- CD20+ BCL6+ EBV-	Frequent **L and H (popcorn) cell** in a background of follicular dendritic cells and reactive B cells	Young males with cervical or axillary lymphadenopathy Excellent prognosis

Clinical Course

Both HL and NHL present with painless enlargement of lymph nodes commonly neck nodes

One rare paraneoplastic symptom specific to HL **is pain in the involved node on consumption of alcohol**

Cyclical high grade fever **(Pel-Epstein fever)**

HL	NHL
More often localized to a single group of nodes (cervical, mediastinal, para-aortic)	More frequent involvement of multiple peripheral nodes
Orderly spread by contiguity	Noncontiguous spread
Mesenteric nodes and Waldeyer's ring rarely involved	Commonly involved
Extranodal involvement uncommon	Common

Treatment

- **ABVD** regimen: Adriamycin, bleomycin, vinblastine, dacarbazine
- **MOPP** regimen: Mechlorethamine, vincristine (oncovin), procarbazine, prednisone

BLEEDING DISORDERS

- Factors involved exclusively in intrinsic pathway-Factor XII, XI, IX, VIII, PREKALLIKREIN, HMW kininogen.
- Factors involved exclusively in extrinsic pathway-Factor VII, tissue thromboplastin (formerly called factor III).
- Factors involved in common pathway-Factor X, V, II, I, XIII.

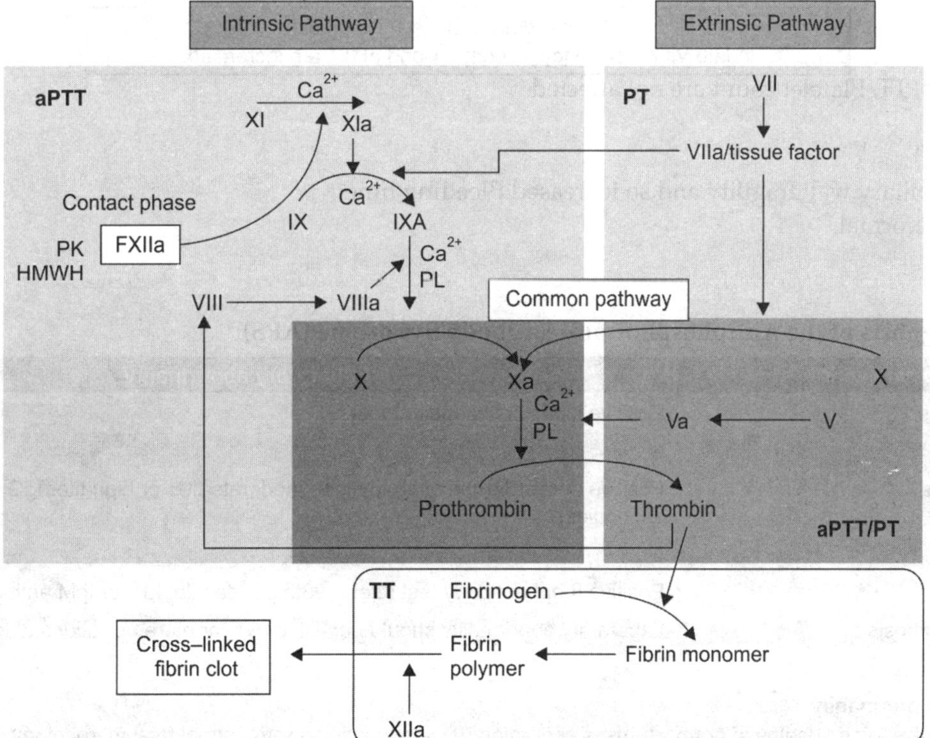

Isolated aPTT prolongation with bleeding manifestations	Isolated aPTT prolongation without bleeding manifestations
• Factor VIII, IX, XI defect • Factor VIII, IX, XI inhibitors	• Factor XII defect, prekallikrein and HMW Kininogen defect (contact factors) • Presence of Lupus anticoagulant

Isolated PT prolongation	Causes of prolonged PT and APTT
• Vitamin K deficiency • Liver disease • Warfarin therapy • F VII deficiency	• Coagulation factor deficiency (Factor X, V, II, Fibrinogen) • Use of oral anticoagulants (Warfarin) • Disseminated intravascular coagulation • Severe vit K deficiency • Liver disease (hepatic insufficiency) • Heparinised sample

Thrombin time is the time taken for the blood to clot when thrombin is added to it.

Thrombin time is raised in
Afibrinogenemia
Dysfibrinogenemia
DIC
Heparin usage

Vit K dependent factors- Factor II, VII, IX, X, protein C and protein S

Vitamin K is needed for γ carboxylation of these factors.

- Of these the **t1/2 of the factor VII is 3–6 hrs**. so factor VII (extrinsic pathway) abnormalities starts early in vit K deficiency.
- Whereas long standing vit K deficiency causes all the other factors to decrease.

> In early Vit K deficiency → PT increases
> In late Vit K deficiency → both PT and aPTT are increased.

Fibrinogen levels, TT, Platelet count are not affected

Vitamin C deficiency

- Increased capillary wall fragility and so increased Bleeding time
- PTT, PT, TT- Normal

APLA

Criteria for Diagnosis of the Antiphospholipid-Antibody Syndrome (APS)

Clinical event	Laboratory abnormality
Venous thrombosis	Positive lupus anticoagulant test
or	or
Arterial thrombosis	Positive anticardiolipin antibody test (moderate-titer or high-titer IgG or IgM antibodies)
or	or
	Positive $\beta_2$gpI antibody test (titer > 99th per-centile, IgG or IgM antibodies) and
Small-vessel thrombosis	Laboratory abnormality should persist for two or more occasions at least 12 wk apart
or	
Complications of pregnancy • One or more unexplained deaths of normal fetuses at or after 10 wk of gestation with normal fetal morphology • One or more premature births of normal neonates before 34 wk of gestation • Three or more unexplained consecutive spontaneous abortions before 10 wk of gestation, excluding anatomic, hormonal, and chromosomal abnormalities	

Contd...

Contd...

Laboratory Diagnosis of Lupus Anticoagulant: International Society on Thrombosis and Haemostasis Criteria
• Prolongation of at least one phospholipid-dependent coagulation test with the use of platelet-poor plasma (e.g., the activated partial thromboplastin time, dilute prothrombin time, **dilute Russell viper venom time**, kaolin clotting time)
• Failure to correct the prolonged coagulation time by mixing patient and normal plasma • Confirmation of lupus anticoagulant by demonstrating correction of the prolonged coagulation time by addition of excess phospholipids or freeze-thawed platelets • Exclusion of alternative coagulopathies using specific assays (e.g. factor VIII antibodies)

(If there is no bleeding history, but only APTT is prolonged, the most likely cause of prolonged APTT is a lupus anti coagulant.)

HEMOPHILIA

Hemophilia A	Hemophilia B (Christmas disease)
Deficiency of coagulant subunit of factor VIII (VIII c) (Factor VIII= VIIIc + VWF)	Deficiency or absence of factor IX
Whole blood clotting time- ↑ APTT- ↑ PT, BT, platelet count- normal	

Hemophilia A

- < 1% activity of factor VIII - severe disease; 2-5% - moderate disease; 6-50% - mild disease
- Hemarthroses +
- Petechiae are characteristically absent
- Treatment involves infusion of recombinant factor VIII or Cryoprecipitate

Pseudotumor Syndrome

Retroperitoneal hemorrhages can accumulate large quantities of blood with formation of masses with calcification and inflammatory tissue reaction and also result in damage to the femoral nerve

Chronic hemarthroses are debilitating, with synovial thickening and synovitis in response to the intraarticular blood. After a joint has been damaged, recurrent bleeding episodes result in the clinically recognized **"target joint,"** which then establishes a vicious cycle of bleeding, resulting in progressive joint deformity that in critical cases requires surgery as the only therapeutic option.

von Willebrand Disease

- Caused by deficiency of VWF

VWF- normal function	In VW disease
VWF is required for normal platelet adhesion and aggregation	Bleeding time-prolonged
It acts as a plasma carrier for factor VIII	Clotting time- prolonged, APTT- prolonged
This acts a cofactor for ristocetin induced aggregation	Impaired platelet aggregation in response to ristocetin

Types of VWD

- **Type 1:** AD, reduced quantity of circulating vWF
- **Type 2:** Type 2A is AD, qualitative defects in vWF. Otherwise called Autosomal hemophilia
- **Type 3:** AR, quantitative deficiency

Hemophilia A	von willebrand disease
X-linked recessive	Autosomal dominant
Factor VIII c decreased	Decreased
vWF normal	Decreased
Ristocetin cofactor normal	Decreased
Presents with features of clotting disorder (hemarthrosis++)	Presents with features of bleeding with clotting disorder (**skin and mucosal bleeding+**, hemarthrosis+)
Lab Investigations	
Bleeding time- normal	BT- prolonged
APTT- Prolonged	APTT- prolonged or normal
Platelet aggregation in response to ristocetin- normal	Platelet aggregation in response to ristocetin- decreased
PT- normal Thrombin time- normal Fibrinogen- normal	

Treatment of Hemophilia

Transfusion therapy	Nontransfusion therapy
Cryo-precipitate fraction Each bag contains 80 IU of factor VIII, fibrinogen, VWF FVIII dose (IU) = Target FVIII levels–FVIII baseline levels x body weight (kg) x 0.5 unit/kg **Target factor levels**: • Mild bleeds- factor level of 30–50% • Large hematomas- 50% • Serious bleeds- 50 to 100 % for 7 to 10 days	DDAVP- synthetic vasopressin analogue causes transient increase in factor VIII and VWF. Oral antifibrinolytic EACA or tranexamic acid to control local hemostasis. Not used for hematuria because of intra renal clot

Complications

Inhibitor formation: The formation of alloantibodies to FVIII or FIX is currently the major complication of hemophilia treatment. Amount of antibodies is expressed as betheda units.

Infectious disease: Hepatitis C viral (HCV) infection is the major cause of morbidity and the second leading cause of death in hemophilia patients exposed to older clotting factor concentrates.

Platelet Function Disorder

Disorders of Platelet Function

Disorders of adhesion	• von Willebrand disease • Bernard-Soulier syndrome (defect in GP Ib)
Disorders of aggregation	• Congenital afibrinogenemia • Glanzmann thrombocytopenia
Disorders of platelet-platelet interaction	• Storage pool deficiency • Quebec platelet disorder • Chediak-higashi syndrome • Gray-platelet syndrome • Wiskott-Aldrich syndrome
Disorders of platelet coagulation-protein interaction	• Scott syndrome

Bernard soulier syndrome	Glanzmann thrombasthenia
• Autosomal recessive • Deficiency of Gp Ib/Ix- platelet adhesion • Platelets cannot adhere	• Autosomal recessive • Deficiency of Gp IIb/IIIa complex • Platelets cannot aggregate
• Aggregation normal in response to standard agonists (collagen ADP, thrombin/but platelets fail to aggregate to ristocetin • Other lab parameters • Thrombocytopenia may be present • Abnormal large platelets • Prolonged bleeding time • VWF normal	• Platelet fail to aggregate to standard agonists but aggregate normally to ristocetin Other lab parameters **Bleeding time prolonged**
Recurrent episodes of severe mucosal hemorrhage	

Wiskott Aldrich syndrome- Classic TRIAD
• **Eczema → Eczematoid rash** • **Thrombocytopenia → Bleeding episodes** – ↓ platelet count – Small sized platelet – Impaired platelet aggregation response • **Immunodeficiency → Repeated infections** – ↓Ig M – ↑Ig E – Ig A and Ig G - Normal – Acquired T cell deficiency

Idiopathic Thrombocytopenic Purpura

- Antibody mediated platelet destruction
- Secondary antibody mediated destruction occurs in - SLE
  - AIDS
  - Viral infections
  - Drug induced
- Antibodies against GP IIb IIIa or GP Ib–IX

Two forms

Features	Acute	Chronic
Age	2–6 yrs	20–40 yrs
F:M	4:1	1:1
H/O infection	+	None
Eosiniophilia	+	–
Lymphocytosis	+	–
Spontaneous remission	+(2–6 wks) in 80% cases	–

Laboratory Features

Prolonged bleeding time

- Normal PT
- Normal APTT
- Normal fibrinogen
- Normal FDP
- Normal levels of coagulation factors

- **Treatment modalities**
  - Corticosteroids
  - IV immunoglobulins
  - Rituximab(anti CD20)
  - Splenectomy
- Differentiate between TTP and HUS

Features	HUS	TTP
Age	Childhood	Adult
Fever	Absent	Present
Neurological	Absent	Present
Neurological	Absent	Present
Infection	Present	Absent
Diarrhea	Present	Absent
Treatment	Supportive	Plasmapheresis
ADAMTS13	Normal	deficient

ENDOCRINOLOGY

Pituitary

- All the pituitary hormones are under stimulatory control of hypothalamus except PROLACTIN.
- Prolactin is under inhibitory control.

What is the substance which inhibits Prolactin secretion?

DOPAMINE

Pituitary apoplexy is associated with

- Pituitary adenoma
- Postpartum (sheehan's syndrome)
- DM
- HT
- Sickle cell anemia
- Acute shock

Pituitary apoplexy present as

- Headache
- Meningeal signs
- B/L visual changes
- Ophthalmoplegia
- Hypoglycemia
- Cvs collapse
- Death

Treatment of apoplexy presenting with

- Visual changes–surgical decompression
- Without visual changes - Glucocorticoids

Sheehan's Syndrome

All hormones need to be replaced. But steroids are essential to prevent CVS collapse.

Kallmann Syudrome

- Defective GnRH syunthesis
- Anosmia or hyposmia due to olfactory bulb agenesis or hypoplasia.
- Color blindness, optic atrophy, nerve deafness, cleft palate, renal defects, cryptorchidism and neurologic abnormalities such as MIRROR MOVEMENTS.
- Males; delayed puberty and micropenis
- Females: primary amenorrhea and failure of secondary sexual development.
- Low LH and FSH levels and low levels of testosterone-hypogonadotrophic hypogonadism.

Most common in pituitary

- MC cause for pituitary dysfunction (hyper/hypo)–Adenoma
- MC pituitary adenoma is–non functioning adenoma
- MC hypersecretoryadenoma–prolactinoma
- MC secondaries in pituitary is–CA breast (100% post pituitary)
  - < 10 mm microadenomas
  - > 10 mm macroadenomas

Tests for Pituitary insufficiency

Growth Hormone	Prolactin	ACTH
• Insulin tolerance test, • L-arginine test • L-dopa test • GHRH test	• TRH test	• Insulin tolerance test • CRH test • Metyrapone test

CRANIOPHARYNGIOMA

- Benign **suprasellar** tumor
- Derived from **Rathke's pouch**.

Clinical Features

Headache, vomiting, visualdefect, papilloedema, hypopituitarism, stalk compression,

CT, MRI: Cystic changes with **partial calcification**

Treatment: Transcranial orTranssphenoidal removal followed by radiotherapy (without R T 75% recur)

HYPERPROLACTINEMIA

- Prolactin is under the inhibitory control of hypothalamus
- Dopamine secreted by hypothalamus act on the D2 receptors of lactotrophs and inhibit Prolactin secretion
- Doaminergic drugs inhibit prolactin secretion
- Anti-dopaminergic drugs causes hyperprolactinemia.

Drugs causing Hyperprolactinemia

Dopamine antagonists	Dopamine synth inhibitor	Dopamine depletors	Others
• Phenothiazine • Metocloppramide • Risperidone	• Alfa-methyl dopa	• Reserpine	• Opiates • H2 blockers • Imipramine

Contd...

Contd...

Dopamine antagonists	Dopamine synth inhibitor	Dopamine depletors	Others
• Butyrophenone • Thioxanthine, sulpride			• SSRI (Fluoxetine) • CCB (Verapamil) • Estrogens • TRH • VIP

Visual defects in pituitary lesions

- **Bitemporal hemianopia + galactorrhea**
- **Craniopharyngioma-inferior temporal quadrontanopia-** bitemporal hemianopia
- **Pituitary mass -superior temporal quadrantonopia-** bitemporal hemianopia

Prolactinoma

- Serum prolactin level normal 10–25 mcg/l
- Most common cause of hyperpituitarism is an adenoma arising in anterior lobe
- Microadenomas are < 1 cm diameter and macroadenomas are > 1 cm diameter

Treatment of Prolactinoma (micro and macroadenoma)

Medical	Indications for surgery (Trans sphenoidal)
• Dopamine agonist - cabergoline, bromocriptine	• If prolactin levels are not controlled • If tumor growth continues • If tumor does not shrinks

Growth Hormone

Confirmatory test for Acromegaly

Demonstrating the failure of GH supression to < 0.04 mcg/l within 1-2 hour of 75 gm oral glucose 100 ml.

- Other tests for GH- **Insulin induced hypoglycemia test**
  - **Serum IGF -1 level-screening test**
  - **TRH mediated GH release**

In Acromegaly TRH paradoxically increases GH secretion. But this is not used for diagnosis of Acromegaly.

Diabetes Insipidus

- Syndrome with urine volume > 50 mg/kg/day
- Urine osmolarity < 300 mosm/l

Nephrogenic DI

Drugs (Calm Fraud)	Metabolic
• Cisplatin • Aminoglycosides • Lithium • Methotrexate • Foscarnet • Rifampicin • Amphotericin B • Demeclocycline	• Hypercalcemia • Hypokalemia • Sickle cell anemia • Genetic • Sarcodosis

Approach to polyuria

Step 1: Confirm polyuria.

24 hrs urine output > 50 ml/kg body weight

Step 2: Classify osmotic or non osmotic diuresis

Urine osmolarity > 300 mosm/l osmotic diuresis

Step 3 : Classify polydipsia or DI

Water deprivation test

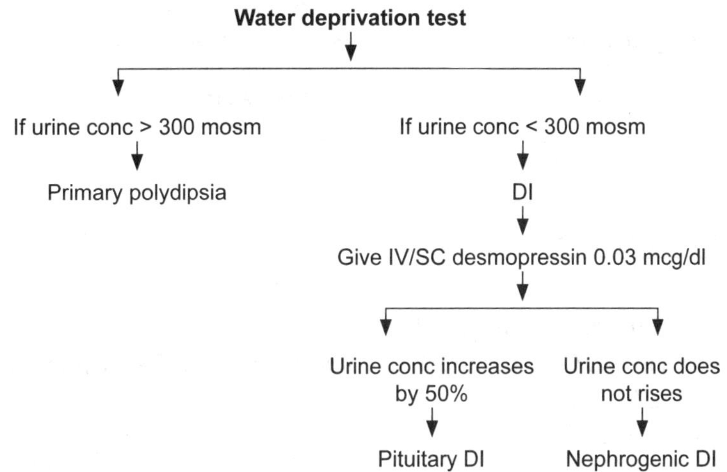

Treatment

- Pituitary DI–desmopressin
- Nephrogenic DI–Thiazide + K- sparing diuretic
  - Indomethacin

Primary Polydipsia–pt education to reduce water intake

Uses of Vasopressin

- DI
- Variceal bleeding vessel
- Nocturnaleneuresis
- Von willibrand disease
- Hemophilia

V1 receptor	V2 receptor
• Vasoconstriction • ACTH release • Glycogenolysis–liver	• Antidiuresis-kidney • Release of factor VIII-liver • Release of VWF-endothelium

SIADH

Causes of SIADH

Infections	Drugs	Malignancies
• TB • Cavity(aspergillosis) • Abscess(lung, brain) • Meningitis	• Vasopressin • Chlorpropamide • Vincristine • Carbamazepine	• CA lung, duodenum, bladder, uterus, ovary, Pancreas, thymoma, mesothelioma

Contd...

Contd...

Infections	Drugs	Malignancies
• Encephalitis • AIDS	• Cyclophosphamide • TCA • MAO inhibitors • SSRIs • Phenothiazines	• Bronchial adenoma, carcinoid, gangliocytoma • Ewing's sarcoma

Features	Treatment
• Hyponatremia • Hyperosmolar urine (150 mosm/lr) • Decreased serum osmolality (< 280 mosm) • ↓ BUN • ↓ S.creatinine • ↓ Uric acid • ↓ S.magnesium	• Fluid restriction • Demeclocycline • IV hypertonic saline • Fludrocortisone • Conivaptin

Endocrine Paraneoplastic Syndrome

- SIADH → small cell CA
- Cushing's syndrome → small cell CA, carcinoid
- Hypercalcemia → non small cell CA (suamous), CA breast, renal cell CA, myeloma
- Acromegaly → small cell CA, carcinoid

Adrenal

- Mineralocorticoids and glucocorticoids
- Mineralocorticoids- aldosterone

Actions	Deficient (Addison's disease)	Excess
• ↑ Na+ reabsorption in DCT and mainly on the P cells of Collecting ducts, water and chloride passively follow leading to increased ECF volume. • ↑ K+ and H+ ion excretion. • ↑ Na+ absorption in sweat glands, salivary glands, stomach and intestines **Net Effect** • ↑ ECF volume, plasma volume, blood volume, Cardiac output and hypertension	Due to TB/Auto-immune • ↑ Excretion of Na+, Cl, water • ↓ **K+** excretion • ↓ GFR and RPF leading to renal failure **Net Effect** • Hyponatremia, Hyperkalemia, Hyponatremia, Hyperkalemia, Hypoglycemia, hypotension, Dehydration and metabolic acidosis. **Addisonian crisis** • Severe circulatory shock, precipitated by stress	**Primary hyper aldosteronism (Conn's syndrome):** • **Tumors of Zona glomerulosa** • **Hypokalemia, Hypernatremia,** ↑ ECF volume, hypertension, polyuria, Alkalosis Secondary hyper aldosteronism • Due to extra-adrenal causes likes Cirrhosis, CCF, Nephrotic syndrome and Hypertension

- **GRA:** Mineralocorticoid secretion under the influence of ACTH stimulation
- **AME:** Mutation in 11β 2 HSD leading to mineralocorticoid activity of cortisol
- **Cushing's syndrome:** Excess cortisol overcomes the 11 β 2 HSD activity
- **Licorice ingestion:** Blocks 11 β 2 HSD activity
- **Liddle's syndrome:** ENaC (β/ϒ) sub unit mutation leading to excess action of Aldosterone

The diagnosis of primary hyperaldosteronism is

- ↑↑Serum aldosterone
- ↓Plasma renin activity

Glucocorticoids

Actions	Excess
• **Carbohydrate metabolism:** • ↑ blood sugar by – ↑**ing** gluconeogenesis and glycogenolysis in liver – ↓ing peripheral glucose utilization and insulin sensitivity. **(Adrenal diabetes)** • **Protein metabolism:** – ↑ Catabolism, ↑**N2** excretion and negative N2 balance. • **Fat metabolism:** – lipolysis, Ketosis • *Beneficial effects for the* actions of catecholamines, glucagon. • *Muscular efficiency.* • *Stress resistance.* • *Blood cells:* – Reduce the number of Basophils, Eosinophils, Lymphocytes (BEL), – Decrease the size of lymph nodes, – Thymic atrophy. • *Immunosuppression* • *Anti-inflammatory:* – By inhibiting the release of mediators • *Connective tissue:* – Reduces fibroblastic activity. • *Anti-allergic action:* • Inhibits the secretion of CTH, MSH, TSH, GH	• MC cause of Cushing's syn–latrogenic • MC cause of non iatrogenic Cushing's syn–pituitary adenoma • Cushing's disease –cushing syndrome due to pituitary adenoma May be due to primary adrenal tumor with low ACTH, or due to primary pituitary tumor due to excess ACTH secretion. **Clinical features:** • Centripetal fat distribution with obesity of the trunk (Buffalo hump), moon face • Thin and paper like skin, visible capillaries • Osteoporosis • Increased protein catabolism • Hyperglycemia and glycosuria – Hypertension **Nelson's syndrome:** • Development of ACTH secreting pituitary tumor following adrenalectomy for Cushing's disease.

Diagnosis

Screening test: overnight dexamethasone suppression test. 1 mg dexa given at midnight, plasma Cortisol measured next day at 8 am is < 140 nmol/L in normal individuals

Definitive diagnosis: measuring urine and plasma Cortisol after 0.5 mg of dexa every 6th hour for 2 days

Congenital Adrenal Hyperplasia

Types	Enzyme function	Mineralo corticoid activity	Gluco-corticoid activity	Androgen activity	Features
3 β-hydroxylase deficiency	Aldosterone and Cortisol synthesis	↓	↓	↑	Male hermaphrodite
11-β hydroxylase deficiency	Cortisol synthesis	↑	↓↓	↑	Hypertension Virilisation andprecocious puberty in Females
17-α hydroxylase deficiency	Cortisol and androgen synthesis	↑	↓	↓↓	Male hermaphrodite Hypertension
21-β hydroxylase deficiency	**Aldosterone and Cortisol synthesis**	↓	↓↓	↑	Hypotension **Virilisation in Females and precocious puberty in males**

For rememberance

- **Hypertension:** 11-hydroxylase deficiency and 17-hydroxylase deficiency.
- **Male hermaphroditism:** 3 β-hydroxylase deficiency and 17-hydroxylase deficiency
- **Female hermaphroditism:** 11-hydroxylase deficiency and 21-hydroxylase deficiency
- **21-hydroxylase deficiency: MC cause for ambiguous genitalia of newborn (virilisation) and primary amenorrhea.**

MEN I (Werner's syndrome)	MEN IIA (Sipple's syndrome)	MEN IIB
Pituitary adenoma/hyperplasia	Parathyroid adenoma/hyperplasia	Pheochromocytoma
Parathyroid adenoma/hyperplasia	Pheochromocytoma	Medullary carcinoma of thyroid
Pancreatic adenoma/hyperplasia/ carcinoma	Medullary carcinoma of thyroid Cutaneous lichen amyloidosis Hirschprung disease	Mucosal and GI neuromas Ganglioneuromas Marfanoid habitus

Diabetes Mellitus

- Type 1 DM is due to autoimmune mediated destruction of β cells.
- Destruction is mediated by T cells
- They have absolute insulin deficiency
- Type 1 is associated with HLA - DR3 and DR4

Virus associated with type 1 DM are

- Measles
- Mumps
- Coxsakie
- Rubella
- EBV

These viruses cause DM by triggering auto antibodies against B cells.

	Type 1	Type 2
Age of onset	< 20 years	> 30 years
Obesity	–	+
Family H/o of DM	Negative	Positive
HLA	DR3, DR4	-
Pathogenesis	Autoimmune destruction of B cells	Insulin resistance
Insulin level	markedly decreased	Not Markedly decreased
Symptoms	More common	Less common
DKA	common	Less common
HONK	Less common	More common
Insulin dependens	+	–

Level of insulin in type 2 DM

- The pathogenesis in DM2 is insulin resistance.
- Therefore initially there will be increased insulin secretion to overcome the resistance.
- This is the stage of Hyperinsulinemia.

Hyertriglyceridemia is common in type 2

Classical diabetic dyslipidemia is a triad of–Elevated LDL, Low HDL, Elevated triglycerides

Maturity onset diabetes in young

- Noninsulin dependent DM
- Occurs in pts younger than 25 yrs
- Patients are nonobese
- Easily under control of OHA
- H/o of similar DM in at least 2 generations.

It is an autosomal dominant transmission.

Diagnosis of DM–anyone of the below

- FBS ≥ 126 mg%
- PPBS ≥ 200 mg% (2 hrs after 100 g oral glucose)
- RBS ≥ 200 mg% with classical symptoms of DM
- HbA1C ≥ 6.5%

As per ADA 2012 guidelines

	Normal	Pre DM	DM
FBS	< 100	100–125	≥ 126
PPBS	< 140	140–199	≥ 200
HbA1C	< 5.8%	5.8–6.4	≥ 6.5%

HbA1C

HbA1C or glycosylated hemoglobin indicates the control of blood sugar for the past 8–12 weeks. The lifespan of RBC is 120 days. Any conditions which makes the RBC to lyse early will affect the reliability of HbA1c, e.g.

Hemolytic anemia–Hemoglobinopathies

Normal HbA1c is 5.8–6.4%

Fructosamine

- S.fructosamine–glycated albumin is another glycated protein
- Half life of albumin is 20 days. So S.fructosamine is useful to know the sugar control of past 2 weeks
- It is useful to monitor treatment during pregnancy where a strict control of DM is needed
- Also in hemolytic anemia and uremia where HbAic is not feasible.

Targets of DM management

- FBS < 130 mg%
- PPBS < 180 mg%
- HbA1c < 7%
- No episodes of hypoglycemia
- Bp < 130/80 mm Hg
- Bp < 125/75 mm Hg if nephropathy is present.

DKA

Clinical features of DKA	Biochemical parameters
• Nausea/vomiting • Poor appetite • Thirst • Polyuria • Dehydration	• Hyperglycemia • Hyperkalemia • Hyponatremia • Hypophosphatemia • Osmolality–increased slightly

Contd...

Contd...

Clinical features of DKA	Biochemical parameters
• Kussmal's breathing • Abdominal pain/tenderness • Hypotension • Tachycardia	• Sr.creatinine–increased slightly • Increased anion gap metabolic acidosis IN DKA • Urine ketone–positive • pH of blood–reduced

Serum measurements of ketone bodies (β -hydoxybutrate) is most specific and useful investigation in DKA

Indications of insulin in type 2 DM

- High blood sugar with symptoms at presentation.
- Secondary failure of OHA
- Any acute illness (infectious/non- infectious)
- Hospitalization, surgery
- Pregnancy
- DKA
- Hyper osmotic non ketotic coma
- Renal failure
- Hepatic failure

DM Neuropathy

Burning sensation of foot with diminished sensation for all sensory modalities.

'a painful painless foot'

Mononeuropathy

Most common–III cranial nerve with pupillary sparing.

Others–IV, VI, VII

Drugs in painful DM neuropathy

- TCA
- Gabapentin
- Pregabalin
- NSAID, Tramadol
- Mexiletne
- Phenytoin, CBZ
- Capscaicin cream

Rx of autonomic neuropathy

Nonpharmacological	Pharmacological
• Adequate salt intake • Avoid dehydration	• Fludrocortisone, yohimbine • **Mitodrine, clonidine, octreotide**

DM Retinopathy

- Nonproliferative DR
- Prolifertaive DR

NPDR	PDR
• Microaneurysm • Dot and Blot hemorrhages	• Hall mark–new vessel formation (neovascularization) • Retinal detachment
• Cotton wool spots (soft exudates) • Earliest change–micro aneurysm • MCC loss of vision in NPDR–macular edema	• Vitreous hemorrhage • Rubeosis iridis

Screening for DR

- Type 2–at diagnosis
- Type 1–5 yrs after diagnosis and yearly thereafter

Treatment

'Laser photocoagulation'

Macular edema–focal photocoagulation

Proliferative DR–pan retinal photocoagulation

Other ophthalmic complications in DM

- 3rd nerve palsy with pupillary sparing
- 4th and 6th nerve palsy
- Myopia due to change in refractive index of lens in acute hyperglycemia (not hypermetropia).

Diabetic Nephropathy

Stages of Diabetic Nephropathy

Stage I	Hyper functioning nephrons GFR–increased, Sr. creatinine low
Stage II	Thickening of GBM
Stage III	Stage of microalbuminuria (reversible)
Stage IV	Stage of macroalbuminuria (irreversible)
Stage V	ESRD

- Microalbuminuria = 30–300 mg of albumin per day
- It is also an indicator of high CVS risk.

Nodular glomerulosclerosis also known as

- Intercapillary GS
- Kimmensteil Wilson disease

Pathology of DM nephropathy

- Capillary BM thickening
- Diffuse mesangial matrix deposition
- Nodular glomerulosclerosis

Fibrin caps–hyaline material in capillary loops

Capsular drops–hyaline material in Bowman's capsule

Protein Excretion

- Normal < 150 mg/day
  - Proteinuria > 150 mg/day
- Significant proteinuria > 500 mg/day
- Nephritic/sub-nephrotic proteinuria > 2 g/day
- Nephrotic range proteinuria > 3 g/day

Albumin Excretion

- Normal < 30 mg/day
- Microalbuminuria 30–300 mg/day
- Macroalbuninuria/overt proteinuria > 300 mg/day
  - Protein creatinine ratio < 0.2/day–normal
  - Albumin creatinine ratio < 0.02/day–normal

Rx of DM Nephropathy

- Strict glycemic control
- Strict control of HT
- Dietary protein restriction
- Drugs–reno protective

ACE inhibitors

ARB's

Other drugs (somereno protection)

- β blockers, Non–DHP CCB's
- Aspirin–low dose
- Statins
- Avoid

Nephrotoxic drugs: NSAID's, Aminoglycosides, radio contrast agent, DHP CCB's and Diuretics as for as possible.

Hypoglycemia

Symptoms of Hypoglycemia

Autonomic response They are early symptoms They are mediated by counter regulatory hormones	Neuroglycopenic response They are late symptoms These are due to decreased nutrition to the neurons of brain
• Palpitation • Tremors • Sweating • Hunger • Parasthesia	• Behavioral changes • Confusion • Fatigue • Seizure • LOC, coma • Death

Causes of Hypoglycemic Unawareness

- Autonomic neuropathy
  - B blockers
- Recurrent hypoglycemia

Only the Autonomic response are blurred

Causes of Hypoglycemia

Critical illness	Endocrine deficiency	Endogenous hyperinsulinemia	Other malignancies	Drugs
• Hepatic failure • Renal failure	• Cortisol • Growth hormone	• Insulinoma	• Fibrosarcoma, • mesothelioma	• Insulin • OHA
• Sepsis • Starvation	• Glucogon and epinephrine		• Rhabdomyosarcoma • Liposarcoma • Hepatoma • Adrenocortical tumor, carcinoid • Leukemia, lymphoma, melanoma, teratoma	• Ethanol • Pentamidine, quinidine

Bone and Calcium

Hyperparathyroidism

Primary	Secondary
• Adenoma • Hyperplasia • Carcinoma	• CRF • Malsbsorption syndrome • Vit D deficiency • Medullary ca thyroid

- Hypocalcemia and hyperphosphatemia are the stimulus for secondary hyper PT

Skeletal changes in hyperPT

- Diffuse bone resorption
- Brown tumors
- Osteitisfibrosacystica
- Bending of long bones
- Cod fish vertebra
- Pathological fracture
- Fibrosis of marrow

X-Ray shows

- Osteoporosis
- Subperiosteal resorption
- Tufting of phalanges
- Pinhead stippling/pepper pot skull
- Absence of lamina dura in dental X-rays

PseudohypoPT

PseudohypoPT is a hereditary disorder characterized by insensitivity of peripheral tissues to PT action Therefore there are symptoms and features of hypoPT inspite of increased S.PT levels.

Features include

- ↑ PTH
- Hypocalcemia
- Hyperphosphatemia
- ↓ cAMP response to exogenous PTH

- Albright hereditary osteodystrophy
  - Short stature
  - Round face
  - Skeletal anomalies
  - Heterotrophic calcifications
  - Brachydactyly
  - Short 4th, 5th MC/MT

Vit D deficiency

	Rickets	Renal Osteo Dystrophy
Calcium	↓ or N	↓
Phosphate	↓	↑
PTH	↑	↑

Vitamin D and Analogs

Vitamin D2	Ergocalciferol
Vitamin D3	Cholecalciferol
25 OH Vitamin D3	Calciferol
1, 25 (OH)2 Vit D3	CALCITRIOL
24, 25 (OH)2 Vit D3	Secalcifediol

Osteoporosis

- Characterized by
- Reduced bone mineral density (BMD)
- Microarchitectural deterioration of bone tissue
- Increased risk of fracture (vertebra and hips)
- Common in postmenopausal women.

Treatment

Antiabsorptive agents	Bone forming agents
• Bisphosphonates • Estrogen and SERM • Calcium salts • Vitamin D and analogs • Calcitonin Thiazide diuretics	• Fluoride • Androgen and Anabolic Steroid • Parathormone • hPTH 1-34)

RHEUMATOLOGY

Inflammatory arthritis	Noninflammatory arthritis
• Rheumatoid arthritis • SLE • GOUT, Pseudogout • Infectious • Reactive arthritis	• Osteoarthritis • Fibromyalgia • Pigm. villonodular sinovitis • Bursitis, tendonitis • Rotator cuff tear

Clinical features

Inflammatory arthritis	Noninflammatory arthritis
• Signs of inflammation • Systemic symptoms • ↑ESR, CRP, thrombocytosis, anemia of chronic disease • Morning stiffness	• Pain without warmth • Day time clumsiness (gel phenomena) • Loose bodies or osteophytes

Pattern of joint involvement

Rheumatoid arthritis (distal sparing)	Osteoarthritis (proximal sparing)	Psoriatic
• PIP • MCP • CMC • Wrist • Distal IP joint spared	• DIP • PIP • I st carpo-metacarpal joint • Spared–MCP, CMJ – (except 1st), wrist	• DIP • PIP • MCP, CMJ, Wrist may be involved

Spine is spared in RA, except cervical spine.

Only cervical spine is involved in RA, of it atlanto-axial subluxuation is common.

Rheumatoid arthritisL: C1, C2

Judicial hanging: C2, C3 or C3, C4

Cervical spondylosis: C5, C6

Rheumatoid Arthritis

Classification Criteria for Rheumatoid Arthritis		
Joint involvement	1 large joint (shoulder, elbow, hip, knee, ankle) 2–10 large joints 1–3 small joints (MCP, PIP, Thumb IP, MTP, wrists) 4–10 small joints > 10 joints (at least 1 small joint)	**0** **1** **2** **3** **5**
Serology	Negative RF and negative ACPA Low-positive RF or low-positive anti-CCP antibodies (3 times ULN) High-positive RF or high-positive anti-CCP antibodies (> 3 times ULN)	**0** **2** **3**
Acute-phase reactants	Normal CRP and normal ESR Abnormal CRP or abnormal ESR	**0** **1**
Duration of symptoms	< 6 weeks 0 ≥ 6 weeks	**0** **1**

These criteria are aimed at classification of newly presenting patients who have at least 1 joint with definite clinical synovitis that is not better explained by another disease.

Application of the newly revised **New 2010 ACR-EULAR criteria** yields a score of 0–10, with a score of 6 fulfilling the requirements for definite RA.

HLA and Rheumatoid arthritis

- Major genetic risk factor–HLA DR 4
- Aggressive disease–HLA DR 4–01, 04 subtypes
- Juvenile Rh.A–HLA DR 5, HLA DR 8

HLA associations

Juvanile RA	DR 5, 8
Diabetes mellitus Type 1	DR 3, 4 (DR 2 Negative association)
Narcolepsy	DR 2
Behchet's disease	B51
Sjogrens syndrome	DR 3
Dermatitis Herpitiformis	DR 3
Psoriasis Vulgaris	CW 6
Pempigus Vulgaris	DR 4, DQ 1
Celiac Disease	DQ 2

Extraarticular Manifestation of RA

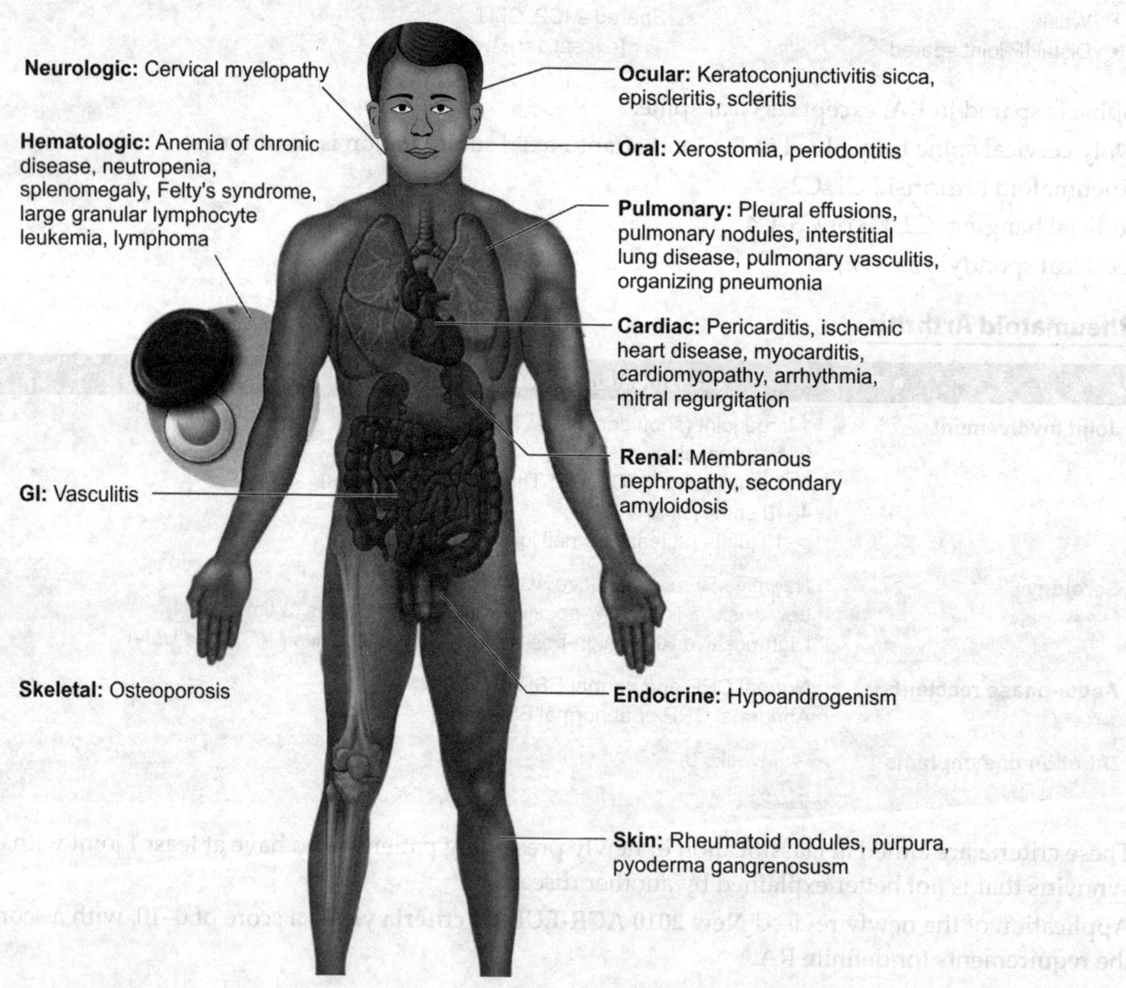

FELTY'S syndrome

- Chronic rheumatoid arthritis
- Splenomegaly
- Neutropenia

Focus of attack: Articular cartilage.

Rheumatoid factor

IgM antibody against the Fc portion of IgG
Seen in 75–80% of pts with RA
Not an useful screening test/diagnostic test
Good prognostic indicator, quantitative marker of disease activity
Level correlates with extraarticular manifestations, subcutaneous nodules, vasculitis.

False positive Rh.factor

Autoimmune causes	Infectious causes	
• SLE (coombs positive) • Sjogrens • Sarcoidosis • Chronic liver disease • Interstitial pulmonary fibrosis	• Infectious mononucleosis • Hepatitis B • TB • Leprosy • Syphilis	• SABE • Visceral Leismaniasis • Schistosomiasis • Malaria

Most specific test for RA

- Anti CCP antibodies
- Same sensitivity, but better specificity than RF
- Prognostic significance

Poor prognostic indicators

- Positive Rh.Factor and high titre
- Positive Anti CCP antibodies and high titre
- High CRP, ESR
- Severe clinical disease, extraarticular menifestations

Plain X ray

- **JA osteopenia**
- Soft tissue swelling
- Joint space loss
- Subchondral erosion
  - MRI–more sensitive for detecting synovial jt effusion, early bone, marrow changes
  - USG–detects erosion better than X-ray
  - Juxtra articular osteopenia.

Rheumatoid arthritis treatment

- Drugs for Rheumatoid arthritis
- NSAIDs
- Glucocorticoids
- DMARDs: Coventional
- DMARDs: Biologicals

Indications for systemic steroids in Rh.A

- To achieve disease control
- Acute flares management
- Chronic low dose for maintenance
- Specific indications
- Mononeuritis multiplex

- Endocarditis
- Pericarditis
- Scleritis
- ACR has recommended Bisphosponates in all patients receiving Prednisolone mg/day for > 3 months

RA-Treatment

- **DMARD-Conventional**
  - Hydroxy chloroquine
  - Sulfasalazine
  - MTX
  - Leflunamide
  - Minocycline
  - MTX is the initial choice–7.5 mg weekly once to 25 mg weekly once
  - Then add SAAZ or Leflunamide
  - Then add the third drug
- **DMARD-biological**
  - **Anti-TNF agents**
  - Infliximab
    - Etanercept
    - Adalimumab
    - Golimumab
    - Certolizumab pegol
- Anakinra–IL-1 receptor antagonist
- Abetacept-fusion product with CTLA-4, F8
- Rituximab-anti CD 20
- Tocilizumab–IL 6 antagonist

CRYSTAL ASSOCIATED ARTHROPATHY

Gout

Disease	Crystals	Appearance
• Gout	• Monosodium urate	• Needle shape
• Pseudogout	• Ca Pyro Phosphate dehydrate	• Rhomboid
• Oxalosis	• Ca Oxalate	• Bi pyramidal
• Ca. appetite deposit disease	• Ca. appetite	• Needle shape only in electron microscope

Treatment

- **Acute Gout**
  - NSAID
  - Colchicine
  - Glucocorticoids
- **Chronic Gout**
  - Uricosuric drugs- Probenacid, Benzbromarone
  - XO inhibitor–Allopurinol, Febuxostat
  - URATE lowering biological agent-Progliticase

CPPD DEPOSITION DISEASE

- MC in elderly
- Mutation in ANKH gene
- Associated with primary hyperparathyroidism, hemochromatosis, hypophosphatasia, hypomagnesemia, Gitelmans synd
- Pseudogout–active CPPD-D
- MC jt involved is knee jt
- **Chondrocalcinosis** is a feature of CPPD-D

CALCIUM APPETITE

- Associated with Milwaukee shoulder
- Hemorrhagic effusion in elderly

CALCIUM OXALATE

- Seen in CRF pts with hemodialysis
- Ascorbic acid supplementation

SLE

- Autoimmune disorder in which organs and cells undergo damage mediated by
  - Auto antibodies
  - Immune complexes
- 90% of pts are **women of child bearing age**

Risk Factors

- Female sex OCP
- HRT Klinefelter's synd
- UV light EBV
- Silica exposure soap powder dust

> = 4 of 11 Criteria Should be Positive

- **Malar rash**
- **Discoid rash**
- **Serositis**
- **Oral ulcer**
- **Arthritis**
- **Photosensitivity**
- **cns lupus** –seizures, psychosis
- **Hematological**-HA, leukopenia < 4000, lymphopenia < 1500, Thrombocytopenia < 1000000
- **ANA**
- **Immunological**–Anti DS, SM
- **Renal lupus** –proteinuria > 0.5g/dl/3+

Autoantibodies in SLE

Antibodies	Features	Pattern of fluorescence
ANA-M.C. antibody (98%)	• Best screening test for SLE • Repeated negative ANA–SLE unlikely	Homogenous or diffuse nuclear staining
Anti-ds ab	• SPECIFIC test for SLE in high titre • Correlate with disease activity	Rim or peripheral staining
Anti–SM	• SPECIFIC for SLE • Doesn't correlate with disease activity	Speckled pattern
Anti–Ro (SSA)	• Associated with sicca synd • SCLE–subacute cutaneous lupus • Neonatal lupus with congenital block • Decreased risk for renal lupus	Speckled pattern
Anti–La (SSB)	• Decreased risk for renal lupus	Speckled pattern
Antihistone	• Drug induced lupus	Homogenous or diffuse nuclear staining

- **Antiribosomal**–psychosis associated with cns lupus (serum)
- **Antineuronal**–CNS lupus (csf)
- **Anti–jo1** - myositis

Clinical Features

Musculoskeletal	• **M.c. symptom** • Erosions are rare • Hands, wrist, knee • Deformities 10% • Myositis
Cutaneous	• DLE: dermal appendages are permanently destroyed • Disfigurity • **SCARRING ALOPECIA** • About 50% are +ve for ANA • About 20 % of SLE have DLE
Malar Rash	• MC Rash in SLE, PHOTOSENSITIVE • Butterfly shaped
Subcutaneous Lupus Erythematous	• Scarly red circular flat red rimmed psoriasis like lesions • Photosensitive, +ve for anti –Ro (SSA) • **LUPUS PROFUNDUS**–Panniculitis
Diffuse CNS Lupus	• Cognitive dysfunction Headache • **Seizures Psychosis** • Myelopathy • **Responds POORLY to steroids**
Vascular:	• TIA • Stroke
Pulmonary	• Pleuritis • Shrinking lung syndrome • Intra alveolar He
Cardiac	• **Pericarditis (M.C)** • Myocarditis • Endocarditis- fibrinous, LIBMANSACKS • Increased risk of MI

Contd...

Contd...

Hematological:	• Anemia (MC)- N/N, hemolysis • Leukopenia < 4000 • Lymphopenia < 1500 • Thrombocytopenia < 1 lac
GIT:	• Autoimmune peritonitis • Interstitial vasculitis • Raised liver enzymes
Ocular	• SJOGREN synd (Anti –Ro ab)
	• Conjunctivitis, retinal vasculitis, optic neuritis • Cataract
Lupus Nephritis 30–50 %	• Most serious manifestation • **Nephrits and infections are most common cause of death in first decade of disease** • Urine analysis is needed for all patients • Renal biopsy useful for planning treatment

LN- Treatment

SLE Treatment

Non Life-Threatening

- Anti malarials-HCQ, DHEA
- Topical steroids, sunscreens, antimalarials
- Methotrexate

Life-Threatening

- High dose steroids
  - Cyclophosphamide
- Azathioprine
  - Rituximab
- Mycophenolate mofetil,
  - Belimumab

Pregnancy and Lupus

- **Usually well tolerated** but small proportion may cause a flare
- **Increased fetal loss**
- **11–beta dehydrogenase 2**–a placental enzyme derivatives glucocorticoids except fluorinated glucocorticoids (dexa and betamethasone)
- **Breastfeeding is not indicated** when mother is on immunosupressants
- **LBW babies**
- **Maternal anti–Ro** abs increases the risk of neonatal lupus (rash, cong heart block), monitor FHR when mother is anti Ro +ve

Poor Prognosis

- S. Creatinine > 1.4 mg%
- Hypertension
- Nephrotic synd (24 hr urine protein > 2.6 g)
- Anemia (< 12.4 g/dl)
- Hypoalbuminemia
- Hypocomplimentemia
- aPL
- Male sex
- Ethnicit y(african, american, hispnic)

Drug Induced Lupus

- Less female prediction
- Rarely involves kidney and brain

Antibody to histone

Antiarrhythmics	• Procainamide • Disopyramide • Propafenone
Antihypertensives	• Hydralazine • ACE I • Beta blockers
Antithyroid	• Propylthiouracil
Antipsychotics	• CPZ, Li
Antibiotics	• INH, minocycline, macrolides
Antirheumatic-	• Sulfasalazine
Diuretic	• Hydrochlorthiazide
Hypolipidemic drugs	• Lovastatin, simvastatin

VASCULITIS

Vasculitis - Classification (also called CHAPELL-HILLS classification)

Primary	Secondary
	• Drug induced • Serum sickness • Infections • Malignancy • Rheumatic disease

Classification based on size of blood vessels

Large vessel vasculitis	Medium vessel vasculitis	Small vessel vasculitis
• Giant cell arteritis • Takayasu arteritis	• PAN – Kawasaki • Burger's disease	• Wegeners • Microscopic PAN • Churg strauss synd • HSP • Essential cryoglobulinemia • Cutaneous leucocytoclastic arteritis • Drug induced vasculitis

Pathological Classification

Granulomatous	Necrotizing	Necrotizing and Granulomatous
• Giant cell • Takayasu • WG • Churg strauss	• PAN • Microscopic PAN • WG • Churg strauss synd	• WG • Churg strauss synd

- **Churg strauss:** Eosinophil rich granulomas
- **HSP:** IgA dominant immune deposit
- **Essential cryoglobulinemia:** Cryoglobulin immune deposits
- **Cutaneous vasculitis:** Leukocytoclastic angitis

ANCA

ANCA: Antibodies against certain proteins in the cytoplasmic granules of neutrophils and monocytes

C- ANCA	Diffuse, granular staining	Wegeners granulomatosis-antibodies against PROTEINASE-3
P ANCA	Localized perinuclear	**Myeloperoxidase** • Microscopic PAN • Cutaneous vasculitis • Crescentic GN • Chrug strauss **Non myeloperoxidase** • Rheumatic diseases • Auto immune diseases • IBD • IE • Cystic fibrosis

WEGENERS GRANULOMATOSIS

Granulomatosis with Polyangitis

- Small arteries
- Necrotising vasculitis
- Granuloma formation

TRIAD

Upper RST (95%)	Pulmonary (85–90%)	Renal (71%)
• Sinusitis • Septal perforation • Serous otitis media • Subglottic tracheal stenosis	• Necrotizing granuloma/cavity formation	• FSGN-may rapidly progress

Biopsy

- Granulomatous inflammation with necrosis
- Renal–pauci immune GN
- Granuloma rarely involves kidney

MICROSCOPIC PAN

Small Vessel Vasculitis

Clinical Features

- Fever, myalgia, wt loss
- Hemoptysis (alveolar Hage)
- Glomerulonephritis
- Mononeuritic multiplex

PAN

Necrotising vasculitis of medium sized arteries

Not involved in PAN

- Glomerular involvement–but renal arteries are involved
- Pulmonary arteries–but bronchial vessels are involved
- Eosinophilia, allergy
- Venule involvement

Associated with Hep .B and Hairy cell leukemia

Clinical features

Skin	Cardiac	CNS	Others
• Rashes, purpura, cutaneous infarcts • Livedo reticularis	• CCF • MI • Pericarditis	• CVA • Seizure	• Musculoskeletal • Renal–renal failure, **hypertension** • GIT, bowel, liver, pancreas infarction

WG	Microscopic pan
GRANULOMA + Upper airway + Pulmonary nodules Pauci immune GN without vasculitis in renal biopsy 90% c-ANCA + ve	----- ----- ------ Pauci immune GN with vasculitis without granuloma 79 % p-ANCA +ve

Classical pan	Microscopic pan
• Medium sized vessels involved • Doen't involve lungs • GN –rare • Renin mediated HT • ANCA negative	• Small sized vessel • Common • Common • HT–rare • P–ANCA posive

CHURG STRAUSS SYND

Allergic angitis and granulomatosis
Asthma
Eosinophilia (peripheral/tissue)
Granuloma (extravascular)
Vasculitis (multiple organ)

Clinical Manifestations

- **MC manifestation is pulmonary, severe asthmatic attacks, pulmonary infiltration**
- **Mononeuritis multiplex-** 2nd MC symptom
- Allergic rhinitis/sinusitis
- Cardiac disease–myocarditis **(important cause of mortality)**
- Purpura, cutaneous nodules

HENOCH SCHONLEIN PURPURA

Other name: Anaphylactoid Purpura

Palpable purpura (Due to vasculitis, not thrombocytopenia) seen in buttocks and lower extremities.
Arthralgia/arthritis-non-deforming, involves large joints, migratory
GI symptom-bleeding, Intussusception, passage of blood and mucus per rectum)
GN-microscopic hematuria
More common in **CHILDREN**
Ig A immune complex in renal biopsies

- Diagnosis–skin biopsy-leucocytoclastic vasculitis with Ig A and C3 deposits
- Prognosis–excellent
- Treatment-prednisolone

GIANT CELL ARTERITIS

Cranial arteritis (or) Temporal arteritis.
Closely associated with **polymyalgia rheumatica**
Occurs almost exclusively in age > 50 yrs
Women more commonly affected.

Clinical Features

- Fever
- Headache
- Features of polymyalgia
- Tender, thick, nodular palpable arteries
- Ischemic optic neuropathy–loss of vision
- Stroke
- **Scalp or tongue infarction**

Lab

↑ESR, ↑SAP, Normocytic normochromic anemia

Diagnosis

- BIOPSY of temporal artery
- **Segmental involvement** is there, so take 3-5 cm biopsy and do serial sectioning.
- HPE: Pan-arterial mononuclear infiltrates- giant cell granuloma
- USG of temporal artery
- Clinical response to a trial of steroids

Rx

- Exquisitely sensitive to steroids
- Aspirin 81 mg/day.

KAWASAKI DISEASE

- Mucocutaneous lymph node syndrome.
- Age < 5 yrs
- Characterized by
  - Nonsuppurative cervical adenitis
  - Conjunctival congestion, erythema
  - Desquamation of skin in finger tips
  - Coronary artery aneurysm (25%)
  - Vasculitis of coronary arteries
    - (MC cause for mortality)
- Rx–IV Ig and Aspirin

TAKAYASU ARTERITIS

Aortic arch syndrome

Pulseless disease

- Adolescent girls and young women
- Pan-arteritis with inflammatory mononuclear infiltrates–occasional giant cells
- Intimal–proliferation fibrosis
- Media–scarring vasculitis
- Elastic lamina–disruption and degeneration
- **Subclavian** most common artery involved 93%
- Common carotid 58%
- Renal artery involvement 38%, hypertension 32–93%
- Coronary < 10%
- Arteriography
  - Stenosis
  - Aneurysm formation

SYSTEMIC SCLEROSIS

	Limited	Diffuse
Skin	Hands and face	Trunk
Reynauds' phenomenon	Precedes by 1 year	Coincides with disease
Joint involvement	Arthralgia	Carpel tunnel syndrome
Pulmonary fibrosis	Less	More
PAH	More	Less
Renal crisis	Less	More
calcinosis	More	Absent
Antibodies	Anti centromere Ab	Anti topho-isomerase I Anti RNA polymerase III

MIXED CONNECTIVE TISSUE DISORDER

- Features of SLE, Polymyositis, RA
- u1RNP Ab
- Presents with Raynaud's phenomenon.

GIT AND MISCELLANEOUS

Liver Function Tests

Excretory function tests	Tests for Hepatocellular damage	Tests for Cholestasis	Biosynthetic function tests
• S.Bilirubin • U.Bilirubin • B.Ammonia • U.Urobilinogen_	• ALT • AST	• SAP • 5'–Nucleotidase • GGT	• S.Albumin • S.Globulin • Prothrombin time

- ALT → more specific for liver.
- AST/ALT ratio < 1 in nonalcoholic liver disease.
- Low levels of ALT is due to alcohol induced deficiency of **Pyridoxal phosphate.**

Markers of Alcoholic Hepatitis

- AST/ALT > 1
- AST/ALT > 2 suggestive of alcoholic hepatitis.
- AST/ALT > 3 highly suggestive
- GGT increased
- Marked elevation of serum bilirubin inspite of moderate elevation of SAP
- PMN > 5500/UL

Discriminant Function

- DF = 4.6* [prolongation of PT] + S.Bilirubin
- DF > 32 indicates poor prognosis in alcoholic hepatitis.

Prognostic indicators in liver disease

Child pugh scoring	Meld scoring	Peld scoring
• S.Bilirubin – S.Albumin – PT – Ascites – HE	• S.Bilirubin • PT • S.Creatinine	• S.Bilirubin • PT • S.Albumin • Age • Nutritional status

Hereditary Hyperbilirubinemias

Criggler Najjar Syndrome

	CN I	CN II
UGT1A1	Absent	Reduced < 10%
Bilirubin	20	< 20
Kernicterus	Usual	Rare
Bile color	Colorless	Pigmented
PBT	No response	25% decrease in bilirubin

Disorder	Defects	Pathology
Unconjugated hyperbilirubinemia		
Criggler-Najjar syndrome type I AR	Absence of UGT1A1 activity	• Liver normal • Usually fatal in the neonatal period • No response to phenobarbitone • Kernicterus in the newborn period
Criggler-Najjar syndrome type II AD		• Liver normal • Generally mild, occasional kernicterus • Phenobarbitone can improve bilirubin glucuronidation by inducing hypertrophy of hepatocellular EPR • Kernicterus rare
Gilbert syndrome AD	Decreased UGT1A1 activity	• Liver normal • Asymptomatic, detected during adolescence, jaundice precipitated by stress, fasting or infections • Phenobarbitone normalizes bilirubin
Conjugated hyperbilirubinemia		
Dubin-Johnson syndrome AR	Impaired biliary excretion of bilirubin glucuronides due to mutation in canalicular multidrug resistance protein 2 (MRP-2)	• Lliver darkly pigmented • Lysosomes contain polymers of **epinephrine** metabolites
Rotor syndrome AR	Decreased hepatic uptake and storage, decreased bilirubin excretion	• Liver normal

Bromosulphalein (Sulpho Bromophthalein) test

BSP is anionic chole cystographic contrast agent which utilizes MRP2 for excretion.

In patients of DJS, BSP shows a characteristic rise in plasma concentration at 90 min due to reflex of conjugated BSP from hepatocytes.

Viral Hepatitis

Virus	Hepatitis A	Hepatitis B	Hepatitis C	Hepatitis D	Hepatitis E
Type of virus	ssRNA	Partially dsDNA	ssRNA	Circular defective	ssRNA
Viral family	Hepatovirus: related to picornavirus	Hepadnavirus	Flaviridae	Subviral particle in Deltaviridea	Calcivirus
Rout of transmission	Fecal-oral (contaminated food or water	Parenteral, sexual contract, perinatal	Parental; intranasal cocain use is a risk factor	Parenteral	Fecal-oral
Mean incubation period	2–4 weeks	1–4 months	7–8 weeks	Same as HBV	4–5 weeks
Frequency of chronic liver disease	Never	10%	~80%	5% (coinfection; $\leq$70% for superinfection	Never
Diagnosis	Detection of serum IgM antibodies	Detection of HBsAg or antibody HBcAg	PCR for HCA RNA; 3rd-generation ELISA for antobody detection	Detection of IgM and IgM antibodies; HDV RNA serum; HDAg in liver	PCR for HEV RNA; detection of serum IgM and IgM antibodies

Acute hepatitis	Chronic hepatitis
Enlarged, reddened liver; greenish if cholestatic **Parenchymal changes:** • Hepatocyte injury: swelling (ballooning degeneration) • Cholestasis: canalicular bile plugs • HCV: mild focal fatty change of hepatocytes • Hepatocyte necrosis: isolated cells or clusters • Cytolysis (rupture) or apoptosis (shrinkage) • If severe: bridging necrosis (portal-portal, central-central, portal-central) • Lobular disarray: loss of normal architecture • Regenerative changes: hepatocyte proliferation **Sinusoidal cell reactive changes:** • Accumulation of phagocytosed cellular debris in Kupffer cells • Influx of mononuclear cells into sinusoids **Portal tracts:** • Inflammation: predominantly mononuclear • Inflammatory spillover into adjacent parenchyma, with hepatocyte necrosis	**Changes shared with acute hepatitis:** • Hepatocyte injury, necrosis, and regeneration • Sinusoidal cell reactive changes **Portal tracts:** • Inflammation: • Confined to portal tracts, or • Spillover into adjacent parenchyma, with necrosis of hepatocytes ('interface hepatitis'), or • Bridging inflammation and necrosis **Fibrosis:** • Portal deposition, or • Portal and periportal deposition, or • Formation of bridging fibrous septa • HBV: 'ground-glass' hepatocytes, 'sanded] nuclei • HCV: bile duct epithelial cell proliferation, lymphoid aggregate formation **Cirrhosis: The end-stage outcome**

- Most common epidemic in children–A
- Most common epidemic in adults–E
- Most common mortality in pregnancy–E
- DNA virus–B

Hepatitis B

Gene	Gene products
S	HBs Ag
C	HBc Ag
P	DNA polymerase
X	HBx Ag

Hepatitis 'B'markers

Seropatterns of HBV Infection

HBsAg	Anti-HBs	Anti-HBc	HBeAg	Anti-HBe	Interpretation
+	–	IgM	+	–	Acute infection
–	–	IgM	+/–	+/–	Acute infection, anti-HBc window
+	–	IgG	+	–	Chronic infection, high infectivity
+	–	IgG	–	+	Chronic infection, low infectivity
+	–	+/–	–	–	Precore infection/core mutant infection
+	–	IgG	–	+/–	Hepatitis B carrier
–	+	IgG	–	+/–	Recovery from infection
–	+	–	–	–	Immunization, false positive, infection in remote past

Markers of Viral Replication

- Viral DNA
- DNA polymerase
- HBeAg (qualitative marker)

Molecular Mutants

- Pre core mutant
  - Mutation in pre C region
  - HBeAg could not be synthesized
  - Anti HBe Ab will be present.
- Escape mutants
  - Mutation in position 145 of HBsAg (glycine to arginine)
  - This is the immuno determinant region.
  - This leads to HBV infection inspite of Anti HBsAg antibodies

Chronic Hepatitis

- Persistence of HBsAg beyond 6 months
- Anti HBcAg IgG
- Absent Anti HBsAg Ab

Chronic Rreplicative	Chronic nonreplicative
• HBeAg positive • HBV DNA $(10)^5$ –$(10)^6$/ml	• HBeAg negative • HBV DNA < $(10)^3$

Markers Of HBV

Acute

- Incubation period 30–180 days
- HBsAg - first marker–appears in 8–12 weeks

- HBeAg–appears along with or following HBsAg
- Transaminases increases
- IgM Anti HBc appears 1–2 weeks following HBsAg
- HBeAg returns to normal
- Anti HBe appears
- HBsAg returns to normal (6 months)
- IgM Anti HBc converted to IgG Anti HBc (window period)
- Anti HBsAg increases.

Chronic

- HBsAg does not reduce beyond 6 months
- Anti HBsAg not formed

Pre Core Mutant

- HBeAg absent but Anti HBe Ab present

Extrahepatic Manifestation of Hep B

- GN with Nephrotic syndrome
- PAN
- Essential mixed cryoglobinuria
- Arthritis
- Cutaneous vasculitis

Extrahepatic Manifestation of Hep C

- Essential mixed cryoglobinuria
- Lichen planus
- Sjogrens
- Porphyria cutanea tarda

Treatment of Hepatitis B

- Parameters to be considered
  - HBeAg–reactive/negative
  - Clinical presentation
    - Asymptomatic
    - Chronic hepatitis
    - Compensated cirrhosis
    - Decompensated cirrhosis
  - HBV DNA
    - Increased
    - Not increased
  - ALT
    - Increased 2x
    - Not increased

Asymptomatic patients

	HBeAg reactive	HBeAg negative
If both DNA and ALT are negative	No Rx	No Rx
If DNA is + ve, ALT < 2x	No Rx	Liver biopsy
If DNA is + ve, ALT > 2x	Liver biopsy	Treat

Chronic hepatitis

	HBeAg reactive	Negative
Both + ve	Treat	Treat
DNA + ve, ALT - ve	Observe	Liver biopsy

- **Compensated cirrhosis**
  - Treat if any one (ALT/DNA) is positive, for both HBeAg positive and negative
- **Decompensated cirrhosis**
  - Treat even DNA is detectable

Drugs

- Injectable
  - IFN α
  - PEG–INF
- Not used in compensated/decompensated cirrhosis
  - Oral
    - Lamivudin - Entacavir
    - Tenofovir - Adefovir dipivoxil
    - Telbevudine

Treatment of HCV

Indications for Treatment

- Positive HCV RNA (with or without ALT rise)
- Portal or bridging fibrosis in biopsy

So in this patient if HCV RNA is negative, go for liver biopsy.

Treatment of relapse after IFN mono therapy, Treatment of non responders to IFN mono therapy

PEG–IFN + Ribavirin

Factors associated with reduced response to IFN - ribavirin

- SND–T allele at 1L28B locus
- Genotype I
- High RNA titre
- Long duration of disease
- Age > 40
- Immunosuppression
- DM2
- Obesity
- Fatty liver
- African american, Latino ethnicity

Cirrhosis

Micronodular cirrhosis	Macronodular cirrhosis	Both
• Primary biliary cirrhosis	• Post necrotic	• Alcoholic
• Hemochromatosis	• Post viral	• Tyrosinemia
• Laennec cirrhosis (alcoholism)	• Wilson's disease	• α1 antitrypsin deficiency
Indian childhood Cirrhosis	Crytogenic	

Microvesicular fatty change	Macrovesicular fatty change	Granualoma formation	Fibrosis/cirrhosis
• Valproate	• Ethanol	• Sulfonamides	• Ethanol
• Tetracyclines	• Methotrexate	• Methyldopa	• Methotrexate
• Salicylates	• Amiodarone	• Quinidine	• Aminodarone
• Yellow phosphorus		• Phenylbutazone	• Other drugs causing hepatitis
• Ethanol		• Hydralazine	
		• Allopurinol	

Nonalcoholic fatty liver disease

Amino transferase are elevated only mildly (1.5–2 times) ALT > AST

- Associated with insulin resistance–syndrome X
- S.Ferritin is increase in 50% of the cases
- To diagnose NASH
  - Alcohol consumption should be < 20 g/day
  - Lab testing to R/O other liver disease
- Biopsy
  - Macro + micro vesicular steatosis
  - Mixed inflammation
  - Mallory bodies
  - Fibrosis–periventricular and perisinusoidal
- It is the most common cause of cryptogenic cirrhosis
- Once cirrhosis develops the biopsy will not show steatosis.

Treatment

- Weight loss and exercise
- Orlistat
- Bariatric surgery
- Thiazolininediones (PPAR gamma inhibitor)
  - Pioglitazone
  - Rosiglitazone
- Antoxidants
- Vitamin E
- Betaiene
- Statins
- UDCA(urso deoxy cholic acid)

Fulminant Hepatitis

Defined as HE occurs within 8 weeks of onset of precipitating illness in the absence of pre-existing liver disease.

Causes
- Drugs–paracetamol MCC
- Viral hepatitis–HDV (most common virus)
- Budd Chiari syndrome
- Reyes syndrome
- Acute fatty liver of pregnancy
- Carbon tetra chloride
- Wilson's disease
- Weils disease

Presentation

- Fetor hepaticus
- Hepatic encephalopathy
- Hepatorenal syndrome
- Cerebral edema
- Hypoglycemia
- Enzymes are mildly/moderately elevated
- S.Bilirubin is very high

Rx

- IV Mannitol
- IV Dextrose
- Liver transplantation

Hepatic Encephalopathy

Factors Precipitating H.E

Increased N_2 load	Electrolyte and metabolic	Drugs	Miscellaneous
• GI bleed • Excess dietary protein • Azotemia • Constipation	• Hypokalemia • Alkalosis • Hypoxia • Hyponatremia • Hypovolemia	• Narcotics • Tranquilizers • Sedatives	• Infection • Surgery • Acute or chronic liver disease • Porto systemic shunts • Massive transfusion • Recurrent diarrhea

Stages	CF	Astrixis	EEG
Stage I	Altered sleep pattern, euphoric Mild confusion	–	Triphasic waves
Stage II	Lethargy, moderate confusion	+	Triphasic waves
Stage III	Sleepy–aurosable Marked confusion	+	Triphasic waves
Stage IV	coma	–	Delta waves

EEG

- Symmetric
- High voltage
- Triphasic
- Slow wave (2–5/sec)

Treatment

- Supportive–nutritional
- Replace animal fat with vegetables
- Lactulose (2–3 stools/day)
- Neomycin
- Mebendazole

- Rifaximin 550 mg bd
- Zinc supplement
- Coenzyme Q 20

PORTAL HYPERTENSION

Site of Obstruction

Presinusoidal	Sinusoidal	Postsinusoidal
Portal vein thrombosis	Cirrhosis	Veno occlusive disease
Schistosomiasis	Acute alcoholic hepatitis	Jamaican bush tea
Idiopathic portal HT	Cytotoxic drugs	Pyrolizidine alkaloids
Congenital hepatic fibrosis	Vitamin A intoxication	Budd Chiari syndrome

Hypopnatremia

Hypovolemic hyponatremia/depletional hyponatremia (Na deficit with small water deficit)	Euvolemic hyponatremia/dilutional hyponatremia (Water retention alone)	Hypervolemic hyponatremia(Na retention + water retention)
Renal Na losses • Diuretic therapy • Adrenocortical failure GI Na losses • Vomiting • Diarrhea Burns	Primary polydipsia Water infusion SIADH Hypotthyroidism	CCF Cirrhosis Nephritic syndrome Chronic renal failure

D/D of Hyponatremia

Urine sodium	Urine osmolality	Possible diagnoses
Low (< 30)	Low (< 100)	• Primary polydipsia • Malnutrition • Beer excess
Low	High (> 150)	• Salt depletion • Hypovolaemia
High (> 40)	Low	• Diuretic action (acute phase)
High	High	• SIADH • Cerebral salt-wasting • Adrenal insufficiency

Pseudohyponatremia

Normal plasma osmolality	Increased plasma osmolality
Hyperlipidemia	Hyperglycemia
Hyperproteinemia	Mannitol
Post TURP	

QUESTIONS

1. A middle aged woman presents with black nasal discharge, right globe fixation and proptosis. Investigations reveal elevated blood sugar and positive urinary ketones. What is the appropriate therapy for this condition? (2014)

a. Amphotericin
b. Itraconazole
c. Broad spectrum antibiotic
d. Ketoconazole

2. Patient presents to emergency room with edema of tongue, stridor, dyspnea, hoarseness and itching following peanut consumption. Most likely cause is: (2014)

a. Foreign body larynx
b. Foreign body bronchus
c. Angioneuritic edema
d. Arapharyngeal abscess

3. An obese, diabetic patient with hypertension who is also a smoker, currently on antihyper-tension who is also a smoker, currently on anti-hypertensive and OHA drugs presents with complains of apnea during night. Polysomnography reveals 5 apneic episodes and 1 hypoapneic episode in one hour. What will be best next line of management is:

a. Nasal CPAP (2014)
b. Uvulopharyngopalatoplasty
c. Mandibular sling
d. Diet and weight reduction

4. Criteria for transudate pleura effusion:

a. WBC > 15000 (2013)
b. RBC 1000
c. Protein 3.5
d. Sp gravity 1.020

5. True statement regarding Heparin given in pulmonary embolism is: (2013)

a. Promptly dissolve clot
b. Increases lipoxigenase activity
c. HIT is a risk factor
d. Heparin given thrice a day

6. Rasmussen's aneurysm is seen in: (2013)

a. Bronchial artery
b. Pulmonary
c. Vertebral artery
d. Internal carotid artery

7. All are true about ARDS except: (2013)

a. Hypercapnia
b. Pulmonary infilatrates
c. Hypoxemia
d. Dyspnea

8. Spirometry finding in Restrictive lung disease profile: (2013)

a. Increased FEV1/FVC Decreased compliance
b. Increased FEV1/FVC increased compliance
c. Decreased FEV1/FVC Increased compliance
d. Decreased FEV1/FVC Decreased compliance

9. All are features of Obstructive sleep apnea except: (2013)

a. EVF
b. LVF
c. Hypoxia
d. Hypercarbia

10. Cystic fibrosis-Which of the following is not true? (2012)

a. Sweat sodium level < 50 meq/lit
b. Recurrent LRI
c. Sweat chloride level > 70 meq/l
d. Infertility

11. Transudative pleural effusion is seen in all except: (2012)

a. Uremia
b. Nephotic syndrome
c. Congestive heart failure
d. Liver cirrhosis

12. True statement regarding bronchiectasis are all except: (2012)

a. Upper lobe involvement seen in 'dry' bronchiectasis
b. Antibiotic may be used during exacerbation
c. Mucolytic has proven action in relief of secretions
d. HRCT is gold standard for diagnosis

13. Bronchial asthma is a: (2012)

a. Ventilation perfusion mismatch defect
b. Diffusion defect
c. Hypoventilation
d. Reversible airflow obstruction

14. Community acquired pneumonia is caused by all except: (2012)

a. Acinetobacter baumanii
b. H influenza
c. Staph aureus
d. Mycoplasma pneumonia

15. Alveolar haemorrhage is seen in all except: (2012)
a. Idiopathic pulmonary hemosiderosis
b. Good Pasture's Syndrome
c. Isolated Pulmonary Capillaritis
d. Idiopathic pulmonary fibrosis

16. Difference between bronchial asthma and COPD: (2011)
a. Reversible bronchoconstriction
b. Hyperventilation in Chest X-ray
c. Acute exacerbation following URI
d. Decreased FEV1/FVC

17. Absence of which of following makes a diagnosis of pulmonary embolism unlikely? (2011)
a. Pleuritic chest pain
b. Hemoptysis
c. Tachypnoea
d. Wheezing

18. Kussmaul breathing is seen in: (2011)
a. Metabolic acidosis
b. Metabolic alkalosis
c. Respiratory acidosis
d. Respiratory alkalosis

19. Hypoxemia in emphysema is due to all except: (2011)
a. Alveolar destruction
b. Increased anatomical dead space
c. Increased physiological dead space
d. Decreased elastic recoil

20. Kartagener's syndrome includes all except: (2010)
a. Situs inversus
b. Bronchiectasis
c. Lobar emphysema
d. Sinusitis

21. Following cranial nerve is most commonly involved in patients with sarcoidosis: (2009)
a. II cranial nerve
b. III cranial nerve
c. VII cranial nerve
d. IX cranial nerve

22. All are true regarding Pulmonary embolism except: (2008)
a. T wave inversion V1 to V4
b. Sinus bradycardia
c. Sight ventricular strain
d. S1Q3TS sign

23. Interleukin involved in asthma: (2008)
a. IL5
b. IL-1
c. IL-2
d. INF-alpha

24. Which of the following drug decreases the clearance of theophylline? (2008)
a. Rifampicin
b. Smoking
c. Phenobarbitone
d. Cimetidine

25. Criteria for transudate pleura effusion all except: (2007)
a. WBC < 1000/cmm
b. RBC < 5000/cmm
c. Protein < 3 g/dL
d. Glucose < 60 mg/dL

26. Residual volume of in an average adult male is: (2007)
a. 3.0 L
b. 0.9 L
c. 1.2 L
d. 1.9 L

27. Which of the following is not characteristic of benign murmur? (February 2014)
a. Diastolic murmur
b. Diastolic murmur
c. Grade 3 murmur
d. Mammary soufflé

28. Defibrillator failed in stopping ventricular fibrillation following cardiac arrest. What is the next line of action? (February 2014)
a. Amiadarone
b. Lidocaine
c. Verapamil
d. Propafenone

29. All the following ECG features indicates ventricular tachycardia except: (February 2014)
a. Capture beats
b. Similar QRS in all leads
c. Left axis deviation
d. Broad complex tachycardia

30. All are ECG features seen in hyperkalemia except: (February 2014)
a. Sine wave pattern
b. Tall T waves
c. Widening of QRS complex
d. U wave

31. First marker to rise in myocardial infarction is: (February 2014)
a. Myoglobin
b. CPK-MB
c. Trop-T
d. Trop C

32. Best scan for assessing myocardial viability: (February 2013)
a. Thallium
b. MIBI

c. Tc99 pyrophosphate scan
d. FDG PET

33. Gaint 'a' wave is in all except: (February 2013)
a. Complete heart block
b. Tricuspid stenosis
c. Pulmonary hypertension
d. MR

34. Rasmussen's aneurysm is seen in: (February 2013)
a. Bronchial artery
b. Pulmonary
c. Vertebral artery
d. Internal carotid artery

35. Exercise/Stress ECG is absolutely contraindicated in: (February 2013)
a. Aortic stenosis
b. 1 week post MI
c. Unstable angina
d. HOCM

36. Subclavian steal phenomenon is due to: (February 2012)
a. Block in the first part of the subclavian artery
b. Block in the second part of subclavian artery
c. Block in the third part of the Subclavian artery
d. Vertebral venous thrombosis

37. A patient is in ventricular tachycardia with hypotension, unresponsiveness, peripheral pulses are not felt. What would be the initial management of this patient? (February 2011)
a. Lignocaine push
b. Amiodarone push
c. Epinephrine
d. 200 Joule Defibrillation

38. Obstruction at the bifurcation of aorta leads to: (February 2011)
a. Claudication of buttocks and thigh
b. Retrograde ejaculation
c. Gangrene
d. Pallor of lower limb

39. Antibiotic prophylaxis is indicated in: (February 2011)
a. Cardiac catheterization
b. Prosectomty
c. Cystoscopy
d. Dental procedures

40. ECG change seen in hypocalcemia: (February 2010)
a. QT prolongation
b. Prolonged PR interval
c. Shortened PR interval
d. QT shortening

41. Reverse splitting of S2 seen in: (February 2010)
a. VSD
b. Severe AS
c. RBBB
d. ASD

42. Dicrotic pulse is seen in: (February 2010)
a. AS with AR
b. HOCM
c. Dilated cardiomyopathy
d. Aortic dissection

43. All are true regarding rheumatic chorea except: (February 2010)
a. Absent in sleep
b. May cause eurolgoic sequelae
c. Lasts for 4 to 10 wks
d. Common in girls

44. Tall 'T' waves are seen in: (February 2010)
a. Hyperkalemia
b. Hypocalcemia
c. Hypercalcemia
d. Hypokalemia

45. True statement regarding pulse oximetry in Methemoglobinemia: (February 2010)
a. No effect
b. Falsely high value in mild cases
c. Falsely low values in severe cases
d. Falsely high values in severe cases

46. Antibiotic prophylaxis is indicated in: (February 2009)
a. Cardiac catheterization
b. Prostectomy
c. Cystoscopy
d. Dental procedures

47. Roth spots are seen in: (February 2008)
a. Infective endocarditis
b. Central retinal vein occlusion
c. Retinitis pigmentosa
d. Diabetic retinopathy

48. Pulses bisferiens is seen in: (February 2008)
a. AR
b. AS
c. MR
d. MS

49. Exaggerated physiological splitting of S2 seen in: (February 2008)
a. VSD
b. Severe AS
c. RBBB
d. ASD

50. Gaint 'a' wave is in all except:
a. Complete heart block
b. Tricuspid stenosis
c. Pulmonary hypertension
d. MR

51. All of the following drugs are indicated in immediate post MI period except:
a. CCBs
b. Morphine
c. Enalapril
d. Aspirin

52. The agent used to chelate aluminum is:
a. Succimer (2014)
b. Desferoxamine
c. Dimercapol
d. D penicillamine

53. Which of the following is a feature of contrast induced nephropathy? (2014)
a. Increased bilirubin
b. Increased creatinine
c. Decreased creatinine
d. Decreased blirubin

54. Not a complication of total parenteral nutrition:
a. Hyperammonemia (2014)
b. Hypercholesterolemia
c. Neutrophil dysfunction
d. Hyperphophatemia

55. Which of the following with asymptomatic bacteruria dose not need treatment? (2014)
a. Neutropenic patient
b. During pregnancy
c. Catheterized patients
d. Urological procedures

56. Hypertension with alkalosis and hypokalemia are seen in all except: (2014)
a. Conn's syndrome
b. Liddle's syndrome
c. Bartter's syndrome
d. Fanconi syndrome

57. All are true regarding Tumor lysis syndrome except: (2013)
a. Hypercalcemia
b. Hypocalcemia
c. Hyperphosphatemia
d. Hyperkalemia

58. Not a side effect of TPN: (2013)
a. Hyperammnonemia
b. Decreased neutrophil fucniton
c. Hyperphosphatemia
d. Hypercholesterolemia

59. Hypertonic hyponatremia is found in:
a. Mannitol infusion (2012)
b. Diuretic therapy
c. CRF
d. Diarrhea

60. Which among the following causes 'Euvolvemic hyponatremia'? (2012)
a. Nephritic syndrome
b. SIADH
c. Diarrhea
d. Vomiting

61. Causes of Type 2 renal tubular acidosis are all except: (2012)
a. Cystinosis
b. Lowe syndrome
c. Essential fructosuria
d. Galatosemia

62. Nephritic syndrome is a complication of malaria cause by: (2012)
a. Plasmodium falciparum
b. Plasmodium ovale
c. Plasmodium malariae
d. Plasmodium vivax

63. Which of the following is an early sign of Hypermagnesemia? (2011)
a. Hypotension
b. Diminished DTR
c. Muscle weakness
d. Hypocalcemia

64. Patient presents with rhabdomyolysis and acute renal failure. What should be done next?
a. Mannitol (2011)
b. Forced alkaline dieresis
c. Dopamine
d. Hemodialysis

65. A patient presents with hypotension in confused state and metabolic alkalosis. Which of the following tests will suggest the diagnosis?
a. Urine ph (2011)
b. Urine Na+
c. Urine Cl-
d. Urine K+

66. Most common cause of End stage renal disease is:
a. Diabetes (2011)
b. Hypertension
c. Chronic GN
d. Polycystic kidney disease

67. Post Kidney transplantation complication caused by CMV is? (2011)
a. Parotitis
b. Cholecystitis
c. Pyelonephritis
d. Hepatitis

68. Urinary stone formed in patients with regional bowel enteritis is: (2011)
a. Calcium oxalate
b. Urate

c. Phosphate
d. Cysteine

69. Decreased erythropoietin levels are seen in:
a. End stage renal disease (2010)
b. Heart failure
c. Polycytic kidney disease
d. Advanced Liver failure

70. All are causes of acute tubulointerstitial nephritis except: (2009)
a. Methicillin
b. Sjogren syndrome
c. SLE
d. Down's syndrome

71. Patient presents with rhabdomyolysis and acute renal failure. What should be done next?
a. Mannitol (2009)
b. Forced alkaline dieresis
c. Dopamine
d. Hemodialysis

72. Causes of Type 2 renal tubular acidosis are all except: (2009)
a. Cystinosis
b. Lowe syndrome
c. Essential fructosuria
d. Galatosemia

73. Urine turns dark on standing in: (2008)
a. Alkaptonuria
b. Maple syrup urine disease
c. Phenyl ketonuria
d. Acute intermittent porphyria

74. All the following commonly cause nephritic syndrome except: (2008)
a. Tuberculosis
b. HIV
c. Malaria
d. Hepatitis C

75. Stage 5 chronic kidney disease is diagnosed when GFR falls below: (2008)
a. 5 mL/min per 1.73 m2
b. 10 mL/min per 1.73 m2
c. 15 mL/min per 1.73 m2
d. 20 mL/min per 1.73 m2

76. The most common class of lupus nephritis is:
a. Class 2 (2008)
b. Cass 3
c. Class 4
d. Class 5

77. All are indications for dialysis in a case of acute renal failure except: (2008)
a. Uremia
b. Hyponatremia
c. Hyperkalemia
d. Metabolic acidosis

78. Ringer's lactate does not contain: (2007)
a. Sodium
b. Potassium
c. Chloride
d. Bicarbonate

79. Drug of choice for low excretors of uric acid in renal failure is: (2007)
a. Bromobenzene
b. Allopurinol
c. Febuxostat
d. Probenecid

80. All are seen is tumor lysis syndrome except:
a. Hypercalcemia (2006)
b. Hypocalcemia
c. Hyperphosphatemia
d. Hyperklemia

81. Hypernatremic hypovolemia causes all except:
a. Cerebral haemorrhage (2006)
b. Cerebral thrombosis
c. Pontine mylinolysis

82. Urine a UTI patient has a PH of more than 8, the probable organism is: (2006)
a. E coli
b. Proteus
c. Klebsiella
d. Candida

83. True about neuroplaxia is: (2014)
a. Blocage of axon
b. Physiological block
c. Incomplete transaction of nerve
d. Complete transaction of nerve

84. All are features of Wernicke enecephalopathy except: (2014)
a. Ataxia
b. External ophthalmoplegia
c. Memory loss
d. Tinnitus

85. All are proximal myopathy except:
a. Myotonic dystrophy (2013)
b. Duchenne Muscular Dystrophy
c. Becker Muscular Dystrophy
d. Polymyositits

86. Xanthochromia of CSF seen in all except:
a. Blood tap (2013)
b. Carotene
c. Increased antibodies
d. Increased proteins

87. Homonymous diplopia is caused by:
a. Exotropia **(2013)**
b. Heterotropia
c. Hypotrpia
d. Esotropia

88. Clinical manifestation of thalamus lesion hemorrhage: (2013)
a. Head bobbing
b. Gaze palsy
c. Miosis
d. Ataxia

89. An industrial worker presents with blue lines on gums and tremors. What is the most probable diagnosis? (2013)
a. Arsenic poisoning
b. Lead
c. Mercury
d. Carbon monoxide

90. Inorganic lead toxicity does not cause:
a. Wrist drop **(2012)**
b. Insomnia
c. Anemia
d. Blue line

91. Herpes zoster most commonly involves:
a. Facial nerve **(2012)**
b. Ophthalmic division of trigeminal
c. Mandibular division of trigeminal
d. Maxillary division of Trigeminal

92. Lacunar infarct will not produce: (2012)
a. Pure sensory stroke
b. Ataxic hemiparesis
c. Hemiplegia
d. Aphaisa

93. True about modified Glasgow coma scale:
a. Highest score means bad prognosis **(2011)**
b. It includes measuring papillary size
c. Includes measurement of intra cranial pressure
d. It includes verbal response

94. Which antiepileptic drug is indicated in pregnancy? (2011)
a. VALPROIC ACID
b. Carbamazepine
c. Trimethadione
d. Phenytoin

95. A 25-year-old male complains of paroxysm of unilateral head ache, associated with nasal discharge and tearing of eyes on the side of head ache, precipitated by bouts of alcohol. Most likely diagnosis is: (2011)
a. Cluster head ache
b. Migraine
c. Sinusitis
d. Tension Headache

96. In amyotrophic lateral sclerosis, which of the following tests are likely to be positive?
a. CSF cytology **(2011)**
b. CT Brain
c. Nerve conduction study
d. Electromyography

97. Earliest clinical sign of raised intracranial pressure is: (2011)
a. Hypotension
b. Tachycardia
c. Dysnea
d. Altered behavior

98. A young female presents with olfactory hallucinations and automatisms. What is the most probabe site of lesion? (2011)
a. Frontal lobe
b. Parietal lobe
c. Temporal lobe
d. Occipital lobe

99. All are features of rabies encephalitis except:
a. Tonic spasm of the body **(2010)**
b. Hypersalivation
c. Sound Phobia
d. Hypotonic paralysis

100. Dorsal column lesions are associated with loss of: (2010)
a. Ankle jerk
b. Knee jerk
c. Proprioception
d. Superficial abdominal reflexes

101. Wernicke hemianopic pupil is seen in lesion of:
a. Optic radiation **(2010)**
b. Optic tract
c. Optic chiasma
d. Afferent tract

102. All are true regarding rheumatic chorea except:
a. Absent in sleep (2010)
b. May cause eurolgoic sequelae
c. Lasts for 4 to 10 wks
d. Common in girls

103. The minimum possible score in "Glasgow coma scale" is: (2009)
a. 0
b. 1
c. 3
d. 5

104. Clinical manifestation of thalamus lesion hemorrhage: (2009)
a. Head bobbing
b. Gaze palsy

c. Miosis
d. Ataxia

105. Which of the following is not seen in Parkinsonism? (2009)
a. Preserved postural reflexes
b. Hypokinesia
c. Rigidity
d. Static tremors

106. All the following are features of Guillian-Barre syndrome except: (2009)
a. Predominant motor involvement
b. Facial nerve involvement
c. Absence of pleocytosis in CSF
d. Bladder and bowel involvement

107. Dorsal column lesions are associated with loss of:
a. Ankle Jerk (2009)
b. Knee jerk
c. Proprioception
d. Superficial abdominal reflexes

108. Features of 'Brainstem death' are all except:
a. No respiration for 15 secs after disconnecting from ventilator (2008)
b. Absent papillary response
c. Absent DTR
d. Isoelectric EEG

109. Man coughed and developed sudden severe headache and fainting. The most probable diagnosis is:
a. Subarachnoid hemorrhage (2008)
b. Migraine
c. Cluster Headache
d. Posterior fossa hemorrhage

110. H. influenza causes hydrocephalus due to:
a. Gliosis (2008)
b. Fibrosis
c. Adhesion of subarachnoid villi
d. None of the above

111. All the following are characteristic feature of cluster headache except: (2008)
a. Periodic pain
b. Conjunctival injection
c. Bilateral photophobia
d. No response to oral sumatriptan

112. Inorganic lead toxicity does not cause: (2008)
a. Wrist drop
b. Insomnia
c. Anemia
d. Blue line

113. Which of the following causes distal myopathy:
a. Myotonic dystrophy (2008)
b. Duchenne Muscular Dystrophy
c. Becker Muscular Dystrophy
d. Polymyositits

114. Xanthochromia of CSF seen in all except:
a. Bloody tap (2007)
b. Carotene
c. Increased antibodies
d. Increased proteins

115. All the following are present on the ipsilateral side in Lateral medullary syndrome except:
a. Diplopia (2007)
b. Impaired pain sensation in the body
c. Horner syndrome
d. Facial pain

116. Which is not a characteristic feature of pseudo tumor cerebri?
a. Headache (2007)
b. Dilated ventricles
c. Increasing opening pressure during LP
d. Papilledema

117. All are following are affected in the middle cerebral artery involvement except: (2007)
a. Hemiplegia
b. Hemianaesthesia
c. Broca aphasia
d. Amnesia

118. A 55-year-old male presents with renal failure, bone pain for 7 years and osteolytic lesions on X-ray. Serum electrophoresis shows M spike and 35% plasma cells with aberrant protein expression. What is the diagnosis? (2014)
a. MGUS
b. Multiple myeloma
c. Smoldering myeloma
d. Plasma cell leukemia

119. In anemia due to lead poisoning, bone marrow will characteristically show: (2014)
a. Dwarf megakaryocyte
b. Ring sideroblasts
c. Pelger huet anomaly
d. Basophilic stippling

120. Palpable purpura is seen in all the following except:
a. HSP (2014)
b. Giant cell arteritis
c. Drug induced vasculitis
d. Cryoglobinemia

121. All are true regarding amyloidosis except:
a. Dystrophic clacification is seen (2013)
b. Renal deposition can cause Renal failure
c. Causes restrictive cardiomyopathy
d. Abdominal fat biopsy is diagnostic

122. False regarding Multiple myeloma is:
a. It is a clacified protein (2014)
b. Bence Jones protein in urine
c. Lytic boen lesions
d. Roulex formation of RBCs

123. Regarding hereditary spherocytosis, all the following are true except: (2012)
a. RBC membrane defect
b. Spherocytes disappear after splenectomy
c. Extravascular hemolysis
d. Young cells are less affected

124. Strawberry gums are seen in: (2012)
a. Wegener's granulomatosis
b. Kawasaki syndrome
c. Phenytoin Therapy
d. Scarlet fever

125. All are seen in iron deficiency except:
a. Decreased serum iron (2012)
b. Decreased serum ferritin
c. Increased RBC protoporphyrin
d. Increased transferring saturation

126. Pinch purpura is seen in: (2012)
a. Primary systemic amyloidosis
b. Vitamin C deficiency
c. Henochschoenlein purpura
d. Purpura fulminans

127. Strawberry tongue is seen in: (2012)
a. Wegener granulomatosis
b. Kawasaki toxicity
c. Phenytoin toxicity
d. Polyarteritis nodosa

128. In Graft-versus –Host reaction monitor all except:
a. Skin (2012)
b. Lung
c. Liver
d. Intestine

129. Transfusion of stored blood causes:
a. Hypekalemia (2012)
b. Hyponatremia
c. Hypercalcemia
d. Hypokalemia

130. Multiple myeloma is best diagnosed by:
(2012)
a. 24 hour urine protein estimation
b. Renal biopsy
c. >10% plasmacytoma
d. Rouleaux formation in blood

131. Defect in Glycoprotein IIb/IIa causes:
a. Glanzmann's thrombasthenia (2012)
b. Bernard-soulier syndrome
c. von willebrand disease
d. Scott's syndrome

132. Which of the following is affected in Megaloblastic anemia? (2011)
a. DNA
b. RNA
c. Globin
d. Iron absorption

133. Common complication seen in polycythemia vera is: (2011)
a. Infection
b. Hemolysis
c. Renal failure
d. Myelofibrosis

134. Not a complication of major blood transfusion:
a. Hypercalemia (2010)
b. Hyperkalemia
c. Volume overload
d. Hypocalcemia

135. Microcytic anemia is seen in deficiency of:
a. Vitamin B2 (2009)
b. Vitamin B5
c. Pyridoxine
d. Folic acid

136. Most common Ig seen in multiple myeloma:
a. IgG (2009)
b. IgM
c. IgA
d. IgE

137. Non-erosive arthritis is characteristic of:
a. SLE (2008)
b. Psoriasis
c. RA
d. Gout

138. Martel's sign is seen in: (2008)
a. Rheumatoid arthritis
b. Gonococcal arthritis
c. Gout
d. TB arthritis

139. Immunological mucocutaneous syndrome is similar to infection caused by: (2008)
a. Staph aureus
b. Pheumococcus
c. Coxsackie
d. Herpes

140. Erythropoietinis increased in all except:
a. EML (2008)
b. MDS
c. Essential thrombocytosis
d. Polycythemia vera

141. Splenomegaly is a feature of all except:
a. Aplastic anemia (2007)
b. CML
c. Thalessemia
d. Hypersplenism

142. All of the following can cause Aplastic anemia except: (2007)
a. Fancon's anemia
b. Wiskotta-aldrich syndrome
c. Dyskeratosis congenital
d. Reticular dysgenesis

143. Pancytopenia is seen in all except: (2007)
a. wiskott-aldrich syndrome
b. fanconi's anaemia
c. schwartzmann diamond syndrome
d. kostman's syndrome

144. Most common Ig seen multiple myeloma:
a. IgG (2007)
b. IgM
c. IgA
d. IgE

145. All are seen in alkaptonuria except: (2006)
a. Cardiac disease
b. Ochronosis
c. Arthritis
d. Seizures

146. All are true about systemic sclerosis except:
a. Genetic component (2006)
b. Calcinosis cutis
c. Pulmonary artery hypertension
d. Anicentromere antibodies

147. Priapism is seen all except: (2006)
a. Sickle cell anemia
b. Megaloblastic anaemia
c. Scorpion sting
d. Spinal injury

148. Not a symptom of hyperthyroidism:
a. Hyperactivity (2014)
b. Palpitation
c. Diarrhea
d. Hair loss

149. Which of the following is characteristic of cushing's disease: (2013)
a. Increased ACTH, increased cortisol
b. Decreased ACTH, increased cortisol
c. Increased ACTH, decreased cortisol
d. Decreased ACTH, decreased cortisol

150. Which of the following statements regarding Diabetic ketoacidosis is true? (2011)
a. Urine output may be misleading
b. Initial Hyperkalemia
c. Phosphaturia leads to phosphate deficiency
d. Soda bicarb is used to treat acidosis

151. An adolescent girl presents with extrapyramidal symptoms. Blood tests reveal hemolytic anemia and liver dysfunction. What is the diagnosis?
a. Hemochromatosis (2011)
b. Riley day syndrome
c. Huntington's disease
d. Wilson's disease

152. Polyglandular syndrome (Schmidt syndrome) is associated with adrenocortical deficiency and which of the following conditions?
a. Graves disease (2011)
b. Hypoparathyroidism
c. Hashimoto's thyroiditis
d. Islet cell adenoma

153. Which of the following is not seen in Non-ketotic hyperosomolar coma? (2010)
a. Insidious onset
b. Kussmaul's breathing
c. Seen in elderly
d. Seen in type 2 DM

154. Episodic hypertension is characteristic of:
a. Carcinoid tumor (2010)
b. Insulinoma
c. Pheochromocytoma
d. Zollinger Ellison syndrome

155. Kartagener's syndrome includes all except:
a. Situes inversus (2010)
b. Bronchiectasis
c. Lobar emphysema
d. Sinusitis

156. Endocrine causes for hypertension are all the following except: (2009)
a. Cushing's syndrome
b. Hypopituitarism
c. Hyperaldosteronism
d. Gigantism

157. In type 1DM all true except : (2008)
a. Decreased Gluconeogenesis
b. Increased Glycogenolysis
c. Increased Lipolysis
d. Increased Ketogenesis

158. In Hyperthyroidism increased cardiac output is due to all the following except: (2008)
a. Increased afterload
b. Increased ventricular contractility
c. Decreased total peripheral resistance
d. Peripheral vasodilatation

159. All the following are causes of hyperthermia except: (2008)
a. Hypothyroidism
b. Cerebral hemorrhage
c. Succinyl Choline
d. Pheochromocytoma

160. A female patient presents with amenorrhea, galactorrhea and bitemporal hemianopia. Most likely diagnosis is: (2008)
a. Cushing's disease
b. Empty sella syndrome
c. Prolactinoma
d. Hypothyroidism

161. All the following tumors are seen in MEN 1 syndrome except: (2007)
a. Pituitary adenomas
b. Parathyroid tumors
c. Insulinoma
d. Medullary Ca of thyroid

162. Photosensitivity is seen in: (2007)
a. SLE
b. Kawasaki disease
c. Rheumatoid arthritis
d. Polyarteritis nodosa

163. Poems syndrome is associated the all except: (2006)
a. Osteolytic multiple myeloma
b. Hypertrichosis
c. papilledema
d. amenorrhea

164. Asthenospermia means: (2006)
a. Immotile sperms
b. Absent sperms
c. Dead sperms
d. dysmorphic sperms

165. Pretransfusion testing does not decrease the incidence of hepatitis. Possible reason could be: (2014)
a. Most carriers do not have HBsAg
b. Post-transfusion hepatitis is caused by CMV
c. Present screening test is not sensitive for HBsAg
d. HCV not screened

166. Patient presents to emergency room with edema of tongue, stridor, dyspnea, hoarseness and itching following peanut consumption. Most likely cause is: (2014)
a. Foreign body larynx
b. Foreign body bronchus
c. Parapharyngeal abscess

167. True statement regarding management of ileocecal Crohn's disease (CD) is: (2014)
a. Avoid antibiotics
b. Avoid steroids in 1st week
c. 5ASA is used reduces small bowel obstructions
d. Cholestyramine improves diarrhea worsens steatorrhoea

168. Delayed clotting in abetalipoproteinemia is due to: (2013)
a. Decreased VLDL
b. Reduced clotting factor synthesis
c. Decreased cylomicrons
d. Decreased fatty acid synthesis

169. Inheritance of familial hypercholesterolemia: (2013)
a. AR
b. AD
c. XR
d. XD

170. All are true in Kawasaki except: (2013)
a. Exudative conjunctivitis
b. Pedal edema
c. Strawberry tongue
d. Thrombocytosis

171. Gold standard test for diagnosis GERD: (2013)
a. Ambulatory pH monitoring
b. Esophageal manometry
c. Endoscopy
d. Barium Swallow

172. All are true regarding Crohn's disease except: (2013)
a. Infertility
b. Risk of CA
c. Medial treatment includes antibiotics, probiotics and TNF alpha blockers
d. ANCA-positive

173. A single retrocardiac air-fluid level on a chest radiography typically implies the presence of: (2013)
a. Sliding hiatal hernia
b. Gastric volvulus
c. Pericardial effusion
d. Lung abscess

174. An industrial worker presents with blue lines on gums and tremors. What is the most probable diagnosis? (2013)
a. Arsenic poisoning
b. Lead
c. Mercury
d. Carbon monoxide

175. Acute alcohol consumption causes: (2013)
a. Inhibits ketogenesis
b. Lactic acidosis
c. Increased gluconeogenesis
d. Decreases brain GABA

176. Primary infertility with a normal karyotype is seen in: (2012)
a. Androgen Insensitivity syndrome
b. Mullerian agenesis

c. Turner syndrome
d. Congenital Adrenal Hyperplasia

177. High SAAG (serum-ascites albumin gradient) ascites is seen in all except: (2012)
a. Cirrhosis of liver
b. Congestive heart failure
c. Chronic renal failure
d. Nephritic syndrome

178. A patient presents within 12-16 hours after consuming home canned vegetables and smoked fish with vomiting and diarrhea. What is the cause of food poisoning? (2012)
a. Clostridium botulinum
b. Bacillis cereus
c. Salmonella
d. Staphylococcus

179. Organism that causes emphysematous cholecystitis is: (2012)
a. Salmonella typhi
b. Cytomegalovirus
c. Clostridium perfringens
d. Bacteroides

180. Prognostic factor in acute liver failure is:
a. Alpha fetoprotein (2012)
b. Prothrombin time
c. Albumin
d. Globulin

181. Poor prognostic factor in a patient with pancreatitis is: (2011)
a. Leucocytosis > 20, 000
b. Elevated serum amylase
c. Elevated serum lipase
d. Diastolic BP > 90 mm Hg

182. A man presents with weakness, pain in upper abdomen, hyperpigmentation, arthritis, hyperglycemia and an enlarged palpable liver. Most probable diagnosis is: (2011)
a. Hemochromatosis
b. Addison's disease
c. Insulin Dependent DM
d. Cushings syndrome

183. Post Kidney transplantation complication caused by CMV is? (2011)
a. Parotitis
b. Cholecystitis
c. Pyelonephritis
d. Hepatitis

184. Urinary stone formed in patients with regional bowel enteritis is: (2011)
a. Calcium oxalate
b. Urate
c. Phosphate
d. Cysteine

185. An adolescent girl presents with extrapyramidal symptoms. Blood tests reveal hemolytic anemia and liver dysfunction. What is the diagnosis?
a. Hemochromatosis (2011)
b. Riley day syndrome
c. Huntington's disease
d. Wilson's disease

186. All except are features plummer vision syndrome: (2010)
a. Hypertrophy of oral mucosa
b. Dysphagia
c. Glossitis
d. Iron deficiency of oral mucosa

187. Skip lesions are seen in: (2010)
a. Crohn's disease
b. Ulcerative colitis
c. Ischemic bowel disease
d. Typhoid colitis

188. MENKES disease due to defective absorption of:
a. Zinc (2009)
b. Manganese
c. Copper
d. Selenium

189. Recurrent meningococcal meningitis occurs in:
a. C1 esterase deficiency (2009)
b. C2 deficiency
c. C3 deficiency
d. C5-9 deficiency

190. 68 years old chronic alcoholic presents with ecchymotic patches in the lower extremities. He also has perifollicular hemorrhages, fragmented hairs, splinter hemorrhages in nail beds and multiple red tender swellings in the muscle. What is the likely diagnosis? (2009)
a. Vitamin K deficiency
b. Vitamin C deficiency
c. Pyridoxine deficiency
d. Chronic myelogenous leukemia

191. All the following are supplemented in cystic fibrosis with gastrointestinal disease except:
a. Vitamin E (2009)
b. Vitamin K
c. Vitamin B12
d. Pancreatic lipase

192. A single retrocardiac air-fluid level on a chest radiography typically implies the presence of:
a. Sliding hiatal hernia (2009)
b. Gastric golulus
c. Pericardial effusion
d. Lung abscess

193. Anti-Saccharomyes cerevisiae antibodies (ASCA) are seen in which of the following condition: (2009)
a. Ulcerative colitis
b. Behcet's syndrome
c. Primary biliary cirrhosis
d. Cryoglobulinemia

194. Features of large orange tonsils and very low HDL levels are characteristic of: (2009)
a. Familial hypobetalipoproteinemia
b. Abetalipoproteinemia
c. Hypoalphalipoproteinemia
d. Tangier disease

195. All except are features of Plummer-Vison syndrome: (2010)
a. Hypertrophy f oral mucosa
b. Dysphagia
c. Glossitis
d. Iron deficieny anemia

196. Niacin deficiency occurs in: (2009)
a. Prolonged antibiotic use
b. Hartnups disease
c. Carcinoid syndrome
d. Isoniazid use

197. Loss of gastric acidity increases the risk of infection due to: (2008)
a. Salmonella species
b. Staph aureus
c. Giardiasis
d. Candida

198. All are true regarding crohn's disease except: (2007)
a. Infertility
b. Risk of Ca
c. Medical treatment includes antibiotics, probiotics and TNF alpha blockers
d. ANCA-positive

199. All the following causes micronodular cirrhosis except: (2007)
a. Laennec's cirrhosis
b. Primary biliary cirrhosis
c. Indian childhood cirrhosis
d. Wilson's disease

200. Drug of choice for low excretors of uric acid in renal failure is: (2006)
a. Bromobenzene
b. Allopurinol
c. Febuxostat
d. Probenecid

201 All of the following causes cirrhosis except: (2006)
a. Wilson's disease
b. Hemochromatosis
c. Paracetamol
d. Cystic fibrosis

202. Angiokeratoma is seen in: (2006)
a. Fabry's disease
b. Pompe's disease
c. Hurler's disease
d. Gaucher's disease

203. Artemesinin is best used for: (2006)
a. Relapse of malaria
b. Cerebral malaria
c. Chronic malaria
d. Recrudescent malaria

ANSWERS AND EXPLANATIONS

1. **Ans. a. Amphotericin** *Ref: Harrison's Principles of Internal Medicine, 18/e p1661–1664*
2. **Ans. c. Angioneurotic edema**
3. **Ans. d. Diet and weight reduction** *Ref: Harrison's Principles of Internal Medicine, 18/e p2188*
4. **Ans. b. RBC 1000**

Ref: Harrison's Principles of Internal Medicine, 18/e p2178, George Mathew prep manual 1st edition

Explanation

Test	Transudate	Exudate
Protein	< 3 g/dl	> 3 g/dl
Pleural/serum protein ratio	< 0.5	> 0.5
LDH	< 200 IU/L	> 200 IU/L
Pleural/serum LDH ratio	< 0.6	> 0.6
Glucose	> 60 mg/dL	< 60 mg/dL

Contd...

Contd...

Test	Transudate	Exudate
Leucocytes	< 1000/cmm	> 1000/cmm
RBC	< 5000/cmm	Variable
Causes	CCF, CRF, Nephrotic syndrome, cirrhosis, hypoproteinemia	Pneumonia, TB, malignancy, pulmonary infarction, Rheumatoid arthritis, pancreatitis

5. **Ans. c. HIT is a risk factor** *Ref: Harrison's Principles of Internal Medicine, 18/e p993, 2175*
6. **Ans. b. Pulmonary** *Ref: American journal of Roentology, Jan 2000, Vol 174, 262–263*
7. **Ans. a. Hypercapnia** *Ref: CMDT 2013 pg 322, 333, Harrison's principles of internal medicine, 18/e p2205*
8. **Ans. a. Increased FEV1/FVC Decreased compliance** *Ref: Davidson 21/e p651*
9. **Ans. b. LVF** *Ref: CMDT 2013, pg. 318–319*
10. **Ans. a. Sweat chloride levels - < 50 meq/lit**
Ref: Nelson's Textbook of Pediatrics 18/e p1803–1809
11. **Ans. a. Uremia**
Ref: Nelson's Textbook of Pediatrics 18/e p1799 & Garrison's principles of internal medicine, 18/e
12. **Ans. c. Mucolytic has proven action in relief of secretions**
Ref: Fishman's pulmonary diseases and disorders 4/e p2186–2189, Harrison's textbook of internal medicine 17/e chapter 252
13. **Ans. d. Reversible airflow obstruction**
Ref: Global initative for bronchial asthma [GINA] guidelines, Harrison's textbook of internal medicine 17/e chapter 248
14. **Ans. a. Acinetobacter baumanii**
Ref: Harrison's principles of internal medicine 17/e chapter 251, British thoracic society guidelines for pneumonia 2009
15. **Ans. d. Idiopathic pulmonary fibrosis** *Ref: Harrison's 18/e*
16. **Ans. a. Reversible bronchoconstriction** *Ref: Harrison's Principles of Internal Medicine, 18/e*
17. **Ans. c. Tachypnoea**
Ref: Harrison's Principles of Internal Medicine, 18/e Chapter 262. Deep Venous Thrombosis and Pulmonary Thromboembolism.
18. **Ans. a. Metabolic acidosis** *Ref: Harrison's Principles of Internal Medicine, 18/e*
19. **Ans. b. Increased anatomical dead space**
Ref: Harrison's Principles of Internal Medicine, 18/e and Robbins Pathologic Basis of Disease, 8/e
20. **Ans. a. Situs inversus** *Ref: Harrison's Principles of internal Medicine, 18/e and Medscape*
21. **Ans. c. VII Cranial nerve** *Ref: Harrison's Principles of internal Medicine, 18/e 2012, Chapter 329 Explanation*
22. **Ans. b. Sinus bradycardia** *Ref: Harrison's Principles of internal Medicine, 18/e*
23. **Ans. a. IL-5** *Ref: Harrison's Principles of internal Medicine, 18/e and Nelson Textbook of Pediatics, 9/e*
24. **Ans. d. Cimetidine** *Ref: Harrison's Principles of internal Medicine, 18/e 2012 chapter 254 (textbook 254-4)*
25. **Ans. d. Glucose < 60 mg/dL**
Ref: Harrison's Principles of internal Medicine, 18/e p2178, George Mathew prep manual 1/e
26. **Ans. c. 1.2L** *Ref. Davidson 21/e p651*
27. **Ans. b. Diastolic murmur**
Ref: Harrison's principles of internal medicine, 18/e p1826, chaptere 13, Approach to a patient with a heartnmurmum; Bedside cardiology, by Ahyut sarkar, 1/e p167

Explanation

Unless otherwise proved diastolic murmur is always organic.

Extra edge: Diastolic murmur which is not organic: transient solitary diastolic murmur of newborn.

Features of benign murmur:
- Should not be more than grade 3
- Never loud at apex
- Never radiates to neck
- Mostly systolic never diastolic
- Never associated with click
- No chamber enlargement clinically

Benign murmurs
- Still's murmur
- Functional murmur in adults
- Pulmonary branch murmur
- Supraclavicular murmur
- Venous hum
- Mammary soufflé.

28. Ans. a. Amiadarone and b. Lidocaine *Ref: Harrison's principles of internal medicine, 18/e p1893*

Explanation

After initial unsuccessful defibrillation or persisitent electrical instability, anti arrhythmic therapy should be instituted. Intravenous amiadarone as initial treatment (150 mg over 10 min, followed by 1 mg/min for up to 6 hours and 0.5 mg/min thereafter.

Lignocaine may be used in early ACS related VT with cardiac arrest or if amiadarone is unsuccessful.

29. Ans. c. Left axis deviation *Ref: Harrison's principles of internal medicine, 18/e p1891–1893*

Explanation

Broad complex tachycardia	
SVT with aberrancy	**VT**
• No AV dissociation • QRS < 140 ms	• AV dissociation(fusion beats or capture beats) • QRS > 140 ms • Extreme QRS axis- 90^0 to 180^0 • Delayed activation of initial phase of QRS wave • Bizarre QRS • Concordance of QRS • RSR' with taller R > R'

30. Ans. d. U wave *Ref: Schamroth and Harrison's Principles of Internal Medicine, 18/e p1838*

In short ECG changes of electrolyte abnormalities

Hyperkalemia	Hypokalemia	Hypercalcemia	Hypocalcemia
• Tall tented T wave • P wave disappear • Prolong PR • Wide QRS(sine wave pattern)	• Disappearance of T waves • Prominent U waves • Prolong PR • ST sagging	• Short QT interval	• Long QT interval

31. Ans. a. Myoglobin

Ref: Harrison's Principles of Internal Medicine, 18/e p2023 and Robbins Pathologic Basis of Diseae, 8/e, http://path.upmc.edu/cases/case178/dx.html and Illustrated Textbook of Cardiovascualr Pathology By P. Chopra, R.Ray A. Saxena

Explanation:

Enzyme	Seen at	Peaks at	Returns to normal	Other features
Creatinine phosphokinase	2–4 hours	24 hours	48–72 hours	• Very sensitive • CPKMB isoenzyme increases the specificity
Lactate dehydrogenase	24 hours	4-5 days		

32. Ans. d. FDG PET *Ref: Harrison's Principles of Internal Medicine, 18/e p1846*

33. Ans. d. MR

Ref: Braunwald 5/e p1073; The Jugular Venous Pressure and Pulse Contour-Clinical Methods, 3rd HK walker

34. Ans. b. Pulmonary *Ref: American journal of Roentology, Jan 2000, Vol 174, 262–263*

35. Ans. c. Unstable angina *Ref: Harrison's Principles of Internal Medicine, 18/e p2004*

36. Ans. a. Blok in the first part of the Subclavian artery *Ref: Harrison's 18/e and Wikipedia*

37. Ans. d. 200 Joule Defibrillation *Ref: Harrison's Principles of Internal Medicine, 18/e*

38. Ans. a. Caludication of buttocks and thigh

Ref: Harrison's Principles of Internal Medicine, 18/e and Nelson Textbook of Pediatircs, 19/e

39. Ans. d. Dental procedures

Ref: Harrison's Principles of Internal Medicine, 18/e and http://emedicine.medscape.com/article/Antibiotic Prophylactic Regimens for Endocarditis

40. Ans. a. QT prolongation *Ref: Harrison's Principles of internal Medicine, 18/e*

41. Ans. b. Server AS *Ref: Hutchison's Clincial Methods, 22/e*

42. Ans. c. Dilated cardiomyopathy *Ref: Harrison's Principles of internal Medicine, 18/e*

43. Ans. b. May cause Neurologic sequlae

Ref: Harrison's Principles of internal Medicine, 18/e and Nelson's textbook of Pediatrics, 19/e

44. Ans. a. Hyperkalemia *Ref: Harrison's Principles of internal Medicine, 18/e*

45. Ans. d. Falsely high values in severe cases

Ref: Harrison's Principles of internal Medicine, 18/e and Emedicine Medscape

46. Ans. d. Dental procedures

Ref: Harrison's Principles of internal Medicine, 18/e and http://emedicine.medscape.com/article/Antibiotic Prophylactic Regimens for endocarditis

47. Ans. a. Infective endocarditis *Ref: Harrison's Principles of internal Medicine, 18/e*

48. Ans. a. AR *Ref: Harrison's Principles of internal Medicine, 18/e*

49. Ans. c. RBBB *Ref: Hutchison's clinical methods, 22/e*

50. Ans. d. MR *Ref: Braunwald 5/e p1073*

51. Ans. a. CCBs *Ref: Harrison's 18/e p2028*

52. Ans. b. Desferoxamine *Ref: Harrison's Priniciples of internal medicine, 18/e p49*

Explanation

In a nutshell

Metal	Chelating agent
Gold	• BAL
Mercury	• Bal • Succimer • Polythiol
Arsenic	• BAL • Succimer • Penicillamine
Lead	• Succimer • Calcium disodium EDTA • BAL
Iron	• Desferrioxamine • Deferiprone
Aluminum	• desferrioxamine

Aluminum toxicity

Serum aluminium levels > 50–60 μg/L suggest aluminium overload used as an indication to start chelation therapy in symptomatic pateients

Typical presentations

- Proximal muscle weakness
- Bone pain
- Multiple non-healing fractures
- Acute or sub acute alteration in mental status
- Premature osteoporosis
- Chronic kidney disease

53. Ans. b. Increased creatinine *Ref: Harrison's principles of internal medicine, 18/e p2300 Table and 3241*

Explanation

Contrast nephropathy

- Rise in serum creatinine atleast 1 mg/dl within next 48 hours of contrast administration
- Risk factors
  - Age > 80 yrs
  - Preexisting renal problems creatinine > 2 mg/dl
  - Diabetes mellitus
  - Dehydration
  - Solitary kidney
  - Paraproteinemia
  - Nephrotoxic drug usage
  - High dose of contrast
- Non ionic low osmolar contrast media prevent this damage
- When e GFR < 45 ml/min/1.73 m^2 avoid iodinated contrast
- Premedication in high risk patients
  - Glucocorticoids
  - H2 blockers (ranitidine)
  - H1 antihistaminics
- High risk patients for anaphylaxis
  - Prior contrast allergy
  - Food allergic to shellfish
  - Atopy or asthma
- MR contrast with gadolinium is less risky.
- When eGFR < 30 ml/min, gadolinium should be avoided.

54. Ans. d. Hyperphosphatemia *Ref: Harrison 18/e p617–620*

Explanation

- Parental nutrition is infusion of complete nutrient solutions into blood stream via central/peripheral vein.
- Indications
  - Patients unable to ingest/absorb nutrients.
  - To support them during acute infection/inflammation of extended critical illness period.
  - Permanent loss of intestinal length or function.

Common clinical conditions

- Major burns
- Trauma
- Acute pancreatitis
- Severe sepsis
- Closed head injury
- Inflammatory bowel disease
- Patients on ventilator
- Cancer patients
- HIV
- Severe hyperemesis gravidarum

Complications

Mechanical	Metabolic	Infectious
• Pneumothorax • Accidental arterial puncture • Thrombosis • Catheter infections • Catheter block	• Hyperglycemia/hypoglycemia • Fluid overload • Refeeding syndrome • Hypernatremia • Hypocalcemia • Hypochloremic metabolic alkalosis due to nasogastric aspiration • Metabolic acidosis • Hyperaminoacidemia • Hypophosphatemia • Neutrophil dysfunction • Thrombocyte dysfunction • Metabolic bone disease • Vitamin deficiencies • Trace element deficiencies • Anemia • Hyperammonemia • Cholestasis-hepatic dysfunction	• Candida albicans • Staphylococcus epidermis

55. Ans. c. Catheterized patients *Ref: Harrison's principles of internal medicine, 18/e p2390-4*

Explanation

Asymptomatic bacteriuria

- Criteria for diagnosis of Asymptomatic bacteriuria
  - Positive urine culture–CFU > 10^5/ml
  - No clinical features of UTI
- Treatment is indicated in
  - Pregnancy
  - Urological surgeries
  - Neutropenic patients
  - Renal transplant patients
- Two different phenomenas

Catheter associated asymptomatic bacteriuria	Catheter associated UTI
No symptoms	Symptoms of UTI

56. Ans. c and d. *Ref: Harrison's Principles of Internal Medicine, 18/e p2949, 2051, 2361, 368*

57. Ans. a. Hypercalcemia *Ref: Harrison's Principles of Internal Medicine, 18/e p2274*

58. Ans. b. Decreased neutrophil function and c. Hyperphosphatemia

Ref: Harrison's Principles of Internal Medicine, 18/e p

59. Ans. a. Mannitol infusion *Ref: Nelson's Textbook of Pediatrics 18/e p275 and Harrison's 18/e*

60. Ans. b. SIADH *Ref: Nelson's Textbook of Pediatrics 18/e p275 and Harrison's 18/e*

61. Ans. c. Essential fructosuria *Ref: Nelson's Textbook of Pediatrics 18/e p2197*

62. Ans. c. Plasmodium malariae *Ref: Harrison's 18/e and Nelson's Textbook of Pediatrics*

63. Ans. a. Hypotension *Ref: Harrison's Principles of Internal Medicine, 18/e*

64. Ans. b. Forced alkaline diruesis *Ref: Harrison's Principles of Internal Medicine, 18/e*

65. Ans. b. Urine Na+ *Ref: Harrison's Principles of Internal Medicine, 18/e*

66. Ans. a. Diabetes *Ref: Harrison's Principles of Internal Medicine, 18/e*

67. Ans. d. Hepatitis *Ref: Harrison's Principles of Internal Medicine, 18/e*

69. Ans. a. Calcium oxalate *Ref: Harrison's Principles of Internal Medicine, 18/e*

69. Ans. a. End stage renal disease *Ref: Harrison's Principles of internal Medicine, 18/e*

70. Ans. d. Down's syndrome *Ref: 2012. Chapter 285. (Table 285-1)*

71. Ans. b. Forced alkaline dieresis *Ref: Harrison's Principles of internal Medicine, 18/e 2012*

72. Ans. c. Essential fructosuria *Ref: Nelson's Textbook of Pediatrics 18/e p2197*

73. Ans. a. Alkaptonuria

Ref: Harrison's Principles of internal Medicine, 18/e & Harper's illustrated Biochemistry, Chapter 29, 28/e p254

74. Ans. a. Tuberculosis

Ref: Harrison's Principles of internal Medicine, 18/e & Nelson textbook of Pediatrics, 19/e

75. Ans. c. 15 mL/min per 1.73 m2

Ref: Harrison's Principles of internal Medicine, 18/e 2012 Chapter 44. p334 (Table 52-1)

76. Ans. c. Class 4

77. Ans. b. Hyponatremia *Ref: Harrison's Principles of internal Medicine, 18/e 2012 Chapter 279*

78. Ans. d. Bicarbonate *Ref: Washington Manual of Medicine*

79. Ans. a. Bromobenzene *Ref: Harrison's 18/e p1382*

80. Ans. a. Hypercalcemia *Ref: Harrison's principles of internal medicine, 18/e p2274*

81. Ans. b. Cerebral thrombosis *Ref: Harrison's 18/e p349*

82. Ans. b. Proteus *Ref: Harrison's 18/e p1245*

83. Ans. a. Blockage of axon

Ref: Current therapy in neurologic disease, volume 1 edited by Richard tiaball Johnson, W. Griffin, Justin c. Mc Arthur, page 247

Neuropraxia	Axonetmesis	Neurotmesis
• Physiological block of nerve conduction within axon without anatomical interruption • Eg. Brachial plexus injury at birth which recovers spontaneously by 4 to 6 weeks	• Anatomical interruption of the axon with no interruption of connective tissue framework • Needs time to regrowth of axon to target muscle • Scar formation will prevent regrowth • Takes months to recover	• Complete anatomical disruption and surrounding connective tissue • Complete nerve rupture • No chance of spontaneous recovery • Needs early surgical intervention

84. Ans. d. Tinnitus *Ref: Harrison's Principles of Internal Medicine, 18/e p2260*

Explanation

Salient points

- Caused by thiamine deficiency
- Thiamine is a cofactor for enzymes
  - Transketolase
  - α-keto glutarate dehydrogenase
  - Pyruvate dehydrogenase
- Thiamine deficiency occurs in
  - Alcoholics
  - Malnourishment due to hyperemesis, starvation, dialysis, AIDS and cancer.
- Clinical features
  - Global confusion
  - Ataxic gait
  - Ophthalmoplegia
  - Memory loss

- Polyneuropathy
- If untreated- stupor, coma and death.
- MRI brain shows Mammilary body enhancement
- Treatment is 100 mg thiamine intramuscular administration
- Untreated leads to Korsakoff's syndrome.

85. Ans. a. Myotonic dystrophy *Ref: Harrison's Principles of Internal Medicine, 18/e p3499–350*

Explanation

Proximal myopathies	Distal myopathies
• Polymyositis • Dermatomyositis • Mitochondrial myopathies • Toxic myopathies • Metabolic • Endocrinal	• Myotonic dystrophy • Welander's myopathy • Tibial muscular dystrophy • Merkesby- Griggs dystrophy • Laing's Nonaka's • Miyoshi myopathy • Myofibrillar myopathy

86. Ans. a. Bloody tap *Ref: Harrison's Principles of Internal Medicine, 18/e p46–1*

Explanation

Xanthochromia is yellowish discoloration of CSF supernatant.

Causes

SAH Jaundice Increased proteins Froin's syndrome (spinal subarachnoidal block) Carotene addiction

87. Ans. d. Esotropia

Ref: Parson, 20th edition pg 401, 403; Khurana 4/e p321, 326; Sunitha Agarwal, Textbook of Opthalamologym p434

Refer opthal section

88. Ans. b. Gaze palsy and C. Miosis *Ref: Harrison's Principles of Internal Medicine, 18/e p3295*

Common site of ICH is Putamen (most common)

Thalamic hemorrhage	Putamen bleed	Pontine haemorrhage	Cerebellar
• Contralteral hemiparesis • Hemisensory loss • Aphasia	• Contraleral hemiparesis, facial palsy, slurring	• Deep coma with quadriplegia, decerebrate rigidity	• Occipital headache • Eyes- ipsilateral gaze palsy, ipsilateral 6th nerve palsy
• Constructional apraxia • Mutism • Ocular features: unequal pupils, skew deviation, ipsilateral Horner's syndrome, absence of convergence, paralysis of vertical gaze, retr	• Deviation of eyes away from the side of hemiparesis • Coma due to brainstem involvement • Dilated and fixed ipsilateral pupil, decerebrate rigidity	• Pin point pupils, absent doll eye movements • Hyperpnea, hypertension & hyperhidrosis	• Blepharospasm, ocular bobbing, • Dysarthria, dysphagis, hydrocephalus due to 4 th ventricle obstruction coma

89. Ans. b. Lead *Ref: Harrison's Principles of Internal Medicine, 18/e p49*

90. Ans. b. Insomnia *Ref: Harrison's 18/e p49*

91. Ans. b. Ophthalmic division of Trigeminal nerve *Ref: Harrison's 18/e*

92. Ans. d. Aphasia *Ref: Harrison's 18/e*

93. Ans. d. It includes verbal response *Ref: Harrison's Principles of Internal Medicine, 18/e*

Explanation

	1	2	3	4	5	6
Eye	Does not open eyes	Opens eye to painful stimuli	Opens eyes in response to voice	Opens eye simultaneously	NA	NA
Verbal	Makes no sounds	Incomprehensible sounds	Utters inappropriate words	Confused, disoriented	Oriented, converses normally	NA
Motor	Makes no movements	Extension to painful stimuli	Abnormal flexion to painful stimuli	Flexion/withdrawal to painful stimuli	Localizes painful stimuli	Obeys commands

94. Ans. b. Carbamazepine

Ref: Harrison's Principles of Internal Medicine, 18/e p and Hernandez-Diaz S, Smith CR, Shen A, Mittendorf R, Hauser WA, Yerby M et al. Comparative safety of antiepileptic drugs during pregnancy. Neurology. 2012 may 22;78(21): 1692-9

95. Ans. a. Cluster headache *Ref: Harrison's Principles of Internal Medicine, 18/e*

96. Ans. d. Electromyography

Ref: Harrison's Principles of Internal Medicine, 18/e and Harrison's Online > Chapter 374. Amyotrophic Lateral Sclerosis

97. Ans. d. Altered behavior *Ref: Harrison's Principles of Internal Medicine 18/e*

Early manifestations are

- Headache
- Projectile vomiting
- Extraocular muscle palsy
- Altered behavior
- Back pain
- Papilledema

98. Ans. a and c

Ref: Harrison's Principles of Internal Medicine, 18/e and The Neurology of Olfaction by Christopher H. Hawkes, Richard L. Doty and Chabolla DR. Characteristics of the epilepsies. Mayo Clin Proc. 2002 Sep; 77(9): 981–90

Explanation

Olfactory hallucinations were initially considred to arise from temporal lobe, now its clear that it arises from orbito frontal complex.

99. Ans. c. Sound Phobia *Ref: Harrison's Principles of internal Medicine, 18/e*

Two acute neurologic form of rabies are seen in humans

- Encephalitic in 80%
- Paralytic in 20%

Encephalitic	Paralytic
• Hyper excitabitiy followed by periods of complete lucidity that become shorter • Early brainstem involvement- classical features of hydrophobia and aerophobia • Rapid progression to death • Cardiac arrhythmias • Mods	• Muscle weakness • Cardinal features of encephalitic rabies are lacking • Sphincter involvement • Milod sensory involvement

100. Ans. c. Proprioception *Ref: Harrison's Principles of internal Medicine, 18/e*

101. Ans. b. Optic tract *Ref: Harrison's Principles of internal Medicine, 18/e*

102. Ans. b. May cause Neurologic sequlae

Ref: Harrison's Principles of internal Medicine, 18/e and Nelson's textbook of Pediatrics, 19/e

103. Ans. c. 3 *Ref: Harrison's Principles of internal Medicine, 18/e 2012 chapter 267 (Table 267-1)*

104. Ans. b and d. Gaze palsy and misosis *Ref: Harrison's Principles of internal Medicine, 18/e p3295*

105. Ans. a. Preserved postural reflexes

Ref: Harrison's Principles of internal Medicine, 18/e 2012. Chapter 372 (Table 372-3)

106. Ans. d. Bladder and bowel involvement

Ref: Harrison's Principles of internal Medicine, 18/e 2012. Chapter 385 (Table 385-3)

107. Ans. c. Proprioception *Ref: Harrison's Principles of internal Medicine, 18/e*

108. Ans. c. Absent DTR *Ref: Harrison's Principles of internal Medicine, 18/e*

109. Ans. a. Subarachnoid hemorrhage *Ref: Harrison's Principles of internal Medicine, 18/e*

110. Ans. d. None of the above

Ref: Internet Article international Federation For Hydrocephalus and Spina Bifida. Post infections hydrocephalus

111. Ans. c. Bilateral photophobia *Ref: Harrison's Principles of internal Medicine, 18/e 2012. Chapter 14 p112*

112. Ans. b. Insomnia *Ref: Harrison's 18/e*

113. Ans. a. Myotonic dystrophy *Ref: Harrison's Principles of internal Medicine, 18/e p3499, 3500*

114. Ans. a. Bloody tap *Ref: Harrison's Principles of internal Medicine, 18/e p46–1*

115. Ans. b. Impaired pain sensation in the body *Ref: Harrison's textbook of internal medicine, 18/e*

116. Ans. b. Dilated ventricles *Ref: Harrison's textbook of internal medicine, 18/e*

117. Ans. d. Amnesia *Ref: Harrison's textbook of internal medicine, 18/e*

118. Ans. b. Multiple myeloma

Ref: Harrison's Principles of Internal Medicine, 18/e p937–942; CMDT 2013, p527–529

119. Ans. d. Basophilic stippling *Ref: Harrison's Principles of Internal Medicine, 18/e p49*

120. Ans. d. Cryoglobinemia *Ref: Harrison's Principles of Internal Medicine, 18/e p421*

121. Ans. a. Dystrophic calcification is seen

Ref: Harrison's Principles of Internal Medicine, 18/e p945–950, CMDT 2013 p531

122. Ans. a. It is a calcified protein *Ref: Harrison's Principles of Internal Medicine, 18/e*

123. Ans. b. Spherocytes disapper after splenectomy

Ref: Chapter 14. Red blood cell and bleeding disorders; page: 644; Robbins and Cotran Pathologic Basis of Disease: 8/e

124. Ans. a. Wegener's granulomatosis *Ref: Harrison's 18/e*

125. Ans. d. Increased transferrin saturation *Ref: Harrison's 18/e*

126. Ans. a. Primary systemic amyloidosis *Ref: Rook's Textbook of Dermatology*

127. Ans. b. Kawasaki disease *Ref: Nelson's Textbook of Pediatrics 18/e p1799*

128. Ans. b. Lung *Ref: Harrison's 18/e*

129. Ans. a. Hyperkalemia *Ref: Harrison's 18/e*

130. Ans. c. > 10% plasmacytoma *Ref: Harrison's Principles of Internal Medicine, 18/e*

131. Ans. a. Glanzmann's thrombasthenia *Ref: Harrison's 18/e*

132. Ans. a. DNA *Ref: Harrison's Principles of Internal Medicine, 18/e*

133. Ans. d. Myelofibrosis *Ref: Robbins Pathologic Basis of Disease, 8/e & Harrison online 18/e*

134. Ans. a. Hypercalcemia *Ref: Harrison's Principles of internal Medicine, 18/e*

135. Ans. c. Pyridoxine *Ref: Davidson 21/e p127*

136. Ans. a. IgG *Ref: Harrison's Principles of internal Medicine, 18/e*

137. Ans. a. SLE *Ref: Harrison's Principles of internal Medicine, 18/e p2728*

138. Ans. c. Gout *Ref: Harrison's 18/e*

139. Ans. d. Herpes *Ref: Harrison's 18/e p390, 1456*

140. Ans. d. Polycythemia vera *Ref: Rison's 18/e p456, 898*

141. Ans. a. Aplastic anemia *Ref: Harrison's 18/e p467*

142. Ans. b. Wiskott-aldrich syndrome *Ref: Harrison's 18/e p887*

143. Ans. a. Wiskott-aldrich syndrome *Ref: Harrions's 18/e p887*

144. Ans. a. IgG *Ref: Harrison's principles of Internal medicine, 18/e*

145. Ans. d. Seizures *Ref: Harrison's 18/e p3219*

146. Ans. a. Genetic component *Ref. Harrison's 18/e p2757*

147. Ans. b. Megaloblastic anemia *Ref: Harrison's 18/e p375, 855*

148. Ans. d. Hair loss *Ref: Harrison's Principles of Internal Medicine, 18/e p2922–2930*

Explanation

Signs and symptoms of hyperthyroidism

Symptoms	Signs
• Hyperactivity • Irritability • Dysphoria • Heat intolerance and sweating • Palpitations • Fatigue and weakness • Weight loss with increased appetite • Diarrhea • Polyuria • Oligomenorrhea • Loss of libido	• Tachycardia • Atrial fibrillation in elderly • Tremor • Goiter • Warm, moist skin • Muscle weakness (proximal myopathy) • Lid retraction • Gynecomastia

Signs and symptoms of hypothyroidism

Symptoms	Signs
• Tiredness • Weakness • Dry skin • Feeling cold • Hair loss • Difficult concentrating and poor memory • Constipation • Weight gain with poor appetite • Dyspnea • Hoarse voice • Menorrhagia • Paresthesia • Impaired hearing	• Dry coarse skin • Cool peripheral extremities • Puffy face hands and feet (myxedema) • Diffuse alopecia • Bradycardia • Peripheral edema • DTR • Carpal tunnel syndrome • Serous cavity effusions

149. Ans. a. Increased ACTH, increased cortisol *Ref: Davidson 21/e p771*

Explanations

Cushing's syndrome refers to clinical features due to chronic exposure to excess of glucocorticoids of any etiology.

2 types

ACTH dependent Cushing's	ACTH independent Cushing's
• Pituitary adenoma secreting ACTH • Ectopic ACTH syndrome (lung carcinoid, small cell ca, medullary ca thyroid, pheochromocytoma)	• Iatrogenic (chronic glucocorticoid therapy) • Adrenal adenoma, adrenal carcinoma

Cushing's disease is due to a pituitary adenoma secreting ACTH
Pseudocushing's causes

- Alcohol excess
- Chronic depression
- Primary obesity

Screening tests: 24 hr urinary free cortisol
Treatment: Surgery for adrenal tumors
Oral agents for cushing's syndrome- metyrapone, ketoconazole, mitotane
IV etimodate in severe cases.

150. Ans. b. Initial Hyperkalemia *Ref: Harrison's Principles of Internal Medicine, 18/e & Nelson Textbook of pediatrics*

Explanation

Due to secondary acidosis, serum potassium may be mildly elevated
Lab abnormalities in DKA
Dka is characterized by

- Hyperglycemia
- Ketosis
- Metabolic acidosis

Serum bicarbonate is frequently < 10 mmol/L
Arterial pH 6.8 to 7.3
Total body stores of sodium, chloride, phosphorus, and magnesium are reduced in DKA but are not accurately reflected by their levels in the serum because of dehydration and hyperglycemia.
Differential diagnosis

- Starvation ketosis
- Alcoholic ketoacidosis (bicarbonate usually > 15 meq/L)

151. Ans. d. Wilson's disease

Ref: Harrison's Principles of Internal Medicine, 18/e p and Harrison's Online > Chapter 360. Wilson's Disease

Explanation

Wilson's disease
Mutations in ATP 7 B gene.
Excess hepatic copper is initially bound to metallothionein, but as this storage capacity is exceeded, liver damage begins.
Clinical features

- Hepatitis
- Cirrhosis
- Hepatic decompensation
- In severe hepatic failure, hemolytic anemia may occur.

152. Ans. a. Graves disease

153. Ans. b. Kussmaul's breathing

Ref: Harrison's Principles of internal Medicine, 18/e & Nelson Textbook of Pediatrics, 19/e

154. Ans. c. Pheochromocytoma *Ref: Harrison's Principles of internal Medicine, 18/e*

155. Ans. a. Situs inversus *Ref: Harrison's Principles of internal Medicine, 18/e and Medscape*

156. Ans. b. Hypopitutarism

Ref: Harrison's Principles of internal Medicine, 17/e 2008 Chapter 241 Pg. 1554. Table 241–3

157. Ans. a. Decreased Gluconeogenesis *Ref: Harrison's Principles of internal Medicine, 18/e & Nelson*

158. Ans. a. Increased afterload

Ref: Harrison's Principles of internal Medicine, 18/e and DeGroot WJ, Leonard JJ.Hyperthyroidism as a high cardiac output state. Am Heart J. 1970 Feb; 79(2): 265–75

159. Ans a. Hypothyroidism *Ref: Harrison's Principles of internal Medicine, 18/e 2012. Chapter 16 p143*

160. Ans. c. Prolactinoma *Ref: Harrison's Principles of internal Medicine, 18/e*

161. Ans. d. Medullary Ca of thyroid *Ref: Harrison's textbook of internal medicine, 18/e*

162. Ans. a. SLE *Ref: Harrison's textbook of internal medicine, 18/e*

163. Ans. a. Osteolytic multiple myeloma *Ref: Harrison' 18/e p3080*

164. Ans. a. Immotile sperms *Ref: Harrison's 18/e*

165. Ans. b. Post transfusion hepatitis is caused by CMV

Ref: Harrison's Principles of Internal Medicine, 18th edition, page 956

Explanation

Reasons for post-transfusion hepatitis inspite of screening

CMV can cause aymptomatic infection

Transfusion transmitted CMV can cause problems in premature neonates, allograph recipients, splenectomised patients.

Hbs Ag is not detected during window period between disappearance of HBs Ag and appearance of IgM Ab Anti HBc (IgM) is detected in this window period, which is not used in screening methods.

166. Ans. c. Parapharyngeal abscess *Ref: Harrison's 18/e p2711*

Explanation

ANGIONEUROTIC EDEMA

- Life threatening allergic condition
- Rapid edema of deep layers of skin
- Characteristic presentation
  - Intense bronchospasm
  - Vascular collapse
  - Shock without antecedent events
- Symptoms develop within seconds to minutes
- Laryngeal edema
- Cutaneous manifestations
  - Utricaria
  - Pruritis
  - Flushing
  - Feeling of warmth
- GI MANIFESTATIONS
  - Nausea
  - Vomiting
  - Crampy abdominal pain
  - Diarrhea
- Known triggers
  - Agents responsible–hormones, enzymes, pollen dust mites animal dander
  - Food: peanuts, milk, egg, seafood, nuts, grains, beans
  - Rubber latex, ETO
  - Hymenoptera venom
  - Thiomersal
  - Dextran
  - Antibiotics- penicillin, cephalosporins, amphotericin B
  - Anesthetics- lidocaine, procaine
- Treatment
  - Adrenaline-0.3 to 0.5 ml of 1;1000 sc/im
  - IV diphenhydramine 50-100mg IM
  - Nebulised salbutamol
  - IV glucocorticoids

167. Ans. c. 5-ASA is used prevents/reduces small bowel obstruction

Ref: Harrison's Principles of Internal Medicine, 18/e p2477–2495

Explanation

Drugs used in inflammatory bowel disease

Antibiotics	Glucocorticoids
• Drugs- ciprofloxacin and metronidazole • Indications – Active CD(crohns disease) – Inflammatory CD – Perianal CD – Fistulous CD • No role in active or quiescent UC • Used to treat pouchitis following IPPAA and colectomy in UC	• Active CD and UC • No role in maintanence of UC or CD

Aminosalicylates	Other drugs
• Drugs – Mesalazine – Olsalasine – Sulfasalasine – Balsalaside • 5-ASA-mainstay for inducing remission in UC • 5-ASA had doubtful role in inducing remission in CD • Available as oral or topical • Cholestryamine improves choleric diarrhea and steatorrhea	• Azathioprine and 6-mercaptopurine-management of glucocorticoid dependent IBD • Methotrexate –inducing remission and reducing glucocorticoid dosage and effective in maintaining remission in active CD • Cyclosporine is effective in severe UC refractory to IV glucocorticoids • Tacrolimus has shown efficacy in children refractory IBD and in adults with extensive involvement of small bowel. also used in adults with steroid dependent or refractory UC and CD as well as fistulising CD • Infliximab-approved for moderately to severely active UC. • Adalizumab- treatment of moderate to severe CD • Natalizumab- treatments of patients with CD refractory or intolerant to anti-INF therapy

168. Ans. b. Reduced clotting factor synthesis *Ref: Harrison's Principles of Internal Medicine, 18/e p3153*

Explanations

Abetalipoproteinemia

- Autosomal recessive disorder
- Mutation in microsomal triglyceride transfer protein needed for transport of lipids and cholesterol and fat-soluble vitamins.
- Low VLDL and chylomicrons
- Fat malabsorpton causing vitamin K deficieny- coagulopathy
- Severe vitamin E deficiency-neurological manifestations
- Acanthocytosis
- Hypocholesterolemia
- Retinitis pigmentosa, posterior column neuropathy and myopathy
- Treated with high doses of vitamin E and other vitamins

169. Ans. b. AD *Ref: Harrison's Principles of Internal Medicine, 18/e p3148*

170. Ans. a. Exudative conjunctivitis *Ref: CMDT 2013, p1417-1418*

171. Ans. a. Ambulatory pH monitoring

Ref: Harrison's Principles of Internal Medicine, 18/e p2428 Confirmatory test for GERD is 24-48 hr pH monitoring to show pH < 4 for > 5% of duration.

172. Ans. d. ANCA-positive *Ref: Harrison's Principles of Internal Medicine, 18/e p2486*

173. Ans. a. Sliding hiatal hernia *Ref: Canadian Asso Radiology journal, 1986*

174. Ans. b. Lead *Ref: Harrison's Principles of Internal Medicine, 18/e p49*

175. Ans. b. Lactic acidosis *Ref: Harrison's Principles of Internal Medicine, 18/e p3546*

176. Ans. b. Mullerian agenesis *Ref: Harrison's 18/e*

177. Ans. d. Nephrotic syndrome *Ref: Harrison's 18/e*

178. Ans. a. Clostridium botulinum
Ref: Nelson's Textbook of Pediatrics 18/e p1606–1608 and Garrison's 18/e

179. Ans. a. Clostridium perfringens *Ref: Harrison's 18/e*

180. Ans. b. Prothrombin time *Ref: Harrison's 18/e*

181. Ans. a. Leucocytosis > 20, 000 *Ref: Harrison's Principles of Internal Medicine, 18/e*

182. Ans. a. Hemochromatosis *Ref: Harrison's Principles of Internal Medicine, 18/e*

183. Ans. d. Hepatitis *Ref: Harrison's Principles of Internal Medicine, 18/e*

184. Ans. a. Calcium oxalate *Ref: Harrison's Principles of Internal Medicine, 18/e*

185. Ans. d. Wilson's disease
Ref: Harrison's Principles of Internal Medicine, 18/e p and Harrison's Online > Chapter 360

186. Ans. a. Hypertrophy of oral mucosa *Ref: Harrison's Principles of internal Medicine, 18/e*

187. Ans. a. Crohn's disease *Ref: Harrison's Principles of internal Medicine, 18/e*

188. Ans. c. Copper *Ref: Harrison's Principles of internal Medicine, 18/e 2008 chapter. 71 p449*

189. Ans. d. C5-9 deficiency
Ref: Harrison's Principles of internal Medicine, 17/e 2008. Chapter 136 p911

190. Ans. b. Vitamin C deficiency *Ref: Harrison's Principles of internal Medicine, 18/e 2012. Chapter 74*

191. Ans. c. Vitamin B12 *Ref: Harrison's Principles of internal Medicine, 18/e 2012 Chapter 259*

192. Ans. a. Sliding hiatal hernia *Ref: Candadian Asso Radiology Journal, 1986*

193. Ans. b. Behcet's syndrome *Ref: Harrison's Principles of internal Medicine, 18/e 2012 chapter 327*

194. Ans. d. Tangier disease *Ref: Harrison's Principles of internal Medicine, 18/e 2012. Chapter 356*

195. Ans. a. Hypertrophy of oral mucosa *Ref: Harrison's Principles of internal Medicine, 18/e*

196. Ans. b. Hartnups disease *Ref: Harrison's Principles of internal Medicine, 18/e*

197. Ans. a. Salmonella species
Ref: Harrison's Principles of internal Medicine, 18/e 2012 chapter 153/chapter 119 (Table 119-1)

198. Ans. d. ANCA-positive *Ref: Harrison's Principles of internal Medicine, 18/e p2486*

199. Ans. d. Wilson's disease *Ref: Harrison's textbook of internal medicine, 18/e*

200. Ans. a. Bromobenzene *Ref: Harrison's 18/e p1382*

201. Ans. d. Cystic fibrosis *Ref: Harrison's 18/e p2592*

202. Ans. a. Fabry's disease *Ref: Harrison's 18/e p2349, 3191*

203. Ans. b. Cerebral malaria *Ref: CMDT 2013, p1492*

QUESTIONS 2015

1. True about ankylosing spondylitis:
a. More in female
b. 50% associated with HLA-B27
c. Heart is affected
d. No association with plantar fascitis

2. Hypercalcemia is caused by:
a. Adrenocortical insufficiency
b. Amyloidosis
c. Hyperthyroidism
d. Vitamin C intoxication

3. True regarding diabetic ketoacidosis:
a. Glucose and Ketone cause diuresis
b. More common in type 2 DM
c. Sodium nitroprusside test is used to detect ketones
d. Serum bicarbonate usually > 10 mmol/L

4. Patient is having mutism and akinesia but he is awake and alert:
a. Stupor
b. Oneroid
c. Delirium
d. Twilight

5. A girl with mild von willebrand disease and molar tooth extraction who had previous history of bleeding episode. The most appropriate step would be:
a. Desmopressin
b. FFP
c. Cryoprecipitate
d. Packed cells

6. A patient with decreased pH with increased pCO_2 with decreased bicarbonate:
a. Partially compensated Respiratory acidosis
b. Uncompensated Respiratory acidosis
c. Respiratory alkalosis
d. Metabolic acidosis

7. In increased intracranial tension, which nerve is affected?
a. 6th
b. 3rd
c. 5th
d. 10th

8. Heart muscle specific disease is associated with:
a. Scleroderma
b. Amyloidosis
c. Sarcoidosis
d. All the above

9. True about hyperthyroidism:
a. T3 T4 TSH all increase
b. T3 T4 TSH all decrease
c. T3 increase T4 increase TSH decrease
d. T3 T4 BOTH decrease TSH increase

10. Which the following is true about glycosylated hb?
a. Increase in diabetic patient with sickle cell anemia
b. It is not a poor indicator of long term diabetic status in a patient with renal disease
c. Contain Hb with a sugar moiety
d. Half life is 80 days in adults

11. Patient with lung cancer was operated and lobectomy was done. After surgery which parameter increases?
a. Dead space
b. Inspiratory reserve capacity
c. Tidal volume
d. Forced vital capacity

12. Which of following ass with decrease in DLCO:
a. Asthma
b. Pulmonary hemorrhage
c. Exercise
d. Lobectomy

13. ARDS is associated with all except:
a. Pulmonary embolism
b. Acute pancreatitis
c. Sepsis
d. Aspiration

14. A boy having acute right iliac fossa pain, fever. Which cell is not seen?
a. Neutrophil
b. Monocyte
c. Macrophage
d. Lymphocyte

ANSWERS AND EXPLANATIONS

1. Ans. c. Heart is affected *Ref: Harrison 19/e ebook p2171*

- Option a: Male :female preponderance is 2:1 to 3:1
- Option b: AS shows a striking correlation with the histocompatibility antigen HLA-B27 and occurs worldwide roughly in proportion to the prevalence of B27 (Chap. 373e). In North American whites, the prevalence of B27 is 7%, whereas it is 90% in patients with AS, independent of disease severity. In population surveys, AS is present in 1–6% of adults inheriting B27, whereas the prevalence is 10–30% among B27+ adult first-degree relatives of AS probands.
- Option c: Heart is affected - Aortic insufficiency, sometimes leading to congestive heart failure, occurs in a small percentage of patients, occasionally early. Third-degree heart block may occur alone or together with aortic insufficiency. Subclinical pulmonary lesions and cardiac dysfunction may be relatively common
- Option d: Associated with plantar fasciitis

Contd...

ASAS criteria for classification of axial spondyloarthritis (to be applied for patients with back pain ≥ 3 months and age of onset, 45 years)[0]		
Sacroilitis on imaging plus ≥ 1 SPA features	or	HLA-B27 plus ≥ 2 other SPA features
Sacroilitis on imaging		SPA features
• Active (acute inflammation on MRI highly suggestive of SPA-associated sacroilitis[b]		• Inflammatory back pain[d]
and/or		• Arthritis
• Definite radiographic sacroollitis according to modified New York criteria[c]		• Enthesitis (heel)[f]
		• Anterior uveitis[g]
		• Dactylitis[e]
		• Psoriasis[e]
		• Crohn's dosease or ulcerative colitis[e]
		• Good response to NSAIDs[h]
		• Family history of SpA[i]
		• HLA-B27
		• Elevated CRP

[a]Sensitivity 83%, specific 84%. The imaging arm (sacroilitis) alone has a sensitivity of 66% and a specific of 97%. [b]Bone marrow edema and/or osteitis on short tau inversion 3 or 4. [d]See text for criteria. [e]Past or Present, diagnosed by a physician. [f]Past or Present pain or tenderness on examination at calcaneus insertion of Achilles tendon tendon or plantar fascia. [g]Past or present, confirmed by an opthalmologist. [h]Substantial relief of back pain at 24–48 h after a full dose of NSAID. [i]First-or second-degree relatives with ankylosing spondylitis (AS), psoriasis, iveitis, reactive arthritis (ReA), or inflammatory bowel disease (IBD). [j]After exclusion of other cause of elevated CRP.

2. Ans. c. Hyperthyroidism *Ref: Harrison 19/e p2477*

Classification of cause of Hypercalcemia	
1. Parathyroid-Related	• Primary hyperparathyroidism – Adenoma(s) – Multiple endocrine neoplasia – Carcinoma • Lithium therapy • Familial hypocalciuric hypercalcemia
2. Malignancy-Related	• Solid tumor with metatases (breast) • Solid tumor with humoral mediation of hypercalcemia (lung kidney) • Hematologic malignancies (multiple myeloma, lymphoma, leukemia)
3. Vitamin D-Related	• Vitamin D intociation • ↑ 1, 25 $(OH)_2D$; sarcoidosis and other granulomatous disease • ↑ 1, 25 $(OH)_2D$; impaired 1, 25 $(OH)_2D$ metabolism due to 24-hydroxylase deficiency
4. Associated with High Bone Turnover	• Hyperthyroidism • Immobilization • Thiazides • Vitamin A intoxication • Fat necrosis
5. Associated with Renal Failure	• Severe secondary hyperparathyroidism • Aluminium intoxication • Milk-akali syndrome

3. **Ans. a. Glucose and ketone causes diuresis** *Ref: Harrison 19/e p2418*
   - Option a: Glucose and ketones will exert an osmotic effect leading to diuresis
   - Option b: Most commonly seen in type 1 Diabetes Mellitus
   - Option c: Nitroprusside test is used to test ketones
   - Option d: Serum bicarbonate is less then 10mmol/L (as it is acidosis)
4. **Ans. a. Stupor** *Ref: Harrison 19/e p1771*
5. **Ans. a. Desmopressin** *Ref: Harrison 19/e p730*
6. **Ans. b. Uncompensated respiratory acidosis** *Ref: Nephrology book by Dr Sanjay Pandya*
7. **Ans. a. Sixth nerve** *Ref: Harrison 19/e p2583*
8. **Ans. d. All the above** *Ref: Harrison 19/e p1563*
9. **Ans. c. T3 and T4 increase and TSH decrease** *Ref: Harrison 19/e p2295*
10. **Ans. c. It contains hemoglobin with sugar moiety** *Ref: Harrison 19/e p2401*
11. **Ans. a. Dead space** *Reference internet not sure*
12. **Ans. d. Lobectomy** *Ref: Harrrison 19/e p chapter 306*

Decrease in DLCO	Increase in DLCO
• Diseases that thicken or destroy pulmonary membrane – Pulmonary fibrosis – Emphysema • Diseases that curtail pulmonary vasculature – Pulmonary hypertension • Diseases that reduce alveolar capillary hemoglobin anemia	• Asthma • Polycythemia • Acute CCF • Pulmonary hemorrhage

13. **Ans. a. Pulmonary embolism** *Ref: Harrison 19/e chapter 322*

Causes

Direct lung injury	Indirect lung injury
• Pneumonia • Aspiration of gastric contents • Pulmonary contusion • Near drowning • Toxic inhalation injury	• Sepsis • Severe trauma – Multiple bone fractures – Head trauma – Flail chest – Burns • Multiple transfusions • Drug overdose • Pancreatitis • Post cardiopulmonary bypass

14. **Ans. d. Lymphocytes** *Ref: Robbins 9/e*

Lymphocytes are seen in chronic inflammation.

Chapter

12

Surgery

Rajamahendran R

Author's Note: Dear friends: In this Chapter I have covered the High yield Areas in Surgery asked in JIPMER exams as Theory initially in Chapter wise manner which will help you to brush up the surgery already read by you. Following which I have added the Previous Year questions and Explanatory Answers. I wish this part of the material will boost up the points you have already learnt from Surgery. All the best.

HIGH YIELD CONCEPTS FOR JIPMER

General

Types of Ulcer

- Sloping ulcer: Healing ulcer
- Undermined edge: Tuberculosis
- Punched out: Syphilitic gumma ulcer and trophic ulcer (due to end arteritis)
- Raised and beaded: Basal cell carcinoma (Rodent ulcer)
- Everted and rolled out: Squamous cell carcinoma.

Oneliners

- **Cock's peculiar tumor:** Sebaceous cyst surface gets ulcerated leading to painful fungating mass in head
- **Sebaceous horn:** Hardening of slow discharge sebum via the punctum
- **Gardners syndrome:** Familial adenomatous polyposis associated with multiple sebaceous cysts
- **Fordyce's disease:** Ectopic sebaceous glands in lip and oral mucosa
- **Dercum's disease:** Multiple painful lipomas (adiposis dolorosa)
- **Hiadrenitis Suppurativa:** Infection of Apocrine sweat glands in Axilla
- **Pott's Puffy tumor:** Frontal Bone Osteomyelitis
- **Milian's Ear sign:** Seen in Erysipelas
- **Acute paronychia:** Subcuticular infection caused by Staphylococcal aureus
- **Chronic paronychia:** Chronic nail infection caused by Candida
- **Felon:** Terminal pulp space infection
- **Deep Palmar abscess:** Abscess beneath flexor tendons (Frog Hand)
- **Dupuytrens contracture:** Thickening of Palmar/Plantar Fascia.

Blood products

Whole blood:	Packed red cells:
• Rich in coagulation factors than packed cells and more metabolically active than stored blood	• The cells are spun down and concentrated. • Each unit is 330 ml* • Hematocrit = 50-70% • Packed cells are stored in SAG-M solution (saline adenine glucose mannitol) to increase their shelf life to 5 weeks* at 2-6 degrees C. • Older storage regimens-Citrate phosphate dextrose giving cells shelf life 2-3 weeks*

Contd...

Contd...

Fresh frozen plasma:	Cryoprecipitate:
• Rich in coagulation factors • Stored at –40 to -60 degrees C. (2 year shelf life)* • Rh D positive FFP can be given to Rh D negative women	• Supernatant precipitate of FFP and is rich in factor VIII* and fibrinogen. • Stored at –30 degree C with a 2 year shelf life*
Platelets: • They are available as pooled platelet concentrate containing 250 x 109 cells/litre • Platelets are stored on a special agitator at 20-24 degrees c. Half life only 5 days* • Useful in patients with thrombocytopenia	**Prothrombin complex concentrates: (PCC)** • Highly purified concentrates prepared from pooled plasma. • They contain factors II, IX, X. Factor VII may be included or produced separately.

Organ Transplantation

- First successful kidney transplant-Murray (1954)*
- First successful liver transplant-Starzl (1963)*
- First heart transplant-Barnard (1967)
- First lung transplant-Derom (1968)
- First pancreatic islets transplant-Sutherland and Najarin (1974)

- ➢ ***Allograft:*** An organ or tissue transplanted from one individual to another
- ➢ ***Xenograft:*** A graft performed between different species
- ➢ ***Orthotopic graft:*** A graft placed in its normal anatomical site
- ➢ ***Heterotopic graft:*** A graft placed in a site different from that where the organ is normally located

Cold storage time:**

Organ	Optimal storage time	Maximum storage time
Kidney	< 24 hours*	48 hours*
Liver	< 12 hours*	24 hours*
Pancreas	< 10 hours	24 hours
Small Intestine/Heart/Lung	< 3 hours	8 hours

HEAD AND NECK

- 90% of oral cancers are squamous cell carcinoma**
- **First echelon nodes of oral cancers:** Supraomohyoid triangle (level I, II, III)
- Skip mets without first echelon nodes: 15 % tongue cancers
- Tongue cancer has poorer prognosis
- M/c oral cancer in India–Gingivobuccal complex (ca. cheek)**
- M/c oral cancer in world–Tongue
- M/c oral cancer in west–lip (2nd common–tongue)

Syphilis in oral cavity

- Primary–Chancre on lip or tongue
- Secondary:
  - Mucous patches–lip, cheeks, fauces
  - **Hutchinson's warts****–condyloma over midline of tongue
  - **Snail track ulcers****–common over pillars of fauces
- Tertiary–gumma (m/c on tongue–anterior 2/3) Glossitis (premalignant).

Branchial sinus

Failure of fusion of the second branchial arch with sixth branchial arch and persistence of cervical sinus results in this condition. In most cases the internal opening is not found, so this is better called a sinus rather than a fistula.

- **Congenital:** Persistent cervical sinus
- **Acquired:**

External opening

Congenital: Typically located in lower 1/3rd of neck at the anterior border of sternocleidomastoid.
Acquired: Typically located at upper 1/3rd to middle 1/3rd junction.

Internal opening

Behind the tonsil and anterior to posterior pillar of the fauces in the lateral wall of the pharynx lies the interior opening.
Treatment: Excision of fistulous tract

CYSTIC HYGROMA

- Sequestration of a portion of jugular lymph sac from lymphatic system accounts for the appearance of these swellings in the neck
- It's a swelling in the **posterior triangle** of neck in the lower third
- **Earliest swelling** one can see in the neck
- Cystic hygroma **presents in neonate** or in early infancy
- May also present at birth as obstructed labor
- Swelling is **brilliantly translucent** and **partly compressible, cough impulse is also positive**
- Cysts are **filled with clear lymph** and lined with a single layer of epithelium.

Complications

- Respiratory difficulty due to rapid growth
- Swelling may become infected as a result of nasopharyngeal infection
- Spontaneous recovery may occur as the swelling becomes inflamed and subsequent fibrosis occur.

Definitive Treatment

- **Conservative neck dissection along with excision of all lymphatic bearing tissues is the ideal treatment of choice.**
- Recently sclerosants like BLEOMYCIN and streptococcal pyogenes derivatives like PICIBANIL (OK432) injected into the lesions. But since the lesion is multicystic and extensive subsequent surgery is needed.
- Radiotherapy is not of any use as the swelling is radioresistant.
- Incomplete removal may result in infection, recurrence, Fluid and electrolyte loss from the open cysts with dehydration.

Salivary Gland Tumors:

- M/c benign parotid tumor in ADULTS–Pleomorphic adenoma
  - Children–Hemangioma
- M/c malignant parotid tumor–mucoepidermoid carcinoma
- M/c benign submandibular gland tumor–pleomorphic adenoma
- M/c malignant submandibular gland tumor–adenoid cystic carcinoma
- M/c site for squamous cell carcinoma salivary gland–submandibular gland
- M/c minor salivary gland tumor -adeno carcinoma
- Tumor that spreads via neural sheath–adenoid cystic carcinoma
- Best diagnostic modality for parotid swelling–FNAC
- Open incisional biopsy in contraindicated
- Best imaging investigation for salivary tumor–MRI

Frey's Syndrome

- Damage of the Auriculotemporal nerve of salivary gland during dissection.
- Injury of Auriculotemporal nerve (postganglionic parasympathetic nerve) from otic ganglion results in its fibres getting united with sympathetic fibres of superior cervical ganglion which supplies vessels and sweat glands over skin of parotid gland.
- **Manifests 2-3 months after surgery****

Clinical Features

- Sweating/erythema over the parotid gland's surgical bed as a consequence of autonomic stimulation of salivation by smell or taste of food
- **Starch iodine test**:** Paint the affected area with iodine, allow it to dry then apply starch. In the presence of sweat starch turns blue.

Prevention

- Barrier kept between skin and parotid bed to minimize appropriate regeneration of autonomic nerve fibers during surgery
- Sternomastoid muscle flap
- Temporalis facial flap
- Insertion of artificial membrane.

Treatment

- Anti perspirants–astringents as aluminium chloride
- Denervation–tympanic neurectomy (Jacobson's)
- (Surgical division of tympanic branch of glossopharyngeal nerve below the round window of middle ear)
- Recent–Botolinum toxin injection in affected skin.

Thyroid Cancers

- Best prognosis-papillary ca
- Cancer that may produce thyrotoxicosis-follicular cancer [1%]
- Bony mets from thyroid are osteolytic
- Bony mets in medullary cancer-osteoblastic
- Pulsatile bony mets-follicular ca thyroid and renal cell ca.
- Cancer associated with dystrophic calcification-papillary ca
- Long standing MNG leads to-follicular ca and rarely anaplastic ca
- Lung involvement m/c in papillary ca and bone involvement m/c in follicular Carcinoma.

Facts from Papillary Cancer

- Most common thyroid malignancy in Iodine sufficient areas–Papillary carcinoma
- Most common thyroid malignancy in Iodine deficient areas–Follicular carcinoma
- Papillary carcinoma has good prognosis
- Most common in females, 30–50 years (F:M ratio = 2.5:1)
- Papillary carcinoma is multicentric in nature
- Papillary carcinoma can arise from Thyroglossal cyst
- Papillary carcinoma produces dystrophic calcification
- Papillary carcinoma–Lateral aberrant thyroid: A metastatic node from occult papillary carcinoma
- Papillary carcinoma m/c way of mets-Lymphatic
- Papillary carcinoma is identified on FNAC-Psammoma bodies, Papillary projections and orphan Annie eyed nuclei
- Papillary carcinoma after surgery is followed up with thyroglobulin level** (Marker)
- Papillary carcinoma treatment: Total thyroidectomy + Lateral neck dissection if nodes are present.
- AGES scoring and AMES scoring are used to know the prognosis of Papillary cancer
- AGES–Age, Grade, Extrathyroidal invasion and size, M in AMES stands for mets.

Breast Concepts

- ➢ Screening mammography age: 40–49 years every 1–2 years and annually after 50 years
- ➢ Popcorn calcification is seen in fibroadenoma
- ➢ Macrocalcifications are seen in benign disorders
- ➢ Microcalcification is finding that favour malignancy
- ➢ Architectural distortion is highly suggestive of malignancy.

BRCA 1 gene mutation -chromosome 17q**	BRCA-2 gene mutation -Chromosome 13q**
• Poorly differentiated* • Invasive ductal type • Hormone receptor negative* • Associated with ovarian, prostate and colon cancers	• Well differentiated • Invasive ductal carcinomas • Express hormone receptors • Associated with ovarian, colon, prostate, pancreas, gallbladder, bile duct, stomach cancers and melanoma

Modified Radical Mastectomy (MRM)

Removal of all breast tissue, nipple -areolar complex, skin, level I and level II axillary nodes.

- **Patey's modification**:
  - Divide and remove the pectoralis minor**.
  - Level I, II, III nodes can be removed.
  - **IN PATEY'S and other types of MRM Pectoralis major not removed****
- **Auchincloss modification:** Retract pectoralis minor superomedially. Level I and II only removed.
- **Scanlon modification:** Divide the tendon at its insertion at coracoid process and put it back. Level I, II, III nodes removed.

Preserve the following structures in MRM**

Axillary Vessels
Bells nerve
Cephalic vein
Nerve to latissmus dorsi
Pectoralis major

Hormone therapy for breast cancers:

Estrogen Receptor Status

- Measured from tumor tissue by Histopathological examination
- If the tumour is ER positive it has good prognosis
- Should be given for 5 years
- Should be given only in cases of Estrogen receptor positive status**

Tamoxifen

- Partial agonist/antagonist
- Antagonist to oestrogen only in breast

Advantage

- As it is estrogen agonist in other regions, it **decreases osteoporosis*** and Blood Cholesterol.

Adverse Effects

- Bone pain, hot flushes, nausea, vomiting
- Thromboembolic manifests**
- Hypercalcemia
- Endometrial carcinoma**
- Increased cataract surgeries

Dose: 10 mg BD for five years

Serm: (Selective Estrogen Receptor Modulators)

- Agonist antagonist with differing spectra of activity

Ideal SERM

- Blocks the ER in breast, neutral or inhibitory in endometrium, lack procoagulant activity. Acts like estrogen in CVS, CNS, skeletal muscle.
- Egs: Raloxifene, Idoxifene, Toremifene
- Tamoxifen is also considered as SERM

Pure Antiestrogen: Fulvestrant–single IM injection every month is enough

Ovarian ablation for Premenopausal patients

- Medical–LHRH agonists (Buserelin, Goserelin)
- Surgical–Oopherectomy
- Radiation Induced.

Aromatose inhibitors for Postmenopausal patients

- Reversible Nonsteriodal : Anastrazole, letrozole
- Irreversible Steroidal : Formestane, exemestane
- Nonselective : Aminoglutathemide (inhibits the conversion of androstenedione to estrogen in peripheral tissues).

GASTROINTESTINAL TRACT

Tracheoesophageal Fistula

- **Mostly associated with Esophageal atresia**

The five major varieties of EA and TEF

- Most common type: EA with distal TEF (type C)–85%**
- The next most frequent is pure EA (type A)–8–10%

- TEF without EA (type E)–8%–Known as H type fistula**
- EA with fistula between both the proximal and distal ends of the esophagus and trachea (type D) is seen in approximately 2% of cases
- Type B, EA with TEF between the proximal esophagus and trachea, is seen in approximately 1% of cases.

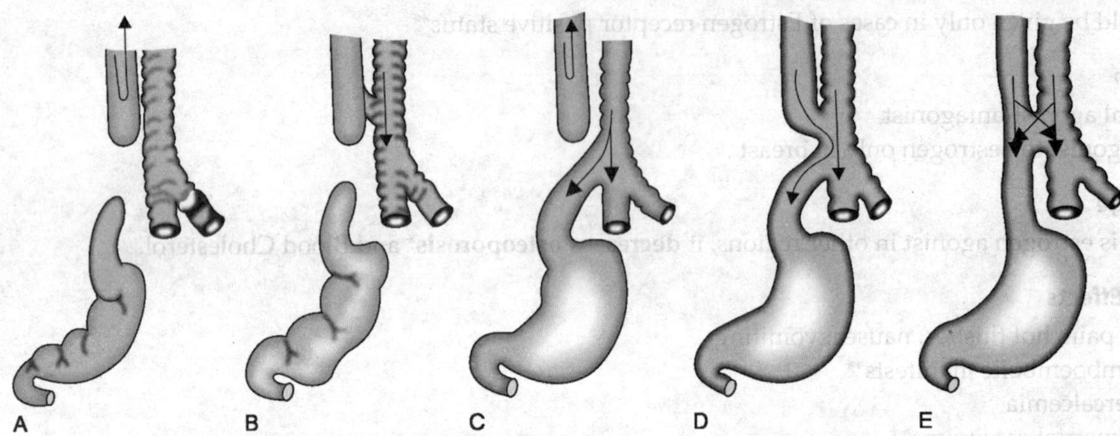

Fig. 12.1: Esophageal atresia and tracheo esophageal fistula

Clinical Features

- Newborn baby regurgitates all of its first feeds, saliva pours continuously from mouth
- Repeated coughing, cyanosis, choking
- Suspect TEF in mothers with polyhydramnios*
- Downs syndrome is associated with TEF*

Diagnosed –by coiling of Ryles tube on insertion goes to stomach

VACTERL anomalies

- Vertebral anomalies, Anal atresia, CVS defects, TRACHEO OESOPHAGEAL FISTULA, renal anomalies, Limb anomalies.

BOERHAAVE SYNDROME {BAROTRAUMA}

- Spontaneous perforation due to vomiting against a clossed glottis
- **M/c site: Lower third towards posterior and left side*,** 2 nd m/c site-mid esophagus
- Complete tear with spillage of highly infective contents into mediastinum

COMPLICATIONS: Hydro pneumothorax, pneumo mediastinum, pleural effusion

Mackler's triad:

- **Vomiting**
- **Chest pain**
- **Subcutaneous emphysema**

Treatment [Surgery is must]

PERFORATION < 24 *Hours*

- Primary closure and external drainage

PERFORATION > 24 *Hours*

- Primary closure not possible, surgical resection is must followed by proximal esophagostomy, distal end closure and feeding jejunostomy along with external drainage. Colonic interposition in a later date.

Achalasia Cardia

Motor disorder of esophageal smooth muscle in which LES does not relax normally with swallowing and esophageal body undergoes non peristaltic contractions.

Pathology

- Degeneration of ganglion cells of **Auerbachs plexus (myenteric plexus) only*** or degeneration of extra esophageal vagus
- Esophagus gets massively dilated **[dilated segment lacks ganglionic cells]***

DD:Hirschsprungs disease;*
- Dilated sigmoid colon contains normal ganglion cells whereas the constricted distal segment is devoid or lack ganglion cells.
- Absence of ganglion cells in **both Auerbach's (Myentric) and Submucosal (Meissner's plexus)***

Clinical Features

- Sex: m = f
- Age 30–50 years
- Progressive dysphagia both solids and liquids [more for liquids]
- Dysphagia worsened by stress
- Regurgitation and pulmonary aspiration
- Pain is infrequent

Investigations

- **First most investigation for dysphagia is barium swallow -Birds beak appearance***
- X ray chest appearance in Achalsia-**Absent fundus gas, air fluid level in mediastinum***
- Endoscopy-to r/o secondary causes like carcinoma,stricture
- Most confirmatory investigation (IOC) for Achalasia cardia-manometry*

Manometry findings in Achalasia:**
- **LES will be hypertensive**
- **LES fails to relax with deglutition**
- **Body of Esophagus has increased pressure**
- **No evidence of progressive peristalsis**
- **Low amplitude wave forms**

Treatment

The aim is to relieve the functional obstruction at cardia:
- Forceful dilatation
- Hellers cardiomyotomy with toupet or dor fundoplication-GOLD STANDARD
- Botulinum toxin injection [short term benefit]
- Drugs: Calcium channel blockers, sublingual nifedipine, nitroglycerine and nitrates.
- RECENT: POEM-Per oral Endoscopic Myotomy**

PSEUDOACHALASIA:
- Adenocarcinoma cardia
- Oat cell bronchogenic cancer
- Pancreatic cancer

Inhalation of amyl nitrate causes sphincter relaxation in true achalasia but not in others
- **TRYPANASOMA CRUZI**-mega oesophagus, chagas disease
- **VARICELLA ZOSTER**-achalasia cardia

Oneliners

- M/c site of iatrogenic perforation-cervical esophagus
- M/c site for barotrauma-lower third posterior and left side
- Best substitute after Esophagectomy-stomach
- Intraluminal pressure of esophagus-5 to + 5 mm Hg

- LES resting pressure-10 to 25 mm Hg.
- Malignant Tracheo Esophageal Fistula best treated nowadays by Covered Sems (Self expanding metallic stents)

Cancer Esophagus

- Most common site-Middle 1/3 rd in India
- Most common site world wide-Middle 1/3 rd
- Most common type: Squamous cell ca
- Most common type in lower 1/3 adeno ca. [m/c type in USA]

Predisposing factors

For squamous cell ca

- Alcohol
- Cigarette
- Carcinogens-nitrates, opiates smoked, fungal toxins
- Physical agents-hot tea, lye ingestion, radiation strictures, chronic achalasia

Note: In Achalasia the MC cancer is SCC, but adenocarcinoma can develop below the air fluid level in mediastinum in middle third Esophagus**

- Plummer vinson syndrome
- Tylosis palmaris et plantaris
- Dietary deficiency of molybdenum, zinc, vitamin a.
- Coeliac sprue

For adenocarcinoma

- Barrets esophagus

Clinical Features

- Dysphagia-m/c symptom but occurs when only **2/3 of circumference is involved***

Treatment

Surgical

Transthoracic Esophagectomies

Ivor Lewis two stage procedure	Mc Keown three stage procedure
• Subtotal esophagectomy • Two Incisions-Abdominal and thoracic (Two regional nodes removed) • Intrathoracic anastomosis • Leak percentage is less • Mortality if leaks is high	• Total esophagectomy • Three incisions-Abdominal, Thoracic and Cervical (Three regional nodes removed) • Neck Anastomosis • Leak percentage is more • Mortality is less as the contamination into the mediastinum never happens and secretions can be drained out.

Transhiatal Esophagectomy (THE): ORRINGER'S OPERATION:

- Two incisions-Neck and abdominal
- Neck anastomosis
- Mortality is less as thorax is not opened
- Nodal clearance is less.
- Post Op radiotherapy is given after THE

Schatzki's ring;
- Occurs at lower end near squamo columnar junction*
- Intermittent dysphagia (EPISODIC DYSPHAGIA**)
- Treatment-Balloon esophageal dilatation
- Surgery must not be done and absolutely contraindicated.

Complications of GASTRIC Surgeries

Post Cibal Syndrome (Dumping Syndrome)

Early Dumping

- After meals; small bowel gets filled with food stuff. Osmotic overload leads to sequestration of fluid from circulation into gastrointestinal tract. This leads to vasomotor and abdominal symptoms **due to hypovolemia***
- Occurs immediately.
- Diagnosed by **increased packed cell volume***

Treatment

- Small, dry meals
- Octreotides (analogues of somatostatin)
- Revision surgery: Roux -en -y reconstruction.

Late Dumping

- After meals; carbohydrate load causes a rise in plasma glucose level; results in increased insulin release that leads to **reactive hypoglycemia***
- 2nd hour after meals.
- Diagnosed by measuring **blood glucose level***
- **Treatment**
- Octreotide is effective. (Side effect: gall stone formation).
- Same as for early dumping.

	Early Dumping	Late Dumping
Incidence	5–10%	5%
Relation to meals	Immediately	Second hour
Duration	30 minutes	30 minutes
Relief	Lying down	Food
Aggravated by	More food	Exercise
Clinical Features	Epigastric fullness, sweating, diarrhea	Tremor, faintness, prostration.

Oneliners:
- Osteomalacia is a complication after GJ because Calcium is not absorbed
- (MC site of calcium absorption is Duodenum)
- **Hypocalcemia** can occur after in similar way after Billroth 2 gastrectomy
- **Duodenal stump blowout** happens usually on 4th Post op day after Billroth 2 surgery. It is managed conservatively by USG guided drainage.
- **Afferent loop syndrome*** is obstruction of the afferent loop (Loop that comes to stomach bringing Bile and pancreatic secretion) in GJ which results in Bilious vomiting without food particles. Can be managed Conservatively.
- **Efferent loop syndrome*** is obstruction of efferent loop (Loop that goes away from stomach carrying food particles) in GJ which results in Vomiting of bile mixed with food. Has to be treated as emergency by Surgery.

Lauren's classification of gastric cancer

Histology	Intestinal	Diffuse
	Areas of intestinal metaplasia	Normal gastric mucosa
Early cancer	Protruding	Flat (depressed/excavated)
Infiltration	Localized	Diffuse
Peritoneal dissemination	Infrequent	Frequent
Hepatic metastasis	Nodular	Diffuse
Sex incidence	Males more common	**Females more common**
Age incidence	Elderly	**Young**
Group A	-	+
Pernicious anemia	-	+
Genetic predisposition	-	+
H.Pylori association	+	+
Prognosis	Good	Bad*
Genetics*	APC gene mutation P53 and P16 inactivation Microsatellite instability	**Decreased E-Cadherin****

- MC type of polyps in stomach-Hyperplastic polyps
- Pacemaker of stomach is located along greater curvature at the proximal body.
- MC cause of Upper GI Bleeding–Peptic Ulcer disease. (Duodenal ulcer > Gastric ulcer)
- Trichobezoar-Consuming her own hair and causing Gastric outelet obstruction. (phytobezoar-Vegetables)-Common in psychiatric patients.
- **Rapunzel Syndrome***-Gastric tricho bezoars with a long extension of hairs that trails into duodenum.

Borchardt's Triad

- Seen in gastric volvulus.
- Stomach can rotate and go for volvulus either in organo axial or mesentrico axial.
- Characterized by **absence of vomiting**** and triad of symptoms (Borchardt's triad)
- **TRIAD: Sudden onset of constant retching epigastric pain+ Inability to vomit +Inability to pass the Ryles tube****

Dieulafoy's lesion:

- Characterized by dilated **submucosal artery (a branch from left gastric artery)** most commonly in the lesser curvature about 6 cm from cardia*
- Presents with severe hemorrhage
- Treatment is by endoscopic elecrocoagulation, angiographic embolisation with surgery as last resort

GAVE (Gastric Antral Vascular Ectasia)-Watermelon stomach

- Most common in antrum
- Dilated venules in the antrum giving the appearance of watermelon
- Presents with iron deficiency anemia and chronic melena. (not with severe bleeding)*
- Treatment is Argon plasma laser coagulation.

Bariatric Surgery

Indications for Obesity or Bariatric surgery:

- BMI > 40 kg/sq.m or 35 kg/sq.m with associated medical co morbidity worsened by obesity
- Failed dietary therapy

- Psychiatrically stable
- Knowledgeable enough about surgery.

Types of Bariatric surgery

Malabsorptive
- Jejunoileal and jejunocolic bypasses (no longer recommended)

Restrictive
- Vertical banded gastroplasty
- Adjustable silicone gastric banding
- Sleeve gastrectomy

Mostly restrictive (and partly malabsorptive)
- Short-limb (50–100 cm) Roux-en-Y gastric bypass
- Long-limb (150 cm) Roux-en-Y gastric bypass

Mostly malabsorptive
- Biliopancreatic diversion with or without duodenal switch.

Meckels Diverticulum**

- Meckels is true diverticulum, located in anti mesentric border*
- M/c congenital anomaly of GIT*
- M/c ectopic mucosa-m/c is gastric (60%)*, pancreatic, colonic, Brunners glands, Endometriosis
- RULE OF 2-prevalence2%, **2 inch length**, located 2 feet proximal to IC VALVE, presents m/c in < 2 years age
- M/c complication in adults-obstruction*, children-bleeding*, overall–bleeding*
- **LITTRES hernia-**Meckels as content in the sac (Amyand's hernia-appendix*)
- **Tc99m pertechnate scan*-**Used to diagnose Meckels Preoperatively. Diagnosis based on the presence of ectopic gastric mucosa. As the age advances the sensitivity decreases as the ectopic mucosa disappears.
- Angiography can diagnose at times of active bleed only.
- Resection of ileum with anastomosis is done if-peptic ulcer in ileum, gangrene affecting base, rarely if malignancy associated
- Incidentally found Meckels during other surgery: Two different opinion given in books. **Sabiston says the life time incidence of Complications in Meckels is 6.8% and hence it should be resected if found incidentally during other surgeries.****

Diverticular Disease

- Diverticulosis–multiple diverticula
- Diverticulitis–perforated diverticulum due to inflammation
- Diverticulosis–Best diagnosed by barium enema (Saw tooth appearance*). Barium Enema should not be done in acute settings
- Diverticulitis–best diagnosed by CT SCAN*
- False divericula-are m/c*
- Left side [sigmoid]colon-m/c site*
- Bleeding diverticula are m/c from right side*
- In small bowel-Duodenum is m/c site, m/c on mesentric side, false diverticula.
- Most sensitive test for SI diverticula-Enteroclysis
- Small bowel diverticula are associated with **Blind loop syndrome**–bacterial overgrowth, B 12 deficiency-megaloblastic anemia.

BLIND LOOP SYNDROME-a condition in which a segment of Small intestine if goes for stagnation without peristalsis bacterial overgrowth happens and the patient gets Vitamin B12 deficiency as the bacteria utilises the vitamin for its growth.
It is easily diagnosed by SCHILLING test**.. Reversability of Schilling test to normal after antibiotics confirms the diagnosis.

Small Bowel Carcinoids

- Most common site of carcinoids now in intestine-**Bronchus > Ileum > Rectum > Appendix (BIRA).**
- Primary–Usually small
- Secondary–Those metastasized produces many symptoms together known as Carcinoid Syndrome

Features

- Arise from enterochromaffin like cells (ECL) also known as kulchisky**/argentaffian cells.
- Produces–5HT (serotonin), ACTH, Somatostatin and Peptide YY.
- 80% are asymptomatic.
- Only when serosa is invaded they produces intense desmoplastic reaction presenting with abdominal pain, intusussception and diarrhea (mainly due to partial obstruction and not due to serotonin.)

Location	Predominant Hormone
Foregut	5-HTP or ACTH (Low serotonin)*
Midgut	Serotonin
Hindgut	Somatostatin or Peptide YY

APUD omas:

- Amine precursor uptake are derived from neural crest tissue as they migrate to different parts of the body.
  - GIT–carcinoids
  - Pancreas–insulinomas
  - CNS-neuroblastomas
  - Adrenal–pheochromocytoma
  - Lungs–small cell carcinoma.

Metastatic carcinoids (secondary)

- Metastasis depends on
  - Size: < 1 cm (< 2%) ; > 2 cm (90%)
  - Site: Appendix (3%) ; ileal (35%) Least With Appendix.
  - Depth of invasion.

*** Malignant carcinoid syndrome develops only liver mets develop; because all the above listed hormones are detoxified in liver.**

Carcinoid syndrome:

- Vasomotor symptoms (80%)-cutaneous flushing
- GIT–explosive diarrhea. Due to serotonin.
- Cardiovascular–**The three most common cardiac lesions are pulmonary stenosis (90%), tricuspid insufficiency (47%), and tricuspid stenosis (42%).**
- Asthmatic attacks-broncho spasm
- Malabsorption and Pellagra (dementia, diarrhea, dermatitis) due to excessive diversion of tryptophan.
  - **Types of Flushing:** Diffuse erythematous, Violaceous, Prolonged flushes and Bright red patchy
  - **MC type of Flushing seen in Gastric carcinoids-Bright red patchy.**

Investigations

- 24 hours urinary 5 hydroxy indole acetic acid (5HIAA)** are highly specific.
- Neuroendocrine tumour marker-chromogranin A
- Pentagastrin provocative tests
- Small bowel carcinoids–difficult to diagnose pre operatively.
- Recently–**somatostatin receptor scintigraphy with indium-111 labelled pentreotide** has shown higher sensitivity than CT scan.

Treatment

- If size < 1 cm–segmental intestinal resection
- If size > 1 cm, nodes+ or if there are multiple metastasis-wide excision along with mesentry.
- Terminal ileum–Right hemicolectomy.
- Liver mets-resection, hepatic artery ligation or embolization or RFA.
- Recent advance: **SMART BOMBS**-Radiolabelled Somatostatin Analogues that deliver radiation specifically to carcinoid cells.

Clinical Features	Ulcerative Colitis	Crohns Disease
Location	Colon only	Anywhere in the alimentary tract
Anatomic distribution	Continuous, beginning distally	Asymmetrical **skip lesions**
Rectal involvement	> 90%	Occasionally
Diarrhea/gross bleeding	Severe, often bloody with mucus	Less severe, infrequent bleeding
Abdominal pain	Yes	Occasionally
Perianal fistulas	Rare	Common
Abdominal mass (palpable)	Rare	Common
Strictures and obstructions	Uncommon	Common
Fistulas and perforations	Rare	Common
Extraintestinal manifestations	Common	Common
Recurrence after surgery	If retained rectal mucosa	Yes

- **Lead pipe* or Hose Pipe appearance:** Loss of haustrations in Colon is a feature of Ulcerative colitis
- **String Sign of Kantor*:** Is seen in terminal ileum in Crohns Disease. Also seen in Hyperplastic Tuberculosis

One liners

- Mucosa is least resistant to ischemia*
- If main trunk of SMA is involved infarction occurs from duodenojeunal flexure to splenic flexure
- **Classically the pain is central and out of proportion to physical findings** in Acute SMA Occlusion**
- **Presence of gas bubbles in mesentric vein is pathognomonic**
- **MC cause of Chronic Mesentric Ischemia is-Thrombosis***
- **Arc of Riolan–Collateral between SMA and IMA at the origin**
- **Marginal Artery of Drummond-Collateral between SMA and IMA at the margin of the Colon.**
- M/C SITE of Ischemic Colitis-SPLENIC FLEXURE*
- **Griffith Point:** Splenic Flexure where ischemic Colitis is common
- **Sudeck's Point:** Sigmoid Colon where ischemic Stricture is common
- **Ischemic Colitis shows: Thumb Print Sign** on Plain X-ray*

Stomas

Ileostomy	Colostomy
Created in Right iliac fossa	Created in Transverse colon or Sigmoid colon
Types: End or loop	Types: End or loop
Ileostomy is sprouted to surface	Colostomy is flushed
Content is liquid	Content is solid stools

Ileostomy

Temporary:

- Loop ileostomy used for allowing the distal anastomosis to heal. (e.g. Following Low anterior resection in Cancer rectum or in Postradiotherapy/Immunocompromised cases)
- Advantage with loop ileostomy is its easy to reclose without doing a laparotomy.

Permanent:

- Its usually an End ileostomy which is sprouting.
- Brooke type is commonly used sprouting one.
- Kock's Ileostomy is continent type having a valve.
- Done following Total Proctocolectomy in Ulcerative colitis.

Complications of Ileostomy:

- Early complication-Stoma necrosis
- Stoma retraction may be early or late complication (M/c in obese patients)
- Fluid and Electrolyte loss (Ileostomy output must be less than 1500 ml)
- Skin irritation
- Parastomal hernia (less common than after colostomy***)
- Stomal prolapse is a late complication**

Colostomy:

- Usually end Colostomy is done.
- Loop colostomy is difficult because of the bulkiness
- Parastomal hernia is a late complication.

MCQ's Asked in Stomas:

- Ileostomy the mc Complication: Necrosis (22%), prolapse (22%), skin irritation (17%), and stenosis (17%)
- ***Parastomal hernia is most common after -Colostomy than ileostomy and after end colostomy***
- ***Stomal Prolapse is more common after transverse loop Colostomy.***

Mesentric Cysts

Types: Chylolymphatic [M/C Type]** and Enterogenous Cyst

Chylolymphatic Cyst	Enterogenous Cyst
Usually congenital as a result of sequestration of lymphatics	Derived from diverticulum of mesentric border that has become sequestrated
Cyst wall is thin, lacks muscular wall, not lined by mucosa	Thick wall lined by mucosa
Usually solitary,often unilocular with clear lymph or chyle	Content is mucinous
Most frequently seen in mesentry of ileum	
Independent blood supply	Common blood supply as adjacent bowel
Enucleation is enough**	**Resection anastomosis needed****

CLINICAL FEATURES

Tillaux Triad

- **Central area of dullness with zone of resonance all around**
- **Swelling moves perpendicular to mesentry freely**
- **Soft fluctuant swelling in the umbilical region**

➢ Recurrent attacks of abdominal pain with or without vomiting due to obstruction
➢ Acute abdominal pain due to torsion of mesentry, rupture of cyst, hemorrhage into cyst, infection of cyst.

HEPATOBILIARY AND PANCREATIC SURGERY

Gallbladder and Biliary Tract

- **Crypts of Luschka*:** mucous folds in GB.
- Common hepatic duct-2.5 cm*
- Common bile duct-7.5 Cm*
- CBD enters the duodenum at ampulla located posteriorly 10 cm from pylorus*
- **Cystic artery***-arises from Right hepatic artery behind common hepatic duct
- **Accessory cystic artery-**From Gastroduodenal artery*
- **Valves of Heister*-**Valves present in the Neck of Gallbladder and Cystic duct.
- M/c anomaly of Gallbladder–**Phrygian cap*** [Fundus is constricted and turned back on itself]
- Normal size of CBD-6 mm*
- Cystic node of Lund -sentinel node of GB. Present in Calot's triangle
- Sphincter of ODDI is made up of 4 sphincters**
- Sphincter ODDI -Basal resting pressure is 13 mm Hg more than duodenum

Moynihans Hump [Cater Pillar Turn]

- Right hepatic artery takes a tortuous course in front of origin of cystic duct and enters the Calot's triangle.
- May be damaged in Calot's triangle

CALOTS TRIANGLE

Formed between
- Inferior-Cystic duct and GB
- Medial-Common hepatic duct
- Above-Inferior liver surface.

Gallstones

M/c type of stone–mixed stone

Types of Stones
- Cholesterol stones
- Brown pigment stones
- Black pigment stones
- Mixed

LITHOGENIC BILE:

Bile salts and phospholipids in bile keep cholesterol in solution by forming micelles.

Cholesterol is insoluble in water which is made soluble by bile salts and phospholipids.

Normal ratio
- Bile acids: cholesterol = 20:1*
- Critical ratio = < 13:1 at which crystallization occurs.

Pigment Stones

Name given when contains cholesterol < 30 %

Black Pigment	Brown Pigment
M/c in hemolytic states • Hereditary spherocytosis, sickle cell disease • Heart valves [mechanical] • Liver cirrhosis • Gilbert's syndrome • Cystic fibrosis • Ileal resection	• Rare in gallbladder • Primary bile duct stone formation** • Due to bile stasis and infection** • M/C–E.COLI* • M/C IN presence of FB, stents, parasites** • MC recurrent type of recurrent stone • MC type of stone seen in Hepatolithiasis (Oriental Cholangiohepatitis)

Acalculus Cholecystitis

- Highest mortality*
- Most commonly missed diagnosis
- M/c in patients recovering from major surgery and burns, trauma*
- **Best treatment is Open cholecystectomy. If unfit for surgery-Cholecystotomy (USG drainage of Gallbladder)**

Complications

Mucocele: Obstruction of stone at **neck** of gallbladder*
Treatment-Early cholecystectomy*

Mirrizi Syndrome

- It refers to the obstruction or stricture of the common hepatic duct as result of extrinsic compression by a gallstone in the cystic duct or Hartman's Pouch in Gallbladder.

Fistulas from Gallbladder

- M/C site duodenum [CHOLECYSTOENTERIC FISTULA]
- Diagnosis suspicious by presence of air in bile duct
- Complication-Gallstone ileus**
- Other sites of fistula-colon.

Gallstone Ileus

- Characterised by Tumbling Intermittent Small intestine obstruction by the Gall stone which has passed via the Choledocho Duodenal Fistula
- **Rigler's triad:** Pneumobilia, Intestinal obstruction and Cholecystoenteric fistula
- Duodenal obstruction due to gallstones usually in the bulb is known as **Bouveret's syndrome***

*Saints Triad***

- Gallstones
- Diverticulosis of colon
- Hiatus hernia

MEDICAL TREATMENT

- ***Useful only for cholesterol Gallstones not for pigment stones****
- Mechanism is by inhibiting HMG CO –A reductase in cholesterol synthesis, thus decrease cholesterol Super saturation.

Useful only in**

- Radiolucent
- Size < 10 mm
- Functioning gallbladder
- Non acute symptoms

Charcot's Triad*

CBD stone causing cholangitis

- Pain
- Jaundice
- Rigors

Reynaulds Pentad*

Includes Charcots triad + Septic shock+ Mental status changes
Management of CBD Stone:

In Presence of Cholangitis

- ERCP with sphincterotomy and stone extraction [Treatment of choice]**
- PTC drainage: ERCP failed cases
- *Surgery:* Only when above two procedures not possible
  Decompression of CBD with T tube.

In Absence of Cholangitis

- Lap cholecystectomy with Lap CBD exploration (or)
- Lap cholecystectomy with ERCP stone removal

CBD Exploration and T Tube Removal *(Ref: Blumgart Page 524)*

- Post op Cholangiogram-on day 14–21
- Remove T tube-14 to 21 days

Carcinoma Gallbladder

- M/c malignancy of biliary tract*
- M/c female elderly
- 70 to 80% cases are gallstones associated*.

Risk Factors

- Gallstones
- Polyps [>10 mm]
- Porcelain GB
- Choledochal cyst
- Anomalous pancreato bile duct junction
- Typhoid carriers*
- Sclerosing cholangitis
- Ulcerative colitis
- Cholecysto enteric fistula
- Drugs-estrogens [not OCP]*
- Carcinogens [nitrosamines, azo dyes, rubber industry chemicals]

Clinical Features

- Pain [73%}
- Anorexia and weight loss{63%}
- Jaundice [54%]-poor prognostic sign*
- Fever
- Vomiting [mechanical obstruction or malignant gastro paresis]
- O/E-mass palpable [50%], hepatomegaly, ascites

Pathology: Adenocarcinoma (90%),undifferentiated, squamous cell carcinoma.

Investigations

- USG: Localized excessive thickening of gallbladder [normal GB thickness is < 3 mm]
- CT contrast [CECT]-lymph nodes > 10 mm visible
- **MRI + MRCP + MRA-is most useful than all above-helps in planning management**
- **FNAC:** Contraindicated in operable tumors [risk of dissemination via tract]
  FNAC is indicated only in inoperable tumors

- **Diagnostic laparoscopy is must:** 38% cases found inoperable among those cases planned for curative resection after all the investigations.
- Tumor markers CEA, CA 19–9

Contraindications for Surgery

- Poor general condition
- Liver mets
- Extrahepatic mets
- Peritoneal spread
- Distant nodes [coeliac, sup mesentric, para aortic]
- Portal vein or hepatic artery involved
- Bilateral involvement of secondary biliary radicles
- Extensive duodenal involvement.

Treatment

- Limited to muscular layer (T1): **simple cholecystectomy**
- Reaching muscular layer but not extending to serosa (T2): **Extended cholecystectomy:** Liver segments IVB and V, and lymphadenectomy of the cystic duct, and pericholedochal, portal, right celiac, and posterior pancreatoduodenal lymph nodes.
- For tumors that grow beyond the serosa or invade the liver or other organs (T3 and T4 tumors), there is a high likelihood of intraperitoneal and distant spread.
- If no peritoneal or nodal involvement is found, complete tumor excision with an **extended right hepatectomy (segments IV, V, VI, VII, and VIII)** must be performed for adequate tumor clearance.

Cancers diagnosed in cholecystectomy specimens

Except for tumors confined to mucosa re do laparotomy is advised with resection as per staging along with lap port sites excision.

Courvoisier's Law:

- For Cases with Obstructive jaundice
- If gallbladder is Palpable it is not due to stones
- Explanation: Because if the CBD stone causes obstruction the gallbladder would have been already thick and fibrosed due to cholecystitis and hence cant expand in cases of Obstructive Jaundice)
- To say in simple: CBD stone-Gallbladder not palpable: Cancer in Periampulla or Distal CBD-Gallbladder is palpable.

Exceptions:

- Double stone–One in CBD and other in Cystic duct-Gallbladder becomes palpable due to Mucocele
- Hilar cholangiocarcinoma (Klatskin Tumor)-Tumor above cystic duct origin so GB not palpable.

PSEUDO CYST PANCREAS

- Most common site of pseudo cyst-body and tail*
- Most common cause of Pseudocyst -Pancreatitis*
- Second Common cause-Trauma*
- Most common cause in children-Trauma.*

Intervention for Pseudocyst:

- Persists > 6 weeks
- Size > 6 cm
- Complications develop
- Secondary infection

Complications:

- Obstruction
- Hemorrhage
- Rupture
- Pseudoaneurysm of splenic artery
- Infection

Ransons criteria for Acute pancreatitis: [LAGAW BUCHOW]*

On admission

- Age > 55 years
- WBC count > 16000/ mm^3
- Blood glucose > 10mmol/l
- LDH > 700u/l
- AST > 250 sigma frankel units %

Within 48 hours

- BUN > 5 mg%
- Arterial 02 saturationPaO_2 < 60 mm Hg
- Serum calcium < 2.0 mmol/l
- Hematocrit fall > 10%
- Base deficit > 4 mmol/l
- Fluid sequestration > 6l

If Scoring is more than 3 it is Severe Pancreatitis.

Pancreatic Tumors

- Exocrine
- Endocrine

M/c type: Adenocarcinoma
M/c site: Head**

Periampullary CA: Tumors in region of ampulla, lower CBD, duodenum
**M/c presentation is painless intermittent jaundice

Courvoisiers Law:
In a patient with obstructive jaundice if there is a palpable gallbladder it is not due to stones.

Exceptions

- Double impacted stone. (a stone where GB palpable due to mucus collection in it)
- Klatskin's tumor

- *Trousseau's Sign: Migratory thrombophlebitis
- *Troisier's Sign: Left supraclavicular node

WHIPPLES PROCEDURE

- Radical pancreaticoduodenectomy

Removal of:

- Pancreas head
- Duodenum
- Stomach
- Portion of jejunum
- Gallbladder and Distal Bile duct

Indications for Whipples procedure:

- Distal CBD growth
- Periampullary growth
- Pancreatic head cancer

Triple anastomosis:

- Choledocho jejunostomy
- Pancreato jejunostomy
- Gastro jejunostomy.

Endocrine Neoplasms

- Insulinoma [beta cells
- Glucogonomas [alpha cells]
- Gastrinomas [G CELLS]
- Somatostatatinomas [D CELLS]
- Vipomas (Vasoactive Intestinal Polypeptide).

Insulinomas

- Most common type of endocrine tumor in pancreas.
- Common site: Head = Body = Tail (Equally distributed)**

Beta Cell Tumor

- Mostly Solitary
- Mostly Benign* [10–15% malignant]
- M/c Symptom-hypoglycemia [confusion, irritation and disorientation]

Whipples Triad

- Signs and symptoms of hypoglycemia
- Blood glucose < 2.8 mmol/l
- Relief of symptoms by IV glucose
- **Gold Standard Investigation to diagnose:** 72 Hours fasting Blood Sugar Level and Blood Insulin level
- **Characteristic symptom is weight gain instead of weight loss***
- **Most sensitive investigation–INTRA OP USG***
- Best investigation to diagnose preoperatively: **Selective arteriography**

Treatment: Surgical Excision

Gastrinomas

- **MC endocrine neoplasm of Pancreas in MEN 1 Syndrome is gastrinoma**
- The majority (60%) of these tumors are malignant
- Gastrinoma give rise to Zollinger Ellison Syndrome which consist of triad*
  - Hypersecretion of gastric acid
  - Severe peptic ulceration
  - Presence of non-beta cell tumour of the pancreas or duodenum.

Zollinger Ellison Syndrome

- Presents with complaints of PEPTIC ULCER-Refractory ulcer, unusual sites and unusual recurrence
- MC site is Passaro Triangle. (If not given in choice-MC site is duodenum)

Passaro Triangle*

- Junction of CBD and cystic duct
- Junction of neck and body of pancreas
- Junction of 2nd and 3rd part duodenum

Diagnosis

- Normal gastrin level < 150 pg/ml
- BAO > 15 meq/hour
- Secretin stimulation-increases the gastrin secretion > 200 pg/ml
- FASTING GASTRIN > 1000 pg/ml is highly suggestive.

- ➢ Investigation of choice to localize the tumor-somatostatin receptor scintigraphy (SRS)
- ➢ Drug of Choice: Proton pump inhibitors.

Vipomas [Verner Morrison Syndrome]

- WDHA SYNDROME*-Watery Diarrhea Hypokalemia Achlorhydria
- Characterized by severe intermittent watery diarrhea
- Most sensitive investigation-EUS

Glucagonomas

(Diabetes + Dermatitis)

- **Necrolytic migratory erythema*-**perianal, lower abdomen, perinIum, foots.

One liners:

- Pancreatogenic diabetes (Type 3) is ***M/c after surgical resection for chronic pancreatitis***
- Double bubble sign-Duodenal atresia, annular pancreas.
- Triple bubble sign-Jejunal atresia.
- Failure of fusion of ventral and dorsal buds of pancreas is called as Pancreas divisum. Treatment is ERCP of minor papilla.
- Failure of complete rotation of ventral bud during development results in Annular pancreas.
- Annular pancreas is associated with Duodenal atresia and Downs Syndrome.
- Annular pancreas is treated by Duodeno duodenostomy.
- **Double duct sign** is an ERCP finding in Ca head of pancreas in which the Distal CBD and Pancreatic duct appears separated and narrowed.
- **Tunnel of Love*** is seen posterior to the neck of pancreas through which Superior mesenteric vein enters and forms Portal vein.

LIVER

Functional Anatomy (Coiunaud's Segments)

- **Cantlie's Line:** An imaginary line running from gallbladder to left side of IVC.
- Right liver–segments 5, 6, 7, 8
- Left liver–segments 1, 2, 3, 4
- Caudate lobe is segment 1.
- **Reidel's lobe-a tongue like extension from the right liver inferiorly.**
- Segments to the left of falciparum segment-segment 2 and 3*
- CAUDATE LOBE* is the lobe that is not affected in Budd Chiari syndrome and cirrhosis of liver because of its direct drainage into IVC.
- Quadrate lobe is the fourth lobe*

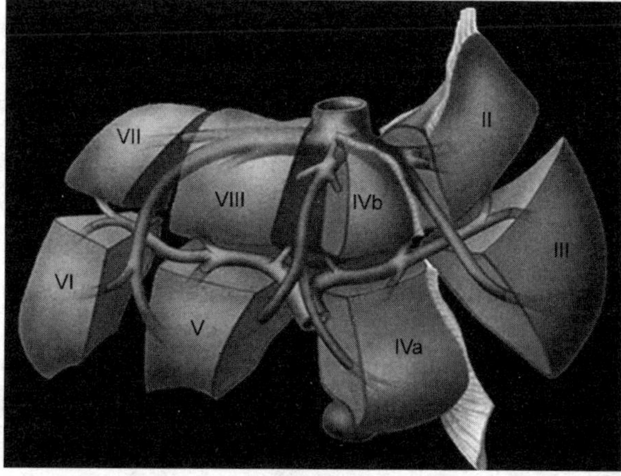

Fig. 12.2: Segments of liver

Types of Hepatectomy:

- Removal of segments 2–4 (left hepatectomy)
- Removal of segments 5–8 (right hepatectomy)
- Removal of segments 5–8 along with 4 (extended right hepatectomy)
- Removal of segments 2–4 along with 5 and 8 (extended left hepatectomy)

Modified Child Pugh Classification

Clinical**	1	2	33
Encephalopathy	None	1 or 2	3 or 4
Ascites	None	Mild	Moderate
Bilirubin (mg/dl)	1–2 mg/dl	2.1–3 mg/dl	≥ 3.1 mg/dl
Albumin (gm/dl)	≥ 3.5 gm/dl	2.8–3.4 gm/dl	≤ 2.7 gm/dl
Prothrombin time (increase in seconds)	1–4	4.1–6	≥ 6

- Grade A: 5–6
- Grade B: 7–9
- Grade C: 10–15 points.

MELD: Modified End Liver Disease Scoring:

Based on: CBI

- Creatinine
- Bilirubin
- INR

Portal Hypertension and Cirrhosis

Related anatomy:

- Portal vein is formed by the confluence of superior mesentric vein and splenic vein behind the neck of pancreas.
- Left gastric (coronary) vein* enters the portal vein at its origin.
- Splenic vein is joined by inferior mesentric vein just before it's confluence with superior mesentric vein.
- Portal vein length: 6-8 cm*
- Normal pressure in portal venous system-3–5 mm Hg* and 10–12 cm H_2O.

MCQ Points

- M/c cause of death in portal hypertension-hepatic failure
- 2nd common cause of death–variceal hemorrhage
- M/c cause of portal hypertension–alcoholic cirrhosis.

Left Sided Portal Hypertension

- Due pancreatic neoplasm or inflammation the splenic vein gets thrombosed and results in left sided portal hypertension
- The superior mesentric and portal venous pressure is normal.
- Left gastroepiploic becomes the major collateral and hence GASTRIC varices develop rather than OESOPHAGEAL.
- Easily reversed by splenectomy.

Bleeding in Portal Hypertension

- The most common cause of bleeding in PHT patients is from esophagogastric varices*
- (esophagus 80% and gastric 20%)
- Isolated gastric varices must raise the suspicion of splenic vein thrombosis**.
- The only nonvariceal cause of portal hypertensive bleeding is Portal Hypertensive Gastropathy** (m/c after eradication of varices)

Treatment

Esophagogastric varices will not bleed until the pressure exceeds 12 mm Hg**

Resuscitation

Interventional

- Endoscopic banding is advantageous because it doesn't lead to necrosis or ulceration of esophagus but both are equally effective in controlling bleeding.
- Sclerosants used-Ethanolamine oleate, Cyano acrynalate, Sodium morrhuate or Sodium tetra decyl sulfate.

Sengstaken Blakemore Tube:

- Modified sengstaken Contains ***FOUR lumens**** *(old sengstaken Blakemore tube contains 3 tubes*)*-one for aspiration from stomach, one from esophagus, one for esophageal balloon dilatation and last one for gastric balloon dilatation.
- The gastric balloon inflated to 250 ml of air and esophageal balloon to a pressure of **40 mmHg using Air****
- The potentially lethal complication is accidentally inflating gastric balloon inside the esophagus resulting in *perforation of esophagus**.
- Balloons should be temporarily deflated after 12 hours to prevent esophageal necrosis.

Pharmacotherapy

- Octreotide (long acting analogue of somatostatin) and somatostatin are effective like endoscopy.
- Vasopressin previously used is also effective but nitroglycerine must be given along with it to prevent coronary vessels constriction.

Transjugular Intrahepatic Portal Shunt: (Tips)**

- Short term Bridge to liver transplant.
- Inserted via IJV by interventional radiologist*.
- Access the portal vein inside the liver via a branch of hepatic vein and dilate the tract to 10 mm* through which expandable metallic stent is inserted.
- It's not used as initial therapy but can be used if endoscopy and pharmacotherapy fails.
- It's a type of **non selective shunt***.

Complications

- Main early complication* is perforation of liver capsule and fatal intraperitoneal hemorrhage.
- Post shunt encephalopathy* is the confusional state due to the toxic metabolites bypassing the metabolism in liver.
- Long-term complication is Shunt stenosis* which may occur in < 1 year.

Contraindications

Absolute

- Right side heart failure
- Polycystic liver disease

Relative

- Portal vein thrombosis

- Hypervascular liver tumours
- Encephalopathy

Prevention of Recurrent Bleed

- Drug used is non selective beta blockers-Propranolol has shown to reduce rebleed.
- Combination of ISDN and propranolol has been shown to be more effective than variceal ligation.

Shunting Surgeries

Nonselective shunts:
- End to side portocaval shunt (Ecks fistula)
- Side to side portocaval shunt
- Large diameter interposition shunts (> 16 mm)
- Conventional splenorenal shunts
- TIPS

Conventional splenorenal shunt:

- Involves removal of spleen** and insertion of proximal splenic vein into renal vein.

  Complication:
  - Portal shunt encephalopathy is more common in this procedure.

  Advantages:
  - This type of shunt also decompresses the splanchnic venous system and intrahepatic sinusoidal network hence side to side shunts are the effective in controlling ascites and preventing rebleed.

Selective Shunts

- Splenorenal shunt: Distal (Warrens)
- **Inokuchi*:** Left gastric vena caval shunt. Vein graft interposed between the left gastric vein and inferior vena cava.

Distal Splenorenal Shunt: (Warrens Shunt)

- Anastomosis of distal end of splenic vein to the left renal vein along with interruption of all collaterals.
- This shunt aggravates the ascites** because sinusoidal and mesentric hypertension is maintained and important lymphatic pathways are transected during dissection.

Nonshunt Operations

- Simplest nonshunt operation is transection and re anastomosis of the distal esophagus with a stapling device.
- Extensive esophagogastric devascularization combined with splenectomy and esophageal transection **(Sugiura Operation)***
- Main indication for this surgery is distal splanchnic venous thrombosis* and for patients with distal splenorenal shunt thrombosis*.

Transplant Candidates

- Non alcoholic cirrhosis and abstinent alcoholic cirrhotics with CHILD B OR C.
- Patients with poor quality life style due to encephalopathy, fatigue of CHILD A will also be indicated.

Hydatid Cyst

- Echinococcus granulosus is m/c. others E.multilocularis, E.oligartus.
- **Dogs are definitive hosts*** in which adult tapeworm is attached in villi of small intestine.
- **Sheeps are intermediate hosts*** that consume the ova passed by the feces of dog over grasses.
- *Humans are accidental hosts* consuming these eggs that coverts to embryo in duodenum and releases an oncosphere containing hooklets that penetrate the mucosa and reach the bloodstream.

- The oncosphere reaches the liver (m/c), or lungs where the parasite develops into larval stage called as hydatid cyst.
- Remember *humans are end stage host.*

Clinical Feature

- M/c in right lobe of liver**
- Most frequent sign-hepatomegaly
- M/c symptoms-abdominal pain, dyspepesia and vomiting.
- Complications: rupture into biliary tree, bronchial tree, pleural, peritoneal and pericardial cavity.

Investigations

- USG: *rosette like appearance* or water lilley appearance.* **Calcifications** in the wall are highly diagnostic.
- Serological tests: ELISA, arc 5 test, IHA test, *Immunoblast test where available is the test of choice*.*
- **Casoni's test:** Intradermal injection of sterile hydatid fluid produces a wheal of 5 cm in half hour.

Gharbi et al Classification of Hydatid Cysts:

- Type 1: Unilocular cyst
- Type 2: Floating membrane (water lilly sign)
- Type 3: Multiseptated (Honey comb/Rosette like)
- Type 4: Heterogenous cysts
- Type 5: Calcified wall

Type 1, 2, 3 are active cysts

Type 4, 5 are Inactive and dead cysts

Treatment

- Primarily surgical but introduction of PAIR has totally replaced it.
- Surgical procedures:
  - Pericystectomy
  - Marsupialization
  - Omentoplasty
  - Total cystectomy
  - Partial hepatectomy
- Remember surgery is now preferred where PAIR is not possible or when it doesn't respond to PAIR or when there is any communication to biliary tree.

PAIR:
- **Percutaneous Aspiration, Infusion of scolicidal agents and Reaspiraion.**
- Given with prophylactic cover of albendazole.
- Scolicidal agents-20% hypertonic saline, 0.5% silver nitrate, 95% ethanol, absolute alcohol, mebendazole 2.4 microgram/ml.

Contraindications for PAIR:
- Superficially located cyst (chance of rupture)
- Honey combing of cysts (multiple thick internal septae)
- Communication with biliary tree.
- Dead or inactive cysts

Budd Chiari Syndrome

- Young females* are affected commonly
- Venous drainage is occluded by either a venous thrombosis or obstruction by a venous web.
- M/c presentation–ascites* and abdominal discomfort

- As a result of venous outflow obstruction the liver gets congested with development of impaired liver function with subsequent portal hypertension, ascites and esophageal varices
- R/O underlying etiology-myeloprolifertaive disorder or procoagulant state like Protein C,S deficiency or Antithrombin deficiency.
- CT scan-ascites with large congested liver or a small cirrhotic liver in which there is **gross enlargement of segment 1 (caudate lobe)***–because only segment 1 has direct drainage to IVC.
- Confirmation of diagnosis-Hepatic venography via transjugular route
- Treatment
  - Cirrhotic liver/fulminant liver failure-liver transplant
  - Noncirrhotic-portocaval shunting.

Liver Transplant

- M/c indication in children-biliary atresia
- M/c indication in adults-cirrhosis from Hepatitis C virus
- 2nd MC indication in adults-Alcoholic cirrhosis
- MC indication in Metabolic disorder-Alpha 1 Antitrypin deficiency
- MC indication after acute liver failure-Acetaminophen Toxicity
- **Starzl (1963)-**First liver transplant
- First split liver transplant-Pichlmayr
- First live donor liver transplant-**Tanaka (1991)** using left lobe

Absolute Contraindications

- Active untreated sepsis
- Advanced cardiopulmonary disease
- Extrahepatic malignancy
- Metastasis in liver
- AIDS
- Life threatening systemic diseases

Expanded criteria for liver donor

The shortage of liver donor has made us to relax the criteria for liver transplant donors.

This criteria is called as **'Marginal donor or Expanded criteria' donor.**

Age even up to 75-80 years

Hepatitis B core ab positive and Hepatitis C positive

Steatosis in the range of 10-30%.

Types of Graft

- **Orthotopic graft:** A graft placed in its normal anatomic site, e.g. liver
- **Heterotopic graft**: A graft placed in a site different from it's normal location, e.g. kidney kept in iliac fossa

Procedure

- The donor cadaveric liver is removed with coeliac trunk and aortic cuff, IVC, common duct.
- Place the donor liver in orthotopic place and anastomosis done in following order
  - Donor and recepient **suprahepatic vena cava**
  - Donor and recepient **infrahepatic vena cava** in end to end fashion
  - **Portal vein anastomosis** is done next (results in reperfusion syndrome-hypotension, bradycardia, arrythmias, cardiac arrest.
  - Aortic carrel patch of donor anastomosed to **hepatic artery** at level of gastro duodenal artery bifurcation of recipient.
  - Last will be **duct anastomosis** of donor liver to duct of recipient with or without T tube.

MCQ Points in Liver Transplant

- **Hepatic artery thrombosis*** may occur spontaneously or as a part of* acute graft rejection*. It may present as fever, bile leak or rise in serum transaminase level. This complication requires immediate re transplantation.
- **Portal vein thrombosis:** Occurs insidiously and doesn't require retransplant
- **Paediatric liver transplant:** Using adult lateral segment of left liver.
- **Chronic liver graft rejection occurs due to vanishingbile duct syndrome**.**
- **Liver is resistant to hyper acute and chronic rejection***

Complications of Splenectomy

- M/c infection after splenectomy–streptococcus pneumonia*

OPSI

Bacterial infection:
- Streptococcus pneumonia
- Hemophilus influenza type B
- Meningococcus
- Group A streptococcus

Protozoan infection after splenectomy:
- Babesia
- Malaria

No increased risk of viral infection*

Before elective splenectomy is planned:

The following vaccination are given:

Two weeks before planned splenectomy:
- Pneumococcal vaccine: boosted every 5years
- H.influenza type B (Hib) vaccine
- Influenza vaccine -annually
- Meningococcal vaccine

Postsplenectomy prophylaxis:

Antibiotic prophylaxis with Penicillin V 250 mg bd (or) erythromycin 250mg bd for longer of the following
- 2 years postsplenectomy (or)
- Up to age of 16 years
  - Risk of development of OPSI is high for hematologic indications then those who undergo splenectomy for trauma.

Immediate

- Hemorrhage
- Gastric dilatation
- Hematemesis

Intermediate

- Left basal atelectasis **(m/c complication after splenectomy–16%)***
- Pancreatic fistula,pancreatitis, pseudocyst
- Gastric fistula (due to perforation as small gastric vessels are cut during surgery)
- Subphrenic abscess/hematoma.

Delayed

- Thromboembolic episodes (due to thrombocytosis as greater than seven and half lakhs platelets gets added after splenectomy)
- OPSI (Overwhelming post splenectomy infection)
- Portal vein thrombosis

HEMATOLOGIC EFFECT OF SPLENECTOMY

- **Immediately after splenectomy**
  - Leucocytosis
  - Thrombocytosis

  ← Return to normal within 2–3 weeks
- **Chronic manifestations**
  - Anisocytosis and poikilocytosis
  - Howel jolly bodies (nuclear remnants)
  - Heiz bodies (denatured hemoglobin)
  - Basophilic stipling

- Liver is the most common organ injured in abdominal injuries (Combining Blunt and penetrating trauma)
- Spleen is the most commonly injured organ in Blunt abdominal inuries.
- MC organ injury necessitating surgery-Splenic injury**
- MC cause of prehepatic portal hypertension-portal vein thrombosis.*
- Isolated Splenic vein thrombosis (left Side portal hypertension) is due to pancreatitis.
- MC cause of intrahepatic presinusoidal portal hypertension-Schistosomiasis**
- MC cause of Portal hypertension-Alcoholic cirrhosis (MC cause of sinusoidal Portal HT)
- MC cause of posthepatic portal hypertension-Budd Chiari syndrome.

UROLOGY

Types of Renal Calculus

- **Calcium oxalate calculus (Most common*)**
  - They have hard, small and jagged surface
- **Phosphate calculus**
  - Usually Calcium phosphate but sometimes is combined with ammonium and magnesium to form the **triple phosphate** calculus ammonium magnesium phosphate
  - Also k/a **struvite stone**
  - Smooth and dirty white and solitary
  - Seen in **alkaline urine** especially with **proteus infection** which split urea to ammonia
  - This type of calculus may enlarge to fill all or most of renal collecting system forming a **staghorn** calculus**
- **Uric acid and urate calculus**
  - These are **radiolucent**
- **Cystine stones**
  - Uncommon, seen in cystinuria
  - Appear only in **acid urine***

Renal Cell carcinoma:

Renal cell carcinoma/Grawitzs tumor/Hypernephroma/Golden tumor	
• A renal cell carcinoma that has spread to renal vein, IVC or even upto the thorax (heart) is operable • A pre op biopsy is not necessary as a **RCC is the most common malignant neoplasm of kidney (90–95%)** and any solid renal mass is considered to be RCC until unless proved otherwise • A chest X-ray should be done to rule out pulmonary metastasis as it will make the Ca of stage IV with worst prognosis and also decide the t/t plan	
More about Renal cell carcinoma	**Risk factors**
• It's the MC malignant neoplasm of kidney (90-95%) • MC site of origin is Proximal Convoluted tubules* • RCC originates in the cortex and tends to grow out into perinephric tissue • Usually situated at poles (commonly at upper pole)* • Male female ratio is 3:2 • Age–6th–7th decade of life	• Cigarette smoking* • Obesity* • Hypertension • Familial (2–3%) • von-Hippel lindau syndrome (cerebellar hemangioblastoma, retinal angiomatosis and B/l renal cell Ca) **Most common sporadic**

Contd...

Contd...

Renal cell carcinoma/Grawitzs tumor/Hypernephroma/Golden tumor

- **Histologically RCC is an adenocarcinoma.** It has been reclassified into subtypes of which Clear cells Ca is the MC type.

Cytogenetics of various subtypes of Renal Cell Ca

Clear cell carcinoma	Papillary carcinoma
• Is the most common type (70-80) • These tumors can be – Familial – Associated with VHL disease or – Sporadic (95%) • Almost all (-98%) of clear cell carcinomas are associated with loss of sequences **on short arm of chromosome 3.** The lost sequences include the VHL gene. • The VHL gene acts as tumor-suppressor gene the loss of which is associated with clear cell Ca.	• Also occurs in both familial and sporadic forms, commonly multicentric • The cytogenetic abnormalities associated with papillary Ca are – Trisomies 7, 16 and 17 and loss of Y is male patients for Sporadic form – Trisomy 7 in the familial form – Familial form is associated with MET protooncogene.

Classical triad of RCC consist of

- Hematuria*
- Flank pain*
- Palpable flank mass*
  - Earliest and MC presenting feature is hematuria*

Paraneoplasitc syndromes

- Fever of unknown origin*
- Anemia*
- Erythrocytosis* (d/t secretion of erythropoietin* by RCC)
  - (but anemia is a more common finding)*

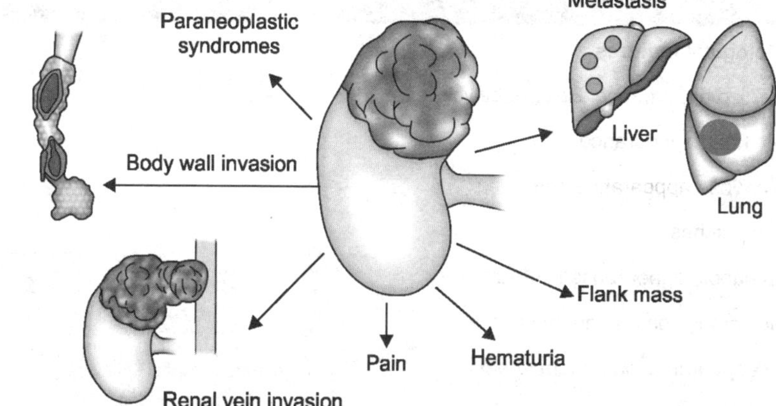

• Hypertension • Abnormal liver function (**stauffers syndrome*** ie non metastatic hepatic dysfunction)	• Hypercalcemia* • Neuromyopathy* • Amylodosis* • **Increased ESR (MC paraneoplastic syndrome)*** • Dysfibrogenemia	• Cushing syndrome* • Galactorrhoea • Feminization and masculanization

Important points in RCC

• MC route of metastasis is **hematogenous** • MC site of distant metastasis is **lung*** • (canon ball secondaries, secondaries may be pulsatile)	• Investigation Of choice → **CT scan*** • Treatment of choice → Radical nephrectomy • Radiotherapy, Chemotherapy or Hormonal therapy have little role in RCC t/t

Treatment

- Partial nepherectomy is now being used as primary surgical therapy for patients with tumour less than 4 cm in size.

• **For tumor < 4 cm-partial nephrectomy (Score used–** RENAL score, PADUA Score) • **For tumor > 4 cm-radical nephrectomy**	**Radical nephrectomy includes removal of:** • Kidney and Gerota's fascia • Ipsilateral adrenal • Renal hilar lymph nodes • Proximal half of ureter

- The Renal cell Ca is prone to grow into the renal vein. Produce cannon ball mets in lung and mets are highly vascular which may pulsate (also in follicular ca thyroid)

MC points
• MC site of distant metastasis from lung Ca → Adrenals*next is Liver, Brain
• MC site for distant metastasis from Breast Ca → Vertebrae
• **MC site for distant metastasis from Bladder Ca → Lung***
• MC site for distant metastasis from Colorectal Ca → Liver*
• MC site for distant metastasis from Melanoma (cutaneous) → Skin/subcutaneous tissue Lung*
• MC site for distant metastasis from Melanoma (ocular) → Liver*
• **MC site for distant metastasis from Prostate → Bones***
• MC site for distant metastasis from Soft tissue sarcoma → Lung*
• **MC site for distant metastasis from Testis Ca → Lung***
• MC site for distant metastasis from Thyroid Ca → Bone*, Lung*
• Metastasis to lung is most commonly from → Breast Ca*

Some important appearances	
Radiological features	**Seen in**
Spider leg appearance, Bell like calyces	Polycystic kidney
Cobra head appearance	Ureterocele
Flower vase appearance on ureters	Horse shoe kidney
Sandy patches	Schistosomiasis of bladder
Soap bubble appearance/RIM sign	Hydronephrosis
Apple core lesion on barium enema	Ca colon
Claw appearance on barium enema	Intussusceptions
Saw tooth appearance	Diverticula of colon
Birds beak appearance of esophagus on barium meal	Achalaisa
Cork screw appearance of esophagus on barium meal	DES
String sign of kantor	Crohn's disease
Thumb printing sign	Ischemic colitis

Bladder calculi

- In general most of the bladder calculi are formed within the bladder itself. Only some stones are formed in the kidney and pass into the bladder, where they grow by additions of crystals

- **Etiology of bladder calculi**
  - Bladder outlet obstruction is the most common cause of vesical in adults
  - Other causes are
    - Neurogenic bladder leading to urinary stasis
    - A foreign body eg. Foley catheter and forgotten DJ stent, which serve as nidus for stones
    - Bladder diverticula.
- Bladder stones are commonly seen in **older men (> 50 years)** usually because of bladder outlet obstruction
- **Common vesical stones** are
  - Uric acid stones and
  - Struvite stones
- Other less common stone type are
  - Oxalate stones
  - Cystein stones
- **Struvite stones are also know as 'jack stones'** because of their rough surface as against the smooth surface of uric acid stones.

Contd...

Contd...

Bladder calculi	
Based on origin	**Clinical features**
• **Primary bladder** stone is one that develops in sterile urine and originates in kidney and passes down the ureters to the bladder,where it enlarges • **Secondary bladder stones** occur in presence of some infections, bladder outflow obstruction, impaired bladder emptying or a foreign body such as non absorbable sutures, metal staples or catheter fragments • **Most of the bladder stones are secondary.** Only some stones are primary. Kidney stones which are small enough to pass through the ureters into bladder are easily passed out through the urethra • Most bladder stones contain calcium and are therefore **radiopaque.**	• **Frequency is the earliest symptom** • Hematuria is common and this may be *characterized by few drops of blood at the end of micturition* • Pain (strangury) may occur because of speculated oxalate stone. It usually occurs at the end of micturition and is usually referred to the tip of penis or to the labia majora. In young boys, screaming and pulling at the end of penis with hand at the end of micturition are indicative of bladder stone. • **Uric acid stones** are primarily formed in bladder. • It is **oxalate stones are dropped** from above
• **Treatment off vesical calculus** – Small stones can be removed or crushed transurethrally (cystolitholapaxy) – Larger stones are often disintegrated by transurethral electrohydraulic lithotripsy (shock wave generating probe), or may require suprapubic transvesical removal (vesiolithotomy)	

Rupture of bladder	
• Bladder rupture is of two types: – Extraperitoneal–80% of cases – Intraperitoneal–20% of cases - **Classic extraperitoneal bladder rupture. IVU:** The pattern of contrast extravasation is **'flame shaped'** and 'whispy' in appearance. Treatment is with catheter drainage.	• Urethral rupture is also of two types: – Bulbar urethral injury–MC – Membranous urethral injury
Extravasation of urine in bladder and urethral injuries	
• **Extravasation of urine (+ blood) in bulbar urethral injury** – It is a superficial extravasation – If the buck's fascia remains intact, extravasation of blood and urine are confined to the penile shaft. – Disruption of buck's fascia–perineal butterfly hematoma	• **Extravasation of urine in membranous urethral Injury and extraperitoneal bladder rupture.** – Extravasation is same in both – It is a deep extravasation – Urine extravasates in the layer of the pelvic fascia and the retroperitoneal tissues – Urine collects in the **perivesical space**
• **Intraperitoneal rupture** – Usually occurs with a direct blow to lower abdomen with full bladder – Blood and urine will extravasate into the peritoneal cavity producing signs of peritonitis	
More about bladder and urethral injuries	
• Bladder injuries are usually associated with pelvic # • Bladder ruptures assoc. with pelvic # is **extraperitoneal type**	• Urethral inj. Assoc. With # pelvis → **membranous urethral inj.** • Urethral inj. causing high riding prostate → **membranous urethral inj.** • Single layered closure of bladder rent with 2/0 absorbable suture

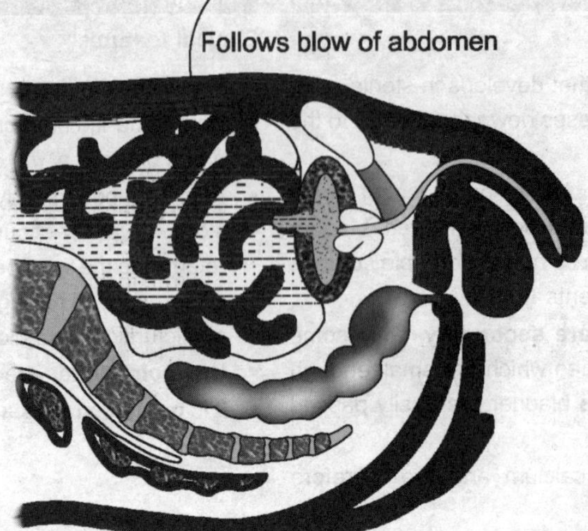

Fig. 12.3: Intraperitoneal rupture

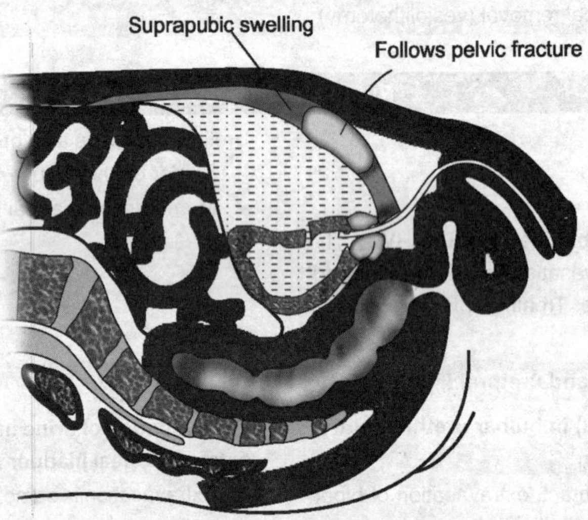

Fig. 12.4: Extraperitoneal rupture

Priapism

- **Priapism** is a rare disorder in which prolonged painful erection occurs > 4 hours
- Types: Ischemic/nonischemic
- Associated with sickle cell anemia, leukemia, metastatic carcinoma and trauma.
- **Treatment:** If erection doesn't subside needle aspiration of blood, then injection of alpha adrenergic agents such as phenyl ephrine done.
- **WINTER shunt:** Fistula created between corpora cavernosa and spongiosum at <u>distal</u> penis near glans.
- **SACHER'S shunt:** Similar fistula at *proximal* cavernospongiosal shunt.
- **GRAYHACK shunt:** Anastomosis of one of corpora cavernosa to saphenous vein (proximal shunt)

Seminal Vesicles

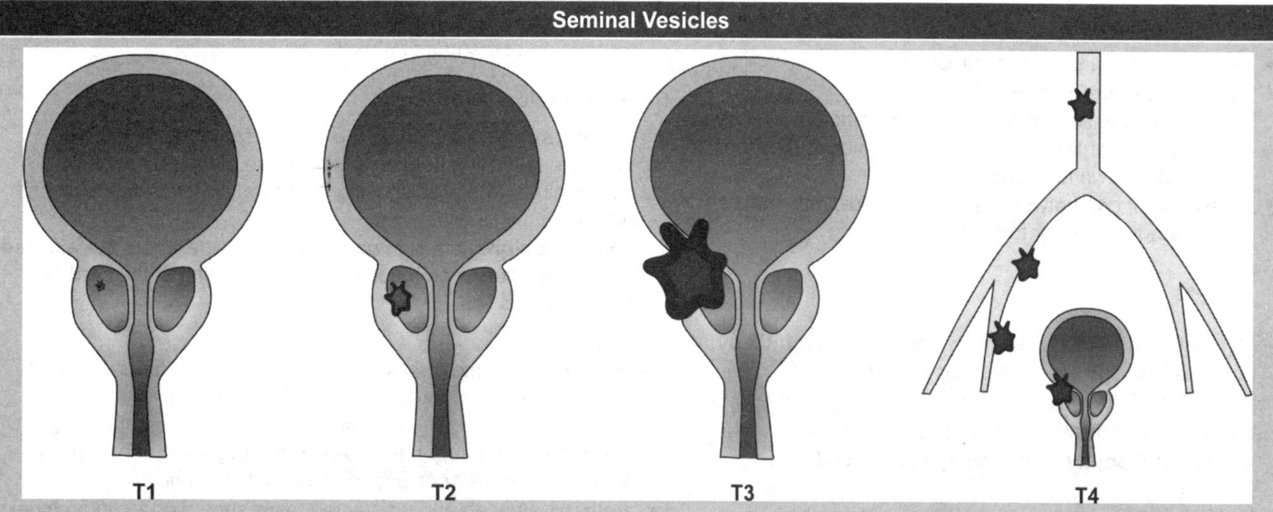

- Sperms are produce in testls and then stored and mature within the epididymis.
- Vas deferens carries the sperms from epididymis to the urethra where they open by separate openings into the prostatic urethra.
- Just before opening vas deferens is joined by ducts of seminal vesicles. Vas deferens and seminal vesicle ducts join to form the ejaculatory duct.
- The secretions of seminal vesicles form a large part of seminal fluid and contain fructose and a coagulating enzyme called the vesiculase (Seminogelin)

Semen analysis forms a important part of infertility assessment

• **Low ejaculatoy volume is caused by** – Retrograde ejaculation into the bladder or – Obstruction of the vas deferens or the ejaculatory duct.	• Azoospermia may be seen in – Testicular failure or – Obstruction of vas deferens	• **Absence of fructose suggests** – Seminal vesicle agenesis or obstruction

- **Semen that is low in volume with azoospermiaand absence of fructose suggests** → either obstruction of the ejaculatory ducts or congenital absence of the vas deferens and seminal vesicles.
- The anatomy of the vas deferens and seminal vesicles can be vasography (where contrast medium is injected into the vas deferens) or TRUS (trans rectal ultrasonography),
  - however TRUS is superior to vasography and is the investigation of choice.

- **Also know**
  - Semen specimen should be obtained following at **least 3 days of abstinence** and examined within 1 or 2 *hours* at least 2 specimens are examined several weeks apart.

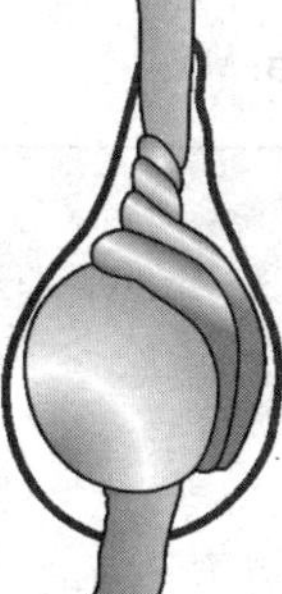

Intravaginal torsion

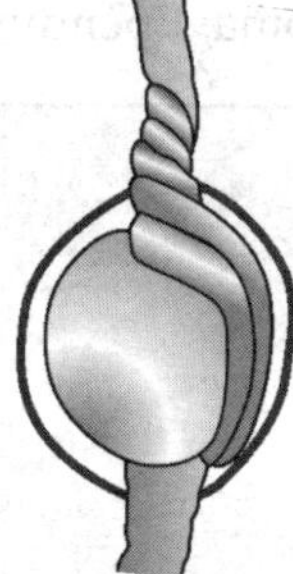

Extravaginal torsion

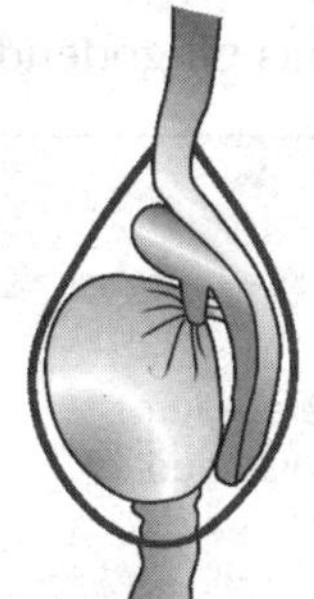

Torsion due to long mesorchium

Torsion of testis

- **Torsion of testis** is the torsion of the spermatic cord causing strangulation of the blood supply to the testis and unless it is t/t within 6 *hours*, testicular atrophy is inevitable
- It is seen commonly in adolescent (10-25 years)
- **Symptoms** → it presents sudden agonising pain in the groin and the lower abdomen. Nausea and vomiting are very common
- Absent testis or Vanishing testis: seen in Prenatal torsion

Predisposing factors	• Heavy straining often precipitates torsion due to vigorous contraction of cremaster muscle
• Inversion of testis–Most common factor • **Bell clapper deformity:** High investment of tunica vaginalis forming a mesentry like structure for testis (mesorchium) which makes the testis hang down horizontally. • Presence of gap between testis and epididymis makes testis hang and go for torsion.	**Signs in torsion testis** • **Angel's sign:** It's a sign on the normal side (unaffected side). Opposite testis lies horizontally because of the presence of mesorchium. (the predisposing factor for torsion is same on both sides) • **Deming's sign:** Its a sign on the affected side where the affected testis is positioned high because of the twisting of the cord and spasm of muscles.
• It must be **differentiated from epididymo-orchitis by:** – **Prehns sign** → on elevation of testis - Pain increases → in torsion - Pain decreases → in epidydimo-orchitis – **Color Doppler** → detects the decreased blood flow to testis in torsion. **It is the inv. Of choice** to exclude torsion from the epididymo-orchitis – **Tc 99m pretechnate scan** → it demonstrates decreased blood flow **Torsion of testicular appendage:** Blue dot sign (Most common appendix of testes)	**Treatment** • In the 1st hour the torsion can be treated by manipulation (but later on surgery has to be done to fix the testis) • If not correctable by manipulation or more than one hour has passed then surgery has to be done. **Surgery must be done within 6** *hours*. Otherwise the testis will be dead • Both the affected and unaffected testis should undergo orchipexy because the anatomical variation responsible for torsion is likely to be bilateral (bell–clapper deformity)

SPECIALITY SURGERIES

High Yield Points from Tumors of CNS

- VHL syndrome (3p gene)-Associated with Hemangioblastoma of Retina, Cerebellum and Spinal cord
- NF-1 is associated with Malignant Glioma
- **Turcot's Syndrome** associated with medulloblastoma and malignant glioma
- **Tuberous sclerosis** associated with Astrocytoma*
- Depression and Psychiatric Symptoms are more common with frontal lobe tumors. (Personality changes are also common with frontal lobe tumors)**
- Tumors that grow rapidly during pregnancy-Meningiomas, Gliomas and Neurofibromas
- CNS tumors showing calcification-Meningiomas (Psammoma bodies)* and Ependymoma
- Stereotactic Radiosurgery means delivery of concentrated doses of Radiation to a defined volume in Brain.
- Lesions treated by Sterotactic radiosurgery-Metastatic tumors, AV malformations, Trigeminal neuralgia and Benign lesions of Cranial nerve.
- **Gliomas: MC type is Astrocytoma****. Others types of gliomas-Oligodendroglioma, Ependymoma.

Astrocytomas:
- MC primary brain tumor of both children and Adults*
- MC type in adults is **Glioblastoma multiforme****
- Mostly supratentorial in adults and intratentorial in Children
- Astrocytoma is the **MC Posterior Fossa tumor in Children**** (Cerebellum)
- Most astrocytomas are low grade in Children and High grade in Adulthood
- Types of Astrocytoma:
  - Grade 1: Pilocytic: MC type in Children. Curable by resection
  - Grade 2: Astrocytomas: Young Children. Not curable by surgery.
  - Grade 3: Anaplastic: Cytoreductive surgery
  - Grade 4: Glioblastoma Multiforme: MC Primary Brain tumor**, Surgery+ EBRT+ Cisplatin. Poor survival–Less than 1 year

Medulloblastomas:
- Highly malignant tumor in Cerebellum and infratentorial location
- MC in Children (peak age-3-4 years)
- MC site is VERMIS* (Adults-Lateral Cerebellum)
- Drop Mets-Dissemination via CSF* is seen
- Mets outside to Bones, Liver and Lymphnodes is seen (Tumor dissemination is important prognostic factor*)
- Most Radiosensitive Tumor in Brain**
- Surgical excision+ RT+ Chemotherapy is given

Meningiomas:
- MC Intracranial Extra axial Dural Based neoplasm
- MC benign tumors in adults and MC in women
- MC site-Along superior sagittal sinus
- Calcification present due to psammoma bodies**
- C/F-Motor deficit (90%)-Spasticity and lower limb weakness and sensory deficit (60%) with Bladder dysfunction

Hemangioblastoma:
- MC primary intra axial tumor in posterior fossa (Cerebellum*)
- 20% cases associated with VHL
- Solid or cystic with a mural Nodule*
- Erythrocytosis may be seen*
- Histologically benign.
- Surgical excision is treatment of choice

Oligodendroglioma:
- 10% of gliomas and involve Frontal lobe in 50-65% cases
- Characteristic histology-Fried egg cytoplasm and Chicken wire vasculature and Microcalcification**
- MC presentation-Seizures
- Calcification in CT-90%
- Surgery+ Chemotherapy is the treatment modality

High Yield Points

- Craniopharyngiomas-Suprasellar calcification and Polyuria
- Craniopharygiomas are benign cystic lesions that most frequently occur in children. There is a second peak incidence in the 50s
- Hypopituitarism+ Diabetes Insipidus+ Growth retardation are all features of Craniopharyngiomas
- Surgery alone is not curative. In the absence of RT-75% cases will recur in Craniopharyngiomas
- MC cause of Hyper pituitarism-Pituitary adenoma*
- MC functional Pituitary adenoma is Prolactinoma
- MC tumors in brain-Metastasis* (70% are multiple)
- MC site of Mets-Cerebral hemispheres.
- MC primary to produce Brain secondary-LUNG > BREAST
- MC Suprasellar mass in Children-Craniopharyngioma
- MC suprasellar mass in adults-Pituitary adenoma
- Most preferred route for Pituitary surgery now is-Trans sphenoidal
- MC Spinal tumor-Mets
- MC Primary spinal tumor-Nerve sheath tumor
- MC intramedullary tumor-Astrocytoma
- MC site of primary Spinal tumor-Intradural extramedullary
- Dumbbell tumor is seen in-neurofibroma
- Witzelsucht (Pathological Joking) is seen in Frontal lobe tumors
- Enlargement of pituitary tumor after Bilateral adrenalectomy is known as-NELSON syndrome

- Most common anterior mediastinal mass-Thymoma**
- Most common mediastinal mass-Neurogenic tumors**
- Most common malignant mass of middle mediastinum -Lymphomas
- Most common mediastinal mass in children-Neurogenic tumor
- Mc mass of middle mediastinum-Pericardial cyst

Bronchogenic Cyst

- They originate as sequestrations from ventral foregut.
- Composed of Pathognomonic inner layer of ciliated Respiratory epithelium**
- Most of them arise in middle mediastinum; but 15% occur in pulmonary parenchyma.
- In lungs most common in right lung, lower lobes.
- Those arising from Mediastinum has no communication with trachea bronchial tree whereas those from the parenchyma has communication**

Complications of bronchogenic cyst

- Infection
- Atelectasis
- Tension pneumothorax

Lung sequestration

A sequestration consists of normally developed bronchioles and alveoli supplied by *systemic* rather than pulmonary arteries

- 95% of time this blood supply is from aorta.
- M/c in lower lobes, Left more common than right.

Extralobar sequestration	Intralobar sequestration
25%	75%
Drain via azygous vein	Drain via pulmonary vein
Do not communicate with lung	Are in communication with tracheo bronchial tree
Associated with Congenital diaphragmatic hernia	Prone to infection and lung abscess

Pancoast tumor

- It is a tumor of the apex of lung (squamous cell or epidermoid cancer)
- Causes destruction of 1st and 2nd ribs.
- May grow to cause-shoulder pain, erosion of ribs and Horner's syndrome

High yield points:

- Ideal place for Chest tube insertion-in the triangle of safety (4th–6th ICS, Anterior to midaxillary line)-Triangle is bounded by–lateral border of P.major, Anterior border of Latissmus dorsi, superior border of 5th or 6th rib
- Malignant pleural effusions are Exudative* -Most common malignancies causing this are Breast and Lung cancer.
- MC cause of Chylothorax-Trauma (Most commonly following surgery)
- Chylothorax is diagnosed by milky fluid and Triglycerides level > 110 mg/dl
- VATS-Stands for Video Assisted Thoracoscopic surgery
- NOTES: Stands for Natural Orifice Transluminal Endoscopic Surgery (e.g. Transoral Appendicectomy, Transvaginal Appendicectomy, etc.)
- Most common route for access to thorax-Posterolateral thoracotomy-Muscles cut are-Lattisimus dorsi, Trapezius, Serratus anterior, IC muscles

Burns

Assessing the area of a burn

- **The patient's whole hand is 1% TBSA, and is a useful guide in small burns**
- **The Lund and Browder chart is useful in larger burns**

- **The rule of nines is adequate for a first approximation only**

Rule of nine (Alexander Wallace rule)
• Each upper limb-9% TBSA
• Each lower leg-18% TBSA
• Anterior or Posterior Trunk-18% TBSA
• Head and neck-9% TBSA
• Perineum–1% TBSA

- Lund and browder chart gives different percentage for head based on the age.
- The Berkow formula is used to determine burn size accurately in children** (Sabiston)
- In children head and neck is relatively large may account for 18-21%
- Infants-21% TBSA

Degrees of burns
First degree: Involves only epidermis
Second degree: Involves epidermis and some part of dermis.
(also known as partial thickness burns)
Further divided into
• Superficial second degree or superficial partial thickness-involves upper part of dermis
• Deep second degree or deep partial thickness-extends up to reticular layer of dermis.
Third degree or Full thickness burns-involves full thickness of dermis
Fourth degree burns-involves subcutaneous fat and deep structures.

First degree	Second degree superficial	Second degree deep	Third degree
No blister formation	**Blisters formed****	Blisters seen	**Eschar formation****
Blanch to touch	Blanch to touch	Mottled pink and white color because of varying blood supply to dermis	Black or brown
Painful	Painful	**Pain is absent****	Painless
Heal without scarring in 5–10 days	Heal without scarring in 7–14 days	**Heals with scar 3–9 weeks**	Heals with wound contracture only or by SSG only.

Fluids for resuscitation

- Children with burns over 10% TBSA and adults with burns over 15% TBSA, consider the need for intravenous fluid resuscitation
- If oral fluids are to be used, salt must be added
- Fluids needed is calculated from a standard formula
- The key is to monitor urine output

Ideal fluid

There are three types of fluid used. The most common is crystalloids:

- Crystalloids:Ringer's lactate or Hartmann's solution;
- Colloids: human albumin solution or fresh-frozen plasma,
- Some centres use hypertonic saline.

About crystalloids

- Ringer's lactate is the most commonly used crystalloid. Crystalloids are said to be as effective as colloids for maintaining intravascular volume.
- They are also significantly less expensive.
- Another reason for the use of crystalloids is that even large protein molecules leak out of capillaries following burn injury; however, non burnt capillaries continue to sieve proteins virtually normally.

Colloids

- Plasma proteins are responsible for the inward oncotic pressure that counteracts the outward capillary hydrostatic pressure.
- Without proteins, plasma volumes would not be maintained as there would be edema.
- **Proteins should be given after the first 12 hours of burn** because, before this time, the massive fluid shifts cause proteins to leak out of the cells.

Parkland formula

- TBSA% × weight (kg) × 4 = volume (ml) needed
- Half this volume is given in the first 8 hours, and the second half is given in the subsequent 16 hours
- The volume replacement is by crystalloids.

Muir and Barclay formula

- The commonest colloid-based formula is the Muir and Barclay formula:

Oneliners from BURNS:
- MC cause of death in Burns: Sepsis
- MC cause of early death: Hypovolemic shock
- MC cause of late death: Sepsis
- MC cancer arising from Burns: SCC (Known as Marjolins Ulcer)
- Best method to assess burns in children < 5 years-Lund and Browder chart
- Hyperglycemia is seen in early burns
- Pus in burns is seen in 3–5 days
- Berkow diagram/formula is one new method to estimate burn size% in an isolated Body part.

Partial thickness (Theirsch)	Full thickness (Wolfe)
• Easy uptake and survival • Large grafts can be derived • Same site graft can be taken • Cosmetically unacceptable • Donor site heals without contraction • m/c site-thigh	• Uptake is difficult • Only small grafts can be taken • Cosmetically good • Donor site has to be closed or else it will heal with contracture. • m/c site-behind ear

Cleft Lip/Palate

The typical distribution of cleft types is:

- Cleft lip alone: 15%;
- Cleft lip and palate: 45%;**
- Isolated cleft palate: 40%.
  - Cleft lip with palate predominates in **males***
  - Whereas cleft palate alone appears to be more common in **females.**
  - In unilateral cleft lip the deformity affects the left side in 60% of cases.

Timing of surgery

- Closure of cleft palate should be done at **6 months** age as it aids in child feeding.
- Pharyngeal flap operation is operation of choice.
- Langenbach's operation and Wardill's operation

Rule of 10 lip for cleft lip repair

- Weight of baby is 10 pounds
- Hemoglobin is 10 gm%
- Age of 10 weeks

Timing of repair-Cleft lip alone

Cleft lip alone	Timing
Unilateral (one side)	One operation at 5–6 months
Bilateral (both sides)	One operation at 4–5 months

Timing of repair-Cleft palate alone

Cleft palate alone		
Soft palate alone	One operation at 6 months	
Soft and hard palate	Two operations	Soft palate-6 months Hard palate-15–18 months

Cleft Lip and Palate

Type		
Unilateral	Two operations	Cleft lip and soft palate at 5–6 months Hard palate with gums with or without revision of lip at 15–18 months
Bilateral	Two operations	Cleft lip and soft palate at 4–5 months Hard palate with gums with or without revision of lip at 15–18 months

VENOUS ULCER: (Stasis Ulcer)

- Site: Lower 1/3 medial side of leg
- Size: Variable
- Shape: Oval to circular
- Margin: Well defined
- Edge: Sloping edge (healing)
- Floor: Formed by deep fascia
- Surrounding: Pigmentation, Eczema, varicosity
- Base: Extend up to periosteum.
- Deformity: Talipes Equino varus

Complications of venous ulcer

Ulcer complicates varicose vein in about 5% of the people.

- **Marjolin's ulcer*:** Malignant change in long standing venous ulcer to squamous cell ca.
- **Periosteitis tibia:** Occurs in long standing ulcer on medial surface of tibia.
- **Equinus deformity:** Walking on toe relieves pain, so he continues walking resulting in shortening of tendoachilles

Lipodermatosclerosis*

Progressive sclerosis of the skin and subcutaneous tissue may occur due to fibrin deposition, tissue death and scarring due to chronic venous hypertension.

- Nerve at risk during **GSV stripping**-saphenous nerve*.
- Nerve at risk at **stripping of SSV** is sural nerve*.

Surgeries for Perforator incompetence

- **Subfascial Ligation of Cockett and Dodd:**
  Preferable in cases of lipodermatosclerosis.
  Long incision made to open the deep fascia and the perforators are ligated deep to deep fascia.
- **Suprafascial Ligation of Linton:**
  There should not be lipodermatosclerosis.
  Perforators are ligated above the deep fascia
- **Seps:** Subfascial endoscopic perforator surgery

One liners:

- The Compression stockings used for varicose veins-**Class 2 stockings** with 30 mmhg at ankle and 10-15mmhg at knee level.
- Most commonly used drug for injection sclerotherapy-**Sodium tetra decyl sulfate*.**
- Best agent for foam sclerotherapy-**Polidocanol**
- M/c anomaly of GSV-double saphenous vein
- M/c complication of varicose vein surgery-recurrence.
- M/c site of aplasia of venous system is IVC
- M/c site of deep vein thrombosis is **calf veins***
- **May Thurner cockett syndrome-**also called as iliac vein compression syndrome: Membranous occlusion of left common iliac vein when it passes behind the right common iliac artery.

Arterial System

Aneurysm

- M/c site of large vessel aneurysm-abdominal aortic aneurysm
- M/c site of peripheral aneurysm-popliteal artery*

Abdominal aortic aneurysm

- 95% aneurysms are infra renal*
- Site of rupture: m/c site = postero lateral (80%)*
- 2nd m/c site = anterior

Indications for surgery

- All symptomatic aneurysm (m/c symptom is back and abdominal discomfort)
- Aneurysms size **greater than 55 mm*** on USG anteroposteriorly.

Arterial stenosis and occlusion

- M/c cause–atheroma
- Characterized by Intermittent Claudication pain.
- M/c site of claudication-calf
- Lerich syndrome* = buttock claudication + sexual impotency due to saddle shaped embolus in Bifurcation of aorta.

CHOICE OF PROCEDURES

- **Aortofemoral**
- **Femoropopliteal**
- **Femorodistal**
- **Axillo bifemoral bypass:**
  - Salvage procedure for poor risk patients with bilateral iliac artery occlusion using a long prosthetic graft.
  - Remember it should not be done for intermittent claudication. It is advised only for impending gangrene cases.

GRAFT MATERIAL

Best grafts

- Superficial femoral artery occlusion-saphenous vein*
- Infrapopliteal occlusions-saphenous vein*
- Aortoiliac–Dacron*

Best materials

- Aorta-2/0 and 3/0 prolene
- Femoral–4/0 and 5/0
- Infrapopliteal-7/0 prolenes

Ainhum**

- Usually affects black men
- Barefoot walkers
- A fissure appears at the level of inter phalangeal joint of a toe, little toe**.
- Complication = Necrosis
- Z-plasty and amputation.

Seldinger technique

- Retrograde seldinger technique is used to enter the vessel by percutaneous puncture technique.
- Used for various diagnostic and therapeutic techniques.
- Especially for Percutaneous transluminal angioplasty (PTA) for occlusion and stenosis
- The catheter used during this technique for dilatation of vessels is FOGARTY CATHETER**

Buerger's disease (Thromboangitis obliterans)

Shionaya criteria:

- H/o smoking
- Onset before age of 50 years
- Infrapopliteal arterial occlusion*
- Either arm involvement or phlebitis migrans
- Absence of risk factors for atherosclerosis other than smoking.

Clinical features

- m/c in young males* (40–45 years)
- Claudication of feet, legs or arms, hands
- Superficial thrombophlebitis (40%)*
- **There will be involvement adjacent veins and nerves***
- On examination**–popliteal pulse is present and there will be absent dorsalis pedis and anterior tibial on both sides (bilateral)*

Investigations

- **Absence of other risk factors** like diabetes, hypertension and hypercholesterolemia must be ruled out.
- Angiography shows–tree root/spider leg or cork screw collaterals.*

Lumbar sympathectomy

Principles

- Increase blood flow (by vasodilatation)
- Nutritive value for small ulcers
- Reduces ischemic rest pain
- No effect on collateral circulation

Indications

- Rest pain*
- Ulcers*
- Superficial gangrene*
- Not useful for intermittent claudication**
- Contraindicated if ABPI > 0.3 and in diabetics**
  (Diabetics have autonomic neuropathy already so there won't be any benefit on sympathectomy)

Ganglia removed

- L2 and L 3 ganglionectomy advised
- If L1 is removed preserve it for atleast for one side (retrograde ejaculation occurs)

Cervicodorsal sympathectomy

- *Treatment of palmar hyperhydrosis**.
- T1, T2 and T3 removed preserving the stellate ganglion* (Horners syndrome-ptosis, miosis, enophthalmosis and anhydrosis on removal of stellate ganglion**)

RAYNAUD'S DISEASE
- Primary–idiopathic (Raynaud's disease)**
- Secondary–Raynaud's phenomenon secondary to scleroderma, SLE and rheumatoid arthritis.
- Vibrating white finger–secondary raynaud's syndrome follow using vibrating tools in factory.

Clinical features
- 70-90% in young females
- Upper limb* m/c affected
- Abnormal sensitivity to cold

Stages:
- Local syncope-white,
- Local asphyxia–blue
- Recovery–crimson red

Treatment
- Raynaud's disease-protect from cold, avoid nail infections, nifedipine and cervicodorsal sympathectomy
- Raynaud's syndrome-Treat the cause.

Lymphatic system

Lymphedema

- M/c cause of lymphedema in India/all over world = filariasis*
- M/c cause of upper limb lymphedema = filarial*
- Classified–primary and secondary

Types of primary Lymphedema:

Congenital	Lymphedema praecox	Lymphedema tarda
Onset < 1 year m/c bilateral* Involve whole leg **Milroy's disease***	Onset 1-35 years m/c primary lymph edema m/c in women m/c unilateral* Mostly involve below knees only **Meig's disease***	Onset > 35 years

- **Stemmers sign*-**inability to pinch subcutaneous tissue in lymphedema.

Treatment of established lymphedema

Types of stockings used for lymph edema:
- Class 3: 40-50 mm Hg stockings
- Class 4: 50-60 mm Hg stockings are used

Drugs:
- In UK only drug approved for **venous disease is oxerutin (paroven)** and no drug is approved for lymphedema
- Benzypyrones are natural drug used for lymphedema.

Bypass procedures	Limb reduction procedures
• Neibulouwitz–anastomosis of nodes to vein (Lymphovenous anastomosis) • Kinmonth-using ileal mucosal patch • Gillies–skin bridge	• **Charles:** Whole subcutaneous and slim excused upto deep fascia and SSG done. • **Sistrunk:** Wedge excision of skin and subcutaneous tissue and wound closed primarily. • **Thompson:** Buried dermal flap. Common complication of this procedure is pilonidal sinus • **Homans:** Skin flap raised, subcutaneous tissue removed. – Most satisfactory operation. – Main complication is skin flap necrosis – Contraindicated in presence of venous obstruction and malignancy.

- Butchers thigh is due to injury to Femoral Artery in Femoral Triangle**

Malignant Melanoma

- 4% of skin cancer
- 79% of skin cancer deaths
- 1.4% of all cancer deaths.
  - ***Melanoma is the leading cause of death in women 25–35 years.***
  - ***M/c cancer in age group from 20–39 years-malignant melanoma.***

Risk factors

- Sunlight
- Xeroderma pigmentosa
- Past/family history of melanoma
- Dysplatic naevi (10% life time risk)
- Immunocompromised-HIV, cyclosporin A therapy, Hodgkin's disease.

Types of Malignant Melanoma:

SUPERFICIAL SPREADING (70%)	**NODULAR MELANOMA (16%)**
• M/C type occurring in white population • Melanomas arising in preexisting Dysplastic naevus are usually SSM. • M/C Sites: – Males: Trunk – Females: Lower legs and back	• Second most common • Can occur on any surface of the body, 50–70 years • M/C site: Head,neck and trunk • Only vertical growth, no radial spread. • High Risk group and **POOR PROGNOSIS**
ACRAL LENTIGENOUS MELANOMA (10%) (PALMS, SOLES, MUCOSAL SURFACES, SUBUNGUAL) • Most common in dark skinned individuals • Because of the location, diagnosed very late • **POOR PROGNOSIS** **Subungual type:** • Arise from nail matrix • m/c -great toe/thumb nails • Diagnostic biopsy includes nail matrix • **Extension of pigment onto the proximal lateral nail fold (HUTCHINSON'S SIGN)**	**LENTIGO MALIGNA MELANOMA: (5%)** • Older age individuals. • Previously called as Hutchinson's melanotic freckle. • Common in face. • *Most commonly affects women than men* • Insitu variant is called lentigo maligna. • *Lowest metastatic potential*

Prognostic factors

- Depth (most important)
- Ulceration
- Lymph node status

Others:

- Site-Extremities (good)
- Sex-Female (good)
- Histology-Lentigo maligna (good)

BRESLOW'S THICKNESS:	**CLARK'S LEVEL:**
Based on thickness of invasion by optical micrometer I : Less than 0.75 mm II : Between 0.76 to 1.5 mm III : 1.51 mm to 4 mm IV : Greater than 4 mm	• Level I: Only in Epidermis • Level II: Into papillary dermis • Level III: Filling of papillary dermis completely up to the junction. • Level IV: Into reticular dermis • Level V: Extension into subcutaneous tissue

Soft tissue sarcomas

Highlighted Points

- M/c soft tissue tumor in a child is Rhabdomyosarcoma
- M/c type: embryonal rhabdomyosarcoma
- Resection is the treatment of choice
- Soft tissue sarcomas mostly spread hematogeneously
- But lymphatic metastasis is seen in embryonal rhabdomyosarcoma
- Lower extremity is the commonest site
- Grade of tumor detects prognosis
- Liposarcoma is the mc retroperitoneal tumor*
- Lymphoma and retroperitoneal sarcoma are mc retroperitoneal malignant lesions.

Named Nodes:

- Rotters nodes: Interpectoral nodes (Ca. Breast)
- Rouviers nodes: Retropharyngeal nodes (Nasopharyngeal Ca)
- Delphian Nodes: Pretracheal nodes (Thyroid cancers)
- Irish Nodes: Left axillary nodes (Ca. Stomach)
- Virchows Nodes: Left Supraclavicular nodes (Intra abdominal malignancy)
- Cloquet Node: Deep Inguinal node in Femoral Canal
- Lund Node: Calots triangle node–Cystic Node
- Krouse Node: Jugula fossa node
- Cabana Node: Sentinel node of Cancer penis-It's a superficial Inguinal node.

One liners from Oncosurgery:

- MC tumor to produce Cervical nodal mets-Nasopharyngeal carcinoma
- MC site of primary for bone mets-Prostate
- MC cause of osteoblastic Secondaries–Male (prostate) Female (Breast)
- MC tumor to metastasize to bone in females-Breast
- MC site of Mets in sarcomas of extremities-LUNGS
- MC site of mets in retroperitoneal sarcomas-LIVER
- Purely osteolytic bone mets-Kidney
- Purely osteoblastic bone mets-Prostate
- MC site of primary for brain secondary-Lungs > breast
- MC cancer in males-Prostate > Lung > Colorectal
- MC cancer in females-Breast > Lung > Colorectal
- Cancer deaths in males-Lung > Prostate
- Cancer deaths in females-Lung > Breast
- Most sensitive phase of cell cycle to Radiation-G2 M > G2
- Most resistant phase of cell cycle to radiation-End of S phase

Congenital Diaphragmatic Hernia

- **Anteromedial:** Space of larrey* (foramen of Morgagni)
  - M/c on right side**
  - Causes no symptom.
- **Posterolateral**: Commonest type of CDH**. Occurs via foramen of Bochdalek.
  - M/c on left
  - Cause respiratory distress and death of infant due to abdominal visceral herniation.
- **Mortality is related to the degree of pulmonary hypoplasia**** and the **presence of congenital anomalies****, neither of which are correctable by Extra corporeal Membrane Oxygenation (ECMO).

Operative repair

- The timing of diaphragm repair is controversial. In patients that are not placed on ECMO, most surgeons perform repair once the hemodynamic status has been optimized.
- Operative repair of the diaphragmatic hernia is best accomplished by an abdominal approach.

Author's Request

Dear friends-Just answer the questions given below without reading the Explanatory answers and mark in a separate sheet of the answers you feel....This will help you train and avoid the mistakes you will do in the exams.

QUESTIONS

1. Indirect inguinal hernia arises: (2007)
a. Medial to inferior epigastric artery
b. Lateral to inferior epigastric artery
c. Medial to medial umbilical ligament
d. Lateral to medial umbilical ligament

2. Anterior Diaphragmatic hernia is known as:
a. Morgagni's hernia (2007)
b. Bochdalek's hernia
c. Eventration of the diaphragm
d. Para esophageal hernia

3. Most common cause of Idiopathic Intussusception is: (2007)
a. Hyperplastic polyp
b. Carcinoma of colon
c. Lymph nodes of Peyer's enlarges
d. Meckel'sdiverticulum

4. HLA typing is not needed in: (2007)
a. Bone marrow transplantation
b. Renal transplantation
c. Liver transplantation
d. Pancreas transplantation

5. The Abdominal approach for rectal prolapse is:
a. Delormes (2007)
b. Altemeiers
c. Ripstein
d. Theirsch

6. Visceral traumatic aneurysm commonly occurs in: (2007)
a. Splenic artery
b. Superior mesenteric artery
c. Inferior mesenteric artery
d. Gastroduodenal artery

7. Hidradenitis suppurativa occurs due to the involvement of: (2008)
a. Eccrine sweat gland
b. Mammary gland
c. Cutaneous apocrine gland
d. Sebaceous gland

8. The blood supply to the liver includes: (2008)
a. 80% from portal vein, 20% from hepatic artery
b. 80% from hepatic artery 20% from portal vein
c. 50% from hepatic artery, 50% from portal vein
d. Entire blood supply from hepatic artery only

9. Most common benign tumour of the parotid:
a. Oncocytoma (2008)
b. Hemangioma
c. Pleomorphic adenoma
d. Warthin's tumour

10. Borders of Hessel-Bach's triangle include all except: (2008)
a. Inferior epigastric vessels
b. Inguinal ligament
c. Vas deferens
d. Rectus abdominis

11. Skin flap with many unnamed small vessels is:
a. Axial flap (2008)
b. Fasciocutaneous flap
c. Randomized flap
d. Myo cutaneous flap

12. Splenectomy is beneficial even though spleen is not enlarged in: (2008)
a. ITP
b. CML
c. Henoch Schonlein purpura
d. Sickle cell anaemia

13. Which drug is not useful in decreasing raised intra cranial pressure after trauma? (2008)
a. Lasix
b. Glycerol
c. Mannitol
d. Dexamethasone

14. Which polyp has malignant potential? (2008)
a. Hyperplastic polyp
b. Hamartomatous polyp
c. Adenomatous polyp
d. Mucus retention polyp

15. The edge of a Venous ulcer is? (2008)
a. Everted
b. Sloping
c. Undermined
d. Pearly

16. GCS (Glasgow Coma Scale) tests for all the following parameters except? (2008)
a. Verbal
b. Eye

c. Bladder
d. Motor

17. Venous thrombosis is best assessed by? (2008)
a. Doppler USG
b. I131 fibrinogen studies
c. Duplex USG
d. Contrast phlebography

18. Breast carcinoma most; commonly affects? (2008)
a. Upper inner quadrant
b. Upper outer quadrant
c. Inner lower quadrant
d. Central region involving the nipple

19. Schatzki's rings refer to? (2009)
a. Spasms of lower esophagus
b. Constriction ring at lower esophagus
c. Convolutions in upper esophagus secondary to tumor
d. Diverticulations in mid esophagus

20. The commonest cause of bile duct stricture is? (2009)
a. Sclerosing cholangitis
b. Post Cholecystectomy
c. Malignancy
d. Ascending cholangitis

21. Commonest indication for surgery in chronic pancreatitis is? (2009)
a. Pain
b. Infection
c. Malignant transformation
d. Duodenal obstruction

22. Congenital atresia's are commonest in? (2009)
a. Distal colon
b. Duodenum
c. Proximal colon
d. Ileum

23. A Rectal polyp in an adult are associated with which of the following? (2009)
a. Hypokalemia
b. Familial adenomatous polyposis coli
c. Irritable bowel syndrome
d. Peutz Jeghers syndrome

24. Internal hernia that can be associated with a sac is: (2009)
a. Trans mesenteric
b. Trans' mesocolon
c. Epiploic foramen
d. Broad ligament

25. Extravasation of urine Occurs in all the spaces in rupture of bulbar urethra, except in? (2009)
a. Penis
b. Scrotum
c. Anterior abdominal wall
d. Ischiorectal fossa

26. Branchial cysts shows all of the following except: (2009)
a. Trans illuminant
b. Contains cholesterol
c. Lined by columnar epithelium
d. Arises from second bronchial cleft

27. The benign prostatic hyperplasia all of the following are seen except: (2009)
a. Detrusor overactivity
b. Narrowing of urethra
c. Increased trabeculation in bladder
d. Enlargement of lateral lobes of prostate

28. Splenic Disease for which splenectomy is effective: (2009)
a. Thalassemia
b. Sickle cell disease
c. Aplastic anaemia
d. Idiopathic thrombocytopenic purpura

29. About ectopic vesicae, following is true, EXCEPT: (2010)
a. Ca bladder may occur
b. Ventral curvature of penis
c. Incontinence of urine
d. Visible uretero -vesicle efflux

30. HLA matching is not necessary in which of the following organ transplanted: (2010)
a. Liver
b. Kidney
c. Pancreas
d. Bone marrow

31. The most cost-effective management of three vessel coronary disease is: (2010)
a. CABG
b. Cardiac transplant
c. GpIIb-IIIa inhibitor
d. Percutaneous transluminal angioplasty

32. The usual site for branchial cyst is: (2010)
a. Ant. border, upper 3rd of sternomastoid
b. Post. Border, upper 3rd sternomastoid
c. Ant. border, lower 3rd sternomastoid
d. Post. Triangle of neck

33. Complication of bilateral lumbar sympathectomy: (2010)
a. Retrograde ejaculation
b. Inability to sustain an erection
c. Dry ejaculation
d. Dribbling micturition

34. All of the, fallowing regarding papillary carcinoma thyroid is true except: (2010)
a. Multicentric origin
b. Secondaries to nodes common

c. Slow growing
d. Only metastasis in early stage

35. The main cause of endogenous Cushing's syndrome is: (2010)
a. Adrenal Carcinoma
b. ACTH-pituitary tumor
c. Adrenal Hyperplasia
d. Adrenal Adenoma

36. Most common cause of subarachnoid hemorrhage is: (2010)
a. Hypertension.
b. Berry aneurysm
c. Intracranial tumors
d. Arterio-venous malformations (AVM)

37. First ever surgeon to do a liver transplantation was: (2010)
a. Christian Bernard
b. Karl Starz
c. Thomas Hudson
d. George Hewlitt

38. Abdominal distension in intestinal obstruction is due to: (2010)
a. Intestinal bacterial fermentation
b. Swallowed air
c. Strangulation
d. Constipation

39. Continuous vomiting leads to: (2010)
a. ↓K, ↓Cl alkalosis
b. ↓K, ↓Cl acidosis
c. ↓K ↑Cl alkalosis
d. ↑K,↑Cl acidosis

40. Hypercalcemia is not seen in: (2011)
a. Squamous cell carcinoma of lung
b. Parathyroid carcinoma
c. Multiple myeloma
d. Gastric carcinoma

41. Most common type of intracranial hemorrhage: (2011)
a. Intra ventricular
b. Extradural
c. Subdural
d. Cerebellar

42. Strangury is due to: (2011)
a. Mid ureter
b. Urethra
c. Inflamed bladder
d. Stretching of renal capsule

43. Tumor staging and grading in early bladder cancer is usually done with following: (2011)
a. USG
b. CT Scan
c. Cystography
d. Transurethral resection

44. A 10 mm calculus in the right lower ureter associated with proximal hydroureteronephrosis in 45 year old best treated withL (2011)
a. Open ureterolithotomy
b. Extracorporeal shockwave lithotripsy
c. Antegrade percutaneous access
d. Ureteroscopic retrieval

45. Aniline dyes are commonly the etiological agent for: (2012)
a. Ca. Thyroid
b. Ca. Prostate
c. Ca. Kidney
d. Ca. Urinary bladder

46. Thimble bladder is seen in: (2012)
a. Cystitis cystica
b. Chronic tubercular cystitis
c. Neurogenic bladder
d. Acute tubercular cystitis

47. Commonest cause of bilateral spider leg deformity of calyces seen on excretory urography is:
a. Hypernephroma (2012)
b. Polycystic kidney
c. Hydronephrosis
d. Wilm'stumor

48. The Most common malignant testicular neoplasm is: (2012)
a. Teratoma
b. Seminoma
c. Choriocarcinoma
d. Lymphoma

49. Commonest cause of blood discharge from the nipple is: (2012)
a. Duct carcinoma
b. Duct-papilloma
c. Chronic cystic mastitis
d. Cystosarcoma phyllodes

50. Villous adenoma of the rectum usually presents with: (2012)
a. Rectal prolapsed
b. Intestinal obstruction
c. Mucous diarrhea with hypokalemia
d. Massive hematochezia

51. Carcinoma prostate most commonly metastasizes to: (2012)
a. Lungs
b. Liver
c. Bones
d. Brain

52. Treatment of choice in severe flail chest is: (2012)
a. Strapping
b. Intercostal block
c. Fixation of fractured ribs with wire
d. Intermittent positive pressure ventilation

53. The commonest tumor of urinary bladder is:
a. Papilloma **(2012)**
b. Adenocarcinoma
c. Transitional cell carcinoma
d. Squamous cell carcinoma

54. Prostatectomy was done in a 80 years old man. Histology revealed a 'Focal area' of well differentiated adenocarcinoma. Future Management should consist of: (2012)
a. Radiotherapy to prostatic area
b. Stilbestrol therapy
c. Orchidectomy
d. No further treatment

55. A child presents with partially compressible, cystic, lobulated and translucent swelling in the posterior triangle of neck. The most-likely diagnosis is: (2012)
a. Aerocele
b. Branchial cyst
c. Pharyngeal pouch
d. Cystic hygroma

56. Warthin's tumor is: (2012)
a. Also known as mucoepidermoid tumor
b. Common in elderly females
c. Seen as a hot spot on isotope scan
d. A relatively malignant tumor

57. The following statement about keloids is correct: (2012)
a. They are more common in whites than in blacks
b. They do not extent into normal skin
c. Local recurrence is common after excision
d. Thus often undergo malignant changes

58. A 24-year-old man is brought into the emergency department after a fall from a ladder. His breathing is labored and he is cyanotic.
No breath sounds can be heard, even in the right lung field, which is resonant to percussion. The first step in his management should be: (2012)
a. Cricothyroidotomy
b. Obtaining a stat chest X-ray
c. Passing an oral endotracheal tube
d. Tube thoracostomy

59. Successful antibiotic penetration of a burn eschar can be achieved with: (2012)
a. Mafenide acetate
b. Neomycin
c. Povidone-iodine
d. Silver nitrate

60. A serum tumor marker correlated with recurrence after management of colon cancer is: (2012)
a. α-fetoprotein
b. Calcitonin
c. Carcinoembryonic antigen (CEA)
d. CA 15-3

61. In the prevention of graft rejection, cyclosporine: (2011)
a. Blocks transcription of IL-l and TNF-a
b. Inhibits lymphocyte nucleic acid metabolism
c. Inhibits RNA and DNA synthesis
d. Selectively inhibits T –cells activation

62. Newman and SeaBrock's surgery is done for:
a. Cleft palate **(2011)**
b. Cleft lip
c. Repair of parotid fistula
d. Chronic Lymphoedema

63. Which statement best describes lymphatic drainage from the breast? (2011)
a. All quadrants of the breast drain into both the axillary and the parasternal nodes
b. The areolar area of the breast drains into retrosternal internal mammary nodes (internal mammary)
c. The lateral area of the breast drains into axillary nodes
d. The medial area of the breast drains into parasternal nodes

64. A 30 year old woman presents with a 1.5 cm mass below her right earlobe. She has been aware of the mass for 4 years. Physical examination reveals firm, non-tender, movable mass and intact facial nerve function; cervical nodes are not palpable. The most likely diagnosis is: (2011)
a. Papillary cystadenoma' (Warthin's tumor)
b. Low-grade mucoepidermoid carcinoma
c. Benign mixed tumor (pleomorphic adenoma)
d. Malignant mixed tumor

65. A 60-year-old woman with a mass in the right pulmonary hilum is found by sputum cytology to have a small cell carcinoma. At this "time, appropriate management is to: (2011)
a. Begin chemotherapy and radiation therapy
b. Curry out u metastatic workup including CT scans of the head and the liver
c. Perform mediastinoscopy
d. Perform thoracotomy and pneumonectomy

66. Which structure is left in simple mastectomy? (2012)
a. Pectoralis major
b. Pectoralis minor
c. Both of the above
d. None of the above

67. True about Paget's disease all except: (2012)
a. Incidence 1:1000
b. Has underlying intralobular carcinoma
c. May have underlying carcinoma
d. Blood stained discharge

68. Choledochal cyst: (2012)
a. Mostly presents in adulthood
b. Excision is infrequently done
c. Presents as slowly progressive jaundice
d. Can lead to carcinoma

69. Lucid interval is seen in: (2012)
a. Subdural hemorrhage
b. Extradural hemorrhage
c. Parenchymal hemorrhage
d. None of the above

70. For hiatus hernia IOC is: (2013)
a. Barium meal follows through
b. Barium meal upper GI
c. Barium meal upper GI in Trendelenburg's position
d. barium meal double contrast

71. Regarding RCC all are true except: (2013)
a. Renal lump, pain abdomen, hematuria
b. Associated with anemia and low ESR
c. Propensity to invade IVC
d. Invasion of renal vein is C/I for surgery

72. Acute pancreatitis is associated with all except: (2013)
a. Steatorrhea
b. Epigastric tenderness
c. Upper abdominal pain
d. Cullen's sign

73. Thumb printing on barium enema is seen in: (2013)
a. Ulcerative colitis
b. Crohn's disease
c. Ischemic colitis
d. None of the above

74. Retrosternal goiter is characterized by: (2006)
a. Stridor
b. Always malignant
c. Bilateral
d. None of the above

75. Bowen's disease is: (2006)
a. Mimics chronic dermatosis
b. Premalignant condition
c. Presents with pruritus
d. All of the above

76. Palpable fibrous plaque on dorsal penile shaft indicates: (2006)
a. Paget's disease
b. Peyronie's disease
c. Hard sore
d. None of the above

77. Subcapsular orchidectomy is done for cancer of: (2006)
a. Testis
b. Prostate
c. Penis
d. Male breast cancer

78. Burns in which part of body are nursed without occlusive dressing? (2006)
a. Hands
b. Legs
c. Head and Neck
d. Chest

79. Thiersch graft is: (2006)
a. Full thickness graft
b. Partial thickness graft
c. Muscle flap
d. Pedicle graft

80. Most common type of hernia in female is: (2007)
a. Femoral
b. Ventral
c. Inguinal
d. Epigastric

81. Felon is: (2007)
a. Mid palmer space infection
b. Terminal pulp space infection
c. Infection of ulnar bursa
d. Infection of radial bursa

82. The most common malignancy found in Marjolin's ulcer is: (2007)
a. Basal cell carcinoma
b. Squamous cell carcinoma
c. Malignant fibrous histiocytoma
d. Melanoma

83. A patient presents with sudden headache and vomiting and unconsciousness. The diagnosis is: (2011)
a. Subarachnoid hemorrhage
b. Intracerebral hemorrhage
c. Subdural hemorrhage
d. Extradural hemorrhage

84. Dentigerous cyst arises from: (2011)
a. The root of a caries tooth
b. The periosteum of the fractured mandible
c. An unerupted permanent tooth
d. The sequestrum of osteomyelitis of mandible

85. A 21 years old woman has 3 cm node in the lower deep cervical chain on the left. The biopsy is interpreted as revealing normal thyroid tissue in a lymph node. The most likely diagnosis is: (2009)

a. Subacute thyroiditis
b. Metastatic carcinoma thyroid
c. Hashimoto's disease
d. Lateral aberrant thyroid

86. The most important prognostic factor in carcinoma breast is: (2009)

a. Size of tumor
b. Skin involvement
c. Involvement of muscles
d. Axillary gland involvement

87. Commonest benign tumor of the esophagus: (2009)

a. Leiomyoma
b. Papilloma
c. Adenoma
d. Hemangioma

88. A patient present with dysphagia of 4 weeks duration. Now he is able to swallow liquid food only. Which of the following is the one investigation to be done? (2009)

a. Barium studies
b. Upper GI endoscopy
c. CT Scan
d. Esophageal manometry

89. Minimum amount of GI bleed to cause melena is: (2010)

a. 10 ml
b. 40 ml
c. 60 ml
d. 115 ml

90. Liver biopsy is done through 8th midaxillary line to avoid injury to: (2010)

a. Lung
b. Pleural cavity
c. Sub diaphragmatic
d. Gallbladder

91. Commonest complication of Pseudocyst of the pancreas is: (2010)

a. Rupture into peritoneum
b. Rupture into colon
c. Hemorrhage
d. Infection

92. Which of the following is a delayed absorbable synthetic suture material? (2010)

a. Chronic catgut
b. Vicryl
c. Silk
d. Nylon

93. Most Common motility disorder leading to dysphagia: (2010)

a. Nut cracker esophagus
b. Esophageal web
c. Diffuse esophageal spasm
d. Achalasia cardia

94. Most Common site of carcinoma of stomach is: (2010)

a. Proximal stomach
b. Gastric antrum
c. Lesser curvature
d. Greater curvature

95. All are causes of dynamic intestinal obstruction except: (2010)

a. Gallstones
b. Bands
c. Intussusception
d. Mesenteric vascular occlusion

96. Most common tumor occurring in appendix: (2010)

a. Melanoma
b. Carcinoid tumor
c. Adenocarcinoma
d. Mucinous carcinoma

97. Treatment of choice for squamous cell carcinoma of anal canal not involving deep structures: (2010)

a. Chemoradiation
b. Wide local excision + chemoradiation
c. Wide local excision + radiotherapy
d. Abdomino perineal resection

98. Not a complication of gallstones: (2010)

a. Mucocele
b. Diverticulosis
c. Acute cholangitis
d. Empyema of the gallbladder

99. Charcot's triad: (2010)

a. Fever, abdominal pain, jaundice
b. Fever, vomiting, jaundice
c. Fever, jaundice, abdominal distension
d. Fever, diarrhea, jaundice

100. Klatskin tumor is: (2010)

a. Merkel cell carcinoma of skin
b. Primitive neuroectodermal tumor of chest wall
c. Common hepatic duct tumor
d. Adenocarcinoma of anal canal

101. Acute emphysematous cholecystitis is caused by: (2010)

a. Pseudomonas aeruginosa
b. Staphylococcus aureus
c. Clostridium perfringens
d. Streptococcus pyogenes

102. Most common cause of pancreatic pseudocyst:
a. Blunt abdominal trauma (2012)
b. Pancreatic carcinoma
c. Acute Pancreatitis
d. Postpancreatic surgery

103. Least recurrence rate in inguinal hernia repair is following: (2013)
a. Lichtenstein mesh repair
b. Intraperitoneal mesh repair
c. Inlay mesh repair
d. Shouldice repair

104. True statement regarding Warthin's tumor: (2013)
a. Common in females
b. Most malignant
c. Hot spots on Tc 99 scan
d. Most common tumor of minor salivary gland

105. Parkland formula is: (2013)
a. Percentage of burns × weight (kg) × 4 = volume in ml
b. Percentage of burns × weight (kg)/2 = 1 ration
c. Percentage of burns × weight (kg) X × = volume in ml
d. 5000ml/m^2 burned + 1500 m^2 = volume in ml

106. Treatment of Cystosarcoma phylloides in a young woman: (2013)
a. Wide excision with a margin
b. Wide excision with chemotherapy
c. Wide excision with radiotherapy
d. MRM

107. BRCA 1 positive woman have __ % increased risk of breast carcinoma: (2013)
a. 10
b. 20
c. 40
d. 60

108. Which of the following about direct inguinal hernia is correct? (2013)
a. Swelling medial to inferior epigastric artery
b. Most common hernia in females
c. Treatment is opening ligation at neck of the sack and repairing
d. Often descends to bottom of scrotum

109. Medial boundary of femoral ring is formed by:
a. Inguinal ligament (2013)
b. Pectineal ligament
c. Lacunar ligament
d. Septum separating it from femoral vein

110. A patient with autoimmune thyroiditis presents with hypothyroidism. Which of the following is true? (2013)
a. Thyroid peroxidase antibodies
b. Painless enlargement of thyroid
c. Common in men
d. No malignant risk

111. Allen's test is used to diagnose: (2013)
a. Thoracic outlet syndrome
b. Palmar arch insufficiency
c. Superior vena cava syndrome
d. Varicose veins

112. The following about thoracic outlet syndrome is true: (2013)
a. Median nerve of brachial plexus is commonly involved
b. Surgical decompression of brachial plexus is the best treatment
c. Often associated with cervical rib abnormalities
d. Arteriography can rule out disease

113. Type of renal stone formed in a patient with .... regional enteritis: (2013)
a. Calcium oxalate
b. Cysteine
c. Struvite
d. Urate

114. Genitourinary TB in a male patient presents with:
a. Painful and tender epididymis (2013)
b. Bacteriuria without Pyuria
c. Renal cysts (unilateral)
d. Microscopic hematuria

115. Treatment of choice for grade superficial bladder carcinoma: (2013)
a. Local excision
b. Radical cystectomy
c. Intravesical BCG
d. Chemotherapy

116. True about hypospadias: (2013)
a. Associated with chordee
b. 50% associated with undescended testis
c. Due to failure of fusion of posterior wall of urethra
d. Circumcision done immediately

117. A 20-year-old male presents with scrotal mass. The first investigation to be done is: (2011)
a. Clinical evaluation
b. USG

c. Biopsy
d. AFP

118. H. pylori is associated with __ % of gastric ulcers: (2011)
a. 5
b. 20
c. 40-60
d. 80

119. A patient who has undergone partial gastrectomy presents with neurological symptoms. Most probable diagnosis: (2011)
a. Folic acid deficiency
b. Thiamine deficiency
c. Vitamin B12 deficiency
d. Iron deficiency

120. Most common complication of end colostomy: (2013)
a. Parastomal hernia
b. Prolapse
c. Perforation
d. Bleeding

121. Anorectal anomalies are commonly associated with: (2013)
a. Cardiac anomalies
b. Urologic Abnormalities
c. CNS malformations
d. Abdominal wall defects

122. Treatment of choice for squamous cell carcinoma of anal canal: (2013)
a. Abdomino-Perineal-Resection
b. Chemoradiation
c. Wide local excision
d. CO_2 laser

123. Most common organ involved in blunt injury to the abdomen: (2013)
a. Spleen
b. Liver
c. Intestines
d. Kidney

124. 65-year-old male presents with tachycardia, sweating, palpitation, giddiness which improves on taking food. Diagnosis: (2012)
a. Insulinoma
b. Zollinger Ellison syndrome
c. Carcinoma pancreas
d. Carcinoid

125. Poor prognostic factor In a patient with acute pancreatitis: (2011)
a. Leucocytosis > 20000/μ
b. ↑serum amylase
c. ↑serum lipase
d. Diastolic BP > 90 mm Hg

126. Retroperitoneal fibrosis most commonly presents with: (2012)
a. Pedal edema
b. Ascites
c. Ureteric obstruction
d. Back pain

127. Intussusception is caused by: (2011)
a. Submucous lipoma
b. Intramuscular lipoma
c. Subfascial lipoma
d. Subserosal lipoma

128. Earliest symptom of carcinoma rectum: (2013)
a. Constipation
b. Pain
c. Bleeding
d. Alternating constipation and diarrhea

129. Emphysematous cholecystitis is seen in infection with: (2013)
a. Pseudomonas aeruginosa
b. Clostridium perfringens
c. Escherichia coli
d. Salmonella typhi

130. The following renal stone is radiolucent: (2007)
a. Calcium oxalate
b. Struvite
c. Uric acid
d. Cysteine

131. In an infant with undescended testis, spontaneous descent will not occur after: (2008)
a. 2 months
b. 3 months
c. 5 months
d. 6 months

132. Most common presenting feature of fibroadenosis: (2013)
a. Pain
b. Discharge from nipple
c. Lump
d. Nodularity

133. Most common type of malignant melanoma: (2014)
a. Superficial spreading
b. Amelanotic melanoma
c. Lentigo maligna
d. Nodular melanoma

134. Ganglion in hand arises due to: (2014)
a. Degeneration of tendon sheath
b. Degeneration of nerve capsule

c. Degeneration of joint capsule
d. Degeneration of periosteum

135. Commonest surgical procedure for soft tissue sarcoma: (2014)
a. Marginal excision
b. Enucleation
c. Wide local excision
d. Compartmental excision

136. Subclavian steal syndrome is due to: (2014)
a. Blockage of first part of subclavian artery
b. Blockage of second part of subclavian artery
c. Blockage of third part of subclavian artery
d. Thrombosis of subclavian vein

137. Acute paronychia is treated by: (2014)
a. Incision and drainage
b. Lifting the paronychium
c. Partial nail excision
d. Total nail excision

138. The procedure contraindicated in diabetics: (2014)
a. Ray amputation
b. Forefoot amputation
c. Syme's amputation
d. Below knee amputation

139. Thiersch graft is also known as: (2014)
a. Full thickness graft
b. Partial thickness graft
c. Wolfe's graft
d. Plastic graft

140. Resection of adjacent gut is most often required in: (2014)
a. Chylolymphatic cyst
b. Enterogenous cyst
c. Mesenteric dermoid cyst
d. Simple cyst

141. A 45-year-old lady is having persistent reflux symptoms. Most accurate investigations in establishing diagnosis before surgical treatment is: (2014)
a. An UGI series
b. Endoscopy
c. Esophageal manometry
d. Ambulatory pH monitoring

142. Barrett's esophagus–true statement: (Nov 2014)
a. Endoscopic surveillance with biopsy every 2 years
b. Helicobacter pylori triple therapy
c. Proton pump inhibitor
d. Histamine antagonist

143. Neo-adjuvant chemotherapy used esophageal carcinoma: (Nov 2014)
a. Doxorubicin
b. Cisplatin
c. 5-Fu-Leucovarin
d. Mitomycin C

144. Benign small bowel tumors most commonly present as: (Nov 2014)
a. Gastrointestinal bleeding
b. Incidental finding on laparotomy
c. Small bowel obstruction
d. Persistent loss of weight

145. The layer responsible for strength of an intestinal anastomosis is: (2010)
a. Mucosa
b. Submucosa
c. Muscularis propria
d. Serosa

146. Least common site of volvulus in children: (2010)
a. Midgut
b. Small bowel
c. Ileocolic
d. Large bowel

147. True fact regarding Crohn's disease: (Nov 2014)
a. Entero enteric fistula is an indication for urgent surgery
b. Medical management includes antibiotics, immunosuppressive agents and biologic agents
c. No increased risk for colonic cancer
d. No effect on fertility

148. A patient with abdominal wall desmoids tumor should be screened for: (Nov 2014)
a. Lung cancer
b. Breast cancer
c. Colonic Polyps
d. Pancreatic cancer

149. Initial investigation for obstructive jaundice: (2013)
a. USG
b. CT scan
c. ERCP
d. MRI

150. Colovesical fistula: (Nov 2014)
a. Most commonly presents with pneumaturia
b. More common in females
c. Most commonly caused by colon cancer
d. Readily diagnosed on barium enema

151. Induration of seminal vesicle is seen most often in: (Nov. 2014)
a. Tuberculosis
b. Gonorrhea
c. Syphilis
d. Lymphogranuloma venereum

152. The following statement is false regarding Grave's disease: (Nov 2014)
a. Hypertrophy/hyperplasia is due to TSH-RAbs
b. Cardiac failure is common
c. Goiter is diffuse and vascular
d. Remissions and exacerbations are not infrequent

153. Medullary carcinoma of thyroid–all are true except: (Nov. 2014)
a. It is tumor arising from C cells
b. Secrete high levels of calcitonin
c. It is not dependent on TSH
d. Most cases are familial

154. Follicular carcinoma of thyroid: (2014)
a. The most common thyroid cancer
b. Readily diagnosed thyroid cancer
c. Spreads through hematogenous route
d. Commonly multifocal

155. Hernia most likely to recur after primary surgery: (2014)
a. Epigastric hernia
b. Spigelian hernia
c. Incisional hernia
d. Femoral hernia

156. Burns with injury to epidermis and superficial dermis is categorized as: (2014)
a. First degree burns
b. Second degree superficial burns
c. Second degree deep burns
d. Third degree burns

157. Not a complication of total parenteral nutrition: (Nov 2014)
a. Hyperammonemia
b. Hypercholesterolemia
c. Neutrophile dysfunction
d. Hyperphosphatemia

158. A child has circumferential burns involving both buttock and thigh, face including scalp with singeing of hairs. What is the approximate percentage of area involved? (Nov 2014)
a. 25
b. 27
c. 37
d. 45

159. Early complication of ileostomy is: (Nov 2014)
a. Necrosis
b. Obstruction
c. Prolapsed
d. Diarrhea

160. Intussusceptions is frequently associated with: (Nov 2014)
a. Subserosal lipoma
b. Intramural lipoma
c. Sub mucosal lipoma
d. Subfascial lipoma

161. Which of the following parotid gland tumor shows hot spot in 99Tc Pertechnate scan? (Nov 2014)
a. Adenoid cystic carcinoma
b. Adenolymphoma
c. Acinic cell carcinoma
d. Adenocarcinoma

162. Nerve damaged during sentinel node biopsy of breast carcinoma is? (Nov 2014)
a. Intercostobrachial nerve
b. Lateral pectoral nerve
c. Long thoracic nerve
d. Nerve to latissimus dorsi

163. True regarding 'Damage control surgery' is: (Nov 2014)
a. Done during damage control surgery
b. Done during triage
c. Minimal intervention to stabilize patient so that definitive surgery can be done later on
d. Maximum possible surgical intervention considering the event

164. An elderly male presents with 4x5 cm lump in right neck. FNAC revealed it to be squamous cell carcinoma. No primary was found. A diagnosis of unknown primary was made. According to AJCC system of classification, the TNM staging of the tumor would be: (Nov 2014)
a. T1 N2 Mo
b. T0 N2a M1
c. T1 N2c Mo
d. T0 N2a Mx

ANSWERS AND EXPLANATIONS

Author's Note:

Dear friends-I have given only 100 percent authenticated answers for the questions. For controversial answers-I have given statements then and there.. So trust me and go ahead...

Answers are Based on

- Schwartz's Principles of Surgery-10th Edition
- Bailey and Love-26th Edition
- Sabiston–19th Edition
- Blumgart's Surgery of Liver and Pancreatic Diseases-5th edition
- Shackelford's Surgery of Alimentary tract-7th Edition

1. **Ans. B. Lateral to inferior epigastric artery**

   Explanation
   - Direct hernia-Medial to inferior epigastric artery
   - Indirect hernia-Lateral to inferior epigastric artery

   Shape of
   - Indirect hernia-Pyriform shaped
   - Direct hernia-Globular

   Indirect hernia comes out via Deep ring which is a defect in Fascia transversalis
   Direct hernia comes out via Hesselbach triangle

2. **Ans. a. Morgagni's hernia**

   Congenital Diaphragmatic Hernia

   Antero medial-Space of larrey's* (foramen of Morgagni)
   - M/C on right side**.
   - Causes no symptom.

   Postero lateral-Commonest type of CDH**.Occurs via foramen of Bochdalek.
   - M/c on left.
   - Cause respiratory distress and death of infant due to abdominal visceral herniation

3. **Ans. c. Lymph nodes of Peyer's enlarges**

   Explanation
   - **Intussusception**
     - Entering tube-intussusceptum
     - Returning-middle tube
     - Outer tube-intussuscipiens**

   M/c cause of intestinal obstruction*-age 3 months to 6 years**

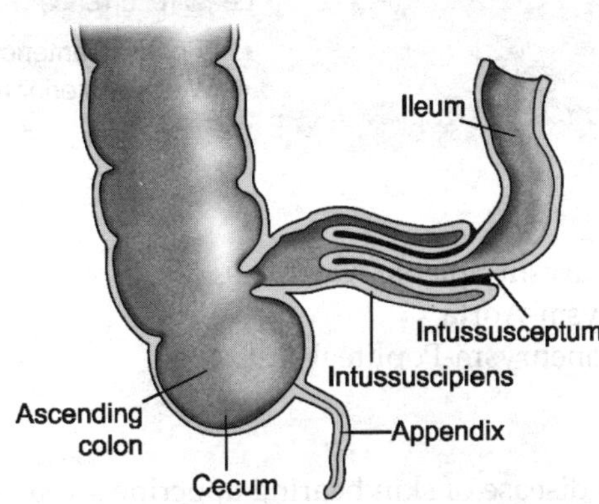

Fig 12.5: Intussusception

Clinical features
- M/c type-ileocolic*
- Characterized by -severe crampy abdominal pain
- Vomiting
- Red currant jelly stool*
- P/A-sausage shaped mass
- Le dance sign-empty right iliac fossa*
- P/R-apex may seen protruding

Types
- Ileocolic [77%]
- Ileoileal colic [12%]
- Ileoileal [5%]
- Colocolic [2%]-More common in Old age due to Cancers.

Investigation
- Barium enema: Claw sign, Coiled spring sign
- Ultrasound: Target sign, Pseudo kidney sign and Bulls eye sign
- X-ray plain: Target sign [soft tissue mass with concentric area of lucency due to mesentric fat]

CAUSES

Paediatric
- Idiopathic [70-90%]
- Hypertrophied Peyer's patch [m/c]
- Respiratory infection, gastroenteritis, urinary infection are associated in 30%
- RARELY-HenochSchonleinPurpura

OLDER INFANTS-Meckel's diverticulum [M/C]*

ADULTS-Tumors, polyps, submucosallipomas.

**Colo colic variety is common in adults

Treatment

Hydrostatic reduction by contrast agent or air enema is diagnostic and therapeutic
Such procedure is contraindicated in peritonitis and hemodynamic instability

4. **Ans. c. Liver transplantation**

Explanation
- HLA typing is not needed for Liver transplant and Heart transplant

5. **Ans. c. Ripstein operation**

Rectal Prolapse Approaches

Perineal approach	Abdominal approach
Useful in very old age who cannot withstand abdominal operation	Used in young age
Recurrence is more	Least recurrence
• Delormes operation • Thiersch operation • Altemier's procedure	• Ripsteins anterior rectopexy • Well's posterior rectopexy

6. **Ans. a. Splenic artery**

Explanation
- M/c site of visceral artery aneurysm-Splenic A
- M/c site of large vessel aneurysm-Aorta
- M/c Site of peripheral artery aneurysm-Popliteal A

7. **Ans. a. Eccrine sweat gland**

Explanation
- Chronic fibrous and infective disease of skin bearing apocrine sweat glands.

- Apocrine glands are those which open into hair follicle
- M/c in diabetics
- M/c in axilla
- M/c due to staphylococci
- Treatment excision with grafting.

8. **Ans. a. 80% from portal vein, 20% from hepatic artery**
   - 80% from portal vein and **20% from hepatic artery***
   - Left hepatic duct has longest extra hepatic course*-2 cm is accessible outside liver.
   - Relations in the porta hepatitis from behind forwards-Portal Vein (posterior), Hepatic Artery (Left) and Hepatic Ducts (right)**
   - **Tumors in the liver receive the major blood supply from the Hepatic artery.**
     - Oxygenated blood is received in majority by Hepatic Artery.

9. **Ans. c. Pleomorphic adenoma**
   - m/c benign parotid tumor in ADULTS–Pleomorphic adenoma
   - m/c malignant parotid tumor–mucoepidermoid carcinoma
   - m/c benign submandibular gland tumor–pleomorphic adenoma
   - m/c malignant submandibular gland tumor–adenoid cystic carcinoma
   - m/c site for squamous cell carcinoma salivary gland–submandibular gland
   - m/c minor salivary gland tumor -adenocarcinoma
   - Tumor that spreads via neural sheath–adenoid cystic carcinoma

10. **Ans. c. Vas deferens**

    Hessel Bach Triangle

    Weak spot in anterior abdominal wall through which direct hernia appears
   - Medial Outer border of rectus abdominis
   - Lateral Inferior epigastric vessels
   - Below Medial part of inguinal ligament
   - Floor Fascia transversalis

11. **Ans. c. Randomized flap**

    Axial and Random flaps
   - If the blood supply is not derived from a recognized artery but, rather, comes from many little unnamed vessels, the flap is referred to as a Random flap. Many local cutaneous (skin) flaps fall into this category.
   - If the blood supply comes from a recognized artery or group of arteries, it is referred to as an axial flap. Most muscle flaps have axial blood supplies.

12. **Ans. a. ITP**

    Splenectomy

    Indications:
   - **Trauma:** Immediate, delayed, spontaneous rupture
   - **Neoplasms:** Lymphomas, leukemias, hemangiomas
   - **As part of other surgeries:** D2 resection (gastreetomy): pancreatectomy, splenorenal shunt
   - **Miscellaneous:** Abscess, infarct, anecrysm, cyst, to prevent graft rejection.
   - **Hematological:**
     - For anemia
     - For purpura
     - Hypersplenism
     - Myelo fibrosis.

Splenectomy always indicated
• Primary splenic tumor
• Hereditary spherocytosis

Splenectomy not indicated for:
- Asymptomatic hypersplenism
- Splenomegaly with infection
- Splenomegaly associated with elevated Ig M
- Hereditary hemolytic anemia of moderate degree
- Acute leukemias
- Agranulocytosis.

- M/c indication for splenectomy–splenic trauma*
- M/c indication for splenectomy in elective setting–ITP*.

Idiopathic Thrombocytopenic Purpura:
- Autoimmune disorder
- Present with low platelet count and mucocutaneous and petechial bleeding.
- Low platelet is due to the **antiplatelet IgG auto antibodies*** produced in spleen.
- Platelet count less than 10,000/mm cube* are at risk of internal bleeding.
- In addition to low platelet count presence of immature (megathrombocytes) is pathognomonic* of ITP.
- **Most common indication for elective splenectomy**
- For patients with low platelet count should have platelets available at surgery but should be infused **only after ligating the pedicle****.
- Should not be given preoperatively*

  The treatment of choice is medical-**oral prednisolone 1mg/kg** produces dramatic response in 50-70% cases.
- Intravenous immunoglobin is indicated for internal bleeding.

  Splenectomy is indicated for
  - Failure of steroids
  - Undesirable effects due to long use of steroids
  - Most cases of first relapse

13. Ans. d. Dexamethasone

Primary treatment for head injury
- The principle aim is to prevent secondary brain injury and best achieved by avoidance of hypoxia and hypotension.
- Positioning head up 20-30 degrees reduces ICP. (Reverse Trendelenburg if spine injured)
- 0.5 ml/kg of 20% mannitol will temporarily reduce ICP.
- Increase ICP can be suggested by pupillary dilatation.

Though it's a controversial Question the Answer is correct as per Sabiston Page 441
- Free water (as dextrose solutions) should NOT be administered
- Elevated blood sugar levels are associated with a worsening of neurologic injury after episodes of global cerebral ischemia.
- Ischemic brain metabolizes glucose to lactic acid, lowering tissue pH and potentially exacerbating ischemic injury.
- Hypertonic solutions and osmotic diuretics such as mannitol will have the opposite effect
- There is no single best fluid for patients with traumatic brain injury, but isotonic crystalloids are widely used and have good scientific basis. Normal saline or lactated Ringer's solution should be the standard resuscitation fluid until further studies show a clear benefit from other therapies.
- Regardless of the fluid type chosen, normovolemia must be maintained and episodes of hypotension avoided.

14. Ans. c. Adenomatous polyp
- Pseudopolyps are not premalignant
- Non neoplastic polyps-hyperplastic, juvenile, Peutz-Jeghers polyps
- Neoplastic polyps-Tubular adenomas, Villous adenomas, Familial polyposis coli, Gardner's syndrome, Turcot's syndrome

15. **Ans. b. Sloping**
    - Sloping ulcer-healing ulcer
        - Inner part is red
    - Undermined edge-tuberculosis
    - Punched out–syphilitic gumma ulcer
        - Trophic ulcer
        - Due to end arteritis
    - Raised and beaded–BCC (rodent ulcer)
    - Everted and rolled out-squamous cell carcinoma

16. **Ans. c. Bladder**

    Glasgow coma scale (EVM-456)

    Eye opening
    - Spontaneous–4
    - To verbal command-3
    - To pain stimuli-2
    - Do not open-1

    Verbal
    - Normal oriented-5
    - Confused-4
    - Inappropriate words-3
    - Sounds only-2
    - No sounds-1

    Motor
    - Obeys commands-6
    - Localizes to pain-5
    - Withdrawal flexion-4
    - Abnormal flexion-3 (decorticate)
    - Extension-2 (decerebrate)
    - No motor response-1

17. **Ans. c. Duplex USG**

    Deep Vein Thrombosis
    - m/c cause-hospital admission for medical or surgical conditions.
    - E-thrombosis: Thrombosis developing in people sitting at their computer for long time.
    - Bilateral DVT is seen in 30% cases.

    Signs of DVT*
    - Homan's sign-forced dorsiflexion
    - Mosse's sign-calf tenderness
    - Pratt's sign-calf tenderness on pressing from sides
    - Modified perthe's test-elastocrepe bandage test to diagnose DVT.

    VIRCHOW'S TRIAD**
    - Endothelial damage
    - Stasis
    - Increased coagulability of blood

    Clinical features

    M/c presentation-pain and swelling in calf

    Treatment:
    - Treatment: start heparin immediately, followed by warfarin 10 mg day 1,2 and 5 mg from day 3
    - Thrombolysis is indicated If there is iliac vein involvement.
    - Surgical treatment: PALMA OPERATION**

    In cases of DVT of the external iliac vein on one side the contralateral saphenous vein is anastomosed to the femoral vein on the affected site below the level of occlusion or stenosis.

18. **Ans. b. Upper outer quadrant**
Incidence of carcinoma in each quadrant
- Upper outer 60%
- Upper inner 12%
- Lower outer 10%
- Lower inner 6%
- Central 12%

19. **Ans. b. Constriction ring at lower esophagus**
- Occurs at lower end near squamocolumnar junction*
- Intermittent dysphagia
- Treatment-esophageal dilatation

20. **Ans. b. Post Cholecystectomy**
- Incidence of Bile duct injury is m/c with Lap cholecystectomy than Open cholecystectomy
- Percentage of Bile duct injuries in Lap Cholecystectomy = 0.4–0.7%
- Bile duct Injuries:

Lap Cholecystectomy associated with higher percentage of injuries [0.16 TO 2.31] compared to OPEN SURGERIES [0.1 TO 0.1]*

Classifications

Bismuth classification based on location	Strausberg classification (Depending on patterns of injury)
TYPE 1: Low common hepatic duct stricture. stump > 2cm	TYPE A: Minor hepatic duct or cystic duct leaks
TYPE 2: Proximal stricture. Stump< 2 cm	TYPE B: Aberrant right hepatic duct or sectoral duct divided and LIGATED
TYPE 3: Hilar stricture. Confluence intact	
TYPE 4: Destructed confluence. Right and left ducts separated	TYPE C: Same as B but BILE LEAK
TYPE 5: Involvement of right aberrant sectoral duct alone or along with stricture at CHD	TYPE D: Lateral injury to CBD or CHD
	TYPE E: Circumferential injury to main ducts

Management
- Early repair not attempted. Only drainage procedures carried out
- Ideal time of repair is 8 to 12 weeks to allow inflammation to subside**
- Roux en y hepatico jejunostomy is ideal repair

21. **Ans. a. Pain**
- Intractable pain due to ductal obstruction is the m/c indication of surgery

SURGERIES;
- **Modified puestow's**: Duct > 8 mm anastomosed to Roux en y jejunum.
- **Frey's procedure**: Head coring anastomosis pancreatico Jejunostomy.
- **Beger's procedure**: DPPHR (Duodenum Preserving Pancreatic Head Resection and Anastomosis)

22. **Ans. b. Duodenum**
- M/c site of intestinal atresia-Duodenal atresia
- Treatment of Duodenal atresia-Duodenoduodenostomy > Duodenojejunostomy
- Double Bubble appearance

23. **Ans. b. Familial adenomatous polyposis coli**
M/c presentation of rectal polyp is bleeding
Other choices:
- Villous Polyps can be associated with Hypokalemia
- IBS does not produce polyps-Infact IBS is a definition used when there is no pathology
- Peutz Jeughers polyps-Seen in jejunum
- FAP will have 100s of polyps all over colon including Rectum

24. Ans. b. Trans mesocolon *Ref: Sabiston1/9e p1107*

Paraduodenal (mesocolic hernias)

- Mesocolic hernias are unusual congenital hernias in which the small intestine herniates behind the mesocolon.
- They result from abnormal rotation of the midgut and have been categorized as right or left.

A right mesocolic hernia occurs when the prearterial limb of the midgut loop fails to rotate around the superior mesenteric artery. This results in most of the small intestine remaining to the right of the superior mesenteric artery. Normal counterclockwise rotation of the cecum and proximal colon into the right side of the abdomen and its fixation to the posterolateral peritoneum cause the small intestine to become trapped behind the mesentery of the right side of the colon. The ileocolic, right colic, and middle colic vessels lie within the anterior wall of the sac** and the superior mesenteric artery courses along the medial border of the neck of the hernia.

Left mesocolic hernias are thought to be caused by in utero herniation of the small intestine between the inferior mesenteric vein and posterior parietal attachments of the descending mesocolon to the retroperitoneum. The inferior mesenteric artery and vein are integral components of the hernia sac**. Approximately 75% of mesocolic hernias occur on the left side.

Other choices:

- Transmesentric hernia occurs through the defects in the mesentry from previous surgery, Naturally will not have sac.
- Epiploic foramen also lets contents to enter the Lesser sac which is the space behind the stomach but has no definite sac.

25. Ans. d. Ischiorectal fossa

Extravasation of urine (+ blood) in bulbar urethral injury

- It is a superficial extravasation
- If the buck's fascia remains intact, extravasation of blood and urine are confined to the penile shaft.
- Extends to the Scrotum and anterior abdominal wall on disruption of buck's fascia–perineal butterfly hematoma**

26. Ans. c. Lined by Columnar Epithelium *Ref: Bailey and Love 700/26/e p700*

- A branchial cyst, thought to develop from the vestigial remnants of the second branchial cleft, is usually lined by squamous epithelium, and contains thick, turbid fluid full of cholesterol crystals.
- The cyst usually presents in the upper neck in early or middle adulthood and is found at the junction of the upper third and middle third of the sternomastoid muscle at its anterior border.
- It is a fluctuant swelling that may transilluminate and is often soft in its early stages so that it may be difficult to palpate.
- It passes superficial to the hypoglossal and glossopharyngeal nerves, but deep to the posterior belly of the digastric. These structures and the spinal accessory nerve must be positively identified to avoid damage** (Nerves at risk during Surgery)**

27. Ans. b. Narrowing of Urethra *Ref: Bailey and Love 26/e p1342*

- Carcinoma of prostate arises most commonly in à the peripheral zone
- Benign prostatic hyperplasia originates in à the transition zone
- BPH arises in Median Lobe, carcinoma is common in posterior lobe

Points Directly from Bailey and Love:

- Pathophysiologically, BOO may be caused in part by increased smooth muscle tone, which is under the control of a-adrenergic agonists.

Anatomically, the effects are as follows:

- The prostatic urethra is lengthened, sometimes to twice its normal length, **but it is not narrowed anatomically.****
- When only one lateral lobe is enlarged, distortion of the prostatic urethra occurs. **(means usually Both Lateral Lobes are enlarged)**
- If BPH causes BOO, the musculature of the bladder hypertrophies to overcome the obstruction and appears **more trabeculated****

- The bladder may become more irritable during filling with a decrease in functional capacity partly caused by detrusor overactivity.

28. Ans. d. Idiopathic thrombocytopenic purpura (Discussed before)

29. Ans. b. Ventral Curvature of penis *Ref: Bailey and Love 26/e p1310*

- Ca bladder is common due to constant irritation of bladder wall.
- In males, the completely epispadiac penis is broader and shorter than normal and bilateral inguinal herniae may be present. There is uretero vesical efflux and incontinence but no ventral curvature of penis.

30. Ans. a. Liver *Ref: Bailey and Love 26/e p1413*

In the case of liver transplants, HLA matching does not confer an advantage and, although it is beneficial in cardiac transplantation, it is not practicable because of the relatively small size of the recipient pool and the short permissible cold ischaemic time.

31. Ans. a. CABG

Coronary artery bypass grafting:

Anatomy of coronary artery:

Coronary arteries are branches of ascending aorta. Right from anterior sinus and left from left posterior sinus.

Left coronary artery:

- Worst prognosis in terms of survival without surgery
- Left main stem disease
- Branches: LAD (left anterior descending) or Anterior interventricular artery and Obtuse/Marginal branches of circumflex artery.
- LAD is the most frequently diseased artery and most often bypassed during CABG (coronary artery bypass grafting)

Right coronary artery:

- Continues as posterior descending artery or inter ventricular artery.

Invasive methods of diagnosis:

- Gold standard for imaging is coronary angiography*.
- Demonstrates extent, severity and location of Stenosis.
- Reduction in diameter > 70% is considered as severe.
- Evaluates suitability of surgery
- Aids in prognostic assessment.

Indications for surgery:

Surgery is indicated for symptomatic or prognostic reasons.

- > 50% Stenosis of the left main stem (critical left main disease)*
- > 70% Stenosis of the proximal left anterior inter ventricular artery.
- All three main coronary arteries diseased. (Triple vessel disease)
- Poor ventricular function associated with coronary disease.

Chronic stable angina:

- Percutaneous transluminal Coronary Angiplasty (PTCA) and stenting is more commonly used than CABG now.

Acute coronary syndrome:

- Unstable angina become asymptomatic within 48 hours of medical anti angina drugs.
- If the patient develops recurrent angina and ecg changes -thrombolysis and ptca is used more than surgery.
- If surgery is to be done elective CABG to be done at least after 6 weeks.

Contraindications for Surgery:

- Small diffusely diseased arteries
- Diffuse disease and heart failure
- Acute MI over 6 hours old.
- Moribund patients after resuscitation

Selection of conduit:

Venous grafts	Arterial graft
• **Long saphenous vein*** is the most commonly used vein as a conduit. • 10 year patency rate for long saphenous vein grafts is reported to be 50–60% with 10-15% occluding in 1 year. • Alternative veins are short saphenous vein and cephalic vein.	• **Left Internal mammary artery or Internal thoracic artery has become the conduit of choice** for LAD. • 10 year patency rates are 90%.* • Internal mammary arteries have some limitations like sternal wound infections in diabetes. • Radial artery is used in those cases as second or alternative arterial bypass graft.

Postoperative complications:
- Bleeding
- Arrythmias (sinus tachycardia is m/c followed by atrial fibrillation)
- Poor cardiac output state
- Neurological dysfunction
- Wound infection
- Mortality (2–3%)

Survival:
- 95%-at 1 year
- 90% at 5 years
- 75% at 10 years
- 60% at 15 years.

32. **Ans. a. Ant. border, upper 3rd of sternomastoid (Discussed Before)**
33. **Ans. a. Retrograde ejaculation (discussed before)**
34. **Ans. d. Only metastasis in early stage**

Papillary Carinoma
- 60% of all thyroid malignancies
- Mean age of presentation 30 to 40 years.
- More common in females
- More common in iodine -sufficient areas

Predisposing Factors
1. Irradiation
2. Hashimoto's thyroiditis
3. Thyroglossal cyst

Clinical Features
- Slow growing painless mass
- Lymph nodal metastasis is more common
- Lateral aberrant thyroid -denotes a cervical lymph node from an occult papillary carcinoma.
- Hard in consistency (may be cystic, firm or variable)

Wolman's Classification
- Occult < 1.5 cm
- Intrathyroidal
- Extrathyroidal
- m/c in females
- m/c age group 30–40 years
- Lymph node metastasis is more common than blood borne metastasis
- Better prognosis than all cancers

Pathology
1. Papillary projections

2. Psammoma bodies [concentric calcifications]
3. Pale empty (orphan Annie) nuclei-Finely dispersed chromatin imparts an empty appearance
4. **Intranuclear grooves and nuclear characteristics are diagnostic of papillary ca.**
5. Multifocality is common in papillary carcinoma.

TSH levels are high; tumors are TSH dependent, hence follow up with TSH**

Prognosis

- Excellent prognosis: 95% 10 year survival rate.
- AGES Scoring: Age, Histologic Grade, Extrathyroidal invasion, Size of tumor
- MACIS Scale: Metastasis, Age, Completeness of \original resection, Invasion of Extrathyroidal tissues, Size of lesion in centimeters.

Treatment

- Near total or total thyroidectomy with Modified Radical Neck dissection (Functional) for nodes.
- Suppressive dose of L-thyroxine 0.3 mg once daily life long.
- Berry picking means removal of involved nodes only. It is not followed nowadays.

35. Ans. b. ACTH-pituitary tumor

- **Cushing's disease:** Pituitary tumor that leads to bilateral adrenal hyperplasia and hypercortisolism
- **Cushing's syndrome:** Complex symptoms resulting from Hypersecretion of cortisol

Incidence

- M/c cause of Cushing's syndrome-iatrogenic steroids for inflammatory disorders.
- Pituitary source (75%) Cushing's disease**
- Adrenal source (15%) primary adrenal Cushing's syndrome.
- Ectopic ACTH source < 10%

Causes

Acth dependent

1. Cushings disease [70%]
2. Ectopic acth production: Carcinoids, bronchial adenoma
3. Ectopic crh production: Pheochromocytoma, bronchial carcinoids

ACTH INDEPENDENT CUSHING'S SYNDROME (15% CASES)

1. Adenoma (solitary adrenal adenoma-90%)
2. Adrenal carcinoma (10%)
3. Adrenal hyperplasia-micro or macro nodular (< 1%)

Differentiating the etiologies

- **Cushings syndrome (Adrenal source)** is characterized by increased glucocorticoids that are not suppressible by exogenous steroids and loss of diurnal variation.
- **Pituitary source (Cushing's disease)** is characterized by increased glucocorticoids that are suppressible by exogenous steroid hormones and maintenance of diurnal variation.

DIURNAL VARIATION (circadian rhythm) ACTH peaks in early morning from 4 am to 10 am

Investigations

- First investigation 24 *hours* urinary cortisol 100% sensitive

Plasma ACTH

- In cushings disease increased [15–500 pg/ml]
- But in cushings syndrome it will be suppressed [< 5 pg/ml]
- In ectopic sources-abnormally high increase [> 1000 pg/ml]

Dexamethasone suppression test

- Low dose dexamethasone suppression test-in Cushings disease no suppression of ACTH
- High dose dexamethasone suppression test-causes decrease in ACTH level in Cushing's disease.

- Ectopic ACTH sources are completely lacking feedback inhibition and hence ACTH level doesn't decrease with high dose dexamethasone suppression.

Features	Cushing's syndrome (adrenal source)	Cushing's disease (pituitary adenoma)	Ectopic ACTH
First test Diurnal variation	Urinary cortisol Lost	Urinary cortisol Maintained	Urinary cortisol
ACTH level	< 5 pg/ml	15–500 pg/ml	> 1000pg/ml
High dose dexa Suppression test	not suppressed	Suppression of ACTH	No response
Imaging	CT abdomen	Pituitary MRI Inferior petrosal venous sampling	Abdomen and chest CT, Somatostatin receptor scintigraphy.

36. Ans. b. Berry aneurysm *Ref: 317/Bailey and love 26/e p317*

- Trauma is the most common cause of subarachnoid hemorrhage and this is managed conservatively.
- It is not usually associated with significant vasospasm, which characterises aneurysmal subarachnoid hemorrhage

Author's Warning:

So friends this is a changing concept-Please note if you have Trauma in Choice go for it in cases of Subarachnoid hemorrhage in Future.

So the Ans. will be like this:

- MC cause of SAH: Trauma
- MC cause of Spontaneous SAH: Berry aneurysm rupture

37. Ans. b. Karl Starz

- Starzl (1963): First liver transplant
- First split liver transplant: Pichlmayr
- First live donor liver transplant: Tanaka (1991) using left lobe

38. Ans. a. Intestinal bacterial fermentation *Ref: Bailey and Love 26/e p1180*

The distension proximal to an obstruction is caused by two factors:

- **Gas:** there is a significant overgrowth of both aerobic and anaerobic organisms, resulting in considerable gas production. Following the reabsorption of oxygen and carbon dioxide, the majority is made up of nitrogen (90 per cent) and hydrogen sulphide.
- **Fluid:** this is made up of the various digestive juices (saliva 500 mL, bile 500 mL, pancreatic secretions 500 mL, gastric secretions 1 litre–all per 24 hours). This accumulates in the gut lumen as absorption by the obstucted gut is retarded

39. Ans. a. ↓, K, ↓, Cl alkalosis

Hypochloremic, hyponatremic, Hypokalemic metabolic alkalosis with paradoxical renal aciduria.

40. Ans. d. Gastric carcinoma

Characteristics	Hypercalcemia	Hypocalcemia
1. Definition 2. Etiology	• Serum calcium > 5.5 meq/L • Milk alkali syndrome • Sarcoidosis • Multiple myeloma • Ca-breast, kidney, bronchus • Lithium excess • Hyperthyroidism • Hyperparathyroidism	• Serum Ca+-< 4.5 meq/L • Tumor lysis syndrome • Hypoparathyroidism • Chronic renal failure • Heparin, protamine, glucagon • Acute pancreatitis • Hypoalbuminemia

Contd...

Contd...

Characteristics	Hypercalcemia	Hypocalcemia
3. Clinical presentation	• Fatigue • Depression • Mental confusion • Lethargy • Anorexia, nausea, vomiting • Constipation • Polyuria • Stupor and coma (sever cases) • Decreased QT interval • Nephrocalcinosis	• Increased neuromuscular excitability • Muscle spasm • Laryngeal spasm and convulsion (in severe cases) • Chvostek's, trousseau's sign • Increased QT interval
4. Treatment	• Diuresis • Calcitonin andBiphosphonates. • Glucocorticoids • Dialysis	• Vit D + IV Cagluconate • Thiazide

41. Ans. c. Subdural *Ref: Intracranial bleeding in patients with traumatic brain injury: A prognostic study; British Medical Journal -Emergency Medicine*

Types of head injury
- Extradural hematoma
- Acute subdural hematoma
- Subarachnoid hemorrhage
- Chronic subdural hematoma
- Cerebral contusions

- Almost 46% of patients had at some type of IB. Subdural hemorrhages were present in 30% of the patients, with epidural and intraparenchymal present in approximately 22% each.

Extradural hematoma
- M/c in young male patients
- Always associated withskull fracture
- Injured vessel-middle meningeal artery
- m/c site of injury is temporal bone at pterion (most thinnest part of skull) which overlies the middle meningeal artery
- The hematoma is located between bone and dura mater.

Classical presentation of EDH (in less than 1/3rd cases only)
- Initial injury followed by lucid interval when patient complains of headache only. After minutes to hours a rapid deterioration occurs leading to contralateral hemiparesis, reduced conscious level and ipsilateral pupillary dilatation as a result of herniation.

CT scan-*lentiform (lens shaped or biconvex)* hyperdense lesion between brain and skull.

Treatment
- Immediate surgical evacuation via craniotomy.
- Overall mortality = 18% for all cases of EDH
- But only 2% for isolated EDH.

Acute subdural hematoma
- Differs from EDH in following points
- Accumulates in space between dura and arachnoid
- Associated with cortical vessel disruption and brain laceration.
- Associated with primary brain injury
- Presents with impaired consciousness from the impact time itself.
- CT scan–hyperdense but hematoma spreads diffusely and have a concavo convex appearance.

Treatment:

Evacuation via craniotomy

Mortality rate = 40%

42. Ans. c. Inflamed bladder *Ref: Bailey and love 26/e p1320*

- Stretching of renal capsule gives pain in the loin which is deep seated sickening aching pain.
- Ureteric colic gives pain which radiates from loin groin, the more distal the stone, the more the pain radiates to the groin.
- Severe inflammation of bladder causes wrenching discomfort at end of micturition (strangury)
- Urethral pain is scalding or burning during voiding felt in the vulva or penis.

Pain (strangury) is most often found in patients with a spiculated oxalate calculus in Bladder. It occurs at the end of micturition and is referred to the tip of the penis or to the labia majora; more rarely, it is referred to the perineum or suprapubic region.

43. Ans. d. Transurethral resection of Tumor *Ref: Bailey and love 26/e p1331*

- Non-muscle-invasive pTa and pT1 tumours account for 70 per cent of all new cases; the previous terminology of 'superficial' bladder cancer in this category has now been abandoned; it is important to distinguish however 'low-risk' uothelial cancers which are unlikely to progress, such as well differentiated (G1) pTa tumours (not invading lamina propria), from 'high-risk' cancers such as poorly differentiated (G3) pT1 cancers (invading lamina propria), which should be followed up carefully and treated aggressively as necessary. This can be determined by careful histological examination.
- Cystoscopy and resection of tumour with separate resection of the tumour base is essential for accurate analysis of invasion into detrusor muscle.

44. Ans. d. Ureteroscopic retrieval

- 'Ureteroscopic stone extraction is highly efficacious for lower ureteral calculi' -Smith's Urology.
- A ureteroscope is a long endoscope that can be passed transurethrally across the bladder into the ureter. The stones can be caught in baskets or endoscopic forceps. Those that cannot be removed via baskets or endoscopic forceps are fragmented using ureteroscopic lithotrities.
- Any renal calculi that is 4 mm or less in size, is allowed some time (approx. 4 weeks) to pass spontaneously.
- Indications for surgical removal of a ureteric calculus -Stone is too large to pass spontaneously
  - Urine is infected
  - Repeated attacks of pain and the stone is not moving
  - Stone is enlarging
  - Stone is causing complete obstruction
  - Stone is obstructing solitary kidney or there is bilateral obstructions.

45. Ans. d. Ca. Urinary bladder

Carcinoma bladder		
• There are three common histological types of bladder cancer		
✓ Transitional cell ca–~ 90%	✓ Squamous cell ca -~5-10 %	✓ Adenocarcinoma -~2%
Risk factor for transitional cell ca of bladder		
1. Cigarette smokingà is the main etiological factor and accounts for about 50% of bladder cancers		
2. Occupational chemicals		
✓ 2 naphthylamine → combustion gases and soot from coal ✓ 4 aminobiphenyl → chlorinated aliphatic hydrocarbons ✓ 4 nitrobiphenyl → certain aldehydes such as acrolein ✓ 4-4 diaminobiphenyl → aniline dyes	• Occupation reported to be associated with increased risk of bladder cancer	

Contd...

Contd...

Carcinoma bladder		
	✓ Autoworker ✓ Painters ✓ Truck drivers ✓ Drill press operator ✓ Leather workers ✓ Metal workers	✓ Textile workers ✓ Dye workers ✓ Petrol workers ✓ Rodent exterminators and sewage worker
3. Schistosoma haematobium → Risk factor for both transitional cell ca and squamous cell ca (Mainly SCC) 4. Drugs such as phenacetin and chlornaphazine 5. Cyclophosphamide therapy 6. Pelvic irradiation		
Risk factor for squamous cell ca of bladder		
• Schistosoma hemotobium	• Chronic irritation from urinary calculi, Long-term indwelling catheters, chronic urinary infections	
Also remember		
• MC primary tumor which gives secondary to penis → bladder carcinoma • Commonest tumor of urinary bladder → transitional call ca • Commonest tumor of U.B. in a child → rhabdomyosarcoma • MC symptom of renal cell Ca → painless hematuria	• MC symptom of wilm's tumor → mass in abd. • MC symptom of bony metastasis → pain • MC symptom of renal stone → pain • Earliest symptom of vesical calculus → frequency • Cardinal symptom of renal trauma → hematuria • MC symptom of acute arterial occlusion → pain	

46. Ans. b. Chronic tubercular cystitis
- Thimble bladder: Chronic TB
- Golf hole ureter: Chronic TB
- Putty Kidney: Chronic TB

47. Ans. b. Polycystic kidney
- Spider leg appearance: PCKD
- Horse shoe kidney: Flower vase appearance

48. Ans. b. Seminoma
- Seminomas represent about 50% of all Germ cell tumors of testis
- Median age is 4th decade (Non seminomas are most frequent in the 3rd decade).
- Seminomas follow a more indolent course.
- Most seminomas (70%) present with stage I disease (disease limited to testis),
- About 20% with stage II disease (with retroperitoneal metastases),
- And 10% with stage III disease (spread beyond retroperitoneum)
- Seminomas as well as non-seminomas typically metastasize through lymphatics (except Choriocarcinoma which demonstrates early hematogenous spread)
- Seminomas are one of the most radiosensitive tumors (Nonseminomas are insensitive to radiation).

49. Ans. b. Duct-papilloma

Discharges from Nipple
- BLOOD: Duct papilloma (m/c cause) carcinoma breast
- PUS: Breast abscess
- MILK: Lactation, Galactocele, Mammary Fistula
- SEROUS/GREENISH: Fibroadenosis and Duct ectasia

Green discharge is m/c from duct ectasia.

Treatment of intraductal papilloma
- Microdochectomy: If bleeding is from single duct
- Hadfield's operation: Cone excision of major duct if exact origin of ductal papilloma is difficult to identify.

50. **Ans. c. Mucous diarrhea with hypokalemia (Discussed before)**
51. **Ans. c. Bones**

One liners from Oncosurgery:
- MC tumor to produce Cervical nodal mets-Nasopharyngeal carcinoma
- MC site of primary for bone mets-Prostate
- MC cause of osteoblastic Secondaries–Male (prostate) Female (Breast)
- MC tumor to metastasize to bone in females-Breast
- MC site of Mets in sarcomas of extremities-LUNGS
- MC site of mets in retroperitoneal sarcomas-LIVER
- Purely osteolytic bone mets-Kidney
- Purely osteoblastic bone mets-Prostate
- MC site of primary for brain secondary-Lungs > breast
- MC cancer in males-Prostate > Lung > Colorectal
- MC cancer in females-Breast > Lung > Colorectal

52. **Ans. d. Intermittent positive pressure ventilation**

Flail chest
- Three or more ribs fractured in two or more places.
- Here a segment of chest wall does not have continuity with rest of thoracic cage.
- On inspiration ***paradoxical movement*** of chest occurs. (segment moves inside on inspiration) and hence less air enters lungs.
- It's a clinical diagnosis and not radiological diagnosis.
- Traditionally the treatment is mechanical ventilation.
- But current treatment is only oxygen administration, adequate analgesia and physiotherapy. Mechanical ventilation is reserved for cases that develop respiratory failure.
- Surgery and internal fixation of ribs are in use again.

53. **Ans. c. Transitional cell carcinoma (Discussed before)**
54. **Ans. d. No further treatment**

Management plan
- Curative treatment can only be offered to patients with early disease **(ie., T1 and T2) → radical prostatectomy of radical radiotherapy (both are equally effective)**
- Radical retropubic prostatectomy is performed for Ca Prostate
- Hemorrhage is the most common intraoperative complication and the most commonly injured vessel is dorsal venous complex
- The treatment for advanced disease (i.e. T3, T4 or any metastasis) is only palliative. Hormone ablation is the line therapy for palliation

T1a disease
- These tumors found incidentally at TURP is by the definition low volume (≤ 5%) and usually well differentiated and associated with very slow growth rate
- They are managed by **watchful waiting** (regular follow up is done by DRE and PSA)

T1b, T1c and T2 disease
- Management depends on patient's age, life expectancy, performance status, and patient's preferences
- In younger, fitter men (< 70 years), May be treated by radical prostatectomy or radical radiotherapy.
- Watchful waiting is an option for elderly with low life expectancy (< 10 years). Even younger patients may choose watchful waiting when counselled about risk versus benefit.

Advanced disease (T3, T4 or any metastasis)
- **Only palliative t/t is the option**
- **Androgen ablation is the first line therapy**

It can be achieved by
- Orchidectomy or
- Drugs (medical castration)

- Palliative radiotherapy
- Androgen ablation is the mainstay of therapy for advanced prostatic cancer (T3, T4 ds or any metastasis)
- Most prostatic carcinomas are hormone dependent and large no. of men with advanced disease show response to androgen ablation therapies
- Surgical orchidectomy is the 'gold standard' approach but least acceptable.

55. Ans. d. Cystic hygroma (Discussed in theory)

56. Ans. c. Seen as a hot spot on isotope scan

Warthin's tumor (adeno lymphoma) (Papillarycystadenomalymphomatosum)

- M/c in males ; incidence 6-10% of tumor of parotid
- Age 40 -70 year
- Bilateral often (10%)
- It occurs due to trapping of jugular lymph sacs in parotid during development period.

High lights in Warthin's tumor

- Malignant transformation is rare (nerve occurs)
- Multicentric/bilateral occurrence is more common
- M/c occurs in lower pole (at angle of mandible)
- M/c in smokers
- Adeno lymphoma–name is a misnomer (not a lymphoma)
- Hot spot in technetium 99m scan
- **Godwin's tumor–benign lympho epithelial tumor of parotid gland.**

57. Ans. c. Local recurrence is common after excision.

Character	Hypertrophic scar	Keloid
Race	-	Black
Genetic	-	Yes
Sex	male = female	Female > Male
Age	Children	10–30 years
Border	Confined to wound	Outgrows wound
Site	Flexor	Triangle–sternum, right and left shoulder
Cause	Tension	Unknown
Natural	Subsides with time	Rarely subsides

58. Ans. d. Tube thoracostomy

- From the history the patient is cyanosed and Tachypneic. No breath sounds heard in right lung with Resonant note implies a case of Closed–Tension Pneumothorax.
- Patient needs emergent intervention to relieve the pressure in Chest.
- ICD inserted in 6th ICS in **mid axillary line** for hydro, haemo, and pyothorax.
- ICD inserted 3rd or 4th space in **mid clavicular** line for pneumothorax.
- Needle Thoracocentesis for Emergency Pneumothorax decompression at 2nd IC space along Mid clavicular line.

59. Ans. a. Mafenide acetate

60. Ans. c. Carcinoembryonic antigen (CEA)

Colonic cancer: Salient Points:

MANAGEMENT

- Malignant obstruction is the **m/c cause of large bowel obstruction***
- **Right colon**
  - Stable case: Right hemicolectomy ileocolic anastomosis in a single stage
  - Unstable/perforated colon-two stage, resection with ileostomy, later anastomosis

- **Left colon**
  - Traditionally and most commonly performed Emergency surgery is resection of lesion and proximal diversion **(Hartmanns Operation)**
  - Stable patient with no peritonitis, resectable tumours-primary resection and anastomosis or subtotal colectomy and ileorectal anastomosis
  - Depth of penetrance is an important predictor for distant mets
  - CEA-marker for recurrence
  - TNM Staging is used for Colorectal Cancer now. Previously used ANN ARBOR, Modified Duke's staging are all not used nowadays.

61. Ans. d. Selectively inhibits T–cells activation *Ref: Bailey and Love 26/e p1414*

- Ciclosporin and tacrolimus (Calcineurin Blockers) are the mainstay of most modern immunosuppressive protocols for organ transplantation.
- Although structurally distinct, they exert their principal immunosuppressive effect through the same intracellular pathway.
- Each of the two agents binds within the T cell to a cytoplasmic protein or immunophilin (ciclosporin binds to cyclophilin and tacrolimus to FK-binding protein). The resulting immunophilin– drug complex then blocks the activity of calcineurin (a phosphatase) within the cytoplasm of the T cell.
- Ciclosporin sometimes causes cosmetic side effects (hirsutism and gingival hypertrophy) that may be distressing, particularly in younger female recipients.

62. Ans. c. Repair of parotid fistula *Ref: Annals of Surgery 1949*

- Chronic lymphedema-Charles Thompson and lympho venous anastomosis surgeries.
- Cleft lip -Millard's Rx, Lemesurier's surgery and Tennessean's Surgery
- Cleft palate -Hynes and Wardills pharyngoplasty.
- Parotid fistula following laceration is repaired using Tantalum wire in 1946 by-Newman's' and SeaBrock's Surgery.

63. Ans. a. All quadrants of the breast drain into both the axillary and the parasternal nodes *Ref: Bailey and Love p799)*

The **lymphatics** of the breast drain predominantly into the axillary and internal mammary lymph nodes. The axillary nodes receive approximately 85 per cent of the drainage and are arranged in the following groups:

- **Lateral,** along the axillary vein;
- **Anterior**, along the lateral thoracic vessels;
- **Posterior**, along the subscapular vessels;
- **Central**, embedded in fat in the centre of the axilla;
- **Interpectoral**, a few nodes lying between the pectoralis major and minor muscles;
- **Apical**, which lie above the level of the pectoralis minor tendon in continuity with the lateral nodes and which receive the efferents of all the other groups.
  - The apical nodes are also in continuity with the supraclavicular nodes and drain into the subclavian lymph trunk, which enters the great veins directly or via the thoracic duct or jugular trunk.

64. Ans. c. Benign mixed tumor (pleomorphic adenoma)

65. Ans. a. Begin chemotherapy and radiation therapy

Histological types

Small cell cancer-oat cell cancers 20%

- Early metastasis to lymph nodes and by blood borne spread
- Median survival in months
- Respond to chemotherapy
- Surgery has little place

Adenocarcinoma

- Most common of NSCLC having overtaken squamous cell cancer now
- Increased incidence in women

Squamous cell cancer

- Appears as well cavitating cancer

Large cell undifferentiated
- Type of NSCLC and is included in neuro endocrine tumor.

Bronchioalveolar carcinoma
- Distinct architecture with less density and appears as patch shadow (Ground glass appearance)

*Lung 'Ca' is the leading cause of cancer death in both male and female.
- Mc site of metastasis is -Liver.
- Mc endocrine organ involved is -adrenal.
- Lung Ca is Mc tumor metastasizing to heart.
- Brain metastasis may present with neurological deficit.

Squamous cell Ca	Adenocarcinoma	Small cell Ca	Large cell Ca
Mc variant in Indian subcontinent • Pancoast tumor is histologically SCC. • Mostly central in distribution • It can cavitate • Best prognosis • M/c associated paraneoplastic syndrome is hypercalcemia and hypophosphatemia* . T/t by surgical excision.	• Overall Mc histological type. • Mc type in non-smoker, young and female. • Mostly peripheral in distribution • Overall prognosis is good. • May metastasize to opposite lung. (this is due to aerosol • Transmissionand is seen more frequently in bronchoalveolar type).	Most aggressive form of lung 'Ca'. (rapidly growing) Mostly central in distribution. It respond best to chemotherapy and radiotherapy. Worst prognosis. (Least resectability) Mc type causing extra thoracic metastasis. Strong association with smoking.	• It may cause gynaecomastia • Galactorrhea due to ectopic prolactin Secretion.

66. Ans. c. Both of the above

Simple mastectomy involves removal of skin, nipple, areola and breast tissue including the tumor. It does not include node removal

67. Ans. b. Has underlying Ductal carcinoma and not lobular carcinoma

PAGET'S DISEASE
- Present as chronic eczematous eruption of the nipple, which may be subtle, but may progress to an ulcerated, weeping lesion.
- Paget's disease is usually associated with extensive DCIS and may be associated with an invasive cancer.
- Palpable mass may or may not be seen.
- Pathognomonic of this cancer is the presence of large, pale, vacuolated cells (Paget's cells) in the rete pegs of the epithelium.
- Surgical therapy may involve lumpectomy, mastectomy or modified radical mastectomy depending on the extent of involvement and presence of invasive cancer.

68. Ans. d. Can lead to carcinoma

Choledochal cysts*
- Congenital dilatation of intra and extra hepatic ducts
- Associated with anomalous pancreatic and biliary duct junction (APBDJ)

Clinical features
- M/c in females*
- M/c age of presentation infancy
- **Classic triad [seen only in 10%]***–Pain, Lump and Intermittent jaundice.

Types of cysts
- Type 1: Most common*. Fusiform dilatation of bile duct
- Type 2: Diverticulum from CBD
- Type 3: [Choledochocele]–dilatation of biliary tract within duodenum
- Type 4: a–Multiple dilatation of intra and extrahepatic ducts

- Type 5: b–Multiple dilatation of extra hepatic ducts
- Type 6: [Carolis disease]* Multiple dilatation of intra hepatic ducts.

Complications
- Recurrent cholangitis
- Pancreatitis
- Gallstones
- Cholecystitis
- Cirrhosis with Portal Hyper tension.
- Portal vein thrombosis
- Malignancy-Risk factor for carcinoma bile duct, GB, pancreas, liver, duodenum.

Treatment
- Types 1 and 2: Cyst excision with roux en y reconstruction with jejunum
- Type 3: Trans duodenal sphincteroplasty
- Type 4 and 5: Liver transplantation.

69. Ans. b. Extradural hemorrhage EDH (Discussed before)

70. Ans. c. Barium meal upper GI in Trendelenburg's position
- Trendlenberg (head down) barium meal will clearly demonstrate the dye flowing back into the herniated contents.

71. Ans. d. Invasion of renal vein is C/l for surgery (Discussed in theory)

72. Ans. a. Steatorrhea

Steatorrhea is a manifestation of Chronic Pancreatitis.

Features of Acute Pancreatitis

Symptoms:
- Pain
- Nausea
- Vomiting
- Retching
- Hiccough
- Severe abdominal pain which gets relieved by leaning forward **[Mohammed prayer sign]****

Signs...
- Tachypnoea
- Tachycardia
- Hypotension
- Icterus
- Facial flushing
- Cyanotic marbling of anterior abdominal wall
- **Grey-Turner's sign****-hemorrhagic pigmentation around the flanks*
- **Cullen's sign****-pigmentation around umbilicus.*
- Tender red nodules in limbs
- Abdominal distension-ileus
- Ascites

Radiology Findings
- No specific radiological sign,Sentinal loop of jejunum
- **Colon cut-off sign*** (gas filled hepaticand splenic flexures separated by gaseless transverse colon)
- Calcified gallstones.

Investigations
- Serum Amylase
- Serum Lipase -most specific*
- Serum Trypsin [EXCLUSIVELY BY PANCREAS]
- Hypocalcemia

73. Ans. c. Ischemic colitis

- Ischemic colitis m/c site is Splenic flexure
- Griffith Point is the Place in splenic Flexure where Ischemic Colitis is Common
- Sudecks Point is the place in Sigmoid Colon where Ischemic Strictures are common.
- Watershed area-Splenic Flexure

74. Ans. d. None of the above

- Usually Retrosternal goiter is asymptomatic. Rarely may cause Superior Vena caval obstruction
- Pemberton sign is used to elicit this compression
- **Surgery for intrathoracicgoitre**
- 99% removed from the neck
- Division of isthmus helps mobilization
- Traction and blunt dissection (Toboggansmaneuver)
- Rarely requires sternotomy

75. Ans. b. Premalignant condition

Premalignant conditions of Skin cancers:

1. **Bowen's disease:** It is an intradermal precancerous condition. It presents as brownish induration with well defined edge. {*'Erythroplasia of queyrat'*: penis}
2. Paget's disease of nipple:
3. Leukoderma, Erythroplakia
4. Senile (or) solar keratosis
5. Radiation
6. Arsenic
7. Chronic scars: Marjolin's
8. Xeroderma pigmentosa
9. Chronic lupus vulgaris
10. Prolonged irritation of skin by dyes, tar, soot, etc.
11. HPV 5 and 16.

76. Ans. b. Peyronie's disease

- Peyronie's disease is usually seen over 40 years of age
  Important points about Peyronie's disease
- It is also k/a penile fibromatosis
- It is due to fibrous plaques in one or both corpus cavernosum. They may later calcify or ossify
- Fibrous plaques leads to pain and curvature of the penis on erection
- Palpable induration or mass appears usually on the dorsolateral aspect of the penis
- Palmar fibromatosis (Dupuytren's contracture), plantar fibromatosis and penile fibromatosis (Peyronie's ds.) are components of the same pathological process called superficial fibromatosis
- The aetiology is uncertain, but it may be a result of past trauma
- Treatment is difficult but some cases may show spontaneous regression
- In the penile deformity is distressing, **Nesbitt's operation can be performed to straighten the penis.**

77. Ans. b. Prostate

- As prostatic cancer is Androgen Dependent-Advanced Prostate cancer Surgical Androgen ablation by means of Bilateral orchidectomy is Gold standard. For Pyschological point of View-Testicular substance may be removed leaving the Tunica Vaginalis (Sub Capsular Orchidectomy).

78. Ans. c. Head and Neck

- **I got reference only from Internet Journal. Couldn't get a Book reference**
- This type of treatment is known as 'Exposure Treatment'–Commonly done for Face and Scalp Burns.

79. Ans. b. Partial thickness graft

Two types of skin graft

1. Full thickness-upto the full dermis-**Wolfe graft***
2. Partial thickness-Upto superficial layer of dermis-**Thiersch graft***

80. **Ans. c. Inguinal**

MC hernia in Females = Inguinal Hernia

- Femoral hernia is MC in Females than Males
- In Males MC hernia = Inguinal hernia

81. **Ans. b. Terminal pulp space infection**

82. **Ans. b. Squamous cell carcinoma**

- Marjolin's ulcer is a long standing venous ulcer or burns scar turning into a Squamous Cell carcinoma.
- Important Point is it will not produce Lymphnode metastatis because of Obstruction of Lymphatics due to previous inflammation.

83. **Ans. a. Subarachnoid hemorrhage (Discussed before)**

84. **Ans. c. An unerupted permanent tooth**

- Dental cyst arises from an infected Erupt tooth
- Dentigerous cyst from an Unerupted tooth

85. **Ans. d. Lateral aberrant thyroid**

- Metastasis from a papillary Carcinoma thyroid occult to neck node is called as Lateral aberrant thyroid

86. **Ans. d. Axillary gland involvement**

- The best prognostic marker for Ca breast-Lymph node involvement

87. **Ans. a. Leiomyoma** *Ref: Sabiston 19/e p1047*

- Leiomyomas constitute 60% of all benign esophageal tumors. They are found in men slightly more often than women and tend to present in the fourth and fifth decades.
- They originate from the mesenchymal layer of embryologic development and are found in the **distal two thirds of the esophagus more than 80% of the time.**
- They are usually solitary and remain intramural, causing symptoms as they enlarge.
- They have been classified as a gastrointestinal stromal tumor (GIST). A true leiomyoma, or a non-GIST (c-KIT–negative) tumor, is rare. All leiomyomas are benign; malignant transformation occurs rarely.

88. **Ans. b. Upper GI endoscopy**

- History of rapid progression of Dysphagia is Commonly seen in carcinoma Esophagus.
- So Endoscopy can provide tissue diagnosis.
- Also for any Dysphagia the First Investigation of Choice in Modern Era is Endoscopy.

89. **Ans. c. 60 ml**

- Melena is presence of Black Tarry stool which cannot be washed out easily from the Latrine even on Pouring huge amounts of water. The stool sticks to the sink as like Tar.
- This is very Common in Upper GI bleed-Bleeding Proximal to ligament of treitz-And the amount must be less than 60 ml. (Its due to Digestion of RBC by the Enzymes of the GUT)
- In Upper GI bleeding if the amount is more than 60 ml-the mainifest will be HEMATOHEZIA-Stool mixed with Frank Blood.
- Any amount of bleeding distal to the Ligament of treitz will manifest as Hematochezia**

90. **Ans. a. Lung injury**

- Liver biopsy via Transcostal Mid axillary approach must be done at 8th ICS and beyond to prevent injury to the lung.
- Pleura may get injured and most of the time settles without intervention.
- CHIBA needle is used for Liver biopsy
- Before Liver biopsy-Prothrombin time/INR must be done and it must be normal
- In Cirrhotics with Bleeding tendency–Transjugular or Lapraoscopic Biopsy must be taken

91. **Ans. d. Infection** *Ref: Shackel ford 1159/7/e p1159*

- A review of the literature reveals that complications develop in up to 40% of patients with untreated pseudocysts, although most series report complication rates of 10% to 20%.
- The most frequently reported complications include infection, hemorrhage, obstruction or compression of adjacent structures, and rupture.

92. Ans. b. Vicryl

Different types of suture material

Non absorbable suture materials	Special properties
• Silk	Natural derived from silkworm*
• Linen	
• Surgical steel	
• Nylon (polyamide polymer)	
• Polyester	
• Polybutester	Monofilament
• Polypropylene (Prolene)	Monofilament
Absorbable suture materials	**Time of absorption**
• Plain catgut	7–10 days (Derived from sheep's intestine)*
• Chromic catgut	90 days
• Polyglactin	60–90 days
• Polyglyconate	180 days
• Polyglycolic acid (Vicryl)	60–90 days
• Polydiaxonone (PDS)	180 days (longest absorbable suture material)
• Polyglycaprone	90–120 days

Biological suture

- Catgut, collagen, cotton, linen, silk.

Monofilament

- Polyamide
- Polyethylene
- Steel
- Polypropylene
- Catgut
- For vascular anastomosis -Prolene is used
- For rectal and esophageal anastomosis -unabsorbable suture IS best.
- Good for bowel anastomosis -Vicryl
- Good for closing peritoneal cavity -PDS (Poly dioxane)
- For circumcision in children -Catgut is used.
- For suturing muscle, fascia -Chromic catgut is used.
- For hernioplasty -Prolene

Preservation of suture

- Isopropyl alcohol -used as preservative while packing suture.
- Ethylene oxide -Used in pasteurization of suture material.

93. Ans. d. Achalasia cardia

Motility Disorders

Manometry

Index	Normal	Abnormal
LES pressure	**10–26 mm Hg***	< 10 or > 26 mm Hg
HPZ relaxation	Relaxes when primary wave reached by primary wave	No relaxation with swallowing
Esophageal body contractions	Primary peristaltic waves	> 10% aperistaltic waves
Amplitude	**30–140 mm Hg***	< 30 or > 140
Duration	2–10 s	> 15 secs
Waveforms	Mostly single or double peaked	Abnormal and multiple peak wave forms
Additional contractions	Secondary peristaltic waves	Tertiary and non peristaltic

Classification

Specific

1. Diffuse esophageal spasm
2. Achalsia cardia
3. Vigorous achalsia
4. Nutcracker esophagus

Nonspecific

1. Hypertonic LES
2. Aperistalsis

Incidence of Achalasia cardia-6/1 lakh Population

- **Others are less common than Achalasia cardia**
- **Among the Hypermotility Disorders–Nut Cracker Esophagus is the MC type**

DIFFUSE ESOPHAGEAL SPASM (DES)

- MANOMETRY

Multi phasic, repetitive, repetitive and often high amplitude contractions

Clinical feature:

- Chest pain mimics angina
- Symptoms are more during emotional stress
- Cold liquids and foods aggravate it

Investigations:

- Barium study-**Cork screw esophagus***
- Manometry

Treatment:

Esophageal dilatation

Long Esophagomyotomy [from OG junction to above aortic arch)

Nutcracker esophagus

- INCREASED AMPLITUDE [>180 mm Hg] AND DURATION [> 6 S]
- Characterised by-Chest pain, dysphagia, odynophagia

Vigorous achalsia

- Repetitive simultaneous contractions in body [as in DES]
- Partial or absent LES RELAXATION [as in achalasia]

94. Ans. b. Gastric antrum

SITE

- Most common in the antrum lesser curve side
- Higher Socioeconomic groups it is most common in the proximal stomach.
- In Pernicious anemia-M/C site is proximal stomach

95. Ans. d. Mesenteric vascular occlusion

Dynamic Obstruction (organic Obstruction) is characterized by the Four cardinal features of Obstruction

- Colicky Pain
- Abdominal Distension
- Severe Vomiting (May be less in Colonic Obstruction with patent Ileo cecal Valve)
- Obstipation (Not passed motion and Flatus).

In Nondynamic Obstructions Obstipation and Colicky Pain may not be much evident-Egs. Mesentric ischemia, Paralytic Ileus, etc.

96. Ans. d. Mucinous Carcinoma

Don't wonder with Answer I am not wrong, Other books would have not updated.

See the points from 19/e Sabiston:

- Although it was previously believed that carcinoid tumors were the most common appendiceal neoplasms, analysis of the Surveillance, Epidemiology, and End Results (SEER) database indicates that mucinous tumors of the appendix are more common.

- Mucoceles that have ruptured are more likely to be associated with the spread of epithelial cells within mucoid fluid throughout the peritoneal cavity, so-called pseudomyxoma peritonei, or mucinous carcinomatosis of appendiceal origin. The appendix is the most common source of mucoid fluid collections in the abdomen.

Author's Note: Order of carcinoid Tumors-BIRA-Bronchus (MC), Ileum (M/C in GIT), Rectum, Appendix (Is the fourth now), Bailey and Love has not updated this concept...

97. Ans. a. Chemoradiation

Anal Cancer

- m/c type-squamous cell ca [also known as epidermoid carcinoma]
- 2nd m/c type-basal cell carcinoma.
- Chemoradiation is the treatment of choice **(Nigro regimen)**
- More than 80% cases are cured by chemoradiation. If any residual tumour is present APR is done
- Chemo used are 5-FU, mitomycin c
- Other agents are bleomycin, cisplatin, doxorubicin

Types of anal carcinoma:

Anal margin-distal to dentate line*	Anal canal-proximal to dentate line*
• Bowen's disease • Paget's disease • Basal cell carcinoma • Anal margin squamous cell carcinoma • Verrucous carcinoma (buschke lowenstein)	• Epidermoid carcinoma-tumours arising in transitional zone share a similar behaviour–cloacogenic, basaloid, squamous cell or muco epidermoid epithelial. • Melanoma • Adenocarcinoma

98. Ans. b. Diverticulosis (Already Discussed in theory)

- Saint's triad-Hiatus hernia, Gallstones and Diverticulosis is a combination. Diverticulosis is not a complication of Gallstones

99. Ans. a. Fever, abdominal pain, jaundice

Charcot's Triad*

CBD stone/Any obstruction causing cholangitis

- Pain
- Jaundice
- Rigors

Reynaulds Pentad*

Includes Charcot's triad + Septic shock+ Mental status changes

100. Ans. c. Common hepatic duct tumor

- Adenocarcinoma at bifurcation of Hepatic duct
- MC site of Bile duct cancers-Klatskin tumor (Hilar Cholangiocarcinoma)
- Hilar Carcinomas are classified by Bismuth classification**

101. Ans. c. Clostridium perfringens

Emphysematous cholecystitis

- Acute emphysematous cholecystitis associated with infection by gas forming organisms like Clostridium welchii or perfringens.
- This condition occurs most frequently in elderly men and in patients with diabetes mellitus.
- Can be seen on plain X-ray.
- The condition is very aggressive, may go for gangrene and perforation.
- Emergency cholecystectomy must be done.

102. Ans. c. Acute Pancreatitis

Pseudocyst Pancreas

- Most common site of pseudo cyst-body and tail*
- Most common cause-pancreatitis*
- 2nd cause-trauma*
- Most common cause in children-trauma.*

103. Ans. a. Lichtenstein Repair *Ref: Shwartz 10/e p1516*

Points from Recurrence and Hernia Repairs:

- The type of anesthetic does not affect the recurrence rate
- The recurrence rate for the laparoscopic repair was lower compared with open nonmesh repairs; however, open and laparoscopic mesh repairs had similar recurrence rates.
- In experienced hands, the overall recurrence rate for the Shouldice repair is about 1%.
- Lichtenstein technique, with an overall recurrence rate of 0.2%

Lichtensteins

We use **PROLENE MESH** to bridge the gap between inguinal ligament and conjoint tendon.
The preferred approach for all hernia*

Shouldice technique

He gave additional strength to the posterior wall by double breasting the fascia transversalis.
Best among all anatomical repairs (Herniorrhaphy]
Least recurrence among herniorrhaphy*

Stoppas procedure

For bilateral direct hernia's, a modified Pfannenstiel incision made in the lower abdomen and a huge mesh placed in between the peritoneum and the fascia transversalis (PREPERITONEAL MESH repair).
Also called as GPVRS-giant prosthetic visceral reinforcement surgery

104. Ans. c. Hot spots on Tc 99 scan (Discussed Already)

105. Ans. a. Percentage of burns × weight (kg) × 4 = volume in ml

Parkland formula

- TBSA% × weight (kg) × 4 = volume (ml) needed
- Half this volume is given in the first 8 hours, and the second half is given in the subsequent 16 hours
- The volume replacement is by crystalloids.

106. Ans. a. Wide excision with a margin

Phyllodes Tumor

(Serocystic disease of Brodie or Cystosarcoma phyllodes)

Classified into

- Benign,Borderline,Malignant
- Present at age > 40 years.
- Gross examination Massive tumor with unevenly bosselated surface with areas of infarction and necrosis.
- Mobile on the chest wall
- Skin ulceration may occur
- Most malignant phyllodes contain Liposarcomatous or rhabdomyosarcomatous elements.
- Treatment
  - Small phyllodes are excised with 1cm margin of normal breast tissue and
  - Large phyllodes require mastectomy
- No axillary dissection needed as there is no axillary metastasis

107. Ans. d. 60 *Ref: Schwartz 10/e [515*

BRCA 1 mutation: (17 q)

- Average lifetime risk has been reported to lie between **60%–70%.**
- Breast cancer susceptibility in these families appears as an autosomal dominant trait with high penetrance.
- Approximately 50% of children of carriers inherit the trait.
- In general, *BRCA1*-associated breast cancers are invasive ductal carcinomas, are poorly differentiated, are in the majority hormone receptor negative and have a triple receptor negative (immunohistochemical profile: ER-negative, PR-negative and *HER-2*-negative).

BRCA 2 mutation: (13 q)

- The breast cancer risk for *BRCA2* mutation carriers is close to **85%,** and the lifetime ovarian cancer risk, while lower than for *BRCA1*, is still estimated to be close to 20%.

- Breast cancer susceptibility in *BRCA2* families is an autosomal dominant trait and has a high penetrance. Approximately 50% of children of carriers inherit the trait.
- Unlike male carriers of *BRCA1* mutations, men with germline mutations in *BRCA2* have an estimated breast cancer risk of 6%, which represents a 100-fold increase over the risk in the general male population.

108. Ans. a. Swelling medial to inferior epigastric artery

Direct hernia in Hesselbach triangle

- Weak spot in anterior abdominal wall through which direct hernia appears
  - **Medial:** Outer border of rectus abdominis.
  - **Lateral:** Inferior epigastric vessels
  - **Below:** Medial part of inguinal ligament
  - **Floor:** Fascia transversalis
- Inguinal hernia MC on right side
- Direct hernia never occurs in females and rarely gets strangulated
- Femoral hernia is MC in females than males
- Indirect inguinal hernia is the MC type of hernia in females
- Cryptorchidism is associated with indirect hernia 90%
- Of all hernias femoral is the one most liable for strangulation because of narrow neck

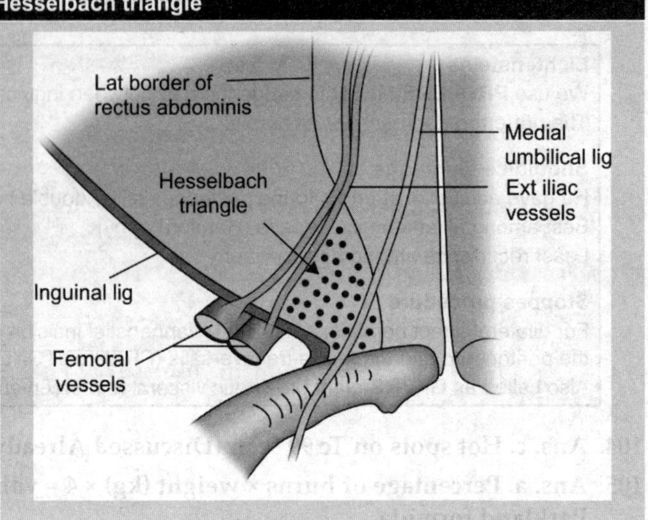

109. Ans. c. Lacunar ligament

Femoral Hernia

- Femoral Canal 2 x 2 cm size
- Medial compartment of femoral sheath

Walls of femoral canal

- Above-Femoral ring
- Below-saphenous opening
- Anteriorly -Inguinal ligament
- Posteriorly -Cooper's ligament
- Medially -Lacunar ligament
- Laterally -femoral vein

Contents Cloquet's node
Lymphatics
Areolar tissue

110. Ans. a. and b. Thyroid peroxidase antibodies and Painless enlargement of thyroid *Ref: Schwartz 10/ep1534*

Hashimotos Thyroiditis

- Transformation of thyroid tissue to lymphoid tissue
- M/c thyroiditis
- **Autoimmune process**
- Cd4+ helper cells directed against thyroglobulin, thyroid peroxidase [m/c], TSH-Receptor
- Microscopy lymphocytes present, hurthle cells/ashkenazi cell
- Risk of lymphoma, papillary carcinoma***

Clinical Features

M: F ratio = 1:10 to 1:20

- Painless anterior neck mass
- Hypothyroidism-20%
- Hyperthyroidism-5%

LAB Investigations
- Increased TSH
- Decreased T3/T4

Thyroid Autoantibodies-confirmatory
FNAC

Treatment
- Hypothyroidism-thyroxine
- Surgery-Suspicion of malignancy,pressure symptoms and cosmetics

111. Ans. b. Palmar arch insufficiency

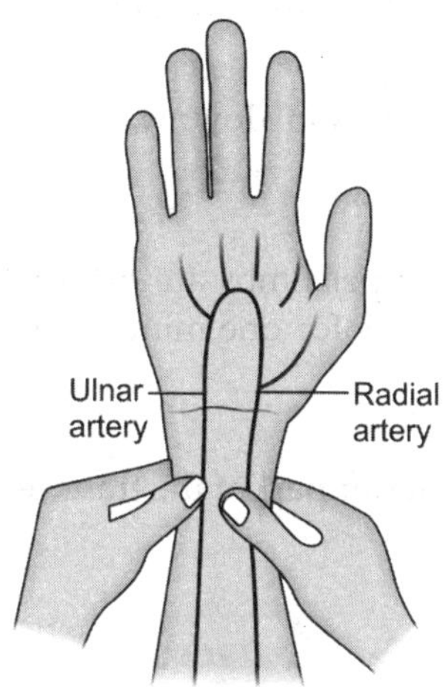

Fig. 12.6: Allen's test

- It's a test to look for the patency of Ulnar and radial Communication for the palmar arches.
- This test must be done before doing hemodialysis Shunt at the wrist.

112. Ans. c. Often associated with cervical rib abnormalities
Causes of thoracic outlet syndrome

Congenital	Acquired
Osseous Cervical rib Long C7 transverse process Abnormal 1st rib	Fracture Clavicle, callus and pseudo arthrosis Fracture 1st rib Exostosis/tumors
Soft tissue Anomalous scalene insertion Scalene muscle hypertrophy Congenital bands and ligaments **Postural** Heavy breast Sagging shoulders	Scalene muscle injury previous surgery/scar Soft tissue tumor Direct brachial plexus injury

Pathology	Symptoms
Neurogenic TOS (m/c) Brachial plexus compression at lower end (C8, T1) m/c–ulnar nerve involved	Pain, paresthesia, along ulnar nerve distribution Hall mark–pain in arm, shoulder, forearms Occipital headache–referred pain from tight scalene muscle
Vascular TOS Intermittent/temporary occlusion of subclavian artery Post stenotic aneurysm Emboli may dislodge into peripheral circulation and produce ischemic fingers Intermittent Raynaud's phenomenon	Claudication Ischemic ulcers Gangrenous tips Cold hands, color changes

Features:
- M/c in 20–40 years
- 70 % are females

O/E:
- Pulsatile supraclavicular mass
- Tinel's sign overbrachial plexus
- Hard and fixed lump in lower part of posterior triangle

Adson's test
- Ask the patient to take deep inspiration and extend his head backwards and turn to affected side. Feel for radial pulse which becomes absent or decreased than before

Costoclavicular compression (Halsted test)
- Patient throws his shoulder backwards and downwards as an exaggerated military position. Feel for disappearance of radial pulse

Elevated arms test (Roos test)
- Abduct the shoulder to 90 deg and upper limbs are externally rotated, elbow flexed to 90 degrees. The patient now opens and closes his fingers for one minute. TOS cases will have fatigue, pain, tingling and numbness in digits

Cervical Ribs:
- Costal element may develop from anterior part of the transverse process of C7 vertebra. This may develop into cervical rib
- M/c in (R) side
- Incidence0.45%
- 50% bilateral cases

Types:

Complete Rib articulation anteriorly with manubrium sterni or 1st rib

Incomplete
- Rib ends as large bony mass
- Rib ends tapering with a fibrous band to scalene tubercule
- Fibrous band only that incorporates into scalene medius

Symptoms:
- Neurological symptoms are less common in cervical rib than vascular symptoms
- If neurological symptoms predominate always rule out disc prolapsed and carpal tunnel syndrome

Surgical treatment
- Excision of cervical rib (extra periosteal excision)
- Scalenotomy

113. Ans. a. Calcium oxalate
- Kidney Stones are probably the most commonly encountered kidney complications of IBD—particularly oxalate stones**
- Kidney stones are more common in Crohn's patients with disease of the small intestine than in the general population because of fat malabsorption.

Mechanism:
- Fat binds to calcium, leaving oxalate (a type of salt) free to be absorbed and deposited in the kidney, where it can form into stones. The risk for developing kidney stones of this type is higher in people who have had a number of small bowel resections and are therefore more prone to dehydration. Their urine is more concentrated, a condition that is more likely to lead to stone formation.

Prevention:
- Kidney stone treatment calls for an increased fluid intake together with a low-oxalate diet (one that's rich in juices and vegetables).

114. Ans. d. Microscopic hematuria *Ref: Bailey and Love 26/e p1302*

Tuberculosis of testis
The disease **first effects the epididymis*** while causing orchitis. The body of testis may remain uninvolved for years, but the contralateral epididymis often becomes diseased**
Lower pole of epididymis involve first due to retrograde spread
Frim and craggy epididymis, Not associated with Severe pain**
Beaded vasdeferens**
Urine and semen examined for TB bacilli
If this does not resolve, epididymectomy is indicated
Treatment is ATT
Note: Syphilis will not affect the epididymis while causing orchitis.**

Genitourinary TB	
• Genitourinary tuberculosis is always secondary to pulmonary infection, though in many cases has healed or is quiescent. • Infection occurs via the **hematogenous route** to Kidney • **Ureter and Bladder**–Secondary to Renal TB • **Most common site**–UV junction** • **In early renal tuberculosis**, the only radiological abnormality may be irregularity (Fussy calyx), Moth eaten calyx, Phantom calyx. • **most sensitive modality to detect it is IUV as it can show detailed calyceal anatomy for early lesion**	**Changes are:** • **TB kidney:** Putty kidney, autonephrectomy, moth eaten appearance, Kerr's kink, irregular cavity, phantom calyx Also: Putty kidney–caseous necrosis, Cement kidney–calcified one and Pseudo calculi • TB ureter: Corkscrew ureter, beaded ureter, pipe stem ureter • TB bladder: Golf hole ureter, thimble bladder
• Computed tomography: shows advanced changes well but is less sensitive in early stages as it cannot detail calyceal anatomy. • 'Sterile pyuria' is the rule** – But about 15-20% of patients with tuberculosis have secondary pyogenic infection, obscuring the clue pyuria – The tubercle bacilli can be identified on AFB staining of 24 hr urine specimen or the first morning urine collected on 3 successive days. – AFB staining is positive in about 60% of cases. • Most common site of genitourinary tuberculosis is → **Kidney** • **TB Bladder:** The fibrosis which usually starts around the ureters, contracts to cause a pull at the ureters. This either leads to a stricture or displaced, dilated and rigid wide mouthed ureters **k/a golf hole ureters. This almost always leads to ureteral reflux**	

115. Ans. c. Intravesical BCG (Discussed Already)

116. Ans. a. Associated with chordee

Hypospadias

Hypospadias is a condition in which the urethral meatus opens on the underside of penis or the perineum, i.e. ventral surface of penis proximal to the tip of the glans penis.

There are several types of hypospadias according to location

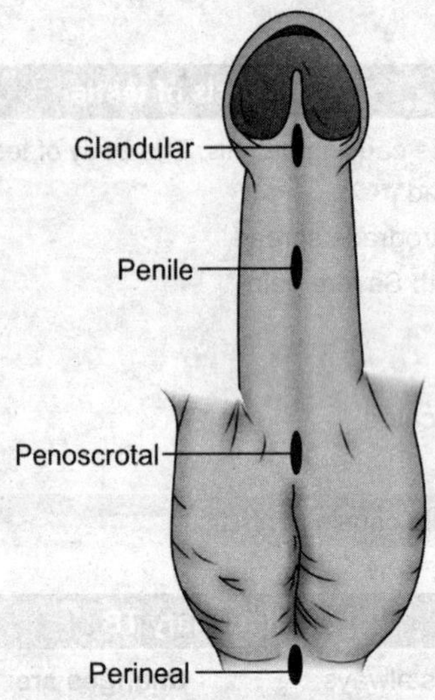

Fig. 12.7: Hypospadias

Types of hypospadias
• Glandular–Opening is in the glans penis, proximal to the tip • Coronal–Opening on the coronal sulcus • Penile • Penoscrotal • Perineal–This is the most severe abnormality. The scrotum is split and the urethra opens between its two halves. There may be testicular mal descent, which may make it difficult to determine the sex of child.

- **Glandular hypospadias is the most common type.**

Also know

- **Hypospadias is the most common congenital malformation of the urethra.**
- In epispadias: The urethra opens on the dorsum of penis. It's a rare congenital anomaly that is commonly associated with bladder exstrophy.

Associated features:

- **Dorsal Hood**
- **Ventral Chordee**
- **Ventral Opening of Urethra in the penis**
- Remember that cryptorchidism is not a feature of hypospadias. But it may be seen associated with hypospadias in 8–9% of cases

Complications of hypospadias

- Difficulty in directing the urinary stream.
- Due to presence of chordee, erection is difficult and painful and the intercourse may be difficult or impossible.
- Infertility can occur (usually associated with penoscrotal and perineal variety)

Surgery for Hypospadias:

- Best time for surgery for hypospadias is between 6–12 months of age
- Operation can be done in one stage or two stage surgeries. Nowadays one stage surgeries are more popular.
- In the first stage chordee is corrected
- Circumcision is not done** in patients with hypospadias as the prepuce can later be used in surgical repair.

117. **Ans. a. Clinical evaluation (Palpation and transillumination)**

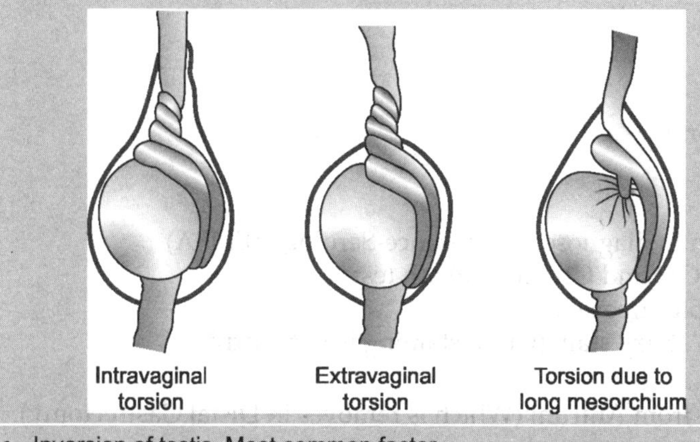

Torsion of testis

- Torsion of testis is the torsion of the spermatic cord causing strangulation of the blood supply to the testis and unless it is t/t within 6 hours, testicular atrophy is inevitable
- It is seen commonly in adolescent (10–25 years)
- **Symptoms** → it presents sudden agonising pain in the groin and the lower abdomen. Nausea and vomiting are very common
- Absent testis or Vanishing testis: seen in Prenatal torsion

- Inversion of testis–Most common factor
- **Bell clapper deformity:**
- High investment of tunica vaginalis forming a mesentry like structure for testis (mesorchium) which makes the testis hang down horizontally.
- Presence of gap between testis and epididymis makes testis hang and go for torsion.

Signs in torsion testis:

- **Angel's sign**: It's a sign on the normal side (unaffected side).Opposite testis lies horizontally because of the presence of mesorchium. (the predisposing factor for torsion is same on both sides)
- **Deming's sign:** Its a sign on the affected side where the affected testis is positioned high because of the twisting of the cord and spasm of muscles.

- It must be **differentiated from epidydimo-orchitis by:**
  - **Prehns sign** → on elevation of testis
    - Pain increases → in torsion
    - Pain decreases → in epidydimo-orchitis
  - **Color Doppler** → detects the decreased blood flow to testis in torsion.

It is the inv. of choice to exclude torsion from the epididymo-orchitis

  - **Tc 99m pretechnate scan** → it demonstrates decreased blood flow

Torsion of testicular appendage–Blue dot sign (Most common appendix of testes)

- **Treatment**
  - In the 1st hour the torsion can be treated by manipulation (but later on surgery has to be done to fix the testis)
  - If not correctable by manipulation or more than one hour has passed then surgery has to be done. **Surgery must be done within 6 hours**. Otherwise the testis will be dead
  - Both the affected and unaffected testis should undergo orchipexy because the anatomical variation responsible for torsion is likely to be bilateral (bell–clapper deformity)

118. **Ans. c. 40–60**

- More with duodenal ulcers-90%
- Gastric ulcers up to 70%

H. Pylori Infection

- Gram-negative spiral shaped bacilli
- Organism gets localised deep beneath the mucus layer closely adherent to the epithelial surface.
- Urease enzyme produces ammonia from urea and raises the pH (alkaline) around bacterium. Hence gastric secretion is increased stimulating the acid level though local alkalinity maintained.
- H.Pylori exclusively colonises gastric type epithelium and is only found in the duodenum in association with patches of gastric metaplasia.
- Around 90% patients of duodenal ulcer and 70% of gastric ulcer are infected with H.Pylori.

*Associations of H. Pylori:**

1. Peptic ulcer (Gastric and duodenal)
2. Ca.Stomach (Intestinal variant)

3. Lymphoma
4. Non ulcer dyspepsia
5. Type `B' gastritis

Not associated with:

1. Type `A' gastritis
2. Ca.Stomach in fundus area (OG junction Tumors)
3. Ca.stomach-Diffuse gastric cancer type.

Repeat MCQ's from H.pylori:

- For H.pylori the best non invasive investigation to diagnose the presence-Serology (ELISA)
- The best investigation to diagnose eradication-C13 and C14 urea breath test
- The best invasive investigation to diagnose-Rapid urease test
- The stain used for H. pylori-Giemsa or warthin starry stain (Gram staining is not used)*

119. Ans. c. Vitamin B12 deficiency

- Due to decreased production of Intrinsic factor from Antrum (Which is removes in Distal Gastrectomy)

Complications of Gastric surgeries:

Post Cibal Syndrome (Dumping Syndrome)

Early Dumping:

- After meals; small bowel gets filled with food stuff. Osmotic overload leads to sequestration of fluid from circulation into gastrointestinal tract. This leads to vasomotor and abdominal symptoms *due to hypovolemia**
- Occurs immediately.
- Diagnosed by increased packed cell volume*

Treatment:

- Small, dry meals
- Octreotides (analogues of somatostatin)
- Revision surgery: Roux-en-y reconstruction.

Late Dumping

- After meals; carbohydrate load causes a rise in plasma glucose level; results in increased insulin release that leads to *reactive hypoglycemia**
- 2nd hour after meals.
- Diagnosed by measuring *blood glucose level**

Treatment

- Octreotide is effective. (Side effect: gallstone formation).
- Same as for early dumping.

	Early Dumping	Late Dumping
Incidence	5 -10%	5%
Relation to meals	Immediately	Second hour
Duration	30 minutes	30 minutes
Relief	Lying down	Food
Aggravated by	More food	Exercise
Clinical Features	Epigastric fullness, sweating, diarrhea	Tremor, faintness, prostration.

Oneliners:

Osteomalacia is a complication after GJ because Calcium is not absorbed (MC site of calcium absorption is Duodenum)

Hypocalcemia can occur after in similar way after Billroth 2 gastrectomy

Duodenal stump blow out happens usually on 4th Post op day after Billroth 2 surgery. It is managed conservatively by USG guided drainage.

Afferent loop syndrome* is obstruction of the afferent loop (Loop that comes to stomach bringing Bile and pancreatic secretion) in GJ which results in Bilious vomiting without food particles. Can be managed Conservatively.

Efferent loop syndrome* is obstruction of efferent loop (Loop that goes away from stomach carrying food particles) in GJ which results in Vomiting of bile mixed with food. Has to be treated as emergency by Surgery.

120. Ans. a. Parastomal hernia

MCQ's Asked in Stomas:

- ***Ileostomy the mc Complication: Necrosis (22%), prolapse (22%), skin irritation (17%), and stenosis (17%).***
- ***Parastomal hernia is most common after -Colostomy than ileostomy and after end colostomy***
- ***Stomal Prolapse is more common after transverse loop Colostomy.***

121. Ans. b. Urological Abnormalities *Ref: Schwartz 10/e p1626*

Anorectal Anomalies:

- Anorectal malformations describe a spectrum of congenital anomalies that include imperforate anus and persistent cloaca.
- Incidence = 1 in 5000 live births: M = F population.
- Anatomic description of imperforate anus has been characterized as either 'high' or 'low' depending on whether the rectum ends above the **levator ani muscle****
- The Rectum ends as a fistula into the **membranous urethra in males* and Vestibule* in females**
- **Approximately 60% of patients have an associated malformation.**** The most common is a **urinary tract defect**, which occurs in approximately 50% of patients** Other Anomalies-Skeletal defects (Sacrum is Commonly involved)Gastrointestinal anomalies occur, most commonly Esophageal atresia. Cardiac anomalies may occur as part of the VACTERLL syndrome.
- **Posterior sagittal anorectoplasty (PSARP) procedure**, as described by **Pena**** and DeVries is the treatment of Choice

122. Ans. b. Chemoradiation (Already Discussed)

123. Ans. a. Spleen

Abdominal trauma

Diagnostic peritoneal lavage	FAST-Focused abdominal sonogram of trauma
• Insert a cannula below the umbilicus. About 1000 ml of warmed ringer lactate is instilled into the abdomen and is then drained out. • *Result: presence of > 1 lakh red cells/microlitre or > 500 white cells/micro litre is positive. It's equivalent to 20 ml of blood in peritoneal cavity.* • DPL has sensitivity about 97-98%.	• To assess presence of blood in peritoneum or pericardium. • ***Focuses on four areas only: pericardial, splenic, hepatic, pelvic areas.*** • It will detect blood more than 100 ml only • It will not detect hollow viscus injury

Oneliners in Blunt injury Abdomen:

- CT is the gold standard to diagnose intra abdominal injuries in stable patients.
- USG is used to diagnose intrabdominal injuries in Unstable patients
- M/c injured organ in Penetrating trauma-***small intestine.***
- M/c organ injured in blunt trauma-***Spleen***
- **Pringle's manoeuvre**-direct compression of portal triad inflow by digitally or soft clamp at the level of Epiploic Foramen

124. Ans. a. Insulinoma (Explained in theory)

- **Whipple's triad is a feature of Insulinoma**
- **Insulinoma is the only tumor associated with weight gain**

125. Ans. a. Leucocytosis > 20000/μ

Based on Ranson's scoring the prognosis is made

Ransons criteria [Code-LAGAW BUCHOW]*

On admission

- Age > 55 years
- WBC count > 16000/mm^3
- Blood glucose > 10mmol/l
- LDH > 700 μ/l
- AST > 250 sigma Frankel units %

Within 48 hours

- BUN > 5 mg%
- Arterial O_2 saturationPa O_2 < 60 mmHg
- Serum calcium < 2.0 mmol/l
- Hematocrit fall > 10%
- Base deficit > 4 mmol/l
- Fluid sequestration > 6l

126. Ans. d. Back pain (page 1460/Scwartz-10th edition. Bailey and Love-Page 985)

- Retroperitoneal fibrosis is a class of disorders characterized by hyperproliferation of fibrous tissue in the retroperitoneum.
- Primary: Ormond's disease
- Secondary: list of causes like malignancy and Drugs
- MC: men, 40-60 years
- The clinical presentation may be one of ill-defined chronic backache or may occur as a result of compromise to involved structures, e.g. lower limb or scrotal oedema secondary to venous occlusion, or chronic renal failure secondary to ureteric obstruction.
- **M/c common organ involved in RP fibrosis is ureter.**

127. Ans. a. Submucous lipoma (discussed before)

128. Ans. c. Bleeding *Ref: Bailey and Love 26/e p1227*

Cancer Rectum

- Earliest and m/c symptom-bleeding*
- 2nd m/c symptom alteration in bowel habits
- Early morning spurious diarrhea is characteristically seen*
- Annular cancer at pelvirectal junction presents with constipation and obstruction

- Best investigation for diagnosis-Sigmoidoscopic biopsy
- Best investigation for local spread-Trans rectal USG
- Best investigation for local T and N staging-Transrectal MRI

Treatment:

- **Rectal cancer needs a clearance atleast 2 cm distally.**

Surgeries for Rectal cancer:

- APR is performed when the sphincter cannot be preserved*
- Complete excision of rectum and anus along with permanent colostomy
- Also known as MILES PROCEDURE*
- For tumours involving upper 1/3rd-Anterior resection and for tumours involving middle 1/3rd low anterior resection
- Even lower 1/3rd tumours are taken up for sphincter saving low anterior resection.

Hartmanns Procedure is done if there is too much sepsis or obstruction, also if the patient is very elderly and unsuitable for any type of resection.

Transanal excision of cancer rectum

- T1N0 or T2N0 lesion < 4 cm in diameter
- < 40% circumference of the lumen
- < 10 cm from dentate line
- Well to moderately differentiated histology
- No evidence of lymphatic or vascular invasion on biopsy.

129. Ans. b. Clostridium perfringens (discussed before)

130. Ans. c. Uric acid (Explained in theory)

131. Ans. b. 3 months *Ref: Bailey and Love 26/e p1377*

Lines Directly From Bailey and Love…

- About 4 percent of boys are born with one or both testes incompletely descended.
- About two thirds of these reach the scrotum during the first three months of life, but full descent after that is uncommon.
- The incidence of testicular maldescent at the age of one year is around 1 per cent

Testis and Scrotum:

Testes develop in the retroperitoneum below the kidney at around 10th Thoracic level.

Descent of testes is facilitated by Gubernaculum, Mullerian inhibiting substance, Maternal Chorionic gonadotrophin.

Undescended testis

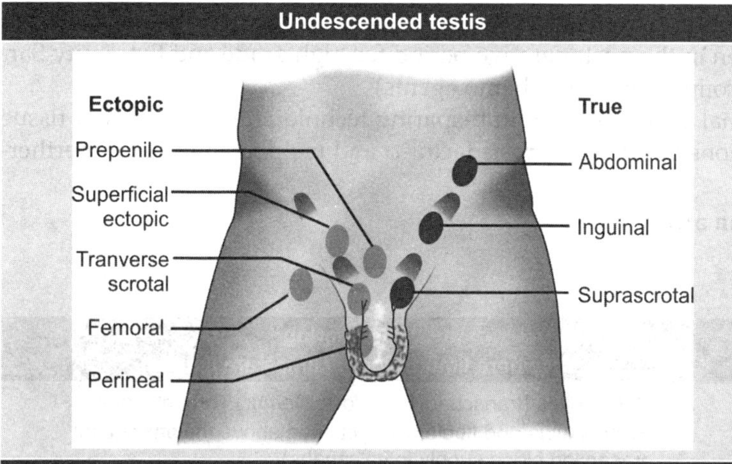

- In **undescended testis**–the testes are arrested in some part of its path to the scrotum. 1% incidence at 1 year of age
- Approx 2/3rd UDT will descend, usually by 3 months of age
- More common in preterm, small for gestational age, LBW and twin neonates
- UDT: More common on **Rt.side**, 20% bilateral
- Secondary sexual characteristics are normal

Complications of incomplete descent

- Torsion of testis
- Epididymo-orchitis
- Atrophy
- Inferility–if the condition is bilateral
- Pain–a testis situated in the ingunial canal is often liable to trauma and give rise to pain in the groin
- Hernia–90% Processus vaginalis
- Malignancy–risk is 5 -10 times more than a normally placed testis

'Definitive treatment of the undescended testis should **occur before 1 year of age**'

- Sub dartos pouch
- Ombredann's technique-mobilised testis is left in opposite scrotum.
- Ladd and gross technique-testis left in scrotum. A stitch is made in the tunica albuginea and brought through the scrotal skin and fixed to medial side of thigh.
- Keetley and torek operation-testis is mobilised and the testis itself is left in the medial aspect of thigh.
- Silbar procedure-orchidopexy by micro vascular anastomosis.
- Fowler stephen procedure-two staged procedure

132. Ans. a. Pain *Ref: Bailey and Love 26/e p807*

- Fibroadenosis are kept under the group of benign diseases of breast known as–ANDI-Aberrations of normal Development and Involution.
- Fibroadenosis presents with Dull aching pain and on examination as sense of lumpiness is present.

133. Ans. a. Superficial spreading (explained in theory)

134. Ans. a. Degeneration of tendon sheath

135. Ans. c. Wide local Excision *Ref: Scwartz, 10/e p1472*

Lines directly from Schwartz...

- Margin status after surgical resection has been shown to be an independent prognostic factor.
- The goal of surgical resection is to achieve a complete resection because microscopically positive or grossly positive resection margins are associated with increased risk of local recurrence and death
- If an unexpected positive margin is found on pathologic examination of the resection specimen, re-excision should be performed.
- The preferred treatment for extremity sarcomas is wide local excision that includes resection of the biopsy site. The goal of wide local excision is to remove the tumor with approximately 1 to 2 cm of surrounding normal soft tissue, but narrower margins may be necessary to preserve uninvolved critical neurovascular structures and may be adequate for patients undergoing radiation therapy.

- For some massive tumors of the extremities, wide local excision entails a radical or complete anatomic compartment resection. Surgical clips should be placed to delineate the extent of the resection bed for patients likely to require postoperative radiation therapy.

Other modalities of Treatment:

- Amputation is needed in near 5% of extremity Sarcomas
- Radiotherapy and Chemotherapy are given in the postoperative period for high grade and Extremity Sarcomas. (Doxo rubicin and Ifosfamide are commonly used Chemo agents)
- **Isolated Limb Perfusion*:** Isolated regional perfusion Is a limb-sparing technique in which a soft tissue sarcoma is perfused with high concentrations of tumor necrosis factor-α and melphalan under hyperthermic conditions.

136. Ans. b. Blockage of second part of subclavian artery

137. Ans. a. Incision and drainage

138. Ans. c. Syme's amputation

Cone bearing (prosthesis possible)	End bearing (where limb fitting facilities are limited)
• Below knee (stump = 8 cm preferably 10–12 cm below knee) • Above knee (stump = 20 cm above knee)	• Gritti stokes (transcondylar at lower femur) Through knee • Syme's (tibia and fibula are sectioned above the ankle joint preserving blood supply to calcaneus)

The flap necrosis may occur if Symes amputation is done in diabetics

Amputation:

- Through Ankle (Syme)-notsuitable for severely ischaemic atheromatous limbs because of poor healing of flap. Contraindicated in Diabetics**
- Lisfranc's (Tarso–Metatarsal)

139. Ans. b. Partial thickness graft (Discussed Already)

140. Ans. b. Enterogenous cyst (Discussed in theory)

141. Ans. d. Ambulatory pH monitoring

Gastroesophageal Reflux Disease

Loss of competence of LES leads to GERD. Dyspepsia with fatty food is more common with GERD than Gallstones:

- Medical treatment-Proton pump inhibitors,
- Surgical treatment-Nissens Floppy fundoplication (360 degrees)-Posterior wrap

Investigations for GERD:

- Ambulatory 24 hours pH monitoring (probe placed 5cm above the OG junction)-**gold standard to diagnose esophageal reflux disease***
- Double probe 24 hours pH monitoring-used to diagnose laryno pharyngeal reflux of GERD.
- **Demeester Score*** is the Score based on 24 hours pH monitoring. If it is more than 14, the patient is having GERD.

Other surgeries done for GERD

- Toupet posterior fundoplication-270 degrees wrap
- Dor anterior fundoplication-180 degrees wrap
- Hills procedure
- Belsey mark 4 operation and **Angelchik prosthesis****

Complications-Stricture, Shortening of esophagus, Barrets esophagus

142. Ans. a. Endoscopic surveillance with biopsy every 2 years

In this question 2 option are correct-Endoscopic surveillance and PPI will be given

Barrets Esophagus

- Metaplastic change of normal squamous to columnar epithelium in response to GERD
- Hall mark of intestinal metaplasia: **Intestinal goblet cells***

- May predispose to adeno carcinoma within 2 cm from junction of squamo columnar epithelium [m/c site]
- Complications-Peptic ulcer, Stricture, Cancer.
- 40 fold increased risk for adenocarcinoma**

Investigation: Diagnosed by endoscopy and biopsy (Endoscopic biopsy)*

Treatment

- Same as reflux esophagitis
- Regular follow-up and biopsy is must
- **In absence of dysplasia-biannual surveillance****
- In presence of low grade dysplasia-annual surveillance
- In presence of high grade dysplasia-subtotal Esophagectomy or Vagal Sparing Esophagectomy or Laser ablation.

143. Ans. b. Cisplatin *Ref: Scwartz 10/e p1012*

- For adenocarcinomas of the distal esophagus and proximal stomach, preoperative Neoadjuvant **5-fluoro-uracil (5-FU) and Cisplatin** chemotherapy has been shown to provide a survival advantage over surgery alone in a well-powered study from the United Kingdom (MRC trial).
- In a second trial from the United Kingdom (MAGIC trial) of distal esophageal and proximal gastric adenocarcinomas, the use of Epirubicin in combination with cisplatin and 5-FU also demonstrated a survival advantage.

144. Ans. c. Small bowel Obstruction *Ref: Schwartz 10/e p1160*

Lines from Scwartz...

- Most small-intestinal neoplasms are asymptomatic until they become large. Partial small bowel obstruction, with associated symptoms of crampy abdominal pain and distention, nausea, and vomiting, is the most common mode of presentation**
- Obstruction can be the result of either luminal narrowing by the tumor itself or intussusception, with the tumor serving as the lead point. Hemorrhage, usually indolent, is the second most common mode of presentation.

Small Bowel Tumors

- M/c benign symptomatic neoplasm of Small intestine-Leiomyoma
- M/c benign neoplasm in Small intestine in Autopsy series-Adenoma
- M/c malignant primary neoplasm of Small Intestine-Based on both the Surveillance, Epidemiology and End Result (SEER) program and National Cancer Data Base (NCDB), small bowel malignancies, in order of frequency, include carcinoid, adenocarcinoma, lymphoma, and GIST.
- M/C Extra abdominal primary to produce small bowel metastasis-Cutaneous melanoma > breast and Lung
- Duodenum is m/c site of small bowel tumours*
- Adenocarcinoma doesn't have good prognosis
- In small and large bowel tumours the liver mets per se is **not a contraindication*** for primary curative resection
- Chemotherapy is not a proven treatment for small bowel cancers*

Site	Most common Lesions
Duodenum	Adenocarcinoma,atresia, Diverticulum
Jejunum	Angiodysplasia, Pneumatosis Intestinalis
Ileum	Small bowel duplication, Adenoma, Lipoma, Leiomyoma, carcinoid.

145. Ans. b. Submucosa

- The strongest layer in Intestinal wall is SUBMUCOSA**

146. Ans. d. Large bowel (Searching...... But Ans. is authentic from Experienced Paediatric GI surgeons)

147. Ans. b. Medical management includes antibiotics, immunosuppressive agents and biologic agents (Discussed in theory)

148. Ans. c. Colonic Polyps

Familial Cancer Syndromes:

- **Familial adenomatous polyposis:** Autosomal dominant [AD] disorder, APC gene (long arm of Chromosome 5), Colorectal cancer develops in all patients at age before 40 years if untreated. Prophylactic colectomy is needed
- **Turcots syndrome:** FAP+ brain tumors like glioma, medulloblastoma, Autosomal recessive.
- **Gardners syndrome:** FAP + Osteomas, Epidermoid cysts, Congenital hypertrophy of retinal pigment epithelium, Desmoid tumour, Retroperitoneal fibrosis, Polyps of stomach, small intestine, adenomas in pancreas, thyroid, adrenal, parathyroid.
- **Peutz jeghers syndrome-Hamartamatous polyps in jejunum*** and other part, pigmentation of lips, tumors of ovary, breast, endometrium, pancreas.
- **Cronkite canada syndrome:** Juvenile polyps are noted along with alopecia, cutaneous pigmentation, atrophy of nails and toe nail.

Hereditary Non Polyposis Colorectal (CRC) Cancer (HNPCC)

- AD inherited syndrome
- Defective MMR genes-Chromosome 2, 3, 7
- Responsible for 3-5% of Colon cancers (FAP only 1%)
- Polyps in HNPCC develop at younger age and larger than general population and distributed equally throughout the colon
- Predominant Right colon cancer**
- Increased synchronous/metachronous tumors
- Diagnosis is by GERMLINE MUTATION in MMR gene.

  Lynch 1: CRC only

  Lynch 2: CRC+ Extraintestinal cancers

Associated tumors in HNPCC:

- Endometrial cancer-MC (40–60%)
- Gastric-13-19%
- Ovarian-6-12%
- Small intestine, Pancreatic, thyroid, TCC of urinary tract, Brain cancer
- CNS tumor–Glioblastoma (In Turcot-Medulloblastoma)

Screening Protocols for Familial Cancer syndromes:

FAP	HNPCC
• For CRC screening colonoscopy screening starts at 10-12 years* • For Periampullary cancer and Duodenal cancer screening starts at 25 years	• CRC screening starts at 20 years • Endometrial cancer screening at 25–35 years

Oneliners:

- Most common cause of death after total procto colectomy for a case of FAP is Duodenal and periampullary cancer*
- 2nd Common cancer in LYNCH syndrome is Endometrial cancer
- Amsterdam and Bethesda criteria are used to diagnose HNPCC syndrome
- Haggit's Criteria is to assess the level of cancer in Pedunculated and sessile Colorectal Polyps.

149. Ans. a. USG

- **USG: First investigation for GB and bile duct.**
- **HIDA SCAN (TC 99 m labelled iminodiacetic acid):** Gold Standard** to diagnose Acute cholecystitis. (There will be non-visualization of Gallbladder)
- **CT scan:** Only in ca gallbladder and bile duct
- **MRCP:** Most accurate non invasive
- ERCP-gold standard to diagnose CBD stones. In modern world only used for interventional purposes*. MRCP has largely replaced it.

150. Ans. a. Most commonly presents with pneumaturia *Ref: Bailey and Love 26/e p1325*

Vesicointestinal Fistulas:

- **The most common cause is diverticulitis of the colon****
- Fistulae may also follow Crohn's disease, appendix abscess or pelvis sepsis after acute salpingitis, or pelvic surgery.
- The onset of a fistula from diverticular disease may well be treated as a simple urinary infection. The diagnosis can be difficult to make, but on cystoscopy a patch of oedema on the left side of the vault is suggestive and bubbles of gas may be seen
- A **cystogram** may reveal the fistula.
- **The passage of gas per urethram in a patient is most suggestive**** (provided that diabetes resulting in urinary infection with a gas-forming organism is excluded).

151. Ans. a. Tuberculosis *Ref: Bailey and love 26/e p1357*

- Tuberculosis of one or both seminal vesicles may be found when examining a patient with chronic tuberculous epididymitis, no symptoms being referable to the internal genitalia.
- On rectal examination, the affected vesicle is found to be nodular***

152. Ans. b. Cardiac failure is common

- In Graves disease-Cardiac toxicity is less and CNS toxicity is more. Its only in secondary thyrotoxicosis cardiac toxicity is more common.

153. Ans. d. Most cases are familial

Medullary Carcinoma

- 5% of all thyroid malignancies
- Arise from parafollicular `C' cells
- Associated with MEN2A and MEN2B syndromes
- RET -proto oncogene mutation is seen in familial variety.

{Ret gene located in centomere region of chromosome 10}

Sporadic

- U/L
- 50-60 years
- No family h/o
- Total thyroidectomy with or without central node dx.

Familial

- B/L
- Young age
- Family h/o +
- Total thyroidectomy with MRND

Pheochromocytoma if associated to be Rx first.

Pathology:

- Sheets of infiltrating neoplastic cells separated by collagen and amyloid. Cells are polygonal or spindle shaped. Amyloid is diagnostic.

Diagnosis

- Immunohistochemistry for calcitonin
- S.Calcitonin, also for follow-up
- FNAC– Amyloid
- CT/MRI in select cases
- CEA is better for prognosis
- Calcitonin better for follow-up

Clinical Features

- Cervical lymphadenopathy (15 to 20%)
- Distant blood borne metastasis to liver, bone, lung.

- Medullary carcinoma secretes calcitonin, carcinoma embryonic antigen (CEA), histaminases', prostaglandins E2 and F2α and serotonin.
- Diarrhea is seen in about 30% cases due to vasoactive intestinal peptides.
- Cushing's syndrome is seen in about 2 to 4% cases due to ectopic Adrenocorticotrophic hormone (ACTH).

MCQ Points

- Sporadic variety — 80% unilateral [M/C TYPE]
- Familial variety — 90% bilateral and multicentric
- FNAC — Shows amyloid stroma
- Tumor Marker — Serum calcitonin (> 0.08 ng/ml)
- Investigate for pheochromocytoma -24 hours urinary VMA, catecholamines, and metanephrine
- Investigate for hyperparathyroidism -serum calcium.

Treatment

If the patient has associated pheochromocytoma operate it first to avoid hypertensive crisis during surgery for thyroid

- Total thyroidectomy with Bilateral central neck node dissection should be performed routinely.
- Tumors larger than 1.5 cm must undergo ipsilateral modified radical neck node dissection.
- External beam radiotherapy is controversial, but is recommended for unresectable residua or recurrent tumor.
- No effective chemotherapy available.
- Prophylactic Total Thyroidectomy is indicated in RET mutation carriers. This procedure is to be done in patients before age of 6 years in MEN 2A and prior to age one in MEN 2B patients.

154. Ans. c. Spreads through hematogenous route

Follicular Cancer

- 20% of thyroid malignancies
- More common in iodine deficient areas

Clinical Features

1. Predisposed by long standing multinodular goiter
2. Hematogenous metastasis is more common than lymph nodal metastasis. Pulsatile secondaries may be seen in skull, ribs, pelvis
3. Malignancy is defined by the presence of capsular and vascular invasion. Hence FNAC cannot differentiate between follicular adenoma and carcinoma
4. Follicular tumors > 4 cm size are more likely to be malignant
5. Follow-up can be done using I^{123} scan or by thyroglobulin estimation. Thyroglobulin levels in patients who have undergone total thyroidectomy should be below 2 ng/ml.

Treatment

- Total thyroidectomy
- Prophylactic nodal dissection is not needed because nodal involvement is infrequent
- But if nodal involvement is seen functional block dissection must be done
- If FNAC shows follicular adenoma; lobectomy is enough because 80% of cases are benign. If the biopsy report becomes positive for malignancy based on angio or capularinvasion Completion Total thyroidectomy must be done.

Other Treatment Modalities

- I131 therapy: Metastatic follicular cancer can be detected by I131 and treated by therapeutic dose. It is also used for recurrent thyroid follicular neoplasms.

External beam Radiotherapy

- Control unresectable, recurrent, invasive disease.
- Secondaries in the bone to prevent fracture and relieve pain.

Chemotherapy Adriamycin and taxanes are used

HURTHLE CELL CARCINOMA
- Variant subtype of follicular carcinoma.
- Malignancy is indicated by vascular and capsular invasion like follicular type, hence FNAC cannot differentiate benign and malignant.

Differ from Follicular carcinoma by
- Derived from oxyphil cells of thyroid gland
- More often multifocal and bilateral
- Do not take up radioactive iodine
- More likely to metastasize through lymph nodes
- Higher mortality (20% at 10 years).

Treatment
Total thyroidectomy with Routine central neck node dissection as done in medullary carcinoma.
Modified radical neck dissection done only if the lateral neck nodes are palpable

155. Ans. c. Incisional hernia *Ref: Bailey and Love 26/e p965*

156. Ans. b. Second degree superficial burns (Explained in theory)

157. Ans. c. Neutrophile dysfunction

Complications
1. Catheter related
2. Infection
3. Injuries-Pneumothorax, Hydrothorax
   Cardiac tamponade
   Injury to artery and vein
   Injury to thoracic duct, nerves.
4. Thrombosis
5. Air embolism, catheter embolism
6. Postcannulation

Metabolic complications
Azotemia
Essential fatty acid deficiency
Fluid overload
Metabolic bone disease
Liver dysfunction
Glucose imbalance (hyperglycemia, hypoglycemia)
Trace element and vitamin deficiency.

Electrolyte abnormalities
Electrolyte abnormalities
Hyper/hyponatremia
Hyper/hypokalemia
Hyper/hypophosphatemia
Hyper/hypomagnesemia
Hyper/hypocalcemia
High/low serum zinc
High/low serum copper
Hyperchloremic metabolic acidosis.

158. Ans. c. 37 *Ref: Sabiston Textbook of Surgery, 19/e p522*

Children have a relatively larger portion of the body surface area in the head and neck, which is compensated for by a relatively smaller surface area in the lower extremities.
Infants have 21% of the TBSA in the head and neck and 13% in each leg, which incrementally approaches the adult proportions with increasing age.
- The Berkow formula** is used to determine burn size accurately in children.

Berkow Formula to Estimate Burn Size (%) Based on Area of Burn in Isolated Body Part

	Age (Yr)					
Body Part	0–1	1–4	5–9	10–14	15–18	Abult
Head	19	17	13	11	9	7
Neck	2	2	2	2	2	2
Anterior trunk	13	13	13	13	13	13
Posterior trunk	13	13	13	13	13	13
Right buttock	2.5	2.5	2.5	2.5	2.5	2.5
Left buttock	2.5	2.5	2.5	2.5	2.5	2.5
Genitalia	1	1	1	1	1	1
Right upper arm	4	4	4	4	4	4
Left upper arm	4	4	4	4	4	4
Right lower arm	3	3	3	3	3	3
Left lower arm	3	3	3	3	3	3
Right hand	2.5	2.5	2.5	2.5	2.5	2.5
Left hand	2.5	2.5	2.5	2.5	2.5	2.5
Right thigh	5.5	6.5	8	8.5	9	9.5
Left thigh	5.5	6.5	8	8.5	9	9.5
Right leg	5	5	5.5	6	6.5	7
Left leg	5	5	5.5	6	6.5	7
Right foot	3.5	3.5	3.5	3.5	3.5	3.5
Left foot	3.5	3.5	3.5	3.5	3.5	3.5

As per findings: (Assuming child age < 5 years)

- Both Buttocks = 2.5+2.5 = 5
- Both Thigh = 6.5+6.5 = 13
- Face and Scalp = 17
- Neck = 2%

Total Burns = 37

Author's Note = Definitely a tough one to remember-But Jipmer is always funny in keeping some questions like this... most of the time Luck only plays here.

159. Ans. a. Necrosis (already Discussed)

160. Ans. c. Submucosal lipoma (already Discussed) *Ref: Bailey and Love's Short Practice of surgery, 26/e*

161. Ans. b. Adenolymphoma (already Discussed)

- The other name of Adenolymphoma is Warthins tumor
- It appears as Hot spot on Tc 99 m scan

162. Ans. a. Intercostrobrachial nerve *Ref: Fischer JE et al. master of Surgery, Lippincott, 2006, 5/e p514*

163. Ans. c. Minimal intervention to stabilize patient so that definitive surgery can be done later on

Ref: Scwartz 10/e p192

- The bloody vicious cycle in trauma is the lethal combination of coagulopathy, hypothermia, and metabolic acidosis.
- The purpose of DCS (Damage Control Surgery)is to limit operative time so that the patient can be returned to the SICU for physiologic restoration and the cycle thereby broken.
- The goal of DCS is to control surgical bleeding and limit GI spillage.

164. Ans. d. T0N2a Mx *Ref: Shwartz 581/10/e p581*

TNM Staging in Head and Neck:

- **Tis**–carcinoma in site
- **T1**–tumor ≤ 2 cm
- **T2**–tumor > 2 cm but ≤ 4 cm
- **T3**–tumor > 4 cm
- **T4** -tumor invades adjacent structures
- **N1**–single node ≤ 3 cm
- **N2a**–single node > 3 cm and < 6 cm
- **N2b**–multiple ipsilateral nodes, all < 6 cm
- **N2c**–Bilateral or contralateral nodes, all nodes < 6 cm
- **N3**–metastasis in a lymph node > 6 cm in greatest diameter
- **M1**–metastasis
- **The patient described here-Occult Primary-T0, Nodal mass 4X5 cm (N2a), MX (metastasis to be assessed).**

Author's Conclusion:

Dear friends, I have given the maximum input needed for JIPMER exams from Surgery in a concised manner... Hope you enjoyed reading. Join in Facebook group 'Final MBBS and MS General Surgery Help group' and get any surgical doubt you cleared from a team of experts. All the best for your exams.

QUESTIONS 2015

1. **Perianal pain, bleeding, unable to do PR or proctoscopy due to pain:**
   a. Hemorrhoids
   b Fissure in ano
   c. Fistula in ano
   d. Solitary rectal ulcer
2. **Bleeding PR, weight loss, lump in LIF, altered bowel habitus-Feature of:**
   a. Ca sigmoid colon
   b. Divericulum colon
   c. Angiodysplasia colon
   d. Ulcerative colitis
3. **An Alcoholic patient admitted in ICU with Acute abdominal pain and periumbilical discoloration. The diagnosis is:**
   a. Liver failure
   b. Acute pancreatitis
   c. Perforation
   d. Ascites
4. **Following injury to perineum a patient presenting with scrotal swelling on micturition. The common site of urethral tear is:**
   a. Bulbar
   b. Membranous
   c. Penile
   d. Prostatic urethra
5. **Swelling in anterior triangle of the neck in a middle aged female. FNAC can detect which of the following:**
   a. Follicular carcinoma
   b. Papillary carcinoma
   c. Carotid body tumor
   d. Anaplastic carcinoma
6. **Ulcerative colitis—The following is seen on barium enema:**
   a. Loss of haustrations
   b. Thumb print sign
   c. Stricture in colon
   d. Apple core appearance
7. **Lucid interval in head injury is due to injury of:**
   a. Middle meningeal artery
   b. Cortical veins tear
   c. Berry aneurysm rupture
   d. Vertebral artery injury
8. **Child need circumcision in:**
   a. Epispadias
   b. Phimosis

c. Hypospadias
d. All the above

9. H.Pylori screening before gastroscopy:
a. Urea breath test
b. Rapid urease
c. Elisa
d. Culture

10. Keratoacanthoma-False statement is:
a. Premalignant skin lesion
b. Has central Crater
c. MC site is Face
d. Asymmetrical lesion

11. Sebaceous cyst-MC site:
a. Scalp
b. Palms
c. Back
d. Extremities

12. Bladder malignancy which is common in smokers:
a. Transitional cell ca
b. Squamous cell ca
c. Adenocarcinoma
d. Papillary

13. Fluctuant well localized breast mass in peri menopausal lady is due to:
a. Breast cyst
b. Breast fibroadenoma
c. Cancer
d. Duct ectasia

14. Investigation in PVD or DVT:
a. Arteriography
b. Duplex scan
c. Hand held Doppler
d. Venography

15. MC complication of subclavian vein cannulation:
a. Injury to pleura
b. Injury to Subclavian artery
c. Shock
d. Fracture cervical spine

16. Right shoulder pain+ fever following duodenal ulcer repair on 3rd Postoperative day is due to:
a. Pleural affusion
b. Subphrenic abscess
c. Diaphragm injury
d. Phrenic nerve injury

17. Modified Astler Coller Staging in Ca colon–node Positive with invasion of tumor to adjacent organ is called:
a. B1
b. B2
c. C1
d. C2

18. Male with multiple soft non fixed swellings over body and positive family history:
a. Dercums disease
b. WEN
c. Muir torre syndrome
d. Piere robbin

ANSWERS AND EXPLANATIONS

1. Ans. b. Fissure in ano *Ref: Bailey and Love p1249*

- Fissure in ano is characterised by Perianal pain, Bleeding Per rectum and pain during defecation associated with Constipation.
- MC site of Fissure in Posterior position in anal orifice, Anterior fissure is MC in women.
- Multiple fissures–Think of Crohns disease
- Per rectal examination is contraindicated in Acute fissure.
- Sentinel Tags are seen in Chronic Fissure
- The Best surgical treatment is Lateral Sphinterotomy in which internal sphincter is cut partially.

2. Ans. a. Colon Cancer *Ref: B and L-26/e p1164*

Tumors of the left side of the colon which are far more common usually present with a change in bowel habit or rectal bleeding, while more proximal lesions typically present later with iron deficiency anemia or a mass.

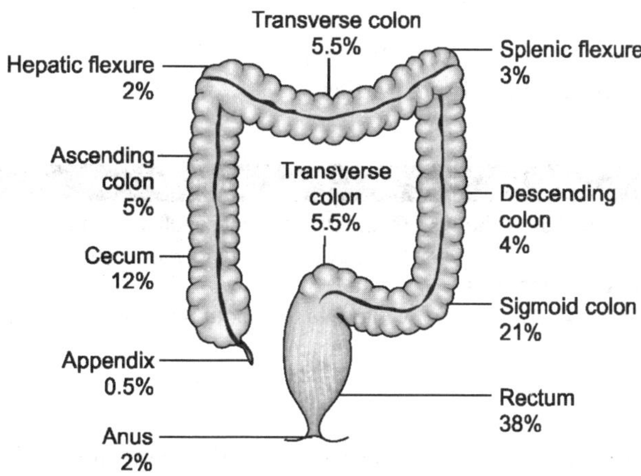

Fig. 12.8: Site of colonic cancer-relative incidence

3. **Ans. b. Acute Pancreatitis (Discussed in Theory)**
   - Periumbilical pigmentation in Acute Pancreatitis-Cullen Sign
   - Flank Discoloration in Acute hemorrhagic pancreatitis-Grey Turner's Sign
4. **Ans. a. Bulbar Urethra** *Ref: B and L 26/e p1361*
   - There is a history of a blow to the perineum, usually due to a fall astride injury/Straddle injury/Cycle bar/Manhole injuries
   - The bulbar urethra is crushed upwards onto the pubic bone, typically with significant bruising.
   - Extravasated urine collects in the scrotum and penis and beneath the deep layer of superficial fascia in the abdominal wall.
   - The signs of a ruptured bulbar urethra are perineal bruising and haematoma, typically with a butterfly distribution.
   - There is usually bleeding from the urethral meatus and retention of urine is also typically present.
   - The optimal treatment is delayed anastomotic urethroplasty after the swelling and bruising have settled down (typically 8–12 weeks later), with excision of the traumatised section and spatulated end-to-end reanastomosis of the urethra.
5. **Ans. b. Papillary Carcinoma (Explained in Theory)**
   - FNAC cannot differentiate between Follicular adenoma and Carcinoma
   - FNAC shows typical Orphan Annie eyed nuclei, Psammoma bodies in papillary carcinoma
   - FNAC must not be done in suspected Carotid Body tumor.
   - FNAC cannot collect representative tissue in anaplastic carcinoma
6. **Answer. a. Loss of Haustrations** *Ref: B and L-26/e p1147*
   - Loss of haustrations is a classic feature of Ulcerative colitis which is seen as LEAD PIPE or HOSE PIPE appearance in X-ray.
7. **Ans. a. Middle meningeal Artery injury** *Ref: B and L /23/e p315*

   Extradural hemorrhage:
   - Typically, it is damage to the middle meningeal artery under the thin temporal bone.
   - A low energy injury mechanism, perhaps with brief loss of consciousness, is sufficient to start the extradural bleeding. The patient may then present in the subsequent lucid interval with headache, but without any neurological deficit. At this stage, the increase in the intracranial volume is not yet causing a significant rise in intracranial pressure because compensation is occurring. However, once the limits of compensation have been reached after as long as some hours (as per Monro Kellie doctrine) rapid deterioration follows.
   - There is contralateral hemiparesis, reduced conscious level and ipsilate al pupillary dilatation, the cardinal signs of brain compression and herniation. Although this classical presentation occurs in only one third of cases, it emphasises the potential for rapid avoidable secondary brain injury in patients with minimal primary injury.

8. Ans. b. Phimosis
- Circumcision is the treatment of choice in Phimosis.
- Circumcision is Contraindicated in Hypospadias

9. Ans. c. ELISA *Ref: Schwartz 10/e p1051*

Noninvasive	Invasive
• **Serology: ELISA-test of choice for initial diagnosis*** • **Urea breath test: (C13 and C 14) method of choice to document eradication**	• Rapid urease test-result in hours • Histology by staining with silver, giemsa or genta • Culture takes about 3-5 days for result.

10. d. Asymmetrical lesion *Ref: Bailey 26/e p588*
- It is a premalignant lesion in Skin.
- Classically, this is a **symmetrical****, cutaneous growth with a central crater filled with a keratin plug.
- It is twice as common in men and is usually found on the face of 50–70 year olds.
- The aetiology of keratoacanthoma is unclear but may be caused by a papilloma virus in a hair follicle during the growth phase. It has also been associated with smoking and chemical carcinogen exposure.
- Keratoacanthoma can grow to between 1 and 3 cm in a 6-week period and then typically resolve spontaneously over the subsequent six months.
- Removal of the central keratin plug may speed resolution. Excision is recommended as the differential diagnosis includes anaplastic SCC and the excision scar is often better than that which remains after resolution.

11. Ans. a. Scalp *Ref: B and L 26/e p584*
- Sebaceous cyst MC in Scalp(90%) and 70 percent are multiple.
- Sebaceous cysts also known as Epidermal cysts
- Sebaceous cyst never occurs in Palms and Soles and Mucosa (as Sebaceous glands are absent in these sites)
- Sebaceous glands present abnormally in Lips is known as Fordyce disease
- Sebaceous glands present multiple in Scrotum is known as WEN
- Punctum is Pathognomonic but may be absentin 30% cases due to chronic friction
- Punctum is the site of Obstruction of Sebaceous Duct.
- Meibomian cysts are epidermal cysts found on the free edge of the eyelid. A chronic Meibomian cyst is called a chalazion.

12. Ans. a. Transitional cell Cancer *Ref: Bailey and Love 26/e p1330*
- Histological types of bladder cancer include urothelial, squamous and adenocarcinoma
- Over 90 percent are urothelial (transitional Epithelium) in origin.
- Pure squamous carcinoma is uncommon (approximately 5 percent)
- Primary adenocarcinoma, which arises either from the urachal remnant or from areas of glandular metaplasia, accounts for 1–2 percent of cases.

Etiological Factors:
- Cigarette smoking is the main aetiological factor (40 percent of cancers). Occupational exposure to dyes is the other important risk factor
- Schistosomiasis and Stones predisposes to Squamous cell cancer.

13. Ans. a. Breast Cyst *Ref: B and L 26/e p807*
- These occur most commonly in the last decade of reproductive life** as a result of a non-integrated involution of stroma and epithelium.
- They are often multiple, may be bilateral and can mimic malignancy. Diagnosis can be confirmed by aspiration and/or ultrasound.
- They typically present suddenly and cause great alarm; prompt diagnosis and drainage provides immediate relief.

- A solitary cyst or small collection of cysts can be aspirated. If they resolve completely, and if the fluid is not blood-stained, no further treatment is required. However, 30 percent will recur and require reaspiration.
- If there is a residual lump or if the fluid is blood-stained, a core biopsy or local excision for histological diagnosis is advisable, which is also the case if the cyst reforms repeatedly. This will exclude cystadenocarcinoma, which is more common in elderly women.

14. Ans. b. Duplex Scan *Ref: B and L 26/e p881*

- The best Noninvasive investigation to diagnose Deep vein thrombosis and also Peripheral Vascular disease is Color Doppler scan. (Duplex Scan)
- It's a B–mode USG which provides images of the vessels.
- Different colours indicate changes in direction and velocity of flow with areas of high flow usually indicating a stenosis.
- In experienced hands, Duplex scanning is as accurate as angiography and has the advantages of cost-effectiveness and safety.

15. Ans. a. Injury to Pleura *Ref: 270/ B and L-26/e p270*

- Subclavian Line and Internal Jugular vein are the two commonly used Central vein access. Subclavian line approach is the best of the two.
- Hickmann Lines are Subcutaneous tunnelled Central vein catheter which helps in reducing catheter related sepsis due to repeated handling.

Complications of parenteral nutrition

- **Related to nutrient deficiency:**
  - Hypoglycemia
  - **Hypocalcemia/hypophosphatemia/hypomagnesemia**** (refeeding syndrome)
  - Chronic deficiency syndromes (essential fatty acids, zinc, mineral and trace elements)
- **Related to overfeeding:**
  - **Excess glucose**: Hyperglycemia, hyperosmolar dehydration, hepatic steatosis, hypercapnia, increased sympathetic activity, fluid retention, electrolyte abnormalities
  - **Excess fat**: Hypercholesterolemia and formation of lipoprotein X, hypertriglyceridaemia, hypersensitivity reactions
  - **Excess amino acids:** Hyperchloremic metabolic acidosis, hypercalcemia, aminoacidemia, uremia.
- **Related to sepsis**
  - Catheter-related sepsis
  - Possible increased predisposition to systemic sepsis
- **Related to line**
  - **On insertion**: pneumothorax, damage to adjacent artery, air embolism, thoracic duct damage, cardiac perforation or tamponade, pleural effusion, hydromediastinum
  - **Long-term use**: occlusion, venous thrombosis.

16. Ans. b. Subphrenic abscess *Ref: B and L 26/e p978*

Right Subphrenic Abscess:

- There is sometimes epigastric fullness and pain, or pain in the shoulder on the affected side due to irritation of sensory fibres in the phrenic nerve, this being referred along the
- descending branches of the cervical plexus. Persistent hiccoughs may be a presenting symptom. A swinging pyrexia is usually present.
- This space lies between the right lobe of the liver and the diaphragm.

17. Ans. d. C2

Though there were lots of named Colonic Cancer staging used... All are replaced by only TNM staging now.. For exam point of view we still read those outdated stagings.

Dukes	AC	MAC	Description
A	A	A	Limited to mucosa, N0
	B1	B1	Penetration into Submucosa, not through Muscularis propria, N0
B	B2	B2	Penetration through Muscularis Propria, N0
		B3	Adherence to adjacent organs, N0
C	C1	C1	N+, Limited to bowel wall(B1)
	C2	C2	N+, Penetrates through Muscularis propria (B2)
		C3	N+. Adherence to adjacent organs (B3)
D			Distant Mets

- AC–Astler Coller
- MAC–Modified Astler Coller
- N0–Node negative
- N+–Node positive
- Remember Stage C means Lymphnode involvement.

18. Ans. c. Muir Torre syndrome *Ref: Sabiston 19/e p1346*

- It's a type of HNPCC (Lynch Syndrome)
- Autosomal Dominant inheritance
- Characterised by Multiple Sebaceous Adenomas all over the body
- Strong Familial tendency is there.
- The typical skin changes found in Muir-Torre syndrome are sebaceous adenomas, sebaceous epitheliomas, sebaceous carcinomas, and keratocanthomas.
- Predisposed to all cancers as in LYNCH syndrome.

Chapter

13 Obstetrics

Anuradha Dhanasekharan

MATERNAL PELVIS AND FETAL SKULL

Maternal pelvis—3 parts—inlet
Midpelvis
Outlet

CaldwellMoloy Classification

- Gynecoid (50%)
- Anthropoid (25%)
- Android (20%)
- Platypelloid (5%)

Features	Gynecoid	Anthropoid	Android	Platypelloid
Inlet	Round	AP-oval	Triangular	Transversely oval
Sacrosciatic notch	Wide and shallow	More wide and shallow	Narrow and deep	Slightly narrow and small
Ischial spines	Not prominent	Not prominent	Prominent	Not prominent
Pubic arch	Curved	Long and curved	Long and straight	Short and curved
Subpubic angle	Wide (85°)	Slightly narrow	Narrow	Very wide (more than 90°)
Bituberous diameter	Normal	Normal or short	Short	Wide

		Gynecoid	Anthropoid	Android	Platypelloid
Inlet	Diameter of engagement	Transverse or oblique	Anteroposterior	Transverse or oblique	Transverse
	Engagement	No difficulty. Usual mechanism	No difficulty except flexion is delayed	Delayed and difficult	Difficult by exaggerated parietal presentation
Cavity	Internal rotation	Easy anterior rotation	Non-rotation common	Difficult anterior rotation. Does not occur early above the ischial spines, chance of arrest deep transverse arrest	Anterior rotation usually occurs late.
Outlet	Delivery	No difficulty	More incidence of face-to-pubis delivery	Difficult delivery with increased chance of perineal injuries	No difficulty

Anteroposterior diameters/conjugates of the inlet

Anatomical conjugate-A	11 cm
Obstetrical conjugate-O	10 cm
Diagonal conjugate-D	12 cm

Obstetrical conjugate = Diagonal conjugate-2 cm

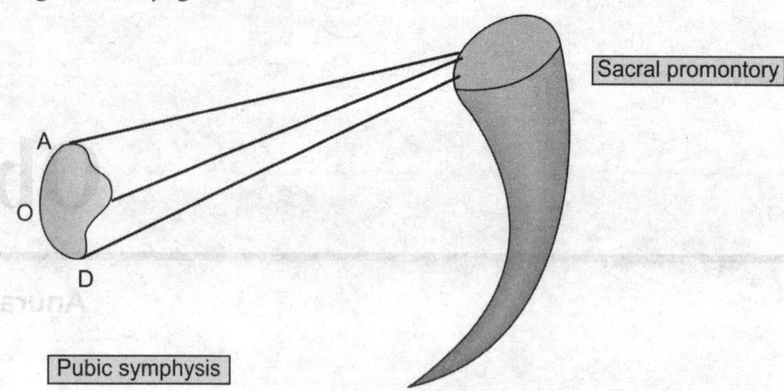

Fig. 13.1: Anteroposterior diameters/conjugates of the inlet

Fetal Skull

Engaging diameters of the fetal skull with respect to various presentations

Diameter	From	To	Measurement	Attitude of the head	Presentation
Suboccipito-bregmatic	Nape of the neck	Center of the bregma	9.5 cm	Complete flexion	Vertex
Suboccipito frontal	Nape of the neck	Anterior end of the anterior fontanelle or center of the sinciput	10 cm	Incomplete flexion	Vertex
Occipito frontal	Occipital eminence	Root of the nose (Glabella)	11.5 cm	Marked deflexion	Vertex
Mento vertical	Midpoint of the chin	Highest point on the sagittal suture	14 cm	Partial extension	Brow
Submentovertical	Junction of the floor of the mouth and neck	Highest point on the sagittal suture	11.5 cm	Incomplete extension	Face
Submentobregmatic	Junction of the floor of the mouth and neck	Center of the bregma	9.5 cm	Complete extension	Face

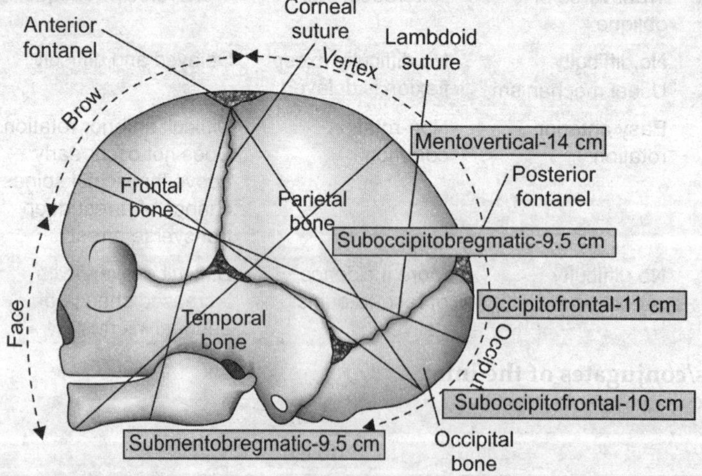

Fig. 13.2: Fetal Skull

Transverse diameters of the fetal skull

Diameter	Extent	Measurement	Remarks
Biparietal	Between two parietal eminences	9.5 cm	In whatever be the position of the head, this diameter nearly always engages
Bitemporal	Between the anteroinferior ends of the coronal suture.	8 cm	
Bimastoid	Between the tip of two mastoid processes.	7.5 cm	Incompressible diameter, impossible to reduce the length of the diameter by obstetrical operations.

Methods to Assess CPD

Munro Kerr-Muller Method

Bimanual method

- Vaginal fingers introduced to the level of ischial spine to know the descent of head
- Abdomen palpation done
- Pelvic assessment done elaborately
- Better than abdominal method

Ian Donald Method

- In dorsal position
- Left hand catches the fetal head and pushes the fetus into the pelvis
- The index and middle fingers of right hand placed over the pubic symphysis
- Inference obtained of how much head pushed into the pelvis

PHYSIOLOGICAL CHANGES IN VARIOUS SYSTEMS DURING PREGNANCY

CVS	RS	Hematological
Increased – CO – HR – Stroke volume – Blood flow Decreased – PVR – Pulmonary VR	Increased – TV – Minute ventilation – Conductance Unchanged – Respiratory vital capacity – Maximum breathing capacity Decreased – TLC – Residual volume – FRC	Increased – Blood volume – Red cell mass – Plasma volume – Hemoglobin mass – Plasma transferrin – **TIBC** – **Fibrinogen** Decreased – Viscosity – Hb concentration – Iron
Renal	**Plasma proteins**	**Nutrition**
Increased – Renal blood flow – GFR by 50% – Urea clearance – Uric acid clearance – Creatinine clearance	Increased – Alpha globulin Decreased – Albumin – A : G ratio Total plasma protein increases but due to hemoconcentration, plasma protein concentration decreases	Increased – Lipids – Triglycerides – Phospholipids – Calorie requirement – Protein requirement – Requirement of folate, Mg, iron, vitamins- A and C

Changes in the Blood

	Nonpregnant	Pregnancy near term	Total increment	Change
Blood volume (ml)	4000	5500	1500	+30–40%
Plasma volume (ml)	2500	3750	1250	+40–50%
RBC volume (ml)	1400	1750	350	+20–30%
Total Hb (gm)	475	560	85	+18–20%
Hematocrit	38%	32%		Diminished

Endocrine Changes in Pregnancy

Pituitary	Thyroid	Adrenal cortex	Pancreas
Increased – GH – Prolactin – ACTH, CRH – Size of gland	Increased – Size – Thyroxine-binding globulin – Total T3 and T4 – BMR	Increased – Aldosterone – Deoxycortisone – Corticosteroid Binding globulin – Cortisol – Testosterone – Androstenedione	Increased – Insulin resistance leads to hyperinsulinemia
Decreased – FSH – LH	Decreased – iodine	Decreased – DHEAS	
Unchanged – TSH	Unchanged – Free T3 and T4 – Euthyroid patient		

Physiological Changes in the Vagina

- Increased vascularity and hyperemia
- Mucosal thickness and smooth muscle hypertrophy of vaginal wall
- Vaginal pH decreases. Acidic–3.5–6
- **Increase in lactobacilli acidophilus** which acts on glycogen and causes increased production of lactic acid, thereby acidic environment
- **As pH becomes acidic, it inhibits growth of other bacteria**

NORMAL LABOR

Stages of labor

- **First stage (cervical stage)**–onset of true labor pain and ends with full dilatation of cervix (12 hours in primi and 6 hours in multi)
- **Second stage**–starts from full dilatation of cervix and ends with expulsion of fetus (2 hours in primi and 30 minutes in multi)
- **Third stage**–expulsion of fetus to expulsion of placenta (15 minutes in primi and multi)
- **Fourth stage**–one hour postexpulsion.

Mechanism of labor in occipitolateral position.

Diameter of engagement: available transverse diameter of the inlet.

Engaging diameter of the head: Suboccipitobregmatic (9.5 cm Suboccipitofrontal 10 cm).

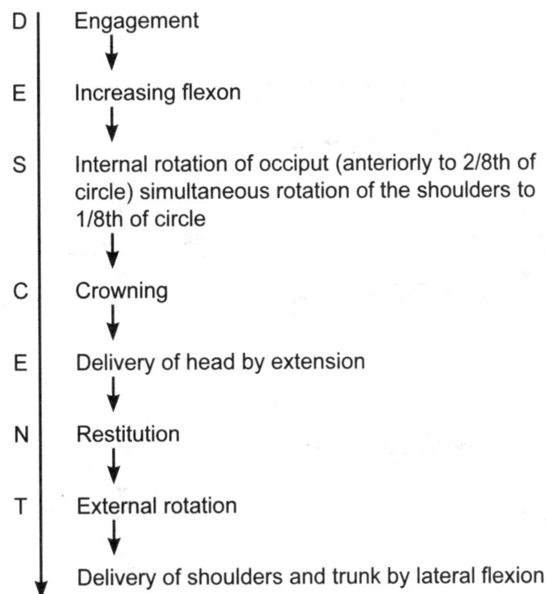

Fig. 13.3: Mechanism of Labor

Engagement

- The entry of greatest **transverse diameter** of presenting part into the pelvis.
- Biparietal diameter in cephalic presentation.

Bishop's Scoring

- Quantitative method for prediction of successful induction of labor.
- It includes the following five parameters:
  - Cervix 4-dilatation, position, effacement and consistency.
  - Fetal head station.

Bishop scoring

Score	Dilatation (cm)	Efface (%)	Station	Cervical consistency	Position
0	Close	0–30%	–3	Firm	Posterior
1	1–2	40–50%	–2	Medium	Mid
2	3–4	60–70%	–1, 0	Soft	Anterior
3	>5	>80%	+1, +2	–	–

Modified Bishop's score-effacement = instead of %, length is used, i.e., 3 cm–score is 0, 2 cm–1, 1 cm–2, 0 cm–3.

Favorable score—6–13

Unfavorable score—0–5

Components of partogram

- Best parameters for assessing progress are cervical dilatation and descent of head— they are plotted on Y–axis.
- Time in hours—X–axis.

WHO modifications of the partograph are:

- No latent phase
- Active phase starts from 4 cm dilatation

Management of Third Stage of Labor

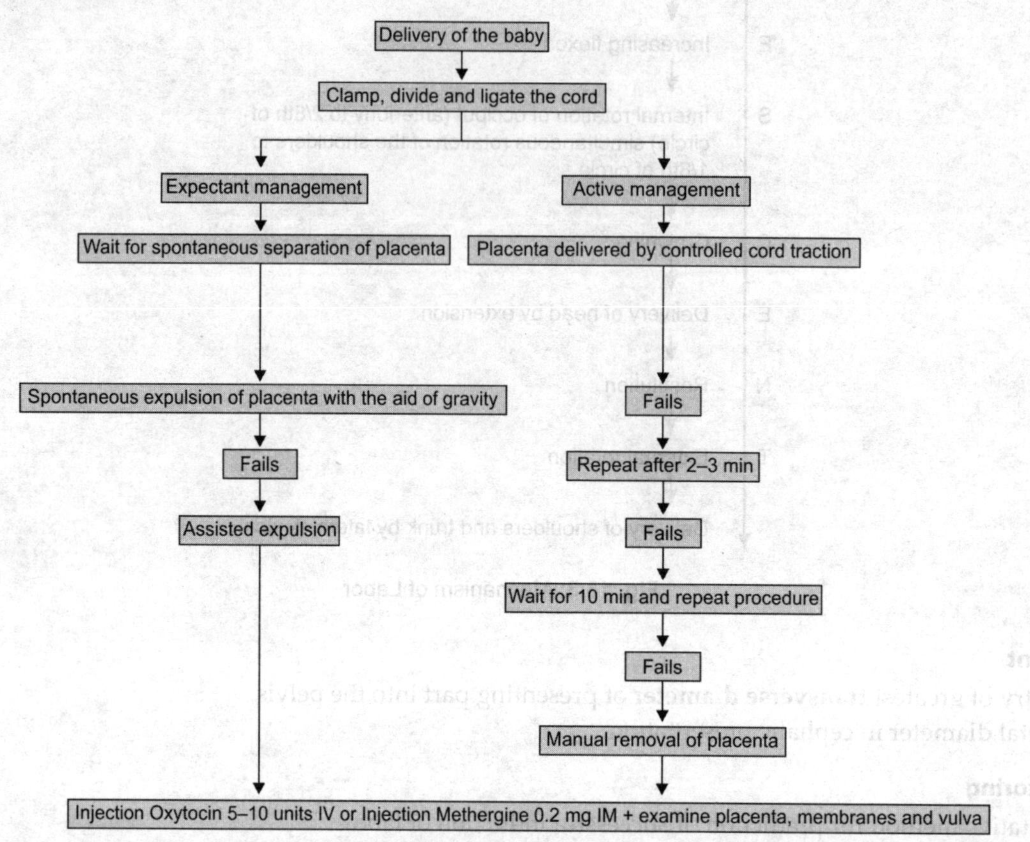

Fig. 13.4: Management of 3rd Stage of Labor

ABNORMAL PRESENTATIONS

Occipitoposterior Presentation

- **Occiput**-placed over sacroiliac joint/directly over the sacrum
- Right OP is 5 times more common than the left OP
- Associated with anthropoid/android pelvis.

Mechanism of Labor

Diameter of engagement—right or left oblique diameter of the inlet

Engaging diameter—sub—occipitofrontal (10 cm)

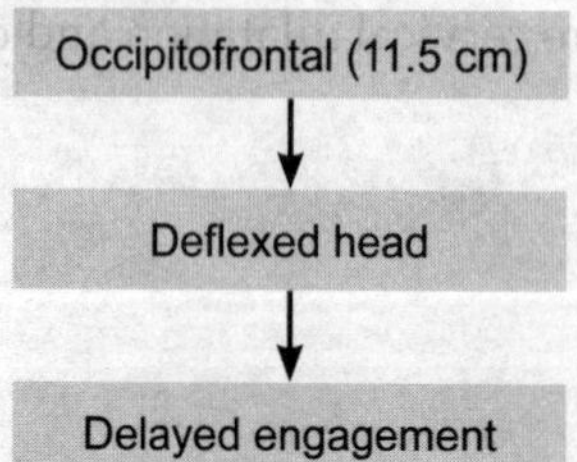

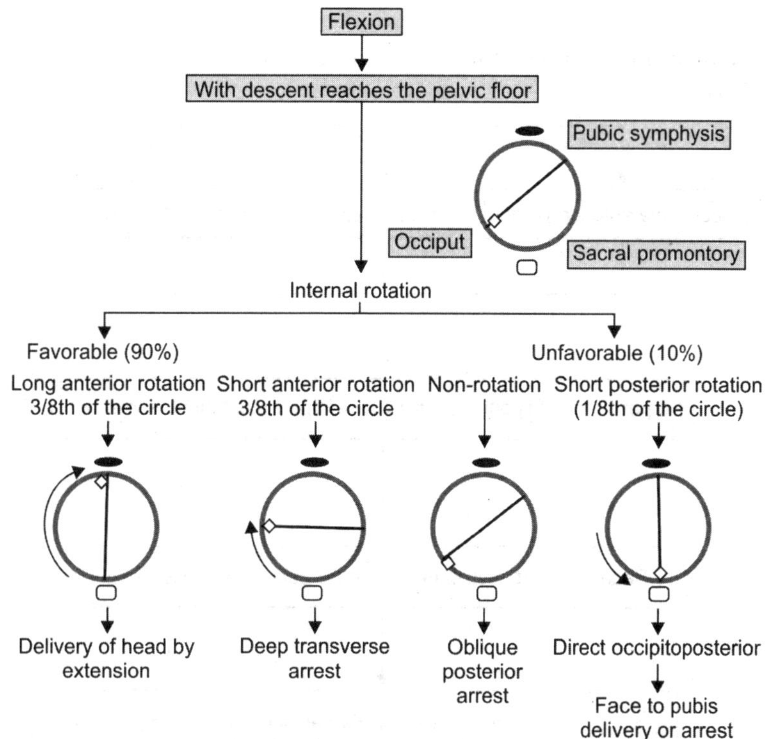

Fig. 13.5: Mechanism of Labor

Brow Presentation

Diameter of engagement—oblique diameter of the inlet
Engaging diameter—Mentovertical (14 cm).
No mechanism of labor in an average sized baby with normal pelvis.
Exception: Small baby, roomy pelvis and mentoanterior brow.

- Mechanism of labor in such cases is similar to face presentation.
- No mechanism is posterior brow presentation.

Management-cesarean section.

Face Presentation

Attitude of the head—complete extension
Denominator—Mentum
Commonest position—left mento—anterior
Diameter of engagement—oblique diameter of the inlet
Engaging diameter—Sub—mento bregmatic (9.5 cm).

Mechanism of Labor (LMA)

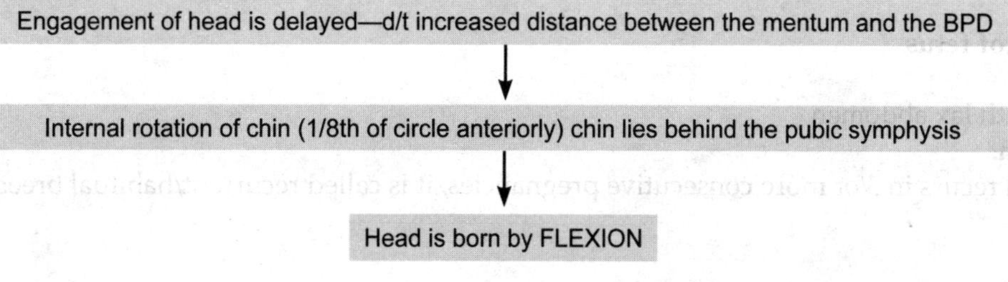

In Mento-posterior:

- Anterior rotation of the mentum occurs in only 20–30% of the cases
- In the remaining 70–80%

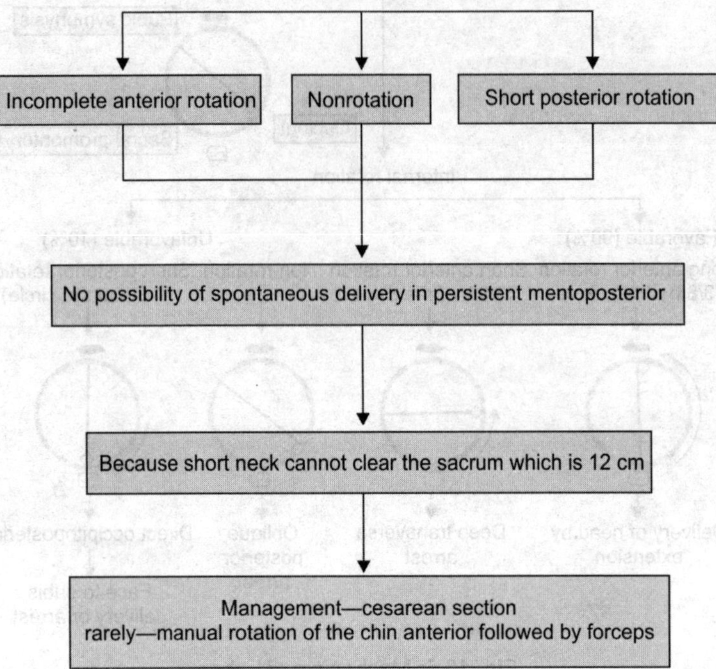

Fig. 13.6: Management of Mentoposterior Presentation

Breech Presentation

Causes for breech:

- m/c cause is prematurity
- Anomalies of uterus (septate/bicornuate)
- Anomalies of fetus (trisomy 13, 18, 21)
- Short cord
- Intrauterine death
- Breech with extended legs
- Oligohydramnios
- Twins.

Other causes

Favorable adaptation:

- Hydrocephalus
- Placenta previa
- Cornufundal attachment of placenta
- CPD

Undue mobility of fetus

- Hydramnios
- Multipara with lax abdomen

Recurrent breech:

- When breech recurs in 3 or more consecutive pregnancies, it is called recurrent/habitual breech

Etiology:

- Congenital malformation of uterus
- Repeated cornufundal attachment of placenta

Types of breech

Complete breech	Incomplete breech
The normal attitude of full flexion is maintained	**Types:** **Frank**–thighs are flexed on trunk but legs are extended at knee. **Footling**–both thighs and legs are partially extended, bringing the legs to pelvic brim **Knee**–thighs extended bringing knees down to pelvic brim.

Engaging diameter

- Breech- bitrochanteric (10 cm)
- Shoulder- bisacromial (12 cm)

Examination of a breech

Type	m/c in	P/V
Flexed breech	Multipara	Ischial tuberosities, sacrum, anus and feet.
Extended breech	Primi	Buttocks with genitalia, feet are not felt
Footling presentation		Feet are presenting

Management of breech

External cephalic version:

- Done after completing 35 weeks
- Ideal time 36 weeks.

Contraindications for ECV

- APH
- Preeclampsia
- Multiple pregnancy
- Obesity
- BOH
- Elderly primigravida
- Ruptured membranes
- Oligohydramnios
- CPD
- Congenital anomalies of uterus
- Significant fetal anomalies/dead fetus
- IUGR.

Indications for elective LSCS (>38 weeks)

- Fetal weight <1500 or >3500 gm
- All complicated pregnancies like APH, oligohydramnios, fetal distres, CPD
- If breech has hyperextended head **(star-gazing sign)**, footling, knee, complete breech
- Previous LSCS.

Assisted breech delivery

Delivery of head:

- Burns Marshall method,
- Mauriceau Smellie Veit method,
- Piper's forceps

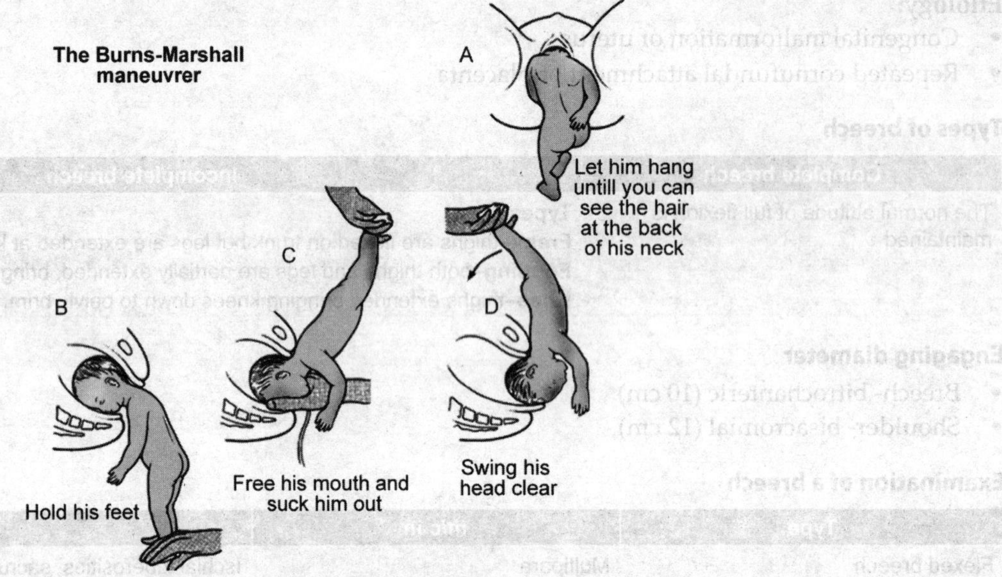

Fig. 13.7: Burns Marshall Technique

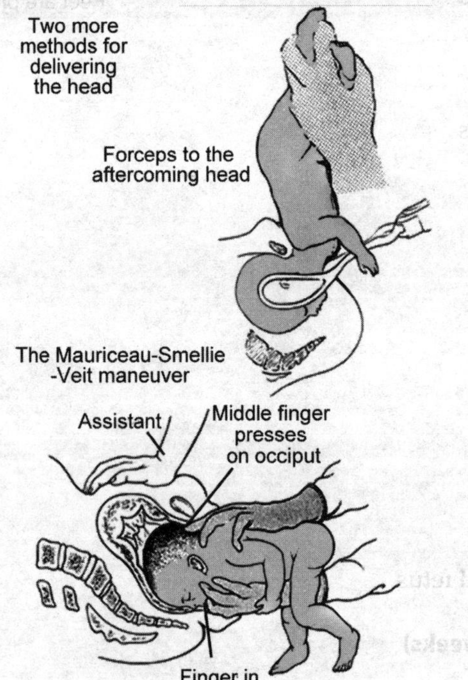

Fig. 13.8: Mauriceau Smellie Veit

- Extended legs—Pinard's maneuver
- Extended arm—Lovset's maneuver

Transverse Lie

ECV should be done in all cases beyond 35 weeks, provided there is no CI. If lie fails to stabilize at 36 weeks, then do it again at early labor after 37 weeks followed by ARM and vaginal delivery.

Early labor	Late labor
ECV–if there is enough amount of liquor; must be tried in all cases. LSCS–if version fails or is contra indicated Baby dead–destructive operation	Baby alive–LSCS

No mechanism of labor in transverse lie.

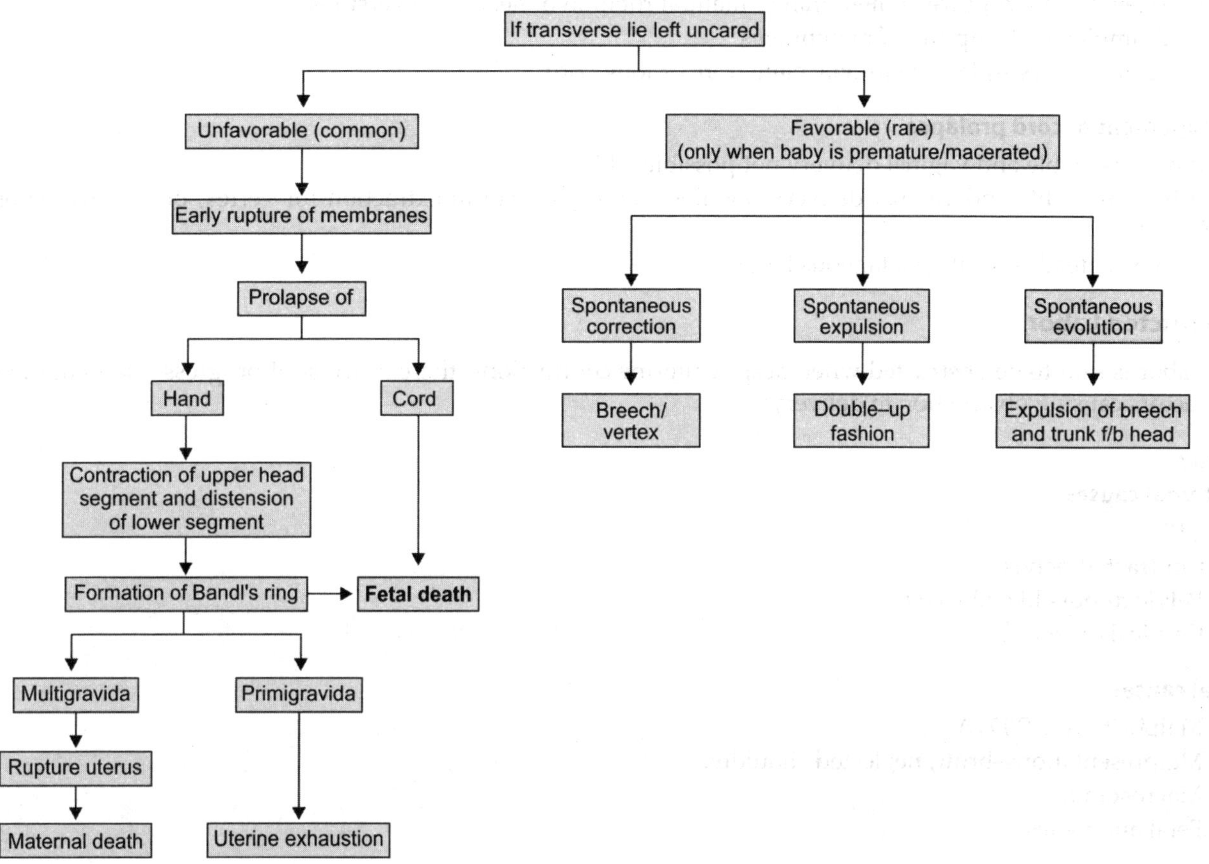

Fig. 13.9: Transverse Lie

Compound Presentation

When cephalic presentation is complicated by the presence of a hand or a foot or both alongside the head or presence of one or both hands by the side of the breech, it is called compound presentation.

Commonest one–head with hand.

Rarest one–head with hand and foot.

Management

Mature fetus with contracted pelvis/cord prolapsed-delivered by cesarean section.

Expectant treatment–elevation of the prolapsed limb with descent of the presenting part takes place spontaneously.

Cord Prolapse

- **Cord prolapse**—condition where umbilical cord lies below the presenting part after rupture of membranes.
- **Cord presentation**—membranes intact.

Causes of cord prolapse

- Malpresentations—more common in transverse lie followed by (flexed or complete breech> footling> frank breech)
- Twins
- Prematurity
- Contracted pelvis
- Iatrogenic—low rupture of membranes, manual rotation of head with versions.
- Hydramnios with rupture of membranes
- Placental factors—placenta previa, battledore or long cord.

Management of cord prolapse

- If baby is viable and vaginal delivery not possible—LSCS
- If baby is viable and vaginal delivery possible—Forceps/vacuum extraction for vertex, breech extraction for breech.
- If baby is dead—await spontaneous labor.

Obstructed Labor

- Labor is said to be obstructed when despite uterine contractions, there is arrest of progress due to mechanical factors causing obstruction to delivery.

Causes

Maternal causes

- CPD
- Contracted pelvis
- Pelvic tumors like fibroids
- Cervical dystocia.

Fetal causes

- Malposition–OP/DTA
- Malpresentations–brow, neglected shoulder
- Macrosomia
- Fetal anomalies.

On examination

On abdomen

- Uterus tonically contracted
- Difficult to palpate the fetus
- Bandl's ring
- Sharp demarcation between upper and lower segments
- Fetal distress.

On P/V

- Vagina is hot/dry
- Cervix is fully dilated
- Membranes absent
- Presenting part jammed in pelvis.

Treatment for obstructed labor

- Fetus alive–immediate LSCS
- Fetus dead–modern days LSCS, in olden days, they did destructive procedures.
- At LSCS–we can look for rupture uterus.

Bandl's ring

Also called pathological retraction ring.

- The thick and shorter upper segment and thinn and stretched lower segment are demarcated by the ring-Bandl's ring.
- It runs obliquely and is always at the junction between the two segments.

DD between

Nature	Constriction ring Schroeder's ring	Retraction ring Bandl's ring
Nature	Manifestation of localized incordinate uterine contracton due to uterine irritability	End state of tonic uterine contraction and relaxation due to obstructed labor
Situation	m/c between US/LS junction. But may be anywhere	Always between US/LS junction
	Once formed it won't move	Progressively moves upward
Uterus	US–contracts and retracts with relaxation in between	US–tonically contracted, no relaxation
	LS–thick and loose	LS–thinned and distended
Maternal	Unaffected	Exhausted and sepsis seen

Rupture Uterus

Incidence of scar rupture

- Classical cesarean section — 4–9%
- T-shaped incision — 4–9%
- Low vertical–1–7%
- Low transverse (LSCS) — 0.2–1.5%
- In 1/3rd cases of classical CS scar, rupture occurs before labor. Spontaneous rupture at pregnancy in the upper segment of the uterus.

Features of impending rupture

- Abdominal pain
- Slight vaginal bleeding
- Maternal tachycardia
- Falling BP
- Fetal distress/absent FHS–passage of meconium
- Tenderness on uterine palpation and ballooning of LUS
- Bladder tenesmus–desire to micturate frequently.

Features of ruptures uterus

- Sense of something giving away
- Collapse, shock, dehydration
- Absent FHS
- Palpation of fetal parts superficially
- *Shortening of cord immediately after delivery is pathognomonic of uterine rupture*
- Hematuria due to bladder rupture.

Scar rupture/dehiscence

- **Scar rupture** refers to separation of old uterine incision throughout most of its length with rupture of fetal membranes. Resulting in communicating uterine and peritoneal cavity.
- **Scar dehiscence** refers to the separation which does not involve the whole of the previous uterine scar. The peritoneum overlying is intact, fetal membrane has not ruptured. It precedes the scar rupture.

- Hematuria is not a sign of scar dehiscence/impending rupture.
- But it is a sign of ruptured uterus.

	Features	Constriction ring	Retraction ring
P/A	Uterus	Firm/non tender	Tense and tender
	Fetal parts	Easily felt	Not felt
	Ring	Not felt	Felt
	Round ligament	Not felt	Felt
	FH	+	Absent
P/V	Ring	Felt	Not felt
	Obstructed labor features	Absent	Present
End	Maternal/fetal	Maternal exhaustion/fetal distress are late	Early features
	Uterus	No chance of uterine rupture	Uterine rupture at lower segment
	Treatment principle	To relax the ring followed by delivery of baby To cut the ring during LSCS	To relieve the obstruction

CONDITIONS COMPLICATING PREGNANCY AND DELIVERY

Antepartum Hemorrhage

Causes for APH

APH is defined as bleeding from or into genital tract after 28th week of pregnancy but before the birth of baby. (1st and 2nd stage labor included)

- Placenta previa
- Abruptioplacenta
- Local causes—cancer cervix, polyp, varicose veins, trauma
- Circumvalate papilla
- Vasa previa—velamentous insertion of placenta
- Unclassified.

Placenta Previa

Implantation of the placenta partially or completely in the lower uterine segment

Risk factors:

- Prior surgery–LSCS
- Previous curettage
- Endometritis
- Increased maternal age (>35 years)
- Increased parity
- Placental size increased (twins)
- Placental anomaly (succenturiate).

Degrees of placenta previa (Browne's):

Type 1. (Low-lying)—Major part of placenta is attached to upper segment and only the lower margin encloses onto lower segment. But not upto os.

Type 2. (Marginal)—Placenta reaches to the margin but not covers the os.

Type 3. (Incomplete or partial central)—Covers the internal os when closed, but not so when fully dilated.

Type 4. (Central or total)—Placenta completely covers the internal os even on full dilatation.

Grading of placenta previa

Mild—type 1 and type 2 anterior

Major—type 2 posterior and type 3 and type 4

Anterior and posterior based on the wall it lies.

Posterior is m/c

Dangerous placenta previa–type 2 posterior:

- It overlies sacral promontory and diminishes AP diameter of inlet and, hence engagement of presenting part.
- Placenta more likely to be compressed if vaginal delivery allowed.
- Cord compression and cord prolapse occur.
- Leads to fetal anoxia and death.

Spontaneous control occurs by:

- Thrombosis of open sinuses.
- Mechanical pressure of presenting part.
- Placental infarction.

Symptoms

Sudden onset of painless vaginal bleeding, causeless and recurrent.

First bout of bleeding will not be so major but may be heavier in subsequent conditions.

On examination:

- Uterus is of size corresponding to GA
- No localized tenderness in uterus
- Persistence of malpresentation like breech or transverse or unstable lie
- Floating head and cannot be pushed into pelvis
- FHS–present
- Stallworthy's sign–slowing of FH rate on pressing the head into pelvis which recovers on releasing
- Vulval examination–shows bright red blood
- No vaginal examination to be done. Can do only in OT.

Complications of placenta previa

Maternal:

- Bleeding with varying degrees of shock
- Malpresentation
- Premature labor
- Early rupture of membranes
- Cord prolapse
- Slow dilatation
- Postpartum hemorrhage-imperfect retraction of lower segment, associated with adherent placenta
- Retained placenta
- Puerperal sepsis, subinvolution and embolism

Fetal

- Low birthweight
- Asphyxia
- Intrauterine death
- Birth injuries
- Congenital malformation

Expectant management

- No active bleeding
- Pregnancy <37 weeks
- Patient hemodynamically stable
- FHS–good
- CTG–reactive fetus.

Active interference

- Bleeding continues
- Pregnancy >37 weeks
- Patient in labor
- Exsanguinated
- FHS–absent
- Gross fetal malformation
- Steroid therapy (if duration of pregnancy <34 weeks)

Cesarean section

- Type 2 (posterior)
- Type 3
- Type 4
- Lesser degree of placenta previa where amniotomy fails to stop bleeding or fetal distress appears
- Complicating factors with lesser degrees of placenta previa where vaginal delivery is unsafe.

Types of placenta previa and management

- Type 1, 2 (anterior)–Artificial rupture of membrane +/– oxytocin
  - Bleeding continues–cesarean section.
- Type 3 (posterior), 3, 4–LSCS.

Management

Between 32–36 weeks if lung maturity is not yet obtained:

- Blood trasfusion
- Close monitoring
- Betamethasone–to accelerate lung maturity.

Done for 24–48 hours.

If it impoves-expectant treatment.

If not-terminate pregnancy.

Vasa previa

- **Velamentous insertion**–the cord inserts into the membranes at some distance from the placenta.
- Fetal vessels traverse the membrane, hence can rupture and result in vasa previa—fetal hypoxia.
- Causes rupture of fetal blood vessels.
- Remember the bleeding is of fetal origin.

To detect fetal blood

- **Wright's stain**
- **Singer's alkali denaturation test**

On Wright's stain-Fetal RBCs appear nucleated.

On Singer's alkali denaturation test-fetal HB is more resistant to denaturation.

Abruptioplacenta (premature separation of placenta)

It is one form of antepartum hemorrhage where bleeding occurs due to premature separation of normally situated placenta.

Varieties

- Revealed–m/c type
- Concealed
- Mixed.

Etiology

- High birth order pregnancy > gravida 5 and above.
- Malnutrition, smoking, previous abruptio placenta, cocaine abuse
- Hypertension in pregnancy is m/c risk factor
  - Preeclampsia, gestational hypertension and essential hypertension
- Trauma–ECV, RTA or needle puncture at amniocentesis
- Sudden uterine decompression-following delivery of first twin, liquor in polyhydramnios and PROM
- Short cord
- Folic acid deficiency
- Thrombophilia
- Supine hypotension syndrome.

Pathogenesis–premature separation of placenta in initiated by hemorrhage into decidua basalis.

The blood can collect in any of the below sites:

- Retroplacental hematoma-depression found on maternal surface of placenta
- Complete accumulation behind the placenta.
- Blood may dissect downward and escape out
- May rupture into amniotic cavity.

Couvelaire uterus

(Uteroplacental apoplexy)

- Massive extravasation of blood into uterine musculature
- Can be diagnosed only by laparotomy
- The myometrial hematoma does not interfere with uterine contraction and hence it is not an indication for hysterectomy while doing LSCS.

Changes in other organs

- Liver fibrin knots in hepatic sinusoids
- Kidneys acute cortical necrosis or acute tubular necrosis shock proteinuria disappears in 2 days (not in pre-eclampsia)
- Blood coagulopathy- due to consumption of fibrinogen
  - (decreased blood fibrin < 150 mg/dl and elevated fibrin degradation products and D-dimer).

Clinical Examination

Grade 0—Clinical feature may be absent.

Grade 1—External bleeding is slight, shock is absent, FHS–good.

Grade 2—External bleeding is mild or moderate, uterine tenderness is always present, shock is absent, *fetal distress/death occurs.*

Grade 3—Bleeding is moderate to severe or may be concealed. Uterine tenderness, *shock is pronounced*, fetal death is rule, coagulation defect and anuria.

Clinical features

- m/c-vaginal bleeding (may be profuse)
- Severe and constant pain abdomen

O/E

- Pallor- signs out of proportion to bleeding.
- Uterine tenderness. (uterus may be woody hard)
- Uterus will be larger than period of gestation
- Difficult to palpate fetal parts
- Fetal distress or absent FHS
- Preterm labor/high-frequency contractions.

Treatment

'Immediate delivery'

Vaginal delivery	Cesarean section
Mild degree	Persistent fetal distress
No evidence of fetal distress	Fetus is in good condition but there is progressive placental separation
Extensive placental separation where fetus is dead	Uncontrolled hemorrhage from a contracting uterus
	Rapidly expanding uterus with concealed hemorrhage
	Uterine apoplexy
	Amniotomy could not be done or fails to control bleeding

Placenta previa (warning hemorrhage)	Abruptio placentae (accidental hemorrhage)
Painless, causeless, recurrent bleeding Fresh bleed (revealed bleeding always) May be associated with malpresentation (esp. breech) Placenta in lower segment/low-lying Diagnosis: USG Prognosis: hemorrhage is rarely fatal Feel of uterus soft and relaxed, non-tender Rx: if presents at 34 weeks–rest and sedation (Per vaginal examination is delayed up to 37 weeks to avoid premature labor) after which PV should be performed in OT–fully prepared for emergency LSCS (double set up)	Painful, continuous bleeding with toxemic features Usually concealed bleed (may be mixed) Signs of fetal distress (absent FHS & shock/hypotension or fetal demise) Placenta in upper segment. Diagnosis: clinical Bad prognosis Tender, tense, rigid Rx: if patient presents at 37 weeks: Correction of hypovolemic shock is first priority [tocolytics not used to arrest premature delivery] After giving dexamethasone, deliver the baby by induction.

Also note that if concealed variety of Abruption is noted you must transfer minimum 1 liter of blood.

Management of abruptio placenta:

Step 1: Resuscitation: Blood and ringer lactate

Step 2: Patient in labor: AROM and oxytocin

patient not in labor: > 37 weeks- induction by AROM/oxytocin

Step 3: Patient < 37 weeks:

No bleeding–reactive fetus–continue pregnancy up to 37 weeks.

Bleeding continues–ARM + oxytocin.

Postpartum Hemorrhage

Definition

Any amount of bleeding from delivery of baby to end of puerperium which adversely affects the general condition of the patient evidenced by rise in pulse rate and falling blood pressure.

Quantitatively–more than **500 ml blood loss.**

Types

Primary–bleeding occurs in < 24 hours following birth. Majorly, it is less than 2 hours.

Subtypes:

- Third stage hemorrhage–bleeding before placenta expulsion
- True postpartum hemorrhage–bleeding after placenta expulsion

Secondary–beyond 24 hours upto puerperium.

Etiology–primary PPH

- Atonic uterus (80%) *flabby uterus*
- Traumatic—genital tract injuries, rupture uterus–*firm uterus*
- Mixed
- Blood coagulopathy–DIC and hypofibrinogenemia.

Predisposing factors for atonic uterus

- Grand multipara
- Overdistension of the uterus
- Malnutrition and anemia
- Ante-partum hemorrhage
- Prolonged labor
- Deeper anesthesia and agents like ether, halothane, and cyclopropane
- Persistent uterine distension
- Malformation of the uterus
- Uterine fibroid
- Mismanaged third stage labor
- Constriction ring formation
- Precipitate labor.

Etiology–secondary PPH

Usually occurs between 8th–14th day of delivery

- Retained bits of cotyledons or membranes [commonest]
- Infections
- Endometritis and subinvolution of the placental site
- Secondary hemorrhage from the LSCS wound (10–14 days)
- Withdrawl bleeding following estrogen therapy for lactation suppression
- Chorioepithelioma, Ca. cervix, fibroids, polyps, etc.

Management-third stage bleeding

Placental site bleeding	Traumatic bleeding
• Palpate the fundus and massage the uterus • Ergometrine 0.25 mg or methergine 0.2 mg IM • Blood transfusion if necessary • Sedation with morphine IM if needed • Removal of placenta under GA, if not separated	• Exploration of the vaginal canal under GA, after placental expulsion and wound suturing.

Management of atonic uterus

Step–I

- Massage the uterus
- Injecation methergine 0.2 mg IV
- Injecation oxytocin 10 units in 500 ml NS at the rate of 40 drops/min
- Examine the expelled placenta
- Catheterize the bladder.

Step–II

- Exploration of the uterus under GA
- Blood transfusion
- If still refractory: 15 methyl PGF 2α–250 μg IM/intra myometrial or Misoprostol 800 μg per rectum.

Step–III: Uterine massage and bimanual compression.

Step–IV (Uterine tamponade)

- Uterine tamponade by a tight intrauterine packing under anesthesia (or)
- Insertion of a Sengstaken-Blakemore tube and inflation.

Step–V (Uterine devascularization procedures)

- Ligation of uterine artery-especially the ascending branch.
- Ligation of ovarian and uterine artery anastomosis.
- Ligation of anterior division of internal iliac artery.
- B-Lynch brace suture and hemostatic suturing.
- Alternative to vessel ligating technique in which the anterior and posterior walls of the uterus opposed leading to compression of fundus and lower uterine segment, thereby controlling hemorrhage.
- Angiographic arterial embolization.

Step–VI (hysterectomy)

Placenta Accreta

Morbidly adherent placenta

- Rare form where placenta is directly anchored to uterine myometrium partially or completely without any intervening decidua.

Degrees

- Placenta increta-upto muscle bundles (partial)
- Placenta percreta-upto serosal layer. (complete)

Risk factors for accreta

- Usually associated with placenta previa, previous CS, D and C, myomectomy, synechiolysis.
- Multiparity
- Advanced maternal age.

Management

Treatment

- Partial–Remove as much as possible. In multi, go for hysterectomy
- Total hysterectomy
- If invade bladder methotrexate. Do not remove placenta as it may necessitate cystectomy along with hysterectomy.

Accreta–female has not completed the family

- Conservative approach
- Cut the cord as high as possible and leave the placenta as such
- Antibiotics and methotrexate in hope of autolysis
- Beta-hCG is used to monitor those cases.

Inversion of Uterus

Uterus is turned inside out partially or completely.

Degrees

- First–dimpling of uterus, but still above internal os
- Second–fundus passes through the cervix but inside vagina
- Third–completely lies out of vagina.

Etiology and complications

Spontaneous–40% (fundal attachment of placenta, short cord, accreta, localized atony).
Iatrogenic–Credés technique, pulling the cord.

Complications

- Neurogenic shock
- Hemorrhage
- Pulmonary embolism
- Left untreated–infection, slough and chronic prolapse.

Management

- Prevention–do not employ any method of placenta removal when uterus is relaxed.
- Replace the inverted uterus, keep the hand in the uterus until it gets contracted by oxytocin/PGF2 alpha.
- Replacement can also be done by O'Sullivan's hydrostatic method.
- Failed cases–HAULTAIN'S operation-abdominal operation.

Overdistended Uterus

Large for gestational age

- **Multiple fetuses**
- Elevation of uterus with distended bladder
- Inaccurate menstrual history
- **Hydramnios**
- Hydatidiform mole
- Uterine myomas
- Closely attached adnexal masses
- Fetal macrosomia (in late gestational age).

Multiple pregnancy

Incidence
Incidence: 1 in 62 (Chennai); 1 in 80 (India).

Hellin's rule

Twins–1 in 80
Triplets–1 in 80 square [n^2]
Quadruplets–1 in 80 cube [n^3]

Highest in Nigeria:
Frequency of uniovular twins is constant throughout the world = 1/250
Types of twins

	Uniovular (identical)	Binovular (fraternal)
1. Placenta	One	Two (fused)
2. Communicating vessels	+	–
3. Intervening membrane	Two amnions and one chorion	2 amnions/2 chorions
4. Sex	**Same (always)**	**Differ (may)**
5. Genetic features (blood group)	Same	**Differ**
6. Skin graft (terminal)	Accept	Reject

Different types of twins

Depending on division of fertilized ovum

- **< 72 hours** of fertilization (3 days)–diamniotic dichorionic
- 4th–8th day–diamniotic monochorionic

- **>8 days**–monoamniotic monochorionic
- **After development of embryonic disc after 2 weeks**–conjoined (Siamese) twins.
  - Thoracophagus (m/c), pyophagus, craniophagus and ischiophagus

MCQ points

Dizygotic twins is m/c–2/3rd
Monozygotic twins 1/3rd.

After delivery

You can diagnose what type of twin it is by examining the placenta and membranes.

Dizygotic twin	Monozygotic twin
Two placentas are Completely separated	Placenta is single
Each fetus is covered by separate amnion and chorion	Each fetus is separated by separate amnion but common chorion
Intervening membrane contains 4 layers A-C-C-A	Intervening membrane contains 2 layers only A-A

Etiology for twins

- Race
- Hereditary
- Advancing age (30–35 years)
- Inversing party (> 5th para).
- Iatrogenic
- Ovulation inducing drugs
  - Clomiphene citrate
  - Gonadotropins
- Following discontinuation of OCP–within one month if she gets conception (due to increased levels of gonadotropin).

Superfecundation

- Fertilization of two separate ova by separate acts of coitus within short periods of time.

Superfetation

- Two ova released in two different menstrual cycles.

Fetus papyracus/compressus

- One fetus dies early. The dead fetus is flattened and compressed.
- m/c in monozygotic twins.

Vanishing twin

- Occasional death of one baby and continuation of pregnancy in the other.
- If death occurs in <14 weeks, the fetus completely vanishes.

Lambda or twin peak sign

- To diagnose the chorionicity of placenta USG at 6–9 weeks.
- In dichorionic twins, there will be **thick septum of 4 layers between the chorionic sacs.**
- Best seen at the base where there will be a triangular projection seen.
- This is known as lambda or twin peak sign.
- Implies there is **dichorionic placenta.**

Complications–maternal

- Nausea, vomiting
- Preeclampsia (25%) due to overdistension
  - Anemia (increased requirement by 2 fetuses)
  - Hydramnios (10%)
- Increased renal perfusion
- Increased urinary output
- Hypervolemia in larger twin
- APH: placenta previa/abruptio placenta
- Malpresentation
- Preterm labor (30%)
- Mechanical distress
- Maternal complications.

During–labor

- Early rupture of membrane and prolapse of
- Prolonged labor
- Operative interference increased
- PPH (real danger).

During puerperium

- Subinvolution
- Infection
- Failing lactation.

Fetal complications

- Increased abortion
- Prematurity (80%)
- Growth problem: discordant growth where weight difference > 25%, due to twin transfusion syndrome, IUGR, anomalies in one fetus.
- **Fetal anomalies**
  - Asphyxia and stillbirth–PIH, operative interference, abruptio placenta, malpresentations.
  - Intrauterine death of one fetus.

Twin transfusion syndrome/discordant

- Exclusively seen in monozygotic twins.
- One twin bleeds into the other via some placenta vascular anastomoses.
- Receptor twin becomes larger, hydramniotic, polycythemic, hypertensive and hypervolemic at the expense of the other.
- Difference in Hb between two exceeds 5 gm% and fetal weight discrepancy is 25% or more.

Twin reversed arterial perfusion (TRAP)

- 'Acardiac-perfused' twin having blood supply from normal co-twin via large arterio-arterial anastomosis.
- In majority, co-twin dies (in perinatal period) due to high output failure.

Management

- 1st twin cephalic–normal delivery
- 1st twin breech–cesarean section
- 2nd twin cephalic–arm ± syntocinon–deliver
- 2nd twin breech/transverse lie–ECV/IPV
  - After ECV–deliver as head
  - After IPV–deliver as breech extraction.

Multifetal pregnancy reduction

- Done in high-order pregnancy (> 4 fetus) to minimize the complications
- Done at 10–12 weeks GA
- Intracardiac injection of KCL
- Two fetuses are left undisturbed and others reduced
- Selective fetal reduction is done if one fetus is selectively abnormal.

Indication of elective cesarean section

- First twin as nonvertex (breech/transverse)
- Both twins nonvertex
- Monoamniotic twins
- Chronic twin-twin transfusion syndrome
- Conjoined twins
- Severe IUGR of one or both fetus
- Previous LSCS
- Discordant twin; weight of smaller one < 1500 gm
- Obstetric indications like CPD, placenta previa, cord prolapse.

Polyhydramnios

Volume of amniotic fluid

- 12 weeks–50 ml
- 20 weeks–400 ml
- 26–38 weeks–1 liter
- Term–600–800 ml
- Postdated–200 ml at 43 weeks
  - **Pale straw colored, 250 mosm/liter**
  - Main function is to protect the fetus.

Amniotic fluid

Theories for formation

- Transudate from maternal serum
- Transudate across umbilical cord, fetal circulation in placenta or amniotic epithelium
- Transudate from fetal skin before keratinization (20 weeks)
- Fetal urine–400–1200 ml, swallows about 200–500 ml/day at term.

Certain abnormal colors of amniotic fluid

- Golden yellow-Rh incompatibility
- Saffron (greenish yellow)–Postmaturity
- Tobacco juice–Intrauterine death.

Causes of polyhydramnios

- Incidence–0.5–1%
- Polyhydramnios is a state where liquor amnii exceeds more than 2000 ml
- U/S-AFI–> 25 cm (>95th percentile) = polyhydramnios/single vertical pocket > 8 cm.

Etiology

Fetal anomalies

Anencephaly

- Transudation from exposed meninges
- Suppression of antidiuretic hormone
- Absence of fetal swallowing.

Open spina bifida–increased transudation.
Esophageal/duodenal atresia.
Facial clefts/neck masses–decreased swallowing.
Hydrops fetalis:
Rh isoimmunization
Cardiothoracic anomalies
Fetal cirrhosis
Placenta: Chorioangioma tumor.

Multiple Pregnancy

Maternal causes

- Diabetes mellitus-increased diuresis in fetus due to increased blood sugar
- Cardiac and renal diseases-transudation from edematous placenta

Complications

Maternal

Pregnancy

- Premature rupture of membranes
- Preterm labor
- Malpresentation
- Weak uterine contractions
- Preeclampsia (25%).

Labor

- Early rupture of membranes
- Uterine inertia
- Cord prolapse
- Abruptio placenta
- PPH/shock
- Retained placenta.

Fetal

- Prematurity
- Congenital
- Cord prolapse
- Hydrops fetalis.

Treatment

- Diuretic-little value.
- **Indomethacin 25 mg** every 6 hours may decrease the amniotic fluid.
- **If unresponsive to treatment:**
  - < 37 weeks: amniocentesis at the rate of 500 ml/hour
  - > 37 weeks: high rupture of membrane using Drew Smythe catheter.

Amniocentesis

- Slow decompression at the rate of 500 ml/hour
- Maximum–1.5–2 liters
- Less than 37 weeks.

Indomethacin

- Decreases the fetal urine production leading to amelioration of symptoms.
- 1.5–3 mg/kg/day
- **Side effect**-premature closure of fetal ductus arteriosus, hence contraindicated beyond 32 weeks of GA.

OLIGO HYDRAMNIOS

Definition

Decrease of fluid < 200 ml

On USG:

- maximum vertical pocket < 2 cm
- AFI is less than 5 cm (< 10th percentile).

Etiology

- Fetal chromosomal anomalies
- Intrauterine infection
- Drugs like PG inhibitors, ACE inhibitors
- Renal agenesis or obstruction of urinary tract (PUV in males)
- IUGR associated with placental insufficiency
- Amnion nodosum—failure of secretion of amniotic fluid by cells of amnion
- Post maturity

Amnioinfusion

Technique to increase the intrauterine fluid volume with normal saline (500 ml).

Indications:

- Treatment of variable or prolonged deceleration (fetal distress)
- Oligohydramnios
- To dilute or wash out thick meconium
- PROM
- Renal agenesis.

Infused at temperature–37 degrees, 250 ml at 30 minutes, intrauterine pressure < 25 mm Hg at any time.

Hypertension in pregnancy

Causes for hypertension

- Gestational hypertension
- Preeclampsia
- Eclampsia
- Chronic hypertension
  - Essential hypertension
  - Chronic renal disease
  - Coarctation of aorta
  - Pheochromocytoma
  - Thyrotoxicosis
  - Connective tissue disorder.

Pre–eclampsia

Definition

- Multisystem disorder of unknown etiology characterized by development of hypertension to the extent of 140/90 mm Hg or more with proteinuria after 20th week in a previously normotensive and nonproteinuric patient.

In Hydatiform mole and acute polyhydramnios

- Preeclampsia feature appears before 20th week.

Incidence: **10% in primigravida** and 5% in multigravida.

Classification

Primary: 70%

- Preeclampsia
- Eclampsia (with convulsion).

Secondary: 30%

- Preeclampsia–eclampsia superimposed on chronic hypertension
- Preeclampsia–eclampsia superimposed on chronic renal disease.

Diagnostic Criteria of Preeclampsia

- **Hypertension**
  - Absolute rise of blood pressure of atleast 140/90 mm Hg.
  - Measure BP at 2 occasions atleast 6 hours apart.
  - Diastolic BP should measure disappearance of sounds (Korotkoff-V)
  - Mean arterial pressure (MAP) = SP+ (DP*2)/3;
  - A rise of 20 mm Hg MAP over previous reading or when MAP is 105 mm Hg or more should be considered significant.
- **Edema**

Physiological–disappear after rest in bed for 8–12 hours and confirmed to ankles/feet.

Pathological

- Persist even after 12 hours of bed rest,
- Present over face, hands, abdominal walls, labia
- **Weight gain**
  - Weight gain : > 0.5 kg/week is significant
  - (i.e) 1 pound/week or more than 5 pounds a month in later months of pregnancy may be the earliest evidence.
- **Proteinuria**
  - ≥ 300 mg in 24 hour's urine collection (or)
  - ≥1+ in a sample of midstream urine on dipstick
    (In the absence of urinary tract infection, it significant.)

Features of PIH.

Order of Appearance of Signs

- First–hypertension
- Second–edema (may also be first)
- Third–proteinuria

Risk factors for Preeclampsia

Maternal factors	Obstetrical factors	Medical factors	Placental factors
Nulliparous	Previous H/O preeclampsia	Chronic hypertension	Poor placentation
New paternity	Multiple pregnancy	Antiphospholipid syndrome	Placental ischemia
Age <20 years and >35 years	Hydrops fetalis with large placenta	Inherited thrombophilias (protein C,S, factor V leiden deficiency)	
Obesity	Molar pregnancy	Diabetes	
African and American ethnicity		Renal disease	
		Thyroid disease	
		Collagen vascular	

Tests predictive of PIH

- Serum uric acid is a biochemical marker of preeclampsia-value >4.5 mg/dl indicates PIH.
- Urinary calcium-preeclampsia is associated with hypocalciuria
- Angiotensin sensitivity test
- Rollover test–28–32 weeks
- Doppler velocimetry of uterine artery
- Fibronectin–elevated.

Pathology

- Deficiency of vasodilator PG I2–vasodilator
- Increased synthesis of TX A2–vasoconstrictor
- Increased vascular sensitivity to Angiotensin–II, pressor agent; which is destroyed by angiotensinase liberated from placenta
- Deficiency of nitric oxide (vasodilator)
- Inflammatory mediators–TNF alpha, Interleukin-6.
- *Finally there is endothelial damage and vasospasm*

Pathophysiology

Vasospasm leads to

- ↓ plasma volume
- ↓ GFR
- ↓ renal blood flow
- Aldosterone secretion increased
- Sodium and water retention and hence edema.

Organ Damage

Liver

- Periportal hemorrhagic necrosis
- Subcapsular hemorrhage
- Fatty degeneration of liver.

Heart

- Petechial hemorrhage
- Focal necrosis in myocardium.

Lungs

- Bronchopneumonia
- Pulmonary edema
- Organ damage.

Kidney

Glomerular endotheliosis.

Brain

- Perivascular hemorrhages
- Tissue hypoxia
- Small petechial hemorrhage
- Convulsions and coma.

Adrenal gland

- Increased secretion → deoxycortisone (DOC) in 3rd Δ

HELLP

- Rare complication on PIH
- c/o nausea, vomiting, epigastric pain, right upper quadrant pain (liver)
- Hemolysis.
- Elevated liver enzymes–↑ SGOT, SGPT
- Low platelet count (< 100,000/microliter).

Complications of PIH

Maternal			Fetal
Pregnancy	Labor	Puerperium	
– Eclampsia – Accidental hemorrhage – Oliguria and anuria – Dimness of vision Blindness – Preterm labor – HELLP syndrome	– Eclampsia – PPH	– Eclampsia – Shock – Sepsis	– IUD – IUGR – Asphyxia – Prematurity

Mild PIH	Severe PIH
BP>140/90 mm Hg Less than 160 systolic or 110 diastolic BP	BP>160 mm Hg or diastolic BP >110 mm Hg
+/– proteinuria (300 mg/24 hours urine or 1+ on dipstick)	Proteinuria >2 gm/day
	HELLP syndrome
	Retinal hemorrhages
	Visual disturbance
	Oliguria <400 ml/hr
	Pulmonary edema
	IUGR of fetus
	C/F–epigastric pain
	Serum creatinine > 1.2 mg/dl

Symptoms

- **Headache**–frontal or occipital
- **Epigastric pain/RUQ pain**–hemorrhagic gastritis or subcapsular hemorrhage in liver
- **Visual symptom**–m/c-scotoma, blindness or blurred vision
- Others–disturbed sleep, diminished urine output.

Drugs used for preeclampsia

Name	Mode of action	Side effect
Labetalol (drug of Choice)	Combined alpha + beta blocker	Postural hypertension
Hydralazine	Peripheral vasodilator	Headache, flushing, tachycardia
Nifedipine	Calcium channel blocker	Headache, flushing and palpitation
Alpha methyldopa	Central action	Postural hypotension, hemolytic anemia
Atenolol	Beta blocker	Bradycardia, hypotension, hypoglycemia

Drugs that must not be used

- ACE inhibitors-impair renal function resulting in oliguria and oligohydramnios, congenital defects.

- Diuretics
- Losartan
- Reserpine
- Nonselective beta blocker (propranolol)
- Sodium nitroprusside.

Drugs used in hypertensive crisis

- Hydralazine
- Labetalol
- Nifedipine/nimodipine/verapamil
- Ketanserin.

Eclampsia

- Fits occurring in eclampsia are Generalized tonic clonic seizures.
- Most seizures are self-limited, lasting less than 2 minutes.
- The first priority in management of seizures is to ensure airway and prevent aspiration of gastric contents.
- Incidence of fits–50% antepartum, 30% intrapartum and 20% postpartum.
- In postpartum, it is usually < 48 hours; if beyond 7 days, it is not eclampsia.

Pritchard regimen

- DOC for management of convulsions-magnesium sulfate
- Therapeutic range— 4–7 meq/l
- Mechanism of action—peripheral action at NM junction, competes with calcium for entry into cells and may have a central action
- Schedule — 4 g of mag sulf 20% soln given IV over 4–5 min f/b, 5 g of 50% soln given IM in each buttock (total 10 g as IM), f/b 5 g of 50% soln given as IM every 4 hours
- Monitor urine output — atleast 30 ml/hr, deep tendon reflex must be present and RR must be >12/minute
- Previously used lytic cocktail (Menon) Regimen is not used now-contains pethidine, Chlorpromazine and phenergan
- **Zuspan/Sibai Regimen**— 4–6 g of mag sulf in 100 ml of IV fluid over 15–20 min (loading dose) f/b, 1–2 g in 100 ml IV fluid/hour.

Obstetric management

- Terminate pregnancy immediately if fits occur.
- Termination must be by LSCS except if fetus is demise and cervix is fully ripe.

Eclampsia cases peculiar management at delivery

- No prophylactic ergometrine
- Anesthesia of choice–spinal or epidural
- Only contraindication for epidural is low platelet count < 50,000
- For status epilepticus–thiopentone sodium is given
- Postpartum continue Mag. sulf for 24 hours
- Diuretics must be given after delivery.

Complications of eclampsia

- M/c cause of maternal death-Intracranial bleeding and acute renal failure caused by abruptio placenta
- M/c cause of fetal death prematurity and asphyxia.

HELLP

Hemolysis

Elevated liver enzymes.

Low platelet count

- M/c symptom-epigastric/RUQ pain
- Hallmark-Microangipathic hemolysis leading to elevated LDH and fragmented RBC
- Treatment–immediate termination of pregnancy/steroids and FFP
- M/c cause of death in HELLP-Abruptio placenta and DIC.

Drugs used for prophylaxis of preeclampsia

- Lowdose aspirin-maintains normal balance of TX and PG
- Calcium supplements-synthesis of Nitrous oxidevasodilator
- Antioxidants–vitamin- C, E and lycopene-scavenges free radicals which cause preeclampsia
- Folic acid-hyperhomocysteinemia is associated with early onset of preeclampsia (FA inhibits homocysteine)

Medical Disorders in Pregnancy

- Rh incompatibility
- Anemia
- Heart disease
- Diabetes
- Infections.

Rh Incompatibility

- If the mother is Rh-negative and the father is Rh-positive, and if fetus is to be Rh-positive-isoimmunization occurs.
- After a latent period, there will be production of maternal IgM antibodies against fetal Rh-antigen.
- IgM antibodies will not cross placenta hence will not affect the first fetus.
- On subsequent exposure of the mother to Rh antigens, there will be production of IgG antibodies due to previously primed B cell.
- With only small amount of fetal antigen, excessive amount of IgG anti-Rh-antibodies is produced which will cross placenta and affect the fetus.

Maternal response to circulating fetal RBC depends on

- Strength of antigen
- Maternal inborn responsiveness about 1/3rd are unresponsive
- Volume of feto maternal hemorrhage- critical sensitising volume = 0.1ml.
- **ABO compatibility:** ABO incompatibility protects the Rh isoimmunization because when incompatible fetal RBCs enter's mothers bloodstream they will be immediately neutralized by available anti-A/B agglutinins.

Rhesus blood group antigens

- Contains 5 antigens, C, c, D, E, e. on short arm of chromosome 1.
- Most immunogenic is D antigen.

Conditions predisposing to Rh isoimmunization

- Abortion
- Amniocentesis
- Attempted version
- Manual removal of placenta
- Chorionic villus sampling
- Antepartum hemorrhage
- Cesarean section
- Post dated pregnancy (increased crossing of fetal RBC across placenta).

Antibody titres can be measured by indirect Coombs test

- Titre < 4IU/l is safe

- Titre > 4 IU/l or 1 : 8 implies iso immunization
- Titre > 10 IU/l or 1 : 16 (critical titre) implies severe hemolysis.

Perform indirect Coombs test

- In primi–at 12 weeks, if negative, then at 28th and 36th weeks.
- In multi–at 12 weeks, then at monthly intervals.

Kleihauer Betke test

- Performed in maternal blood to assess the fetomaternal bleed amount.
- Citric acid phosphate buffer is used.

Rh negative mother (non immunized)
- ICT at 12 weeks-In primi
- ICT at 12 weeks-In multi

ICT is negative
- Repeat at 28 week, 34 week-ICT negative
- Repeat every month-ICT negative

Delivery at 40 weeks
- If baby is Rh-positive and Coombs test negative Anti-D immunoglobin within 72 hours of delivery

Rh-negative mother (Immunized)
- ICT positive → Antibody Titre >4 IU/l or 1 : 8 → Amniocentesis

Amniocentesis

- At 20 weeks or as early as 16 weeks, if the mother has a high Titre or a previous baby with hydrops or died in utero or ultrasound shows early signs of fetal hydrops.
- Amniotic fluid containing bilirubin pigment is measured at 450 nm wavelength using spectrophotometry.
- The result of amniocentesis is plotted at Liley's chart.

Amniocentesis–Liley's Chart

Zone	Management
Zone 1 (fetus mildly affected)	Repeat amniocentesis at 2–4 weeks or Deliver at 38–40 weeks
Zone 2 (fetus is moderately affected)	Repeat amniocentesis 1–2 weeks or deliver at 38 weeks
Zone 3 (fetus is severely affected)	Cordocentesis → Intrauterine transfusion if hematocrit <30% or deliver at 34 weeks

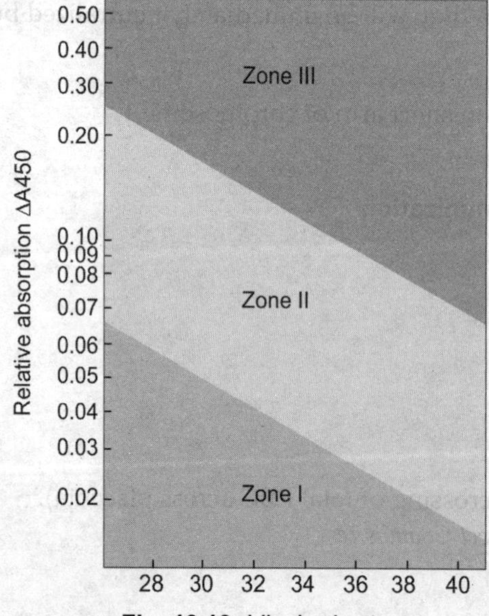

Fig. 13.10: Liley's chart

Intrauterine transfusion

- Where there is severe affection of fetus in utero prior to 34 weeks
- group Rh-negetive Blood is transfused
- Types–intraperitoneal and Intravascular transfusion.

Exchange transfusion of new born

Indications:

Rh + positive baby with direct Coombs test positive babies

a. Having cord blood Hb <11 gm/dl or Bilirubin > 4 mg/dl
b. Rising Titres of bilirubin >1 mg/dl/hour despite phototherapy
c. Total bilirubin >20 mg/dl or more.

Indications of Anti-D immunoprophylaxis

First trimester	Later pregnancy
Miscarriage	Miscarriage
Ectopic pregnancy	Amniocentesis
Hydatidiform mole	Fetal blood sampling
Threatened abortion	Antepartum hemorrhage
Medical or surgical MTP	External cephalic version
Chorionic villus sampling	Routine antepartum prophylaxis
	Delivery
	Manual removal of placenta

Dose

- Calculate it based on the volume of fetomaternal bleed
- Gestational age <12 weeks–50 microgram
- Also for abortions/CVS/ectopic–dose is 50 microgram
- Beyond 12 weeks–dose is 300 microgram.
- Antepartum prophylaxis where antibodies are not detected and ICT is negative-anti-D 300 microgram given as prophylaxis.

Complications in mother and fetus

Mother	Fetus
Preeclampsia	Immune hydrops–most serious
Polyhydramnios	Icterus gravis neonatorum–less severe
Big size baby and its hazards	Congenital hemolytic anemia–mildest
Hypofibrinogenemia Due to retained dead fetus	
PPH due to big placenta and coagulopathy	
Maternal syndrome-generalized edema, proteinuria and pruritus due to cholestasis	
APH is not a direct complication but may occur due to hypofibrinogenemia	

Fetal Hazards

Immune hydrops fetalis

- Skin edema, pericardial effusion, pleural effusion and huge placenta. Fetus is in buddha position with halo around the head on USG.
- Main pathology–severe anemia, hypoproteinemia, increased capillary permeability and cardiac failure.

Nonimmune hydrops fetalis

- It is due to causes other than Rh incompatibility
- Accumulation of fluid in tissues and serous cavities without evidence of circulating antibodies.
- M/c than hydrops fetalis.

Many causes are there; few are given:

- Trisomy 21 (m/c), Turner syndrome
- Cardiac defects,
- Hematological problems-thalassemia, G6PD deficiency
- Diaphragmatic hernia
- Chorioangioma and umbilical vein thrombosis
- Idiopathic
- Infections.

Infectious causes of nonimmune hydrops.

PRATSCHEC causes hydrops except–AIDS and Rubella:

- Parvovirus (m/c)
- Rubella
- AIDS
- Toxoplasma
- Syphilis
- CMV
- Herpes
- Echovirus
- Coxsackie virus.

Anemia Complicating Pregnancy

According to WHO, anemia in pregnancy is diagnosed when hemoglobin is less than 11 gm%

ICMR grades of anemia in pregnancy:

- Mild anemia — 10–10.9 gm%
- Moderate anemia — 7–9.9 gm%
- Severe anemia — 6.9–4 gm%
- Very severe anemia — < 4 gm%.

Features of iron-deficiency anemia

Stages of iron deficiency	
Depletion of iron store	• Serum ferritin-decreased (<20 mg/ml) • Normal hemoglobin/hematocrit • Normal RBC
Iron deficiency without clinical manifests	• Decreased serum ferritin • Decreased transferrin saturation <25% • Decreased serum iron <60 mg/dl • Increased free serum protoporphyrin • Increased TIBC
Frank iron-deficiency anemia	• Decreased MCV/MCH • Hematocrit fall (<28%) • Red cell distribution width > 14.5%

Iron-deficiency anemia

- Red cells are hypochromic and microcytic
- Anisocytosis and poikilocytosis
- Target cells, elliptical forms in severe cases
- Polychromatic cells.

Dimorphic anemia

- Cells may be normocytic, microcytic and macrocytic (anisocytosis-variation in size of RBC seen)
- Hypochromia or normochromia.

Types of Anemia

Dimorphic anemia

- Commonest type of anemia in underprivileged sections
- Results from Vitamin B_{12}, folic acid and iron-deficiency anemia
- Bone marrow is megaloblastic
- Treatment is both iron and folic acid.

Total iron requirement: in pregnancy: 1000 mg.

- Fetus: 300 mg
- Placenta: 300 mg
- Expanded RBC mass: 400 mg.

There is net gain of about 300 mg of iron due to amenorrhea in 10 months.

A minimum of about 4–6 mg of iron should be absorbed in the body per day during pregnancy which can be had only from 40–60 mg of dietary iron.

Iron requirement

- 2.5 mg/day–upto 20 weeks
- 5.5 mg/day–upto 20–32 weeks
- 6–8 mg/day–32 weeks onwards.

Treatment of iron-deficiency anemia.

Arbitrary hemoglobin level for admission 7.5 mg/dl.

Oral

- For prophylaxis–100 mg iron/ 0.5 mg FA
- For treatment–180 mg iron/4 mg FA
- Each ferrous sulfate tablet is 200 mg
- *1 tablet of 200 mg ferrous sulfate releases only 60 mg elemental iron*
- 3 tablets of ferrous sulfate is given for treatment
- Patient feels good with better appetite
- Increased reticulocyte count increases in 5–10 days
- Rise in hemoglobin-0.3–1 gm/week; seen after 3 weeks of initiation of therapy.

Iron therapy should be continued for 100 days after delivery.

Formulas to calculate total iron requirement.

- 4.4 × body weight in kg × Hb deficit (gm/dl)
- 0.3 × weight in lb × % of Hb deficit
- Wt in kg = wt in pound × 2.2.

Parenteral iron therapy

Indications

- Contraindications of oral therapy-severe anemia/intolerance
- Poor compliance to oral therapy
- Case seen for the first time during the last 8–10 weeks with severe anemia.

Advantage: Dose adjustments to fix up the iron store.

Rate of improvement: Increase Hb concentration at the rate of about 0.7 g to 1 g/100 ml per week.

Parenteral Injections

Intravenous route	Intra muscular route
– Iron dextran (2 ml ampoule) is used which contains 50 mg of elemental iron in 1 ml. – Iron sucrose (5 ml ampoule) contains 100 mg of elemental iron Iron ferricarboxymaltose. **Advantages:** Eliminates repeated and painful IM injections Cheaper, out-patient procedure. **Limitations:** Mostly suitable to 30–36 weeks.	Iron dextran and Iron sorbitol complex are used. **Limitations:** – Pain in the injection site. – Skin discoloration and abscess formation – Allergic reactions

Indications for blood transfusion

- Correction of anemia due to blood loss and PPH
- Patient with severe anemia seen beyond 36 weeks of pregnancy
- Refractory anemia
- Improvement is expected after 3 days of transfusion.

Complications

Pregnancy	Labor	Puerperium
Heart failure Preterm labor Intercurrent infection Preeclampsia	Postpartum hemorrhage Cardiac failure Shock	Puerperal venous thrombosis Puerperal sepsis Failing lactation Pulmonary embolism Subinvolution

HEART DISEASE IN PREGNANCY

Physiological changes in CVS

- Cardiac output: 6.7 l/min by 10th week
- Heart rate: increase 10–15 beats/min by 14th and 20th weeks
- Systolic blood pressure: Inchanged or lowered until 20th week, then rises to prepregnancy level
- Diastolic blood pressure: Slightly reduced
- Plasma and blood volume:
  ↑by 40–50% between 12 and 34 weeks
  (and continue at that level till term)
- Red cell mass: by 18–20% (between 8 and 40 week)
- Vital capacity: by 15% (by 20th week) declines by 5% (by 40th weeks).

Diagnostic criteria of heart disease

- Diastolic murmur
- Unequal cardiac enlargement
- Systolic murmur (of marked intensity) with thrill
- Arrhythmias
- Pericardial rush.

Newyork Heart Association (NYHA)–dyspnea

Grade I: But without limitation of ordinary physical activity.

Grade II: Slight limitation of physical activity (comfort at rest).

Grade III: Marked limitation of physical activity (comfort at rest).

Grade IV: Unable to carryout any physical activity without discomfort (Cardiac insufficiencies are present even at rest).

Antepartum management

Hospitalize: Class 1 at 36 weeks
Class 2 at 28 weeks.

Class 3/4 should avoid pregnancy; if seen in 1st trimester MTP is must. If diagnosed late-admit as early as possible.

Intrapartum management

- No spontaneous labor, but if required induction with PG E2 gel is safe in heart disease
- No place for trial labor-go for elective LSCS
- Vaginal delivery is allowed if there is no specific obstetric contraindication.
- Only heart disease where vaginal delivery is contraindicated–coarctation of aorta
- Cut short second stage with outlet forceps
- 40 mg frusemide can be given immediately after the baby is born.

3rd stage and puerperium management

- Ergometrine and methergine are contraindicated
- Oxytocin must be used in 3rd stage by IV infusion
- Give prophylactic antibiotics for infective endocarditis
- Early ambulation and lactation.

Period of high risk in cardiac failure

- Between 12–16 weeks of gestation (when hemodynamic changes just began)
- Between 28 and 32 weeks (when hemodynamic changes are maximum)
- During delivery
- Immediate postpartum
- Finally, 4–5 days after delivery when changes start reverting back
  - M/c heart disease in India-rheumatic. Followed by congenital heart disease.
  - M/c RHD = Mitral stenosis.
  - M/c heart disease in western countries-congenital heart disease (ASD).

Contraindications for pregnancy

- Eisenmenger's syndrome
- Primary pulmonary hypertension
- Uncorrected severe coarctation
- Marfan's with aortic involvement
- Severe MS with complications
- Pulmonary hypertension of any cause (absolute indication for termination).

Diabetes Mellitus.

Definition of GDM

The term includes cases with abnormal carbohydrate intolerance with onset or first detected during present pregnancy.

Potential candidates for GDM

- Positive family history
- Previous overweight baby of > 4 kg
- Previous stillbirth with pancreatic islet hyperplasia on autopsy.

- Unexplained perinatal loss
- Presence of polyhydramnios, recurrent vaginal candidiasis in present pregnancy.
- Age >30 years
- Obesity
- Ethnicity (East Asian Pacific Island ancestry).

Glucose challenge test

- Administer 50 g glucose and measure blood plasma glucose 1 hour later
- >140 mg/dl–further testing by GTT
- <140 mg/dl–further testing not required
- >200 mg/dl–no further testing needed because this confirms GDM.

3 hours glucose tolerance test

O'Sullivan and Mahan method

Modified by **Carpenter and Couston**

- Give 100 g oral glucose
- Fasting–95 mg/dl
- 1 hour–180 mg/dl
- 2 hours–155 mg/dl
- 3 hours–140 mg/dl
- GDM is diagnosed when 2 values are elevated.

Who GTT

- Give 75 g oral glucose
- Fasting: >110 and <126 (normal)
- 2 hours post glucose:
- >140 and <200 (impaired).

Overt diabetes

- FBS> 126 mg/dl
- 2-hour plasma glucose (75 g) value exceeds 200 mg/dl.

White's classification of diabetic pregnant women

Class	Age of onset, duration (years), vascular disease, insulin need
A	Gestational diabetes, any age onset or duration A1-dietary management A2-Insulin needed
B	Onset >20 years, duration <10 years
C	Age of onset 10–19 years, duration 10–19 years
D	Onset of age <10, duration >20 + Background retinopathy
F	Nephropathy with proteinuria >500 mg/day
H	Coronary disease
R	Retinopathy-proliferative/vitreous hemorrhage
T	Renal transplant

Complications of GDM

At pregnancy

- Preeclampsia
- Hydramnios
- Preterm labor
- Stillbirth

- Intercurrent illness
- Pyelonephritis
- DKA and coma
- Retinopathy and nephropathy in overt diabetes cases.

During labor and puerperium

- Prolongation of labor due to big baby
- Shoulder dystocia
- Perineal injuries
- PPH
- Operative interventions
- Puerperal sepsis
- Lactation failure.

Fetal complications

Congenital malformation:

- Related to the severity of diabetes during organogenesis in 1st trimester

Fetal macrosomia

- Maternal hyperglycemia—hypertrophy and hyperplasia of fetal islets-stimulates fetal insulin leading to increased carbohydrate metabolism and fat deposition
- Elevated maternal FFA—transfers to fetus

Major birth defects in infants of diabetic mothers

CNS and skeletal	Cardiac	Renal	GI	Others
• Neural tube defects • Anencephaly • Microcephaly • Sacral agenesis	• VSD/ASD • Coarctation of aorta • TGA • Cardiomegaly	• Renal agenesis • Hydronephros • Ureteral duplication	• Duodenal atresia • Anorectal atresia	Single Umbilical artery

Early detection of fetal anomalies

- Glycosylated Hb (HbA1c)–before 14 weeks reflect past 3 month's glycemic control (N < 6%). Chance of fetal anomalies is more if > 9.5
- MSAFP at 16 weeks
- USG
- Fetal echocardiography.

Principal causes of neonatal mortality

- Hypoglycemia
- Respiratory distress
- Polycythemia
- Jaundice (hyperbilirubinemia)
- Hypocalcemia
- Hypomagnesemia
- Cardiomyopathy.

Management

- Prepregnancy counselling
- Good glycemic control
- Switch over from OHA to insulin
- Folic acid supplementation
- Retinopathy and nephropathy screening

- Stop ACE inhibitors
- Nutritional therapy.

Maternal glucose homeostasis

Early pregnancy
- Basal glucose and insulin levels remain unchanged
- Fasting glucose reduces.

Advancing gestation
- Basal and postprandial insulin secretion increases due to human chorionic somatomamotropin (HCS), estrogen, progesterone, prolactin, cortisol
- Net effect–Reduced FBS and sustained in PPBS.

Gestational DM

Insulin secretion and basal production of glucose is the same
- Insulin is less effective in suppressing hepatic gluconeogenesis
- Increased peripheral resistance to insulin

Fetal glucose homeostasis
- Glucose crosses placenta by facilitated transport
- Insulin does not cross placenta.

Pedersen hypothesis

Hyperglycemic hyperinsulinism
- Leads to macrosomia, organomegaly of liver and heart
- Increased erythroprietin production and decreased surfactant production.

Reasons for switching from OHA to insulin
- Insulin never crosses the placenta
- Insulin requirement is increased during pregnancy which cannot be met by OHA
- OHA crosses placenta and causes teratogenicity, especially ear defects
- OHA causes severe fetal hyperinsulinemia and neonatal hypoglycemia.
- OHA aggravates neonatal hyperbilirubinemia by competing for albumin-binding sites.

Glyburide
- Sulfonylurea acts by stimulating insulin released from storage granules of beta cells of pancreas
- Also decreases the insulin resistance
- Nonteratogenic
- The only drug used in pregnancy.
- Hyperglycemia at early pregnancy results in spontaneous abortion and miscarriage
- At late pregnancy results in macrosomia, hypocalcemia, polycythemia, respiratory difficulties, CCF and cardiomyopathy.

Route of Delivery

- Diabetes per se is not an indication of LSCS
- Vaginal delivery is allowed unless there are any maternal or fetal complications
- Continuous CTG needed
- Anticipate shoulder dystocia
- Macrosomic fetus > 4500 g adviced LSCS
- Weight between 4000 and 4500, vaginal delivery or LSCS depends on the obstetrician.

Shoulder Dystocia

This term is used if there is a delay of more than one minute in the delivery of the shoulders after the delivery of the head.

Risk factors

- Fetal macrosomia
- Maternal DM
- Maternal obesity
- Post-term
- Anencephaly
- Fetal ascites
- Mid-pelvic instrument delivery.

Management of shoulder dystocia

- Discourage maternal push
- Apply liberal episiotomy
- No fundal pressure as it may result in uterine rupture
- Moderate suprapubic pressure can be applied. This reduces the bisacromial diameter and rotates the shoulder into oblique pelvic diameter
- Manoeuveres–Robert's, woods, rubins, zavanelli.

McRoberts maneuver

- Flexion and abduction of maternal thighs on her abdomen.
- It straightens the lumbo sacral angle, rotates the maternal pelvis cephalad and is associated with an increased uterine pressure and amplitude of contractions.

Wood's manoeuver

- If the above measures fails
- Progressively rotate the posterior shoulder to 180 degrees so that the impacted anterior shoulder is released.

Rubin's: reverse Wood's.

Thirdline measures

- Cleidotomy (bending the clavicle by surgical/hand)
- Symphysiotomy
- Zavanelli maneuver-replace the head into pelvis, go for LSCS.

Complications of shoulder dystocia

Maternal: Lacerations of birth canal, ruptured uterus, PPH.

Fetal

- Fetal asphyxia and death
- Meconium aspiration
- Erb's palsy-injury to spinal nerves–C5, 6, 7 resulting in hanging upper arm–arm is internally rotated, adducted at shoulder and pronated at elbow
- Klumpke's paralysis–injury to C8, T1 resulting in claw hand
- Fractured clavicle and humerus
- Sternocleidomastoid hematoma.

Infections in Pregnancy

Vertical transmissions

Agent	Infections
Rubella	**80% at first 12 weeks** 54% at 13–14 weeks 25% at the end of second trimester

Contd...

Contd...

Agent	Infections
Toxoplasmosis	6% at first trimester 72% at 36 weeks
Syphilis	T. pallidum enters fetal circulation only after 20 weeks with disappearance of Langerhans' layer (cytotrophoblast) in villi.
Hepatitis	10% in first trimester 90% in third trimester

Toxoplasmosis in pregnancy

Women who are seropositive before pregnancy usually are protected against acute infections and do not give birth to the congenitally infected fetus.

Timing of infection	Risk of transmission
In previous pregnancy	No
> 6 months before conception	No
< 6 months before conception	Risk increases as interval between infection and conception decreases
In first trimester	Risk is less (15%) but severity is more
In third trimester	Risk is more (60%) but disease is mild

HIV transmission from mother to child can occur at:

- Antepartum (transplacental)
- Peripartum (exposure to maternal blood and body fluids)
- Postpartum (breastfeeding)

In the absence of any intervention:

- 15–30% risk of transfer during pregnancy and delivery
- 10–20% will transmit through breastfeeding.
- Most (50–70%) transmission occurs at intrapartum period.

Zidovudine

- Antepartum to be started at 14–34 weeks and continued throughout pregnancy (100 mg 5 times a day)
- Given IV during labor and therafter 2 mg/kg is given to neonate every 6 hours for 6 weeks commencing 8–12 hours after birth
- This therapy reduces the perinatal and intrapartum transmission from 22% to 5%.

Intrapartum management of HIV mothers

- Elective LSCS for all HIV-positive mothers with HIV RNA load >1000 copies.
- Cord clamp done early
- Amniotic fluid and placenta are highly infectious
- Postpartum no breastfeeding must be given, as it increases the rate by 14%. But in the developing countries, the risk of not breastfeeding overweighs, so give breastfeed in India.
- All babies to be treated by ART. Accurate diagnosis can be established only by PCR and DNA analysis.
- A negative HIV antibody test only at 18 months confirms that the child is not affected.

About vaginal delivery

- ARM must not be done
- Schedule the time of delivery by LSCS or induction of labor at 38 weeks. To avoid rupture of membranes before labor
- Vaginal can be done if viral copies <100/ml.

Infections causing congenital malformation:

- Rubella
- Varicella
- CMV
- Parvovirus
- Toxoplasmosis.

Congenital rubella syndrome

- It affects all the organs
- M/c manifestation is mental retardation
- Most severe congenital infection
- Risk is high in 1st trimester and gradually diminishes in 3rd trimester
- In late 2nd and 3rd trimesters malformations are uncommon, but MR and hearing loss alone can occur.

Features

- Sensorineural hearing loss
- Eye-cataract, glaucoma
- Congenital heart disease-PDA, Pulmonary artery stenosis
- CNS defects-microcephaly, develomental delay and mental retardation
- Thrombocytopenia
- Hepatosplenomegaly
- **Extended rubella syndrome-**includes panencephalitis and diabetes developing in 2nd/3rd decade of life.

CMV

- Most common cause of fetal and perinatal infections but asymptomatic in 90%
- Fetal infection can also occur with reactivation of infection in pregnancy, So previous infection does not prevent congenital infection
- No relation to gestational age.

Features of congenital CMV

- Stillbirth
- Microcephaly
- Choroidoretinitis
- Deafness
- Hemolytic anemia (blood dyscrasia)
- Thrombocytopenia with petechia
- IUGR
- Hepatosplenomegaly
- Icterus
- Mental retardation
- Pneumonitis and intracranial calcifications.

MCQ	Answer
Fetal infection is nil in 1st trimester	Syphilis
Maximum risk if infection occurs after 20 weeks	Syphilis
Maximum risk if infection occurs before 20 weeks	Varicella zoster
Maximum risk if transmission in 1st trimester	Rubella
Rate of transmission increases as pregnancy advances	Toxoplasma/hepatitis
No relation to GA	CMV

Contd...

Contd...

MCQ	Answer
Maximum risk of transmission at delivery LSCS is indicated for infections with	HIV and herpes
Most common congenital infection	CMV
Most severe congenital infection	Rubella
Congenital infection with no teratogeniecity	HIV

Preterm labor, PROM, Postdatism and IUD

Preterm labor

Definition

- Defined as labor (regular, painful frequent uterine contractions causing progressive effacement and dilatation of cervix) occuring before 37 completed weeks of gestation.

Causes

- Chorioamnionitis (main cause)
- M/c organism responsible–Ureoplasma urealyticum and gardenella vaginalis causing bacterial vaginosis.
- Pregnancy complications–preeclampsia, antepartum hemorrhage, premature rupture of membranes and polyhydramnios.
- Medical and surgical illnesses.

Diagnosis of preterm labor

- Regular uterine contractions with or without pain (atleast one in every 10 minutes)
- Dilatation >2 cm and effacement 80% of cervix
- Length of cervix (measured by TVS) < 2.5 cm and funneling of internal os.
- Pelvic pressure, backache or vaginal discharge.

At 24 weeks

- If cervix length is < 2.5 cm, there is increased risk of preterm delivery (mean cervical length = 3.5 cm)
- About fetal glycoprotein–**Fetal fibrinogen**
- Normally, it is found in cervicovaginal discharge before 22 weeks and again after rupture of membranes.
- If by ELISA-value of it is > 50 ng/ml, it is considered as positive and predisposes to preterm delivery.

Explanation on translabial USG

- T-shaped internal os–labor has not begun
- Y-shaped internal os–early effacement
- U/V-shaped (funneling) = complete effacement.

Contraindications for TVS

- Established preterm labor
- In patients with PROM (due to risk of chorioamnionitis)
- In patients with placenta previa (risk of bleeding)
- In cases of PROM, translabial USG can be done.

Drugs used for preterm labor

- Tocolytics
- Prostaglandins
- Diazoxide.

Tocolytics

- Betamimetics: Ritodrine, salbutamol, terbutaline and Isoxsuprine.
- Indomethacin/sulindac

- Glyceryl trinitrate
- Magnesium sulfate
- Atosiban
- Nifedipine/Nicardipine.

Others

- Progesterone–tocolytic property is due to its antagonistic effect on PGF2 alpha.
- Diazoxide–thiazide diuretic used to arrest preterm labor.
  Adverse effects–hypotension, tachycardia, hyperglycemia and decreased uteroplacental flow.

Management of a case of preterm labor

- Tocolytics
- Steroids for fetal lung maturity
- Phenobarbitone–to prevent intraventricular bleeding in newborn (especially if fetal weight < 2 kg and weeks < 32)
- Antibiotics
- Vitamin K1–to prevent intraventricular bleeding.

Steroid therapy

Recommended for women to deliver before 36 weeks
Dose: 2 doses intramuscular—12 mg 24 hours apart. Betamethasone is steroid of choice.

Advantages

- Reduces respiratory distress syndrome
- Decreases intraventricular hemorrhage in a newborn.

Side effects of betamimetics

- Tachycardia, hypotension
- Pulmonary edema
- Myocardial ischemia
- Hyperglycemia
- Hypokalemia.

Fetal side effects

- Tachycardia, hyper-or hypoglycemia, ileus, increased intraventricular hemmorhage.

PREMATURE RUPTURE OF MEMBRANES

Definition

- Spontaneous rupture of membrane before the onset of labor is called PROM
- Preterm premature rupture (PPROM)-defined as premature rupture before 37 weeks
- The most probable cause is reduction in membrane tensile strength caused by bacterial proteases or by repeated uterine contraction causing stretching.

Complications of PROM

- Predominant risk between 32 and 36 weeks chorioamnionitis
  Here the aim is to deliver the patient
- Predominant risk between 28 and 32 weeks hyaline membrane disease
  Here the aim is to prolong the latent phase and administer glucocorticoids and antibiotics.

Tests to detect PROM

- Visualization of amniotic fluid in vagina
- Nitrazine test

- Fern test-drying salts in amniotic fluid
- Evaporation test-endocervical samples are heated and if a white residue is left, it is amniotic fluid
- Following substances in amniotic fluid can be detected-diamine oxidase, fetal fibrinogen and alpha feto protein.

Nitrazine test-principles

- Vaginal pH is 4.5–5.5, amniotic fluid is 7–7.5
- Nitrazine paper is smeared with vaginal secretions
- Will turn deep blue if amniotic fluid is present in vagina-becomes alkaline
- False result- antiseptic solution, urine, blood and vaginal infections.

Prolonged Labor

Definition

Said to be prolonged

- When combined duration of 1st and 2nd stage is more than 18 hours
- Cervical dilatation is less than 1 cm/hour
- Descent of presenting part is < 1 cm/hour for a period of 4 hours.

Causes prolonged labor

Fault in power	Fault in passage	Fault in passenger	Others
• Uterine inertia	CPD	Malposition	Sedatives
• Constriction ring	Cervical dystocia	Malpresentation	Analgesics
• Epidural anesthesia	Pelvic tumor	Hydrocephalus	
	Full bladder	Deflexed head	
	Old scarring	Big baby	

Prolonged labor

- **Latent phase**
  - 20 hours in nullipara
  - 14 hours in multipara.
- **Active phase**

Nulliparous: <1.2 cm/hour dilatation
< 1 cm/hour descent
Multiparous: <1.5 cm/hour dilatation
< 2 cm/hour of descent.

Precipitate labor

Nulliparous: dilatation/descent >5 cm/hour
Multiparous: dilatation/descent >10 cm/hour

Postdated Pregnancy

Postdatism

- A pregnancy continuing beyond 42 weeks or 294 days is called as postmaturity/postdatism.

Causes of postdatism

- Wrong dates
- Hereditary
- Maternal factors–primi, elderly multi, past h/o prolonged pregnancy, sedentary
- Fetal factors–anencephaly, adrenal hypoplasia
- Placental–low estrogen leading to sulfatase deficiency

Complications of Postdatism

- Ageing of placenta-placental insufficiency leads to fetal hypoxia and acidosis, stillbirth
- Liquor decrease-oligohydramnios, cord compression, shoulder dystocia
- Meconium aspiration syndrome
- Operative intervention
- Genital injuries due to big baby.

Neonatal complications

- Chemical pneumonitis
- Atelectasis
- Pulmonary hypertension
- Hypoxia, respiratory failure
- Hypoglycemia, polycythemia.

Intrauterine Death

- Death of fetus in utero after the period of viability (after 28 weeks in the developing countries and 20 weeks in developed countries).

Clinical features of IUD

- Size of uterus decreased
- Liquor decreased
- FHS absent
- Fetal movements absent
- Egg-shell crackling feel of fetal head (late feature)
- Earliest diagnosis is possible by USG.

USG–features

- Absent fetal cardiac activity
- Decreased liquor amnii
- Spalding's sign (overlapping of skull bones) due to shrinkage of cerebrum after fetal death.

X-ray features

- Robert's sign-presence of gas in fetal large vessels (earliest sign-within 12 hours of death)
- Ball sign-hyper flexion of spine
- Spalding's sign.

Buddha position of fetus-Halo around the scalp-Rhesus incompatibility, hyrops.

Management of IU dead baby

- The treatment for transverse lie is cesarean section. It is best in those who are not skilled in destructive operations.
- Decapitation and evisceration are destructive operations. Today they are rarely done.

Complications of IUD

- Psychological upset
- Uterine infections
- Blood coagulation disorder-if dead baby retained more than 4 weeks, there is possibility of hypofibrinogenemia and silent DIC
- During labor–uterine inertia, retained placenta and PPH.
- **LSCS done only for transverse lie, placenta previa and previous LSCS.**

Indications for interference

- Psychological upset
- Uterine infections
- Falling fibrinogen level
- Tendency for prolongation of labor beyond 2 weeks
- But this expectant management is not done nowadays
- Labor induced with oxytocin drip+ PGE2 gel.

Destructive operations:

Operation	Indication	Procedure
Craniotomy	• Delivery of dead fetus with cephalic presentation • Delivery of arrested aftercoming head in breech • Interlocking of twins' heads	Fetal skull is perforated And contents are evacuated. Perforate at: • **Vertex**–parietal bone • **Brow**–frontal bone • **Face**–orbit/roof of mouth • Aftercoming head in breech-occipital bone
Craniocentesis	• Hydrocephalus	• Per abdomen reduction of hydrocepahlic head using large bore needle
Decapitation	• Neglected shoulder • Interlocking head of twins	Fetal head is separated from body and delivered

QUESTIONS

1. **The reagent used in Apt test is: (2014)**
   a. Sodium bicarbonate
   b. KCL
   c. Sodium hydroxide
   d. Sodium chloride
2. **Which of the following is useful in first trimester screening for Down's syndrome? (2014)**
   a. Inhibin
   b. Estradiol
   c. PAPP-A
   d. Acetylcholinesterase
3. **Fetal and maternal blood can be differentiated by: (2014)**
   a. Kleihauer-Betake test
   b. Apt test
   c. Bubbling test
   d. Osmotic fragility test
4. **Most accurate method to detect pregnancy at 6 weeks' gestation is: (2014)**
   a. USG fetal cardiac activity
   b. Doppler
   c. Urine hCG
   d. Clinical examination
5. **Best method for termination of pregnancy at 11 weeks' gestation is: (2014)**
   a. Hysterectomy
   b. D and C
   c. Prostaglandin + Mifepristone
   d. Manual vacuum aspiration
6. **According to WHO, what is given to prevent PPH by active management of third stage of labor? (2014)**
   a. IV PGF2 alpha agonist
   b. IM oxytocin
   c. IV ergometrine
   d. Per rectal prostaglandins
7. **Deep transverse arrest occurs in which type of pelvis: (2013)**
   a. Platypelloid
   b. Gynecoid
   c. Android
   d. Anthropoid
8. **Prostaglandin used to control bleeding in post partum hemorrhage is: (2013)**
   a. Carboprost
   b. Alprostadil
   c. PGE2
   d. PGI2
9. **Longest fetal skull diameter is: (2013)**
   a. Mentovertical
   b. Submentovertical
   c. Submentobregmatic
   d. Occipitofrontal

10. Placenta in which vessels divide before reaching margin is called: (2013)
a. Marginal
b. Velamentous
c. Battledore
d. Circumvallate

11. Important factor which determines the outcome in twin pregnancy is: (2013)
a. Chorionicity
b. Placenta
c. Lie of first twin
d. Lie of second twin

12. Least chance of cord prolapse is seen in: (2013)
a. Frank breech
b. Complete breech
c. Knee presentation
d. Footling presentation

13. All are done in quadruple test in downs syndrome except: (2013)
a. AFP
b. hCG
c. PAPP
d. Inhibin A

14. APLA is associated with all except: (2013)
a. Recurrent fetal loss
b. Thrombosis
c. Bleeding
d. Coagulation

15. Which is not done for shoulder dystocia? (2013)
a. McRoberts' maneuver
b. Wood's maneuver
c. Mauriceau Smellie Kiet technique
d. Zavanelli maneuver

16. Which is false regarding hCG? (2012)
a. It is a glycopeptide
b. Synthesized by cytotrophoblast
c. Doubling time is 2 days
d. High levels are seen in multiple pregnancies

17. Primordial follicles are maximum at: (2012)
a. 4 weeks
b. 20 weeks
c. At birth
d. Puberty

18. Bleeding of fetal origin: (2012)
a. Vasa previa
b. Circumvallate placenta
c. Placenta previa
d. Abruptio placenta

19. In placenta previa, separation of placenta will not occur by: (2012)
a. Per vaginal
b. Per speculum
c. Rupture of membranes
d. External cephalic version

20. Impending signs of rupture of uterine scar are all except: (2012)
a. Abdominal pain
b. Fetal tachycardia
c. Fetus in peritoneal cavity
d. Scar tenderness

21. Which of the following regarding cardiovascular changes in pregnancy is not true? (2011)
a. Increased blood volume
b. Increased heart rate
c. Increased cardiac output
d. Increased blood viscosity

22. Best sonological marker for diagnosis of Down's in 1st trimester: (2011)
a. Nuchal translucency
b. Fetal heart
c. Microcephaly
d. Polyhydramnios

23. Fetus is called an embryo until: (2011)
a. 6 weeks
b. 8 weeks
c. 10 weeks
d. 12 weeks

24. Pathological contraction ring is due to: (2011)
a. Obstructed labor
b. Uterine inertia
c. Preterm labor
d. Oligohydramnios

25. Progesterone causes stimulation of: (2011)
a. Myometrial activation
b. Myometrial quiescence
c. Increases oxytocin receptors
d. Causes cervical ripening

26. Modified biophysical profile includes: (2011)
a. Fetal tone and breathing
b. Fetal movements and tone
c. NST and AFI
d. AFI

27. Antepartum bleed of fetal origin is: (2011)
a. Vasa previa
b. Circumvallate placenta
c. Abruptio placenta
d. Placenta previa

28. Most common site of ectopic pregnancy is: (2011)
a. Ampullary portion of fallopian tube
b. Isthmus

c. Interstitium
d. Abdomen

29. An eclamptic pregnant woman receives intravenous magnesium sulfate. What is the first sign of hypermagnesemia? (2011)
a. Loss of tendon reflex
b. Respiratory depression
c. Hypotonia
d. Hypotension

30. Proteinuria in preeclampsia is due to: (2011)
a. Glomerular damage
b. Degree of hypertension
c. Release of vasoconstrictors
d. Liver failure

31. Recurrent breech presentation is due to: (2011)
a. Placenta previa
b. Hydrocephalus
c. Septate uterus
d. Short cord

32. Magnesium sulfate is contraindicated in: (2010)
a. Placenta previa
b. Preeclampsia
c. Epilepsy
d. Myasthenia gravis

33. Most common cause of spontaneous abortion in first trimester is: (2010)
a. Chromosomal anomalies
b. Uterine anomalies
c. Antiphospholipid antibody syndrome
d. Hypothyroidism

34. Which is not a complication specific to monochorionic twins? (2010)
a. Malpresentation
b. Conjoint twins
c. Twin-to-twin transfusion
d. Growth retardation of one fetus

35. A pregnant woman presents with a placenta previa of a major degree. The fetus is malformed. Which of the following will be the best line on management? (2009)
a. Cesarean section
b. Oxytocin drip
c. Rupture of membranes
d. Instillation of PGE2

36. Transverse lie is most likely to occur in: (2009)
a. Subseptate uterus
b. Uterus didelphys
c. Hypoplastic uterus
d. Unicornuate uterus

37. What is Osiander's sign? (2009)
a. Pulsation in the lateral vaginal fornix
b. Bluish color change in the vagina
c. Softening of the cervix
d. On bimanual palpation, the fingers can be approximated as if nothing is in between

38. In 'aftercoming head', best forceps used for delivery is: (2009)
a. Piper's forceps
b. Kielland's forceps
c. Wrigley's forces
d. Kocher's forceps

39. Longest diameter of the skull is: (2009)
a. Suboccipital bregmatic
b. Occipital frontal
c. Bitemporal
d. Biparietal

40. Bishop score is used to evaluate: (2009)
a. Cervix status
b. Uterine contraction
c. Fetal well-being
d. Pelvic assessment

41. The management of eclampsia includes all except: (2009)
a. Control of convulsion
b. Prolongation of pregnancy
c. Control of BP
d. Delivery of fetus

42. The most common cause of vesicovaginal fistula in the developing countries is: (2009)
a. Pressure necrosis of urethra during obstructed labor
b. Forceps delivery
c. Abdominal hysterectomy
d. Tuberculosis

43. Engaging diameter in fully extended head: (2008)
a. Submentobregmatic
b. Suboccipitobregmatic
c. Mentovertical
d. Suboccipitofrontal

44. Deep transverse arrest occurs in which type of pelvis? (2008)
a. Platypelloid
b. Gynecoid
c. Android
d. Anthropoid

45. Which is the most common complication during vaginal delivery in diabetic women? (2008)
a. Uterine inertia
b. Shoulder dystocia
c. Obstructed labor
d. Post partum hemorrhage

46. Polyhydramnios is seen in all except: (2008)
a. Diabetes mellitus
b. Anencephaly
c. Tracheoesophageal fistula
d. Renal agenesis

47. Sher's classification is done in cases of: (2008)
a. Uterine prolapse
b. Puerperal sepsis
c. Abruption
d. Placenta previa

48. Shortest fetal skull diameter is: (2008)
a. Bimastoid
b. Submentovertical
c. Submentobregmatic
d. Occipitofrontal

49. Modified biophysical profile includes: (2008)
a. Fetal tone and breathing
b. Fetal movements and tone
c. NST and AFI
d. AFI

50. Human placenta is: (2007)
a. Hemochorial
b. Endothen-esdothelima
c. Chorio-endothelial
d. Non-Discoidal

51. All are sonological markers for downs syndrome except: (2007)
a. Nuchal transluscency
b. Short femur
c. Echogenic bowel
d. Hydronephrosis

52. The most common breech presentation in a nulliparous woman is: (2007)
a. Frank breech
b. Complete breech
c. Footling
d. Incomplete breech

53. Shoulder dystocia occurs in delivery of fetus with: (2007)
a. Anencephaly
b. Hydrocephalus
c. Fetal ascites
d. Breech

54. Magnesium sulfate as an uterine relaxant is contraindicated in the following except: (2007)
a. Premature rupture of membrane
b. Intrauterine infection
c. Myasthenia gravis
d. Renal failure

55. A pregnant woman with mitral stenosis is most likely to develop cardiac failure in which period? (2007)
a. 16 weeks
b. 24 weeks
c. 20 weeks
d. 28 weeks

56. Incidence of scar rupture in a pregnant lady with previous LSCS is: (2007)
a. 0.2
b. 0.5
c. 0.7
d. 0.9

57. True statement regarding transverse lie is: (2007)
a. Cord prolapse is common
b. 3rd degree perineal tear is common
c. Deep transverse arrest can occur
d. More common in primi

58. Variable deceleration indicates: (2007)
a. Head compression
b. Cord compression
c. Fetal hypoxemia
d. Maternal sedation

59. Regarding monozygotic twins, which of the following is not true? (2007)
a. USG is more useful in the first half of pregnancy
b. Sex discordance can occur rarely
c. Always monochorinonic
d. More common following ovulation induction

60. The placenta is formed from: (2007)
a. Decidua basalis
b. Decidua vera
c. Chorion laeve
d. Decidua capsularis

61. Which is the most common complication during vaginal delivery in diabetic women? (2007)
a. Uterine inertia
b. Shoulder dystocia
c. Obstructed labor
d. Postpartum hemorrhage

62. Most common cause of spontaneous abortion in first trimester: (2007)
a. Chromosomal anomalies
b. Uterine anomalies
c. Antiphospholipid antibody syndrome
d. Hypothyroidism

63. The level of hCG us maximum during which day of pregnancy? (2007)
a. 50–60
b. 60–70
c. 70–80
d. 80–90

64. AP diameter is more than transverse diameter in the following: (2006)
a. Anthropoid pelvis
b. Android pelvis
c. Platypelloid pelvis
d. Gynecoid pelvis

65. True about amnion are all except: (2006)
a. No lymph supply
b. Rich blood supply
c. No nerve supply
d. Dilates cervix during labor

66. Antihypertensive of choice in pregnancy is:
a. Hydralazine (2006)
b. Propranolol
c. Alpha methyldopa
d. Labetalol

67. Ventouse is contraindicated in: (2006)
a. Preterm
b. Post-term
c. Prolonged second stage
d. Cardiac disease

68. Monoamniotic monochorionic fetus is formed when fertilization occurs: (2006)
a. <2 days
b. 2–8 days
c. >8 days
d. >2 weeks

ANSWERS AND EXPLANATIONS

1. Ans. c. Sodium hydroxide

Ref: Nelson's Textbook of Paediatrics, Alkali Denaturation test, www.Wikipedia.org,19/e

Apt test/Apt-Downey test	Kleihauer Betke test
• Used to detect the presence or absence of fetal blood in a vaginal discharge to rule out vasa previa • Also used in neonatal bloody vomiting whether it is a genuine upper GI hemorrhage or swallowed maternal blood during delivery or from cracked nipple	Sample is maternal peripheral smear used to see how much of fetal blood has been transfused into the maternal serum in order to assess the risk of isoimmunization
Qualitative	Quantitative

Apt test method-blood + sterile water = cause hemolysis releasing the free hemoglobin
- Sample centrifuged and supernatant mixed with 1 ml of 1% sodium hydroxide for each 5 ml of supernatant
- Color of the fluid is assessed after 2 minutes
- Fetal Hb-stays pink
- Adult Hb-turns yellowish-brown due to conversion to hematin.

2. Ans. c. PAPP-A

Ref: Dutta's Textbook of Obstetrics, 7/e p106; Williams Obstetrics, 23/e

Down's syndrome
- Increased nuchal translucency
- Decreased PAPP–A (pregnancy-associated plasma protein)
- Decreased MSAFP
- Decreased unconjugated estriol
- Increased beta hCG
- Increased Inhibin.

Test and their timings
- Amniocentesis 14–16 weeks
- CVS 10–14 weeks
- Cordocentesis 24 weeks
- Nuchal translucency of value only <14 weeks.
- Beyond 14 weeks, the test to be performed is QUAD test (triple test+inhibin level).

For Down's syndrome

	<14 weeks	>14 weeks
Screening test	Combined test (Nuchal transclucency + Free beta hCG + PAPP-A)	Quad test (triple test + inhibin)
IOC	Chorionic Villus sampling	Amniocentesis

3. **Ans. b. Apt test**

Ref: Cloherty's Manual of Neonatal Care, 6/e

Apt test–It is a qualitative test which helps us differentiate fetal cells and maternal red cells.

Kleihauer–Betke test–is a quatitative test which identifies the amount of fetal blood cells in the maternal serum. (Also refer Q1)

4. **Ans. a. USG fetal cardiac activity**

Ref: Williams obstetric, 23/e and Daftary's Manual of Obstetrics, 3/e

Ultrasound fetal cardiac activity–is seen as early as 6 weeks by a trans vaginal ultrasound. Gestational sac and yolk sac by 5 weeks and embryonic movements at 7 weeks.

This is a definitive sign of a viable ongoing intrauterine pregnancy.

Doppler's effect of ultrasound–It can pick up fetal heart rate reliably by 10th week. It is a hand-held device. Disadvantages are: uterine souffle can be mistaken for a heartbeat and in maternal abdominal wall obesity, Doppler's test may not be able to detect FHS.

Urine hCG–tests done are:

Test	Sensitivity	Time taken	Inference	Positive on
Agglutination inhibition test	0.51 IU/ml	2 min	Absence of agglutination	2 days of missed period
Direct latex agglutination test	0.2 IU/ml	2 min	Presence of agglutination	2–3 days of missed period
Two-site sandwich immunoassay	30–50 mIU/ml	4–5 min	Colorbands in the control and test window	In the first day of a missed period

Clinical examination–There are certain signs like Hegar's, Palmer's, Goodell's, Mcdonald's signs, which can be elicited at the time of 6 weeks, but they are not definitive in the diagnosis.

5. **Ans. B, C and d**

Ref: Daftary's Manual of Obstetrics, 3/e p458 and 655, Dutta Textbook of Obstetrics 6/e p174–76

Methods of termination of pregnancy

First trimester (upto 12 weeks)	Second trimester (13–20 weeks)
Surgical • MVA • Suction and evacuation • D and C Medical • Mifepristone • Mifepristone and Misoprostol • Methotrexate and Misoprostol • Tamoxifen and Misoprostol	• Dilatation and evacuation • Intrauterine instillation of hypertonic solutions • Prostaglandins-PGE1, PGF2-alpha, PGE2–used intramuscular, intravaginal, intra-amniotic • High-dose oxytocin infusion • Hysterotomy

Of all the options, options b, c and d can be used for 1st trimester abortions, though the best option is b.

6. **Ans. b. IM oxytocin**

Ref: Manual of WHO Recommendations for Prevention of PPH ISBN 978-92-4-154850-2

Recommendations for the prevention of PPH

- Routine use of uterotonics is recommended in the 3rd stage of labor
- Oxytocin IV/IM 10 units recommended uterotonic
- If oxytocin unavailable, then, methylergometrine/oral misoprostol 600 mcg is recommended

- Controlled cord traction (CCT) for the delivery of placenta only if delivery conducted by a skilled birth attendant; if not, CCT is not advocated
- Late cord clamping (after 1–3 minutes after birth) recommended for all births while simultaneously initiating essential newborn care
- Early cord clamping (<1 min) is not recommended unless the neonate is asphyxiated and needs to be moved for immediate resuscitation
- Postpartum uterine tone assessment for early identification of uterine atony
- Sustained uterine massage is not recommended, if the patient has received oxytocin
- In cesarean section, oxytocin IV/IM is the preferred uterotonic and CCT is the preferred method of removal of placenta.

7. Ans. c. Android pelvis

Ref: Dutta's Textbook of Obstetrics 6/e p346 & p372, Williams' Obstetrics 23/e p480

Android pelvis:
- Inlet is triangular
- Posterior segment is short
- Cavity is narrow and deep
- Convergent side walls
- Prominent ischial spines
- Narrow subpubic angle
- Short bituberous diameter
- Results in–Delayed engagement
  - Difficult anterior rotation and deep transverse arrest (DTA)
  - Difficult delivery with more chances of perineal injuries

Management of DTA:
- Ventouse
- Manual rotation of head and forceps
- Forceps rotation and delivery with Keilland's forceps rotation
- If vaginal delivery not safe, then cesarean section
- Craniotomy if baby is dead.

8. Ans. a. Carboprost

Ref: Dutta DC 6/e p417

In the management of PPH–the following prostaglandins are used:
Carboprost (15-methyl PGF2α) 250 μg intramuscular/intramyometrial
Misoprostol (PGE1 analogue) 1000 μg per rectum
Other options:
Alprostadil (PGE1 analogue) used in erectile dysfunction in males, It increases the blood flow to the penis and causes erection.

PGE2 analogue–It is dinoprostone (trade names-cervidil, cerviprime). It is used to soften the cervix and causes uterine contraction. Mainly used in induction of labor

PGI2–It is also known as prostacyclin. Its chief function is to prevent platelet plug formation in primary hemostasis. It is an effective vasodilator. Its function is opposite to that of thromboxane A2 (TXA2).

9. Ans. a. Mentovertical

Ref: Dutta DC 5/e p85

Diameter	From	To	Measurement	Attitude of the head	Presentation
Suboccipito-bregmatic	Nape of the neck	Center of the bregma	9.5 cm	Complete flexion	Vertex

Contd...

Contd...

Diameter	From	To	Measurement	Attitude of the head	Presentation
Suboccipitofrontal	Nape of the neck	Anterior end of the anterior fontanelle or center of the sinciput	10 cm	Incomplete flexion	Vertex
Occipitofrontal	Occipital eminence	Root of the nose (Glabella)	11.5 cm	Marked deflexion	Vertex
Mentovertical	Midpoint of the chin	Highest point on the sagittal suture	14 cm	Partial extension	Brow
Submentovertical	Junction of the floor of the mouth and neck	Highest point on the sagittal suture	11.5 cm	Incomplete extension	Face
Submento-bregmatic	Junction of the floor of the mouth and neck	Center of the bregma	9.5 cm	Complete extension	Face

10. Ans. b. Velamentous

Ref: Dutta DC 6/e p219, 220

Velamentous–cord is attached to the membranes and divides before reaching the placenta.

When present over the internal os, it can rupture and cause APH, the blood lost is of fetal origin leading to fetal distress and even death.

Placenta marginata–a thin fibrous ring is present at the margin of the chorionic plate where fetal vessels appear to terminate.

There are increased chances of abortion, hydrorrhea gravidarum (excessive watery vaginal discharge), APH, IUGR, preterm labor, retained placenta or membranes.

Battledore placenta–the cord is attached to the margin of the placenta.

If present in the lower segment, it can cause cord compression during delivery and fetal anoxia

Circumvallate placenta–the fetal surface has a central depressed zone surrounded by thickened white ring which is usually complete. Vessels radiate from the cord insertion till the ring and disappear from the view. The peripheral zone outside is thicker and edge is elevated and rounded. Clinical significance is the same as placenta marginata.

11. Ans. a. Chorionicity

Ref: High-risk Pregnancy & Delivery by Fernando Arias 3/e p295

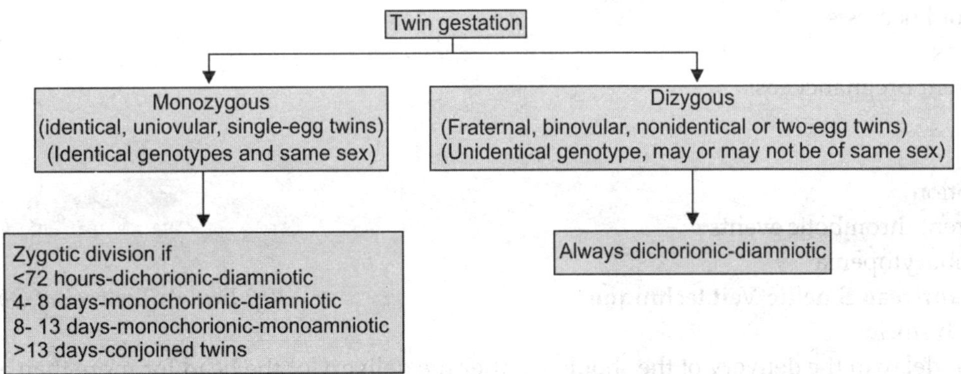

The diagnosis of chorionicity is important because it is more specific than monozygosity as a risk factor for adverse perinatal outcome.

Chorionicity can be determined antenatally and used for clinical management, while zygosity cannot be assessed before birth.

Monochorionic twins are at a higher risk than dichorionic twins for neurological morbidity, birthweight discordance and death.

12. Ans. a. Frank breech

Ref: Dutta DC 6/e p399

Factors favouring cord prolapse

- Malpresentations-most common is transverse (1 in 5), breech with flexed legs, i.e., complete breech (1 in 20) or footling/knee presentation
- Contracted pelvis
- Prematurity
- Twins
- Hydramnios
- Placental factor-minor degrees of placenta previa, marginal insertion of the cord or long cord
- Iatrogenic-low rupture of membranes, manual rotation of head and version

Frank breech–In this legs extended at the knees legs are therefore only the buttocks occupy the lower segment of the uterus and not complicated but in the presence of legs as in other types of breech, the chances of cord prolapse are less in Frank breech compared to other types of breech.

13. Ans. c. PAPP *Ref: Dutta DC 6/e p107*

Screening tests for Down's syndrome

< 14 weeks	Double screening/combined test	Nuchal translucency scan + free β HCG + PAPP-A
> 14 weeks (around 15–18 weeks)	Triple test	MSAFP + hCG and unconjugated estriol (UE3)
	Quadruple test/Quad test	Triple test + Inhibin A

Nuchal translucency and PAPP-A has no role after 14 weeks in detecting Down's syndrome.

14. Ans. c. Bleeding *Ref: Dutta DC Obstetrics 6/e p343*

APLA syndrome:

Pathology– It includes the production of antiphospholipid antibodies LA (Lupusanticoagulant) and ACAS (Anticardiolipin antibodies). They are IgG or IgM, bind to the phopholipids and prevent the physiological changes in the decidual vessels. There is a subsequent decrease in the production of prostacyclin (vasodilator) and increase in the level of thromboxane (vasoconstrictor).

It causes:

- Placental vascular atherosis
- Intervillous thrombosis
- Decidual vasculopathy
- Fibrinoid necrosis

↓

Recurrent pregnancy loss
IUGR
PIH
Abruption
Recurrent thrombotic events
Thrombocytopenia

15. Ans. c. Mauriceau Smellie Veit technique *Ref: Dutta's Textbook of Obstetrics 6/e p406*

Shoulder dystocia

Definition- delay in the delivery of the shoulders after the delivery of the head for more than a minute.

Dos

- Suprapubic pressure–is the pressure applied by the assistant slightly towards the side of the fetal chest. This will reduce the bisacromial diameter and rotate the anterior shoulder towards the oblique diameter.
- McRobert's maneuver–abduct the maternal thighs and hyperflex them onto her abdomen. There is rotation of the symphysis pubis upwards and decrease in angle of pelvic inclination.
- Wood's maneuver–done under GA. The posterior shoulder is rotated to the anterior position (180°) by a screwing movement. This helps in easy entry of the bisacromial diameter into the pelvic inlet.

- Extraction of posterior arm–the operator's hand is introduced into the vagina along the fetal posterior humerus. The arm is then swept across the chest and delivered by gentle traction. If this fails, baby is likely to be dead by this time.
- Cleidotomy–one or both of the clavicles are cut with scissors to reduce the shoulder girth.
- Zavenelli's maneuver–fetal head is flexed and replaced into the uterus followed by delivery of the baby by emergency cesarean section.

Don'ts

- Don't panic
- No traction over baby's head
- No fundal pressure

Mauriceau Smellie Viet technique is used in the delivery of the aftercoming head in a vaginal breech delivery. Baby is placed on the supinated left forearm with limbs hanging on the sides and the middle and index fingers are placed over the malar bones and the head is flexed and delivered.

Other methods employed in the delivery of the after coming head in breech are:

Burns-Marshall technique–where baby is allowed to hang by its own weight

Piper's forceps.

16. Ans. b. Synthesized by cytotrophoblast: *Ref: Dutta's Obstetrics, 7/e p58*

hCG measurement.

True statement regarding hCG is:

(a) Half-life is 7 days

(b) Doubling time in plasma is 1.4 to 2 days (ans.)

(c) Can be detected only after 4 weeks

(d) It has a specific α unit and a nonspecific β unit.

HCG

- Glycoprotein made of 2 subunits–nonspecific alpha and a specific beta unit.
- Produced by the syncytiotrophoblast of the placenta and Half-life is about 24 hours.
- Values related to HCG
- By radioimmunoassay, it can be detected in the maternal serum or urine as early as 8–9 days following ovulation.
- In the early pregnancy, the doubling time of hCG in plasma is 1.4–2 days.
- The blood and urine values reach maximum levels ranging 100 iu and 200 iu/ml between 60 and 70 days of pregnancy.

Disappears from the circulation within 2 weeks following delivery.

Levels of hCG in different conditions DCH MR increased

Increased	Decreased
Multiple pregnancy	Ectopic pregnancy
Rh incompatibility	Impending spontaneous abortion
Down's syndrome	
Chorio carcinoma	
Hydatidiform mole	

Hormones produced by placenta:

Synctiotrophoblast	Cytotrophoblast
• HCG – HPL – Human chorionic thyrotropin – Pregnancy-specific beta 1 glycoprotein – Pregnancy-associated plasma protein A	• Corticotropin releasing hormone • GnRH • Growth hormone-releasing hormone • Thyrotropin-releasing hormone • Neuropeptide Y

Contd...

Contd...

Synctiotrophoblast	Cytotrophoblast
– Growth factors-inhibin, activin, EGF – Estrogen – Progesterone – Relaxin – Leptin (both synctiotophoblast/cytotrophoblast)	

17. Ans. b. 20 weeks *Ref: Dutta's Obstetrics 6/e p17*

Oogenesis:

- Primitive germ cells take origin in the yolk sac and at the end of 3rd week, they migrate into the gonadal ridges

↓

Undergo mitosis, and differentiate to oogonia

↓

At 20 weeks it is maximum–7 million

↓

They enter the first meiotic division and get arrested in the prophase–**they are called primary oocytes**

↓

At birth, there is no more mitosis or meiosis and the number of primary oocytes is **2 million**

↓

At puberty, only 400,000 primary oocytes are left behind

↓

Out of it only **400** are required to ovulate during the entire reproductive period

↓

First meiotic division is complete and **Secondary Oocyte** is formed after which ovulation occurs

↓

The second meiotic division is completed by the secondary oocyte only after fertilization, and results in the formation of a mature ovum.

18. Ans. a. Vasa previa *Ref: Dutta Textbook, of obstetrics 7/e p260*

Antepartum hemorrhage

APH is defined as bleeding from or into genital tract after 28th week of pregnancy but before the birth of baby. (1st and 2nd stage labor included)

- Placenta previa
- Abruptio placenta
- Local causes–cancer cervix, polyp, varicose veins, trauma
- Circumvalate papilla
- Vasa previa–velamentous insertion of placenta
- Unclassified.

Placenta previa:

Degrees of placenta previa (Browne's):

Type 1: (Low-lying). Major part of placenta is attached to upper segment and only the lower margin encloses onto the lower segment. But not upto os.

Type 2: (Marginal)–placenta reaches to the margin but does not cover the os.

Type 3: (Incomplete or partial control)–covers the internal os when closed, but not so when fully dilated.

Type 4: (Central or total)–Placenta completely covers the internal os even on full dilatation.

Grading of placenta previa

Mild–type 1 and type 2 anterior

Major–type 2 posterior and type 3 and type 4

Anterior and posterior based on the wall it lieson.

Posterior is m/c

Causes for Antepartum hemorrhage in placenta previa:

- As placental growth slows down in later, life the lower segment progressively dilates, So the inelastic placenta shears out leading to opening of uteroplacental vessels and episode of bleeding.
- This separation of placenta may be evoked by coitus, vaginal examination, external version or during high rupture of membranes.
- Blood is always maternal.

Abruptio placenta:

(Premature separation of placenta)

It is one form of antepartum hemorrhage where bleeding occurs due to premature separation of normally situated placenta.

Varieties:

- Revealed–m/c type
- Concealed
- Mixed.

Pathogenesis–premature separation of placenta in initiated by hemorrhage into decidua basalis.

The blood can collect in any of the below sites

- Retroplacental hematoma–depression found on maternal surface of placenta
- Complete accumulation behind the placenta
- Blood may dissect downwards and escapes out
- May rupture into the amniotic cavity
- Blood is of maternal origin.

Circumvallate placenta:

Circumvallate placenta–the fetal surface has a central depressed zone surrounded by thickened white ring which is usually complete. Vessels radiate from the cord insertion till the ring and disappear from the view. The peripheral zone outside is thicker and edge is elevated and rounded. Clinical significance is the same as placenta marginata.

There are increased chances of abortion, hydrorrhea gravidarum (excessive watery vaginal discharge), APH, IUGR, preterm labor, retained placenta or membranes.

Vasa previa:

Velamentous insertion–the cord inserts into the membranes at some distance from the placenta.

Fetal vessels traverse the membrane; hence can rupture and result in *vasa previa*–fetal hypoxia.

Causes rupture of fetal blood vessels.

Remember the bleeding is of fetal origin.

To detect fetal blood:

- **Wright stain**
- **Singers'alkali denaturation test**
  - On Wright's stain- fetal RBC appear nucleated.
  - On Singer's alkali denaturation test-fetal HB is more resistant to denaturation.

19. Ans. b. Per peculum *Ref: Dutta's Textbook of Obstetrics, 7/e p245, 249, 380*

Causes of bleeding in placenta previa

- During later months of pregnancy and in labor, the lower segment progressively dilates, the inelastic placenta is sheared off the wall of the lower segment. This leads to opening up of the utero-placental vessels and leads to an episode of bleeding. This is the physiological phenomenon of cause of bleeding in placenta previa.
- It is also provoked by:
  - Trauma
  - Vaginal examination
  - Coital act
  - External version
  - During high rupture of membranes
  - Clinical confirmation by:

Double set-up examination
- Less frequently done
- Indications are–inconclusive USG report:
  - USG revealed type I placenta previa,
  - USG facilities are not available
- Done in operation theater
- Where patient is put under GA
- Blood kept ready
- All facilities kept ready for an emergency cesarean section
- Per speculum examination is done using Cusco's speculum
- Followed by index finger gently introduced and the fornices palpated for any boggy mass felt between the presenting part and the finger
- If head is felt throughout, the slowly the finger is introduced into the cervical canal past the internal os
- Once the placenta is felten the examination is stopped
- Otherwise the lower segment is explored by sweeping the finger 360 degrees around the internal os before declaring that there is no placental tissue
- In that case, ARM is done to induce labor.

20. Ans. c. Fetus in peritoneal cavity *Ref: Dutta's Textbook of Obstetrics 6/e p431*

Scar dehiscence
- Disruption of part of the scar and not the entire length
- Fetal membranes are intact
- Bleeding is nil or minimal.

Scar rupture
- Disruption of the entire length of the scar
- Rupture of the membranes
- Varying amount of bleeding from the margins or from its extension.

Signs of impending scar rupture
- Dull abdominal pain over the scar with slight vaginal bleeding
- Varying degrees of tenderness on uterine palpation
- FHR is irregular or absent
- CTG shows a nonreactive trace
- Maternal tachycardia and hypotension.

Signs of scar rupture
- Patient in exhaustion and shock
- Cessation of uterine contraction
- Superficial fetal parts felt (fetus in peritoneal cavity)
- Absence of uterine contour
- Two separate swellings-one is contracted uterus and the other is fetal ovoid
- P/V–recession of presenting part and varying degrees of bleeding.

21. Ans. d. Increased blood viscosity *Ref: Ian Donald 6/e p103*

CVS changes in pregnancy

***Increase in blood volume**

Plasma volume increase–40–50%

Red cell mass increase–30%

Hemodilution–5–15%

***Increase in cardiac output 30–40%**

Begins at about 5th week and peaks at 20–24 weeks and continues to increase till 32 weeks and then plateaus. This is achieved by increase in stroke volume and heart rate of about 10–20 beats/minute.

***Systemic vascular resistance is reduced**

This helps to decrease BP in spite of an increase in cardiac output.

Diastolic BP decreases more than the systolic BP, leading to widening of pulse pressure.

***Increase in the size of the heart** d/t increased work and by 3rd trimester, it is displaced more outwards.

- These changes are mediated by **estrogen normal prostacyclins and locally produced nitric oxide.**

Effect of the changes in the CVS:

Hemodilution

↓

Decrease in viscosity of blood

Increased placental flow and also mid-trimester opening of placental sinuses contribute to decreased peripheral resistance.

22. Ans. a. Nuchal translucency *Ref: Ian Donald 6/e p47*

Tests for Down's syndrome

1st trimester

USG marker–Nuchal translucency (NT)–is the most sensitive marker

@13 weeks–NT is 1.4–1.5 mm

Combination of NT with maternal age is the most sensitive marker for Down's syndrome

When NT is combined with biochemical markers (Beta hCG and PAPP-A), the detection rate is increased to 80–88% for Down's syndrome, 100% for Trisomy 18 and 95% for all aneuploidies.

2nd trimester

Triple test–Maternal serum alpha fetoprotein (MSAFP) + free beta hCG + Unconjugated estriol (UE3)

In Down's syndrome–↑ in MSAFP and UE3 and ↓ βhCG

Quadruple (Quad) test–Triple test + Inhibin A.

23. Ans. c. 10 weeks *Ref: Dutta's Textbook of Obstetrics 7/e p41*

There are 3 periods distinguished in the prenatal period:

Ovular/Germinal period–lasts for 2 weeks following ovulation; despite the ovum is fertilized, it is still called the ovum.

Embryonic period–begins at 3rd week following ovulation and extends upto 10 weeks of gestation (8 weeks postconception). The CRL of the embryo is 4 mm.

Fetal period-starts from 10 weeks of gestation (8 weeks postconception) and ends till delivery. The chronology in the fetal period is henceforth expressed in terms of menstrual age and not in embryonic age.

24. Ans. a. Obstructed labor

Ref: Dutta's Textbook of Obstetrics 6/e p363

Nature	Constriction ring Schroeder's	Retraction ring Bandl's
Nature	Manifestation of localized incoordinate uterine contraction due to uterine irritability	End state of tonic uterine contraction and relaxation due to obstructed labor
Situation	M/c between US/LS junction. But may be anywhere	Always between US/LS junction
	Once formed would not move	Progressively moves upward
Uterus	US-contracts and retracts with relaxation in between	US-tonically contracted, no relaxation
	LS-thick and loose	LS-thinned and distended
Maternal	Unaffected	Exhausted and sepsis seen

	Features	Constriction ring	Retraction ring
P/A	Uterus	Firm/non tender	Tense and tender
	Fetal parts	Easily felt	Not felt
	Ring	Not felt	Felt
	Round ligament	Not felt	Felt
	FH	+	Absent

Contd...

Contd...

	Features	Constriction ring	Retraction ring
P/V	Ring	Felt	Not felt
	Obstructed labor features	Absent	Present
End	Maternal/fetal	Maternal exhaustion/fetal distress are late	Early features
	Uterus	No chance of uterine rupture	Uterine rupture at lower segment
	Treatment principle	To relax the ring followed by delivery of baby To cut the ring during LSCS	To relieve the obstruction

25. Ans. b. Myometrial quiescence

26. Ans. c. NST and AFI *Ref: Dutta's Textbook of Obstetrics 7/e p109*

Manning's scoring Fetal biophysical profile (BPP)

Parameters	Minimal normal criteria	Score
1. NST	Reactive pattern	2
2. Fetal breathing movements	1 episode >30 seconds	2
3. Gross body movement	3 discrete body/limb movements	2
4. Fetal muscle tone	1 episode extension with return of flexion	2
5. Amniotic fluid	1 pocket measuring 2 cm in two perpendicular planes	2

BPP SCORE-8–10: no fetal asphyxia

Modified BPP-NST and AFI alone are used

27. Ans. a. Vasa previa *Ref: Q3 of 2012 paper*

28. Ans. a. Ampullary portion of the fallopian tube *Ref: Shaw's Textbook of Gynaecology, 15/ed*

Extra uterine
Tubal (m/c) • Ampulla (55%) • Isthmus (25%) • Infundibulum (18%) • Interstitial (2%)
Ovarian (0.5%)
Abdominal (1%) • Primary (rare) • Secondary – Intraperitoneal – Extraperitoneal – Broad ligament

- Isthmus ruptures at 6–8 weeks
- Ampullary rupture at 8–12 weeks
- Interstitial rupture at 4 months

29. Ans. a. Loss of deep tendon reflexes *Ref: Williams' Obstetrics*

Magnesium Sulfate

It is the DOC in the control of ecclamptic seizures and also for the prevention of impending ecclampsia

Regimens for magsulf

Pritchard regimen–total loading dose 14 g

4 g IV (20 ml of 20% solution) given over 15–20 minutes + 10 g deep IM, 5 g in each buttock (10 ml of 50% solution).

This is f/b 5 g IM every 4 hours

- **Zuspan/Sibai Regimen**–4 g IV over 15–20 minutes f/b IV infusion of 1–2 g/hour

- **Mechanism of action:**
  - Decreases ACH release from nerve endings and decreases the sensitivity of motor nerve end-plate
  - Blocks calcium channel
  - Causes vasodilatation–increases cerebral, uterine and renal blood flow.
  - Decreases intracranial edema.
- Therapeutic dose:
  4–7 meq/l or 1.8–3 mmol/l.
- Magnesium toxicity causes:
  - Respiratory paralysis
  - Cardiac conduction defects
  - Cardiac arrest.
- Toxicity monitored by is:
  - Presence of deep tendon reflexes
  - Respiratory rate of > 12/minutes
  - Urine output >30 ml/hour or > 100 ml/4 hours
- At 10 meq/l = patellar reflexes disappear.
- At 12 meq/l = respiratory paralysis and arrest follows.
- To treat magnesium toxicity
  - 10 ml of 10% calcium gluconate solution infused slowly over 3 minutes
  - Withold further doses of magsulf

Other facts of magsulf:
- Category B drug
- IV–Onset of action is immediate and lasts for 30 minutes
- IM–Onset of action is about 1 hour and lasts for 3–4 hours
- Excretion is solely by kidney.

Not used to treat hypertension.

Uses:
- Prevention and control of seizures in preecclampsia and ecclampsia
- Tocolytic in preterm labor
- In Torsades de pointes
- IV magsulf used during spinal anesthesia (Br J Anaesth. 2010 Jan; 104(1):89–93) and general anesthesia (The Internet Journal of Anesthesiology, Vol 30, No.2) improves postoperative analgesia
- In TPN, added to the nutrient mixture to correct or prevent hypomagnesemia.

MCQ Points
- 1st sign of hypermagnesemia- loss of deep tendon reflexes–@10 meq/l
- Proteinuria in pre-ecclampsia is d/t–release of vasoconstrictors from the placenta
  - Causes endothelial dysfunction, vasoconstriction and increased vascular permeability
- Contraindication of magsulf–myasthenia gravis and impaired renal function.

30. Ans. c. Release of vasoconstrictors

Ref: Previous question, Robbins Pathologic Basis of Disease, 8/e

Also asked in PGI.

31. Ans. c. Septate uterus *Ref: Ian Donald 6/e p429*

Etiology for breech presentation
- Prematurity (main cause of breech)
- Multiple pregnancy
- Congenital fetal malformations
- Fetal growth restriction
- Contracted pelvis
- Mullerian anomalies
- Placenta previa/cornuofundal placenta

- Hydramnios
- Oligohydramnios
- Pelvic tumors
- Nulliparity
- Extended legs.

Etiology of recurrent breech presentation-factors which are permanently present in all pregnancies like.

- Contracted pelvis
- Mullerian anomalies.

In the options given in the MCQ, all are factors responsible for a breech presentation, but the recurrent cause for a breech presentation is only option c, septate uterus (Mullerian anomaly).
Incidence of breech in Mullerian anomaly is 46–61%.

32. Ans. d. Myasthenia gravis *Ref: Dutta's Textbook of Obstetrics 7/e p508, 509, 234*

For explanation refer Q8 of 2011 paper.

33. Ans. a. Chromosomal anomalies *Ref: Dutta's Textbook of Obstetrics 7/e p160*

Causes for 1st trimester abortion

- Genetic factors (50%)–autosomal trisomy, polyploidy, monosomy
- Endocrine disorders (10-15%)–Luteal phase defect, thyroid abnormalities, diabetes)
- Immunological disorders (5–10%)–autoimmune (anti-nuclear antibodies, APLA) and alloimmune
- Infection (5%)
- Unexplained (40–60%).

34. Ans. a. Malpresentation *Ref: Dutta's Textbook of Obstetrics 6/e p209*

Complications of monochorionic twins

- **Twin to Twin transfusion syndrome, TTTS:**
  - One twin appears to bleed into the other through some kind of placental vascular anastomosis. As a result, the receptor fetus becomes larger with hydramnois, polycythemic, hypertensive and hypervolemic. The donor twin becomes smaller with oligohydramnios, anemic, hypotensive and hypovolemic.
  - The donor twin may appear stuck due to severe ologohydramnios
  - Difference in hemoglobin concentration > 5 g%
  - Difference in fetal weight > 25%
  - Management-diagnosis is ultrasound with Doppler.

Treatment:

Serial amniocentesis to control polyhydramnios in recipient twin. This will prevent preterm labor and placental abruption.

Laser photocoagulation to interrupt the anastomotic vessels

Selective feticide–of one twin is done when survival of both fetuses is at risk. The smaller twin has a better outcome. The plethoric twin runs the risk of congestive cardiac failure and hydrops.

Perinatal outcome in TTTS is 70%.

- **Dead fetus syndrome:**
  - Death of one twin is associated with poor outcome of the surviving twin. It runs the risk of cerebral palsy, microcephaly, renal cortical necrosis and DIC
- **Twin reversed arterial perfusion, TRAP:**
  - Characterized by an acardiac perfused twin having blood supply from the normal co-twin via large arterioarterial anastomosis. The surviving twin dies due to high output cardiac failure.
- **Monoamniocity**–high mortality is due to cord entanglement
- **Conjoint twins**
  - Malpresentation–common in twins than in singleton pregnancies. This is not a specific complication for monochorionic twins alone.

35. Ans. a. Cesarean section *Ref: Dutta's Textbook of Obstetrics 6/e p252*

Indications for cesarean section in placenta previa

- Severe degrees of placenta previa (Type-II posterior, Type III and IV) - indicated for maternal interest even if the fetus is dead.
- Lesser degrees of placenta previa where amniotomy fails to stop bleeding or fetal distress appears.
- Complicating factors associated with lesser degrees of placenta previa where vaginal delivery is unsafe.

36. Ans. a. Subseptate uterus *Ref: Dutta's Textbook of Obstetrics 7/e p395*

Arcuate or a subseptate uterus favours a transverse lie

Septate or a bicornuate uterus favours breech presentation.

37. Ans. a. Pulsation in the lateral vaginal fornix *Ref: Dutta's Textbook of Obstetrics 6/e p65*

Chadwick's sign/Jacquemier's sign

- Dusky hue of vestibule and anterior vaginal wall due to local vascular congestion
- 8th week of pregnancy
- Also in pelvic fibroids.

Osiander's sign

- Increased pulsations felt through lateral fornices
- At 8th week
- Also in PID.

Goodell's sign

- Softening of cervix like lip of mouth
- 6th week of IUL
- Also in those who use OCP.

Hegar's sign

- Because of softening of the isthmus which you can bimanually palpate the fingers which can be opposed
- 6–10 weeks.

Palmer's sign

- Rhythmic contractions in uterus on bimanual examination
- 4–10 weeks.

Mc Donald's sign

- Uterus is flexible at uterocervical junction
- 4–8 weeks.

Clinical examination of a pregnant lady at second trimester

- Chloasma–24 weeks
- Breast–appearance of secondary areola
- Secretion of colostrum–12 weeks
- Thickening of colostrum–16 weeks
- Linea nigra
- Striae.

38. Ans. a. Piper's forceps *Ref: Dutta's Textbook of Obstetrics 6/e p384*

Assisted breech delivery

Delivery of head:

- Burns Marshall method,
- Mauriceau-Smellie Veit method,
- Piper's forceps- specially designed for this with absent pelvic curve
  - Extended legs-Pinard's maneuver
  - Extended arm-Lovset's maneuver.

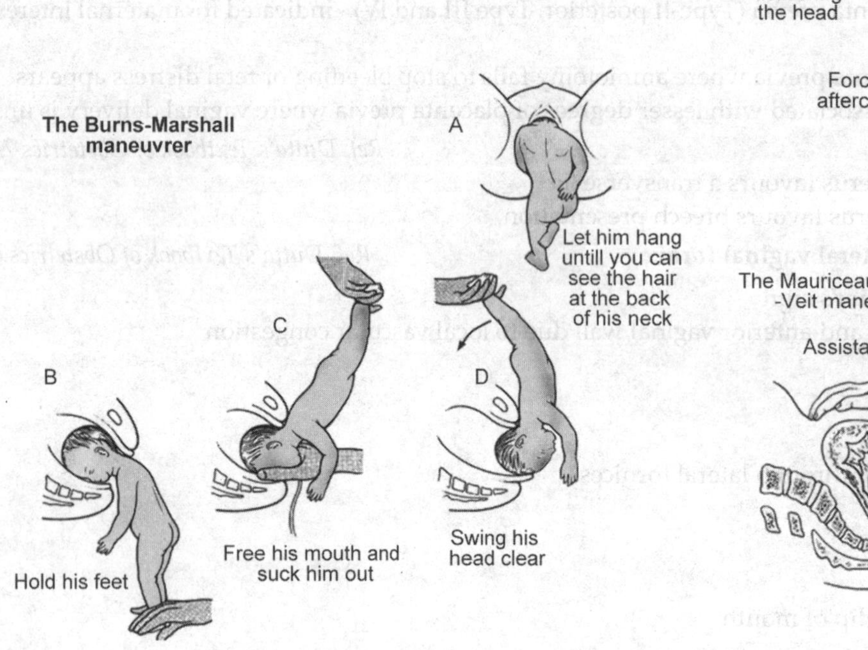

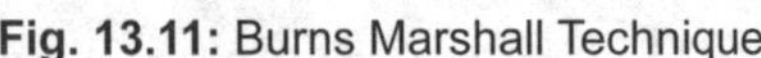

Fig. 13.11: Burns Marshall Technique

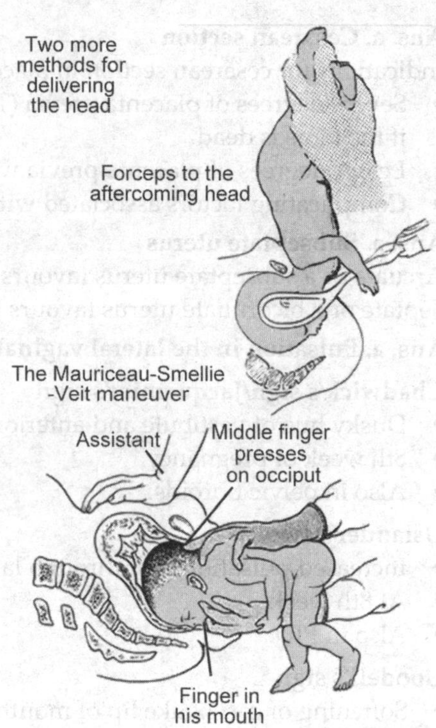

Fig. 13.12: Mauriceau Smellie Veit Method

39. Ans. b. Occipitofrontal *Ref: Dutta's Textbook of Obstetrics 7/e p85*

Dear friends, I do not mind repeating this table for you, because of its high yield. There have been lot of MCQ's from this area, so be through with this table. You can crack many!

Diameter	From	To	Measurement	Attitude of the head	Presentation
Suboccipito-bregmatic	Nape of the neck	Center of the bregma	9.5 cm	Complete flexion	Vertex
Suboccipitofrontal	Nape of the neck	Anterior end of the anterior fontanelle or center of the sinciput	10 cm	Incomplete flexion	Vertex
Occipitofrontal	Occipital eminence	Root of the nose (Glabella)	11.5 cm	Marked deflexion	Vertex
Mentovertical	Midpoint of the chin	Highest point on the sagittal suture	14 cm	Partial extension	Brow
Submentovertical	Junction of the floor of the mouth and neck	Highest point on the sagittal suture	11.5 cm	Incomplete extension	Face
Submentobregmatic	Junction of the floor of the mouth and neck	Center of the bregma	9.5 cm	Complete extension	Face
Diameter	**Extent**		**Measurement**	**Remarks**	
Biparietal	Between two parietal eminences		9.5 cm	Whatever be the position of the head, this diameter nearly always engages	
Diameter	**Extent**		**Measurement**	**Remarks**	
Bitemporal	Between the anteroinferior ends of the coronal suture		8 cm		

Contd...

Contd...

Bimastoid	Between the tip of the two mastoid processes	7.5 cm	Incompressible diameter, impossible to reduce the length of the diameter by obstetrical operations

In the options given, occipitofrontal is the longest diameter of the skull. But the actual longest diameter is the mentovertical which is 14 cm, but not given as an option.

40. Ans. a. Cervix status *Ref: Dutta's Textbook of Obstetrics 7/e p522*

Bishop's scoring

- Quantitative method for prediction of successful induction of labor.
- It includes the following five parameters:
  - Cervix 4–dilatation, position, effacement and consistency
  - Fetal head station.

Bishop scoring

Score	Dilation (cm)	Efface (%)	Station	Cervical consist	Position
0	Close	0–30%	–3	Firm	posterior
1	1–2	40–50%	–2	Medium	Mid
2	3–4	60–70%	–1,0	Soft	Anterior
3	>5	>80%	+1, +2	–	–

Modified Bishop's score–effacement = instead of %, length is used, i.e. 3 cm–score is 0, 2 cm–1, 1 cm–2, 0 cm–3
Favorable score–6–13
Unfavorable score–0–5.

41. Ans. b. Prolongation of pregnancy *Ref: Dutta's Textbook of Obstetrics 7/e p232*

Eclampsia

- Fits occurring in eclampsia is generalized tonic clonic seizures
- Most seizures are self-limited are lasting less than 2 minutes
- The first priority in, management of seizures is to ensure airway and prevent aspiration of gastric contents
- Incidence of fits–50% antepartum, 30% intrapartum and 20% postpartum
- In postpartum the it is usually <48 hours; if beyond 7 days, it is not eclampsia.

Pritchard's regimen:

- DOC for management of convulsions- magnesium sulfate
- Therapeutic range–4–7 meq/l.
- Mechanism of action peripheral action at NM junction, competes with calcium for entry into cells and may have a central action
- Schedule–4g of magsulf 20% solution given IV over 4–5 min f/b, 5 g of 50% soln given as IM in each buttock (total 10 g as IM), f/b 5 g of 50% soln given as IM every 4 hours
- Monitor urine output–atleast 30 ml/hours, deep tendon reflex must be present and RR must be >12/minutes
- Previously used lytic cocktail (Menon) regimen is not used now-contains pethidine, chlorpromazine and phenergan
- Zuspan/Sibai regimen–4–6 g of magsulf in 100 ml of IV fluid over 15–20 minutes (loading dose) f/b, 1–2 g in 100 ml IV fluid/hour.

Obstetric management

- Terminate pregnancy immediately if fits occurs
- Termination must be by LSCS except if fetus is dead and cervix is fully ripe.

Eclampsia cases, peculiar management at delivery

- No prophylactic ergometrine
- Anesthesia of choice–Spinal or epidural
- Only contraindication for epidural is low platelet count <50,000.

- For status epilepticus–thiopentone sodium is given
- Postpartum continue $MgSO_4$ for 24 hours
- Diuretics must be given after delivery.

Complications of eclampsia

- M/c of maternal death–Intracranial bleeding and acute renal failure caused by abruptio placenta
- M/c of fetal death–prematurity and asphyxia.

HELLP

Hemolysis

Elevated liver enzymes

Low platelet count

- M/c symptom–Epigastric/RUQ pain
- Hallmark–Microangipathic hemolysis leading to elevated LDH and fragmented RBC
- Treatment–Immediate termination of pregnancy/steroids and FFP
- M/c cause of death in HELLP–Abruptio placenta and DIC.

Drugs used for prophylaxis of preeclampsia

- Low dose aspirin- maintains normal balance of TX and PG
- Calcium supplements–synthesis of nitrous oxide-vasodilator
- Antioxidants–vitamins C, E and lycopene-scavenges-free radicals which cause preeclampsia
- Folic acid-hyperhomocysteinemia is associated with early onset of preeclampsia (FA inhibits homocysteine).

42. Ans. a. Pressure necrosis of the urethra during obstructed labor *Ref: Dutta Gynecology 6/e p401*

Fistulae

Causes:

Obstetrical (most common)

- Ischemia 3–5 months following delivery
- Traumatic instrumental delivery-operation.

Gynecological:

- Operative injury
- Traumatic
- Malignancy
- Radiation (1–2 years following RT)
- Infective
- Most common urinary fistula – vesicovaginal (VVF)
- Most common cause of VVF – obstructed labor
- Most common cause of ureterine VF – gynecological operations esp. wertheim's operation
- Most common of Vesico uterine F – cesarian section
- Most common of Recto vaginal F – complete perineal tear.

JIPMER 2008

43. Ans. a. Submentobregmatic

Ref: Dutta's Textbook of Obstetrics 7/e p85, also refer to the explanation of Q5 of 2009 paper

As I told you this is a high-yield area, you can see that you almost get at least one MCQ from this area. Through the table.

44. Ans. c. Android pelvis *Ref: Dutta's Textbook of Obstetrics 6/e p346, Williams' Obstetrics 23/e p480*

	Inlet	Cavity	Outlet
Gynecoid	Engage in transverse/oblique diameter No difficulty in engagement	Easy anterior rotation	No difficulty in delivery

Contd...

Contd...

	Inlet	Cavity	Outlet
Anthropoid	Engage in A-P diameter (occipito-posterior) Can be a delayed flexion	Long anterior rotation/non-rotation is common	Delivery is face-to-pubis (head is delivered by flexion)
Android	Engage in transverse/oblique diameter Engagement is delayed and difficult	Difficult anterior rotation (deep transverse arrest)	Difficult delivery with increased incidence of perineal injuries
Platypelloid	Engage in transverse diameter Engagement can be difficult by exaggerated parietal presentation	Anterior rotation usually occurs late in the perineum	No difficulty in delivery

45. Ans. b. Shoulder dystocia *Ref: Current Diagnosis & Treatment-Obstetrics and Gynecology 10/e p316*

Complications of GDM

At pregnancy

- Preeclampsia
- Hydramnios
- Preterm labor
- Stillbirth
- Intercurrent illness
- Pyelonephritis
- DKA and coma
- Retinopathy and nephropathy in overt diabetes cases.

During labor and puerperium

- Prolongation of labor due to big baby
- Shoulder dystocia–most common complication
- Perineal injuries
- PPH
- Operative interventions
- Puerperal sepsis
- Lactation failure.

Fetal complications

Congenital malformation:

- Related to the severity of diabetes during organogenesis in 1st trimester.

Fetal macrosomia

- Maternal hyperglycemia-hypertrophy and hyperplasia of fetal islets-stimulates fetal insulin, leading to increased carbohydrate metabolism and fat deposition
- Elevated maternal FFA-transfers to fetus.

46. Ans: d. Renal agenesis

Ref: Ian Donald: Practical Obstetric Problems 6/e p366, DC Dutta's Textbook of Obstetrics, 7/e p211, 215

Etiology of polyhydramnios

Fetal Anomalies:

Anencephaly

- Transudation from exposed meninges
- Suppression of antidiuretic hormone
- Absence of fetal swallowing.

Open spina bifida–increased transudation

Esophageal/duodenal atresia

Facial clefts/Neck masses–decreased swallowing
Hydrops fetalis:
Rh isoimmunization
Cardiothoracic anomalies
Fetal cirrhosis.
Placenta: Chorioangioma tumor
Multiple pregnancy:
Maternal causes
- Diabetes mellitus-increased diuresis in fetus due to increased blood sugar
- Cardiac and renal diseases–transudation from edematous placenta.

Etiology of oligohydramnios
- Fetal chromosomal anomalies
- Intra uterine infection
- Drugs like PG inhibitors, ACE inhibitors
- Renal agenesis or obstruction of urinary tract (PUV in males)
- IUGR associated with placental insufficiency
- Amnion nodosum-failure of secretion of amniotic fluid by cells of amnion.
- Postmaturity

47. Ans. c. Abruption *Ref: Practical Guide to High-risk Pregnancy & Delivery: Fernando Arias 3/e p344*
Sher's classification for abruption placenta.

Grade I	Mild retroplacental clot of vol <150 ml
Grade II	Classical features of abruption are present Fetus is alive Most of them have abnormal FHR patterns Perinatal mortality is high Retro-placental clot is 150–500 ml
Grade III	Features of grade II with fetal demise A-Presence of coagulopathy B-Absence of coagulopathy

48. Ans. a. Bimastoid *Ref: Q5 of 2009 JIPMER paper for explanation*
49. Ans. c. NST and AFI *Ref: Dutta's Textbook of Obstetrics 7/e p109*
This question is also a repeat.
You can refer the explanation of Q6 of JIPMER 2009 paper.
50. Ans. a. Hemochorial *Ref: Dutta's Textbook of Obstetrics 7/e p28*
Human placenta is
- Discoid–shape
- Hemochorial–because of direct contact with maternal blood
- Deciduate–because some maternal tissue is shed.

51. Ans. d. Hydronephrosis *Ref: DC Dutta's Textbook of Obstetrics, 7/e p106, 649, Williams' Obstetrics, 23/e*
USG markers of Down's syndrome:
- Nuchal translucency >3 mm
- Heart anomalies–VSD, ASD
- Bilateral dilatation of renal pelvis
- Clinodactyly, short femur
- Duodenal atresia
- General growth restriction.

52. Ans. a. Frank breech *Ref: Dutta's Textbook of Obstetrics 7/e p374*
Complete breech (Flexed breech)–the normal attitude of full flexion is maintained. The thighs are flexed at hip and the legs at the knees. The presenting part consists of 2 buttocks, external genitalia and 2 feet.

Commonly seen in multiparae
Incomplete breech–varying degrees of extension of thighs or legs at the podalic pole.
Frank breech (with extended legs)–thighs are flexed at the hip and legs are extended at the knee joints. The presenting part is 2 buttocks and external genitalia only.
Common in primigravidae (about 70%).
Footling presentation–both thighs and legs are partially extended bringing the feet down.
Knee presentation–the thighs are extended at the hip and knees flexed (kneeling down position).
Latter two varieties are uncommon.

53. Ans. a. Anencephaly *Ref: Dutta's Textbook of Obstetrics 7/e p406*

Shoulder dystocia

This is term used if there is a delay of more than one minute in the delivery of the shoulders after the delivery of the head.

Risk factors

- Fetal macrosomia
- Maternal DM
- Maternal obesity
- Post-term
- Anencephaly
- Fetal ascites
- Midpelvic instrument delivery.

In this MCQ, both the options a and c are right, but anencephaly causing shoulder dystocia is more common than fetal ascites, Hence I chose option a.

54. Ans. a. Premature rupture of membranes

Ref: Practical Guide to High Risk Pregnancy & Delivery: Fernando Arias 3/e p224

Magnesium sulfate acts by blocking the neuromuscular junction. Hence, it is contraindicated in myasthenia gravis.
It is excreted through kidneys; hence Cautiously used in renal failure patients.
Tocolysis as such is contraindicated in chorioamnionitis or intrauterine infection.
Options b, c and d are ruled out.
Tocolysis can be given in preterm PROM after ruling out chorioamnionitis.

Complications of magnesium sulfate

- Muscular weakness
- Pulmonary edema
- Respiratory depression
- Neurotoxicity
- Neonatal depression
- Neonatal hypotonia
- Neonatal hypocalcemia
- Intraventricular hemorrhage.

Drugs used for tocolysis

- Nifedipine
- Magnesium sulfate
- Beta-adrenergic drugs like isoxsuprine, ritodrine, terbutaline
- Indomethacin
- Nitroglycerine
- Diazoxide.

Safest tocolytic with least side effects: Nifedipine

55. Ans. d. 28 weeks *Ref: Dutta's Textbook of Obstetrics 7/e p276*

Period of high risk in cardiac failure:

- Between 12 and 16 weeks of gestation (when hemodynamic changes just began)
- Between 28 and 32 weeks (when hemodynamic changes are maximum)
- During delivery
- Immediate postpartum
- Finally 4–5 days after delivery when changes start reverting back

When the hemodynamic changes are maximum that is the time when the risk of cardiac failure is more in a patient with cardiac disease; in this case, mitral stenosis.

56. Ans. b. 0.5 *Ref: Williams' Obstetrics, 23/e and www.cesarean.org.uk/articles/VBACMM.html*

The incidence of scar rupture in a previous LSCS for VBAC is 0.5% or 1 in 200 chances.

Risk of scar rupture

Type of incision	Incidence of scar rupture
Low transverse	0.2–1.5%
Low vertical	1–7%
T shaped	4–7%
Classical	4–7%

57. Ans. a. Cord prolapse is common *Ref: Dutta's Textbook of Obstetrics 6/e p394*

Etiology for transverse lie

- Multiparity–lax and pendulous abdomen, imperfect uterine tone and extreme uterine obliquity
- Prematurity–center of gravity is in the middle of the body
- Twins–2nd of the twin
- Hydramnios
- Contracted pelvis
- Placenta previa
- Pelvic tumors
- Congenital malformation of the uterus–arcuate/subseptate
- Intrauterine death.

Clinical course in labor

- Unfavorable events-early rupture of membranes
  - prolapsed of the hand or cord
  - obstructe labor
  - rupture uterus and maternal death
  - maternal exhaustion especially in a primigravida
- Favorable events (rare)-spontaneous correction to vertex or breech
  - spontaneous expulsion
  - spontaneous evolution (expulsion of breech and trunk followed by head)

58. Ans. b. Cord compression *Ref: Dutta's Textbook of Obstetrics 6/e p609*

FHR pattern	Features	Seen in
Early deceleration	Coincides with uterine contraction Uniform onset and recovery	Head compression
Late deceleration	Begins at or after contraction Peaks and touches base only after contraction	• Maternal hypotension • Maternal DM/HTN/collagen vascular diseases • Acute late deceleration is placental disruption
Variable deceleration	Ragged waveform	Cord compression

59. Ans. c. Always monochorionic *Ref: Dutta's Textbook of Obstetrics 7/e p201*

Dizygotic twin	Monozygotic twin
Two placentas Completely separated	Placenta is single
Each fetus is covered by separate amnion and chorion	Each fetus is separated by separate amnion but common chorion
Intervening membrane contains 4 layers A-C-C-A	Intervening membrane contains 2 layers only A-A

60. Ans. a. Decidua basalis *Ref: Dutta's Textbook of Obstetrics 7/e p30*

Placenta anatomy

- Diameter–15–20 cms
- Thickness–2.5 cm
- Weight–500 g
- Volume of blood = 500 ml
- Ratio of placenta : fetus = 1 : 6 in weight
- Placenta separates after delivery of baby-through the line of decidua spongiosum
- Phagocytic cells seen in placenta are called *Hofbauer cells.*

Placenta

Maternal surface	Fetal surface
Formed by decidua basalis	Formed by chorion frondosum and chorionic plate
Dull red color	Fetal surface covered by blood vessels
15–20 lobes of cotyledon	

61. Ans. b. Shoulder dystocia

Ref: Current Diagnosis & Treatment-Obstetrics and Gynecology 10/e p316

It is a repeat question. Refer to Q3 of JIPMER 2008 for explanation.

62. Ans. a. Chromosomal anomalies *Ref: Dutta's Textbook of Obstetrics 7/e p160*

This is repeated question too. Refer to Q2 of JIPMER 2010 paper for explanation

63. Ans. b. 60–70 *Ref: Dutta's Textbook of Obstetrics 7/e*

Level of hCG is highest at 60–70 days of pregnancy.

hCG is produced by the syncyitiotrophoblasts.

It is responsible for the rescue and maintenance of corpus luteum in the first 6 weeks

hCG: MR-DCH Increased

Increased	Decreased
Multiple pregnancy	Ectopic pregnancy
Rh Incompatibility	Impending spontaneous abortion
Down's syndrome	
Choriocarcinoma	
Hydatidiform mole	

64. Ans. a. Anthropoid pelvis *Ref: Dutta's Textbook of Obstetrics 6/e p346*

Caldwell-Moloy Classification

- Gynecoid (50%)
- Anthropoid (25%)
- Android (20%)
- Platypelloid (5%)

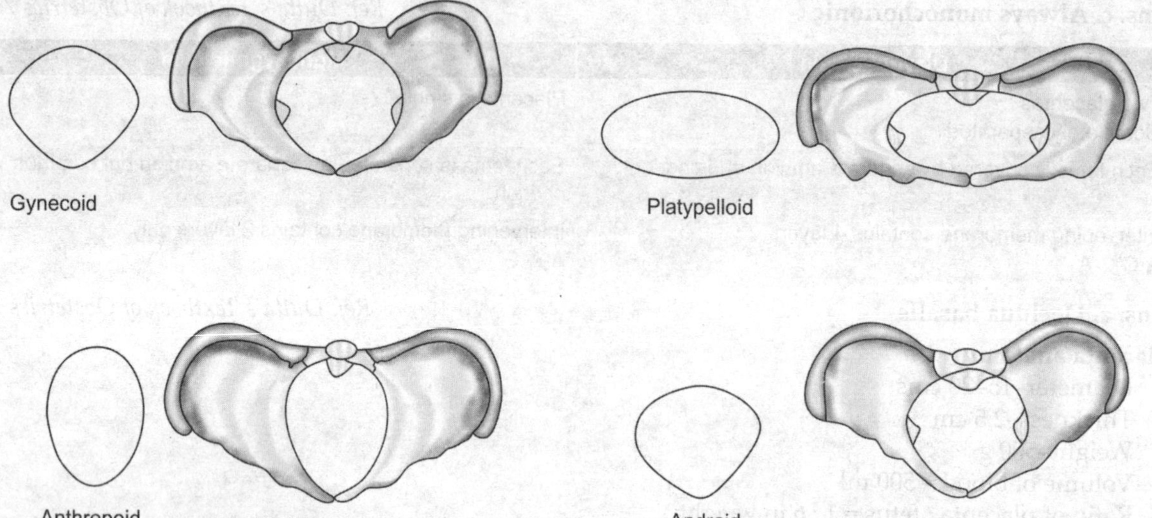

Features	Gynecoid	Anthropoid	Android	Platypelloid
Inlet	Round	AP–oval	Triangular	Transversely oval
Sacrosciatic notch	Wide and shallow	More wide and shallow	Narrow and deep	Slightly narrow and small
Ischial spines	Not prominent	Not prominent	Prominent	Not prominent
Pubic arch	Curved	Long and curved	Long and straight	Short and curved
Subpubic angle	Wide (85°)	Slightly narrow	Narrow	Very wide (more than 90°)
Bituberous diameter	Normal	Normal or short	Short	Wide

Composite measurement of diameters

	Inlet	Cavity	Outlet
Anteroposterior	11	12	13
Oblique	12	12	–
Transverse	13	12	11

65. Ans. b. Rich blood supply *Ref: Dutta's Textbook of Obstetrics 6/e p37*

Amnion

- Single layer of cuboidal epithelium
- Basement membranes
- Compact layer of reticular structure
- Fibroblastic layer
- Spongy layer
- No blood, nerve or lymphatic supply
- Helps cervical dilatation during labor.

66. Ans. c. Alpha-methyldopa *Ref: Dutta's Textbook of Obstetrics 6/e p506*

Friends, this is a tricky question. The older edition of *Dutta's Textobook of Obstetrics* quotes that alpha-methyl dopa is the safest antihypertensive in pregnancy, but the latest edition says both alpha-methyldopa and labetalol are first line drugs.

Looking into the literature.

Alpha-methyl dopa–is a Class B drug and is the drug of choice according to NHBEP. Safety of the drug after first trimester is well-documented, including 7 years' follow-up of the offspring.

Labetalol–is a Class C drug, which states that human studies are lacking and animal studies are either positive for fetal risk or not, the drug is given only when the benefits outweigh the risk to the fetus. This drug may be associated with fetal growth restriction.

Therefore, the drug of choice in hypertension in pregnancy is alpha-methyl dopa

Drugs used for preeclampsia

Name	Mode of action	Side effect
Labetalol (drug of choice)	Combined alpha + Beta blocker	Postural hypertension
Hydralazine	Peripheral vasodilator	Headache, flushing and tachycardia
Nifedipine	Calcium channel blocker	Headache, flushing and palpitation
Alpha-methyldopa	Central action	Postural hypotension and hemolytic anemia
Atenolol	Beta blocker	Bradycardia, hypotension and hypoglycemia

Drugs that must not be used

- ACE inhibitors–impair renal function resulting in oliguria and oligohydramnios and congenital defects
- Diuretics
- Losartan
- Reserpine
- Nonselective beta blocker (propranolol)
- Sodium nitroprusside.

Drugs used in hypertensive crisis

- Hydralazine
- Labetalol
- Nifedipine/nimodipine/verapamil
- Ketanserin.

67. **Ans. a. Preterm** *Ref: Dutta's Textbook of Obstetrics 6/e p580*

Ventouse/Vacuum Extraction

Ventouse is an instrument which assists in delivery by creating a vacum between it and scalp.

Prerequisite:

- Bladder empty
- Cervix should be atleast 6 cm
- Vertex presentation
- Head should be engaged
- No bony resistance below head/no evidence of CPD.

Indications of ventouse

- As an alternative to forceps operation
- Alternative to rotational forceps in O-P or O-transverse position
- Delay in descent of head in case of second twin
- Delay in late first-stage labor
- Deep transverse arrest.

Contraindications

- Prematurity
- Fetal coagulopathy
- Macrosomia
- Unengaged head
- Distress of fetus
- CPD
- Nonvertex presentations.

Complications

Maternal	Fetal
Less than that of forceps in mother Soft tissue injuries Annular detachment of cervix Traumatic PPH	M/c is retinal hemorrhage Scalp injury Cephalhematoma* Subgaleal hemorrhage* Neonatal jaundice Asphyxia Shoulder dystocia* * M/c with ventouse

Vaccum	Forceps
Advantages • No anesthesia • Less maternal injuries • Promotes auto rotation-can be used in unrotated or malrotated O-P cases • Does not require full cervical dilatation (> 6 cm is enough) • Less traction force needed	**Disadvantages** Requires anesthesia More injuries No autorotation Requires full dilatation More traction needed
Disadvantages • Requires maternal effort • Takes time in fetal distress • More cephalhematomas/subgaleal • Can't be used in preterm • Can't be used in other presentations	**Advantages:** No maternal effort *Quick in fetal distress* Less cepha hematoma Can be used in preterm Can be used in face and breech

68. Ans. c. > 8 days *Ref: Dutta's Textbook of Obstetrics 6/e p203*

Different types of twins,

Depending on division of fertilized ovum

- **< 72 hours** of fertilization (3 days)–diamniotic dichorionic
- **4th–8th day**–diamniotic monochorionic
- **> 8 days**–monoamniotic monochorionic
- **After development of embryonic disc after 2 weeks**–conjoined (Siamese) twins.
  - Thoracophagus (m/c), pyophagus, craniophagus and ischiophagus.

QUESTIONS 2015

1. **Which of the following causes greatest risk of ectopic pregnancy?**
   a. PID
   b. IUD use
   c. Previous ectopic pregnancy
   d. Previous MTP
2. **Breast cancer in pregnancy. Which one of the following is correct?**
   a. Better prognosis
   b. Radiotherapy can be given in first trimester
   c. TT is mastectomy and radical node dissection
   d. Surgery for breast cancer should be done
3. **HELLP syndrome is associated with:**
   a. Lower abdominal pain
   b. Elevated platelets
   c. Preeclampsia
   d. Lower liver enzymes

ANSWERS AND EXPLANATIONS

1. **Ans. a. PID** *Ref: Dutta's Textbook of Obstetrics 6/e p179*

Tubal pregnancy-etiology

Factors that prevent migration of fertilized ovum to uterine cavity	Factors facilitating nidation of fertilized ovum in tubal mucosa
PID Chlamydia trachomatis is m/c risk factor	Early resumption of trophoblastic activity
Iatrogenic – IUD – Sterilization operation – Progestin only pills – Tubal surgeries – Pelvic surgeries – Ovulation induction – IVF/GIFT techniques	Increased decidual reaction
Previous ectopic	Tubal endometriosis

2. **Ans. d. Surgery for breast cancer should be done** *Ref: www.cancer.gov/types/breast/patient*

Breast cancer in pregnancy.

Treatment options depend on the stage of the disease and the age of the fetus.

Three types of standard treatment used are:

- Surgery
- Radiotherapy
- Chemotherapy.

New modalities in treatment are:

- Hormone therapy
- Immunotherapy.

Surgical modalities are:

- Simple mastectomy
- Modified radical mastectomy with LN dissection
- Breast conservation surgery like lumpectomy, partial mastectomy.

Radiotherapy:

- Early stage disease (stage I and II)—contraindicated
- Late stage disease (stage III and IV)—contraindicated during the 1st 3 months of pregnancy.

Chemotherapy:

- Shouldn't be given during the first 3 months of pregnancy
- Can be given after 3 months, but may cause early labor and low birthweight.

Hormone therapy:

- The effectiveness and safety of it in pregnant women is not yet known.

Prognosis:

Breast cancer in pregnancy has a poor prognosis due to the rapidity of growth caused by the endogenous ovarian hormones (estrogen and progesterone).

3. **Ans. c. Preecclampsia** *Ref: Dutta's Textbook of Obstetrics 6/e p224*

HELLP

- Rare complication on PIH
- C/o nausea, vomiting, epigastric pain, right upper quadrant pain (liver)
- Hemolysis
- Elevated liver enzymes—↑ SGOT, SGPT
- Low platelet count (< 100000/microliter)
- M/c symptom—epigastric/RUQ pain

- Hallmark—microangipathic hemolysis leading to elevated LDH and fragmented RBC
- Treatment—immediate termination of pregnancy/steroids and FFP
- M/c cause of death in HELLP—Abruptio placenta and DIC.

Mild PIH	Severe PIH
BP> 140/90 mm Hg Less than 160 systolic or 110 diastolic BP	BP> 160 mm Hg or diastolic BP >110 mm Hg
+/– proteinuria (300 mg/24 hours urine or 1+ on dipstick)	Proteinuria > 2 g/day
	HELLP syndrome
	Retinal hemorrhages
	Visual disturbance
	Oliguria <400 ml/hr
	Pulmonary edema
	IUGR of fetus
	C/F–epigastric pain
	Serum creatinine > 1.2 mg/dl

Chapter

14 Gynecology

Anuradha Dhanasekharan

ANATOMY AND PHYSIOLOGY

Vagina

Walls: anterior, posterior and two lateral walls

Relations:

- **Anterior:** upper 1/3rd—Base of the bladder, lower 2/3rd—Urethra
- **Posterior:** upper 1/3rd—Pouch of Douglas, middle 1/3rd—Rectum, lower 1.3rd—Anal canal
- **Lateral:** pelvic diaphragm

Uterus

- **Body/corpus:** made of fundus–the part which lies above the openings of the uterine tubes
- **Isthmus:** constricted part between body and the cervix. Measures 0.5 cm
- **Cervix:** cylindrical in shape, measures 2.5 cm normal length of uterine cavity: 6.5–7 cm

Fallopian Tubes

- Measures 4 inches (10 cm) or more in length and approximately 8 mm in diameter
- The fallopian tube is divided anatomically into four parts:

The interstitial portion

- Innermost, shortest and narrowest part
- No longitudinal muscle fibers here but the circular fibers are well developed

The isthmus

- One-third of the total length contains both longitudinal and circular fibers and covered by peritoneum except for a small inferior bare area related to the broad ligament
- It is relatively straight. Site of sterilization.

The ampulla

- Lateral, widest and longest part of the tube comprising roughly 2/3rd of the tube, measuring 2.5 inches (60–75 mm) in length
- Mucosa is arborescent with many complex folds
- Fertilization occurs in the ampullary portion of fallopian tube

The fimbriated extremity or infundibulum

- The part where the abdominal ostium opens into the peritoneal cavity
- The epithelium consists of three types of cells:

- **Ciliated (M/C):** either columnar or cubical in type. Its function is to transport the inert ovum
- **Goblet-shaped cell:** not ciliated, which does not give the his to chemical reaction of mucin. It functions as a lubricant and is possibly nutritive to the ovum
- Intermediate small rod-shaped cells called 'peg' cells whose purpose is not known

Physiology

Pulsatile GnRH initiates secretion of FSH and LH.

UTERINE ENDOMETRIUM

The proliferative phase or oestrogenic phase:

- Starts when regeneration of menstruation endometrium is complete
- The maximum peak oestrogen secretion is seen about 48 hours before ovulation
- Lasts until the 14th day of a 28-day cycle

The secretory phase

- Progesterone induces secretory changes only if the endometrium is primed by oestrogen which produces progesterone receptors in the endometrial cells
- The secretory phase of the endometrium begins on the 15th day and persists until the onset of menstruation
- The secretory phase reaches its peak by the 22nd day of the cycle after which no further growth ensues
- About the 24th day of the cycle some shrinkage of the glands is apparent, partly due to the dehydration of the stroma
  - LH surge occurs 24–36 hours before ovulation
  - LH peak occurs 10–16 hours before ovulation
  - Ovulation occurs 14 days prior to next cycle

AVERAGE AMOUNT OF BLOOD LOSS IN NORMAL MENSTRUATION: 50 ML

- **Menorrhagia:** excessive blood loss (increase in duration of bleeding, >5 days/heavier blood flow, >80 ml/cycle) without any change in the cycle length
- **Polymenorrhea or epimenorrhea:** frequent menstrual cycles as a result of shortening of the cycle length (<21 days)
- **Polymenorrhagia:** characterized by shorter duration of the cycles coupled with heavier flow or prolongation in the duration of flow
- **Oligomenorrhea:** infrequent menses, >35 days apart (the cycle length is prolonged without affecting the duration and amount of flow)
- **Hypomenorrhea:** the cycle length remains unaltered; however the duration of bleeding or the amount of blood loss, or both substantially reduced
- **Amenorrhea:** complete cessation of menstruation: Metrorrhagia–occurrence of intermenstrual bleeding

Cornification index is the percentage of the cornified cells in vaginal cytology

The vaginal cytology during the different phases of menstrual cycle:

Menstruation	Early proliferative phase	Late proliferative phase	Early secretory phase	Late secretory phase
Minimum	Rises	Highest	Falls	Lack of cornification

- Brown staining of the vagina, with Lugol's iodine, gives a rough indication of the glycogen content of the cells lining the vaginal epithelium, and thereby the oestrogenic titer of the patient's blood
- The maximum glycogen content in the vaginal epithelium is found in the vaginal fornices, where it is present to the extent of 2.5 to 3.0 mg%, and it is at its lowest in the lower third, where its value is 0.6 to 0.9%

In girls, the sequence of events during puberty is:

- The first event is the development of breasts, thelarche*
- Followed by pubarche, the development of axillary and pubic hair

- Then by menarche, the first menstrual period

Hence the sequence is Thelarche-Pubarche-Menarche (T→P→M)

Adrenarche: rise in secretion of the adrenal androgens during puberty. Occurs at 8–10 years in girls and 10–12 years in boys

INFECTIONS IN GYNECOLOGY

Vaginal pH

Newborn infant	4.5–7	Reproductive age group	4–5.5
6-weeks-old child	7	Pregnancy	3.5–4.5
Puberty	Changes from alkaline to acidic	Late postmenopausal	6–8

- Adults—stratified squamous epithelium
- Newborn—transitional epithelium
- Squamous epithelium is resistant to gonococcal infection

  Doderlein's bacillus (lactobacilli)—breaks down glycogen of the vaginal epithelium into lactic acid—pH is acidic (4–5.5)

Vaginitis	M/C Organism	Symptom	Signs	Diagnosis	Rx
Trichomonas vaginitis (mc)	Trichomonas vaginalis, flagellated protozoa	Profuse frothy yellowish green discharge with itch	pH- 5.5–6.5, strawberry or angry looking vagina	Wet mount microscopy-motile flagellated trichomonads, culture—Feinberg-whittington media	Metronidazole-500 mg BD/2 g single dose, both partners treated, pregnancy—DOC
Candidiasis	Candida albicans, G+ve, fungus	Intense pruritus, curdy white discharge, dysuria, dyspareunia	Cottage cheese like app, pH< 4.5, inflamed genitals	Adding 10% KOH-fungal elements seen—WHIFF test negative, culture-Sabouraud's media	Azoles- fluconazole, miconazole topical/oral, both partners treated, pregnancy-only topical
Bacterial vaginosis	Gardnerella mycoplasma, peptostretococci, bacteroides	Foul-smelling dirty white discharge with no itch	50% asymptomatic, thin grey foul-smelling discharge, pH> 4.5	Amsel's criteria • Any 3 of the following should be present: • Thin homogenous greyish white discharge • pH> 4.5 • Wet film microscopy—clue cells • Whiff test—positive	Metronidazole—500 mg BD for 7 days 2 g single dose not useful for BV no need to treat partner

50% vaginitis is due to bacterial vaginosis, 20–25% due to candidiasis and 15–20% due to trichomoniasis

- Most common vaginal infection: candidiasis
- M/C vaginal infection in clinical practice: Trichomoniasis

Gardnerella (Bacterial) Vaginosis

- Alteration in the normal vaginal flora than infection
- **Agents:** *Haemophilus vaginalis, gardnerella, mobiluncus and mycoplasma hominis*. The mobiluncus is a gram positive curved rod with a characteristic corkscrew spinning anaerobe
- The bacterial vaginosis is therefore a polymicrobial condition
- It is not sexually transmitted with a variable incubation period

Treatment

- Metronidazole/Ampicillin/Cephalosporin/Ornidazole 500 mg vaginal tablet daily for 7 days
- Clindamycin 2% cream locally
- Lactel is protein-free acidifying lactate gel which neutralizes the vaginal pH (lactic acid 5% W/V, 0.1% glycogen)-5 ml is applied daily for 7 days
- The infection recurs in 30%

Candidial (Monilial) Vaginitis

- The commonest species causing human disease is C. albicans, which is gram positive and grows in acid medium
- It may be sexually transmitted. Almost 25% of women harbor Candida in the vagina and are often asymptomatic

Risk Factors

- Promiscuity, immunosuppression, pregnancy, steroid therapy, following long term antibiotic therapy, OCPs, DM, poor personal hygiene and obesity

Treatment

- Local intravaginal applications of antifungal agents like imidazole, miconazole, clotrimazole or terconazole vaginal pessaries or creams used for 3–6 days is very effective
- A single dose of fluconazole 150 mg is also very effective. Ideally, both partners should be treated
- Recurrent infection requires fluconazole–150 mg every 72 hours for 3 doses and then weekly for a few weeks

Trichomoniasis

- The trichomonas organism is a protozoon, actively motile, slightly larger than a leukocyte and is anaerobic

Treatment

- Metronidazole is effective in 85% of patients. Recent modality → 2g Metronidazole for 1 day only
- During pregnancy, vinegar douche to lower the pH, trichofuran suppositories and Betadine gel are useful
- Recurrent infection is treated with tinidazole 500mg q.i.d. and vaginal pessary 500mg b.d for 14 days

Chlamydial Infection

- Chlamydia trachomatis—obligate intracellular organism
- Infects the columnar and transitional epithelial cells
- MC sexually transmitted bacteria
- Often asso with Nesseria gonorrheae

Clinical Features

- Asymptomatic in 80%
- Mucopurulent endocervical discharge
- Urethral syndrome—dysuria, frequency, pyuria, no bacteria
- Pelvic pain
- Postcoital/intermenstrual bleeding

Investigations

- Nucleic acid amplification test (NAAT)-preferred
- PCR
- Tissue culture on McCoy or Hela cells

Treatment

- Doxycyline 100 mg BD for 7 days or

- Azithromycin 1 g single dose
- Treat partners simultaneously
- In pregnancy—Azithromycin 1 g single dose or Amoxycillin 500 mg TID for 7 days

Neisseria Gonorrhoea

- 50% are asymptomatic
- MC symptom—vaginal discharge
- Lower abdominal pain, dysuria

Investigations

- Gram stain
  - G-ve intracellular diplococci
- Gold standard
  - Culture-Mod Thayer Martin medium
- Widely used
  - NAAT

Treatment

Single dose–Ceftriaxone 125 mg IM or

– Cefixime 400 mg oral or–Ciprofloxacin 500 mg oral

+

– Doxy/Azithro to treat chlamydia (because of high rate of coinfection)

Complications

- Acute salpingitis, PID
- Fitz-Hugh-Curtis syndrome (liver capsule infection)
- Reiter's syndrome-arthritis, conjunctivitis, urethritis
- Infertility-tubal obstruction
- Ectopic pregnancy
- Chronic pelvic pain
- Perinatal infection- conjunctivitis, pneumonia

PID

Organisms causing are:

Primary	Secondary
Gonococci	*E. coli*
Chlamydia	*Group B streptococcus*
Mycoplasma	*Klebsiella*
	Anerobes

- **Cervicitis and vaginitis are not part of PID**
- Microorganisms colonizing the endocx ascends to endometrium and fallopian tubes
- Upper genital tract infection
- Includes endometritis, salpingitis and peritonitis

Syndromic Approach

- Treatment based on signs and symptoms rather than the lab tests
  CDC 2006 criteria for diagnosing PID

Minimum Criteria

- Lower abdominal tenderness
- Adnexal tenderness
- Cervical motion tenderness

Additional Criteria

- Oral temp >38.3 degrees C (101 degrees F)
- Abn Cx/vaginal mucopurulent discharge
- Pr of abundant WBC on saline mount of vaginal secretion
- ESR >15 mm/hr
- Elevated CRP
- Lab documentation of *N. gonorrhea*/Chlamydia infection

Definitive Criteria

- HPE E/O endometritis on endometrial Bx
- TO abscess on U/S or radiological tests
- Laparoscopic abnormalities consistent with PID

CDC guidelines for treatment of PID

- Outpatient treatment

  Regimen A

  1. Cefoxitin 2g IM + Probenicid 1g oral, or
  2. Ceftriaxone 250 mg Im, or
  3. Equivalent cephalosporin + Doxy 100 mg BD–14 days + Metro 500 mg BD—14 days

  Regimen B

  1. Ofloxacin 400 mg BD—14 days
  2. Levoflox 500 mg OD—14 days +/– Metro 500 mg BD—14 days

- Inpatient treatment

  Regimen A

  1. Cefoxitin 2g IV Q6H, or
  2. Cefotetan 2g IV Q12H + Doxy 100 mg PO/IV Q12 H

  Regimen B

  1. Clindamycin 900 mg IV Q8 H + Gentamycin- Loading dose–2 mg/kg BW Maint dose–1.5 mg/kg BW Q8 H

Indications for inpatient treatment, CDC 2006

- Surgical emergencies like appendicitis cannot be ruled out
- Patient is pregnant
- HIV positive
- Doesn't respond to oral antibiotics (within 72 hrs)
- Pt unable to follow OP regimen
- Severe illnessnausea, vomiting and high fever
- Patient has TO abscess

Sequelae of PID

- Infertility seen in 6–60% patients
- Ectopic pregnancy
- Chronic pelvic pain, dysparunia
- Fitz-Hugh-Curtis syndrome

Genital Ulcers

- M/C causes of ulcers in young women are
  - Herpes simplex virus (HSV)
  - Treponema pallidum (Syphllis)
  - Hemophilus ducreyi (Chancroid)
- Number
  - Multiple—Herpes
  - Chancroid
  - Single—Primary Syphillis
- Edges
  - Raised—Syphillis
  - Erythematous—Herpes
  - Undermined—Chancroid
- Base
  - Smooth, nonpurulent, nonerythematous—Sphyllis
  - Erythematous nonvascular—Herpes
  - Purulent and bleeds on touch—Chancroid
- Induration
  - Firm—Syphllis
  - Undermined—Chancroid
- Pain
  - Present—Herpes
  - Chancroid
  - Absent—Syphillis
- Lymph node enlargement
  - B/L and nontender LNs—Syphillis
  - B/L and tender LNs—Herpes
  - Unilateral and tender LNs—Chancroid

HSV

- 90% = HSV 2; 10% = HSV 1
- HSV 1 = cause disease above the belt
- HSV 2 = disease below the belt
- Lesion = appears as erythematous plaque-later forms vesicles-small ulcers with erythematous halo and yellow base
- Ulcers are extremely tender and inguinal nodes enlarged
- DOC—acyclovir
- Gold standard for diagnosis—tissue culture

Syphillis

- Causative agent—treponema pallidum

Stage	Lesion seen
Primary	Chancre/ulcer
Secondary	Condyloma lata-coarse flat topped moist necrotic lesion
Tertiary	Gumma-punched ulcer with rolled out margins

- DOC-benzathine penicillin
- Tubes are not affected in primary syphillis and infertility doesn't occur.

Genital Tuberculosis

- Mostly secondary to primary infection elsewhere
- Primary focus in lungs-50%
- Fallopian tube is the most frequently involved part (100%). Followed by uterus (70–80%), ovaries (30%)
- The lesions are often bilateral
- Initial site-submucosal layer of ampulla
- Commonest symptom: infertility
- Commonest menstrual disturbance: Menorrhagia

Investigations

- Diagnostic curettage in premenstrual period. Hysteronsalpingo gram: contraindicated

Features

- Lead pipe appearance
- Cornual block and calcification of the tube
- **Tobacco pouch appearance**
- Honey comb appearance of uterine cavity due to adhesions
- Adhesive type of peritonitis with intestinal adhesions. → 'Frozen pelvis'

Prognosis

- 90%: cured with chemotherapy but fertility is restored only in 10% cases
- Of those who conceive: 50% have a tubal pregnancy, 20–30% abort
- Only 2% women with genital TB will have live births

Treatment

- Cat 1—for 6 months
- HRZE—2 months; HR—4 months
- Surgery for restoration of fertility (tuboplasty)—CI in genital TB
- IVF after ATT is the treatment for infertility

Urogynecology

Classification and Causes of Urinary Incontinence

- **Genuine stress incontinence**
  - Bladder neck displacement
  - Intrinsic sphincter dysfunction (ISD)
- **Detrusor instability/urge incontinence**
  - Idiopathic
  - Neurologic detrusor hyperreflexia
- **Mixed incontinence (genuine stress and detrusor instability combined)**
- **Overflow incontinence with urinary retention**
  - Obstruction
  - Bladder hyporeflexia
- **Bypass incontinence**
  - Genitourinary fistulas
- Urethral diverticulum
- Congenital urethral abnormalities (e.g. epispadiasis, bladder exstrophy, ectopic ureter)
- Functional and transient incontinence
  - Infection
  - Pharmacologic

- Restricted mobility
- Dementia/delirium
- Excessive urine production (diabetes mellitus, diabetes insipidus, resorption of extravascular fluid as with lower extremity edema)
- Stool impaction

Genuine Stress Incontinence

- Involuntary loss of urine that occurs, when, in the absence of a detrusor contraction, the intravesical pressure exceeds the maximum urethral closure pressure

  Different investigations used for stress incontinence are
  - Stress test
  - Cotton swab stick test/Q-tip test
  - Marshall and Bonney's test
  - Urethroscopy
  - Urodynamic evaluation

Bonney's test—two fingers are placed in the vagina at the urethra-vesical junction on either side of urethra and bladder neck elevated. On straining or coughing, absence of leakage of urine indicates a positive test.

- Importance–in patients with positive test, absence of leakage of urine following bladder neck elevation is indicative of beneficial outcome, following surgical repair.

Treatment of Stress Urinary Incontinence

Conservative: Kegel's pelvic floor exercise, vaginal cone and electric stimulation

Medical methods: Estrogen and alpha adrenergic agonists

Surgical repair:

- **Vaginal operation:** These include anterior colporrhaphy, anterior colporrhaphy with placation of the bladder neck (Kelly's repair), or opposing the medial fibers of the puborectalis muscles in the midline under the bladder neck region to elevate the same (Pace's repair)
- **Abdominal operations:** retropubic colposuspension by Marshall-Marchetti-Krantz operation
- Combined abdominal and vaginal operations
- Bruch colposuspension
- Laparoscopic colposuspension
- Intravesical bladder neck plication
- Tension-free vaginal T-type (TVT)
- Periurethral collagen injection

Urge Incontinence (Detrusor Instability)

- Involuntary loss of urine associated with a strong desire to void
- Usually associated with involuntary contractions of the bladder or detrusor contractions

  Synonyms: bladder dyssynergia, overative bladder, detrusor hyperreflexia, uninhibited detrusor and unstable bladder

Fistulas

- Commonest genito urinary fistula—Vesicovaginal fistula
- **Causes:**

  Obstetrical (commonest)
  - Ischemia 3–5 months following delivery
  - Traumatic instrumental delivery—operation

  Gynecological:
  - Operative injury
  - Traumatic

- Malignancy
- Radiation (1–2 years following RT)
- Infective
- Most common urinary Fistula – vesicovaginal (VVF)
- Most common cause of VVF – obstructed labor
- Most common cause of Uretero VF – gynecological operations, esp. Wertheim's operation
- Most common of Vesico Uterine F – Cesarian section
- Most common of Recto Vaginal F – complete perineal tear

Three Swab Test

- **Ureterovaginal fistulae**
  Uppermost swab soaked with urine but unstained with dye. The lower two fistula swabs remain dry
- **Vesicovaginal fistulae**
  Upper and lower swabs remain dry but the middle swab stained with the dye
- **Urethrovaginal fistulae**
  Upper two swabs remain dry but lower swab stained with the dye

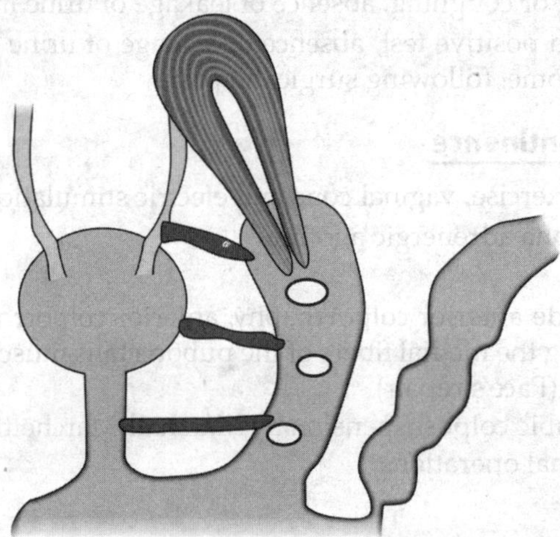

Fig. 14.1: Fistulas

- **Latzko procedure and Chassar—Moir techniques are used for VVF repair**
  If primary repair fails, one should wait at least 3 months before attempting a second repair*

Ureteral injury associated with gynecological surgery (The Most Commons)

- **Most common site**—Pelvic brim near the infundibulopelvic ligaments
- **Most common procedure**—Simple abdominal hysterectomy
- **Most common type of injury**—Obstruction
- **Most common activity leading to injury**—Attempts to obtain hemostasis

Prolapse of uterus

Supports of the Uterus

Primary supports:

Muscular/Active supports	Fibromuscular or mechanical support
• Pelvic diaphragm (formed by levator ani) • Perineal body • Urogenital muscle (deep transverse perineal muscle)	• Uterine axis • Pubocervical ligament • Transverse cervical ligament/cardinal ligament/Mackenrodt's ligament • Uterosacral ligament

Main support that prevents prolapse: Mackenrodt's ligament and its posterior extension: Uterosacral ligament

Delancey threelevel system of uterine support:

Level–I	Uterosacral and cardinal ligaments-support the uterus and vaginal vault
Level–II	Endopelvic fascias and paracolpos-connect the vagina to the white line on lateral pelvic wall via arcus tendinosus
Level–III	Perineal muscle, body and the membrane-support the lower 1/3rd of vagina

Uterine Prolapse

- Nulliparous prolapse—2%
- Vault prolapse–0.5%

Etiology

- Most important cause: Atonicity and asthenia of uterus (menopause).
- Birth injury (reduced by perineal tear)
- Peripheral nerve injury-pudendal nerve
- Home deliveries
- Spina bifida occulta, split pelvis
- Ventouse extraction of fetus before cervical dilatation
- Delivery of big baby
- Rapid succession of pregnancies
- Smoking and chronic cough and elevated intra-abdominal pressure
- Abdominoperineal resection and radical vulvectomy

Classification

Anterior vaginal wall: (Cystourethrocele)

- Upper 2/3rd—Cystocele
- Lower 1/3rd—Urethrocele

Posterior vaginal wall:

- Upper 1/3rd—Enterocele
- Lower 2/3rd—Rectocele

Uterine descent—Anatomical classification

First degree: descent of the cervix into the vagina

Second degree: descent of the cervix upto the introitus

Third degree: descent of the cervix outside the introitus

Procidentia: the entire uterus outside the introitus

Role of pessary:

Current indications	Limitations
• Young woman planning for pregnancy • During early pregnancy • Puerperium • Woman unfit/refusing for surgery • Temporary use for infections and decubitus ulcer	• Only palliative/not curative • Causes vaginitis and dyspareunia • Difficulty in retention, needs to be changed every 3 months • Does not cure stress urinary incontinence • Forgotten pessary can cause ulcer, Ca. vagina and a vesicovaginal fistula

Surgeries for Uterine Prolapse

Fothergill's repair (Manchester operation):

- Operative treatment for uterine prolapse in a woman who completed the family but which to retain the menstrual function

- In this operation, the surgeon combines an anterior colporrhaphy with amputation of cervix, sutures the cut ends of the Mackenrodt's ligaments in front of the cervix, covers the raw area on the amputated cervix with vagina mucosa and follows it up with a colpoperineorrhaphy.

Other modalities

- Anterior colporrhaphy
- Posterior colporrhaphy and colpoperineorrhaphy
- Shirodkar's procedure
- Vaginal hysterectomy with pelvic floor repair
- **Lefort's repair:** done in old age if the patient is unfit for prolonged surgeries
- **Abdominal sling operations:**
  - Abdomino cervicopexy
  - Shirodkar's abdominal sling operation
  - Khanna's abdominal sling operation

Vault Prolapse

- Vault prolapse is a delayed complication of both abdominal and vaginal hysterectomy when the supporting structures at level 1 become weak and deficient.

Treatment

Vaginal approach:

- Sacrospinous colpopexy—attaching vaginal vault to sacrospinous ligament
- McCall's culdoplasty—approximation of the uterosacral ligaments and vault to uterosacral ligaments
- Iliococcygeus colpopexy—vaginal vault to iliococcygeus muscle
- Uterosacral ligament suspension—vault to the uterosacral ligaments

Abdominal approach:

- Abdominal sacrocolpopexy—vault to the anterior sacral ligament
- Abdominal uterosacral suspension—vault to uterosacral ligament

Laparoscopic approach:

- Laparoscopic sacrocolpopexy—vault to anterior sacral ligament

Abnormal Uterine Bleeding (DUB)

- Menstrual blood loss is controlled by interaction between PGE_2, PGF_2a, PGI_2 secreted by the endometrium

Etiology

- Organic causes:
  - Diseases of the genital tract
  - Systemic diseases
- Dysfunctional uterine bleeding

Dysfunctional Uterine Bleeding

- Menorrhagia without any structural abnormality, pelvic disease or other general or endocrine disease
- Etiology:
  - Altered HPO function
  - Local changes in prostaglandin production

Anovulatory (80%)	Ovulatory (20%)
• Puberty menorrhagia (Threshold bleeding) • Metropathia hemorrhagica • Premenopausal menorrhagia	• Irregular ripening • Irregular shedding (Halban's disease)—due to persistent corpus luteum • Following IUCD insertion and sterilization operation

Puberty Menorrhagia

- M/C cause: hypothalmo-pituitary-ovarian dysfunction
- Due to excess oestrogen and unopposed progesterone due to anovulation

Metropathia Hemorrhagica (Dub in prepubertal age and perimenopause)

- Specialized form of DUB
- The endometrium is thick and polypoidal and ovary contains a cystic follicle
- Prevalent in women over the age of 40 (40–45 years), not related to parity
- M/C complaint: continuous vaginal bleeding without pain

Irregular ripening: due to deficient corpus luteal function, deficient progesterone
Irregular shedding: due to persistent corpus luteum

Treatment

Medical	Surgical
Combined oral pills, MIRENA, Progestogens, Danazol, NSAID, Antifibrinolytics, GnRH analogoes anemia treatment	D and C, hysteroscopic minimal invasive surgery-endometrial ablation, radiofrequency-induced thermal endometrial ablation, Balloon therapy-hysterectomy

- Danazol is contraindicated in puberty menorrhagia, due to androgenic side effects

Medical Methods

Hormone therapy

- Duphaston (10 mg daily) does not suppress ovulation → useful in young women desirous of pregnancy
- Norethisterone: 5 mg given TDS till bleeding stops. After 2–4 days of stopping the drug, withdrawal bleeding occurs. This is called Medical Curettage
- Medroxyprogesterone acetate (MDPA) 10 mg
- Gestrinone, a derivative of 19–nortestosterone, is effective in a dose oral 2.5 mg twice weekly for 6 months
- Progesterone-impregnated IUCDs (Progestasert, MIRENA)—reduces blood loss in 97% cases
- OCPs reduce blood loss by 50% and eliminate dysmenorrhea
- Clomiphene is advocated if pregnancy is desired, and if cycles are anovulatory

Nonsteroidal anti-inflammatory drugs (NSAIDs): Mefenamic acid for 5 to 6 days controls menorrhagia in 70%

Antifibrinolytic agents

- Tranexamic acid and epsilon amino-acid–50% success with 50% reduction in the blood loss
- Ethamsylate with tranexamic acid is also effective but contraindicated in renal failure
- Ethamsylate reduces the capillary fragility; reduces menorrhagia by 50%

GnRH: GnRH is used as a last drug when others fail

Newer drugs

- **Ormeloxifene** (selective oestrogen receptor modulator): effective in 50%. It is antagonist to uterine and breast tissue by antioestrogenic effect and does not cause cancer. It is agonist to bone and CVS, and therefore cardiovascular and bone-protective unlike GnRH.
- Seasonale (combined estrogen and progestogen) is used daily for 84 days+gap of 6 days for 3 months
- Recombinant-activated factor VII (RF VII a) called Novo Seven
- Mirena

Operative Procedures

Curettage

Hysterectomy

Minimal invasive surgeries (MIS)

- **Hysteroscopic endometrial ablation** by Nd: YAG laser
- Transcervical resection of endometrium (TCRE)
- **Radiofrequency-induced thermal endometrial ablation (RITEA)**
  - Radiofrequency electromagnetic thermal energy destroys the endometrium at 66°C
  - Cheaper and simpler procedure compared to TCRE
- **Cava term balloon therapy:** mainly done for premenopausal women who completed their family
- **Microwave endometrial ablation (MEA):** utilizes magnetic energy and works at the frequency of 9.2 GHz. It is a simple OPD procedure with no need for preoperative endometrial thinning. Temperature of 80°C is maintained for 3 minutes
- **Uterine tamponade:** Novasure is the recent safe procedure, completed in 90 seconds
- **Endometrial laser intrauterine thermotherapy (ELITT)**
- **Bilateral uterine artery embolization:** is the latest technology used in intractable menorrhagia
- **Hysterectomy** if all the modalities fail

Uterine Artery Embolization (UAE)

- Menorrhagia was relieved in 80–90%, pressure symptoms in 40–70% and the volume decreased by 50%

Endometriosis

Presence of functional endometrium (endometrial glands and the stroma) in sites other than uterine mucosa.
Incidence: 10%: in infertile women: 20%

Theories

- Coelomic metaplasia (Mayer and Ivanhoff)
- Retrograde menstruation (Sampson's implantation theory)
- Lymphatic theory (Halban/Metastatic)
- Direct implantation
- Histogenesis by induction (Merill)
- Hematogenous spread
- Hereditary and immunological factors
- Activation of embryonic cell nest
- Activation of Wolffian rest
- Metaplasia of urothelium

Sites: Common sites are the ovaries, the pouch of Douglas (2nd commonest)
Following LSCS, scar endometriosis occurs in 0.2%
Symptoms: The classic symptoms are dysmenorrhea (commonest), dyspareunia, menorrhagia and infertility

Pelvic examination

- Nodules in the pouch of Douglas
- Cobblestone feel of the uterosacral ligament
- Bluish sports in posterior fornix
- Pelvic tenderness and Fixed retroverted uterus
- Bilateral adnexal mass

Investigation of choice-Laparoscopy

Pathological findings

- Vary with duration of the lesion, size and location
- 'Powder-burn'-puckered black spots, red flame shaped areas, vascular, bluish, blackish cysts, chocolate cyst and dense adhesions in the pelvis as well as yellow brown peritoneal fluid are the findings
- 'Match stick spots' seen on the peritoneum of Pouch of Douglas

Chocolate cysts of the ovaries

- Most important manifestation of endometriosis

Treatment

- Pseudopregnancy state-Medroxyprogesterone acetate, Dudrogesterone, Norethisterone
- Pseudomenopausal state: Danazol and Gestrinone
- Medical castration: GnRH analogues like Buserelein, Naferelin, Goserelin
- Aromatase inhibitors like letrozole, anastrazole and roficoxib
- Mifepristone
- Minimal invasive surgery-for infertility

LUNA-laser uterosacral nerve ablation-for midline pain in endometriosis

Infertility

Definition: Failure of a couple of reproductive age to conceive after at least 1 year (<35 years) or 6 months (>35 years) of regular coitus without contraception

- **Fecundability**—probability of achieving pregnancy within one menstrual cycle. For a normal couple, it is 25%
- **Fecundity**—ability to achieve a live birth within one menstrual cycle

Causes of infertility

- Male factor (30–40%)
- Female factor (40–50%)
- Combined (10%)
- Unexplained (10%)
  - Primary infertility
    - A couple that has never conceived
  - Secondary infertility
    - Infertility that occurs after previous pregnancy regardless of outcome

TESTS FOR INFERTILITY

Postcoital Test (Sims' or Huhner's test)

- Cervical mucus is aspirated and examined two hours after intercourse around ovulation time
- Normally 10–50 motile sperms are seen per hpf
- The sperms show progressive, but not rotator movements
- The presence of antispermal antibodies in the cervical mucus imparts shaky or rotator movements to the sperms or may totally immobilize them
- The advantage of this test is that the cervical mucus can be simultaneously studied for estrogenic effect and ovulation

Miller-Kurzrok Test

- Placing ovulation mucus on a glass slide with specimen of husband's sperms
- Penetration < 3 cm at 30 minutes is abnormal

Sperm penetration test: The physiological profile of the sperms can be studied in vitro by using the zona-free hamster egg which resembles the human ovum

Semen-cervical mucus contact test:

- Equal quantity of semen and mucus is mixed, so there is no interface
- In presence of antibodies more than 25% sperms show jerky or shaky movements by 30 minutes
- The cross check with the donor semen will indicate the source of antibodies, whether it is cervical or seminal antibodies

Fern Test (Test for Ovulation)

- Cervical mucus during the estrogenic phase shows a characteristic pattern of fern formation, due to the presence of sodium chloride. This ferning disappears after ovulation
- At the time of ovulation, mucus has the property of great elasticity and will withstand stretching up to 10 cm. This phenomenon is called spinnbarkeit or the thread test for oestrogen activity
- Insler devised a scoring system which took into account the various cervical mucus properties such as amount, spinnbarkeit, ferning, viscosity and cellularity
- The maximum score is 15 and a score less than 10 is considered unfavorable

Semen Analysis

- Done after abstinence of 3 to 5 days
- The seminal fluid is normally viscous with pH of 8, and contains fructose
  - Aspermia → means no semen
  - Azoospermia → implies no sperm
  - Oligospermia → low sperm count
  - Asthenospermia → no motile sperm or diminished motility
  - Necrospermia → dead sperms
  - Teratospermia → abnormal morphology of sperm

Normal Semen Parameters

Parameter	1992 Guidelines	2010 Guidelines
Volume	2 ml	> 1.5 ml
Sperm concentration	20 million/ml	> 15 million/ml
Sperm motility or > 25% rapidly progressive	50% progressive	> 32% progressive
Morphology (strict criteria)	> 15% normal forms	> 4% normal forms
WBC	< 1 million/ml	1 million/ml
Immunobead/mixed antiglobulin RN test	< 10% coated with antibodies	< 50%

Tests for Tubal Patency

- Usually done in the preovulatory phase (usually the tenth day of the cycle)
- If performed in the postovulatory period, it may disturb a fertilized or implanted ovum → endometriosis

Hysterosalpingography/Laparoscopic Chromotubation

- Indicated in patients with blocked fallopian tubes prior to undertaking tubal microsurgery
- Invasive procedure and requires hospitalization
- Advantages of laparoscopy–can proceed with therapeutic procedures if adhesions or block is recognized

Sonosalpingography

- Popularized as the **'Sion test'**, a safe and practical method of evaluation tubal patency
- The ultrasound scan also shows the presence of free fluid in the pouch of Douglas if **the tubes are patent**
- Sonosalpingography is a good technique of detecting the sub mucous fibroid polyp and intrauterine lesions

New modalities

- **Falloscopy and hysteroscopy**
- **Ampullary and fimbrial salpingoscopy**

In Vitro Fertilization

- Today, IVF and embryo transfer are offered to women in whom tuboplasty has failed or to women with extensive and irreparable tubal damage

- The success rate of 20 to 30% is obtained. This is very expensive
- Contraindications to IVF: extensive pelvic adhesions and inaccessible ovaries due to adhesions–ova retrieval in such cases may be impossible or dangerous to the bowels
- Normally, three trials are given and if IVF fails, other micro-assisted fertilization processes offered

Gamete Intrafallopian Transfer Technique (GIFT)

- Aspiration of oocytes following ovulation induction either laparoscopically or under US-guided transvaginally
- Success rate of 40%

Others:

- Microassisted fertilization (MAF) process in vitro
- Intracytoplasmic semen insemination
- Epididymal or testicular aspiration

CONTRACEPTIVES

Pearl index: The failure rate of any contraceptive is calculated in terms of pregnancy rate per hundred women years (H.W.Y.) of use.

It is calculated according to the following formula (Pearl index).

- Pregnancy failure rate/100 WY = $\frac{\text{No. of accidental pregnancies} \times 1200}{\text{No. of patients observed} \times \text{months of use}}$

  (1200 = number of months in 10 years)
- When the pregnancy rate is below 10, the effectiveness of the particular method is considered to be high and if it is more than 20, it is said to be low.
- **Methods of contraception**

  Permanent

  Female—Tubectomy

  Male—Vasectomy

  Temporary

  Barrier methods

  Natural methods

  OCP's

  Injectables

  Implants

  LNG-IUS

  Natural Methods: Aims at avoiding sexual intercourse at around the time of ovulation
- Rhythm method
- Standard days method
- Basal body method
- Billing's cervical mucus method
- Symptothermal method

Rhythm method

- Based on *Ojjino Knauss* theory
- States that ovulation occurs on 14+/– 2 days in a female with regular 28 day cycle (i.e. avoid sex b/w 12th and 16th day)
- Fertilizable span for sperm is 48–72 hours and ova is 12–24 hours
- Therefore unsafe period is 8–18th day (Failure rate is 25–35%)
- Failure rate is reduced to 10% if sex is avoided from 7–21 days
- So safe sex is only the first and last 7 days of a cycle.

- In irregular cycle–safe period = shortest cycle–18 (gives the 1st day of fertile period), longest cycle–11 (gives the last day of fertile period)
  High failure rate–9/100 WY

Standard days method (Ritumala method in India)

- Developed by Georgetown University's Institute for Reproductive Health
- More effective than rhythm method
- Uses Cyclebeads to keep track of estimated high and low fertility points during her menstrual cycle
- Can be used if only the cycles are between 26 and 32 days.
- In this:
  - days 1–7—infertile
  - 8–19—fertile
  - from day 20, infertility resumes
- Failure rate-2/HWY
- **Cycle Beads**

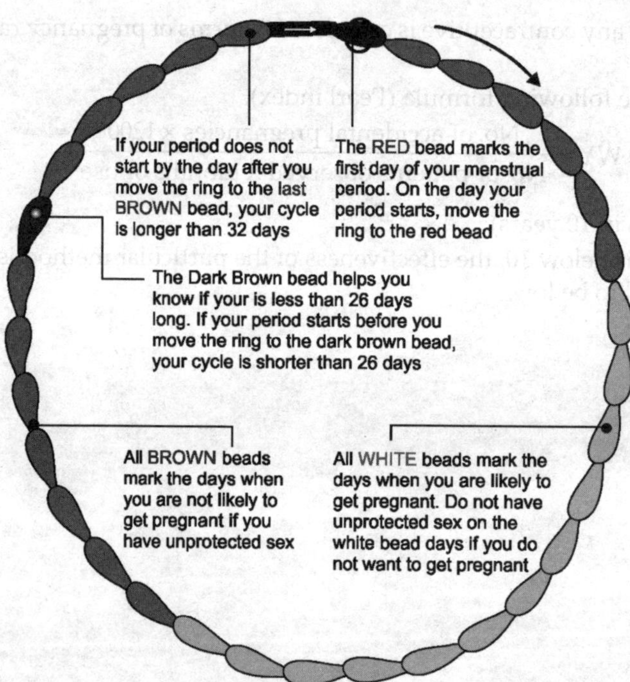

Fig. 14.2: Cycle beads

Basal body temperature

- At ovulation drop in temperature of 0.2–0.4 degree fahrenheit is present
- Luteal phase 0.2–0.4 degree fahrenheit increase
- This persists for atleast 3 days after ovulation
- Hence safe pd starts 4th day to the last day of the next period
- To use this, a BBT chart has to be maintained

Billing's/cervical mucus method

- Based on the observation of changes in the characteristic of cervical mucus
- During flow—unsafe pd
- After flow—there is no mucus-dry days-safe
- At the time of ovulation—cervical mucus becomes watery, clear, smooth, profuse and slippery—d/t influence of estrogen—Spinbarkeit (Peak Day)

- After ovulation–mucus thickens and lessens in quantity—d/t influence of progesterone-Tack
- The couple must abstain until the 4th day after the peak day

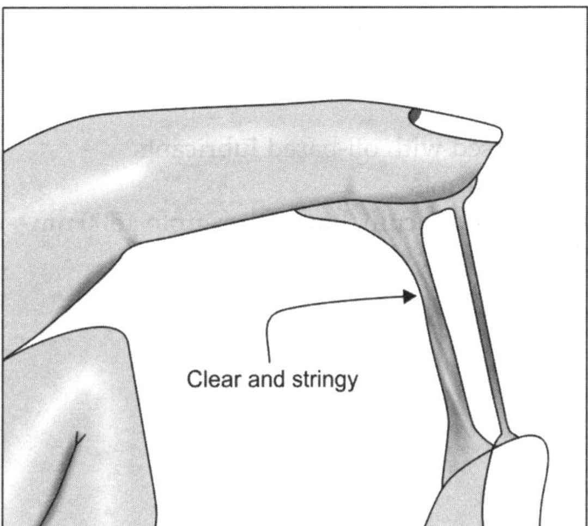

Fig. 14.3: Spinbarkeit

Symptothermal method

- Uses two methods to identify the fertile period
- Usually the cervical mucus method and the BBT chart.

Withdrawal/coitus interruptus

- Means discharge of semen outside the female genitalia at the time of intercourse

Lactational amenorrhea (LAM)

MOA:

- Frequent intense suckiling
- Prolactin is released
- Disrupts secretion of GnRH
- Interferes with release of LH and FSH
- Disrupts follicular development
- Anovulation and amenorrhea

Three prerequisites for LAM:

- Exclusive breastfeeding
- Baby < 6 months of age
- There is amenorrhea (menses should not have resumed)
  Failure rate = 5/HWY

Natural methods not suitable for the following conditions:

- With irregular cycles (< 21 days)
- In adolescents, lactation and premenopausal age
- Who have had a cervical surgery (cautery/conization)
- With vaginal infection
- Who had STD/PID in the last three months
- Who had a recent abortion
- Non-cooperative husbands and who have a casual sex

Barrier Methods

Males

- Condoms

Females

- Female condom (Femshield)
- Vaginal sponge (Today)
- Vaginal diaphragm/cervical cap

Condoms

- Polyurethane has a longer shelf life, used with oil-based lubricants
- Latex get damaged with oil based lubricants
- Natural-membrane condoms-using lamb cecum, have pores upto 1500 nm—doesn't allow sperms to pass, but can allow HIV and Hep B virus.

Advantages

- Easily available
- Cheap
- Easy to carry
- Free from side effects
- Requires no instructions
- Protects against HIV, STIs

Disadvantages

- Latex sensitivity
- Condom breakage
- Condom slippage
- Interruption
- Decreased pleasure
- May only be used with water-based lubricant

Spermicides

- Failure rates 0–50% for typical users
- Cost
- Nonoxynol-9 destroys sperm cell membrane
- OTC
- Can be used as a 'back-up method' along with a barrier contraceptive

Female condom

- One-time use
- Proper placement

Contraceptive sponge

- Contains spermicidal
- One size
- Continuous protection up to 24 hours
- Marketed as today

Diaphragms and cervical caps

- Rubber cup with a flexible rim
- Used with spermicide
- Can stay in place up to 6 hours
- Must be in place for 6 hours after IC and not more than 24 hours
- Perfect Effectiveness Rate = 94%
- Typical Effectiveness Rate = 80%
- Latex barrier placed inside vagina during intercourse
- Fitted by physician

Contraindications for use of a diaphragmj
- Prolapse, cystocele, rectocele
- Retroversion
- VVF/RVF
- Badly eroded/lacerated cervix
- Recurrent UTI

IUCD

Mechanisms of Action
- Inhibition of sperm transport;
- Increased tubal motility causing failure of implantation of immature zygote;
- Inhibition of implantation secondary to endometrial inflammation;
- Phagocytic destruction of sperm and blastocyst; and
- Alteration of cervical mucus (only progesterone IUSs).

Noncontraceptive benefits of LNG—IUD
- Significant reduction in menstrual blood loss, **menorrhagia, dysmenorrhea, and PMS**
- It can be used in the treatment of **endometrial hyperplasia, adenomyosis, uterine leiomyoma, endometrial carcinoma**
- It can be used as an **alternative to hysterectomy for menorrhagia**
- It provides excellent **benefits of HRT** when used over the transition years of reproduction to menopause.

Side effects of IUCD:
- **The commonest complaint of women fitted with IUD (inert or medicated) is increased vaginal bleeding**
- Pain is the second most common side effect leading to IUD removal Bleeding can take the following forms
- Greater risk of blood loss
- Longer menstrual period
- Mid-cycle bleeding—Usually it settles between 1–2 months.
- **Previous ectopic pregnancy is an absolute contraindication for IUD insertion.**

Timing of insertion of IUCD
- A convenient time for IUD insertion is 6–8 weeks after delivery (postpuerperal infection). It has several advantages:
- IUD insertion during 1st week after delivery (immediate postpartum)
  - Greater risk of perforation
  - Associated with high expulsion rate
- **Expulsion of IUD** occurs in 5–15% and is due to small size of IUD. It is common during the puerperal period or following MTP of a large gestation size.
- It can also be taken up immediately after a legally induced 1 st trimester abortion.
- **Note: IUD insertion immediately after the 2nd trimester abortion is not recommended. Also, IUD insertion after an illegal abortion is not approved of.**

Absolute contraindications of IUD
- Mnemonic: **Please do not ever put condom**
- **P**regnancy
- **D**UB
- H/O **E**ctopic pregnancy
- Current **P**ID/STD or within the past 3 months
- **C**ancer cervix/endometrium

Relative contraindications of IUD
- Abnormal uterine size or shape
- Medical conditions (e.g. on corticosteroid, valvular heart disease, any immunosuppression)
- Nulligravidity
- H/O ectopic pregnancy
- Abnormal pap smear

'Hysteroscopic removal' is the treatment of IUCD inserted intra myometrially

Life span of IUD's
- Cu T 200, Multiload Cu 250, Cu T 220—3 years
- Nova T—5 years
- Cu T 380 A–10 years
- Progestasert—1 year
- Levonova—5 years

Mirena (Lng-Ius)—5 Years

Hormonal contraceptives
- Oral Contraceptives (Birth Control Pill)
- Injections (Depo-provera)
- Implants (Norplant I and II)

OCPs

Mechanism of action
- Suppresses LH surge (E > P)
- Suppresses ovulation (E > P)
- Produces atrophy of the endometrium (P)
- Creates a hostile cervical mucus (P)

Types of OCPs
- Monophasic
  - Have same estrogen and progestrone in the 21 pills
- Biphasic
  - 1st 10 pills have one dosage of E+P
  - Next 11 pills have other dosage
- Triphasic
  - 1st 7 pills–EE–30 mcg, LNG–50 mcg
  - 2nd 7 pills–EE–40 mcg, LNG–75 mcg
  - 3rd 7 pills–EE–30 mcg, LNG–125 mcg

Composition of the available OCPs
- Mala D
  - EE–30 mcg
  - Norgestrel–0.15 mg
- Mala N
  - EE–30 mcg
  - LNG–0.15 mg
- Loette
  - EE–20 mcg
  - LNG–0.10 mg
- Femilon
  - EE–20 mcg
  - Desogestrel–0.15 mg

Estrogen in OCP

- Based on the dosage of estrogen in the pill
- Standard dose–EE–50 mcg
- Low dose-EE–30–35 mcg
- Very low dose–EE–20 mcg
- M/C estrogen used is **Ethinyl estradiol**

Progesterone in OCP

- First generation
  - Norethisterone
  - Norethindrone
  - Norethinodrel
  - Lynestrenol
- Second generation
  - Levonorgestrel
  - Norgestrel
- Third generation
  - Desogestrel
  - Gestodene
  - Norgestimate
- Fourth generation
  - Drospirenone
  - Spirinolactone
  - Cyproterone acetate

Benefits of 3rd generation progesterone

- Desogestrel/Gestodene/Norgestimate
  - Increase SHBG
    - Decrease the free testosterone concentration–decreases acne, hirsutism,
    - PMS and has a favorable lipid profile
  - Less BTB
  - Do not increase body weight
  - Slightly increased chance of VTE

Contraindications of Combined Oral Pills

Absolute

- Circulatory diseases (past or present)
- Arterial or venous thrombosis
- **Severe hypertension**
- Valvular heart disease, ishcaemic heart disease, angina
- **Hyperlipidemia**
- **Focal migraine**
- Diseases of the liver
- Active liver disease[Q]
- History of cholestatic jaundice
- Liver adenoma, [Q]carcinoma
- Others
- Pregnancy
- Undiagnozed genital tract bleeding
- Estrogen-dependent neoplasm–breast cancer

Relative Contraindications

- Hypertension
- Migraine
- Diabetes mellitus
- Epilepsy
- Obstructive jaundice in pregnancy
- Gallbladder disease
- Surgery with prolonged immobilization
- Sickle-cell disease

Protective against

- Ectopic pregnancy
- Ovarian CA (40%)
- Endometrial CA (50%)

Progestin only pill (mini pill)–[Q]

- No adverse effect on lactation and hence can be suitably presented to lactating women and so it is often called **Lactation Pill**
- A frequent side effect is **break-through bleeding.**

Low-dose progestational contraceptive primarily acts on–Cervix"

The main **mechanism** of action of progestin only pill or minipill is:

- **Thickening of cervical mucous secretion** which is hostile to sperm penetration
- It also has some **antiovulatory** action due to LH inhibition.
- Endometrium becomes atrophic, so blastocyst implantation is also hindered

DMPA

- **The standard dose of DMPA** is an i.m. injection of 150 mg every three months. It gives protection from pregnancy in 99% of women for at least three months.
- Shaws writes—monthly injection of DMPA 25–50 mg combined with 5 mg estrogen is considered to be effective
- Frequent side effects are:
  Osteoporosis
  Irregular, unpredictable bleeding
  Prolonged return of fertility
  Weight gain

Progestin-only subcutaneous implant

- Trade name of **Norplant**
- **Levonorgestrel** as the active ingredient.
- The continuous release continues for 5 years.
- A frequent side effect is **break-through bleeding.**
- Norplant I–6 capsules, 5 years
- Norplant II–2 capsules, 3 years

Lactation and OCPs

- Lactation is suppressed with combined pills. The combined oral contraceptives are therefore contraindicated in a lactating mother. It has effect on milk secretion and increases the thromboembolic phenomenon. The estrogen component adversely affects the quantity and constituents of breast milk and less frequently causes premature cessation of lactation
- Progestin only pill—is safe in lactating women and can be started 6 weeks onwards
- Progestogen implants—can be prescribed 6 weeks onwards after delivery
- IUD—should not be prescribed to puerperal women, as the risk of infection, perforation and expulsion is high. It should be inserted 3 months after delivery.

According to WHO study decrease in milk production after 18 weeks is:

- Combined oral contraceptive—42%
- Progestogen only pill—12%
- Non- hormonal—0.16%

EMERGENCY CONTRACEPTION

Emergency contraception prevents pregnancy by all of the following mechanism

- Delaying/inhibiting ovulation
- Inhibiting fertilization
- Interfering with implantation

Emergency contraception is a method used to prevent pregnancy after an unprotected intercourse within 72 hours. They are used after rape, unprotected intercourse or accidental rupture of condom during coitus taking place around ovulation.

Different methods of emergency contraception are:

Hormones:

- Morning after pill—Ethinyl estradiol 2.5 mg and Premarin (conjugated estrogen 15 mg)
- **Yuzpe method**—(combined hormonal regimen)

  EE 0.1 mg with 1 mg of dl-norgestrel repeated after 12 hours

  EE 50 mcg and 250 mcg LNG two tablets are taken within 72 hours of unprotected intercourse repeated 2 tablets after 12 hours

  EE 30 mcg and 150 mcg LNG four tablets are taken instead of two in the above schedule
- **LNG (progestin only pill)**

  0.75 mg LNG two tablets 12 hours apart (or)

  1.5 mg of LNG single dose

  Mode of action—ovulation is either prevented or delayed when the drug is taken Immediately[Q]

  - Fertilisation is interferred
  - Implantation is prevented as the endometrium is rendered unfavourable
  - Interferes with the function of corpus luteum or may cause luteolysis

  IUD—can be **introduced within a maximum period of 5 days**[Q]

  Mode of action—Prevents implantation[Q]

  RU-**486**—Antiprogesterone[Q]

Mode of action—Binds competitively with the progesterone receptor and nullifies the effect of endogenous progesterone and it causes sloughing and shedding of deciduas and prevents implantation.[Q]

Note: RU-486 also causes interruption of early pregnancy. This agent can be used for MTP upto 7 weeks. This use is however not termed as emergency contraception.

Advantages of LNG as an emergency contraceptive:

- It has no estrogen and no associated side effects
- It can be offered to HTN, cardiac and diabetic women
- It can be offered to a lactating women
- **It can be given as late as 120 hours after unprotected intercourse**
- Single-dose therapy is an advantage

PERMANENT METHODS

Female sterilization:

Postpartum sterilization- within 1 week of delivery

Interval sterilization–after 6 weeks of delivery—Preovulatory period

Eligibility criteria

- Should be married
- Age- Female- between 9 and 22 years, Male–< 60 years
- Couple should have atleast 1 child more than 1 years of age unless medically indicated
- Should be mentally sound
- Mentally ill pts, must be certified by a psychiatrist and consent given by legal guardian/spouse

Mini laparotomy:

- **Pomeroy's technique:** Isthmus is tied at its base with catgut and excised. Failure rate- 0.4%
- **Madlener method:** Middle third portion of tube is crushed at the base and tied with silk.
- **Irving operation:** ligation and burying the proximal tubal end in the serosa of the post uterine wall. Irreversible
- **Uchida method:** ligation and burying the medial end in the mesosalpinx. No failure rate
- **Madlener's fimbriectomy:** Middle third portion of tube is crushed at the base and tied with silk. Failure rate is high–0.3–2/100 surgeries
- **Parkland technique:** Tube separated from the mesosalpinx and 2 cm tube is excised. Both cut ends are tied and buried in the mesosalpinx.

Lap. Sterilization

Recent advance

Essure

- Permanent birth control device
- Dynamically expanding microinsert made of stainless steel (inside) and outer dynamic coil
- Occlusion of fallopian tubes by local tissue reaction

Male sterilization-vasectomy

- Simple, safe and effective
- Consists of dividing and excising a part of the vas deferens and disrupting the passage of sperms
- Done under LA
- 2 methods–conventional and non scalpel vasectomy
- Occlusion is done by different methods
  - Ligation and excision (done in India)
  - Electrocautery
  - Thermal cautery
  - Clips
  - Open ended vasectomy

Nonscalpel Vasectomy—NSV

- Introduced in China by Dr. Lishungiang
- Instead of scalpel, he uses 2 instruments
  - ringed clamp
  - dissecting forceps
- Smaller incision than conventional tech, hence no sutures req
- Early resumption of sexual activity
- Failure rate- 0.1–0.5%
- Reversibility-possible with microsurgery
  - 90% return of sperms
  - 50% pregnancy rate
- Sterility does not occur immediately after vasectomy
- Sperm remain in the semen for 15–20 ejaculations for about 3 months
- Contraception needed for 3 months
- Semen analysis performed thrice in these 3 months, once azoospermia results no need for anymore contraception

Cancers of the Genital Tract

Vulval cancers

- May arise from the skin, subcutaneous tissues, glandular elements of the vulva, or the mucosa, or the mucosa of the lower third of the vagina
- Primary a disease of postmenopausal women, with a peak incidence in the 60's

Preinvasive lesions	Invasive lesions
• Intraepithelial cancers VIN, I, II, III • Bowen's disease • Paget's disease • Microinvasive	• Squamous cell carcinoma or epidermoid cancers (90%, most common) • Melanoma–3–5% • Adenocarcinoma (1%) and Sarcoma–2% • Rodent ulcer or basal cell carcinoma–1% • Carcinoma of Bartholin's gland and Basal cell carcinoma

- **Epidermoid cancer: frequently involves the anterior half of the vulva**

International federation of gynecology and obstetrics (FIGO) Staging of Invasive Cancer, 2008	
Stage	
Stage 0	Carcinoma in situ, intraepithelial carcinoma
Stage I	Tumor confined to the vulva or perineum, no nodes Ia–size < 2 cm, stromal invasion <1 mm Ib–size > 2 cm, stromal invasion >1 mm
Stage II	Tumor of any size, spread to lower urethra, vagina/ anus; no nodal metastasis
Stage III	Tumor of any size with or without spread to adjacent perineal structures with positive inguinofemoral LNs IIIa–one LN ≥ 5 mm or 1–2 LNs < 5 mm IIIb–2 or more LNs ≥ 5 mm or 3 or more LNs < 5 mm IIIc–positive nodes with extracapsular spread
Stage IV Tumor invades other regional or distant structures	
Stage IVa	Tumor invades any of the following: upper urethra, bladder mucosa, rectal mucosa, pelvic bone or bilateral regional node metastasis (fixed/ulcerated), or a combination
Stage IVb	Any distant metastasis including pelvic lymph nodes

Treatment of vulval cancer:

Stage Ia–radical local excision

Stage Ib–

Lateral lesions—radical local excision + ipsilateral inguinofemoral lymphadenectomy

Midline lesions—radical local excision + B/L inguinofemoral lymphadenectomy

Stage II, IIIa—radical local excision/partial vulvectomy + B/L inguinofemoral lymphadenectomy

Advanced disease (IIIb-IVb)—chemoradiation

CARCINOMA CERVIX

Risk Factors

- Age of first pregnancy less than 20 years and Multiparity with poor birth spacing
- Early intercourse, poor personal hygiene and Multiparity sexual partners
- STD: HPV-16 (high risk), 18 (commonly leads to adeno Ca,), HPV-6 (Verrucous Ca), HSV2, HIV
- OCPs and progestogens usageover 8 year period can cause Adeno carcinoma of the endocervix (double the risk)
- DES exposure in childhood
- Low socio economic status, smoking, alcohol, drug abuse, immunocompromised
  - Low risk type: Subtype HPV 6,11
  - High risk: type 16, 18, 31, 33, 45, 58

Precancerous Lesions

A. Cervical intraepithelial neoplasia (stage 0)

- Intact basement membrane with dysplasia of the stratified squamous epithelium

B. Metaplasia

- Process starts at squamo-columnar junction. (Transformation zone)
- Normal cells without nuclear atypia and do not become malignant
- Atypical metaplasia is the precursor of dysplasia and malignancy
- Aneuploidy is the hallmark of malignant potential of these cells and diploidy or polyploidy is seen in benign/reparative cells

C. Dysplasia

Mild dysplasia (CIN–I): undifferentiated cells occupy the lower third of the epithelium. The cells are more differentiated toward the surface.

Moderate dysplasia (CIN–II): undifferentiated cells occupy the lower 50–75% of the epithelial thickness. Mostly intermediate cells with moderate nuclear enlargement, hyperchromasia, irregular chromatin and multiple nucleations

Severe dysplasia and Carcinoma in Situ (CIN–III): entire epithelium is replaced by abnormal cells

- **Tadpole cells:** seen in invasive cancers
- **Koilocytes:** cells with perinuclear halo in the cytoplasm, seen in young women with human papilloma virus infection, disappear as dysplasia advances

Investigations

- **Pap smear:** detects the abnormal cells
- **Endocervical scrap cytology**
- **HPV DNA testing by hybridization or PCR:** improves the predictive value of Pap smear by 95%
- **Visual inspection of acetowhite areas (VIA):** application of 5% acetic acid dehydrates the abnormal areas containing increased nuclear material and protein which turns white. The abnormal areas are biopsied
- **Visual inspection with Lugol's Iodine (VILI):** normal areas containing glycogen take up iodine and turn mahogany brown and abnormal (Schiller's test), unstained areas are biopsied
- **Speculoscopy and Spectroscopy**
- **Colposcoy:** locates the abnormal lesion. Oestrogen cream for 7–10 days and 400 mg misoprostol 3–4 hours before colposcopy expose the ectocervix better
- **Cervicography**
- **Cone biopsy:** both diagnostic and therapeutic. A wide cone excision including the entire outer margin of the lesion and the entire endocervical lining is obtained using cold knife technique under GA/LLETZ/laser excision
- **AgNOR:** new molecular tumor marker stands for Silver stained Nucleolar Organizer Regions

Modalities for management of CIN

Ablative procedures	Cryotherapy, laser vaporization therapy	Major drawback: tissue destruction, no specimen for HPE
Excisional procedure	Loop Electrosurgical Excision Procedure (LEEP)/ Large Loop Excision of Transformation Zone (LLETZ) Needle Excision of Transformation Zone (NETZ)	Both diagnostic and therapeutic (done in OP) Procedure of choice for CIN II and CIN III Complications: Bleeding, infections
Surgery	Conization, Hysterectomy	

Prophylaxis

- Given before exposure to virus, about 70% protection is expected
- Bivalent vaccine against HPV 16,18 (Cervarix) and Quadrivalent vaccine (Gardsil) against HPV 6, 11, 16, 18 are available
- First dose: 0.5 ml, before sexual exposure

- Second dose: 2 months after first dose
- Third dose: 6 months after first dose
- Contraindicated during pregnancy

Invasive Cancer

Pathology

- Commonest type → squamous cell cancer of ectocervix → appearing as cauliflower like growth
  - Spread is by contiguity or continuity or lymphatic spread or vascular embolisation
- Small cell → poor prognosis
- Adenoma malignum → well differentiated adeno carcinoma–good prognosis, but more prone for ovarian metastasis

Symptoms

Bleeding (most common): post coital bleeding/post menopausal bleeding. and vaginal discharge

Staging-Clinical

- **Stage I**—Carcinoma confined to cervix
  IA–preclinical carcinoma (diagnosed only by microscopy)
  - IA-1-Minimal stromal invasion ≤ 3mm and width ≤ 7 mm
  - IA-2- > 3 mm, not > 5 mm and not wider than 7 mm
  - I B-1-lesion not exceeding 4 cm in size
  - 1B-2 > 4 cm in size
- **Stage II**—Extend beyond cervix, but not upto pelvic wall: involves vagina but not lower 1/3rd
  - IIA-no obvious parametrial involvement
  - IIA-obvious parametrial involvement
- **Stage III**—tumor extends to the pelvic wall or to the lower third of the vagina
  - IIIA–no extension to pelvic wall but lower 1/3rd of vagina involved
  - IIIB–extension to pelvic wall or hydronephrosis or non functioning kidney
- **Stage IV**—extends beyond true pelvis or involves the mucosa of bladder or rectum
  - IVA–spread to adjacent organs
  - IVB–spread to distant organs
- Involvement of pelvic nodes: 5% in stage I, 15% in stage II and 25% in stage III
- Para aortic nodes: 20% in stage II ans 30% in stage III
- Ureteric obstruction (leading to uremia) occurs in 30% in stage III and 50% in stage IV
- Hypercalcemia indicates bone metastasis

Sentinel node: Obturator node. Blue dye is injected before surgery to delineate

Staging is clinical and requires investigations recommended by FIGO

Physical Examination	Radiological Studies	Procedure
Palpate lymph nodes	CXR	Biopsy
Examine vagina	Skeletal X-ray	Conization
Bimanual rectovaginal examination	IVP	Endocervical curettage ECC
	Barium enema	Colposcopy
		Hysteroscopy
		Cystoscopy
		Proctoscopy

U/S, MRI, CT scan, Laparoscopy, Laparotomy/Lymphangiography are not recommended by FIGO for staging

Mneumonic for FIGO approved procedures

- BS4C Exam
- Biopsy
- Scopies 4 = hysteroscopy/colposcopy/cystoscopy/proctoscopy
- Conization
- Endocervical curettage

Treatment

- **Stage IA1 (Microinvasive)**—conization with clear margin
- **Stage**—IA2, Modified Radical hysterectomy lymph node dissection. Vaginal trachelectomy with peliclymphadenectomy
- **Stage**—IB1, IIA, IB2: Wertheim's (Meig-Obayshi) Hysterectomy or Shauta vaginal hysterectomy (Mitra's operation)/primary radiotherapy. In IB2-combined surgery and radiotherapy
- Stage IIB–IVB—chemoradiation
- Uremia is the most common cause for death in complications related to Ca, Cervix

Brachytherapy for Carcinoma Cervix

Two important points in RT

- Cervical cancer requires a radiation dose of 6000 cGy
- Tolerance dose: for rectum—5000cGy, for bladder–6000cGy

	Point A	Point B
Location	2 cm above and 2 cm lateral to the external os	2 cm above and 5 cm lateral to the external os
Structure present	Paracervical/parametrial LN	Obturator LN
Dose of radiation	7000–8000 cGy	4000–6000 cGy

Comparison between surgery and RT

	Surgery	Radiation
Survival	85%	85%
Serious complications	Urological fistulas 1–2%	Intestinal and urinary strictures and fistulas 1.4–5.3%
Vagina	Shortened in length	Fibrosis and possible stenosis
Ovaries	Can be conserved	Destroyed
Chronic effects	Bladder atony–3%	Radiation fibrosis of bowel and bladder 6–8%
Surgical mortality	1%	1% d/t pulmonary embolism during brachytherapy

Endometrial Carcinoma

Etiology

- Advanced age, nulliparity, late menopause
- Corpus cancer syndrome (DM+HT+Obesity)
- Unopposed estrogen stimulation like Anovulation, PCOD, estrogen secreting ovarian tumors, exogenous estrogen as in unsupervised HRT.
- Tamoxifen
- Family history-Lynch II syndrome

Symptoms

- Postmenopausal bleeding
- Vaginal discharge
- Simpson's pain—Pelvic pain

Investigations

- Pap smear
- Fractional curettage
- USG
- Hysteroscopy
- Cystoscopy-snow hill pattern, von Brunn epithelial islets
- CT, MRI, CEA, Cytogenetic analysis

FIGO Staging of Endometrial Cancer, 2008

- **Stage I: cancer confined to the corpus uteri.**
  - IA G123–no or < half of myometrial invasion
  - IB G123–invasion ≥ than half of the myometrium
- **Stage II G123: Tumor involves cervical stroma but not beyond the uterus**
- **Stage III local and/or regional spread**
  - IIIA G123–involves serosa and/or adnexa
  - IIIB G123–vaginal and/or parametrial involvement
  - IIIC–metastasis to pelvis and para-aortic lymph nodes
  - III C1 G123–positive pelvic nodes
  - III C G123–positive para aortic nodes with or without positive pelvic nodes
- **Stage IV: Tumor invades bladder, bowel or distant sites**
  - IVA G123–Tumor involves bladder or bowel
  - IVB G123–Tumor shows distant metastasis (intra-abdominal and inguinal lymph nodes)

Endocervical glandular involvement is considered stage I positive peritoneal cytology is reported separately Without changing the stage, surgical staging is mandatory for all women. Steps are

- Adequate abdominal incision (vertical)
- Peritoneal washing for cytology
- Exploration of the pelvis and abdomen
- Total abdominal hysterectomy
- B/L salpingoophorectomy
- Open the uterus
  - assess the size and site of tumor
  - depth of myometrial invasion
  - ervical extension
- Pelvic and para-aortic lymphadenectomy
- Advanced stage-cytoreductive surgery

Treatment of Ca Endometrium

Stage-0: endometrial hyperplasia: older women–TAH+BSO
Young women-progesterone therapy and MIRENA IUCD
Transcervical resection of Endometrium (TCRE) is contraindicated
Stage I: surgery +
Follow up: Ia-Grade: 1 and 2–close follow up
Ia–Grade 3-vaginal brachytherapy
Ib G123-External pelvic radiation + vaginal brachytherapy
Stage II: surgery + external pelvic radiation + vaginal brachytherapy
Stage IIIa, IIIb, IIIc1: G123-surgery + external pelvic radiation + vaginal brachytherapy
Stage IIIc2: G123 surgery + extended field radiation + vaginal brachytherapy
Stage IV: Surgery + whole abdomen radiation + pelvic radiation + vaginal brachytherapy
Chemotherapy and hormone therapy–stage III and IV disease and recurrence

Ovarian tumors:

WHO Classification of Ovarian Tumors

- **Common epithelial tumors**
  - Serous tumors
  - Mucinous tumors
  - Endometrioid tumors
  - Clear cell (mesonephroid tumors)
  - Brenner tumors (transitional cell tumor)
  - Mixed epithelial tumors
  - Undifferentiated carcinoma
  - Unclassified carcinoma
  - Unclassified epithelial tumors
- **Sex cord (gonadal stroma) tumors**
  - Granulose—stromal cell tumors, theca cell tumors
  - Androblastomas—Sertili-Leydig cell tumors
  - Gynandroblastomas
  - Unclassified
- **Lipid (lipoid) cell tumors**
- **Germ cell tumors**
  - Dysgerminoma
  - Endodermal sinus tumors (yolk sac tumor)
  - Embryonal carcinoma
  - Polyembryoma
  - Choriocarcinoma
  - Teratoma
  - Mixed forms
- **Gonadoblastoma**
  - Pure
  - Mixed with dysgerminoma or other germ cell tumors
- **Soft tissue tumors not specific to ovary**
- **Unclassified tumors**
- **Secondary (metastatic) tumors**

Table: International Federation of Gynecology and Obstetrics (FIGO) staging of overian neoplasma
Stage I. Growth limited to the ovaries
Ia—one ovary involved
Ib—both ovaries involved
Ic—Ia or Ib and ovarian surface tunor, ruptured capsule, malignant ascites, or peritoneal cytology positive for malignant cells
Stage II. Extension of the neoplasm from the ovary to the pelvis
IIa—extension to the uterus or fallopian tube
IIb—extension to other pelvic tissues
IIc—IIa or b and ovarian surface tumor, ruptured capsule, malignant ascites, or peritoneal cytology positive for malignant cells
Stage III. Disease extension to the abdominal cavity
IIIa—abdominal peritoneal surfaces with microscopic metastases
IIIb—tumor metastases < 2 cm in size
IIIc—tumor metastases > 2 cm in size or metastatic disease in the pelvic, para-aortic, or inguinal lymph nodes
Stage IV. Distant metastatic disease
Malignant pleural effusion
Pulmonary parenchymal metastases
Liver or splenic parenchymal metastases (not surface implants)
Metastases to the supraclavicular lymph nodes or skin

Investigations

- Ultrasound
- Doppler flow studies–resistance index
- CA 125 > 35—postmenopausal > 200—premenopausal
- CT scan—detects 1.5–2 cm
- MRI—detects > 1 cm
- Paracentesis
- Fine needle aspiration cytology/biopsy

Risk categorization in early stage ovarian carcinomas

Low Risk	High Risk
Stage I A/B	Stage I A/B, stage I C
Nonclear cell tumors	Clear cell tumors
Grade ½	Grade 3
No dense adhesions	Dense adhesions
No intraoperative rupture	Intraoperative rupture
Diploid tumor	Aneuploid tumor

Treatment

Surgical staging is done the same way as in endometrial carcinoma + infracolic omentectomy + pelvic and para aortic lymphadenectomy

Adjuvant therapy in early stage disease

- Chemotherapy—3–6 cycles cisplatin/carboplatin + paclitaxel } stage I-high risk, Stage II
- Stage I-low risk-no need for adjuvant therapy

Advanced stage

- Primary cytoreduction + post op ChemoT

  or
- Neoadjuvant ChemoT—f/b Surgery-post op ChemoT
- Chemotherapy—IV + Intraperitoneal

Germ Cell Tumors

- **Mnemonic—YES PCT**

  Y = Yolk sac (endodermal sinus) tumor

  E = Embryonal ca

  S = Seminoma = Dysgerminoma

  P = Polyembryoma

  C = Chorioca

  T = Teratoma = Dermoid
- **Treatment of early stage dysgerminoma Stage IA**
  - Surgery alone/fertility preserving surgery with F/U
  - No chemotherapy
- Rest of the stages–Surgery + Chemotherapy
- M/C used regimens for GCT
  - BEP–bleomycin, etoposide, cisplatin
  - VBP–vinblastin, bleomycin, cisplatin
  - VAC–vincristine, actinomycin, cyclophosphamide

Gestational Trophoblastic Disease

Classification:

- Hydatidiform mole (vesicular mole)
  - Complete (more common)
  - Partial
- Invasive mole
- Placental site trophoblastic tumor
- Choriocarcinoma
  - Nonmetastatic
  - Metastatic
    - Low risk (good prognosis)
    - High risk (poor prognosis)

Hydatidiform Mole (Vesicular Mole)

Abnormal proliferation of placental tissue involving both cytptrophoblast and/or synctiotrophoblast

Features	Complete mole	Partial mole
Fetus	Absent	Present, malformed or IUGR
Fetal vessels	Absent	Present
Hydropic changes	Diffuse and placenta not present	Focal
Trophoblastic hyperplasia	Marked	Mild to moderate
Beta-hCG level	Very high	Comparatively low
Karyotype	46XX mostly and paternally derived	69XXY
Malignant potential	15–20%	Rare

Protocol for management of H Mole

Investigations {Serum Beta HCG levels, USG, Chest X-ray

↓

Suction evacuation/curettage

(It is the treatment of choice in molar pregnancy irrespective of uterine size)

↓

Products of conception to be sent for histopathological examination

↓

Regular followup serum β–hCG

FIGO scoring system 2008

	0	1	2	4
Age	<40	≥40	–	–
Prior pregnancy	Mole	Abortion	Term pregnancy	–
Pregnancy (months)	<4	4–6	7–12	≥ 13
Pretreatment ß-hCG	<1000 IU	1000–10,000	10,000–100,000	>10,00,000 mIU/ml
Size of tumor (cm)	< 3 cm	3–5 cm	> 5 cm	Including uterus
No. of metastasis	–	1–4	5–8	> 8
Site of metastases	Lung	Spleen, kidney	GIT	Liver, brain
Prior chemotherapy	–	–	Single	Multiple
< 6-low risk; ≥ 7-high risk				

FIGO Staging of GTDs

- Stage I: disease confined to uterus
- Stage II: extends outside uterus, but confined to genital structure
- Stage III: lung metastasis with or without genital involvement
- Stage IV: other metastasis
  - IVA: no risk factor
  - IVB: one-risk factor (serum β-hCG level > 100,000 IU/ml or disease duration > 6 months)
  - IVC: two-risk factor (serum β-hCG level > 100,000 IU/ml and disease duration > 6 months)

Signs and Symptoms

- Persistent or irregular uterine hemorrhage
- Offensive vaginal discharge
- When amenorrhea occurs, it is due to high levels of hCG secreted by the metastatic growth outside the uterus
- Dyspnea and hemoptysis are noticed with lung metastasis
- Neurological symptoms like hemiplegia, epilepsy, headache and visual disturbances suggest brain metastasis
- On examination, a vaginal metastasis appears as a bluish red vascular tumor which bleeds easily on touch

Ultrasound—'Snowstorm Appearance'

Treatment

Suction evacuation

Chemotherapy:

- Since β-hCG is a very specific marker, the chemotherapy can be administered based on this alone
- The most effective chemotherapeutic agent is the folic acid inhibitor methotrexate
- Combined chembined chemotherapy is recommended for high-risk cases
- A variety of combinations of chemotherapeutic agents are being used, such as:
  - Methotrexate, actinomycin-D and chlorambucil (MAC)
  - Methotrexate, actinomycin-D and adriamycin (MAA)
  - EMA-CO—is the currently recommended regimen for high-risk cases
    - Etoposide
    - Methotrexate
    - Actinomycin D
    - Cyclophosphamide
    - Vincristine (Oncovin)

Surgery

- Hysterectomy is indicated in:
  - High-risk cases over 40 years, multiparous
  - Chemotherapy ineffective
  - Hemorrhage due to uterine perforation
  - Large size growth in the uterus
  - Placental site trophoblastic disease (Do not respond to any chemotherapy)

Hormones in Gynecology

- **GnRH**
- Natural-glycoprotein, produced by the arcuate nucleus of the hypothalmus
  - short ½ life
  - secreted in a pulsatile manner

- Synthetic
  - MOA—given continously—bind to GnRH receptor in the pituitary and cause competitive inhibition of endogenous GnRH
  - initial increase in FSH and LH f/b decrease
- Preparations
  - Buserelin Leuproline
  - Nafarelin Goserelin
  - Triptorelin Historelin
- Indications—Mnemonic A-F and HIP
- A—Adenomyosis
- B—IBD (under trial)
- C—Ca breast
- D—DUB
- E—Endometriosis
- F—Fibroid uterus
- H—Hirsuitism
- I—Infertility
- P—Precocious puberty
- Adverse effects
  - Allergicrns
  - Menopausal symptoms
  - Osteoporosis
- **FSH/LH**
- Promotes gametogenesis
- Production of estrogen
- **Prolactin**
- Acts on breast–causes milk secretion
- Acts on pituitary-dec FSH secrn-anovulation
- **Estrogen**

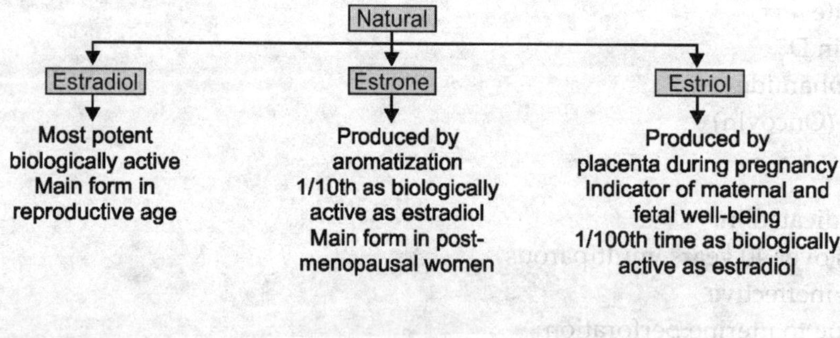

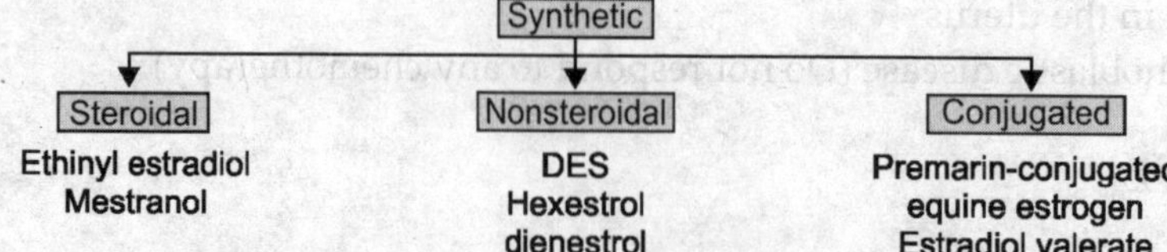

Functions

- Growth and development of FGT
- Negative feedback on FSH and LH

- Increased risk of Ca breast, endometrium and cervix
- Stimulates CTZ—causes vomiting
- Increased predisposition of DVT and PE
- Glucose intolerance, Na+ and water retention
- Maintain bone mass
- Vasodilatation—by increasing the release of NO
- Delayed puberty
- Lactation suppression
- DUB, Polymenorrhea
- Menopausal symptoms
- Oral contraception
- Senile vulvovaginitis
- In intersex for growth of seconadary sexual characters

SERMs

- Estrogen agonist and antagonist
- Used to provide beneficial effects of EZ and counter the adverse effects
- Clomiphene—used in OI
- Raloxifene—used in osteoprosis
- Ormeloxifene—contraception, DUB

Progesterone

- Secreted by the corpus luteum of ovary
- Synthetic
- Pregnanes
- Estranes
- Gonanes
- 19–Norprogest derivatives
- Spirinolactone derivatives

Uses

- Progesterone challenge test
- Contraception
- DUB
- Dysmenorrhea and PMS
- Postponement of menses
- LPD
- Endometriosis
- Endometrial hyperplasia and Ca
- HRT

Antiprogesterone-Mifepristone RU486

- Derivative of 19–nortestosterone

Uses

- Postcoital pill
- To induce abortion upto 7 weeks
- Ripening of Cx
- Management of fibroid

QUESTIONS

1. A 40-year-old multiparous woman was detected to have CIN-2 by PAP smear. What is the next line of management? (2014)
a. Conization
b. Hysterectomy
c. Colposcopy
d. Repeat PAP smear

2. Whiff test is useful in the diagnosis: (2014)
a. Trichomonas
b. Bacterial vaginosis
c. Candida
d. PID

3. A female presents with 3 cm painless ulcer with raised edges on labia majora. Most common cause is: (2014)
a. Syphilis
b. Gonorrhea
c. Herpes
d. Chlamydia trachomatis

4. A 45-year-old multipara presents with dysmenorrhea and menorrhagia. Uterus is symmetrically enlarged upto 14 weeks. What is the probable diagnosis? (2014)
a. Intramural fibroid
b. Adenomyosis
c. Endometrial hyperplasia
d. Pelvic inflammatory disease

5. Advantage of lap sterilization over mini laparotomy sterilization is: (2014)
a. Less failure rate
b. Less blood loss
c. Less post operative stay
d. Easy procedure

6. Hormone Replacement Therapy (HRT) in postmenopausal women is beneficial in all thee except: (2014)
a. Vasomotor symptoms
b. Osteoporosis
c. Prevention of CAD
d. Vaginal atrophy

7. Schiller-Duval bodies are seen in: (2013)
a. Endodermal sinus tumor
b. Embryonal carcinoma
c. Dermoid cyst
d. Brenner tumor

8. Choice of contraception in recently delivered lactating mother: (2013)
a. Safe period
b. OCP
c. IUCD
d. Depot provera

9. Barrier type of contraception among the following: (2013)
a. OCPD
b. IUD
c. Spermicidal jelly
d. Symptothermic method

10. All cause endometrial carcinoma except: (2013)
a. Fibromyoma
b. HRT
c. OCPs
d. Corpus Cancer Syndrome

11. Whiff test is done in: (2013)
a. Bacterial vaginosis
b. Trichomonas vaginalis
c. Vaginal candidiasis
d. Chlamydial infection

12. Hirsutism is cased by all except: (2013)
a. Testicular feminization syndrome
b. PCOD
c. CAH
d. Obesity

13. Absent uterus with normal breast and scanty pubic hair is: (2013)
a. Androgen insensitivity syndrome
b. Meyer rokitansky syndrome
c. Turner syndrome
d. Klinefelter syndrome

14. True about Halban's disease are all except: (2013)
a. Malignant ovarian tumor
b. Irregular shedding
c. Persistent cropus luteum
d. Ovulatory DUB

15. Sentinel lymph node biopsy is done in all except: (2013)
a. Ca vulva
b. Ca cervix
c. Ca breast
d. Choriocarcinoma

16. Most common organism causing carcinoma cervix: (2013)
a. HPV 33
b. HPV 18
c. HPV 16
d. HPV 31

17. Drug of choice for Chlamydia urethritis in pregnancy: (2013)
a. Azithromycin
b. Erythromycin

c. Tetracycline
d. Doxycycline

18. MIRENA life is: (2013)
a. 3 years
b. 1 year
c. 5 years
d. 10 years

19. Anterior colporrhaphy and colpoperineorrphy is known as:
a. Ward-Mayo surgery
b. Shirodkar repair
c. Manchester repair
d. Pelvic floor repair

20. Ovarian cause of hirsutism: (2012)
a. PCOD
b. Ovarian carcinoma
c. Dysgerminoma
d. Endometriotic cyst

21. Progesterone only pills carry the risk of: (2012)
a. Hypertension
b. Venous embolism
c. Irregular bleeding
d. Ectopic pregnancy

22. Which of the following is false regarding partial mole: (2012)
a. Malignant potential is rare
b. It has diploid karyotype
c. Fetal parts are present
d. USG shows fetus and placenta with cystic spaces

23. Drug of choice for maternal toxoplasmosis: (2012)
a. Spiramycin
b. Pyrimethamine
c. Doxy + sulfadiazine
d. Trimethoprim sulfamethoxazole

24. All are correct regarding estrogen except: (2012)
a. Responsible for preovulatory LH surge
b. Causes negative feedback on FSH
c. Produces proliferative ednometrium
d. Secreted by theca cells

25. All are correct regarding IUCD except: (2012)
a. Reduces fertility after removal
b. Increases risk of ectopis pregnancy
c. Causes menorrhagia
d. Can be used for emergency contraception

26. 16-year-old girl presented with primary amenorrhea. Her karyotype is normal. On USG-uterus and cervix are absent, ovaries are normal. What is the probable diagnosis? (2012)
a. Turner's syndrome
b. Mullerian agenesis
c. Testicular feminizing syndrome
d. Imperforate hymen

27. 52-year-old postmemopausal woman presented with mass in the lower abdomen. The patient underwent hysterectomy and bilateral oophorectomy. Biopsy showed endometrioid carcinoma. This type of tumor is predisposed by: (2012)
a. HPV
b. Adenomyosis
c. OCPs
d. Oestrogen excess

28. OCPs do not protect against: (2012)
a. Ca cervix
b. Ca endometrium
c. Ca ovary
d. Ca breast

29. The angle of anteflexion occurs at the level of: (2012)
a. Internal os
b. External os
c. Upper vagina
d. Cervix

30. Sertoli cells secrete: (2012)
a. FSH
b. Androgen-binding protein
c. Testosterone
d. LH

31. Which of the following is an example for transplacentation carcinogenesis? (2012)
a. Vaginal Ca
b. Pancreatic Ca
c. Colon Ca
d. Breast Ca

32. Placental alkaline phosphatase is secreted by: (2012)
a. Endogenous sinus tumor
b. Choriocarcinoma
c. Granulose cell tumor
d. Dysgerminoma

33. Cervix-to-body ratio in a prepubertal girl is: (2011)
a. 1 : 1
b. 2 : 1
c. 1 : 2
d. 3 : 1

34. Best IUCD for a woman with menorrhagia is: (2011)
a. Lippes loop
b. Cu-T 375
c. Cu-T 200
d. Levonorgestrel IUCD

35. Clue cell is seen in: **(2011)**
a. Trichomonas vaginalis
b. Bacterial vaginosis
c. Candidiasis
d. Herpes

36. Antiprogestin used for emergency contraception is: **(2011)**
a. Mifepristone
b. Misoprostol
c. Methotrexate
d. Norethisterone

37. OC pills have been shown to be useful in the prevention of which of the following malignancies?
a. Ca colon **(2011)**
b. Ca endometrium
c. Ca breast
d. Ca cervix

38. Lactating mother's best contraceptive is: **(2011)**
a. Monophasic pill
b. Biphasic pill
c. Triphasic pill
d. Mini pill

39. In which condition is there a pain before the onset of menstruation, which is relieved after the beginning of menses? **(2011)**
a. Spasmodic dysmenorrhea
b. Congestive dysmenorrhea
c. Membranous dysmenorrhea
d. Menorrhagia

40. Endometrial Ca with poor prognosis: **(2011)**
a. Adeno grade 2
b. Adenosquamous
c. Adenoacanthoma
d. Clear cell

41. Main support of the uterus is formed by: **(2011)**
a. Mackendrot's ligament
b. Broad ligament
c. Fallopian tubes
d. Round ligament

42. Marker of endodermal sinus tumor is: **(2011)**
a. Alphafetoprotein
b. hCG
c. LDH
d. CA-125

43. Vaginal adenosis precedes: **(2011)**
a. Clear cell carcinoma
b. Endometrial Ca
c. Cervical Ca
d. Squamous cell Ca of vagina

44. Fibrocystic disease is due to high levels of:
a. Estrogen **(2011)**
b. Progesterone
c. LH
d. Testosterone

45. Pseudomyxoma peritonei occurs due to: **(2010)**
a. Mucinous cystadenoma ovary
b. Ca colon
c. Adenoma stomach
d. Pancreatic adenocarcinoma

46. Most ideal site for sterilization by tubectomy is:
a. Ampulla **(2010)**
b. Isthmus
c. Fimbriated extremity
d. Interstitial portion

47. Most common site of fertilization is: **(2010)**
a. Interstition
b. Isthmus
c. Ampulla
d. Infundibulum

48. How will you prevent bleeding after IUCD insertion? **(2010)**
a. Aspirin
b. Progesterone-only pill
c. Combined oral pills
d. Tranexamic acid

49. Not an epithelial tumor: **(2010)**
a. Hilus cell tumor
b. Clear cell carcinoma
c. Transitional cell tumor
d. Endometrioid carcinoma

50. Which is the most common ovarian tumor in pregnancy: **(2010)**
a. Serous cystadenoma
b. Mucinous cystadenoma
c. Dermoid tumor
d. Solid teratoma

51. Tumor marker for dysgerminoma: **(2010)**
a. LDH
b. CEA
c. CA 19
d. CA 125

52. Vasectomy leads to all except: **(2010)**
a. Decreased libido
b. Sperm granuloma
c. Antisperm antibody
d. Infection

53. Most common cause of vesicovaginal fistula is:
a. Laparoscopy **(2010)**
b. Abdominal hysterectomy
c. Obstructed labor
d. Cystoscopy

54. Clue cells are seen in: (2010)
a. Bacterial vaginosis
b. Moniliasis
c. Trichomoniasis
d. Gardenella vaginalis

55. Ca cervix with involvement of upper 1/3rd vagina but not the parametrium is: (2010)
a. Stage IIA
b. Stage IIIA
c. Stage IIB
d. Stage IIIB

56. Schiller duval bodies seen in: (2010)
a. Endodermal sinus tumor
b. Embryonal carcinoma
c. Dermoid cyst
d. Brenner tumor

57. Least common tumor in vagina among the following is: (2010)
a. Metastasis from cervix
b. Metastasis from endometrium
c. Metastasis from choriocarcinoma
d. Primary vaginal carcinoma

58. OC pills prevent all except: (2010)
a. Ca colon
b. Ca endometrium
c. Ca breast
d. Ca cervix

59. Primary amenorrhea is seen in all except:
a. Kallman's syndrome (2010)
b. Rokitansky's syndrome
c. Ashermann's syndrome
d. Turner's syndrome

60. Which of the following is the most common cause of urethritis with leucorrhea? (2009)
a. Chlamydia tranchomatic
b. *H. vaginalis*
c. Trichomonas
d. Candida

61. The most common cause of vesicovaginal fistula in developing countries is: (2009)
a. Pressure necrosis of urethra during obstructed labor
b. Forceps delivery
c. Abdominal hysterectomy
d. Tuberculosis

62. Treatment of primary ovarian failure is: (2009)
a. FSH
b. GnRH
c. LH
d. Estrogen/progesterone

63. The characteristic symptom of dysmenorrheal, menorrhagia, recurrent abdominal pain and infertility is suggestive of: (2009)
a. Endometriosis
b. Ectopic pregnancy
c. Endometritis
d. Endometrial carcinoma

64. Anteversion of uterus is due to the following ligament: (2009)
a. Uterosacral ligament
b. Mackenrodt's ligament
c. Round ligament
d. Pubocervical ligament

65. A nulliparous female aged 30 years develops IInd degree UV prolapsed. The operative procedure done is: (2009)
a. Cervicopexy
b. LeForte repair
c. Manchester repair
d. Ward-Mayo surgery

66. In minilap procedure, the most common method successfully used is: (2009)
a. Uchida's
b. Pomeroy's
c. Irving's
d. Parkland's

67. Mesonephric duct remnant presenting as swelling in anterior vaginal wall is: (2009)
a. Nebothian cyst
b. Gartner's cyst
c. Bartholin's cyst
d. Inclusion cyst

68. All are symptoms of molar pregnancy except:
a. Amenorrhea (2008)
b. Symptoms of Hypothyroidism
c. Abnormal vaginal bleeding
d. Expulsion of grape-like vesicles

69. Choice of contraception in a recently delivered lactating mother: (2008)
a. Safe period
b. OCP
c. IUCD
d. Depot provera

70. Clue cells are seen in: (2008)
a. Gardenella vaginitis
b. Trichomoniasis
c. Moniliasis
d. Pelvic inflammatory diseases

71. IUD of choice in menorrhagia: (2008)
a. Lippes loop
b. Cu-T 375
c. Cu-T 200
d. Levonorgestrel IUCD

72. Most common site for fibroids in uterus is: (2008)
a. Subserous
b. Intramural
c. Submucous
d. Cervical

73. All are true regarding adenomyosis except:(2008)
a. Occurs in a parous woman aged around 40 years
b. Menorrhagia
c. Uterus symmetrically enlarged
d. Uterus not tender on palpation

74. Genital prolapsed in a female can be due to all except: (2007)
a. Ascites
b. Complete perineal tear
c. Chronic cough
d. Obesity

75. Evidence of ovulation has occurred in all except:
a. 10 mm Graffian follicles on USG (2007)
b. Progesterone >5 ng/ml
c. Corpus luteum
d. Biphasic increase in temperature

76. All cause endometrial carcinoma except: (2007)
a. Fibromyoma
b. HRT
c. OCPs
d. Corpus Cancer Syndorme

77. Cervix to body ratio in a postpubertal adolescent girl is: (2007)
a. 1 : 1
b. 2 : 1
c. 1 : 2
d. 3 : 1

78. Least common cause of malignancy in vagina is:
a. Choriocarcinoma (2006)
b. Cervical ca
c. Primary vaginal ca
d. Endometrial ca

79. PID does not include: (2006)
a. Cervicitis
b. Endometritis
c. Peritonitis
d. Salpingitis

80. Highest failure rate is seen in: (2006)
a. Laparoscopic method
b. Irwin method
c. Pomeroy method
d. Madlener method

81. Which is not true about pregnancy and TB?
a. No difference in prognosis of pregnancy (2006)
b. Congenital TB is rare
c. Active TB can be transmitted by transplacental route
d. Concomitant HIV infection increases the risk

82. Alpha fetoprotein is decreased in: (2006)
a. Spinal bifida
b. Down's syndrome
c. Dead fetus
d. Abdominal wall deficiency

83. In case of carcinoma cervix, hydronephrosis or renal involvement is seen in:
a. Stage 3a (2006)
b. Stage 3b
c. Stage 2
d. Stage 4

84. Cysts seen in vagina are all except: (2006)
a. Nebothian cyst
b. Gartner's cyst
c. Bartholin's cyst
d. Inclusion cyst

85. Call-Exner bodies are found in: (2006)
a. Granulose cell tumor
b. Sertoli leydig cell tumor
c. Gynandroblastoma
d. Thecoma

86. Invasive mole differs from choriocarcinoma in all the following except: (2006)
a. Absence of villi
b. No evidence of muscle necrosis
c. Diagnosed < 6 months following an abortion
d. Invasive mole follows an abortion or molar pregnancy

87. Menopausal flushing is due to: (2006)
a. LH
b. FSH
c. Estrogen
d. Progesterone

88. Contraindications for OCPs are all except:
a. Headache (2006)
b. Jaundice
c. Diabetes
d. Varicose veins

89. Sex cord stromal tumors are all except: (2006)
a. Granulose cell tumor
b. Leydig cell tumor
c. Yolk sac tumor
d. Sertoli cell tumor

ANSWERS AND EXPLANATIONS

1. **Ans. c. Colposcopy** *Ref: Sakala EP, High-Yield Obsterics and Gynecology, 2/e p169*

Cervical Intraepithelial Neoplasia (CIN)

- Presence of atypical cells within squamous epithelium
- CIN graded as I to III depending on the extent to which these cells are present in the epithelium
- CIN I (mild dysplasia)—Atypical cells are present in lower 1/3rd of epithelium
- CIN II (moderate dysplasia)—atypical ells are present in lower 2/3rd of epithelium
- CIN III (severe dysplasia)—Atypical cells occupy the full thickness of epithelium, but basement membrane is intact—carcinoma in situ
- LSIL—Low-grade squamous intraepithelial lesion—New terminology for CIN-1 (According to Bethesda system)
- HSIL—High-grade squamous intraepithelial lesion—New terminology for both CIN-2 and CIN-3 (According to bethesda system)

American College of Obstetrics and Gyneocology (ACOG) guidelines for cervical cancer screening

PAP smear finding	Intervention	Treatment
Unsatisfactory	Repeat PAP smear in 6–12 weeks	
Negative for CIN or malignancy	Follow with PAP smear according to guidelines	
Atypical squamous cells-cannot exclude high-grade lesion (ASC-H)	Colposcopy-directed biopsy	
CIN-1 (LGSIL)	Any of the following: • Repeat PAP in 4–6 months • Obtain HPV DNA testing • Colposcopy-directed biopsy (Preferred)	**a. Satisfactory colposcopy** • Follow-sup (or) • Ablation procedure – Electrocautery – Cryotherapy – Laser
		b. Unsatisfactory colposcopy • Excision procedure – Conization – Loop electrosurgical excision procedure (LEEP)
CIN-2 and CIN-3 (HGSIL)	Colposcopy-directed biopsy	For both satisfactory and unsatisfactory colposcopy Excision procedure is indicated: • Conization • Loop electrosurgical excision procedure (LEEP) • Large loop excision of transformation zone (LLETZ)

ACOG Screening guidelines

Age	Recommended screening	Comment
Less than 21	No screening	
Age 21–29	Pap smear alone every 3 years	
Age 30–65	Pap smear and HPV co-testing every 5 years or pap smear alone every 3 years	Screening HPV testing alone is not recommended
Age 65 and older	No screening after adequate negative prior screening results	Women with a history of high grade pap smear should continue age based screening for at least 20 years

Contd...

Contd...

Age	Recommended screening	Comment
Women who have had hysterectomy	No screening necessary	Applies to women without a cervix and without a history of high grade pap smear or can cer in the past 20 years
Women vaccinated against HPV	Same as vaccinated	

2. Ans. b. Bacterial vaginosis *Ref: Shaw's Textbook of Gynecology, 15/e p131*

Gardnerella vaginalis

- Alteration in normal vaginal flora
- Decrease in number of lactobacilli in vaginal discharge—lactobacilli reduce pH and release hydrogen peroxide toxic to other bacteria
- *Hemophilus vaginalis, Gardnerella, Mobiluncus and Mycoplasma hominis*-polymicrobial cause.
- White, milky non-viscous discharge, pH of discharge more than 4.5.
- Whiff Test—Fishy odor when vaginal discharge is mixed with 10% KOH-due to release of amino metabolites from various organisms
- Presence of Clue Cells—epithelial cells with granular cytoplasm caused by gram-negative bacilli adhering on the surface
- Wet smear, gram stain and culture are investigations.

Amsel Criteria for Diagnozing Bacterial Vaginosis

- Thin, white, yellow, homogenous discharge
- **Clue cells** on microscopy
- **pH** of vaginal fluid > 4.5
- Release of a fishy odor on adding alkali-10% potassium hydroxide (KOH) solution
  - **at least three of the four criteria** should be present for a confirmed diagnosis

Nugent's Criteria for Diagnozing BV

- **Grade 1 (Normal):** *Lactobacillus* morphotypes predominate
- **Grade 2 (Intermediate):** Mixed flora with some Lactobacilli present, but Gardnerella or *Mobiluncus* morphotypes also present
- **Grade 3 (Bacterial Vaginosis):** Predominantly Gardnerella and/or *Mobiluncus* morphotypes. Few or absent Lactobacilli.

Treatment

- Metronidazole 500 mg bd for 7 days
- Ampicillin 500 mg or cephalosporin 500 mg bd for 7 days
- Tetracycline 500 mg 4 times a day
- Dozycycline 100 mg bd
- Sulphafurazole 1 g 4 times daily for 10–14 days
- Clindamycin 300 mg daily for 7 days
- Clindamycin 2% cream locally
- Ornidazole 500 mg vaginal tablet for 7 days
- Lacteal is protein free acidifying lactate gel neutralizes vaginal ph 5 ml applied for 7 days

3. Ans. a. Syphilis *Ref: Essentials in Dermatology, 1/e*

Syphilis

- Causative agent—*Treponema pallidum*

Stage	Lesion seen
Primary	Chancre/ulcer
Secondary	Condyloma lata-coarse flat topped moist necrotic lesion
Tertiary	Gumma-punched ulcer with rolled-out margins

- DOC—benzathine penicillin

Tubes are not affected in primary syphillis and infertility doesn't occur

4. Ans. b. Adenomyosis *Ref: Shaw's Textbook of Gynecology, 15/e p474*

- Common in **women above 40 years**
- Often **coexists with fibroid, endometriosis** and **endometrial cancer**
- Uterus is **symmetrically enlarged to not more than 14 week's size**
- **Histology—Islands of endometrial glands** surrounded by **stroma** seen in the **myometrial tissue beyond** the **endomyometrial junction.**
- The **distance** between **basal endometrium** and the **endometrial gland** should be >2.5 mm.
  - Common complaint—**Menorrhagia** and **progressive dysmenorrhoea**
  - Clinical examination reveals **symmetrical enlargement of uterus** and **tender uterus**
  - Treatment is localized excision, hysterectomy.
  - Medical treatment includes **Danazol, GnRH, Mirena IUD.**

5. Ans. c. Less postoperative stay *Ref: 'Practice of Fertility Control' by SK Chaudhuri, 6/e p246*

Minilaparotomy

Advantages	Disadvantages
OP procedure done with minimal training	High chances of wound and pelvic infections
Can be done in a peripheral setting with minimal training	Longer duration and severity of postoperative pain
Doesn't require special equipment	Longer convalesence
Performed after puerperium and 1st and 2nd trimester abortions	Longer incisional scar
Can be done for interval sterilization	
Doesn't require special training	

Laparascopic Sterilization

Advantages	Disadvantages
As effective as minilap with less complication rate	Compliocations low but if occurs can be life threatening
Done in a peripheral setting as outpatient procedure	Costly equipment and requires expertise
Small scar with less post operative pain	Increased risk of postoperative shoulder pain, cardiorespiratory distress, air embolism and sudden cardiac arrest during insufflations
Shorter convalescence	Cannot be done after 2nd trimester abortions and in puerperium
Highly reversible especially when clips are used	Relatively contraindicated in obesity, pelvic adhesions and previous abdominal surgeries

6. Ans. c. Prevention of CAD *Ref: Shaw's Textbook of Gynecology, 15/e*

Hormone Replacement Therapy

Hormone Replacement Therapy (HRT) in Menopause

- Medical treatment in surgically menopausal, perimenopausal and postmenopausal women
- Goal—To mitigate discomfort caused by diminished circulating estrogen and progesterone hormones in menopause
- **Combination HRT is often recommended normal** it decreases the amount of endometrial hyperplasia and cancer associated with unopposed estrogen therapy

The 2002 Women's Health Initiative (WHI) of the National Institutes of Health (NIH) found disparate results for all cause mortality with hormone replacement

- There was an increased incidence of breast cancer, heart attacks and stroke
- **Reduced incidence of colorectal cancer and bone feature**
- Some of the **WHI findings were** again **found in a larger national study** done in the UK, known as **The Million Woman Study**

Benefits and Risks

- Relief of menopausal symptoms
- **↓Hot flushes**
- **↓Vaginal dryness**

7. Ans. a. Endodermal sinus tumor *Ref: Dutta Textbook of Gynecology 5/e p368*

Ovarian Tumors and their Specific Features

- **Schiller Duval bodies:** Endodermal sinus tumor
- **Signet ring cells:** Krukenberg's tumor
- **Coffee bean cells/Call Exner bodies:** Granulosa cell tumor
- **Sertoli and Leydig cells:** Arrhenoblastoma
- **Psammoma bodies:** Papillary serous cytadenoma
- **Rokitansky's protuberance:** Dermoid cyst (Mature teratoma)
- **Hobnail cells:** Clear cell Ca (mesonephroid Ca)
- **Reinke's crystal:** Hilus cell tumor
- **Walthard cell nest:** Brenner tumor

8. Ans. d. Depot provera *Ref: Williams Obsterics 23/e p652 table 30–4*

Lactation and OCPs

- Lactation is suppressed with combined pills. The combined oral contraceptive are therefore contraindicated in a lactating mother. It has effect on milk secretion and increases the thromboembolic phenomenon. The estrogen component adversely affects the quantity and constituents of breast milk and less frequently causes premature cessation of lactation
- Progestin only pill—is safe in lactating women and can be started 6 weeks onwards
- Progestogen implants/injectable (depot Provera)—can be prescribed 6 weeks onwards after delivery
- IUD—should not be prescribed to puerperal women, as the risk of infection, perforation and expulsion is high. It should be inserted 3 months after delivery.

According to WHO study, decrease in milk production after 18 weeks is:

- Combined oral contraceptive—42%
- Progestogen only pill—12%
- Non-hormonal—0.16%

9. Ans. c. Spermicidal jelly *Ref: Dutta Textbook of Gynecology 5/e p534*

Barrier methods

- **Males**
  - Condoms
- **Females**
  - Female condom (Femshield)
  - Vaginal sponge (Today)
  - Vaginal diaphragm/cervical cap
  - Spermicidal jelly

Spermicides

- Failure rates 0–50% for typical users
- Cost
- Nonoxynol-9 destroys sperm cell membrane
- OTC
- Can be used as a 'back-up method' along with a barrier contraceptive
- Allergy
- Failing to wait long enough after inserted
- Using too little

10. Ans. c. OCPs *Ref: Shaw's Textbook of Gynecology 15/e p416*

Endometrial carcinoma

Risk factors

- **Mnemonic—Family Has OLD AUNTI**
- Family—Family history
- Has—Hypertension, Heriditary HNPCC

- O—Obesity
- L—Late menopause/early menarche
- D—Diabetes
- A—Atypical endometrial hyperplasia
- U—Unopposed estrogen/increased estrogen—HRT, fibroid, PCOD, feminizing ovarian tumors
- N—Nulliparity
- T—Therapy—tamoxifen, radiation
- I—H/O infertility/menstrual irregularity

Protective factors

- OCPs—E + P
- Smoking—as it decreases the levels of estrogen, decreases wt and asso with early age of menopause OCP disease risk

Cervical cancer—relative risk 2–4 times Ovarian cancer—50% reduction in risk Endometrial cancer—40% reduction in risk

11. Ans. a. Bacterial vaginosis *Ref: Shaw's Textbook of Gynecology 15/e p131*

Repeat question—Refer to JIPMER 2014 Q2.

12. Ans. a. Testicular feminization syndrome *Ref: Dutta's Textbook of Gynecology 5/e p546*

Refer to Q2 of JIPMER 2012 paper

13. Ans. a. androgen insensitivity syndrome *Ref: Dutta's Textbook of Gynecology 5/e p424*

Amenorrhea

HYPER gonadotropic (FSG>40 miU/ml)	Abnormal sex chromosome	Turner's syndrome, Abnormal X chromosome
	Normal sex chromosomes	46XX pure gonadal dysgenesis 46XY gonadal dysgenesis-Swyer's syndrome, testicular feminizing syndrome Ovarian failure (Savage syndrome)
Eugonadotropic	Absence of Mullerian development	Androgen insensitivity syndrome (testicular feminization) Mullerian agenesis: absence of uterus/vagina Rokitansky-Kuster-Hauser syndrome
	Normal Mullerian development	Female or true intersex, PCOD, adrenal or thyroid disorders, TB endometritis
	Cryptomenorrhea	Imperforate hymen, vaginal septum
Hypogonadotropic	Hypothalamic	Delayed puberty, obesity, Kallman's syndrome, weight loss, malnutrition, anorexia nervosa
	Pituitary	Short stature, obesity, genital dystrophy, mental retardation, polydactyly, retinitis pigmentosa
		Neoplasms: Prolactinomas, craniopharyngiomas, adenomas, empty sella turicica Hypoituitary states: Simmond's disease, Chiari-Frommel syndrome, firbes Al bright syndrome, pineal gland tumor, Laurence-Moon Biedl syndrome
	Systemic diseases	Tuberculosis, syphilis
	Endocrinal	Adrenal or thyroid disorders

Note: Though all the four given options can cause primary amenorrhea, PCOD usually causes secondary amenorrhea than primary amenorrhea

Easy way to remember the causes of primary amenorrhea

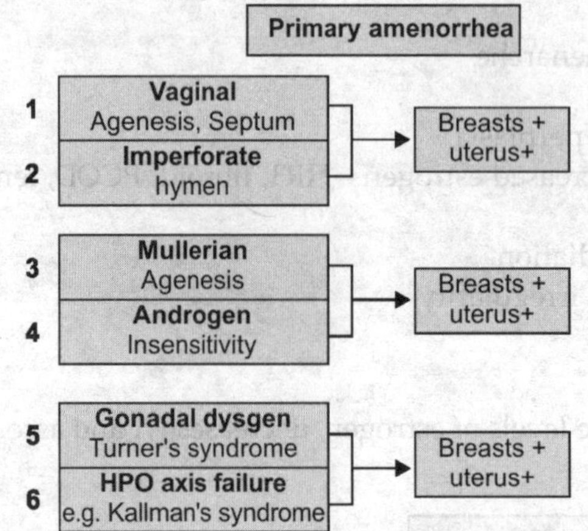

Testicular feminizing syndrome (Androgen Insensitivity syndrome)

Etiology:

In this condition, there is a defect at the testosterone receptor level. The fetal karyotype is 46XY and has a testis. The testis produces testosterone and MIF (Mullerian inhibiting factor), which causes the growth of the wolffian structures and the regression of the mullerian structures.

But in AIS, since there is a problem at the receptor level, the testosterone produced is unable to bind to the wolffian structures to cause the male internal organs to develop and the MIF binds to the mullerian structures causing it to regress, hence no internal structures develop (NO uterus) and the external genitalia is that os a female and patient presents with primary amenorrhea and O/E—there is only a blind vagina (Phenotypically Female)

Breast–present Uterus–absent	Mullerian agenesis 46 XX	Androgen insensitivity 46 XY
Uterus absent due to	Idiopathic causes	MIF
Gonads are	Ovaries	Testes
Pubic hair	Present	Absent
Testosterone levels	Female	Male
Treatment	No hormones Create vagina for sexual function IVF–Surrogacy	Estrogen replacement Create vagina Remove testes Donor oocyte-surrogacy

14. Ans. A. Malignant ovarian tumor *Ref: TeLinde's 9/e p461, 596*

DUB

Anovulatory (80%)	Ovulatory (20%)
• Puberty menorrhagia (Threshold bleeding) • Metropathia hemorrhagica • Premenopausal menorrhagia	• Irregular ripening • Irregular shedding **(Halban's disease)**–due to persistent corpus luteum • Following IUCD insertion and sterilization operation

15. Ans. d. Choriocarcinoma *Ref: Dutta's Textbook of Gynecology 5/e p328*

Sentinel lymph node—is the first lymphnode to receive drainage from malignancy.

When isosulfan blue dye or radiolabelled dye is injected into the tumor, the 1st node that receives the lymphatic drainage, called the sentinel node, can be identified intra operatively.

If the biopsy of this node is negative on frozen section, a full lymphadenectomy can be omitted, there by reducing morbidity.

Usefulness if this procedure is being evaluated

Sentinel node for Ca cervix—paracervical/ureteric LN

Contd...

Sentinel node for Ca vulva—inguinal node
Sentinel node for Ca breast—axillary LN

16. Ans. c. HPV 16 *Ref: Dutta's Textbook of Gynecology 5/e p312*

- 'Only certains type of HPV counts for about 90% of high-grade intraepithelial lesions and cancer (HPV-16, 18, 31, 33, 35, 39, 45, 51, 52, 56 and 58). Type 16 is the most common HPV found in invasive cancer and in CIN2 and 3 and it is found in 47% of women with cancer in these stages.'
- 'Unfortunately, HPV-16 is not very specific, it can be found in 16% of women with low grade lesions and in upto 14% of women with normal cytology.'
- 'HPV-18 is found in 23% of women with invasive cancers, 5% of women with CIN2 and CIN3, 5% of women with HPV and CIN1 and fewer than 2% of patients with negative finding.'
- 'Therefore, HPV-18 is more specific than HPV-16 for invasive tumors.'

Hence,
Most common HPV subtype causing Ca Cervix—HPV 16
Most specific HPV subtype causing Ca Cervix—HPV 18

17. Ans. b. Erythromycin *Ref: Dutta's Textbook of Gynecology 5/e p146, Lakshmi Seshadri 1/e p174*

Treatment of Chlamydia trachomatis–of the urogenital infections
DOC—Azithromycin 1g single dose OR Doxycycline 100 mg BD for 7 days
In pregnancy:
Erythromycin 500 mg QID for 7 days OR Tablet with Amoxycillin base

18. Ans. c. 5 years *Ref: Dutta's Textbook of Gynecology 5/e p538, 539, 543*

LNG containing IUCD

Device	Content of progesterone (LNG)	Amount of release/day	Life span
Progestasert	38 mg	65 mcg	1 year
Levonova	60 mg	20 mcg	5 years
Mirena	52 mg	20 mcg	5 years

19. Ans. d. Pelvic floor repair

Ref: Dutta's Textbook of Gynecology, 5/e p211 & Shaw's Textbook of Gynecology, 15/e p338

Anterior colporrhaphy and colpoperineorrhaphy is known as **pelvic floor repair**

Components of Ward-May Surgery

- Anterior colporrhaphy
- Colpoperineorrhaphy
- Vaginal hysterectomy

Fothergill's Repair/Manchester Repair

- Anterior colporrhaphy
- Amputation of cervix
- Suturing cut ends of Meckendrodt's ligaments in front of cervix
- Covering the raw area on amputated cervix with vaginal mucosa
- Colpoperiniorrhaphy

Shirodkar's Repair (Modified Forthergill's Repair):

- No cervical amputation
- POD is opened
- Uterosacral ligaments identified and divided close to cervix and the stumps are crossed and situated together in front of cervix
- High closure of POD

20. Ans. a. PCOD *Ref: Shaw's Textbook of Gynecology, 15/e p115*

- Ovarian causes of hirsutism:
  - PCOD
  - Hyperthecosis
  - Masculinizing ovarian tumor

- Arrhenoblastoma
- Hilus cell tumor

Causes of Hirsutism

- Genetic and ethnic
- **Excess androgen or increased sensitivity of the pilosebaceous unit** to testosterone
- Liver disease when the level of SHBG level drops
- Ovarian
  - PCOD (polycystic ovarian disease)
  - Hyperthecosis
  - Masculinizing ovarian tumors, e.g. arrhenoblastoma
  - Hilus cell tumor
- **Adrenal**
  - Congenital adrenal hyperplasia
  - Cushing's syndrome
  - Adrenal tumor (1–2% cases)
- **Drugs**
  - Androgens
  - Progestogens with androgenic effect
  - Levonorgestrel
  - Anabolic steroids
  - Phenytoin
  - Danazol
  - Minoxidil
- **Others**
  - Obesity
  - Hypothyroidism
  - Anovulatory hypo-oestrogenism
  - Idiopathic—15%
  - Hyperprolactinemia
- Hirsutism occurs early in CAS, around puberty in PCOD and at menopause.

21. Ans. c. Irregular bleeding *Ref: Shaw's Textbook of Gynecology, 15/e p233*

Irregular bleeding per vaginum is the most common side effect of POP (20%)

Advantages with minipill are:

- No increase in
  - Coagulability
  - Glucose tolerance
  - B.P.
  - Cardiovascular complications
- Do not interfere with lactation

Disadvantages with minipill are:

- High failure rate (2–3/100 WY)
- Irregular bleeding (20%)
- Functional ovarian cysts
- Weight gain
- Depression

22. Ans. b. It has diploid karyotype

Ref: Shaw's Textbook of Gynecology, 15/e p253 and Novak's Textbook of Gynecology, 14/e p1585

Refer text for the comparison table

23. Ans. a. Spiramycin *Ref: Textbook of Obstetrics by DC Dutta, 7/e p297*

Treatment of choice for toxoplasmosis during pregnancy:

- **Spiramycin 3 g/day**
- **Pyrimethamine 25 mg+sulphadiazine** 1 g QID for 4–6 weeks

- Pyrimethamine is not given in 1st trimester
- Mode of infection: eating raw, uncooked meat/through cat feces/through placenta
- Effects on baby:
  - Hydrocephalus
  - Chorioretinitis
  - Cerebral calcifications
  - Microcephaly
  - Mental retardation

24. Ans. d. Secreted by theca cells *Ref: Shaw's Textbook of Gynecology, 15/e p46, 47*

Function of estrogens in menstrual cycle
- **Produces proliferative changes** in the **endometrium**
- **Secretes inhibin** and **inhibits FSH production** by anterior pituitary
- The **maximum peak of estrogen** secretion is seen about 48 hours before ovulation
- Whereas **LH peak** occurs 24–36 hours before ovulation
- FSH → Granulosa cells → Estrogen
- LH → Theca cells → Progesterone

25. Ans. a. Reduces fertility after removal *Ref: Shaw's Textbook of Gynecology, 15/e p46, 47*
- There is no evidence of reduced fertility following removal of IUCD

Complications of IUCD are:
- Expulsion
- Perforation
- Vaginal infection: Actinomycosis, PID
- Menorrhagia, dysmenorrhea
- Ectopic pregnancy
- Pregnancy 1–3/100 W.Y.

26. Ans. b. Mullerian agenesis *Ref: Shaw's Textbook of Gynecology, 15/e p290, Fig. 21.8*
Refer to Q7 of JIPMER 2013 for explanation

27. Ans. d. Oestrogen excess
Ref: Novak's Text book of Gynecology, 14/e p1463 and Shaw's Textbook of Gynecology, 15/e p422

Endometrioid carcinoma:
- It constitutes 6–8% of epithelial ovarian tumors
- Endometroid ovarian cancer is associated with 15–20% of cases of endometrial cancer

Risk factors for ovarian cancer are:
- Age 45–60 years
- Nulliparity/Low parity
- H/o PCOD
- Tamoxifen therapy, prolonged HRT
- Late menopauses
- High-calorie, high-fat diet
- BRCA 1, BRCA 2 genes
- Breast and genital ca
- HPV is associated with cervical cancer but not with ovarian cancer
- The malignant change in endometriosis is rare and manifests as endometriod cancer
- Malignant changes are not reported in adenomyosis
- Oral contraceptives reduce the risk of epithelial ovarian cancer
- Hence, estrogen excess could be the best option in this question

28. Ans. a. Ca Cervix *Ref: Shaw's Textbook of Gynecology, 15/e p231*

Noncontraceptive benefits of OCPs are:

- Protection against
  - Ovarian cancer
  - Uterine cancer
  - Benign breast neoplasia
  - Anorectal cancer
- Reduces the incidence of
  - PID
  - Ectopic pregnancy
  - PCOD
  - Endometriosis
- Protects against **rheumatoid arthritis**
  - Prolonged use of OCPs (more than 8 years) is associated with risk of endocervical cancer
  - The role of OCP in breast cancer is controversial. But lately evidence-based data fail to prove its adverse role on breast disease
  - Both options a and d are correct
  - But as the role of OCP in breast cancer is still controversial, option a can be taken as the relatively better option.

29. Ans. a. Internal os *Ref: Shaw's textbook of gynecology, 15/e p8*

Normal position of the uterus

Anteversion and Anteflexion

- The body of the uterus is bent forwards on the cervix at the level of the internal os
- The forward inclination of the body of the uterus on the cervix constitutes anteflexion
- In antversion-external os is directed downwards and backwards, the anterior lip of cervix is first felt on P/V
- In retroversion-external os is directed downwards and forwards, the posterior lip of the cervix is first felt on P/V

30. Ans. b. Androgen binding protein *Ref: Ganong's Review of Medical Physiology 22/e p424–425*

Testes has 2 types of cells:

- **Leydig cells:** produce testosterone, insulin-like factor 3 and estradiol
- **Sertoli cells:** inhibin B, anti Mullerian hormone and androgen-binding protein

Androgen binding protein (ABP)

- binds to the testosterone and dihydrotestosterone
- makes them less lipophilic and become concentrated within the luminal fluid of the seminiferous tubules
- has the same aminoacid sequence as the sex hormone binding globulin (SHBG)
- ABP's production is regulated under influence of FSH on sertoli cells.

31. Ans. a. Vaginal Ca *Ref: Shaw's Textbook of Gynecology, 15/e p52*

Transplacental carcinogenesis is the possibility of development of vaginal carcinoma (clear cell adenocarcinoma) seen in younger females who were exposed to diethyl stilbesterol (DES) in utero.

32. Ans. d. Dysgerminoma *Ref. Shaw's textbook of gynecology, 15/e p52*

Tumor Markers

Epithelial ovarian tumors	Serous	CA-125
	Mucinous	CA 19–9, CEA
	Serous and mucinous	OCCA, OCA
Germ cell tumors	Endodermal sinus/yolk sac tumor	AFP
	Chorioca	HCG
	Dysgerminoma	LDH, PLAP
	Teratoma	Nil
SCST	Granulosa cell tumor	Inhibin

- Very High Yield Table for Exam

33. Ans. b. 2 : 1 *Ref: Shaw's Textbook of Gynecology, 15/e p8*

Relationship between the length of cervix and the body of uterus:
- Before puberty—2 : 1
- After puberty—1 : 2
- During reproductive period—1 : 3

34. Ans. d. Levonorgestrel IUCD *Ref: Shaw's Textbook of Gynecology, 15/e p230*

- Levonorgestrel IUCD is progesterone impregnated IUCD and is recommended to control bleeding in menorrhagia

Other noncontraceptive benefits of LNG IUCD:
- DUB
- Endometrial hyperplasia

Intrauterine contraceptive devices (IUCD)
Biologically inert devices: Lippe's loop
Copper-containing devices: Copper T
Hormonal IUCDs: Progestasert, Levonova, MIRENA
Hormonal IUCDs
Also refer to Q12 of 2013 JIPMER Paper

35. Ans. b. Bacterial vaginosis *Ref: Shaw's Textbook of Gynecology, 15/e p131*

Repeat Question

36. Ans. a. Mifepristone *Ref: Shaw's Textbook of Gynecology, 15/e p237*

Mifepristone (RU 486)
- It is an anti-progesterone which blocks the action of progesterone on the endometrium and causes sloughing and shedding of the deciduas
- Failure rate—0.9%

Other drugs that can be given for emergency contraception:
- **Yuzpe regime:** ethinyl estradiol 0.1 mg+dl—norgestrel 1 mg X 2 doses 12 hours apart starting within 72 hours of unprotected intercourse
- **Levonorgestrol 0.75 mg X 2 doses 12 hours apart or 1.5 mg single dose**
- **IUCD** with 5 days of intercourse.

37. Ans. b. Ca endometrium *Ref: Shaw's Textbook of Gynecology, 15/e p232*

- CA endometrium is the right option
- **Combined OC pills** reduce the incidence of ovarian cancer by 40% and uterine cancer by 50% if taken for 1 year. Risk of anorectal cancer is reduced by 30–40%
- Regarding breast cancer, the role of combined pills is still controversial. Some studies reported that women who took combined pills for more than 4 years are at risk of breast cancer. But the risk disappears after 10 years of stopping the drug. But, lately evidence based data fail to prove the adverse role of pills on breast cancer
- Regarding cervical cancer, risk of endocervical cancer has been reported in women who used combined pills for more than 5 years

Benefits of combined OC pills:
- Menorrhagia
- Polymenorrhea
- Dysmenorrheal
- Premenstrual tension
- Benign breast neoplasia
- Functional ovarian cysts
- PID
- Rheumatoid arthritis
- Acne
- PCOD

- Endometriosis
- Ovarian cancer
- Anorectal cancer

38. Ans. d. Minipill *Ref: Shaw's Textbook of Gynecology, 15/e p233*

- Minipill (progesterone only pill) is the right option
- Monophasic, biphasic and triphasic pills are all varieties of combined pills. Combined pills suppress lactation and, therefore, not recommended during lactation

Advantages of minipills:

- Lactation women
- Women over 35 years and smokers
- Those with migraine
- Diabetic women
- Hypertensive women
- Sickle cell anemia
- Those who are intolerant to estrogen or in whom estrogen is contraindicated.

39. Ans. b. Congestive dysmenorrhea *Ref: Shaw's Textbook of Gynecology, 15/edition*

- **Congestive dysmenorrhoea** presents as pelvic pain a few days before menses begins. After the onset of menses, patient is relieved of pain
- Causes: PID, pelvic endometriosis, fibroids
- **Spasmodic dysmenorrhoea** presents as cramping pain most pronounced on the first and second day of menses
- Primary dysmenorrhoea is the one which is not associated with any pelvic pathology. Occurs due to the prostaglandins released by progesterone in the endometrium

40. Ans. d. Clear cell *Ref: Novak's Gynecology, 14/e p1359*

The following cases have poor prognosis in endometrial cancer and required pelvic and paraaortic lymph node dissection during surgery.

- Tumor histology clear cell, serous, squamous, or grade 2–3 endometrioid
- Myometrial invasion ?1/2
- Isthmus-cervix extension
- Tumor size >2 cm
- Extrauterine disease

41. Ans. a. Mackendrot's ligament *Ref: Shaw's Textbook of Gynecology, 15/e p18*

Supports of uterus are triradiate condensation of endo pelvic fascia:

- **Anterior** spoke—**Pubocervical** ligament
- **Lateral** spoke—**Mackenrodt** ligament
- **Posterior** spoke—**Uterosacral** ligament

Supports of the Genital Tract

DeLancey's three-level systems of support
• Level I—Uterosacral and cardinal ligaments support the uterus and vaginal vault
• Level II—Pelvic fascias and paracolpos which connects the vagina to the white line on the lateral pelvic wall through arcus tendineus
• Level III—Levator ani muscle supports the lower one-third of vagina

42. Ans. a. Alpha fetoprotein *Ref: Robbins Pathologic Basis of Disease, 8/edition*

Endodermal Sinus (Yolk Sac) Tumor

- This tumor is rare but is the **second most common malignant tumor of germ cell origin**
- Derived from differentiation of malignant germ cells along the extra-embryonic yolk sac lineage
- Similar to the normal yolk sac, the tumor is rich in α1-antitrypsin
- Its characteristic histologic feature is a glomerulus-like structure composed of a central blood vessel enveloped by germ cells within a space lined by germ cells (Schiller-Duval body) Conspicuous intracellular and extracellular hyaline droplets are present in all tumors, and some of these stain for αfetoprotein by immunoperoxidase techniques.

- Most patients are children or young women presenting with abdominal pain and a rapidly developing pelvic mass
- The tumors usually appear to involve a single ovary but grow rapidly and aggressively
- These tumors were once almost uniformly fatal within 2 years of diagnosis, but combination chemotherapy has measurably improved the outcome

43. Ans. a. Clear cell carcinoma *Ref: Robbins Pathologic Basis of Disease, 8/edition*

Vaginal adenosis

- It is a **remnant of embryonal columnar, endocerivcal-type epithelium**
- During emboryonal development this epithelium extends from the endocervix and covers the extocervix and upper vagina
- It is replaced by the squamous epithelium advancing upwardly from the urogenital sinus
- Small patches of unreplaced glandular epithelium my persist focally into adult life
- Adenosis presents clinically as red, granular areas contrasting with the normal pale-pink vaginal mucosa
- On microscopic examination, adenosis consists of columnar mucinous epithelium indistinguishable from endocervical epithelium
- Adenosis, while normally present in a small percentage of adult women
- It has been reported in 35% to 90% of women exposed to DES in utero
- Rare cases of clear cell carcinoma arising in DES-related adenosis were recorded in teens and young women, resulting in discontinuation of DES treatment

44. Ans. a. Estrogen *Ref: Robbins Pathologic Basis of Disease, 8/edition*

Fibrocystic breast disease

- Aka nonproliferative breast changes/fibrocystic changes/fibrocystic breast
- Affects 30–60% of women and at least 50% of women of childbearing age
- These lesions are termed nonproliferative to distinguish them from "proliferative" changes, which are associated with an increased risk of breast cancer.

Etiopathogenesis

- Not fully understood
- Related to hormone levels, as lesions subside after menopause
- There are also cyclical symptoms in relation to menstrual cycle
- The most important of these hormones are estrogen, prolactin and progesterone
- These hormones directly affect the breast tissues by causing cells to grow and multiply

Histopathology

There are three principal morphologic changes:

- Cystic change, often with apocrine metaplasia
- Fibrosis
- Adenosis

45. Ans. a. Mucinous cystadenoma ovary *Ref: Shaw's Textbook of Gynecology, 15/e p375*

Mucinous Tumors of Ovary

- Multiloculated cyst lined by **columnar epithelium**
- Cut surface shows multilocular and **honeycomb appearance**
- Can grow to large size 5 to 10 kgs, pedunculated
- Usually unilateral (Bilateral in 5% cases)
- Usually benign (5 to 10% malignant)
- Bilateral—metastasis from GI tract, mucocele of appendix, primary adenoca appendix
- In women 30 to 60 years
- Has a glistening surface
- If tumor ruptures it may lead to formation of pseudomyxome peritonei and vicera show extensive adhesions
- Appendicectomy prevents this condition as mucocele of appendix often causes this complication

46. Ans. b. Isthmus *Ref: Dutta's Textbook of Obstetrics, 7/e p554*

- Most ideal site for tubectomy consists mainly of **isthmus** and **ampullary part of tube** [Proximal and middle 3rd]

Other MCQ Points

- M/C used method—pomeroy
- Irreversible methods—irving and fimbriectomy
- Good potential for reversibility—Pomeroy and Uchida
- Asso with ectopic—Madlener

  Best chances for reversibility in recanalization is seen in:
  - Isthmo- isthmic type
  - Laparoscopic clips (best)
  - yoon falope ring/band
  - Pomeroy and Uchida methods

47. Ans. c. Ampulla *Ref: Dutta's Textbook of Obstetrics, 7/e p21, 22*

Fertilisation

- Process of fusion of sperm with ovum forming zygote
- Fertilization occurs in the ampullary end of the tube
- Complete dissolution of **corona radiate** occurs by chemical action of **hyaluronidase** liberated from **acrosomal cap** of hundreds of **sperm** present at the site

48. Ans. d. Tranexamic acid *Ref: Dutta's Textbook of Obstetrics, 7/e p540*

- The excessive bleeding after IUCD insertion involves increased menstrual blood loss, prolongation of duration of periods, intermenstrual bleeding
- Tranexamic acid may be given for short term relief

Adverse Effects or Complications from IUDs

- Cramping
- Displaced threads
- Ectopic pregnancy
- Embedment or fragmentation of IUD
- Expulsion
- Infertility
- Pelvic infections
- Septicemia during pregnancy
- Tubo-ovarian damage
- Uterine or cervical perforation
- Vaginal bleeding, with or without anemia
- Vasovagal reaction (on insertion)

49. Ans. a. Hilus cell tumor *Ref: Shaw's Textbook of Gynecology, 15/e p367*

- **Hilus cell (similar to leydig cells) tumor** is a **virilising mesenchymoma**
- Clear cell is otherwise mesonephroid tumor of epithelial origin
- **Transitional cell Ca** includes **benign and malignant Brenner tumor**

Refer to table in the text

50. Ans. c. Dermoid tumor *Ref: Dutta's Textbook of Obstetrics, 7/e p310*

Dermoid Tumor in Pregnancy

- Incidence—1 in 2000
- Incidence of dermoid cyst increased two folds in pregnancy
- **Effects of tumor:**
  - Retention of urine
  - Malpresentation
  - Mechanical distress
  - Non engagement of head

- Effects on tumor:
  - Torsion
  - Hemorrhage
  - Rupture
  - Infection
- Diagnosis-abdominal examination to detect swelling
- Vaginal examination-**Hingorani Sign**—a groove felt in between uterus and tumor
- Investigations—**USG**
- Treatment-surgery best **14 to 16 weeks** if umcomplicated
- If complicated, surgery is performed irrespective of gestation

51. Ans. a. LDH *Ref: Dutta Textbook of Gynecology 5/e p367*

Dysgerminoma

- Most common **malignant germ cell tumor**
- Arises from undifferentiated form of germ cells
- Majority occurs before 30 years
- HCG assays are positive
- 20 to 30% occurs in pregnancy
- May be associated with endodermal sinus tumor or choriocarcinoma
- 5 to 15 cm diameter
- Micro—Uniform large round cells
- Treatment—Laparotomy, surgical staging and unilateral salpingooopherectomy [for stage 1] with chemotherapy
- Chemotherapy—Carboplatin, BEP, VBP, VAC regimens [bleomycin, etoposide, cisplatin, vinblastine, actinomycind, cyclophosphamide]
- Combination chemotherapy for recurrent disease—POMB-ACE [Vincristine, Bleomycin, Methotrexate, Cisplatin, Etoposide, Actinomycin D, Cyclophosphamide]
- Tumor markers—HCG, AFP,LDH

52. Ans. a. Decreased libido *Ref: Bailey and Love's Short Practice of Surgery 25/edition*

Sterilization	Tubectomy	Vasectomy
Removal of	Portion of the tube	Portion of the vas deferens
Performed in	Operation theatre	Office procedure
Anaesthesia	Regional/GA	Local
Failure rate	1 in 200	1 in 500
Success criteria	None	Azzospermia after 12 ejaculations
Complications	None	Antisperm antibodies, sperm granuloma, local infection

53. Ans. c. Obstructed labour *Ref: DC Dutta's Textbook of Gynecology 6/e p401*

Vesicovaginal Fistula

- **MC type** of genitor urinary fistula
- **Causes**

A. Obstetrcal:

- Accounts for **80% cases of VVF in developing countries**
- 5–15% cases in developed countries
- VVF may result from
  - **Ischemia**
    - Obstructed labour: Ischaemic necrosis of the bladder base following prolonged compression of the bladder base between fetal head and pubic symphysis—infection-sloughig-fistula
    - **Take 3–5 days following delivery to roduce ischaemic fistula**
    - MC in developing countries

- **Traumatic**
  - Instrumental vaginal delivery
    - Forceps-specially with Kielland's forceps
    - Destructive operations
    - Instruments used for craniotomy procedure-perforators and carniocalsts
    - Injury may be inflicted by bony spicule of fetal skull
  - Abdominal surgeries
    - Hysterectomy for rupture uterus
    - LSCS
    - **Traumatic injuries manifest soon after delivery**

B. Gynecological causes:

- Accounts for 80% fistulas in developed countries
- MC type of VVF in developed countries
- Casues
  - Operative injury-anterior colporrhapy, TAH
  - Traumatic-illegal abortions, pelvic fractures
  - Advanced malignancies of genital tract organs
  - **Radiation therapy** for Ca cervix
    - Instrumental
    - Due to end arteritis obliterans
    - Takes long time to develop—1–2 years
  - Infective—vaginal TB, LGV, Schistosomiasis, Actinomycosis
  - **Ureterovaginal fistula**
    - **2nd common cause** of urinary fistula
    - MC site of injury to ureter
      - In hysterectomies-ureteric tunnel in mackenrodt's ligament
      - In radical surgery for Ca cervix-near crossing of pubocervical ligament

54. Ans. a. Bacterial vaginosis *Ref: Shaw's Textbook of Gynecology, 15/e p131*

Repeat question

55. Ans. a. Stage IIA *Ref: Shaw's Textbook of Gynecology p412*

Refer text

56. Ans. a. Endodermal sinus tumor *Ref: Dutta's Textbook of Obstetrics, 7/e p368*

- **Schiller duval bodies** are characteristic histological feature of **endodermal sinus tumor**
- They are tuft of vascular tissue inside cystic spaces lined by flattended epithelium.

Endodermal Sinus Tumor

- Originate from multipotential embryonal tissue as a result of selective differention of yolk sac structures
- Peak—15 to 20 years of age
- Second most common malignant germ cell tumor of ovary
- Unilateral, solid >10 cm diameter
- Micro-schiller duval bodies, eosinophilic hyaline bodies containing alphaprotein
- Associated with dysgerminoma
- Treatment—surgical staging and unilateral salpingo oopherectomy
- Combination chemotherapy-POMB-ACE regimen (cyclophosphamide, vincristine, methotrexate, bleomycin, actinomycin D, cisplatin, etoposide (VAC regimen, VBP regimen
- Tumor marker—alphafetoprotein >20 microgm/ml, elevated alpha 1 antitrypsin
- Respond well to chemotherapy and good survival rate

57. Ans. d. Primary vaginal carcinoma *Ref: Dutta's Textbook of Obstetrics, 7/e p325*

Primary Vaginal Carcinoma

- Incidence very rare 0.6 per 100000 women [1% of genital malignancies]
- Etiology:

- HPV
- VAIM [vaginal intraepithelial neoplasia]
- Diethyl stilboesterol
- Irradiation
- Pessary usage
- White race

• **Upper 3rd** of vaginal **posterior** wall
• **MC-Squamous cell Ca 90%,** adenoca, melanoma, sarcoma
• **Spread-lymphatic, direct and blood borne**
• C/f-abnormal vaginal bleeding, foul smelling discharge
• Investigations-cytolgy, colposcopy, biopsy
• Treatment-surgery and radiotherapy

Secondary Vaginal Ca

• Follows Ca of cervix, vulva, urethra by direct spread
• Metastasis in **lower 3rd vagina** or **vault** occurs in choriocarcinoma or endometrial Ca
• Commoner than primary Ca

58. Ans. d. Ca cervix *Ref: Shaw's Textbook of gynecology 15/e p232*

Infact, OCPs are associated with increased risk of endocervical cancer

OCPS and malignancy

• **Combined OC pills** reduce the incidence of **ovarian cancer** by **40%** and **uterine cancer** by 50% if taken for 1 year
• **Risk of** colonic **and** anorectal **cancer is reduced by 30–40%**
• Regarding breast cancer, the role of combined pills is still controversial. Some studies reported that women who took combined pills for more than 4 years are at risk of breast cancer. But the risk disappears after 10 years of stopping the drug. But, lately evidence based data fail to prove the adverse role of pills on breast cancer.
• Regarding cervical cancer, risk of endocervical cancer is increased has been reported in women who used combined pills for more than 5 years
• OCPs are also associated with Hepatocellular Carcinoma

59. Ans. c. Asherman's syndrome *Ref: Dutta's Gynecology p433*

Asherman's syndrome or fritsch syndrome

• It is characterized by **adhesions** and **fibrosis** of the **endometrium**
• Most often associated with **dilation** and **curettage** of the **intrauterine cavity**
• Patients present with **secondary amenorrhea.**

60. Ans. a. Chlamydia trachomatis *Ref: DC Dutta's Textbook of Gynecology 6/e p144*

• **Chlamydial** and **gonococcal infections** are the most common infections that cause **vulvovaginitis and urethritis**
• **Chlamydia** affects the **columnar and transitional epithelium** of the genitourinary tract
• **Chlamydia** causes
  - Urethritis
  - Bartholinitis
  - Cervicitis
  - Endometritis
  - Salpingitis
  - Perihepatitis
• **Tubal scarring** caused by **Chlamydia results** in infertility and ectopic pregnancy
• **Fitz-Hugh-Curtis syndrome-perihepatitis** caused by **Chlamyda trachomatis** (violin string adhesions)

61. Ans. a. Pressure necrosis of urethra during obstructed labor

Ref: DC Dutta's Textbook of Gynecology 6/e p401
Ref: 2010 Obsterics and Gynaecology question explanation

62. Ans. d. Estrogen/progesterone *Ref: DC Dutta's Textbook of Gynecology 6/e p401*

Hypergonadotropic hypogonadism

Causes

- **Primary ovarian failure/premature ovarian failure**
  - Ovarian failure before 40 years
  - Failure of germ cell migration or accelerated germ cell deplation
  - Causes
    - Genetic turner's
    - Gonadal dysgenesis
    - Autoimmune disorders
    - Infections: mumps, TB
    - Latrogenic: RT, Chemotherapy
    - Metabolic: galactosemia (follicles destroyed by toxic effects of galactose)
- **Resistant ovarian syndrome**
  - FSH receptor defect or absence (savage syndrome)
  - Follicles are present

Diagnosis

- History of amenorrhea in <35 years
- **Increased FSH levels**
- **Decreased E2 levels**
- Karyotyping abnormality (Turner's)
- Organ specific Ab (anti-thyroid Ab most common)
- Ovarian biopsy
  - Autoimmune disorders-perifollicular infiltration
  - Premature ovarian failure—follicles are absent
  - Resistant ovarian syndrome—follicles are present (FSH rec. defect)
  - Menopausal symptoms

Management:

- **HRT**
  - To prevent/minimize post menopausal symptoms
  - Prevention of osteoporosis
  - Specific group of women for prescription of HRT
    - Premature ovarian failure
    - Gonadal dysgenesis
    - Surgical or radiation menopause
  - **Preparations for HRT**
    - Estrogen + Progesterone combination
    - Estrogen: conjugated estrogen/micronized estradiol
    - Progestins: mpa/micronized p/dydrogesterone

63. Ans. a. Endometriosis *Ref: DC Dutta's Textbook of Gynecology 6/e p293*

Refer to text

64. Ans. a. Uterosacral ligament *Ref: DC Dutta's Textbook of Gynecology 6/e p192*

Support of Uterus

- Condensation of endopelvic fascia-triradiate ligament-at pericervical ring
  - Mackenrodt's or cardinal ligaments or transcervical ligament—lateral spoke
  - Uterosacral ligament—posterior spoke
  - Pubocervical ligament—anterior spoke (least developed)
  - The above three ligaments have string of Hammock arrangement and prevents uterine descent

65. Ans. a. Cervicopexy

Ref: DC Dutta's Textbook of Gynecology 5/e p211; Shaw's Textbook of Gynecology 15/e p338

Surgeries for prolapse

- **Ward-Mayo's operation**
  - Women >40 years
  - Completed family
  - Not desirous or retaining menstruation
- **Components of Ward-Mayo surgery**
  - Anterior colporraphy
  - Colpoperineorraphy
  - Vaginal hysterectomy
  - Anterior colporraphy and colpoperineorraphy is known as pelvic floor repair
- **Manchester/Fothergill's operation**
  - Women <40 years
  - Completed family
  - Desirous of retaining menstrual function
- **Fothergill's repair/Manchester repair**
  - Anterior colporraphy
  - Amputation of cervix
  - Suturing cut ends of Meckendrodt's ligaments in front of cervix
  - Covering the raw area on amputated cervix with vaginal mucosa
  - Colpoperineorraphy
- **Shirodkar's repair (modified Fothergill's repair)**
  - No cervical amputation
  - POD is opened
  - Uterosacral ligaments identified and divided close to cervix and the stumps are crossed and situated together in front of cervix
  - High closure of POD
- **Abdominal sling surgery (cervicopexy)**
  - Young women
  - Nulliparous prolapsed
  - Desirous of retaining child bearing function
    - Shirodkar's sling-to anterior longitudinal ligament of sacrum
    - Khanna's sling-to ASIS
    - Purandrare's sling-to rectus sheath
- **Lefort's repair**
  - Very elderly post menopausal bedridden patients
  - Approximation of anterior and posterior vaginal flaps with two channels in vagina for drainage
- **Pregnancy with prolapse**
- Pessary inserted
- Surgery 3–4 months after delivery

66. **Ans. b. Pomeroy's** *Ref: DC Dutta's Textbook of Gynecology 6/e p476*

Tubectomy methods

a. **Abdominal Methods**
   1. **Conventional laparotomy**—abdominal incision 3–5 cms
   2. **Minilaparotomy**—abdominal incision 2–2.5 cms

- Techniques
  - **Modified Pomeroy's**
    - Recommended by Govt. of India
    - Most common method
    - 1–1.5 cms tube excised
    - Isthmus portion of tube
    - No. 1–0 chapter. Catgut used for ligation of tube

  - Advance:
    - Failure rate: 0.1-0.5%
    - Simple procedure
- Parkland method-another commonly employed method with similar success rates
- Other uncommon methods
  - Uchida method
  - Irving's method
  - Madlener method
  - Kroener's method

3. Laparoscopy
- Single/double puncture
- C/I dring Puerpereum
- Fallope ring (silicon rubber with 5% barium sulphate)
- Filshie clip (titanium lined with silicon rubber)
- Hulka-Clemens spring clip
- Electrosurgical method—bipolar cautery preferred over unipolar

b. Vaginal Methods
- Through posterior colpotomy incision
- Hysteroscopic electrocoagulation of tubes
- Essure—4 cms long, 2 mm dm microcoil made of nickel titanium steel alloy containing polyethylene fibers within it
- Tubes blocked permanently by scar tissue growing into the device
- Additional contraceptive method used for first 3 months

67. Ans. b. Gartner's cyst *Ref: Shaw's Textbook of Gynecology 15/e p136*

Vaginal cysts
- Vaginal cysts are rare and are located more commonly in **anterior vaginal wall**
- **Gartner's cyst**
  - Arises from remnants of mesonephric duct
  - Lies in anteriolateral aspect of vaginal wall
  - Small cyst is asymptomatic
  - Large cyst causes dyspareunia
  - Large symptomatic cysts require excision
- **Inclusion cyst**
  - Seen in lower end of vagina on its posterior surface
  - It is casued by tags of mucosa embedding inside the scar that later forms a cyst
- **Bartholin cyst-extends into vagina**
- **Endometriotic cyst**
  - Bluish bulge in posterior fornix
  - It is treated with either danazol or surgical excision

A Nabothian Cyst (or Nabothian Follicle)
- It is a mucus-filled cyst on the surface of the cervix
- They are most often caused when stratified squamous epithelium of the ectocervix grows over the simple columnar epithelium of the endocervix (Metaplasia)
- This tissue growth can block the cervical crypts, trapping cervical mucus inside the crypts.

68. Ans. b. Symptoms of Hypothyroidism *Ref: Shaw's Textbook of Gynecology 15/e p253*

Clinical features of hydatidiform mole
- Most common symptom is **bleeding prior to 16 weeks'** gestation and passage of vesicles from the vagina.
- 3Hs
- Hypertension
- Hyper-thyroidism
- Hyperemesis gravidarum

- Most common sign
  → fundus larger than dates
- Fetal heart tones
  Absence
- Bilateral cystic enlargements of ovary
  → **Theca-lutein cysts**
- Most common site of distant metastasis
  Lungs-dyspnea and hemoptysis present
- Neurological symptoms like hemiplegia, epilepsy, headache and visual disturbances suggest brain metastasis
- On examination, a vaginal metastasis appears as a bluish red vascular tumor which bleeds easily on touch

Ultrasound—'Snowstorm Appearance'

69. Ans. d. Depot provera *Ref: Williams Obstetrics 23/e p652 table 30–4*

In the above options, appropriate choice would be depot provera.

Contraceptive Prescription

- **Conventional contraceptives can be safely prescribed during the entire reproductive period.**
- Advice on the usage of pill or IUCD during different phases of reproductive life

1. Postpartum

- **Contraception for lactation women**
  - **Progestin only pill** to be started at 2–3 weeks postpartum (best choice)
  - Depot **medroxyprogesterone acetate** initiated at **6 weeks postpartum**
  - **Hormonal implants** inserted at **6 weeks postpartum**
  - **POP** contains LNG 75 microgm taken from day of cycle at same time every day-failure rate 0.5–2 per HMY
  - **Deport provera** dose 150 mg every 3 months within 5th day of cycle, administered i.m-failure rate 0–0.3 per HWY
  - **Norplant** contains 75 microgram LNG, releases 50 microgram/day for 3 years-failure rate 0.1 per HWY
  - **LNg-IUD** contains 58 mg LNG releases 20 microgram/day
- **Nonlactating**
  - Contraception started as early as 3 weeks following delivery
  - OCPs/IUCD/DMPA inj./implanon

2. Adolescent girls

- LD OCPs–most effective
- Alternatives-DMPA, Norplant

3. Newly married

- OCPs-most effective

4. Postabortal

- Started immediately following abortion
- OCPs/IUCD

5. Women at risk of STDs

- Need dual protection against pregnancy and STDs
- Condom with spermicides/condom with any other contraceptive method

6. Women using enzyme inducers

- **High-dose OCPs,** if prescribed/IUCD/DMPA inj.

70. Ans. a. Gardenella vaginits *Ref: Dutta's Gynae p156*

Repeat question

71. Ans. d. Levonorgestrel IUCD *Ref: Shaw's Textbook of Gynecology 15/e p230*

Repeat question

72. Ans. b. Intramural *Ref: Shaw's Textbook of Gynecology 15/e p352*

Uterine Fibroids

- Fibroids are the **most common** benign solid tumors in females

- Most common tumor of uterus
- Fibroids are estrogen dependent for growth
- **Progesterone inhibits their growth**
- **GnRH shrinks size of fibroid**
- **Increases in size** during **pregnancy and OCP intake**
- **Decreases** in size after menopause
- The presence of myoma causes hyperplasia of the myometrial wall
- The cavity of the uterus is often distorted and enlarged
- The endometrium tends to be thicker due to endometrial hyperplasia
- The ovaries at times are enlarged, cystic and hyperemic with evidence of salpingoophoritis in about 15% cases
- Distribution of fibroid in the body of uterus:
  - Intramural 75%
  - Submucus 15%
  - Subserous 10%
- Most common site is body of uterus
- A typical myoma is a well-circumscribed tumor with a pseudocapsule
- The vessels which supply blood to the tumor lie in the capsule and send radial branches into the tumor. Because of this arrangement of blood supply, the central portion of the tumor receives the least blood supply, and degeneration is noticable early and most often in this part of the tumor. On the other hand, calcification begins at the periphery and spreads inwards along the vessels

Points to be Remembered in Fibroid

- Most common complication of fibroid during pregnancy red degeneration
- Incidence of sarcomatous change in fibroid—0.5%
- Most common presenting symptom is menorrhagia
- Metrorrhagia is caused by—submucous fibroid
- Most common degeneration-Hyaline degeneration
- Recurrent pregnancy loss is associated with submucous fibroid
- Polycythemia in myoma is due to extramedullary erythropoisis within the substance of myoma
- Danazole, GnRH and RU 486 reduces the size of fibroids

73. Ans. d. Uterus not tender on palpation *Ref: Shaw's Textbook of Gynecology 15/e p474*

Adenomyosis

- Common in women aged 40 years and above
- Often co-exists with fibroid, endometriosis and endometrial cancer
- Uterus is symmetrically enlarged to not more than 14 weeks size
- Histology-islands of endometrial glands surrounded by stroma seen in the myometrial tissue beyond the endomyometrial junction
- The distance b/w basal endometrium and the endometrial gland should be >2.5 mm
- Common complaint-menorrhagia and progressive dysmenorrhoea
- Clinical examination reveals symmetrical enlargement of uterus and tender uterus
- Treatment is localized excision, hysterectomy
- Medical treatment includes danazol, GnRH, Mirena IUCD

74. Ans. b. Complete perineal tear *Ref: DC Dutta's Textbook of Gynecology 6/e p413*

Complete Perineal Tear

- Symptoms
- Inability to hold flatus and faeces
- Soreness over perianal region due to constant iriitation by stool
- Inspite of deficit of perineum, women with CPT do not develop prolapse. This is because of overactivity of levator ani muscles

Etiology of pelvic organ prolapse

- Trauma of vaginal delivery to ligaments, endopelvic fascia, levators and perineal body

- Congenital weakness of upporting structures
- Postmenopausal atrophy
- Increased intraabdominal pressue
  - Chronic cough
  - Constipation
  - Ascitis
  - Mass abdomen
- Heavy work—weightlifting
- Obesity

75. Ans. a. 10 mm Graafian follicles on USG *Ref: DC Dutta's Textbook of Obstetrics, 7/e p224*

Diagnosis of ovulation

- **Indirect methods**
- **Menstrual history**
  - Regular menstrual cycle
  - Mittelschmerz
  - Premenstrual syndrome/primary dysmenorrhoea
- **Basal body temperature**
  - **Biphasic pattern of temperature (0.5 °C) in ovulatory cycles**
  - Rise in temperature following ovulation is due to progesterone
- **Cervical mucus method**
  - Proliferative phase-mucous thin, copious, stretchable (Spinnarkeit test)
  - Disappearance of fern pattern of mucous beyond 22nd day of cycle suggests ovulation
- **Vaginal cytology**
  - Maturation index shifts to left in 2nd half of the cycle due to progesterone effect
- **Hormonal estimation**
  - Serum progesterone ↑
  - Serum LH-LH surge at time of ovulation
    - **Ovulation occurs 34–36 hours following LH surge**
  - Serum estradiol
    - Peaks 24 hours prior to LH surge
    - Coincides 24–36 hours prior to ovulation
- **Endometrial biopsy**
  - Biopsy done on 21st–23rd day of cycle-secretory endometrium
  - Subnuclear vacuolation-earliest evidence
    - Appears 36–48 hours following ovulation
- **USG**
  - Serial TVS during midcycle
  - Precisely measures Graafian collicle
  - Just prior to ovulation measures 18–20 mm
  - Following ovulation features of recent ovulation in USG
    - Collapsed follicle
    - Fluid in PID
- **Direct method**
  - **Laparoscopy**
    - Laparoscopic visualization of recent corpus luteum
    - Detection of ovum in aspirated peritoneal fluid

76. Ans. c. OCPs *Ref: Shaw's Textbook of Gynecology 15/e p416*

Predisposing Factors for Endomentrial Carcinoma:

- Hormone replacement therapy after menopause
- Chronic nonovulatory cycles in DUB
- Familial predisposition-familial lynch II syndrome

- Tamoxifen given breast cancer
- Corpus cancer syndrome-obesity, diabetes and hypetension-30%
- PCOD
- Fibroid-3%
- Feminizing ovarian tumor
- OCPs have a protective effect and reduces the risk by 40–50% and also adding progestogens for 12 days each cycle to oestrogen in HRT reduces its risk to 2%

77. Ans. c. 1 : 2 *Ref: Shaw's Textbook of Gynacology 15/e p8*

Relationship between the length of cervix and the body of uterus:
- Before puberty—2 : 1
- After puberty—1 : 2
- During reproductive period—1 : 3

78. Ans. c. Primary vaginal Ca *Ref: Dutta's Textbook of Gynecology 5/e p325*

Repeat question

79. Ans. a. Cervicitis *Ref: Dutta's Textbook of Gynecology 5/e p124*

Pelvic Inflammatory Disease (PID)
- Infection of upper genital tract involving
  - Endometrium
  - Fallopian tubes
  - Ovaries
  - Pelvic peritoneum and surrounding structures
- **Cerivicitis is not included in PID**

80. Ans. d. Madlenea's method *Ref: Dutta's Gynecology p455, Shaw's Textbook of Gynecology p240*

Failure rates

Method	Failure Rate
Laparoscopic sterilization	0.2 to 0.6%
Pomeroy's method	0.1 to 0.5%
Madlener's method	1.5 to 7%
Rhythm method	24 pregnancy rate per HWY
Coitus interruptus	19
Lactational amenorrhoea	2
Condom	14
Diaphragm	20
IUCD	0.1 to 3
OCPs	0.1
POP	1
DMPA and NET injectables	0.3
Norplant	0.1
Vasectomy	0.15
Tubectomy	0.5

81. Ans. a. No difference in prognosis of pregnancy *Ref: Dutta's Textbook of Obstetrics p293*

Tuberculosis in Pregnancy
- Incidence—1 to 2%
- **Risk factors**
  - Positive family history
  - Low SE status
  - HIV infection

 - Alcohol
 - IV drug abuse
 - Diabetes
 - Jejunostomy bypass
 - Underweight
- **Diagnosis**
 - Manteaux test
 - Chest x-ray
 - Sputum smear
 - Gastric washings
 - Diagnostic bronchoscopy
 - PCR
- **Congenital TB** is rare-noted in first week of life, **Cavitating hepatic granuloma,** HIV increases risk
- In untreated patients, increased changes of:
 - Preterm labour
 - IUGR
 - Perinatal morality
- Treatment
 - With no active disease, INH 300 mg/day after 1st trimester for 6 to 9 months
 - With active disease, INH 300 mg, RMP 600 mg, EMB 2.5 gm, PYZ 2gm
- **Breast feeding is not contraindicated** when mother is taking drugs
- In active disease baby isolated and given INH prophylaxis 20 mg/kg/day for 3 months But if mother is on ATT for 2 weeks there is no need to isolate baby. BCG given as soon as possible.
- Contraception-pregnancy avoided atleast for 2 years. OCPs not used with RMP because of contraceptive failure. Barrier method is used.

82. Ans. b. Down's syndrome *Ref: Dutta's Textbook of Obstetrics p106*

Maternal Serum AFP
- AFP is oncofetal protein with molecular weight 70000
- It is produced by Yolk sac and fetal liver
- Highest level of AFP in fetal serum and amniotic fluid is seen around 13 weeks and thereafter decreases
- Maternal serum AFP reaches a peak around 32 weeks
- MSAFP level is elevated in:
 - Wrong gestational age
 - Open NTD
 - Multiple pregnancy
 - Rh isoimmunisation
 - IUFD
 - Anterior abdominal wall defects
 - Renal anomalies
- **MSAFP is low in:**
 - Down's syndrome
 - GTD [Gestational trophoblastic disease]
- Test is done between 15 to 20 weeks

83. Ans. b. Stage 3b *Ref: Shaw's Textbook of Gynecology p412*

Refer to text for staging

84. Ans. a. Nebothian cyst *Ref: Shaw's textbook of gynecology 15/e p136*

Repeat question

85. Ans. a. Granulosa cell tumor

Granulosa Cell Tumor
- Accounts for 2% of ovarian neoplasms
- Originates from rest of **primitive granulose cells**

- **Most common ovarian stromal tumor**
- 2% bilateral, slow growing
- Solid/cystic
- Cut section-yellow/orange due to lipid content
- Histopath
  - Cells polygonal or round with granular eosinophilic cytoplasm with ill defined borders with coffee bean nuclei
  - Granulose cells are arranged in small clusters around a central cavity called call exner bodies
- Tumor marker-Inhibin
- Unopposed estrogen secretion → endometrial hyperplasia → endometrial Ca
- C/F—due to hyperestrogenism
  - Precocious puberty
  - AUB
  - Postmenopausal bleeding
  - May rupture and cause acute abdomen
- Treatment-Laparotomy and surgical stanging, Unilateral salpingooopherectomy
- Chemotherapy
  - **VAC Regimen** [vincristing+adriamycin+cyclophosphamide]
  - **BEP Regimen** [bleomycin, etoposide, cisplatin]

86. Ans. a. Absence of villi *Ref: Dutta Textbook of Gynecology 5/e p348; Shaw's Textbook of Gynecology 5/e p253*

Invasivemole	Choriocarcinoma
Evidence of chorionic villi	Villous formation lost
Follows abortion/mole	Following full-term pregnancy
Diagnozed <6 months following	>6 months to be diagnozed
Abortion/mole	

87. Ans. b. FSH *Ref: Dutta's Textbook of Gynecology 5/e p57, Shaw's Textbook of Gynecology 15/e p62*

Menopausal Flushing

- Characteristic vasomotor symptom of menopause
- Hot flush is sudden feel of heart followed by sweating
- Decreased estrogen causes GnRH pulse secretion lasting for 1 to 10 min
- Thermoregulatory center in association with GnRH-center in hypothalamus is involved in etiology
- Decreased estrogen causes rebound increase in secretion of FSH and LH by anterior pituitary
- FSH level may rise as much as 50 fold and LH 3–4 fold

88. Ans. d. Varicose veins *Ref: Dutta Textbook of Gynecology 5/e p466*

Refer to text for list of contraindications for OCPs

89. Ans. c. Yolk sac tumor *Ref: Shaw's textbook of gynecology 15/e*

Refer text

QUESTIONS 2015

1. Genuine stress incontinence is diagnozed by:

a. Cystometry
b. Cystoscopy
c. Methylene blue 3 swab test
d. None of the above

2. Regarding vasectomy the false statement is:

a. Done under local anaesthesia
b. Disrupting the vas deferens
c. Sterility is immediate
d. Ligation and excision is done in India

3. Regarding ovarian anatomy the statement is:

a. The number of oogonia reaches maximum at the 20th week
b. Germ cells are ectodermal in origin

c. The gonads are undifferentiated and bipotential until 10th week

d. The ovary is attached to the uterus by the infundibulo pelvic ligament

4. Stress incontinence is seen associated with:
a. Prolapse
b. Cervical malignancy
c. Bladder stone
d. Complete perineal tear

ANSWERS AND EXPLANATIONS

1. Ans. a. Cystometry *Ref: Dutta's Gynecology 5/e p382*

- **Genuine stress incontinence**
  - Bladder neck displacement
  - Intrinsic sphincter dysfunction (ISD)
- Involuntary loss of urine that occurs, when, in the absence of a detrusor contraction, the intravesical pressure exceeds the maximum urethral closure pressure
- Normally, while at rest the intraurethral pressure is greater than the intravesical pressure
- The pressure difference between the bladder and the urethra is known as the urethral closure pressure
- **Cause:**
  - Intrinsic sphincteric deficiency is frequently an important cause of urinary incontinence
  - Anatomic descent of the proximal urethra below its normal intra-abdominal position
  - Altered anatomic relationships between the urethra and bladder

Failure of neuromuscular and connective tissue components

Different investigations used for stress incontinence are:

- Stress test
- Cotton swab stick test/Q-tip test
- Marshall and Bonney's test
- Urethroscopy
- Urodynamic evaluation/cystometry
- Normal findings of cystometry:
  - Residual volume: 0–50 ml
  - First sense of voiding: 150–200 ml
  - Capacity: 400–600 ml
  - Intravesical pressure on filling and standing: 0–15 cm H_2O
  - Absence of systolic detrusor contraction
  - No leakage on cough
  - Able to interrupt the flow
  - Peak urinary flow rate >15 ml/sec.
  - Maximum detrusor pressure during voiding <70 cm H_2O

2. Ans. c. Sterility is immediate *Ref: Dutta's Gynecology 5/e p473*

Vasectomy

- Simple, safe and effective
- Consists of dividing and excising a part of the vas deferens and disrupting the passage of sperms
- Done under LA
- 2 methods—conventional and non scalpel vasectomy
- Occlusion is done by different methods
  - Ligation and excision (done in India)
  - Electrocautery
  - Thermal cautery
  - Clips
  - Open-ended vasectomy

Advantages:
- Operative technique is simple with minimal training
- OP procedure
- Complications are few and immediate
- Failure rate is minimal—0.15%
- Reversal rates are high—50%
- Overall expenditure is less

Disadvantages:
- Additional contraceptive for next 3 months, sterility is not immediate (>12 ejaculations or >3 months)
- Frigidity or impotency mostly psychological

3. Ans. a. The number of oogonia reaches maximum at the 20th week *Ref: Dutta's Gynecology 5/e p11*

Ovary: concerned with:
- Germ cell maturation, storage and its release
- Steroidogenesis
  - Measures—3*2*1 cm
  - They are intraperitoneal structures
  - Gonads remain undifferentiated and bipotential until the end of 7th week
  - Germ cells are endodermal
  - By 20th week in utero—the oogonia are maximum—7 million
  - By birth—they are 2 million
    - Ovary consists of cortex and medulla
    - Cortex–has the germinal epithelium and below is the stromal cells
    - Medulla–has the hilus cells-homologous to the interstitial cells of the testes
    - Arterial supply-ovarian artery-branch of abdominal aorta
    - Attachments—by the ovarian ligament to the uterus and by the infundibulopelvic ligament to the pelvic wall

4. Ans. a. Prolapse *Ref: Dutta's Gynecology 5/e p383*

Risk factors for genuine SUI
- Developmental weakness-genetic variation in the collagen and other connective tissues
- Childbirth trauma-denervation to the smooth and the striated components of the sphincter mechanism. More common in gynecoid pelvis and least in android pelvis
- Pregnancy-functional due to high preogesterone
- Postmenopausal-estrogen deficiency
- Trauma
- Following repair of VVF, Bladder neck surgery
- Obesity

Chapter

15 Pediatrics

Subramani Seenivasan

GROWTH, DEVELOPMENT AND BEHAVIOR

Periods of Growth

Prenatal period	
Ovum	0 to 14 days
Embryo	14 days to 9 weeks
Fetus	9 weeks to birth
Perinatal period	22 weeks to 7 days after birth
Postnatal period	
Newborn	0–28 days
Infancy	First year
Toddler	1 to 3 years
Preschool child	3–6 years
School age child	6–12 years
Adolescence	
Early	10–13 years
Middle	14–16 years
Late	17–20 years

Laws of Growth

- Growth and development are continuous and orderly process.
- Growth pattern of every individual is unique.
- Different tissues grow at different rates.
- In postnatal life, growth velocity is high during first few months of life and during puberty.
- Order of growth is cephalocaudal and distal to proximal. (cephalocaudal-head grows before neck, arms grow before legs; proximal to distal–hands increase in size before upper arms)
- Neonatal head size is 65–70% of adult size; 90% at 2 years.
- Lymphoid growth is most notable in mid childhood (4–8 years)

Age	Weight (kg)	Length/Height (cm)	Head circumference (cm)
Birth	3	50	34
6 months	6	65	43
1 year	9	75	46
2 years	12	90	48
3 years	15	95	49
4 years	16	100	50

- A child gains 2 kg every year between 3 and 7 years and 3 kg per year after that till puberty.
- A child grows by 6 cm every year from 4 to 12 years.
- Head circumference at 12 years is 52 cm.
- Chest circumference is 3 cm less than HC at birth and HC = CC at 1 year.
- From 3–12 months, wt (kg) = [age (months) +9]/2.
- 1 to 6 years, wt (kg) = 2A + 8. A is age in years.
- From 7–12 years, wt (kg) = (7A–5)/2.
- Height in cm from 2–12 years is 6A + 77.
- Lower segment is from pubic symphisis to floor. Upper segment is Height minus lower segment.

Age	US/LS ratio
Birth	1.7:1
3 years	1.3:1
7 years	1:1

- A newborn sleeps 16.5 hours a day. It is 10 hours in 9 years, 9 hours in 14 years and 8.25 hours in 18 years.

Developmental Milestones

Gross Motor

S. No	Milestone	Average age in months
1.	Holds head steadily while sitting	2
2.	Pulls to sit with no head lag	3
3.	Brings hand together in midline	3
4.	Asymmetric tonic neck reflex gone	4
5.	Sits with support	6
6.	Rolls backs to stomach	6.5
7.	Walks alone	12
8.	Runs	16

Fine Motor

S. No.	Milestone	Average age in months
1.	Grasps rattle	3.5
2.	Reaches for objects	4
3.	Palmar grasp gone	4
4.	Transfers object from hand to hand	5.5
5.	Thumb finger grasp	8
6.	Turns pages of book	12
7.	Scribbles	13
8.	Builds tower of 2 cubes	15
9.	Builds tower of 6 cubes	22

Communication and Language

S. No.	Milestone	Average age in months
1.	Smiles in response to face, voice	1.5
2.	Monosyllabic babble	6
3.	Inhibits to 'no'	7
4.	Follows one step command to gesture	7

Contd...

Contd...

S. No.	Milestone	Average age in months
5.	Follows one step command without gesture	10
6.	Saya 'mama', ' dada'	10
7.	Points to objects	10
8.	Speaks first real word	12
9.	Speaks 4–6 words	15
10.	Speaks 10–15 words	18
11.	Speaks 2 word sentence	19

Cognitive

S. No.	Milestone	Average age in months
1.	Stares momentarily at spot where object disappeared	2
2.	Stares at own hand	4
3.	Bangs 2 cubes	8
4.	Uncovers toy (after seeing it hidden)	8
5.	Egocentric Symbolic play (pretends to drink from cup)	12
6.	Uses stick to reach toy	17
7.	Pretends play with doll	17

Other Important Milestones

S. No.	Milestone	Average age in months
1.	Follows moving object	1
2.	Follows moving object to 180°	2
3.	Social smile	2
4.	Moro disaappears	3
5.	Rolls over	7
6.	Crawls (with chest on the ground)	7
7.	Pivots	7
8.	Reaches out for objects	7
9.	Prefers mother, stranger anxiety	7
10.	Enjoys mirror	7
11.	Sits with support	7
12.	Sits without support	10
13.	Creeps (chest off the ground)	10
14.	Grasps with thumb and forefinger	10
15.	Plays "pat a cake or peek a boo"	10
16.	Waves "bye bye"	10
17.	Plays simple ball game	12
18.	Walks alone, crawls upstairs	15
19.	Jargon	15
20.	Feeds self	18
21.	Puts 3 words together (subject, verb, object)	24
22.	Goes up stairs alternating feet	30
23.	Uses pronoun "I", knows full name	30

Contd...

Contd...

S. No.	Milestone	Average age in months
24.	Knows age and sex	36
25.	Rides tricycle, stands momentarily at one foot	36
26.	Hops on one foot, uses scissors	48
27.	Skips	60
28.	Names colors	60

Drawing

S. No.	Pattern	Average age in months
1.	Vertical stroke	18
2.	Horizontal stroke	24
3.	Circle	36
4.	Square, rectangle, cross, man with 2-4 parts	48
5.	Triangle	60

Building Tower of Cubes

S. No.	No. of cubes	Average age in months
1.	3	15
2.	4	18
3.	6	21
4.	7	24
5.	9	30
6.	10	36
7.	Gate of 5 cubes	48

Eruption of Tooth

Primary Dentition–Time of eruption (approximated for easy remembrance)

• Central incisor	6–9 months
• Lateral incisor	9–12 months
• First molar	14 months
• Canine	18 months
• Second molar	24–30 months

Secondary Dentition–Time of eruption

• First molar	6 years
• Central incisor	7 years
• Lateral incisor	8 years
• First premolar	10 years
• Canine	11 years
• Second premolar	12 years
• Second molar	13 years
• Third molar	18 years

First primary tooth to erupt is lower central incisor. First secondary tooth to erupt is first molar. First and second molars in primary dentition are replaced by first and second premolars respectively in secondary dentition. Delayed eruption of primary dentition is said if no tooth erupt in 13 months of age.

Causes of delayed eruption

- Familial (most common)
- Hypothyroidism
- Hypoparathyroidism
- Idiopathic.

Causes of early exfoliation

- Histiocytosis X
- Cyclic neutropenia
- Leukemia
- Trauma
- Idiopathic.

Radiographs to assess age of a child is as follows:

3 to 9 months–Shoulder

1 to 13 years–Hands and wrist

12 to 14 years–Elbow and hip.

Behavior and Psychiatric Disorders

Rumination

Rumination disorder is defined as the repeated regurgitation and rechewing of food for a period of at least 1 month following a period of normal functioning. The rumination is not due to an associated gastrointestinal illness or other general medical condition (e.g., esophageal reflux). It does not occur exclusively during the course of anorexia nervosa or bulimia nervosa. Malnourishment with resultant weight loss or growth delay is a hallmark of this disorder.

Etiology–disturbed relationship with primary caregivers.

DD

- Congenital gastrointestinal system anomalies,
- Pyloric stenosis,
- Sandifer's syndrome,
- Increased intracranial pressure,
- Diencephalic tumors,
- Adrenal insufficiency, and
- Inborn errors of metabolism.

Treatment

Self-stimulation, reinforcing correct eating behavior, minimizing attention to rumination. No drug therapy is recommended.

PICA

Pica involves the persistent eating of nonnutritive substances (e.g., plaster, charcoal, clay, wool, ashes, paint, earth). The eating behavior is inappropriate to the developmental level. It is more common in children with mental retardation, pervasive developmental disorders, obsessive-compulsive disorders, and other neuropsychiatric disorders. It can occur in adolescence and adulthood. Geophagia (eating earth) is associated with pregnancy. Children with pica are at **increased risk for lead poisoning, iron-deficiency anemia, obstruction, dental injury, and parasitic infections.** Treatment is combined medical and psychosocial approach. Specific treatment of lead poisoning, IDA, etc.

Enuresis

Enuresis is defined as the repeated voiding of urine into clothes or bed at least twice a week for at least 3 consecutive months in a child who is **at least 5 year of age**. The behavior is not due exclusively to the direct physiologic effect of a substance (e.g., a diuretic) or a general medical condition (e.g., diabetes). *Primary enuresis* occurs in children who have never been consistently dry through the night, whereas *secondary enuresis* refers to the resumption of wetting after at least 6 months of dryness. *Monosymptomatic enuresis* has no associated daytime symptoms (urgency, frequency, daytime enuresis), and *nonmonosymptomatic enuresis*, which is more common, often has at least one subtle daytime symptom. Monosymptomatic enuresis is rarely associated with significant organic underlying abnormalities.

Etiology

Primary–biological, emotional, social, familial

Secondary–UTI, chronic kidney disease, hypercalcemia, hypokalemia, chemical urethritis, constipation, diabetes mellitus or insipidus, sickle cell anemia, seizures, pinworm infection, spinal dysraphism, neurogenic bladder, hyperthyroidism, sleep-disordered breathing, drugs (selective serotonin reuptake inhibitor, valproic acid, clozapine) and giggle or stress incontinence.

Treatment

- Behavior therapy
- Application of alarm (75–95% success, 40% relapse)
- Desmopressin (high relapse rate)
- Imipramine, Oxybutinin and tolterodine.

Encopresis pneumonic BAD TOI (LET)

Voluntary or involuntary passage of feces into inappropriate places at least once a month for **3 consecutive months** once a chronologic or developmental **age of 4 years** has been reached. Encopresis is not diagnosed when the behavior is due exclusively to the direct effects of a substance (e.g., laxatives) or a general medical condition.

Rretentive encopresis–with constipation and overflow incontinence (representing 65–95% of cases)

Nonretentive encopresis–without constipation and overflow incontinence.

Encopresis can persist from infancy onward (primary) or can appear after successful toilet training (secondary). It is 4–5 times more common in boys than in girls.

Treatment - clearance of impacted fecal material, mineral oil or laxatives to prevent further constipation, high-fiber diet and family support for behavioral change.

Rapid rectal disimpaction	Slow oral disimpaction
Glycerine suppositories,	Polyethylene glycol
Phosphate enema	Milk of magnesia
Milk of molasses enema	Lactulose, Sorbitol

Habit Disoeders–Bruxism, thumb sucking, trichotillomania.

Bruxism

Also called teeth grinding.

Occurs in first 5 years of life.

Can cause dental occlusion.

Can manifest as muscular/temperomandibular joint pain.

Thumb sucking is normal in infancy and toddlerhood. Treatment is simple reinforcement or noxious stimulus (bitter salves).

Trichotillomania is the repetitive pulling of hair resulting in loss and strand breakage of hair. Onset is around 13 years. Sense of tension present. Often remits spontaneously. SSRI–Fluoxetine maybe used.

Tic disorder–a tic is defined as a sudden, rapid, recurrent, nonrhythmic, stereotyped motor movement or vocalization that is experienced as irresistible, but can be suppressed for varying lengths of time. Markedly diminished during sleep.

Tourette's syndrome (TS) is characterized by multiple motor and vocal tics. Multiple tics and complex vocal sounds, such as barking and grunting, develop over time and peak in severity by age 10–12 years. Shouting obscene words **(coprolalia)** is characteristic. Often jeopardize patients' social interaction with other children, is a life long disorder.

Criteria for the diagnosis

- Multiple motor and vocal tics lasting > 1 year, with no tic-free interval lasting > 3 months,
- Onset before age 18 years, and
- No medical causes (drugs, central nervous system disease).

Treatment–Haloperidol, Pimozide, Risperidone, Clonidine.

DSM-IV-TR diagnostic criteria for major depressive episode

- Five (or more) of the following symptoms have been present during the same 2 week period and represent a change from previous functioning; at least one of the symptoms is either (1) depressed mood or (2) loss of interest or pleasure.
  - Depressed most of the day
  - Markedly diminished interest or pleasure in all
  - Significant weight loss when not dieting or weight gain (> 5% of body weight in a month), or decrease or increase in appetite nearly every day.
  - Insomnia or hypersomnia nearly every day.
  - Psychomotor agitation or retardation
  - Fatigue or loss of energy nearly every day.
  - Feelings of worthlessness or inappropriate guilt
  - Diminished ability to think or concentrate, or indecisiveness
  - Recurrent thoughts of death, recurrent suicidal ideation/attempt

Treatment of depression–SSRI

Anorexia nervosa (AN) involves significant overestimation of body size and shape, with a relentless pursuit of thinness that typically combines excessive dieting and compulsive exercising in the **restrictive** subtype; in the **binge-purge** subtype, patients might intermittently overeat and then attempt to rid themselves of calories by vomiting or taking laxatives, still with a strong drive for thinness.

Bulimia nervosa (BN) is characterized by episodes of eating large amounts of food in a brief period, followed by compensatory vomiting, laxative use, and exercise or fasting to rid the body of the effects of overeating in an effort to avoid obesity.

Diagnostic criteria for anorexia nervosa

- Refusal to maintain body weight at or above a minimally normal weight for age and height (body weight < 85% of that expected)
- Intense fear of gaining weight or becoming fat, even though underweight.
- Disturbance in the way one's body weight or shape is experienced, undue influence of body weight or shape on self-evaluation, or denial of the seriousness of the current low body weight.
- In postmenarcheal females, amenorrhea

Specify Type:

Restricting Type: during the current episode of anorexia nervosa, the person has not regularly engaged in binge-eating or purging behavior

Binge-Eating/Purging Type: during the current episode of anorexia nervosa, the person has regularly engaged in binge-eating or purging behavior

Incidence

Anorexia Nervosa–0.5 to 1%.

Bulimia Nervosa–3 to 5%.

Treatment–A **nurturant-authoritative** approach using the **biopsychosocial** model is useful.

AN–Food is more useful than SSRI.

BN–SSRI is very effective.

Cognitive Behavioral therapy, Dialectical Behavioral therapy, Group therapy, EFamily based treatment.

PERVASIVE DEVELOPMENTAL DISORDERS AND AUTISM SPECTRUM DISORDERS

Autism	Asperger's syndrome	Rett's syndrome	Childhood disintegrative disorder	Pervasive developmental disorder—not otherwise specified
Delayed and disordered communication Atypical social interaction Restricted range of interests Onset before 3 years of age	Similar to autism except language skills relatively intact Usually not cognitively delayed	Almost always affects girls Regression in skills between 6 and 18 months of age	Clinically significant regression in skills (language, social skills, bowel and bladder control, play motor skills) before 10 years of age	Features of 1 of the other autism spectrum disorders, but insufficient for a specific diagnosis

Autism

The core features of autistic disorder (AD) include impairments in 3 symptom domains: social interaction; communication; and developmentally appropriate behavior, interests, or activities. Stereotypical body movements, a marked need for sameness, and a very narrow range of interests are also common. Head circumference is normal at birth. AD show an abnormally rapid increase in head circumference from 6–14 months of age, increased brain volume in 2–4 years olds, increased volume of the cerebellum, cerebrum, and amygdala, and marked abnormal growth in the frontal, temporal, cerebellar, and limbic regions of the brain.

Treatment– Speech,occupational, physical therapy, Cognitive behavior therapy and drugs

Drugs:

- SSRI (fluoxetine, fluvoxamine, citalopram, escitalopram, paroxetine, sertraline)
- Methylphenidate, dextroamphitamine, atomoxetine
- Atypical antipsychotic agents–risperidone, aripiprazole, olanzapine, quetiapine, ziprasidone
- α agonists–clonidine, guanfacine
- Mood stabilizers–Levetiracetam, valporic acid, topirramate.

Aspereger's disorder— Children with Asperger's disorder have a qualitative impairment in the development of reciprocal social interaction. They show restrictive, repetitive patterns of behavior, interests, or achievements with other people. These disturbances must cause significant impairments in social or occupational functioning. They have a history of normal language milestones with single words used by age 2 years and communicative phrases used by age 3 years. They have deficits in nonverbal and pragmatic aspects of communication (facial expressions, gestures) but do not have the severe language delays.

Childhood disintegrative disorder (also termed Heller's syndrome, dementia infantilis, or disintegrative psychosis) is a marked regression in multiple areas of functioning following a period of at least 2 years of apparently normal development.

The DSM-IV-TR criteria for this disorder includes apparently normal development for at least the 1st 2 years after birth as manifested by the presence of age-appropriate verbal and nonverbal communication, social relationships, play, and adaptive behavior along with the clinically significant loss of previously acquired skills (before age 10 years) in at least two of the following areas: expressive or receptive language, social skills or adaptive behavior, bowel or bladder control, play, and motor skills. They face permanent disability and require long-term care.

Treatment–behavior therapy and antipsychotic medication.

Diagnostic Criteria for Schizophrenia

- Characteristic symptoms: Two (or more) of the following, each present for a significant portion of time during a 1 month period (or less if successfully treated):
  - Delusions
  - Hallucinations
  - Disorganized speech (e.g., frequent derailment or incoherence)
  - Grossly disorganized or catatonic behavior
  - Negative symptoms, i.e., affective flattening, alogia, or avolition

For at least 6 months duration

Attention-deficit/hyperactivity disorder (ADHD) is the most common neurobehavioral disorder of childhood, among the most prevalent chronic health conditions affecting school-aged children, ADHD is characterized by **inattention, hyperactivity, impulsivity**. (including increased distractibility and difficulty sustaining attention; poor impulse control and decreased self-inhibitory capacity; and motor overactivity and motor restlessness).

Prevalence–5 to 10% in school aged children. Features must begin before age 7. Have smaller prefrontal cortex and basal ganglia. **Dopamine hypothesis** (low levels of Dopamine activity) explains pathogenesis.

Treatment–Methyphenidate, Dexmethyphenidate, Dextroamphitamine, Mixed amphetamine salts, Atomoxetine, Bupropion, Imipramine, Desipramine, Nortryptyline, Clonidine, Guanfacine.

Dyslexia is characterized by an unexpected difficulty in reading in persons who otherwise possess the necessary intelligence and motivation that should permit accurate and fluent reading. Dyslexia is the most common of the **learning disabilities,** constitutes 80% of learning disabilities. They display an effortful approach to decoding and recognizing single words, an approach in children characterized by hesitations, mispronunciations, and repeated attempts to sound out unfamiliar words.

EMERGENCY AND CRITICAL CARE

- Hallmark of refeeding syndrome is severe hypophosphatemia.
- Rapid correction of hyponatremia leads to central pontine myelinosis.
- Maple syrup urine disease is caused by deficiency of branched chain amino acis α ketoacid dehydrogenase.
- Most common cause of shock in children world wide is hypovolemic shock.
- ECG changes in hyperkalemia are tall T-waves, prolonged PR, wide QRS, flat P-waves and sine wave.
- ECG changes in hypokalemia are falt T-waves, ST depression and appearance of U-waves.
- ECG finding in Tricyclic antidepressant posinonin is wide QRS (> 100 ms).
- Antidote for sulfonylurea poisoning is Octreotide
- Rumack–Mathew nomogram is used in Paracetamol poisoning.
- Pao2/Fio2 ratio in acute lung injury is < 300 (for ARDS < 200).
- Subgaleal bleed in a newborn occurs beneath the aponeurosis of occipitofrontalis muscle.
- Size of uncuffed ET tube in children is Age in years/4 + 4.
- In Prader–willi syndrome uniparental disomy of maternal chromosome occurs (missing paternal chromosome 15) and in Angelman syndrome, uniparental disomy of paternal chromosome occurs (missing maternal chromosome 15).
- Total body water in a term newborn is 75% of body weight.
- Osmolality = 2[Na] + [Glucose]/18 + [Urea]/2.8
- Na (corrected) = Na (measured) + 1.6 [(Glucose–100)/100].
- Pseudohyponatremia is seen in hyperlipidemia and hyperproteinemia.
- Mnimum urine osmolality in children is 30–50 mOsm/kg where as maximum urine osmolality is 1200 mOsm/kg.
- Electrolte abnormality in diabetes insipidus is hypernatremia.
- Sodium correction in hyponatremia is done at the rate of < 12 mEq/L/day or < 0.5 mEq/L/hr.
- Rapid correction of hyponatremia may lead to **central pontine myelinolysis.**

Diagnostic Criteria for Syndrome of Inappropriate Antidiuretic Hormone Secretion

Absence of:
- Renal, adrenal, or thyroid insufficiency
- Heart failure, nephrotic syndrome, or cirrhosis
- Diuretic ingestion
- Dehydration

Urine osmolality > 100 mOsm/kg (usually > plasma)
Serum osmolality < 280 mOsm/kg and serum sodium < 135 mEq/L
Urine sodium > 30 mEq/L

- Diagnostic criteria for Diabetes Insipidus is Urine osmolality < 300 mOsm/kg and serum osmolality > 300 mOsm/kg.
- The electrolyte abnormalities in **Hungry Bone Disease** are hypocalcemia, hypophosphatemia and hypomagnesemia.
- The electrolyte/biochemical abnormalities in **Tumor Lysis Syndrome** are hyperurecemia, hyperkalemia, hyperphosphatemia and hypocalcemia.
- Normal serum Magnesium is 1.5–2.3 mg/Dl.
- Familial hypomagnesemia with hypercalciuria and nephrocalcinosis , known as **Michelis-Castrillo syndrome,** an autosomal recessive disorder, is due to mutations in the gene for claudin 16 (paracellin-1), which is located in the tight junctions of the TAL of the loop of Henle.
- **EAST syndrome** is due to mutations in a potassium channel, and patients with this autosomal recessive disorder have hypokalemia, metabolic alkalosis, and hypomagnesemia.
- **Fanconi syndrome** is a generalized defect in the proximal tubule leading to urinary wasting of bicarbonate, phosphorus, amino acids, uric acid, and glucose.
- **Normal values of arterial blood gases**

pH	7.35–7.45
$[HCO_3^-]$	20–28 mEq/L
Pco_2	35–45 mm Hg

By Winter's formula, PCO2 = 1.5 $[HCO_3^-]$ +8 ± 2.

- Diarrhea is the most common cause of metabolic acidosis in children.
- The goals of maintenance fluids are
  - Prevent dehydration
  - Prevent electrolyte disorders
  - Prevent ketoacidosis
  - Prevent protein degradation
- 100% of maintenance fluids will give only 20% of required calories.
- Body weight method for calculating daily maintenance fluid volume

Body weight	Fluid per day
0–10 kg	100 mL/kg
11–20 kg	1,000 mL + 50 mL/kg for each kg >10 kg
>20 kg	1,500 mL + 20 mL/kg for each kg >20 kg*

*The maximum total fluid per day is normally 2,400 mL.

Hourly maintenance water rate

For body weight of 0–10 kg: 4 mL/kg/hr
For body weight of 10–20 kg: 40 mL/hr + 2 mL/kg/hr × (wt − 10 kg)
For body weight of >20 kg: 60 mL/hr + 1 mL/kg/hr × (wt − 20 kg)*

*The maximum fluid rate is normally 100 ml/hr.

Composition of intravenous solutions

Fluid	[Na]	$[Cl^-]$	$[K^+]$	$[Ca^{2+}]$	$[Lactate^-]$
Normal saline (0.9% NaCl)	154	154	–	–	–
Half-normal saline (0.45% NaCl)	77	77	–	–	–
0.2 normal saline (0.2% NaCl)	34	34	–	–	–
Ringer lactate	130	109	4	3	28

- Normal plasma osmolality is 285–295 mOsm/kg.
- Compression: breath ratio in Pediatric resuscitation 30 : 1 for one rescuer and 15 : 1 for 2 rescuer and in newborn, it is 3 : 1. For both 1 or 2 rescuers
- High quality CPR

- Rate 100 perminute
- Compression depth 1/3 to ½ AP diameter of chest wall (4 cm in infants and 5 cm in children)
- Allow complete chest recoil after each compression
- Minimize interruption in chest compression
- Avoid excessive ventilation.

- In CPR, pulse should be checked in 10 seconds (not 1 minute).
- High dose Insulin therapy is the considered the antidote of choice for Calcium channel blocker poisoning.
- Serotonin syndrome is a triad of altered mental status, autonomic instability, and neuromuscular hyperactivity (hyperreflexia, tremors, clonus in the lower extremities more than the upper extremities).
- Methemoglobinemia is suggested by the classic "chocolate brown" blood and confirmed via co-oximetry. Methemoglobinemia is treated with methylene blue. Co-oximetry is also used in Cyanide toxicity.
- Antidote of cyanide toxicity is cyanide kit (Amyl nitrate, Sodium nitrate and Sodium thiosulphate). Hydroxy cobalamine is also used.
- Cerebral Perfusion Pressure (CPP) = Mean Arterial Pressure (MAP)–Intra Cranial Pressure (ICP)
- The 3 key components of clinical brain death diagnosis are demonstrations of irreversible coma/unresponsiveness, absence of brainstem reflexes, and apnea.
- During Apnea test, absence of respiratory efforts with a $PCO_2 > 60$ mm Hg or more that 20 mm Hg above an elevated baseline value is consistent with brain death.
- Inotrope for cold septic shock is Epinephrine and for warm septic shock is Norepinephrine.
- **Typical localizing signs for pulmonary pathology**

Site of pathology	Respiratory rate	Retractions	Audible sounds
Extrathoracic airway	↑	↑↑↑↑	Stridor
Intrathoracic extrapulmonary	↑	↑↑	Wheezing
Intrathoracic intrapulmonary	↑↑	↑↑	Wheezing
Alveolar interstitial	↑↑↑	↑↑↑	Grunting

- **Simplified consensus definition of acute lung injury**

> - Acute onset (<7 days)
> - Severe hypoxemia ($Pao_2/Fio_2 < 300$ for acute lung injury, or <200 for acute respiratory distress syndrome)
> - Diffuse bilateral pulmonary infiltrates on frontal radiograph consistent with pulmonary edema (these can be patchy and asymmetric, and pleural effusions can be present)
> - Absence of left atrial hypertension (pulmonary artery wedge pressure <18 mm Hg if measured)

- Estimation of Body Surface Area in Burns.

	Newborn	3 years	6 years	>12 years
Head	18%	15%	12%	6%
Trunk	40%	40%	40%	38%
Arms	16%	16%	16%	18%
Legs	26%	29%	32%	38%

- Pain measurement tools in children are
  - Visual Analog Scale (VAS)
  - Likert scale
  - Faces scales (FACES-R, Wong Baker, Oucher, Bieri, McGrath scales)
  - Behavioral/combined behavioral-physiologic scales.
  - Autonomic (HR, BP, HR spectral analysis)
  - Hormonal-metabolic measures (e.g. Cortisol, Epinephrine).
- Indications for genetic counselling
  - Maternal age ≥ 35 years.
  - Paternal age ≥ 50 years.

- Enzyme replacement therapies are available for Gaucher disease and Fabry disease, some mucopolysaccharidoses (I, II, VI), Niemann-Pick disease type C, and Pompe disease.

NEONATOLOGY

APGAR Evaluation of Newborn Infants*

Sign	0	1	2
Heart rate	Absent	Below 100	Over 100
Respiratory effort	Absent	Slow, irregular	Good, crying
Muscle tone	Limp	Some flexion of extremities	Active motion
Response to catheter in nostril (tested after oropharynx is clear)	No response	Grimace	Cough or sneeze
Color	Blue, pale	Body pink, extremities blue	Completely pink

Factors Affecting the APGAR Score*

False-positive (no fetal acidosis or hypoxia; low apgar score)
• Prematurity • Analgesics, narcotics, sedatives • Magnesium sulfate • Acute cerebral trauma • Precipitous delivery • Congenital myopathy • Congenital neuropathy • Spinal cord trauma • Central nervous system anomaly • Lung anomaly (diaphragmatic hernia) • Airway obstruction (choanal atresia) • Congenital pneumonia and sepsis • Previous episodes of fetal asphyxia (recovered) • Hemorrhage-hypovolemia
False-negative (acidosis; normal apgar score)
• Maternal acidosis • High fetal catecholamine levels • Some full-term infants

Normal newborn HR is 120–160 beats/min and RR 30–60/min.

- An extraordinary division of the body from the forehead to the pubis into red and pale halves is known as **harlequin color change**, a transient and harmless condition.
- Mongoloid spots–Slate-blue, well-demarcated areas of pigmentation are seen over the buttocks, back, and sometimes other parts of the body, disappear by 1 year of age.
- Erythema toxicum may persisit for 1 week; contains esinophils.
- Pustular melanosis–vesiculopustular eruption around the chin, neck, back, extremities, and palms or soles; it lasts 2–3 days. DD–Herpes simplex, Staph aureus

Disorders Associated with a Large Anterior Fontanel

- Ac hondroplasia
- Hypothyroidism
- Prematurity
- IUGR
- Trisomies 13, 18, 21

- Cleidocranial dysostosis
- Osteogenesis Imperfecta
- Hydrocephalus
- Congenital Rubella Syndrome
- Vitamin D deficient Rickets.
- **Pupillary reflexes** are present after 28–30 weeks of gestation.
- **Leukokoria** (white pupillary reflex) suggests cataracts, tumor, chorioretinitis, retinopathy of prematurity, or a persistent hyperplastic primary vitreous

Drugs Contraindicated in Breastfeeding

Amphetamines	Doxorubicin
Antineoplastic agents	Ergot
Bromocriptine	Gold salts
Chloramphenicol	Heroin
Clozapine	Immunosuppressants
Cocaine	Iodide
Corticosteroids	Lithium
Cyclophosphamide	Methimazole
Diethystilbesterol	Radiopharmaceuticals

- A reactive (normal) NST (Non Stress Test) result demonstrates two fetal heart rate accelerations of at least 15 beats/min lasting 15 sec.
- The full **BPP** (Bio Physical Pofile) assesses fetal breathing, body movement, tone, heart rate, and amniotic fluid volume, and it is used to improve the accurate and safe identification of fetal compromise. A score of 2 is given for each observation present. A total score of 8–10 is reassuring; a score of 6 is equivocal, and retesting should be done in 12–24 hours; and a score of 4 or less warrants immediate evaluation and possible delivery.
- Feta bradycardia, HR 110/min; Fetal tachycardia HR > 160/min.
- Fetal HR deceleration
  - Early deceleration–Head compression
  - Variable deceleration–Cord compression
  - Late deceleration–Fetal hypoxemia/uteroplacental insufficiency.
- Fetal scalp pH < 7.25 indicates fetal distress.
- Zero dose Hepatitis B vaccine is given to all newborns > 2 kg at birth.
- Inj. Vitamin K1 (not k2 or k3) is administered 1 mg IM to all newborn to prevent hemorrhagic disease of the newborn.
- Not a contraindication to breastfeeding–Hepatitis B, C, E, CMV, HSV, HZV (unless breast lesions), HIV, active TB in developing countries.
- Contraindication to breastfeeding–HIV, active TB in developed countries.
- According to WHO/NACO–National AIDS Control Organization, maternal HIV is not a contraindication to breastfeeding. Pregnant women/post natal mother has to take triple drug Anti Retroviral Therapy (ART) irrespective of HIV staging/CD 4 counts and baby should be given daily Nevirapine syrup depending upon weight of the infant. DNA PCR is done to baby at 6 weeks of life. ART is given to positive infants irrespective of HIV staging/CD 4 counts.
- Hepatitis B vaccine 0.5 ml and Anti Hepatitis B immunoglobin 100 IU is given on separate thighs, to all newborn to HBsAg positive women within 12 hours of birth but not later than 72 hours.
- Polyhydromios. 2000 ml, oligohydromnios < 500 ml.
- Conditions associated with high maternal serum α feto protein
  - Open neural tube defects
  - Gastoschisis

- Omphalocele
- Congenital nephrosis
- Twin pregnancy
- Conditions associated with low maternal serum α feto protein
  - Incorrect gestational age.
  - Trisomy 18, 21
  - IUGR
- Screening in Down's syndrome
  - Nuchal translucency ≥ 6 mm
  - Maternal serum AFP–decreased
  - Serum unconjugated Oestriol-decreased
  - Total and free β HCG–increased
  - Inhibin A–increased
  - Pregnancy associated plasma protein A-decreased.
- Absent fetal nasal bone–Trisomy 21.
- Teratogenic drugs

Accutane (isotretinoin)	Facial-ear anomalies, heart disease, CNS anomalies
Alcohol	Congenital cardiac, CNS, limb anomalies; IUGR; developmental delay; attention deficits; autism
Carbamazepine	Spina bifida, possible neurodevelopmental delay
Carbimazole	Scalp defects, choanal atresia, esophageal atresia, developmental delay
Carbon monoxide	Cerebral atrophy, microcephaly, seizures
Chloroquine	Deafness
Cigarette smoking	LBW baby
Danazol	Virilization
17 α ethinyl testosterone	Masculinization of female fetus
Hyperthermia	Spina bifida
Lithium	Ebstein's anomaly, macrosomia
Methy mercury	Minamata disease, microcephaly, deafness, blindness, mental retardation
Penicillamine	Cutis laxa syndrome
Phenytoin	Congenital anomalies, IUGR,Neuroblastoma, bleeding (vitamin K deficiency)
Prednisone	Oral clefts
Progesterone	Masculinization of female fetus
Statins	IUGR, limb deficiencies, VACTERAL
Diethylstibosterol	Vaginal adenocarcinoma in adolescence
Stretomycin	Deafness
Tetracycline	Retarded skeletal growth, pigmentation of teeth, hypoplasia of enamel, cataract, limb malformations
Thalidomide	Phocomelia, deafness
Valporate	CNS (spina bifida), facial and cardiac anomalies, limb defects, impaired neurologic function
Vitamin D	Supravalvular aortic stenosis, hypercalcemia
Warfarin	Fetal bleeding and death, hypoplastic nasal structures

- The estimated radiation dose for most radiographs is less than 0.1 rad, and for most CT scans it is less than 5 rad. Large doses of radiation (20–50 rad) may cause fetal death (the most sensitive period is the 3rd and 4th post-conception week) as well as microcephaly, severe mental retardation, and growth retardation (the most sensitive period is 4th to 15th week).
- Amniocentesis is usually done between 15th and 16th week.

Small for Gestational Age (SGA)-Less than 10th Percentile

Problems associated with SGA/IUGR babies

Intrauterine fetal demise	Hypoxia, acidosis, infection, lethal anomaly
Perinatal asphyxia	↓ Uteroplacental perfusion during labor ? chronic fetal hypoxia-acidosis; meconium aspiration syndrome
Hypoglycemia	↓ Tissue glycogen stores, ↓ gluconeogenesis, hyperinsulinism, ↑ glucose needs of hypoxia, hypothermia, large brain
Polycythemia-hyperviscosity	Fetal hypoxia with ↑ erythropoietin production
Reduced oxygen consumption/ hypothermia	Hypoxia, hypoglycemia, starvation effect, poor subcutaneous fat stores
Dysmorphology	Syndrome anomalads, chromosomal-genetic disorders, oligohydramnios-induced deformation, TORCH (toxoplasmosis, other agents, rubella, cytomegalovirus, herpes simplex) infection

- New Ballard scoring in preterm newborn

Physical maturity- skin, lanugo, plantar surface breast, eye/ear, genitals

Neuromuscular maturity–Posture, square window, arm recoil, popliteal angle, scarf sign, heel to ear

Each 5 points represent 2 weeks of age. The gestational age for scores are

Score	Gestational age (weeks)
–10	20
0	24
40	40
50	44

NEONATAL PROBLEMS ASSOCIATED WITH PREMATURE INFANTS

Respiratory
• Respiratory distress syndrome (hyaline membrane disease)* • Bronchopulmonary dysplasia • Pneumothorax, pneumomediastinum; interstitial emphysema • Congenital pneumonia • Apnea*
Cardiovascular
• Patent ductus arteriosus* • Hypotension • Bradycardia (with apnea)*
Hematologic
• Anemia (early or late onset)
Gastrointestinal
• Poor gastrointestinal function—poor motility* • Necrotizing enterocolitis • Hyperbilirubinemia—direct and indirect* • Spontaneous gastrointestinal isolated perforation
Metabolic-endocrine
• Hypocalcemia* • Hypoglycemia* • Hyperglycemia* • Late metabolic acidosis • Hypothermia* • Euthyroid but low thyroxine status

Central nervous system
• Intraventricular hemorrhage* • Periventricular leukomalacia • Seizures • Retinopathy of prematurity • Deafness • Hypotonia*
Renal
• Hyponatremia* • Hypernatremia* • Hyperkalemia* • Renal tubular acidosis • Renal glycosuria • Edema
Other
• Infections* (congenital, perinatal, nosocomial: bacterial, viral, fungal, protozoal)

- Large for Gestational Age (LGA) is more than 90th percentile for gestational age.
- Difference between caput saccedaneum, cephalhematoma and subgaleal bleed

	Caput succedaneum	Cephalhematoma	Subgaleal bleed
Swelling	Edema of soft tissue	Hemorrhage beneath periosteum	Hemorrhage beneath galea aponeurotica
Cross midline/sutures	Yes	No	Yes
Extension to neck	No	No	Yes
Underlying skull #	No	Yes	Yes
Underlying coagulopathy	No	No	Possible
Hyperbilirubinemia	Rarely occur in eccymotic swelling	Yes	Yes
Resolve in	Few days	2 weeks 3 months	2–3 weeks

- **HYPOXIC–ISCHEMIC ENCEPHALOPATHY:** Causes permanent CNS damage to the newborn which may lead to death, cerebral palsy or mental retardation. More common with fetal pH, 6.7 or base deficit > 25 mmol/L.

Etiology

- Maternal hypoxia
- Maternal hypotension
- Uteroplacental insufficiency
- PIH
- Postmaturity
- Neonatal respiratory distress
- Shock in the newborn

Pathophysiology

Decreased cerebral blood flow

↓

Hypoxia, Ischemia

↓

↑ lactate and inorganic phosphate

↓

↑ toxic excitatory aminoacids, free radicals, nitric oxide

↓

Cerebral edema, tissue sweeling and damage

Term infants–Neuronal necrosis of cortex, focal/multifocal cortical infarcts, seizures common, hemiplegia
Preterm infants–Periventricular leukomalacia, spastic diplegia
Clinical features–Altered sensorium (hyperalert, lethargic, coma), pupillary chages, tone abnormalities depending upon clinical staging (Sarnat and Sarnat staging I, II, III). Seizures are present in stage II.

Treatment

Supportive care, Selective head/systemic cooling, treatment of seizures (Phenobarbitone DOC)
Prognosis
Stage I–good
Stage II–Variable
Stage III–50 % mortality, remaining 50% severe sequelae.

Neonatal Resuscitation

- Primary apnea–responds to stimulation by establishing normal respiration.
  Secondary apnea–due to asphyxia or neuromuscular disorder
- Indications for Bag and mask ventilation–Apnea/inadequate respiration gasping and HR < 100/min
- Indications for Chest compression–HR < 60/min. despite adequate ventilation.
- Indication for Epinephrine–HR < 60/min despite BMV and chest compression.
- Compression–ventilation ration in newborn is 3 : 1.
- IV Epinephrine dose is 0.01 mg/kg or 0.1 ml/kg of 1: 10,000. The ET dose is 10 times the IV dose
- Contraindication to bag and mask ventilation–Diaphragmatic hernia.
- Non vigorous baby in Meconium stained amniotic fluid–poor respiratory effort, poor muscle tone or HR < 100. Needs endotracheal intubation and suctioning.
- Abdominalm wall defects–Gastroschisis (more common, not covered by membrane), Omphalocele (covered by membrane).
- Most common bone fractured in the newborn during delivery is clavicle.
- Apnea is defined as cessation of breathing for longer than 20 sec or for any duration if accompanied by cyanosis and bradycardia. Types–obstructive, central, mixed. Mixed is the most common type. Recurrent apnea of prematurity maybe treated with theophylline or caffeine.

Respiratory Distress Syndrome

Primarily in preterm infants. (60–80 % in < 28 weeks), rarely in > 37 weeks.
Etiopathogenesis:

Surfactant deficiency (decreased production and secretion) is the primary cause of RDS. The major constituents of surfactant are dipalmitoyl phosphatidylcholine (lecithin), phosphatidylglycerol, apoproteins (surfactant proteins SP–A, SP–B, SP–C, and SP–D), and cholesterol. Surfactant is produced by type II pneumocytes.

Abnormalities in surfactant protein B and C genes as well as a gene responsible for transporting surfactant across membranes (ABC transporter 3 *[ABCA3]*) are associated with severe and often lethal familial respiratory disease. Due to surfactant deficiency lung are not able to maintain FRC.

Alveolar atelectasis, hyaline membrane formation, and interstitial edema make the lungs less compliant in RDS

Clinical features

RDS usually appear within minutes of birth. Tachypnea, retractions, grunting, nasal flaring, cyanosis may occur. **Downe's scoring and Silverman scoring** are used in assessing respiratory distress in newborn.

- **X-ray findings in Neonatal diseases**

Disease	CXR finding
RDS	• Low lung volume • Reticulogranular pattern, air bronchogram • Ground glass opacities • White out lungs

Contd...

Disease	CXR finding
TTN (Transient tachypnea of newborn)	• Normal/hyperinflated lungs • Prominent minor interlobar fissure • Mild cardiomegaly • Prominent hilar, pulmonary markings • Flat diapharagm • Small pleural effusion.
MAS (Meconium Aspiration Syndrome)	• Hyperinflation • Areas of patchy atelectasis
Congenital pneumonia	• Low to normal lung volume • Patchy atelectasis
PPHN (Persisitent pulmonary Hypertension)	• Pulmonary oligemia • Features of underlying lung disease
Air leaks	• Pleural air • Mediastinal shift

Treatment–O_2, CPAP, Surfactant, ventilatory care.

Long term complication–Bronchopumonary dysplasia (treatment with > 21% O_2 for atleast 28 days). Vitamin A prophylaxis reduces the incidence of BPD, death.

Treatment of BPD includes furosemide, thiazide diuretics, salbutamol, iptratropium, theophylline etc.

Transient Tachypnea of Newborn

- Usually follows uneventful preterm or term vaginal delivery or caesarean section.
- Recovery is rapid within 3 days.
- Minimal retraction needing not more than 40% O_2.
- Hypercapnea and acidosis uncommon
- Secondary to slow absorption fetal lung fluid.
- Treatment is supportive.
- Malignant TTN–severe morbidity and mortality may occur in some case due to pulmonary hypertension.

Meconium Aspiration Syndrome

- Occurs in term and post term infants.
- Fetal distress → Meconium passage → meconium stained liquor → inuterogasping and postpartum aspiration → proximal and distal airway obstruction, chemical pneumonitis → lead to atelectasis, air traping and air leak, V/Q mismatch, pulmonary vascular remodeling, PPHN (Persisten Pulmonary Hypertension) finally lead to → hypoxia, hypercapnea, acidosis.
- Respiratory distress in first hour of life-tachypnea, retractions, cyanosis, grunting.
- Can be prevented by early induction of delivery in late deceleration or poor beat to beat variability of HR. Aminoinfusion and intrapartum suctioning not recommended.
- Tracheal suction is recommended for non-vigorous baby. Supportive care, ventilator support, Sildenafil for PPHN are treatment modalities.
- Air leaks (pneumothorax, pneumomediastinum) and PPHN are common complications.
- Treatment of PPHN–O_2, inotropes (**Dopamine**, dobutamine, epinephrine, milrinone), ventilator support, Nitric oxide, Sildenafil and ECMO (Extra Corporeal Menbrane Oxygenation).

Congenital Diaphragmatic Hernia

- Bokdalek hernia accounts for 90% and Morgagni 2–6%. Left side hernia is common (85%).
- Less than 5% are bilateral.
- **Pulmonary hypoplasia** is a major limiting factor for survival.
- Can be diagnosed in > 50% of cases in prenatal USG between 16–24 weeks.

- Findings on ultrasonography may include polyhydramnios, chest mass, mediastinal shift, gastric bubble or a liver in the thoracic cavity, and fetal hydrops.
- DD–pulmonary sequestration, cystadenoid malformation
- Respiratory distress can occur soon after birth or after 48 hours.
- Scaphoid abdomen and mediastinal shift are clues to diagnosis.
- Inotropes, ventilator support, ECMO are supportive treatment. Corrective surgery is the treatment of choice usually done at 48 hours after stabilization of the infant and resolution of pulmonary hypertension.
- Lung Head Ratio(LHR) in prenatal USG (24–26 weeks) is a good prognostic indicator. There were no survivors when the LHR was <1, and all babies with LHR >1.4 survived. Presence of liver in thorax is a poor prognostic sign.
- Treatment of meconium ileus is Gastrografin enema.

Necrotizing Enterocolitis (NEC)

Most common life threatening emergency of GIT in newborn. Etiology is multifactorial. Mucosal and transmural necrosis of intestine occurs.

Pneumatosis intestinalis–accumulation of gas in submucosa occurs which may progress to necrosis, perforation, sepsis and death.

About 90% occur in preterm infants.

The triad of intestinal ischemia (injury), enteral nutrition (metabolic substrate), and bacterial translocation has classically been linked to NEC.

Imaging(USG/ X-ray)–pneumatosis intestinalis, portal venous gas, pneumoperitonium.

Three staging by Bell.

Stage I–Suspect

Stage II–Definite

Stagee III–Advanced

Treatment includes–NPO, Nasogastric aspiration, antibiotics and surgery (resection with enterostomy or primary anastomosis).

Neonatal Jaundice

Diagnostic features of the various types of neonatal jaundice

Diagnosis	Nature of van den bergh reaction	Jaundice		Peak bilirubin concentration		Bilirubin rate of accumulation (mg/dl/day)	Remarks
		Appears	Disappears	Mg/dl	Age in days		
'Physiologic jaundice'							Usually relates to degree of maturity
Fullterm	Indirect	2–3 days	4–5 days	10–12	2–3	<5	
Premature	Indirect	3–4 days	7–9 days	15	6–8	<5	
Hyperbilirubinemia due to metabolic factors:							Metabolic factors: hypoxia, respiratory distress, lack of carbohydrate
Fullterm	Indirect	2–3 days	Variable	>12	1st week	<5	Hormonal influences: cretinism, hormones, Gilbert syndrome
Premature	Indirect	3–4 days	Variable	>15	1st week	<5	Genetic factors: Crigler-Najjar syndrome, Gilbert syndrome Drugs: vitamin K, novobiocin

Contd...

Contd...

Diagnosis	Nature of van den bergh reaction	Jaundice		Peak bilirubin concentration		Bilirubin rate of accumulation (mg/dl/day)	Remarks
		Appears	Disappears	Mg/dl	Age in days		
Hemolytic states and hematoma	Indirect	May appear in 1st 24 hours	Variable	Unlimited	Variable	Usually >5	Erythroblastosis: Rh, ABO, Kell Congenital hemolytic states: spherocytic, nonspherocytic Infantile pyknocytosis
							Drugs: vitamin K Enclosed hemorrhage–hematoma
Mixed hemolytic and hepatotoxic factors	Indirect and direct	May appear in 1st 24 hours	Variable	Unlimited	Variable	Usually >5	Infection: bacterial sepsis, pyelonephritis, hepatitis, toxoplasmosis, cytomegalic inclusion disease, rubella, syphilis Drugs: vitamin K
Hepatocellular damage	Indirect and direct	Usually 2–3 days; may appear by 2nd week	Variable	Unlimited	Variable	Variable, can be >5	Biliary atresia; paucity of bile ducts, familial cholestasis, galactosemia; hepatitis and infection

Kernicterus

- Kernicterus, or bilirubin encephalopathy, is a neurologic syndrome resulting from the deposition of unconjugated (indirect) bilirubin in the basal ganglia and brainstem nuclei.
- Occurs in 30% if serum bilirubin is 25–30 mg%.
- Occurs after 2–5 days in term infants and up to 7 days in preterm infants.
- Lethargy, poor feeding, and loss of the Moro reflex are common initial signs.
- Opisthotonos with a bulging fontanel, twitching of the face or limbs, and a shrill high-pitched cry, convulsions and spasm occur later. Rigidity is rare at late stage.
- After 1 year, movement disorders (choreoathetosis, ballismus, tremor), upward gaze, sensorineural hearing loss may occur.

Anemia

Term cord bilirubin is 16.8 g% (14–20).

Anemia of prematurity occurs in LBW infants 1–3 months after birth, Hb levels <7–10 g/dL.

Delayed cord clamping (≈1–2 min or after cessation of cord pulsation) maybe beneficial in preventing anemia in full-term well newborn.

Swallowed maternal blood in newborn can be differentiated by APT test (using 0.25 N NaOH) which detects fetal Hb (alkali resistant). Kleihauer-Betke test and flow cytometer also differentiate fetal and maternal Hb.

Term umbilical cord length is 55 cm.

Treatment of umbilical granuloma is cauterization with silver nitrate.

Umbilical Hernia

Usually disappear by 6 months to 1 year.

Even large hernias (5–6 cm in all dimensions) disappear spontaneously by 5–6 years of age.

Strangulation is rare.
Strapping is ineffective.
Surgery is indicated if

- hernia persists to the age of 4–5 year,
- causes symptoms,
- becomes strangulated, or
- becomes progressively larger after the age of 1–2 year.

Defects exceeding 2 cm are less likely to close spontaneously.

Infant of Diabetic Mother

Maternal hyperglycemia → Fetal hyperglycemia → Fetal hyperinsulinemia → ↑ lipogenesis and protein synthesis.
Complications

- Macrosomia, birth trauma
- Hypoglycemia
- Hypocalcemia
- Hyperbilirubinemia
- Polycythemia
- Respiratory Distress Syndrome.
- Renal vein thrombosis
- Lazy left colon syndrome
- Cardiac–Asymmetrical septal hypertrophy-MC, VSD, ASD, TGA, Truncus arteriosus, Ticuspid Atresia, DORV, COA.
- Lumbosacral agenesis, Neural tube defect
- Hydronephrosis, Renal agenesis, double ureter
- Duodenal/anorectal atresia
- Situs inversus, holoprosencephaly

Indications for Karyotyping

- At least one major and two minor malformations
- At least two major malformations
- Developmental or growth retardation with two or more major or minor anomalies
- Gold standard test for the evaluation of a dysmorphic child is karyotyping.

Handwashing

Single most important means of preventing nosocomial infection.

2 minutes handwashing (6 steps) to be done before entering the newborn unit and **20 seconds** before and after touching the babies.

Steps of handwashing.

Roll sleeves above elbow. Remove wrist watch, bangles, rings etc. Use plain water and soap with the following sequence.

- Palms and fingers and web spaces
- Back of hands
- Fingers and knuckles
- Thumbs
- Finger tips
- Wrist and forearm up to elbow.

Kangaroo Mother Care

Two components of KMC—

- Skin–skin contact
- Exclusive breastfeeding

Two prerequisites of KMC

- Support to mother in hospital and home
- Post discharge follow up

Benefits of KMC

- Temperature maintenance with reduced risk of hypothermia
- Increased breastfeeding rates
- Early dischare from health facility
- Less morbidities such as apnea and infections
- Less stress (for mother nad baby)
- Better infant bonding

Eligibility criteria

All stable LBW babies are eligible for KMC

- Birth wt > 1800 g–soon after birth
- Birth wt 1200–1799 g–after a few days
- Birth wt < 1200 g–after days to weeks

Positioning

- Baby should be placed between the mother's breasts in an upright position
- Head should be turned to one side in a slightly extended position keeping airway open and allows eye contact between baby and mother
- Hips are flexed and abducted (frog position) and arms flexed
- Baby's abdomen at mother's epigatrium–mother's breathing stimulates baby and reduces apnea

Support baby's bottom with sling/binder

Duration–At least 1 hour session, up to 24 hours/day.

Mother, father or any relative can provide KMC.

KMC can be provided to babies on OG feeds, IV fluids or oxygen or the when mother is sleeping in semi-recumbent position.

ALLERGY, ASTHMA, IMMUNOLOGY

Atopic individuals respond to allergen exposure with rapid expansion of **T helper type 2 (Th2)** cells. Th1 cells are typically involved in the eradication of intracellular organisms, such as mycobacteria.

Chronic allergic reactions are characterized by infiltration of Th1 and **Th17 cells**

Formal evaluation of asthma exacerbation severity in the urgent or emergency care setting*

	Mild	Moderate	Severe	Subset: respiratory arrest imminent
Symptoms				
Breathlessness	While walking	While at rest (infant–softer, shorter cry, difficulty feeding)	While at rest (infant–stops feeding)	
	Can lie down	Prefers sitting	Sits upright	
Talks in	Sentences	Phrases	Words	
Alertness	Maybe agitated	Usually agitated	Usually agitated	Drowsy or confused
Signs				
Respiratory rate	Increased	Increased	Often >30 breaths/min	
Use of accessory muscles; suprasternal retractions	Usually not	Commonly	Usually	Paradoxical thoracoabdominal movement

Contd...

Contd...

	Mild	Moderate	Severe	Subset: respiratory arrest imminent
Wheeze	Moderate; often only end-expiratory	Loud; throughout exhalation	Usually loud; throughout inhalation and exhalation	Absence of wheeze
Pulse rate (beats/min)	<100	100–120	>120	Bradycardia
Pulsus paradoxus	Absent <10 mm Hg	Maybe present 10–25 mm Hg	Often present >25 mm Hg (adult) 20–40 mm Hg (child)	Absence suggests respiratory muscle fatigue
Functional assessment				
Peak expiratory flow (value predicted or personal best)	≥70%	Approx. 40–69% or response lasts <2 hours	<40%	<25% [?]
Pao_2 (breathing air) and/or	Normal (test not usually necessary)	≥60 mm Hg (test not usually necessary)	<60 mm Hg; possible cyanosis	
Pco_2	<42 mm Hg (test not usually necessary)	<42 mm Hg (test not usually necessary)	≥42 mm Hg; possible respiratory failure	
Sao_2 (breathing air) at sea level	>95% (test not usually necessary)	90–95% (test not usually necessary)	<90%	
	Hypercapnia (hypoventilation) develops more readily in young children than in adults and adolescents			

Lung function abnormalities in asthma

Spirometry (in clinic):
Airflow limitation:
- Low FEV_1 (relative to percentage of predicted norms)
- FEV_1/FVC ratio <0.80

Bronchodilator response (to inhaled β-agonist):
- Improvement in FEV_1 ≥12% and ≥200 mL*

Exercise challenge:
- Worsening in FEV_1 ≥15%*

Daily peak flow or FEV_1 monitoring: day to day and/or am-to-pm variation ≥20%*

Acute Atopic Dermatitis skin lesions are characterized by **spongiosis,** or marked intercellular edema, of the epidermis.

Chronic Atopic Dermatitis is characterized by
- Lichenification
- Thckening of skin
- Fibrotic papules (prurigo nodularis).

Treatment of AD

- Cutaneous hydration
- Topical steroids
- Topical calcineurin inhibitors
- Tar preparations
- Antihistamines
- Systemic steroids
- Cyclosporine
- PUVA therapy

Rheumatic Diseases of Childhood

Criteria for the classification of juvenile rheumatoid arthritis

Age at onset: <16 years Arthritis (swelling or effusion, or the presence of 2 or more of the following signs: limitation of range of motion, tenderness or pain on motion, increased heat) in ≥1 joints Duration of disease: ≥6 weeks Onset type defined by type of articular involvement in the 1st 6 months after onset: Polyarthritis: ≥5 inflamed joints Oligoarthritis: ≤4 inflamed joints Systemic disease: arthritis with rash and a characteristic quotidian fever Exclusion of other forms of juvenile arthritis

Juvenile Dermatomyositis

- Shawl sign–erthema over chest and neck
- Heliotrope rash–blue–violet discoloration eyelid ± periorbital edema
- **Gottron papules**–bright pink or pale, shiny, thickened or atrophic plaques over the proximal interphalangeal joints and distal interphalangeal joints
- **Mechanic's hands**–thickened erythematous and scaly rash develops in children over the palms

Diagnostic criteria for juvenile dermatomyositis

Classic rash	Heliotrope rash of the eyelids Gottron papules
Plus three of the following:	
Weakness	Symmetric Proximal
Muscle enzyme elevation (≥1)	Creatine kinase Aspartate aminotransferase Lactate dehydrogenase Aldolase
Electromyographic changes	Myopathy Denervation
Muscle biopsy	Necrosis Inflammation

Amyopathic JDM–Some children present with classic rash but no apparent muscle weakness or inflammation.

Kawasaki disease (formerly known as **mucocutaneous lymph node syndrome** and **infantile polyarteritis nodosa)**

Epidemiologic case definition (classic clinical criteria)*
Fever persisting **at least 5 days** Presence of at least 4 principal features: Changes in extremities: Acute: Erythema of palms, soles; edema of hands, feet Subacute: Periungual peeling of fingers, toes in weeks 2 and 3 Polymorphous exanthem Bilateral bulbar conjunctival injection without exudate Changes in lips and oral cavity: Erythema, lip cracking, strawberry tongue, diffuse injection of oral and pharyngeal mucosa Cervical lymphadenopathy (>1.5 cm diameter), **usually unilateral** Exclusion of other diseases with similar findings
Cardiovascular findings: Congestive heart failure, myocarditis, pericarditis, valvular regurgitation Coronary artery abnormalities Aneurysms of medium-sized noncoronary arteries Raynaud phenomenon Peripheral gangrene Musculoskeletal system: Arthritis, arthralgias

Contd...

Contd...

Laboratory findings in acute kawasaki disease
Leukocytosis with neutrophilia and immature forms
Elevated erythrocyte sedimentation rate (ESR)
Elevated C-reactive protein (CRP)
Anemia
Abnormal plasma lipids
Hypoalbuminemia
Hyponatremia
Thrombocytosis after week 1
Sterile pyuria
Elevated serum transaminases
Elevated serum gamma glutamyl transpeptidase
Pleocytosis of cerebrospinal fluid
Leukocytosis in synovial fluid

ECHO is done at diagnosis and 2–3 weeks of illness.

Coronory artery aneurysms have been defined with use of absolute dimensions by the Japanese Ministry of Health and are classified as small (<5 mm internal diameter), medium (5–8 mm internal diameter), or giant (>8 mm internal diameter).

Treatment

- Acute stage–IV Ig, High dose Aspirin
- Convalascent stage–Low dose aspirin
- Long term therapy–Low dose aspirin, Clopidogrel, LMW Heparin, Warfarin.

TNF inhibitor Infliximab is used in IV Ig resistant cases.

GIT, LIVER

- Most commn cause of emesis in children–Gastroenteritis.
- Acid-base/electrolyte abnormalities in vomiting are metabolic alkalosis, hypochloremia, hyponatremia and hypokalemia.
- Acute diarrhea–excessive loose stools of >10 mL/kg/day in infants and >200 g/24 hours in older children, which lasts <14 days.
- Chronic diarrhea– > 14 days. Constipation–a hard stool passed with difficulty every 3rd day.
- MC cause of GIT bleeding in children–Bacterial enteritis.
- MC cause of massive upper GI bleeding in children–EHPVO (Extra hepatic portal vein obstruction).
- **Anodontia** or absence of teeth, occurs when no tooth buds form (e.g. ectodermal dysplasia, or familial missing teeth).
- **Twinning**–2 teeth are joined together.
- **Gemination**–division of 1 tooth germ to form a bifid crown on a single root with a common pulp canal.
- **Amelogenesis imperfecta**–hereditary condition that manifests in enamel defects of the primary and permanent teeth without evidence of systemic disorders.
- **Fluorosis** (mottled enamel–results from systemic fluoride consumption >0.05 mg/kg/day during enamel formation, residing in an area of high fluoride content of the drinking water (>2.0 ppm).

Primary mechanism	Defect	Stool examination	Examples	Comment
Secretory	Decreased absorption, **increased secretion,** electrolyte transport	Watery, normal osmolality with ion **gap <100 mOsm/kg**	**Cholera, toxigenic Escherichia coli; carcinoid, VIP, neuroblastoma,** congenital chloride diarrhea, *Clostridium difficile,* cryptosporidiosis (AIDS)	**Persists during fasting;** bile salt malabsorption can also increase intestinal water secretion; no stool leukocytes

Contd...

Contd...

Osmotic	Maldigestion, transport defects, ingestion of **unabsorbable substances**	Watery, acidic, and **reducing substances** +; increased osmolality with ion gap >100 mOsm/kg	**Lactase deficiency,** glucose-galactose malabsorption, **lactulose,** laxative abuse	**Stops with fasting;** increased breath hydrogen with carbohydrate malabsorption; no stool leukocytes

Surgical condition	Time of surgery
Cleft lip	3 months
Cleft palate	Before 1 year.
Congenital Inguinal hernia	Soon after diagnosis in infants
Hypospadiasis	6–12 months
Congenital Hydrocele	12–18 months

MC organism associated with dental carries–Streptococcus mutans.

Parulis (gum boil)–soft reddish papule located adjacent to the root of a chronically abscessed tooth. In the most common form of Esophageal Atresia/Tracheo-Esophageal Fistula, the upper esophagus ends in a blind pouch and the TEF is connected to the distal esophagus.

Triad of Achalasia, Alacrima, and ACTH corticotropin insensitivity is known as **Allgrove syndrome (AAA Syndrome).**

Spontaneous esophageal rupture **(Boerhaave syndrome)** is caused by sudden increases in intraesophageal pressure in situations such as vomiting, coughing, or straining at stool.

Portal hypertension is defined as an elevation of portal venous pressure to levels 10–12 mm Hg higher than pressures present in the inferior vena cava.

Asymptomatic foreign bodies (blunt objects and coins) lodged in the esophagus can be observed for up to 24 hours in anticipation of passage into the stomach.

Infantile Hypertropic Pyloric Stenosis

Risk factors

- First born males
- H/O IHPS in the mother
- White race, rare in Asians.
- B and O blood group.
- Tracheo Esophageal Fistula
- Hypoplasia of inferior labial frenulum.

Etiology

- Idiopathic
- Monozygotic twins
- Use of Erythromycin in first 2 weeks of life.
- Use of macrolide antibiotics in mothers during pregnancy and breastfeeding
- Reduced levels of neuronal nitric oxide synthase (nNOS)

Clinical features

- Non bilious vomiting
- Usually after 3rd week of life (1 week to 5 months)
- Baby hungry after vomiting
- Asso. with unconjugated hyperbilirubinemia (icteropyloric syndrome)
- Firm olive shaped mass on left side of abdmen
- Visible gastric peristalysis.

Diagnosis

- USG–pyloric thickness 3–4 mm, length 15–19 mm, diameter 10–14 mm.
- Contrast - elongated pyloric channel (string sign), a bulge of the pyloric muscle into the antrum (shoulder sign), and parallel streaks of barium seen in the narrowed channel–"double tract sign".
- Metabolic alkalosis, hyponatremia, hypochloremia, hypokalemia.

Treatment

- Surgical procedure of choice is pyloromyotomy–Ramstedt procedure

Meckel's Diverticulum

- Most common GIT anomaly in infants.
- Remnant of embryonic yolk sac.
- Also known as persistent omphalomesentic duct/vitellointestinal duct.
- Between the 5th and 7th weeks of gestation, the duct attenuates and separates from the intestine.
- 3–6 cm outpouching of the ileum along the antimesenteric border 50–75 cm from the ileocecal valve.

Intussusception

- Most common cause of intestinal obstruction between 3 months and 6 years of age
- Most common abdominal emergency in children <2 years.
- Male predominance (3 : 1)

Etiology

- Idiopathic (90%)
- Asso. with Aenovirus type C respiratory infection
- Was receiving a tetravalent rotavirus vaccine within 2 weeks of immunization (now banned).
- Swollen Peyer patches in the terminal ileum, Lymphoid nodular hyperplasia are risk factors.
- **Recognizable lead points** for the intussusception are Meckel diverticulum, intestinal polyp, neurofibroma, intestinal duplication cysts, hemangioma, or malignant conditions such as lymphoma. Lead points are more common in children >2 years of age.
- The upper portion of bowel, the **intussusceptum,** invaginates into the lower, the **intussuscipiens.**

Clinical features

- The classic triad of pain, a palpable sausage-shaped abdominal mass, and bloody or currant jelly stool is less common.
- Previously will child has coliky abd. Pain.
- Straining efforts with legs and knees flexed and loud cries
- Normal in between
- Lethargy,vomiting, fever, shock can occur
- **Recurrent intussusception** is noted in 5–8% and is more common after hydrostatic than surgical reduction.

Diagnosis

- X-ray–density in the site of intussception
- USG–Doughnut or Target appearance in transverse view
- Contrast enema–coiled spring sign

Treatment

- Surgical reduction
- Hydrostatic reduction under fluoroscopic or ultrasonic guidance (recurrence present)

Traveller's diarrhea–Enterotoxigenic E.coli

Pediatric Appendicitis Scores

Feature	Score
Fever >38 °C	1
Anorexia	1
Nausea/vomiting	1
Cough/percussion/hopping tenderness	2
Right lower quadrant tenderness	2
Migration of pain	1
Leukocytosis >10,000 (10^9/L)	1
Polymorphonuclear-neutrophilia >7,500 (10^9/L)	1
Total	10

Score ≤2 -> less likely appendicitis

Scores ≥ 8 highly asso with appendicitis

Score between 3 and 7 needs further evaluation.

The ultrasound criteria for appendicitis include wall thickness ≥6 mm, luminal distention, lack of compressibility, a complex mass in the RLQ, or a fecalith.

Treatment of Rectal mucosal prolapse

- Delorme mucosal sleeve resection
- Frykman-Goldberg procedure
- Ripstein procedure and
- Altemeier perineal rectosigmoidectomy

Pancreatitis–A bluish discoloration seen around the umbilicus (***Cullen*** sign) or in the flanks (***Grey Turner*** sign).

Alagille syndrome (arteriohepatic dysplasia) is the most common syndrome with intrahepatic bile duct paucity

Byler disease–Progressive familial intrahepatic cholestasis type 1 (PFIC 1) or FIC1 disease is a severe form of intrahepatic cholestasis. Presents steatorrhea, pruritus, vitamin D–deficient rickets, gradually developing cirrhosis, and **low** γ-glutamyl transpeptidase (GGT) levels. The absence of bile duct paucity and extrahepatic features differentiate this disorder from Alagille syndrome.

Caroli disease–Intrahepatic cholestasis due to embryonic ductal plate malformation.

Neonatal iron storage disease (NISD; neonatal hemochromatosis)– ↑ iron deposition in the liver, heart, and endocrine organs without increased iron stores in the reticuloendothelial system. Alloimmune disorder with maternal antibodies directed against the fetal liver. Laboratory findings include hypoglycemia, hyperbilirubinemia, hypoalbuminemia, and profound hypoprothrombinemia. Treatment is exchange transfusion and IV Ig. Liver transplant maybe curative. Prognosis is poor.

Biliary atresia–Gallbladder either is not visualized or is a microgallbladder in USG. Triangular cord sign is seen. Hepatobiliary scintigraphy differentiates biliary atresia from non obstructive causes. Treatment is **hepatoportoenterostomy (Kasai) procedure.** Success rate is 90% if done before 8 weeks of life.

Liver Biopsy

Biliary atresia–bile duct proliferation, biliary plug, portal or periloblar edema and fibrosis,but basic lobular architecture is intact.

Neonatal hepatitis–severe hepatocellular disease, distortion of lobular structure, marked infiltration with inflmatory cells, focal hepatocellular necrosis, bile ductules show little alteration.

Wilson Disease

Hepatolenticular degeneration, Autosomal recesseive, Chromosome 13(13q14). (Retinoblastoma gene RB 1 is also located in 13q14).

Defect in copper transporting ATPase ATP 7B which respsible for biliary copper excretion and incorporation of copper into ceruloplasmin.

Copper is accumulated in liver, brain and kidneys.

Liver involvement more common in young patients. (M:F = 1:3). After 20 years of age, neurological symptoms predominate.

Neurological symptoms–intention tremor, dysarthria, rigid dystonia, parkinsonism, choreiform movements, motor incoordination, deterioration in school performance, or behavioral changes.

Kayser-Fleischer rings maybe absent in young patients with liver disease but are always present in patients with neurologic symptoms.

Coomb's negative anemia is present.

Serum Ceruloplasmin < 20 mg/Dl.

Urine copper > 100 μg/day

Hepatic copper > 250 μg/g of dry weight.

Treatment

- Restrict copper intake < 1 mg/day.
- D Penicillamine
- Ammonium tetrathio molybdate (for neurological disease)
- Zinc
- Liver transplant is curative in 85-90%.

Fulminant hepatic failure–

- biochemical evidence of acute liver injury (**usually <8 weeks duration**);
- no evidence of chronic liver disease; and
- hepatic-based coagulopathy defined as a prothrombin time (PT) >15 sec or international normalized ratio (INR) >1.5 not corrected by vitamin K in the presence of clinical hepatic encephalopathy, or a PT >20 sec or INR >2 regardless of the presence of clinical hepatic encephalopathy.

Fulminant hepatic failure can be a complication of viral hepatitis (A, B, D, E) not C.

RESPIRATORY SYSTEM

Interpreting the clinical signs of respiratory disease

Sign	Extrathoracic airway obstruction	Intrathoracic-extrapulmonary airway obstruction	Intrapulmonary airway obstruction	Parenchymal pathology
Tachypnea	+	+	++	++++
Retractions	++++	++	++	+++
Stridor	++++	++	–	–
Wheezing	–	+++	++++	–
Grunting	–	–	++	++++

Pickwikian syndrome–chronic alveolar hypoventilation and right heart failure in children with marked obesity.

MC cause of common cold–Rhinovirus.

Common bacteria causing sinusitis in children and adolescents are Streptococcus pneumoniae (~30%), nontypable Hemophilus influenzae (~20%), and Moraxella catarrhalis (~20%).

Lemierre disease–characteristic infection of the parapharyngeal space, in which infection from the oropharynx extends to cause septic thrombophlebitis of the internal jugular vein and embolic abscesses in the lungs. The causative pathogen is *Fusobacterium necrophorum.* Manifests with fever, toxicity, neck pain and stiffness, and respiratory distress due to multiple septic pulmonary emboli. Treatment-Ampicillin-sulbactam, clindamycin, penicillin, or ciprofloxacin and heparinizationli.

Most common cause of bacterial infection in the pharynx–Group A β-hemolytic streptococcus (GABHS)

Most episodes of acute pharyngotonsillitis are caused by viruses.

Most common cause of stridor in infants–Laryngomalacia.

Most common cause of acute upper airway obstruction in children–Croup, Acute Larygotracheobronchitis (ALTB). X ray finding in ALTB is narrowing of subglottis(Steeple sign).

MC cause of ALTB–Parainfluenza virus.

MC cause for acute epiglottitis–H. Influenza type b. X-ray finding in acute epiglottitis is "Thump sign".

MC cause of bacterial tracheitis–Stauph aureus. X-ray shows pseudomembrane detachment in trachea.

Prophylaxis for house hold contacts of H. Influenza infection–Rifaampcin.

Prophylaxis for house hold, day care, school contacts of N. meningitides infection–Rifampicin, Cefriaxone and Ciprofloxacin.

MC respiratory tract neoplasm in children–Papilloma

MC cause of acute bronchiolitis–Respiratory Syncytial Virus.

MC site of Congenital Lobar Emphysema–Left upper lobe.

Radiographic features that may help differentiate cardiogenic from noncardiogenic pulmonary edema

Radiographic feature	Cardiogenic edema	Noncardiogenic edema
Heart size	Normal or greater than normal	Usually normal
Width of the vascular pedicle*	Normal or greater than normal	Usually normal or less than normal
Vascular distribution	Balanced or inverted	Normal or balanced
Distribution of edema	Even or central	Patchy or peripheral
Pleural effusions	Present	Not usually present
Peribronchial cuffing	Present	Not usually present
Septal lines	Present	Not usually present
Air bronchograms	Not usually present	Usually present

Measurement of brain natriuretic peptide (BNP), often elevated in heart disease, can help differentiate cardiac from pulmonary causes of pulmonary edema. A BNP level >500 pg/mL suggests heart disease; a level <100 pg/mL suggests lung disease.

Silo filler disease (also known as **silage gas poisoning** or **silo filler pneumoconiosis)** is caused by nitrogen dioxide toxicity.

Paraquet poisoning presents with vomiting, diarrhea, and caustic injury to the oral or esophageal mucosa and may develop renal failure, hepatic dysfunction, and progressive pulmonary fibrosis, resulting in respiratory failure and death.

Primary eosinophilic lung diseases include simple pulmonary eosinophilia (Loffler syndrome), acute eosinophilic pneumonia, chronic eosinophilic pneumonia, and idiopathic hypereosinophilic syndrome.

Secondary eosinophilic lung diseases include tropical pulmonary eosinophilia, pulmonary eosinophilia with asthma, polyarteritis nodosa, Churg-Strauss syndrome, allergic bronchopulmonary aspergillosis (ABPA), and drug-induced eosinophilic lung disease.

Most common cause of under 5 mortality in the world is pneumonia (19%) followed by diarrhoea (17%).

Pneumonia organisms w.r.t. age

3 weeks to 4 years–Streptococcus pneumonia

>5 years–Mycoplasm Chlamidia.

Recurrent pneumonia is defined **as 2 or more** episodes in a single year **or 3 or more** episodes ever, with radiographic clearing between occurrences.

Differentiation of Pleural Fluid

	Transudate	Empyema
Appearance	Clear	Cloudy or purulent
Cell count (per mm^3)	<1000	Often >50,000 (cell count has limited predictive value)
Cell type	Lymphocytes, monocytes	Polymorphonuclear leukocytes (neutrophils)
Lactate dehydrogenase	<200 U/L	>1000 U/L
Pleural fluid/serum LDH ratio	<0.6	>0.6
Protein >3g	Unusual	Common
Pleural fluid/serum protein ratio	<0.5	>0.5
Glucose	Normal	Low (<40 mg/dL)
pH	Normal (7.40–7.60)	<7.10
Gram stain	Negative	Occasionally positive (less than one-third of cases)

Few syndromes associated with Bronchiectasis

- William–**C**ampell syndrome–congenital absence of annular bronchial **c**artilage.
- **M**arnier–Kuhn syndrome–congenital tracheobroncho**m**egaly
- Right middle lobe syndrome–chronic extrinsic compression of right middle lobe bronchus by hilar lymph nodes.
- Yellow nail syndrome–pleural effusion, lymphedema, discolored nails.

Treatment of Pulmonary abscess is conservative. Two to three weeks of IV antibiotics followed by oral drugs for total 4–6 weeks. Surgery is reserved for seriously ill children who fail after 7–10 days of IV antibiotics.

cystic fibrosis transmembrane conductance regulator protein (CFTR) has more than 1500 mutations of which Δ F 508 is the most common(50%).

The common presentations of Cystic Fibrosis are (most common to less common)

- Acute or persistent respiratory symptoms (45%)
- Failure to thrive, malnutrition
- Abnormal stools
- Meconium ileus, intestinal obstruction (20%)

Acid–base imbalance in CF is hypochloremic alkalosis.

DIAGNOSTIC CRITERIA FOR CYSTIC FIBROSIS (CF)

Presence of typical clinical features (respiratory, gastrointestinal, or genitourinary)
OR
A history of CF in a sibling
OR
A positive newborn screening test
PLUS
Laboratory evidence for CFTR (CF transmembrane regulator) dysfunction:
Two elevated sweat chloride concentrations obtained on separate days (Cl− ≥ 60 mEq/L)
OR
Identification of two CF mutations
OR
An abnormal nasal potential difference measurement

Conditions associated with false-positive and false-negative sweat test results

With false-positive results
Eczema (atopic dermatitis) Ectodermal dysplasia Malnutrition/failure to thrive/deprivation Anorexia nervosa Congenital adrenal hyperplasia Adrenal insufficiency Glucose-6-phosphatase deficiency Mauriac syndrome Fucosidosis Familial hypoparathyroidism Hypothyroidism Nephrogenic diabetes insipidus Pseudohypoaldosteronism Klinefelter syndrome Familial cholestasis syndrome Autonomic dysfunction Prostaglandin E infusions Munchausen syndrome by proxy
With false-negative results
Dilution Malnutrition Edema Insufficient sweat quantity Hyponatremia Cystic fibrosis transmembrane conductance regulator (CFTR) mutations with preserved sweat duct function

Forms of bronchopulmonary dysplasia (BPD)

Features of all BPD	Additional features of mild BPD	Additional features of moderate BPD	Additional features of severe BPD
<32 weeks postmenstrual age (PMA) Oxygen requirement first 28 days	Breathing room air at 36 week PMA	<30% supplemental oxygen at 36 week PMA	>30% supplemental oxygen at 36 week PMA and mechanical support, continuous positive airway pressure (CPAP), or ventilation
>32 weeks PMA Oxygen requirement first 28 days of life	Breathing room air at 56 days of life	<30% supplemental oxygen at 56 days of life	>30% supplemental oxygen at 56 days of life and mechanical support, CPAP, or ventilation

CARDIOLOGY

Primitive cardiac tube is formed at 22 days of gestation.

The **total fetal cardiac output**—the combined output of both the left and right ventricles—is ≈450 mL/kg/min. (65% flows to placenta and 35% perfuses fetal organs and tissues).

Newborn cardiac output is 350 mL/kg/min and that of adult is 75 mL/kg/min.

The foramen ovale is functionally closed by the 3rd mo of life.

Functional closure of the ductus arteriosus is complete by 10–15 hours. The ductal wall begins to constrict when PO2 is 50 mm Hg.

Tall P-waves → 2.5 mm indicates Right atrial enlargement. For example, Congenital pulmonary stenosis, Ebstein's anomaly, Tricuspid atresia, Cor pulmonale.

Broad P-waves (or bifid, biphasic)–Left atrial enlargement. For example, VSD, PDA, MS, MR.

T-wave is normally inverted in V1 in children up to 8 years of life. Positive T-wave in V1 signifies RVH.

MC congenital cardiac lesion–VSD (35%), followed by ASD (6–8%), PDA (6–8%), COA (5–7%) and TOF (5–7%).

Mutation in Di George syndrome–Ch 22q11.2

Incidence of Congenital heart disease in general population–0.8%

Incidence of CHD if one sibling or parent has CHD–2–6%

Incidence of CHD if two 1 st degree relatives affected–20–30%.

Hyperoxia test is a bed side test that helps to differentiate right to left shunt from pulmonary diseases. If pO_2 rises > 150 mm Hg with 100 % O_2, intra cardiac right to left shunt is unlikely. It is not a confirmative test.

MC type of ASD–Ostium secondum.

MC type of ASD in Down syndrome–Ostium primum.

MC heart disease in Down syndrome–Endocardial cushion defect.

Chamber not enlarged in ASD- LV.

Timing of closure in ASD–After 1 year and before school entry.

Scimitar syndrome– a type of partial anomalous pulmonary venous return where pulmonary vein drains in IVC and produces a crescentic shadow along right border of heart.

Indications for surgery in VSD

- Pts with large defect at any age in whom clinical symptoms and failure to thrive cannot be controlled medically.
- Pts 6 months to 12 months with large defect and pulmonary hypertension even of symptoms controlled medically.
- Pts more the 2 years with Qp : Qs ratio greater than 2 : 1.
- Supracristal VSD of any size (risk of AR)
  - Severe pulmonary vascular disease nonresponsive to pulmonary vasodilators is a contraindication to closure of a VSD.
  - Indications for closure of PDA
  - Aymptomatic patients before 1 year of life.
  - Irrespective of age, patients with PDA need surgical or device closure.
  - Small PDA–Intravasular coil closure.
  - Mod to large PDA–Umbrella device.
  - Pulmonary hypertension is not a contraindication for closure of PDA if shunt is predominantly left to right.
- MC cardiac abnormality in Noonan syndrome–pulmonary stenosis.
- Cardiac abnormality in Alagille syndrome (arterio hepatic dysplasia)–pulmonary stenosis.
- Williams syndrome–supravavular aortic stenosis, Elfin facies (full face, broad forehead, flattened bridge of the nose, long upper lip, and rounded cheeks), mental retardation, idiopathic hypercalcemia of infancy.
- Shone complex–left sided obstructive lesions–COA, subaortic stenosis, MS
- COA–notching of inferior border of ribs due to pressure erosion by enlarged collaterals.

Complications in TOF

- Cerebral thrombosis (in < 2 years)
- Cerebral abscess(in > 2 years)
- Bacterial endocarditis
- Heart failure (rare, except in pink Fallot, asso, anemia, endocarditis, myocarditis, severe obstructive lesion etc.)

Cardiac abnormality	CXR finding
TOF	Boot shaped heart (with normal heart size), coer en sabot
Ebstein's anomaly	Massive cardiomegaly (wall to wall heart)
TAPVC total anomalous pulmonary venous connection	Snow man's appearance, Figure of "8", cottage leaf appearance
PAPVC partial anomalous pulmonary venous connection	Scimitar sign
TGA transposition of great arteries	Egg on end appearance
Tricuspid atresia	Box shaped appearance

Contd...

Contd...

Cardiac abnormality	CXR finding
Pulmoary hypertension	Jug handle appearance, pruned tree appearance
Constrictive pericarditis	Egg in cup appearance
COA	Inferior notching of ribs, "3" like appearance
Pulmonary edema	Bat wing appearance
Pericardial effusion	Leather bottle or money bag appearance

Procedure	Anastomosis	Indications
Foton shunt	SVC and IVC to right ppulmonary artery	Pulomnary atresia, Tricuspid atresia, Hypoplastic left heart, hypoplastic right heart, Ebstein's anomaly
Glenn shunt	SVC to right pulmonary artery	Pulmonary atresia, Tricspid atresia
Norwood procedure	Proximal pulmonary artery to aorta and right subclavian to right pulmonary artery	Hypoplastic left heart
Rastelli operation	A valved homograft conduit between right ventricle and pulmonary artery.	• TGA/VSD/PS • DORV/VSD/PS
Jantene	Arterial switch	TGA
Mustard, Senning operation	Atrial switch	TGA
Damus-Stansyl-Kaye operation	Proximal pulmonary artery to side of ascending aorta	Single ventricle
Sano shunt procedure	Conduit between RV and pulmonary artery	Hypoplastic left heart
Modified Blalock–Taussig shunt	Gore tex conduit anastomosingsubclavian artery to ipsilateral branch of pulmonary artery.	TOF
Waterston shunt (not done nowadays)	Ascending aorta to right pulmonary artery	TOF
Pott shunt (not done nowadays)	Descending aorta and left pulmonart artery	TOF
Intra cardiac repair	Resection of obstruction, valvotomy of pulmonary annulus and patch closure of VSD.	TOF

CCHD associated with WPW syndrome/SVT–Epstein's anomaly.

Truncus aretiosus is associated with Di George syndrome (deletion of Ch22q11).

Heterotaxia–two variations

- Asplenia syndrome–right isomerism–bilateral right sidedness
- Polysplenia syndrome–left isomerism–bilateral left sidedness.

Feature	Asplenia syndrome (right isomerism)	Polysplenia syndrome (left isomerism)
Spleen	Absent	Multiple
Lungs	B/L trilobar with eparterial bronchi	B/L bilobar with hyparterial bronchi
Sex	M > F	F > M
Right stomach	Yes	Less common
Symmetrical liver	Yes	Yes
Partial intestinal rotation	Yes	Yes
Pulmonary blood flow	Decreased	Increased
Severe cyanosis	Yes	No
TGA	More common	Less common
TAPVR	More common	Less common
Common AV valve	More common	Less common
Single ventricle	More common	Less common

Contd...

Contd...

Feature	Asplenia syndrome (right isomerism)	Polysplenia syndrome (left isomerism)
Absent inferior vena cava with azygos continuation	No	Characteristic
B/L SVC	Yes	Yes
Risk of sepsis	Yes	No
Absent gall bladder/biliary atresia	No	Yes

Treatment of pulmonary hypertension

- Prostacyclin analogue (PGI2)–Epoprostenol, Iloprost, Trepostinil
- Endothelin receptor antagonist–Bosenton
- PDE 5 inhibitor–Sildenafil
- Ca channel blockers–Diltiazem, Nifedipine.

Most common tumor of heart in children–Rhabdomyoma.

MC association of Rhabdomyoma of heart–Tuberous scelosis.

HEMATOLOGY

Hematopoisis begins in yolk sac at 10–14 days of gestation which is taken over by fetal liver by 6–8 weeks of gestation.

Stage	Hemoglobin	Hb chains
Adult	Hb A	• $\alpha_2\beta_2$
	Hb A2	• $\alpha_2\delta_2$
Fetal	Hb F	• $\alpha_2\gamma_2$
Embryonic	Gower 1	• $\zeta_2\varepsilon_2$
	Gower 2	• $\alpha_2\varepsilon_2$
	Portland	• $\zeta_2\gamma_2$

Monoclonal antibody used in autoimmune hemolytic anemia–Rituximab.

Most common gene mutation of membrane protein in Hereditary spherocytosis is **Ankyrin-1,** followed by band-3, β spectrin, α spectrin and protein 4.2.

Tests used in Hereditary spherocytosis

- Osmotic fragility test
- Cryohemolysis test.
- Osmotic gradient ektacyometry
- Eosin–5 maleimide test.

Causes of spherocytosis

- Hereditary spherocytosis
- Autoimmune haemolytic anemia
- Thermal injury
- Clostridial sepsis
- Wilson disease.

Ovalocytosis is caused by deficienct of Protein 3 and is seen in Southeast Asia. Protein 3 is one of the malarial receptor and hence pts with ovalocytosis have protection against falciparum malaria. The affected patients may also have distal renal tubular acidosis.

MC globin mutation world wide is Hb Eβ.

Blood sample of methhemoglobinemia is chocolate brown in color.

"Heinz bodies" and "bite cells" are characteristic of G6PD deficiency.

WHO diagnostic criteria for Polycythemia Vera

Major criteria

- Hb > 18.5 g/dL(men) or > 16.5 g/dl(women) or
  Hb or Hct > 99th percentile for age, sex or altitude. Or
  Hb > 17 g/dl(men) or >15g/dl (women) if asso. With a sustained increase of ≥ 2 g/dl from base line than cannot be attributed to correction of iron deficiency anemia or
  Elevated red cell mass > 25% above predicted normal.
- Presence of JAK2 or similar mutation.

Minor criteria

- Bone marrow trilineage myeloproliferation.
- Subnormal serum erythropoietin level.
- Endogenous erythroid colony growth.

Diagnosis–Both major and one minor criteria or first major and 2 minor criteria.

Hemophilia C is the bleeding disorder associated with reduced levels of factor XI.

Reduced levels of the *contact factors* (factor XII, high molecular weight kininogen, and prekallikrein) are associated with significant prolongation of activated partial thromboplastin time but are not associated with hemorrhage.

Parahemophilia–deficiency of Factor V.

The most common hereditary bleeding disorder is von Willebrand disease.

Autosomal hemophilia–von Willibrand disease type 2N weak binding of factor VIII to VWF.

VWD asso. with thrombocytopenia–Type 2B VWD and Platelet type (Pseudo) VWD.

Kasabach–Merritt syndrome–giant hemangioma with localized intravascular coagulation causing thrombocytopenia and hypofibrinogenemia.

Congenital thrombocytopenic syndrome

- Throbocytopenia–Absent Radius (TAR) syndrome
- Wiskott–Aldrich syndrome
- MYH9 related thrombocytopenia.

Platelet function disorders

- Bernard–Soulier syndrome
- Glanzmann throbasthenia
- Dense body deficiency
- Gray platelet syndrome

CANCER AND BENIGN TUMORS

MC childhood malignancy–Leukemia.

Factors predisposing to childhood Leukemia

Genetic factors	Environmental factors
BD FANS Bloom syndrome Down syndrome Diamond Blackfan anemia Fanconi anemia Ataxia telengiectasia Neurofibromatosis type–I Schwachman–Diamond syndrome Severe Combined Immuno Deficiency	Ionizing radiation Alkylating agents Benzene exposure Nitrosourea Epipodophyllotoxin Advanced maternal age.

Contd...

Contd...

Favorable prognosis	Unfavorable prognosis
ALL	
• Trisomy 4, 10, 17	• t(4,11)
• t(12,21)	• t(9,22)
• Hyperdiploidy	• Hypodiploidy
• Age 1–10 years	• Age > 10 years
• Initial WBC count < 50,000/mm^3	• Initial WBC count > 50,000/mm^3
AML	
• t(8,21)	Del(7)
• t(5,17)	11q23
• Inv (16)	

Juvenile myelomonocytic leukemia (JMML), formerly termed **juvenile chronic myelogenous leukemia,** typically affects children **<2 years of age**.

Infections that maybe associated with Hodgkin Lymphma–Epstein Bar virus, Cytomegalovirus and Human Herpes virus 6.

New WHO/Revised European American classification of HL (Hodgkin Lymphoma)

- Nodular lymphocyte predominance
- Classical Hodgkin Lymphoma
  - Lymphocyte rich
  - Lymphocyte depletion
  - Mixed cellularity
  - Nodular sclerosis

Four major pathological subtypes of Non Hodgkin Lymphoma are

- Burkitt lymphoma
- Lymphoblastic lymphoma
- Diffuse Large B Cell Lymphoma
- Anaplastic Large Cell Lymphoma

Syndromes associated with Pediatric Brain tumors

- NF–1
- NF–2
- von Hippel Lindau syndrome
- Tuberous sclerosis
- Li-Fraumeni syndrome
- Cowden syndrome
- Turcot syndrome
- Nevoid basal cell carcinoma

MC brain tumor in children–gliomas (of which Pilocytic astrocytoma is most common).

MC solid tumor in children–Glioma

Medulloblastoma (35–40%) and Cerebellar astrocytoma (35–40%) are the most common posterior fossa tumors in children.

MC malignant tumor in infants–Neuroblastoma.

MC extracranial solid tumor in children–Neuroblastoma.

MC primary malignant renal tumor in children–Wilm's tumor.

MC intra ocular tumor in children–Retinobastoma.

Parinaud syndrome is seen with pineal region tumors. It is manifested by paresis of upward gaze, pupillary dilation reactive to accommodation but not to light, nystagmus to convergence or retraction, and eyelid retraction.

Rosenthal fibers are characteristic of Pilocytic astrocytoma.

Small round blue cell tumors–Neuroblastoma, rhabdomyosarcoma, Ewing sarcoma and non-Hodgkin lymphoma.

Syndromes associated with neuroblastoma

Eponym	Features
Pepper syndrome	Massive involvement of the liver with metastatic disease with or without respiratory distress.
Horner syndrome	Unilateral ptosis, myosis, and anhidrosis associated with a thoracic or cervical primary tumor. Symptoms do not resolve with tumor resection.
Hutchinson syndrome	Limping and irritability in young child associated with bone and bone marrow metastases.
Opsoclonus-myoclonus-ataxia syndrome	Myoclonic jerking and random eye movement with or without cerebellar ataxia. The condition is likely immune mediated, may not resolve with tumor removal, and often exhibits progressive neuropsychological sequelae.
Kerner-Morrison syndrome	Intractable secretory diarrhea due to tumor secretion of vasointestinal peptides.
Neurocristopathy syndrome	Neuroblastoma associated with other neural crest disorders, including congenital hypoventilation syndrome or Hirschsprung disease.

Worse prognosis in Neuroblastoma

- N-MYC amplification
- Loss of Heterozygosity of 1p, 11q, 14q
- Gain of 17q
- Segmental chromosomal aberrations.

Good prognosis

- Hyperdiploidy
- Age at diagnosis < 1 year
- Stage 4S
- Whole chromosome gains.

Diagnosis of Neuroblastoma

- CT/MRI to localize the tumor
- Elevated rine VMA and HMA
- Small blue round cells, rosette formation in bone marrow aspiration
- Iodine–123 labelled Metaiodobezylguanidine (123I-MIBG) to detect dissemination.

Syndromes associated with wilms tumor

Syndrome	Clinical characteristics	Genetic anomalies
Wilms tumor, aniridia, genitourinary abnormalities, and mental retardation (WAGR syndrome)	Aniridia, genitourinary abnormalities, mental retardation	Del 11p13 (WT1 and PAX6)
Denys-Drash syndrome	Early-onset renal failure with renal mesangial sclerosis, male pseudohermaphrodism	WT1 missense mutation
Beckwith-Wiedemann syndrome (BWS)	Organomegaly (liver, kidney, adrenal, pancreas) macroglossia, omphalocele, hemihypertrophy	Unilateral paternal disomy, duplication of 11p15

Four histological subtypes of Rhabdomyosarcoma

- Embryonal–MC type, intermediate prognosis
- Botryoid–seen in vagina, uterus, urinary bladder, nasopharynx, middle ear
- Alveolar–asso with chromosomal translocations
- Pleomorphic–adult form, rare in children.
  - Sarcoma botryoides–vaginal rhabdomyosarcoma presents as grape like mass bulging through vaginal orifice.

- Osteosarcoma in X-ray–Sunburst pattern
- Ewinng sarcoma in X-ray–Onion peel appearance
- Retinoblastoma gene–RB1–Ch 13q14.
- Knudson "two hit" model of oncogenesis–Retinoblastoma.
- Trilateral retinoblastoma–Pineal tumor with hereditary Retinoblastoma.

Causes of Leukocoria (white eye reflex)

- Retinoblastoma
- Persistent hyperplastic primary vitreous
- Coats disease
- Cataract
- Toxocara canis endophthalmitis
- Choroidal cloboma
- Retinopathy of prematurity.

Increased risk for germ cell tumor

- Down syndrome
- Klinefelter syndrome (mediastinal GCT)
- Undescended testis
- Infertility
- Testicular atropy
- Inguinal hernia
- GCT in first degree relative
- Monozygotic twins

Classification of Childhood Histiocytosis

Class I–Langerhan cell histiocytosis–Langerhan cells, CD 1a, CD 207 positive, Birbeck granules.

Class II

- Familial erythrophagocytic lymphohistiocytosis
- Infection associated hemophagocytic syndrome

Class III

- Malignant histiocytosis
- Acute monocytic leukemia

Clinical entities of Class I or Histiocytosis X

- Esinophilic granuloma
- Hand–Schuller–Chistian disease
- Lettrer–Siwe disease

Diagnostic guidelines for Hemophagocytic Lypho Histiocytosis (HLH or Class II Histiocytosis)

The diagnosis of HLH is established by fulfilling 1 or 2 of the following criteria
• A molecular diagnosis consistent with HLH (e.g., PRF mutations, SAP mutations) OR • Having 5 out of 8 of the following: – Fever – Splenomegaly – Cytopenia (affecting ≥2 cell lineages; hemoglobin ≤9 g/dL (or ≤10 g/dL for infants <4 weeks of age, platelets <100,000/?L, neutrophils <1,000/?L) – Hypertriglyceridemia (≥265 mg/dL) and/or hypofibrinogenemia (≤150 mg/dL) – Hemophagocytosis in the bone marrow, spleen, or lymph nodes without evidence of malignancy – Low or absent NK cell cytotoxicity – Hyperferritinemia (≥500 ng/mL) – Elevated soluble CD25 (IL-2Rα chain; ≥2,400 U/mL)

NEPHROLOGY

- Heme positive urine without RBCs in urine microscopy–Hemoglobinuria or myoglobinuria.
- Hemoglobinuria without hematuria–Hemolysis.
- Myoglobinuria without hematuria–Rhabdomyolysis.
- Significant hematuria > 50 RBCs/μL.
- MC common cause for gross hematuria in children–UTI.
- MC chronic glomerular disease in children–Ig A nephropathy.
- Ig A deposits are present in mesangium of Ig A nephropathy but serum Ig A levels are normal in 85% of patients.
- Hereditary hematuria with bilateral sensorineural deafness and anterior lenticonus–Alport syndrome.

Poststrepptococcal Glomerulonephritis

Caused by Group A β hemolytic streptococci in association with throat (serotype 12) and skin (serotype 49) infections.

Pathology

- Kindneys are symmetrically enlarged.
- Glomeruli–enlarged and relatively bloodless, with mesangial proliferation and neutrophilic infiltration. Crescent maybe seen.
- Immunoflurescence shows "lumpy-bumpy" deposits of immunoglobins and complements over glomerular basement membrane (GBM).
- On electron microscopy, electron dense deposits (humps) seen on epithelial side of GBM.

Clinical features

- Age group–5 to 12 years.
- Develops 1–2 weeks after streptococcal pharyngitis or 3–6 weeks after streptococcal pyoderma.
- Presents as microscopic hematuria or gross hematuria, edema, hypertension, oliguria or altered sensorium (hypertensive encephalopathy).
- Associated nephrotic syndrome in 5% of cases.
- Usually resolves in 6–8 weeks.
- Hypertension and proteinuria resolve b 4–6 weeks whereas microscopic hematuria may persist upto 1–2 years.

Diagnosis

- Urine analysis shows RBCs, RBC casts, protein, neutophils.
- Serum C3 decreased in > 90% of patients. Serum C4 is usually normal.
- Positive streptococcal throat culture or elevated ASO, anti DNase B level, positive Streptozyme test gives evidence of streptococcal infection.

Indications for renal biopsy

- Acute renal failure
- Nephrotic range of proteinuria
- Absence of evidence of streptococcal infection.
- Normal complement levels
- Persistent low complement levels beyond 2 months.

Treatment

- Salt restriction, diuretics, anti hypertensives, treatment of renal failure, antibiotics. (antibiotics do not alter the history of glomerulonepritis).
- C3 nephritic factor which activates alternate complement pathway, is present in type II MPGN (dense deposit disease).
- MC small vessel vasculitis in children–Henoch Schonlein purpura.

Hemolytic Uremic Syndrome

Characterised br triad of

- Acute onset microangiopathic hemolytic anemia.
- Renal injury
- Low platelet count

Thrombotic Thrombocytopenic Purpura TTP is characterised by above three plus

- CNS involvement
- Fever

Laboratory criteria

- Anemia with microangiopathic changes (schistocytes, burr cells, helmet cells) in peripheral smear.
- Renal injury evidenced by hematuria, proteinuria, elevated creatinine ≥ 1 mg/dl in children , 13 year or ≥ 1.5 mg/dl in children > 13 year or > 50% rise from base line.

Case classification

Probable

- An acute illness diagnosed as HUS or TTP that meets the laboratory criteria in a patient who does not have a clear history of acute or bloody diarrhea in the preceding 3 weeks, or
- An acute illness diagnosed as HUS or TTP that (a) has onset within 3 weeks after onset of an acute or bloody diarrhea and (b) meets the laboratory criteria except that microangiopathic changes are not confirmed.

Confirmed

An acute illness diagnosed as HUS or TTP that both meets the laboratory criteria and began within 3 weeks after onset of an episode of acute or bloody diarrhea.

Infections associated with HUS

- Verotoxin producing E. Coli
- Shiga toxin-producing Shigella dysentereriae type 1
- Neuraminidase-producing Streptococcus pneumoniae
- Human immunodeficiency virus Hypercalciuria is 24 hours urine calcium excretion more than 4 mg/kg or spot calcim–creatinine ratio of > 0.2 in children and > 0.8 in infants < 7 months.

Polycystic Kidney Disease

Autosomal recessive PKD	Autosomal dominant PKD
Affects newborn or infants	Commonly adults, less common in children
Fibrocystin is the affected protein	Polycystin 1(PKD1-Ch 16) and Polycystin 2(PKD 2-Ch 4)
May affect a sibling (AR)	First degree relative commonly affected (AD)
Presents with oligohydomnios, pulmonary hypoplasia, resp. distress in neonates	Presents as hematuria, flank mass, abdominal pain, UTI. Neonatal presentation may mimic ARPKD.
Asso with hepatic dutal proliferation/fibrosis	Asso cysts in liver, pancreas, spleen, ovaries
Intracranial aneurysm is not seen	Intracranial aneurysm in 5%
Hernia and intestinal dverticula may not be seen	Hernia and intestinal diverticula maybe seen
Renal cell carcinoma is not associated	Renal cell carcinoma maybe associated.
USG shows small cysts and loss of corticomedullary differentiation.	USG shows large cysts in kidneys, liver, pancreas etc.
IVP shows characteristic mottled nephrogram with brushlike medullary opacification.	IVP shows spder–leg configuration.

Normal proteinuria ≤ 4 mg/m2/hr, abnormal proteinuria 4–40 mg/m2/hr and nephritic range is > 40 mg/m2/hr.
Normalm urine protein/creatinine ratio is < 0.5 in children < 2 years and < 0.2 in children > 2 years.
In nephritic syndrome spot urine protein/creatinine ratio > 2 (some books > 3).

Causes of transient proteinuria

- Fever
- Exercise
- Heart failure
- Seizures
- Dehydration
- Cold exposure
- Stress

Nephrotic Syndrome

Characterised by nephritic range of proteinuria, hypoalbuminemia, edema and hyperlipidemia.
Causes of typical nephritic syndrome

- Finnish type congenital nephritic syndrome (absence of nephrin)
- Focal Segmental Glomerulo Scelrosis (mutations of podocin, α actinin 4)
- Diffuse mesangial scelrosis (mutations in laminin β 2 chain)
- Denys Drash syndrome (mutations in WT1 transcripter factor)

Idiopathic NS

- Minimal change NS
- FSGS
- Membranous nephropathy

Drugs causing NS

- Gold
- Heroin
- Interferon
- Lithium
- Mercury
- NSAID
- Pamidronate
- Penicillamine

Infections causing NS (HMT Syphilis)

- Hepatitis B,C
- HIV
- Malaria
- Toxoplasma
- Syphilis

Steroid resistant NS

Gene	Name	Chromosome	Inheritance	Renal disease
NPHS 1	Nephrin	Ch 19	Recessive	Finnish type NS
NPHS 2	Podocin	Ch 1	Recessive	FSGS
FSGS 1	α actinin 4	Ch 19	Dominant	FSGS
FSGS 2	Unknown	Ch 11	Dominant	FSGS

Pathophysiology

Increased permeability of glomerular capillary is the primary defect. The hallmark of idiopathic NS is extensive effacement of podocyte foot processes.

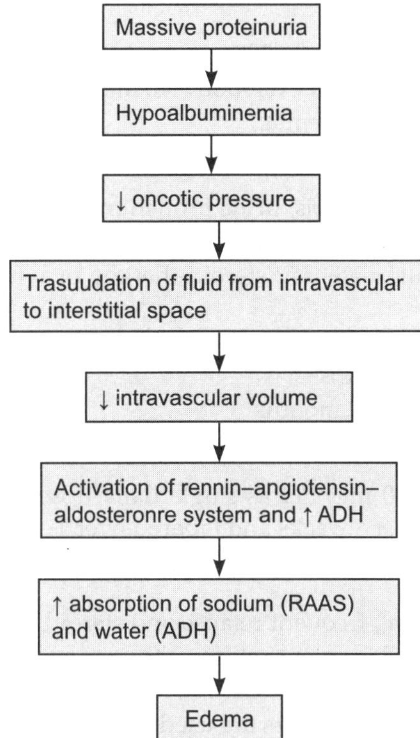

Increased renal avidity for sodium and water maybe the cause in some patients with increased intravascular volume.

Hyperlipidemia is due to increased protein synthesis (including lipoproteins) due to hypoalbuminemia and reduced synthesis of lipoprotein lipase enzyme (due to loss in urine).

Increased risk of infection with capsulated organisms (Pneumococcus and H. Influenza) due to loss of complement c3b, properdin factor B and immunoglobins in urine.

NS is a hypercoagulable state due to increased fibrinogen, clotting factors, decreased serum anticoagulants, increased platelets and increased platelet aggregation.

Hisological types of Idiopathic NS

	Minimal change NS	Mesangial proliferation	FSGS
Light microscopy	Goleruli normal or ↑in mesangial cells	Diffuse ↑in mesangial cells and matrix	Mesangial proliferation, segmental scarring
Immunoflurescence	Negative	Mesangial IgM/IgA staining	IgM and C3 staining
Electron microscopy	Effacement of epithelial foot process	↑ in mesangial cells, matrix and effacement of epithelial foot process	Segmental scarring, obliteration of glomerular capillary lumen
Response to steroids	95%	50%	20%

Clinical presentation

- Age group 2–6 years, twice more common in boys.
- Minimal change NS 85% in < 6 years whereas 20–30% in adolescents.
- FSGS more common in older age group.

Periorbital edema and lower limb edema are the presenting features. Anorexia, irritability, abdominal pain, diarrhoea are common. Gross hematuria and hypertension are characteristically absent. Ascites, pleural effusions and genital edema are seen in severe cases.

Diagnosis

- Urine protein 3+ or 4+, microscopic hematuria in 20%.
- Spot protein/creatinine ratio > 2, urine protein excretion > 40 mg/m²/hr.
- Hypoalbuminemi < 2.5g/dl, hypercholesterolemia.

Terminology

- Response to steroids–clinical remission, diureis, urine protein trace or negative for 3 consequtive days.
- Relapse–3+ or 4+ proteinuria and edema after remission.
- Steroid dependent–relapse during alternate day steroid therapy or within 28 days after successful course of steroid therapy.
- Steroid resistant–who donot respond after 8 weeks of steroid therapy.
- Frequent relapses – ≥ 4 relapses in 12 months
- Infrequent relapses–3 or less relapses in 12 months

Treatment

Prednisolone 60 mg/m²/day (maximum 80 mg) PO as single daily dose for 4–6 consecutive weeks followed by 40/mg/m²/day on every other day for atleast 4 weeks and tapered over 1–2 months and stopped.

Alternative drugs

- Cyclophosphamide–steroid depentdent, frequent relapse and steroid resistant NS
- Mycophenolate–Steroid dependent and frequent relapse NS
- Tacrolimus–Steroid resistant NS.
- ACE inhibitors and Angiotensin receptor blockers are used as adjuvants to reduce proteinuria.

Complications

- Spontaneous bacterial peritonitis, cellulitis, pneumonia, sepsis,
- Thromboembolism–both arterial and venous–renal vein thrombosis, pulmonary embolus, sagittal sinus thrombosis, thrombosis of arteral venous catheters.
- Renal Tubular Acidosis Type II (Proximal RTA)

Common causes

- Sporadic (most common)
- Cystinosis
- Lowe syndrome
- Galactosemia
- Hereditary fructose intolerance
- Tyrosinemia
- Wilson disease
- Dent disease (X linked nephrolithiasis)

Clinical and laboratory features

Growth failure in first year of life.

Polyuria, dehydration, vomiting, anorexia, constipation, hypotonia are other features.

Normal anion gap metabolic acidosis, urine pH < 5.5.

Phosphaturia (rickets), glycosuria, aminoaciduria, uricosuria, elevated urine Na and K.

CKD maybe present.

Lowe syndrome–Oculocerebrorenal syndrome–X linked recessive, cataract, mental retardation, Fanconi syndrome. Blindness and renal failure may develop.

Cystinosis–defective metabolism of cystine–accumulation of cystine crystals in kidneys, liver, eyes and brain. Presents in 2 years of life with growth failure, fair blond skin, dehydration, hepatosplenomegaly, photophobia, impaired visual acuity, retinopathy, Fanconi syndrome and renal failure. Diagnosis is by detection of cornealcystine crystals and measurement of leukocyte cystinecontent in cornea. Treatment is with **Cysteamine.**

Type I RTA (Distal RTA)

- Defect in acidification process in distal tubule (H^+/ATPase, HCO_3^-/Cl^-).
- **Urine pH > 5.5** despite metabolic acidosis.
- Hypokalemia, **hypercaluria, nephrocalcinosis**, nephrolithiasis, hypocitraturia.
- Presents with growth failure and non anion gap metabolic acidosis.
- Phosphaturia and bicarbonateuria are absent.(present in Type I RTA).
- Urine anion gap = [urine Na^+ + urine K^+]–Urine Cl^-.
- Positive urine anion gap–distal RTA and negative urine anion gap–proximal RTA.

Type IV RTA

Due to impaired aldosterone production (hypoaldosteronism) or impaired renal response to aldosterone (pseudohypoaldosteronism). **Hyperkalemia** is characteristic.

Treatment of RTA

Bicarbonate replacement. Phosphate replacement in proximal RTA. Thiazide diuretics for treatment of hypercalciuria in distal RTA. Treatment of hyperkalemia in Type IV RTA.

Bartter syndrome

Bartter syndrome is a group of disorders characterized by hypokalemic metabolic alkalosis with hypercalciuria and salt wasting.

Antenatal Bartter syndrome (types I, II, IV) (also called hyperprostaglandin E syndrome) Classical Bartter–Type III

Defect in Na/Cl/K channel in thick ascending loop of Henle. Autosomal recessive disorder.

Presents with polyhydrominos, prematurity, dysmorphic facies (triangular facies, protruding ears, large eyes), polyuria, dehydration, failure to thrive. BP is usually normal or maybe low. Classical hypokalemic metabolic alkalosis with hypercalciuria is seen. Renal function is normal. Nephrocalcinosis is present in types I, II, III and V.

Treatment is preventing dehydration, maintaining nutritional status, and correcting hypokalemia. Indomethacin is effective.

Bartter syndrome	Gitelman syndrome
Autosomal recessive	Autosomal recessive
Defect in Na/Cl/K channel in thick ascending loop of Henle	Defect in Na-Cl cotransporter in DCT
Resembles chronic use of loop diuretics	Resembles chronic use of thiazide diuretics
Presents in infancy	Late childhood and adolescent
Recurrent dehydration present	Recurrent dehydration absent
Hypercalciuria, nephrocalcinosis	Hypocalciuria
Hypomagnesemia in 20%	Hypomagnesemia in 100%
Indomethacin is useful	Magnesium, Amiloride useful

Gordon syndrome–defect in distal convoluted tubule, gain-of-function mutations in *WNK1* and loss-of-function mutations in *WNK4*, lead to excessive NCCT-mediated salt reabsorption with the clinical picture of pseudohypoaldosteronism type 2 (familial hyperkalemic hypertension [FHH].

Liddle syndrome–defect in collecting duct, gain-of-function mutations of the gene that encodes the epithelial sodium channel causes an inherited form of hypertension. Patients have constitutive sodium uptake in the collecting duct, with hypokalemia and suppressed aldosterone.

The juvenile nephronophthisis (JN)–medullary cystic kidney disease complex (MCKD) is a group of inherited cystic renal diseases that share a common histologic phenotype of chronic Tubular Interstitial Nephritis. JN is inherited as an autosomal recessive trait. JN causes 10–20% of pediatric end-stage renal disease (ESRD) in Europe. JN presents with polyuria, growth failure, "unexplained" anemia, and chronic renal failure in late childhood or adolescence. Variants of JN with extrarenal involvement include **Senior-Loken syndrome** (retinitis pigmentosa), **Joubert syndrome,** and **oculomotor apraxia type Cogan. MCKD** is an autosomal dominant disease that manifests in adulthood.

Pediatric-Modified Rifle (Prifle) Criteria

Criteria	Estimated CCI	Urine output
Risk	eCCl decrease by 25%	<0.5 mL/kg/hr for 8 hours
Injury	eCCl decrease by 50%	<0.5 mL/kg/hr for 16 hours
Failure	eCCl decrease by 75% or eCCl <35 ml/min/1.73 m^2	<0.3 mL/kg/hr for 24 hours or anuric for 12 hours
Loss	Persistent failure >4 weeks	
End-stage	End-stage renal disease (persistent failure >3 months)	

eCCl, estimated creatinine clearance

Urinalysis, urine chemistries and osmolality in acute renal failure

	Hypovolemia	Acute tubular necrosis	Acute interstitial nephritis	Glomerulo nephritis	Obstruction
Sediment	Bland	Broad, brownish granular casts	White blood cells, eosinophils, cellular casts	Red blood cells, red blood cell casts	Bland or bloody
Protein	None or low	None or low	Minimal but maybe increased with NSAIDs	Increased, >100 mg/dL	Low
Urine sodium, mEq/L	<20	>30	>30	<20	<20 (acute) >40 (few days)
Urine osmolality, mOsm/kg	>400	<350	<350	>400	<350
Fractional excretion of sodium %	<1	>1	Varies	<1	<1 (acute) >1 (few days)

Standardized terminology for stages of chronic kidney disease

Stage	Description	GFR (mL/min/1.73 m^2)
1	Kidney damage with normal or increased GFR	>90
2	Kidney damage with mild decrease in GFR	60–89
3	Moderate decrease in GFR	30–59
4	Severe decrease in GFR	5–29
5	Kidney failure	<15 or on dialysis

MC cause for renal transplant is Renal hypoplasia/dysplasia followed by obstructive uropathy.

Mayer-Rokitansky-Kuster-Hauser syndrome–unilateral renal agenesis or ectopia, ipsilateral Mullerian defects, and vaginal agenesis.

UTI

More common in girls (10 : 1) in > 1 years. In infants, UTI is more common in boys.

E.coli is the most common organism followed by Klebiella, Proteus, Staphylococcus saphrophyticus, enterococcus.

Acute hemorrhagic cystitis often is caused by *E. Coli,* adenovirus types 11 and 21. Adenovirus cystitis is more common in boys; it is self-limiting, with hematuria lasting approximately 4 days.

Asymptomatic bacteriuria refers to a condition in which there is a positive urine culture without any manifestations of infection. It is more common in girls. (incidence <1% in preschool and school-age girls). Incidence declines with increasing age. This condition is benign and does not cause renal injury, except in pregnant women.

Risk factors for UTI

• Female gender	• Tight underwear
• Uncircumcised male	• Pin worm infestation
• Vesicoureteric reflux	• Constipation
• Toilet training	• Bacteria with fimbriae
• Voiding dysfunction	• Labial adhesion
• Obstructive uropathy	• Neuropathic bladder
• Urethral instrumentation	• Sexual activity
• Wiping from back to front in girls	• Pregnancy

Pyuria is leukocytes in urine. It suggests infection. Infection can occur without pyuria and conversely pyuria can occur without infection.

Causes of sterile pyuria (positive leukocytes, negative culture)

- Partially treated UTI
- Viral infection
- Renal TB
- **Renal abscess**
- UTI with urinary obstruction
- Urethritis due to STD
- Inflamation near ureter or bladder (appendicitis, crohn's disease)
- Interstitial nephritis (esinophils).

A child is considered to have UTI if colony count is > 1,00,000 for a single organism or > 10,000 in a symptomatic child.

Indications for Ultrasonogram for 1st episode of UTI

- Febtile UTI
- UTI in infants
- Positive culture
- Associated systemic illness

Next a DMSA scan is performed to assess whether the child has pyelonephritis. If the DMSA scan is positive and shows acute pyelonephritis or renal scarring, VCUG (Voiding Cysto Urethro Gram).

NICE (National Institute of health and Clinical Excellence, UK) guidelines for imaging in UTI

- < 6 months–Renal sonogram and DMSA
- 6 months to 3 years–DMSA for atypical or recurrent UTI
- > 3 years–DMSA only for recurrent UTI.

Grading of Vesico Ureteric Reflux (VUR)

Grade I–Reflux into a nondilated ureter.

Grade II–Reflux in to upper collecting system without dilatation.

Grade III–Reflux into a dilated ureter and/or blunting of calyces

Grade IV–Reflux into a grossly dilated ureter.

Grade V–Massive reflux with significant ureter dilatation and tortusity and loss of papillary impression.

Antibiotic prophylaxis is given to most children with reflux. The drugs used are Trimethoprim–Sulfamethoxazole, Nitrifurantoin, Cephalexin at dose 25–30 5 of normal dose as daily single dose. Surgery is recommended for children who fail medical management (breakthrough UTI, persistent reflux) and those with high reflux that are unlikely to resolve.

Hinman syndrome–Non neurogenic Nerugenic bladder–due to failure of external sphincter to relax during voiding in children without neurological abnormalities. This condition is also known as **detrusor–sphincter dyssnergia**. Presents with staccato stream, day–night wetting, recurrent UTI, constipation, encopresis. Treament includes anticholinergic and α-adrenergic blocker therapy, timed voiding, treatment of constipation, behavioral modification, biofeedback, encouragement of relaxation during voiding, botulinum toxin.

Pollakiuria-or daytime frequency syndrome of childhood–Some children(4–6 years) have abrupt onset of severe urinary frequency, voiding as often as every 10–15 min during the day, without dysuria, UTI, daytime incontinence, or nocturia. It is self limited in 2–3 months. Anticholinergics maybe useful.

Micropenis–stretched penile length less than 1.9 cm.

Radioluscent stones–Cystine, Xanthine and Uric acid stones.

ENDOCRINOLOGY

Differentiation between SIADH, Cerebral salt wasting and Central Diabtes Insipidus

Clinical parameter	SIADH	Cerebral salt wasting	Central DI
Serum sodium	Low	Low	High
Urine output	Normal or low	High	High
Urine sodium	High	Very high	Low
Intravascular volume status	Normal or high	Low	Low
Vasopressin level	High	Low	Low

Causes of Childhood Tall stature

- Familial Tall Stture
- Cerebral gigantism
- Beckwith-Wiedemann syndrome
- Exogenous obesity
- Excess GH secretion (pituitary gigantism)
- McCune-Albright syndrome or MEN associated with excess GH secretion
- Precocious puberty
- Marfan syndrome
- Klinefelter syndrome (XXY)
- SHOX excess syndromes
- Weaver syndrome
- Fragile X syndrome
- Homocystinuria
- XYY
- Hyperthyroidism

Sotos syndrome (Cerebral Gigantism) are above 90th percentile for length and weight at birth. Also have macrocrania at birth. Accelerated growth continues upto 4–5 years and normalizes. Bone age corresponds to chronological age. Have increased risk of carcinoma of liver, ovary and Wilm's tumor.

Precocious puberty is defined by the onset of secondary sexual characters before the age of 8 years in girls and 9 years in boys.

MC cause of congenital hypothyroidism is thyroid dysgenesis (aplasia, hypoplasia, ectopic gland, 80–85%)

Pendred syndrome–autosomal recessive–defect in chloride–iodide channel protein. Have impaired iodide organification and a positive perchlorate discharge. Presents with sensorineural deafness and goitre.

X-ray findings in Hypothyroidism

- Distal femoral epiphysis is absent at birth.
- Delayed bone age
- Epiphyseal dysgenesis-epiphyses have multiple foci of ossification
- Beaking deformity of 12th thoracic or 1st or 2nd lumbar vertebra.
- Skull has large fontanels and sutures.

- Wormian (intersutural) bones are common
- Sella turcica enlarged and round.
- Delayed eruption of tooth.

Causes of acquired hypothyroidism

- Autoimmune thyroid disease
- Down syndrome
- Turner syndrome
- Type 1 Diabetes mellitus
- William syndrome
- Irradiation
- Drugs–iodides, amiodarone, lithium, prophythiouracil, methimazole
- Nephropathic cystinosis
- Hepatitis C infection
- Hemangioma of liver
- Langerhan cell histiocytosis

Subclinical hypothyroidism–normal free T4 and elevated TSH

MC organism causing suppurative thyroiditis–viridians streptococci

Idiopathic hypoparathyroidism–low parathyroid hormone, hypocalcemia, elevated phosphorus.

Pseudoparathyroidism (Albright hereditary Osteodystriphy)–defect in hormone receptors–elevated parathyroid levels, hypocalcemia, elevated phosphorus. Affected patients are short and stocky, round face, brachydactyly, wide phalanges, bowing and thickend calvaria.

Pseudopseudohypoparathyroidism–physical features of psudohypoparathyroidism, elevated parathyroid level and normal levels of calcium and phosphorus.

Type I Autoimmune polyendocrinopathy–(APS–1)–APECED–Autoimmune Poly Endorinopathy, Candidiasis, Ectodermal Dysplasia. Chronic mucocutaneous candidiasis is the most common presentation followed by hypoprathyroidism, Addison's disease.

Congenital Adrenal Hyperplasia

Congenital Adrenal Hyperplasia due to 21 hydroxylase deficiency presents in newborn at 10–14 days of life with progressive weight loss, anorexia (poor feeding), vomiting, dehydration, weakness, hypotension, hypoglycemia, hyponatremia and hyperkalemia.

Afffected female newborn have enlarged clitoris and paritial complete labial fusion.

Affected males are normal at birth and hence easily missed until they develop signs of adrenal insufficiency.

17 hydroxy progesterone level is markedly elevated.

Trement includes hydrocortisone and fludrocortisone.

Klinefelter syndrome (47XXY)

- MC sex chromosomal aneuploidy in males.
- Have learn disabilities (mainly language), normal IQ
- Are anxious, immature, excessively shy
- Tall(longer legs), slim and underweight.
- Delayed pubertal development
- Normal testosterone levels with elevated LH, FSH
- Have gynecomastia, sparse facial hair
- Azoospermia and infertility common
- Testicular sperm extraction and intracytoplasmic sperm injection (ICSI) can result in birth of healthy infants.
- Increased risk of varicose veins, ca male breast, leukemia and lymphoma.
- Treatment–Testosterone replacement. Gynecomastia is treated with aromatase inhibitors.

Turner syndrome(45X0)

At birth–Low birth weight and decreased length, edema of dorsum of hands and feet, loose skin folds at nape of neck.

Sexual infantism, webbed neck, cubitus valgus, short stature, low posterior hair line, small mandible, prominent ears, epicanthal folds, high arched palate, broad chest with illusion of widely spaced nipples, hyperconvex fingers.

Mean adult height 143–144 cm.

Bicuspid aortic valve, dialation of ascending aorta, coarctation of aorta, aortic stenosis, partial anomalous pulmonary venous connection are the cardiac anomalies.

Renal anomalies include pelvic kidney, horse shoe kidney, double collecting system, complete absence of one kidney, pelviureteric junction obstruction.

Autoimmune thyroiditis, type 2 diabetes, hypercholesterolemia, inflammatory bowel disease maybe present in adolescents and adults.

Skeletal deformities include sterna malformations, scoliosis, congenital hip dysplasia.

Eye findings include keratoconus ans anterior segment dysplasia.

Recurrent bilateral otitis media and sensorineural deafness are common.

Intelligence is normal except in patients with ring chromosome. [45X0, 46X, r(X)].

Growth hormone replacement increases height velocity and ultimate stature. Oxandrolone is also useful. Ostrogen replacement is indicated at 12–13 years of age.

Noonan syndrome

- Can occur in both males and females with normal chromosomes.
- Phenotypic features are similar to that of females with Tturner syndrome.
- Short stature, webbing of neck, pectus carinatum or excavatum, right sided heart disease occur.
- Characteristic facies include hypertelorism, epicanthic folds, downward slanting palpebral fissure, ptosis, micrognathia, ear abnormalities.
- Clinidactyly, hernia, vertebral anomalies are less common.
- Sensorineural hearing loss is common.
- Pulmonary valvular stenosis is most common cardiac defect followed by hypertrophic cardiomyopathy and ASD.
- Hepatospelomegaly may occur.
- Low clotting factors XI, XII, Acute lymphoblastic leukemia and chronic myelomonocytic leukemia may occur.
- Male have crptorchidism and small testes. Testosterone level may low or normal. Spermatogenesis maybe affected.
- Human growth hormone may accelerate growth.

NEUROLOGY

- Anterior fontanelis 2 × 2 cm in size. It close from 9–18 months of age.
- Visual acuity in term newborn is 20/150 and reaches the adult value of 20/20 at 6 months.
- Allen's chart for visual acuity can be used from 2.5 to 3 years of age.
- Neural tube defects occur when neural tube fails to close between 3rd and 4th week of intrauterine life.
- Neural tube defect can be prevented by taking 0.4 mg 400 microgram of Folic acid (and 4 mg for previous affected child) from 1 month before planning pregnancy.
- MC site of myelomeningocele is lumbosacral region (75%).
- MC associated anomaly with myelomeningocele–type II Chiari malformation (80%).
- **Lissencephaly**–agyria-absence of cerebral convolutions and a poorly formed sylvian fissure.
- **Schizencephaly**–Presence of unilateral or bilateral clefts in the cerebral hemispheres.
- **Porencephaly** is the presence of cysts or cavities within the brain that result from developmental defects or acquired lesions.

- **Polymicrogyria–**an augmentation of small convolutions separated by shallow enlarged sulci. **Holoprosencephaly** results from defective formation of the prosencephalon and inadequate induction of forebrain structures.
- **Aicardi syndrome**–X linked dominant–mental retardation, chorioretinal lacunae, agenisis of corpus callosum, seizure, infantile spasms.
- **Mobius syndrome**–bilateral facial weakness, associated abducent nerve palsy, normal development and mentation.
- **Chiari malformation**–small posterior fossa with herniation of cerebellar tonsils through foramen magnum. MC malformation of posterior possa and hind brain.
- **Dandy–Walker malformation**–cystic dilatation of the fourth ventricle, hypoplasia of the cerebellar vermis, hydrocephalus, and an enlarged posterior fossa with elevation of the lateral venous sinuses and the tentorium.
- **Joubert syndrome**–autosomal recessive–cerebellar vermis hypoplasia and the pontomesencephalic **molar tooth sign.**
- **Lhermitte-Duclos** disease is–dysplastic gangliocytoma of the cerebellum leading to focal enlargement of the cerebellum and macrocephaly, cerebellar signs, and seizures.

Timing of Selected Primitive Reflexes

Reflex	Onset	Fully developed	Duration
Palmar grasp	28 weeks	32 weeks	2–3 months
Rooting	32 weeks	36 weeks	Less prominent after 1 months
Moro	28–32 weeks	37 weeks	5-6 months (some books - 3 months)
Tonic neck	35 weeks	1 month (postnatal)	6–7 months
Parachute	7–8 months	10-11 months (postnatal)	Remains throughout life

Causes of Microcephaly

A. Primary causes

- Familial
- Syndromes–CRESD
  - Cri–du chat (5p) syndrome
  - Cornelia de Lange syndrome
  - Rubinstein–Taybi syndrome
  - Edward syndrome
  - Smith–Lemli- Opitz syndrome
  - Down's syndrome

B. Secondary causes

- TORCH infections (CMV, Rubella, Toxoplasmosis)
- Fetal alcohol syndrome
- Fetal Hydantoin syndrome
- Radiation (before 15 weeks of gestation)
- Maternal diabetes/hyperphenylalaninemia
- Meningitis/encephalitis
- Hypoxic Ischemic Encephalopathy
- Hyperthermia

Causes of Hydrocephalus

A. Communicating (B CAMP)

- Benign enlargement of subarachnoid space
- Basilar impression
- Choroid plexus papilloma
- Achondroplasia

- Meningitis
- Meningeal malignancy
- Posthemorrhagic

B. Noncommunicating (ADMK CM)

- Aqueductal stenosis
- Autosomal dominant
- Autosomal recessive
- Dandy Walker syndrome
- Mitochondrial
- Klippel–Feil syndrome
- Chiari malformation
- Mass lesion
  - Abscess
  - Hematoma
  - Tumor
  - Vein of Galen malformation
  - Walker–Warburg syndrome

A **simple febrile seizure** is a primary generalized, usually tonic-clonic, attack associated with fever, lasting for a maximum of 15 min, and not recurrent within a 24–hour period.

A **complex febrile seizure** is more prolonged (>15 min), is focal, and/or recurs within 24 hour. **Febrile status epilepticus** is a febrile seizure lasting >30 min.

Risk for recurrence of Febrile Seizures

Major

- Age < 1 year
- Duration of fever < 24 hours
- Fever 38–39 °C

Minor

- Family history of febrile seizure
- Family history of epilepsy
- Complex febrile seizure
- Day care
- Male gender
- Low serum sodium.

Risk of subsequent epilepsy

- Simple febrile seizure–1%
- Complex febrile seizure–6%
- Neuroevelopmental abnormalities–33%.

CT/MRI is not recommended for evaluation of simple febrile seizure.

Intermittent prophylaxis for febrile seizure includes

- Clobazam
- Clonazepam
- Nitrazepam
- Diazepam
- Phenobarbitone
- Sodium valporate

Antipyretics can decrease the discomfort of the child but do not reduce the risk of having a recurrent febrile seizure.

Rasmussen's encephalitis–a form of chronic encephalitis that manifests with unilateral intractable partial seizures, epilepsia partialis continua, and progressive hemiparesis of the affected side, with progressive atrophy of the contralateral hemisphere.

West syndrome starts between the ages of 2 and 12 months. It consists of a triad of infantile spasms, developmental regression, and a typical EEG picture called **hypsarrhythmia.**

Status epilepticus is defined as continuous seizure activity or recurrent seizure activity without regaining of consciousness lasting for >30 min. (Nelson–30 min, some authors–5 min).

MC type of recurrent headache in children–Migraine.

Difference between ADEM and first episode of MS

	ADEM	MS
Age	<10 year	>10 year
Stupor/coma	+	–
Fever/vomiting	+	–
Family history	No	20%
Sensory complaints	+	+
Optic neuritis	Bilateral	Unilateral
Manifestations	Polysymptomatic	Monosymptomatic
MRI imaging	Widespread lesions: basal ganglia, thalamus, cortical gray-white junction	Isolated lesions: periventricular white matter, corpus callosum
CSF	Pleocytosis (lymphocytosis)	Oligoclonal bands
Response to steroids	+	+
Follow-up	No new lesions	New lesions

ADEM–Acute Disseminated Encephalo Myelitis, MS-Multiple Scelrosis.

Inborn Errors of Metabolism (IEM)

IEM associated with peculiar odor

Inborn error of metabolism	Urine odor
Glutaric acidemia (type II)	Sweaty feet, acrid
Hawkinsinuria	Swimming pool
3-Hydroxy-3-methylglutaric aciduria	Cat urine
Isovaleric acidemia	Sweaty feet, acrid
Maple syrup urine disease	Maple syrup
Hypermethioninemia	Boiled cabbage
Multiple carboxylase deficiency	Tomcat urine
Oasthouse urine disease	Hops-like
Phenylketonuria	Mousey or musty
Trimethylaminuria	Rotting fish
Tyrosinemia	Boiled cabbage, rancid butter

Wolman disease–Autosomal recessive lysosomal storage diseases due to deficiency of acid lipase and the accumulation of cholesterol esters and triglycerides in histiocytic foam cells of visceral organs. Presents in newborn with failure to thrive, relentless vomiting, abdominal distention, steatorrhea, hepatosplenomegaly, hyperlipidemia, hepatic dysfunction. **Calcification of the adrenal glands** is pathognomonic.

Glycogen storage disease	Enzyme deficiency
I a/von Gierke disease	Glucose-6 phosphatase
Ib	Glucose-6 phosphate translocase
II/Pompe's disease	Acid maltase (Acid α–glucosidase)
IIIa/Cori or Forbe's disease	Debranching enzyme-amylo 1, 6, glucosidase
IV/Anderson disease	Branching enzyme
V/**M**c Ardle's disease	**M**uscle phophorylse
VI/**H**er's disease	Liver (**H**epatic) phosphorylase
VII/Tauri's disease	Phosphofructokinase

Phenylketonuria

Caused by deficiency of Phenylalanine hydroxylase or its co factor Tetrahydro biopterin (BH4). It leads to accumulation of phenylalanine in body fluids and brain. Excess phenylalanine is metabolised to phenylketones (phenylpyruvate and phenyllactate) which are excreted in urine. Tyrosine becomes an essential amino acid.

Clinical features–Affected babies are normal at birth. Present with vomiting, seizures, purposeless movements, athetosis, spasticity, tremors, hyperreflexia, micocephaly, prominent maxilla with widely separate teeth, enamel hypoplasia and growth retardation. Skin is fair complexioned, may have sebborheic or ecchymatic rashes. Children have unpleasant mousey or musty odour due to phenyllactic acid.

Diagnosis–Ferric chloride test and Guthrie's test are outdated. Quantitative tests (flurometric and tandem mass spectroscopy) are currently used.

Treatment–Phenylalanine restricted diet (not phenylalanine free diet). Tyrosine is supplemented in adequate quantities.

Deficiency of BH4 should be treated with low phenylalanine diet, supplementation of BH4 and precursors of neurotransmitters (L-dopa and 5-hydroxytryptophan).

Pregnant women with hyperphenylalaninemia who are not on a phenylalanine-restricted diet have a very high risk of having children with mental retardation, microcephaly, growth retardation, and congenital heart disease.

Homocystinuria

Inborn error of methionine metabolism. Folic acid and vitamin B12 are used as co factors in methionine metabolism. Classical homocystinuria is caused by deficiency of Cystathionine β synthase

Clinical features–Affected infants are normal at birth. Presents as failure to thrive and developmental delay. Other important clinical features are

- **Ectopia lentis** (subluxation of lens)
- Myopia
- **Iridodonesis**
- Astigmatism
- Glaucoma
- Cataract
- Retinal detachment
- **Progressive mental retardation**
- **Skeletal abnormalities resembling Marfan syndrome**
- **Fair complexion, blue eyes**
- **Thromboembolic episodes**

Diagnosis is by enzyme assay in liver biopsy and cultured fibroblasts.

Treatment is with high dose Vitamin B6 (and Vitamin B12 for Methycobolamine cofactor deficiency).

MAPLE SYRUP URINE DISEASE (MSUD)

Caused by defective decarboxylation of branched chain aminoacids (leucine, isoleucine and valine).

Clinical features

- Normal at birth
- **Vomiting**
- **Lethary**
- Refusal of feeds
- Hypoglycemia (not improving with glucose)
- **Hypertonia, rigidity, opithotonus alternating with flaccidity**
- **Convulsion**
- Cerebral edema, coma
- **Mousy or musty odour of urine and cerumen**

Diagnosis–Marked elevation in plasma and urine of leucine, isoleucine, valine and their ketoacids in urine. On adding a few drops of DNPH (2, 4, Dinitrophenyl Hydeazine) to urine, it gives a yellow precipitate (positive test). Neuro imaging shows cerebral edema in acute state, and hypomyelination and cerebral atropy later.

Treatment includes hydration, peritoneal dialysis and a diet low in branched chain aminoacids. Prgnosis is guarded.

MULTIPLE CARBOXYLASE DEFICIENCY

The early infantile form is caused by holocarboxylase synthetase deficiency whereas the late juvenile form is caused by biotinidase deficiency.

In the early form, the newborn is normal initially.

Symptoms include

- Respitatory distress
- Feeding problems.
- Vomiting
- Hypotonia
- **Exfoliative dermatitis**
- **Alopecia**
- Failure to thrive
- Immunodeficiency
- Irritability, lethargy
- Seizures
- Coma
- Peculiar odor of urine **(Tom cat urine)**

Investigations show metabolic acidosis, ketosis, hyperammonemia. Lyphocyte enzyme assay confirms the diagnosis.

Treatment with **Biotin** improves clinical features.

The late form also presents in a similar manner with neurological and dermatological symptoms.

SOME HIGH YIELDING POINTS

- Handedness appears by 3rd year.
- Bed wetting is normal up to 4 years in girls and 5 years in boys.
- Characteristics of Narcolepsy include profound daytime sleepiness, cataplexyhypnogogic/hypnopompic hallucinations and sleep paralysis.
- Treatment of Tourette's syndrome includes risperidone and clonidine.
- Language development is normal in Asperger's disorder.

- Secondry enuresis refers to resumption of wetting after at least 6 months of dryness.
- Obesity is defined as BMI > 30.
- Bayley scale of Infant development and Wechsler scale are most commonly used psychological testing scale in infants ans children more than 3 years respectively.
- Vineland scale is the most commonly used test of adaptive behavior.
- Most common fractures in child abuse are metaphyseal lesions, posterior rib fractures, fractures of scapula, sternum and spinous process.
- Characteristic autopsy finding in SIDS is none (no characteristic finding).
- Retinal hemorrhages are an impotant marker of abusive head trauma.
- First immunization of newborn is Colustrum milk.
- Nutrients deficient in vegetarian diet are iron, vitamin B12, essential fatty acids, calcim and zinc.
- Noma is chronic necrotizing ulceration of gingival and cheek caused any Fusobacterium nacrophoram and Prevotellla intermedia.
- RUTF Ready to Use Therapeutic Food F75 and F100 are used in the initial and rehabilitation phase of treating malnutrition, respectively
- Stunting refers to chronic malnutrition whereas wasting refers to acute malnutrition
- Hyperostosis of long bones occurs in Hypervitaminosis A.
- Stoss therapy is used in Vitamin D deficiency.
- Angiokeratomas are seen in Fabry disease.
- Hallmark of refeeding syndrome is severe hypophosphatemia.
- Rapid correction of hyponatremia leads to central pontine myelinosis.
- Maple syrup urine disease is caused by deficiency of branched chain amino acis α ketoacid dehydrogenase.
- Most common cause of shock in children world wide is hypovolemic shock.
- ECG changes in hyperkalemia are tall T-waves, prolonged PR, wide QRS, flat P waves and sine wave.
- ECG change sin hypokalemia are falt T-waves, ST depression and appearance of U waves. ECG finding in Tricyclic antidepressant posinonin is wide QRS (> 100 ms).
- Antidote for sulfonylurea poisoning is Octreotide
- Rumack–Mathew nomogram is used in Paracetamol poisoning.
- Pao_2/Fio_2 ration in acute lung injury is < 300 (for ARDS < 200).
- Subgaleal bleed in a newborn occurs beneath the apponeurosis of occipitofrontalis muscle.
- Size of uncuffed ET tube in children is Age in years/4 + 4.
- In Prader–willi syndrome uniparental disomy of maternal chromosome occurs (missing paternal chromosome 15) and in Angelman syndrome, uniparental disomy of paternal chromosome occurs (missing maternal chromosome 15).
- Total body water in a term newborn is 75% of body weight.
- Osmolality = 2[Na] + [Glucose]/18 + [Urea]/2.8
- Na (corrected) = Na (measured) + 1.6 [(Glucose–100)/100].
- Pseudohyponatremia is seen in hyperlipidemia and hyperproteinemia.
- Mnimum urine osmolality in children is 30–50 mOsm/kg where as maximum urine osmolality is 1200 mOsm/kg.
- Electrolte abnormality in Diabetes Insipidus is hypernatremia.
- Sodium correction in hyponatremia is done at the rate of < 12 mEq/L/ day or < 0.5 mEq/L/hr.
- Rapid correction of hyponatremia may lead to **central pontine myelinolysis**.

Diagnostic criteria for syndrome of inappropriate antidiuretic hormone secretion

Absence of:
Renal, adrenal, or thyroid insufficiency
Heart failure, nephrotic syndrome, or cirrhosis
Diuretic ingestion
Dehydration
Urine osmolality > 100 mOsm/kg (usually > plasma)
Serum osmolality < 280 mOsm/kg and serum sodium < 135 mEq/L
Urine sodium > 30 mEq/L

- Diagnostic criteria for Diabetes Insipidus is Urine osmolality < 300 mOsm/kg and serum osmolality > 300 mOsm/kg.
- **Pseudoporphyria** is characterized by small hypopigmented depressed scars occurring in areas of minor skin trauma, such as fingernail scratches, or after small spontaneous vesicular lesions. It occurs more commonly in Naproxen than in NSAIDs.

QUESTIONS

1. Object permanence in a child is seen after: (2014)
a. 6 months
b. 9 months
c. 12 months
d. 15 months

2. High anion gap acidosis is seen in all except: (2014)
a. Diarrhea
b. Salicylate poisoning
c. Acute renal failure
d. Lactic acidosis

3. An infant presents with irritability, increased tone of extremities and recurrent seizures. Tissue examination reveals globoid cells in parenchyma around blood vessels. What is the most probable diagnosis? **(2014)**
a. Taysach's disease
b. Krabbe disease
c. Adrenoleukodystrophy
d. Kanavan's disease

4. An 8-year-old mentally retarded child presents with left side flank pain. On ultrasound hyperechoic lesion is seen in right kidney and multiple lesions in the liver. CT scan of abdomen shows-50-to-60 HU density of the lesion in kidney and liver. The most probable diagnosis is: **(2014)**
a. Familial angiolipomatosis
b. ADPKD
c. VHL
d. Tuberous sclerosis

5. Breastfeeding should be avoided by a mother on ATT for how many weeks? **(2014)**
a. 1 b. 2
c. 3 d. 4

6. Perecentage of sucrose solution used for newborn analgesia is: **(2014)**
a. 5% b. 10%
c. 24% d. 50%

7. An infant presents with lethargy, frontal bossing and bowing of legs, X-ray shows widening of epiphysis. What is the diagnosis? **(2014)**
a. Scurvy
b. Rickets
c. Osteomalacia
d. Osteopetrosis

8. What is the dose of adrenaline given to a child with cardiac arrest? **(2014)**
a. 0.1 ml/kg of 1:1000 solution
b. 1 ml/kg of 1:1000 solution
c. 0.1 ml/kg of 1:10000 solution
d. 1 ml/kg of 1:10000 solution

9. All affect effectiveness of phototherapy except: (2014)
a. Skin pigmentation
b. Initial level of serum bilirubin
c. Spectral irradiance
d. Type of lamp used

10. Most dangerous sign in LRTI in children is: (2014)
a. Abdominal breathing
b. Chest retraction
c. Grunting
d. Tachypnea

11. 24 hours after fever, maculopapular rash and erythema appears on the face of infant. This organism can also cause: **(2014)**
a. ALL
b. CML
c. Pure red cell aplasia
d. Hairy cell leukemia

12. True about ischemic stroke in children: **(2014)**
a. Spontaneous parenchymal bleed is common
b. Intracranial arterial aneurysms are common
c. Basal ganglia infarct by VZV
d. ?

13. A child came to casualty after seizures. On examination, respiratory rate is 5 per min, pulse 54 per min and cyanosis is present. What should be the next step of management? **(2014)**
a. Give diazepam (seizures) and then give adrenaline and chest compression
b. Intubation followed by ventilation with O_2 and give chest compression
c. O_2 chest compression and adrenaline, LMA
d. IV Midazolam stat followed by LMA

14. An 18 months child came with LRTI with Respiratory Rate of 50/min. Child was not lethargic but irritable and has stridor. Examination reveals bilateral rhonchi. SpO_2 88%. What is next best management? (2014)

a. Give O_2 by mask with child on the lap of the mother, along with beta agonist and adrenaline nebulization
b. Examine throat, give O_2 by mask along beta agonist nebulization with one dose of steroid
c. Immediate intubation and ventilate the child and establish IV/IO access
d. Urgent referral to tertiary care

15. Lecithin/Sphingomyelin ratio is done to assess the maturity of: (2014)

a. Lung
b. Fetal circulation
c. Brain
d. Gonad

16. A 4 year child with bronchial asthma presents history of with and 3 and more episodes during daytime in a week and 2 wheezing episodes during night in a month. How will you grade this asthma? (2013)

a. Mild Persistent
b. Moderate persistent
c. Severe persistent
d. Mild intermittent

17. Hutchison triad all seen except: (2013)

a. Interstitial keratitis
b. Cataract
c. Deafness
d. Notched incisors

18. Definition of low birth weight: (2013)

a. Wt < 2.5 kg
b. Wt < 2 kg
c. Wt < 1.5 kg
d. Wt < 1 kg

19. Nocturnal enuresis is abnormal after: (2013)

a. 2 years b. 3 years
c. 4 years d. 5 years

20. Amount of Protein present in 100 ml of breast milk is: (2013)

a. 2.2 g b. 1.1 g
c. 0.55 g d. 3.3 g

21. All are radiologic signs in scurvy except: (2013)

a. White line in Metaphysis
b. Cupping and fraying
c. Ground glass appearance
d. Zone of rarefaction

22. Most common cause of congenital hypothyroidism: (2013)

a. Thyroid dysgenesis
b. Dyshormonogenesis
c. Antithyroid antibodies
d. Maternal Hypothyroidism

23. What percentage of weight loss in children constitutes severe dehydration? (2013)

a. >4% loss of body weight
b. >6% loss of body weight
c. 5% loss of body weight
d. 7% loss of body weight

24. A 7 days old neonate present with recurrent seizures. On examination, tachycardia and S3 gallop, bruit in anterior fontanelle. Blood investigations are normal. Neurosonogram shows a hypoechoic lesion. What is the diagnosis? (2013)

a. Arachoid cyst
b. Vein of Galen malformation
c. Dilated ventricles
d. Intraventricular hemorrhage

25. Fatty liver in kwashiorkor is due to: (2013)

a. Decrease in carbohydrates
b. Decrease in protein substrates
c. Abnormal protein synthesis
d. Reduced synthesis of lipoprotein carrier

26. An infant presents with cardiac failure. Examination reveals a weaker femoral pulse when compared to the radial pulse. What is the probable diagnosis? (2013)

a. PDA
b. COA
c. Aortoilliac vasculitis
d. VSD

27. Common cause neonatal mortality among high-risk newborns are all except: (2013)

a. Diarrhea
b. Prematurity
c. Low birth weight
d. Birth asphyxia

28. Non immune fetal hydrops caused by all except: (2013)

a. Parvovirus B19 infection
b. Rh incompatibility
c. Congenital heart block
d. Twin-twin transfusion syndrome

29. Total body irradiation is routinely done before which of the following transplantation? (2013)

a. Lungs
b. Liver
c. Bone marrow
d. Pancreas

30. A 2 year old child presents with loose stools. On examination she has signs of severe dehydration. If her weight is 10 kg, what would be the volume of fluid to be given in the first 4 hours? (2012)
a. 1000 ml
b. 100 ml
c. 200 ml
d. 500 ml

31. You order a wrist X-ray for a 2 months old child. Which carpal bone are you expecting to be present? (2012)
a. Capitates
b. Scaphoid
c. Lunate
d. Trapezoid

32. How many permanent teeth will be present in an 8 year old child? (2012)
a. 20
b. 24
c. 12
d. 16

33. Two months old child presented with fever, respiratory distress, recurrent apnea followed by bradycardia and cyanosis. What is the probable diagnosis? (2012)
a. Congenital heart block
b. Whooping cough
c. Tracheobronchiomalacia
d. Epiglotitis

34. Most common ausative organism for sepsis in newborn is: (2012)
a. Streptococcus agalactiae
b. Klebsiella pneumonia
c. Streptococcus pyogenes
d. H.influenzae

35. Breast milk is rich in_ when compared to cow's milk: (2012)
a. Lactose
b. Protein
c. Fat
d. Vitamin K

36. Abnormality in Crigler Najjar syndrome: (2012)
a. Uptake of bilirubin
b. Defect in hepatic conjugation
c. Canalicular Release
d. Reduced bile excretion

37. In a Rh negative Mother with Rh positive baby, exchange transfusion is not indicated if: (2012)
a. Cord blood Hemoglobin less than 11 gm/dl
b. Bilirubin increases 1 mg/hour despite phototherapy
c. Increase in total bilirubin level more than 10 mg/24 hours
d. Cord blood bilirubin >4 mg/dl

38. Which sinus will be absent in a newborn? (2012)
a. Forntal sinus
b. Maxillary
c. Anterior ethmoidal
d. Posterior ethmoidal

39. Pulmonary plethora is not seen in: (2012)
a. VSD
b. TOF
c. Trauncus arteriosus
d. TAPVC

40. Sagittal sutures overlapping causes: (2012)
a. Oxycephaly
b. Dolicocepaly
c. Plagiocepaly
d. Cephalocephaly

41. Diplegia means: (2012)
a. Weakness of upper limbs
b. Weakness of lower limbs
c. Weakness of unilateral upper and lower limbs
d. Weakness of the all four limbs

42. A child with prolonged aPTT underwent laparotomy and still did not develop any bleeding complications. Which of the following clotting factors is most likely to be deficient? (2012)
a. Factor VII
b. Factor XII
c. Factor X
d. Factor XIII

43. Administration of which of the following can prevent neural defects in newborn? (2011)
a. Folic acid
b. Vit B12
c. Pyridoxine
d. Vitamin C

44. Which of the following is a feature of marasmus and not kwarshiorkor? (2011)
a. Voracious appetite
b. Fatty change in liver
c. Hypoalbuminemia
d. Edema

45. Jeune syndrome is transmitted as: (2011)
a. Autosomal recessvie
b. Autosomal Dominant
c. X linked Dominant
d. X linked Recessvie

46. Definitive sign of scurvy in X-ray is: (2011)
a. Ringed epiphysis
b. Ground glass appearance
c. White line in metaphysic
d. Pencil thin cortex

47. Which of the following manifestation of rheumatic fever disappears completely? (2011)
a. Carditis
b. Arthritis
c. Chorea
d. Subcutaneous nodules

48. Which of the following is a risk factor for developing type 1 Diabetes mellitus? (2011)
a. Male Gender
b. Old age
c. Gestational diabetes
d. HLA DR3

49. Grasp reflex is fully developed at: (2011)
a. 24 weeks
b. 28 weeks
c. 32 weeks
d. 36 weeks

50. Killed vaccine among the following is: (2011)
a. Oral Polio Vaccine
b. Hepatitis B
c. Yellow fever
d. Japanese encephalitis

51. All are true regarding SCID except: (2011)
a. Due to deficiency of adenosine deaminase
b. Toxicity of leucocytes due to accumulation of cAMP
c. Both cellular and humoral immunity affected
d. Bone marrow transplantation is the treatment

52. Daily maintenance fluid for a child weighing 10 kg is: (2011)
a. 1000 ml/day
b. 800 ml/day
c. 500 ml/day
d. 1200 ml/day

53. Most common cause of Acute otitis media in children is: (2010)
a. Strep pneumoniae
b. Strep pyogenes
c. Staph aureus
d. Pseudomonas

54. Child with recurrent fractures and wormian bones is most likely to have: (2010)
a. Osteogenesis imperfecta
b. Rickets
c. Battered baby syndrome
d. Shaken baby syndrome

55. Cleft lip is repaired at: (2010)
2–4 months
1–4 weeks
6–12 months
12–18 months

56. Parkland formula is: (2010)
a. Percentage of burn area × body wt × 4
b. Percentage of burn area × body wt/4
c. Percentage of burn area × body surface area × 4
d. Percentage of burn area × body surface area/4

57. Surfactant is produced by: (2010)
a. Type 2 pneumocytes
b. Type 1 pneumocytes
c. Clara cells
d. Endothelium

58. First sinus to develop in a growing fetus: (2010)
a. Maxillary
b. Frontal
c. Ethmoidal
d. Sphenoidal

59. Maintenance IV fluids per day for child weighing 10 kg: (2010)
a. 400 ml
b. 500 ml
c. 800 ml
d. 1000 ml

60. Pincer grasp is seen at: (2010)
a. 5–6 months
b. 7–8 months
c. 9–11 months
d. >12 months

61. Most common complication of mumps in children: (2010)
a. Orchitis
b. Aseptic meningitis
c. Myocarditis
d. Pancreatitis

62. Max limit of cardiothoracic ratio in children below 2 years: (2010)
a. 0.40 b. 0.45
c. 0.50 d. 0.55

63. False about hartnup's disease: (2010)
a. Defect in neutral aminoacid transport
b. Mental retardation is the common presentation
c. Most children are asymptomatic
d. Photosensitivity

64. Hyaline membrane deposition is seen in: (2010)
a. ARDS
b. RDS
c. Pulmonary hemorrhage
d. Interstitial lung disease

65. Patient with VSD develops pulmonary hypertension. Which of the following will be present? (2010)
a. Cyanosis
b. Initial resolution of symptoms
c. Clubbing
d. Ejection systolic murmur in pulmonary area

66. In which of the following tubercular infection steroid is used? (2010)
a. TB Lymphadenitis
b. TB Osteomylitis
c. Endobronchial TB
d. Neurotuberculosis

67. Most common cause of congenital hypothyroidism:
a. Thyroid dysgenesis (2010)
b. Maternal antibodies
c. Inborn errors of thyroid hormone defects
d. Maternal iodine deficiency

68. Juvenile idiopathic arthritis includes all the following categories except: (2009)
a. Psoriatic arthritis
b. Enthesitis related arthritis
c. Systemic arthritis
d. Reactive arthritis

69. An infant presents with cardiac failure. Examination reveals a weaker femoral pulse when compared to the radial pulse. What is the probable diagnosis? (2009)
a. PDA
b. COA
c. Aortoilliac vasculitis
d. VSD

70. What percentage of weight loss in infants constitutes severe dehydration? (2009)
a. >10% loss of body weight
b. >6% loss of body weight
c. 5% loss of body weight
d. 7% loss of body weight

71. All the following are indicated in the long-term therapy of children with coronary abnormalities in kawasaki disease except: (2009)
a. Intravenous immunoglobulins
b. Aspirin
c. Clopidogrel
d. Warfarin

72. All the following drugs are indicated in the treatment of complicated typhoid fever in children except: (2009)
a. Ceftriaxone
b. Oral azithromycin
c. Ciprofloxacin
d. Chloramphenicol

73. A 6-year-old boy presents with complaints of hyperactivity, excessive shoulder shrugging, throat clearing and eye blinking. During examination, he is not cooperative, uses obscene words and runs around in the consulation room. What is the most probable diagnosis? (2009)
a. Attention deficit hyperactivity disorder
b. Tic disorder
c. Psychomotor seizures
d. Childhood psychosis

74. Areola and papilla forming secondary mound in adolescent girls is classified under which stage of sexual maturity rating (SMR)? (2009)
a. SMR stage 2
b. SMR stage 3
c. SMR stage 4
d. SMR stage 5

75. Daily maintanence fluid for a child weighing 10 kg is: (2009)
a. 1000 ml/day
b. 800 ml/day
c. 500 ml/day
d. 1200 ml/day

76. Definition of extremely low birth weight: (2009)
a. Wt <2.5 kg
b. Wt <2 kg
c. Wt <1.5 kg
d. Wt <1 kg

77. Nocturnal enuresis should be investigated and treated after: (2009)
a. 2 years
b. 3 years
c. 4 years
d. 5 years

78. Child with recurrent fractures and wormian bones is most likely to have: (2009)
a. Osteogenesis imperfecta
b. Rickets
c. Battered baby syndrome
d. Shaken baby syndrome

79. Cleft palate is repaired at: (2009)
a. 2–4 months b. 1–4 weeks
c. 6–12 months d. 12–38 months

80. Kopilk spot is located: (2008)
a. Opposite to first molar
b. Opposite to premolar
c. Opposite to incisor
d. Opposite to canine

81. Grasp reflex begins at: (2008)
a. 24 weeks
b. 28 weeks
c. 32 weeks
d. 36 weeks

82. Cystic fibrosis is associated with: (2008)
a. Meconium ileus
b. Short bowel syndrome
c. Hirschprung disease
d. Congenital pyrolic stenosis

83. Amount of fluid to be given to 8 months baby weighing 10 kg with severe dehydration: (2008)
a. 100 ml
b. 800 ml
c. 400 ml
d. 1000 ml

84. All are true regarding Hypereosinophilic syndrome in children except: (2008)
a. Eosinophilia of > 1500 cells/microliter
b. Persistent eosinophilia for 6 months
c. Absence of any specific organ involvement
d. Corticosteroids are first line therapy

85. All are causes of eosinophilia except: (2008)
a. Allergic Rhinitis
b. Trichinosis
c. Corticosteroid therapy
d. Rheumatoid arthritis

86. Children can reach for objects by: (2008)
a. 4 months
b. 6 months
c. 8 months
d. 10 months

87. Which of the following symptoms of rheumatic fever be the only isolated manifestation? (2008)
a. Carditis
b. Arthritis
c. Chorea
d. Subcutaneous nodules

88. Which of the following is a risk factor for developing Type 1 Diabetes mellitus? (2008)
a. Male Gender
b. Old age
c. Gestational diabetes
d. HLA DR3

89. False about Hartnup's disease: (2008)
a. Defect in neutral aminoacid transport
b. Mental retardation is the common presentation
c. Most children are asymptomatic
d. Photosensitivity

90. A 15-month-old child is able to do all the following except: (2007)
a. Crawl upstairs
b. Make a tower of 5 cubes
c. Name familiar objects
d. Point to familiar things

91. All the following are true regarding the management of asymptomatic close contacts of whooping cough except: (2007)
a. Azithromycin is the drug of choice
b. Drug therapy not required in an adequately immunized child
c. Isolation is not required
d. Booster dose is given for under-immunized children

92. All are true regarding osmotic diarrhea except: (2007)
a. Due to highly osmotic substances in lumen
b. Fasting may improve symptoms
c. Stool reducing substances are present
d. Can be mediated by bacterial toxins

93. All are true regarding subacute combined immunodeficiency except: (2007)
a. Due to deficiency of adenosine deaminase
b. Toxicity of leucocytes due to accumulation of cAMP
c. Both cellular and humoral immunity affected
d. Bone marrow transplantation is the treatment

94. How many permanent teeth will be present in an 8-year-old child? (2007)
a. 20
b. 24
c. 12
d. 16

95. Breast milk is rich in _ when compared to cow's milk: (2007)
a. Lactose
b. Protein
c. Fat
d. Vitamin K

96. Most common complication of mumps in children: (2007)
a. Orchitis
b. Aseptic meningitis
c. Myocarditis
d. Pancreatitis

97. Least useful antirachitic: (2006)
a. 1, 25-hydroxy cholecalciferol (calcitriol)
b. Cholecalciferol
c. 25-hydroxy cholecalciferol
d. Calcium

98. Subperiosteal hemorrhage is seen in: (2006)
a. Vit C deficiency
b. Vit A deficiency
c. Vit E deficiency
d. Vit B2 deficiency

99. Arnold chiari malformation is associated with:
a. Meningomyelocele **(2006)**
b. Leptomeningeal cyst
c. Agenesis of corpus callosum
d. Dandy-Walker anomaly

100. LBW is defined as birth weight less than: (2006)
a. 2 kg
b. 1 kg
c. 1.5 kg
d. 2.5 kg

101. Alkaline phosphatase level are not elevated in:
a. Renal rickets **(2006)**
b. Nutritional rickets
c. Hypophosphatasia
d. Hypophosphatemic rickets

102. Suture of skull fuse by: (2006)
a. 5 years b. 1 year
c. 3 years d. 8 years

103. Incubation period of pertussis is: (2006)
a. Three days
b. Three weeks
c. Two weeks
d. Four weeks

104. Hallmark of uncompensated shock in a child is imbalance between O_2 delivery and O_2 consumption. This is manifested by all except:
a. High anion gap metabolic acidosis **(Dec. 2014)**
b. Increased lactic acid production
c. Decreased oxygen extraction in the tissues
d. Low mixed venous oxygen saturation

105. An 11 year child with failure to thrive, metabolic acidosis with increased anion gap. Not true regarding the differential diagnosis: (Dec. 2014)
a. Insulin dependent diabetes mellitus
b. Chronic renal failure
c. Renal tubular acidosis
d. Inborn errors of metabolism

106. Not an indication to administer anti-snake venom to a child at early morning 4 am is:
a. Local swelling with fang marks **(Dec. 2014)**
b. Severe abdominal pain without fang marks
c. Gum bleeding or prolonged 20 minutes whole blood clotting time (WBCT)
d. External ophthalmoplegia with inability to lift the head

107. Most common organ involved in blunt trauma in children: (Dec. 2014)
a. Spleen
b. Kidney
c. Liver
d. Small intestine

108. A coin is loaded in the esophagus of an asymptomatic 3 years female child, Treatment is:
a. Endoscopic removal within 24 hours
b. Immediate endoscopic removal **(Dec. 2014)**
c. Wait for 48 hours
d. Dislodge the coin to the stomach by inserting Ryle's tube

109. A child with upper gastro intestinal bleed due to varices. Line of management is: (Dec. 2014)
a. Octreotide is reserved for situations where immediate endoscopy is not available
b. Sengstaken Blackmore tube is preferred than pharmacotherapy
c. Lavage is given in room temperature
d. Target of haemoglobin for blood transfusion is 10g/dl.

110. Invertogram in a newborn with imperforate anus is done: (Dec. 2014)
a. After 2 hours
b. After 4 hours
c. After 6 hours
d. Immediately

111. Intussusception is caused by: (Dec. 2014)
a. Submucous lipoma
b. Subfascial lipoma
c. Subserous lipoma
d. Intramural lipoma

112. The normal gain in length in a full term baby, at first 6 months of life is: (Dec. 2014)
a. 6 cm
b. 9 cm
c. 15 cm
d. 24 cm

113. Bed wetting is normal upto what age in girls and boys respectively? (Dec. 2014)
a. 3 years and 4 years
b. 4 years and 5 years
c. 5 years and 5 years
d. 5 years and 6 years

114. Molar ratio of Sodium and Glucose in WHO ORS is: (Dec. 2014)
a. 1 : 1
b. 1 : 2
c. 1 : 4
d. 2 : 1

115. According to WHO, severe acute malnutritionin children is defined as: (Dec. 2014)
a. Weight for height Z score < -3
b. Weight for height Z score < -2
c. Weight for height Z score < -1
d. Weight for height Z score between -2 and -3

116. To prevent acute rheumatic fever, acute pharyngitis due to group A streptococci should be treated with antibiotics before: (Dec. 2014)
a. 7 days of illness
b. 8 days of illness
c. 9 days of illness
d. 10 days of illness

117. Not a typical localizing sign indicative of involvement of intrathoracic extra pulmonary site in children with respiratory infections:
a. Stridor **(Dec. 2014)**
b. Wheezing
c. Tachypnoea
d. Chest retraction

118. Neonatal liver failure is uncommonly associated with: (Dec. 2014)
a. Hereditary fructose intolerance
b. Congenital hepatic fibrosis
c. Galactosemia
d. Hemophagocytic lympho histiocytosis.

119. Phenylketonurla–true statement: (Dec. 2014)
a. Urine phenyl alanine metabolites are increased
b. Deficiency of tyrosine hydroxylase
c. Serum tyrosine levels are decreased
d. Mental retardation does not occur if patient is advised to have phenyl alanine free diet

120. Component of initial impression in Pediatric Advanced life Support (PALS)-2010 are all except: (Dec. 2014)
a. Airway
b. Breathing
c. Color
d. Consciousness

121. USG in 18–20 weeks is done to: (Dec. 2014)
a. Detect maturity
b. Detect anomalies
c. Detect the sex of the fetus
d. Estimate the liquor

122. Myelination begins at: (Dec. 2014)
a. 20 weeks
b. 25 weeks
c. 30 weeks
d. 35 weeks

123. A child presents with tuberculosis. Steroids are not indicated in: (Dec. 2014)
a. Tuberculoma
b. Endobronchial tuberculosis
c. Pleural effusion
d. Progressive primary pulmonary disease

124. Paratid enlargement in a HIV infected child is characterized in which stage of AIDS, according to WHO: (Dec. 2014)
a. Stage 1
b. Stage 2
c. Stage 3
d. Stage 4

ANSWERS AND EXPLANATIONS

1. Ans. b. 9 months *Ref: Nelson's Texbook of Pediatrics, 19/e p27*

Object permanence (constancy) is the understanding that objects continue to exist, even when not seen. e.g. A hidden toy. It is a major Milestone that is achieved at 9 months of age.

2. Ans. a. Diarrhea *Ref: Nelson's Texbook of Pediatrics, 19/e p231*

Anion gap is difference between measured cations (Na^+, K^+, etc) and anions (Cl^-, HCO_3^-). For simplicity, K is not included. Anion gap signifies the amount of unmeasured anions in blood.

Anion gap = $[Na^+]-[Cl^-]-[HCO_3^-]$

Normal anion gap is 4 to 11. This normal anion gap is mainly due to albumin. Normal anion gap metabolic acidosis mostly occurs due to GIT or renal loss of HCO_3^-.

Common causes of normal anion gap metabolic acidosis are
- Diarrhoea
- Renal tubular acidosis
- Urinary tract diversions
- Ammonium chloride intake

Common causes of High anion gap metabolic acidosis are (MUDPILES)

- Methanol poisoning
- Uremia
- Diabetic ketoacidosis
- Phenformin, Paraldehyde poisoning
- In born error of metabolism, Iron/Isoniazid overdose
- Liver failure, Lactic acidosis
- Ethanol poisoning
- Statvation ketoacidosis

3. **Ans. b. Krabbe disease** *Ref: Robbins, Genetic Metabolic Disease; Nelson's Textbook of Pediatrics, 19/e p490*

Krabbe disease is also known as globoid cell leukodystrophy caused due to defiency of the enzyme galactocerebrosidase (β galactosidase). It is inherited as autosomal recessive fashion. In this disease both central and peripheral myelin are affected. The early infantile form presents with **irritability, hypertonia , seizures and mental impairment.** Death occurs before 3 years of age. The late infantile form occurs after 2 years of age. Diagnosis is by demonstration of enzyme defiency in WBCs and cultured skin fibroblasts. Treatment is umbilical cord stem cell transplant.

P–Pompe's–α glucosidase deficiency
G–Gaucher's–β glucocerebrosidase deficiency
F–Fabry's–α galactosidase deficiency
K–Krabbe's–β galactocerbrosidase deficiency

4. **Ans. d. Tuberous sclerosis** *Ref: Nelson's Texbook of Pediatrics, 19/e p2049 and 2052*

The diagnosis is Tuberous sclerosis Complex (TSC). TSC presents with renal angiomyolipoma which may bleed causing flank pain. On ultrasound these lesions are hyperechoic when compared to anechoic lesion of ADPKD (Autosomal ominant Polycystic Kidney Disease). Familial angiolipomaosis presents with benign subcutaneous masses on arms, trunk and legs. von Hippel Lindau (vHL) Disease may present as cystic lesions of kidneys, liver, pancreas, epididymus but the cysts are anechoic. Mental retardation occurs in about 40% of TSC whereas it is rare in vHL.

Tuberous Sclerosis Complex is inherited as an autosomal dominant trait with an extremely heterogenous clinical spectrum. The major features of TSC are cortical tuber, subependymal nodule, subependymal giant cell astrocytoma, facial angiofibroma, ungual/periungual fibroma, hypomalanotic patches (>3), Shagreen patch, multiple retinal hamartomas, cardiac rhabdomyoma, renal angiomyolipoma, pulmonary lymphangiomyomatosis. Clinical features together with MRI of brain usually confirms diagnosis. Genetic testing for TSC_1 and TSC_2 mutations may considered when clinical criteria are not met. Treatment is supportive.

5. **Ans. None** *Ref: Tran JH, Montakantikuk P. The safety of antibuberculosis medications during breastfeeding. J Hum Lact 1998; 14(4): 337–40. Elizabeth 4/e p13. Indian J Med Res, 140 July 2014, pages 32–39.*

Recent IAP and WHO guidelines (2014) do not recommend avoiding breastfeeding to the infant born to mother with active TB. Baby should be given Isoniazid prophylaxis for 6–9 months. Baby should given BCG which decreases the risk of TB infection in the exposed infant. Mother should observe appropriate cough hygiene. Maternal ATT makes the baby less likely to be infected, after 2 weeks of intensive course. Maternal ATT neither produces a therapeutic effect nor adverse drug effect in the breast fed infant.

Contraindications for Breastfeeding

Absolute

- Congenital Lactose Intolerence
- Galactosemia

Relative

- Antimalignant drugs
- Anti thyroid drugs
- Lithium

Note: Propylthio uracil and Warfarin are safe in lactating mothers.

Breastfeeding is contraindicated in infant of HIV positive mother in western countries, as HIV transfers through breast milk. However, as the mortality due to pneumonia and diarrhea in non breast fed children is more than that of HIV, WHO and NACO (National AIDS Control Organization) advise exclusive breastfeeding in infants of HIV positive mothers. Mixed feeding (breastfeeding and formula feeding) should not be practiced as the transmission rate is more than breastfeeding alone. Breastfeeding is not contra indicated in HBs Ag positive mothers.

6. **Ans. c. 24%** *Ref: Cloherty's Manual of Newborn Care, 7/e p879*

For minimally invasive procedures in neonates, like drawing blood, 24% Sucrose solution is used. For neonates undergoing invasive and very painful procedures, narcotics (Morphine and Fentanyl) and sedatives (Midazolam and Phenobarbital) are used. For circumcision in newborn, 24% Sucrose and Parcetmol 15 mg/kg/ dose preoperatively along with ring or dorsal penile block with 0.5% Lidocaine for procedure are used. Note: Maximum concentration of Dextrose given intravenously through a peripheral vein in newborn is 12.5%. A higher concentration has to be given via a central line.

7. **Ans. b. Rickets** *Ref: Nelson's Texbook of Pediatrics, 19/e p205*

The clinical features of lethargy, frontal bossing, bowing of legs (genu varum) alongs with widening of epiphysis leads to the diagnosis of Rickets. The radiographic changes in Rickets are:

- Decreased calcification
- Loss of sharp borders of metaphysis (cupping and fraying)
- Edge of metaphysic is more convex or flat rather than normal concave shape.
- Widening of distal end of metaphysis
- Coarse trabeculation of Diaphysis
- Generalised rarefaction

The radiological features of Scurvy are:

- Ground glass appearance
- Thin and dense cortex (Pencil line cortex)
- White line of Frenkel at metaphysis
- Zone of rarefaction (Trumer feld zone)
- Pelkan spur
- Subperiosteal hemorrhage (not seen in acute stage)

The scorbutic rosary are more angulated and tender where as the rickety rosary are more rounded and painless.

8. **Ans. c. 0.1 ml/kg of 1:10000 solution** *Ref: Nelson's Textbook of Pediatrics, 19/e p288–294*

The dose of Adrenaline (Epinephrine) in Pediatric cardiac arrest is 0.01 mg/kg or 0.1 ml/kg of 1:10,000. The dose of Adrenaline through ET tube is 10 times the IV dose (0.1 mg/kg). The drugs that are administered through ET tube are LEAN (Lignocaine, Epinephrine, Atropine, Naloxone).

9. **Ans. Skin pigmentation** *Ref: OP Ghai and Nelson's Textbook of Pediatrics, 19/e p610 and Rossi's Principles of Transfusion Medicine, Simon TL et al., 4/e Cloherty 7/e p325–329*

Phototherapy is given with special blue lamps with wave lenths 450 to 475 nm are most efficient. However, cool white lamps with peak wave length 550 to 600 nm are usually adequate for treatment. Phototherapy is effective when the irradiance is in the range of 6 to 12 Mw/cm^2/. If initial level of serum bilirubin high,phototherapy is very effective and bilirubin falls rapidly.

During phototherapy, toxic bilirubin is converted in to non toxic isomers which are excreted in bile and urine. The three photochemical reactions that occur during phototherapy are

- **Photoisomerization** (bilirubin converted in to less toxic polar isomer that is excreted in bile without conjugation),
- **Structural isomerization** (bilirubin converted in to lumirubin that is excreted in bile and urine without conjugation) and
- **Photooxidation** (bilirubin converted into small polar compounds that are excreted in urine). Structural isomerization is the most important pathway for lowering serum bilirubin.

Phototherapy is usually contraindicated in conjugated hyperbilirubinemia where it may lead to **"bronze baby syndrome"**

10. **Ans. c. Grunting** *Ref: Pediatric Advanced Life Support 2011, pages 16–17*

Abdominal breathing maybe seen in normal infants. Tachypnea and chest reactions are seen in respiratory distress. Grunting indicates progression of respiratory distress to respiratory failure. Grunt occurs as child exhales against a partially closed glottis. It is sign of lung tissue disease resulting from small airway collapse, alveolar collapse or both.

Grunting occurs in pneumonia, pulmonary contusion, ARDS, pulmonary edema, also in abdominal pathology like bowel obstruction, perforated viscus, appendicitis or peritonitis.

11. Ans. c. Pure red cell aplasia *Ref: Nelson's Texbook of Pediatrics, 19/e p1094–97*

Fever, maculopapular rash and erythema on the face of infant is characteristic of Fifth disease (**Erythema Infeciosum**). It is caused by Parvo virus B 19. The characteristic facial flushng is described as "**slapped cheek appearance**". Parvo virus B19 also causes **RBC aplasia** to transient aplastic crisis. Parvo Virus B19 in mother can cause intra uterine fetal demise or **Non immune fetal hydrops**.

Sixth disease (also known as **Exanthum subitum or Roseola Infantum**) is another self limiting illness caused by Human Herpes Virus type 6 (HHV–6). The characteristic ulcers seen at the uvulopatoglossal junction are termed as **"Nagayama spots"**

12. Ans. c. Basal ganglia infarct by VZV

Ref: Nelson's Texbook of Pediatrics, 19/e p2080 and Askalan R et al. Chickenpox and stroke in childhood; A study of frequency and causation. Stroke 2001; 32(6): 1257–62

Unilateral hemiparesis in ischemic stroke may occur due to basal ganglia infarct 1 to 4 months after Varicella Zoster infecrion. Etiology is due to spasm of Lenticostriate arteries. Prognosis is good as neurological deficits improve over time. Varicella infection has 3 fold increase in arterial ischemic stroke in children than in general population.

13. Ans. c. O_2, chest compression and adrenalin, LMA. *Ref: Nelson Textbook of Pediatrics, 19/e p287–8*

The PALS (Pediatric Advanced Life Support) 2010 guidelines recommend CAB (Chest compression, airway and breathing) rather than ABC. A child with impending respiratory failure and HR of 54 (< 60) is an indication for CAB resuscitation. O_2, chest compression, adrenaline and LMA (Laryngeal Mask Airway) is the best treatment for this child. Anticonvulsants in a child with cardiopulmonary compromise will kill a child. Intubation in a child with HR 54 is not recommended immediately.

14. Ans. a. *Ref: Nelson Textbook of Pediatrics, 19/e p287–8*

An 18 months old child with respiratory rate of 50 (tachypneic) and stridor is probably having ALTB (Acute Laryngo Tracheo Bronchitis). The treatment is giving O_2 in a non threatening manner with child on mothers lap. Adrenaline nebulization is recommended (beta agonist maybe added as this child is having bilateral wheeze). IM Dexamethazone can be given in ALTB but throat examination should not be done in this child as this would agitate the hypoxic infant and worsen the condition. Immediate intubation should not be done in any child with suspected upper air way obstruction without the help of an expert or an ENT surgeon, in the Pediatric Emergency Room. Urgent referral of any critically ill child should not be done without stabilization.

15. Ans. a. Lung *Ref: Cloherty's Manual of Newborn Care, 7/e p406–407*

Lecithin/Phingomyelin ratio is to assess fetal lung maturity. It is done by thin layer chromatography. A value of > 2 indicates the risk of Respiratory Distress Syndrome is very less (exceptins are infant of diabetic mother, erythroblastosis fetalis and intrapartum asphyxia). Contamination of blood and meconium affects the interpretation of the test. The other test to assess fetal lung maturity are

- TDx–FLM II,
- Lamellar body counts and
- Presence of Phosphatidylglycerol.

16. Ans. a. Mild Persistent *Ref: Nelson's Texbook of Pediatrics, 19/e p790*

S. No.	Component of severity	Mild intermitent	Mild persistent	Mod persistent	Severe persistent
1.	Day time symptoms	≤ 2 days/week	>2 days/week but not daily	daily	Throughout the day
2.	Night awakenings 0–4 years	0	1–2/months	3–4/months	>1/week
3.	Night awakenings ≥5 years	≤ 2/months	3–4/months	>1/week	Often 7/week

17. Ans. b. Cataract *Ref: Nelson's Texbook of Pediatrics, 19/e p1017*

Hutchinson triad includes

- Hutchinson teeth (peg shaped upper central incisors with a notch along the biting surface),
- Interstitial keratitis and
- Eighth nerve deafness.

18. Ans. a. Wt < 2.5 kg *Ref: Nelson's Texbook of Pediatrics, 19/e Cloherty 7/e p76*

Normal birth weight is 2500 to 4000 g
Low birth weight (LBW) is < 2500 g (includes both term and preterm neonates)
Very low birth weight (VLBW) is < 1500 g
Extremely low birth weight (ELBW) is < 1000 g
Preterm is < 37 completed weeks (gestational age) or < 259 days
Late preterm is 34 to 36 weeks (238 to 258 days)
Term is 37 to 40 weeks (260 to 294 days)
Post term is 42 weeks (295 days) or more.

19. Ans. d. 5 years *Ref: Nelson's Texbook of Pediatrics, 19/e p71*

Enuresis is defined as thee repeated voiding of urine into clothes or bed at least twice a week for at least 3 consecutive months in a child who is at least 5 year of age. Diurnal enuresis refers to wetting while awake and nocturnal enuresis refers to voiding during sleep. Primary enuresis occurs in children who have never been considered dry through the night whereas secondary enuresis refers to the resumption of wetting after at least 6 months of dryness.

At 5 years, 7% of boys and 3% of girls have enuresis. Primary enuresis accounts for 85% of cases. It is common in low socioeconomic groups, in larger families, and in institutionalized children. Iurnal enuresis is more common in girls. The etiology of enuresis includes

- Familial
- Low Arginine Vasopressin secretion
- Sleep apnea
- Psychological stress (parental divorce, school trauma, sexual abuse, hospitalization)
- UTI
- Chronic Kidney Disease
- Spinal cord disorders
- Constipation
- Diabetes

Treatment includes behavior therapy, urine alarm, drugs (Desmopressin DDAVP, Imipramine)

20. Ans. b 1.1 g *Ref: Nelson 19/e p161. Elizabeth 4/e p18*

Comparison between Human milk and Cow's milk (per 100 ml)

	Human milk	Cow's milk
Protein	1.1 g	3 g
Casein: whey	40 : 60 (lactabumin, lactoferrin)	80 : 20 (lactoglobin)
Lactose	7 g	4.5 g
Fat	3.8 g	3.7 g
EFA	13%	2%
P/S ratio	1.2 : 1	1 : 2
Ash/mineral	0.25 g	0.75 g
Ca: P ratio	>2	<2
Sodium	0.7 mEq	2.2 mEq
Potassium	1.4 mEq	
Vitamin K	15 μg	60 μg
Vitamin E	2 mg	0.4 mg
Osm	7.9 mOsm	22.1 mOsm
Energy: Protein	70 : 1	25 : 1
Calories	67 cal	67 cal

Note:

Carbohydrate–Breast milk > Cow's milk

Protein–Breast milk < Cow's milk

Fat–Breast milk = Cow's milk

Conditions for which breastfeeding has protective effect.

- Acute conditions
  - Diarrhoea
  - Otitis media
  - UTI
  - Necrotizing enterocolitis
  - Septicemia
  - Infant botulism
- Chronic disorders
  - Type 1 DM
  - Celiac disease
  - Crohn's disease
  - Lymphoma, Leukemia
  - Recurrent otitis media
  - Allergy
- Others
  - Obesity
  - Hospitalization
  - Infant mortality

Components in Breast milk protective against microorganisms

Lactoferrin	E.coli
Bile salt stimulated Lipase (BSSL)	Ameba and Giardia
PABA (Para amino benzoic acid)	Malarial parasite

Drugs that suppress lactation: Pneumonic: NO BP

- Nicotine
- OC Pills
- Bromocriptine
- Pyridoxine

21. **Ans. b. Cupping and fraying** *Ref: Nelson's Texbook of Pediatrics, 19/e p198*

Also refer Q6, 2014

22. **Ans. a. Thyroid dysgenesis** *Ref: Nelson's Texbook of Pediatrics, 19/e p1895*

The most common cause of congenital hypothyroidism is thyroid dysgenesis (aplasia, hypoplasia, ectopic gland), accounting for 80–85% of cases. Fifteen percent are caused by inborn error of thyroxine synthesis (dyshormonogenesis)and 2% are the result of transplacental maternal thyrotropin–receptor blocking antibodies (TRBAb). In the thyroid dysgenesis group, 33% are due aplasia whereas the remaining 66% are due to ectopic thyroid (lingual thyroid) anywhere from the base of tongue and normal position in the neck.

23. **Ans. b. >6% loss of body weight** *Ref: Nelson's Texbook of Pediatrics, 19/e p245 Chapter on 'Deficit Therapy'.*

Dehydration in Infants and children (% of body weight)

S.No.	Severity	Infants	Children/Adult	Clinical features
1.	Mild	< 5%	< 3%	N or ↑HR, ↓urine output, thirsty, normal physical finding
2.	Moderate	5–10%	3–6%	HR ↑, little or no urine output, irritanle/lethary, sunken eye/ fontanel, ↓ tears, dry mucous memb, mld delay in skin turgor, CRT > 1.5 sec, cool and pale
3.	Severe	>10%	>6%	Peripheral pulses weak, ↓BP, no urine output, very sunken eyes/ fontanel, no tears, parched mucous memb, poor skin turgor, CRT > 3 sec, cold, mottled, limp, depressed consciousness.

24. Ans. b. Vein of Galen malformation *Ref: Nelson's Texbook of Pediatrics, 19/e p1639*

Vein of Galen is present under the cerebral hemispheres that drains the anterior and central regions of the brain into the venous sinuses of posterior cranial fossa. Vein of Galen malformation is a choroidal type of AV malformation that presents in neonates with congestive cardiac failure (tachycardia, S3 gallop), bruit over anterior fontanel and seizures. It may also present as developmental delay and as hydrocephalus. The congenital malformation develops during weeks 6–11 of fetal development as a persistent embryonic prosencephalic vein of Markowski; thus, VGAM is actually a misnomer. The vein of Markowski actually drains into the vein of Galen. It is diagnosed by its typical clinical features along with imaging (Canial USG, CT or MRI). In USG it is hypoechoic. Treatment includes management of CCF, shunt procedures for hydrocephalus, vaso occlusive therapy,endovascular embolization etc.

Aracnoid cyst and dilated ventricle may neither present with CCF nor have a bruit over AF. Intraventricular hemorrhage is a hyperechoic lesion in cranial USG and may have abnormal blood investigations like ↓Hb, prolonged PT/PTT, thrombocytopenia, etc.

25. Ans. d. Reduced synthesis of lipoprotein carrier *Ref: OP Ghai 8/e p99*

Common differences between Marasmas and Kwashiorkar

S.No.	Clinical finding	Marasmas	Kwashiorkar
1	Occurrence	More common	Less common
2	Edema	Absent	Present
3	Activity	Active	Apathetic
4	Appetite	Good	Poor
5	Liver enlargement	Absent	Present
6	Mortality	Less than Kwashiorkar	High in early stage
7	Recovery	Early recovery	Slow recovery
8	Infections	Less prone	More prone

In the management of Severe malnutrition, hypoglycemia, hypothermia, dehydration, electrolyte imbalance, infections are treated immediately whereas, iron supplementation should be started after 1 week only.

26. Ans. b. COA *Ref: Nelson's Texbook of Pediatrics, 19/e p1568*

The classical sign of coarctation of aorta (COA) is a disparity in pulsation and blood pressure in the arms and legs. The femoral, popliteal, posterior tibial and dorsalis pedis are weak (or absent) in contrast to the bounding pulses of arms and carotids. A radiofemoral delay occurs due to blood flow to descending aorta coming through the collateral circulation. Normally, systolic BP in legs is 10–20 mm Hg greater than that in the arms. However, in COA, blood pressure in legs is lowerlimbs than in the arms.

27. Ans. a. Diarrhea

Ref: Nelson's Texbook of Pediatrics, 19/e p532 & Million Death Study Collaborators, Bassani DG, Kumar R, Awashi S, Morris SK, Paul VK et al. Causes of neonatal andchild mortality in India: a nationally representative mortality survey. Lancet. 2010 Now 27; 376(9755): 1853–60

Common Neontal mortality in India in 2010 (in no./1000 live births) are

- Prematurity and low birth weight (12.0),
- Infections (9.9),
- Birth asphyxia (7.0),
- Non communicable diseases (1.8),
- Congenital anomalies (1.2),
- Diarrhea (1.2),
- Tetanus (1.2),
- Injuries (0.2) and
- Other causes (2.4).

The causes of post neonatal mortality in 1–59 months of age are (in no./1000 live births)

- Pneumonia (13.5),
- Diarrhea (11.1),

- Measles (3.3),
- Non communicable diseases (3.2),
- Injures (2.9),
- Malaria (2.0),
- Meningitis/encephalitis (1.9),
- Nutritional diseases (1.5),
- Acute bacterial sepsis (1.4),
- Other infections (1.2),
- Other causes (6.9).

28. Ans. b. Rh incompatibility *Ref: Nelson's Texbook of Pediatrics, 19/e p615*

Rh and Kell incompatibily will lead to Immune hydrops fetalis while other three lead to non immune hydrops fetalis.

The other cases of Non Immune Hydrops fetalis are

- Anemia–α thalassemia, G6PD deficiency, Diamond Blackfan syndrome, Twin–twin transfusion
- Cardiac–Supraventricular tachycardia, congenital heart block, hypoplastic LV, cardiomyopathy
- Vascular–Angioma of umbilical cord, umbilical cord aneurysm, true knot of umbilical cord, thrombosis of renal, umbilical vein, IVC
- Lymphatic–Cystic hygroma, chylothorax
- CNS–Absent corpus callosum, intracranial hemorrhage
- Congential infections–Parvovirus, TORCH infections
- Trisomies 13, 15,16, 18, 21

29. Ans. c. Bone marrow

Ref: Adkins DR, DiPersion JF. Total body irradiation before allogeneic stem cell transplantation: is there a magic dose? Curr Opin Hematol. 2008 Now: 15(6): 55–60. & Nelson Textbook of Pediatrics, 19/e p757

Total body irradiation (TBI) is a form of **radiotherapy** used primarily as part of the preparative regimen for **haematopoietic stem cell (or bone marrow) transplantation.** As the name implies, TBI involves irradiation of the entire body, though in modern practice the **lungs** are often partially shielded to lower the risk of radiation-induced lung injury. Total body irradiation in the setting of bone marrow transplantation serves to destroy or suppress the recipient's immune system, preventing **immunologic rejection** of transplanted donor **bone marrow** or **blood stem cells.**

There are three types of bone marrow transplant.

- Autologous–stem cells are removed from the patient before aggressive radiotherapy or chemotherapy, cryopreserved and transfused after that.
- Allogenic–stem cells are harvested from another HLA matched person.
- Umblical cord transplant–a type of allogenic transplant where stem cells are removed from umbilicus of a newborn soon after birth.

Bone marrow is removed (Bone marrow harvest) from the iliac crest of the donor or from peripheral blood (Leukapheresis). The harvested stem cells are transfused to the HLA matched recipient through the peripheral vein(not into bone marrow). HLA matching is not indicated in Liver transplant.

30. Ans. a. 1000 ml *Ref: OP Ghai, Textbook of Pediatrics; 7/e p267*

Treatment of severe dehydration is 100 ml/kg of crystalloid given as follows.

S.No.	Volume of fluid	< 1 year of age	>1 year
1.	First 30 ml/kg	1 hour	½ hour
2.	Next 70 ml/kg	5 hours	2½ hours

Treatment of some dehydration is 75 ml /kg of ORS given orally over 4 hours.

31. Ans. a. Capitate *Ref: Nelson's Texbook of Pediatrics, 19/e p27*

Epiphyseal centres at distal Femur and proximal Tibia are usually present at birth, while that of head of Humerus ossified at 3 weeks of life. Among the carpal bones, Capitate is ossified first at 2 months followed by Hamate at 3 months.

Capitate–2 months

Hamate–3 months
Triangular–30 months
Lunate–42 months
Trapezium–67 months
Trapezoid–69 months
Scaphoid–66 months
Pisiform–variable
Head of Femur–4 months
Patella–46 months
The corresponding ages in females is earlier.

32. Ans. c. 12 *Ref: OP Ghai, Textbook of Pediatrics; 8/e p11*

Secondary Dentition–Time of eruption

• First molar	6 years
• Central incisor	7 years
• Lateral incisor	8 years
• First premolar	10 years
• Canine	11 years
• Second premolar	12 years
• Second molar	13 years
• Third molar	18 years

From the above tables, by 8 years of age, first molar, central and lateral incisors would have erupted in each quadrant. So there would be 12 (3 × 4 = 12) permanent teeth present at 8 years.
First primary tooth to erupt is Lower central incisor. First secondary tooth to erupt is first molar. First and second molars in primary dentition are replaced by first and second premolars respectively in secondary dentition. Delayed eruption of primary dentition is said if no tooth erupt in 13 months of age.

33. Ans. b. Whooping cough *Ref: Nelson 19/e p945*

The classical stages of Whooping cough are

- **Catarrhal stage (1–2 weeks)**–consisting of low grade fever, sneezing, lacrimation and conjuntival suffusion.
- **Paroxysmal stage (2–6 weeks)**–cough marks the onset of this stage. The cough is dry, intermittent, irritative hacking which becomes inexorable paroxysmsms which is the hall mark of pertusssis. A well appearing toddler with insignificant provocation suddenly expresses an axious aura and may clutch a parent before beginning a machine- gun burst of uninterrupted cough on a single exhalation. As cough ceases, a loud whoop follows as inspied air traverses through still partially closed airway. Post tussive emesis is common and exhaustion is universal.
- **Convalescent stage (next ≥ 2 weeks)**–number, severity and duration of episodes diminish.

In infants < 3 months, the classic stages are not seen. The catarrhal phase is usually unnoticed. Cough may not be prominent. A well appearing infant on stimulus due to light, sound, stretching may choke, gasp, gag and flail the extremities with face reddened. Apnea and cyanosis may occur without cough. Convalescence includes several paroxysms throughout first year of life.
Congenital heart block may present as cardiac failure or even hydrops fetalis and not with fever, apnea, cyanosis. Trachebronchomalacia presents with stridor and respiratory distress. Epiglottitis presents with high fever, stridor, hot potato voice in 2–7 years of age.

34. Ans. b. Klebsiella pneumonia *Ref: OP Ghai, Textbook of Pediatrics; 7/e p136*

35. Ans. a. Lactose

Ref: Care of The Newborn by Meharban Singh 7/e p163 Preventive and Social Medicine by K. Park, 18/e p398

36. Ans. b. Defect in hepatic conjugation *Ref: Nelson's Texbook of Pediatrics, 18/e p1666–67. Cloherty 7/e p307–311*

Crigler Najjar syndrome is due to defective hepatic conjugation of bilirubin (bio transformation), Type I due to complete enzyme (UDP glucoronyl transferase) deficiency and Type 2 due to partial enzyme deficiency.

Crigler–Najjar syndrome is inherited as autosomal recessive. Phenobarbitone is useful in Type 2, as about 10% enzymes are available

Physiological jaundice occurs in both term and preterm infants which peaks in 3–5 days and then falls. The level may go upto 12 in term and 10–12 in preterm babies. Levels up to 15 may occur occasionally. The bilirubin value reaches, 2 mg/dl by 1 month of life. Causes for physiological jaundice are

- Increased RBC volume per kg and decreased RBC survival (90 days)
- Increased enterohepatic circulation
- Defective uptake due to decreased ligandin
- Defective conjugation due to decreased UGT activity
- Decreased hepatic excreation of bilirubi.

Factors that suggest non physiological jaundice

- Onset of jaundice before 24 hours of life
- Bilirubin level that warrants phototherapy
- Rise in bilirubin level of > 0.2 mg/hour
- Signs of underlying illness (vomiting, lethargy, wt loss, poor feeding,apnea, temperature instability)
- Jaundice presenting after 8 days in term and 14 days in preterm infants.

Causes of Direct hyperbilirubinemia

- Hepatitis
- Intrauterine infections
- Toxoplasmosis
- Biliary obstruction
- Sepsis
- Galactosemia
- α–1 antitrypsin deficiency
- Cystic fibrosis
- Tyrosinosis
- Cholestasis
- Hyperalimentation
- Syphilis
- Hemochromatosis
- **Dubin Johnson syndrome**
- **Rotor syndrome**

Causes of Indirect hyperbilirubinemia

Normal RBC morphology and reticount	Abnormal RBC morphology and reticount
Enclosed hemorrhage	Spherocytosis
Increased enterohepatic circulation	Ellipocytosis
Breast milk	Stomatocytosis
Hypothyroidism	Pyknocytosis
Crigler–Najjar syndrome	ABO incompatibility
Infant of Diabetic mother	Red cell enzyme deficiency
RDS	Alpha thalassemia
Asphyxia	Drugs(Penicillin)
Infection	DIC
Gilbert syndrome	
Drugs(Novobiocin)	

Breastfeeding Jaundice is due to decreased intake of milk that leads to slower bilirubin elimination and increased enterohepatic circulation. Bilirubin level may reach > 12 mg/dl. It usually occurs after day 3 of life.
Breast milk jaundice is due to 3 α 20 β pregnendiol and other unidentified factors in breast milk that interfere

with bilirubin metabolism. Bilirubin levels may reach 20 to 30 mg/dl by 14 days if no treatment is started. The bilirubin level falls after 2 weeks to reach normal value by 4 to 12 weeks. If breastfeeding is stopped, bilirubin level will fall rapidly in 48 hours. If breastfeeding is restarted, bilirubin may rise by 2 to 4 mg/dl but not to previous high values.

37. Ans. c. Increase in total bilirubin level more than 10 mg/24 hours

Ref: Manual of Neonatal Care by John P. Cloherty 7/e p329

The indications for double volume exchange transfusion are

- Cord bilirubin > 4.5 mg/Dl and cord Hb < 11 g%
- Bilirubin level rising more than 1 mg/dl/hour despite phototherapy
- When Hb is between 11 and 13 g/dl, bilirubin rising > 0.5 mg/dl/hour despite phototherapy.
- Bilirubin level is 20 mg/dl or it appears that the level will reach 20 mg/dl at the rate it is rising.
- There is progression of anemia in the face of adequate control of bilirubin by phototherapy.

In Rh incompatibility, O Rh negative blood is used, crossed matched against the infant after delivery. In ABO incompatibility, O Rh negative or Rh compatible with the mother and the infant. Double volume exchange is done with 160 ml/kg of blood (newborn blood volume is 80 ml/kg) which replaces 87% of infant blood with new blood.

38. Ans. a. Frontal sinus *Ref: Nelson's Texbook of Pediatrics, 19/e p1436*

Both ethmoidal and maxillary sinuses are present at birth but only ethmoid sinuses are pneumatised. The maxillary sinuses are pneumatised at 4 years of age.

The sphenoidal sinuses are present at 5 years of age.

The frontal sinuses begin development at age 7–8 years and not completely developed until adolescence.

The paranasal sinuses are normally sterile, maintained by the mucociliary clearance. Here, frontal sinus is the best answer.

39. Ans. b. TOF *Ref: Pediatric Cardiology by Myung K. Park 5/e p217*

VSD, Trunchus Arteriosus and TAPVC have increased pulmonary blood supply and hence pulmonary plethora whereas TOF has decreased blood supply (pulmonary oligemia) due right ventricle outflow tract obstruction.

40. Ans. b. Dolicocephaly *Ref: Nelson's Texbook of Pediatrics, 18/e p2456*

Early fusion or overlapping of sagittal suture causes arrest of growth perpendicular to the suture and hence long head called Dolichocephaly. Early fusion of coronal suture causes short head head or Brachycephaly.

41. Ans. d. Weakness of all four limbs. *Ref: Nelson's Texbook of Pediatrics, 19/e p2062–63*

Weakness of one limb is known as monoparesis. (paresis-weakness, plegia–paralysis). Weakness of both lower limbs is paraparesis. Diplegia is symmetrical weakness of all 4 limbs with lower limb involvement more than the upper limb. Quadriparesis or tetraparesis is weakness of all 4 limbs, not necessarily symmetrical.

42. Ans. b. Factor XII *Ref: Nelson's Texbook of Pediatrics, 19/e p1703–04*

Deficiency of "contact factors" (Factor XII, prekallikrein, high molecular weight kininogen) cuases prolonged PTT but no clinical symptoms. Plonged PTT in these patients is due to the fact that these contact factors function at the initiation of the intrinsic clotting system by the reagent used to measure PTT.

Factor XIII (Fibrin stabilizing factor or Transglutaminase) is responsible for the cross–linking of fibrin to stabilize the fibrin clot. Deficiency of factor XIII causes delayed hemorrhage secondary to instability of the clot. Patients have trauma on day 1 have a bruise/hematoma on the next day. In these patients there would be delayed separation of umbilical stump beyond 4 weeks of age. (another cause is Leucocyte Adhesin factor deficiency type 1, LAD–1). Women may have recurrent spontaneous abortions. Hemarthoses and intracranial hemorrhages are rarely found. Screening test with 5 M urea shows increased solubility in these patients. FFP or cryoprecipitate will correct the defiency.

The most common hereditary bleeding disorder is von Willebrand disease and not Hemophilia.

43. Ans. a. Folic acid *Ref: Nelson's Texbook of Pediatrics, 19/e p2001*

To prevent neural tube defect, all women of child bearing age capable of becoming pregnant should take 0.4 mg of Folic acid daily. If pregnancy is planned in high risk women (previously affected children), 4 mg (10 times the normal dose) of Folic acid should be taken daily, beginning 1 month before time of planned conception.

44. Ans. a. Voracious appetitie

Ref: Nelson's Texbook of Pediatrics, 19/e p174–79. Robbins Pathologic basis of disease, 8/e page: & Vishnu Bhat's Protein Energy Malnutrition, 1/e p121, 135., OP. Ghai 8/e p99

45. Ans. a. Autosomal recessive

Ref: Nelson's Texbook of Pediatrics, 19/e page & http://emedicine. Medscape.com/article/945537-overview

Jeune syndrome also known as Asphyxiating Thoracic Dystrophy is a genetic cause of dwarfism inherited as autosomal recessive manner. It is a disease of infancy with no sex predilection. The affected children have short limbs, narrow thoracic cage and renal and hepatic problems. The major problem in this disease is hypoventilation due to narrow thoracic cage due to short ribs. Microcystic renal disease may occur which may lead to tubular atropy and eventually renal failure. Radiography

- Small and bell-shaped thorax with reduced transverse and anterior-posterior diameter
- Short and horizontally oriented ribs with irregular costochondral junctions and bulbous and irregular anterior ends
- Short squared iliac wings
- Trident appearance of acetabular margin
- Short limbs relative to trunk
- Variable limb shortening
- Short phalanges, metacarpals, or metatarsals with or without polydactyly
- Premature ossification of the capital femoral epiphyses

Pulmonary function test may show restrictive lung disease pattern. Treatment is supportive. Parents of an affected child have a 25% chance of recurrence.

Autosomal dominant	Autosomal recessive	X linked dominant	X linked recessive
Familial Hypercholesterolemia	Sickle cell disease, Thalassemia	Vitamin D resistant rickets	Duchenne muscular dystrophy
Polycystic kidney disease	Cystic fibrosis	Hypophosphatemic rickets	Becker muscular dystrophy
Neurofibromatosis type 1	Tay sachs disease	Rett syndrome	Hemophilia A, B
Hereditory sperocytosis	Phenyketonuria	Incontentia pigmenti	Color blindness
Hereditory elliptocytosis			Fragile X syndrome
von Willibrand's disease	Mucopolysacchridoses except Hunters, Mucolipidosis	Aicardi syndrome	Hunter's disease
Marfan syndrome	Galatosemia	Klinefelter's syndrome	Male pattern baldness
Huntington's disease	Glycogen storage disease	Alport syndrome	Vitamin D dependent rickets type 1 and 2
Acute Intermittent Porphyria	Lysosomal acid lipase deficiency		G6PD deficiency
Porphria cutanea tarda	17 β hydroxyl steroid dehydrogenase deficiency		Fabry disease
Varigate porphyria	Abetalipoproteinemia		Lesch-Nyhan syndrome
Peutz Jegher syndrome	Albinism		Ornithine transcarbamaylase deficiency
Di George syndrome	Alkaptinuria		Ocular albinism
Hawkinsinuria	Aldolase deficiency		Menke's syndrome
Noonan syndrome	Bloom syndrome		Testicular feminisattion syndrome
Nail patella syndrome	Canavan disease		
Multiple endocrine neoplasia	Carbamoyal phosphate synthatase deficiency		
Spinocerebellar ataxia	Chediak Higashi syndrome		

Contd...

Contd...

Autosomal dominant	Autosomal recessive	X linked dominant	X linked recessive
Tuberous scelosis	Congenital adrenal hyperplasia		
von Hippel-Lindau syndrome	Cystinuria		
	Ellis van crevald syndrome		
	Essential fructosuria		
	Fanconi anemia		
	Familial Mediterranean fever		
	Friedreich's ataxia		
	Gaucher's disease		
	Hartnup disease		
	Homocystinuria		
	Infantile Refsum disease		
	Krabbe disease		
	Maple syrup urine disease		
	Niemann pick disease		
	Orotic aciduria		
	Xeroderma pigmentosm		
	Tyrosinemia		
	Wilson disease		

Note: The list is enough. Please do not learn by heart the autosomal recessive conditions. It is better to exclude them when you know the other three.

46. Ans. a. Ringed epiphysis *Ref: Nelson's Texbook of Pediatrics, 19/e p198. Also refer Q6, 2014*

47. Ans. b. Arthritis *Ref: Nelson's Texbook of Pediatrics, 19/e p920–25*

Arthritis in Rheumatic Fever occurs in 75% of the patients. The joint involvement is characteristically migratory in nature, **severely inflamed joints can become normal in 1–3 days without treatment**, as 1 or more large joints become involved. Monoarticular joint involvement is unusual. A dramatic response occurs even to small doses of aspirin and the absence of such response should suggest an alternative diagnosis. Rheumatic arthritis is typically non deforming. Arthritis is the earliest manifestation of acute rheumatic fever and may temporarily correlate with peak streptococcal antibody titers. There is often an inverse relationship between severity of arthritis and severity of cardiac involvement.

The major consequence of rheumatic carditis is chronic, progressive valvular disease. Chorea may rarely lead to permanent neurologic sequelae.

48. Ans. d. HLADR3

Ref: Nelson's Texbook of Pediatrics, 19/e p1969–72

HLA DR3/DR 4 DQ2/8 genotype have getic risk of 1/20 compared to a population risk of 1/300. This risk of developing T1 DM is even higher when HLA haplotypes are shared with a sibling or a parent.

T1 DM affects both boys and girls equally with a slight female preponderance in Japan. Peaks of presentation occurs in 2 age groups–5 to 7 years and at puberty, not in old age.

49. Ans. d. 36 weeks

Ref: Fanaroff and Martin's Neonatal-Perinatal Medicine, Disease of the Fetus and Infant, Eighth Edition & Fenichel GM: Neonatal Neurology, 2/e New York, Churchill Livingstone, 1985

Grasp reflex begins at 28 weeks of gestation whereas it is fully developed at 36 weeks.

50. Ans. d. Japanese encephalitis

Ref: Ananthanaryan, Pankier CJ. Textbook of Microbiology. 8/e p88, 451. London: John Wiley & Sons; 2009

S. No.	Live vaccines	Killed/Inactivated vaccines	Subunit/conjugate vaccines
1	BCG	Polio vaccine (Salk,IPV)	Hepatitis B
2	Oral polio vaccine	Typhoid vaccine	Pneumococcal
3	Measles	Pertusis vaccine	Meningicoccal
4	Mumps	Influenza vaccine (Injectable)	Hib
5	Rubella	Plague vaccine	Pertusis (part of DTaP)
6	MMR	Cholera vaccine	HPV (Human papilloma virus)
7	Varicella	Rabies	Conjugated Typhoid
8	Ty21 a(Typhoid)	Japanese Encephalitis	
9	Yellow fever vaccine		
10	Influenza (nasal spray)		
11	Japanese Encephalitis		

51. **Ans. b. Toxicity of leukocytes due to accumulation of cAMP** *Ref: Nelson's Texbook of Pediatrics, 19/e p730–31*
    Severe Combined Immuno Deficiency is one of the most severe forms of immunodeficiency that has both cellular and antibody defects. It is due to defective mutations that encode components of lymphoid cell development. Patients with SCID have very small thymus. Lymph nodes, tonsils, adenoids and peyer patches are absent or underdeveloped. Disease presents within first few months of life with persistent or recurrent diarrhea, pneumonia, otitis media, sepsis and cutaneous infections. Adenosine deaminase levels maybe decreased. Treatment of choice is bone marrow transplant.

Characteristic	Predominant T-cell defect	Predominent B-cell defect	Granulocyte defect	Complement defect
Age at onset	2–6 months	5–7 months, children, adulthood	Early onset	Any age
Pathogens	Common Gram + and Gram–bacteria, mycobacteria, CMV, EBV, adenovirus, enterovirus, Candida, Pneumocystitis	Pneumococci, streptococci, Staphylococci, Hib, Campylobacter, Mycoplasma, enterovirus, giardia, cryptococcus	Staphylococci, Pseudomonas, Klebsiella, Serratia, Salmonella, Candida, Nocardia, Aspergillus	Pneumococci, Nisseria
Manifestations	Mucocutaneous candidiasis, lung infections, failute to thrive, protracted diarrhoea	Recurrent sinopulmonary and GIT infections, malabsorption, arthritis, enterovirus meningitis	Abscess, cellulitis, Impetigo, adenitis, gingivitis, osteomyelitis	Meningitis, arthritis, sinopulmonary infections, septicemia

52. **Ans. a. 1000 ml/day** *Ref: Nelson's Texbook of Pediatrics, 19/e p243*
    Daily maintenance fluid is calculated from Holliday–Segar formula as follows.
    First 10 kg–100 ml/ kg
    10 to 20 kg–50 ml/kg
    More than 20 kg–20 ml/kg.
    For example a child weighing 25 kg,
    First 10 kg = 10 × 100 = 1000 ml
    10 to 20 kg = 10 × 50 = 500 ml
    Next 5 kg = 5 × 20 ml = 100
    1000 + 500 + 100 = 1600 ml/24 hours.
    Maintenance fluid is also calculated by ml/hr.
    First 10 kg = 4 ml/kg/hr
    10 to 20 kg = 2 ml/kg/hr
    More than 20 kg = 1 ml/kg/hr

For example, a child of 25 kg needs
First 10 kg = 10 × 4 = 40
10 to 20 kg = 10 × 2 = 20
Next 5 = 5 × 1 = 5
40 + 20 + 5 = 65 ml/hour.
The maximum fluid requirement in a child is 100/hour. The dextrose concentration in maintenance fluid in a child is 5%.

53. Ans. a. Strep pneumoniae *Ref: Nelson's Texbook of Pediatrics, 19/e p2201*
The three common organisms causing Acute otitis media are Strptococcal pneumonia, Non typeable Hemophilus influenza, Moraxella catarrhalis.

54. Ans. a. Osteogenesis imperfecta *Ref: Nelson's Texbook of Pediatrics, 19/e p2437–2440*
Wormian bones, also known as intra sutural bones, are extra bone pieces that occur in the cranial sutures. These are isolated irregular bones that appear in addition to usual ossified bones of cranium. They are frequently seen along the lambdoid suture. The causes of wormian bones are " PORKCHOPS"
- Pyknodysostosis
- Osteogenesis imperfect
- Rickets
- Kinky hair Menke's syndrome
- Cleidocranial dysostosis
- Hypoparathyroidism and hypophosphatasia
- Otopalatodigital syndrome
- Primary acro osteolysis
- Syndrome–Down's

Among the options provided, recurrent fractures is most common in Osteogenesis imperfect and is the best answer.
Osteogenesis Imperfecta (OS), also known as the brittle bone disease, is the most common genetic cause of osteoporosis. It is inherited as autosomal dominant fashion (recessive form in type VII and VIII). The triad of OS includes fragile bones, blue sclera and early deafness. The bone matrix contains structurally abnormal collagen type 1 fibrila and relatively increased levels of type III and V collagen. The various types are
Ttype I–Mild
Type II–Perinatal lethal
Type III–Progressive deforming
Type IV–Moderativelly severe
Type V–Hyperplastic callus
Type VI–Mineralization defect
Type VII, VIII–Recessive form.
Complications include cardiopulmonary failure, recurrent pneumonia, basilar invagination, brain stem compression, hydrocephalus, syringohydromelia etc. There is no cure for OS. Treatment is supportive for non lethal types, to maintain higher functional level with orthopedic management.

55. Ans. a. 2–4 months *Ref: Nelson's Texbook of Pediatrics, 19/e p1252–53*
Cleft lip is surgical closure is usually done at 3 months of age when the infant has satisfactory weight gain and is free from oral, respiratory and systemic infection. Modified Millard rotation advancement technique is the most common technique used. The initial repair maybe revised at 4 or 5 years of age. Closure of cleft palate is usually done before 1 year to enhance normal speech development. When it is delayed beyond 3 years of age, contoured speech bulb is used to develop intelligible speech.

56. Ans. a. Percentage of burn area × body wt × 4 *Ref: Nelson's Texbook of Pediatrics, 19/e p352*
For example a 20% burn in a 10 kg child requires 20 × 10 × 4 = 800 ml. The first 50% of the calculated fluid is given within 8 hours of burn whereas the next 50% of the calculated fluid is given in next 16 hours. Maintenance fluid is given in addition to this.

57. Ans. a. Type 2 pneumocytes *Ref: Nelson's Texbook of Pediatrics, 19/e p1497*

58. Ans. a. Maxillary *Ref: Nelson's Texbook of Pediatrics, 19/e p1436*

59. Ans. d. 1000 ml/day *Ref: Nelson's Texbook of Pediatrics, 19/e p243. Also refer Q10, 2011*

60. Ans. c. 9–11 months *Ref: Nelson's Texbook of Pediatrics, 19/e p27*

61. Ans. b. Aseptic meningitis *Ref: Nelson's Texbook of Pediatrics, 19/e p1080*

The most common complication of Mumps is aseptic meningitis with or without encephalitis followed by orchitis/oopheritis. The uncommon complications are conjunctivitis, optic neuritis, pneumonia, nephritis, pancreatitis, myocarditis, arthritis, thyroiditis and thrombocytopenia.

Mumps virus is neurotropic and it enters CNS via choroid plexus. Smptomatic CNS involvement occurs in 10–30% of infected individuals. CSF pleocytosis occurs in 40–60% of patients with mumps parotitis. Though orchitis is extremely rare in prepubescent boys, it occurs in 30–40% of infected males. Orchitis is bilateral in 30% of cases. Atropy of testes may occur but sterility is rare even with bilateral involvement.

62. Ans. c. 0.50 *Ref: Nelson's Texbook of Pediatrics, 19/e p1537. & Park's Pediatric Cardiology for Practitioners*

When the maximal cardiac width is more than half of the maximal chest width (cardiothoracic ratio > 50%), the heart is said to enlarged. The cardiac size should be evaluated only when the film is taken during inspiration with the patient in upright position.

63. Ans. b. Mental retardation is the common presentation *Ref: Nelson's Texbook of Pediatrics, 19/e p429–30*

Harnup disease is an autosomal disorder due to defect inn the transport of neutral amino acids (including tryptophan) by intestinal mucosa and renal tubules. Decreased absorption of tryptophan in conjugation with increased renal loss is believed to cause reduced availability of tryptophan for niacin synthesis. Most children with Hartnup defect remain asymptomatic. The major clinical manifestation in the rare symptomatic patient is cutaneous photosensitivity. Skin becomes rough and red on exposure to sun and maybecome pellagra–like. Some patients may develop intermittent ataxia. Mental development is usually normal. The main laboratory finding is aminoaciduria restricted to neutral aminoacids. Plasma concentrations of neutral aminoacids are usually normal. Treatment is with nicotinamide and a high protein diet.

64. Ans. b. RDS *Ref: Nelson's Texbook of Pediatrics, 19/e p581*

65. Ans. d. Ejection systolic murmur in pulmonary area *Ref: Nelson's Texbook of Pediatrics, 19/e 1556–58*

66. Ans. c. Endobronchial TB and d. Neurotuberculosis

Ref: Harrison's Priniples of Internal Medicine,, 18ed. & Nelson's Texbook of Pediatrics, 19/e p1009

Corticosteroids are useful in tubercular meningitis, endobronchial tuberculosis, pericardial effusion, pleural effusion with mediastinal shift and in military tuberculosis. The most common prescribed regimen is prednisolone 1–2 mg/kg/day in 1–2 divided doses given orally for 4–6 weeks followed by gradual tapering.

67. Ans. a. Thyroid dysgenesis *Ref: Nelson's Texbook of Pediatrics, 19/e p1895. Also refer Q7, 2013*

68. Ans. d. Reactive arthritis *Ref: Nelson's Texbook of Pediatrics, 19/e p830*

International League Association for Rheumatology (ILAR) characteristics of Juvenile Idiopathic Arthritis are

- Age – < 16 years
- Minimum duration – ≥ 6 weeks
- ≤ 4 joints in first 6 months of presentation–Oligoarticular
  - Persistent < 4 for course of disease
  - Extended > 4 joints after 6 months
- > 4 joints in first 6 months of presentation–Polyarticular (Rheumatoid factor positive and negative)
- Fever, rash , arthritis–**systemic**
- Other characteristics included–**Psoriatic arthritis, Enthesitis-related arthritis**, undifferentiated
- Inclusion of psoriatic arthritis, inflammatory bowel disease, ankylosing spondylitis–yes.

69. Ans. b. COA *Ref: Nelson's Texbook of Pediatrics, 19/e p1567. Also refer Q11, 2013*

70. Ans. a. >10% loss of body weight

Ref: Nelson's Texbook of Pediatrics, 19/e Chapter on 'Deficit Therapy'. Page 245. Also refer Q8, 2013

71. Ans. a. Intravenous immunoglobulins *Ref: Nelson's Texbook of Pediatrics, 19/e p867*

Acute stage

- IV Immunoglobin and
- High dose Aspirin (80–100 mg/kg/day)

Long term therapy
- Low dose Aspirin 3–5 mg/kg/day
- Clopidogrel
- Warfarin
- Low molecular weight Heparin

72. Ans. d. Chloramphenicol *Ref: Nelson's Texbook of Pediatrics, 19/e p958*

Uncomplicated	Drugs
• Fully sensitive	Chloramphenicol, Amoxicillin
• Multidrug resistent	Fluroquinolone, Cefixime
• Quinolone resistant	Azithromycin, Ceftriaxone
Complicated	
• Fully sensitive	Ampicillin, Ceftriaxone
• Multidrug resistant	Fluroquinolone
• Quinolone resistant	Ceftriaxone

73. Ans. b. Tic disorder *Ref: Nelson's Texbook of Pediatrics, 19/e p76*

Tic is defined as sudden, rapid, recurrent, nonrhythmic, stereotyped motor movement or vocalization that is experienced as irresistible, but can be suppressed for varying lengths of time. They are usually diminished during sleep.

Tics involve face, neck, shoulder, trunk or hand muscles.

Simple tics–eye blinking, neck jerking, shoulder shrugging, cough

Complex tics–facial gestures, grooming bahaviours

Simple vocal tics–throat clearing, grunting, barking, sniffing

Complex vocal tics–coprolalia (obscene words), palilaia (repetition of patient's words), echolalia (repetition of words said to patient).

Tics maybe associated with obsessions, compulsions, hyperactivity, distractibility, impulsivity, social discomfort, anxiety and depression. Though they have normal intelligence, learning difficulties are common. Treatment includes cognitive behavioral therapy, clonidine, guanfcine, haloperidol, pimozide and risperidone.

74. Ans. c. SMR stage 4 *Ref: Nelson's Texbook of Pediatrics, 19/e p651–52*

SMR Stage	Pubic hair	Breasts
1	Preadolescent	Preadolescent
2	Sparse, lightly pigmented, straight, medial border of labia	Breast and papilla elevated as small mound, diameter of areola increased
3	Darker, begining to curl, increased amount	Breast and areola enlarged, no contour separation
4	Coarse, curly, abundant but less than in adult	Areola and papilla form secondary mound
5	Adult feminine triangle,spread to medial surface of thigh	Mature, nipple projects, areola part of general breast contour

SMR Stage	Pubic hair	Penis	Testes
1	Preadolescent	Preadolescent	Preadolescent
2	Scanty, long, lightly pigmented	Minimal change/enlarement	Enlarged scrotum, pink, texture altered
3	Darker, starting to curl, small amount	Lengthens	Larger
4	Coarse, curly, less than adult	Larger, glans and breath increase in size	Larger, scrotum dark
5	Adult distribution, sprea to medial surface of thigh	Adult size	Adult size

75. Ans. a. 1000 ml/day *Ref: Nelson's Texbook of Pediatrics, 19/e p243. Also refer Q10, 2011*

76. Ans. d. Wt <1 kg *Ref: Q3, 2013*

77. Ans. d. 5 years *Ref: Nelson's Texbook of Pediatrics, 19/e p71. Refer Q4, 2013*

78. Ans. a. Osteogenesis imperfecta *Ref: Nelson's Texbook of Pediatrics, 19/e 2437–2440. Refer Q2, 2010*

79. Ans. c. 6–12 months *Refer Q3, 2010*

80. Ans. b. Opposite to premolar *Ref: Nelson's Texbook of Pediatrics, 19/e p1070*

In lymphoid tissue, multinucleated giant cell called **Warthin Finkeldy giant cells pathognomic for Measles**.

- Common questions in viral infections are Cytomegalic inclusion disease–Symptomatic congenital CMV infection
- Treatment of CMV infection–Ganciclovir, Foscarnet, Cidofovir
- Best method of diagnosis of congenital CMV infection–Viral isolation or DNA PCR in first week of life
- Heterophile Antibody test is done for–Epstein Bar virus
- EBV immunological disease–X linked lymphopriliferative disease (Duncan syndrome)
- IAP recommendation for Varicella vaccine–15 months
- Oka strain–Varicella
- Jerry–Lynn strain–Mumps
- RA 27/3–Rubbella
- 17D vaccine–Yellow fever
- Conenital varicella syndrome–cacatrial skin lesions, limb hypolpasia, microcephaly, seizures, mental retardation, chorioretinitis, cataract, microphthalmia
- Scrum pox–Herpes in rugby players
- Herpes gladiatorum–Herpes in wrestlers
- Herpetic whitlow–HSV infection of fingers and toes
- PPGSS–Papular purpuric gloves and socks syndrome–Parvo virus B19
- Slapped cheek appearance–Fifth disease–Parvo virus B19
- Roseola infantum, Exanthum subitum, sixth disease–HHV 6
- Nagayama spots–Sixth disease, HHV 6
- Break through varicella–varicella in vaccinated individuals
- Hand–foot–mouth disease most commonly caused by Coxsackie virus A16, followed by Enterovirus 71, Coxsackie A 5, 7, 9 Herpangina is caused by–Enterovirus 71 and Coxsackie A virus
- Post polio syndrome–after an interval of 30–40 years!, 30–40% of persons who survived paralytic polio develop muscle pain and exacerbation of existing weakness or even new weakness
- Rope sign–angulation between chin and larynx caused by weakness of hyoid muscles in bulbar polio.
- Paralytic polio occurs in 0.1% and non paralytic polio in 1% of patient infected with wild polio virus
- Mumps is caused by Paramyxoviridae family, genus Rubula virus
- Treatment of Measles–Vitamin A
- Fever blisters or cold sores are the most common manifestation of recurrent HSV infection
- Neonatal varicella occurs when mother has rashes 5 days prior and 2 days after delivery
- Peliosis hepatis and Bacillary angiomatosis are caused by Bartonella hensela and Bartonella quintana
- Classiccal triad of botulism includes acute onset of symmetric descending paralysis with clear sensorium, no fever and no paresthesia
- Pupura fulminans is caused by N. meningitidis

81. Ans. b. 28 weeks

Ref: Fanaroff and Martin's Neonatal-Perinatal medicine, Diseases of the Fetus and Infant, Eighth Edition & Fenichel GM: Nonatal Neurology, 2/e New York, Churchill Livingstone, 1985. Refer Q8, 2010

82. Ans. a. Meconium lieus

Ref: Nelson's Texbook of Pediatrics, 19/e 1481–1497 & Harrison's 18/e p2149

The common presentations of Cystic Fibrosis are (most common to less common)

- Acute or persistent respiratory symptoms (45%)
- Failure to thrive, malnutrition

- Abnormal stools
- Meconium ileus, intestinal obstruction (20%)

83. Ans. d. 1000 ml *Ref: Nelson's Texbook of Pediatrics, 19/e & OP GHAI, Textbook of Pediatrics; 7/e p267. Refer Q1, 2012*

85. Ans. c. Absence of any specific organ involvement *Ref: Nelson's Texbook of Pediatrics, 19/e p740*

85. Ans. c. Corticosteroid therapy *Ref: Nelson's Texbook of Pediatrics, 19/e p740. Corticosteroid therapy is associated with esinopenia and not esinophila.*

86. Ans. a. 4 months *Ref: Nelson's Texbook of Pediatrics, 19/e p27*

Milestone	Age
Grasps rattle	3.5 months
Reach for objects	4 months
Palmar grasp gone	4 months
Trnsfer object from one hand to other	5.5 months
Thumb-finger grasp	8 months

87. Ans. c. Chorea *Ref: Nelson's Texbook of Pediatrics, 19/e p922*

Sydenham chorea occurs in 10–15% of patients with acute rheumatic fever. **It often presents as an isolated frequently subtle, neurological behavior disorder.** Emotional liability, incoordination, poor school performance, uncontrollable movements and facial grimacing that are exacerbated by stress and disappear with sleep are characteristic. Chorea is occasionally unilateral. The latent period between streptococcal infection and Chorea is longer often months. Antibody levels maybecome normal. Rarely, chorea leads to permanent neurologic sequelae.

88. Ans. d. HLA DR3 *Ref: Nelson's Texbook of Pediatrics, 19/e Please refer Q6, 2011*

89. Ans. b. Mental retardation is the common presentation. *Please Q11, 2010*

90. Ans. b. Make a tower of 5 cubes *Ref: Nelson's Texbook of Pediatrics, 19/e p. Please refer Q1, 2014*

At 15 months, a child can crawl upstairs, can name familiar objects (4–6 words). A child can point objects at 10 months. However, a child could make a tower of 4 cubes at 18 months an a tower of 6 cubes at 21 months. b is the answer here.

91. Ans. b. Drug therapy not required in an adequately immunized child > c. Isolation is not required. *Ref: Nelson's Texbook of Pediatrics, 19/e p947*

A macrolide agent should be given promptly to all household contacts and other close contacts, such as those in daycare, **regardless of age, history of immunization, and symptoms**. The same age-related drugs and doses used for prophylaxis are used for treatment. Azithromycin and Erythromycin are the primary agents for treatment and prophylaxis whereas Clarithromycin and Cotrimoxazole are alternative agents. Booster dose is given for under-immunized children. Visitation **and movement of coughing family members in the hospital must be assiduously controlled (isolation)** until erythromycin has been taken for 5 days.

Close contacts of invasive H. influenza and Meningococcal infections should receive Rifampicin prophylaxis. Alternative drugs for prophylaxis for contacts Meningococcal disease are ceftriaxone and Ciprofloxacin

92. Ans. d. Can be mediated by bacterial toxins *Ref: Nelson's Texbook of Pediatrics, 19/e p1245*

Osmotic diarrhea occurs after ingestion of a poorly absorbed solute. The solute maybe the one which is normally not well absorbed 9 magnesiun, phosphate, lactulose, or sorbitol) or one that is not well absorbed because of a disorder of the small bowel (lactose with lactase deficiency or glucose with rota virus diarrhea). Malabsorbed carbohydrate is fermented in the colon and short chain fatty acids (SCFAs) are produced. The SCFAs increase the osmotic solute load and cause diarrhea. This type of diarrhea produces lesser volume than a secretory diarrhea and stops with fasting. Stool reducing substances maybe present. In osmotic diarrhea stool anion gap > 100 mOsm.

The common causes of secretory diarrhea are actase deficiency, glucose–galactose malabsorption, lactulose therapy, laxative abuse. The common cause of secretory diarrhea are cholera, toxigenic E.coli, carcinoid, VIPoma, neuroblastoma, congenital chloride diarrhea, Clostridium diffficle, Cryptosporidisis.

93. Ans. b. Toxicity of leucocytes due to accumulation of cAMP *Ref: Nelson's Texbook of Pediatrics, 19/e p730–33*

94. Ans. c. 12 *Ref: OP Ghai, Text book of Pediatrics: 7/e p4. Please refer 3, 2012*

95. Ans. a. Lactose *Ref: Care of The Newborn by Meharban singh 7/e p163 preventive and social medicine by K. Park, 8/e p398. Please refer Q5, 2013*

96. Ans. b. Aseptic meningitis *Ref: Nelson's Texbook of Pediatrics, 19/e p. Please refer Q9, 2010*

97. Ans. b. Cholecalciferol *Ref: Nelson's Texbook of Pediatrics, 19/e p200–208, and CRC Desk Reference for Nutrition, Second Edition, By Carolyn D. Berdanier*

1, 25, cholecalciferol (Calcitriol) is useful in acute phase of rickets as it is the active form, reversing hypocalcemia immediately. 25-hydroxy Cholecaliferol is preferred in secondary vitamin D deficiency (rickets due to malabsorption, liver diseases, defective bile acid metabolism, pancreatic dysfunction, cystic fibrosis etc.), because of its better absorption. Calcium is part of treatment of rickets, some patients even need intravenous calcium in the acute stage, followed by oral supplementation. In fact, rickets can occur secondary to inadequate dietary calcium. Cholecalciferol is the best answer of exclusion.

98. Ans. a. Vitamin C deficieny *Ref: Nelson's Texbook of Pediatrics, 19/e p198. Please refer Q6, 2014*

99. Ans. a. Meningomyelocoele *Ref: Nelson's Texbook of Pediatrics, 19/e p1522*

Arnold chiari malformation is associated with myelomeningocele, hydrocephalus, and herniation of the cerebellar tonsils, caudal brainstem, and the fourth ventricle through the foramen magnum

100. Ans. d. 2.5 kg *Ref: Nelson's Texbook of Pediatrics, 19/e. Please refer Q3, 2013*

101. Ans. c. Hypophosphatasia *Ref: Nelson's Texbook of Pediatrics, 19/e 454, 1922*

Hypophosphatasia is associated with mild to moderate hypercalcemia. Serum levels of phosphorus are normal, and those of **alkaline phosphatase are subnormal**. The bones exhibit rachitic-like lesions on radiographs. All other three conditions are associated with increased alkaline phosphatase.

102. Ans. c. 3 years

Ref: http://www.nlm.nih.gov/medlineplus/ency/article/caranial sutures and Cunningham ML, Heike CL (December 2007). "Evaluation of the infant with an abnormal skull shape". Curr. Opin. Pediatr. 19(6): 645–51

103. Ans. c. Two weeks *Ref: Nelson's Texbook of Pediatrics, 19/e 944–948*

Disease	Incubation period
Diphtheria	2–5 days
Pertusis	7–14 days
Tetanus	2–14 days
Measles	8–12 days
Mumps	16–18 days
Rubella	14–21 days
Polio	8–12 days
Varicella	14–16 days
Cholera	1–3 days
Shigella dysentery	12 hours
Typhoid fever	7–14 days

104. Ans. c. Decreased oxygen extraction in the tissues *Ref: Nelson Textbook of Pediatrics pages 305–306*

Shock is a syndrome characterized by the body's inability to deliver adequate oxygen to meet the metabolic demands of vital organs and tissues. Patient in shock have insufficient oxygen at tissue level resulting in shift to anaerobic metabolism and increased lactic acid production. Increased lactic acid production causes high anion gap metabolic acidosis. As a compensatory mechanism increased extraction of oxygen in the tissues (not decreased oxygen extraction) occurs which leads to low mixed venous oxygen. In fact one of the goals of shock is to maintain mixed venous saturation(SVC O_2) > 70%.

105. Ans. c. Renal tubular acidosis *Ref: Q2, July 2014*

106. Ans. a. Local swelling with fang marks

National Snake Bite Management protocols 2009, Govt of India.

Indications for Antisnake Venom:

- Whole blood clotting time more than 20 minutes or signs of spontaneous bleeding.
- Evidence of neurotoxicity–Ptosis, diplopia, inability to lift the head, stridor, respiratory distress, neuroparalysis.
- Swelling extending
  - 15 cm or more within 1 hour.
  - Swelling reaching the knee or elbow in < 4 hours.
  - Swelling involving the entire imb in 8 hours
  - Extension to trunk
  - Swelling causing air way compromise or shortness of breath
  - Compartment syndrome or vascular involvement
- CVS abnormalities–hypotension, shock, arrhythmia, abnormal ECG patterns.
- Persistent severe vomiting and abdominal pain.

Feature	Cobra	Krait	Russell Viper	Saw scaled Viper	Hump nosed Viper
• Local pain/Tissue damage	Yes	No	Yes	Yes	Yes
• Ptosis/Neurological signs	Yes	Yes	Yes!	No	No
• Hemostatic abnormalities	No	No	Yes	Yes	Yes
• Reanl complications	No	No	Yes	No	Yes
• Response to Neostigmine	Yes	No	No	No	No
• Response to ASV	Yes	Yes	Yes	Yes	No

DOs and DONOTs in snake bite

I. Dos–RIGHT

- Reassure–70% snakes are non poisonous
- Immobilize the limb
- Get to the Hospital.
- Tell the doctor any systemic symptoms.

II. DONOTs

- Do not wash the wound
- Do not apply tourniquet
- Do not incise the wound
- Do not apply suction to the wound
- Do not apply electric shock or cryotherapy to wound
- Avoid pressure immobilization.

Note: Test dose is not required for ASV. Any allergy or anaphylaxis occurring, should be treated accordingly. ASV is stopped temporarily and restarted at a slower rate.

107. Ans. a. Spleen *Ref. Nelson textbook of Pediatrics 19/e p338*

Frequency of abdominal organ injury by injury mechanism

Blunt		Penetrating	
Organ	%	Organ	%
Spleen	30	Gastrointestinal tract	70
Liver	28	Liver	27
Kidneys	28	Blood vessels	19
Gastrointestinal tract	14	Kidneys	10
Bladder/urethra/ureters	4	Spleen	9
Pancreas	3	Bladder/urethra/ureters	8
Blood vessels	3	Pancreas	6

108. Ans. c. Wait for 48 hours. *Ref. Nelosn textbook of Pediatrics 19/e p1271.*

Treatment of esophageal foreign bodies merits endoscopic visualization of the object and underlying mucosa and removal of the object; therapeutic endoscopy is most conservatively done with an endotracheal tube protecting the airway. **Sharp objects in the esophagus, disk button batteries, or foreign bodies associated with respiratory symptoms mandate urgent removal.** Button batteries, in particular, must be expediently removed because they can induce mucosal injury in as little as 1 hour of contact time and involve all esophageal layers within 4 hour. **Asymptomatic blunt objects and coins lodged in the esophagus can be observed for up to 24 hour** in anticipation of passage into the stomach.

109. Ans. c. Lavage is given at room temperature *Ref. Nelson Textbook of Pediatrics, 19/e p1415*

The stepwise management of Variceal bleeding in children is given below.

- Volume resuscitation–crtstalloids (NS, RL), blood
- Correction of coagulopathy–Vitamin K, fresh frozen plasma, platelets
- Vasopressin (or its analogs–Octreotide)
- Endoscopic scelrotherapy, banding
- Mechanical compressin by Sengstaken–Blackmore tube (poorly tolerated in children)
- Shunt sugeries/TIPS
- Liver transplantation

Octrotide or Vasopressin can be used before endoscopy. Sengstaken Blackmore tube is poorly tolerated in children and may often need sedation. In fact, it is used in children who continue to bleed despite pharmacotherapy. Lavage is given in room temperature. Target hemoglobin for blood transfusion is 8 g/dl.

110. Ans. c. After 6 hours *Ref. Nelosn textbook of Pediatrics 19/e p600 & 1358*

Normally, air can be demonstrated by radiographs in the jejunum by 15–60 min, in the ileum by 2–3 hour, and in the colon by 3 hour after birth. Absence of rectal gas at 24 hour is abnormal.

The invertogram or upside-down x-ray is of little value now, but a prone cross-table lateral plain x-ray at 24 hour of life (to allow time for bowel distention from swallowed air) with a radio opaque marker on the perineum can demonstrate a low lesion by showing the renal gas bubble <1 cm from the perineal skin.

111. Ans. a. Submucous lipoma *Ref: Nelson Textbook of Pediatrics page 1287–89*

Intussusception

- Most common cause of intestinal obstruction between 3 months and 6 years of age
- Most common abdominal emergency in children <2 years.
- Male predominance (3 : 1)

Etiology

- Idiopathic (90%)
- Asso. with Aenovirus type C respiratory infection
- Was receiving a tetravalent rotavirus vaccine within 2 week of immunization (now banned).
- Swollen Peyer patches in the terminal ileum, Lymphoid nodular hyperplasia are risk factors.
- **Recognizable lead points** for the intussusception are Meckel diverticulum, intestinal polyp, neurofibroma, intestinal duplication cysts, hemangioma, or malignant conditions such as lymphoma. Lead points are more common in children >2 years of age.
- The upper portion of bowel, the **intussusceptum,** invaginates into the lower, the **intussuscipiens.**

Clinical features

- The classic triad of pain, a palpable sausage-shaped abdominal mass, and bloody or currant jelly stool is less common.
- Previously will child has coliky abd. Pain.
- Straining efforts with legs and knees flexed and loud cries
- Normal in between
- Lethargy,vomiting, fever, shock can occur
- **Recurrent intussusception** is noted in 5–8% and is more common after hydrostatic than surgical reduction.

Diagnosis

- X ray–density in the site of intussception
- USG–Doughnut or Target appearance in transverse view
- Contrast enema–coiled spring sign

Treatment

- Surgical reduction
- Hydrostatic reduction under fluoroscopic or ultrasonic guidance (recurrence present)

112. Ans. c. 15 cm *Ref: Nelson Textbook of Pediatrics page 39*

Normal length of infants:
Term newborn–50 cm
6 months–65 cm
1 year–75 cm
Normal gain in length in a full term baby at first 6 months is 15 cm and in the next 6 months is 10 cm.

113. Ans. b. 4 years and 5 years respectively. *Ref: Nelson Textbook of Pediatrics page 71–73*

114. Ans. a. 1 : 1 *Ref: Nelson Textbook of Pediatrics page 1335*

The compoments of WHO ORS are
Glucose 75 mmol/L
Sodium 75 mmol/L
Potassium 20 mmol/L
Chloride 65 mmol/L
Bicarbonate 10 mmol/L
Toatal = 245 mmol/L.
Molar ration of Sodium and Glucose is therefore 1 : 1.

115. Ans. a. Weight for height Z score < –3. *Ref: Nelson Textbook of Pediatrics, page 172*

Definitions of Malnutrition

Classification	Definition	Grading	Criteria
Gomez	Weight below % median WFA	Mild (grade 1)	75%–90% WFA
		Moderate (grade 2)	60%–74% WFA
		Severe (grade 3)	<60% WFA
Waterlow	z scores (SD) below median WFH	Mild	80%-90% WFH
		Moderate	70%–80% WFH
		Severe	<70% WFH
WHO (wasting)	z scores (SD) below median WFH	Moderate	−3 ≤ z score <−2
		Severe	z score <−3
WHO (stunting)	z scores (SD) below median HFA	Moderate	−3 ≤ z score <−2
		Severe	z score <−3
Kanawati	MUAC divided by occipitofrontal head circumference	Mild	<0.31
		Moderate	<0.28
		Severe	<0.25
Cole	z scores of BMI for age	Grade 1	z score <−1
		Grade 2	z score <−2
		Grade 3	z score <−3

116. Ans. c. 9 days of illness *Ref: Harrison*

117. Ans. a. Stridor *Ref: Nelson Textbook of Pediatrics page 315*

Typical localizing indicative of intrathoracic extra pulmonary site are tachypnea, chest retractions and wheezing. Stridor occurs in extra thoracic airway obstruction.

118. Ans. a. Hereditary fructose intolerence *Ref: Nelson Textbook of Pediatrics page 503, 1413*

Hereditary Fructose Intolerence is an inborn error of fructose metabolism caused by deficiency of 1,6, Bisphosphate Aldolase (Aldolase B). The infants are asymptomatic until fructose or sucrose (table sugar) is given in the form of fruit, fruit juice or sweetened cereal. Clinical features resemble galactosemia. It includes jaundice, hepatomegaly, vomiting, irritability, lethary and convulsion. If fructose ingestion continues, hypoglycemic episodes recur followed by liver and renal failure. However, liver failure is rare in the neonatal period.

All other three conditions Congenital hepatic fibrosis, Galactosemia, Hemophagocytic lympho histiocytosis can cause neonatal liver failure.

Common causes of Liver failure in children are

- Infections
  - Hepatitis (A, B, D, E)
  - Cyto Megalo Virus
  - Ebstein Bar virus
  - Adenovirus
  - Enterovirus
  - Parvovirus B19
  - Varicella zoster
  - Human herpes virus 6
  - Lepto spirosis
- Auto immune
- In born errors of metabolism
  - Galactosemia
  - Hereditory tyrosinemia
  - Hereditory fructose intolerance
  - Neonatal iron storage disease
  - Defects in β oxidation of fatty acids
  - Defect in mitochondrial electron transport
- Hemophagocytic Lympho Histocytosis (HLH)
- Hepatotoxic drugs/ toxins–Sodium valporate, paracetamol, INH, Rifamipicin, Pyrazinamide, Carbon tetrachloride, Halothane, *Amantia phalloids* mushroom.
- Metabolic–Wilson's disease
- Ischemic – Hepatic vascular occlusion, CCF, Shock, Congenital cyanotic heart disease
- Idiopathic

119. Ans. a, c, d. *Ref: Nelson Textbook of Pediatrics page 418–22*

Phenyketonuria is caused by the deficiency of **Phenylalanine hydroxylase** (not Tyrosine hydroxylase) and several other enzymes, including **deficiency of Biopterin.** Urine levels of phenyl ketones (phenylpyruvate and phenyl lactate) are increased. Serum tyrosine levels maybe decreased and tyrosine becomes an essential amino acid. All children should be treated with Phenylalanine restricted diet should be started as soon as diagnosis and probably continued for life as stopping even in adulthood may decrease IQ.

120. Ans. d. Consciosness *Ref: Nelson Textbook of Pediatrics page 279–81*

The components of initial impression in Pediatric Advanced Life Support (PALS) are ABC–Airway, Breathing and Circulation (assessed by skin color and temperature).

121. Ans. b. Detect anomalies

122. Ans. c. 30 weeks *Ref. Nelson Textbook of Pediatrics page 27*

Myelination begins prenatally at 30 weeks gestation.

123. Ans. d. Progressive primary pulmonary tuberculosis

Ref: Nelson Textbook of Pediatrics page. Refer Q.14, JIPMER 2010

In progressive primary pulmonary tuberculosis, steroids are contra indicated because it may flare up TB. All other condions are indications for steroid.

124. Ans. b. Stage 2 *Ref: Nelson Textbook of Pediatrics page 1163*

Clinical Stage 1

- Asymtomatic
- Persistent generalized lymphadenopathy

Clinical Stage 2
- Hepatosplenomegaly
- Papular purpuric eruptions
- Seborrheoic dermatitis
- Extensive human papilloma virus infection
- Extensive molluscum contagiosum
- Fungal nail infections
- Recurrent oral ulcerations
- Lineal gingival erythema
- Angular cheilitis
- Parotid enlargement
- Herpes zoster
- Recurrent or chronic RTIs (otitis media, otorrhoea, sinusitis)

Clinical Stage 3
- Moderate unexplained malnutrition not adequately responding to standard therapy
- Unexplained persistent diarrhea (14 days or more)
- Unexplained persistent fevet (one month or more, intermittent or constant)
- Oral candidiasis (outside neonatal period)
- Oral hairy leukoplakia
- Acute necrotizing ulcerative gingngivitis/periodontitis
- Pulmonary TB
- Severe recurrent presumed bacterial pneumonia
- Chrnic HIV associated lung disease including bronchiectasis
- Lymphoid interstitial pneumonia (LIP)
- Unexplained anemia (< 8 g/dl), neutropenia (< 1000 /mm^3) or thrombocytopenia 9 < 50,000/ mm^3) for more than one month.

Clinical Stage 4
- Unexplained severe wasting or malnutrition not responding to standard therapy.
- Pneumocystis pneumonia
- Recurrent severe presumed bacterial infections (e.g. empyema, pyomyositis, bone or joint infection, meningitis, but excluding pneumonia)
- Chronic herpes simplex infection; (orolabial or cutaneous of more than one month's duration)
- Extrapulmonary TB
- Kaposi's sarcoma
- Oesophageal candidiasis
- CNS toxoplasmosis
- HIV encephalopathy
- CMV infection (CMV retinitis or infection of organs other than liver, spleen or lymph nodes; onset at age one month or more)
- Extrapulmonary cryptococcosis including meningitis
- Any disseminated endemic mycosis (e.g. extrapulmonary histoplasmosis, coccididiomycosis, penicilliosis)
- Cryptosporidiosis
- Isosporiasis
- Disseminated non-tuberculous mycobacteria infection
- Candida of trachea, bronchi or lungs
- Visceral herpes simplex infection
- Acquired HIV associated rectal fistula
- Cerebral or B cell non-Hodgkin lymphoma
- Progressive multifocal leukoencephalopathy (PML)
- HIV-associated cardiomyopathy or HIV-associated nephropathy.

QUESTIONS 2015

1. **Intervention in congenital deafness is ideal before:**
   a. 3 months
   b. 6 months
   c. 12 months
   d. 24 months
2. **Abdominal wall defect with protrusion of abdominal viscera, in a newborn along the umbilicus covered by a membrane is:**
   a. Exomphalos
   b. Umbilical hernia
   c. Gastoschisis
   d. None
3. **Which of the following is associated with good prognosis in congenital diaphragmatic hernia?**
   a. Lung head ratio < 1
   b. Detection of CDH in first trimester scan
   c. Symptoms develops after 48 hours
   d. Liver herniated in to thorax
4. **An infant with a solid abdominal mass was found to have calcifications in X-rays. The likely diagnosis is**
   a. Neuroblastoma
   b. Wilm's tumor
   c. Polycystic kidney disease
   d. Renal cell carcinoma
5. **Immediate change in the fetal circulation after birth is**
   a. Reversal of flow in the ductus arteriosus
   b. Closure of flap valve of foramen ovale
   c. Closure of ductus venosus
   d. Increase in LV wall thickness and mass
6. **Newborn with umbilical hernia—the likely diagnosis is**
   a. Congenital Hypothyroidism
   b. Down's syndrome
   c. Turner's syndrome
   d. Noonan syndrome

ANSWERS AND EXPLANATIONS

1. **Ans. b. 6 months** *Ref: Nelson Textbook of Pediatrics page 2188-96*

In congenital deafness, identification and amplification before age 6 months makes a very significant difference in the speech and language abilities of affected children, compared with cases identified and amplified after the age of 6 months. Infants and young children with profound congenital or prelingual onset of deafness have benefited from **multichannel cochlear implants.** Pneumococcal vaccine is recommended in children with cochlear implants.

Congenital infections associated with sensorineural hearing loss
- Cytomegalo virus—most common
- Lymphocytic choriomengitic virus
- Rubella virus
- Toxoplasma gondii
- Treponema pallidum (Syphilis)

Common types of syndromic sensorineural hearing loss

Autosomal dominant:
- Waardenberg syndrome (Dystopia cantorum, congenital hearing loss, heterochromic irises, white fore lock)
- Brachio-otorenal syndrome (hearing loss, preauricular pits,brachial, renal and external ear abnormalities)

Autosomal recessive:
- Pendred syndrome (hearing loss, dilatation of vestibular aqueduct, cochlear hypoplasia, goiter
- Usher syndrome (hearing loss, vestibular areflexia, retinitis pigmentosa)

Bilateral neural hearing loss is categorized as mild (20–30 dB), moderate (30–50 dB), severe (50–70 dB), or profound (>70 dB).

Types of hearing loss
- Central or retrocochlear
- Peripheral

- Conductive
- Sensorineural
- Mixed

Conductive hearing is the most common hearing loss in children and middle ear fluid is the most common cause of conductive hearing loss. The recommended hearing screening techniques are either otoacoustic emissions (OAE) testing or auditory brainstem evoked responses (ABR).

2. Ans. a. Exomphalos *Ref: Cloherty's manual of Neonatal Care, 7/e p821–22*

Exomphalos	Gastroschisis
• Midline defect	Paramedian defect
• Abdominal wall defect with intact sac (peritoneum, amnion or wharton jelly)	Abdominal wall defect with no covering on the viscera
• Associated with other anomalies (70%) like cardiac, GIT or genitourinary tract	Less common (8–16%). May have associated GIT anomalies only
• Insertion of umbilical cord is broad	Insertion of umbilical cord is normal sized
• Contents include small bowel, liver, stomach	Content is usually small bowel and liver is very rarely present
• Associated with chromosomal anomalies	Not associated with chromosomal anomalies

3. Ans. c. Symptoms develop after 48 hours *Ref: Cloherty's manual of Neonatal Care, 7/e p 815–16*

Factors associated with good prognosis in congenitl diaphragmatic hernia are

- Herniation of bowel into chest after 2nd trimester
- Absence of liver herniation
- Absence of co existing anomalies
- Lung head ratio > 1.4 (less pulmonary hypoplasia)
- Symptoms develop later. (Later the symtoms better the prognosis)

Among these things, the major limiting factor for survival of CDH is pulmonary hypoplasia.

4. Ans. a. Neuroblastoma *Ref: Nelson Textbook of Pediatrics page 1753–54.*

An infant with solid abdominal mass with calcification is a neutoblatoma. Neuroblatoma is associated with calcification and hemorrhage whereas Wilm's tumor is associated with necrosis and hemorrhage. Polycustic kidney disease is a cystic mass and is not associated with calcification. Renal cell carcinoma is very rare in children.

- MC malignant tumor in infants—Neuroblastoma
- MC primary malignant renal tumor in children—Wilm's tumor.
- MC brain tumor in children—gliomas (of which Pilocytic astrocytoma is most common).
- MC solid tumor in children—Glioma
- Medulloblastoma (35–40%) and Cerebellar astrocytoma (35–40%) are the most common posterior fossa tumors in children.
- MC extracranial solid tumor in children—Neuroblastoma.
- MC intraocular tumor in children—Retinobastoma.

5. Ans. a. Reversal of flow in ductus arteriosus. *Ref: Nelson Textbook of Pediatrics page 1529*

The order of events that occur in transitional circulation(fetal to neonatal circulation) are

- Reversal of flow in ductus arteriosus as the pulmonary vascular resistance decreases (due to increase in PO_2) and systemic vascular resistance increases.
- Closure of flap valve of foramen ovale to increase in left atrial pressure
- Closure of ductus venosus after the removal of the placenta
- Increase in LV wall thickness and mass due to increase in the work load as systemic vascular resistance and LV output increase.
- Decrease in RV wall thickness and mass due to decrease in work (neonatal RV pumps blood only to lungs whereas the fetal RV pumps both to lungs and to aorta through the ducus arteriosus).

6. Ans. a. Congenital hypothyroidism *Ref: Nelson Textbook of Pediatrics pages 1895–1901*

Common causes of umbilical hernia in the newborn are

- Preterm
- Congenital hypothyroidism
- Down's syndrome
- Ascites

The clinical features of Congenital hypothyroidism are

- Asymptomatic
- Normal birth weight and length
- Feeding difficulties
- Prolonged physiological jaundice
- Respiratory distress
- Large tongue
- Apnea
- Little cry
- Increased sleepiness
- Poor appetite
- Large abdomen
- **Umbilical hernia**–usually present
- Hypothermia
- Edema of genitals and extremities

The clinical features of Down's syndrome in the newborn are **(Hall's Criteria)** (in decreasing order of frequency)

- Poor moro reflex
- Hypotonia
- Flat facial profile
- Upward-slanting palpebral fissures
- Simple, small round ears
- Redundant loose neck skin
- Single palmar crease
- Hyperextensible large joints
- Pelvis radiograph abnormal
- Hypoplasia of fifth-finger

Umbilical hernia is common in Congenital Hypothyroidism. It can occur Down's syndrome but is not so common and is also not a part of Hall's Criteria.

Key messages in neonatal umbilical hernia

- Umbilical hernias are common in neonates.
- Uncomplicated umbilical hernias maybe safely observed in the first few years of life, with spontaneous regression occurring in most cases.
- Most cases require no surgical intervention
- Dressings to cover the hernia (e.g. coins, strapping) are ineffectual and may traumatise surrounding skin.
- Umbilical hernias which cause serious complications are rare. O_2

Chapter

16 Anesthesia

Prem Kumar

HISTORY

- 1846–termed anesthesiology: **Oliver Wendell Holmes**
- Demonstrated general anesthetic effects of ether: **William T.G. Morton**–October 16,1846 **(world ether day)**
- **Carl Koller**–1884–introduced cocaine as an ophthalmic anesthetic
- **Joseph Priestley**–produced Nitrous oxide-1772
- **Horace wells**–demonstrated use of Nitrous oxide for tooth extraction-1844
- **August bier**–1898-first spinal anesthesia
- **John Simpson**–first to use chloroform
- **John Lundy** first used IV anesthetic thipentone-1934
- **Ferdinade Cathelin**–1901-caudal epidural anesthesia
- **Fidel pages**–1921-Lumbar epidural anesthesia
- **Alexander wood**–1855-invented needle and syringe
- **Harold Griffith**–1942-used curare
- **Lofgren**–1943-introduced Lidocaine
- **John Lundy and Ralph waters**–coined 'balanced anesthesia'
- **Ketamine**–first used by Domino and Corsen
- Succinyl choline–synthesized by **Bovet**
- **First Boyle's machine**–Edmund Gaskin Boyle in 1917
- **First endotracheal intubation**–Ivan Magill
- **First nasal intubation**–Stanlers Rowbothom

ANESTHESIA MACHINE

- Consists of high, Intermediate and low pressure systems
- The high pressure system includes cylinder, bourdon pressure gauge and yoke assembly
- The intermediate pressure system is from pressure regulator to flow control valve
- Low pressure system is downward from the flow meter to common gas outlet.

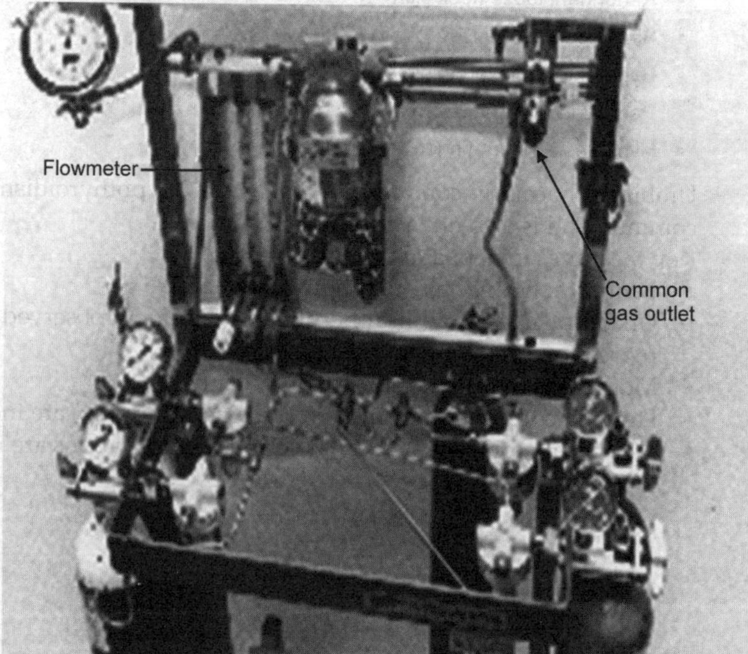

Fig. 16.1: Anesthesia machine

Flow diagram of anesthesia machine

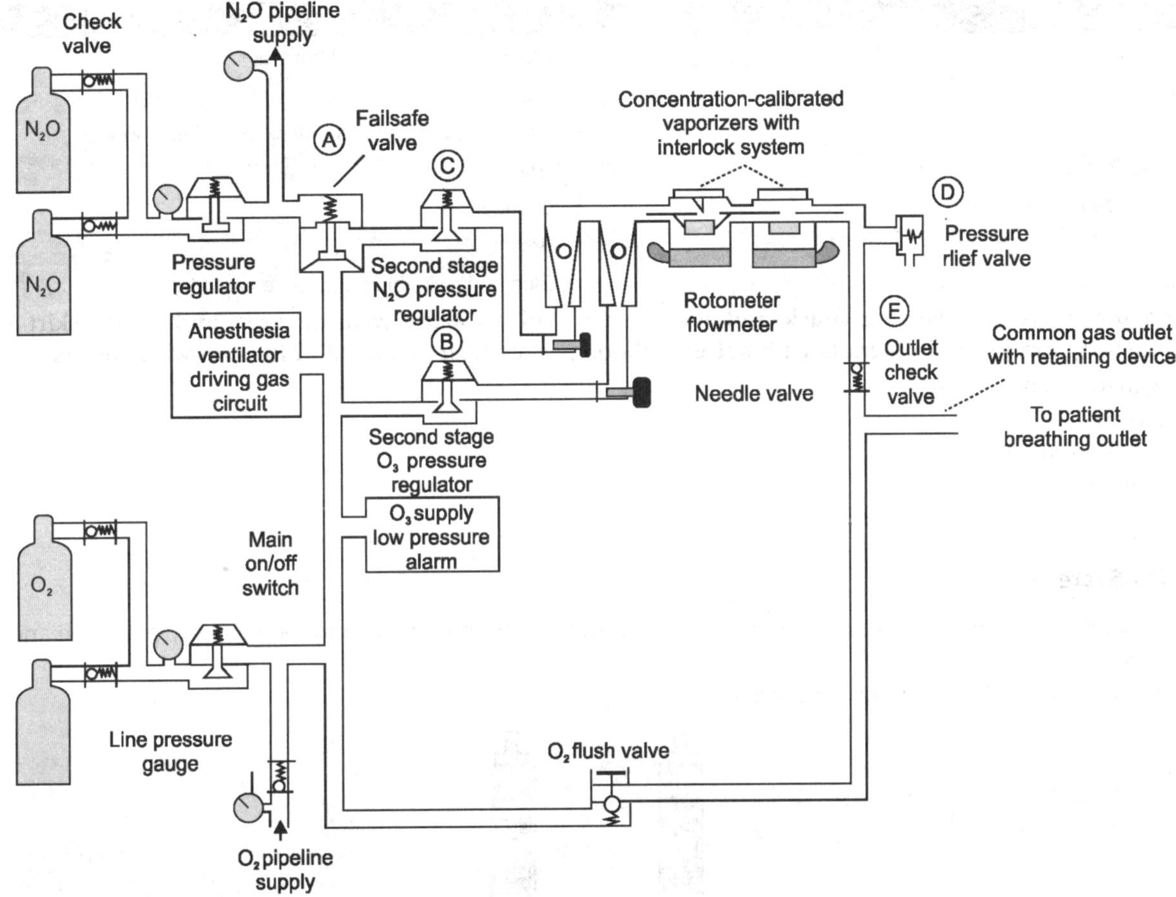

Cylinders in Anesthesia

- Cylinders in anesthesia are made of Molybdenum steel. It helps to withstand high Pressures.
- Chromium is added to decrease the weight of cylinders.
- Aluminium cylinders are MRI compatible
- Cylinders are attached to the machine via hanger-yoke with a pin index safety system to prevent errors
- The yoke assembly includes index pins, a washer, a gas filter, and check valve that prevents retrograde gas flow
- Cylinder pressure is usually measured by a Bourdon pressure gauge
- A flexible tube within this gauge straightens when expose to gas pressure, causing a gear mechanism to move a needle pointer

Oxygen Cylinder–Black body with white shoulders

- Pressure is 2000 psi
- MC used cylinder type used in anesthesia machines is type E, type H is used in manifold
- Liquid O_2–1 ml of liquid O_2 = 840 ml of gas
- Liquid O_2 is stored at–119 °C

N_2O cylinders–Blue color cylinder

- Pressure is 745 Psi
- The central supply of O_2 and N_2O is at 60 Psi
- Critical temperature of nitrous oxide is–36.5 degree Celsius , so it can be stored At room temperature in liquid form without refrigeration

Color Coding of Cylinders

Cylinder	Color
• Oxygen	• Black body with white shoulder
• Nitrous Oxide	• Blue
• Air	• Grey or black body with black and white shoulder
• Carbon Dioxide	• Grey
• Cyclopropane	• Orange
• Helium	• Brown
• Entonox	• Blue body with blue and white shoulder

Mnemonic: Oviyan wearing **black and white** shirt had an **artist** wearing **grey and white** skirt riding **greycar**carrying **orange** and **bluen**uts with **helium**balloon parked near an **ox** with **blue** and **white** horns

- Oviyan–oxygen
- Artist–air
- Car–carbon dioxide
- Balloon–brown
- Ox- entonox

Pin Index System

- It is a safety mechanism for gas cylinders used in anesthesia so that one cannot be wrongly placed in another's position.
- 2 pins of 4 mm and 6 mm long are present

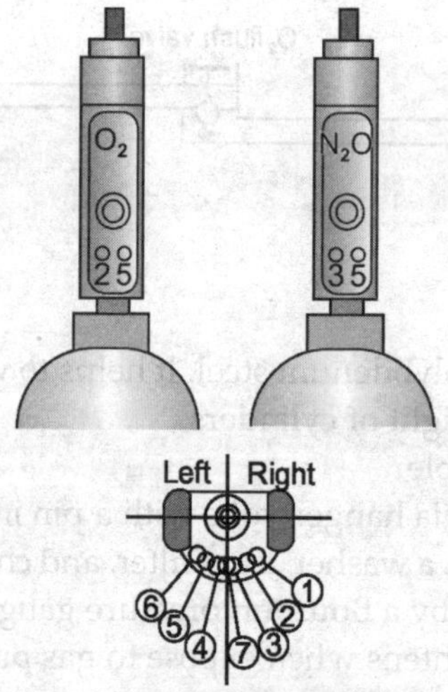

Fig. 16.2: Pin index system

Gas	Pin Index
• Air	1, 5
• Oxygen	2, 5
• Nitrous Oxide	3, 5
• Nitrogen	1, 4
• Carbon Dioxide (>7.5%)	1, 6
• Carbon dioxide (<7.5%)	2, 6
• Cyclopropane	3, 6

Mnemonic–AON, CCC–arranged in ascending order.

Pin Index Safety System [Piss]

- Present In high pressure system [valve outlets of cylinders]
- Can be violated if wrong gas is filled in cylinder
- Pin is present in the machine end
- Holes are in the cylinder end.

Cylinder Pressures

O_2	137 bar/2000 psi
Air	137 bar/2000 psi
Helium	137 bar/2000 psi
Nitrous oxide	745 psi

Intermediate pressure system

- It includes pipeline, pressure regulator, oxygen pressure failure device (fail safe valve), flow control valve, oxygen flush
- Gas pipes are made of seamless copper tubing
- Oxygen, nitrous oxide, and often air are delivered to the operating room through a piping network
- Pressure regulator ensures constant flow irrespective of pressure fluctuations and it reduces the cylinder gas pressure to 55–60 psig before it enters the flow valve
- Oxygen pressure failure device cuts off nitrous oxide flow in case of fall in oxygen pressure to avoid hypoxic mixture
- Oxygen flush–when activated, the flow rate is 35–75 litres/min, it shouldn't be activated during the inspiratory phase of ventilatory cycle, it may cause barotrauma, dilution of gases causing awareness in case of accidental activation.
- Oxygen is reduced to 14 psig and nitrous oxide is reduced to 26 psig at flow control valve.

Diameter Index Safety System [DISS]

- Present on the machine end where pipeline is attached.
- The tubing is color coded and has a diameter-index safety system (DISS) fitting that prevents incorrect hose attachment.

Low Pressure System

- It includes flowmeter, anti hypoxic device, back bar, vaporizer, common gas outlet.

Flow Meters

- **Flowmeters are classified as either constant-pressure variable-orifice or electronic flowmeters**
- To reduce the risk of providing a hypoxic gas mixture in vase of leak, oxygen flowmeters are always positioned downstream to all other flow meters (nearest to the vaporizer)

Order of Flowmeter

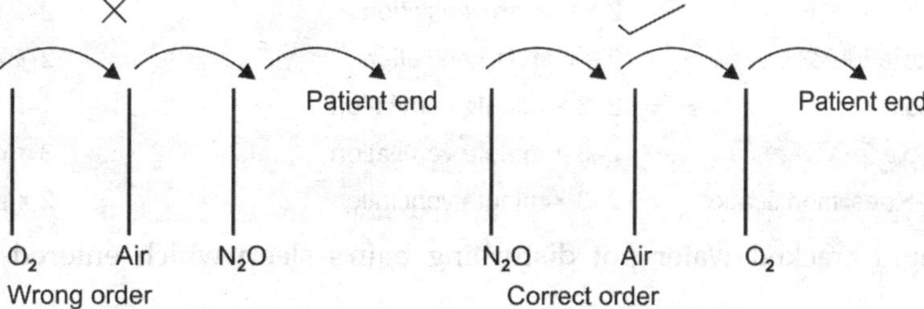

Fig. 16.3: Order of flowmeter

- It contains bobbin or marker to indicate the flow rate of gas
- Cause of inaccurate readings include static electricity and dirt.

Breathing Systems

1. Open Breathing System:

- It is by a mask or gauss piece applied over the nose and mouth
- Open breathing system was used with Ether (or) Chloroform but nowadays obsolete. This requires a special mask (Schimmelbusch's mask).

2. Semi Closed/semi open Breathing System (Mapleson'S Circuit):

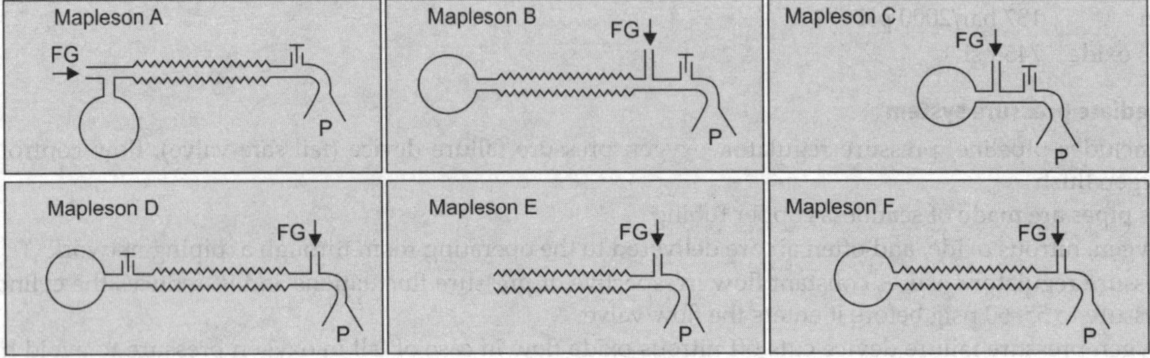

Fig. 16.4: Mapleson's circuit

Mapleson A/magill system Modified variant: LACK system (coaxial)	Efficient for spontaneous ventilation because fresh gas flow equal to minute volume is sufficient to prevent re–breathing.
Mapleson C system/water's system	Post operative recovery, CPR
Mapleson D system	Most efficient for controlled ventilation, since fresh gas flow forces air away from patient and towards pressure relief valve
Mapleson E system/ayre's T piece system	Primarily used in infants and young children. Main advantage of T piece is absence of resistance to expiration, a factor of crucial importance to children
Mapleson's F system/Jackson-Rees modification of Ayre's T piece	Popular in pediatric anesthesia, requires 2-3 times minute ventilation
Efficiency of system with spontaneous respiration: A > d > and e > c > b mnemonic–adeb	
Efficiency of system with controlled respiration: D > F > E > B> C > A mnemonic–debca	
Most commonly used version of Mapleson-D: Bain Coaxial system	
Universal circuit–bain's circuit since it can be used for both spontaneous and controlled ventilation and for both adults and children.	

		Required Fresh Gas flows	
Mapleson Class	Other names	Spontaneous	Controlled
A	Magill	Equal to minute ventilation (80 mL/kg/min)	Very high and difficult to predict
B		2 × minute ventilation	2–2 1/2 × minute ventilation
C	Water's to-and-fro	2 × minute ventilation	2–2 1/2 × minute ventilation
D	Bain circuit	2–3 × minute ventilation	1–2 × minute ventilation
E	Ayre's T-piece	2–3 × minute ventilation	3 × minute ventilation (I:E=1:2)
F	Jackson-Rees' modification	2–3 × minute ventilation	2 × minute ventilation

Mnemonic–arrogant magill cracked water pot disturbing bain's sleep which entered ayre's ears and wetting jackson' s feet.

3. Closed Breathing System: Rebreathing system

- It is a circle system in which the CO_2 is absorbed by soda lime and the exhaled gases can be reused.
- **Components of Soda lime**–Ca (OH)2 (94%), , NaOH (5%) as catalyst, KOH (1%)
- Granule size is 4–8 mesh
- Absorbs 23–25 L of CO_2/100g
- With trilene, soda lime forms phosgene gas which produces ARDS and dicholoroacetylene (neurotoxic)
- Sevoflurane reacts with soda lime to produce compound A (i.e.Pentafluoroisopropenyl–fluoromethyl ether) which is nephrotoxic but not at clinical concentration.
- Hence trilene is contraindicated with soda lime.
- Desflurane reacts with Bara lime and sodalime to produce CO. lowest concentration of CO is produced by halothane and sevoflurane.
- Methoxyflurane and halothane reacts with rubber tubing of closed circuit.
- Silica is added to make soda lime harder. Indicators are used which indicates exhaustion of soda lime by color changes
- Phenolphthalein is a indicator which is white when fresh and converts to pink on exhaustion.
- Water content is 14–18%.

Components of Bara lime–80% Ca $(OH)_2$ + 20% Ba $(OH)_2$

- Granule size is 4–8 mesh
- Absorb up to 18 L CO_2/100 g

Dura sorb is pink when fresh and becomes white when exhausted

Other signs of exhaustion of Soda lime–Tachycardia, Hypertension and entitled CO_2 on capnography

Sterilization of Anesthetic Instruments

- Laryngoscopes, stylet and Magill's forceps can be autoclaved
- Other instruments are sterilized by ethylene oxide gas
- 2% glutaraldehyde is also effective

PHARMACOLOGY

Stages of Anesthesia (Guedel's staging based on ether)

- **Stage I: Analgesia:** Loss of pain sensation results from interference with sensory transmission in the spinothalamic tract. The patient is conscious and conversational. Amnesia and reduced awareness of pain occur as Stage II is approached
- **Stage II: Excitement:** The patient experiences delirum and possibly violent, combative behavior. There is a rise and irregularity in blood pressure. The respiratory rate may increase. To avoid this stage of anesthesia, a short-acting barbiturate, such as thiopental, is given intravenously before inhalation anesthesia is administered.
- **Stage III: Surgical anesthesia:** Regular respiration and relaxation of the skeletal muscles occurs in this stage. Eye reflexes decrease progressively, until the eye movements cease and the pupil is fixed. Surgery may proceed during this stage. Stage III is divided into 4 planes.
  Laryngeal reflexes and spontaneous respiration are lost during Plane III and the patient can be safely intubated. Plane IV is diaphragmatic paralysis. Stage III, Plane III is the best stage for surgery
- **Stage IV: Medullary paralysis:** Severe depression of the respiratory and vasomotor centers occurs during this stage. Death can rapidly ensue unless measures are taken to maintain circulation and respiration.

Inhalational Anaesthetics

Can be used for both induction and maintenance of anesthesia

Classification of General Anesthetics

- Halogenated ether (isoflurane, sevoflurane, desflurane, enflurane)

- Alkane (halothane)
- Gaseous anesthetics (nitrous oxide and xenon).

Mechanism of action of inhaled anaesthetics:

- The potency of general anesthetics correlates with their solubility in oil, indicating the importance of their interaction with hydrophobic targets.
- The immobilizing effect of inhaled anesthetics involves a site of action in the spinal cord, whereas sedation/ hypnosis and amnesia involve supraspinal mechanisms
- Volatile inhaled anesthetics enhance inhibitory synaptic transmission postsynaptically by potentiating ligand-gated ion channels activated by γ-aminobutyric acid (GABA) and glycine, extrasynaptically by enhancing GABA receptors and leak currents, and presynaptically by enhancing basal GABA release.
- Inhaled anesthetics suppress excitatory synaptic transmission presynaptically by reducing glutamate release (volatile agents) and postsynaptically by inhibiting excitatory ionotropic receptors activated by glutamate (gaseous agents).

Properties of Specific Inhaled Anesthetics

- Anesthesia protocols include several agents in combinations.
- Inhaled anesthetics have varying potency in proportion to their lipid solubility.
- MAC (minimal alveolar anesthetic concentration) is defined as the concentration of inhaled anesthetic, as a % of inspired air, at which 50% of patients do not respond to a surgical stimulus.
  - MAC is a measure of potency: ED50
  - The more lipid soluble the anesthetic, the lower the MAC and the greater the potency.
  - MAC values are additive.
  - MAC values are lower in the elderly and in the presence of sedative–hypnotics.
- Rate of onset and recovery depend on the blood-gas ratio.
  - The more soluble the anesthetic in the blood, the slower the anesthesia.
  - Anesthetics with high blood–gas ratios are associated with slow onset.
  - Anesthetics with high blood–gas ratios are associated with slow recovery.
  - Anesthetics with low blood–gas ratios have fast onset and recovery.

Minimum Alveolar Concentration (MAC Value)

- It is measure of potency of inhalational agent. It is the minimum alveolar concentration of an inhalational agent required to produce unresponsiveness to noxious stimuli like skin incision in 50% of pt.
- Greater the MAC value, lesser is the potency
- Methoxyflurane is the most potent having least MAC value (0.16%)
- N_2O has maximum MAC value (104%) and is the least potent inhalationalanaesthetic

Gas	MAC Value
Methoxyflurane	0.16
Trilene	0.2
Halothane	0.74
Isoflurane	1.15
Enflurane	1.68
Ether	1.92
Sevoflurane	2.05
Desflurane	6.0
Cyclopropane	9.2
XENON	71
N_2O	104

Factors Affecting MAC Value

Factors Decreasing MAC Value

- Hypothermia
- Pregnancy
- IV anesthetics
- Local anesthetics
- Hypoxia
- Hyperthermia up to 42 °C
- Alcohol intoxication
- Anemia
- Hyponatremia
- Hypercarbia
- Hyper calcemia
- Hypermagnesemia

Factors Increasing MAC Value

- Hypernatremia
- Hyperthermia > 42 °C
- Increased Barometric pressure
- Chronic alcoholism

No Change in MAC Value

- Thyroid disease/sex of pt.

Blood Gas Partition Coefficient

- It is indicator of blood solubility. It determines the speed of onset and recovery of anesthetic drug
- Greater the blood gas partition coefficient, lesser the solubility slow speed of onset and recovery.

Gas	Blood Gas Partition Coefficient
Xenon	0.115
N_2O	0.47
Desflurane	0.42
Sevoflurane	0.69
Ether	12
Methoxyflurane	15
Isoflurane	1.38
Halothane	2.4

- Fastest Induction and Fastest recovery is seen with Desflurane and is the inhalational agent of choice for day care surgery in adults.
- Methoxyflurane has the slowest induction
- Halothane has slower induction compared to most other used anesthetics
- In Pt's with low cardiac output as in shock, Inhalational agent with low blood gas partition coefficient is preferred.

Effect of Inhalational Agents on Body

Respiratory System

- All Inhalational agents are bronchodilators. Max. Bronchodilation is by Halothane hence preferred in patients with obstructive lung disease.

- All inhalational agents depress the respiratory system.
- Max. Blunting of ventilatory response is with halothane

Cardiovascular System

- All inhalational agents decrease cardiac output except isoflurane
- Max. decrease in CO is with halothane
- CO is best maintained by isoflurane
- N_2O is pulmonary vasoconstrictor
- All inhalational agents reduce mucociliary activity of airways except ether.
- Max. Inhibition of baroreceptor reflexes is with Halothane
- All inhalational agents reduce BP except cyclopropane which increases BP
- Isoflurane is the agent of choice for controlled hypotension. Isoflurane is agent of choice for cardiac pt's because of maintenance of CO and min. response on
- baroreceptor reflexes
- Halothane sensitizes the heart to arrhythmogenic action of adrenaline.
- Halothane is CI in pt's with Pheochromocytoma.
- isoflurane is agent of choice for pheochromocytoma.

Effect on CNS

- All inhalational agent increase intracranial tension because of cerebral vasodilation.
- All inhalational agent increase cerebral metabolic rate and O_2 consumption of brain.
- Max. reduction of cerebral metabolic rate and O_2 consumption is with isoflurane.
- Min. increase in ICT is isoflurane and Desflurane < 6%
- Inhalational agent of choice for neurosurgeries is Isoflurane
- Halothane produces hepatocellular damage or toxicity (Halothane is not used in Pheochromocytoma)

Effect on Kidneys

- Nephrotoxicity of inhalational is because of fluoride content
- Anaesthetics are fluorinated to make them non-inflammatory
- Max. fluoride content is seen in methoxyflurane, hence max. nephrotoxicity with methoxyflurane
- Methoxyflurane produces vasopressin resistance, polyuric renal failure.

Action on Blood

- N_2O can cause bone marrow suppression, megaloblastic anemia and Vit B_{12} deficiency
- All inhalational agents relaxes the uterus. Max. with halothane and thus halothane is agent of choice for internal version and manual removal of placenta
- Hyperglycemia is produced by ether, cyclopropane and Desflurane > 6%

Nitrous Oxide (N_2O)

- It is stored in blue color cylinders
- It is also known as laughing gas
- It is stored as liquid at a pressure of 745 Psi
- It is a nonirritant gas, not metabolized by body. It is colorless, nonirritating and noninflammable.
- Mainly eliminated through lungs (95%) and 5% through skin
- N_2O is a good analgesic but weak anesthetic and poor muscle relaxant. Hence not a complete anaesthetic.
- N_2O has blood gas coefficient of 0.47 and has fast induction
- It has MAC value of 104; Hence Potency is low
- N_2O is used as a carrier gas given in a mixture of 33% O_2 and 66% N_2O
- Entonox is a mixture of 50% O_2 and 50% N_2O

- Poynting effect: Entonox (50% O_2 and 50% N_2O) and mixture of gases (O_2 and N_2O) keeps them in gaseous form. If temperature is altered, one of the gas turns to liquid.
- **Concentration Effect:** The inspired anesthetic concentration influences both the rate of rise and the height of the Fa/Fi ratio. Increasing the inspired concentration accelerates the rate of rise.
- **2nd Gas Effect:** The loss of volume associated with the uptake of nitrous oxide concentrates the potent anesthetic. Replacement of the gas taken up by an increase in inspired ventilation augments the amount of potent anesthetic present in the lung
- **Diffusion Hypoxia:** On recovery from anesthesia, the outpouring of large volumes of nitrous oxide can produce what Fink called diffusion anoxia. These volumes may cause hypoxia in two ways. First, they may directly affect oxygenation by displacing oxygen. Second, by diluting alveolar carbon dioxide, they may decrease respiratory drive and hence ventilation. Diffusion hypoxia is prevented by giving 100% O_2 before discontinuing N_2O
- Methemoglobinemia and laryngospasm can occur due to presence of impurities like NO and NO_2
- N_2O produces bone marrow suppression, megaloblastic anemia due to B12 deficiency can lead to subacute combine degeneration of spinal cord.
- N_2O is CI in
  - Middle ear surgeries and tympanoplasty
  - Laparoscopic surgeries
  - Acute intestinal obstruction and volvulus
  - Microlaryngeal surgeries
  - Pneumothorax, pneumoperitonium
  - Eye surgeries
  - Pneumoencephalos.

N_2O reacts with O_2 to form nitric oxide which could damage the ozone

Xenon

- Properties: inert gas, normal atmospheric constituent, not an environmental pollutant, no ozone depletion global warming effect
- Manufactured by fractional distillation of air → costly
- MAC → 71% [more potent that N_2O]
- Blood gas partition coefficient → 0.14 [emergence is rapid than with desflurane/propofol]
- Minimal cardiovascular and hemodynamic side effects
  - Cardioprotective
  - Neuroprotective
  - Nonteratogenic
  - Nonmetabolized in liver/kidney
  - No malignant hyperthermia
- Density of xenon → 5.887g/dl (more than N_2O and air)
  - Increases pulmonary resistance and breathing
  - Cautiously used in moderate to severe COPD, morbidly obese and premature infants.

Halothane

- Least expensive and least pungent
- Potent anesthetic, no analgesia
- Dissolve rubber and corrodes metals
- Contains **0.01% thymol** for stability
- Decomposed by light but is stable when in amber coloured bottles
- **May persist in the liver for as long as 12 days after administration and is usually not given in same patient within 3 months (potent hepato toxic)**

- Relaxes both skeletal and uterine muscle and blood vessels
- In pediatric patients and combined with its pleasant odor, suitable in children for inhalation induction
- Halothane results in Postanesthetic chills and shivering A/K Halothane shakes
- It sensitizes the heart to the arrhythmogenic action of adrenaline
- It produces max. suppression of baroreceptor mechanism
- It produces max. suppression of ventilatory responses to hypercapnia and hypoxia
- The halothane hepatitis is immunological mediated occurs 1 in 35,000 pt's. MC in pt's with autoimmune disease
- Repeated use of halothane should be avoided in the same pt.
- C.I–Previous pt. of hepatitis, pt's with head injuries and ICT, in pt's with cardiac diseases and pheochromocytoma.

Isoflurane

- It is isomer of enflurane. It is mildly irritant, colorless with pungent odor.
- MAC value–1.15
- It is not a good analgesic
- Baroreceptor reflexes are preserved with isoflurane. CO is maintained and is inhalational agent of choice for cardiac surgeries and cardiac disease.
- Isoflurane produces least increase in Intracranial pressure and is the agent of choice for neuro surgeries
- It is inhalational agent of choice for producing controlled hypotension.

Enflurane

- It is an ether derivative
- It is epileptogenic
- Enflurane is CI in pt. with Epilepsy and renal failure

Desflurane

- It is a ether derivative, Colorless pungent liquid, boils at room temperature with very high vapor pressure.
- Desflurane is fastest inducing agent and less MAC value–0.42
- Desflurane is agent of choice for Day care surgery in adults
- Induction is unpleasant with desflurane with coughing and laryngospasms.
- It has similar cardiac property as isoflurane but does not produce coronary steal phenomenon.
- It has low metabolism and fluoride production
- Agent of choice in old patients and obese patients is desflurane
- desflurane > 6% stimulates sympathetic activity
- tec 6 vaporizer is exclusively used for desflurane.
  - Desiccated carbon dioxide absorbent and inhaled anesthetic interactions can lead to the production of carbon monoxide in the anesthesia circuit (desflurane ⋙ enflurane > isoflurane). Negligible amounts of carbon monoxide are formed from halothane and sevoflurane.

Sevoflurane

- It has smooth induction and agent of choice for induction in children
- It has poor analgesic effect
- It should not be used with very low flow (< 2L/min)in closed circuit because it reacts with soda lime to produce compound A which is nephrotoxic.

Methoxyflurane

- It is the most potent inhalational agent with least MAC Value. It has slow induction and slow recovery because of highest blood gas partition coefficient.
- It should not be used in closed circuits because it reacts with rubber tubing of closed circuit.
- It has max. fluoride production produces high output renal failure (vasopressin resistant polyuria)

Cyclopropane

- It is no longer used.
- It is highly inflammable and explosive. Stored in orange color cylinders.
- It stimulates sympathetic system and increases BP.
- It inhalational agent of choice in pt. with hemorrhagic shock in olden days of anesthesia administration.
- It can also sensitizes the heart to adrenaline and should not be discontinued abruptly since it produces cyclopropane shock.

Trilene

- Also called Trichloroethylene
- It has max. analgesic property
- C.I in closed circuit since it reacts with soda lime and produce dichloroacetylene which is neurotoxic and phosgene which produces ARDS.

Chloroform

- No more used
- Highly cardiotoxic, produces Ventricular fibrillation
- Also hepatotoxic, can produce hyperglycemia
- Adrenaline is not given with chloroform
- Chloroform is more hepatotoxic than halothane so both are contraindicated in liver disease

Ether

- It is a complete anesthetic nearer to ideal anaesthetic. It is highly inflammable, highly volatile and explosive
- It is an irritant, pungent smelling liquid
- It has slow induction and is very unpleasant
- Ether does not affect the mucociliary action and is good bronchodilator.
- Ether has good anaesthetic, good analgesic, good skeletal muscle relaxant
- Ether does not depress respiration but rather it is stimulated
- It increases respiratory secretion and salivation thereby anticholinergic should always be given before giving ether to prevent these reactions.
- Ether has highest incidence of nausea and vomiting among inhalational agents.
- Ether causes hyperglycemia and is C.I in diabetes
- Guedel's 4 stages of anesthesia were based on ether. Ether should not be used with cautery.
- Ether is safe in unskilled professionals and is very economical
- Ether derivatives–Enflurane, Isoflurane, Desflurane, sevoflurane.

CO_2

- 5 % CO_2 is used for creating pneumoperitoneum during laparoscopy
- Has analgesic property too

Helium

- It is very low density gas lighter than air
- A mixture of 80% helium and 20% O_2 is used for tracheal obstruction.

O_2

- Stored at pressure of 2000 Psi
- Excess of O_2 produces retrolental fibroplasias

Hepatotoxicity of Anesthetic Agents

Depends on

- Gender (Female > male)
- Age (middle age adults)
- Obesity
- Enzyme induction
- Prior anesthetic exposure
- Genetics

- Hepatotoxicity of inhalational agents is due to TFA [Tri flour acetyl] metabolite.
- Therefore, hepatotoxicity is proportional to the percentage of metabolism
- % metabolism: halothane (20%) > Sevoflurane (2–5%) > Enflurane (2–4%) > Isoflurane (0.2%) > desflurane (0.02%)
- Bet sevoflurane does not cause hepatotoxicity because its metabolite is HFIP (not TFA).

Intravenous Agents

IV anesthetics are used in induction of anesthesia in adults

Barbiturates

1. Thiopentone

Ultra short acting barbiturate used for induction

Actions:

CNS:

- Cerebroprotective
- Decreases cerebral blood flow and intracranial tension
- Decreases cerebral O_2 consumption and increases the perfusion pressure
- Antianalgesic
- It has anticonvulsant/antiepileptic property
- It can produce hyperalgesia by reducing the threshold of pain

Musculoskeletal system: Tremors, twitching, respiratory excitation including cough, hiccup

Respiratory system: Respiratory depression [double apnea], upper airway obstruction

- CVS–hypotension
- It is not a muscle relaxant. Thiopentone has antithyroid properties bcos it has thiourilene structure

- It is available as amorphous yellow powder, reconstituted just by use.
- Ringer lactate should not be used for reconstitution as it gets precipitated with it.
- Thiopentone is highly alkaline with pH of 10.4
- Mechanism of action–Thiopentone like other barbiturate acts by facilitating GABA mediated chloride channel opening.
- It produces unconsciousness in one arm brain circulation time (about 15 sec)
- It is 90% protein bound mainly to arginine, highly lipid soluble and has fast action. The action of drug is terminated very quickly due to redistribution.
- IV agent of Choice for neurosurgery and head injury patients.
- It crosses BBB and Placental barrier.

Complications

- It induces ALA synthetase which may precipitate acute intermittent porphyria.
- Perivenous and IM injections cause tissue necrosis and ulcerations due to highalkalinity.
- Prevention is done by using 2.5% solution, injecting very slowly and in incremental doses.
- Stop the injection if pt. complains pain. It is preferably given on dorsum of hand.

- Accidental injection of thiopentone in arteries produces thrombosis and vasoconstriction progressing to ischemia and gangrene. Treatment of this condition is done by leaving the needle inside, diluting the needle with saline, immediate heparinization and papaverine injection to relief spasm.
- Vasodilators like phenoxybenzamine are also given.
- Brachial plexus or stellate ganglion block can be given to relief vasospasm.
- Treatment of extravasation is done by giving 1% lignocaine and 100 units of hyaluronidase in the area.
- Other complications–thrombophlebitis, respiratory depression and laryngospasm.
- Thiopentone should be avoided in asthmatics, pt's with hypotension, shock, pts on B blockers, Pt's with hypokalemia, heart blocks, valvular stenosis and dystrophia myotonia.
- Thiopentone like other barbiturates have enzyme induction properties.

2. Methohexitone

- Ultra short acting barbiturate. More potent than thiopentone Induces seizures and is the agent of choice for electroconvulsive therapy.

Propofol

- It is a milky–white powder, preservative free, should be used within 6 hours.
- It is an oil-based preparation and injection is painful because it contains soyabean oil, egg lecithin and glycerol
- 1% xylocaine is also given along with it to reduce pain on injection.
- Mechanism of action is GABA mediated. Onset within 15 sec and also shows redistribution.
- Propofol has strong antiemetic and antipruritic action
- It is IV anesthetic of Choice for Day care surgery
- IV anesthetic of choice in pt's with malignant hyperthermia
- Propofol with alfentanil is used as anesthetic of choice for total IV anesthesia.
- Propofol does not have muscle relaxant property instead produces myoclonic jerking and muscle twitching.
- Propofol has rapid and smooth induction, rapid and smooth recovery, no active metabolites and strong antiemetic property.
- Improve neurologic outcome and reduce neuronal damage by depressing cerebral metabolism and cerebral oxygen consumption.
- Water-soluble phosphorylated prodrug: fospropofol [hy drolyzed by endothelial cell surface alkaline phosphatases]
  - The rapid recovery of neurologic status makes it a good sedative in ICU patients
  - Bolus dose: 1 to 2 mg per kg induces loss of consciousness with 30 seconds
  - Maintenance infusion rate: 100 to 200 μg per kg per minute are adequate in younger subjects, whereas doses should be reduced by 20% to 50% in elderly individuals.

Propofol Infusion Syndrome

- Occurs if given at the rate of 4 mg/kg/hour or more for 48 hours or longer
- Lethal disorder as it interferes with mitochondrial oxidation
- Features:
  - Acute refractory bradycardia leading to asystole
  - Metabolic acidosis
  - Rhabdomyolysis
  - Hyperlipidemia
  - Enlarged/fatty liver
  - Cardiomyopathy with acute cardiac failure, skeletal myopathy.

Ketamine

- Ketamine interacts with the N-methyl-D-aspartate receptor
- Causes profound analgesia, dissociative anesthesia.

- Complete anesthetic as it induces analgesia and unconsciousness. It is the Agent of choice in shock
- It is associated with emergence psychoto mimetic side effects 'DISSOCIATIVE ANESTHESIA' (delirium, illusions, and hallucination) it is less common in children and after pretreatment with benzodiazepines
- Can be used as an adjunct in regional anesthesia
- Only IV anesthetic agent with both anesthetic and analgesic activity
- **It is a sympathetic stimulant so it causes** Cardiac stimulation (sensitizes the heart to adrenaline) → Increased HR, BP, Oxygen demand and cardiac output
- Increases all pressure → BP, IOT, ICT
- Increased muscle tone → myalgia
- Potent bronchodilator → AOC in bronchial Asthma, Upper airway reflexes are intact (Beneficial in patients with either hypovolemic or cardiogenic shock as well as in patients with asthma.)
- Has strong analgesic property and used for burn dressings.
- IV agent of choice in Burns pts.
- Ketamine does not suppress pharyngeal and laryngeal reflexes
- It is IV agent of choice for shock
- It is potent bronchodilator IV anesthetic of choice for asthma patients.
- It can be given by IV, IM, Oral or rectal methods
- It is preferred in patients with Rt to lt. shunts, congestive heart failure, asthma and COPD.
- Action of ketamine starts in 30–60 sec. and terminates within 15–20 mins because of redistribution
- Ketamine is therefore used when circulatory depression is undesirable
- Contraindicated in raised intracranial pressure and intracranial pathology with mass effect
- Dosage: intravenous (2 mg/kg BW); intramuscular (5–10 mg/kg BW)
- **Avoided in:** CGF, coronary Artery disease, hypertension, CVA and Arterial aneurysm
- Salivation is increased so anticholinergic (atropine) is always given in premedication.

Etomidate

- It is most cardiostable IV agent. Agent of choice for cardiac disease.
- S/E–Max. incidence of nausea and vomiting is seen with etomidate.
- It suppress the adrenal cortex.
- Injection of Etomidate is painful and produces thrombophlebitis
- It also produces myoclonus and vitamin C deficiency.

Droperidol

- It is a D2 receptor blockers. It produces extrapyramidal side effects.
- Neurolept analgesia = Droperidol + fentanyl
- Neurolept anesthesia = Droperidol + fentanyl + N_2O

Benzodiazepines

- Acts on the frequency of opening of GABA mediated chlorine channels.
- Midazolam is MC benzodiazepine used in premedication
- It is used with ketamine to prevent hallucinations
- Benzodiazepines have anxiolytic, anticonvulsant, sedative hypnotic properties.
- Benzodiazepines are centrally acting muscle relaxants.

1. Diazepam

- It is oil-based and injection is painful
- It has highest incidence of dysphoria and the sleep is not smooth
- It produces active metabolites which can cause postoperative respiratory depression.

2. Midazolam

- It is MC used benzodiazepine intraoperatively
- It is water based painless injection
- It is benzodiazepine of choice for day care surgery because of its short duration of action
- It can be given IV, IM, Oral or nasal and is a preferred premedication in children.

3. Lorazepam

- It is preferred premedication in adults, longest amnesia with highest receptorbinding.
- The action of lorazepam cannot be completely reversed with flumazenil.

Opioids

- Mainly used for analgesia during intraoperative and postoperative period.
- Derived from Papaver somniferous
- Opioid receptors–3 receptors
  - mu-receptor–Sedation, analgesia, Constipation, respiratory depression, euphoria, meiosis (SACRUM)
  - K (Kappa) receptor–Dysphoria (Psycho mimetic effects), hallucination night mares, constipation and analgesia.
  - delta receptor–Spinal analgesia.
- Endogenous opiate peptides represented by endorphins, enkephalins, and dynorphins
- Three receptor families: μ, k, and δ
- Presynaptic and postsynaptic inhibition through G_1 coupling
- Mu pharmacology most important
- Morphine is the prototype μ agonist
- Pharmacology of **morphine:**
  - Analgesia: ↑ pain tolerance and ↓ perception and reaction to pain
  - Sedation
  - Respiratory depression
  - Cardiovascular: minimal effects on heart, but vasodilation (avoid in head trauma)
  - Smooth muscle
    - Longitudinal relaxes
    - Circular constricts
      G1: ↓ peristalsis, constipation, cramping
      GU: urinary retention, urgency to void
      Biliary: ↓ pressure
      Pupils: miosis
    - Cough suppression: antitussive action, independent of analgesia and respiratory depression
    - Nausea and vomiting: stimulation of the chemoreceptor trigger zone (CTZ) in the area postrema
    - ↑ histamine release
- Pharmacokinetics of morphine:
  - Glucuronidation
  - Morphine-6-glucuronide is highly active
  - Caution in renal dysfunction
- Other opioids and analgesics
- Side effects of opioid analgesics;
  - Acute toxicity: classic triad
    - Pinpoint pupils
    - Respiratory depression, chest wall rigidity
    - Coma

- Management of acute toxicity:
  - Supportive
  - IV naloxone
- Abuse liability of opioid analgesics:
  - Tolerance: pharmacodynamic; occurs to all effects, except miosis and constipation
  - Dependence: physical and psychologic
  - Withdrawal:
    - Yawning
    - Lacrimation, rhinorrhea, salivation
    - Anxiety, sweating goose bumps
    - Muscle cramps, spasms, CNS–originating pain
  - Management of withdrawal:
    - Supportive
    - Methadone
    - Clonidine
- Opiate–related drugs with specific indications
  - Loperamide: diarrhea
  - Dextromethorphan: cough

Opioid Antagonists

- Naloxone is given parenterally and is short acting
- Nalmefene is also given parenterally but is short acting
- Naltrexone is long acting, orally effective opioid antagonists
- These drugs precipitate withdrawal symptoms in opioids dependent pt's
- Naloxone has highest antagonist properties and is a drug of choice for acute opioid poisoning
- Naloxone also antagonizes the action of diazepam, barbiturates, alcohol and N_2O
- Naloxone reverses the action of all opioids except buprenorphine
- Naloxone is also used in neonatal resuscitation to treat neonatal asphyxia of any cause.
- Naltrexone is used in maintenance drug for opioid poisoning
- Naltrexone prevents relapse after opioid de-addiction and is also used to decrease craving in chronic alcoholics.

Local Anesthetics

Mechanism of action: Blocks voltage gated Na+ channels from inside of cell membrane by binding to a-subunit of Na K pump

	Local anesthetic	
	Ester linked	Amide linked
Shorter duration (< 30 min)	Procaine (low potency) Chlorprocaine (intermediate potency)	
Intermediate duration and potency (30–90 min)	–	Lidocaine, Mepivacaine, Prilocaine
Long duration and potency (> 120 min)	Tetracaine, Benzocaine	Bupivacaine, Ropivacaine, Dibucaine Etidocaine

Mode of Action of Local Anesthetics

- Local anesthetics provide regional anesthesia.
- Drugs:
  - **Esters:** procaine, cocaine, benzocaine are metabolized by plasma and tissue esterases
  - **Amides:** lidocaine, bupivacaine, mepivacaine are metabolized by liver amidases

- **Mechanisms**
  - Nonionized form crosses axonal membrane
  - From within, ionized form blocks the inactivated Na^+ channel
  - Slows recovery and prevents propagation of action potentials
- **Nerve fiber sensitivity**
  - Nerve fibers most sensitive to blockade are of smaller diameter and have high firing rates

Classification of Peripheral Nerves According to Anatomy, Physiology, and Function

Fiber Class	Subclass	Myelin	Diameter (μm)	Conduction Velocity (msec)	Location	Function	Susceptibility to Local Anesthetic Block
A	α	+	6–22	30–120	Efferent to muscles	Motor	++
	β	+	6–22	30–120	Afferent from skin and joints	Tactile, proprioception	++
	γ	+	3–6	15–35	Efferent to muscle spindles	Muscle tone	++++
	δ	+	1–4	5–25	Afferent sensory nerves	Pain, cold temperature, touch	+++
B		+	< 3	3–15	Preganglionic sympathetic	Various autonomic functions	++
C	sC	-	0.3-1.3	0.7–1.3	Postganglionic sympathetic	Various autonomic functions	++
	dC	-	0.4-1.2	0.1–2.0	Afferent sensory nerves	Various autonomic functions Pain, warm temperature, touch	+

- **Absorption**
  - Vasoconstrictors, usually epinephrine (5 μg/mL or 1: 200,00), are frequently included in local anesthetic solutions to decrease the rate of vascular absorption, thereby allowing more anesthetic molecules to reach the nerve membrane and thus improve the depth and duration of anesthesia, as well as to provide a marker for inadvertent intravascular injection.
  - The addition of sodium bicarbonate to a solution of local anesthetic applied to an isolated nerve accelerates the onset and decreases the minimum concentration (Cm) required for conduction blockade. Increase in the pH of the local anesthetic solution increases the amount of drug in the uncharged base form, which should enhance the rate of diffusion across the nerve sheath and nerve membrane and result in a more rapid onset of anesthesia.
- **Side effects**
  - Neurotoxicity
  - Cardiovascular toxicity
  - Allergies (esters via PABA formation)
- Esters are metabolized by pseudocholinesterase in the plasma (except cocaine)
- Amines are metabolized by liver
- Esters have high allergic reaction due to production of Para amino benzoic acid
- Amines have low incidence of allergy.

Cocaine

- It was 1st local anesthetic used, is an ester that is not metabolized by pseudo Cholinesterase
- It is potent vasoconstrictor
- It is metabolized in liver, prevents the reuptake of noradrenaline and is never given I.V (or) with adrenaline.

Chloroprocaine

- It is shortest acting local anesthetic, most acidic and most neurotoxic
- Neurotoxicity is due to presence of Na^+ metabisulphite as preservative
- Chloroprocaine is C.I for spinal anesthesia.

Tetra Caine

- a/k amethocaine, Tetracaine and cocaine can cause ventricular fibrillation

Prilocaine

- Causes the max. methemoglobinemia
- It is the safest local anesthetic as it is metabolized by extrahepatic tissues like kidney, lung, amylases
- It is the preferred local anesthetic for Bier's block

Bupivacaine

- It is the long acting local anesthetic with high protein binding
- Bupivacaine is the most cardiotoxic and should not be used for Bier's block
- Bupivacaine produces ventricular fibrillation
- Procainamide is the DOC for bupivacaine induced arrhythmias. Amiodarone is the 2nd DOC.

Ropivacaine

- It is less cardiotoxic and derivative of Bupivacaine.

Dibucaine

- It is the most potent, longest acting and most toxic local anesthetic
- Dibucaine is used to determine the levels of atypical pseudocholinesterase.

Lignocaine

- a/k lidocaine (or) Xylocaine
- 4% lignocaine is used for topical (or) surface anesthesia
- 1–2% lignocaine is used for nerve blocks
- 0.5% is used for IV regional anesthesia
- 5% for spinal anesthesia
- 2% jelly is used for urethral procedures.

Eutectic Mixtures

- It is 2.5% prilocaine + 2.5% lignocaine
- Eutectic mixture is used to anesthetize intact skin
- Lignocaine should not be used in patients with history of malignant hyperthermia
- Lignocaine is used for ventricular fibrillation specially after MI
- Lignocaine can produce cauda equina syndrome
- Preservative free lignocaine called xylocard is preferred for IV injection
  - Shortest acting LA-chlorprocaine
  - Intradural injection is contra indicated and may cause paraplegias-chlorprocaine
  - Longest acting LA-Dibucaine
  - Only naturally occurring LA-cocaine
  - All LA are vasodilators except Cocaine (vasoconstrictor)
  - Safest LA and causes maximum Methemoglobinemia–prilocaine
  - Best LA for regional block and isobaric spinal analgesia–bupivacaine
  - Dibucaine is longest acting L.A followed by Tetracaine > Bupivacaine
  - Shortest acting L.A is chlorprocaine (mnemonic–Dibucaine - chloroprocaine) (Delhi to Chennai)

LA used in surface anesthesia	Never used as surface anesthetic
Hexycline, Lignocaine Dibucaine, Tetracaine Prilocaine, Cocaine	Procaine Mepivacaine Bupivacaine

- Bupivacaine: racemic mixture of → and (S) isomers while Levobupivacaine: single (S) stereoisomer, both containing butyl groups
- The most common ECG finding with bupivacaine intoxication is slow idioventricular rhythm with broad QRS complexes and eventually, electromechaincal dissociation.
- Recent recommendation for treatment of bupivacaine induced cardiotoxicity: 20% intralipid [4 ml/kg followed by 0.5 ml/kg/min infusion]
- O-Toludine metabolites of prilocaine, accumulates aften large doses and convert hemoglobin to methemoglobin
- Treatment of Methemoglobinemia is IV methylene blue (1–2 mg/kg of 1% solution) which reduces methemoglobin (Fe^{3+}) to hemoglobin (Fe^{2+})
- Bupivacaine causes differential blockade (autonomic 2 segments higher > sensory > motor)
- Repeated doses of 5% lidocaine and 0.5% tetracaine neurotoxicity (cauda equine syndrome)
- LA's are myotoxic (bupivacaine > liodcaine > procaine, Least with Ropivacaine), if injected directly into a muscle.

Adverse effects of chloroprocaine:

- When injected into the subarachnoid space leads to prolonged neurological deficit, d/t preservative, sodium bisulfate (now replaced with an antioxidant, a derivative of EDTA)
- Severe back pin following epidural administration

Different fiber types are also differentially sensitive to local anesthetic blockade. In vivo experiments in which continuous superperfusion of peripheral nerve allows equilibration with drug and experiments in which a drug bolus is delivered by percutaneous injection, analogous to clinical peripheral nerve block, show unequivocally that small myelinated axons (Aγ motor and Aδ sensory fibers) are the most susceptible to impulse annihilation. Next in order of block are the large myelinated (Aα and Aβ) fibers, and the least susceptible are the small, nonmyelinated C fibers. In fact, in this last group, impulses in the slowest conducting population (conduction velocity of 0.5 to 0.8 msec) are the most resistant to local anesthetic. The generalized notion that local anesthetics block the smallest fibers first or most is clearly wrong.

Among sensory fibres temperature (cold > heat) > pain > touch > deep pressure > proprioception

Intravenous regional anesthesia involves the intravenous administration of a local anesthetic into a tourniquet-occluded limb (i.e. Bier block). Drug of choice is prilocaine. Lignocaine can be used. Bupivacaine should be avoided b'cos of cardiotoxicity.

Skeletal Muscle Relaxants

Classification of nondepolarizing neuromuscular blockers

Class of Blocker	Clinical Duration			
	Long-Acting (> 50 min)	Intermediate-Acting (20–50 min)	Short-Acting (15–20 min)	Ultrashort-acting (<10–12 min)
Steroidal compounds	Pancuronium Pipecuronium	Vecuronium Rocuronium		
Benzylisoquinolinium compounds	*d*-Tubocurarine Metocurine Doxacurium	Atracurium Cisatracurium	Mivacurium	
Others				
Asymmetrical mixed-onium chlorofumarates				Gantacurium
Phenolic ether	Gallamine			
Diallyl derivative of toxiferine	Alcuronium			

Directly acting–Dantrolene, Quinine

Centrally acting agent

Acts on cerebrospinal axis without altering consciousness

- Benzodiazepine
- Mephensin
- GABA derivatives as Baclofen
- Tizanidine

	Depolarizing block	Non depolarizing block
Effect on single twitch height	Depression	Depression
Train of four fade	Absent	Present
Tetanic fade	Absent	Present
Post tetanic facilitation	Absent	Present
Effect of anti cholinesterase	Potentiation of block	Reversal of block

Muscle Relaxants

- **Maximum histamine release, Contraindicated in Asthma: d-TC**
- **Minimum histamine release, used in Asthma: Vecuronium**
- Metabolized by pseudo cholinesterase: Succinyl choline
- Muscle relaxant which increases BP and heart rate–Pancuronium
- Muscle relaxant with ganglion block: d-tc (highest), Galamine, Trimethaphan.
- Muscle relaxant with highest histamine release–d-tc > mivacurium, atracurium
- Highest vagolytic effect–pancuronium
- Gallamine is least potent whereas most potent and longest acting skeletal muscle relaxant doxacurium
- Fastest acting nondepolarising skeletal muscle relaxant is Rocuronium
- Shortest acting non depolarizing agent is gantacurium > mivacurium.
- Shortest acting (both onset and duration) muscle relaxant–succinylcholine
- Muscle relaxant of choice for full stomach patients, rapid sequence induction–succinylcholine

Sequence of Muscle Blockade after muscle relaxants therapy

- First muscle to be blocked: Central muscles (Muscles of face) followed by jaw → pharynx → larynx → respiratory muscles-small muscles.
- Then peripheral muscles are involved
- Recovery occurs in the same order
- **Muscle monitored for activity during blockade: Adductor pollicis**

Succinylcholine

- **It is the only depolarizing (noncompetitive) muscle relaxant in use**
- **It has rapid onset of action (30–60 seconds) and has over all shortest duration of action** (3–5 min) due to rapid hydrolysis by pseudo choline esterase
- **Scoline is metabolized completely into succinic acid+choline**
- Dibucaine inhyibits pseudo choline esterase activity. The percentage of inhibition of pseudo choline esterase activity is termed the dibucaine number
- Percent of abnormal/normal pseudo choline esterase is determined by Dibucaine number and fluoride number
- Normal Dibucaine no = 75–85
- Succinylcholine Causes dual or biphasic block with large or repeated doses
- Succinylcholine is avoided till 2–3 months after trauma, 6 months after hemiplegia and 2 years after burns.
- Also C.I in pt's with muscle diseases like muscular dystrophy, myasthenia gravis, gush injury, burns and rhabdomyolysis.
- Prolonged apnea after succinylcholine is due to low pseudocholinesterase levels, atypical pseudocholinesterase

and phase II block.

- Rx of prolonged apnea–continue intermittent positive pressure ventilation and wait for spontaneous recovery. Given frozen plasma (2nd choice)
- Rx–IPPV intermittent +ve pressure ventilation and spontaneous recovery.
- Neostigmine can also reverse phase II block.

Phase I Block	Features of classical depolarization block
Phase II Block	Results from desensitization of receptor to Ach. and resembles competitive/non–depolarization block and partially antagonized by Anticholinesterases

Clinical characteristics of phase 1 and phase 2 neuromuscular blockade during succinylcholine administration

Characteristic	Phase 1	Transition	Phase 2
Tetanic stimulation	No fade	Slight fade	Fade
Post-tetanic facilitation	None	Slight	Yes
Train-of-four fade	No	Moderate fade	Marked fade
Train-of-four ratio	> 0.7	0.4–0.7	< 0.4
Edrophonium	Augments	Little effect	Antagonizes
Recovery	Rapid	Rapid to slow	Increasingly prolonged
Dose requirements (mg/kg)*	2–3	4–5	> 6
Tachyphylaxis	No	Yes	Yes

Side effects: it causes increase in

- Muscle tone
- Muscle fasciculation/Muscle soreness or Ache
- Normally it increases serum potassium by 0.5 meq/l
- Hyperkalemia → diastolic cardiac arrest. More prone are: burns, massive trauma, neurological disorders, tetanus, and extensive soft tissue injury
- Intraocular pressure
- Intra abdominal pressure
- Temperature i.e. Malignant Hyperpyrexia (M.H)–most common agent triggering MH.

Reversal of Muscle Relaxation

- Depolarizing (Noncompetitive) agents are not antagonized
- NonDepolarizing (Competitive) MR are antagonized by Acetyl choline or Anti Choline Esterase-Neostigmine, Pyridostigmine and Edrophonium
- Atropine is given to prevent muscarinic effects

Nondepolarizing agents

Atracurium

- ➢ **Hofmann Elimination: [depends on pH and temperature]**
- Atracurium is inactivated in plasma by spontaneous non enzymatic degradation and by choline esterases
- Cisatracurium is 4 times more potent stereo isomer of Atracurium
- Major metabolite is laudanosine (CNS stimulant) produce epileptiform fits
- Acrylate is another metabolite.
- It's duration of action is not altered in patients with hepatic and renal in sufficiency or hypodynamic circulation
- **Muscle Relaxant of choice in renal failure and hepatic failure patients**
- ➢ **Histamine release leading to flushing of skin**

Cisatracurium

- Undergoes Hoffman elimination predominantly
- 4–5 times more potent than atracurium

- Laudanosine production is 5 times lesser than atracurium
- No histamine release.

Pancuronium

- It is a steroidal compound causes vagal blockade and releases noradrenaline
- It produces tachycardia and hypertension
- It is muscle relaxant of choice in shock and hypotension
- It is metabolized by the kidney, so avoided in renal failure.

Vecuronium

- Most commonly used muscle relaxant for routine surgery
- It is the muscle relaxant of choice for cardiac patients
- It is the most cardio stable, metabolized in liver and excreted through bile. Hence C.I in liver disease and in biliary obstruction
- Causes polyneuropathy on long-term use.

Pipecuronium

- It is long acting steroid analogue of pancuronium with no vagolytic activity (or) ganglion blockade activity.

Rocuronium

- Earliest onset of action among non-depolarising muscle relaxant
- Muscle relaxant of choice for pre-curarization and nondepolarizing muscle relaxant of choice for intubation.

Rapacuronium

- It is not used anymore because of severe bronchospasm

D–Tubocurarine

- It has the highest histamine release–causes asthma attacks, anaphylaxis
- It causes max ganglion blockade and severe hypotension.

Doxacurium

- It is longest acting and Most potent Non-depolarising skeletal muscle relaxant. It doesn't release histamine.

Mivacurium

- It is a short acting non depolarizing skeletal muscle relaxant
- It is metabolized by esterases
- It has quick onset and short duration and is the muscle relaxant of choice for day care surgeries.

Gallamine

- It is the least potent, but has maximum vagolytic action producing severe tachycardia.
- It nephrotoxic and teratogenic
- CI in renal disease and pregnancy

Recent advances in muscle relaxants and reversal agents

- **Asymmetric Mixed-Onium Chlorofumarates (Gantacurium):** Gantacurium is an ultra short acting muscle relaxant and it appears to be degraded by two chemical mechanisms, neither of which is enzymatic: (1) rapid formation of an apparently inactive cysteine adduction product, with cysteine replacing chlorine, and (2) slower hydrolysis of the ester bond adjacent to the chlorine substitution, presumably to inactive hydrolysis products
- **Sugammadex**: Sugammadex (ORG 25969) is the first selective relaxant binding agent. A modified γ-cyclodextrin, sugammadex is a new type of reversal agent. Their three-dimensional structure resembles a hollow truncated cone or a doughnut. The structure has a hydrophobic cavity and a hydrophilic exterior because of the presence

of polar hydroxyl groups. Sugammadex exerts its effect by forming very tight complexes in a 1: 1 ratio with steroidal neuromuscular blocking agents (rocuronium > vecuronium >> pancuronium). It produces rapid and effective reversal of even profound neuromuscular blockade.

Uses of Central Acting Muscle Relaxants

- Muscle Spasms
- Spinal injuries
- Cerebral Palsy
- IV diazepam (is used for tetanus)

Direct Acting Skeletal Muscle Relaxants

- Dantrolene and Quinine
- Dantrolene inhibits release of Ca^{+2} from sarcoplasmic reticulum, by inhibiting Ryanodine receptors.
- Dantrolene is DOC for malignant hyperthermia and neurolept malignant syndrome.
- S/E of Dantrolene–Muscle weakness and hepatitis
- Quinine is used in Rx of nocturnal leg cramps.

PREOPERATIVE ASSESSMENT

Pulmonary Function Test: Measured by spirometry

- Breath holding time in normal people is > 25 sec.
- If breath holding time between 15–25 sec–borderline pulmonary function
- If breath holding time < 15 sec–significant cardio pulmonary depression

Airway Assessment

Mallampati scoring is for assessment of difficult airway

Class I–Soft palate, Uvula, faucial pillars and posterior pharyngeal wall are visible.

Class II–Faucial pillars and soft palate are seen but free edge of Uvula is not seen.

Class–III only soft palate is seen

Class–IV–Only hard palate is seen

Other methods of airway assessment is thyromental distance. Normal thyromental distance is > 6.5 cms.

If < 6 cm–intubation is difficult

American society of Anesthesiology has graded pt's into 6 categories.

American Society of Anesthesiologists Physical Status Classification

ASA 1	Healthy patient without organic, biochemical, or psychiatric disease
ASA 2	A patient with mild systemic disease, e.g. mild asthma or well-controlled hypertension. No significant impact on daily activity. Unlikely to have an impact on anesthesia and surgery
ASA 3	Significant or severe systemic disease that limits normal activity, e.g. renal failure on dialysis or class 2 congestive heart failure. Significant impact on daily activity. Probable impact on anesthesia and surgery
ASA 4	Severe disease that is a constant threat to life or requires intensive therapy, e.g. acute myocardial infarction, respiratory failure requiring mechanical ventilation. Serious limitation of daily activity. Major impact on anesthesia and surgery
ASA 5	Moribund patient who is equally likely to die in the next 24 hours with or without surgery
ASA 6	Brain-dead organ donor

GENERAL ANESTHESIA

Preanesthetic Medication

- Opioids-Morphine
- Anxiolytics-aprazolam, diazepam

- Hypnotic-Barbiturate
- Anticholinergics-Atropine, Hyoscine
- Neuroleptic-chlorpromazine

Fasting guidelines

Adults

Clear fluids–2 hours

Semisolids–4 hours

Solid foods–6–8 hours

Children

Clear fluids–2 hours

Breast milk–4 hours

Formula milk, solid foods–6 hours

Adjuncts for Anesthesia

- H2 blocker-Metoclopramide, Ondansetron: reduce the risk of aspiration pneumonia
- Metoclopramide increase lower esophageal sphincter tone, speeds gastric emptying and lowers gastric fluid volume
- Serotonin 5-HT3 receptor blockers like Ondansetron, granisetron, and dolasetron for anti emetic effects
- Dexmedetomidine is a parenteral selective α2-agonist with sedative properties. It appears to be more selective for the α2-receptor than clonidine
- Patients are at risk if their gastric volume is greater than 25 mL (0.4 mL/kg) and their gastric pH is less than 2.5
- Antacids like omeprazole, Ranitidine reduce gastric secretions night b4 surgery
- Glycopyrrolate is the most preferred anticholinergic drug to reduce Oropharyngeal secretions. It does not cross BBB and devoid of central side effects.

Balanced Anesthesia

- The term Balanced anesthesia consists of 4 components
- Narcosis and Amnesia
- Analgesia
- Muscle relaxation
- Abolishment of reflex with maintenance of Hemostasis

General Protocol of Anesthesia

- Premedication of benzodiazepines
- Premedication with 100% of O_2 for 5 mins
- Induction of anesthesia with IV anesthesia followed by depolarizing or non depolarizing muscle relaxant
- Intubation
- Maintenance of anesthesia with 33% O_2, 66% Nitrous oxide (N_2O) and volatile agent along with Non-depolarizing muscle relaxant.
- Reversal of skeletal muscle relaxation is done by cholinesterase inhibitors like Neostigmine extubation.

Bag and Mask Ventilation

Contraindications–Full stomach

Aspiration Risk (Pregnancy, Hiatus Hernia)

Intestinal Obstruction

Unconscious/Semiconscious patients

Diaphragmatic Hernia

Tracheoesophageal fistula

Meconium aspiration

Management of Pre-existing Drug Therapies During Anesthesia

Oral Hypoglycemic Drugs: Should be continued with omition of morning dose in case of minor surgery. In major surgeries, shift to Insulin 48 hours before surgery.

OCP's: Should be stopped 4 weeks by surgery to — incidence of thromboembolism

Oral Anticoagulants: Should be stopped 4 days before and should be shifted over to low molwt. heparin. Heparin is then stopped one day before surgery.

In case of emergency Vit K is given if at least 6 hours are available and if the surgery is to be performed immediately fresh frozen plasma is to be given.

Unfractionated heparin–stop 6 hours before surgery

LMWH–stop 12 hours before surgery, if high dose stop 24 hours before surgery

Note–Heparin blocks circulating coagulating factors

Warfarin prevents synthesis of coagulating factors.

Anti hypertensive drugs: Should be continued and even the morning dose before surgery should be taken. Except ACE inhibitors and ARB'S whose morning dose is withheld

Anti Anginal Drugs: Should be continued and even the morning dose is given.

Antiplatelet Drugs: Clopidogrel should be stopped 1 week b4 surgery. In emergency platelet transfusion should be given prior to surgery. Aspirin can be continued on the day of surgery.

Antithyroid Drugs: Should be continued b4 surgery and even morning dose is given

Anti Epileptic Drugs: Should be continued b4 Surgery and even morning dose is given.

Levodopa: Should be continued

Anticholinesterases: Should be continued

Lithium: Should be stopped 48–72 hours before surgery because of its of half life of 24–36 hours. Lithium prolongs skeletal muscle relaxants and enhances neuromuscular blockage.

Steroids: If the pt. is on steroids by any route for > 1 week in last one year, intraoperative hydrocortisone replacement is necessary (Dose of steroids should be b4 surgery)

Smoking: Should be ideally stopped 6–8 weeks b4 surgery (complete ciliary recovery)

Antitubercular Drugs: Should be continued with monitoring of liver function test

Aminoglycosides: Have neuromuscular blocking activity so it is shift to another antibiotic 48 hours prior to surgery.

Note: 3 MC side effects of aminoglycosides →
- Ototoxicity
- Nephrotoxicity
- Neuromuscular Blockade

ANESTHESIA FOR CONCURRENT DISEASES

Diseases with altered responses to muscle relaxants

Muscular dystrophy (Duchenne type)	Hyperkalemia and malignant hyperthermia	Hypersensitivity
Myasthenia gravis	Resistance and prone to phase II block	Hypersensitivity
Myasthenic syndrome	Hypersensitivity	Hypersensitivity

Anesthesia for Liver Disease

- Isoflurane is volatile anesthetic agent of choice in patients with liver disease because it has least effect on hepatic blood flow
- Cisatracurium, atracurium is neuromuscular blocking agent of choice owing to its unique nonhepatic metabolism.

Anesthesia for Renal Disease

- Inhalation anesthetics–isoflurane
- IV anesthetics–ultra short acting barbiturates such as thiopental and propofol.

- Opioids–Remifentanil, fentanyl, sufentanil
- Muscle relaxants–Atracurium, cisatracurium–drug of choice.

Anesthesia for respiratory disease

Induction agents of choice –halothane, sevoflurane, ketamine.

Robert Shaw and Carlen tube is used for thoracic surgeries or single lung Ventilation. This tube is used to prevent spillage of pus and malignant cells during bronchopleural lavage and bronchopleural fistulas. The major side effect is hypoxia due to malposition and ventilation perfusion mismatch. Confirmation is done by bronchoscopy.

Anesthesia for cardiac patients

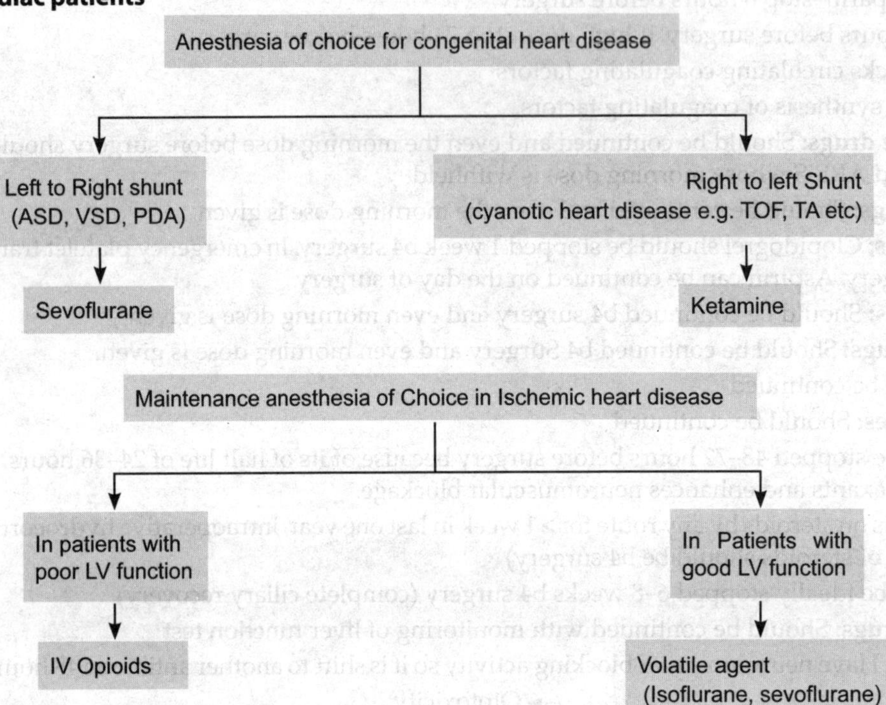

Anesthesia for neurosurgery

Total intravenous anesthesia (TIVA) is preferred–propofol with opioids in anesthetic of choice.

Among volatiles, isoflurane is agent of choice since it causes least increase in CBF.

During sitting craniotomy , venous air embolism can occur which is a dangerous complication.

MALIGNANT HYPERTHERMIA

- MH is a pharmacogenetic clinical syndrome that in its classic form occurs during anesthesia with a volatile halogenated alkane such as halothane and the depolarizing muscle relaxant succinylcholine
- Inheritance of human MH can no longer be considered to be solely autosomal dominant with variable penetrance because more than one MH-linked mutation has been identified in some probands and families
- Vigorous muscle contractions, an abrupt increase in temperature, and subsequent cardiovascular collapse
- Uncontrolled release of Ca^{2+} from the sarcoplasmic reticulum due to defect in the ryanodine receptor (RYR1) is the initiating event.

Drugs known to trigger malignant hyperthermia	Drugs safe in malignant hyperthermia
• Halothane • Succinylcholine (m.c.) • Methoxyflurane	• Nitrous oxide • Barbiturates • Diazepam

Contd...

Contd...

Drugs known to trigger malignant hyperthermia	Drugs safe in malignant hyperthermia
• Enflurane, isoflurane • Decamethonium • Gallamine • Diethyl ether • Ethylene • Ethyl chloride • Trichloroethylene • Ketamine • Phencyclidine • Cyclopropane	• Nondepolarizing muscle relaxants • Opiates • Propofol

- **Triggers:** Stress, excitement, anoxia, viral infections, and lymphoma and conditions of ischemia or hypoxia occurs at any age but is most frequent in young patients; the mean age is 22 years, 65% of patients are male 76% have no family history.
- The two classic clinical manifestations of fulminant MH syndrome may start in one of the following two scenarios.
  - Rigidity after induction with thiopental and succinylcholine but successful intubation, followed rapidly by the symptoms.
  - Normal response to induction of anesthesia and uneventful anesthetic course until onset of the following symptoms:
    - Unexplained sinus tachycardia or ventricular arrhythmias, or both
- Tachypnea if spontaneous ventilation is present
- Unexplained decrease in O_2 saturation (because of a decrease in venous O_2 saturation)
- Increased in end-tidal pCO_2 with adequate ventilation (and in most cases unchanged ventilation)
- Unexpected metabolic and respiratory acidosis
- Central venous desaturation
- Increase in body temperature above 38.8 °C with no obvious cause
- Masseter muscle contracture, metabolic acidosis, supraventricular tachyarrhythmias, and hypertension
- Two signs helpful in making a prehyperthermic diagnosis: increased end-tidal CO_2 and masseter spasm
- Patients with other muscle syndromes or dystonias have an increased frequency of contracture and hyperthermia in the anesthesia setting.

Malignant Hyperthermia Protocol

- Discontinue volatile anesthetic and succinylcholine
- Hyperventilate with 100% O_2 at high flows
- Administer sodium bicarbonate, 1–2 mEq/kg intravenously
- Mix dantrolene sodium with sterile distilled water and administer 2.5 mg/kg iv
- Institute cooling measures (lavage, cooling blanket, cold intravenous solutions)
- Administer inotropes and antiarrhythmic agents as necessary
- Administer additional doses of dantrolene if needed
- Change anesthetic tubing and soda lime
- Monitor urinary output, K^+ Ca^{2+}, blood gases, end-tidal carbon dioxide; perform clotting studies
- Treat severe hyperkalemia with dextrose, 25–50 intravenously, and regular insulin, 10–20 U intravenously (adult dose)
- Consider invasive monitoring of arterial blood pressure and central venous pressure.

Neuroleptic Malignant Syndrome

- Rare complication of antipsychotic therapy, Meperidine and metoclopramide Rx
- Mechanism: dopamine blockade in the basal ganglia and hypothalamus and impairment of thermoregulation

- In its most severe form, the presentation is similar to that of malignant hyperthermia
- Muscle rigidity, hyperthermia, rhabdomyolysis, autonomic instability, and altered consciousness
- Motor and behavioral symptoms: muscular rigidity and dystonia, akineisa, mutism, obtundation, and agitation
- Autonomic symptoms include high fever, sweating, and increased pulse and blood pressure.

Diagnostic criteria

- ➢ Developmental of severe muscle rigidity and elevated temperature associated with use of neuroleptic medication
- ➢ Two or more of the following
- Diaphoresis (sweating)
- Dysphagia
- Tremors
- Tachycardia
- Incontinence
- Mutism
- Change of level of consciousness from confusion to coma
- Elevated or labile BP
- Leucocytosis
- Laboratory evidence of muscle injury (e.g. elevated CPK), renal function test.

Treatment

- Stop neuroleptic drugs
- Dantrolene (drug of choice)
- Bromocriptine/Amantadine.

REGIONAL ANESTHESIA

Spinal Anesthesia

- The local anesthesia is injected in the subarachnoid space between L_3– L_4 in adults and L_4–L_5 in children
- Spinal cord ends at the level of L_1 in adults and L_3 in children

Structures encountered during lumbar punctures

- Skin
- Subcutaneous tissue
- Supraspinous ligament
- Interspinous ligament
- Ligamentum flavum
- Dura Matter and
- Arachnoid matter
- Piamater

Drugs Used for Spinal Anesthesia

- 5% lignocaine in 7.5% dextrose–no longer used nowadays due to neurological complications especially transient neurological syndrome.
- 0.5% Bupivacaine in 8% dextrose
- Cross reactivity occurs among local anesthetics belonging to the same group but not between esters and amines.

Indications of Spinal Anesthesia

All surgeries involving lower abdomen and lower limbs

Complications

The MC intraoperative complication is hypotension

Other complications during intraoperative period

- Bradycardia
- Respiratory depression and
- Cardiac arrest
- Anaphylactic reaction
- Postdural puncture headache

Postdural puncture headache

It occurs 12–24 hours later, mainly occipital which is made worse by sitting on erectposture.

Relationships Among Variables and Postspinal Puncture Headache

Factors that may increase the incidence of postspinal puncture headache	
Age	Younger more frequent
Gender	Females > males
Needle size	Larger > smaller
Needle bevel	Less when the needle bevel is placed in the long axis of the neuraxis
Pregnancy	More when pregnant
Dural punctures (no.)	More with multiple punctures
Factors not increasing the incidence of post–spinal puncture headache	
Continuous spinals	
Timing of ambulation	

- MC cause is leakage of CSF to the hole in duramater
- The Headache can be prevented by using small bore needles
- Treatment of the headache consists of
  - Lying down for 24 hours, bedrest
  - Abdominal compression
  - Oral or intravenous Fluids
  - Caffeine
  - Epidural patch (last resort but > 90% effective)
- Other complications include–Urinary, retention, cranial nerve paralysis (specially abducens nerve), meningitis, Paraplegia and cauda equina syndrome.

Absolute Contraindications of Spinal Anesthesia

- Raised intracranial pressure
- Patient refusal
- Shock
- Bleeding disorders
- pt's on anticoagulants
- Infection of the local site and
- Septicemias

Relative CI

- Aortic and mitral stenosis, MI, Heart block, spinal deformities, psychiatric and CNS disorders.

Epidural Anesthesia

- It is given in the epidural space between the ligamentum flavum an the duramater with Tuohy needle (MC used).

Indications for Epidural Anesthesia

- Epidural anesthesia is mainly used for controlling post–operative pain
- Painless labor
- Can be used for all surgeries done by spinal anesthesia
- Epidural anesthesia can be used for upper abdominal, thoracic and neck surgeries
- They can also be used for chronic cancer pain
- Spinal anesthesia is easier, reliable and has quick onset, whereas epidural anesthesia is difficult to perform less reliable and slower
- Redosing cannot be done with spinal anesthesia. So performed for surgeries of limited duration.

Caudal anesthesia

Done primarily for analgesia in children. Caudal anesthesia requires identification of the sacral hiatus. The sacrococcygeal ligament (i.e. extension of ligamentum flavum) overlying the sacral hiatus lies between the sacral cornua. To facilitate locating the cornua, the posterior superior iliac spines should be located and, by using the line between them as one side of an equilateral triangle, the location of the sacral hiatus should be approximated.

MONITORING

EEG: On EEG if prefrontal area shows beta Waves and Desynchronization of waves, it is called light anesthesia

- Presence of delta–waves indicates deep anesthesia
- Evoked potentials are one of the best guides of depth of anesthesia

Bispectral index is commercially available monitor to see the depth of anesthesia, it uses many parameters like EEG, eye blink etc to calculate a score, A score of 40–60 is considered adequate score for anesthesia (100 fully awake and 0 completely silent brain).

Transesophageal Echocardiography

- It is the most sensitive for wall motion abnormalities and is also used to detect ischemia and air embolism during intraoperative period
- For detecting arrhythmias in ECG lead II is preferred
- For detecting ischemia in ECG lead V_5 is preferred
- Inf. Wall MI shows abnormality in lead II, III and avf.

EtCO$_2$ (capnography)

The most commonly used type of capnograph plots PCO_2 versus time. The tracing is traditionally divided into an inspiratory phase and three expiratory phases. Continuous measurement of end tidal CO_2. Normal expired CO_2 is 35–45 mm Hg. Capnography uses infrared light which is absorbed by CO_2 it has 3 phases and 2 angles (alpha and beta angle)

Phase 0: Inspiratory phase

Phase I: Dead space and little or no CO_2

Phase II: Mixture of alveolar and dead space gas

Phase III: Alveolar plateau, with the peak representing end-expiratory (end-tidal) CO_2 ($PetCO_2$).

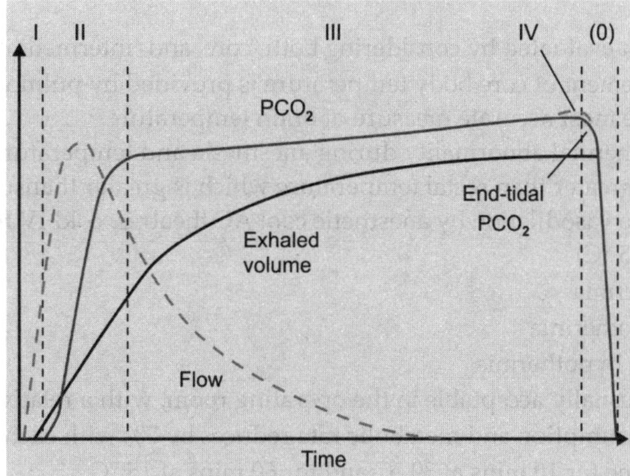

Fig. 16.5: Capnograph

Uses:

- Surest confirmatory sign of correct intubation
- Diagnosis of malignant hyperthermia
- Detecting obstruction of Endotracheal tube
- Indicates cardiac output
- Diagnoses pulmonary embolism

Neuromuscular Monitoring

- M/C muscle used in neuromuscular monitoring is Adductor pollicis supplied by Ulnar nerve.
- Most accurate measurement for NM monitoring is orbicularis oculi supplied by facial nerve.
- Neuromuscular monitoring is done clinically by train of 4 (in this 4 stimuli are given each of 2 Hz with a gap of 0.5 sec between each stimuli and repeated every 10–12 sec, recording are taken. Absence of Train 4 response means 75% receptors and blocked and is sufficient for most surgeries.
- Train of 4 is best utilized during maintenance phase of anesthesia.

  Ex.: Succinylcholine (Depolarizing Blocker)

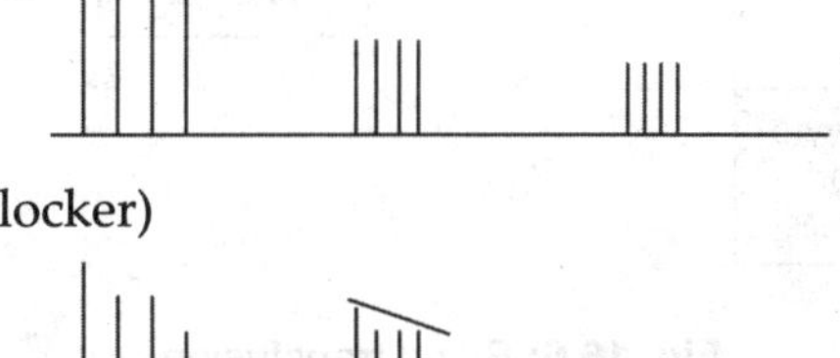

  Tubocurarine (nondepolarizing blocker)

- Train of 4 differentiates depolarizing and nondepolarizing blockers. Fading is property of nondepolarizing blockers
- It a pt on succinyl choline shows fading, It is pathognomic of phase 2 block.

Temperature Monitoring

The core thermal compartment is composed of highly perfused tissues whose temperature is uniform and high in comparison to the rest of the body. Temperature in this compartment can be evaluated in the pulmonary artery, distal part of the esophagus, tympanic membrane, or nasopharynx.

Even during cardiopulmonary bypass, the core temperature–monitoring sites (e.g. tympanic membrane, nasopharynx, pulmonary artery, and esophagus) remain useful. In contrast, rectal temperatures lag behind those measured in core sites. Consequently, rectal temperature is considered an 'intermediate' temperature in deliberately cooled patients.

Adequacy of rewarming is best evaluated by considering both 'core' and 'intermediate' temperatures.

- The most accurate measurement of core body temperature is provided by pulmonary artery.
- Tympanic membrane is the most accurate measure of brain temperature
- Hypothermia is common thermal abnormality during anesthesia and temperature monitoring is mandatory.
- Core body temperature is greater than rectal temperature which is greater thansurface temperature.
- Hypothermia occurs due to vasodilation by anesthetic cool AC theatres, cold IV fluids and by evaporation. (Hypothermia is temp. < 35 °C)

  < 28–35 °C is mild hypothermia

  21–27 °C is moderate hypothermia

  < 20 °C is severe/profound hypothermia

Temperatures of 22–24 °C are usually acceptable in the operating room, with a relative humidity of 50–60%;

Induced Hypothermia: O_2 consumption and metabolic rate reduces by 7% with each degree fall in temperature

- Brain protection can be done for 10 mins at 30 °C and for 60 mins at 15 °C
- Induced hypothermia is specially useful during carotid surgeries and protect against tissue ischemia during cardiac surgeries.

CRITICAL CARE

Blood Transfusion

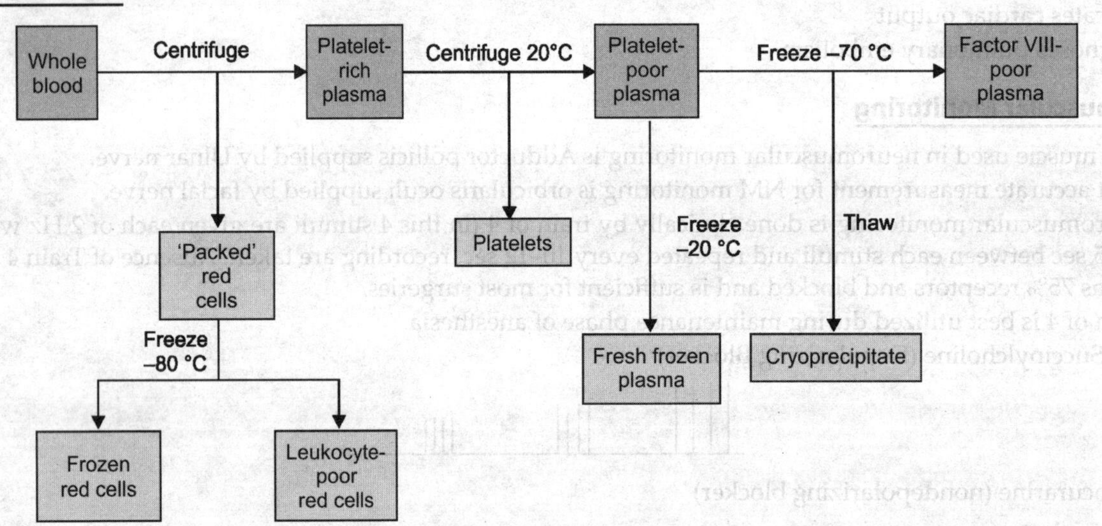

Fig. 16.6: Blood transfusion

- **Whole Blood**: One Unit = 500 ml anticoagulated blood (40% Hematocrit) contains normal concentration of albumin and clotting factors But low levels of factors V and VIII
- **Packed Red Cells**: One unit = 250 ml (60% Hematocrit) contains no platelets One unit of packed cells increases Hb by 1 gm% and Hematocrit by 3%
- **Fresh Frozen Plasma:** It contains all the plasma proteins, particularly factors V and VIII, which gradually decline during the storage of blood. The use of FFP carries with it certain inherent risks that are observed with the use of essentially any blood product. The major risk is transmission of infectious diseases, such as hepatitis B, hepatitis C, and AIDS.
- **Cryoprecipitate** is obtained from FFP contain large quantities of factor VIII, VWF, fibrinogen, fibronectin
- **Platelet Concentrate** = Contains 50–80% platelets in a unit of fresh whole blood one platelet concentrate usually produces an increase of about 7000 to 10,000 platelets/mm^3.

Massive Blood Transfusion

Transfusion of blood more than pt's blood volume (5 lts) in 24 hours.

(or)

Transfusion of > 10% blood volume in < 10 minutes

Complications: Hypocalcemia, Hypothermia, Hyperkalemia, Hyperammonemia, Metabolic alkalosis, ARDS, DIC (MC cause of death).

Monitored Anesthesia

- Initial sedation and anxiolysis with a Benzodiazepine (Midazolam) followed by Propofol then local anesthesia
- For minor procedures, day care procedures which needs sedation e.g. Upper GI Endoscopy.

Brain Death

- It is defined as irreversible cessation of all brain function spinal cord function below C_1 may still be present
- Brain death can be applied only in absence of hypothermia, hypotension, drugdepressing brain function, neuromuscular blocking agent, endocrinal and metabolic abnormalities
- Coma, absence of brain stem, Absence of Motor activity, Absence of ventilatory effort.

Diagnostic Criteria for the Clinical Diagnosis of Brain Death

Prerequisites. Brain death is the absence of clinical brain function when the proximate cause is known and demonstrably irreversible.

- Clinical or neuroimaging evidence of an acute central nervous system catastrophe that is compatible with the clinical diagnosis of brain death
- Exclusion of complicating medical conditions that may confound clinical assessment (no severe electrolyte, acid-base, or endocrine disturbance)
- No drug intoxication or poisoning
- Core temperature ≥ 32 °C (90 °F)

The three cardinal findings in brain death are coma or unresponsiveness, absence of brainstem reflexes, and apnea.

- Coma or unresponsiveness—no cerebral motor response to pain in all extremities (nail-bed pressure and supraorbital pressure)
- Absence of brainstem reflexes
  - Pupils
    - No response to bright light
    - Size: midposition (4 mm) to dilated (9 mm)
  - Ocular movement
    - No oculocephalic reflex (testing only when no fracture or instability of the cervical spine is apparent)
    - No deviation of eyes to irrigation in each ear with 50 mL of cold water (allow 1 minute after injection and at least 5 minutes between testing on each side)
  - Facial sensation and facial motor response
    - No corneal reflex to touch with a throat swab
    - No jaw reflex
    - No grimacing to deep pressure on nail bed, supraorbital ridge, or temporomandibular joint
  - Pharyngeal and tracheal reflexes
    - No response after stimulation of the posterior pharynx with tongue blade
    - No cough response to bronchial suctioning

Helium–O_2 therapy

Heliox (a 70 : 30 helium-oxygen mixture) is about one third as dense as room air and decreases the work of breathing of some asthmatics. Heliox cannot be used if high oxygen concentrations are required.Heliox (70% helium, 30%

oxygen) greatly increases flow for any given pressure gradient, or allows the same flow for a smaller pressure gradient. In contrast with laminar flow, in which resistance depends on gas viscosity during turbulent flow, resistance depends on gas density. Heliox leads to a dramatic decrease in airway resistance and improvement in ventilation. The higher the concentration of helium in the mixture, however, the lower the FiO_2. Used for bronchial asthma, COPD.

THE 2010 AHA GUIDELINES FOR CPR

Recommend a change in the BLS sequence of steps from A-B-C (Airway, Breathing, Chest compressions) to C-A-B (Chest compressions, Airway, Breathing) for adults, children, and infants (**excluding the newly born).**

Adult BLS Algorithm

New Recommendations

Key changes from the 2005 ACLS Guidelines include

- Continuous quantitative waveform capnography is recommended for confirmation and monitoring of endotracheal tube placement.
- Cardiac arrest algorithms are simplified and redesigned to emphasize the importance of high-quality CPR (including chest compressions of adequate rate and depth, allowing complete chest recoil after each compression, minimizing interruptions in chest compressions and avoiding excessive ventilation).
- Atropine is no longer recommended for routine use in the management of pulseless electrical activity (PEA)/ asystole.
- There is an increased emphasis on physiologic monitoring to optimize CPR quality and detect ROSC.
- Chronotropic drug infusions are recommended as an alternative to pacing in symptomatic and unstable bradycardia.
- Adenosine is recommended as a safe and potentially effective therapy in the initial management of stable undifferentiated regular monomorphic wide-complex tachycardia.

Treatable Causes of Cardiac Arrest: The H's and T's

H's	T's
Hypoxia	Toxins
Hypovolemia	Tamponade (cardiac)
Hydrogen ion (acidosis)	Tension pneumothorax
Hypo/hyperkalemia	Thrombosis, pulmonary
Hypothermia	Thrombosis, coronary

External Chest Compression

- CPR of short duration force blood to flow by directly compressing the heart (cardiac pump)
- As CPR continues, the heart becomes less compliant and the increase in intrathoracic pressure (thoracic pump) mechanism becomes more important
- Breaths are delivered slowly (inspiratory time of ½-1s) with a smaller tidal volume [VT] (6–8 ml/kg) than was recommended in the past
- If these breaths cannot be delivered, either the airway is still obstructed and the head and neck need repositioning or a foreign body is present that must be removed.

	Newborn	Infants and children		Adult
Compression	90/min	100/min	100/min	≥100/min
Compression ventilation ratio	3:1	Single rescuer: 30:2	Two rescuer: 15:2	30:2

- Most common cause of inadequate mouth-to-mouth ventilation is insufficient airway control
- Attempts at intubation should not interrupt ventilation for more than 30s
- Cricoids pressure (Sellick maneuver) decreases the possibility of regurgitation and aspiration during intubation

Newborn resuscitation

HR < 100/min –positive pressure ventilation

HR < 60/min–chest compression and consider intubation.

Maternal cardiac arrest

- Perform manual left uterine displacement and do CPR
- If no return of spontaneous circulation within 4 min, do perimortem cesarian section.

Circulation

Cardiac Massage

- Cardiac massage in adults
  - Compressions–over lower third of sternum (2 fingers above xiphoid process)
- Cardiac massage in children–Two thumbs technique for compressions
- Cardiac Massage in newborns–Two thumbs with encircled chest technique for compressions
- Cardiac Massage in pregnant–External cardiac Massage with lateral tilt.

Airway Management

Ambubag: It is an artificial manual breathing unit with a capacity of 2 liters

Facemask: Dead space and chances of aspiration are increased by mask ventilation

O_2 delivery system: 2 Systems

- High flow system consists of venture mask and special nebulizer. High flow system allow accurate delivery of inspired O_2
- Low flow system include nasal cannula and O_2 mask

Reservoir Bags:

For Neonates–250 ml

For infants and children–500 ml

Adults–2000 ml

Airways

- **Guedel's airway:** MC used airway. Length of airway is distance between tip of nose to tragus + 1 inch
- **Laryngeal Mask Airway:** It is easy to insert than intubation. Can be used in cervical instability and it is reusable, it is used for emergency airway, difficult intubations
- Advantage–Does not require any laryngo scope, Visualization and muscle relaxants.
- Disadvantage–It does not prevent aspiration. Can cause laryngospasm and bronchospasm.
- **Combitube** is a double lumen tube used for emergency airway management
- **Laryngoscope:** The most commonly used laryngoscope is macintosh which has curved blades and position of head and neck during laryngoscopy is 'Extension at atlanto occipital Joint 75–85 degrees and flexion at cervical spine 15–25 degrees–magill position'
- Complication–MC injury during laryngoscopy is damage to upper incisors, damage to soft tissue and damage to cervical spinal cord
- **Endotracheal tubes:**
  - In small children < 6 years uncuffed tube should be used but with the advent of newer cuffs, cuffed tubes can be used even for children.
  - Reflex response to intubation–tachycardia, hypertension, Laryngospasm, ↑ Intracranial tension, ↑ Cortisol and catecholamines
  - Methods to inhibit reflex response–xylocaine spray, xylocard injection, Opioids, Ca–Channel blockers
  - The surest sign of intubation is Capnography (etc. O_2)
  - RAE tube–used for oral and dental surgeries like cleft lip and cleft palate

Airway Maintenance

- Endotracheal tube is most definitive method
- In other cases of airway obstruction (laryngeal edema, epiglottitis, laryngotracheobronchitis), tracheostomy is used

Breathing/Ventilation

- Mouth to Mouth
- Mouth to airway–Safar or Brook airway
- Bag and mask–Increases aspiration, increases dead space
- Advanced methods–Endotracheal tube (Best method)
  - Laryngeal mask airway
  - Combitube

Monitoring of CPR

- Capnography–Most reliable, best Indicator
- Palpation of Carotid pulse–Most effective clinical indicator
- Invasive blood pressure
- Central venous oxygen saturation

Complications of CPR

- Rib fracture, pneumothorax, pneumomediastinum, pneumopericardium, Injury to diaphragm, Injury to Stomach, Injury to lungs, Injury to major vessels, Injury to abdominal organs.

Drugs Used in CPR

- Vasopressors–Adrenaline, vasopressin
- Antiarrhythmics

Drugs not routinely used in CPR

- Calcium–The only indication is Hypocalcemia, Hyperkalemia
- Sodium bicarbonate–only indication is metabolic acidosis, Hyperkalemia

Defibrillation

- **DC cardioversion: Rx of choice for ventricular tachycardia and ventricular fibrillation**
- **Ventricular fibrillation**–most common in adults who experience nontraumatic cardiac arrest
- The time from collapse to defibrillation is the most important determinant of survival
- Chances for survival decline 7–10% for every minute without defibrillation
- Shock should be delivered within 3 min (± 1 min) of arrest
- Defibrillators deliver energy in either monophasic or biphasxic waveforms
- Increasingly, biphasic waveforms are recommended for cardioversion
- Biphasic shocks delivering low energy for defibrillation (150–200 joules [J]) have been found to be as effective as 200–360 J monophasic damped sine (MDS) waveform shocks.

Indications	Shocks (J)
Unstable atrial fibrillation	50–100
Unstable atrial flutter/tachycardia	30–50
Monomorphic ventricular tachycardia	100
Polymorphic ventricular tachycardia or ventricular fibrillation	120–200

Anatomy of Upper Airway

Dead Space

- Total physiological dead space = Anatomical dead space (150 ml)
  +
  Alveolar dead space (60–80 ml)
  = 210–230 ml
- Anatomical dead space is constituted by Air in nose, trachea and bronchial tree

Normal value is 150 ml (30% of tidal volume)

Anatomical dead space is increased by	Anatomical dead space is decreased by	Alveolar dead space is increased by
Old age Neck extension Jaw protrusion Bronchodilators (atropine), halothane Increased lung volume Anesthesia mask and circuits IPPV (Intermittent positive pressure ventilation) PEEP (Positive end expiratory pressure)	Intubation Tracheostomy Hyperventilation Neck flexion Bronchoconstrictors Massive pleural effusion	IPPV PEEP General anesthesia Hypotension Lung pathologies affecting diffusion like interstitial lung disease, pulmonary embolism, pulmonary edema, ARDS

QUESTIONS

1. Bradycardia is most common in: (2014)
a. Midazolam
b. Succinylcholine
c. Isoprenaline
d. Dopamine

2. The most potent anti-emetic agent in pre-operative period is: (2014)
a. Ondansetron
b. Metoclopramide
c. Perchlorperazine
d. Chlorpromazine

3. Delivery of high concentration of oxygen (more than 90%) is delivered via: (2014)
a. Partial rebreathing mask
b. Nasal cannula with oxygen flow at 5L/min
c. Simple face mask
d. Non rebreathing face mask with oxygen reservoir

4. A patient on epidural anesthesia with 15 ml of 1.5% lignocaine with adrenaline for hernia surgery develops hypotension and respiratory depression in three min. Most common cause for this clinical condition is: (2014)
a. Systemic toxicity of anesthetic agents
b. Drug allergy
c. Vaso vagal shock
d. Drug entering into sub arachnoid space

5. A 20 year old male patient met with motor vehicle accident and sustained head injuries. BP-90/60 mmHg, Pulse rate-150/min. All the following anesthtic agents are avoided for induction except:
a. Thiopentone **(2014)**
b. Halothane
c. Succinylcholine
d. Ketamine

6. A child with intestinal obstruction and deranged LFT. Anesthetic agent of choice is: (2014)
a. Halothane
b. Enflurance
c. Isoflurane
d. Sevoflurane

7. A 25 years old primi with mitral stenosis and mitral regugitation wants a normal delivery. The appropriate analgesia is: (2014)
a. Inhalational analgesia
b. Spinal anesthesia
c. Neuro axial block analgesia
d. IV opioids

8. True regarding hypothermia during anaesthesia:
a. Body may lose heat by conduction **(2014)**
b. Beneficial to patients in some conditions
c. Always occur irrespective of the type of anaesthesia
d. Prevented by giving warm fluids

9. **Best spontaneous breathing circuit is: (2014)**
   a. Mapleson A
   b. Mapleson D
   c. Mapleson E
   d. Mapleson F
10. **Most metabolized inhaled anesthetic is: (2014)**
   a. Desflurane
   b. Halothane
   c. Isoflurane
   d. Sevoflurane
11. **Which IV anesthetic causes increased cerebral blood flow and cerebral metabolic rate? (2014)**
   a. Thiopentone
   b. Etomidate
   c. Ketamine
   d. Propofol
12. **Drug contraindicated in epilepsy patients posted for general anesthesia is: (2014)**
   a. Midazolam
   b. Ketamine
   c. Thipentone
   d. Propofol
13. **Most potent local anesthetic is: (2014)**
   a. Lignocaine
   b. Procaine
   c. Bupivacaine
   d. Prilocaine
14. **During laproscopic cholecystectomy, patient develops wheezing. What is the next best line of management? (2014)**
   a. IV ketamine
   b. IV lignocaine
   c. Bronchodialators beta 2 agonist and oxygenation
   d. Deepen plane of anesthesia
15. **Not a contraindication for combined spinal and epidural anesthesia: (2014)**
   a. Platelet count < 50,000
   b. Patient on clopidogrel
   c. Local infection
   d. Patient on antihypertensive medication
16. **Regarding celiac plexus block true is: (2014)**
   a. Bilaterally done
   b. Diarrhea and hypotension are common side effects
   c. Done in painful conditions of lower abdomen
   d. Done around L3
17. **Postlumbar puncture headache is minimized by all except: (2014)**
   a. Keep stylet and remove needle
   b. Atraumatic needle
   c. Small diameter needle
   d. Hydration by crystalloid infusion
18. **Hyperkalemia is caused by: (2014)**
   a. N_20
   b. Atracurium
   c. Succinyl choline
   d. Pancuronium
19. **Muscle most resistant to the action of non depolarizing muscle relaxants is: (2014)**
   a. Diaphragm
   b. Head and neck muscles
   c. Upper limbs
   d. Abdomen
20. **Lithium should be stopped how many days before surgery: (2014)**
   a. 1
   b. 2
   c. 3
   d. 4
21. **True regarding hypothermia during anesthesia is: (2014)**
   a. Occurs in all types of anaesthesia
   b. Treated with warm saline
   c. Is beneficial to patients
   d. Mechanism of heat loss is conduction
22. **Which of the following can deliver 90% oxygen? (2014)**
   a. Venture mask
   b. Rebreathing O_2 mask
   c. Nasal prongs
   d. Non-rebreathing mask with O_2 reservoir bag
23. **Anesthetic producing least amount of carbon monoxide is: (2013)**
   a. Isoflurane
   b. Desflurane
   c. Sevoflurane
   d. Enflurane
24. **Most cardiotoxic local anesthetic is: (2013)**
   a. Bupivacaine
   b. Lignocaine
   c. Lidocaine
   d. Ropivacaine
25. **Anesthetic not impairing CNS activity is: (2013)**
   a. Isoflurane
   b. Enflurane
   c. Ketamine
   d. Desflurane

26. What is Mendelson syndrome due to? (2013)
a. Gastric Dilatation
b. Wrong intubation
c. Tracheal inflammation secondary to intubation
d. Chemical pneumonitis following aspiration

27. In spinal anaesthesia, during is deposited between: (2013)
a. Between pia and arachnoid
b. Between dura and arachnoid
c. Between pia and dura
d. Outside dura

28. Intravenous anesthetic Induction agent used in Day care surgery is: (2013)
a. Propofol
b. Ketamine
c. Etomidate
d. Thiopentone

29. Dose Ratio of adrenaline to be used with lidocaine is: (2013)
a. 1: 200
b. 1: 2000
c. 1: 20000
d. 1: 200000

30. Anesthetic which increases intracranial tension:
a. Ketamine (2013)
b. Propofol
c. Etomidate
d. Ether

31. Intravenous anesthetic causing suppression of steroid synthesis: (2013)
a. Etomidate
b. Thiopentone
c. Ketamine
d. Propofol

32. Anesthetic which is least metabolized in the body is: (2013)
a. Xenon
b. Ether
c. Halothane
d. Methoxyflurane

33. Fentanyl at the dose of 5–15 micrograms causes:
a. Ciliary musc contraction (2013)
b. Iris dilator paralysis
c. Muscle stiffiness
d. Reduces sweating

34. Intravenous anesthetic drug that doesn't induce cerebral metabolism: (2013)
a. Thiopentone
b. Ketamine
c. Propofol
d. Methohexitone

35. Stage 2 block (Phase II block) is seen with:(2013)
a. Suxamethonium
b. Isoflurane
c. Sevoflurane
d. Enflurane

36. Malignant hyperthermia is caused by: (2013)
a. Succinyl Choline
b. N_20
c. Atropine
d. Dantolene

37. Mechanism of action of Local anesthetics: (2013)
a. Inhibition of Na^+ channels
b. Inhibition of Na^+ K^+ ATPase
c. Inhibition of K^+ channels
d. Inhibition of Ca^{2+} channels

38. Which of the following Drug has least t1/2?
a. Thiopentone (2012)
b. Propofol
c. Midazolam
d. Ketamine

39. In day care anesthesia 'named' scale (Post anesthetic discharge score) PADDS. Which of the following criteria is not assessed? (2012)
a. Drinking
b. Nausea and vomiting
c. Pain
d. Vitals

40. Which of the following is an ultrashort acting anesthetic? (2012)
a. Propofol
b. Thiopentone
c. Succinyl choline
d. Midazolam

41. Which of the following disease show resistance to succinyl choline? (2012)
a. Myasthenia gravis
b. Polymyositis
c. Eaton lambert myasthenia syndrome
d. Muscular dystrophy

42. Minimum alveolar concentration of an inhaled anesthetic is a marker of: (2012)
a. Potency
b. Efficacy
c. Elimination
d. Distribution

43. In anesthesia, fitting of wrong gas cylinder to the anesthesia machine can be prevented by: (2012)
a. Pin index system
b. Yolk assembly
c. Bodock seal
d. Gas analyser

44. Which of the following is a short acting muscle relaxant? (2012)
a. Suxamethonium
b. Pancuronium
c. Vecuronium
d. Atracurium

45. A patient in ICU is weaned from ventilator. The mode least used for this purpose is: (2012)
a. ASV
b. CPAP
c. SIMV
d. CMV

46. Fixed performance device: (2011)
a. Venturi mask
b. Nasal cannula
c. Simple mask
d. Non rebreathing mask

47. Which gas accumulates in cavities post general anaesthesia? (2011)
a. Nitrous oxide
b. Halothane
c. Ether
d. Sevoflurane

48. Long acting local anaestheic agent: (2011)
a. Procaine
b. Lidocaine
c. Bupivacaine
d. Etidocaine

49. Malignant hyperthermia is common with: (2011)
a. Local anesthetics
b. Succinyl choline
c. Propofol
d. Barbiturates

50. Hypotension is caused by all except: (2011)
a. Halothane
b. Propofol
c. Ketamine
d. Thiopentone

51. Plasma potassium concentration is increased with: (2010)
a. Succinyl choline
b. Atracurium
c. Pancuronium
d. Propofol

52. Drug used to prevent nausea and vomiting:
a. Propofol **(2010)**
b. Fentanyl
c. Nitrous oxide
d. Sevoflurane

53. Drug producing haematological side effect is:
a. Nitrous oxide **(2010)**
b. Halothane
c. Ketamine
d. Sevoflurane

54. Best treatment for relieving pain during intra-partum period is: (2010)
a. Neuraxial block
b. Epidural anesthesia
c. IV ketamine
d. General Anesthesia

55. Drugs used in advanced life support include all except: (2010)
a. Calcium
b. Amiodarone
c. Vasopressin
d. Adrenaline

56. Which of the following mechanism prevents fitting of wrong gas cylinder to the anesthesia machine in operation theatre? (2009)
a. Pin index system
b. Yolk assembly
c. Bodock seal
d. Gas analyser

57. Centrineuraxial anesthesia is not contra-indicated in: (2009)
a. Platelets < 80,000
b. Patients on aspirin
c. Patient on anticoagulants
d. Raised intracranial pressure

58. All are true about ether except: (2009)
a. It has additional sympathomimetic effect
b. Can undergo spontaneous decomposition when exposed to light
c. It has additional bronchodilator and analgesic effects
d. It inhibits salivation

59. Dead space is increased by all except: (2009)
a. Anticholinergic drugs
b. Standing
c. Hyperextention of neck
d. Endotracheal intubation

60. Anesthetic which increases intracranial tension: **(2009)**
a. Ketamine
b. Propofol
c. Etomidate
d. Ether

61. Which is non invasive positive pressure ventilation? **(2008)**
a. CPAP
b. SIMV
c. CMV
d. IMV

62. Anesthetic drug of choice in asthmatic: **(2008)**
a. Ketamine
b. Propofol
c. Etomidate
d. Propofol

63. Neuromuscular blocker of choice in real failure: **(2008)**
a. Atracurium
b. Pancuronium
c. Rocuronium
d. Tubocurare

64. Hoffman's elimination is seen with: **(2008)**
a. Atracurium
b. Pancuronium
c. Suxamethonium
d. Rocuronium

65. Anesthetic agent which can cause massive hepatic necrosis? **(2008)**
a. Halothane
b. Isoflurane
c. Methoxyflurane
d. N_2O

66. Ventilator breath dyssynchrony is maximum with which mode of ventilation? **(2008)**
a. CMV
b. CPAP
c. SIMV
d. PSV

67. Anesthetic not impairing CNS activity is: **(2008)**
a. Isoflurane
b. Enflurane
c. Ketamine
d. Desflurane

68. The following anesthetic drug causes pain on intravenous administration: **(2007)**
a. Midazolam
b. Propofol
c. Ketamine
d. Thiopentone sodium

69. Malignant hyperthermia is caused by: **(2007)**
a. Succinyl choline
b. N_2O
c. Atropine
d. Dantolene

70. Fixed performance device: **(2007)**
a. Venture mask
b. Nasal cannula
c. Simple mask
d. Non rebreathing mask

71. Which of the following agents can be safely used in asthma? **(2006)**
a. Thiopentone
b. Ketamine
c. Etomidate
d. Propofol

72. Which anesthetic agent does not affect blood flow to liver? **(2006)**
a. Halothane
b. Isoflurane
c. Enflurane
d. Sevoflurane

73. Postoperative shivering is treated with: **(2006)**
a. Diazepanm
b. Antihistaminics
c. Anticholinergics
d. Pethidine

HIGH YIELD POINTS

1. Choice for For Day Care Surgery
   Inhalational–Desflurane > sevoflurane
   IV–Propofol
   Opioid– Remifentanil infusions
   Muscle Relaxant–gantacurium
2. Epileptogenic
   Inhalational–Enflurane

3. Cardio Stable
   Inhalational–Isoflurane
   IV–opioids (drug of choice), etomidate
   Muscle relaxant–Vecuronium
4. Shock
   Inhalational–Desflurane > 6%
   IV–Ketamine
5. Asthma
   Inhalational–Halothane
   IV–Ketamine
6. Hepatic and renal disease
   Inhalational–isoflurane
   IV–Remifentanyl
   Muscle relaxant–Atracurium

Anesthetics Causing

Increase ICT	Sevoflurane, Desflurane, Isoflurane, Enflurane, Methoxyflurane, Halothane, Ketamine, Nitrous Oxide (N_2O), Althesin, succinyl choline
Decreased ICT	Barbiturates (e.g: Thiopentone), Cyclopropane, Droperidol, Etomidate, Li docaine, Propofol
Increased IOT	Succinyl choline, Ketamine, N_2O
Increased BP	Ketamine, Pentazocine, Pancuronium
Bronchodilatation	(preferred in asthmatics) Ketamine (most potint), Halothane
Bronchospasm	(contraindicated in asthmatics): Ether, N_2O, thiopentone

Salient points regarding LA's

- All Local anesthetics are vasodilators except cocaine
- All Local anesthetics decrease BP except cocaine
- Cocaine should never be given with IV route or with adrenaline
- Chloroprocaine is the shortest acting local anesthetic
- Dibucaine is the most potent longest acting and most toxic local anesthetic
- Chloroprocaine is neurotoxic should not be used for spinal anesthesia.
- Procaine is the local anesthetic of choice for malignant hyperthermia
- Lignocaine is the MC used local anesthetic
- All Local anesthetics are class IB anti-arrhythmic drugs
- Lignocaine is known to produce malignant hyperthermia.
- Reversal of local anesthetic action is first with motor fibers
- The MC toxicity of local anesthetic action is CNS toxicity in the form of numbness, tremors (or) convulsions

Muscle Relaxants

- **Maximum histamine release, Contraindicated in Asthma: d-TC**
- **Minimum histamine release, used in Asthma: Vecuronium**
- Metabolized by pseudo cholinesterase: Succinyl choline
- Muscle relaxant which increases BP and heart rate–Pancuronium
- Muscle relaxant with ganglion block: d-tc (highest), Galamine, Trimethaphan.
- Muscle relaxant with highest histamine release–d-tc > mivacurium, atracurium highest vagolytic effect-pancuronium
- Gallamine is least potent whereas most potent and longest acting skeletal muscle relaxant doxacurium
- Fastest acting nondepolarising skeletal muscle relaxant is Rocuronium

- Shortest acting non depolarizing agent is gantacurium >mivacurium.
- Shortest acting (both onset and duration)muscle relaxant–succinylcholine
- Muscle relaxant of choice for full stomach patients, rapid sequence induction–succinylcholine

ANSWERS AND EXPLANATIONS

1. **Ans. b. Succinylcholine** *Ref: Miller's anesthesia 7/e ch29*
   The autonomic mechanism involved in sinus bradycardia is stimulation of cardiac muscarinic receptors in the sinus node. This is particularly problematic in individuals with predominantly vagal tone, such as children who have not received atropine. Sinus bradycardia has also been noted in adults and appears more commonly after a second dose of the drug is given approximately 5 minutes after the first. The bradycardia may be prevented by the administration of thiopental, atropine, ganglion-blocking drugs, and nondepolarizing neuromuscular blockers. The implication of this information is that direct myocardial effects, increased muscarinic stimulation, and ganglionic stimulation may all be involved in the bradycardia response. The higher incidence of bradycardia after a second dose of succinylcholine suggests that the hydrolysis products of succinylcholine (succinylmonocholine and choline) may sensitize the heart to a subsequent dose.
2. **Ans. a. Ondansetron** *Ref: Miller's anesthesia 7/e ch86*
   Ondansetron was the first serotonin antagonist, and its introduction was a milestone in the prevention of early chemotherapy-induced nausea and vomiting. It was considerably more effective and had fewer side effects (no extrapyramidal symptoms or sedation) compared with all previous antiemetics. Given its superior efficacy for chemotherapy-induced nausea and vomiting, it is not surprising that ondansetron quickly established a reputation as the most effective antiemetic for prevention of PONV.
3. **Ans. d. Non rebreathing face mask with oxygen reservoir** *Ref: Morgan's clinical anesthesia 5/e p1282*
   Both the options A and D are correct since both rebreathing mask and non breathing mask can deliver 90 % oxygen. The delivery of FiO_2 in these masks are dependent on high flows (10 L/min). if the question was asked with flow rate, then the answer would have been easy. This is a poorly framed question. Now to choose between the options, the addition of reservoir bag increases the FiO_2, IN OPTION A, there is no addition of reservoir bag hence the FiO_2 would not reach 90%. Hence non breathing mask with reservoir bag is the answer.
4. **Ans. d. Drug entering into sub arachnoid space** *Ref: Miller's anesthesia 7/e ch51*
   Since lignocaine is used, the onset is faster. The clinical features are similar to high spinal anesthesia causing hypotension, bradycardia and respiratory depression few minutes after admi nistering the drug, As in any neuraxial block that reaches high levels, arterial blood pressure and heart rate should be supported. The Trendelenburg position should be instituted to maximize venous return. Intravenous atropine and ephedrine are often effective and provide the time to administer a more potent catecholamine, if needed. Ventilation should be supported, and if the entire dose (20 to 25 mL) of local anesthetic has been administered into the CSF, tracheal intubation and mechanical ventilation are indicated because patients may require approximately 1 to 2 hours to maintain adequate spontaneous ventilation consistently.
5. **Ans. a. Thiopentone** *Ref: Miller's anesthesia 7/e ch26*
   Thiopentone similar to other CNS depressants, have potent effects on cerebral metabolism A dose-related depression of cerebral metabolic oxygen consumption rate ($CMRO_2$), produces a progressive slowing of the EEG, a reduction in the rate of adenosine triphosphate consumption, and protection from incomplete cerebral ischemia. With the reduction in $CMRO_2$, there is a parallel reduction in cerebral perfusion, which is seen in decreased cerebral blood flow and ICP. With reduced $CMRO_2$, cerebral vascular resistance increases, and CBF decreases. The ratio of CBF to $CMRO_2$ is unchanged. The reduction in CBF after the administration of barbiturates causes a concurrent decrease in ICP. Even though the MAP decreases, barbiturates do not compromise the overall CPP because the CPP = MAP - ICP. In this relationship, ICP decreases more relative to the decrease in MAP after barbiturate use, preserving CPP. Whereas halothane causes increase in cerebral blood flow causing increased ICT. Ketamine and succinylcholine causes increase in ICT and hence contraindicated in head injury patients.

6. **Ans. d. Sevoflurane** *Ref: Miller 7/e ch26*

All volatile anesthetics decrease hepatic blood flow, but desflurane and sevoflurane have the least significant effect on total hepatic blood flow and hepatic oxygen delivery, whereas halothane induces the most profound reductions in hepatic blood flow. Sevoflurane appears to be the most effective of the inhaled anesthetics for maintaining both blood flow and oxygen delivery to the liver.

7. **Ans. c. Neuro axial block analgesia** *Ref: Miller 7/e ch69*

Epidural or combined spinal epidural analgesia is the best mode of labor analgesia for pregnant patients with heart disease.

8. **Ans. a. Body may lose heat by conduction** *Ref: Miller 7/e ch48*

Inadvertent hypothermia is by far the most common perioperative thermal disturbance during anesthesia. Hypothermia results from a combination of anesthetic-impaired thermoregulation and exposure to a cold operating room environment. Of these two causes, impaired thermoregulation is much more important. Heat can be transferred from a patient to the environment in four ways: radiation, conduction, convection, and evaporation. Among these mechanisms, radiation and convection contribute most to perioperative heat loss. Conductive heat loss is proportional to the temperature difference between two adjacent surfaces and the strength of the thermal insulation separating them. radiation is the major type of heat loss in most surgical patients.

Though radiation is the most common mechanism of heat loss in the intraoperative period, this q is formulated that conduction may cause heat loss in option A. hence optionA is correct. Hypothermia cant be prevented only by giving warm fluids. Patients cannot be warmed by administering heated fluids because the fluids cannot (much) exceed body temperature. On the other hand, heat loss from cold intravenous fluids becomes substantial when large amounts of crystalloid solution or blood are administered.

9. **Ans. a. Mapleson A** *Ref: Dorsch and Dorsch 5/e ch1*

Mapleson A/magill system Modified variant: LACK system (coaxial)	Efficient for spontaneous ventilation because fresh gas flow equal to minute volume is sufficient to prevent rebreathing.
Mapleson C system/water's system	Postoperative recovery, CPR
Mapleson D system	Most efficient for controlled ventilation, since fresh gas flow forces air away from patient and towards pressure relief valve
Mapleson E system/ayre's T piece system	Primarily used in infants and young children. Main advantage of T piece is absence of resistance to expiration, a factor of crucial importance to children
Mapleson's F system/Jackson-Rees modification of Ayre's T piece	Popular in pediatric anesthesia, requires 2–3 times minute ventilation
Efficiency of system with spontaneous respiration: A > d > and e > c > b mnemonic - adeb **Efficiency of system with controlled respiration:** D > F > E > B > C > A mnemonic - debca **Most commonly used version of Mapleson-D: Bain Coaxial system** **Universal circuit–bain's circuit since it can be used for both spontaneous and controlled ventilation and for both adults and children.**	

10. **Ans. b. Halothane** *Ref: Miller's anesthesia 7/e ch24*

Halothane, enflurane, isoflurane, and desflurane are all metabolized to trifluoroacylated hepatic protein adducts that have been reported to induce liver injury in susceptible patients. The propensity to produce liver injury appears to parallel metabolism of the parent drug; thus, halothane (20%) ⪢⪢ enflurane (2.5%) ⪢ isoflurane (0.2%) > desflurane (0.02%).

11. **Ans. c. Ketamine** *Ref: Miller 7/e ch26*

Ketamine increases cerebral blood flow by sympathetic stimulation and causes increased $CMRO_2$. Hence it is contraindicated in patients having increased intracranial tension and head injury.

12. **Ans. b. Ketamine** *Ref: Miller 7/e chapter 26*

Ketamine increases cerebral metabolism, CBF, and ICP. Because of its excitatory CNS effects, which can be detected by generalized EEG development of theta wave activity and by petit mal seizure–like activity in the hippocampus, ketamine increases $CMRO_2$. Hence it is contraindicated in patients with epilepsy.

13. Ans. c. Bupivacaine *Ref: Miller 7/e ch30*

Drug	Relative conduction-blocking potency*	Physiochemical properties	
		pK_a[†]	Hydrophobicity[†]
Low Potency			
Procaine	1	8.9	100
Intermediate Potency			
Mepivacaine	1.5	7.7	130
Prilocaine	1.8	8.0[‡]	129
Chloroprocaine	3	9.1	810
Lidocaine	2	7.8	366
High Potency			
Tetracaine	8	8.4	5822
Bupivacaine	8	8.1	3420
Etidocaine	8	7.9	7320

14. Ans. d. Deepen plane of anesthesia *Ref: stoelting coexisting diseases 5/e ch9*

This patient is under general anesthesia and the patient has developed after general anesthesia was administered. so the patient is intubated and maintained with intravenous or inhalational anesthetics which is not mentioned in the history. Now this scenario indicates the diagnosis as intraoperative bronchospasm. It should be treated promptly, otherwise patient may end up in hypercarbia, hypoxia and cardiac arrest.

Line of management of intraop bronchospasm

Deepen the plane of anesthesia with volatile anesthetics

↓

Intravenous propofol or ketamine

↓

Inhaled beta 2 agonists like albuterol

↓

Intravenous steroids

15. Ans. d. Patient on antihypertensive medication *Ref: Miller 7/e ch51*

Absolute contraindications of neuraxial Anesthesia

- Raised intracranial pressure
- patient refusal
- Bleeding disorders
- pt's on anticoagulants
- Infection of the local site

Relative C.I

- Aortic and mitral stenosis, shock, platelet count < 80,000, patient on antiplatelets

16. Ans. a. and b. *Ref: Lee's textbook of anesthesia 3/e chronic pain management*

Coeliac plexus block is given for painful conditions of the upper abdomen. It is done at the level T12-L1 junction. Celiac gangion is present around the aorta bilaterally, hence the block is given bilaterally. Diarrhea and hypotension are adverse effects and it is done by fluoroscopic guidance or ultrasound.

17. Ans. a. Keep stylet and remove needle

Ref: Miller 7/e ch51

Relationships Among Variables and Post–spinal Puncture Headache

Factors that may increase the incidence of postspinal puncture headache	
Age	Younger more frequent
Gender	Females > males
Needle size	Larger > smaller
Needle bevel	Less when the needle bevel is placed in the long axis of the neuraxis
Pregnancy	More when pregnant
Dural punctures (no.)	More with multiple punctures
Continuous spinals	
Timing of ambulation	

MC cause is leakage of CSF through the hole in duramater

- The Headache can be prevented by using small bore atraumatic needles
- Treatment of the headache consists of
  - Lying down for 24 hours, bed rest
  - Abdominal compression
  - Oral or intravenous Fluids
  - Caffeine
  - Epidural patch (last resort but > 90% effective)

18. Ans. c. Succinylcholine *Ref: Miller 7/e ch29*

Administration of succinylcholine to an otherwise well individual for an elective surgical procedure increases plasma potassium levels by approximately 0.5 mEq/dL. This increase in potassium is due to the depolarizing action of the relaxant. With activation of the acetylcholine channels, movement of sodium into the cells is accompanied by movement of potassium out of the cells. This slight increase in potassium is well tolerated by most individuals and generally does not cause dysrhythmias.

Several early reports suggested that patients in renal failure may be susceptible to a hyperkalemic response to succinylcholine. Severe hyperkalemia may follow the administration of succinylcholine to patients with severe metabolic acidosis and hypovolemia. Patients with any number of conditions that result in the proliferation of extrajunctional acetylcholine receptors, such as neuromuscular disease, are likely to have an exaggerated hyperkalemic response after the administration of succinylcholine.

19 Ans. a. Diaphragm *Ref: Miller 7/e ch29*

Most resistant muscle to neuromuscular blockade is vocal cord. The 2nd most resistant muscle is diaphragm.

20. Ans. b. 2 *Ref: Journal reference*

Lithium has a half life of 48 hours, and its interaction with non depolarizing agents can prolong their duration of action. Hence practically 48 hours is a better answer. Still some journals indicate to stop the drug 72 hours before surgery. To me, 48 hours seems to be a better option. Now the ball is in your court.

21. Ans. a. and b. *Ref: Miller 7/e ch48*

- General anesthetics decrease the thresholds (triggering core temperatures) for vasoconstriction and shivering by 2 °C to 3 °C.
- Anesthetic-induced impairment of thermoregulatory control, combined with a cool operating room environment, makes most patients hypothermic.
- The major initial cause of hypothermia in most patients is core-to-peripheral redistribution of body heat.
- Neuraxial anesthesia impairs both central and peripheral thermoregulatory control and is associated with substantial hypothermia.
- Large randomized trials have proved that even mild hypothermia (i.e. 1.5 °C to 2.0 °C) causes adverse outcomes, including a threefold increase in morbid myocardial outcomes, a threefold increase in risk for wound infection, coagulopathy and need for allogeneic transfusion, prolonged recovery, and prolonged hospitalization.

- Body temperature should be monitored in patients undergoing surgery lasting longer than 30 minutes, and core temperature should be maintained at 36 °C or higher whenever possible. Forced-air warming currently offers the best combination of high efficacy, low cost, and remarkable safety. Fluid warmers can also prevent heat loss. Hence it is obvious that both general and regional anesthesia produces hypothermia. Heat loss mechanism is by conduction, convection, radiation.

22. **Ans. d. Non-rebreathing mask with O_2 reservoir bag** *Ref: morgan's clinical anesthesia 5/e p1282*
Both the options B and D are correct since both rebreathing mask and nonbreathing mask can deliver 90% oxygen. The delivery of FiO_2 in these masks are dependent on high flows (10 L/min). if the question was asked with flow rate, then the answer would have been easy. This is a poorly framed question. Now to choose between the options, the addition of reservoir bag increases the FiO_2, IN OPTION b, there is no addition of reservoir bag hence the FiO_2 would not reach 90%. Hence non breathing mask with reservoir bag is the answer.

23. **Ans. c. Sevoflurane** *Ref: Miller 7/e ch24*
Desiccated carbon dioxide absorbent and inhaled anesthetic interactions can lead to the production of carbon monoxide in the anesthesia circuit (desflurane ⋙ enflurane > isoflurane). Negligible amounts of carbon monoxide are formed from halothane and sevoflurane.

24. **Ans. a. Bupivacaine** *Ref: Miller 7/e ch30*
    - It is the long acting local anesthetic with high protein binding
    - Bupivacaine is the most cardiotoxic and should not be used for Bier's block
    - Bupivacaine produces ventricular fibrillation

25. **Ans. a. Isoflurane** *Ref: Miller 7/e ch20*
Isoflurane produces least increase in Intracranial pressure and least effect on the cerebral blood flow and is the agent of choice for neurosurgeries

26. **Ans. d. Chemical pneumonitis following aspiration** *Ref: Chestnut obstetric anesthesia 2/e ch3*
Mendelson syndrome was originally described in pregnant patients but later the nomenclature was used in all chemical aspiration pneumonitis. Ph < 2.5 volume > 25 ml is criteria.

27. **Ans. a. Between pia and arachnoid** *Ref: Miller 7/e ch51*

    Structures encountered during lumbar punctures
    - Skin
    - Subcutaneous tissue
    - Supraspinous ligament
    - Interspinous ligament
    - Ligamentum flavum
    - Dura Matter and
    - Arachnoid matter
    - Piamater

28. **Ans. a. Propofol** *Ref: Miller 7/e ch26*
Propofol has rapid and smooth induction, rapid and smooth recovery, no active metabolites and strong antiemetic property. Hence it is the intravenous anesthetic of choice for day care surgery.

29. **Ans. d. 1: 200000** *Ref: Miller 7/e ch30*

30. **Ans. a. Ketamine** *Ref: Miller 7/e ch26*
    - Only IV anesthetic agent with both anesthetic and analgesic activity
    - **It is a sympathetic stimulant**
    - Increases all pressure → BP, IOT, ICT
    - Hence Contraindicated in raised intracranial pressure and intracranial pathology with mass effect

31. **Ans. a. Etomidate** *Ref: Miller 7/e ch26*
Even a single dose of etomidate can cause adrenocortical suppression through a dose-dependent reversible inhibition of the enzyme 11 β-hydroxylase

32. Ans. a. Xenon *Ref: Miller 7/e ch24*

- Properties: inert gas, normal atmospheric constituent, not an environmental pollutant, no ozone depletion global warming effect. Because it is inert, it is not metabolized

33. Ans. c. muscle stiffness *Ref: Miller 7/e ch27*

Fentanyl at higher dose or large dose can cause chest wall rigidity also called wooden chest syndrome.

34. Ans. A. Thiopentone *Ref: Miller 7/e ch26*

A dose-related depression of cerebral metabolic oxygen consumption rate ($CMRO_2$), produces a progressive slowing of the EEG, a reduction in the rate of adenosine triphosphate consumption, and protection from incomplete cerebral ischemia. With the reduction in $CMRO_2$, there is a parallel reduction in cerebral perfusion, which is seen in decreased cerebral blood flow and ICP. With reduced $CMRO_2$, cerebral vascular resistance increases, and CBF decreases. The ratio of CBF to $CMRO_2$ is unchanged. The reduction in CBF after the administration of barbiturates causes a concurrent decrease in ICP.

35. Ans. a. Suxamethonium *Ref: Miller 7/e ch29*

When succinylcholine is given at a larger dose, phase 2 block Results from desensitization of receptor to Ach. and resembles competitive/non–depolarization block with fading on TOF (TRAIN OF FOUR)

Characteristic	Phase 1	Transition	Phase 2
Tetanic stimulation	No fade	Slight fade	Fade
Post-tetanic facilitation	None	Slight	Yes
Train-of-four fade	No	Moderate fade	Marked fade
Train-of-four ratio	> 0.7	0.4–0.7	< 0.4
Edrophonium	Augments	Little effect	Antagonizes
Recovery	Rapid	Rapid to slow	Increasingly prolonged
Dose requirements (mg/kg)*	2–3	4–5	> 6
Tachyphylaxis	No	Yes	Yes

36. Ans. a. Succinylcholine *Ref: Miller 7/e ch37*

Drugs known to trigger malignant hyperthermia	Drugs safe in malignant hyperthermia
• Halothane • Succinylcholine (m.c.) • Methoxyflurane • Enflurane, isoflurane • Decamethonium • Gallamine • Diethyl ether • Ethylene • Ethyl chloride • Trichloroethylene • Ketamine • Phencyclidine • Cyclopropane	• Nitrous oxide • Barbiturates • Diazepam • Nondepolarizing muscle relaxants • Opiates • Propofol

37. Ans. a. Inhibition Na^+ channels *Ref: Miller 7/e ch30*

Local anesthetics Blocks voltage gated Na+ channels from inside of cell membrane by binding to a-subunit of Na K pump.

38. Ans. b. Propofol *Ref: Miller 7/e ch26*

Among all these agents, propofol has the least half life.

39. Ans. a. Drinking *Ref: Miller 7/e ch85*

With the increase in number and complexity of outpatient surgeries, discharge criteria have been amended by various authors to include assessment of home readiness. The resulting PADSS, or postanesthesia discharge scoring system, continues to evolve. It was initially based on five criteria: vital signs, ambulation and mental status, pain and nausea/vomiting, surgical bleeding, and fluid intake/output.

Variable evaluated	Score*
Vital Signs (stable and consistent with age and preanesthetic baseline)	
Systemic blood pressure and heart rate within 20% of the preanesthetic level	2
Systemic blood pressure and heart rate 20% to 40% of the preanesthetic level	1
Systemic blood pressure and heart rate >40% of the preanesthetic level	0
Activity Level	
Steady gait without dizziness or meets the preanesthetic level	2
Requires assistance	1
Unable to ambulate	0
Nausea and Vomiting	
None to minimal	2
Moderate	1
Severe (continues after repeated treatment)	0
Pain (minimal to no pain, controllable with oral analgesics)	
Yes	2
No	1
Surgical Bleeding (consistent with that expected for the surgical procedure)	
Minimal (does not require dressing change)	2
Moderate (up to two dressing changes required)	1
Severe (more than three dressing changes required)	0

40. Ans. a. Propofol *Ref: Miller 7/e ch26*

Refer explanation of question no.1.

41. Ans. a. Myasthenia gravis *Ref: Miller 7/e ch35*

Disease	Response to depolarizers	Response to non depolarizers
Muscular dystrophy (Duchenne type)	Hyperkalemia and malignant hyperthermia	Hypersensitivity
Myasthenia gravis	Resistance	Hypersensitivity
Myasthenic syndrome	Hypersensitivity	Hypersensitivity

42. Ans. a. Potency *Ref: Miller 7/e ch21*

- It is measure of potency of inhalational agent. It is the minimum alveolar concentration of an inhalational agent required to produce unresponsiveness to noxious stimuli like skin incision in 50% of pt.
- Greater the MAC value, lesser is the potency
- Methoxyflurane is the most potent having least MAC value (0.16%)
- N_2O has maximum MAC value (104%) and is the least potent inhalational anesthetic

43. Ans. a. Pin index system *Ref: Dorsch and dorsch–anesthesia equipments 5/e ch1*

- It is a safety mechanism for gas cylinders used in anesthesia so that one cylinder cannot be wrongly placed in another's position.
- 2 pins of 4 mm and 6 mm long are present
- Present In high pressure system [valve outlets of cylinders]
- Can be violated if wrong gas is filled in cylinder.
- Pin is present in the machine end.
- Holes are in the cylinder end.

44. Ans. a. Suxamethonium *Ref: Miller 7/e ch29*

- Fastest acting nondepolarising skeletal muscle relaxant is Rocuronium
- Shortest acting non depolarizing agent is gantacurium > mivacurium.
- Shortest acting (both onset and duration) muscle relaxant–succinylcholine
- Muscle relaxant of choice for full stomach patients, rapid sequence induction–succinylcholine

45. Ans. d. CMV *Ref: Miller 7/e ch93*

Initiation modes
- Control mode ventilation (CMV)

Weaning modes
- Synchronized intermittent mandatory ventilation (SIMV)
- Pressure support ventilation (PSV)
- CPAP (continuous positive airway pressure)
- BiPAP (bilevel positive airway pressure)

46. Ans. a. Venturi mask *Ref: morgan's clinical anesthesia 5/e p1282*

Variable performance devices
- Nasal cannula
- Nasal mask
- Simple O_2 mask
- Masks with reservoir bag–partial rebreather, non-rebreather masks

Fixed performance devices
- Anesthesia bag valve mask system
- Venturi mask
- Air entraining nebulizers
- High flow air oxygen system
- Oxygen hood

47. Ans. a. Nitrous oxide *Ref: Miller 7/e ch21*

Nitrous oxide diffuses faster than nitrogen and hence can accumulate in closed spaces and causes distension. Hence it is contraindicated in surgeries like myringoplasty, intestinal obstruction.

48. Ans. c. Bupivacaine *Ref: Miller 7/e ch30*

Drug	Plain solution			Epinephrine-containing solution	
	Concentration (%)	Max Dose (mg)	Duration (min)	Max dose (mg)	Duration (min)
Short Duration					
Procaine	1–2	500	20–30	600	30–45
Chloroprocaine	1–2	800	15–30	1000	30
Moderate Duration					
Lidocaine	0.5–1	300	30–60	500	120
Mepivacaine	0.5–1	300	45–90	500	120
Prilocaine	0.5–1	350	30–90	550	120
Long Duration					
Bupivacaine	0.25–0.5	175	120–240	200	180–240
Ropivacaine	0.2–0.5	200	120–240	250	180–240

49. Ans. b. Succinylcholine *Ref: Miller 7/e ch37*

Most common agents causing MH are succinylcholine > halothane > all fluorinated inhalational agents.

50. Ans. c. Ketamine *Ref: Miller 7/e ch26*

Halothane causes hypotension due to myocardial depression, propofol and thipentone causes hypotension due to vasodilatation. Ketamine causes sympathetic stimulation and causes hypertension and tachycardia.

51. Ans. a. Succinylcholine *Ref: Miller 7/e ch29*

Refer explanation of question no.10 in jipmer 2014.

52. Ans. a. Propofol *Ref: Miller 7/e ch26*

- Propofol has rapid and smooth induction, rapid and smooth recovery, no active metabolites and strong antiemetic property.
- Propofol has significant antiemetic activity at low (subhypnotic) doses. It has been used successfully to treat postoperative nausea in a bolus dose of 10 mg.

53. Ans. a. Nitrous oxide *Ref: Miller 7/e ch24*

- N_2O produces bone marrow suppression, megaloblastic anemia due to B_{12} deficiency which can lead to subacute combine degeneration of spinal cord.

54. Ans. a and b. *Ref: Miller 7/e ch69*

I think that the question is either recollected or framed wrongly because neuraxial block constitutes epidural and spinal anesthesia. In any patient with pregnancy, combined spinal epidural analgesia or epidural analgesia is better for labor analgesia. For LSCS, spinal anesthesia is more commonly preferred.

55. Ans. a. Calcium *Ref: Miller 7/e ch97, www.heart.org*

Calcium gluconate is not routinely recommended for cardiac arrest in ACLS.

56. Ans. a. Pin index system *Ref: dorsch and dorsch 5/e ch1*

- It is a safety mechanism for gas cylinders used in anesthesia so that one cannot be wrongly placed in another's position.
- 2 pins of 4 mm and 6 mm long are present
- Present In high pressure system [valve outlets of cylinders]
- Can be violated if wrong gas is filled in cylinder.
- Pin is present in the machine end.
- Holes are in the cylinder end.

57. Ans. b. Patient on aspirin *Ref: Miller 7/e ch51*

Absolute contraindications of neuraxial Anesthesia

- Raised intracranial pressure
- Patient refusal
- Bleeding disorders
- pt's on anticoagulants
- Infection of the local site

Relative CI

- Aortic and mitral stenosis, shock, platelet count < 80,000, patient on antiplatelets

58. Ans. d. It inhibits salivation *Ref: lee's textbook of anesthesia 2/e ch2*

- It is a complete anaesthetic. It is highly inflammable, highly volatile and explosive
- It is an irritant, pungent smelling liquid
- It has slow induction and is very unpleasant
- Ether does not affect the mucociliary action and is good bronchodilator.
- Ether has good anaesthetic, good analgesic, good skeletal muscle relaxant
- Ether does not depress respiration but rather it is stimulated
- It increases respiratory secretion and salivation thereby anticholinergic should always be given before giving ether to prevent these reactions.
- Ether has highest incidence of nausea and vomiting among inhalational agents.
- Ether causes hyperglycemia and is Contraindicated in diabetes
- Guedel's 4 stages of anesthesia were based on ether. Ether should not be used with cautery.
- Ether is safe in unskilled professionals and is very economical
- Ether derivatives–Enflurane, Isoflurane, Desflurane, sevoflurane.

59. Ans. d. Endotracheal intubation *Ref: nunn's respiratory physiology 2/e–respiratory physiology*

Anatomical dead space is increased by	Anatomical dead space is decreased by	Alveolar dead space is increased by
Old age Neck extension Jaw protrusion Bronchodilators (atropine), halothane Increased lung volume Anesthesia mask and circuits IPPV (Intermittent positive pressure ventilation) PEEP (Positive end expiratory pressure)	Intubation Tracheostomy Hyperventilation Neck flexion Bronchoconstrictors Massive pleural effusion	IPPV PEEP General anesthesia Hypotension Lung pathologies affecting diffusion like interstitial lung disease, pulmonary embolism, pulmonary edema, ARDS

60. Ans. a. Ketamine *Ref: Miller 7/e ch26*

- Only IV anesthetic agent with both anesthetic and analgesic activity
- **It is a sympathetic stimulant**
- Increases all pressure → BP, IOT, ICT
- Hence Contraindicated in raised intracranial pressure and intracranial pathology with mass effect

61. Ans. a. CPAP *Ref: Miller 7/e ch93*

Noninvasive modes are

- CPAP–Continuous positive airway pressure
- BiPAP–Bilevel positive airway pressure
- PSV–Pressure support ventilation

62. Ans. b. Ketamine *Ref: Miller 7/e ch26*

Since ketamine is the only intravenous anesthetic with bronchodilator property, it is the IV anesthetic agent of choice for asthmatics.

63. Ans. a. Atracurium *Ref: Miller 7/e ch29*

Atracurium undergoes hoffmans degradation which is non enzymatic degradation, hence it is not dependent on liver or kidney for metabolism. Hence it is the muscle relaxant of choice for hepatic and renal failure patients.

64. Ans. a. Atracurium *Ref: Miller 7/e ch29*

Refer the explanation of question no.3.

65. Ans. a. Halothane *Ref: Miller 7/e ch24*

Two distinct types of hepatic injury have been associated with the clinical use of halothane. Mild injury occurs in 20% of adults who receive halothane, and laboratory tests show mild elevations in alanine aminotransferase (ALT) and aspartate aminotransferase (AST). The second type of injury is the fulminant form, commonly known as halothane hepatitis, which is characterized by elevated ALT, AST, bilirubin, and alkaline phosphatase levels; massive hepatic necrosis; and a fatality rate ranging from 50% to 75%. Because of the potential for halothane-induced hepatitis, halothane is not generally recommended for use in adults.

66. Ans. a. CMV *Ref: Miller 7/e ch93*

Patient ventilator asynchrony is common in modes which has controlled ventilation for e.g. CMV. It is less seen in WEANING ventilation modes like SIMV, cpap, BiPAP, PSV.

67. Ans. a. Isoflurane *Ref: Miller 7/e ch22*

Isoflurane causes least increase in cerebral blood flow among volatile agents and hence little effect on intracranial tensiom. Hence isoflurane is preferred in neurosurgery patients.

68. Ans. b. Propofol *Ref: Miller 7/e ch26*

- Propofol is an oil-based preparation and injection is painful because it contains soyabean oil, egg lecithin and glycerol
- 1% xylocaine is also given along with it to reduce pain on injection.

69. Ans. a. Succinylcholine *Ref: Miller 7/e ch37*

MH is a pharmacogenetic clinical syndrome that in its classic form occurs during anesthesia with a volatile halogenated alkane such as halothane and the depolarizing muscle relaxant succinylcholine.

Drugs known to trigger malignant hyperthermia	Drugs safe in malignant hyperthermia
• Halothane	• Nitrous oxide
• Succinylcholine (m.c.)	• Barbiturates
• Methoxyflurane	• Diazepam
• Enflurane, isoflurane	• Non–depolarizing muscle relaxants
• Decamethonium	• Opiates
• Gallamine	• Propofol
• Diethyl ether	
• Ethylene	
• Ethyl chloride	
• Trichloroethylene	
• Ketamine	
• Phencyclidine	
• Cyclopropane	

70. **Ans. a. Venture mask** *Ref: morgan's clinical anesthesia 5/e p1282*

Variable performance devices
- Nasal cannula
- Nasal mask
- Simple O_2 mask
- Masks with reservoir bag–partial rebreather, non-rebreather masks

Fixed performance devices
- Anesthesia bag valve mask system
- Venturi mask
- Air entraining nebulizers
- High flow air oxygen system
- Oxygen hood

71. **Ans. b. Ketamine** *Ref: Miller 7/e ch26*

Since ketamine is the only intravenous anesthetic with bronchodilator property, it is the IV anesthetic agent of choice for asthmatics.

72. **Ans. d. Sevoflurane** *Ref: Miller 7/e ch26*

All volatile anesthetics decrease hepatic blood flow, but desflurane and sevoflurane have the least significant effect on total hepatic blood flow and hepatic oxygen delivery, whereas halothane induces the most profound reductions in hepatic blood flow. Sevoflurane appears to be the most effective of the inhaled anesthetics for maintaining both blood flow and oxygen delivery to the liver.

73. **Ans. d. Pethidine** *Ref: Miller 7/e ch26*

Meperidine or pethidine is the most effective pharmacological treatment for postop shivering.

QUESTIONS 2015

1. Structure pierced during spinal anesthesia after interspinous ligament?
a. Ligamentum flavum
b. Aeriolar space
c. Arachnoid space
d. Supraspinous ligament

2. Not a complication of LSCS with regional anesthesia?
a. Delayed respiratory depression
b. Venous air embolism
c. Hypotension
d. Ischemia of lower limbs

3. What is done to reduce pain after administration of local anesthetic ?
a. Alkalinize the LA
b. Add adrenaline
c. Cool the LA
d. All of the above

4. Which is the correct statement regarding esophageal intubation?
a. Cannot be detected by stethoscope
b. It doesn't occur for an inexperienced person
c. Capnography may not detect esophageal intubation during cardiac arrest
d. None of the above

ANSWERS AND EXPLANATIONS

1. **Ans. a. Ligamentum flavum** *Ref. Morgan 4/e ch16*

The following structures are pierced in spinal anesthesia by a spinal needle in order:
- Skin
- Subcutaneous tissue
- Supraspinous ligament
- Interspinous ligament
- Ligamentum flavum

- Epidural space
- Dura
- Arachnoid membrane
- Subarachnoid space
- Piamater
- Vertebral column

2. **Ans. d. Ischemia of lower limbs** *Ref: Morgan 4/e ch16*
   - Hypotension
   - Bradycardia
   - Total spinal anesthesia—respiratory depression-can be early or delayed
   - Venous air embolism has been a reported complication in patients undergoing LSCS.
   - Epidural abscess
   - Meningitis
   - Vertebral canal haematoma
   - Nerve injury
   - Spinal cord ischaemia
   - Wrong route error
   - Cardiovascular collapse

   Ischemia of lower limbs has never been a reported complication after regional anestehesia in lscs.
3. **Ans. a. Alkalinize the LA** *Ref: Morgan 4/e ch14*
   Adding sodium bicarbonate will alkalinise the local anesthetics and fasten the onset of action of LA and reduce the pain of LA after infiltration in tissues.
4. **Ans. c. Capnography may not detect esophageal intubation during cardiac arrest** *Ref: Morgan 4/e ch6*
   Esophageal intubation can be detected by stethoscope but the gold standard to detect oesophageal intubation is with capnography but capnography can miss out tracheal or esophageal intubation during cardiac arrest due to low CO2 levels during cardiac arrest.

Chapter

17 Dermatology

M Garthick Arivudainambi

Skin is the largest organ of the body composed of epidermis, dermis and subcutaneous layer. Skin is derived from ectoderm.

EPIDERMIS

Layers of Epidermis

Stratum corneum	Outermost layer, made of flat, anucleated cells organelles
Stratum lucidum	Transparent layer, seen only in palm and sole
Stratum granulosum	• 2-5 cell thickness, made of Intracellular basophilic Kerato hyaline granules, forms a water impermeable layer; contains abundant Odland bodies • Layer absent in nail bed and matrix
Stratum spinosum/ prickle cells layer [Malpighian layer]	8-10 layers of polyhedral cells with round nuclei, spines made of desmosomes, Langerhans' cells present
Stratum basale /stratum germinatum	• Lies next to the dermis. Single layer of columnar/cuboidal cells, contains mitotically active keratinocytes and melanocytes

- Skin doubling time: 4 weeks
- Epidermal turn over time: 1 month
- Accelerated cell turnover: Psoriasis and ichthyosiform erythroderma (2 to 3 days)
- Lichen planus: The granular cell layer is focally increased
- Adamson's fringe: Beginning of Keratinization
- Abrupt keratinization: Seen in pilomatricoma
- Keratins: capable of absorbing vast amounts of water
- Langerhans cells are found scattered evenly throughout the epidermis
- Merkel cells are normally located in the basal layer, although they are inconspicuous in routine sections. Ultra structurally, they contain dense core neuro secretory granules.

Cells in the Skin

- 80-90% of epidermal cells are Keratinocytes.
- The keratinocytes contain lamellar bodies called as Odland bodies.
- Melanocytes are derived from neural crest cells and are present in stratum basale.. They synthesize Melanin and transfer it to keratinocytes.
- For every 10 stratum basale cells there is one melanocyte.
- Each melanocyte provides melanin to about 36 keratinocytes.
- Albinism is due to decreased production of melanin by melanocytes.
- Vitiligo is due to decreased number of melanocytes.
- Langerhans cells are derived from bone marrow, they are antigen presenting (APC) cells in the epidermis. These cells are present in stratum spinosum. CD marker for Langerhans cell is CD 1. Langerhans cells have Bier beck granules (tennis racket shaped granules). Tumor of Langerhans cells is Histiocytosis X

- Merkel cells are also derived from neural crest and acts as Mechanoreceptors. They are present in stratum basale.
- Grenz zone is a narrow clear zone present between epidermis and dermis.

DERMIS

- It is Mesodermal in origin.
- The major type of collagen is Type I collagen and about 20% is Type III collagen.
- Dermis is further divided into superficial papillary dermis and deep Reticular dermis.
- Scarring occurs when reticular dermis is disrupted.

SUBCUTANEOUS LAYER

- It consists of adipose cells, sweat glands, blood vessels and nerves.
- The nourishment to epidermis is provided by dermis.

SWEAT GLANDS

- They are ectodermal in origin.
- There are 2 main types of sweat glands, i.e. Eccrine and Apocrine sweat glands.
- Eccrine sweat glands are present all over the skin particularly in the palms and soles. They secrete watery hypotonic secretions onto the skin.

Blockade of eccrine sweat glands is k/a **Miliria.**

- Apocrine sweat glands open into hair follicle. They are present in the Axilla, Anogenital region, scalp and near nipples. They start functioning at the time of puberty. Secretions of apocrine glands are sterile. Bacterial action gives these secretions odor.

Modified apocrine sweat glands

- Mammary Glands, Moll glands of eye, cerumen glands (ear wax) of ear are modified apocrine glands.
- Blockade of apocrine sweat glands is called as Fox Fordyce disease.
- Pus containing infection of apocrine sweat glands is called as hidradenitis.

SEBACEOUS GLANDS

- They are present all over the body except palms and soles.
- They produce sebum made of fatty acids, cholesterol esters and wax.
- The major areas of sebaceous glands are scalp, face, interscapular and sternal areas.
- They are holocrine glands that act as a pilo sebaceous unit.

Ectopic sebaceous Glands:

- They are not associated with hair follicles.
- Fox–Fordyce spots are ectopic sebaceous glands on the lips, can be seen in normal healthy people.
- Tyson glands are ectopic sebaceous glands on penis.
- Meibomian glands are ectopic sebaceous glands of eyes.
- Montgomery tubercles are ectopic sebaceous glands of breasts.

Types of Hair

- Lanugo Hair– These are long fine silky hair present in Embryonic life (only on babies).
- Vellus hair are short, fine hair present mainly over malar region of face, Non-pigmented hair.
- Terminal hair are pigmented, long and coarse hair.

Stages of Hair Cycle

- Anagen phase–It is actively growing phase of the hair that constitutes 90% of total hair. Duration of anagen is 3-5 years. It grows at rate of 0.4 mm/day.
- Catagen phase–It is transitional phase of hair constituting 1-3% of total hair.
- Telogen phase–It's a resting phase of the hair, constitutes 8-9% and has a depigmented narrow club.

Nails

- It's a hard plate of keratin with high sulfur content.
- Finger nails grows 0.1 mm/day.
- Mees line are seen in arsenic poisoning.
- Beau's line occurs when nail growth stops and then regrows producing transverse ridges, seen in patients with infections and soon after recovery.
- Half and Half nail is seen in chronic renal failure.
- Terry Nails are seen in cirrhosis.
- Periungual Fibroma is seen in tuberous sclerosis.

Skin Lesions

- Contact dermatitis produces linear skin lesions.
- Koebner phenomenon is development of isomorphic skin lesions on uninvolved skin after trauma, seen in psoriasis, lichen planus and vitiligo.
- Iris/target lesions are seen in Erythema Multiformis.
- Herald patch/circinate patch also k/a mother patch is seen pityriasis Rosea.
- Morbilliform rash is seen in Measles.
- Sheet line rash called as scalariform rash is seen in scarlet fever.
- Macule is change in color of skin < 0.5 cms.
- Patch is macule > 0.5 cms.
- Papule is raised solid lesion < 0.5 cms.
- Plaque is papule > 0.5 cms.
- Vesicle is fluid filled lesion < 0.5 cms.
- Bullae is fluid filled lesion > 0.5 cms.
- Nodule is solid, raised and deeply circumscribed lesion > 0.5 cms.
- Pustule is pus filled vesicle
- Petechia are pin sized macules of blood in skin
- Purpura is extravasation of blood > 2 mm under skin.
- Telangiectasia is visible dilatation of blood vessels.
- Lichenification is thickening of skin with hyperpigmentation and increased skin margins.
- Erythroderma is inflammation of > 90% of BSA along with scaling. It's a dermatological emergency.

Technical Terms

- Acanthosis is increased thickening of stratum spinosum
- Acantholysis is loss of cell adhesions between keratinocytes producing rounded cells, called Tzanck cells.
- Parakeratosis is presence of nuclei in stratum corneum seen in psoriasis
- Hyperkeratosis is proliferation of stratum corneum
- Dyskeratosis is faculty keratinization seen in dariers disease.
- Spongiosis is intra epidermal edema
- Epidermotropism is the extravasation of blood cells into the epidermis.
- Munro-Micro abscess is seen in Psoriasis consisting of neutrophils in the stratum corneum of epidermis.
- Pautrier's abscess is seen in Mycosis fungoides (cutaneous T cell Lymphoma)
- Papillary tip abscess is seen in Dermatitis Herpetiformis.

Clinical Testing

- Diascopy is visualizing the skin through glass slides.
- Wood lamp examination uses 360 nanometers (UV rays). It has **Nickel oxide** filter.

On wood lamp examination	
Tinea capitis	Light Yellow green
pseudomonas	Apple green/golden yellow
Tuberous sclerosis	Blue White
Vitiligo	White
Erythrasma(corynebacterium minutissimum)	Coral Red/Pink
Porphyria cutanea tarda	Red/pink
Pityriasis versicolor	Golden Yellow/apple Green

- Nikolsky's sign is shearing of skin on application of lateral pressure, seen in Pemphigus Vulgaris, Staphylococcal Scalded Skin Syndrome And Toxic Epidermal Necrosis (TEN)
- **Bulla spread** sign is +ve in pemphigus vulgaris.
- **Auspitz sign** is fine bleeding points after removal of scales seen in Psoriasis.
- **Darrier sign** is seen in urticaria Pigmentosa. There is itching, Erythema and edema
- Dermographism /Triple response of Lewis consists of Redness due to vasodilation, Axonal flare and wheal due to extravasation of fluid (RAW)
- Dimple sign is seen in Dermatofibroma.
- Tzanck test is demonstration of Tzanck cells (acantholytic cells) using Giemsa stain. These cells are seen in Herpes zoster, chicken Pox and Pemphigus.
- Apple Jelly nodules are seen in lupus vulgaris (cutaneous TB) and Sarcoidosis
- White dermatographism is seen in atopic dermatitis.
- Patch test is done for contact allergic Dermatitis.
- KOH examination with 10-20% KOH is used for all fungal infections.

BLISTERING DISEASE OF SKIN

Pemphigus Vulgaris

- It is an Intra epidermal break
- It is a supra basal break (occurs in stratum spinosum i.e. above stratum basale)
- It is auto immune disorder with production of IgG antibodies directed against **Desmoglein 3** that are cell adhesion molecules.
- It is the most common type of pemphigus. There is destruction of intracellular cementing substance with loss of cell adhesion molecules producing Acantholysis.
- It is a type II hypersensitivity reaction.

Clinical Features

- Seen in 4th–6th decade. The initial lesion are painful oral mucosal lesions
- Involvement of skin is in the form of non–itchy bullae over the face, scalp, axilla and trunk
- Bulla spread sign also k/a Asboe. Hansen sign is positive and Nikolsky's sign is +ve.
- The bullae ruptures to produce painful eruptions. Pemphigus may be associated with other autoimmune diseases like myasthenia gravis and malignancies like thymoma lymphoma etc.
- Tzanck smear shows Tzanck cells (Acantholytic cells)
- The basal keratinocytes remain attached to basement membrane and form Row of tombstone appearance.
- Immunofluorescence shows fish net pattern with deposition of IgG throughout the epidermis.

Pemphigus Vegetans

- It is a variant of pemphigus vulgaris effecting mainly the flexor areas.

Pemphigus Foliaceous

- It is a sub-corneal break characterized by IgG antibodies directed against Desmoglein -1.
- It is usually seen in seborrheic areas like scalp, face, etc.
- It does not have oral lesions.
- Nikolsky's sign is +ve
- Tzanck smear shows Tzanck cells.
- Immunofluorescence is similar to Pemphigus vulgaris.
- It has a better prognosis than Pemphigus Vulgaris.

Pemphigus Erythematosis

- It's a variant of pemphigus foliaceous having features of pemphigus and lupus Erythematosus.

R_x of Pemphigus

- Steroid pulse therapy (high dose) and antibiotics to prevent secondary infections.
- Drug induced pemphigus: it usually presents as pemphigus foliaceous. Commonly associated drugs are captopril, penicillamine, Rifampicin, penicillin, etc.

Bullous Pemphigoid

- Autoimmune disease with Antibodies (IgG) directed against the basement membrane hemi desmosomes
- It produces subepidermal break.

Clinical Features

Intense Itching with dense bullae especially on the flexor aspects, axilla, abdomen and groin.

- Facial skin and scalp are usually spared.
- The lesions rupture producing erosions and post inflammatory hyperpigmentation.
- Nikolsky's sign is usually negative and mucosal lesions are rare.
- It is commonly associated with gastric carcinoma, diabetes, Rheumatoid arthritis and psoriasis.
- Tzanck cells are not seen. Tzanck smear shows eosinophils.
- Immunofluorescence shows linear IgG and c3 deposits on basement membrane.
- Prognosis of Bullous pemphigoid is better than pemphigus.
- R_x: Systemic steroids.

Dermatitis Herpetiformis

- It is intensely pruritic chronic, recurrent, papulovesicular lesions with underlying gluten sensitive enteropathy
- This is the only condition of vesiculo bullous disease where papules can be seen.
- Usually occurs b/w 25-55 yrs symmetrical involvement with erythematous **papules vesicles.** involving mainly extensors of limbs (elbows and knees)
- Oral lesions are common. Oral lesions are worsened with oral iodides or by iodide patch testing
- Histological examination shows neutrophilic collection at tip of dermal papillae k/a Papillary Tip Abcess.
- Immunofluorescence is diagnostic and performed on normal skin preferably buttocks, shows granular IgA deposits in dermal papillae
- Anti basement antibodies are –ve but anti thyroid and anti gliadin antibodies are present

R_x

Dapsone and gluten free diet.

Herpes Gestationalis

- It is a nonviral autoimmune blistering disease of young women occurring during 21–28 weeks of gestation characterized by pruritis and blisters around Periumbilical area.
- Immunofluorescence shows linear C3 and IgG deposits along the basement membrane.

R_x:

Steroids.

CBDC: Chronic Bullous Dermatitis of Childhood

- It is an autoimmune sub epidermal blistering disease with **IgA** antibodies against the basement membrane.
- Onset is about 5 years of age characterized by perioral blisters with formation of String of Pearls or Cluster of Jewel appearance.
- Immunofluorescence shows linear IgA deposits on the basement membrane.

Psoriasis

- It is a scaling disorder of skin.
- A chronic relapsing inflammatory disorder with presence of erythema.
- Few papules and plaques covered by **silvery** micaceous scales
- They commonly involve extensors of elbows and Knees.
- Lesions tend to be symmetrical.
- Koebner's phenomenon is development of isomorphic lesions after trauma or itching at the uninvolved site.
- Psoriasis have variable pruritis.
- No known causative agent, multifactorial. Has a strong association with HLA CW_6
- HLA–B27 +ve is seen in 70% of patients with Psoriatic arthritis.
- There is rapid epidermal turnover within 3-4 days.
- Intracellular C-GMP levels are and c-AMP levels are ↓.

Types of Psoriasis

- Chronic plaque psoriasis is Mc type of Psoriasis.

Guttate Psoriasis

- Also called as Rain drop Psoriasis. It is seen in children and is precipitated by B-hemolytic streptococcal infections.

Pustular Psoriasis

- It is precipitated by steroidal withdrawal.

Erythrodermic Psoriasis

- In this 90% of skin is involved and is a dermatological emergency.

Precipitating Factors of Psoriasis

- Beta hemolytic streptococcal infection, HIV
- Drugs like Li, B-Blockers, NSAIDS and Iodides.

Inverse Psoriasis

- It is the one involving flexor surfaces. It usually does not producing scaling.

Nail changes in Psoriasis

- MC change is nail pitting.
- Earliest change is nail discoloration.
- Hyperkeratosis and nail dystrophy are present.
- onycholysis is breaking up of nails.

Psoriatic Arthritis

- It is a sero –ve arthritis, oligo articular involving the DIP joints.
- It is erosive arthritis producing pencil in cup deformity.
- Telescopic sign of DIP is +ve.
- Sausage shaped fingers and toes.
- There is involvement of Achilles tendon usually asymmetrical.
- Only about 5% of Psoriasis patients develop Psoriatic arthritis.

Diagnosis

- It is made by clinical characteristics and skin biopsy of the lesion site.
- Histopathology shows parakeratosis, hyperkeratosis, there is elongation of rete ridges, loss of granular cell layer k/a Agranulosis and suprapapillary thinning of epithelium.
- There is intra epidermal presence of neutrophils k/a munro–microabcess.
- There is **Acanthosis.**
- Dilated capillaries are seen in the dermis that are responsible for Auspitz sign. The scales are easily removed in the form of white shining membrane k/a grattage test.

R_x

- Topical steroids [systemic Steroids are C/I in Psoriasis].
- Coal tar has anti inflammatory and anti–mitotic activity and is used in Psoriasis.
- Goeckerman regimen is UV light + coal tar.
- Ingram regimen is UV light + Anthralin.
- PUVA therapy is psoralen + UV A light.
- Immunosuppressants like methotrexate, cyclosporine, mycophenolate.
- Tacrolimus also k/a FK-506 is a T cell modulator.
- Other agents used are Infliximab, Etanercept.
- Retinoids are used in R_x of Pustular Psoriasis.

Impetigo Herpetiformis

- It is pustular Psoriasis in Pregnancy and is treated by giving steroids.
- Indications for Methotrexate therapy in Psoriasis.
- Psoriatic arthritis, Erythrodermic Psoriasis and chronic plaque Psoriasis not responding to R_x.

Lichen Planus

- It's a papulo-squamous scaling disorder characterized by pruritic, polygonal, purple, plain topped papules.
- Etiology is not known, may be associated with Hep B and Hep C virus.
- There could be Pterygium of the nail.
- It commonly involves flexor areas of the wrist, lower back and oral mucosa.
- Scalp is involved leading to hair loss.
- Mucosal Lesions are present as white reticular laces.
- Wickham's Striae is a network of greyish lines characteristic of Lichen planus.
- Nail changes are seen in 10% of patients, it consists of Pterygium formation, longitudinal ridges, splitting of nail plate and onychodystrophy. Involvement of hair produces Cicatricial Alopecia (Scarring Alopecia).

- Diagnosis is made by clinical features i.e. Hyperkeratosis, Hypergranulosis, Acanthosis, Basal cell degeneration produces Civatte bodies and Max Joseph Space. There is a band like infiltration of Lymphocytes at dermo-epidermal junction.
- There is saw toothing of Rete–Ridges.

R_x

- It undergoes spontaneous remission. Topical steroids are mainstay of R_x.
- Topical soothing agents, Vit A derivative, Anti histaminics are also used.
- Oral Dapsone is used for oral Lichen Planus.

Pityriasis Rosea

- It is a papulosquamous disorder seen in children common during spring and fall.
- There is a Herald patch with fine scaling, fine cigarette paper like collaret of scales.
- They have truncal predilection (Christmas tree pattern).

R_x

- No R_x required, it is self limiting.

KERATINIZATION DISORDERS

Ichthyosis

- It's a Keratinization disorder which can be hereditary or acquired characterized by scaling.
- Hereditary Ichthyosis.
- M.C is Ichthyosis vulgaris, autosomal dominant condition involving.
- Extensors surfaces while flexor surfaces like cubital fossa and popliteal fossa are spared.
- X-linked recessive Ichthyosis is common in males and is due to deficiency of sterol sulfatase.
- Lamellar ichthyosis is present at birth and is called collodion baby. or Alligator Boy. There are large thick scales covering the entire body.

Refsum's Disease

- It is due to deficiency of Phytanic acid oxidase, characterized by cutaneous and neurologic manifestations due to accumulation of phytanic acid.
- Skin lesions are similar to Ichthyosis and neurological symptoms include cerebellar Ataxia and Sensory neural deafness.

Acquired Ichthyosis

- It is seen in patients of Hodgkin's Lymphoma, Malabsorption and internal malignancies.

R_x

Emollients are used to remove the scales.

- Topical salicylic acid application which is keratinolytic and oral retinoids.

Pityriasis Rubra Pilaris

- It is characterized by epidermal over activity near hair follicles.
- There is follicular hyper keratosis, Palmo–plantar keratoderma.
- Salmon colored patch over trunk and extremities with areas of uninvolved skin in between.

R_x

Retinoid, Steroids and Methotrexate.

Darrier's Disease

- It is dyskeratosis with dirty, greasy, wart-like papules in the seborrheic areas.
- There is V shape splitting of nails. Presence of corps and Ronds.

R_x

- Retinoids.

Alopecia

- Physiological hair loss is 100/day.
  - Scarring Alopecia
- Its seen due to Burns, Radiations, Mechanical trauma, infections like kerion, favus and also Lichen planus, DLE (discoid)
  - Nonscaling alopecia
    - Androgenetic alopecia
    - Telogen Effluvium
    - Anagen Effluvium
    - Trichotillo mania
    - Alopecia areata.

Androgenetic alopecia (physiological process not a disease) also k/a male pattern baldness. Seen in genetically predisposed. The terminal hair are transformed into vellus hair, this is k/a miniaturization.

- R_x: Minoxidil, finasteride
  - Surgical correction

Alopecia Areata is an auto Immune disease occurs due to viral infection or emotional stress. There is smooth bald patch over eyebrows, scalp or beard. Exclamation mark is present in Alopecia areata.

Trichotillomania occurs in psychologically disturbed females usually in age group 11-17 yrs. The patient twists the hair and pulls it deliberately. The alopecia covers the entire scalp except the margins. It is also called tonsure alopecia / or entrich sign.

Telogen Effluvium is shedding of hair > 100 per day seen in patient undergoing surgeries anemias, acute febrile illness, endocrine disorders

- Hair loss usually occurs 2-3 months after the trigger and there is usually recovery after 6 months.
  - R_x : Assurance and Minoxidil

Anagen effluvium is loss of hair even in Anagen phase seen in patient undergoing cancer therapy.

- Traction Alopecia is seen in females keeping tight pony tail.
- Alopecia Steatoidis is non-scarring occurring due to dandruff.

ACNE

- Acne patient secretes more sebum than normal people.
- Its primarily disease of sebaceous follicles. Occurs mc in adolescents.
- It consists of polymorphic lesion like pustules, comedones, papules.

Pathogenesis of Acne

- ↑ Sebum production, hypercornification of sebaceous duct, microbial infection and inflammation.
- Open comedones are k/a Blackheads

Closed comedones are k/a white heads.

- Comedones represent hyper proliferating ductal Keratinocytes.
- Propionobacter, Malasezzia furfur and staph epidermidis are sometimes isolated.

- Acne is not infectious, predominantly occurs over the face.
- Infraorbital area is usually spared.
- Comedones are pathognomic for Acne.

R_x

- Comedolytic agents like Tretinoin (Retinoids), Adapalene.
- Anti-microbial creams like Benzyl Peroxidase, Erythromycin, and clindamycin.
- Systemic antibiotics like oral Minocycline, Doxycycline and Erythromycin are used.
- Adapalene has good anti-inflammatory activity.
- Isotretinoin is preferred for nodular acne, avoided in pregnancy and lactating women.
- Acne surgeries: Comedo extraction, aspiration of cyst, incision and drainage, intra-steroid injections with Triamcinolone.
- Latest techniques include laser abrasion and Derma abrasion and laser peeling.

Rosacea

- It's a Centro facial disease papulopustular lesions on an erythematous background.
- Its characterized by Telangiectasia, flushing.
- There is hyperplasia and enlargement of sebaceous glands esp. of nose k/a Rhinopyma.

Urticaria/Hives

Its transient, erythematous, edematous eruptions of Dermis.

- Usually associated with Itching.
- Main chemical mediator is histamine.

Angio edema/Quinke's Edema

- It caused due to deficiency of c1 esterase inhibitor.
- Urticaria involving subcutaneous tissues, involving genitalia, lips, eyelids. Involvement of tongue and larynx gives acute onset.
- Itching is absent.

Urticaria Pigmentosa

- It is cutaneous mastocytosis presenting as itchy skin lesions with Erythema and Edema k/a Darriers Sign.
- Histological exam shows mast cell infiltration in dermis.

Pellagra

- Its due to deficiency of Niacin.
- Four D"s of Pellagra are Dermatitis, Dementia, Diarrhea, and Death if untreated.
- Skin lesions in pellagra are symmetrical photosensitive skin eruptions.
- An erythematous rash involving dorsum of hand.
- K/a glove / gauntlet of pellagra.
- On the face it produces lesions similar to LE (lupus).
- Eruption on neck appears like a necklace k/a casal necklace. Also k/a cravat.

Acrodermatitis Enteropathica

- It's due to deficiency of Zinc. It presents with Dermatitis, Alopecia and Diarrhea esp. When baby is shifted from Breast milk to cow's milk.
- There is perioriphyseal acral dermatitis, alopecia and diarrhea
  - Rx : Zinc

Pie Baldism

- Its autosomal dominant condition characterized by white forelock and amelanotic vitiligo like macules.
- Hyper pigmented macules within amelanotic areas can be seen in Pie baldism.

Waardenburg Syndrome

Its autosomal dominant condition with white forelocks, hypomelanotic macules, congenital deafness and Heterochromia iridis.

Albinism

- It's due to deficiency of enzyme tyrosinase. Its autosomal recessive disorder.
- There is reduced synthesis of melanin in melanocytes.

Vitiligo

- Its milky white cutaneous macules devoid of melanocytes.

Pathogenesis

- Multifactorial, auto antibodies to Melanocytes, Genetic factors and other mechanisms.
- Typical vitiligo has a white colored patch with scalloped margins. Disease is usually progressive.
- Mucosal involvement is common in vitiligo.

Associated with Vitiligo

- It is associated with other autoimmune diseases like type I diabetes, Pernicious anemia, Auto immune Thyroiditis, scleroderma, collagen vascular disorders, Alopecia Aerate.

R_x

- PUVA therapy i.e. [UVA + Psoralen).
- Corticosteroids.
- Immunomodulators like Azathioprine and cyclosporine.
- Antioxidants.
- Surgical management should be done only in stable vitiligo by punch grafting and split skin grafting.

Melasma

- Its hyper pigmentation seen in pregnancy also k/a chloasma.

Eczematous Lesions of Skin

- Eczema is inflammatory response of the skin characterized by Erythema
- Vesiculation occur during acute episode.
- Scaling and lichenification in chronic stages.
- Vesiculation is an important feature of Eczema.
- Histologically Eczema shows spongiosis, Acanthosis, perivascular lymphocytic infiltration.

Classification of Eczema

Exogenous: Contact irritant dermatitis, contact allergic dermatitis ; Infective Eczema

Endogenous: Atopic dermatitis, Seborrheic dermatitis.

Nummular Dermatitis, stasis eczema,

Asteatotic eczema (xerotic eczema), Discoid

Eczema, Hand eczema, Pityriasis Alba.

CONTACT IRRITANT DERMATITIS

- Its characterized by burning sensation limited to area of contact.
- The 1st step is Vesiculation.
- Common irritants include detergents, alkalis, acids, soaps.
- Common in people working in printing, painting, hair dressing, agricultural, medicinal professions.

Clinical Features

- There is erythema, vesicular bullous lesions, crustations in acute cases.
- Lichenification (thickening of epithelium) and scaling in chronic cases.

Contact Allergic Dermatitis

- Occurs after a long contact with Allergen.
- There is severe itching going beyond the area of contact.
- Common allergens include rubber, dyes, and cosmetics.

Clinical Features

- Erythema, Swelling, Lichenification with constant Itching.
- MC recognized form is Photodermatitis. Other forms include Photodermatitis.
- Demeclocycline causes Tanning.

Atopic Dermatitis

- Type I hypersensitivity reaction.

Patient has predisposition to develop asthma, allergic rhinitis along with Atopic dermatitis

- 70% of pat have a positive family history. There is eosinophilia in blood.
- It usually manifests in 1st year of life and 90% of time within 5 years.

Major Criteria

- Itching
- Typical Morphology and distribution
- Chronic and relapsing
- Positive family history.

Minor Criteria

- Dry Skin.
- Double infra orbital fold k/a 'Dennie Morgan fold'.
- There is pallor about nose, ear, eyes, its k/a Headlight sign.
- Increased susceptibility to cutaneous infection of staphylococcus Aureus and HSV.
  - White dermatographism is seen with Atopic Dermatitis.
  - Patients can have keratoconus, Pityriasis Alba and other food allergies esp. sea food.
  - Wool and synthetic fibers can exaggerate the lesions.
  - Diagnosis is mainly clinical with a history of asthma.

R_x

- Tacrolimus / picrolimus which is a T cell modifier is DOC.
- Antibiotics for secondary infections.
- Topical steroids.

Seborrheic Dermatitis

- It is chronic erythematous lesions covered by greasy scales. (Stuck on appearene)
- The area of distribution is distinctive, involving scalp, face near the foreheads, eyebrows at upper trunk (sternum and scapula)
- Dandruff is earliest manifestation of seborrheic Dermatitis. Also k/a Pityriasis capitis
- In the infant it could form a cradle cap.

R_x

- Selenium Sulphide
- Itching is prominent feat
- Topical steroids
- Oral Ketoconazole/Itraconazole.

Nummular Eczema/Discoid Eczema

- In these there is single circular Eczema Plague with clearly demarcated edge (coin like lesions):
  - Mainly present on trunks and extensor surface of limbs.

Stasis Eczema

- Occurs in patients with venous incompetence / chronic Edema
- Primarily involving lower limbs in patients of Varicose veins
- Hyperpigmentation of lesion due to Extravasation of blood and Hemosiderin pigment.

R_x

- Elevation of leg.
- Compression stockings.
- Steroids should be cautiously used ,as they delay healing.

Asteatotic Eczema

- Also k/a Xerotic (dry) Eczema / Winter Itch/Eczema craculae
- Lack of skin surface lipids
- Lower leg is commonly inv and MC in elderly.

Hand Eczema

- It's confined to the hands. Pompholyx is crops of clear vesicles with itching developing in palms.

Pityriasis Alba

- Nonspecific superficial dermatitis of unknown origin and can be associated with Atopic dermatitis
- Initially presents with round plaques over the face which on healing produce hypo pigmented scaly patch.

Naevi

- They are congenital lesions / birth marks.
- Melanocytic Naevi are benign tumors derived from melanocyte. They are further classified into junctional naevi, compound naevi and dermal naevi.
- Junctional Naevi are proliferative nevus cells at derma-epidermal junc.
- If the Junctional nevus extends into dermis we call it compound naevi.
- If Junctional component resolves leaving on Dermal part its k/a Intradermal Nevus.

Rx

Surgical excision.

Mongolian Spot

- Mongolian spots are dermal nevus that prod blue greyish macular pigmentation usually seen on sacral region at birth
- They resolve spontaneously on 1st decade of life so no R_x required.

Infantile Hemangioma

- Its benign vascular tumor with high incidence on infancy.
- Mc site for Infantile hemangioma is head and neck.

Salmon Patch

- Its capillary dilatations seen in neonatal period involving nape of neck.

Port Wine Stain

- Its seen Sturge Weber synd.
- Associated with Ipsilateral Leptomeningeal vascular abnormalities, epilepsy, hemiplegia and ipsilateral choroidal lesions.

Glomus Tumor

- Its neuromyo arterial receptor (glomus body tumor)
- These tumors are common on fingers and toes and beneath the nail plates.
- These receptors detect temp changes and regulate Arterial blood flow.

Clinical Features

- Isolated nodule on nail bed with Paroxysmal pain elicited by changes in temp.

R_x

Simple excision is R_x of choice.

Mycosis Fungoides

- Its cutaneous T cell Lymphoma.
- Pruritus is an important Symptom.
- Histology reveals atypical lymphocytes in the epidermis. Pautrier's micro abscess is pathognomic feature.

REACTIVE SKIN DISEASE

Erythema Multiformis

- Its caused by circulating immune complexes (Type III Hypersensitivity reaction). Herpes viruses are strongly associated. Other causes include Mycoplasma, Isoniazid, Anti Epileptic drugs and Malignancies.
- Its common in young adults and pres as vesicles, bullae and target lesions.
- Target lesion / Bull's eye / Iris Lesion has 3 zones a) A central dark zone surrounded by edematous zone and peripheral surrounding edema. It has a centrifugal spread.

R_x

Symptomatic. R_x: give Acyclovir if Herpes is suspected.

Steven–Johnson Syndrome and TEN: (Toxic epidermal necrosis)

- They are acute mucocutaneus intolerance reactions.
- They are caused mainly by drugs and infections

- In SJs the mucosal erosions are < 10%
- In TEN the mucosal erosions are > 30%
- Drugs associated c SJS are sulfonamides, Phenytoin Penicillin, NSAID's and phenobarbitone etc.
- Ulcerative stomatitis and hemorrhagic crusting are the most characteristic features.

R_x

- Withdraw the drug
- Supportive care
- Steroids.

TEN

- It's a life threatening disease characterised by sheets of Erythema, necrosis and epidermal bullae.
- Nickolsky's sign +ve.
- Mucosal and conjunctival erosions are common.
- Septicemia is M/c cause of death in TEN.
- There is sub-epidermal break in TEN.
- In staphylococcal scolded skin syndrome there is sub corneal break.
- The skin lesions in TEN are erythematous, necrotic with wetness.
- In SSSS skin lesions are dry and parchment like with absence of mucosal lesion.

R_x

- Intensive care management c fluid maintenance and electrolyte balance.
- IV Immunoglobulins are helpful but steroids are CI

Erythroderma

- It's also k/a Exfoliative dermatitis.
- Its inflammatory skin disorder affecting > 90% causes are Eczema, Psoriasis and certain drugs like gold, mercury, arsenic, Rifampicin and Isoniazid.
- There is generalized edema with scarring
- It can be seen with cancers like Leukemias and Lymphomas.
- It involves large scales with generalized erythema and scarring.

R_x

- ICU management
- Electrolyte and fluid balance
- Methotrexate is started in Erythrodermic Psoriasis.

Drug Eruptions

- They are sudden in onset, bilateral symmetrical c history of drug intake.
- General rules of drug eruptions :
  - Greatest potency to drug allergies is by Topical route.
  - Common in older people.
  - There is regression of drug eruption on drug withdrawal
  - They are pruritic and similar lesions reappear on re-exposure to drugs.

Fixed Drug Eruptions

- They occur at fixed sites. They are single or multiple c burning sensation.
- Usually unilateral and heal by grayish pigmentation
- Mucocutaneous junctions are often involved.

- FDE can be seen by sulfonamides, Dapsone, captopril, Tetracycline and Phenopthalin.
- The drug started with in one week of onset of eruption is most imp suspect.
- In vivo testing for drug allergies include patch testing and challenge re challenge test.
- In vitro testing is done by radio allego-sorbent assay (RAST), ELISSA, etc.

STD'S

Pathogen	Disease
Treponema Palladium	Syphilis (chancre)
Haemophilus Ducreyi	Chancroid (Chancre like)
Chlamydia Trachomatis	Lympho granuloma Venerum (LGV). Urethritis, Endocervicitis, Pelvic inflammatory disease (PID), Reiter's Syndrome (Reactive arthritis)
Calymmatobacterium granulomatosis	Donovanosis (Granuloma inguinale)
N. Gonorhoea	Gonorrhoea, urethritis
Human Papilloma Virus (HPV)	Anogenital and oral warts (condyloma acuminata)
HSV (Herpes Simplex)	Herpes Genitalia.
Hep B and D	Active and chronic Hepatitis.
HIV	AIDS
Trichomonas Vaginalis	Vaginitis.
Gardnerella	Bacterial Vaginosis.

Chancroid (soft Chancre)

- Its caused by Haemophilus Ducreyi, they are multiple painful ulcers with deep ulceration 3-4 weeks after exposure.
- The ulcer is soft, nonindurated.
- Produces painful, inguinal lymphadenitis k/a Inflammatory Bubo.

Diagnosis

- H. ducreyi forms pool school of fish of gram –ve cocobacilli in the smear taken from ulcer or from the pus from the bubo.
- R_x: Ceftriaxone i.m or Azithromycin 1 gm single oral dose.or alternative is Doxycycline if chlamydia is suspected.

LGV

- Its caused by chlamydia Trachomatis L1, L2, L3
- It has incubation period of 3-30 days produces painless papules / pustules forming asymptomatic, herpetigenous ulcer.
- The ulcer heals without scarring.
- After 2-6 weeks of primary lesions, a 2nd stage, the inguinal stage appears consisting of painful inflammation of inguinal and femoral lymph nodes (painful lymphangitis and lymphadenitis).
- There are enlarged lymph nodes above and below the inguinal ligament producing the sign of groove.
- These heal with ulcerations and puckered scars
- The 3rd stage is k/a genitorectal syndrome occurring a year or 2 later prod genital elephantiasis, proctitis, rectal abscess and strictures.
- Diagnosis is made by isolation of organism on culture.

R_x

- Doxycycline 100mg a day for 21 days.

Granuloma Inguinale (Donovanosis)

- Its caused by Calymmatobacterium granulomatosis a gram –ve obligate intracellular bacillus.
- It prod multiple, painless, beefy red ulcerations with distinct raised rolled up margins after an incubation period of 8-12 days weeks.
- There is enlargement in inguinal region due to subcutaneous granulomas that arise superficially k/a PseudoBubo
- The Beefy red ulcer bleeds on touch.
- Diagnosis: There is presence of intracytoplasmic inclusion bodies k/a Donovan/safety-pin bodies in histiocytes

R_x

- Doxycycline / cotrimoxazole.

Herpes Genitalis

- HSV is MCC of genital ulcerations
- Incubation period is 3-4 days. There is prod of small grouped vesicles that progress and break to ulcerative lesion.
- Painful inguinal lymphadenopathy can occur

R_x

- Acyclovir

Gonorrhea

- It's a gram –ve diplococcus seen with in PN\N (neutrophils) acute anterior urethritis is mc manifestation of gonococcal infection in men and is usually asymptomatic in women.
- Predominant symptoms are mucopurulent urethral discharge from the urethral meatus, dysuria epididymitis. Prostatitis and seminal vesiculitis.
- Testis is usually spared (never inv)
- In females it rarely manifests and can lead to mucopurulent cervical discharge, ascending infection, pelvic inflammatory disease can occur.
- Ophthalmia neonatorum occurs due to perinatal transmission (usually on 2nd day)

Diagnosis

- Identification of gonococci from urethral discharge.
- Pres of more than 5 pus cells per oil emulsion indicates.
- Pres of gram –ve diplococci in pus cells.

R_x

- Ceftriaxone (single I.M dose). If oral 400 mg.
- Nongonococcal urethritis is caused by Ureaplasma and Chlamydia Trachomatis.

R_x

- Doxycycline/Azithromycin.

Fitz Hugh Curtis Syndrome

- **It is perihepatitis with Pelvic inflammatory disorder caused by Chlamydia/gonorrhea presents with upper abdominal pain and violin string adhesions over the liver on laparoscopy.**

- Bacterial Vaginosis
- It's caused by Gardnerella.
- Presence of clue cells, vaginal P^{H}> 2.5, +ve Whiff test on KOH.
- Absence of Lactobacilli

R_x

- Metronidazole. (Does not usually require Partner treatment).

DIFFERENTIAL DIAGNOSIS OF GENITAL ULCERS

Features	Syphilis (1° chancre)	Chancroid	LGV	Donovanosis (Granuloma inguinale)	Herpes genitalis
Organism	Treponema palladium	Hemophilus ducreyi	Chlamydia trachomatis (L1, L2, L3)	Calymmato bacterium granulomatosis	Herpes simplex virus type II (rarely type I)
Incubation period	9-90 days	1-14 days	3 days-6 weeks	1-4 wks (upto 6 months)	2-7 days
No. of attacks	Only one (1)	1 or 2	Only one (1)	Only one (1)	Recurrent
No. of lesions	Usually 1	Usually multiple may coalesce	Usually 1	Variable	Multiple, may coalesce
Early 1° lesion Diameter Depth Edges	Papule 5-15 mm superficial or deep sharply demarcated, elevated, round/oval	Pustule Variable Excavated Undermined, ragged, irregular	Papule, Pustule 2-10 mm Superficial or deep Elevated, round or oval	Papule Variable Elevated Elevated, irregular serpiginous	Vesicle 1-2 mm Superficial Erythematous
Base	Smooth, non-purulent , non-vascular	Purulent, bleeds easily	Variable nonvascular	Red and velvety (beefy red), bleeds easily with exuberant granulation tissue	Serous, Erythematous, Nonvascular
Induration	Firm	Soft	Occasionally	Firm	None
Pain	Uncommon	Usually very tender	Variable	Uncommon	Frequently tender
Lymphadenopathy	Firm, non tender, shotty, bilateral	Tender, may suppurate, loculat ed, usually unilateral (Bubo)	Tender, may suppurate, loculated, usually unilateral (Bubo)	No lymphandenopathy pseudo buboes (subcutaneous nodules in inguinal region, may ulcerate)	Firm, tender often bilateral
Diagnosis	- Dark field Microscopy - Serological tests	-Clinical features -Gram staining (gram-ve cocco-bacilli with rail road appearance)	- Demonstration of LGV as elementary and inclusion bodies - Frie's test - Hyper gamma-globulinemia - Complement fixation +ve	- Tissue smear and histopathological microscopy show 1. Donovan bodies 2. Safety pin appearance	- Multinucleated giant cell on Tzanck smear - Culture is confirmatory
Treatment	Penicillins/ Doxycycline/ tetracycline	- Azithro/ erythromycin - Ceftriaxone - Ciprofloxacin	- Doxy/ tetracycline - Erythromycin	Doxycycline/ tetracycline Azithromycin/ erythromycin (in pregnancy)	Acyclovir

SCABIES

EPIDEMIOLOGY

- Infestation caused by Acarus hominis /Sarcoptes scabies
- Incubation period is 2-4 weeks
- Itching worse at night is most common symptom
- Family history of similar itchy eruptions in close contact

MORPHOLOGY

Primary Lesions

- **Burrow: serpentine (S- shaped) path traversed by parasite in stratum corneum. It is pathognomic lesion.**
- **Papules** and papulo-Vesicles: Are due to hypersensitivity to the mite
- **Fine pin head size follicular papules**

Secondary Lesions

- Pustules due to 2° infection is one of commonest form of presentation
- **Eczematized crusted lesion,** in infants and children are predominant lesions
- **Nodular lesion** are seen on scrotum (m.c.), groin, and anterior axillary fold (N odular scabies).

Variants / Types

- **Crusted Norwegian scabies** is most severe form seen in immune compromised or mentally ill patients, and showing hyperkeratotic crusted lesion on whole body.
- **Scabies incognito** is wrongly treated with steroids.

TREATMENT

- Drug choice: Permethrin (1st) BHC (2nd)
- Oral drug (only): Ivermectin
- Other drugs: Benzyl benzoate 25%, Crotamiton 10%, Malathion, monosulfiram
- In secondary infection: IV antibiotics
- Drug safe in pregnancy and infants <2 months: Precipitated sulfur 5-10%
- Scabicides should be applied to the whole body (below jaw line in adults) to all members of family whether symptomatic or not
- Itching may last for several days and does not require retreatment with Scabicides. Antihistamines are usually adequate
- In unworn clothes, mites die within 7 days.

PEDICULOSIS

- **Macula cerula** (bluish stain on the skin d/t louse bite) **is a typical lesion of Pediculosis**
- **P. capitis (Head louse):** Involves scalp
- **P. Corporis (Body louse):**
  - Causes **vagabond disease.**
  - Macula cerulean is a typical lesion of pediculosis
  - The body louse is responsible for transmission of epidemic typhus, which is due to Ricketessia prowazeki, as well as trench fever and relapsing fever due to Borrelia recurrentis
  - Rx is disinfection of clothes with 10% DDT or 1% Gamma Benzene Hexachloride (BHC or Gamexine)+pediculocide drug application
  - P. Publis (Pubic louse): Is a STD

MOLLUSCUM CONTAGIOSUM

- Caused by virus of pox virus group, transmitted by skin to skin contact and is a STD
- Typical lesion is pink or skin coloured, umbilicated papule containing a grayish central plug
- Face and genitals are commonly involved. Face is most commonly involved in children. And in children groins and genitals are not affected which are usually involved in sexual active adults
- Pathology: Cup shaped epidermal thickening with characteristic degenerative change in granular cell layer and Molluscum bodies on giemsa stain is pathognomic
- Spontaneously resolved after squeezing, curettage, cautery and salicylic acid application.

T. Barbae also called **barber's itch or Tinea sycosis**, caused by T. Mentagrophytes and T. Verruscosum.

TINEA INFECTIONS

Tinea capitis	Microsporum cains or Trichophyton tonsurans	Boggy swelling on scalp with easily pluck hair (kerion)
Tinea corporis	Microsporum, trichophyton	Infection of glabrous or non-hairy skin of the body
Tinea cruris	E.Floccosum T.R ubrum and T. Mentagrophytes	Infection of groin thigh, perineum, perianal area (ringworm of groin/jock itch), adults Males most commonly affected
Tinea pedis		Ringworm of feet (athlete foot), common in shoe and socks wearers
Tinea unguium	T.rubrum	Tie nail mainly involved, involves soft keratin of nail bed and later nail plate (hard keratin)

- **Tinea manuum:** Less common, chronic from, usually involves one palm only, which is usually dull red with silver scales in the palmar creases due to T. rubrum.
- **Tinea incognito:** Extensive ringworm with an atypical appearance due to the inappropriate use of topical corticosteroids.
- **Tinea nigra:** Superficial fungal infection of the stratum corneum caused by Hortaea (Ex ophiala or phaeoannellomyces) werneckii, occurring more commonly in tropical climiates.

Previous Years Questions

Answers are based on references from

- Rook's Dermatology, Essentials in Dermatology, 2nd edition
- Robbins Pathologic Basic of Diseases, 8th edition and Harrison's Online
- Thappa DM, Essentials in Dermatology, 2nd edition
- Nelson Textbook of Pediatrics, 19th ed

QUESTIONS

1. Lepra type 2 reaction is a type of which hypersensitivity reaction? (2014)

a. Type 1 hypersensitivity reaction
b. Type 2 hypersensitivity reaction
c. Type 3 hypersensitivity reaction
d. Type 4 hypersensitivity reaction

2. Most common organism causing Tinea capitis is: (2014)

a. Trichophyton mentagranophyte
b. Trichosporum schleoni
c. Trichosporum tonsurans
d. Trichosporum sudanense

3. Acute contact dermatitis is best treated with: (2014)

a. Cream
b. Ointment
c. Emulsion
d. Moist compress

4. Which is not a fungal infection? (2014)

a. Favus
b. Mycosis fungoides

c. Kerion
d. Piedra

5. Most common subtype of melanoma is:
a. Lentiginous (2014)
b. Superficial spreading
c. Amelanotic
d. Nodular

6. Frie's skin test used to diagnose: (2014)
a. Syphilis
b. Granuloma inguinale
c. LGV
d. Herpes genitalis

7. Donova body is found in: (2013)
a. Granuloma inguinale
b. Lymphogranuloma venereum
c. Chlamydia
d. Chancroid

8. Keratoderma blenorrhagica is found in:
a. Reiters syndrome (2013)
b. Psoriasis
c. Lichen Planus
d. Bechet syndrome

9. Wickham striae is present in: (2013)
a. Lichen Planus
b. Psoriasis
c. Pityriasis rosea
d. Eczema

10. Indurated seminal vesicle is characteristic of:
a. TB (2013)
b. Syphilis
c. Gonorrhea
d. Chlamydia

11. Origin of melanocyte cell causing melanoma is:
a. Neural crest cells (2013)
b. Mesoderm
c. Ectoderm
d. Endoderm

12. All are true regarding Tinea versicolor except: (2013)
a. Orange fluorescence in Wood lamp examination
b. Caused by Malessesia globosa
c. Griseofulvin is the drug of choice
d. Both hypo and hyperpigmented lesions

13. Eye lash infestation by pediculosis is caused by:
a. Pediculosis capitis (2012)
b. Pediculosis corporis
c. Pthirus pubis
d. Hymenoptera

14. Acute paronychia is commonly treated by:
a. I and D (2012)
b. Partial nail avulsion
c. Total nail avulsion
d. 'Nail bed destruction

15. Most common variety of malignant melanoma:
a. Superficial spreading (2012)
b. Nodular type
c. Lentiginous type
d. Alentiginous

16. Koebner's phenomenon is not seen in:
a. Vitiligo (2012)
b. Psoriasis
c. Dermatitis herpertiformis
d. Lichen planus

17. How many bacilli should be there in the tissue for slit skin smear to be positive for Hansen's disease?
a. 10 baccili/ gram of tissue (2012)
b. 10(2) baccili/ gram of tissue
c. 10(3) baccili/gram of tissue
d. 10(4) baccili/gram of tissue

18. Malignant pustule is caused by:
a. Anthrax
b. Pseudomonas infection
c. Bacillary angiomatosis
d. Erysipeloid

19. Antibiotics are indicated in which type of psoriasis?
a. Guttate (2012)
b. Pustular
c. Chronic plaque psoriasis
d. Erythrodermic psoriasis

20. Drug of choice for type II Lepra Reaction is:
a. Thalidomide (2011)
b. Steroids
c. Clofazamine
d. Rifampicin

21. A young lady presents with white lacy lesions in oral cavity and her proximal nail fold has extended onto the nail bed. What is the likely diagnosis? (2011)
a. Psoriasis
b. Geographic tongue
c. Lichen planus
d. Candidiasis

22. Fishnet appearance in immunoflorescence is seen in:
a. Pemphigus vulgaris (2010)
b. Bullous pemphigoid
c. Dermatitis herpetiformis
d. Darier disease

23. A22-year-old sexually active male presents with painful, foul smelling genital ulcer which bleeds easily to touch and has excessive granulation tissue. What is the most probable diagnosis?
a. Chancroid (2010)
b. Herpes
c. Syphilis
d. Donovaniosis

24. Vitiligo is most commonly associated with:
a. Diabetes mellitus (2010)
b. Addisons disease
c. Hypothyroidism
d. Diabetes insipidus

25. PUVA treatment is not used in: (2010)
a. Melasma
b. Vitiligo
c. Psoriasis
d. Cutaneous T cell lymphoma

26. Leukonychia is seen in: (2010)
a. Hypoalbuminemia
b. Onycomycosis
c. Lead Poisoning
d. Psoriasis

27. All are seen in dermatoyositis except: (2010)
a. Calcinosis cutis
b. Heliotropic rash
c. Shawl sign
d. Gottron's rash

28. Epidermolysis bullosa is due to: (2009)
a. Autoimmune disease
b. Atopic disease
c. Infective agent
d. Genetic fragility of skin

29. Ridley-Jopling classification includes all except:
a. Lepromatous leprosy (2009)
b. Borderline borderline
c. Tuberculoid
d. Neuritic

30. Most common nerve affected in leprosy is:
a. Radial nerve (2009)
b. Ulnar nerve
c. Median nerve
d. Axillary nerve

31. Apple jelly nodules are seen in: (2009)
a. Ichthyosis
b. Lichen planus
c. Lupus vulgaris
d. Lupus erythematous

32. Not a fungal infection is: (2008)
a. Mycoses fungoides
b. Tinea nigra Palmaris
c. White Piedra
d. Black Piedra

33. Dermatitis herpeteformis is associated with:
a. Gluten sensitive enteropathy (2008)
b. Celiac disease
c. Protein losing enteropathy
d. Whipple's disease

34. Vesicular lesion is seen in: (2008)
a. Primary syphilis
b. Secondary syphilis
c. Tertiary syphilis
d. Congenital syphilis

35. In chronic folliculitis the treatment of choice is:
a. Topical antibiotics (2008)
b. Systemic antibiotics
c. Both A and C
d. Surgery

36. Condyloma accuminatum is produced by which type of papilloma virus? (2008)
a. HPV 6,16
b. HPV 6,11
c. HPV 16,18
d. HPV 11,18

37. Herald patch is seen in: (2008)
a. Pityriasis rosea
b. Lichen planus
c. DLE
d. Reiter syndrome

38. A 20-year-old woman with past history of enteric fever 4 months back presents with diffuse hair loss for 1 month. The likely causes is:
a. Androgenic alopecia
b. Telogen effluvium
c. Anageneffuvium
d. Alopecia areata

39. Scabies in children differs from that in adults in that it affects: (2007)
a. Webspace
b. Face
c. Genitalia
d. Axilla

40. A smear from a genital lesion shows Donovan bodies. The diagnosis is: (2007)
a. Lymphogranuloma venerium
b. Chancroid
c. Granuloma inguinale
d. Syphilis

41. In urticaria pigmentosa, the cell most commonly seen in skin on microscopy is: (2007)
a. Mast cell
b. Langerhan's cell

c. Plasma cells
d. Lymphocytes

42. **Koebner's phenomenon is seen in all the following except: (2007)**
a. Lichen planus
b. Psoriasis
c. Warts
d. Pityriasis rosea

43. **Airborne contact dermatitis can be diagnosed by:**
a. Skin biopsy (2007)
b. Patch test
c. Prick test
d. Estimation of serum IgE levels

44. **How many bacilli should be there in the tissue for slit skin smear to be positive for Hansen's disease? (2007)**
a. 10 baccili / gram of tissue
b. 10^2 bacilli/ gram of tissue
c. 10^3 bacilli / gram of tissue
d. 10^4bacilli / gram of tissue

45. **Fishnet appearance in immunoflorescence is seen in: (2007)**
a. Pemphigus vulgaris
b. Bullous pemphigoid
c. Dermatitis herpetiformis
d. Darier disease

46. **Gottron's papules are seen in: (2006)**
a. Dermatomyositis
b. Scleroderma
c. Mixed connective tissue disorder
d. Pemphigus vulgaris

47. **Dennie-Morgan fold is seen in: (2006)**
a. Atopic dermatitis
b. Seborrheic dermatitis
c. Contact dermatitis
d. Dermatomyositis

48. **Herpes zoster patient should be isolated for: (2006)**
a. 6 days
b. 3 days
c. 9 days
d. 12 days

49. **Koilonychias is seen in: (2006)**
a. Iron deficiency anemia
b. Hypoalbuminemia
c. Lead poisoning
d. Psoriasis

50. **Stevens-Johnson syndrome is caused by:**
a. Herpes simplex (2006)
b. CMV
c. Chicken pox
d. Toxoplasma

51. **Exfoliative dermatitis is seen in: (2006)**
a. Eczema
b. Epidermolysis bullosa
c. Dermatitis herpetiformis
d. Vitiligo

52. **Typical lesion in hard chancre is: (2006)**
a. Painless and indurated
b. Painful and indurated
c. Painless and non-indurated
d. Painful and non-indurated

53. **Apple jelly nodules on diascopy is seen in:**
a. Lupus vulgaris (2006)
b. Tinea versicolor
c. Erythrasma
d. Vitiligo

ANSWERS AND EXPLANATIONS

1. **Ans. c. Type 3 hypersensitivity reaction**

2. **Ans. c. Trichosporum tonsurans**
Tinea capitis caused by Microsporum cains or Trichophyton tonsurans

3. **Ans. d. Moist compress**
Acute contact dermatitis is best treated by moist compress. No creams or ointment would stay of the skin at this stage

4. **Ans. b. Mycosis fungoides**
Mycosis Fungoides
- Its cutaneous T cell Lymphoma.
- Pruritus is an important Symptom.
- Histology reveals atypical lymphocytes in the epidermis. Pautrier's micro abscess is pathognomic feature

5. Ans. b. Superficial spreading

Superficial spreading melanoma

- Most common subtype accounting for 70% cases

6. Ans. c. LVG

7. Ans. a. Granuloma inguinale

8. Ans. a. Reiters syndrome

9. Ans. a. Lichen Planus

Wickham's Striae is a network of greyish lines characteristic of Lichen planus

10. Ans. a. TB

11. Ans. a. Neural crest cells

12. Ans. c. Griseofulvin is the drug of choice

13. Ans. c. Pthirus pubis

Pthiriasis pubis is transmitted sexually or non sexually by fomites, beddings etc

In children, crab lice may colonize the eyelashes and scalp

14. Ans. a. Acute paronychia is commonly treated by I and D

- Acute paranychia is caused by staphylococcal infection
- Treated commonly by incision and drainage

15. Ans. a. Superficial spreading type

16. Ans. c. Dermatitis herpertiformis

17. Ans. d. 10(4) bacilli/gram of tissue

18. Ans. a. Anthrax

19. Ans. a. Guttate

Guttate psoriasis

- Streptococcal etiology
- Hence antibiotic therapy is indicated

20. Ans. b. Steroids

21. Ans. c. Lichen planus

22. Ans. a. Pemphigus vulgaris

Pemphigus vulgaris

Features

- Seen in 4th–6th decade. The initial lesion are painful oral mucosal lesions
- Involvement of skin is in the form of non–itchy bullae over the face, scalp, axilla and trunk
- Bulla spread sign also k/a Asboe. Hansen sign is positive and Nikolsky's sign is +ve.
- The bullae ruptures to produce painful eruptions. Pemphigus may be associated with other autoimmune diseases like myasthenia gravis and malignancies like thymoma lymphoma etc.
- Tzanck smear shows Tzanck cells (Acantholytic cells)
- The basal keratinocytes remain attached to basement membrane and form Row of tombstone appearance.
- Immunofluorescence shows fish net pattern with deposition of IgG throughout the epi dermis.

23. Ans. a. Chancroid

24. Ans. b. Addisons disease

25. Ans. a. Melasma

26. Ans. a. Hypoalbuminemia

Leukonychia is a white discoloration of nails seen in hypoalbuminaemia of chronic liver disease

27. Ans. a. Calcinosis cutis

Calcinosis cutis is a feature of CREST SYNDROME

C-Calcinosis cutis

R-Raynauds phenomenon

E-Esophageal dysmotility

S-Sclerodactyly
T-Telengiectasia

28. **Ans. d. Genetic fragility of skin**
29. **Ans. d. Neuritic**
30. **Ans. b. Ulnar nerve**
31. **Ans. c. Lupus vulgaris**
32. **Ans. a. Mycoses fungoides**
33. **Ans. a. Gluten sensitive enteropathy**
34. **Ans. d. Congenital syphilis**
35. **Ans. c. Both a and c**
36. **Ans. b. HPV 6,11**
37. **Ans. a. Pityriasis rosea**
38. **Ans. b. Telogen effluvium**
39. **Ans. b. Face**
40. **Ans. c Granuloma inguinale**
41. **Ans. a. Mast cell**
42. **Ans. d. Pityriasis rosea**
43. **Ans. b. Patch test**
44. **Ans. d. 10^4bacilli/gram tissue**
45. **Ans. a. Pemphigus vulgaris**
46. **Ans. a. Dermatomyositis**
    Gottron's papules
    - Violaceous flat topped papules on IP joints and knuckles, also knee, elbow, medial malleoli.
    - Pathognomic feature of dermatomyositis
47. **Ans. a. Atopic dermatitis**
48. **Ans. a. 6 days**
49. **Ans. a. Iron deficiency anemia**
50. **Ans. a. Herpes simplex**
51. **Ans. a. Eczema**
52. **Ans. a. Painless and indurated**
53. **Ans. a. Lupus vulgaris**

QUESTIONS 2015

1. **Premalignant condition is?**
   a. Actinic keratosis
   b. Keratocanthoma
   c. Both a and b
   d. None of the above

2. **True about skin lesion and associated disease**
   a. Erythema infectiosum - Tuberculosis
   b. Erythema chronicum migrans - Lyme disease
   c. Erythema marginatum–parvovirus B19
   d. None of the above

ANSWERS AND EXPLANATIONS

1. **Ans. Both a and b** *Ref: Clin Plast Surg. 1980 Jul;7(3):289-300.Premalignant skin lesions.Pinkus H, Mehregan AH.*
2. **Ans. b. Erythema chronicum migrans - Lyme disease**

- Erythema nodosum: This is characterized by tender red swellings usually over the shins. The most common cause is streptococcal infection. Tuberculosis, sarcoidosis, leprosy, sulphonamides and inflammatory bowel disease are other important causes.
- Erythema marginatum: This is a non-itchy, pale red, macular eruption. It is a major criterion for the diagnosis of rheumatic fever but is also seen in acute glomerulonephritis and drug reactions.
- Erythema multiforme: This is characterized by cutaneous 'target' lesions and mucosal involvement. Children and young adults are more commonly affected. Orf, mycoplasma, and herpes simplex are among the known causes.
- Erythema induratum: Cutaneous tuberculosis. Otherwise known as Bazin's disease.
- Erythema infectiosum: 'Slapped cheeks', caused by parvovirus B19.
- Erythema chronicum migrans: An expanding annular lesion occurring in Lyme disease.
- Erythema gyratum repens: Erythema forming repeated concentric rings. Often there is an underlying malignancy.

Chapter

18 Radiology

K Vino Bharath

RADIODIAGNOSIS AND RADIOTHERAPY

Condition	First line investigation	Confirmatory test	Comments
Head trauma	CT without contrast X-ray–not useful	CT scan	MRI–essential in evaluation of chronic SDH and Diffuse Axonal Injury
Intracranial hemorrhage	CT without contrast–can detect bleed	MRI can stage the bleed	Most Common site for Hypertensive bleed–Putamen
Acute stroke	CT without contrast	MRI with Diffusion weighted Imaging	CT–gold standard for hemorrhage. MRI–gold standard for infarct.
Pneumonia	Chest X-ray	CT/HRCT chest	'Air bronchogram'
Chest mass	X-ray–PA and Lateral projections	CT contrast CT guided FNAC	'Bronchial cut-off' sign/Corona radiata indicates malignancy
Pulmonary embolism	Chest radiograph Ventilation/ perfusion scan (nuclear scan)	CT angio is diagnostic. Conventional angio is gold standard.	'Polo mint ' sign/'Railway track' sign–Partial thrombosis
Aortic aneurysm/dissection	USG, Doppler study	CT/MR aortogram	Intimal tear; double lumen aorta.
Chest trauma	Chest X-ray	CT	Pneumothorax–CT is best
Carotid stenosis	Duplex ultrasound	Duplex ultrasound CT/MR angiogram	ICA PSV and presence of plaque–primary parameters for grading of stenosis
Dysphagia	Barium swallow	Barium Swallow under fluoroscopy. Endoscopy	Rat tail appearance–Carcinoma. Bird beak appearance–Achalasia.
Renal Artery Stenosis	Doppler ultrasound	Catheter angio CT/MR angio	Functional evaluation–Doppler USG, radionuclide study (Tc MAG 3). Anatomical evaluation–Conv./ CT/MR Angio
Bowel perforation	Chest X-ray(free air)	CT	Football sign, Rigler sign, Inverted V sign, Tell-tale triangle sign, Cupola sign, Falciform ligament sign
Blunt Abdominal trauma	'FAST' Ultrasound	CT contrast	Vital signs + imaging decides management

Contd...

Contd...

Condition	First line investigation	Confirmatory test	Comments
Choledocholithiasis	Ultrasound	MRCP–noninvasive, diagnostic. ERCP–invasive, diagnostic and therapeutic.	Double duct sign (dilated CBD and PD)–pancreatic (head)/ ampullary malignancy
Cholecystitis	Ultrasound	Ultrasound. Contrast CT–best modality to evaluate complicated GB disease.	Sonographic Murphy sign. HIDA–problem solving modality, differentiates acute from chronic disease
Intestinal obstruction	Abdominal X-ray (supine and upright)	CT	'string of pearls' sign–pathognomic of SBO.
Appendicitis	Ultrasound	CECT abdomen	Graded compression USG technique of Puylaert
Nephrolithiasis	Ultrasound	Multi slice CT scan	Lucent stones–uric acid, cystine, indinavir, pure matrix stones
Ureteric calculus	Ultrasound	Multi slice CT scan	Comet tail sign–phlebolith. Soft tissue rim sign–ureteric calculus
Diverticulitis	USG/Barium enema	Contrast CT	Presence of diverticula + pericolic stranding. Most common–Sigmoid
Fibroid uterus	Ultrasound (TVS >TAS)	MRI	MRI–usually problem-solving modality
Bone metastasis	X-ray	Bone scan > MRI > CT	MRI-excellent in depicting bone marrow changes
Pregnancy evaluation	Ultrasound (transvaginal detects sooner than transabdominal)	Ultrasound	Fetal MRI–rapidly advancing field CRL–most sensitive biometric parameter
MSK trauma	X-ray	Bone trauma–CT Soft tissue trauma - MRI	Follow-up evaluation–by radiographs
Osteomyelitis (acute)	X-ray	MRI–most sensitive Bone scan–earliest diagnosis	Chronic osteomyelitis–CT
Pyloric stenosis	Ultrasound	Ultrasound	Infant with Bilious vomiting–probably malrotation–barium UGI study. Non-bilious vomiting–IHPS–USG.

FAST–Focused Assessment with Sonography in Trauma.

Chest X-rays

Most X-rays are posterior-anterior (PA) films.

Anterior-posterior (AP) films

Done in patients who are too ill or unstable to stand up, like patients with central venous lines or chest tubes.

Expiratory Films

Done in case of pneumothorax.

Lateral Chest X-ray

Lateral chest X-rays will determine whether a structure in the chest is more anterior or posterior.

(PA view–for detection of mass lesions; Lateral view–for localization of mass lesions).

Lateral X-rays also have a greater sensitivity for the detection of small pleural effusions.

Decubitus Films

Decubitus films help detect the presence of a pleural effusion. These are taken with the patient lying on his or her side.

Lordotic Films

Right middle lobe collapse is better seen.

HRCT

High Resolution CT scan provides greater detail than Conventional CT scan because of 1 mm cut.

Interstitial lung diseases may appear as reticular pattern, nodular pattern or cystic pattern in HRCT.

Types of densities

Linear or reticular densities → thickened interlobular septa, fibrosis

Reticulonodular densities → inflammation in peribronchovascular interstitium

Nodular densities → granulomas

Ground glass opacity → usually represents acute interstitial disease Hazy increase in lung density. Vessels can be clearly seen through haze

Honeycombing → ring shadows 2–10 mm; end-stage lung disease

Specific Views in Radiology

View	Structures seen
Caldwell (Occipitofrontal) view	• Superior orbital fissure, foramen rotundum and superior margin or orbit • Maxillary sinus, ethmoid sinus, frontal sinus
Water (Occipitomental) view	• Maxillary sinus, sphenoid sinus-frontal sinus • Infra Temporal fossa, zygoma and zygomatic arch
Basal submentovertical view	• Sphenoid, posterior ethmoid, maxillary sinus, Zygoma and Zygomatic arch • Mandible along with coronoid and condyloid process

Disease/region of interest	X-ray view
Congenital Dislocation of hip	von Rosen view
Fracture scaphoid	Oblique
Gallbladder calculus	Right anterior oblique view
Skull trauma, Sella turcica	Lateral view
Internal auditory canal (both sides)	Stenver's view
Left atrial enlargement	Right anterior oblique
Mastoid process	Lateral oblique (Schuller's view)
Orbital roof, orbital floor fracture	Water's view (occipitomental view)
Orbital lesions	Caldwell view (15' occipitofrontal)
Optical foramen	Rhese view
Pneumothorax	PA View on expiration
Paranasal sinuses (PNS)	Water's view
Patella	Skyline view
Minimal pleural effusion	Decubitus view (ipsilateral)
Spondylolisthesis intervertebral foramina Sphenoid sinuses	Posterior oblique
Superior orbital fissure	Water's view
Recurrent shoulder dislocation	Caldwell view (occipito-frontal view)
	Stryker's view

MRI

- Based on gyromagnetic property of protons (H+)
- Described first by Bloch and Purchell, applied as human tool by Damadian and Lauterbeur (1972)

- In 1952, Felix Bloch and Edward Purcell were awarded the Nobel Prize in physics for their independent discovery of the magnetic resonance phenomenon in 1946.
- Most common contrast agent used is iv Gadolinium
- Magnetic field used in the range of 0.15–3 tesla
- Relaxation time:
  - T1: time taken to return to original axis (T1 images are used to find out normal anatomical details) It has got high soft tissue discrimination (CSF looks black)
  - T2: Time taken by proton to displace. Used to assess pathological processes (fluid looks white)

MRI T1 and T2 weighted sequences

T1 W

Hypointense	Hyperintense
H2O, CSF, tumor/pathology, calcification, cortical bone, Hemosiderin, ferritin	Fat, blood, melanoma

T2 W

Hypo intense	Hyper intense
Calcification, cortical bone, hemosiderin, ferritin.	H_2O, CSF, fat, blood, tumor pathology

T1 image–For Anatomy–Fat bright

T2 image–For Pathology–Water bright

Gadolinium DTPA–Causes Nephrotoxicity (Nephrogenic Systemic Fibrosis) in pre-existing renal failure

Common Contraindications to MR Imaging

- Cardiac pacemaker or permanent pacemaker leads
- Internal defibrillatory device
- Cochlear prostheses
- Electronic infusion devices
- Intracranial aneurysm clips
- Swann-Ganz catheter

Advantages of MRI

- High intrinsic soft tissue contrast
- Direct transverse, sagittal and coronal imaging
- No bone or air artifact
- No ionizing radiation
- No known biological hazards
- Possibility for tissue characterization and blood flow imaging

Disadvantages of MRI

- Long imaging time
- Poor bone and calcium details
- Reduced spatial resolution especially with body coil.
- Claustrophobia
- Difficulty to manage and monitor patients who critically ill.
- High cost.

Central Nervous System

In general, the most accurate test for evaluating the central nervous system is magnetic resonance imaging (MRI).

	CT Scan	MRI
Best	Hemorrhagic stroke, Head trauma	Detection of stroke, Cancer, multiple sclerosis and infections. Evaluation of the posterior fossa structures, such as the cerebellum and brainstem.

In cases of CVA, CT is taken first to rule out hemorrhage. If there is no hemorrhage, then a MRI should be planned to diagnose thrombotic stroke.

Diffusion weighted imaging in MRI is very sensitive in detecting ischemic focus.

CT perfusion in ischemic stroke–detects the ischemic penumbra that surrounds the infarct core; this ischemic penumbra can be salvaged by intervention (e.g. by thrombolysis or clot retrieval).

Features of Brain Hematoma on CT Scan

Extradural	Subdural	Subarachnoid (SAH)
Limited by sutures Biconvex (Lens shaped/lenticular) Hyperdense in acute cases Hypodense in chronic cases	Crosses sutures Crescent shaped (Concavoconvex) Hyperdense (< 2 weeks) Isodense (2–4 weeks) Hypodense (> 4 weeks)	Four vessels (both carotids and both vertebrals) Digital subtraction angiography (DSA) is the investigation of choice for determining etiology. The hallmark of SAH is blood in CSF detected by lumbar puncture.

- Most common cause of SAH is head trauma
- Most common cause of spontaneous SAH is ruptured berry aneurysm
- Investigation of choice for SAH is Noncontrast CT

Bone Imaging

An X-ray is certainly the first study (and in many cases, the only study) to consider when evaluating trauma and fracture.

Radiological signs in vertebral diseases:

Vertebra plana	Eosinophilic Granuloma (Infection, Metastasis/myeloma, Lymphoma/leukemia, Trauma/ tuberculosis) *mnemonic IMELT*	Loss of almost entire height of a vertebral body
Rugger jersey spine	Secondary hyperparathyroidism of chronic renal failure (differential diagnoses include osteopetrosis and paget's disease)	It indicates the end-plate densities causing alternating opaque-lucent-opaque zones simulating the transverse bands of a *rugby jersey*.
Fish mouth vertebra **Codfish vertebra**	Homocystinuria, Sickle cell anemia	Biconcave appearance of lumbar vertebrae.
Picture frame vertebra, 'Cotton wool,' or osteoporosis circumscripta	Paget's disease	Picture frame appearance caused by overall increased density of the vertebra with sclerosis most marked at the periphery and a relatively lucent center. Osteoporosis circumscripta–welldefined geographic lytic lesion in skull most commonly involving frontal bone.
Ivory vertebra sign	Osteoblastic Metastases from Prostate and breast Lymphoma Paget disease	Homogenous increase in opacity of a vertebral body that otherwise retains its size and contour.
Inverted Napoleon Hat sign	Spondylolisthesis	Seen in frontal radiograph of LS spine. Implies the presence of bilateral spondylolysis and significant spondylolisthesis
Scottie dog sign	Spondylolysis	Oblique view presents a dog like appearance of the vertebra; the neck of the dog represents the pars interarticularis. Spondylolysis is the pars interarticularis defect, i.e. the neck of the scottie dog

Joint Involvement in Arthritis

Osteoarthritis

- DIP (Heberden's node)- most common, PIP (Bouchard's node) and CMC joint of thumb along with hip, knee, spine are involved
- Wrist and MCP joints are spared
  Radiological features
  - Loose bodies
  - Narrowing of joint space
  - Osteophytosis
  - Subchondral cyst
  - Subchondral bone sclerosis.

Rheumatoid arthritis

- Persistent inflammatory synovitis usually involving peripheral joints in a symmetrical distribution
- Involve MCP joint (most common) and PIP joint with sparing of DIP joint
- Swan neck deformity-hyperextension of PIP and hyper flexion of DIP joint
- Boutonniere deformity-hyperextenion of DIP and hyper flexion at PIP
- Hitch Hiker thumb
- Hammer toes
  - Hallmarks—Cartilage damage, Bone erosions, Change in joint integrity

Approach to bone tumor and tumor-like lesions

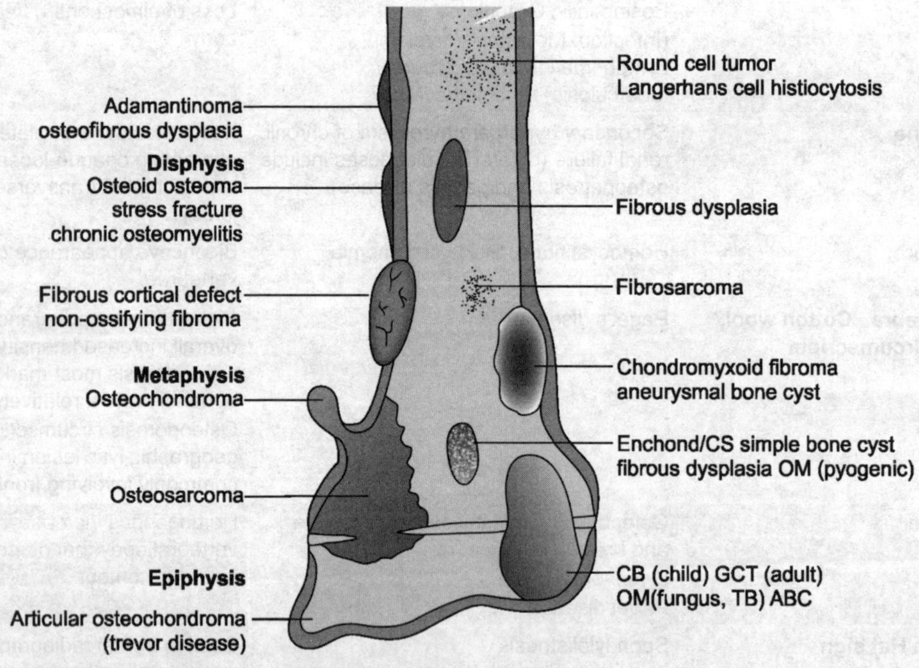

Fig. 18.1: Approach to bone tumor and tumor like lesions

Classical radiological feature	Condition	Description
Sunray appearance, Codman's triangle	Osteosarcoma	Codman's triangle - Triangle area of new subperiosteal bone that is created when a tumor raises the periosteum away from the bone.
Onion peel appearance	Ewing's sarcoma	Multiple concentric parallel layers of new bone adjacent to cortex (similar to the layers of onion).

Contd...

Contd...

Classical radiological feature	Condition	Description
Soap bubble appearance	Osteoclastoma	Subarticular expansile lytic lesion with multiloculated appearance.
Speckled/Mottled/Patchy calcification	Chondrosarcoma	Large osteolytic lesion with endosteal scalloping and rings-and-arcs or popcorn calcification in an elderly person.
Wormian bones	Osteogenesis imperfecta Hypothyroidism Rickets	Abnormal intra-sutural bones that lie between the cranial sutures commonly found around the lambdoid suture.
Trethowan's sign	Slipped capital femoral epiphysis	A line drawn up the lateral edge of the femoral neck (line of Klein) fails to intersect the epiphysis.
Honey comb appearance	Adamantinoma (common tumor of mandible and tibia)	Cortical lucencies combined with sclerosis.
Driven snow appearance	Pindborg tumor (calcifying epithelial odontogenic tumor)	Radiolucent lesion having small radio opacities within it. Commonly seen in posterior mandible in adults.
Hill sach's lesion/sign	Anterior dislocation of shoulder	Cortical depression in the posterolateral head of the humerus.
Bankart's lesion Bony Bankart	Repeated anterior dislocation of shoulder Associated with the Bankart's lesion	Injury of the anterior inferior glenoid labrum of the shoulder. Fracture of the anterior-inferior glenoid cavity of the scapula.

Disease	Radiological feature
Osteosarcoma	Variable mixture of radio opacities and radiolucency (hall mark). New bone formation in the matrix of the tumor Sun burst/sun ray appearance. Codman's triangle (nonspecific)
Osteoclastoma Ewing's sarcoma	Soap bubble appearance Onion peel appearance
Paget's disease	In osteolytic hot phase: Advancing wedge/Blade of grass/candle flame In mixed phase: cotton ball skull, picture frame vertebrae In cool phase: bowing, bone density increased

CARDIOLOGY

Radiological feature	Disorder	Description
Egg on a string/egg on its side appearance	Transposition of great arteries	Malposition of the pulmonary artery; cardiovascular silhouette becomes enlarged and globular
Snow man sign	Total Anomalous Pulmonary Venous Return	The dilated vertical vein on the left, the innominate vein on the top, and the superior vena cava on the right form the head of the snowman; the body of the snowman is formed by the enlarged right atrium.
Scimitar sign	Partial anomalous pulmonary venous return	Anomalous pulmonary vein drains any or all of the lobes of the right lung. The characteristic appearance of the vein has led to its comparison to a scimitar, a Turkish sword.
Goose neck sign	Endocardial cushion defect	Deficiency of both the conus and sinus portions of the interventricular septum, with narrowing of the left ventricular outflow tract. The characteristic shape has been compared to a sitting goose with elongated neck on the anteroposterior projection in left ventricular angiography.
Boot-shaped heart (Coeur-en-sabot)	Tetralogy of Fallot	The heart has the shape of a wooden shoe or boot due to uplifting of the cardiac apex because of the right ventricular hypertrophy and concavity of the main pulmonary artery.
Double cardiac shadow	Mitral stenosis	Left atrial enlargement causing 'shadow in shadow' appearance.

Contd...

Contd...

Radiological feature	Disorder	Description
Figure of 3 sign Reverse figure of 3 sign	Coarctation of aorta	The aortic segment affected by the coarctation has a shape that resembles the number 3 on frontal chest radiographs. The number 3 is formed by dilatation of the left subclavian artery and aorta proximal to the site of coarctation, indentation of the site, and dilatation of the aorta distal to the site. The reverse figure-of-3 sign, a mirror image of the number 3, is observed on the left anterior oblique view during barium esophagography in patients with aortic coarctation.
Box-shaped heart	Ebstein's Anomaly	The most consistent imaging feature is right atrial enlargement; the right atrium may be huge and fill the entire right hemithorax.
Jug handle appearance	Severe pulmonary hypertension	Aneurysmally dilated main and right pulmonary artery.
Hilar dance (pulmonary plethora)	ASD	Pulsation of the central pulmonary arteries on fluoroscopic examination.
Water bottle/flask shaped heart/money bag heart	Pericardial effusion	Symmetrically enlarged cardiac silhouette with small vascular pedicle.
Spade like deformity	HOCM	Echo–best screening technique Cardiac MRI–reference standard
Egg in cup appearance	Constrictive pericarditis	Predominantly right heart failure Square root sign is seen in invasive RV pressure study Cardiac MRI is diagnostic
Inverted moustache sign	Mitral stenosis	Prominent upper lobe veins (Antler's horn sign)

GASTROINTESTINAL TRACT

Sign/Feature	Disease	Comments
Single Air Bubble sign	Pyloric stenosis/obstruction	Solitary air bubble in X-ray abdomen of the infant is diagnostic
Double bubble sign	Ladd band/Malrotation, annular pancreas Duodenal atresia/stenosis/web duplication cyst	Dilatation of stomach and proximal duodenum produces double bubble sign. Can be identified in antenatal ultrasound. 30% of duodenal atresia babies have Down's syndrome.
Multiple air fluid level Triple bubble sign	Ileal obstruction Jejunal obstruction	Radiography is the best initial modality. CT–most sensitive.
Gas under diaphragm Rigler's sign Football sign	Pneumoperitoneum	Upright CXR can detect as little as 1 ml. Both walls of the bowel are seen due to air within and outside the bowel. Massive air gives rise to football sign in pediatric cases.
Bird beak appearance (barium meal) Cork screw appearance (barium meal) Nutcracker esophagus	Achalasia cardia Diffuse esophageal spasm	Absent fundal gas shadow and air-fluid level in esophagus–plain radiographic findings Intermittent contractions of the mid and distal esophageal smooth muscle. Due to high amplitude esophageal contractions; manometric diagnosis, no role for imaging.
Beak sign Double track or Tram track sign Antral nipple sign String sign	Hypertrophic pyloric stenosis	Mass impression upon antrum with streaks of barium pointing toward pyloric channel. Crowding of mucosal folds in pyloric channel. Redundant pyloric channel mucosa protruding into gastric antrum in USG. Passing of small barium streak into the pyloric channel.

Contd...

Contd...

Sign/Feature	Disease	Comments
Seagull/Mercedes Benz/Crow feet sign	Cholelithiasis	Triradiate collection of nitrogen gas within the gall stones; Seen in abdominal radiograph.
Whirl pool sign in USG (Corkscrew sign)	Midgut volvulus Cecal volvulus Closed loop obstruction	Bowel rotates around its mesentery, with the mesenteric vessels creating the whirls. Whirlpool sign is also seen in testicular and ovarian torsion.
Coffee Bean sign, Bent tyre tube sign	Sigmoid volvulus	Sigmoid colon gets dilated when it gets twisted at the root of its mesentry and appears like a coffee-bean.
Lead pipe appearance/pipe stem appearance Stippled appearance Pseudopolyps	Ulcerative colitis	Colon gets shortened due to spasm of longitudinal muscles/fibrosis. Fine granular mucosa and spiculated bowel mucosa due to multiple ulcerations. Scattered islands of edematous mucosa in a sea of ulcerated mucosa.
String sign of Kantor, Cobblestone appearance Bull's eye or Target lesion Comb sign	Crohn's disease (regional Ileitis)	Tubular narrowing due to spasm or stricture. Due to severe mucosal ulceration. Punctate shallow central barium collections surrounded by a halo of edema due to aphthoid ulcerations. Mural thickening with submucosal edema and mesenteric hypervascularity (in CECT)
Thumb printing sign	Ischemic colitis (Also in amoebic and ulcerative colitis)	Due to hypertrophied mucosal islands on barium studies.
Accordion sign	Pseudomembranous colitis	Represents trapped enteric contrast between thickened colonic haustral folds
Saw tooth appearance (on barium enema)/Champagne glass sign	Diverticulum of colon	Pericolic inflammatory stranding is characteristic; notably absent in colorectal cancer.
Apple core lesion and Napkin sign (on barium enema)	Ca-colon	Mucosal destruction and circumferential bowel narrowing with shelf-like overhanging borders.
Pincer sign, Claw sign, Coiled spring appearance, target sign, Meniscus sign, doughnut sign	Intussusception	Due to trapping of contrast between the folds of intussusceptum and intussuscipiens.
Bubbly/frothy/soap bubble/apple sauce appearance	Meconium ileus	Manifestation of cystic fibrosis Microcolon
Pulled up cecum/obtuse ileocaecal angle/filling defect/ incompetent ileocaecal valve	Ileocecal TB	Goose neck deformity, Fleischner sign, Stierlin sign

KUB

Sign/Feature	Disease	Comments
Rim nephrogram Crescent sign Soap bubble appearance	Hydronephrosis	Rim sign refers to the rim enhancement peripheral to the dilated calyceal system. The crescent sign refers to the appearance of concentrated contrast material in collecting tubules, arranged parallel to the margin of a dilated calyx, which produces a thin line of contrast material at the edge of the calices, resembling a crescent. Severe hydronephrosis and paper thin renal parenchyma produces soap bubble appearance in renal arteriogram.

Contd...

Contd...

Sign/Feature	Disease	Comments
Spider leg appearance	Polycystic kidney	Contrast filling of the calyces that are elongated and deformed by the cysts.
Swiss cheese nephrogram	Polycystic kidney	Multiple low-attenuation cystic lesions at the nephrographic phase of IVU has been described as 'swiss cheese'.
Flower vase appearance of ureter	Horseshoe kidney	As each ureter crosses the isthmus (of horseshoe), it curves laterally and then assumes a normal medial course giving rise to the flower-vase appearance.
Yoyo phenomenon	Partial duplication of the collecting system with single distal ureter	It refers to the refluxed contrast first entering one moiety, draining and then entering the other moiety of the duplicated Pelvicalyceal system.
Putty kidney, autonephrectomy, moth eaten appearance, Kerr's kink, irregular cavity, phantom calyx	TB kidney	Putty kidney–tuberculous pyonephrosis from ureteral stricture. Moth eaten calyx–irregular feathery appearance of surface of papilla due to erosion (earliest sign).
Saw-tooth appearance, Pipe stem ureter, Corkscrew or beaded ureter	TB ureter	Dilatation and irregularity of the ureteral lumen. Ureter may become a straight rigid tube. Healing with associated fibrosis.
Drooping lily appearance	Duplicated collecting system (classic sign on IVP of a duplicated collecting system with obstruction).	Deviation of the lower moiety of a complete duplication is seen due to the mass effect from the obstructed upper moiety. This usually occurs due to obstruction of the upper pole moiety ureter at its orifice associated with ectopic insertion or an ureterocele or calculus.
Cobra head appearance/adder head appearance	Ureterocele	Orthotopic ureterocele is seen on IVU as cobra head deformity when the dilated ureterocele is filled with contrast and bulges into the contrast-filled bladder.
Egg in cup appearance	Renal papillary necrosis	Irregular calyces with contrast tracking out from the fornices into the papillae, producing an egg in cup appearance.
Thimble bladder	Tubercular/chronic cystitis	Tuberculosis involvement of the bladder may cause calcification in the wall, which may become thick and reduce the capacity of the bladder; the resultant, very small bladder has been referred to as a thimble bladder.
Fish hook bladder	BPH	Enlarged prostate causes elevation of the bladder floor and lower ureters lifting them medially.
Sun burst nephrogram	Autosomal recessive Polycystic kidney	Striated nephrogram with persistent radiating opaque streaks on delayed images (on IVP).

- Pseudoureterocele: malignant stricture of distal ureter

RADIOISOTOPE USED IN SCINTIGRAPHY

Organ system	Radioisotope
Liver and biliary function	Tc 99, colloidal Au, I (rose Bengal 131)
Kidney	Tc99-DTPA, Tc99- Mag3 ,Tc 99 –DMSA Orthoiodohippurate
Bone scans, bone metastasis	Tc 99
Thyroid scan	I 123 , selenium, T c 99
Brain abscess, ventriculography	Tc99
Lung	Tc99Maceoaggregates
Parathyroid gland scan	Thallium –Tc

Radiotracer uptake in various bone diseases

Increased Uptake	Decreased uptake
• Joint's disease • Metastatic disease • Fractures • Paget' disease • Infection • Metabolic bone disease	• Avascular lesion • Multiple myeloma • Leukemia • Spina bifida • Advanced tumors

Pet Scanning

Positron emission tomography (PET) scans are useful in the detection of cancer.

They are particularly useful in determining whether lesions that are visible on a CT scan of the chest are malignant or benign.

Cancer tissues are typically associated with the increased uptake of fluorodeoxyglucose.

PET scanning is used after chemotherapy to assess for the presence of residual cancer in some patients.

- A cyclotron is required to generate positron-emitting isotopes that can be made from compounds, such as F, C, N and O
- Radiopharmaceuticals for PET imaging: FDG, C methionine and (18) Fa-methyl tyrosine
- Disadvantages of PET: limited availability and high cost due to the necessity of a cyclotron
- 18FDG-informs glucose utilization and is the most frequently used moiety,
- **Indications:**
  - To distinguish radiation necrosis from recurrence
  - To evaluate transformation of brain tumor from low grade to high grade
  - To assess tumor viability and monitor treatment response
  - For diagnosing occult metastasis
  - For diagnosing recurrent cancers
  - To differentiate benign from malignant pulmonary nodules
  - For the diagnosis, staging, and restaging of colorectal, esophageal, head and neck, breast and lung cancers and lymphoma and melanoma
  - In stroke, PET is useful to differentiate viable from nonviable tissue.

Single Photon Emission Computed Tomography

- Detection of emitted gamma rays by a gamma camera
- Requires radiopharmaceuticals that cross the blood-brain barrier
- Radiopharmaceuticals used are 133Xe, 123I isopropyliodoamphetamine (IMP), 99 mTc ethyl cystenate dimer (ECD) or 99 mTc hexamethylpropylene amine oxide (HMPAO)
- Clinical applications include dementia, cerebrovascular disease, epilepsy's, encephalitis, head injury, and other less common disorders that result in abnormal cerebral perfusion
- Many different SPECT radiopharmaceuticals are taken up into intracranial tumors, including 201 TI chloride, 99 mTc MIBI, 123 Ia-methyl tyrosine and 111 in octreotide
- Because of the requirement for lead collimation, SPECT has inherently poorer resolution than PET and absolute quantification is not possible.

RADIOTHERAPY

Radiotherapy is treatment of malignant tumor with ionizing radiation, most commonly by using γ rays; which causes excitation or ionization of electron (ejection of electron from orbit).

It kills tumor cells by producing double strand breaks in DNA (direct) or free radicals (indirect)

- The DNA molecules present along the chromosomes are the critical targets for radiation damage

- Chromosomal abnormalities occur in cells irradiated in G1 phase before doubling of genetic material
- Chromatid aberration occurs in cells irradiated in G2 phase
- Most sensitive phase to radiation is M > G2 M interphase
- Most resistant phase is Late S phase
- Lymphocyte analysis provides evidence of recent total body exposure

Radiation	Content	Penetrating power	Ionizing power	Damaging power	Sources
α-Particle	Helium nuclei (i.e. 2 protons and 2 neutrons	Poorest	Maximum	Most damaging	U-235, PO4-239, Th-232
β-Particle	High energy electron	Greater than α-particle (100)	Lesser than α particle	<α particle	P-32, Sr-90, Co, Cs, I-131, Tc, Y-90, Au
X-ray	Low energy photons	More than β-particles	Lesser than β particle	<β Particle	
γ-Radiation	Very high energy photons	More than X-rays 10000, i.e. most penetrating	Minimum ionizing	Least damaging	Cs, Tc, Ra, I-131, Co

Penetration power: γ-ray > X-ray > β particle > α particle

Ionizing and Damaging Power: α-particle > β-particle > X-ray > γ-ray

- X-rays and gamma rays are the forms of radiation most commonly used to treat cancer
- X-rays are generated by linear accelerator when electron beam strikes the anode
- Gamma rays are produced by decay of atomic nuclei in radioisotopes like Cobalt and Caesium
- For deep seated tumors, X-rays and Gamma rays are used, as high energy penetrating beam deliver a less intense superficial dose and causes less skin damage
- Electron beams have very low penetrance and are used to treat mycosis fungoides
- I-131: emits both beta and gamma rays
- Californium: emits neutron
- Linear accelerator and betatron are used to produced X-ray by accelerating electrons.

Brachytherapy

- First proposed by Forssell in 1931
- Delivered by two methods:
  - Intracavitary therapy, e.g. Manchester system for Rx of Ca. cervix
  - Interstitial implantation, e.g. HDR therapy for Ca. Bronchus and Ca. Esophagus
- Therapeutic radiation is delivered in three ways:
  - Teletherapy, with beams of radiation generated at a distance and aimed at the tumor within the patient
  - Brachytherapy, with encapsulated sources of radiation implanted directly into/adjacent to tumor tissues
  - Systemic therapy, with radionuclide's targeted in some fashion to a site of tumor
- Teletherapy is the most commonly used form of radiation therapy
- Radionuclides used in brachytherapy:
  - Cesium 137, Cobalt 60, Iridium 192, Iodine 125, Radon 222, Strontium 90, Samarium 145, Palladium 103, Gold 198, Yttrium 169
- The characteristic features of Brachytherapy are:
  - Maximum radiation effect can be obtained in diseased tissue
  - Minimum risk to the normal tissue
  - It is often used in brain tumors and cervical cancers
  - Prophylactic Craniospinal irradiation is useful in CNS malignancy which disseminates via CSF or any malignancy with high-risk of CNS spread
  - They are: Medulloblastoma, Glioblastoma, Germinoma, Small cell lung Carcinoma, ALL, Non-hodgkin's lymphoma and Leptomeningeal rhabdomyosarcoma

- The standard treatment for brain metastases has been whole-brain radiotherapy (WBRT) usually administered to a total dose of 3000 cGy in 10 fractions
- This affords rapid palliation; approximately 80% of patients improve with glucocorticoids and radiation therapy.

Radiosensitivity

Very high	High	Intermediate	Low
Bone marrow (most), Testes and ovary, Growing cartilage/growth plate/ epiphysis, Breast, Lens	Skin, growing muscles, bones, Brain, spinal cord, pituitary, thyroid, salivary gland, stomach, small intestine, intestine, colon, rectum, Liver, lung, heart, kidney, cornea	Adult bone, Adult cartilage, Oral mucosa, Oesophagus Urinary bladder	Pancreas, Uterus vagina, Adrenals

Radiosensitizers	Radioprotective agents	Radiation potentiator
• Anti cancer drugs: Cisplatin, 5FU, Hydroxyurea vincristine, Bleomycin • Metronidazole, Misonidazole, Etanidazole, Pimonidazole • Hyperbaric O2 (Most potent) (not-cyclophosphamide)	• Amifostine • Sodium butyrate • IL-1 • GM-CSF	• Doxorubicin • Dactinomycin

Co–60 has the following features:

- Naturally occurring isotope
- Half-life 5.3 years
- Emits β and γ-rays
- Used in both Brachy and Teletherapy

Feature	SI Unit	Non SI Unit
Radioactivity	Becquerel (Bq)	Curie
Absorbed dose	Gray (Cy)	Rad
Dose equivalent	Sievert (Sv)	Rem
Exposure	Coulomb s/kg	Roentgen

Know the inventors

Radioactivity	Henry Becquerel in 1896
Electrons	J.J. Thompson
X-rays	W.K. Roentgen in 1895
Radioactive substances radium, uranium	Madam Marie Curie
Nucleus, alpha and beta rays	Rutherford
Neutrons	Chadwick
Electromagnetic waves	Maxwell

Some Mnemonics

Lymphangitic carcinomatosis	Diaphyseal lesions in general
Certain cancers spread by plugging the lymphatics	**Cement**
Cervix	**C**ysts
Colon	**E**nchondroma
Stomach	**M**etastasis
Breast	**E**osinophillic granuloma (EG)
Pancreas	**N**onossifying fibroma (NOF)
Thyroid	**T**B/infections
Larynx	

Unilateral hyperlucent lung Poems Poland syndrome/Pneumothorax Oligemia/Obstruction (PE) Emphysema Mastectomy Swyer James	Epiphyseal lesions Cigs Chondroblastoma Infection Giant cell tumor/Granuloma (EG) Subchondral cyst
Cavity lesions in lungs **Cavity** Carcinoma-SCC Abscess-fungal/bacterial/TB Vascular-septic emboli Inflammatory-rheumatoid nodule Trauma-resolving contusion Young-bronchogenic cyst	**Erlenmeyer flask deformity** **Chong** Craniometaphyseal dysplasia Hemoglobinopathies (thalassemia, sickle cell disease) Osteopetrosis Niemann-Pick disease Gaucher's disease
Multiple fractures in children **Shot** Scurvy Hypophosphatasia Osteogenesis Imperfecta Trauma	**Egg shell calcification of lymph nodes** **A Silly Cool Surgeon Loves Her Beautiful Theatre assistant** Amyloidosis Silicosis Coal workers pneumoconiosis Sarcoidosis Lymphoma (post irradiation Hodgkin's Disease) Histoplasmosis Blastomycosis Tuberculosis
CP angle lesions **Slow game** Schwanomma: V and VII Lymphoma/lipoma Glomus tumor Aneurysm Meningioma/Metastasis Epidermoid/Ependymoma	**Vertebra plana** **Imelt** Infection Mets/Myeloma EG Lymphoma/Leukemia Trauma
Ring-enhancing lesion in brain **Magic DR** **Immunocompromised** Toxoplasmosis vs lymphoma vs TB **Immunocompetent** Mets Abscess Glioma Infarct Contusion Demyelinating (MS) Radiation Necrosis	**Anterior mediastinal masses** 4 T's Thymoma (most common anterior mediastinal mass) + other thymic lesions Thyroid lesions T cell lymphoma (Hodgkin and NHL) Teratoma and other germ cell tumors (seminoma, choriocarcinorna)

SIGNS AND APPEARANCES IN RADIOLOGY

- **Absent bow tie sign:** Absence of normal bow-tie appearance of meniscus on sagittal MRI of knee in bucket handle tears.
- **Accordion sign:** Seen in pseudomembranous colitis as a result of oral contrast trapped between oedematous haustral folds.

- **Air bronchogram sign:** Normal black airways rendered visible because of surrounding air space disease (thus becoming white) like consolidation.
- **Air crescent sign:** Air inside a pulmonary cavity surrounding a nodular opacity as seen with invasive aspergillosis.
- **Ant-eater's nose sign:** Sign of calcaneonavicular tarsal coalition.
- **Antral nipple sign:** Redundant pyloric mucosa protruding into the gastric antrum in pyloric stenosis.
- **Apple core appearance:** Circumferential narrowing of the lumen secondary to colon cancer.
- **Banana sign:** Seen on antenatal US and refers to a banana-shaped configuration of the cerebellum. Associated with neural tube defects.
- **Bare orbit sign:** Classical frontal radiograph sign of Neurofibromatosis I.
- **Bat wing appearance:** Bilateral Peri-hilar opacity in pulmonary edema.
- **Bat wing 4th ventricle:** Appearance of 4th ventricle that may be seen with Joubert syndrome.
- **Beak sign:** Seen in hypertrophic pyloric stenosis; also seen in arterial dissection.
- **Beer paw sign:** Refers to the CT appearance of the kidney in xanthogranulomatous pyelonephritis which resembles the paw of bear.
- **Bird's beak:** Narrowing of distal esophagus in achalasia as seen in barium swallow.
- **Blade of grass:** Paget's disease.
- **Bone within bone sign:** Appearance of spine that may be seen with osteopetrosis.
- **Boot-shaped heart:** Appearance of heart that may be seen with tetralogy of Fallot (Coeur en sabot).
- **Bulging fissure sign:** Bulging of a pulmonary fissure. Most commonly associated with Klebsiella pneumonia.
- **Bullet shaped vertebra:** anterior beaking of vertebra seen in mucopolysaccharidoses.
- **Bunch of grapes sign:** cystic, dilated bronchi in bronchiectasis; multiple cystic spaces in uterus as a result of hydropic distension of trophoblastic villi in hydatiform mole.
- **Caput medusa appearance:** seen in venous angioma in Contrast CT/MRI and angiography (only in venous phase).
- **Carman meniscus sign:** Lenticular shape of barium seen in barium studies in malignant gastric ulcer.
- **Celery stalking:** Irregular appearance of metaphyses in patients with rubella. Also used to describe metaphyses in patients with osteopathia striata.
- **Central dot sign:** Sign of Caroli's disease; Central dot corresponds to the enhancing portal vein that is surrounded by dilated bile ducts.
- **Cloverleaf skull:** Appearance of the skull that may be seen with thanatophoric dysplasia.
- **Claw sign:** seen in barium enema in intussusception.
- **Cobra head sign:** Dilatation of the distal ureter that may be seen in patients with ureterocele.
- **Cobblestone appearance:** Seen in Crohn's disease due to longitudinal and circumferential fissures and ulcers giving a cobblestone appearance.
- **Coffee bean sign:** Seen in plain abdominal radiograph in sigmoid volvulus.
- **Colon cut off sign:** Gaseous distension in proximal colon associated with narrowing of splenic flexure in cases of acute pancreatitis.
- **Comet tail sign:** Produced by the distortion of vessels and bronchi that lead to an adjacent area of round atelectasis.
- **Continuous diaphragm sign:** Chest radiograph sign of pneumomediastinum/pneumopericardium.
- **Cord sign:** Sign of intracranial dural sinus thrombosis; dural sinus or a cerebral vein appears bright as it is filled with thrombus.
- **Corkscrew sign:** Upper GI series sign of Midgut volvulus.
- **Corduroy appearance:** Appearance of thickening trabeculations seen in intraosseous hemangiomas of the spine. Cf. polka dot sign.
- **Crazy-pavement:** Linear network or reticular pattern with areas of ground-glass opacification. Classically associated with pulmonary alveolar proteinosis.
- **Crescent sign:** Seen in radiographs of avascular necrosis; linear area of subchondral lucency seen in proximal femoral head.

- **CT angiogram sign:** Enhancing branching pulmonary vessels within low-attenuating pulmonary consolidation in CECT in cases of Broncho alveolar carcinoma.
- **Cupola sign:** Seen on a supine chest or abdomen radiograph.
- **Dagger sign:** Radiographic feature in ankylosing spondylitis; single central radio-dense line representing ossification of supraspinous and interspinous ligaments.
- **Dark bronchus sign:** Relatively darker bronchus in the background of diffuse ground glass opacity as seen in Pneumocystis jirovecii pneumonia.
- **Dense MCA sign:** Sign of cerebrovascular accident that represent thrombus in the middle cerebral artery.
- **Deep sulcus sign:** Seen in cases of pneumothorax in supine chest radiograph.
- **Double bubble sign:** Sign of duodenal atresia and other forms of duodenal obstruction.
- **Double decidual sign:** Sign of early normal intrauterine gestation.
- **Double density sign (cardiac):** Sign of left atrial enlargement when right side of the left atrium pushes into the adjacent lung.
- **Double duct sign:** Simultaneous dilatation of the common bile and pancreatic ducts that is generally caused by a tumor in the pancreatic head.
- **Double PCL sign:** MRI sign of a bucket-handle meniscal tear.
- **Double track sign:** Appearance of hypertrophic pyloric stenosis that may be seen on upper GI series.
- **Draped aorta sign:** Sign of contained rupture of an abdominal aortic aneurysm.
- **Dripping candle wax sign:** Appearance of sclerotic cortical thickening in melorheostosis.
- **Dural tail sign:** Reactive dural thickening adjacent to the meningioma.
- **Egg on a string:** Appearance of the heart that may be seen with transposition of great arteries.
- **Empty delta sign:** Sign of intracranial dural sinus thrombosis; thrombosed superior sagittal sinus is seen as a filling defect in contrast CT.
- **Epicardial fat pad sign:** Sign of a pericardial effusion.
- **Eye of the tiger sign:** Low signal intensity circumscribing the globus pallidus in patients with Hallervorden-Spatz syndrome.
- **Fallen fragment sign:** Sign of a pathologic fracture seen with unicameral bone cysts.
- **Figure 3 sign:** Appearance of the aorta that may be seen in patients with coarctation of the aorta.
- **Finger in glove sign:** Sign of mucous plugging seen either allergic bronchopulmonary aspergillosis.
- **Football sign:** Sign of pneumoperitoneum seen on supine radiographs.
- **Golden S sign:** Right upper lobe atelectasis created by a central mass. Should raise the suspicion of a central neoplasm.
- **Gull wing appearance:** Appearance of erosions that may occur in patients with erosive osteoarthritis.
- **Halo sign:** Ground-glass attenuation surrounding a pulmonary nodule or mass on CT images. Represents hemorrhage and is highly suggestive of Aspergillus.
- **Hampton's hump:** Triangular opacity secondary to infraction in the periphery of the lung distal to a pulmonary embolism.
- **High-attenuating crescent sign:** Sign of impending abdominal aortic aneurysm rupture.
- **Keyhole sign:** US appearance that may be seen with posterior urethral valves.
- **Lambda sign:** On a gallium-67 citrate scan, uptake in the hilar and paratracheal lymph nodes gives the appearance of a lambda. This is seen in sarcoidosis.
- **Lead pipe:** Narrowing of colon with loss of haustra that may be seen in patients with ulcerative colitis.
- **Linguine sign:** MRI sign that may be seen in patients with intracapsular breast implant rupture.
- **Lobster claw sign:** Sign of papillary necrosis on IVU.
- **Luftsichel sign:** Sign that may be seen with left upper lobe atelectasis.
- **Mercedes Benz sign:** Appearance of gas within gallstones.
- **Molar tooth sign:** Enlarged and horizontal tubular structure on each side of the midline emerging from the midbrain in patients with Joubert syndrome.
- **Monod sign:** Air surrounding an aspergilloma (also see air crescent sign).

- **Nipple sign:** Appearance of hypertrophic pyloric stenosis that may be seen on ultrasound.
- **Pencil in cup deformity:** Erosion pattern of digits that may be seen in patients with psoriatic arthritis.
- **Picket fence appearance:** Appearance of bowel that may be seen on small bowel series with Whipple disease or gastrointestinal amyloidosis.
- **Polka-dot pattern:** Appearance of thickening trabeculations seen in intraosseous hemangiomas of the spine. Cf. Corduroy appearance.
- **Porcelain gallbladder:** Calcification of the gallbladder wall.
- **Putty kidney appearance:** It may be seen with end-stage renal tuberculosis.
- **Reversed halo sign:** Relatively specific sign of pulmonary nodules in cryptogenic organizing pneumonia.
- **Ribbon ribs:** Appearance of ribs that may be seen with neurofibromatosis 1.
- **Rigler's sign:** Sign of pneumoperitoneum where both sides of a loop of bowel are outlined by air.
- **Ring of fire sign:** US finding. Hypervascular ring in the adnexa that may be seen with either ectopic pregnancy or corpus luteum.
- **Salt and pepper skull:** Appearance of skull that may be seen in patients with hyperparathyroidism.
- **Sausage digit:** Soft tissue swelling of digits in patients with psoriatic arthritis.
- **Shepard's crook deformity:** Appearance of proximal femur that may be seen with fibrous dysplasia.
- **Shoulder sign:** Appearance of hypertrophic pyloric stenosis that may be seen on upper GI series.
- **Signet ring sign:** Sign of bronchiectasis.
- **Snowman appearance of heart:** It may be seen with supracardiac total anomalous pulmonary venous return.
- **Snowstorm pattern (breast):** US pattern for breast implant rupture.
- **Snowstorm pattern (Ob/Gyn):** US pattern for a molar pregnancy.
- **Soft-tissue rim sign:** Appearance of a ureteral edema surrounding a calculus.
- **Spalding sign:** Overlapping cranial sutures. Sign of fetal demise on prenatal ultrasound.
- **Spinnaker sail sign:** Elevation of the thymus by air that may be seen with pneumomediastinum.
- **Split pleura sign:** CT sign of thoracic empyema.
- **Steeple sign:** Appearance of narrowing of the subglottic tracheal lumen that may be seen with croup.
- **Stepladder sign:** US sign that may be seen in patients with intracapsular breast implant rupture.
- **Strawberry skull:** Appearance of skull that may be seen on fetal US with Trisomy 18.
- **String of beads:** Appearance of multiple stenosis that may be seen in patients with fibromuscular dysplasia.
- **String sign:** Appearance of hypertrophic pyloric stenosis that may be seen on upper GI series.
- **String sign of Kantor:** Sign of Crohn's disease.
- **Telephone receiver shaped femora:** Appearance of femora that can be seen with thanatophoric dysplasia.
- **Terry Thomas sign:** Sign of scapholunate ligament disruption.
- **Thumb sign:** Classic lateral radiographic finding for epiglottitis.
- **Thumb printing sign:** Thumb printing sign of bowel wall thickening seen with entities such as ischemic bowel, diverculitis, Crohn's disease, and ulcerative colitis.
- **Tram-track sign (chest):** Sign of bronchiectasis.
- **Tram-track sign (neuro):** Sign of optic nerve meningioma.
- **Tram-track sign (neuro):** Appearance of cortical calcifications that may be seen with Sturge-Weber syndrome.
- **Tree in bud:** Nonspecific pulmonary pattern seen on thin-section computed tomography; also seen in endobronchial tuberculosis.
- **Trident hand:** Appearance of hands that may be seen with achondroplasia.
- **Waterlily sign:** Sign of hydatid cyst.
- **Whirpool sign:** US sign of midgut volvulus in a neonate; ultrasound sign in testicular and ovarian torsion.
- **Wimberger's ring sign:** A circular, opaque, radiologic shadow surrounding epiphyseal centers of ossification in patients with scurvy.
- **Westermark's sign:** Regional pulmonary oligemia secondary to pulmonary embolism.
- **Yin-yang sign:** Swirling blood flow pattern within a pseudo aneurysm.

High yield points:

- Best modality to detect blood/hemorrhage → CT
- Best modality to stage hemorrhage → MRI
- Best modality to diagnose acute infart → Diffusion weighted MRI
- Best modality to detect calculi/calcification → MDCT
- Best modality to detect air containing lesions → CT
- Best modality to detect fat containing lesions → CT
- Best modality to diagnose lesions involving neurovascular bundle → MRI
- Best modality to characterize soft tissue tumors → MRI
- Best modality to characterize acute osteomyelitis → MRI
- Best modality to characterize chronic osteomyelitis → CT
- Earliest modality to diagnose acute osteomyelitis → Radionuclide studies
- Best modality to characterize avascular necrosis of hip → MRI
- Best modality to diagnose intracranial and intraspinal neoplasms → MRI
- Best modality to characterize temporal bone diseases → HRCT
- Best modality to diagnose mediastinal lesions → CECT
- Best modality to characterize lung tumors → CECT
- Best modality to characterize Pancoast tumor → MRI
- Best modality to characterize interstitial lung diseases → HRCT
- Best modality to screen for breast cancers → screening digital mammography
- Problem solving modality in breast lesions → MRI
- Best modality to evaluate pulmonary thromboembolism → CT angiography
- Gold standard modality to evaluate pulmonary thromboembolism → Catheter angiography
- Best modality to diagnose aortic dissection → CT aortography
- Best modality to diagnose in stable aortic dissection/chronic dissection → MR aortography
- Best modality to diagnose aortic dissection in unstable patients → CT > TEE
- Best modality to evaluate acute aortic syndrome → CECT
- Best modality to evaluate focal liver lesions → Contrast MRI
- Best modality to evaluate pancreas → CECT
- Best modality to evaluate Gallbladder → USG
- Best screening modality to evaluate renal artery stenosis → Doppler ultrasound
- Gold standard modality in renal artery stenosis → catheter angiography > MR/CT angiography
- Best screening modality in acute blunt trauma of abdomen → FAST (USG)
- Best modality in evaluation of acute blunt trauma of abdomen → CECT
- Best modality in evaluation of bladder trauma → CT cystography
- Best modality in evaluation of bladder and prostate malignancy → MRI
- Most important use of Transrectal Ultrasound → guided prostatic biopsy
- Best modality to evaluate anterior urethra → Retrograde Urethrogram
- Best modality to evaluate posterior urethra → Micturating cystourethrogram
- Best modality to diagnose vesicoureteric reflux → Micturating cystourethrogram
- Best modality in evaluation of renal tuberculosis → CT urography
- Earliest modality to diagnose renal tuberculosis → IVU
- Best modality to differentiate Fibroid from Adenomyosis → MRI
- Imaging modality of choice for Endometrioma → MRI
- Modality of choice for Diffuse type of endometriosis → Laparoscopy
- Best modality in evaluation of ulcerative colitis → Double contrast Barium enema
- Earliest modality to diagnose ulcerative colitis → Double contrast Barium enema
- Best modality to diagnose transmural inflammation in Crohn's disease → CECT
- Best modality to analyze ventricular function → Cardiac cine MR

- Best modality to evaluate meniscal and labral tears → MRI (MR arthrography)
- Best modality to evaluate ligaments, muscles and bone marrow → MRI
- Best imaging modality to evaluate adrenal lesions → MRI
- Imaging Method of choice for Pheochromocytoma → MRI
- Most common tumor in undescended testis → Seminoma
- Most accurate way of detecting bone mineral density–DEXA (dual energy X-ray absorptiometry)
- Best modality to evaluate Small bowel–MRI and CT enteroclysis
- Most common intramedullary spinal neoplasm in children → Astrocytoma
- Most common intramedullary spinal neoplasm in adults → Ependymoma
- Most common site of ectopic pregnancy → Ampulla of fallopian tube
- Most sensitive modality to evaluate bladder trauma → CT Cystography
- Agent of choice for assessment of Glomerular Filtration → Tc-99m DTPA
- Agent of choice for imaging of functioning cortical mass → Tc-99m DMSA
- Radiotherapy:
- Most common skin manifestation → Erythema
- Most sensitive blood cell → lymphocyte
- Most resistant blood tissue → platelets
- Most sensitive body tissue à bone marrow
- Most resistant body tissue → CNS
- Most sensitive cell in CNS → neuron
- Most sensitive CNS part → mid brain, medulla, spinal cord
- Most sensitive abdominal organ → kidney
- Most sensitive hormone → growth hormone
- Most sensitive mucosa → intestinal mucosa.

QUESTIONS

1. Which of the following is not seen in imaging of acute pyelonephritis? (2014)

a. Grossly enlarged kidney
b. Focal areas of hypoechogenicity
c. Perinephric edema
d. Increased vascularity

2. Symptomatic spinal cord injury without any radiological evidence most commonly found in: (2014)

a. Children
b. Elderly
c. Teenagers
d. Young adults

3. The dose of radiation for point A for early and locally advancing cervical cancer during brachytherapy according to ABS guidelines is: (2014)

a. 70–75 Gy—75–80 Gy
b. 75–80 Gy—80–85 Gy
c. 80–85 Gy—85–90 Gy
d. 85–90 Gy—90–95 Gy

4. 20-year-old male with history of RTA presents with breathlessness. Stratosphere sign on USG with M mode is seen. What is the probable diagnosis? (2014)

a. Hemothorax
b. Pneumothorax
c. Cardiac tamponade
d. Pulmonary embolism

5. Increased pulmonary blood flow radiologically indicated by all except: (2014)

a. Descending pulmonary artery diameter >16 mm
b. Kerley B lines
c. Diameter of 2 peripheral arteries > accompanying bronchus
d. Peripheral arteries more than 6 in outer 1/3rd

6. True statement regarding photoelectric effect:

a. Interaction between low energy incident photon and inner shell electron of atom (2014)
b. Interaction between incident photon and the outer shell electron of an atom
c. Interaction of the incident photon with the nucleus of an atom
d. Interaction between a photon and electric current

7. Best investigation to diagnose H-type tracheoesophageal fistula is: (2014)
a. X-ray
b. Esophagoscopy
c. Tracheobronchoscopy
d. CT scan

8. The braggs peak is found in: (2013)
a. Proton beam
b. Microwave
c. UV Rays
d. Infrared

9. Earliest sign of raised intracranial tension in skull X-ray of infants is: (2013)
a. Sutural diastasis
b. Erosion of dorsum sella
c. Pineal gland ;displacement
d. Copper beaten appearance

10. Drooping water lily sign seen in: (2013)
a. Spleen tumor
b. Liver tumor
c. Supra renal mass
d. Superior pole renal mass

11. Cold lesion on bone scan suggest: (2013)
a. Osteomyelitis
b. Lytic lesion
c. Metastasis
d. Sequestrum

12. 99 m Technetium labeled RBC scintigraphy is used in the diagnosis of: (2013)
a. Hepatoma
b. Hepatic hemangioma
c. Left ventricular function wall motion
d. GI Bleeding

13. Snowstorm appearance in Ultrasound is seen in: (2013)
a. Hydatiform mole
b. Twins
c. Hydronephrosis
d. Downs syndrome in fetus

14. Bamboo spine appearance in lumbar radiograph is seen in: (2013)
a. Ankylosing Spondylitis
b. Rheumatoid Arthritis
c. TB spine
d. Osteoarthritis

15. SI unit of radiation absorption: (2012)
a. Sievert
b. Gray
c. Becquerel
d. Rads

16. The t1/2 of iodine 131 is: (2012)
a. 13 days
b. 8 days
c. 2 days
d. 12 days

17. Which of the following agents is used in renal function testing to measure 'glomerular filtration rate' (GFR)? (2012)
a. Technetium 99 DMSA
b. Technetium 99 DTPA
c. Technetium 99 MAG3
d. Iodohippurate

18. Lyre's sign in CT angiography is seen in: (2012)
a. Carotid body tumor
b. Glomus tympanicum
c. Glomus jugulare
d. Branchial fistula

19. Which does not form the border of heart in PA view of a chest X-ray? (2012)
a. Right atrium
b. Right ventricle
c. Aortic knuckle
d. Left Ventricle

20. Reverse 3 sign in barium swallow is seen in: (2012)
a. Coarctation of Aorta
b. Aberrant right subclavian artery
c. Patent ductus arteriosus
d. Double arotic arch

21. True about PET scan is: (2012)
a. Single photon peak at 511 kev
b. Dual photon peak at 511 kev
c. X-rays are used
d. Lead collimators are used

22. Long-term effect of craniospinal irradiation for medulloblastoma is: (2011)
a. Secondary malignancy
b. Neuroendocrine abnormalities
c. Neurocognitive effects
d. Hearing loss

23. Isotope used to treat bony metastasis is: (2011)
a. Samarium 153
b. Yttrium
c. Palladium-103
d. Iodine 131

24. A 65-year-old male hypertensive presents with bruit in the carotid artery. Which of the following is the investigation of choice? (2011)
a. Doppler ultrasonography
b. Internal carotid angiography
c. Aortic arch angiography
d. Spiral CT angiography

25. Most radio resistant phase in cell cycle: (2011)
a. G1 phase
b. Early S phase
c. Late S phase
d. G2 phase

26. Gamma knife contains: (2010)
a. Cs 127
b. Co 60
c. Iridium 92
d. Tc 99

27. Gold standard test for pulmonary embolism: (2010)
a. CT Angiography
b. MRI
c. PET
d. Echocardiography

28. Which isotope is used to assess myocardial function? (2010)
a. 99m Tc MDP
b. 99m Tc Sestamibi
c. 99m Tc Exametazime
d. 99m Tc Pyrophosphate

29. Spider leg appearance is seen in: (2010)
a. Adult polycystic kidney disease
b. Wilm's Tumor
c. Horse shoe kidney
d. Vesicoureteral reflux

30. String sign of Kantor is seen in: (2010)
a. Crohn's disease
b. Ulcerative colitis
c. Ca Colon
d. Typhoid colitis

31. Thymus is rarely discovered in chest X-ray after the age of: (2009)
a. 6 months
b. 2 years
c. 4 years
d. 8 years

32. Causes of thickened gallbladder wall on ultrasound examination are all except: (2009)
a. Postprandial state
b. Cholecystitis
c. Congestive cardiac failure
d. Kawasaki disease

33. Popcorn calcification in lung is characteristic of: (2009)
a. Congenital adenoid malformation'
b. Hamartoma
c. Small cell Ca lung
d. Bronchial carcinoids

34. All are characteristic radiological features of cardiogenic pulmonary edema except: (2009)
a. Bilateral infiltrates
b. Cardiomegaly
c. Kerley B lines
d. Oligemia

35. Investigation of choice for pulmonary embolism is: (2008)
a. CT angiography
b. Contrast enhanced MRI
c. Pulmonary angiography
d. Echocardiography

36. Best investigation to diagnose calcification is: (2008)
a. CT
b. MRI
c. X-ray
d. USG

37. In chest radiograph, the right border of mediastinum is formed by all except: (2008)
a. SVC
b. Right atrium
c. Right Ventricle
d. Right brachiocephalic vein

38. In a child with coarctation of aorta, all the following are seen in plain chest radiography except: (2008)
a. Rib notching
b. Three sign
c. 'E' Sign or 'reverse Three sign'
d. Prominent ascending aorta

39. Rat tail tapering of lower esophagus in barium swallow is seen in: (2007)
a. Diffuse esophageal spasm
b. Achalasia cardia
c. Ca esophagus
d. Gastrosophageal reflux

40. Rigler's sign in plain abdominal X-ray is seen in: (2007)
a. Perforated peptic ulcer
b. Ascites
c. Intussusception
d. Portal vein obstruction

41. Drooping water lily sign seen in: (2007)
a. Spleen tumor
b. Liver tumor
c. Supra renal mass
d. Superior pole renal mass

42. Cold lesion on bone scan suggest: (2007)
a. Osteomyelitis
b. Lytic lesion
c. Metastasis
d. Sequestrum

43. Cobra head appearance is seen in: (2007)
a. Ureterocele
b. Wilm's Tumor
c. Horse shoe kidney
d. Vesicoureteral reflux

44. String sign of Kantor is seen in: (2007)
a. Crohn's disease
b. Ulcerative colitis
c. Ca Colon
d. Typhoid colitis

45. Investigation of choice in subarachnoid hemorrhage: (2006)
a. Non contrast CT
b. Contrast CT
c. MRI
d. Lumbar puncture

46. Following is used in PET scan: (2006)
a. FDG
b. DTPA
c. MAG-3
d. I131

47. Rotting fence post appearance of femur is seen in: (2006)
a. Fibrous dysplasia
b. Hyperparathyroidism
c. Paget's disease
d. Fracture neck of femur

48. Mega voltage therapy consists of: (2006)
a. Greater than 1000 k volts
b. 5000–1000
c. Less than 500
d. More than 2000

49. T D 50 for kidney is: (2006)
a. 2000 cGy
b. 3000 cGy
c. 2800 cGy
d. 2400 cGy

50. Half life of I 131 is: (2006)
a. 13 days
b. 8 days
c. 2 days
d. 12 hours

ANSWERS AND EXPLANATIONS

1. Ans. d. Increased vascularity

Ref: Cavorsi K, Prabhakar P, Kirby C. Acute pyelonephritis, Ultrasound Q 2010; 26(2): 103-5, Ultrasound: A Practical Approach to Clinical Problems, Edited by Edward I. Bluth, Page 465 and Genitourinary Imaging by Shailendra Chopra, thieme Publishers

Areas of hypoperfusion (decreased vascularity) is characteristic. Rest of the options are classical ultrasound features of acute pyelonephritis.

In general, routine radiologic imaging is not required for diagnosis and treatment of uncomplicated cases in adult patients.

Computed tomography (CT), when performed before, immediately after, and at delayed intervals from contrast material injection, is the preferred modality for evaluating acute bacterial pyelonephritis.

Excretory urography delineates the anatomy of the pelvicaliceal system and provides an overview of the urothelial system from the kidneys to the urinary bladder.

Findings seen in cases of acute kidney infections include
- renal enlargement,
- striated or delayed nephrogram,
- delayed caliceal appearance time and
- dilatation or effacement of the collecting system.

The weaknesses of excretory urography include the inability to characterize masses, (i.e. as cysts, neoplasms, or abscesses), the lack of fine parenchymal detail, and the dependency on functioning kidneys. In addition, several studies have demonstrated that only about 25% of patients with acute pyelonephritis have abnormal findings at excretory urography.

Positive findings of pyelonephritis found at USG
- hydronephrosis,
- renal enlargement,

- loss of renal sinus fat due to edema,
- changes in echogenicity due to both edema (hypoechoic) or hemorrhage (hyperechoic),
- loss of corticomedullary differentiation,
- abscess formation and
- areas of hypoperfusion (visible with power Doppler interrogation).

When imaging is warranted, CT is the modality of choice for evaluating acute bacterial nephritis.

It provides comprehensive anatomic and physiologic information that accurately characterizes both intra- and extrarenal pathologic conditions.

Unenhanced CT is excellent for identifying urinary tract gas, calculi, hemorrhage, renal enlargement, inflammatory masses, and obstruction.

Involved regions occasionally appear with lower attenuation related to edema. The above findings are frequently absent, however, and unenhanced CT images may appear normal.

It is only after contrast material is administered that the diagnostic features of acute bacterial nephritis are revealed.

After administration of contrast material, acute bacterial nephritis most commonly manifests as one or more wedge-shaped areas or streaky zones of lesser enhancement that extend from the papilla to the renal cortex. This pattern of differential enhancement reflects the underlying pathophysiology of tubular obstruction caused by inflammatory debris within the lumen, interstitial edema, and vasospasm.

Tc-99m DMSA scan kidney–Cannot differentiate renal parenchymal disease from perinephric process.

2. Ans. a. Children

Ref: www.wheelessonline.com/ortho sciwora_syndrome_spinal_cord_injury_without_radiologic_abnomality

Spinal cord injury without radiological abnormality (SCIWORA) is defined as the occurrence of acute traumatic myelopathy despite normal plain radiographs and normal computed tomography (CT) studies. SCIWORA is mainly a Diagnosis of Exclusion.

This occurs predominantly among the pediatric population, where its reported incidence ranges from 4%–66% of all spinal cord injuries.

Inherent elasticity in pediatric cervical spine can allow severe spinal cord injury to occur in absence of X-ray findings.

In young children, the pathogenesis of SCIWORA may be related to the mismatch in the elasticity of the tissue of the vertebral column and spinal cord.

MRI is preferred for acute assessment because it is noninvasive, delineates spinal cord and soft tissue abnormalities, and can assess compressive pathology. If MRI facility is unavailable or not possible and acute assessment is indicated then, CT myelography should be performed.

Neurological presentation: SCIWORA can have a wide spectrum of neurological dysfunction, ranging from mild, transient spinal cord concussive deficits to permanent, complete injuries of the spinal cord. The incidence and severity of injury are related to the patient's age. Until the age of 8 years, neurological injuries tend to be severe. Three quarters of the injuries in this group are complete. Over half of the injuries in young children occur in the thoracic spine; almost all of these thoracic injuries are complete. Adolescents sustain less severe, typically incomplete injuries.

3. Ans. c. 80–85 Gy—85–90 Gy

Ref: www.americanbrachytherapy.org/guidelines/cervical_cancer_taskgroup.pdf

Dose of radiation for early and locally advanced cancer cervix at point A during brachytherapy 80–85 Gray and 85–90 Gray.

Dose prescriptions in Carcinoma Cervix

Point A:

- Early stage disease (non bulky stage 1–2): 80–85 Gy.
- Advanced stage disease (bulky or stage 3b): 85–90 Gy.

Pelvic sidewall: LDR equivalent of 50–55 Gy (early stage) or 55–60 Gy (Advanced stage).

- Early stage disease (non bulky stage 1–2): 50–55 Gy.

Advanced stage disease (bulky or stage 3b): 55–60 Gy.

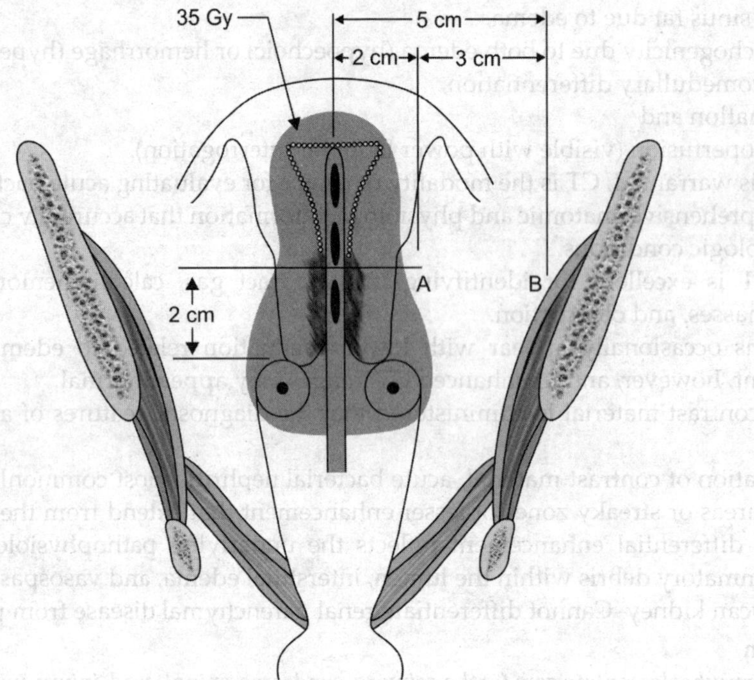

Fig. 18.2: Brachytherapy using a cervical tandem and two vaginal ovoids delivers the highest dose of radiation to the cervical tumor and parametrium (shaded area equaling approximately 35 Gy). Two imaginary points (A and B) are used to describe doses of radiation where the uterine artery crosses the ureter (point A) and at the pelvic side wall (point B). Adapted with permission.

4. **Ans. b. Pneumothorax**

Ref: Stone MB, Ultrasound diagnosis of traumatic pneumothorax, J Emerg Trauma Shock 2008 Jan-Jun; 1(1):19–20

Seashore sign → Ground glass or sandy appearance under the pleural line indicating normal lung tissue.
Stratosphere/barcode sign → absence of normal seashore sign below the pleural line; replaced with multiple small horizontal lines indicating pneumothorax.
M-mode uses acoustic waves to determine a structure's movement overtime.
An important term relating to M-mode use when diagnosing a pneumothorax is the 'seashore sign.'
Normal lung scans produce this characteristic seashore sign. These normal images are viewed as hyperechoic, horizontal lines that run the entire distance from the left side to the right side of the image. Near the top of the image, the bright-white pleural line will be visible. Below the pleural line, the landscape will change to become granular appearing, like ground glass. The image has been described as one of standing on the beach viewing the sea in the distance. The water appears as thin, horizontal lines that traverse the entire top portion of the screen.
The sign associated with air in the pleural layer is the barcode sign or stratosphere sign.
The stratosphere sign is present with a pneumothorax, and the air will produce only the horizontal lines throughout the image.

5. **Ans. b. Kerley B lines** *Ref: Fundamentals of Diagnostic Radiology, William E. Brant, Clyde A. Helms, Pg.375*

Normally, the diameter of the artery is the same as that of the companion bronchus. When redistribution occurs, the artery will appear larger than the accompanying bronchus.
Radiographs obtained from both these patient groups demonstrate redistribution of flow as evidenced by an equalization of vessel size between upper and lower lung fields.
Patients with pulmonary arterial hypertension differ from those with pulmonary venous hypertension in that, in addition to redistribution, they also demonstrate enlargement of their central pulmonary arteries. This particular radiographic appearance is called 'centralized' pulmonary blood flow pattern with peripheral pruning.

- Blood vessels become visible in the outer third of lung field (at least 6 vessels can be traced to the outer third).
- Ratio of right descending pulmonary artery to trachea > 1.
- Right descending pulmonary artery diameter > 14 mm suggests increased blood flow and > 16 mm is very strongly suggestive.
- Prominent end-on vessels seen below crest of diaphragm.
- Ratio of vessel to adjacent bronchus > 2:1.

These are 1–2 cm thin lines in the peripheries of the lung. They are perpendicular to, and extend out to the pleural surface. They represent thickened subpleural interlobular septa and are usually seen at the lung bases. Causes of Kerley B lines include pulmonary edema, lymphangitis carcinomatosa, viral and mycoplasmal pneumonia, interstitial pulmonary fibrosis, pneumoconiosis and sarcoidosis.

6. **Ans. a. Interaction between low energy incident photon and inner shell electron of atom**

Ref: Christensen Physics of Diagnostic Radiology, 4/e p64, 79

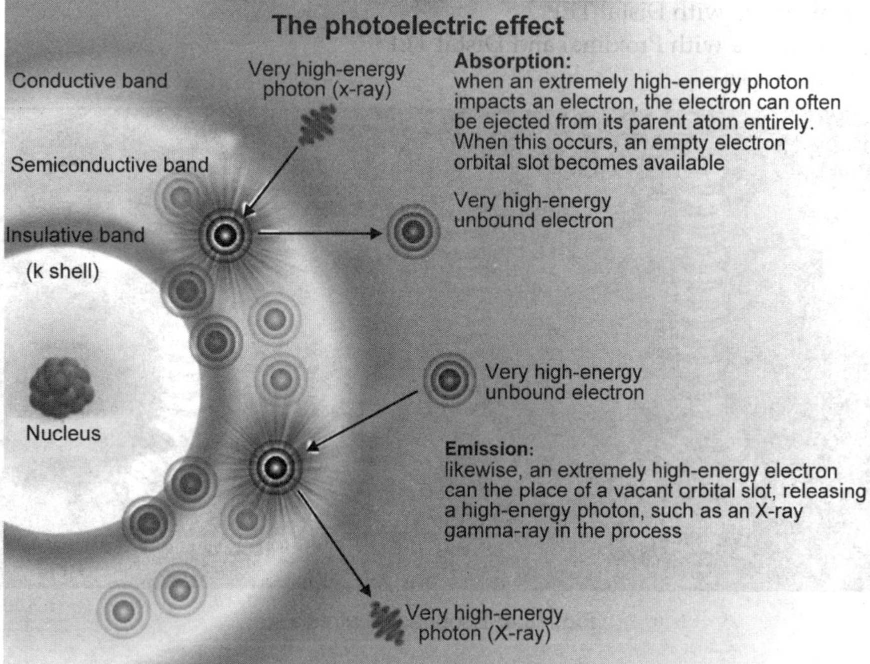

Fig. 18.3: Photoelectric effect

- When an incident photon, with little more energy than the binding energy of k-shell electron (inner shell electron), encounters one of these electrons, it ejects it from orbit and the photon disappears, giving up all its energy to electron.
- This electron now flies into space and is absorbed. Thus the atom is now left with an electron void on the k-shell, which is filled up soon by as an electron from adjacent shell drops into k-shell, giving up energy in the form of X-ray photon. This is photoelectric effect.
- The photoelectric effect is inversely proportional to cube of energy of incident photon and directly proportional to cube of atomic number of interaction material.

Compton Scattering or Compton Effect

- Occurs when an incident X-ray photon interacts with a loosely bound outer–shell electron, removes the electron from the shell and then proceeds in a different direction as a scattered photon.

7. **Ans. b. Esophagoscopy**

Ref: Radiology Review Manual, 7/e Dahnert, p832. Karnak I, Senocak ME, Hicsonmez A, Buyukpamukcu N. The diagnosis and treatment of H-type tracheoesophageal fistula. www.med-ed.virginia.edu

TEF represents complex of congenital anomalies characterized by failed/incomplete formation of the tubular esophagus or an abnormal communication between esophagus and trachea.

Most infants with Esophageal Atresia with TEF have proximal atresia with distal Fistula. They are easily diagnosed soon after birth as to apparent clinical features.

H-type TEF may not be diagnosed for several years because esophagus is patent.

Many diagnostic methods have been advocated for the diagnosis of H-type fistula.

Esophagram is usually a reliable method to identify congenital H-type tracheoesophageal fistula, though often difficult, requiring multiple attempts before the defect is confirmed.

Furthermore, contrast-enhanced studies have the potential risk of aspiration pneumonia and pulmonary injury and should be performed with adequate neonatal emergency resuscitation at hand.

Endoscopic methods like bronchoscopy and esophagoscopy have the advantage of being diagnostic allowing placement of a catheter across the fistula to assist in its localization during surgery.

'Coiled tube' sign–inability to pass feeding tube into stomach indicates esophageal atresia.

Type A–Esophageal atresia without fistula

Type B–Esophageal atresia with Proximal TEF

Type C–Esophageal atresia with Distal TEF

Type D–Esophageal atresia with Proximal and Distal TEF

Type E–TEF without atresia

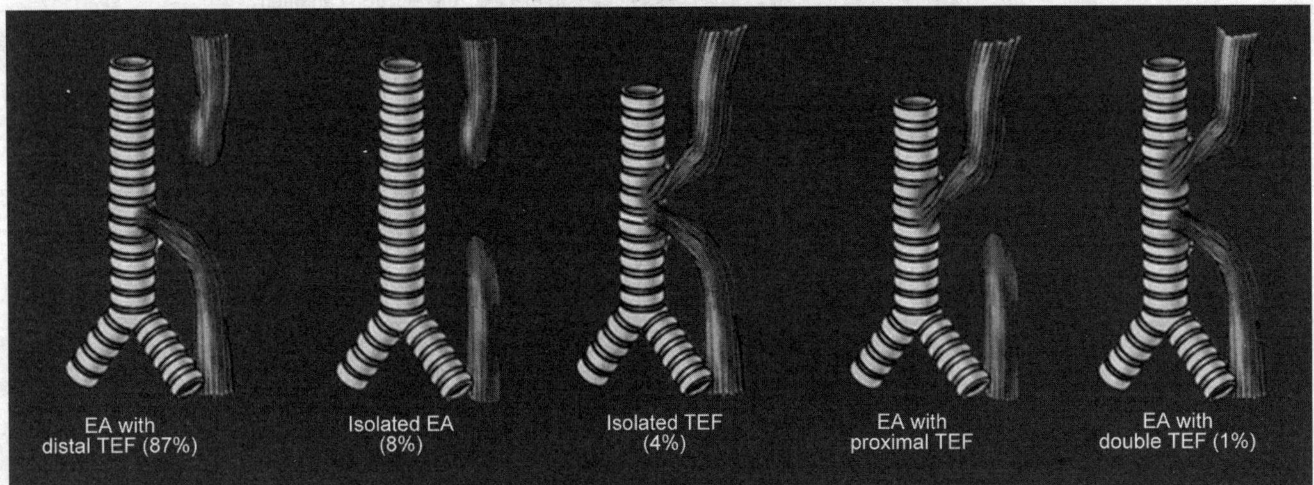

Fig. 18.4: Esophageal atresia

VACTERL

- Vertebral anomalies
- Anorectal anomaly
- Cardiovascular anomalies
- Tracheo-
- Esophageal fistula
- Renal anomalies
- Limb anomalies

8. **Ans. a. Proton beam** *Ref: Internet source: Medscape Radiology*

The plot of specific energy loss (which can be related to specific ionization) along the track of a charged particle is called a *Bragg Curve.*

Proton beam therapy delivers a high dose of radiation to a very localized site. Protons, being mass particles unlike X-rays, slow down faster than photons. They deposit more energy as they slow down, culminating in a peak (the Bragg peak). This allows the majority of radiation to be delivered to the target site with less scattering of radiation around and beyond to the adjacent normal issues.

9. **Ans. a. Sutural diastasis** *Ref: Radiology Review Manual, 7/e p299; Dahnert*

Signs of raised intracranial pressure in skull film

Infants/Newborn

- Sutural diastasis
- Bulging anterior fontanelle
- Copper beaten/silver beaten appearance
- Macrocephaly

Adolescent/Adult

- Erosion/thinning/discontinuity of floor of sella
- Enlargement of sella turcica

10. Ans. d. Superior pole renal mass *Ref: Callahan MJ. The drooping lily sign, Radiology 2001 Apr; 219(1); 226–8*

Drooping lily sign is seen in excretory urography in patients with duplicated collecting system (ureteral duplication).

The sign consists of Inferolateral displacement of a functioning lower pole moiety usually by a non-opacified, hydronephrotic upper pole collecting system.

The appearance of the lower pole collecting system is reminiscent of a drooping lily flower.

An obstructing ureterocele or ectopic insertion of the upper pole ureter is the usual cause of hydronephrosis of the upper pole collecting system.

The enlarged obstructed upper pole moiety exerts a mass effect on the remaining lower portion of the kidney, which results in the inferolateral displacement of lower pole moiety.

The drooping lily sign can also be identified in a nonduplicated collecting system in the presence of an upper pole renal mass, such as a renal abscess or Wilm's tumor.

The drooping lily configuration would not be expected if the entire kidney is displaced by an extra-renal mass (e.g. suprarenal mass) lesion.

Weigert Meyer Rule

This describes the relationship of the upper and lower renal moieties in duplicated collecting systems to their drainage inferiorly.

The upper renal moiety has ectopic insertion medial and inferior to the lower pole moiety ureter and frequently ends in ureterocele.

The lower renal moiety has orthotopic insertion lateral and superior to the ureter draining the upper pole and reflux typically occurs.

11. Ans. c. Metastasis

Ref: Radiology review manual, Dahnert, 7/e p1106. Internet Source; http://radiology.med.miami.edu/documents/2009Bone_Scan_All.pdf

Cold lesions on bone scan are lesions with decreased radiotracer uptake. Metastasis is the most common cause.

Cold Spots may be caused by:

- Malignant Tumors–Lung (2–4%)–Breast (5%)–Renal (10%)–Neuroblastomas (bone marrow metastases)–Thyroid (most cases)–Multiple Myeloma (most cases)
- Bone Abscesses (they are surrounded by activity)
- Bone ischemia (AVN, sickle cell, etc.)
- Hemangiomas (normal or decreased activity)

12. Ans. d. GI Bleeding *Ref: Clinical Nuclear Medicine, 4/e p622*

RBC Scintigraphy detects bleeding as low as 0.1 mL/min.

If GI bleeding is not detectable by RBC Scintigraphy, it will not be detectable by angiography.

Most sensitive imaging method for lower GI bleeding.

In most instances it identifies the bleeding site within first hour of study.

It serves as a test to identify patients who need/benefit from angiography.

RBC Scintigraphy is superior to Sulphur colloid.

13. Ans. a. Hydatiform mole *Ref: Diagnostic Radiology, 5/e p1229, Vol. 2, Grainger & Allison.*

The hydatiform mole can be complete or partial.

Complete moles are associated with the absence of a fetus and partial moles usually occur with an abnormal fetus.

The classical sonographic appearance of a complete mole is that of a large for gestational age uterus with an echogenic soft tissue mass distending the endometrial canal punctuated by multiple small cystic spaces giving a snowstorm appearance.

The term snowstorm sign usually dates back to earlier ultrasound equipment with inferior resolution. On ultrasound, molar tissue demonstrates the bunch of grapes sign which represents hydropic swelling of trophoblastic villi.

The role of imaging in gestational trophoblastic disease has been primarily to document metastatic disease at initial diagnosis or to evaluate persistent disease.

14. Ans: a. Ankylosing Spondylitis *Ref: Radiology review manual, Dahnert, 7/e p203.*

Ankylosing spondylitis–autoimmune disease of unknown etiology primarily affecting axial skeleton.
Location–axial skeleton: sacroiliac joints, thoracolumbar + lumbosacral junctions
Bilateral symmetric Sacroilitis (hallmark)
Square vertebra–Straightened anterior vertebral margins
Shiny corner sign–reactive sclerosis of corners of vertebral body
Bamboo spine–On AP radiograph; undulating contour due to marginal syndesmophytes
Ossification of supraspinous and interspinous ligaments
Dagger sign–single radiodense line of AP view
Trolley track sign–central line of ossification with two lateral lines of ossification on AP view
Atlanto-axial subluxation

15. Ans. b. Gray *Ref: www.ieer.org, Measuring Radiation: Terminology and Units.*

Some units used in measuring ionizing radiation and radiation dose

Unit	Description
Rem (roentgen equivalent man)	A unit of equivalent absorbed dose of radiation which takes into account the relative biological effectiveness of different forms of ionizing radiation, or the varying ways in which they transfer their energy to human tissue. The dose in rem equals the dose in rad multiplied by the quality factor (Q). For beta and gamma radiation, the quality factor is taken as one, that is, rem equals rad. For alpha radiation, the quality factor is taken as 20, that is, rems equal 20 times rads. Rem is essentially a measure of biological damage. For neutrons, Q is typically taken as 10.
Sievert (Sv)	A unit of equivalent absorbed dose equal to 100 rem.
Rad (radiation absorbed dose)	A unit of absorbed dose of radiation. Rad is a measure of the amount of energy deposited in tissue.
Gray (Gy)	A unit of absorbed radiation dose equal to 100 rad. Gray is a measure of deposition of energy in tissue.
Curie (Ci)	The traditional unit of radioactivity, equal to the radioactivity of one gram of pure radium-226.
Becquerels (Bq)	The standard international unit of radioactivity equal to one disintegration per second.

16. Ans. b. 8 days *Ref: Internet Sources*

17. Ans. b. Technetium 99 DTPA *Ref: Radiology by Wolfgang Dahnert 5/e p1113 & Internet Sources*

Technitium-99m DTPA is exclusively excreted by glomerular filtration (similar to inulin) without reabsorption/tubular excretion/metabolism.
Its biological half life is 20 min.
It is the agent of choice for assessment of

- Perfusion
- Glomerular filtration rate
- Obstructive uropathy
- Vesicoureteral reflux

Technitium-99m DMSA is suitable for imaging of functioning cortical mass (to differentiate pseudotumors from tumors)
Technitium-99m MAG3 is suitable for evaluating the renal plasma flow.
ACE inhibitor Scintigraphy is a screening test for Renovascular hypertension.

18. Ans. a. Carotid body tumor

Ref: Radiology by Wolfgang Dahnert 5/e p401 & Internet Sources. http://emedicine.medscape.com/article/1575155-overview

The **lyre sign** refers to the splaying of the internal and external carotid by a carotid body tumor.
Classically described on angiography it is also visible on CT angiography.
It appears as an enhancing oval mass with splaying of ICA and ECA above CCA bifurcation.
Malignant transformation in 6%.

19. Ans. b. Right Ventricle *Ref: Clinical diagnosis cardiovascular system, Rajendran, chapter 65, Radiology by Wolfgang Dahnert 5/e p40 Cardiopulmonary imaging, Kazeeroni, p82*

The right atrium forms the right border of the heart. Above the right heart border lies the edge of the SVC.
The left border of the heart is formed by the aortic knuckle, main pulmonary artery, left atrial appendage and left ventricle.
Both the left atrium and right ventricle are not visible on the normal chest radiograph.
Silhouette sign–Any intrathoracic opacity, (e.g. pneumonia, atelectasis, mass, fluid) that comes in contact with mediastinal or diaphragmatic border will obliterate or silhouette that border.
Recognition of this sign is useful in localising areas of pathology.
For eg, right paratracheal stripe–right upper lobe
Right heart border–right middle lobe
Right hemidiaphragm–right lower lobe
Aortic knuckle–left upper lobe
Left heart border–lingular segment
Left hemidiaphragm–left lower lobe

20. Ans. a. Coarctation of Aorta *Ref: Gastrointestinal Radiology: A Pattern Approach, p30. Ronald L. Eisenberg*

The aortic segment affected by the coarctation has a shape that resembles the number 3 on frontal chest radiographs.
The number 3 is formed by dilatation of the left subclavian artery and aorta proximal to the site of coarctation, indentation of the site, and dilatation of the aorta distal to the site.
The reverse figure-of-3 sign, a mirror image of the number 3, is observed on the left anterior oblique view during barium esophagography in patients with aortic coarctation.
Inferior rib notching involving ribs 3-9.
Second most common cause of congestive heart failure in neonate.

21. Ans. b. Dual photon peak at 511 kev *Ref: Radiology review manual, 7/e p1096, Dahnert*

PET scan is a technique that permits noninvasive in vivo examination of metabolism, blood flow, electrical activity, neurochemistry.
Reaction involves formation of annihilation photons which are emitted in exactly opposite directions (511 keV each).
Serum glucose competes with FDG for entry into tumor cells; trapped intracellularly as FDG-6-phosphate; malignant cells have a high rate of glycolysis.
Hybrid PET/CT imaging–combination of high resolution PET scanner + CT scanner allows acquisition of 3D images.

22. Ans. c. Neurocognitive effects

Ref: Kiltie AE, Lashford LS, Gattamaneni HR. Survival and late effects in medulloblastoma patients treated with craniospinal irradiation under three years old. Med Pediatr Oncol. 1997 May; 28(5): 348–54. & http://www.pedsoncologyeducation.com

The indications for craniospinal irradiation are medulloblastoma, PNET, pure germinoma, germ cell tumors with CSF positive for malignant cells, NHL with CSF positive for malignant cells.
Medulloblastoma is usually treated with craniospinal RT and children who develop this disease are often between 4 and 6 years old, so as a group they suffer from significant treatment related toxicity.
Radiation effects secondary to craniospinal irradiation are classified as early, early delayed and late effects.
The most devastating late effect of therapy for medulloblastoma is usually neurocognitive delay, (e.g. poor short term memory, difficulty with executive function).

23. Ans. a. Samarium 153

Ref: Handbook of radiation oncology: Basic principles and clinical applications, Bruce Haffty, p217

Radiopharmaceutical treatment of bone metastases is well tolerated.

Strontium 89 is given to patients with metastatic prostate cancer and results show significant improvement in pain relief.

Samarium 153 gets accumulated in bone with specifically targeting the osteoblastic lesions and is seen in low concentrations in normal bone.

24. Ans. a. Doppler ultrasonography

Ref: Sonographic examination of the carotid arteries, Radiographics, 2005, volume 25, issue 6. Carotid Artery Stenosis: Gray-Scale and Doppler US Diagnosis—Society of Radiologists in Ultrasound Consensus Conference, November 2003, volume 229, issue 2.

The bruit tends to become more apparent when stenosis is 50% or greater but may actually disappear when stenosis reaches 85–90%.

Doppler US is by far the most common imaging examination performed worldwide to aid in the diagnosis of carotid disease.

This imaging modality is increasingly becoming the only examination performed before surgical intervention.

Ultrasonography (US) of the carotid arteries is the modality of choice for triage, diagnosis, and monitoring of cases of atheromatous disease.

Because stenosis is typically an area of narrowing caused by plaque, with a focal area of increased velocity and a poststenotic disturbed flow, the location and characteristics of plaque in the ICA should be determined.

The intima-media thickness of the carotid arteries is a measurable index of the presence of atherosclerosis.

An important component of carotid US is to adequately document the location, internal characteristics, and surface detail of plaque.

The ICA PSV and the presence of plaque at gray-scale or color Doppler imaging are primary parameters for the grading of ICA stenosis.

Doppler US criteria for Carotid artery stenosis:

	Primary Parameters		Additional Parameters	
Degreeo of Stenosis (%)	ICA PSV (cm/sec)	Plaque Estimate (%)*	ICA/CCA PSV Ratio	ICA EDV (cm/sec)
Normal	< 125	None	< 2.0	< 40
< 50	< 125	< 50	< 2.0	< 40
50–69	125–230	≥ 50	2.0–4.0	4–100
≥ 70 but less than near occlusion	> 230	≥ 50	> 4.0	> 100
Near occlusion	High, low, or undetectable	Visible	Variable	Variable
Total occlusion	Undetectable	Visible, no detectable lumen	Not applicable	Not applicable

25. Ans. c. Late S phase

Ref: S. Biade, C. C. Stobbe, and J.D. Chapman (1997) The Intrinsic Radio-sensitivity of Some Human Tumor Cells Throughout Their Cell Cycles. Radiation Research: April 1997, Vol. 147, No.4, pp.416–421.

The cell cycle is an ordered set of processes by which one cell grows and divides into two daughter cell.

Since cells in different phases exhibit different radio-sensitivity and radiation can effect cell cycle.

The radiosensitivity of cells is dependent on the phase of the cell cycle.

- Cells are most radiosensitive in G2-M phase and most radio-resistant in Late S phase.
- Late S phase radio-resistance is due to Homologous Recombination (HR) repair between sister chromatids that is more likely to occur after DNA has replicated.

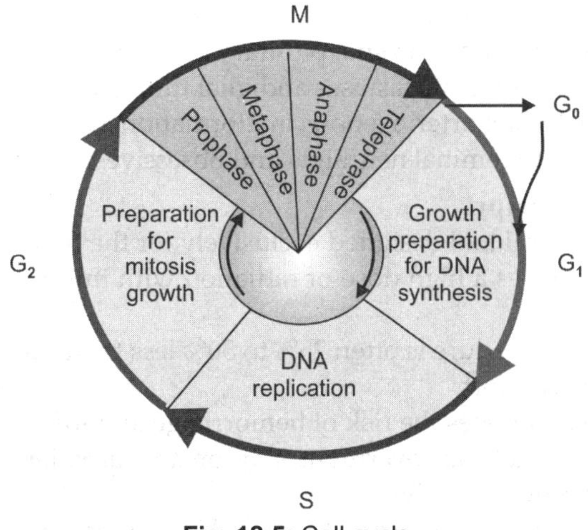

Fig. 18.5: Cell cycle

The cell cycle

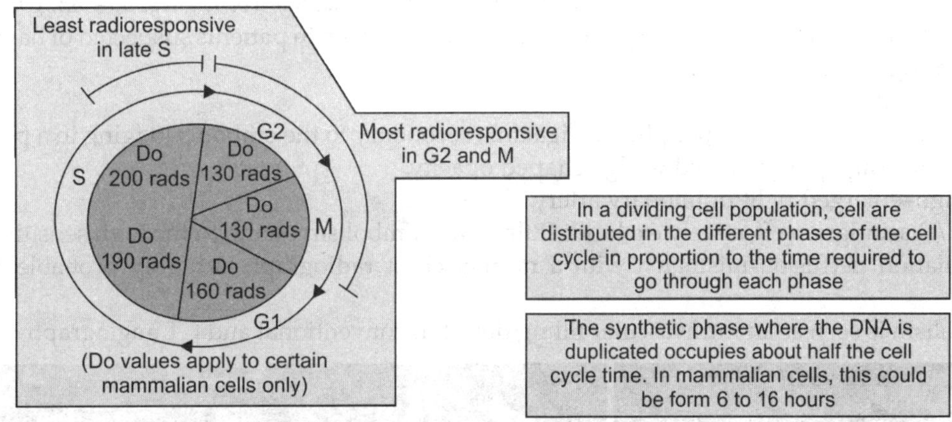

Fig. 18.6: Radiosensitivity of cells

26. Ans. b. Cobalt 60 *Ref: Radiosurgery practice guidelines, www.irsa.org*

Gamma knife radiosurgery is able to accurately focus many beams of high-intensity gamma radiation to converge on one or more tumors.

Each individual beam is relatively low energy, so the radiation has little effect on intervening brain tissue and is concentrated only at the tumor itself.

It is a non-invasive modality.

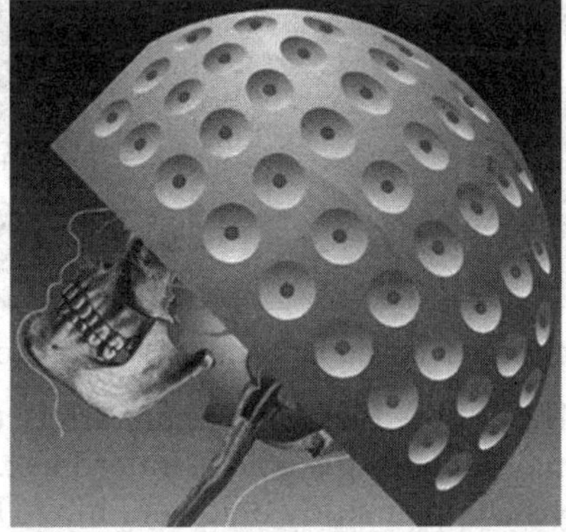

Fig. 18.7: Gamma knife radiosurgery

Conditions for which the Gamma Knife is considered most effective are:

- Intracranial tumors such as acoustic neuroma, pituitary adenoma, pinealoma, craniopharyngioma, meningioma, chordoma, chondrosarcoma, metastases and glial tumors.
- Vascular malformations including arteriovenous malformations.
- Functional disorders such as trigeminal neuralgia and obsessive-compulsive disorder.

Advantages of Gamma knife therapy:

- Gamma Knife is a neurosurgical tool designed exclusively for the treatment of brain disorders.
- The lesion being treated receives a high dose of radiation with minimum risk to nearby tissue and structures.
- The cost of a Gamma Knife procedure is often 25% to 30% less than traditional neurosurgery.
- Patients experience little discomfort.
- The absence of an incision eliminates the risk of hemorrhage and infection.
- Hospitalization is short, typically an overnight stay or an outpatient surgical procedure. Patients can immediately resume their previous activities.
- Gamma Knife technology allows treatment of inoperable lesions. The procedure offers hope to patients who were formerly considered untreatable or at very high-risk during open skull surgery.

27. Ans. a. CT Angiography

Ref: Diagnostic Radiology, Vol.1, 7/e p536–543, Grainger & Allison.

Chest radiography is often the first imaging examination performed in patients suspected of having Pulmonary Embolism; however, it is unreliable.

Characteristic radiographic signs:

- Westermark's sign–localized peripheral oligaemia secondary to the embolus lodging in a peripheral artery.
- Hampton's hump–pleural based wedge-shaped opacity.
- Palla's sign–enlarged right pulmonary artery.

A normal V/Q scintigram effectively excludes Pulmonary Embolism owing to the high sensitivity of the test.

Large ventilation perfusion mismatch with a normal chest radiograph is highly probable for Pulmonary Embolism.

Acute embolism is seen as an intravascular filling defect in conventional and CT angiography.

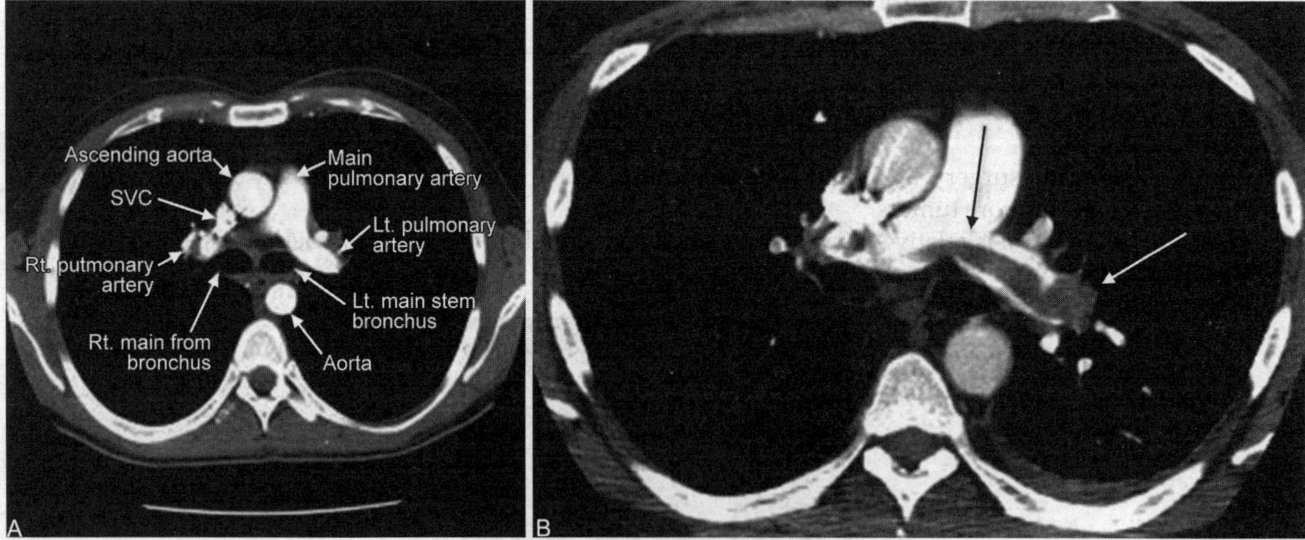

Figs 18.8 (A and B): A: Normal left pulmonary artery, B: Thrombosed left pulmonary artery

Normal left pulmonary artery (a); Thrombosed left pulmonary artery (b).

Conventional pulmonary angiography remains the gold standard test.

Indirect investigation include Venous Doppler study of lower limb to look for deep vein thrombosis.

28. Ans. b. 99 m Tc Sestamibi

Ref: emedicine Medscape

- Technetium (99 m Tc) sestamibi is a lipophilic cation which, when injected intravenously into a patient, distributes in the myocardium proportionally to the myocardial blood flow.
- Single photon emission computed tomography (SPECT) imaging of the heart is performed using a gamma camera to detect the gamma rays emitted by the technetium 99m as it decays.
- Two sets of images are acquired.
- For one set, 99mTc MIBI is injected while the patient is at rest and then the myocardium is imaged.
- In the second set, the patient is stressed either by exercising on a treadmill or pharmacologically.
- The drug injected at peak stress and then imaging is performed.

The resulting two sets of images are compared with each other to distinguish ischemic from infarcted areas of the myocardium.

29. Ans. a. Adult polycystic kidney disease

Ref: Diagnostic Radiology, Vol. 2, 7/e p1556, Grainger & Allison. Radiology Review Manual, Dahnert, 7/e p964.

ADPKD is rarely seen in childhood and commonly presents after the third decade of life.

Extrarenal manifestations:

- Cysts in liver, pancreas or spleen
- Intracranial aneurysm → Subarachnoid hemorrhage
- Colonic diverticulosis
- Mitral valve prolapse

Antenatal ultrasound → Highly reflective kidneys

Bilateral enlarged kidneys with cysts typically scattered throughout both the cortex and medulla.

Swiss cheese nephrogram → multiple lesions of varying size with smooth margins.

Spider leg appearance → Multiple smooth defects in the nephrogram with elongation and deformity of calyces.

Increased incidence of renal cell carcinoma.

Ultrasound is an excellent choice for repeated imaging as it is fast, relatively inexpensive and lacks ionising radiation. IVU has a little role.

Note: When found in a child younger than 5 years of age with no family history, a diagnosis of tuberous sclerosis must also be considered.

30. Ans. a. Crohn's disease

Ref: CT imaging of colitis, Sep. 2006, Volume 240, Issue 3.

Feature	Ulcerative colitis	Crohn disease
Distribution	Continuous	Discontinuous ('skip')
Symmetry	Symmetric	Asymmetric
Fat halo sign location	Colon	Small bowel
Side	Left sided or diffuse	Right sided or diffuse
Rectum	Involved	Often not involved
Ileocecal value	Open	Stenosed
Small-bowel involvement	Terminla ileum only	Any small-bowel segment
Terminla ileum involvement	Backwash ileitis	String sign
Fat	Perirectal fat increased	Mesenteric fat increased
Pericolonig stranding	Rare	Frequent
Lymph nodes	Not enlarged	Usually enlarged
Fistulae	No	Yes
Toxic megacolon	Yes*	Yes
Stricture	Yes	Yes†
Abscess	Yes	Yes†

31. Ans. d. 8 years

Ref: Arthur R. Interpretation of the Paediatric Chest X-ray; Current Paediatrics (2003) 13, 438-447. www.radiopedia.org

The thymus gradually becomes less evident between the ages of 2–8 years, after which it cannot be visualized on the frontal chest radiograph.

At times, the normal thymus can appear very large, and may need to be differentiated from a mediastinal mass or an area of pulmonary consolidation.

Thymic sail sign à thymus is seen as a triangular sail frequently towards the right of the mediastinum.

It has no mass effect on trachea or esophagus.

Spinnaker sign/angel wing sign → sign of pneumomediastinum seen on neonatal chest radiographs. It refers to the thymus being outlined by air.

32. Ans. d. Kawasaki disease

Ref: Manual of Emergency critical care ultrasound, Vicke E Noble. 2/p156; www.radiologyassistant.nl

Thickening of the gallbladder wall is a relatively frequent finding at diagnostic imaging studies. A thickened gallbladder wall measures more than 3 mm, typically has a layered appearance at sonography.

In CT, it frequently appears as a hypodense layer of subserosal oedema that mimics pericholecystic fluid.

Gallbladder wall thickening	
Cholecystitis – acute – chronic – acalculous – xanthogranulomatous Gallbladder carcinoma Adenomyomatosis	Livercirrhosis Hepatitis Congestive right heart failure Renal failure Pancreatitis

33. Ans. b. Hamartoma

Ref: Radiology Review Manual, 7/e p480.

Popcorn calcification → amorphous calcification with rings and arcs that resembled popcorn kernels.

Seen in Pulmonary hamartoma
- Fibroadenoma of breast with calcific degeneration
- Calcified uterine fibroid
- Bone tumor with chondroid matrix

Pulmonary hamartoma
- Most common benign tumor of the lung.
- Smooth lobulated mass
- Popcorn Calcification
- Fat component in 50%

Bronchial Carcinoid is a neuroendocrine tumor. It appears as an exophytic mass in bronchoscopy.

Dense ossification/scattered calcification is characteristic. Low malignant potential.

34. Ans. d. Oligemia

Ref: Harrison's Principles of Internal Medicine 18/e d. www.radiologyassistant.nl

Pulmonary edema–abnormal accumulation of fluid in the extra vascular compartment of lung.

2 Basic types: cardiogenic and non-cardiogenic.

Cardiogenic pulmonary edema is caused by increased hydrostatic pulmonary capillary pressure.

Noncardiogenic edema is caused by either altered capillary membrane permeability or decreased plasma oncotic pressure.

The chest radiograph still remains the most practical and useful method of radiologically assessing and quantifying pulmonary edema.

Stage of congestive heart failure		
Stage 1 Redistribution PCWP 13–18 mm Hg	→	Redistribution pulmonary vessels Cardiomegaly Broad vascular pedicle (non acute CHF)

Contd...

Contd...

Stage of congestive heart failure		
Stage 2 Interstitial edema PCWP 18–25 mm Hg	→	Kerley lines Peribronchial cuffing Hazy contour of vessels Thickened interlobar fissure
Stage 3 Alveolar edema PCWP > 25 mm Hg	→	Consolidation Air bronchogram Cottonwool appearance Pleural effusion

Cephalization of pulmonary vessels is only seen in cardiogenic pulmonary edema and never seen in pulmonary edema of renal failure/overhydration/low oncotic pressure.

Causes of Non-cardiogenic pulmonary edema:
Not Cardiac
N: near drowning
O: O_2 therapy/post intubation pulmonary edema
T: trauma/transfusion (TRALI: Transfusion-Related Acute Lung Injury)
C: CNS: neurogenic pulmonary edema
A: allergic alveolitis
R: renal failure
D: drugs
I: inhaled (toxins)
A: altitude: high altitude pulmonary edema (HAPE), ARDS
C: contusion

Chest X-ray findings in Cardiogenic pulmonary Edema
- Cephalization of the pulmonary vessels
- Kerley B lines or septal lines
- Peribronchial cuffing
- 'Bat wing' pattern
- Patchy shadowing with air bronchograms
- Cardiomegaly

35. Ans. a. CT angiography

Ref: Diagnostic Radiology, Vol. 1, 7/e p536-543, Grainger & Allison.
CT Angiography of Pulmonary Embolism: Diagnostic criteria and causes of misdiagnosis. Radiographics, Sep. 2004, Vol. 24, Issue 5.

Chest radiography is often the first imaging examination performed in patients suspected of having PE; however, it is unreliable.
D-dimer assay–high sensitivity, but poor specificity
Ventilation perfusion Scintigraphy–high sensitivity, but very poor specificity
Pulmonary angiography–diagnostic standard of reference/gold standard; but underused, not universally available.

Characteristic radiographic signs:
- *Westermark's sign*–localized peripheral oligaemia secondary to the embolus lodging in a peripheral artery.
- *Hampton's hump*–pleural based wedge-shaped opacity.
- *Palla's sign*–Enlarged right descending pulmonary artery.

McConnell's sign–regional wall motion abnormalities sparing the RV apex in Echocardiography.
A normal V/Q scintigram effectively excludes PE owing to the high sensitivity of the test.
Large ventilation perfusion mismatch with a normal chest radiograph is highly probable for PE.
Indirect investigation include Doppler study of lower limb to look for deep vein thrombosis.
Acute embolism is seen as an intravascular filling defect in conventional and CT angiography.

Diagnostic criteria in CT angiography

- Arterial occlusion with failure to enhance the entire lumen due to a large filling defect; the artery may be enlarged compared with adjacent patent vessels.
- A partial filling defect surrounded by contrast material, producing the 'polo mint' sign on images acquired perpendicular to the long axis of a vessel and the 'railway track' sign on longitudinal images of the vessel.
- A peripheral intraluminal filling defect that forms acute angles with the arterial wall.

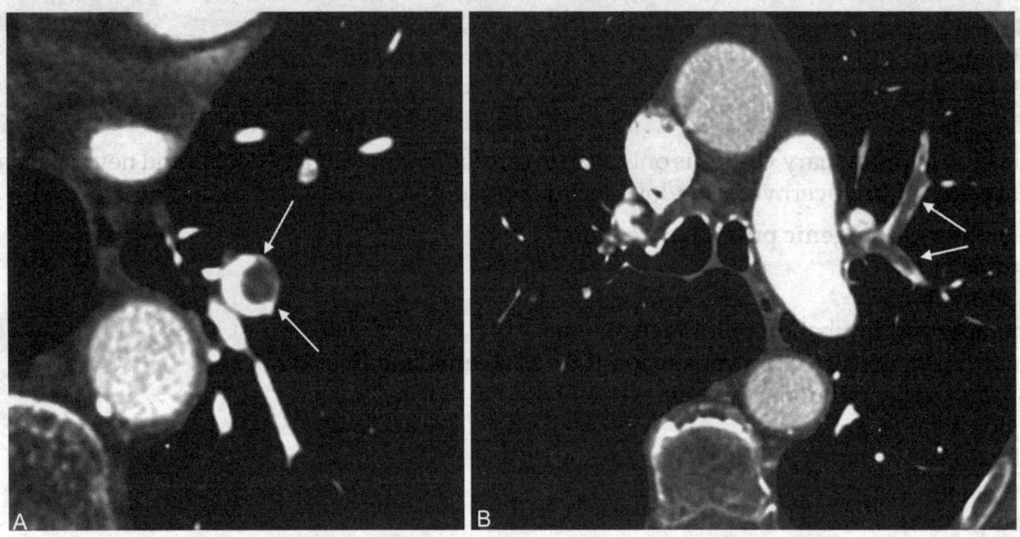

Figs 18.9 (A and B): A: Polo Mint sign, B: Railway track sign

36. Ans. a. CT

Ref: Imaging of Pancreas: Recent advances, Vikas Chaudhary, Encyclopedia of Imaging, Volume 2. Albert Baert, p215.

CT outclasses all imaging modalities in detecting calcifications.

CT is the most sensitive imaging modality while MR imaging is poor at detecting calcification.

USG and X-ray are modalities with lesser sensitivity.

CT is particularly useful in conditions like chronic pancreatitis and ovarian dermoid in which calcification is characteristic.

37. Ans. c. Right Ventricle

Ref: Cardiac X-rays by V. Chockalingam and A. Chockalingam. 1/e Elsevier. 2008 p10

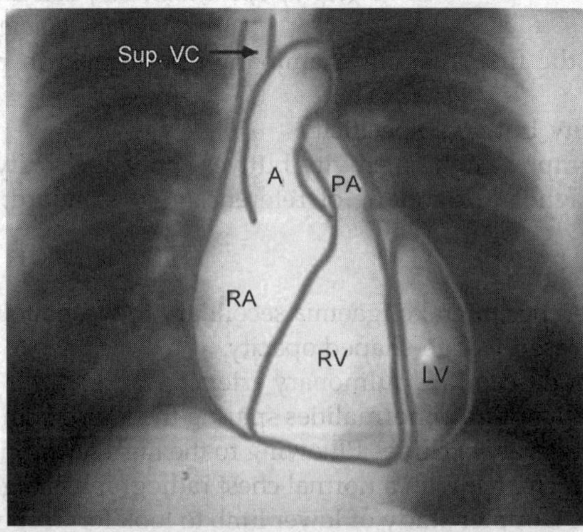

Fig. 18.10 A: Chest X-ray

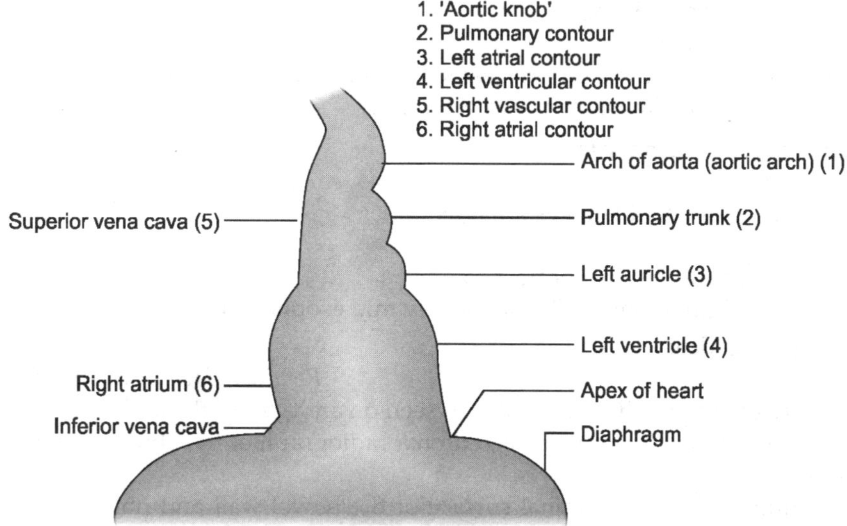

Fig. 18.10 B: Cardiac outline

38. Ans. c. 'E' Sign or 'Reverse Three sign'

Ref: Gastrointestinal Radiology: A Pattern Approach, p.30. Ronald L. Eisenberg

Coarctation of aorta–localized obstruction at the junction of aortic arch and descending aorta secondary to a fibrous ridge protruding into aortic lumen.

Two forms exist:

Adult type–postductal type, localized coarctation; coexistent cardiac anomalies less common.

Infantile type–preductal type, diffuse type; coexistent cardiac anomalies common.

Common associations–bicuspid aortic valve and PDA.

The aortic segment affected by the coarctation has a shape that resembles the number 3 on frontal chest radiographs.

The number 3 is formed by dilatation of the left subclavian artery and aorta proximal to the site of coarctation, indentation of the site, and dilatation of the aorta distal to the site.

The reverse figure-of-3 sign ('E' sign), a mirror image of the number 3, is observed on the left anterior oblique view during barium esophagography in patients with aortic coarctation.

Inferior rib notching involving ribs 3-9 (secondary to dilated intercostal collateral vessels).

1st and 2nd ribs don't participate because they have arteries originating from costocervical trunk (thus proximal to coarctation).

If unilaterally seen on the left side, it suggests an associated aberrant right subclavian artery arising after the coarctation.

If unilaterally seen on the right side, then the origin of the left subclavian artery is distal to the coarctation.

Second most common cause of congestive heart failure in neonate.

39. Ans. b. Achalasia cardia

Ref: Radiology Review Manual, Dahnert, 7/e p812.

- Primary abnormality–failure of organized peristalsis and relaxation at level of lower esophageal sphincter.
- Bird beak/rat tail deformity–V-shaped conical and symmetric tapering of stenotic segment with most marked narrowing OG junction.
- Hurst phenomenon–temporary transit through cardia when hydrostatic pressure of barium column is above tonic LES pressure.
- The mucosal contours remain smooth without nodularity, abrupt contour change, or evidence of intraluminal mass.
- The appearances although classically occurring in primary achalasia, can also occur in pseudoachalasia due to a gastric tumor involving the gastroesophageal junction.
- Radiologic characteristics of achalasia with normal manometric findings is diagnostic of pseudoachalasia.
- Achalasia is primarily a manometric diagnosis.

Manometric characteristics of achalasia

- Absence of primary peristalsis
- Increased or normal resting lower esophageal sphincter (LES) pressures
- Incomplete or absent LES relaxation on swallowing

Chest radiographic signs of Achalasia

- Absent gastric air bubble
- Mediastinal widening due to dilated esophagus
- Air-fluid level
- Anterior displacement and bowing of trachea

Complication–esophageal carcinoma in 2–7% (usually mid esophagus)

40. Ans. a. Perforated peptic ulcer

Ref: Radiology Review Manual, Dahnert, p771–773.

- Rigler sign–also known as the double-wall sign seen on an X-ray of the abdomen.
- Both sides of the bowel wall can be visualized on a radiograph of the abdomen obtained with the patient in the supine position.
- Gas normally outlines only the luminal surface of the bowel wall and not the serosal surface. When at least a moderate amount of free intraperitoneal air exists, however, this free air is more likely to accumulate between bowel loops, thus permitting visualization of the outer walls of the bowel. This is the classic appearance of the Rigler sign.
- A variant of the Rigler sign occurs when only the outside of the bowel wall is visible because the lumen is filled with fluid.
- A false double wall sign can result from two loops of bowel being in contact with one another.
- Foot ball sign–large pneumoperitoneum outlining entire abdominal cavity.
- Tell tale triangle sign–triangular air pocket between 3 loops of bowel.

Rigler's sign should not be confused with Rigler's triad, the Rigler notch sign or Hoffman-Rigler sign.

41. Ans. d. Superior pole renal mass

Ref: Callahan MJ. The drooping lily sign. Radiology. 2001 Apr; 219(1): 226–8. Radiology Review Manual, Dahnert, 7/e p1001–1002.

- Hydronephrotic upper pole displacing the lower pole moiety laterally and inferiorly (i.e. the 'drooping lily' sign).

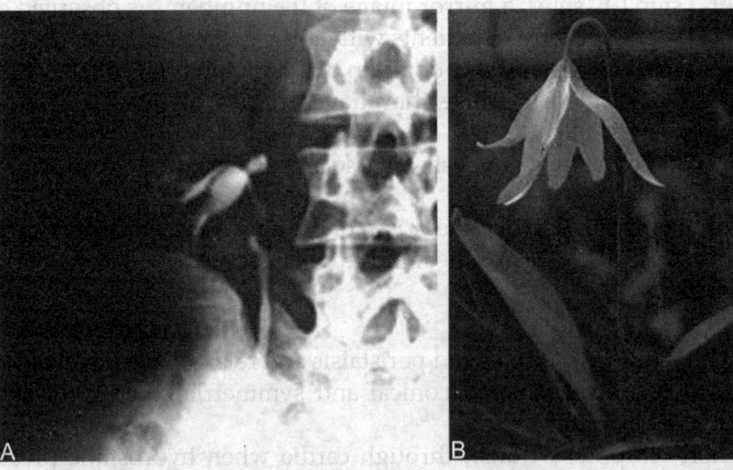

Fig. 18.11: Drooping lily sign

- *Drooping lily sign*–Classically described in urography; in a completely duplicated system, a dilated, obstructed upper moiety collecting system, may produce downward and lateral displacement of the functional lower moiety collecting system.
- The sign is often accompanied by a bladder filling defect, representing an ureterocele, which is associated with the ectopic insertion of the upper moiety ureter.

- As the frequency of excretory urography wanes, the 'classic' drooping lily is less frequently encountered.
- Diagnostic consideration should be given to the presence of a duplication anomaly whenever a process is discovered in only one portion of a kidney.
- *Nubbin sign*–scarring, atrophy and decreased function of lower pole moiety may simulate a renal mass.
- *Weigert-Meyer rule*–Upper pole moiety ureter inserts ectopically inferior and medial to lower moiety ureter (as ureterocele) and is prone for obstructive hydronephrosis. Lower moiety ureter inserts orthotopically and is prone for vesicoureteric reflux.

42. Ans. c. Metastasis *Ref: http://radiology.med.miami.edu/documents/2009Bone_Scan_All.pdf*

Cold Spots may be caused by

- Malignant Tumors
  - Lung (2–4%)
  - Breast (5%)
  - Renal (10%)
  - Neuroblastomas (bone marrow mets)
  - Thyroid (most cases)
  - Multiple Myeloma (most cases)
- Bone Abscesses (they are surrounded by activity)
- Bone ischemia (AVN, sickle cell, etc.)
- Hemangiomas (normal or decreased activity)

43. Ans a. Ureterocele *Ref: The Cobra Head Sign 1, pubs.rsna.org/doi/full/10.1148/radiol.2253011206*

- An ureterocele is a congenital saccular dilatation of the terminal portion of the ureter.
- The **cobra head sign** (or **spring onion sign**) refers to dilatation of the terminal ureter, surrounded by a thin lucent line, which is seen in patients with an adult-type ureterocele.
- The presence of this cobra head appearance is an indicator of uncomplicated ureterocele.
- The terminal ureter dilates in response to restriction of flow at the ureteral orifice in the bladder.
- The lucent hood represents the combined thickness of the ureteral wall and prolapsed bladder mucosa, outlined by contrast material within the bladder lumen.
- This lucent line should be thin and well defined. Any thickening, irregularity, or loss of definition of the cobra's hood should raise concern for the presence of a pseudoureterocele.
- A pseudoureterocele can result from edema related to stone impaction or recent stone passage, or more important, tumor overgrowth of the ureteral orifice.
- If the cobra head appearance is not 'classic,' cystoscopic evaluation should be performed.

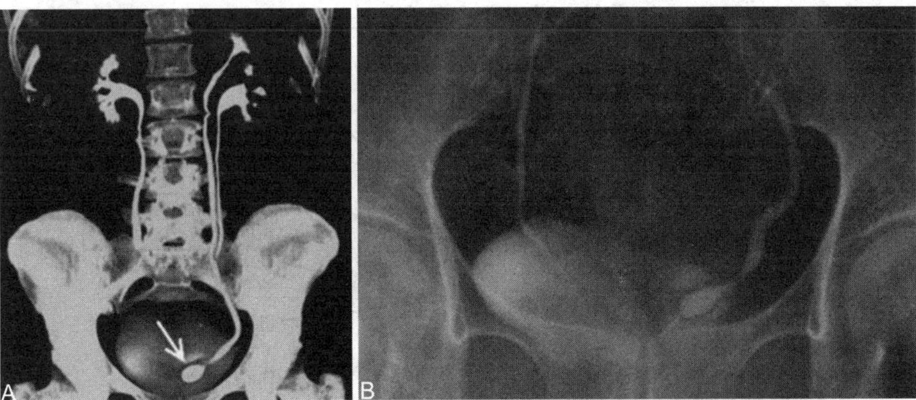

Figs 18.12 (A and B): Cobra head sign

44. Ans. a. Crohn's disease.

Ref: Radiology Review manual, Dahnert, 7/e p834–835. Diagnostic Radiology, Grainger & Allison, 5/e p662–665.

Transmural inflammation leads to decreased luminal diameter and limited distensibility.

This leads to a radiographic string sign (string sign of Kantor) that represents long areas of circumferential inflammation and fibrosis resulting in long segments of luminal narrowing.

Crohn's disease

Chronic, progressive, transmural disease.

Affects any part of GIT; most commonly involves small intestine.

Most characteristic feature–variety of its radiological appearances and the multiplicity of imaging features.

Radiological signs of Crohn's disease:

- Ulceration–discrete ulcers, fissure ulcers, longitudinal ulcers
- Cobble stoning
- Thickening of Valvulae conniventes
- Stenosis
- Dilatation proximal to stenosis
- Asymmetric involvement
- Skip lesions
- Inflammatory polyps (pseudopolyps)
- Featureless outline
- Thickened wall
- Enlarged ileocaecal valve

String sign–irreversible severe narrowing of bowel loop due to marked fibrous thickening of the intestinal wall.

Comb sign–hyperemic engorged tortuous vasa recta adjacent to actively inflamed bowel segment.

Target sign–active inflammation with mural stratification.

Creeping fat sign–massive fibro-fatty proliferation of mesentery.

45. Ans. a. Non contrast CT

Ref: Radiology Review Manual, Dahnert, 7/e p329–330.

- Most common cause of Sub Arachnoid hemorrhage (SAH) is trauma.
- Most common cause of spontaneous SAH is ruptured aneurysm.
- Non contrast CT is diagnostic.
- Accuracy high within 5 days of onset.
- Increased density in basal cisterns, superior cerebellar cistern, sylvian fissure, cortical sulci, along inter-hemispheric fissure and intra-ventricular location.
- Cortical vein sign–visualization of cortical veins passing through extra-axial fluid collection.
- MRI–sulci and cisterns appear hyperintense (bright) on FLAIR sequence.
- MRI is more sensitive than CT (for small SAH).

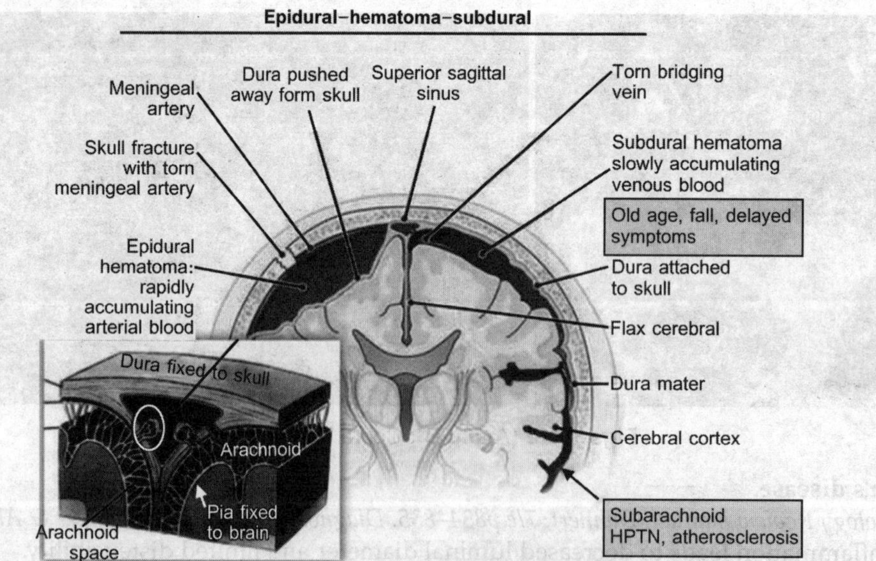

Fig. 18.13: Hematoma

46. Ans. a. FDG

Ref: Radiology by Wolfgang Dahnert 5/e p1113

Positron emission tomography (PET) uses short-lived positron-emitting isotopes, which are produced by a cyclotron immediately before use.

Two gamma-rays are produced from the annihilation of each positron and can be detected by a specialized gamma camera.

The resulting images reflect the distribution of the isotope. Invariably, some form of computer is linked to the gamma camera to enable rapid serial images to be taken and to perform computer enhancement of the images when relevant. The electrical pulse is further amplified and analyzed by a processing unit so that a recording can be made.

In selected cases emission tomography is performed. In this technique, the gamma camera moves around the patient. A computer can analyze the information and produce sectional images similar to CT.

47. Ans. b. Hyperparathyroidism

Ref: Harrison's Principles of Internal Medicine, 18/ed.
Radiology Review Manual, Dahnert, p108–109.

- Metaphyseal changes resembling rickets and cortical erosions giving a 'rotting fence-post' appearance, specially at the femoral neck.
- Renal osteodystrophy is the term applied to the bone changes present in patients with chronic renal failure.
- In CRF, secondary Hyperparathyroidism coexists with rickets, Osteomalacia, osteosclerosis and osteoporosis as part of spectrum of findings called renal osteodystrophy.
- Osteosclerosis is characteristic with predilection for axial skeleton.
- Rugger jersey spine–subchondral deposition of bone in vertebra leading to alternate dark and light bands on radiography
- In children, metaphyseal changes resembling rickets are seen. This together with cortical erosions can give rise to rotting fence post appearance, particularly at the femoral neck

Fibrous dysplasia → two forms: Monostotic (more common) and Polyostotic.

Monostotic form more commonly involves ribs.

Shepherd's crook deformity–extensive involvement of proximal femur results in a characteristic varus deformity which resembles a shepherd's crook.

Cherubism–familial fibrous dysplasia; bilateral expansile cystic mass involving bilateral mandible and maxilla.

Ground glass matrix in bones is characteristic in radiography and CT.

Paget's disease → chronic multifocal skeletal disease with disordered and exaggerated bone remodeling

Three phases–active (osteolytic), mixed and inactive (late, quiescent).

Pelvis more commonly involved than spine.

Osteoporosis circumscripta–well defined lytic lesion involving skull.

Cotton wool appearance–mixed lytic and blastic pattern of skull.

Candle flame/blade of grass Lysis–advancing tip of V shaped lytic defect in diaphysis of long bone.

Picture frame vertebra–bone within bone appearance; enlarged square shaped vertebral body with reinforced peripheral trabeculae with central radiolucency.

Ivory vertebra–uniformly white vertebra with no abnormality of its contours and adjacent disks; Differential diagnosis–osteoblastic metastasis from carcinoma prostate.

Markedly increased uptake in bone scan is characteristic.

May transform to secondary osteosarcoma.

48. Ans. a. Greater than 1000k volts

Ref: Internet source

- Megavoltage X-rays are produced by linear accelerators.
- Operates at voltages in excess of 1000 KV (1MV) range, and therefore have an energy in the MeV range.
- Beams with the voltage range of 4–25 MV are used to treat patients because they penetrate well to deep sites within the body.

49. Ans. c. 2800 cGy

Ref: Emami V. Lyman J, Brown A, Coia L, Goitein M, Munzenrider JE et al. Tolerance of Normal tissue to therapeutic Irradiation. Int J Radiat Oncol Biol Phys. 1991 May 15;21(1):109-22

TD 50–Tolerance dose that within 5 years will cause a maximal 50% complication rate (unacceptable).

50. Ans. b. 8 days

Ref: Internet Source

Iodine 131 is a radio-isotope with a very short half-life of 8.02 days, making it highly radioactive.
Two isotopes of iodine are used in patients with thyroid diseases:
I123–harmless to thyroid cells; I131–destroys thyroid cells.
I-123 is the usual isotope used to take pictures and determine the activity of the intact thyroid gland.
I-131 is given to destroy overactive thyroid tissue.
Large doses of I-131 are used to destroy thyroid cancer cells.

QUESTIONS 2015

1. Difference between light and X-ray:
a. Energy
b. Mass
c. Speed
d. Type of wave

2. Best radiological investigation for insulinoma:
a. PET
b. CECT
c. MRI
d. Radionuclide scan

3. True about PA chest X-ray view:
a. Left dome of diaphragm higher than the right
b. Pulmonary vessels behind heart are not visible
c. Bowel between liver and right hemidiaphragm is abnormal
d. Rotation causes a change in translucency of the lungs

4. Hot spot in heart seen in which scan:
a. Gallium
b. Albumin labelled
c. Thallium
d. Tc Pyrophsophate scan

5. Plain Abdominal X-ray can diagnose:
a. Sigmoid volvulus
b. Cholesterol gallstones
c. Carcinoma Cecum
d. Acute pancreatitis

6. Technique used to counter movement of tumor due to breathing in radiotherapy:
a. Gating
b. Bolus tracking technique
c. Faraday cage
d. Gel dosimetry

7. Which of the following is used for pancreatic scanning?
a. Cr–51
b. Tc–99
c. Se–75
d. I–131

8. Tc99 labelled white cells used for?
a. Ca colon
b. Intra-abdominal mass
c. Terminal ileitis in crohn's disease
d. Stricture

9. Structure superior to male bladder in CT scan:
a. Sigmoid colon
b. Pubic symphsis
c. Rectum
d. Levator ani

10. Gold standard investigation for scarring of kidney:
a. Tc99 DMSA scan
b. Tc99 DTPA scan
c. MIBG scan
d. Sestamibi scan

11. Pathognomonic radiological feature of hyperparathyroidism:
a. Subperiosteal bone resorption
b. Calcific pancreatitis
c. Brown tumor
d. Nephrocalcinosis

12. Which of the following radiological feature of Ulcerative Collitis differentiates it from Crohn's?
a. Loss of haustrations
b. Tracking of contrast in gut wall
c. Rectal sparing
d. Patchy or discontinuous involvement

ANSWERS AND EXPLANATIONS

1. **Ans. a. Energy** *Ref: Squire's Fundamentals of Radiology, Robert A. Noveline, Lucy Frank Squire. Ch.1, p1*
   - X-rays are a type electromagnetic rays. Electromagnetic waves are classified into several regions according to their energy.
   - X-rays are high energy electromagnetic waves, but visible light is medium energy electromagnetic waves.
   - X-rays are a form of radiant energy similar in several respects to visible light.
   - The fundamental difference between X-rays and light rays is their range of wavelengths.
   - Wavelengths of X-rays being shorter than those of visible light.
   - The science of diagnostic radiology is based on this difference since many substance that are opaque to light are penetrated by X-rays.
2. **Ans. b. CECT**

   Ref: Insulinoma: diagnosis and surgical treatment. [Indian J Gastroenterol 2006; 25 : 244–247]
   Pancreatic Endocrine Tumors: Radiologic-Clinicopathologic Correlation. Rachel B. Lewis, LCDR, MC, USN, Grant E. Lattin, Jr, Maj, USAF, MC, and Edina Paal, MD, October 2010, volume 30, issue 6.

   Insulinoma is the most common sporadic endocrine tumors of pancreas.

   These tumors can be relatively small and multiphase contrast enhanced thin slice cross-sectional imaging is ideal.

   Most insulinomas are small (2/3rds less than 2 cm at presentation 3) and hypervascular. Some contain calcification. Malignant tumors tend to be large.

   Sensitivity is higher (as high as 94%) with endoscopic US; however, the procedure requires use of conscious sedation, and endoscopic US may allow only limited evaluation of the pancreatic tail. The sensitivity of intraoperative US is similar to that of endoscopic US, but it requires full mobilization of the pancreas during surgery.

   CT visualizes the exact location of an insulinoma, its relationship to vital structures, and the presence of metastases. Typically, insulinomas are hypervascular and, as a result, demonstrate a greater degree of enhancement than normal pancreatic parenchyma during the arterial and capillary phases of contrast bolus. They typically are hyperattenuating on arterial and venous phase images, a finding due to their rich capillary network. Technical advances have improved the quality of CT, with a recent study reporting that using a multidetector CT enabled visualization of 94.4% of insulinomas. CT is currently accepted as the first-line investigation for the visualization of insulinomas.

   Currently, there is strong evidence emerging for the use of MRI in the imaging of insulinomas, and investigators have shown a high sensitivity for MRI in the detection of insulinomas. If dual-phase CT does not identify a lesion, conventional MRI is unlikely to be of additional help.

   Nuclear medicine imaging may be used to localize a known functioning PET in a patient with a specific clinical syndrome
   - Narrow the differential diagnosis of a pancreatic mass,
   - Evaluate for metastatic disease or recurrence and
   - Assess receptor status for possible radionuclide-based treatment.

   However, for most of these techniques, the PET must be well-differentiated and contain somatostatin receptors. The most frequently used technique is somatostatin-receptor scintigraphy with indium-diethy lenetriaminepenta acetic acid-octreotide 111 (111 In-octreotide).
3. **Ans. d. Rotation causes a change in translucency of the lungs**
   - Left dome is at a lower level due to heart.
   - Pulmonary vessels behind heart are well visualized in optimally taken radiographs.
   - Bowel between liver and right diaphragm is a normal variant called as Chilaiditi syndrome.
   - Rotation leads to changes in lung density due to asymmetry of overlying soft-tissue may be incorrectly interpreted as lung disease.

4. **Ans. d. Tc Pyrophsophate scan**

Tc pyrophosphate is the adjunctive diagnostic agent for detection of acute myocardial infarction.

5. **Ans. a. Sigmoid volvulus**

Ref: 'The Coffee Bean sign', Deborah Feldman, Radiology, July 2000, vol. 216, issue. 1

The coffee bean sign is a classic conventional radiographic finding of sigmoid volvulus.

Plain radiographs show a markedly distended sigmoid loop, which assumes a bent inner tube or inverted *U*-shaped appearance, with the limbs of the sigmoid loop directed toward the pelvis.

The twisted loop of sigmoid colon is said to resemble a coffee bean. The loop of dilated sigmoid colon—or 'coffee bean'—usually points upwards towards the diaphragm.

As the closed loop of the sigmoid colon distends with gas, apposition of the medial walls of the dilated bowel form the cleft of the coffee bean, while the lateral walls of the dilated bowel form the outer walls of the bean.

Cholesterol gallstones are usually radiolucent.

Plain abdominal radiographs are a useful first step in the evaluation of patients presenting with complications of colon cancer, such as large bowel obstruction or perforation.

Acute pancreatitis can show colon cutoff sign but that is not diagnostic.

6. **Ans. a. Gating**

Ref: Respiratory Gating for Radiotherapy: Main Technical Aspects and Clinical Benefits, ISRN Pulmonology, Volume 2013 (2013), Article ID 519602.

Respiratory-gated radiotherapy offers a significant potential for improvement in the irradiation of tumor sites affected by respiratory motion such as lung, breast, and liver tumors.

Five main strategies are used to reduce respiratory motion effects: integration of respiratory movements into treatment planning, forced shallow breathing with abdominal compression, breath-hold techniques, respiratory gating techniques, and tracking techniques.

Respiratory gating techniques use external devices to predict the phase of the breathing cycle while the patient breathes freely.

7. **Ans. c. Se–75** *Ref: Textbook of Radiopharmacy, C.B. Sampson. Pg. 204*

Selenomethionine was developed as a selenium-75 labelled analogue of the amino acid methionine. Its use in pancreas scanning is based on the fact that digestive enzymes produced by the pancreas are secreted with each meal, and to keep up with this turnover, the pancreas must synthesize new protein at a very rapid rate. Selenium-75 can be detected in proteins within an hour of intravenous injection.

8. **Ans. c. Terminal ileitis in crohn's disease**

Ref: World J Gastroenterol. 2009 Jun 14; 15(22): 2693–2700. Role of scintigraphy in inflammatory bowel disease. Ulcerative colitis imaging, www.emedicine.medscape.com

Until recently, gallium-67 (67Ga) was the only radionuclide used in the scanning of inflammatory bowel disease (IBD). However, recent developments in leukocyte labeling have largely replaced the use of gallium because of better dosimetry and resolution and a lower radiation burden to the patient.

With the availability of indium-labeled WBCs, radionuclide-imaging studies have a definite role in the diagnosis and staging of IBD. The indium-111 (111 In) WBC study is particularly helpful in evaluating recurrent disease in patients with severe intercurrent diseases and in screening patients, without the need for barium examinations.

WBCs may be labeled with Technetium-99m HMPAO. Technetium-99m HMPAO leukocyte labeling may be performed in the presence of plasma and appears to have significant selectivity for granulocytes.

Radionuclide-labeled WBC scanning using111. In is an accurate, quantitative, and noninvasive method for assessing the degree of bowel inflammation in cases of IBD; it is also useful in assessing response to therapy.

Studies have indicated that imaging with 99m Tc-labeled leukocytes may be more sensitive than imaging with 111 In-labeled leukocytes for detecting and determining the extent of IBD, especially in the small bowel.

Tc-99m hexamethylpropylene amine oxime white blood cells remain a widely acceptable scintigraphic method for the diagnosis of IBD, as well as for the evaluation of disease extension and severity.

9. **Ans. a. Sigmoid colon**

Relations of bladder–male

Anteriorly—pubic symphysis posteriorly—rectovesical pouch and rectum inferiorly—prostate, obturator internus muscle, levator ani muscle superiorly—peritoneum laterally—ischioanal fossa

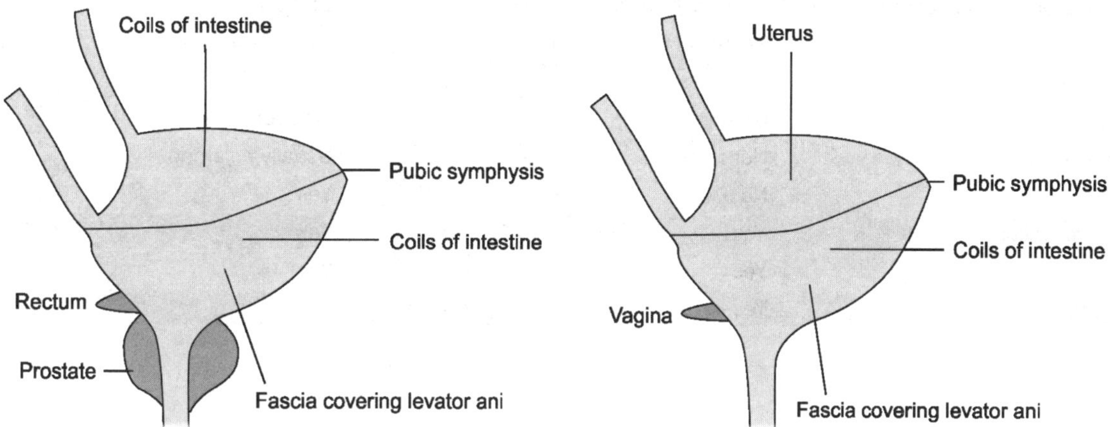

Figs 18.14 (A and B): A: Relations of bladder-male, B: Relations of bladder-female

10. **Ans. a. Tc99 DMSA scan** *Ref: Radiology Review Manual, Dahnert, Pg.1138.*

Renal cortical scarring is the sequela of upper urinary tract infection.

Nuclear medicine renal scanning with a cortical imaging agent (e.g. technetium-99m [99m Tc] dimercaptosuccinic acid) is a better means of detecting and identifying renal scarring.

Agents for renal function—Tc99m DTPA, I–131 Hippuran

Renal cortical agent—Tc99m DMSA

Renal combination agent—Tc99m glucoheptonate

Tc99m DMSA differentiates pseudotumor from neoplasms.

Tc99, DTPA is the agent of choice for assessment of Renal perfusion, glomerular filtration (relativel GFR), obstructive uropathy and vesicoureteric reflux.

11. **Ans. a. Subperiosteal bone resorption** *Ref: Radiology Review Manual, Dahnert, p108.*

Subperiosteal bone resorption of radial aspect of middle phalanx of 2nd, 3rd and 4th finger are considered pathognomonic for hyperparathyroidism.

Brown tumor—expansile lytic cyst like lesion without adjacent reactive bone formation.

Renal stones/nephrocalcinosis and calcific pancreatitis are sequelae of hyperparathyroidism.

Rugger jersey spine—alternating bands of dense-lucent-dense appearance of vertebrae at multiple levels; distinctive for hyperparathyroidism.

12. **Ans. a. Loss of haustrations** *Ref: Radiology Review Manual, Dahnert, p890.*

Loss of haustrations or lead pipe like appearance is seen in UC.

Skip involvement, rectal sparing and transmural involvement are seen in Crohns disease.

Feature	Ulcerative Colitis	Crohn Disease
Distribution	Continuous	Discontinuous ('skip')
Symmetry	Symmetric	Asymmetric
Fat halo sign location	Colon	Small bowel
Side	Left sided or diffiuse	Right sided or diffuse
Rectum	Involved	Often not involved
Ileocecal valve	Open	Stenosed'
Small-bowel involvement	Terminal ileum only	any small-bowel segment

Contd...

Contd...

Feature	Ulcerative Colitis	Crohn Disease
Terminal ileum involvement	Backwash ileitis	String sign
Terminal ileum involvement	Backwash ileitis	String sign
Fat	Perirectal fat increased	Mesenteric fat increased
Pericolonic stranding	Rare	Frequent
Pericolonic stranding	Rare	Frequent
Lymph nodes	Not enlarged	Usually enlarged
Fistulae	No	Yes
Toxic megacolon	Yes*	Yes
Stricture	Yes	Yes†
Abscess	Yes	Yes†

Chapter

19 Orthopedics

P Selvaraj

TRAUMA I

Formation of Skeleton

During early **fetal life** the human skeleton is mostly cartilaginous, but is subsequently largely replaced by bone.

In adults, cartilage persists at the surfaces of synovial joints, in the walls of the larynx and epiglottis, trachea, bronchi, nose and external ears.

Developmental replacement by bone is a complex process: cells in cartilaginous growth plates - which lie between ossifying epiphyses and the diaphyses of long bones - continue to proliferate, increasing the length of the bones concerned until they eventually ossify.

Two Mechanisms of Bone Formation

- The *transformation* of fibrous primitive connective tissue into bone is called ***intramembranous ossification.*** All flat bones viz ***pelvis, skull and clavicle*** are formed by this process.
- The *replacement* of cartilage by bone is called endochondral ossification. All ***long bones*** of the skeletal system are formed by ***endochondral ossification except clavicle***.

FRACTURE HEALING

The fracture healing involves five stages:

- Hematoma
- Inflammation
- Soft Callus Formation
- Hard Callus Formation
- Remodeling.

Hematoma induces attraction of inflammatory infiltrate. Granulation tissue gradually replaces the hematoma, fibroblasts produce collagen.

Abundant new cartilage formation marks the soft callus stage.

During hard callus stage, the callus converts to woven bone.

The ***final stage*** of the healing process involves slow ***remodeling from woven to lamellar bone*** and reconstruction of the medullary canal.

- **Wolff's law:** bone remodels in response to mechanical stress. (Increasing mechanical stress leads to significant bone gain

BONE HEALING

The bone heals by laying of new bone tissues; this is in contrast to other tissues which usually heal by fibrous tissue giving rise to scarring.

Bone healing is important in fracture conditions irrespective of surgical or non-surgical management. There are two types of bone healing.

- **In primary fracture healing**, the fracture unite ***without the formation of callus*** (osteonal or Haversian healing). This occurs when the fracture surfaces are rigidly held in contact by ***ORIF using Plates.***
- ***Secondary fracture healing*** results in the ***formation of callus*** and involves the participation of the periosteum. E.g. Fractures managed by ***casting, intramedullary nailing,*** etc.

When healing progresses more slowly than average, it is referred to as **delayed union**. Failure of bone healing, or **nonunion,** results from an arrest of the healing process.

A nonunion that occurs despite the formation of a large volume of callus around the fracture site is referred to as a **hypertrophic nonunion**, in contrast to an **atrophic nonunion** where little or no callus forms and bone resorption occurs at the fracture site.

In some non-unions, cartilaginous tissue forms over the fracture surfaces and the cavity between the surfaces fills with a clear fluid resembling normal joint or bursal fluid creating a **pseudoarthrosis,** or false joint.

Nonunion: a fracture that fails to show progressive evidence of healing over a ***4 to 6-month*** period can be considered a nonunion.

The common causes are: ***inadequate blood supply, inadequate immobilization of the fracture, soft-tissue interposition, infection.***

Nonunions have been classified according to their radiologic characteristics.

Hypertrophic nonunions have viable bone ends, whereas **atrophic nonunions** have nonviable bone ends. This differentiation has importance both in prognosis and in determining appropriate treatment.

AMPUTATIONS

MESS: ***Mangled Extremity Severity Score*** was designed to predict the likelihood of amputation in cases of fractures and crush injuries. A ***score of*** >7 has been reported to predict amputation accurately.

During amputation surgeries, the muscles usually are divided at least 5 cm distal to the intended bone resection.

The stump may be stabilized by one of these two methods.

- **Myodesis**: suturing muscle or tendon to bone
- **Myoplasty:** suturing muscle to periosteum or to fascia of opposing musculature).

Myodesis is contraindicated in severe ischemia because of the increased risk of wound breakdown.

Complications: Infection, Wound Necrosis, Contractures.

Pain Mechanical low back pain, Residual limb pain, painful neuroma, Phantom limb pain),

Contact dermatitis, Verrucous hyperplasia.

Ideal Bone Stump Length

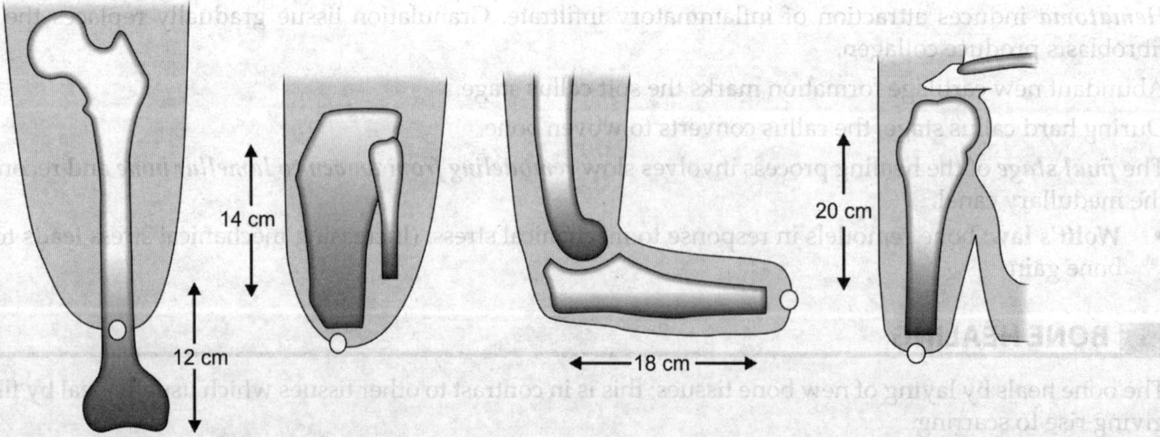

Fig. 19.1: Amputation levels

Femur: Resect 12 cm from knee
Tibia: Leave at least 14 cm
Forearm: 18 cm
Humerus: 20 cm

Midfoot Amputations

- *Lisfranc amputation:* a disarticulation at tarso-metatarsal joint.
- *Chopart amputation:* a midtrasal amputation; removes the forefoot and midfoot and saves only the talus and calcaneus.

Hind Foot Amputations

- *Boyd's amputation* consists of a talectomy and calcaneal-tibial arthrodesis.
- *Pirogoff's ampuation* consists of a talectomy with calcaneal-tibial arthrodesis after the vertical transection of the calcaneus

These two types of hindfoot amputations are done mostly in children to preserve length and growth centers, prevent heel pad migration, and improve socket suspension.

- **Syme's amputation** consists of amputation at the distal tibia and fibula ***0.6 cm*** proximal to the periphery of the ankle joint and passing through the dome of the ankle centrally.

FRACTURES

Fracture is a break in the normal continuity of a bone. The clinical features are ***Severe pain Swelling, Deformity, Abnormal mobility, Crepitus.***

Based on the cause, a fracture may be:

- Traumatic
- Pathological
- Stress

Open fractures are also called as *Compound* fractures.

When the fractured fragments are more than two, it is known as *comminuted* fracture.

The fracture pattern depends on the type of load (force) acting on the bone.

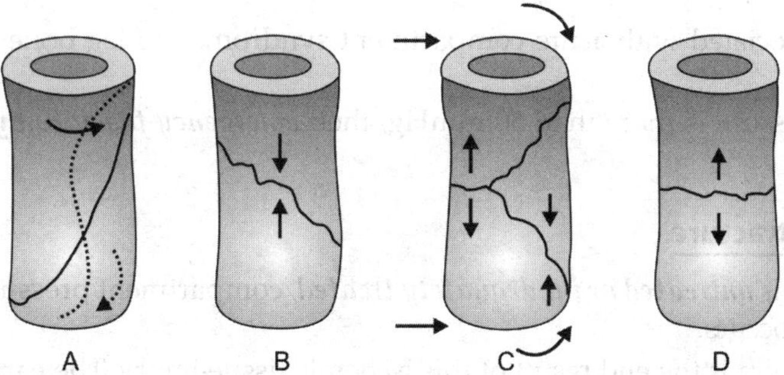

Figs 19.2 (A to D): Types of force and fracture pattern

Fx pattern	Type of force
a. Spiral pattern:	Twisting
b. Oblique pattern:	Compression
c. Triangular 'butterfly' fragment:	Bending
d. Transverse pattern:	Tension/direct

Stress Fractures

Occur in normal bone when the bone is subjected to ***unaccustomed*** stresses.

Commonly seen in young active adults involved in vigorous and excessive exercise, e.g ***army or police recruits***.

Radiographs may be normal in early satege; and may show healing / healed fracture line after a few weeks.

- Radionuclide imaging, CT and MRI can be helpful for occult fractures.
- Treatment is by ***rest, protection in cast***.
- Second metatarsal neck is the most likely site for stress fracture ***(March fractures).***

Other common sites are femoral neck, femoral shaft, tibia (medial tibial stress syndrome), calcaneum, talus and the bones of upper extremity.

Pathological Fractures

Fractures may occur even with normal activity or trivial force if the bone has been ***weakened*** by a pathological process, (e.g.osteoporosis, osteogenesis imperfecta, Paget's disease, bone cyst or a metastasis).

The most common cause is ***osteoporosis,*** and the most common site is ***spine.***

Fat Embolism Syndrome

A unique orthopedic manifestation of ***ARDS*** caused by the release of marrow fat into the circulation following fractures of major bones such as pelvis, femur.

Pathologic examination of the lungs shows fat droplets, usually diffusely distributed throughout the pulmonary vasculature.

It can result in severe pulmonary compromise and death.

Compartment Syndrome

Increased intra compartmental pressures and decreased perfusion resulting in myonecrosis.

5 P's: ***Pain, parathesias, paralysis, pallor, pulselessness*** (all are not needed for diagnosis).

Pain is the earliest and most consistent symptoms; whereas the ***pulse*** may still be palpable even after the syndrome is fully established.

Clinically, the affected limb is very firm and tense on palpation.

In trauma cases, ***fracture*** is the most common cause; and severe soft tissue injury without fracture may too predispose to compartment syndrome.

Most common fractures associated with acute compartment syndrome are leg bone (***tibial)*** *fracture* and ***forearm*** *bone fractures.*

When the compartment pressure is more than 30 mmHg, then ***emergency fasciotomy*** must be performed to save the limb.

Volkmann's Ischemic Contracture

If a compartment syndrome is ***untreated or inadequately treated,*** compartment pressures continue to increase until irreversible tissue ischemia occurs.

Volkmann ischemic contracture is the end result of this ischemic tissue injury. The earliest changes usually involve the ***flexor digitorum profundus*** muscles in the middle third of the forearm.

The typical clinical picture **of established Volkmann contracture** includes elbow flexion, forearm pronation, wrist flexion, thumb adduction, metacarpophalangeal joint extension, and finger flexion.

Clinically, passive extension of fingers is possible only after the wrist is flexed. This is called ***Volkmann's sign.***

Open Fracture (Compound fracture)

The fracture that involve exposure of bone to the outside environment through a traumatic wound.

Gustillo and Anderson Classification: (for open fractures)

Grade I: clean wound less than 1 cm long.

Grade II: laceration is more than 1 cm long, but there is no extensive soft-tissue damage.

Grade III: extensive wounds more than 10 cm in length, significant fracture comminution. Usually a high-energy injury . Grade III injuries are divided into subtypes A, B, and C.

Grade IIIA: open fractures have extensive soft-tissue lacerations, but ***soft-tissue coverage about the fracture is usually well preserved.*** Includes segmental or severely comminuted fractures, regardless of the size of the wound.

Grade IIIB: open fractures have extensive soft-tissue loss with ***periosteal stripping and bony exposure.*** They usually are massively contaminated.

Grade IIIC: open fractures with an ***arterial injury*** that requires repair regardless of the size of the soft-tissue wound.

Open fracture Treatment

Adequate wound irrigation and ***debridement*** are the most important steps in open fracture treatment. The fracture is stabilized with ***External Fixator.***

EPONYMOUS FRACTURES

Jefferson fracture: Burst fractures of atlas C1.

Hangman's fracture: Traumatic Spondylolisthesis of C2 over C3. The mechanisms involved are hyperextension and distraction.

Clay shoveler's fracture: An avulsion of the spinous processes of the lower cervical and upper thoracic vertebrae.

Chance fractures: Seat- Belt injury, due to Flexion-Distraction force involving lumbar spine.

Crescent fracture: Fracture of iliac wing on side of impact due to lateral compression of pelvis.

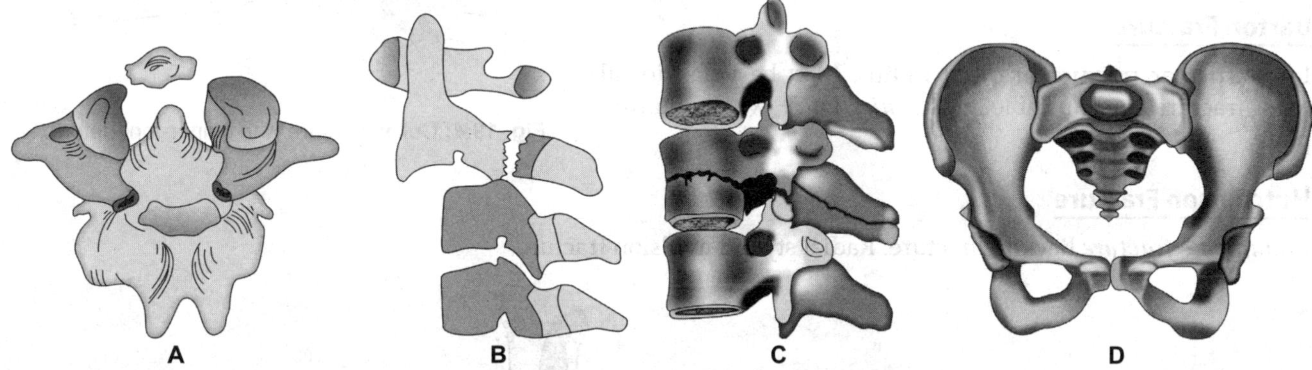

Figs 19.3 (A to D): A. Jefferson Fracture, B. Hangman's Fracture, C. Chance Fractures, D. Crescent fracture

Jumper's Fracture

Dissociation between central and lateral portions of sacrum usually occurs with suicidal jumping on to the floor.

Sentinel Fracture

Fracture through the lamina on either side of the spinous process.

Monteggia Fracture

Fracture of the proximal ulna accompanied by radial head dislocation.

Night Stick Fractures

Result from direct trauma to the ulna along its subcutaneous border, usually by lathi charge.

Galeazzi or Piedmont Fracture

Fracture of the radial diaphysis at the junction of the middle and distal thirds with associated disruption of the distal radioulnar joint.

Reverse Galeazzi Fracture

Denotes a fracture of the distal ulna with associated disruption of the distal radioulnar joint.

Essex-Lopresti lesion: Components are:
- Fracture of the radial head
- Disruption of DRUJ
- Tearing of interosseous membrane.

Laugier's Fracture

Fracture of Trochlea distal humerus.

Colles Fracture

The original description was for extraarticular fractures. Present usage includes both extraarticular and intraarticular distal radius fractures. Dorsal angulation (apex volar), dorsal displacement produce the classical ***dinner fork deformity***.

Treated with cast immobilization in ***cotton-loader position***.

Smith fracture ***(reverse Colles fracture)***: fracture of distal radius with volar angulation (apex dorsal) – ***garden spade deformity***.

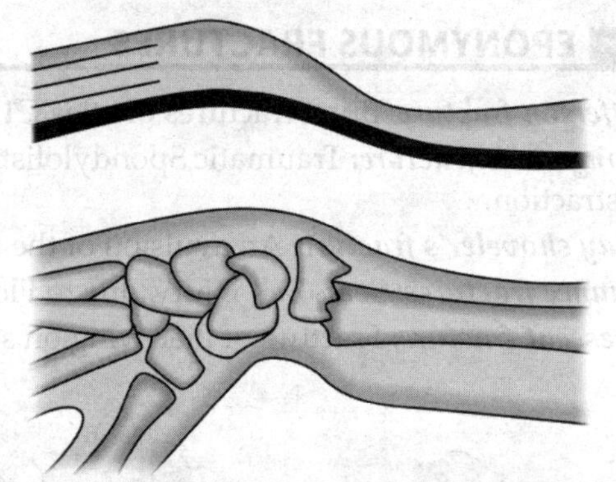

Fig. 19.4: Colles fracture with dinner-fork deformity

Barton Fracture

Intra-articular fracture of distal radius. May be volar/dorsal. Most fractures are unstable and ***require ORIF*** with a buttress plate.

Hutchinson Fracture

Chauffeur's fracture Backfire fracture: Radial styloid avulsion fracture.

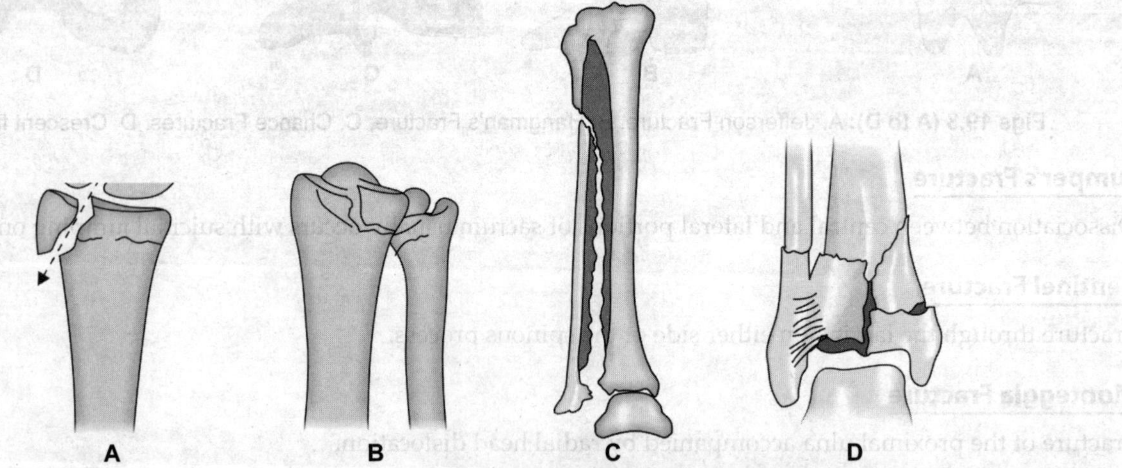

Figs 19.5 (A to D): A. Chauffeur's fx, B. Barton's fx C. Maisonneuve fracture; D. Pilon fracture

Gamekeeper's thumb *or skier's thumb*: Injury to the ulnar collateral ligament thumb MCP joint .

Boxer's Fracture

Fracture at neck of fifth metacarpal bone.

Bennett Fracture

Intraarticular fracture of the base of first metacarpal- the shaft is laterally dislocated by the unopposed pull of ***Abductor Pollicis Longus***. Treated with closed reduction and percutaneous pins or ORIF.

Rolando Fracture

A Y-shaped fracture (a comminuted Bennett fracture) involving the base of the thumb metacarpal. Treated with closed reduction and percutaneous pins or ORIF.

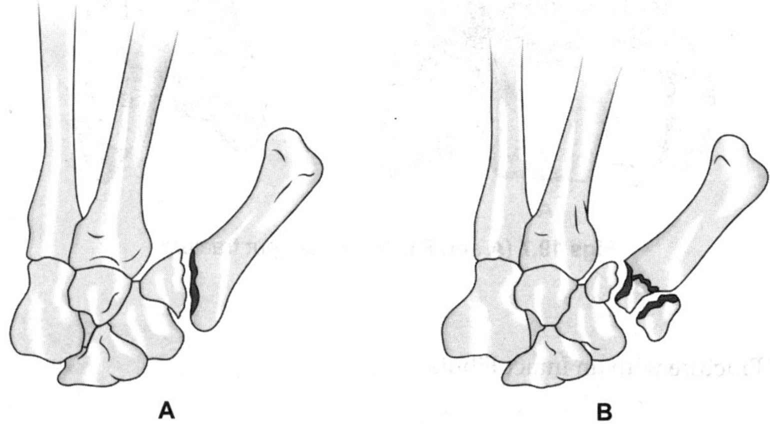

Figs 19.6 A and B: A. Bennett's fx; B. Rolando's fx

Hoffa's Fracture

Coronal plane fracture of the distal femur.

Maisonneuve Fracture

An ankle injury with a fracture of the proximal third of the fibula.

Curbstone Fracture

An avulsion fracture of the posterior tibia is produced by a tripping mechanism.

Pilon Fracture

Intraarticular distal tibial fractures.

Aviator's Fracture

Fracture through neck of talus.

March Fracture

A stress fracture of neck of second mrtatarsal bone.

Pott's Fracture

Bimalleolar (medial and lateral malleoli) fracture.

Cotton's Fracture

Trimalleolar (medial, lateral and posterior) fracture of ankle.

LeForte-Wagstaffe Fracture

Anterior fibular tubercle avulsion fracture by the anterior tibiofibular ligament.

Tillaux-Chaput Fracture

Avulsion of anterior tibial margin by the anterior tibiofibular ligament is the tibial counterpart of the LeForte-Wagstaffe fracture.

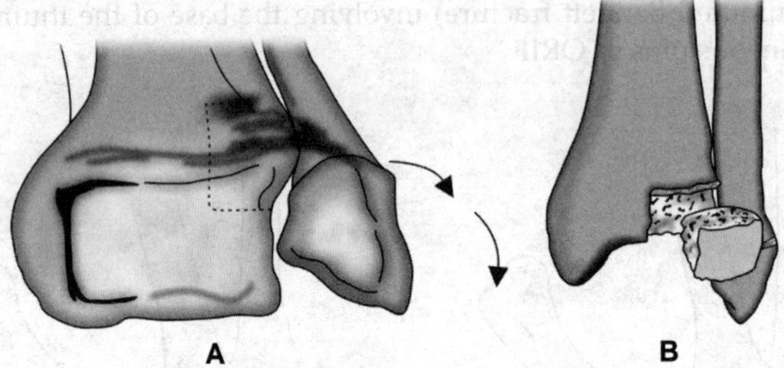

Figs 19.7 (A and B): Tillaux-Chaput fracture

Toddler's Fracture

Oblique or Spiral Tibial Fracture with an Intact Fibula.

Jone's Fractures

Fracture of the base fifth metatarsal. Treated by short-leg cast.

Lisfranc Injury

Fractures / dislocation through tarsometatarsal joint.

COMMON FRACTURE CLASSIFICATIONS

Fracture	Name of the Classification
Open Fractures	Gustilo and Anderson
Supracondylar Humerus	Gartland (based on displacement)
Proximal Humerus	Neer (4 part fractures)
Distal radius	Frykman, Fernandez
Pelvis	Young And Burgess, Tile.
Femoral Neck (pediatric)	Delbet Classification
Femoral Neck (adult)	Pauwel (based on fracture angle), Garden (based on displacement)
Intertrochanteric	Boyd and Griffin, Evans
Femoral Shaft	Winquist and Hansen (based on degree of communition)
Tibial Plateau	Schatzker
Pilon Fracture	Ruedi-Allgower

Fracture	Name of the Classification
Ankle	Lauge-Hansen, Danis-Weber
Talar Neck	Hawkins
Calcaneum	Essex-Lopresti, Sanders(based on CT findings)
Physeal injuries	Salter-Harris Classification

GENERAL FRACTURE MANAGEMENT

General indications for *open reduction and internal fixation*:

- Displaced intra-articular fractures.
- Unstable fractures in which an appropriate trial of nonoperative management has failed.
- Major avulsion fractures.
- Displaced pathological fractures.
- Fractures for which nonoperative treatment is known to yield poor functional results, (femoral neck fractures, Galeazzi fracture, and Montegegia fracture).
- Displaced physeal injuries.
- Fractures with compartment syndromes.
- Nonunions.

ORIF Methods

- Pin and Wire Fixation - small bones fractures, avulsion fractures.
- Screw Fixation - spiral/oblique fractures.
- Plate Fixation - periarticular fractures, humerus, forearm bones etc.
- Intramedullary Nail Fixation - diaphyseal fractures of long bones (tibia, femur).

TRAUMA II

Pelvic Fracture

Occurs with high energy trauma, viz RTA, fall from height, industrial accidents.

Open book fracture: Anteroposterior compression force produces ***diastasis of the pubic symphysis.***

Crescent fracture: lateral compression force causes ***iliac wing fracture*** on the side of impact.

Bucket-handle fracture: severe lateral compression force produces bilateral rotational instability.

Death in pelvic fracture is due to ***hypovolemic shock*** caused by disruption of the venous plexus in the posterior pelvis. It may also be caused by a large-vessel injury, such as external or internal iliac disruption producing marked hemodynamic instability.

Methods of immediate hemorrhage control include:

- Military antishock trousers (MAST),
- Pneumatic antishock garment (PASG)
- Anterior external fixator,
- Wrapping of a pelvic binder
- Pelvic C-clamp.

Open reduction and internal fixation (ORIF): Urgent ORIF for pelvic fractures is ***contraindicated*** because loss of the ***tamponade effect*** may encourage further hemorrhage. Consider angiography or embolization if hemorrhage continues despite closing of the pelvic volume.

FEMORAL NECK FRACTURE

They common in the elderly by trivial injury, due to osteoporosis. In the young, usually by road-traffic accident. Classically the limb is ***shortened and externally rotated.***

Classified as intracapsular and extracapsular:

Sub-types are:
- ***Intracapsular*** – subcapital, transcervical and basicervical.
- ***Extracapsular*** – pertrochanteric (or intertrochanteric) and subtrochanteric.

Neck of femur fracture- Garden's Classification

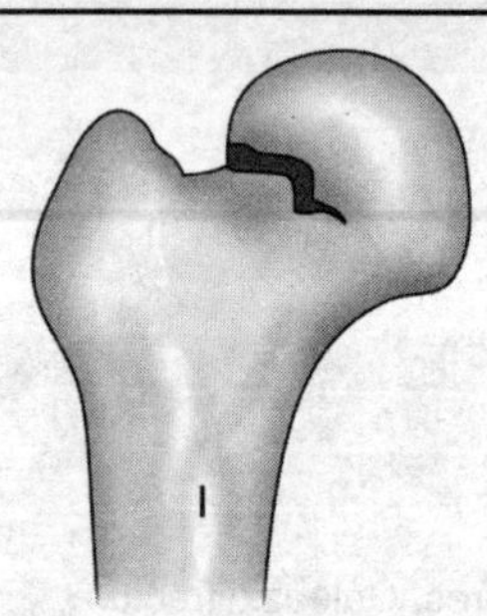

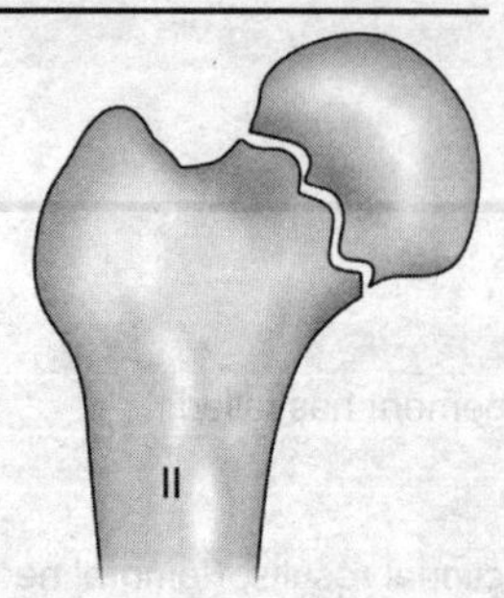

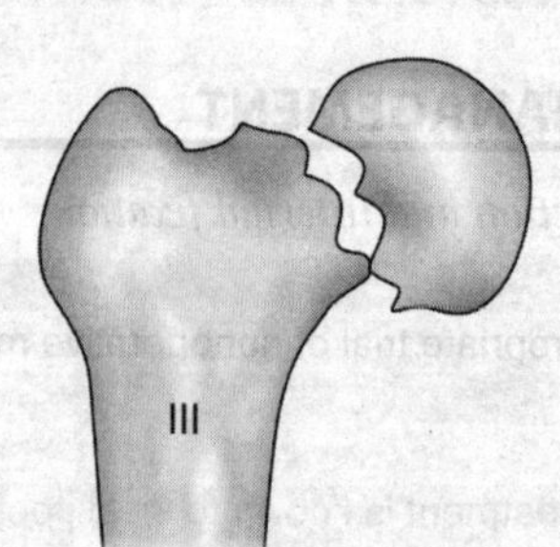

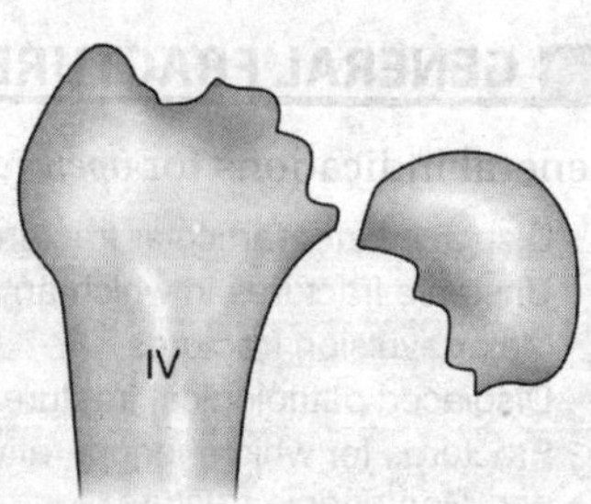

Fig. 19.8: Garden's classification

- Grage I- Incomplete, Valgus impaction.
- Grade II- Complete undisplaced.
- Grade III – complete with partial displacement and angulated trabecular pattern.
- Grade IV- complete with Fully displaced, femoral head trabeculae align with trabecular pattern of acetabulum.

Neck of Femur Fracture- Pauwel's Classification

Based on the angle formed between fracture line and horizontal plane.

Gr I- 30 deg, Gr II- 50 deg, Gr III-70 deg.

Increasing angle lead to more fracture instability, poorer result.

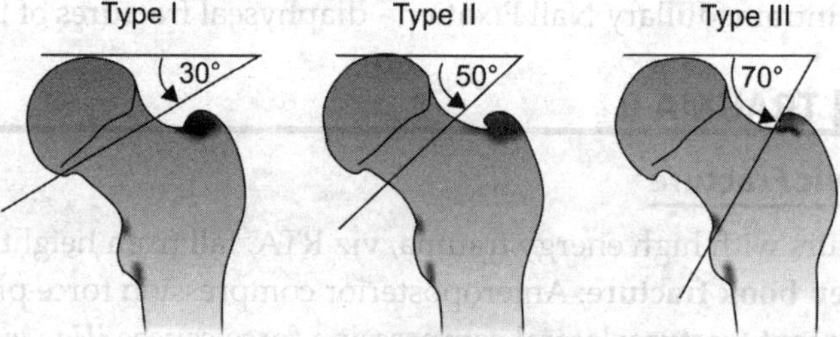

Fig. 19.9: Pauwel's classification

Management

Intracapsular

- In young patients, the femoral head is retained; the fracture is fixed with multiple screws.
- In elderly population, the femoral head is removed and replaced with total hip replacement or hemiarthroplasty.

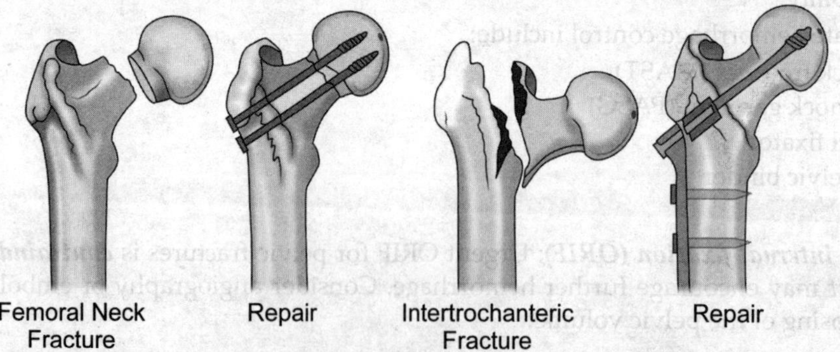

Figs 19.10 (A and B): A. Femur neck Fx treated with multiple Screws B, Intertrochateric Fx , treated with DHS

Extracapsular

- ***Intertrochanteric fracture*** - dynamic hip screw(DHS) or intramedullary hip screw type fixation.
- ***Subtrochanteric fracture*** - DCS (dynamic condylar screw) blade plate, or reconstruction nail.

*(**Tips:** untreated intracapsular fractures end up in nonunion and AVN, whilst the intertrochanteric fractures end up in malunion.)*

PEDIATRIC HIP FRACTURES

Hip fractures in children are very rare.

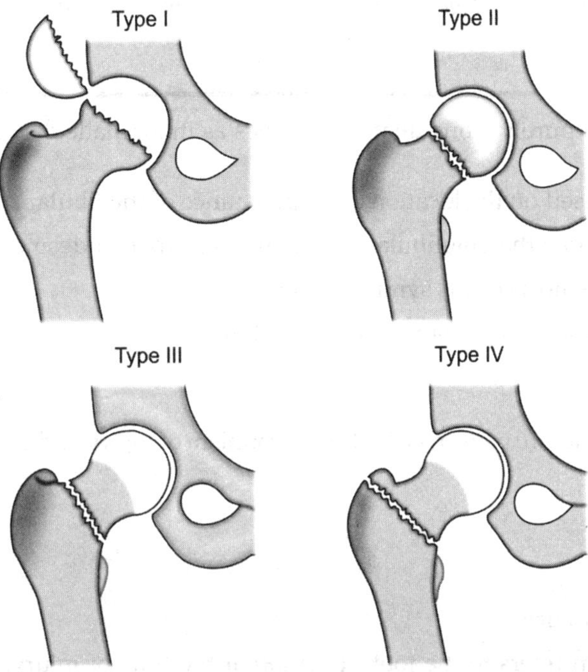

Fig. 19.11: Delbet classification of hip fractures in children

Type I, transepiphyseal (5%)
Type II, transcervical (***most common,*** 50%)
Type III, cervicotrochanteric (25-30%)
Type IV, intertrochanteric(15%).

The treatment of hip fractures in children is different because

- Child tolerates immobilization better
- Variety of treatment methods such as traction, a spica cast, and bed rest, in addition to operative treatment are possible in children.

FEMORAL SHAFT FRACTURE

Result of high-energy trauma. Average blood loss into the thigh is 1200 mL.
Management: according to age group:

- <6 Months: Pavlik harness or splint
- 6 Months to 6 Years: Immediate spica casting
- 6 to 12 Years: Flexible intramedullary nails/ Spica casting - for stable fractures
- 12 to Maturity: Intramedullary fixation with either flexible or interlocked nails is the treatment of choice.

Intramedullary (IM) Nailing: This is the standard of care for femoral shaft fractures in adults.

PATELLA FRACTURE

Transverse Patellar Fracture: result of an *indirect force*, caused by sudden voluntary contraction of the quadriceps muscle or sudden forced flexion of the leg with the quadriceps contracted. Treated by *figure-of-eight tension band wiring.*

Stellate or comminuted fracture: *Direct trauma* to the patella may produce this pattern. Abrasions over the area or open injuries are common. Treated *by cerclage wiring or partial / total patellectomy.*

ANKLE FRACTURES

Ankle fractures can be classified purely along anatomical lines as monomalleolar, bimalleolar **(Pott's fracture)**, or trimalleolar **(Cotton's fracture)**.

Danis-Weber classification is based on the location and appearance of the fibular fracture.

Type A: Fracture of the fibula below the tibiofibular syndesmosis (infra (syndesmotic)

Type B: At the level of the syndesmosis (trans syndesmotic)

Type C: Above the level of the syndesmosis (supra syndesmotic)

Lauge-Hansen Classification

Attempted to associate specific fracture patterns with the mechanism of injury and proposed a detailed classification. This classification includes:

- Supination–external rotation
- Supination–adduction
- Pronation–abduction, and
- Pronation–external rotation injuries.

The first word in the designation refers to the foot's position at the time of injury; the second word refers to the direction of the deforming force.

The most common mechanism is ***supination–external rotation*** which may in most severe cases produce ***trimalleolar fracture.***

In Pronation injuries, the fibula fracture is above the ankle joint (suprasyndesmotic).

CALCANEAL FRACTURE

Commonest (and largest) of the tarsal bones to fracture. Axial loading force, e.g. fall from height, is the commonest mechanism of injury. ***Spine fractures*** are associated with Calcaneal fractures. ***Bohler's Angle, Crucial Angle of Gissane*** indicate posterior facet depression, and are useful in subtle cases.

TALUS FRACTURE

Neck of talus fracture occurs due to Fall from height with ankle in hyper-dorsiflexion Also called as ***Aviator's fracture.***

Complications such as AVN and Non union are the commonest because the talus has no muscle attachment. (Blood supply to the bone usually reaches through muscle attachment).

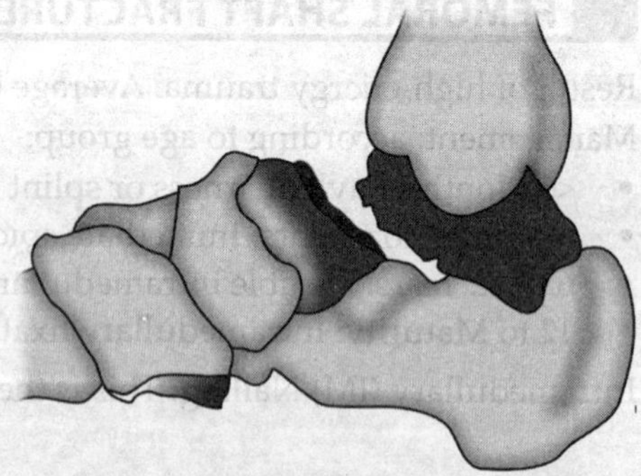

Fig. 19.12: Talar neck fracture

METATARSAL FRACTURES

Fifth metatarsal base fractures fall into two groups:

- Avulsion fracture of the tip is due to to an inversion force. Though peroneus brevis has its attachment to the base of 5th metatarsal, the reduction of the fracture fragment is opposed by the pull of the lateral band of the ***plantar aponeurosis.***
- ***Jones' fracture:*** occurs at ***metaphyso-diaphyseal junction.*** As the risk of non-union and avascular necrosis is high, a nonweight- bearing cast for 6 to 8 weeks is recommended.

SCAPHOID FRACTURE

Commonest carpal bone fracture,occurs following a fall onto out-stretched hand. Fractures ***through the waist*** of scaphoid are by far the commonest.

The major scaphoid blood supply enters distally and thus in waist fractures, vascularity may be compromised risking ***AVN of proximal* fragment.**

Clinically there is tenderness in the anatomical snuff box. X ray may not show subtle injury. Repeat X-ray at 2 weeks used for diagnosis of occult fractures.

Management: immobilise in scaphoid cast in ***glass holding position.*** For displaced ORIF with ***Herbert screw.*** Non-union and AVN are the common complications.

PEDIATRIC FRACTURES

Softer bone in children can lead to unique fracture behavior.

Greenstick fracture: Incomplete fractures, seen as disruption of the cortex on one side with angualtion or bowing on the opposite. Most greenstick deformities will remodel well.

A torus fracture is a small *buckling* or impaction of one cortex with a slight bend on the opposite cortex.

Plastic deformation is a change in the natural shape of a bone without a detectable fracture line.

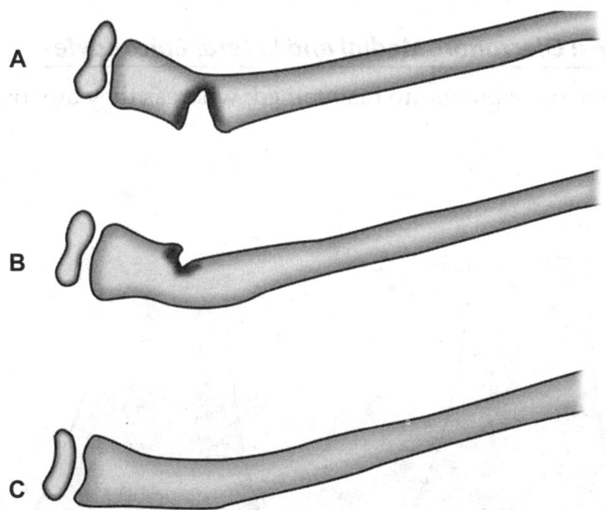

Figs 19.13 (A to C): Pediatric fracture patterns
A. Greenstick fracture; B. Torus fracture; C. Plastic deformation

Salter-Harris Classification of Physeal Injuries

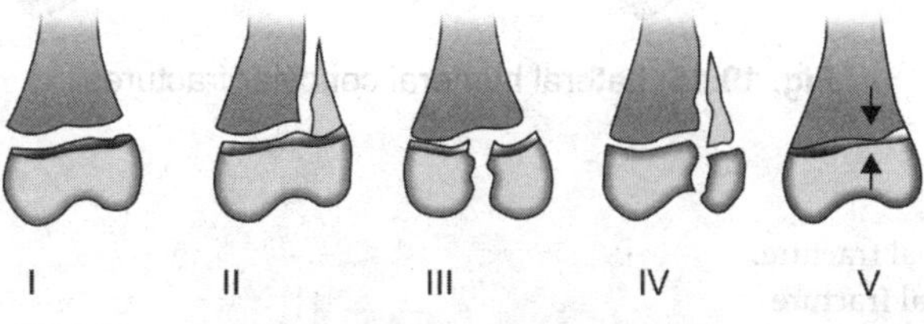

Fig. 19.14: Physeal injury types

- Type I–Fracture line is entirely within the physis.
- Type II–Most common type. Fracture line extends from physis into the metaphysis. Triangular fragment of metaphyseal bone is known as ***Thurston-Holland fragment.***
- Type III–Fracture line extends from the physis into the epiphysis
- Type IV–Fracture line extends through the physis, epiphysis and metaphysis
- Type V–Crush injury to the physis. A retrospective diagnosis. Worst prognosis.

Supracondylar Humerus Fractures (Malgaigne's Fracture)

The most common elbow injury, occurs mostly at 5–8 years of age. Left side most frequently injured.

Extension type: MC (98%), Hyperextension occurs during fall onto an outstretched hand.

Flexion type: comprises 2%.

By direct trauma or a fall onto a flexed elbow.

Treatment

By open or closed reduction and pinning with K-wires

Complications

- ***Neurologic injury***: Most are neuropraxia requiring no treatment. Median nerve/anterior interosseous nerve is most commonly affected. Ulnar nerve is injured in flexion-type supracondylar fractures.
- ***Vascular injury:*** This may represent direct injury to the brachial artery or may be secondary to antecubital swelling.
- ***Myositis ossificans:*** Rare and is seen after vigorous manipulation. Brachilalis muscle is usually affected.
- ***Cubitus varus or* gun stock deformity**: most common late complication. It requires French corrective osteotomy.

Three Bony Point Relationships: *Olecranon, Medial and Lateral Epicondyles*

In supracondylar fracture, all three bony points are maintained; whereas they are disrupted in elbow dislocation.

Lateral Humeral Condylar Fractures

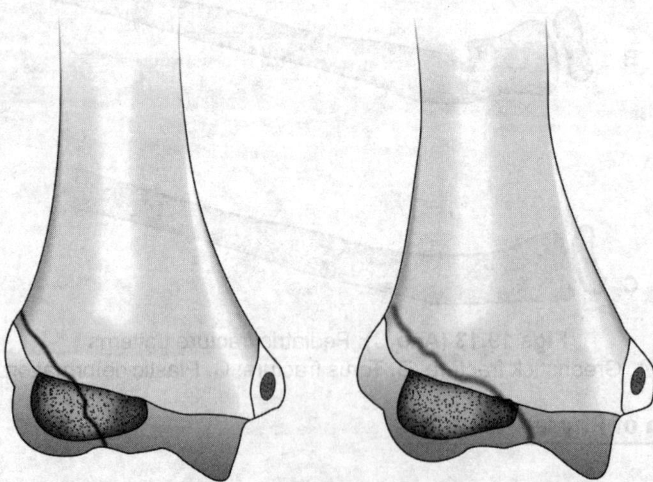

Fig. 19.15: Lateral humeral condylar fractures

Types

- A-Salter-Harris type IV epiphyseal fracture.
- B- Salter-Harris type II epiphyseal fracture

Complications

- Nonunion
- Cubitus valgus
- ***Tardy ulnar nerve palsy.***

RADIAL HEAD SUBLUXATION

Referred to as ***Nursemaid's elbow or pulled elbow.*** Occurs at ages between 6 months to 6 years. Closed reduction is performed. Immobilization is generally unnecessary.

HETEROTOPIC BONE FORMATION/MYOSITIS OSSIFICANS

- Caused by vigorous attempts at reduction. Most commonly seen in ***the elbow joint,*** next common joint is ***the hip joint.***
- ***Brachialis*** muscle is most commonly affected. Forcible manipulation or passive stretching increases soft tissue trauma and should be avoided.
- ***Indomethacin or radiation therapy (7 Gy)*** is recommended as prophylaxis.

Fractures of Child Abuse

Usually, the victims less than 2 years of age. Multiple ***fractures in different stages of healing*** almost always indicate child abuse.

Multiple areas of large ecchymoses in different stages of resolution.

Epiphyseal-metaphyseal ***("corner") fractures*** are almost always pathognomonic of child abuse because the pulling and twisting forces necessary to produce these injuries rarely are accidental. MC sites of fractures caused by child abuse are *the* ***humerus, tibia, and femur.***

DISLOCATIONS

Traumatic Hip Dislocation

Posterior hip dislocation: MC type of hip dislocation (80%). It is a ***dashboard injury*** which tends to occur with the hip flexed and adducted at time of impact *(With hip in abduction at the time of injury, anterior dislocation can occur.)*

Clinically the deformity in Posterior dislocations is ***flexion, adduction and internal rotation.***

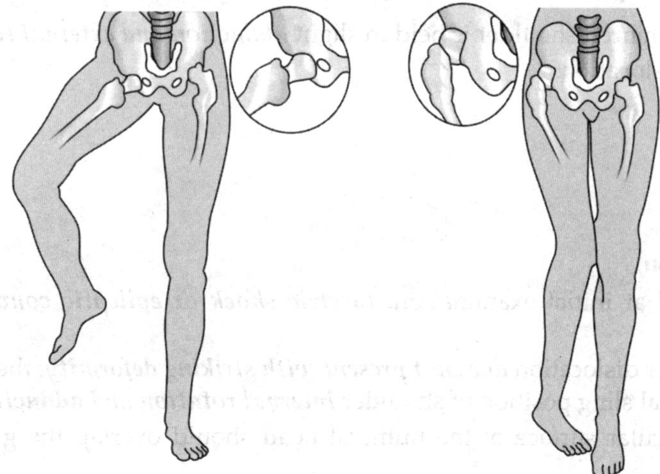

Fig. 19.16: Anterior and posterior hip dislocation

Anterior hip dislocations comprise 10% to 15% of traumatic hip dislocations and present with position of hip *abduction and external rotation* with mild flexion.

Methods of closed reduction: Allis', Bigelow's, Stimson's, Lefkowitz's, East Baltimore lift, etc.

Complications:

- Osteoarthritis is the most common complication after hip dislocation.
- Osteonecrosis (4% to 22%).
- ***Sciatic nerve palsy*** (10% to 20%) (Usually, the peroneal portion of the nerve is affected).

Shoulder Joint Dislocations

Anterior Shoulder Dislocation

It is the commonest (about ***90%***)type in shoulder dislocation; posterior and inferior dislocations are rare. Anterior dislocation is subdivided into:

- ***Subcoracoid (most common)***
- Subglenoid
- Intra thoracic.
- The shoulder joint is ***most common*** joint prone for recurrent dislocation, and is the most common joint to undergo non recurrent (traumatic) dislocation.

The following are the classical lesions described in recurrent anterior dislocation:

- ***Bankart's lesion:*** avulsion of anterior glenoid labrum.
- ***Hill-Sachs lesion*** An impression fracture on the postero-lateral aspect of Humeral head.
- Humeral avulsion of Glenohumeral ligaments (HAGL)

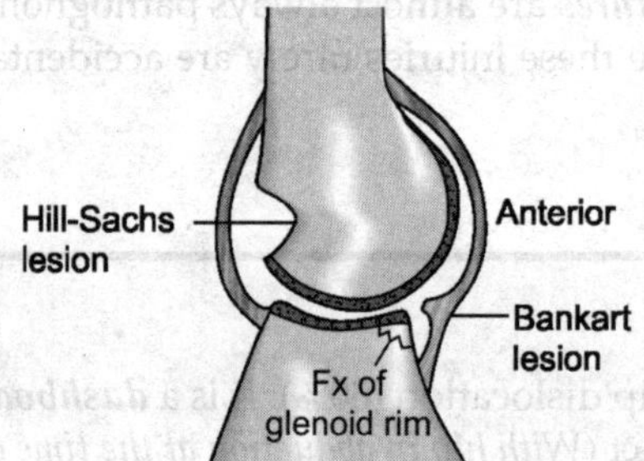

Fig. 19.17: Pathoanatomy of recurrent shoulder dislocation

Clinically, the attitude of the injured shoulder is held in slight ***abduction and external rotation.***

Tests for anterior shoulder dislocation:

- Duga's test
- Hamilton ruler test
- Callaway' test
- Bryant's test

Posterior Shoulder Dislocation

They are often ***unrecognized*** at initial examination. ***Electric shock or epileptic convulsions*** produce posterior dislocations.

Clinically, a posterior shoulder dislocation ***does not present with striking deformity***; the injured upper extremity is typically held in the traditional sling position of shoulder ***internal rotation and adduction.***

In normal shoulder, the articular surface of the humeral head should overlap the glenoid producing elliptical shadow.

A posteriorly dislocated joint shows a ***vacant glenoid sign (or positive rim sign).***

On a standard AP view of the shoulder, signs suggestive of a posterior glenohumeral dislocation include:

- ***Reverse Hill-Sachs lesion***: opposite of anterior dislocation.
- The glenoid appears vacant (***vacant glenoid sign).***

- The humeral head, because it is internally rotated due to posterior dislocation, looks abnormal in shape- like an *electric light bulb*. ***(Light bulb sign).***

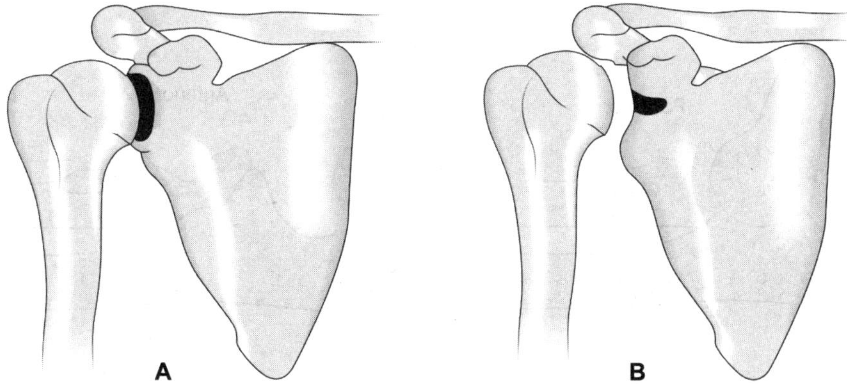

Figs 19.18 (A and B): A. Normal B. Vacant glenoid sign

Inferior Dislocation of Shoulder

It is a rare injury caused by severe hyper abduction of shoulder joint.
Called as ***luxatio erecta*** as the humeral head is subluxated (dislocated inferiorly and shaft points upwards -erected).

Arm locked in almost full abduction/elevation is the common symptom. A potentially serious consequence like neurovascular damage is quite common.

NOTE

Mode of injury of shoulder dislocations:

- ***Anterior dislocation***: Abduction and external rotation force.
- ***Posterior dislocation***: indirect force producing marked internal rotation and adduction.
- ***Inferior dislocation***: Severe hyper abduction force.

Elbow Dislocation

The elbow is a 'modified hinge' joint. The high degree of stability is conferred by:

- Joint morphology
- Tension of triceps and flexors
- Presence of strong ligaments.

There are three separate joints in the elbow region:

- Ulnohumeral (hinge type)
- Radio humeral
- Proximal radio-ulnar.

The elbow is the ***second most commonly dislocated*** joint in adults.
Most commonly, the dislocation is caused by a fall onto an outstretched hand or elbow.
Types: According to the direction of displacement of the ulna relative to the humerus, it is classified as:

- ***Posterior (most common)***
- Posterolateral
- Posteromedial
- Lateral
- Medial
- Anterior.

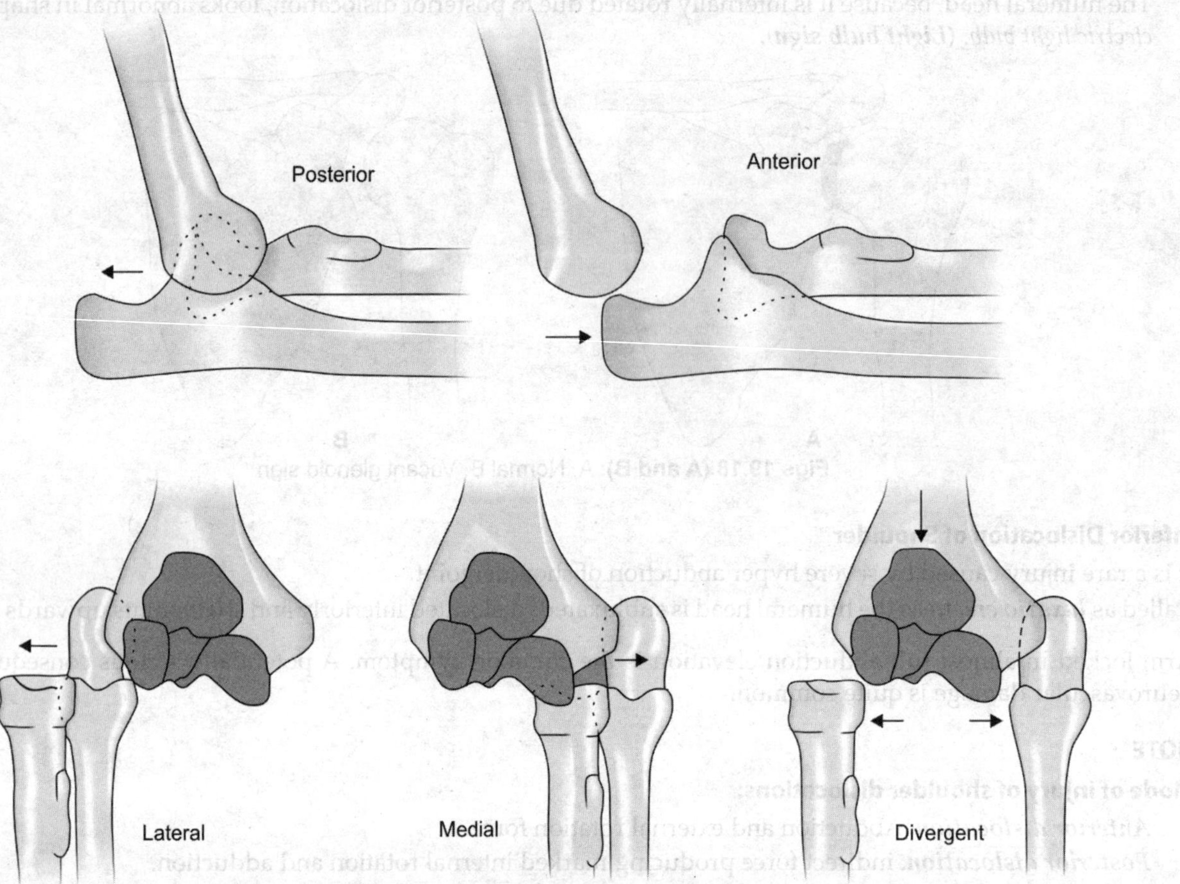

Fig. 19.19: Classification of elbow dislocation

On presentation, the triceps tendon stands out prominently. This is called ***'bowstringing of triceps'.***

The relationships among the ***three bony landmarks are disrupted or reversed.***

Terrible triad injury of elbow: Posterior elbow dislocation + fracture of the radial head + fracture of coronoid process

All acute elbow dislocations are easily reducible by closed method.

Associated Injuries

- Radial head fracture
- Fracture of coronoid process of ulna
- Ulnar nerve and anterior interosseous branches of the median nerve injuries
- Brachial artery may be injured in rare cases.

Usual Methods of Treatment for Common Fractures

Fracture	Usual methods of treatment
Clavicle	Arm sling or a figure "8" strap, plate fixation, hook plates
Proximal humerus	Undisplaced- armsling; Displaced- ORIF. Four part fracture: prosthetic replacement (hemiarthroplasty).
Displaced forearm bones	Plate fixation
Supracondylar humerus in children	Percutaneuos or open reduction and K-wire fixation

Fracture	Usual methods of treatment
Olecranon	Figure-of-eight tension Tension band wiring, screw fixation, hook plates
Colle's fracture	POP cast in cotton loader posiotion (mostly), plate fixation
Scaphoid fracture	Nondisplaced: thumb spica splint (in glass holding position) Displaced: ORIF with Kirschner wires or Herbert's headless screws
Bennett's fracture	k-wire fixation
Intertrochanteric fx femur	Sliding compression hip screws (aka Dynamic Hip screw (DHS))
Subtrochanteric femur	Dynamic condylar screws (DCS)
Intracapsular femoral neck fracture	Young patient: multiple screw fixation Elderly patients: Hemiarthroplasty, total hip replacement.
Femoral shaft fracture	Intramedullary (IM) nailing
Patella	Undisplaced: Cylinder or Tube cast, Displaced transverse fx: tension tension band wiring, Comminuted fx: Cerclage wiring, patellectomy (Partial or Total)
Tibial shaft	Displaced: Intramedullary (IM) Nailing, Undisplaced: Patella tendon bearing (PTB) cast.
Medial malleolus	Cancellous screws or tension band wiring.
Jone's fracture	POP cast

PERIPHERAL NERVE INJURIES

Seddon's Classification of Nerve Injuries

- **Neurapraxia**: simple contusion or compression of a peripheral nerve with preservation of the axon.
- Transmission of impulses is ***physiologically interrupted***; recovery is complete in days-weeks. E.g: Saturday night palsy.
- **Axonotmesis**: ***axon alone is cut;*** endoneurium is intact which allows axon regeneration; recovery is slow, growth 1mm/day, but usually full.
- Associated with ***closed fractures*** / dislocations.
- **Neurotmesis: *complete anatomical severance*** of the nerve or extensive avulsing or crushing injury. Occurs with open fractures, cut injuries.

Spontaneous recovery cannot be expected. Requires surgical repair.

Sunderland classification is more useful, more readily applicable clinically; each degree of injury suggesting a greater anatomical disruption with its correspondingly altered prognosis.

Degree of injury		Histopathological changes					Tinel sign	
Sunderland	Seddon	Myelin	Axon	Endoneurium	Perineurium	Epineurium	Present	Progresses Distally
I	Neurapraxia	±					–	–
II	Axonotmesis	+	+				+	+
III		+	+	+			+	+
IV		+	+	+	+		+	–
V	Neurotmesis	+	+	+	+	+	+	–

Tinel Sign: Elicited by gentle percussion along the course of an injured nerve.
A ***tingling sensation*** should be felt by the patient in the distribution of the injured nerve. Tested in distal-to-proximal direction.
A positive Tinel sign is ***presumptive evidence of nerve regeneration*** that *has not obtained complete myelinization.*

Nerve Supply

Nerves	Segmental Levels	Sensory	Motor
Radial N	C5, C6, C7, C8, T1	Posterior aspect of forearm	Triceps brachii, anconeus, Brachioradialis, Extensor carpi radialis longus
Ulnar N	C7, C8, T1	Medial hand Medial 1½ digit	Flexor carpi ulnaris, medial half of flexor digitorum profundus, All interossei, ***medial 2 lumbricals***, All hypothenar muscles
			Two thenar muscles (adductor pollicis, deep head of flexor pollicis brevis)
Musculocutaneous N	C5, C6, C7	Becomes lateral cutaneous nerve of forearm	Coracobrachialis, biceps brachii, brachialis (dual supply)
Axillary	C5, C6	Lateral shoulder (Regimental badge area)	Teres minor Deltoid
Median	C6, C7, C8, T1	Palmar and distal dorsal aspects of lateral 3½ digits and lateral palm	Flexor carpi radialis, flexor digitorum superficialis, lateral ½ of flexor digitorum profundus, flexor pollicis longus, pronator quadratus, pronator teres. All thenar muscles ***(except adductor pollicis, deep head of flexor pollicis brevis)***, Lateral two lumbricals.
Posterior interosseous N (branch Radial N)	C5, C6, C7, C8, T1	None	Abductor pollicis longus, extensor pollicis brevis, extensor digitorum communis, extensor indicis, extensor digiti minimi

Common Nerve Injuries Associated with Trauma

Nerve injury	Fracture/Dislocation
Radial nerve	Humeral shaft fracture
Ulnar nerve	Medial humeral epicondyle fracture (lateral humeral condyle non-union: tardy ulnar n palsy)
Median nerve	Dislocation of the elbow
Posterior interosseous nerve	Monteggia fracture dislocation
Anterior intersseous nerve	Supracondylar humerus fracture
Axillary nerve	Shoulder dislocation, Surgical neck of humerus fracture
Common Peroneal nerve	Fibular neck fracture
Sciatic nerve	Hip dislocation

Common Nerve Palsies

Nerve palsy	Deformity
Erb's palsy	Police man receiving tips/Waiter's tips posture
Klumpke's palsy	Claw hand
Long Thoracic Nerve	Winging of scapula
Radial Nerve (Crutch palsy, Saturday night palsy)	Wrist drop
Ulnar nerve	Claw hand
Median nerve	Ape thumb deformity
Common peroneal nerve	Foot drop

Contd...

Contd...

Test	Nerve injury	Muscle(s) tested
Froment's sign (Book test)	Ulnar nerve	Adductor pollicis, FPL of thumb, 1st dorsal interossei
Card test	Ulnar nerve	Palmar interossei
Egawa's test	Ulnar nerve	Dorsal interossei of middle finger
Pen test	Median nerve	Abductor pollicis brevis
Oschner clasp test (pointing index), Benediction test	Median nerve	Flexor digitorum profundus of index finger

Long Thoracic Nerve: supplies serratus anterior muscle. When this muscle is paralyzed and the patient attempts to exert forward pushing movements with the hands, ***"winging" of the scapula*** occurs.

Axillary Nerve: injured by ***dislocation*** of the shoulder and fracture of surgical neck of humerus. The deltoid muscle is paralysed. The sensation over ***regimental badge area*** is lost.

Radial Nerve: primarily a motor nerve that innervates the triceps; the supinators and the extensors of the wrist, fingers, and thumb.

Sensory supply: The autonomous zone is between the first and second metacarpals.

- Injured most often ***by fractures of the humeral shaft, fracture of humerus at spiral (radial) groove.***

Ulnar Nerve

When the intrinsic muscles (the lumbricals) are paralyzed, MCP joints are in extension while the IP joints are flexed the hand tends to assume the ***intrinsic minus*** posture, referred to as **a claw hand** (also called **Duchenne's sign**).

Various Signs of Ulnar Nerve Palsy

- ***Wartenberg's sign*** - is the inability to pull in (adduct) the small finger against the ring finger.
- ***Froment's sign*** - is the hyperflexion of the thumb IP joint to substitute for the lack of adductor pollicis muscle action.

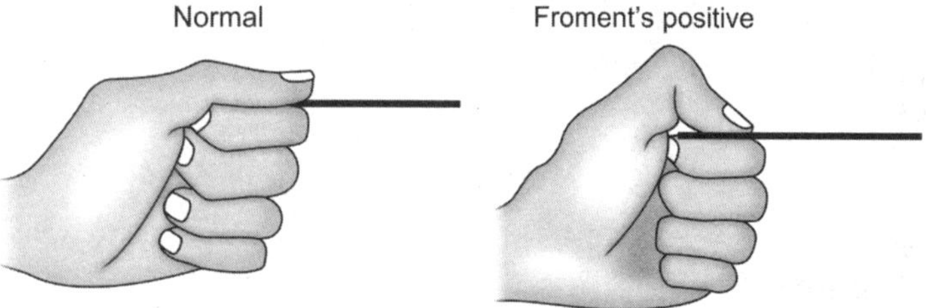

Fig. 19.20: Froment's Sign

- Weakness of DIP joint flexion due to loss of FDP function of the ring and small finger is known *as* ***Pollock's sign.***
- The flattening of the natural metacarpal arch of the hand seen in association with hand muscle wasting is known as ***Masse's sign.***

Median Nerve

It is the ***laborer's nerve***. Most commonly injured at elbow by supracondylar fracrure or elbow dislocation.

At wrist, it gets compressed at the carpal tunnel. It is known as carpal tunnel syndrome.

When paralysed, ***ape-thumb deformity*** results because of wasting of thenar muscles. ***Along with ulnar nerve palsy, a total claw hand produced.***

As FDP of index finger is weak, the patient is unable to flex the index finger. This is the main attitude in the following tests:

- Pointing index
- Oschner's clasp test
- Benediction test.

BRACHIAL PLEXUS INJURY

It is a traumatic injury to the brachial plexus resulting in partial or complete paralysis of the upper extremity, usually occurring secondary to ***obstetric complications***. It can be Erb's or Klumpke's palsy.

Brachial plexus

- **Erb's palsy:** involves *C5, C6* roots. Weakness in shoulder abduction, external rotation, elbow flexion, and forearm supination result in the characteristic ***"waiter's tip" posture*** of the upper extremity.
- **Klumpke's palsy**: involves the lower spinal roots **(*C8-T1*).** Forcible hyperabduction of shoulder joint may end up in injuring C8-T1. Paralysis of small muscle of hand resulting in ***claw hand*** deformity. Severe injury may add injury to sympathetic fibres producing ***Horner's syndrome.***

Sciatic Nerve

L4, L5, S1, S2, S3.

It has two components.

- **Tibial component** supplies:
  - Hamstring muscles,
  - Gastro-soleus,
  - Tibialis posterior ,
  - Long flexors of toes
  - Sensation to sole of the foot
- **Peroneal component:** two divisions:
  - Deep peroneal nerve supplies
    - Tibialis anterior
    - Long extensors of the toes
    - Sensation to first web space
  - Superficial peroneal nerve supplies
    - Peroneus longus
    - Peroneus brevis
    - Sensation to anterolateral leg and dorsum of foot

Sciatic Nerve is Injured by

- Posterior hip dislocation
- Intramuscular injection
- Surgery: total hip replacement
- Compression by piriformis muscle.

TREATMENT OF NERVE INJURIES

- Splinting to prevent muscle contracture and wasting
  - Cock-up splint for wrist drop
  - Knuckle-bender splint for claw hand
- Repair of nerves – neurorrhaphy
- Release of adhesions- neurolysis
- **Nerve** Grafting- sural nerve is commonly used
- Tendon transfers.

Tendon Transfers

For Radial Nerve Palsy

- Transfer of pronator teres (PT) to extensor carpi radialis brevis (ECRB)
- Transfer of flexor carpi radialis (FCR) to extensor digitorum communis (EDC)
- Palmaris longus (PL) to rerouted extensor pollicis longus (EPL).

For Ulnar Nerve Palsy

Low Ulnar Nerve Palsy: The functional deficits caused by low ulnar nerve palsy are weakness of pinch resulting from paralysis of the adductor pollicis and first dorsal interosseous, weakness of grip produced by paralysis of most of the finger intrinsics, and sometimes clawing of the ring and little fingers associated with paralysis of all of their intrinsics.

Normal tightness of the meta carpo phalangeal joints of the ring and little fingers may limit clawing of these fingers and enable the long extensors to extend their inter phalangeal joints. So in claw hand deformity, the purpose of surgery is to stabilize the MCP joints rather than correcting the deformity. This stabilization is achieved by tendon transfer procedures; where extensor tendons are normally used. Whichever tendon is chosen, it has to be passed through lumbrical canal and attached to dorsal (extensor) digital expansions.

So many named procedures have been explained. They are:

- **Bunnell's procedure**: ***flexor digitorum sublimis*** tendon from each finger is detached, split, and passed one slip to each side of the extensor aponeurosis of each finger by way of the lumbrical canals.
- **Fowler's procedure:** Done by splitting the ***extensor indicis proprius tendons*** to form four slips and attach one each to the extensor aponeuroses.
- **Brand's technique:** Done by is using the ***extensor carpi radialis brevis*** tendon lengthened by a free graft from the plantaris tendon.
- **Riordan's procedure:** ECRB tendon can be transferred to the thumb proximal phalanx to provide thumb pinch (adduction).
- **Smith's transfer:** Extensor carpi radialis brevis tendon is transferred to adductor pollicis.
- **Boyes's transfer:** Brachioradialis is transferred to adductor pollicis.

For Median Nerve Palsy

- **Bunnell procedure:** flexor digitorum superificalis of ring finger to opponens pollicis through a pulley of flexor carpi ulnaris.
  - **Camitz procedure:** Palmaris longus extended by a strip of palmar fascia to abductor pollicis brevis.
  - **Burkhalter procedure:** extensor indicis proprius is the tendon donor.
  - **Huber procedure:** abductor digiti minimi is the tendon donor.

For Common Peroneal Nerve Palsy

Foot drop (dynamic equino varus deformity)is caused by weakness of ankle dorsiflexors and evertors. Transfer of ***tibialis posterior*** tendon brings active dorsiflexion of the foot.

NERVE ENTRAPMENT SYNDROMES

Carpal Tunnel Syndrome

Also known as ***tardy median nerve palsy.***

It is the result of compression of the median nerve within the carpal tunnel.

The manifestations include:

- Paraesthesiae and numbness in the distribution of the median nerve in the hand.
- Clumsiness for intricate finger/manual activities.
- Wasting of the thenar eminence.
- Weakness of opposition of the thumb and/or abduction of the thumb.
- Reduced sensation in the distribution of the median nerve.

Though the cause is not known, CTS is commonly associated with the following clinical conditions *(that reduce the space for the median nerve in the carpal tunnel):*

- Rheumatoid arthritis
- Tenosynovitis of the finger flexors
- Pregnancy
- Acromegaly
- Hypothyroidism
- Diabetes
- Amyloidosis
- Space-occupying lesions such as a ganglion.

The specific tests for CTS are:

- Phalen's wrist flexion test
- Durkan's carpal compression test
- Percussion test (Tinel sign).

Anterior Interosseous Syndrome

It occurs due to fascial bands or aberrant blood vessels compressing the anterior interosseous nerve. *(Anterior interosseous nerve is a branch of the medial nerve).*

May also be caused by compression of the nerve by ***Ganzer's muscle*** (accessory head of the flexor pollicis longus).

It presents with weakness of the flexor pollicis longus muscle and the flexor digitorum profundus to the index finger. Patients cannot make an ***"OK" sign*** due to FPL and FDP weakness.

Pronator Syndrome

It is caused from direct compression of the ***median nerve*** by the pronator teres muscle. The site of compression is distal to the branch of the anterior interosseous nerve.

Wartenberg's Syndrome (Chiralgia parasthetica)

The terminal branches of the radial nerve

- Superficial radial nerve
- Posterior interosseous nerve.

Compressive neuropathy of the ***superficial radial nerve*** as it exits the brachioradialis muscle can result in Wartenberg's syndrome.

Posterior Interosseous Nerve Compression

It may occur at five sites, represented by the mnemonic **FREAS**

[Fibrous bands around radiocapitellar joint; Recurrent arterial branches; Extensor carpi radialis brevis, Arcade of Frohse (a thickening at the proximal edge of supinator); distal edge of Supinator]. – Apley.

The posterior interosseous nerve travels around the radial neck and through the interval between the two heads of the supinator muscle.

This opening, which often has an overlying, compressive fibrous arch, is known as the ***arcade of Frosche***. The space beneath the supinator muscle belly and where the PIN travels is known as the radial tunnel.

Ulnar Tunnel Syndrome

The ulnar nerve passes from the forearm into the hand through the ***Guyon's canal***. The anatomic borders of the Guyon canal are the pisiform and pisohamate ligament ulnarly, the hook of the hamate and insertion of the transverse carpal ligament radially, and the volar carpal ligament forming the roof of the tunnel.

Cubital Tunnel Syndrome

The ulnar nerve is most commonly compressed at the cubital tunnel - at the ***elbow*** within the fibro-osseous groove known as the cubital tunnel behind the medial epicondyle. Other sites of potential ulnar nerve compression at the elbow or ulnar include ***the arcade of Struthers,*** the medial intermuscular septum, and ***the ligament of Osborne.***

The nerve is tethered anteriorly with elbow flexion. May manifest as **tardy ulnar nerve palsy** in non-union lateral condylar fracture of humerus.

Tarsal Tunnel Syndrome

Entrapment of the ***posterior tibial nerve*** behind the medial malleolus. Pain and paresthesia at the sole of the foot is the main symptom.

Meralgia Paresthetica

Compression of lateral cutaneous nerve of thigh.

Piriformis Syndrome

It is the compression of the **sciatic nerve** as it passes under the piriformis muscle.

The ***FAIR*** (flexion, adduction, internal rotation) test is positive.

SPORTS INJURY

Knee

Meniscal Injury

Medial meniscus is semicirclular, fixed to medial collateral ligament and ***less mobile*** than lateral meniscus; the medial meniscus can easily get trapped ***(cannot escape)*** in between the femoral and tibial condyles during rotational movement.

So ***tears are more common with medial meniscus.***

Lateral meniscus is smaller, more circular and more mobile.

Vertical longitudinal tear: A complete longitudinal tear is known as ***bucket handle tear*** which is often unstable and common cause of ***locking.*** Mostly seen in young individuals.

Tests for Meniscal Injury

- McMurray's test
- Apley's grinding test
- Duck walk test.

➢ ***Arthroscopy*** is the "gold standard" for diagnosing meniscal disease and intra-articular disorders of the knee.

Treatment methods include:

- Nonsurgical,
- Meniscal repair,
- Partial meniscectomy.

Tears in the ***outer third*** of the meniscus heal with repair by suturing; because this region has better blood supply.

Tears in the ***inner third*** do not heal as this region is avascular. Hence excision is the option.

Young patients who undergo meniscectomy will develop osteoarthritis. So repair is more favored than excision of meniscus.

Anterior Cruciate Ligament Injury

- Anterior cruciate ligament (ACL) travels from the medial border of the lateral femoral condyle to its insertion site anterolateral to the medial tibial spine.

This ligament ***prevents anterior translation*** and rotation of the tibia on the femur.

ACL injuries are the ***most common*** knee ligament injuries seen in all forms of sporting activities.

The tests for ACL tears are:

- **The Lachman test** is the most sensitive; performed with knee in 20–30 deg flexion. Can be done even in acutely swollen knee joint
- **The anterior drawer test:** performed with the knee in 90 deg flexion ; less sensitive than the Lachman test. tability.
- **Pivot shift test:** done in chronic cases with anterolateral knee instability.

In young athletes surgical treatment necessary to restore the knee stability.

The ACL is reconstructed using one of the following grafts:

- Patellar tendon
- Semitendinosus/gracilis hamstring *(latest and most common)*
- Quadriceps tendon.

Unhappy triad of O'Donoghue is combination of injuries of all three following structures

- Medial collateral ligament
- Medial meniscus
- Anterior cruciate ligament.

Posterior Cruciate Ligament Injury

The posterior cruciate ligament (PCL) prevents posterior subluxation of the tibia on the femur.

- It runs from the lateral aspect of the medial femoral condyle to the posterior aspect of the tibia, just ***below the joint line.*** Isolated tears of the posterior cruciate ligament are relatively rare.

The tests for PCL injuries are:

- Posterior sag test,
- Posterior drawer test
- Quadriceps active test
- Reverse pivot shift
- The dial test.

Chondromalacia of Patella

Literally, softening of the patellar articular cartilage. The true aetiology is not known.

It is common in ***female adolescents***.

The pain is localized to anterior part of the knee and is most prominent after sitting in one position for a long time ***("movie sign" or "theater sign.")*** and while descending stairs.

Treatment: Anti-inflammatory medications, quadriceps exercises, and hamstring stretching.

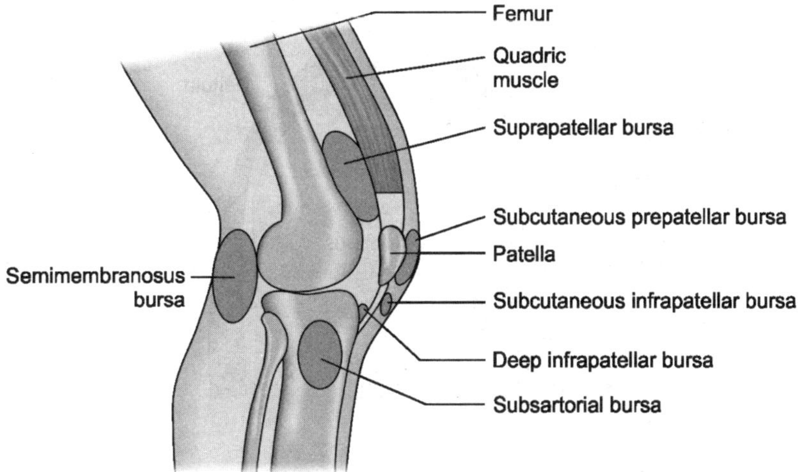

Fig. 19.21: Bursa around the knee

Jumper's Knee

Patellar ligament insertion at the inferior pole of the patella is inflamed. It is caused by repetitive traction or overload injury during sports.

Tips: ***Pes anserinus*** is the term for the conjoined insertion of the ***sartorius, gracilis, and semitendinosus muscles*** at the proximal medial aspect to the tibia.

Tips: ***Ober's test*** is positive in condition which produce tight iliotibial band (ITB), such as cerebral palsy, poliomyelitis and sometimes ITB syndrome

*(**ITB Syndrome** is due to friction and contracture of ITB which occurs during repetitive knee flexion motion)*

Shoulder

Slap Lesions

This acronym stands for **s**uperior **l**abrum **a**nterior-to-**p**osterior) denotes glenoid labral degeneration or rupture involving the origin of the ***long head of the biceps***

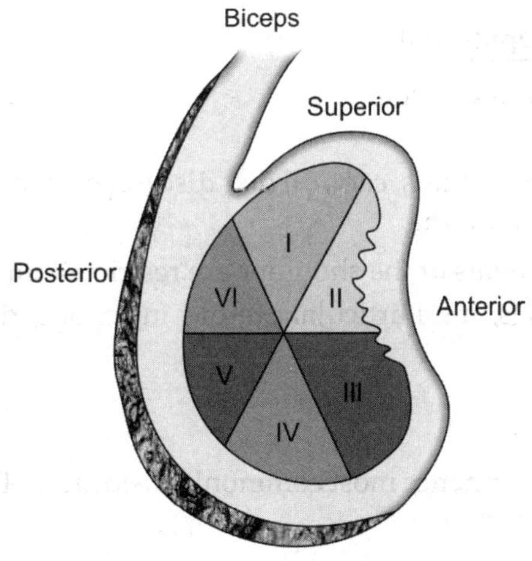

Fig. 19.22: Schematic diagram–SLAP lesion of glenoid labrum

Impingement Syndrome

Can occur with ***repetitive overhead activities*** as a result of mechanical impingement of the rotator cuff and humeral head against the lateral edge of the acromion.

The *supraspinatus tendon* is most susceptible to impingement.

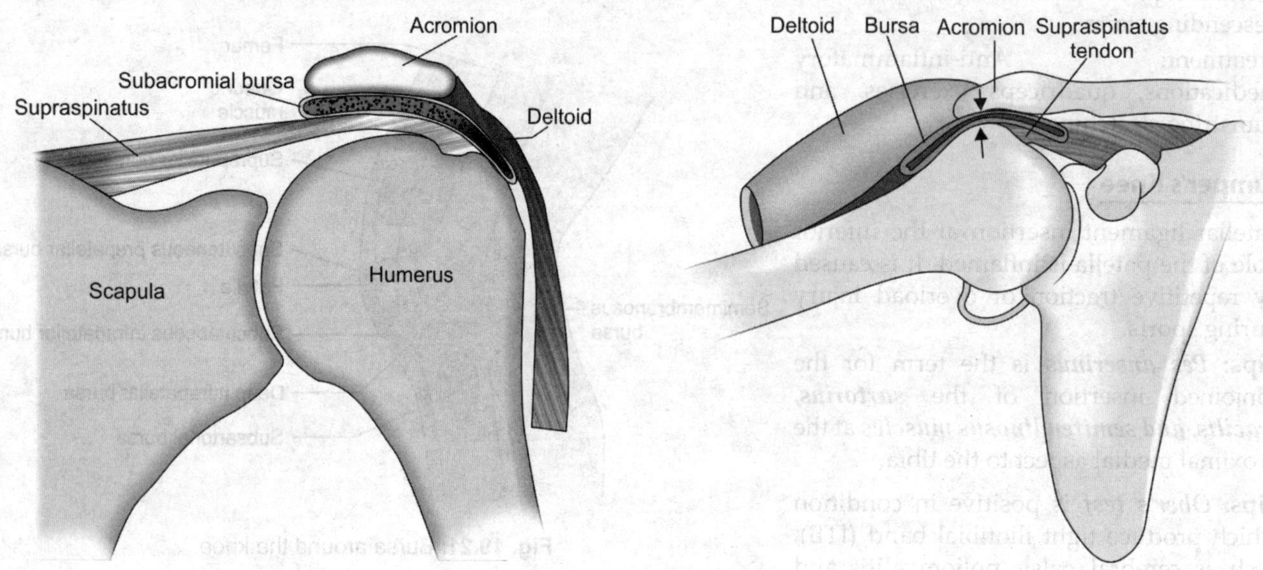

Fig. 19.23: Subacromial space and Impingement

Neer Test and Hawkin's Test: Testing for supraspinatus tendon impingement.

Treatment: analgesics, rest, intra-lesional steroids, deep heat therapy, Physical exercises for rotator cuff strengthening. *Acromioplasty* is tried when conservative measures fail.

Rotator Cuff Tendinitis

Of the four rotator cuff muscles, the *supraspinatus tendon* is most often initially involved.

Rotator cuff tendonitis also results from impingement syndrome and is characterized by pain with overhead activity.

FROZEN SHOULDER (or adhesive capsulitis)

Commonly known as *periarthritis* of the shoulder.

It is a self-limiting condition.

- Seen in female sex, old age, diabetes mellitus, cervical disc disease, prolonged immobilization, hyperthyroidism, stroke or myocardial infarction and trauma.

Internal rotation and abduction movements of the shoulder are restricted initially.

Treated with physical therapy, NSAIDs, intra-articular steroid injections, distention arthrography, closed manipulation under anaesthesia.

Shoulder Instability

The shoulder joint the most unstable joint; hence most commonly dislocated. The following tests are for the shoulder instability:

- Test for *inferior* shoulder instability:
  - The sulcus test.
- Test for *anterior* instability:
  - The apprehension test
  - The fulcrum test
  - The crank test
  - Shoulder relocation test.
- Test for *posterior* instability:
  - The jerk test.

Surgical procedures for shoulder dislocation

- ***Bankart's repair***- detached anterior structures attached to glenoid rim by sutures
- ***Putti platt***- double breasting of subscapularis muscle
- ***Bristow procedure***- transplantation of coracoids process to anterior rim of the glenoid cavity.

Elbow

Lateral Epicondylitis (Tennis Elbow):

It is an inflammation at the common extensor origin at lateral epicondyle of the humerus.

It is the consequence of ***repetitive overuse activities.*** Classically described in the tennis player, now it is more common with manual labourers.

Though all muscles which originate from lateral epicondyle are affected, the ***extensor carpi radialis brevis*** (ECRB) is affected more commonly and more severely.

➢ ***Cozen's test, Mill's maneuvre*** are positive in clinical examination.

Treatment: Majority responds to rest, ice, ***steroid injections, and physical therapy*** with ultrasound, iontophoresis, electrical stimulation and counterforce bracing.

Surgical treatment is for refractory cases. This procedure is to resect the degenerated tissues in the lesion.

Medial Epicondylitis (Golfer's Elbow)

Caused by inflammation at the common flexor origin of medial epicondyle of humerus. It is less common and more difficult to treat than the lateral epicondylitis.

Pronator teres muscle and flexor carpi radialis are the principal muscles involved.

Treatment: bracing, rest, ice, and injections of steroid .

SOBRIQUET ELBOWS

Student's elbow	:	Olecranon bursitis
Nursemaid's elbow	:	Pulled elbow or radial head subluxation.
Golfer's elbow	:	Medial epicondylitis
Tennis elbow	:	Lateral epicondylitis

The Wrist and the Hand

Zones of Flexor Tendons of Hand

Zone I extends from just distal to the insertion of the sublimis tendon to the site of insertion of the profundus tendon.

Zone II is in the critical area of pulleys ***(Bunnell's "no man's land")*** between the distal palmar crease and the insertion of the sublimis tendon.

Zone III comprises the area of the lumbrical muscles.

Zone IV is covered by the transverse carpal ligament (flexor retinaculum).

Zone V is proximal to the transverse carpal ligament and includes the forearm.

Flexor tendon repair is more challenging, in Zone II where both FDS and FDP tendons run together in a tight sheath.

Zone II is called ***'no man's land'*** because injuries in this zone are the most dangerous and most difficult to restore normal function.

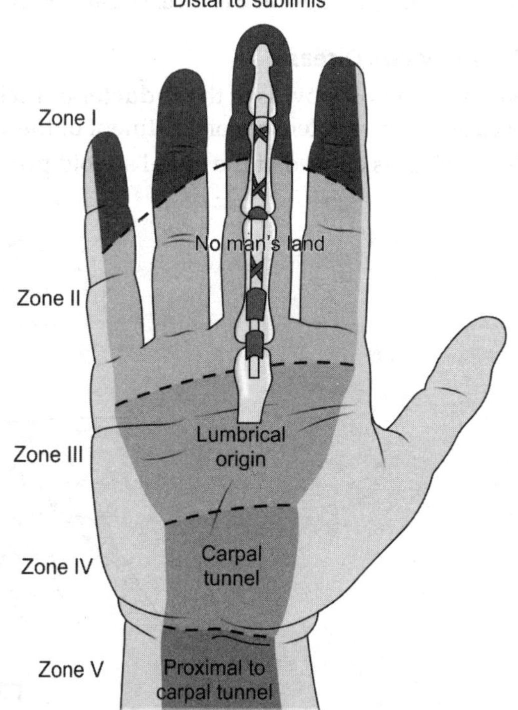

Fig. 19.24: Flexor zones of hand

Contents of Extensor Compartment of Wrist

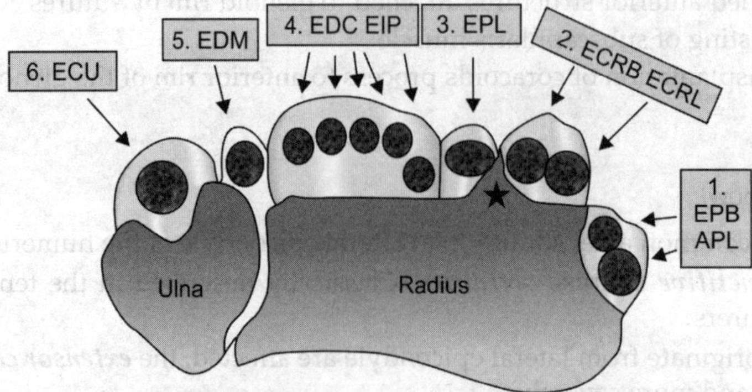

Fig. 19.25: Contents of extensor compartments of wrist

I	Extensor pollicis brevis, abductor pollicis longus
II	Extensor carpi radialis brevis andlongus
III	Extensor pollicis longus
IV	Four tendons of extensor digitorum communis and extensor indicis proprius
V	Extensor digiti quinti
VI	Extensor carpi ulnaris

Trigger Finger (Stenozing Tenosynovitis)

This condition is characterized by thickening of the ***first annular (A1) pulley*** of the fibrous flexor tendon sheath at the level of the metacarpophalangeal joints of fingers.

Patients complain of triggering and clicking. The ***ring finger***, middle finger, or thumb are most commonly affected. Nodules are palpable at the level of MCP joint.

De Quervain's Disease

Stenosing tenosynovitis of the **abductor pollicis longus and extensor pollicis brevis** (APL and EPB) tendons which occupy the first extensor compartment of the wrist.

Tenderness is elicited at the radial styloid process. **Finkelstein's Test** is positive.

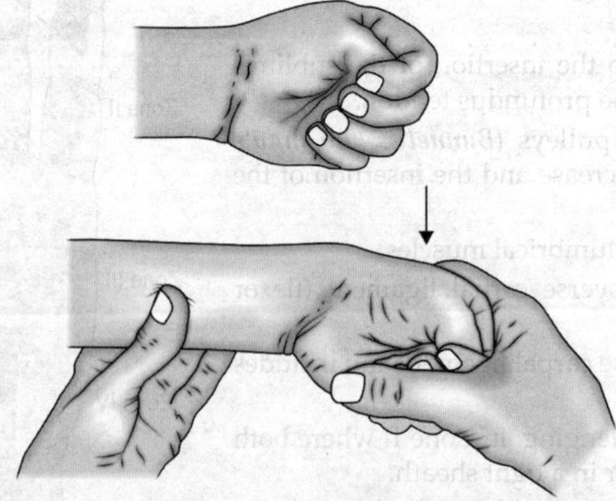

Fig. 19.26: Finkelstein's test

Bowler's Thumb: It is ***perineural fibrosis*** caused by repetitious compression of the ulnar digital nerve of the thumb while grasping a bowling ball.

Gamekeeper's Thumb: Ulnar collateral ligament injury of thumb at MCP joint.

Jersey Finger: It is avulsion of ***Flexor*** tendon of fingers from distal phalanx.

Mallet Finger: It is avulsion central slip of ***extensor*** tendon from distal phalanx. Usually treated with splinting the DIP joint in hyperextension.

TENDON RUPTURES

Tendon ruptures are more common in middle-aged and elderly patients.

Intrinsic weakness of the tendon as a result of ***repetitive microtrauma*** predispose to tendon rupture.

Commonly ruptured tendons are:

- Supraspinatus,
- Biceps,
- Achilles tendons.

Conditions such ***as rheumatoid arthritis, lupus erythematosus, systemic steroids and local injection of steroids*** may also predispose the tendon rupture.

Eponymous Bursae

- Servant maid's Knee : Prepatellar bursitis
- Clergyman's knee : Infra patellar bursitis
- Pes Anserinus bursa : Busra at insertion of Sartorius, Gracilis, Semitendinosus
- Student's elbow : Olecranon bursitis
- Bunion : Bursa and deformity over 1st MTP in Hallux valgus
- Weaver's bottom : Ischial bursitis

Tests/signs	Conditions showing positivity
Neer Impingement test, Hawkins-Kennedy Test, Empty can test	Impingement syndrome /supraspinatous tendinitis
Drop-arm test	Supraspinatus tendon rupture
Sulcus sign/test	Inferior shoulder laxity
Yergason test, Speed test	Bicipital tendinitis
Popeye sign	Biceps tendon rupture
Jobe relocation test	Recurrent shoulder dislocation
Gerber's lift-off test, belly press test	Rupture of the subscapularis
Cozen's test, Mill's maneuver	Lateral epicondylitis (tennis elbow)
McMurray test, Apley's grinding test	Meniscal tears
Finkelstein test	de Quervain's disease
Thompson calf squeeze test	Achillas tendon rupture

BONE AND JOINT INFECTIONS

Bacteria can gain entry into the bone by the following three methods:

- Hematogenous spread
- Direct penetrating injury
- Spread from adjacent sites of infection.

Of these, ***hematogenous route is the most common mode*** of entry.

➢ Infection of bone is called ***osteomyelitis;*** infection of joint is called ***septic arthritis.***

Pathogenesis

In acute osteomyelitis, the ***metaphysis is commonly involved***. Presence of vascular structures in ***hairpin loop pattern*** causes a slow flow of blood at this area.

Also, low oxygen tension in this region leads to ***less phagocytic activity*** of white blood cells. Thrombosis caused by infection results in a region of avascular necrosis that may lead to abscess formation.

As pus accumulates and pressurizes, it can track through the cortex and collect beneath the periosteum. Subperiosteal abscesses may stimulate the formation new bone.

Once out of the cortex, pus can also track through the skin, forming a draining sinus.

Chronic osteomyelitis: As the periosteum is elevated, the cortical bone is deprived of its blood supply and may become necrotic, forming ***sequestrum*** *(dead necrotic bone).*

Because the periosteum retains its blood supply, it remains viable and produces osteoid.

The periosteal new bone formation around the necrotic sequestrum is known as ***involucrum***.

Multiple holes formed in the involucrum are called ***cloacae.***

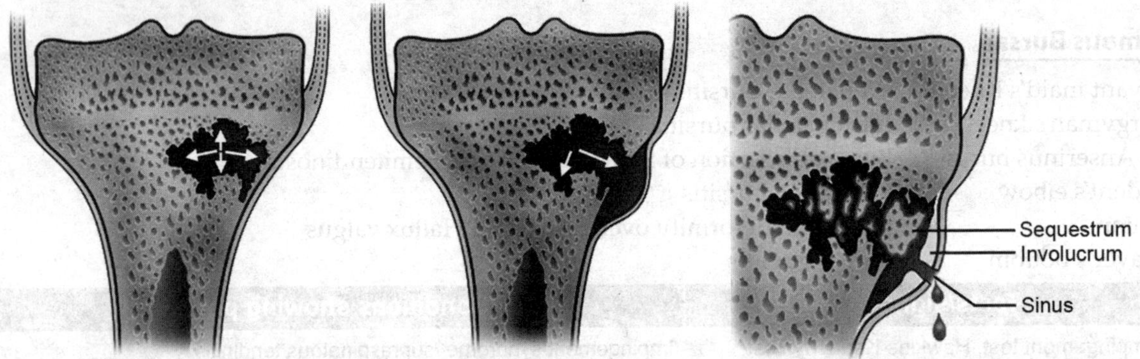

Fig. 19.27: Osteomyelitis

Osteomyelitis is classified based on duration of symptoms:
Acute: <2 weeks
Subacute: Weeks to months,
Chronic: > 3 months.

Organisms: The causal organism in both adults and children is usually

- ***Staphylococcus aureus** is the most common organism*(found in over 70% of cases),
- Less often by Group A beta-hemolytic streptococcus (*Streptococcus pyogenes)* or
- The alpha-hemolytic diplococcus S. *pneumoniae.*

Acute hematogenous osteomyelitis most commonly affects distal femur, proximal tibia and humerus.

[Acute osteomyelitis in adults: usually follows an open injury or complications of surgery.

➢ True haematogenous osteomyelitis is uncommon and it usually affects the ***vertebrae.*]**

Clinical features: Severe pain and restriction of movements-are the most common presenting signs of infection in all age groups.

Symptoms include fever, anorexia, irritability, and lethargy, localized tenderness, swelling, warmth, and erythema.

Diagnosis: Done mostly by ***clinical examination*** alone. Investigations are for confirmation and treatment planning.

Plain Radiographs

- Show ***soft-tissue swelling*** within 3 days of onset of infection;
- Bone changes like destruction and ***periosteal new bone formation*** may take **2 *weeks*** to be visible in X-rays.

CT: It is helpful in determining the extent of bone destruction. Useful to guide needle localization for biopsy, debridement, aspiration.

MRI: Provides better soft-tissue resolution and can be used to identify abscesses as well as to help ***differentiate cellulitis from osteomyelitis***.

MRI is useful in visualizing marrow involvement and differentiating between malignant neoplasm and infection. More ***useful in early diagnosis*** of osteomyelitis.

Radionuclide scanning: Although radiographs and CT scans give a structural or anatomical picture, radionuclide scanning gives a more physiological picture.

[Bone scanning does not detect the presence of infection, but instead reflects inflammatory changes or the reaction of bone to the infection.]

The three most commonly used radioisotopes are ***technetium-99m phosphate, gallium-67 citrate, and indium-111–labeled leukocytes.***

Technetium scanning is relatively ***nonspecific,*** and increased uptake may be caused by any process that increases vascularity or deposition of calcium phosphate. Tumor, trauma, and bone resorption due to disuse may cause increased uptake.

Treatment: Standard evaluation includes needle aspiration for culture and subsequent initiation of empirical antibiotics.

Six weeks of antibiotic therapy are usually indicated. (2 weeks of parenteral antibiotics followed by 4weeks of oral antibiotic therapy.

In acute osteomyelitis, antibiotics and symptomatic treatment alone is adequate in most cases.

- When symptoms do not improve with drugs (which indicates the abscess formation), decompression and drainage pus is warranted.

In chronic osteomyelitis, the successful treatment requires the ***surgical removal of all nonviable tissue and foreign debris.***
Necrotic tissue- sequestrum- shelters bacteria from access by white blood cells and from therapeutic concentrations of antibiotics, the ***sequestrum must be completely removed,*** although the involucrum should be left in place.

Involucrum is viable reactive tissue that has a generous vascular supply and contributes to the mechanical stability of the bone.

Brodie's Abscess

It is a localized subacute osteomyelitis.
The lesion is located eccentrically in the metaphysis.
On X-ray, it appears as a ***lytic lesion with a rim of sclerotic bone;*** easily mistaken for a variety of neoplasms.
S. aureus is cultured in 50% of patients; in 20%, the culture is negative.
It is form of ***subacute osteomyelitis*** is distinctly different from acute or chronic osteomyelitis in that it responds predictably to antibiotic therapy, and surgical debridement is often unnecessary.

Garre's Sclerosing Osteomyelitis

A unifocal form of Chronic Recurrent Multifocal Osteomyelitis (CRMO) and typically presents as an enlarged, painful segment of bone.
The metaphyses of long bones and the mandible are the most commonly involved sites.

- Bone is thickened and distended
- Abscesses and sequestra are absent
- Causative organism is not known.

Caffey's Disease

Also known as ***Infantile Cortical Hyperostosis***.

It presents with painful swelling of ***ulna or mandible*** with no local signs of inflammation. ESR is elevated.

X-ray shows periosteal new bone formation resulting in thickening of the bone. Cause is not known.

Sickle Cell Disease

Acute osteomyelitis in patients with sickle-cell disease differs in two forms: the infection is usually located in the ***diaphysis*** rather than metaphysis. The organism responsible is most frequently ***salmonella,*** although ***S. aureus*** is also common in patients with sickle-cell disease.

Salmonella Osteomyelitis

- Subacute type of osteomyelitis, usually occurring in the ulna, tibia or vertebra.
- Often multiple bones are affected, may be bilaterally symmetrical. Usually occurs during the convalescent phase after an attack of tyhoid.

SEPTIC ARTHRITIS

It is a pyogenic infection of joint.

Hematogenous seeding of the synovium during transient bacteremia is the most common cause of septic arthritis in children.

Other foci of infection, such as otitis media or sinusitis, may be present well in advance of the joint infection.

Septic arthritis may also arise from a contiguous site of infection, such as ***adjacent osteomyelitis, or from a penetrating injury with direct inoculation into the joint.***

Proteases, peptidases, and collagenases are released from leukocytes, synovial cells, and cartilage. These enzymes break down the cellular and extracellular structure of cartilage. This results in rapid destruction of the joint and thereby pathological fusion (***bony ankylosis)***

Clinically, apart from constitutional symptoms, the affected joint will show effusion, warmth, tenderness.

The range of movement is severely restricted. The child will not move the limb because of pain; this is called **pseudoparalysis**.

Treatment: The treatment of septic arthritis is complete surgical evacuation of a purulent effusion.

It is achieved by ***open arthrotomy or arthroscopic drainage***.

The synovial fluid from an infected joint is opaque, light yellow or light gray, and nonviscous. Cell analysis often reveals a white blood count (WBC) of more than 100,000 and more than 90% polymorphonuclear (PMN) leukocytes

[*Tips:* fibous or painful ankylosis is seen in TB and Rheumatoid arthritis; whereas bony or painless ankylosis is usually the end result of untreated septic arthritis.

Note: TB of spine results in bony ankylosis; in other bones and joints TB results in fibrous ankylosis]

Tips: joint fusion by pathological disease process is called as **ankylosis;** fusion achieved by surgical methods is known as **arthrodesis.]**

Tom-Smith Arthritis

It is ***septic arthritis of hip joint in infants***. Because of the cartilaginous nature of femoral head in infantile age, bacterial infection rapidly destroys the femoral head. Since there is no femoral head, bony ankylosis does not occur. These children, if untreated in early stage, present ***with limb shortening and unstable hip joint.***

SKELETAL TUBERCULOSIS

Bone tuberculosis is always a secondary infection, primary being lungs, lymph nodes, GIT. Usually **monoarticular** arthritis.

Isolated osteomyelitis without affecting joint is rare. Any bone or joint may be affected.

Predilection

Spine is the MC affected joint (50%).

Hip (15%), Knee (10%) and rarely Shoulder are also affected.

- ***ATT is the mainstay of treatment in all cases.***

Phemister Triad

- Juxta articular osteoporosis
- Peripheral osseous lesions 3.Gradual narrowing of joint space.

Seen in TB arthritis, fungal disease and rheumatoid arthritis.

Tuberculosis of Hip Joint

It is second most common joint involved.

(Spine-dorsolumbar- is MC site of skeletal tuberculosis- Pott's spine).

Stages of TB of Hip

- ***Synovitis:*** Hip in position of ***flexion, abduction, external rotation.*** There will be apparent lengthening.
- ***Early arthritis:*** Hip in position ***of flexion, adduction, internal rotation***. There will be *apparent shortening.*
- ***Advanced arthritis:*** Exaggeration of flexion, adduction, internal rotation. There is *true Shortening.*
- ***Advanced arthritis with subluxation/dislocation: Migrating or wandering acetabulam*** is seen.

The infectious process leads too resorption of acetabulum; the head may get dislocated from acetabulum to ilium because of the constant pull of hip muscles.

This pseudo-acetabulum formed in the ilium is known as ***'wandering acetabulum' or travelling acetabulum.***

With advanced arthritis and periarticular osteoporosis there is destruction of acetabular roof so the acetabular cavity may get enlarged and deepened giving the ***mortar-pestle appearance***.

Tuberculosis of Knee Joint

Third most common site. It causes the classical ***Triple deformity of knee***:

- Flexion,
- Posterolateral subluxation and
- External rotation.

It is treated by ATT and arthrodesis (done by POP-immobilization/Charnley's method)

Tuberculosis of Shoulder Joint

The pathology of shoulder TB is different from other joints.

Dry ***granular type*** reaction occurs here, hence no effusion of joint or cold abscess is seen.

This dry atrophic form is known as ***- caries sicca.***

Tuberculous dactylitis: May resemble sickle cell dactylitis, with swelling of the phalanges, metacarpals, and metatarsals. This is called ***spina ventosa.***

The treatment of skeletal tuberculosis is medical. Surgical debridement of the bone lesions is not necessary for a cure, although drainage of large abscesses often improves the patient's overall constitutional symptoms.

Causative Organisms for Musculoskeletal Infections

Patient Characteristics	Causative Organisms
Nosocomial infection	*Pseudomonas aeruginosa, Staph aureus,*
Community-acquired infection	*S. aureus (Most common organism in all ages and all clinical conditions)*
Infants	group B streptococcus
Sickle cell disease	*Salmonella species, S. aureus,*
Puncture wound/IV drug addicts	*Pseudomonas aeruginosa, S. aureus*
Immuno-compromised	*Candida, Aspergillus, atypical mycobacteria*

Bacterial Species Associated with Common Conditions

Organism	Common Occurrence
Staphylococcus aureus	Most common organism in osteomyelitis, acute hematogenous osteomyelitis (90%), and infected metal implants
Group B strep	Infants <1 year old
Haemophilus influenza	Children 1-16 years old
Pseudomonas aeruginosa	Nosocomial, puncture wound through shoe
Eikenella corrodens	Animal bite
Salmonella	Sickle cell disease
Candida albicans, Aspergillus, Atypical mycobacteria	Immunocompromized
Escherichia coli	Neonatal
Neisseria gonorrhea	Septic arthritis in young sexually active adult

METABOLIC BONE DISEASES

Vitamin D Deficiency

Vitamin D deficiency can result in rickets and osteomalacia.

- **Rickets** is a disease of **growing children or adolescents,** and is characterized by failure of or delayed mineralization of endochondral new bone at the growth plates.
- **Osteomalacia** is a failure of mineralization of newly formed osteoid at sites of bone turnover **in *adult.***

Rickets

Biochemical Abnormalities in Rickets

Type of Rickets	Calcium	Phosphate	Alkaline Phosphatase	PTH
Nutritional	N	N↓	↑	↑
Vitamin D–resistant (XLH, RTA, Fanconi's)	N	↓	↑	N
Vitamin D–dependent type I (1α hydroxylase)	↓	↓	↑	↑
Vitamin D–dependent type II (receptor insensitivity)	↓	↓	↑	↑
Renal osteodystrophy	N↓	↑	↑	↑↑

(N, normal; PTH, parathyroid hormone; RTA, renal tubular acidosis; XLH, X-linked hypophosphatemia)

Clinical Features

Beading of the ribs- **rachitic rosary'** is due to enlargement of the costochondral junctions.

The pull of the diaphragm on the ribs produces a horizontal depression known as ***Harrison's groove***. Short stature results from insufficient longitudinal growth.

Pectus carinatum is caused by forward projection of the sternum.

Closure of the ***fontanelles is delayed*** and the sutures are thickened, which leads to a skull appearance described as resembling ***hot cross buns***.

The dentition is affected, with **delays in appearance of the teeth**.

As the child begins standing and walking, the softened long bones bow.

- In toddlers, **bowleg, or genu varum**, is one of the most common initial signs. In older children, ***genu valgum*** and coxa vara may be the initial features.

Spine: Kyphoscoliosis may be present.

The bone ends at ***wrists, elbows, and knees are thickened.***

Radiographic features: The hallmark of rickets:

- ***Widening of growth plates.***
- ***Cupping and splaying of metaphysis.***

Osteomalacia

The hallmark **is *Looser zones*** - transverse bands of unmineralized osteoid, which typically appear in the medial aspect of the proximal femur and at the posterior aspect of the ribs.

Also called as ***pseudofractures or Milkman's lines.***

Scurvy

Ascorbic acid deficiency causes failure of collagen synthesis and osteoid formation.

Sub-periosteal haemorrhage, gum bleeding are characteristic.

Scurvy is called ***Barlow's disease*** when present in infants.

X-ray: Generalized osteoporosis/osteopenia

- **White line of Frankel:** is dense ***sclerotic*** edge of the metaphysis.
- **Trummerfeld zone:** Metaphysis shows transverse ***radiolucent*** bands.
- **Wimberger's sign (ring sign):** epiphysis is ring shaped because the central region is demineralized (lucent) with peripheral mineralization (sclerotic).

Osteoporosis

Bone is comprised of cells and extracellular matrices.

Bone is a dynamic entity regulated by ***osteoblasts*** (responsible for bone formation), and ***osteoclasts*** (responsible for bone resorption).

Peak bone mass is established between 20 and 30 years of age.

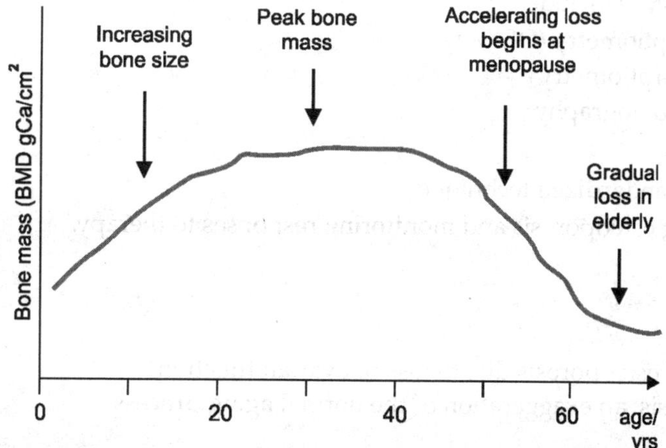

Osteoporosis A systemic skeletal disorder characterized by:

- ***Low bone mass***

- Disruption of the micro-architecture of bone
- Compromised bone strength

which lead to an ***increased risk for fracture.***

Osteoporosis is a decrease in bone mass. (i.e it is a quantitative defect).

Here, the ***mineralization is normal.***

World Health Organization criteria for diagnostic osteoporosis using bone density measurements	
Category	**T-Score**
Normal	Not more than 1.0 standard deviations (SD) below the young adult mean
Osteopenia	Between 1.0 and 2.5 SD below the young adult mean
Osteoporosis	More than 2.5 SD below the young adult mean
Severe or established osteoporosis	More than 2.5 SD below the young adult mean with a fracture

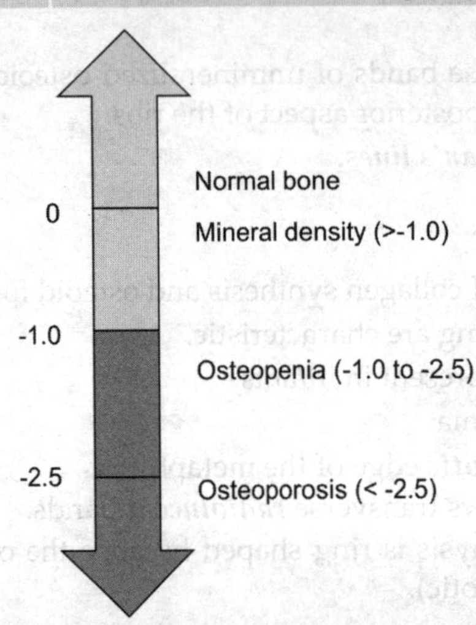

The most common osteoporosis-related **fractures** involve

- Thoraco*lumbar spine: anterior wedge collapse of vertebral body producing* **kyphosis**
- *Hip:* ***Neck of femur fracture***
- *Distal radius:* ***Colle's fracture.***

Bone densitometry (BMD): a major diagnostic tool in osteoporosis.

Techniques for quantifying BMD include:

- Dual-energy X-ray absorptiometry (DEXA)
- Single-energy X-ray absorptiometry
- Quantitative computed tomography
- Quantitative ultrasound.

DEXA: It is by far the ***best*** standardized technique.

It is preferred for diagnosing osteoporosis and monitoring responses to therapy.

Types of Osteoporosis

Primary

- Type 1: ***Postmenopausal*** osteoporosis due to loss of ovarian function.
- Type 2: ***Senile*** osteoporosis, an exaggeration of the normal aging process.

Secondary

Causes of Secondary Osteoporosis

- **Hormonal**

Hypogonadism
Cushing's syndrome
Addison's disease
Hyperthyroidism
Hyperparathyroidism acromegaly

- **Nutritional**
  Severe malnutrition (e.g., anorexia nervosa)
  Malabsorption
  Severe liver disease
- **Hereditary**
  Osteogenesis imperfecta
  Ehlers-Danlos syndrome
  Homocystinuria
  Hypophosphatasia
- **Rheumatological**
  Rheumatoid arthritis and related diseases
  Ankylosing spondylitis
- **Hematological**
  Multiple myeloma
  Hemochromatosis
  Hemophilia
  Mastocytosis
  Thalassemia
  Leukemia and lymphoma
- **Others**
  Paralysis or immobilization
  Chronic obstructive lung disease
  Diffuse metastatic carcinoma
  Hypercalcemia of malignancy.

Management of Osteoporosis:

- Lifestyle modifications:
  Exercise, physical activity
- Nutritional interventions:
  Daily intake of calcium 1000-1500 mg
  Vitamin D 800 IU).

Pharmacologic Therapy:

- ***Bisphosphonates:*** are potent selective ***inhibitors of osteoclastic bone resorption. Commonly used for the treatment and prevention*** of post-menopausal osteoporosis.
- ***Calcitonin***: Although the physiological role of calcitonin in humans has not been established, it is well documented that this hormone can profoundly ***inhibit osteoclast function*** and retard bone loss.
  - *(Salmon calcitonin available as a **nasal spray,** with each metered dose providing 200 IU of the drug has been approved by the FDA for osteoporosis therapy.)*
- **Ipriflavone** is a flavinoid derivative that has recently been demonstrated to have both direct and indirect effects on the skeleton.
  - Not only does this drug *inhibit the differentiation of precursors to osteoblasts and inhibit bone resorption, it also appears to stimulate osteoblast production and activity.*
- **Parathyroid Hormone:**
  - ***Continuous*** treatment by parathyroid hormone (PTH) results in ***increased bone resorption*** and bone loss.
  - By contrast ***intermittent PTH*** treatment in individuals with osteoporosis ***stimulates*** bone formation, increases BMD, and reduces the risk of fractures.

Teriparatide is recombinant human PTH, the newest drug for osteoporosis. It is the ***only drug having anabolic (bone forming)*** action in osteoporosis management.

- ***Hormone replacement therapy*** is helpful at maintaining bone density although it is not preferred because of associated side effects.

Broadly, two group of drugs for osteoporosis:

- Anti-resorptive: Bisphophonates, SERMs, Calcitonin
- Anabolic: Teriparatide.

Renal Osteodystrophy

➢ Renal osteodystrophy is a general term used to describe ***skeletal changes secondary to chronic renal failure***.

Metabolic bone diseases develop in pattients with chronic renal disease because kidney plays major role in metabolism of vitamin D, calcium, phophorus, magnetium, etc.
Clinical features are:

- Rickets or osteomalacia
- Osteoporosis/osteopenia
- Osteosclerosis
- Soft tissue calcifications
- Secondary hyperparathyroidism.

Rickets or osteomalacia is characterized by incomplete mineralisation of the normal bone tissue.

Abnormal phosphate retention in renal osteodystrophy leads to hypocalcaemia with resulting ***secondary hyperparathyroidism***.

Rugger jersey spine: Osteosclerosis of the vertebral end plate may produce a 'rugger jersey' appearance in lateral X-rays of the spine, due to alternating bands of increased and decreased bone density.

Biochemical Features

- Low serum calcium,
- Elevated alkaline phosphatase
- High serum phosphate
- High plasma PTH.

OSTEOPETROSIS (Albers-Schonberg's disease):

It is a sclerosing bone disease (the density of the bone is increased).

➢ Due to reduced bone resorption of bone caused by ***osteoclast defect***.

Patients present with pathologic fractures

They may have ***cranial nerve problems*** including optic nerve compression, facial nerve dysfunction, and sensorineural deafness due to ***narrowing of the skull foramina***.

They may have bone pain related to fractures or stress fractures; and they frequently have ***infections of the bones or mandibles.***

The disease limits the narrow space available, contributes to ***pancytopenia and hepatosplenomegaly***.

Radiographic characteristics:

- The bones are dense white, without medullary cavities, and appear marble-like. (that is why it is called as ***Marble bone disease***)
- A ***bone within bone or endobone*** appearance may be seen within the pelvis.
- Marked sclerosis of the end plates of the vertebral bodies may give vertebrae a ***rugger jersey appearance***.
- Failure of metaphyseal cutback by osteoclasts leads to an ***Erlenmeyer flask shape of the epiphysis***.

Treatment: ***Bone marrow transplantation*** corrects both the skeletal and hematologic abnormalities associated with osteopetrosis.

Most fractures in children with osteopetrosis will heal well if treated with closed means, although ***healing may be delayed***.

PAGET'S DISEASE OF THE BONE

Also known as **Osteitis Deformans.**

Characterized by

- Increased bone turn over
- Enlargement and thickening of bone,
- Internal architecture is altered and weak.

Rare in Asia.

Cause: unknown, viral infection is suggested.

Marked increase in activity of both cells

- Osteoclasts (bone lytic)
- Osteoblasts (bone forming)

So, the ***bone turnover is accelerated.***

Over activity of osteoclast function is the basic defect.

Lab findings:

- ***Alkaline phosphatase is raised*** (due to osteoblastic activity)
- Increased ***excretion of hydroxyproline in the urine*** (due to osteoclastic activity).
- Normal serum phosphorus and calcium

Microscopy: marble / ***mosaic appearance***

Deformities

Pelvis, tibia, femur, skull, spine are commonly affected, in that order.

Skull: enlarged; base become flattened ***(platybasia)***

Cranial nerve compression may lead, facial palsy deafness etc.

(Another cause of deafness in Paget's disease is otosclerosis).

Long bones: ***sabre tibia***, bowing of femur.

Spine: Kyphosis

Radiologic findings:

- Skull: ***Osteoporosis circumscripta,*** and ***cotton wool*** appearance.
- Long bones (Tibia, femur): Lesions are in ***blade of grass*** and ***flame-shaped***
- Spine: ***Picture frame vertebrae.***

Complications

- Osteoarthritis,
- Pathological fractures,
- Protrusio acetabuli
- Cranial nerve palsies
- High-output cardiac failure
- Osteosarcoma

Treatment

- **Bisphosphonate** is the treatment of choice. It inhibits osteoclastic-mediated bone resorption.
- **Calcitonin:** It reduces bone resorption by decreasing both the activity and the number of osteoclasts; it also has ***analgesic*** property.

PAEDIATRIC ORTHOPEDICS

HIP

Developmental Dysplasia of HIP

Previously called as ***congenital dislocation of the hip (CDH)***. Now recognized as a ***developmental*** failure of the acetabulum around the femoral head.

The ***acetabulum is shallow*** and 'vertical' rather than concentrically covering the femoral head.

This allows an increased degree of instability in the hip joint which, in extreme cases, presents as frank dislocation of the hip.

Incidence: 1/1000 live births. ***Female***: male ratio of 7: 1.

Left hip more commonly affected than right; bilateral in 20% cases.

First-born child is more likely to be affected than subsequent children.

Risk factors: include **5 F's** – *F*emale, *F*amily History, *F*rank breech birth, *F*irst born, *Left* side involvement.

Clinical Features

- ***Galleazzi Sign***: also known as ***Allis test***. There is shortening of thigh segment on the affected side when hip and knee are fully flexed in a child lying supine. So the affected side knee is lower than the normal side knee.

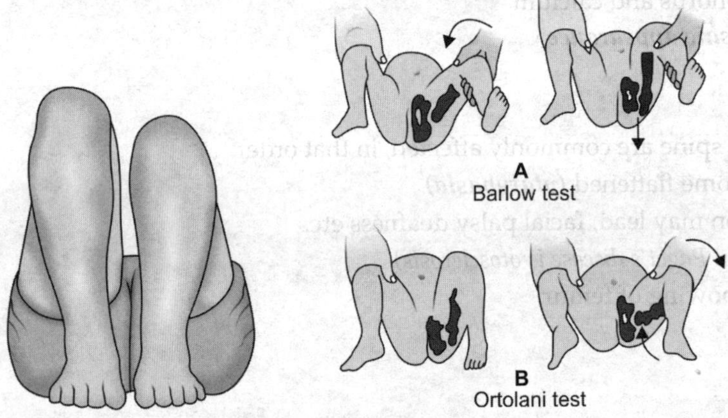

Fig. 19.28: Galeazzi sign

- **Ortolani test:** (click of entry) On flexion and *abduction* of hip will reduce the dislocation. It is felt by palpable click.
- **Barlow's test:** (click of exit) this is a provocative maneuver. The hip is flexed and *adducted* → femoral head is dislocated out of the acetabulum.

Gait Pattern

In Unilateral DDH show ***Trendelenburg gait.*** In Bilateral DDH there is ***waddling gait.***

Diagnosis

- The clinical examination remains the gold standard.
- Radiographs and Ultrasound.

Changes in the radiographic measurements

- ***Perkin's vertical line***: A perpendicular line drawn at the lateral margin of the acetabulum
- ***Hilgenreiner's horizontal line:*** A line through the triradiate cartilages.
- ***Shenton's line:*** A curved smooth line drawn along inferior surface of femoral neck and inferior surface of superior pubic rami.

- ***Wiberg's center-edge angle:*** Angle formed by a line drawn from the center of the femoral head to the outer edge of the acetabular roof, and a verticle line drawn through the center of the femoral head. Normally it is more than 25 deg.
- ***Acetabular index:*** An angle formed by Hilgenreiner's line and a line drawn along the acetabular surface. Normally, it is < 30 deg.
- Normally, femoral epiphysis (head) should lie within the inner lower quadrant formed by Perkin's and Hilgenreiner's lines.

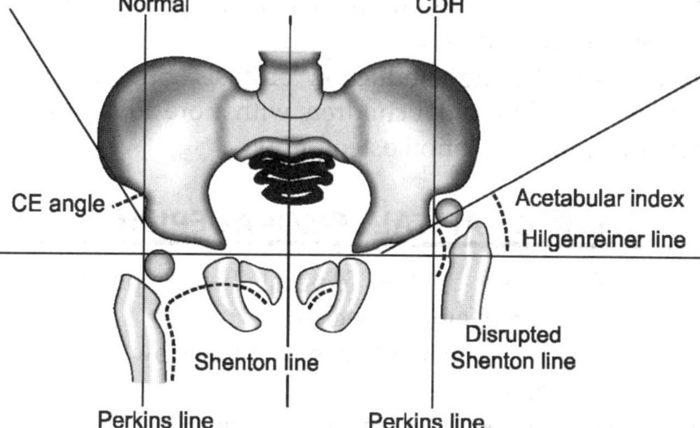

Fig. 19.29: Important lines in the hip radiograph

In DDH

- Upward displacement of femoral head
- Delayed appearance of femoral head ossific nucleus
- Disruption of the Shenton line
- Increase in slope of the acetabular roof, i.e. increased acetabular index
- Decrease in CE angle of Weiberg.

Treatment

- Infants aged 0–6 months: Pavlik harness or von Rosen splint
- Infants 6–15 months: Closed reduction under anesthesia and spica cast application
- Children 15 months to 2 yrs: Open reduction and spica casting
- Older children require osteotomy of femur and pelvis.

Various Osteotomy Procedures for the DDH

Osteotomy	Description
Salter osteotomy	Transverse cut is made above the acetabulum, the acetabular fragment is **rotated** forward and outward to improve acetabular coverage.
Pemberton acetabuloplasty	A pericapsular iliac osteotomy. An osteotomy cut is made above the acetabulum down to the flexible triradiate cartilage.
Steel triple osteotomy	The ischium, the superior pubic ramus, and the ilium all are divided. Then the acetabulum is repositioned and stabilized.
Chiari medial displacement osteotomy	An osteotomy is performed at the superior margin of the acetabulum, and the pelvis inferior to the osteotomy is displaced medially.

TOM-SMITH ARTHRITIS

It is ***septic arthritis of hip joint in infants.*** The infectious process destroys the femoral capital epiphysis which will be cartilaginous during that age.

Because of loss femoral head, the femur becomes shortened; the hip joint becomes ***unstable*** allowing excessive movement in all directions.

- ➢ The same septic pathology in older children and adult ends up with ***bony ankylosis;*** here the joint is fused allowing no movement.

LEGG-CALVÉ-PERTHES DISEASE

A type of ***avascular necrosis of femoral head in children.*** The cause is unknown.

Also called as: ***coxa plana, osteochondritis deformans, coxa juvenilis, pseudocoxalgia.***

Occurs in children 4 to 8 years.

More common in ***boys*** than in girls, ratio of 4 to 1. Affected children are usually ***small for age.*** Presents with a ***painless limp.***

Radiographs: fragmentation, irregularity, collapse of the femoral head.

MRI standard method of early diagnosis and investigation of choice..

Treatment: Bracing- abduction orthosis. Surgery is recommended for older children, with more advanced disease (vaus derotation osteotomy).

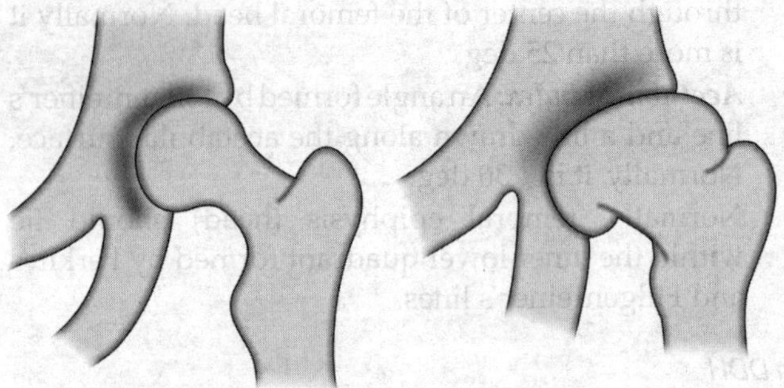

Fig. 19.30: Normal Perthes disease

SLIPPED CAPITAL FEMORAL EPIPHYSIS

- Displacement of the femoral head epiphysis relative to the femoral neck.
- It is a mechanical insufficiency of the growth plate of femoral neck.
- The head slips *backward and downward.*

Etiology: unknown.

But the common predisposing factors are:

- Obesity
- Hypothyroidism
- Panhypopituitarism
- Hypogonadism.

Clinical: Common in ages between 10 - 16 yrs of age.

Male > female.

Presents with ***pain, limp, and decreased range of motion of the hip***.

Radiograph: straight line at the upper surface of neck passes above the femoral head epiphysis. This is ***Trethowon sign.***

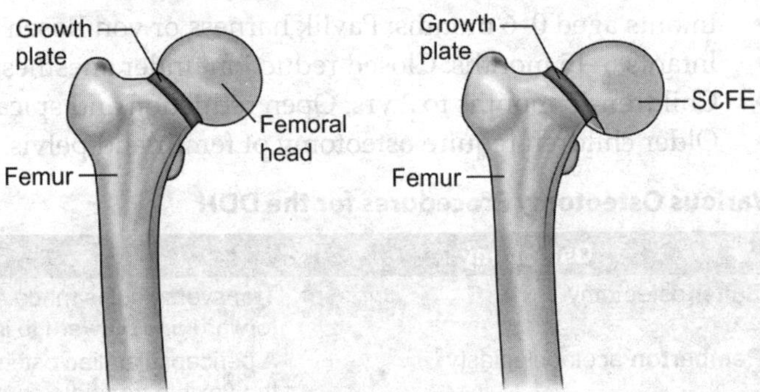

Fig. 19.31: Slipped capital femoral epiphysis

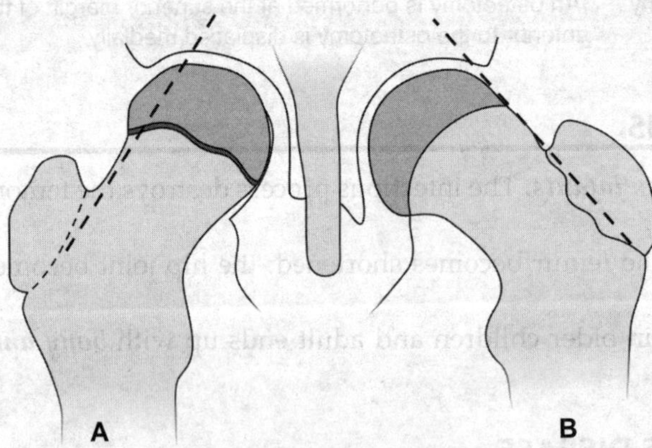

Figs 19.32 (A and B): Normal and Trethowan sign

Management

- In acute stage, the patient is allowed to bear weight.
- The goals of treatment are to prevent further slipping of the epiphysis.
- Methods of operative treatment: Include percutaneous and open in situ pinning, open reduction and internal fixation, epiphysiodesis, osteotomy.

COXA VARA

The normal femoral neck–shaft angle is 160 degrees at birth, decreasing to 125 degrees in adult life.

- An angle of ***less than 120 degrees*** is called coxa vara.

The deformity may be either congenital or acquired.

Common causes of coxa vara are:

- Rickets
- Perthes disease
- SCFE
- Malunion of femoral neck fractures
- Bone dysplasia.

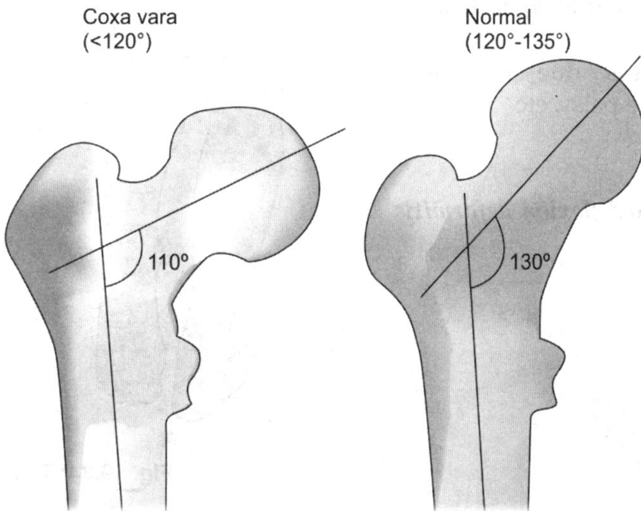

Fig. 19.33: Neck-shaft angle of femur

Fairbank Classification of Coxa Vara

- Idiopathic:
  - Congenital: Mild or severe coxa vara, with associated congenital anomalies
  - Developmental: Progressive, appearing between 2-6 years, with characteristic X-ray features
- Rachitic: Usually associated with active rickets
- Adolescent: Secondary to slipped capital femoral epiphysis
- Traumatic: Usually following # of the femoral neck (rare in children)
- Inflammatory: Secondary to tuberculosis or other infection
- Secondary to other underlying bone diseases such as:
  - Osteogenesis imperfecta
  - Cretinism
  - Dyschondroplasia (s)
  - Paget's disease
  - Osteoporosis
  - Tumor-like conditions (e.g. fibrous dysplasia).

Trendelenburg Test

Abductor mechanism consists of:

- Hip joint
- Neck of femur

- Hip abductors (gluteus medius and minimus).

This structural mechanism is important to keep the pelvis and both hip joints in same level.

Any disturbance in the above structures will produce ***positive Trendelenburg test.***

When the patient stands on affected side and lifts the opposite leg, the pelvis on opposite side drops. That is the ***sound (normal) side sags(SSS).***

The causes of positive test are:

- ***Hip joint:*** congenital dislocation/traumatic dislocation
- ***Neck of femur:*** fracture, reduced neck-shaft angle (coxa vara)
- ***Hip abductors:*** weakness due to polio, muscular dystrophy, nerve palsy, etc.

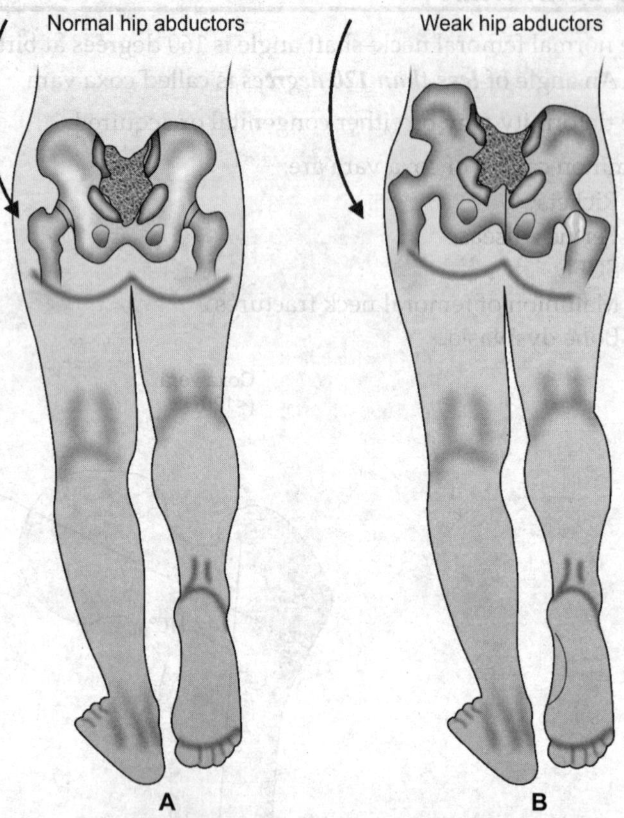

Fig. 19.34: Trendelenburg test

Thomas Test

To measure the degree of ***fixed flexion deformity of hip joint.***

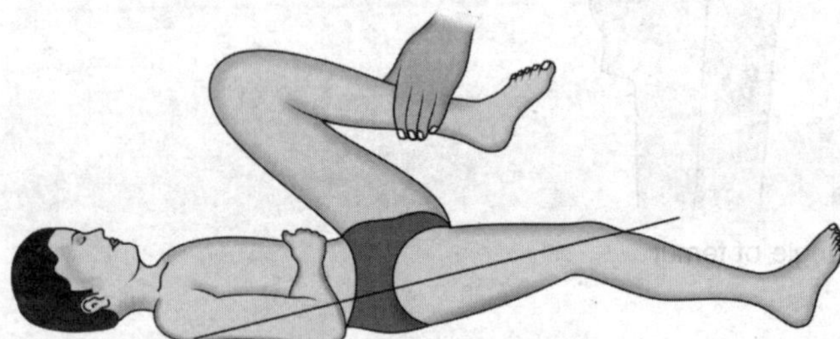

Fig. 19.35: Thomas test

When the hip is fixed in a certain degree of flexion, the patient develops ***excessive lordosis of lumbar spine*** in order to keep straight during erect posture.

This test is to ***unmask and measure the FFD of hip*** by obliterating the lumbar lordosis.

KNEE AND LEG

The common knee deformities are:

- Genu valgum (Knock knee)
- Genu varum (Bow leg)
- Genu recurvatum (Hyperextension deformity)
- Procurvatum (Flexion deformity)
- Wind-sweep deformity (varum one side and valgum the other side)
- Triple deformity (TB).

The above deformities are caused by:

- Infection
- inflammation
- Trauma
- Developmental disorders

- Rickets
- Tumor etc. or
- Simply, physiological.

Normal Physiological Development of Knee Alignment

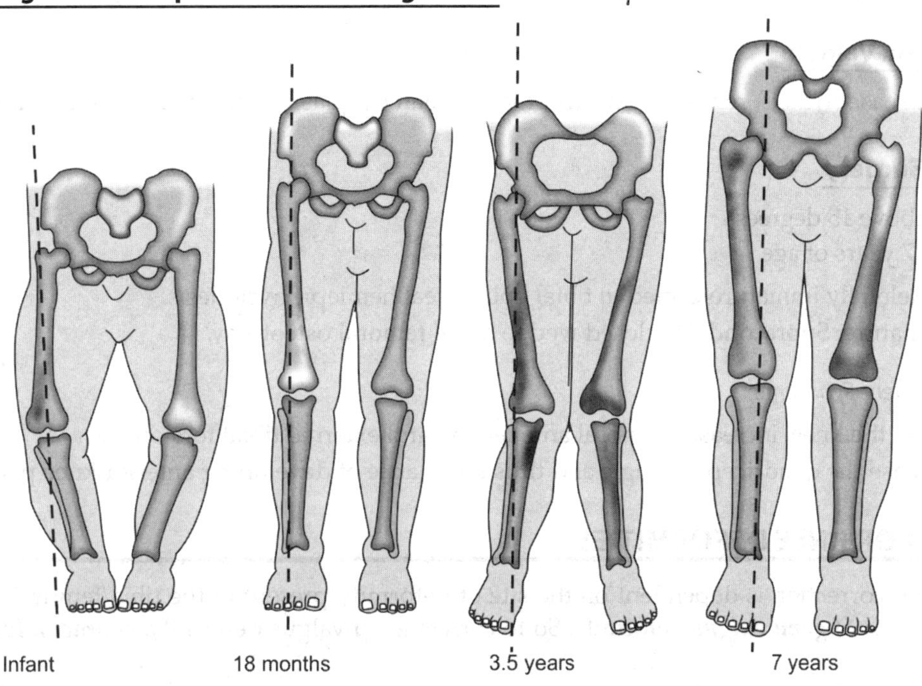

Fig. 19.36: Normal knee alignment pattens in growing children

- Genu varum upto 2 ***years*** of age
- Then genu valgum develops and reaches maximum at ***4 years*** of age.
- Then the amount of valgus reduces to some extent and fixes at 7 ***years*** of age.

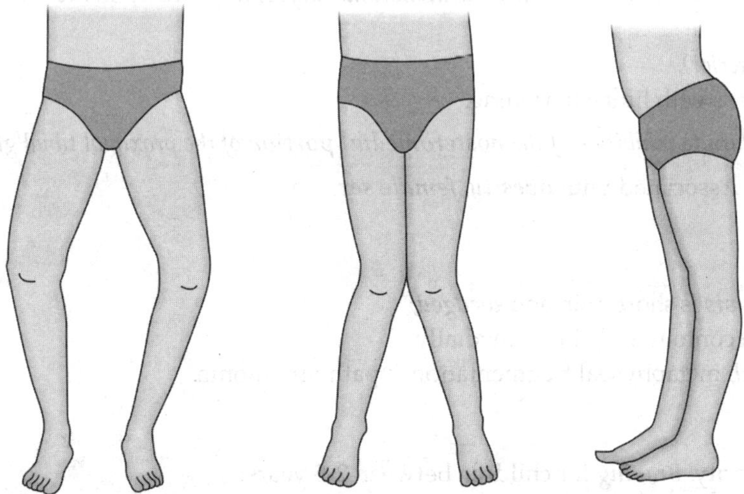

Fig. 19.37: Genu varum-Genu valgum-Genu recurvatum

By definition, at the age of 10 yrs are pathological:

- Tibial intercondylar distance > 6 cm- ***genu varum.***
- Tibial intermalleolar distance > 8 cm- ***genu valgum.***

GENU VALGUM

- The knock-knee is most dramatic at 3-6 years of age ***[physiologic genu valgum]***
- At this time, the anatomic angle may be as high as 15 degrees of valgus and it gradually remodels spontaneously to the adult average value of 5-7 degrees of valgus.

Pathological Genu Valgum

Metabolic bone disease (rickets, renal osteodystrophy), skeletal dysplasia, trauma, tumors, and infection.

Indications for Surgery

- Deformities above 15 degrees
- Patients over 7 years of age

If the patient is skeletally immature ® medial tibial epiphyseal hemiepiphysiodesis.
In the skeletally mature, Supracondylar closed wedge distal femoral osteotomy.

Miserable Malalignment Syndrome

Increased valgus at the knee, increased femoral anteversion and external tibial torsion.

- All three increase the quadriceps Q angle and thus the chance of developing anterior knee pain.

SURGERY FOR KNEE DEFORMITIES

The site of surgical correction is dependent on the site of deformity present in the tibia/femur. ***The femur*** is more often the primary site of ***genu valgus*** deformity. So to correct genu valgus deformity, ***supracondylar osteotomy*** of femur is done.
The ***tibia*** is the primary site correction for ***genu varum*** deformity.

Blount's Disease

Also called ***tibia varum,*** as it was originally thought of single deformity.
Recent investigations find this condtion as ***three-dimensional deformity*** which includes:

- Tibia varum,
- *Procurvatum (apex anterior),*
- *Internal rotation develops* with limb shortening.

These changes are *secondary to inhibition of the* ***posteromedial portion*** *of the proximal tibial growth plate.*

Bilateral in 80% of cases; Associated with ***obesity, female sex.***

X-ray

- Medial half of ***epiphysis*** is short, thin and ***wedged;***
- ***Physis*** is irregular in contour and slopes medially.
- ***Metaphysis*** is ***beaked;*** metaphyseal fragmentation *is* pathognomonic.

Treatment

Depends on age and severity. ***Bracing*** for children between 2-5 years;
if the deformity persists or progresses , it is treated with ***corrective osteotomy.***

OSTEOCHONDRITIS DISSECANS

Here an area of subchondral bone becomes necrotic; ***the necrotic bone and the cartilage overlying it separate*** from parent structures and together become a loose body.

It occurs ***most often in the knee*** joint, but it can occur in ***talus, capitellum*** etc.
It is the ***most common source of loose bodies in the knee joint.***
In the knee, ***medial femoral condyle*** is the most common.

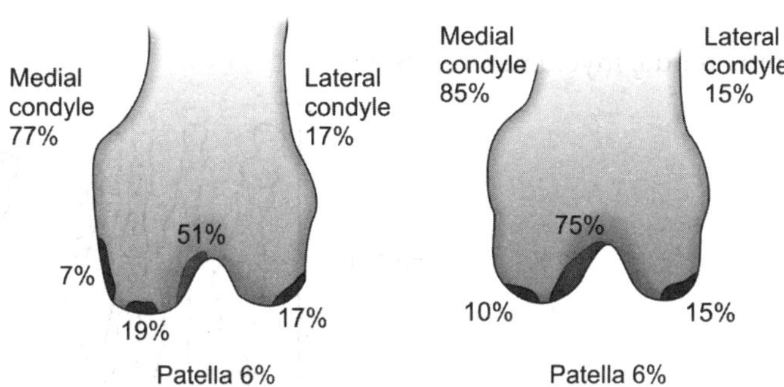

Fig. 19.38: Osteochondritis dessicans

Etiology

It is unclear but ***repetitive microtrauma*** is the postulated factor.
It is more common in males and during adolescence.
A positive ***Wilson's test*** occurs with the knee flexed 90 degrees and internally rotated.

➢ As the knee is extended, the patient complains of pain that is relieved by external rotation.

Radiographic examination with ***the tunnel or intercondylar notch view*** may be the most revealing.

Treatment

- The lesions often heal with conservative treatment in young patient.
- For adult, the surgical treatment such as drilling or excision of the fragment, débridement of the crater, ORIF and bone grafting are needed.

Congenital Pseudarthrosis of Tibia

An anterolateral bowing of leg which is progressive deformity and always require treatment.
Neurofibromatosis occurs in more than 50% of patients.

Treatment

- Bracing
- Intramedullary nail fixation bone graft,
- Circular ring fixation with bone transport,
- Vascularized fibular graft.

FOOT

Congenital Clubfoot (CTEV)

This ***foot and ankle deformity*** is characterized by:

- Plantar flexion of the ankle (equinus),
- Inversion of subtalar joint (varus),
- Adduction of forefoot,

Also called *Congenital Talipes Equino Varus (CTEV).*

Occurs 1 in 1000 births, more commonly in ***males;*** bilateral in 50% of cases. In India, this is the MC congenital skeletal deformity (not DDH).

Although most are isolated and ***idiopathic,*** clubfoot may be present in association with:

- Myotonic muscular dystrophy
- Poliomyelitis
- Cerebral palsy
- Spinal deformities (e.g. spina bifida, myelomeningocele).

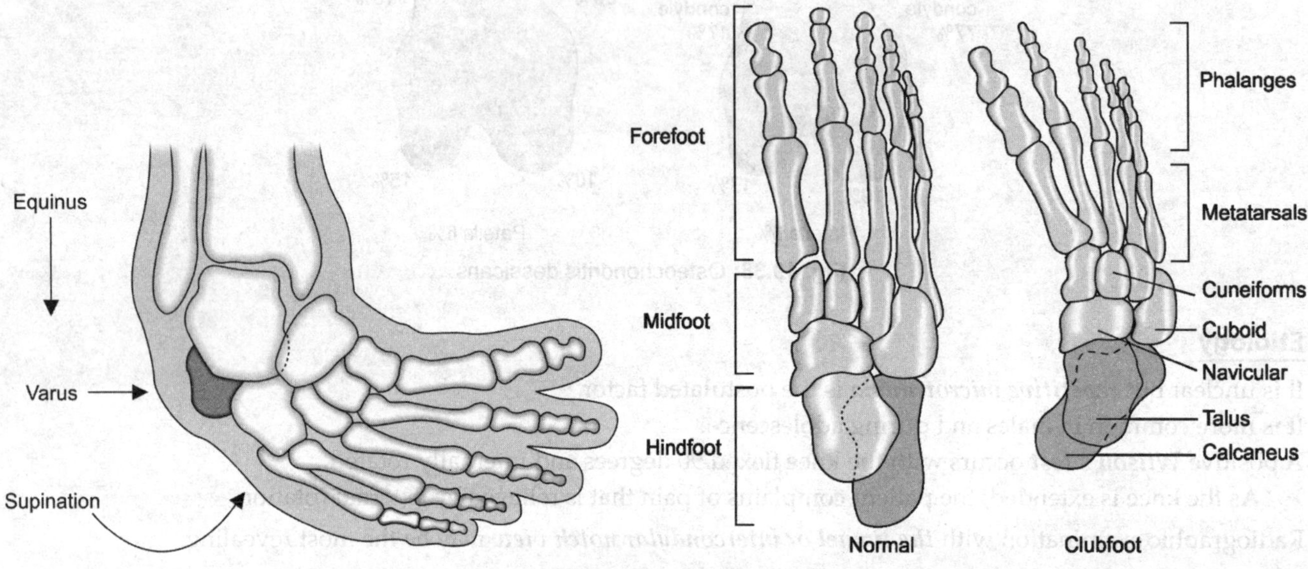

Fig. 19.39: Clubfoot

Treatment

Clubfoot always requires treatment, which should ***begin at birth.***

The initial approach is passive ***manipulation*** and positioning to the corrected position.

When satisfactory correction is not obtained, more extensive ***surgery*** is necessary.

- **Ponseti method** combination of **weekly** manipulation and casting, Achillis tenotomy, and prolonged splinting with ***Dennis-Brown bar.***
  Successful correction: 90% to 98%.

The order of correction: cavus, adduction, varus, and equinus (CAVE). This order prevents development of ***rocker-bottom deformity.***

Treatment of Resistant Clubfoot

Deformity	Treatment
Hindfoot varus	Modified McKay procedure, Dwyer osteotomy, Dillwyn-Evans procedure.
Equinus	Achilles tendon lengthening plus posterior capsulotomy.
All three deformities	> 10 years: triple arthrodesis

(***Triple arthrodesis***: surgical fusion of the subtalar, calcaneocuboid, andtalonavicular joints.)

Congenital Vertical Talus

Rare condition, present at birth; basically subluxation of the talonavicular joint also known as ***rocker bottom foot.***

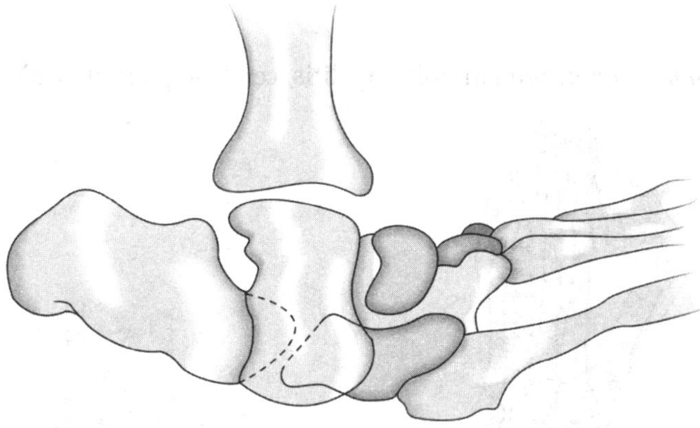

Fig. 19.40: Congenital vertical talus

More than 80% of cases are associated with other syndromes and anomalies (e.g. Marfan syndrome, arthrogryposis, myelomeningocele, etc).

Clinically, ***the plantar surface of the foot is convex,*** instead of normal concave arch.

On lateral X-ray, ***the talus is vertical,*** hence the name.

POP cast treatment is ineffective; so surgical correction is the right method.

PES Planus (Flatfoot)

Refers to loss of normal medial longitudinal arch.

- Types: *flexible and rigid.*

Common causes of ***rigid flat foot*** are:

- Congenital vertical talus
- Tarsal coalition

- ***Flexible flatfoot:*** Physiologic flat foot (hypermobile flatfoot) is characterized by varying degrees of loss of the longitudinal arch of the foot on weight bearing (the foot remains flexible).

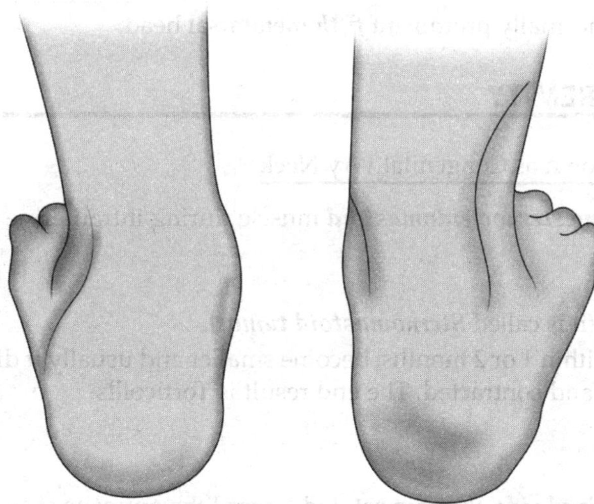

Fig. 19.41: 'Too many toes' sign on right side

In cases of flat foot, more toes are visible (compare with opposite side) when they are viewed from back. It is known as ***"Too many toes"*** sign.

Cavus Foot

It is the opposite of flat foot.

It is a foot with an ***abnormally high arch***. Seen in poliomyelitis, cerebral palsy, HMSN, etc.

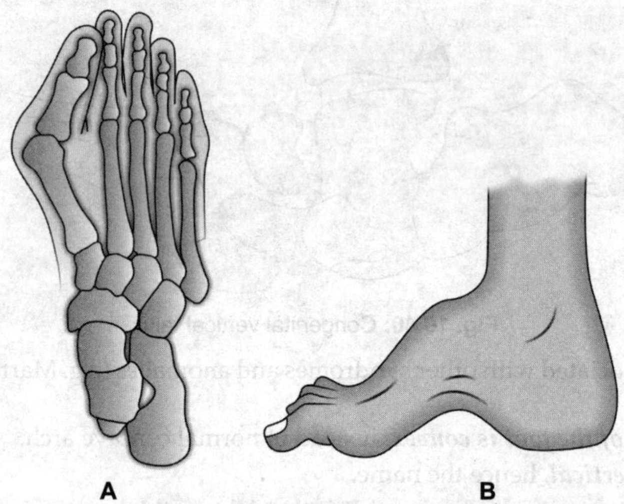

Figs 19.42 (A and B): A. Hallux valgus, B. Cavus foot

Hallux Valgus

Also called ***bunion deformity.***

It is the commonest of the foot deformities, characterized by lateral deviation of the **great toe** with prominence of the first metatarsal head medially.

It is often associated with a flatfoot.

Causes: Congenital, Tight shoes, rheumatoid arthritis etc.

Tailor's Bunion

A painful bunionette over an abnormally prominent ***fifth*** metatarsal head.

NECK AND UPPER EXTREMITY

Congenital Torticollis: Also known as Congenital Wry Neck

It results from ***ischaemia affecting sternocleidomastoid*** muscle during intrauterine life; ischaemia is secondary to abnormal position *in utero*.

More common on the right side.

This condition presents as mass (it is called ***Sternomastoid tumor).***

The mass attains maximal size within 1 or 2 months; become smaller and usually it disappears within 1year leaving the muscle permanently fibrotic and contracted. The end result is Torticollis.

Clinically

The ***head tilted toward the involved side***, the chin rotated toward the opposite side.

Plagiocephaly of skull may develop secondary to abnormal neck posture.

Treatment

Most cases resolve with stretching but, surgical release of the sternocleidomastoid at one or both ends is needed in some cases.

Associated conditions with torticollis ***(packaging disorders)*** are:

- Metatarsus adductus
- Developmental dysplasia of hip
- CTEV

Klippel-Feil Syndrome

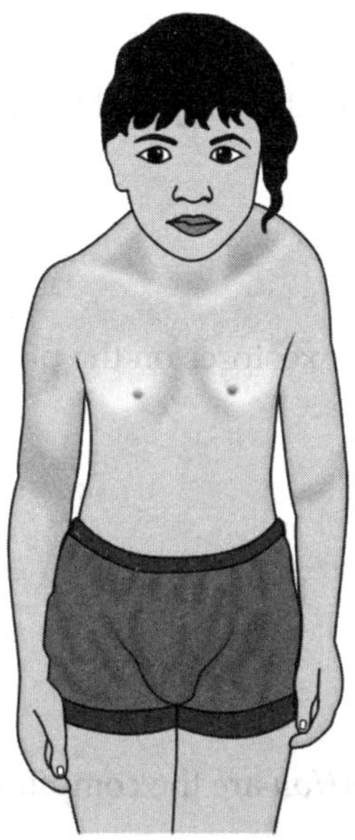
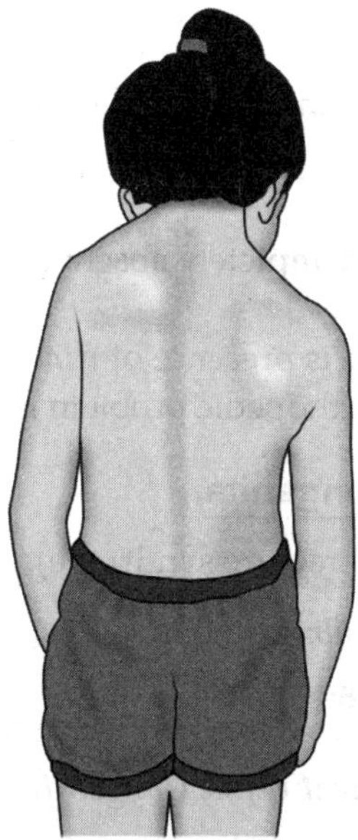

Fig. 19.43: Klippel-feil syndrome

Congenital fusions of the cervical vertebrae, clinically exhibited by ***the triad*** of:

- Low posterior hairline,
- Short neck, and
- Restricted neck movement

About 30% of patients have an associated ***Sprengel deformity***.

Sprengel's Deformity

- Congenital elevation of ***scapula***.
- It is hypoplastic.
- Rarely, one or more scapular muscles are partly or completely absent.

Cleidocranial Dysostosis

- The ***clavicles*** *are partially or completely* ***absent***.
- Pelvis and hip abnormality (coxa vara) is associated.
- The absence of clavicles causes the shoulders to drop and the neck to appear longer.
- The ***classic diagnostic feature*** is that the shoulders can be brought together. (i.e the ***shoulders can touch each other*** in front of chest).

Congenital Radioulnar Synostosis

- Due to ***failure of normal separation*** of the radius and ulna at proximal level these bones fused (synostosis).
- Seen with *fetal alcohol syndrome, DDH, clubfoot and other congenital anomalies.*
- As the forearm fixed in pronated position, the child has ***difficulty to perform forearm supination.***

GENERALIZED DISORDERS

Duchenne Muscular Dystrophy

An X-linked disorder that presents in boys 6–9 years of age.
Progressive muscle weakness, usually involving the ***proximal muscles.***
The ***pseudohypertrophy caused by replacement of calf muscles with fat*** is a classic finding.

Gower's Sign

Inability to rise from the floor without using the hands to walk up the body and legs. *(Climbing up on their own body)*

Nail-Patella Syndrome

- The ***nails and patellae*** are completely absent or hypoplastic.
- ***Radial head*** is dislocated.
- The pathognomonic feature is presence of ***iliac horns:*** bony exostoses on the posterior surface of the ilium.
- The most important non-Orthopedic problem is ***renal failure***.

Arthrogryposis Multiplex Congenita

- (or multiple congenital contracture syndrome):

The limbs are ***featureless and tubular.***
Normal skin creases are lacking.
Muscle mass is reduced.

- ***Club foot, Congenital vertical talus, Congenital hip dislocation*** are the complications of this condition.

Myositis Ossificans Progressiva (Fibrodysplasia Ossificans progressiva)

An autosomal dominant condition: there is ***widespread ossification of muscles of trunk***. Starts in childhood.
Shortening of big toe or thumb is seen.
Genetically, it is caused by ***overexpression of bone morphogenetic protein 4 (BMP 4) gene***.

- Life span is shortened due to respiratory infection and failure.

Treatment is supportive, large dose ***biphophonates*** are tried with limited results.

[Compare with MYOSITIS OSSIFICANS]

- A type of **heterotopic ossification**
- It occurs after trauma to muscles associated with bone fractures
- Most common locations are over the diaphyseal segment of long bones
- Matured lesions show peripheral mineralization with a central lucent area ***(zonal pattern)***
- It is not attached to the underlying bone
- Most common muscles involved are: *brachialis, deltoid, quadriceps.*
- Treatment: rest, gentle active movements, excision of bony mass. *Indomethacin and radiotherapy prevent recurrence.*

Achondroplasia

The most common form of short-limb dwarfism. An autosomal dominant trait.
Femur and humerus *are* most affected.
Mutation is in the fibroblast growth factor receptor 3 ***(FGFR-3) gene*** in chromosome 4.

- **Clinical Features:** The trunk length is normal but the limbs are shorter.
- Intelligence is normal.

Face shows frontal bossing and midface hypoplasia.
The metacarpals and metatarsals of all ***digits are all of almost equal length.***

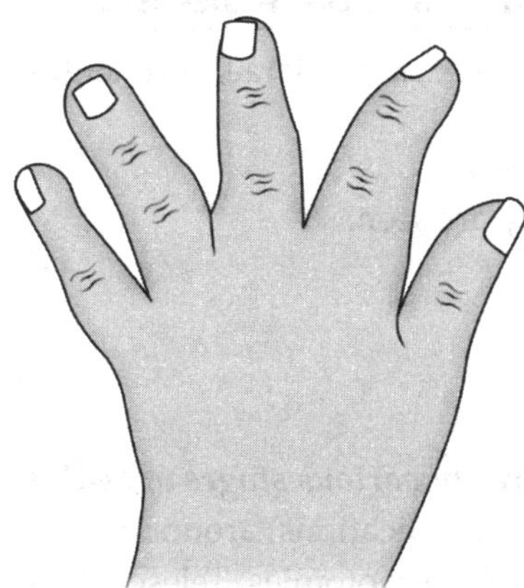

Fig. 19.44: Trident hand

The fingers have extra space between 3rd and 4th metacarpals, so that the digits are separated into three groups *(the trident hand).*

HYPERLAXITY SYNDROMES

- Marfan Syndrome
- Ehlers-Danlos Syndrome
- Osteogenesis Imperfecta.

Marfan's Syndrome

It one among some Hyperlaxity syndromes.
Caused by mutation in the **fibrillin** *gene*.

Characteristic Features

- ***Tall stature***
- ***Arachnodactyly*** (abnormally long and slender digits)
- ***Dolichostenomelia*** (long, narrow limbs)
- Pectus deformities and scoliosis.

There is ***hyperlaxity of skin and subluxation joints.***

- In the cardiovascular system, aortic regurgitation, aortic dilatation, aneurysms, and mitral valve prolapse can occur.
- Ocular findings are myopia and superior displacement of the lens.

Ehlers-Danlos Syndrome

The clinical findings:

- Hyperextensibility of skin
- Hypermobility of joints,
- Easy bruisability of skin and soft tissue,
- Fragility of bone.

Subluxations and ***recurrent dislocations*** of joints are common.

Skin bruises heal with peculiar ***cigarette-paper scars.***

(Children with this condition may be born prematurely because of premature rupture of fetal membranes, because these membranes are derived from the fetus itself!)

Osteogenesis Imperfecta: Also known as Brittle Bone Disease.

Due to ***abnormal or deficient collagen*** - in bone, skin, sclerae, and dentin (all these structures made mainly of type I collagen).

The defect is with ***collagen1A1 and 1A2 genes.***

Ligamentous laxity and joint hypermobility are seen.

The *diagnostic triad*:

- *Blue sclerae,*
- *Dentinogenesis imperfecta,*
- *Generalized osteoporosis.*

The patients presents with ***multiple fractures in various stages of healing***.

Multiple ***wormian bones*** (areas of vicarious calcifications) around the base of the skull are a major finding.

Treatment includes bisphosphonates.Multiple Osteotomies, Telescopic Nail Fixation.

OSTEOCHONDROSES

Osteochondritis designate ***disorders of actively growing epiphyses.***

- Mainly occur in adolescents and young adults during the phases of ***increased physical activity, initiated by trauma or repetitive stress.***
- The mechanisms involved are crushing, splitting and pulling.
- X-ray will show **compression, fragmentation, and separation** of involved bone and cartilage.
- Technetium-99m bone scanning shows increased uptake.

Freiberg's Disease

Osteochondrosis of the Metatarsal Head -the ***second metatarsal head*** is the most commonly involved, although the disease may affect the third or fourth metatarsal head.

Osgood-Schlatter Disease: Osteochondritis of the ***Tibial Tuberosity***. Radiographs of the lateral proximal tibia show the characteristic fragmentation.

Iselin Disease: Traction opsteochondritis of the *Fifth Metatarsal Base.*

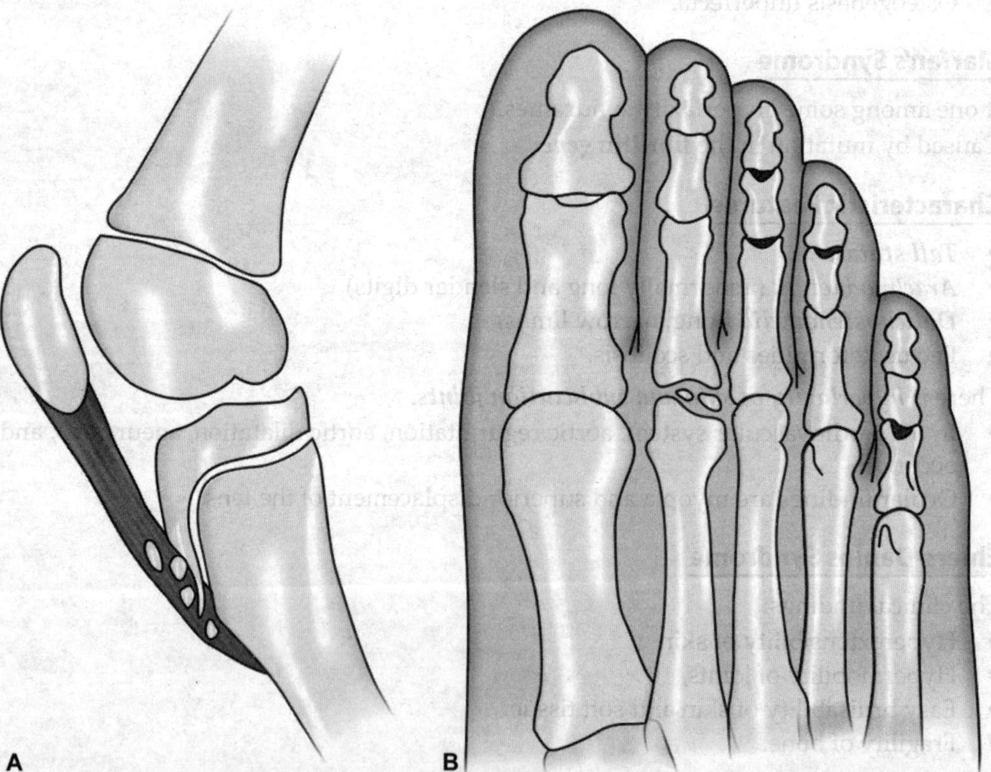

Figs 19.45 (A and B): Osgood-Schlatter disease Freiberg's disease

Köhler Disease: Osteochondrtitis of the Navicular Bone

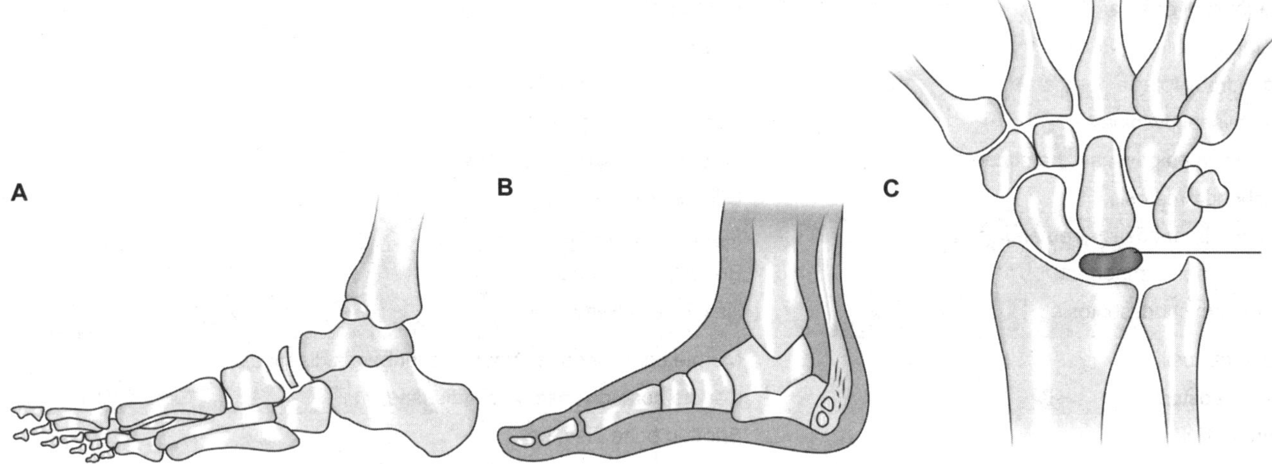

Figs 19.46 (A to C): A. Köhler Disease, **B.** Sever's disease, **C.** Kienböck disease

Sever's disease: A ***calcaneal*** apophysitis *at* ***Achillis tendon insertion****. It* is one of the most common overuse syndromes seen in growing children.

Scheuermann's disease: Vertebral osteochondritis involving the ***peripheral ring*** epiphysis of body.

Panner disease's: Osteochondritis of the ***capitellum*** of distal humerus.

Kienböck disease: Osteonecrosis of the ***lunate bone****.* Seen in ominant wrist of men engaged in manual labor. Predisposed by short ulna (Ulna minus variant)

Perthes disease: *Osteochonritis deformans of femoral head.*

Characterized by varying degrees of ***necrosis of the femoral ossific nucleus.***

Most common in 4 to 8 years, boys > girls, bilateral is 10%.

Signs

- Waldenstrom's sign: Increased medial joint space,
- Caffey's sign: Sub chondral fracture,
- Sagging rope sign: Osteosclerotic line extending from head to trochanter.
- Gage's sign: Metaphyseal radiolucency.

Name	Osteochondritic site
Iselin disease	Fifth metatarsal base
Freiberg's disease	Metatarsal head (2nd MT is most common)
Köhler disease	Navicular
Kienböck disease	Lunate
Osgood-Schlatter disease	Tibial tuberosity
Sinding–Johanssen–Larsen disease	Lower pole of patella
Blount's disease (Tibia Vara)	Medial side of the proximal tibial epiphysis.
Panner's disease	Capitellum
Perthe's disease	Femoral head
Scheuermann's disease:	Ring epiphysis of vertebral body
Calve's disease	Centre bony nucleus of vertebral body
Madelung deformity	Distal radial physis
Sever disease	Calcaneum (at insertion site of tendo achilles)

Disorders	Other names
Chondroectodermal dysplasia:	Ellis-van Creveld Syndrome
Diaphyseal aclasia:	Hereditary multiple exostosis
Metaphyseal dysplasia	Pyle's disease
Chondrodysplasia punctata	Stippled epiphyses, Conradi's disease
Diaphyseal dysplasia,	Camurati or Engelmann's disease
Dysplasia epiphysealis hemimelica	Trevor's disease
Enchondromatosis	Ollier's disease
Enchondromatosis + hemangioma,	Maffucci syndrome
Osteogenesis imperfect	Brittle bone disease
Osteo-onychodysostosis	Nail-Patella Syndrome
Osteopetrosis	Marble bone disease, Albers-Schonberg's disease
Melorheostosis	Candle bone disease, Leri's disease
Osteopoikilosis	Spotted bone disease

BONE TUMORS

Most of the bone tumors and cysts ***arise from metaphysis,*** because of higher growth potential in this region. But some lesions arise from other part of bone. They are:

- **Epiphyseal tumors:**
  - Chondroblastoma (age 10-20)
  - Giant cell tumor (age 20-40)
- **Diaphyseal tumors:**
  - Osteoid osteoma (20-30)
  - Ewing sarcoma (age 5-25)
  - Adamantinoma (20-30)
  - Fibrous dysplasia (age 5-30)

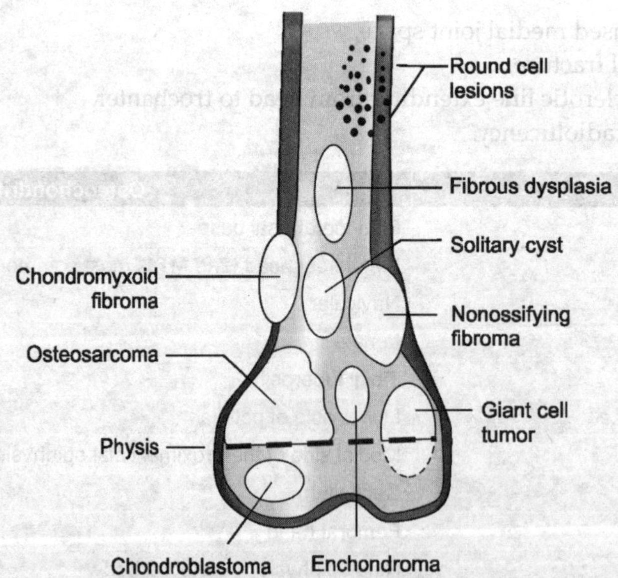

Fig. 19.47: Locations of various tumors

Bone-forming Tumors

Only three lesions produce osteoid.

- Osteoid osteoma
- Osteoblastoma
- Osteosarcoma.

Cartilage forming tumors

- Enchondroma
- Osteochondroma
- Chondroblastoma
- Chondrosarcoma.

OSTEOID OSTEOMA

It is the ***most common true benign tumor***; seen in young males of 20-30 yrs of age.
It arises from **diaphysis** - may involve the medullary cavity, periosteum and cortex.

Most commonly affects ***femur and tibia***.
In the ***spine,*** the typical location for an osteoid osteoma is in the posterior elements, such as the lamina or pedicle.

The classical clinical feature is: ***pain worsens at night and is relieved by aspirin or other NSAIDs.*** The pain, caused by excess prostaglandin E2 produced by the proliferating osteoblasts in the nidus-that is why relieved by aspirin.

The tumor consists of a small radiolucent lesion called ***nidus*** with surrounding bony sclerosis.
The size of the nidus is ***less than 1.5 cm*** in diameter, and not visible with plain radiograph.
CT is the best to identify the nidus and confirm the diagnosis.
The lesions show increased uptake on technetium bone scans.

Treatment is complete removal of nidus.
The latest treatment of choice is ***radiofrequency ablation***.

OSTEOBLASTOMA

It is nothing but a ***giant osteoid osteoma***. Most commonly occurs in the ***spine*** at pedicles, laminae. The pain is dull, achy, and not responsive to salicylate; and it does not induce a marked bony reaction.
X-ray: More lytic and destructive appearance than the osteoid osteoma.
Its nidus is greater than 1–2 cm; it has a less sclerotic reactive bone.
Treatment is same as osteoid osteoma.

OSTEOSARCOMA

It is the ***most common primary malignant tumor of bone*** 2nd only to multiple myeloma.
It is highly malignant.

95% occurs at ***metaphysis*** of long bone.

Histologically **osteoid** is present always and its demonstration is mandatory for diagnosis
Classic Osteosarcoma: *(high grade intramedullary)* typically occurs in *adolescent age group*.

Males > females.
In the **metaphyseal areas** of long bones, with 50% of lesions seen about the knee joint.
The ***distal femur is the most common site,*** followed by the ***proximal tibia*** and then the ***proximal humerus***.

Symptoms

Pain is complained of before a *tumor mass* is noticed. Night pain and rest pain are charaecteristic. Skin- stretched and shiny, dilated veins are seen.

X-ray: Mixed lytic and dense areas.
Breaching of cortex into subperiosteal space which forms the ***Codman's triangle.***

Streaks of new bone radiating-***sunburst appearance***.
In 2–25% of cases, an additional lesion found at a higher level in the femur. It is called as ***skip lesion*** – and should be considered as a true metastatic focus.

Secondary Osteosarcoma: Osteosarcoma can arise from bone diseases such as:
- Paget disease
- Osteochondroma
- Osteoblastoma
- Fibrous dysplasia
- Giant cell tumor
- Bone infarction
- Irradiation
- Chronic osteomyelitis.

Treatment of Osteosarcoma

Combination of neoadjuvant chemotherapy + surgery + adjuvant chemotherapy
- The drugs commonly used: **High-dose methotrexate, doxorubicin, cisplatin, and ifosfamide.** (Given in cyclic intervals of 3–4 weeks for approximately 11–15 weeks prior to surgery).
- Surgery: Amputation or limb-sparing surgery.

➢ Limb-salvage with wide resection of the tumor is the standard approach.

Limb Salvage Techniques

Reconstruction of resected segment of limb by:
- Endoprosthesis
- Structural bony allografts
- Composites of synthetic and allograft materials, etc.

➢ Amputation is reserved for the exceptional or recurrent cases.

CARTILAGINOUS TUMORS

Enchondroma

Benign cartilage forming tumor, most commonly occurs in the small tubular bone of ***hand* and feet**, but can occur anywhere like ***femur or humerus***.
Usually occur at the junction of metaphysis and diaphysis.
Mostly asymptomatic and an incidental radiographic finding or present with ***pathological fracture.***
- **X-ray:** ***stippled or mottled calcification***- pathognomonic feature.
  - **Ollier's disease**: multiple enchondromas.
  - **Maffucci's syndrome**: multiple enchondromas + multiple hemangiomas of skin and soft tissues.

Treatment

Enchondromas generally do not require surgical treatment. If needed, curettage and bone grafting is adequate.
- Ollier's disease and Maffuci's syndrome must be followed carefully because high rate of malignant transformation to ***chondrosarcomas.***

Osteochondroma (Exostosis)

It is the most common benign tumor of bone

- A developmental or hamartomatous process that arises from a defect in the outer edge of the growth plate.

The bony base ***continues with medullary canal*** of the bone from which it arises.

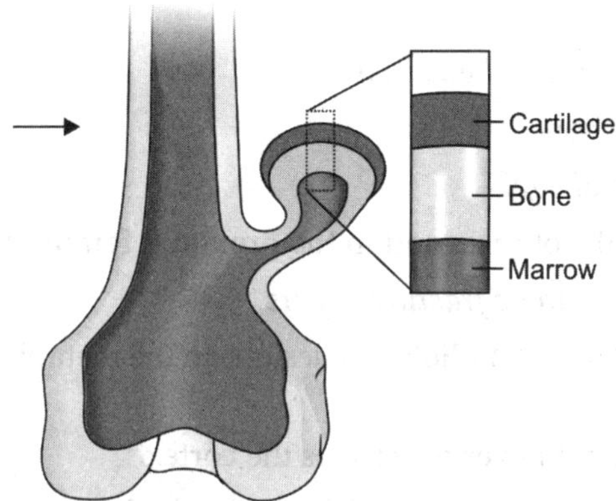

Fig. 19.48: Osteochondroma

The growth of the ***tumors stops at end of growth of the affected individual attaining skeletal maturity.***

- If it enlarges further after the end of the skeletal growth malignant transformation should be strongly suspected and treated accordingly.

Treatment

Pressure symptoms and cosmesis are two indications that warrant excision.

Hereditary Multiple Exostoses

Otherwise known as ***Diaphyseal aclasis.***
It is an autosomal dominant condition.

- Multiple swellings over metaphysis of the long bones, the spine, the ribs, the pelvis, and the scapula.

The patients are ***shorter*** than average and present with deformities such as ***genu valgum, radial bowing.***

- Malignant transformation to chondrosarcoma or osteosarcoma can occur in 2-5% cases.

Chondroblastoma (Codman's tumor)

Occurs in the ***epiphysis*** of long bones in patients of *< 20 yrs of age.*

- The cartilage matrix mineralizes giving a ***"chicken wire" pattern.*** Males > females.
- Locations - **proximal *humeral*** (Most common), distal femoral and proximal tibial epiphysis.
- **Radiograph:** Demonstrates a lytic tumor with central stippled or flocculated calcification.
- **Treatment:** Curettage and bone grafting. Recurrence is common.

Chondrosarcoma

A low-grade, slow growing tumor.
Usually occurs in adults of ***30-60 yrs*** of age. Men > women.
Pelvis and femur are the most common locations, then the ribs, proximal humerus and scapula.

- X-ray: shows ***punctate, popcorn comma shaped calcification.***

Chondrosarcoma may arise secondary to:

- Ollier's disease
- Mafucci's syndrome

- Fibrous dysplasia
- Radiation and
- Diaphyseal aclasis.

CYSTIC LESIONS OF BONE

Simple Bone Cyst

Also called ***solitary bone cyst or unicameral bone cyst.***

It consists of *fluid-filled cavities* within bone.

Most Common in children ***< 15 years*** of age.

Found in the **proximal humerus** in 50% of cases and in the **proximal femur** in 25%.

Patients are asymptomatic until a ***pathologic fracture*** occurs.

Radiographic appearance: ***centrally*** located, radiolucent lesions in the metaphysis, marked thinning of the adjacent cortex.

The cyst may expand ***concentrically***, but never penetrates the cortex.

A thinned cortical fragment may get fractured and fallen into the base of the lesion; this is known as ***"Fallen fragment" sign*** and is pathognomonic of simple bone cyst.

Treatment is curettage and bone grafting. Methyl-prednisolone injection into the cyst gives successful remission in >90% cases.

Aneurysmal Bone Cyst

They are locally destructive, ***blood-filled lesions,*** common before 20 yrs of age.

MC locations: ***Proximal humerus***, distal femur, proximal tibia, and ***spine.***

Radiograph: Shows an ***eccentrically*** located expansile lesion in the metaphysis.

*[To differentiate from simple bone cyst: MRI scan shows a **double-density fluid level** and intralesional septations which indicate an aneurysmal bone cyst.]*

Treatment

Extended curettage and bone grafting.

MISCELLANEOUS TUMORS

GIANT CELL TUMOR (*Osteoclastoma*)

*(Do you remember? Osteoclast is originally **not** a bone cell; instead it is derived from monocyte-macrophage system. Osteoclasts are macrophage giant cell. Hence this tumor bears the name).*

It is a benign but ***aggressive*** lesion consisting of osteoclast-like giant cells.
Patients with GCTs are 30-45 years of age. ***Female*** are more commonly affected.

Most commonly found around the knee-proximal tibia, distal femur and distal radius.
This tumor occurs in the ***epiphysis*** of mature bone (> 20 years).

(Compare with Chondroblastoma: it occurs in the epiphysis of immature bone, <20 yrs of age)
Clinically presents with complains of ***pain*** and slight swelling at the end of a long bone;
Radiographic findings: ***Eccentrically located in the epiphyses*** of long bones, frequently expands and ***breaks through the cortex*** *(Compare with simple and aneurysmal bone cyst)*

Treatment: As simple curettage is associated high rate of recurrence, ***extended curettage*** is preferred.

*(**Extended curettage** means curettage and adding adjuvants, such as liquid nitrogen, phenol, bone cement, electrocautery, or an argon beam coagulator- they kill any remaining tumor cells.)*

For aggressive GCT of the ***distal radius***, primary ***resection and reconstruction*** with a proximal fibular autograft is safe method.

*(**Tips:** all tumors are more common in male except GCT and parosteal osteosarcoma which are preferring females)*

Ewing's Sarcoma

They are thought to arise from the neural crest and are closely related to primitive neuroectodermal tumor (PNET).

The characteristic chromosomal ***translocation [t(11:22) (q24:q12)]*** is present in greater than 90% of cases.

Histologic appearance shows ***small round cell***.

Occurs in 10-20 yrs of age.

Present with pain, swelling and ***fever***.

Laboratory investigations will show: elevated ESR, leukocytosis, anemia.

This tumor ***begins in metaphyses of long bones, extends and presents as a diaphyseal tumor***.

Tibia, femur, humerus, are the common bones affected.

The characteristic periosteal reaction in multiple layers give rise to multilaminated appearance known as ***onion-skin appearance*** .

Treatment: It is ***radiosensitive*** tumor.

The treatment involves a multimodal approach with combination of:

- Multi-drug chemotherapy
- Irradiation and
- Surgical resection.

Hemangioma

Hemangioma of bone is a hamartomatous process, most commonly found in ***vertebral bodies***.

Being asymptomatic, they are usually discovered as incidental finding.

The radiographic appearance in the spine is characteristic: Thickened, vertically oriented trabeculae giving the classic ***"jailhouse" appearance*** or ***"corduroy" appearance***.

In cross sectional CT picture, these thickened trabeculae have a ***"polka dot"*** pattern.

Multiple Myeloma

It is the ***most common primary bone tumor***. Commonly occurs after ***50 yrs*** of age.

It is characterized by a triad of:

- Osteolytic punched-out lesions
- Neoplastic proliferation of plasma cells
- Monoclonal gammopathy.

Spine is the most common location followed by the ribs and pelvis.

Bone pain is the most common complaint.

Lab findings:

Severe anemia, elevated ESR, abnormal ***serum protein electrophoresis*** and immunoelectrophoresis, Bence Jones proteinuria are seen.

The radiographic features multiple ***"punched out"*** *areas* of bone destruction in the skull and pelvis.

Despite being a malignant tumor, the lack of reactive bone formation leads to ***negative (reduced uptake) on bone scan.***

Adamantinoma

They are found in the tibia in 90% of cases; and are usually ***diaphyseal*** in location in ***tibia*** (around 90%).
The cause of adamantinoma remains unknown, newer investigations say it is a tumor of **epithelial *origin*.**
*(The name **adamantinoma** was given to the tibial lesion because its histologic appearance is similar to that of the adamantinoma of jaw bone **(ameloblastoma),** but the two entities have no other relationship clinically.)*
Treatment: Wide resection or amputation.
It is radioresistant and chemoresistant.

Chordoma

It arises from *notochord remnants.*

Most commonly seen in the **sacro-coccygeal region** or at the base of the skull.

Age: 30- 80 yrs.

Microscopy: Large vacuolated cells appear like a signet ring- referred to as ***physaliferous cells.***

Treatment for the sacral lesions is an aggressive wide resection with pre and post op radiotherapy.

Eosinophilic Granuloma

MC in < 10 years old. Has a predilection for the ***thoracic region.***

Classic X-ray picture is **vertebra plana.** (complete collapse of the vertebral body on the lateral view).

Present with pain and swelling. Histologically, the proliferating histioyte with an *indented or grooved nucleus* is the characteristic cell. A self-limited process, it may regress spontaneously.

Treatment options: Observation, low-dose irradiation, curettage and bone grafting.

Fibrous Dysplasia

It is not a true neoplasia but a developmental abnormality, common in children.

Presents with pain, pathologic fracture, or skeletal deformity.

The histologic hallmark is ***replacement of normal bone and marrow by fibrous tissue.***

Any bone may be involved, with ***the proximal femur*** being the most common. May be monostotic (85%) or polyostotic.
X-ray shows areas of decreased bone density having a ground glass appearance.

When proximal femur involved- the resulting weakening of the bone may lead to progressive microfractures and is referred to as **"Shepherd's crook deformity"**.

McCune-Albright syndrome: refers to combination of:

- Polyostotic fibrous dysplasia
- Cutaneous pigmentation
- Endocrine abnormalities
- Precocious puberty.

BONE TUMOR STAGING SYSTEMS

Enneking's Staging of Benign Bone Tumors

Stage	Description	Example
1. Latent	Well-defined margin. Grows slowly and then stops Remains static/heals spontaneously	Osteoid osteoma

Contd...

Contd...

Stage	Description	Example
2. Active	Progressive growth limited by natural barriers Not self-limiting. Tendency to recur	Aneurysmal bone cyst
3. Aggressive	Growth not limited by natural barriers	Giant cell tumor

Enneking's Staging of Malignant Bone Tumors

Stage	Grade	Site	Metastases
IA	Low	Intracompartmental	None
IB	Low	Extracompartmental	None
IIA	High	Intracompartmental	None
IIB	High	Extracompartmental	None
III	Any	Any	Regional or distant metastases

Skeletal Metastases of Unknown Origin

There are 5 primary malignancies which most commonly metastasize to bone.
They are:

- Breast, lung, prostate, kidney, thyroid.

Prostate and breast are the two most common primary sources for bone metastases.

Metastatic deposits most commonly occurs at: Pelvis, vertebral bodies, ribs, femur, proximal humerus, and skull.

- Rare in small bone, distal to elbow and knee.

Pathogenesis explained for frequent occurrence of **spine** is presence of valveless, bidirectional ***Batson's vertebral vein plexus.***

Radiographic Patterns

- Osteoblastic (Osteosclerotic) deposits: Prostate and Breast
- Osteolytic deposits: Renal cell ca, lung Ca, thyroid ca.
  - **Blastic metastases** are frequently ***painless*** and associated with a lower incidence of pathologic fracture because the bone is not as severely weakened.
  - The **lytic** variants are painful and can cause ***pathologic fractures.***

Treatment is palliative and aimed to control pain.

Pathological fractures require internal fixation and prophylactic internal fixation is required for impending pathological fracture.

INVESTIGATIONS IN BONE TUMORS

X-Ray Features of Bone Tumors

Multiple Myeloma: multiple "punched out" areas.

Eosinophilic granuloma: vertebra plana

Giant cell tumor : *Soap bubble appearance*

Ewing's sarcoma : *Onion peel appearance*

Fibrous dysplasia : *Ground glass appearance.*

A: Solid, e.g. Osteoid osteoma

B: Onion peel appearance, e.g. Ewing's sarcoma

C: Sun-ray appearance, e.g. Osteosarcoma

D: Codman's triangle, e.g. osteosarcoma and other malignancies.

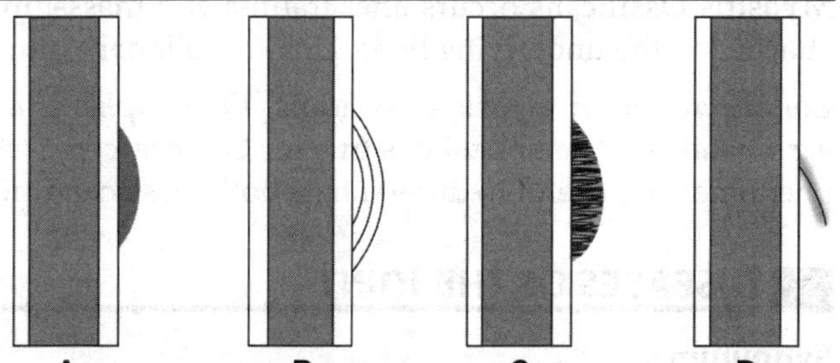

Figs 19.49 (A to D): Patterns of periosteal reaction in bone tumors

CT: It is most helpful in assessing ossification and calcification.

The best imaging study to localize the nidus of an osteoid osteoma.

- CT of the lung: most effective to detect pulmonary metastases.

Technetium Bone Scans

Bone scintigraphy with with 99 mTc-methyl diphosphonate **(99mTc-MDP)** is useful:

- To determine the activity of a lesion
- To detect the presence of multiple lesions
- To detect the presence skeletal metastases.

Most malignant neoplasms of bone show increased uptake. (Except: multiple myeloma does not show increased uptake).

MRI: has replaced CT as the study of choice to determine the size, extent, and anatomical relationships of bone and soft-tissue tumors.

- The most accurate technique for determining the limits of disease within and outside bone.
- MRI is mandatory ***for staging*** the tumors and for surgical planning.

Biopsy: It may be:

- Needle biopsy (fine needle or core needle)
- Open biopsy
- Excisional biopsy.

The biopsy should be the ***final staging procedure***, i.e biopsy should be done ***only after*** clinical, laboratory, and radiographic examinations are complete.

The biopsy ***track gets contaminated*** with tumor cells during the procedure. The biopsy site and incision site is a crucial decision so that ***the biopsy track can to be excised along with the tumor*** during the definitive surgery.

The tissue block is ***removed from the boundary zone***, so that it can include normal and abnormal tissues for comparison and for determining the limits of soft tissue infiltration.

So, the surgeon who performs the biopsy should be the same surgeon who will perform the definitive operative procedure.

[*Non-invasive methods like, Bone scans, CT or MRI should be done before undertaking a biopsy, because the biopsy procedure may distort the imaging appearances.*]

SOME USEFUL POINTS

- **Giant cell tumors and chondroblastoma** are *benign but occasionally aggressive*; they may produce pulmonary metastases.
- **Osteomyelitis:** Can mimic tumors such as Ewing sarcoma, osteosarcoma.

Myositis Ossificans occurs after trauma and massaging. Locations are over the diaphysis oflong bones. It is not attached to the underlying bone. Unlike malignant tumors, this becomes less painful over time.

Zonal pattern: in myositis ossificans, ***the peripheral areas matured by mineralization and central lucent areas are immature***. The opposite is true for Osteosarcoma- the central area shows matured tissues. This is called 'zone phenomenon', useful to differentiate both these conditions.

DISEASES OF THE JOINT

Synovium

It provides nutrients to cartilage and produces lubricants for the joint. The intimal lining of the synovium has two different cells.

- *Type A macrophage-like*
- *Type 2 fibroblast-like synoviocytes.*

Type A synoviocytes: They are bone marrow derived; represent cells of the mononuclear phagocyte system.

Type B synoviocytes: Represent a resident fibroblast population in the synovial lining. They ***produce the essential joint lubricants*** hyaluronic acid (HA) and lubricin. They also synthesize normal matrix components, including fibronectin, laminin, collagens, proteoglycans, etc.

Synovial Fluid Analysis

Group	Appearance	Cell Count/μL	Neutrophils%	Typical Diagnosis
Normal	Clear, colorless to straw colored.	< 100	< 25	None
I (Noninflammatory)	Clear, straw colored, good string	200-2,000	< 25	Degenerative arthritis, internal derangement, trauma, aseptic necrosis
IIA (Mild inflammatory)	Faintly cloudy, moderate string	1,000-10,000	25-50	Systemic lupus erythematosus, rheumatoid arthritis, spondyloarthropathies.
IIB (Severe inflammatory)	Translucent but cloudy, yellow, drops like water	2,000-75,000	50-75	Moderate to severe rheumatoid arthritis, gout, pseudogout, tuberculosis.
III (Septic arthritis)	Creamy, opaque,	>50,000	> 80	Acute gout, bacterial infection

Synovial Fluid Aspirates

- ***A frankly bloody fluid***: tumor, trauma, or hemophilia.
- ***A dark brown fluid*** full of hemosiderin is seen in hemophilia and pigmented villonodular synovitis.
- ***Fat floating*** on a bloody fluid indicates fracture or tumor exposing the marrow cavity to the synovial space.
- Small white clots ***(rice bodies)*** represent tuberculous arthritis.

OSTEOARTHRITIS

A degenerative joint disease of articular hyaline cartilage of synovial joints.

Most common symptom is joint pain exacerbated by activity and relieved with rest; constitutional symptoms are absent.

Pathological changes in the articular cartilage include:

- ***Increased water content,***
- ***Decreased proteoglycan content,***
- ***Altered collagen matrix.***

All leading to the deterioration of articular cartilage integrity and degeneration.

*[**Aging cartilages** show decreased water content, decreased production and increased degradation of proteoglycons. But relative increase in keratan sulphate is observed.]*

Radiographic hallmarks of osteoarthritis:

- Joint space narrowing,
- Osteophytes,
- Subchondral cysts,
- Bony sclerosis (eburnation).

OA is common in the following joints:
first CMC of thumb, DIP, PIP, knee, hip joint and spine.

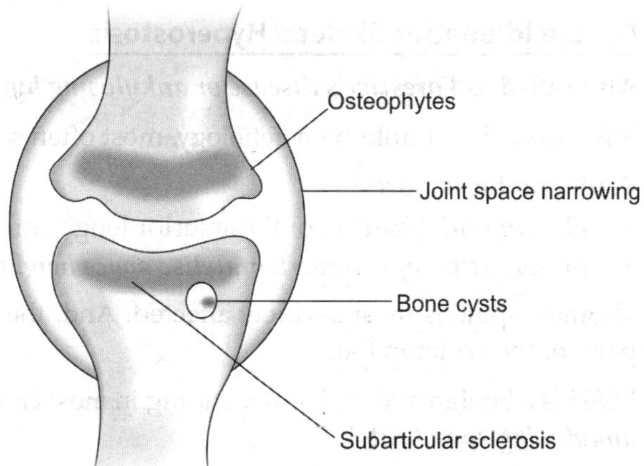

Fig. 19.50: X-ray features of OA of knee joint

Osteophytes that form at DIP joints are known as ***Heberden nodes***.

At PIP joint, such osteophytes are known as ***Bouchard nodes***

Treatment Principles in OA

- **Conservative treatment for early stages:**
  - Physical therapy
  - Avoidance of excessive loading of the joint
  - ***Weight reduction***
  - Analgesics
  - Intra-articular steroid injection
  - Visco-supplementation (injecting hyaluranan into the joint).
- **Surgical treatment for late stages:** The surgical modalities used for patients with OA of knee joint are:
  - High tibial osteotomy (HTO)
  - Arthroscopic debridement
  - Total knee arthroplasty (TKR)
  - Osteochondral or chondrocyte transplantation
  - Arthrodesis.

High tibial osteotomy: Osteotomy performed at the proximal metaphyseal region of tibia.

- Useful for osteoarthritis of the knee when the changes are confined to one compartment of the knee only (***i.e unicompartmental OA***).

The idea is to ***'unload' of the involved joint*** compartment by correcting the malalignment of the knee joint.

The indications for HTO: Young active laborer, with evidence arthritis confined to one compartment with a corresponding varus or valgus deformity.

[Severe deformities are contraindicated for HTO.

- Tibial subluxation of more than 1 cm
- Tibial bone loss of more than 2 or 3 mm
- Flexion contracture of more than 15 deg
- Knee flexion of less than 90 deg
- Rheumatoid arthritis.]

Total Knee Replacement

Indicated in ***severe OA of the knee*** joint in older age group, less physical demand individuals.

Diffuse Idiopathic Skeletal Hyperostosis

Also called as ***Forestier's disease or ankylosing hyperostosis (DISH).***

It is a disorder of unknown aetiology, most often seen in middle/elderly males and principally affecting the ***spine***,

Radiographic features:

- ***Flowing calcification*** of the anterior longitudinal ligament (ALL)
- ***Preservation of intervertebral disc space height***.

Thoracic spine is most severely affected. And, there will be progressive ossification along the ligaments of other parts of the skeleton too.

DISH is a benign and incidental finding in most cases; but should be differentiated from ***osteoarthritis of spine and ankylosing spondylitis***.

Main features	DISH	Ankylosing spondylitis
Age at onset	>50	< 40
Pain	±	++
Sacroiliac joint erosion	-	++
ALL ossification	++	-
Syndesmophytes	-	++

RHEUMATOID ARTHRITIS

An autoimmune inflammatory systemic disease of unknown etiology.

Symptoms: Joint stiffness (worse in morning), pain, swelling.

Laboratory: Anemia, ***elevated ESR*** or CRP, positive rheumatoid factor.

Rheumatoid nodules are seen in approximately 25% of patients with RA, almost exclusively in those patients who are seropositive for rheumatoid factor.

Rheumatoid nodules are ***specific feature*** for RA.

Distribution: Symmetric small joints- MCP, PIP joints. ***(spares DIP).***

- The disease starts in the MCP, PIP, and MTP joints followed by the wrists, knees, elbows, ankles, hips, and shoulders in roughly that order.
- RA almost ***always spares the distal interphalangeal (DIP) joints***
  (In contrast, these joints are often involved in osteoarthritis and psoriatic arthritis).
- **Wrists** are involved in most patients with RA. Early in the course of the disease, synovial proliferation in and around the wrists can compress the median nerve, causing ***carpal tunnel syndrome.***
- Joint symptoms must persist for ***at least 6 weeks.***

ACR diagnostic criteria for RA

- Morning stiffness
- Arthritis in at least three joints
- Arthritis in hands
- Symmetric arthritis
- Rheumatoid nodules
- Serum rheumatoid factor
- Radiographic changes.

Rheumatoid Factor

An autoantibody directed against Fc region of IgG.

- Rheumatoid factor is positive in about 50% of cases at presentation and an additional 20–35% of cases become positive in the first 6 months after diagnosis.

It is not unique to RA and occurs in many other diseases.

Anticyclic Citrullinated Peptide (Anti-CCP) Antibodies

- Anti-CCP antibodies are present in 60–70% of patients with RA at diagnosis
- They are 90–98% specific for RA
- They are present in the serum years before RA is diagnozed
- It correlate strongly with ***erosive disease.***

Rheumatoid Deformities

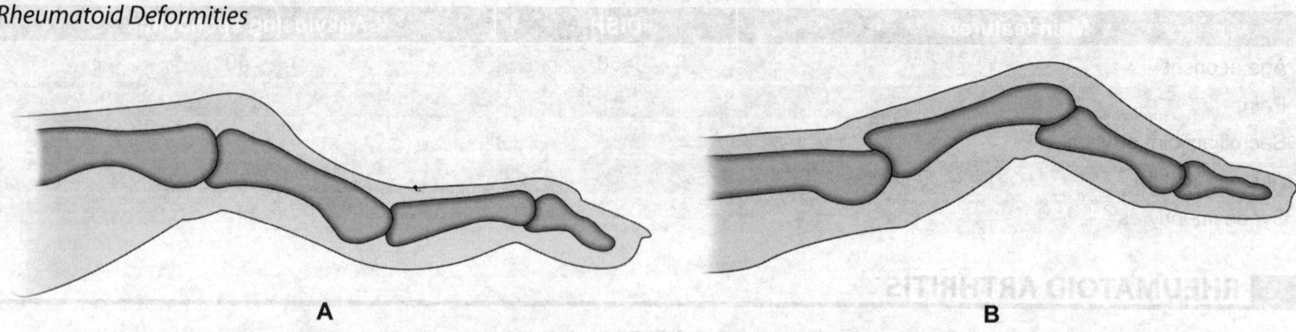

Figs 19.51 (A and B): A. Swan neck deformity; B. Buttonhole deformity

- ***Swan-neck deformity***: flexion posture of the DIP and hyperextension posture of the PIP joints.
- ***Buttonhole or Boutonnière Deformity***: PIP in flexion, DIP in hyperextension.
- **Wind sweep deformity:** hallux valgus on one side and hallux varus on other side- produce deformity which are parallel to each other.
- (A similar Wind sweep deformity is seen in knee joint in cases of rickets: genu varum on one side and genu valgum on the opposite side)
- ***Intrinsic plus deformity:*** caused by tightness and contracture of the intrinsic muscles, seen in RA, Cerebral palsy etc. Here the IP joints are in extension and MCP joints are in flexion. ***(Intrinsic minus deformity:*** IP joints in flexion; MCP joints in hyperextension – known as ***Claw hand.)***
- **Z deformity:** Radial deviation of wrist joint with ulnar deviation of MCP joints.

X-ray Features OA and RA

	Osteoarthritis	Rheumatoid arthritis
1	Joint space narrowing	Joint space narrowing
2	Marginal **sclerosis**	Periarticular **osteoporosis**
3	Subchondral cyst	Erosions
4	Osteophyte formation	Ankylosis

Four broad categories of medical therapies are used for the treatment of RA:

- NSAIDs
- Glucocorticoids
- DMARDs
- Biological therapy.

Conventional DMARDs: Methotrexate, sulfasalazine, gold, antimalarials, leflunomide, azathioprine, penicillamine, and minocycline.

Biologic therapy: Pro-inflammatory cytokines- ***tumor necrosis factor (TNF-α) and interleukin-1***, play a central role in the pathophysiology of RA.

Based on this hypothesis, the following biological agents have been developed and used successfully in RA.

- TNF-α inhibitors: etanercept, infliximab, and adalimumab
- Interleukin-1 inhibitor: Anakinra.
- T-cell co-stimulation Blocker: Abatacept
- B-cells Targeting agent: Rituximab.

SPONDYLOARTHROPATHIES

A group of inflammatory diseases that includes:

- ***Ankylosing spondylitis***
- ***Reactive arthritis***

- ***Psoriatic arthritis***
- ***Arthritis associated with inflammatory bowel disease.***

The common clinical features include:

- Arthritis of the ***axial skeleton*** (sacroiliac joints and spine),
- ***Enthesitis*** *(inflammation at sites where tendons, ligaments, and joint capsule insert onto bone).*
- These are ***not*** associated with rheumatoid factor; referred to as the seronegative spondyloarthropathies.

Ankylozing Spondylitis

More common in ***males***

Classical features:

- Onset ***under age 40***
- Gradual onset
- Symptoms persistent over 3 months
- Morning stiffness
- Symptoms ***better with exercise.***
- HLA-B27 is strongly associated with ankylosing spondylitis

Insidious onset of low back pain due to ***sacroilitis***, the pain worsens with rest, improves with activity.

- ➢ Over time the spine loses mobility (ankylosed- i.e fused).

The **Schober test** is the standard test to assess lumbar spine movement.

Involvement of the costovertebral and costochondral joints commonly leads to impaired chest expansion.

Radiographic Changes

- ***Squaring off*** vertebral bodies
- ***Syndesmophytes***: the most characteristic finding. It is formed by gradual ossification of the edges of the annulus fibrosus of intervertebral disc.
- ***Bamboo spine*** appearance: Due to bridging at multiple levels.

Hip involvement requires total hip replacement (THR) approximately 5% of patients with ankylosing spondylitis.

Spinal Fractures: Most important complication. The fused, osteopototic spine of ankylosing spondylitis is at great risk for fracture.

REITER'S SYNDROME

Also known as **Reactive Arthritis**.

It is an ***aseptic inflammatory arthritis*** associated with non-specific urogenital or bowel infection.

The inflammation is triggered by bacterial infections of the gastrointestinal or genitourinary tracts.

But the cultures of synovial fluid are ***sterile.***

The ***Reiter's triad*** includes

- Arthritis,
- Conjunctivitis and
- *Urithritis.*

Reactive arthritis typically develops after a bout of gastroenteritis caused by:

- *Shigella,*
- *Salmonella,*
- *Campylobacter,*
- *Yersinia,*

or after a genitourinary tract infection with

- Chlamydia trachomatis.

*[These agents **have not been cultured** from synovial tissues despite the presence of significant joint swelling and synovitis, hence the term **reactive arthritis**.]*

PSORIATIC ARTHRITIS

About 5% of psoriatic patients develop arthritis.
DIP joints are characteristically involved.
Cartilage and bone destruction may be severe enough giving rise to ***"arthritis mutilans"***.
Dactylitis: ***sausage digits*** complete swelling of a single digit in the hand or foot.

X-ray features: ***Pencil-in-cup*** **appearance**.

Clinical and Epidemiologic Features of Spondyloarthropathies

Features	Ankylosing Spondylitis	Psoriatic Arthritis	Reactive Arthritis	Enteropathic Arthritis
Male : female ratio	3:1	1:1	9:1	1:1
Axial arthritis	100%	20%	20%	15%
Sacroiliitis	Bilateral	Unilateral	Unilateral	Bilateral
Syndesmophytes	Symmetric	Asymmetric	Asymmetric	Symmetric
Peripheral arthritis	25%	60–95%	90%	20%
Typical affected joints	Hip, knee, ankle	Knee, ankle, DIPs	Knee, ankle	Knee, ankle
Dactylitis	Uncommon	25%	30–50%	Uncommon
Cutaneous findings	None specific	Psoriasis, Onycholysis	Oral ulcerations keratoderma blennorrhagica	Erythema nodosum Pyoderma gangrenosa
HLA-B27 positivity	90%	40%	50–80%	30%

NEUROPATHIC ARTHROPATHY

Also known as **Charcot's Joint**
Charcot joint is a progressive destructive arthropathy associated with numerous diseases that ***produce loss of pain sensation and proprioception.***
So among the arthritic conditions, this is least painful or overtly ***painless.***

Conditions Producing Charcot's Joint

- Diabetes
- Leprosy
- Spinal cord compression
- Syringomyelia
- Syphilis- **tabes dorsalis**
- Congenital insensitivity to pain
- Myelomeningocele
- Alcohol abuse, etc.

Pathology: Osteophyte formation, articular and subchondral fractures and calcification in the surrounding soft tissues.
Marked destruction of joint surfaces, collapse of joint spaces, often with dislocations of one or more joints
(4 Ds: Destruction, Dislocation, Deformity, Debris).
Treatment: Usually not successful. Splintage for early cases and ***Arthrodesis*** for severely unstable joints.

➢ *Presently the most common cause of neuropathic joint is **Diabetes mellitus;** and the most common joint involved is the **joints of foot.***

CRYSTAL ARTHROPATHY

Gout

Caused by deposition of ***uric acid crystals*** and usually associated with hyperuricemia.
Usually begins as acute monarthritis, especially of ***the first metatarsophalangeal joint (MTP joint of great toe).***

Over time, the attacks become more frequent, less intense, and involve more joints.
Diagnosed by ***demonstrating uric acid crystals in joint fluid.***
Extra-articular manifestations include tophi and renal stones.
Arthritis responds to nonsteroidal anti-inflammatory drugs or colchicine.

Hyperuricemia: is defined as a serum urate concentration ***more than 7.0 mg/dL.***

At least 5% of asymptomatic ***normal adult*** males manifest hyperuricemia on at least one occasion.
So hyperuricemia alone is not sufficient for the diagnosis of gout.
During acute attack of gouty arthritis, the serum uric acid level may be low, normal or high.
Hence, **demonstrating *MSU crystals in synovial fluid* is diagnostic.**

Mono Sodium Urate crystals under polarized light microscopy will reveal ***negatively birefringent, needle-shaped crystals*** found within PMNs.
Conditions mimic gout: 1.Septic arthritis 2. Pseudogout.

When serum urate levels exceed the solubility limit, it crystallizes in soft tissues and joints and causes an inflammatory reaction, gouty arthritis.

Apley textbook says:
*"With the passage of time, urate deposits may build up in joints, peri-articular tissues, tendons and bursae; common sites are around the metatarsophalangeal joints of the big toes, the Achilles tendons, the olecranon bursae and the pinnae of the ears. These clumps of chalky material are known as **tophi**".*

Management of Acute Gout

- NSAIDs like Indomethacin are DOC due to better tolerability. Aspirin is not used as it may cause hyperuricemia.
- Colchicines is more effective and faster acting
- Intra-articular corticosteroids can be used in the refractory cases.

Management of Chronic Gout

- Allopurinol: Used during inter-attack periods. Contraindicated in acute gout due to interference with release of cytokines.
- Febuxostat – A xanthine oxidase inhibitor
- Drugs increasing Excretion: Probenecid, Sulfinpyrazole and benzbromarone.
- Recombinant urate exidase is now available as Rasbricase and Pegloticase.

PSEUDOGOUT *(CPPD crystal deposition disease): Cause- unknown.*

Associated metabolic conditions

- Hyperparathyroidism
- Hemochromatosis
- Hypothyroidism, etc.

CPPD crystals are **generally *rhomboid-shaped and positively birefringent*** under polarized microscope.
Radiographic findings: calcification of hyaline articular cartilage-i.e ***chondrocalcinosis***- seen in

- Knee joint (menisci calcification)
- Wrist (triangular cartilage of the radiocarpal joint)

Diagnosis

Made by identification of CPPD crystals in tissue or synovial fluid

Gout	Pseudogout
Smaller joints	Large joints
Pain intense	Pain moderate
Joint inflamed	Joint swollen
Hyperuricaemia	Chondrocalcinosis
Uric acid crystals	Ca pyrophosphate crystals

Milwaukee Shoulder

A chronic destructive arthritis of shoulder joint; seen in ***calcium hydroxyapatite deposition disorders.***)

HEMOPHILIC ARTHROPATHY

Primarily involves the ***knee joint,*** with the elbow and ankle joints affected less frequently.
Recurrent hemarthrosis produces deposits of hemosiderin and synovitis.

In the acute phase, hypertrophy of synovium occurs, causing a higher risk of repeated bleeding.

A pannus may form, as in RA, with underlying cartilage destruction. With time, synovial fibrosis occurs, resulting in joint stiffness.

Skeletal changes are:

- Subchondral sclerosis and cyst formation
- Osteophyte formation
- *Squaring of the patella*
- Widening of intercondylar notch of femur.

Characteristic Joint Involvement in Various Arthritic Conditions

Condition	Joints commonly/characteristically involved
Osteoarthritis	Carpometacarpal joint of thumb, DIP, PIP, Knee
Rheumatoid arthritis	MCP, PIP, wrist, knee, ankles
Ankylosing spondylitis	Sacroiliac joint, whole spine (lumbar MC), hip
Reactive Arthritis	Knee
Psoriatic arthritis	DIP joint
Gout	MTP of great toe
Pseudogout	Knee
Hemophilia	Knee

Radiographic Findings of Various Arthritis

Disease State	Findings
Osteoarthritis	Asymmetric Joint space narrowing, subchondral sclerosis, osteophytes, subchondral cysts
Rheumatoid arthritis	Uniform (symmetric) Joint narrowing, erosion near joint capsule
Ankylosing spondylitis	Osteoporosis, syndesmophytes, squaring of vertebra, bamboo spine, sclerosis of sacroiliac joints
Gout	Tophi, erosions.
Pseudogout	Calcification of menisci and hyaline cartilage (Chondrocalcinosis)
Neuropathic joint	Four Ds: destruction, debris, dislocation, densification (sclerosis, hypertrophy)
Hemophilic arthropathy	Joint space narrowing, Squaring of the patella and widening of intercondylar notch

ARTHROPLASTY

Total Joint Arthroplasty is replacing both sides of the joint using artificial prosthesis.

For example, removing and replacing the following:

- Acetabulum and femoral head in hip joint;
- Distal femoral condyles and proximal tibial condyles in knee joint.

Total replacement of the articular surfaces is ***the ideal way*** of treating the disorders that cause joint destruction.

Indications for total joint replacement: any non-septic, painful, disabling arthritic joint.

- Rheumatoid arthritis
- Juvenile rheumatoid arthritis
- Ankylosing spondylitis
- Osteoarthritis
- Fractures (NOF fracture etc.)
- Osteonecrosis of femoral head
- Gouty arthritis.

Contraindications for Total Joint Replacement

- Recent or current foci of sepsis near or remote to the joint
- Charcot's (neuropathic) joint.

The knee, hip, shoulder and elbow are the common joints totally replaced, in that order.

Other joints such as the ankle, wrist replacement surgeries are less successful.

The Implants

The implant materials used in joint replacement surgery can be classified as:

- Metals
- Polyethelene
- Ceramic.
- **Metals:** The most commonly used metal alloys are:
  - Cobalt-based alloys
  - Titanium-based alloys.
- **Polyethelene:**
  - Ultra high-molecular-weight polyethylene (UHMWPE)
  - Highly cross-linked polyethylene (XLPE)
- **Ceramics:**
  - Aluminum Oxide (Alumina)
  - Zirconium oxide (Zirconia)

The above implants can be fixed to the bone with bone cement ***(cemented)*** or without bone cement ***(un-cemented).***

Bone cement: is made of ***Polymethyl methacrylate*** (PMMA) and is used as a grouting agent. It provides immediate fixation of implant components to the bone.

The bond between bone and the implant is improved by in-growth of bone on the implant or cement. This is known as ***osseo-integration.***

This is important to achieve strong and stable fixation to as to prolong the longevity of the artificial joint.

Methods of Enhancing Osseointegration

- For cemented surgery: Apply the cement under high pressure.
- For uncemented surgery: Implants may be covered with a ***metal mesh or porous coating or hydroxyapatite coating***.

HIP

Sir John Charnley first performed total hip arthroplasty in 1960. He is regarded father of total joint arthroplasty.
Hemiarthroplasty is the replacement of only the femoral side of the hip joint.
It is indicated if displaced fractures of the femoral neck in older individuals.
[*Hemiarthroplasty in a young individual will result in gradual wear and tear and ultimately destruction of the articular cartilage of the acetabulum. Hence hemiarthroplasty is avoided.*]

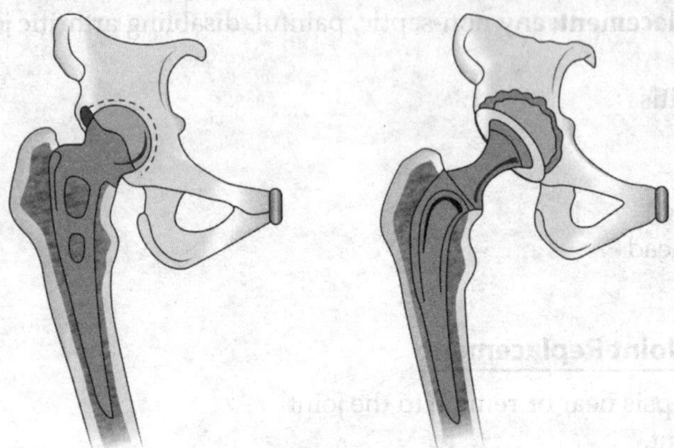

Figs 19.52 (A and B): A. Hemiarthroplasty; B. Total hip arthroplasty

Total Hip Replacement (THR)

The usual combination is a metal femoral made of either titanium or cobalt– chrome alloy; the acetabular socket made of polyethylene. ***(i.e metal -on- poly).***

The UHMWPE produces more debris (wear particles) which induce ***osteolysis*** around the implant and ***loosening.*** This has led to the development of alternative bearing surfaces such as XLPE, ceramic-on-ceramic or metal-on metal combinations.

Ceramic-on-ceramic: They are wettable, have very low wear rates, But , ceramics are brittle and are ***prone to fractures. Metal-on-metal:*** Metal bearing surfaces have very low wear rates and are self polishing.

This combination is durable; it allows patients to return to vigorous recreational activities, and are known as ***'high performance bearings'.***

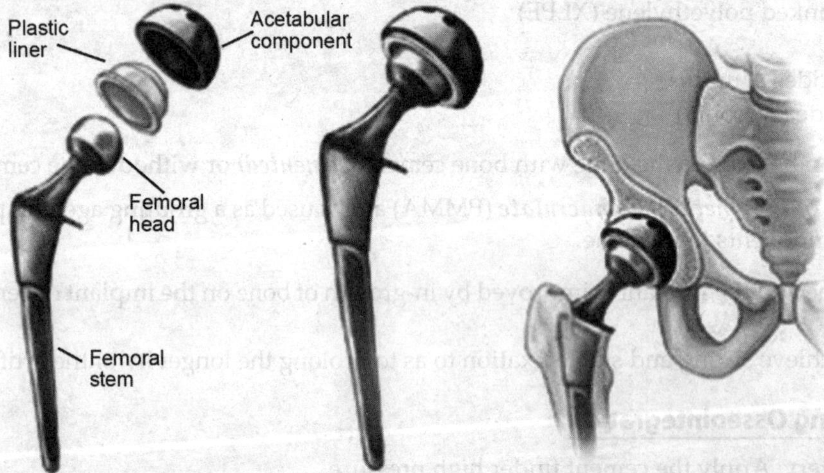

Fig. 19.53: A cemented THR with components marking

Hybrid hip: usually both the hip components are either cemented or uncemented.

A combination of a cemented femoral stem and an uncemented acetabular cup is known as ***hybrid prosthesis.***

Complications of THR

- ***Thromboembolic disease:*** DVT and PE are the one of the most common serious complications arising from total hip arthroplasty. Most common cause of immediate ***post-operative mortality*** along with myocardial infarction and cardio-respiratory arrest.
- ***Sciatic nerve palsy*** more common with a posterior approach .
- ***Periprosthetic Fractures*** of the femur or acetabulum can occur during and after total hip arthroplasty. Femoral fractures are the most common and usually require some form of treatment.
- ***Postoperative dislocation*** is rare if the prosthetic components are correctly placed.
- ***Heterotopic ossification***: The cause is unknown, but patients with skeletal hyperostosis and ankylosing spondylitis are at risk. This can be ***prevented by:***
  - Taking indomethacin 75 mg daily 6 weeks postoperatively or
  - A single dose of irradiation to the hip.
- ***Implant Loosening***: Femoral or acetabular loosening is the most serious long-term complications of total hip arthroplasty: it is the ***commonest cause of long-term failure,*** hence the most common indications for revision surgery.
- ***Osteolysis:*** particles of metal, cement, and polyethylene all can produce osteolysis of the bonearound the implants. But because they are most numerous, ***polyethylene particles seem to be the major culprit.***
- ***Infection*** is the most serious postoperative complication.

KNEE

Most common indications for TKR are ***osteoarthritis and rheumatoid arthritis.***

Unicompartmental Arthroplasty

Done for pure medial compartment osteoarthritis.

Total condylar arthroplasty is the true total knee replacement (TKR) surgery performed in tri-compartmental joint disease (medial tibio-femoral, lateral tibio-femoral and patello-femoral).

The implants are:

- Metal on the femoral side
- Polyethylene insert on a metal tray on the tibial side and
- Polyethylene alone on patella.

They are fixed to the bone with or without the bone cement.

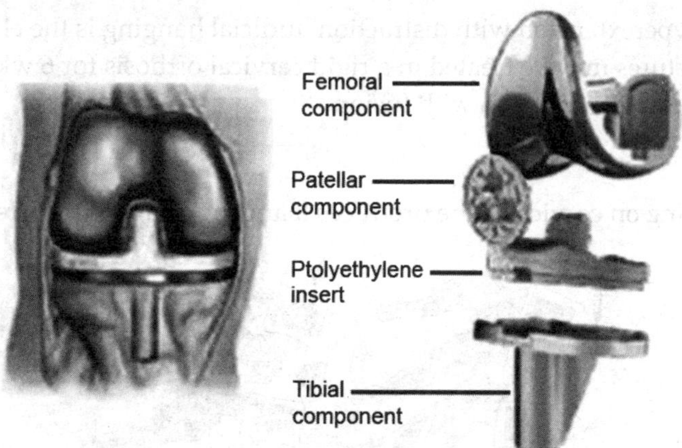

Fig. 19.54: TKR components

Complications of TKR

- ***Thromboembolism:*** The development of DVT may result in ***life-threatening*** pulmonary embolism.
- ***Infection:*** is one of the most dreaded complications. The most common organisms causing postoperative infection are *Staphylococcus aureus, Staphylococcus epidermidis,* and *Streptococcus* species.
- ***Patellofemoral complications*** include patella-femoral instability, patellar fracture and extensor mechanism rupture.
- ***Peroneal nerve palsy*** is commonly reported nerve palsy after TKR.
- ***Periprosthetic Fractures:*** Fracture of tibia or femur around the implant may complicate if the bone is weakened by osteoporosis, rheumatoid arthritis, systemic steroid use, etc.

Overall Advantages and Disadvantages of the Bearing Surfaces

Bearing combination	*Advantages*	*Disadvantages*
Ceramic on ceramic	***Very low wear rate***, Wettable (hydrophilic) High biocompatibility Surface finish smoother than metal. No adverse systemic effects	Implant ***fracture***, High cost
Metal on metal	Low wear, Self–polishing Moderate wear rate ***High performance couples***	Systemic toxic effects of metal ions. Teratogenic problems when used for ***young women***. Contraindicated in ***renal failure.***
Metal on polyethylene	Most commonly used ***Cheaper***	Polyethelene ***wear rate is highest*** and major cause of long term failure

SPINE

Fractures of the Spine

C1 Vertebral Fracture

C1 is also known as the ***Atlas***. When axial compression force acts on C1, it produces ***burst*** fracture. It is called ***Jefferson's fracture***. Neurological deficit is rare.

X-rays may not show all fractures; hence CT is necessary for evaluation.

Most fractures of the atlas can be treated with immobilization in a rigid cervical orthosis or a halo vest. Fusion is required for unstable injuries and with severe neurological symptoms.

Hangman's Fracture

It is traumatic spondylolisthesis of C2. (i.e ***fracture of pars interarticularis of C2***). So the C2 body slips over C3 vertebra.

The mechanism of injury is hyperextension with distraction. Judicial hanging is the classical example.

Treatment: Nondisplaced fractures may be treated in a rigid cervical orthosis for 6 wk.

Severe disruption may require open reduction with fusion.

Tear Drop Fracture

Compressive flexion force acting on cervical spine produces tear drop-shaped fracture fragment.

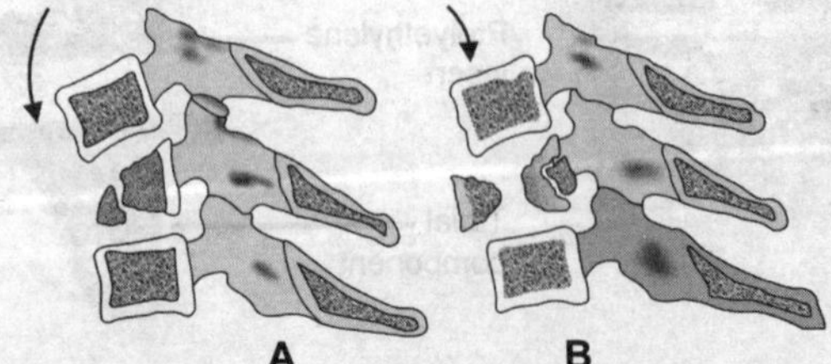

Figs 19.55 (A and B): A. Tear drop fracture; B. Burst fracture

Note:

- **Vertical (axial) compression** produces burst fracture of vertebral body. It is a stable fracture. Here, the peripheral displacement of fragments may enter the neural canal and produce canal compromise.
- **Flexion–rotation** force produces the most ***unstable*** injury. So the risk of displacement or dislocation is more.

Clay Shoveler's Fracture

Avulsion fracture of the spinous processes of the lower cervical or upper thoracic vertebrae. This results from muscular avulsion during shoveling.

Whiplash Injury

The ***cervical*** soft-tissue sprains are common after low velocity ***rear-end collision*** while travelling in cars.

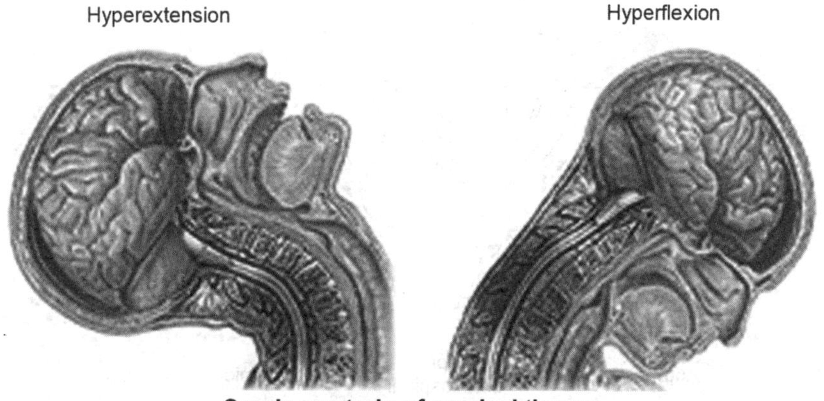

Fig. 19.56: Whiplash Injury

Here the person's trunk is seated and the ***neck is forcibly flexed and hyperextended*** due to elastic recoil of the soft tissues.
Pain and stiffness are the usual complaints. Neurological deficits are rare.

Chance Fracture

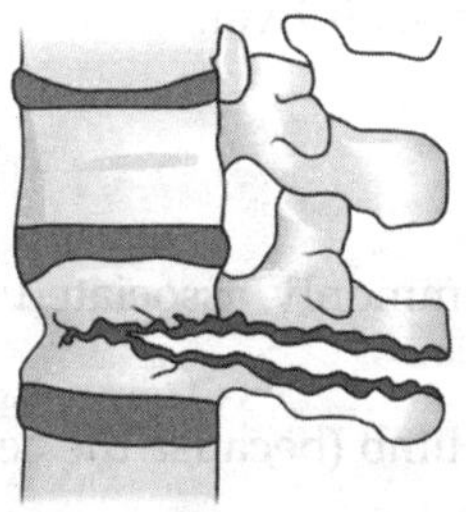

Fig. 19.57: Chance fracture

Also known as ***seat-belt injury***. The mechanism of injury is by flexion- distraction force. Common in ***lumbar*** spine. Here a transverse fracture line passes through the body of vertebra.

SPINAL CORD INJURY

Injury to the spinal cord manifests with variety of symptoms depending on the level and severity of injury.

Classified based on the severity and pattern of neurologic dysfunction:

- Complete injury
- Incomplete injury

The incomplete injuries are subdivided into:
- Anterior cord syndrome
- Central cord syndrome
- Posterior cord syndrome
- Brown-sequard syndrome.

Complete Spinal Cord Injury

Absence of sensation or voluntary motor function caudal to the level of injury. There will be *intact bulbocavernosus reflex*.

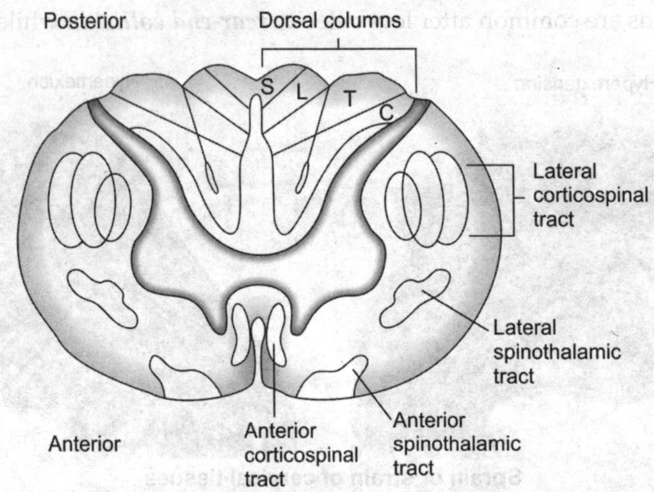

Fig. 19.58: Topography of tracts of spinal cord

Note:
Sacral sparing: It means the presence of:
1. Perianal sensation
2. Voluntary rectal motor function
3. Great toe flexion.

In cases of spinal cord injury after the spinal shock is over.
It indicates incomplete cord injury.

Central Cord Syndrome

Most common type of spinal cord injury. Commonly associated with ***hyper-extension*** of osteoarthritic cervical spine in middle aged persons.

Upper limbs are more affected than the lower limb (because the cervical fibres of corticospinal tracts more central than the lumbosacral fibres).

Anterior Cord Syndrome

Anterior part of the spinal cord carries corticospinal and spinothalamic tracts.

When anterior spinal cord is injured, the ***motor function, pain and temperature sensation are lost***.

There is intact light touch and proprioception which are carried by dorsal columns.

Posterior Cord Syndrome

Injury to posterior columns are rare. It presents with ***loss of touch, proprioception***. There is normal motor power, pain, and temperature sensation which are part of anterior cord.

Brown-Sequard Syndrome

It is a hemicord injury. Features are:

- ***Ipsilateral side:*** muscle paralysis, loss of proprioception and light touch sensation.
- ***Contralateral side:*** hypesthesia to pain and temperature.

Drugs For Spinal Cord Injury

Intravenous methylprednisolone: it is the standard drug for spinal cord injury.

Give loading dose of 30 mg/kg is given as soon as possible.

And then give

- 5.4 mg/kg/hour over the next 24 hours if started within 3 hours of spinal cord injury.
- 5.4 mg/kg/hour over the next 48 hours if started within 8 hours of spinal cord injury.

This infusion is of no benefit, if started more than ***8 hours*** after injury.

Experimental drugs useful for cord injury:

- Naloxone
- Thyrotropin-releasing hormone
- GM_1 gangliosides.

NEUROLOGICAL EXAMINATION

Nerve root	*Test*
C5:	Elbow flexion
C6:	Wrist extension
C7:	Wrist flexion, finger extension
C8:	Finger flexion
T1:	Finger abduction
L1,2:	Hip adduction
L3,4:	Knee extension
L5,S1:	Knee flexion
L5:	Great toe extension
S1:	Great toe flexion

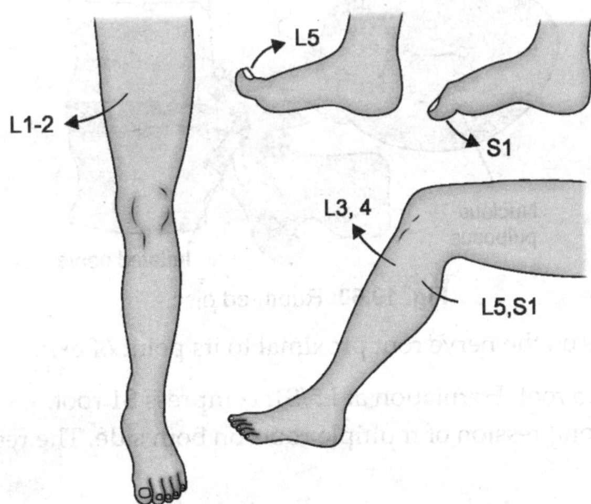

Fig. 19.59: Neurological examination

Root value	*Tendon reflex*
C5	Biceps
C6	Brachioradialis
C7	Triceps
L3,4	Quadriceps (patellar tendon reflex)
L5,S1	Achilles tendon (ankle reflex)

INTERVERTEBRAL DISC

They are made of fibrocartilage.

Each disc consists of an outer lamellated anulus fibrosus and an inner nucleus pulposus.

Annulus fibrosus: *Outside,* type I collagen, connects to vertebral hyaline cartilage.

Nucleus pulposus: *Inside,* type II collagen, high water content until old age.

- Derived from notochord, can prolapse/ herniate through the annulus fibrosus.
- It is avascular.

Intradiscal Pressure Variation

The pressure within the disc varies in different positions.

- It is ***lowest when a person is lying supine.***
- It is increasing from ***supine <standing< sitting < bending forward < weight lifting.***

High pressure situations increase the risk of disc prolapse.

Intervertebral Disc Prolapse

Common in age 20-45 years.

Typical history: sudden onset of severe back pain ***while lifting a weight or stooping.***

The most common levels: ***L4 to L5, L5 to S1,*** In cervical spine **C5-C6 is** most commonly involved.

More commonly, the prolapse occurs in ***posterolateral direction.*** Less commonly ***central*** prolapse can occur.

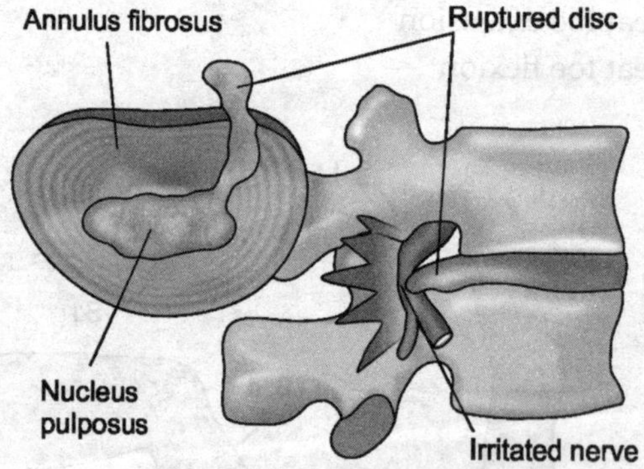

Fig. 19.60: Ruptured disc

- **Posterolateral** rupture presses on the nerve root proximal to its point of exit.

So herniation at L4/5: Compress L5 root. Herniation at L5/S1: compress S1 root.

- **Large central** rupture cause compression of multiple roots on both side. The result is ***cauda equina syndrome.***

Neurological Features of Specific Nerve Root

L4 root Involvement

- Weak quadriceps and tibialis anterior;
- Decreased sensation in medial leg and foot
- Patellar tendon reflex is decreased.

L5 Root Involvement

- Weak extensor hallucis longus
- Decreased sensation over Anterolateral leg, dorsum of the foot, and great toe
- Tibialis posterior reflex is decreased.

S1 Root Involvement

- Weak gastrocnemius
- Decreased sensation in lateral foot
- Achilles tendon reflex is decreased.

A positive straight-leg raise (SLR) test indicates 'sciatic' pain.
Lasegue's test: Foot dorsiflexion during SLRT, worsens the sciatic pain.

Treatment

In >90% of patients, pain resolves by:

- Limited bed rest ***(1–2 days),***
- NSAIDs, and physical therapy;
- Epidural steroid injections

Surgical Treatment

Indications for surgery

- Cauda equina syndrome
- Neurological deterioration
- Persistent sciatic pain

The most widely performed surgery

- *Laminotomy*
- *Microdiscectomy.*

CAUDA EQUINA SYNDROME

When a large central disc prolapsed compress multiple nerve roots produces the following symptoms:

- Bilateral lower limb weakness
- ***Saddle anesthesia***
- Bilateral sciatica
- Bladder and bowel symptoms
- Absent deep tendon reflex.

It is a surgical emergency; requires emergency surgical decompression by laminectomy and discectomy.

Spinal Stenosis

Refers to ***narrowing of the spinal canal or intervertebral foramen.***
Most common cause is secondary to degenerative changes in the lumbar disc and facet joints.

Neurogenic claudication: Most common symptom is ***leg pain precipitated by walking and relieved by rest.***

The treatment of choice for spinal stenosis is surgical decompression of the stenosed area.

Comparing Vascular and Neurogenic Claudication

Evaluation	Vascular	Neurogenic
Walking distance	Fixed	Variable
Relieved by	Standing	Sitting/bending
Aggravated by	Walking	Walking/standing
Walking uphill	Painful	Painless
Bicycle test	Positive (painful)	Negative
Pulses	Absent	Present

Spondylolisthesis

Spondylolysis: Defect or stress fracture (without slippage) in pars interarticularis.

➢ X-ray lumbar spine - oblique view: ***a Scotty dog wearing a collar.***

Spondylolisthesis: Forward slip of one vertebra over the other. Most common at ***L5 – S1*** level.

➢ When spondylolysis progresses to slip of vertebral body, spondylolisthesis results.

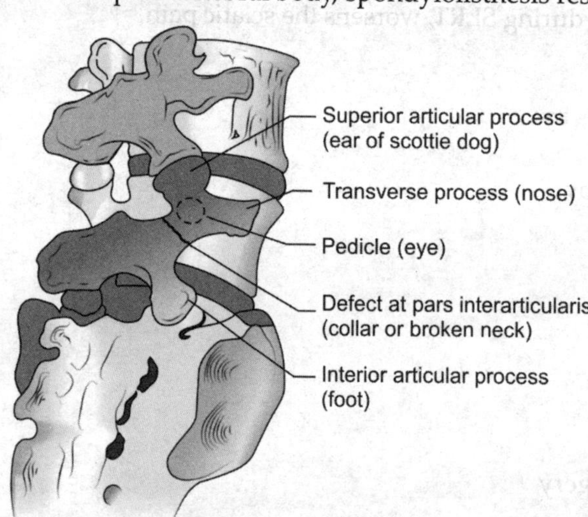

Fig. 19.61: The Scotty dog

X-ray lumbar spine

➢ Oblique view: ***a Scotty dog with a broken neck appearance.***

➢ AP view: ***Napolean hat sign.***

*[**Retrolisthesis:** posterior displacement of one vertebra over the other.*
***Spondyloptosis:** complete displacement of L5 in front of S1].*

Scheuermann's Disease

Usually appears in adolescence.

- Patients have an ***increased kyphosis*** in the thoracic or thoracolumbar spine
- ***Schmorl nodes:*** Herniation of the disk material in to the vertebral endplates.

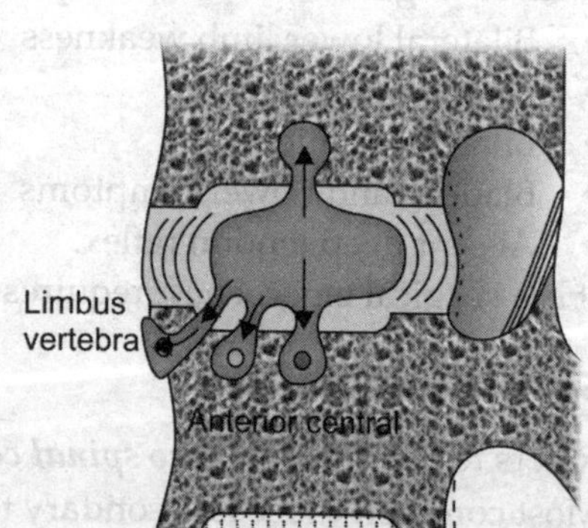

Fig. 19.62: Schmorl's nodes

Criteria for Diagnosis

1. 5 deg of wedging

2. at least three adjacent vertebrae involved
3. thoracic kyphosis is > 50 deg.

SPINAL DEFORMITIES

- The normal thoracic kyphosis: Cobb angle 20- 50 deg (mean 35 deg)
- The normal lumbar lordosis: Cobb's angle 40- 80 deg (mean 60 deg).

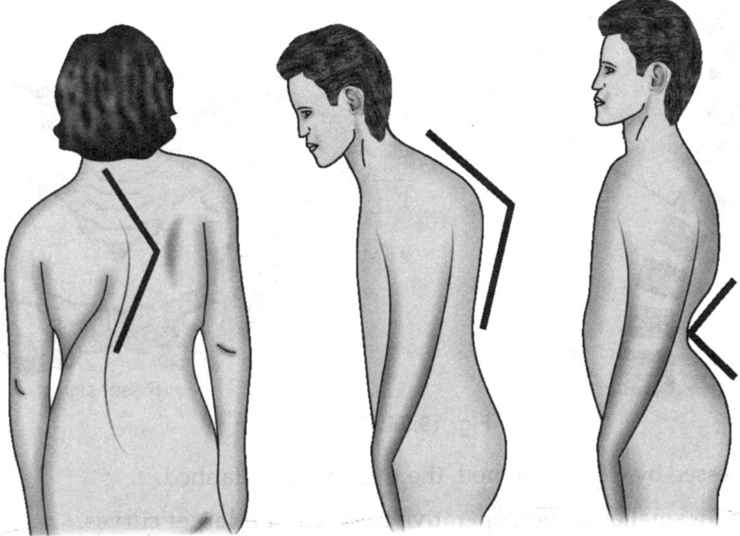

Figs 19.63 (A to C): A. Scoliosis, B. Kyphosis, C. Lordosis

Scoliosis

Abnormal lateral curvature of the spine. The scoliosis may be structural or nonstructural.

➢ A nonstructural scoliosis corrects on ***Adam's forward bending test.***
➢ A structural scoliosis is a fixed lateral curvature with rotation.

Aetiology of Scoliosis

- Congenital: due to bony anomalies
- Neuromuscular conditions
- Idiopathic: ***Most common***

Idiopathic Scoliosis

Can be classified according to the patient's age at the time onset of deformity.

- Infantile: Birth to 3 years
- Juvenile: 3-9 years
- Adolescent: >10 years.

Adolescent Idiopathic Scoliosis

This is the ***commonest*** type, occurring in 90 per cent of cases, mostly in girls.

Most common types of curves in cases of idiopathic scoliosis are the right thoracic curve.

- When the thoracic curves are severe, cardiopulmonary function can become compromised and a secondary ***restrictive lung disease*** may result from the chest deformity.
- Curve progression is most common during continued skeletal growth.

So surgical treatment in children who continue to grow will result in recurrence of deformity.

Degree of curvature is measured by ***Cobb's angle***.

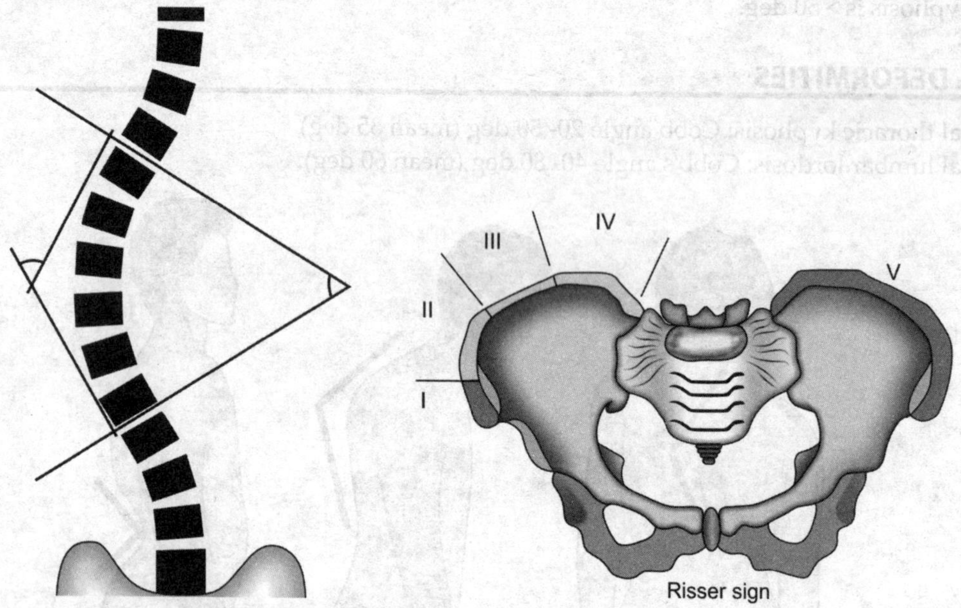

Fig. 19.64: Cobb's angle

Based on the severity assessed by Cobb's method, the treatment is planned.

Non-operative treatment for smaller curves, operative treatment for larger curves.

Skeletal maturity is assessed by the ***Risser's sign.*** It is progressive ossification of the iliac apophysis from lateral to medial direction.

When surgery is performed in immature spine, recurrence is most likely. So surgery will be the best option at grade IV or V.

Treatment Plan as per Cobb's Angle

a. *< 25 deg:* observation for progression.

b. *20-30 deg:* Bracing.

Bracing is used to prevent curve progression and generally does not lead to permanent curve improvement.

The commonly used braces are:

1. Milwaukee brace
2. Boston brace
3. ***Charleston night bending brace***- worn only during the night.

a. *>30 deg:* Surgery constitutes corrective instrumentation and spinal fusion.

Kyphosis

A curvature of the spine in the sagittal plane in which the convexity of the curve is directed posteriorly.

Causes

Increased kyphosis can be one of the following:

- Postural (Taller persons)
- Scheuermann disease
- Congenital defects
- Paralytic (Poliomyelitis)
- Posttraumatic

- Post infective (Pott's spine)
- Metabolic (Osteoporosis)
- Developmental (Achondroplasia).

Vertebroplasty

For acutely painful ***vertebral compression fractures*** can be treated with vertebroplasty.

It is done by placing large spinal needles into the fractured vertebral body through the pedicle and ***injecting bone cement*** into the fractured bone.

This procedure is ***to decrease pain*** and strengthen the bone to prevent further collapse and ***not to restore*** vertebral body height or prevent spinal deformity.

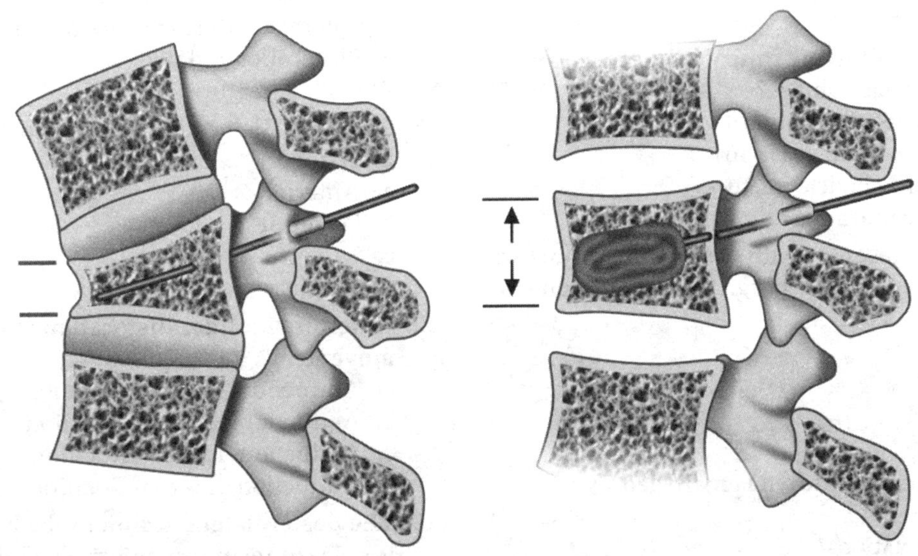

Fig. 19.65: Vertebroplasty

Balloon Kyphoplasty

Evolved as the next step in the treatment of vertebral compression fractures.
A procedure ***to correct kyphosis.***

The procedure is performed by inserting needle into the vertebral body through the pedicle.
A small balloon is inflated ***to restore the height of a collapsed vertebral body*** and create a cavity inside. The cavity is filled with the bone cement.

SOME TESTS IN THE SPINE

Schober's test: Determines the degree of lumbar spine movement. The movement is decreased ***in ankylosing spondylitis.***

FABER test: Acronym for flexion, abduction, external rotation. It is ***figure-of-four test*** to examine for sacroiliac pain.

The wall test: To assess cervical spine movement.

Step-off sign: A step-like feel on palpation of spinous processes in midline of the back. Seen in spondylolisthesis

Coin test: Inability to pick up the dropped coin on the floor due do spasm of parasapinal muscles. Elicited in ***tuberculosis of the spine.***

QUESTIONS

1. March fracture is: **(2010, 2014)**
a. Fracture of neck of 2nd metatarsal
b. Fracture of shaft of 2nd metatarsal
c. Fracture of shaft of 3rd metatarsal
d. Fracture of base of 5th metatarsal

2. Which of the following needs a violent force?
a. Fx Neck of femur **(2011)**
b. Intertrochanteric fracture
c. Clavicle fracture
d. Colle's fracture

3. Which of the following injury is likely to cause a severe vascular damage? **(2013)**
a. Posterior knee dislocation
b. Posterior elbow dislocation
c. Middle third clavicle fracture
d. Tibial plateau fracture

4. A patient presents with compound fracture of tibia with 1 cm opening. What grade does it belong? **(2000)**
a. Grade I
b. Grade II
c. Grade IIIA
d. Grade IIIB

5. Open fracture in children is managed by:
a. Debridement **(2014)**
b. External fixation
c. Open reduction and Internal fixation
d. Intramedullary nail

6. Open fracture is best treated by: **(JIPMER)**
a. Internal fixation
b. External fixation
c. Debridement
d. Tourniquet

7. Which of the following is true about Open reduction and Internal fixation? **(2001)**
a. It is of two types: onlay and inlay
b. In most cases of ORIF require supplementation with external splinting
c. Immobilization in ORIF is less than that of External fixation
d. ORIF is used when closed reduction is impossible, inaccurate and difficult to maintain.

8. Open reduction and internal fixation does all except: **(2007)**
a. Consolidation
b. Stability
c. Better function
d. Better alignment

9. All of the following sites are associated with nonunion of fracture due to avascularity, except:
a. Fracture neck of femur **(2002)**
b. Fracture neck of scaphoid
c. Fracture neck of humerus
d. Fracture neck of talus

10. Volkmann's ischemia is a known complication in:
a. Supracondylar fracture of the humerus
b. Lateral condyle fracture of the humerus
c. Dislocation of knee
d. Colle's fracture **(2012)**

11. Shoulder dislocation occurs most often in which direction? **(2011)**
a. Anterior
b. Posterior
c. Superior
d. Inferior

12. Anterior shoulder dislocation is caused by what movement? **(2013)**
a. Adduction–External Rotation
b. Abduction–External Rotation
c. Abduction–Internal Rotation
d. Adduction–Internal Rotation

13. The posterolateral lesion in the head of humerus is cases of recurrent anterior shoulder dislocation is: **(2014)**
a. Bankart's lesion
b. Hill-Sachs lesion
c. Reverse Hill-Sachs lesion
d. Greater tuberosity avulsion fracture

14. Light bulb sign is seen in: **(2014)**
a. Anterior dislocation of shoulder
b. Posterior dislocation of shoulder
c. Fracture acromion
d. Clavicular fracture

15. Posterior hip dislocation is characterized by:
a. Flexion, adduction, external rotation **(2014)**
b. Flexion, adduction, internal rotation
c. Extension, adduction, internal rotation
d. Extension, adduction, external rotation

16. What is the position of lower limb in anterior dislocation of hip? **(2007)**
a. Flexion, Adduction and Internal rotation
b. Flexion, Adduction and External rotation
c. Flexion, Abduction and Internal rotation
d. Flexion, Abduction and External rotation

17. What is the treatment of choice for 4 week old neck of femur fracture in a 55 yr old man? (2005)
a. Mcmurray's osteotomy
b. Open reduction and internal fixation
c. Hemireplacement arthroplasty
d. Total hip arthroplasty

18. In fracture shaft of femur, which nail is commonly used for ORIF? (2007)
a. Kuntscher nail
b. Austin Moore pin
c. K-wire
d. Smith – Peterson nail

19. Degree of angulation acceptable after reducing tibial fracture is: (2007)
a. 5
b. 10
c. 15
d. 20

20. Fracture subluxation of volar or dorsal rim of distal radius is termed as: (2008)
a. Galeazzi fracture
b. Barton's fracture
c. Smith's fracture
d. Chauffeur's fracture

21. Most common site of clavicle fracture is:
a. Junction of middle and outer 1/3rd (2006)
b. Middle 1/3rd
c. Medial 1/3rd
d. Lateral 1/3rd

22. All of the following are the complications of Colle's plaster except: (2000)
a. Stiffness of wrist
b. Stiffness of shoulder
c. Carpal tunnel syndrome
d. Wrist drop

23. A patient on Colle's cast present after two weeks with inability to extend his thumb, the most likely reason is: (2006)
a. Rupture of extensor pollicis longus tendon
b. Compartment syndrome
c. Carpal tunnel syndrome
d. Sudeck's osteodystrophy

24. Not a complication of Colle's fracture:
a. Malunion (2006)
b. Nonunion
c. Sudeck'sosteodystrophy
d. Carpal-tunnel syndrome

25. A 75 year woman present with h/o fall in the bathroom, unable to walk, or bear weight on her left hip. O/E her left lower limb is externally rotated, hip is tender, active SLR not possible. The most possible diagnosis is: (2006)
a. Osteoarthritis of hip
b. Dislocation of hip
c. Acetabular fracture
d. Fracture neck of femur

26. Fracture of 1st metacarpal bone is:
a. Barton's fracture (2010)
b. Bennet's fracture
c. Chauffeur's fracture
d. Boxer's fracture

27. Conditions requiring open reduction in children is:
a. Intercondylar fracture femur (2011)
b. Fracture both bones of forearm
c. Lateral condylar fracture of humerus
d. Epiphyseal separation of tibia

28. The most common complication of lateral humeral condyle fracture in children is:
a. Valgus deformity (2014)
b. Varus deformity
c. Malunion
d. Hyperextension

29. A 12 year old child presents with tingling sensation and numbness in the little finger. With h/o four years ago the child sustained elbow injury. What would be the most probable fracture at that time? (2005)
a. Injury to ulnar nerve
b. Fracture of lateral condyle
c. Supracondylar fracture
d. Elbow dislocation

30. Which of the following elbow injury results in nonunion? (2001)
a. Intercondylar fracture
b. Fracture of lateral condyle
c. Supracondylar fracture
d. Fracture of medial epicondyle

31. Three point relationship is maintained in which of the following? (2005)
a. Elbow dislocation
b. Fracture of lateral condyle
c. Supracondylar fracture
d. Fracture of medial epicondyle

32. Gunstock deformity occurs as a complication of:
a. Capitulum fracture (2013)
b. Supracondylar fracture
c. Fracture of lateral epicondyle of humerus
d. Fracture of neck of radius

33. In supracondylar fracture, after closed reduction and plaster application, which of the following angles will help in evaluate the quality of reduction? (2010)
a. Q angle
b. Cobb's angle
c. Bohler's angle
d. Baumann's angle

34. Monteggia fracture is a: (2012, 2014)
a. Fracture of atlas
b. Fracture of radial styloid
c. Fracture of proximal 1/3 of ulna with dislocation of proximal radioulnar joint
d. Fracture of distal 1/3 of radius with dislocation of distal radioulnar joint

35. Avascular necrosis is seen in all of the following, except: (2003)
a. Scapula
b. Head of femur
c. Body of talus
d. Head of humerus

36. Carpal tunnel syndrome is due to compression of: (2011)
a. Anterior interosseus nerve
b. Median nerve
c. Radial nerve
d. Ulnar nerve

37. Causes of carpal tunnel syndrome are all except: (2013)
a. Pregnancy
b. Acromegaly
c. Hypothyroidism
d. Tuberculosis

38. Pointing index in a case of supracondylar fracture humerus in children occurs due to involvement of: (2000)
a. Radial nerve
b. Anterior interosseous nerve
c. Musculocutaneous nerve
d. Ulnar nerve

39. Pointing index is a complication seen in: (2014)
a. Lateral humeral condyle fracture
b. Supracondylar fracture of humerus
c. Shoulder dislocation
d. Fracture of shaft of humerus

40. Nerve commonly involved in fracture of distal shaft of humerus is: (2011)
a. Radial n
b. Medial n
c. Ulnar n
d. Circumflex brachial nerve

41. Medial nerve involvement is most commonly with: (2008)
a. Elbow dislocation
b. Supracondylar fracture
c. Lateral condyle fracture
d. Olecranon fracture

42. Inferior shoulder dislocation, the nerve damaged is: (2011)
a. Axillary nerve
b. Radial nerve
c. Ulnar nerve
d. Median nerve

43. Meralgia paresthetica is due to involvement of: (2014)
a. Lateral thoracic nerve
b. Lateral cutaneous nerve of thigh
c. Anterior femoral nerve
d. Gluteal nerve

44. Tardy ulnar nerve palsy is seen in: (2012)
a. Cubitus varus
b. Cubitus valgus
c. Genu varus
d. Genu valgus

45. Meniscal injury occurs during: (2011)
a. Flexion
b. Rotation
c. Extension
d. Flexion and Rotation

46. Housemaid's knee is inflammation of: (2009)
a. Prepattellar bursa
b. Suprapatellar bursa
c. Infrapatellar bursa
d. Anserine bursa

47. Clergyman's knee is due to involvement of: (2011)
a. Semimemranous bursa
b. Infrapatellar bursa
c. Suprapatellar bursa
d. Prepatellar bursa

48. A footballer complains of sudden giving away of knee, which could be due to? (2008)
a. Medial collateral ligament tear
b. Anterior cruciate ligament tear
c. Medial meniscal tear
d. Posterior cruciate ligament tear

49. History of twisting strain and locking of knee joint occurs due to: (2008)
a. Tear of Anterior cruciate ligament
b. Tear of Medial cruciate ligament
c. Meniscal tear
d. Patellar fractures

50. Which of the following is the most common type of meniscal injury? (2002)
a. Anterior horn tear of lateral meniscus
b. Anterior horn tear of medial meniscus
c. Bucket handle tear of lateral meniscus
d. Bucket handle tear of medial meniscus

51. What would be the most reliable test for an acutely injured knee? (2008)
a. Ant. Drawer test
b. Post. Drawer test
c. Lachman test
d. Pivot shift test.

52. Kanavel's sign is seen in: (2013)
a. Flexor tendon sheath infectious inflammation in hand
b. Mid palmar space abscess
c. Ulnar bursitis
d. Web space involvement

53. Painful arc syndrome is due to: (2004)
a. Subacromial bursitis
b. Fracture of greater tubercle
c. Chronic supraspinatus tendinitis
d. All of the above

54. Mallet finger is: (2014)
a. Facture of proximal phalanx
b. Avulsion of extensor tendon
c. Rupture of flexor tendon
d. Capsular rupture of PIP joint

55. Tom Smith arthritis is: (2014)
a. Tuberculous involvement of hip joint
b. Tuberclous involvement of knee joint
c. Syphilitic involvement of hip joint
d. Septic Arthritis of hip joint in infants

56. The earliest radiological manifestation of TB of hip joint is: (2012)
a. Loss of joint space
b. Femoral head loss
c. Periosteal thickening
d. Osteopenia

57. Wandering acetabulum is seen in: (2014)
a. Fracture of acetabulum
b. Hip dislocation
c. Rheumatoid arthritis
d. TB of hip

58. In osteomalacia, all the following seen except:
a. Looser's zone (2001, 2009)
b. High alkaline phosphatase
c. Increased resistance to pathological fractures
d. Diminished urinary excretion of calcium

59. The X-ray findings seen in osteomalacia are all except: (2012)
a. Looser's zone
b. Biconcave vertebrae
c. Absence/rarity of pathological fractures
d. Trefoil pelvis

60. Bone mass is reduced in all of the following conditions, except: (2009)
a. Osteoporosis
b. Osteomalacia
c. Hyperparathyroidism
d. Osteopetrosis

61. All the following cause osteopenia, except:
a. Rickets (2010)
b. Osteomalacia
c. Osteoporosis
d. Osteopetrosis

62. Characteristic feature of rickets is/are: (2004)
a. Decrease in calcium content of bone
b. Widening of growth cartilage
c. Beading of ribs
d. All of the above

63. What is the diagnostic radiological finding in skeletal fluorosis? (2008)
a. Interroseous membrane ossification
b. Sub-periosteal cortical resorption of the middle phalanges
c. Osteoclerosis of vertebral body
d. Ossification of ligaments of knee joint

64. von Rosen splint is used in: (2005)
a. Clubfoot
b. Congenital dislocation of hip
c. Congenital coxa vara
d. Perthes' disease

65. Fixed flexion deformity of hip is assessed by:
a. Barlow's test (2003)
b. Thomas test
c. Trendlenberg's test
d. Lachman's test

66. Recognizing feature of achondroplasia:
a. AR inheritance (2008)
b. Diagnozed radiologically at birth
c. Increased liability for fractures
d. Short spine

67. Rigid flat foot is not seen: (2008)
a. Athlete's foot
b. Rheumatoid arthritis
c. Peroneal spasm
d. Congenital tarsal coalition

68. One of the causes of the recurrence of club foot is due to weakness of: (2005)
a. Tendo achillis
b. Gastrocnemius
c. Plantar fascia
d. Peroneal muscles

69. Trendlenberg's sign is positive in paralysis of:
a. Gluteus maximus (2007)
b. Gluteus medius
c. Quadriceps femoris
d. Quadratus lumborum

70. A 14 year old boy with 78kg wt and hypothyroidism developed sudden onset of severe pain and tenderness on left hip as a result of minor fall. Most likely diagnosis is: (2002)
a. Fx neck of femur
b. SCFE
c. Perthes' disease
d. Hip dislocation

71. Siffert-Katz sign is seen in: (2013)
a. Perthes disease
b. Blount's disease
c. Osteogenesis imperfecta
d. Pulled Elbow

72. What is the best management of CTEV in newborn? (2014)
a. Manipulation alone
b. Manipulation and corrective splint
c. Corrective surgery
d. Wait and watch

73. All are true regarding CTEV, except:
a. Hindfoot varus (2010)
b. Cavus
c. Increased dorsiflexion
d. Forefoot adduction

74. Multiple bone fractures with wormian bones are seen in: (2010)
a. Rickets
b. Osteomalacia
c. Battered baby syndrome
d. Osteogenesis imperfecta

75. Bone tumors arising from diaphysis:
a. Chondromyxoid fibroma (2010)
b. Primitive neuroectodermal bone tumor
c. Osteoclastoma
d. Chondroblastoma
e. Giant cell tumor

76. Osteochondroma is a arises:
a. Metaphysis (2001, 2008)
b. Diaphysis
c. Epiphysis
d. Periosteum

77. A patient with pain in the thigh, relieved by aspirin. X-ray shows a radiolucent mass surrounded by sclerosis. Diagnosis is: (2011)
a. Osteoma
b. Osteoid osteoma
c. Osteoblastoma
d. Osteoclastoma

78. Bone to bone metastasis is commonly seen in:
a. Osteosarcoma (2010)
b. Ewing's sarcoma
c. Chondrosarcoma
d. Reticulum cell carcinoma

79. Soap-Bubble appearance is seen in:
a. Ewing's sarcoma (2007)
b. Giant cell tumor
c. Adamantinoma
d. Osteosarcoma

80. A 30 year man with radiodence mass around elbow with a clear zone between the mass and humerus. What is the probable diagnosis?
a. Paraosteal osteosarcoma (2008)
b. Periosteal osteosarcoma
c. Myositis ossificans
d. Tumor calcinosis

81. Which of the following tumors is a common differential diagnosis of osteomyelitis? (2008)
a. Chondrosarcoma
b. Ewing's sarcoma
c. Osteosarcoma
d. Synovial sarcoma

82. Mafucci syndrome is: (2014)
a. Multiple osteochondromas
b. Multiple enchondromas
c. Multiple enchondromas with soft tissue malignancies
d. Multiple hemangiomas

83. Characteristic histopathological feature of osteosarcoma is: (2014)
a. Codman's triangle
b. Matrix new bone formation with Codman's triangle
c. Malignant cells with osteoid formation
d. Spindle cells

84. A 20 year old female presents with eccentric cystic expansile growth from metaphysis of femur. X-ray shows 'soap-bubble' appearance. What is the probable diagnosis? (2001)
a. Aneurysmal bone cyst
b. Osteochondroma

c. Osteosarcoma
d. Osteoclastoma

85. Osteoblastic metastasis is seen with: (2013)
a. Kidney
b. Prostate
c. Lung
d. Thyroid

86. Which of the following is the most radiosensitive tumor? (2005)
a. Ewing's sarcoma
b. Osteosarcoma
c. Fibrosarcoma
d. Liposarcoma

87. Characterisitic feature of osteoarthritis on X-ray: (1997)
a. Spurring
b. Subchondral sclerosis
c. Diminution of cartilage space
d. All of the above

88. All are true regarding Psoriatic arthritis except: (2001)
a. Arthritis mutilans
b. DIP involvement
c. Ankylosis of small joints
d. Sacroilitis
e. Telescoping of digits.

89. Bamboo spine is characteristic of: (2013)
a. Rheumatoid arthritis
b. Osteoarthritis
c. Ankylosing spondylitis
d. Hyperparathyroidism

90. Haemophilic arthropathy, which is not seen? (2014)
a. Subchondral bone cyst formation
b. Increase in intercondylar distance
c. Juxta articular osteosclerosis
d. Subchondral thinning

91. 58 year old female patient presents with one year history of anterior knee pain on climbing stairs. On examination crepitus was present. There was severe restriction of movements beyond 110 degrees. Examination of hip and back was normal. Diagnosis is: (2014)
a. Osteoarthritis
b. Psoriatic arthritis
c. Osteonecrosis
d. Gout

92. A 60 year old diabetic presents with swelling and pain in ankle and foot. X-ray shows loose bodies and bony sclerosis. What is the diagnosis? (2010)
a. Septic arthritis
b. Osteoarthritis
c. Gouty arthritis
d. Neuropathic joint

93. In a patient with arthritis, examination of synovium aspirate, numerous lymphocytes, plasma cells and histiocytes are found. What type of arthritis it is? (2014)
a. Acute pyogenic arthritis
b. Chronic arthritis
c. Granulomatous arthritis
d. Rheumatoid arthritis

94. The position of the hip in a patient of osteoarthritis is: (2003)
a. Extension, abduction internal rotation
b. Flexion, adduction, internal rotation
c. Flexion, abduction, internal rotation
d. Flexion, adduction, external rotation

95. Which of the following on deposition causes the calcific tendinitis of supraspinatus tendon? (2001)
a. Calcium biurate crystals
b. Calcium pyrophosphate crystals
c. Calcium hydroxylapatite
d. Uric acid

96. Intervertebral dics pressure is lowest in: (2007)
a. Lying supine
b. Lying on side
c. Sitting
d. Standing

97. All are true regarding whiplash injury except: (2007)
a. Lumbar spine commonly involved
b. Sprains and strains without vertebral fracture
c. Hyperextension injury
d. Symptomatically treated

98. After spinal injury, the lower limb power greater than upper limb. The sacral sensation is present. Type of spinal cord lesion is: (2007)
a. Anterior cord syndrome
b. Posterior cord syndrome
c. Central cord syndrome
d. Complete spinal cord injury

99. Jefferson fracture is: (2013)
a. Fracture of C1
b. Fracture of C2
c. Fracture of C1 and C2
d. Fracture of T1

100. Spondylolysis means: (2008)
a. Defect of pars interarticularis
b. Degenerative changes of the spine
c. Arthritic changes in facial joints
d. Fracture of vertebral body

101. A patient is diagnosed with disc prolapse. Examination reveals paralysis of Extensor Hallucis Longus. Which nerve root is affected? (2014)
a. L3
b. L4
c. L5
d. S1

ANSWERS AND EXPLANATIONS

1. **Ans. a. Fracture neck of 2nd metatarsal**
Ref: Maheshwari's Essential Orthopedics 4/e p160.
March fracture is a fatigue fracture of metatarsal, resulting from long continued or often repeated stress. It may occur in army recruits freshly committed to marching – hence the term March fracture.

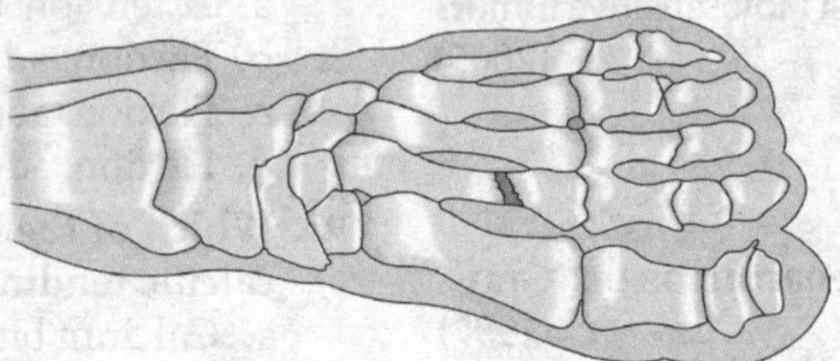

Fig. 19.66: Fracture neck of 2nd metatarsal is the commonest site of stress (march) fracture.

2. **Ans. c. Clavicle fracture** *Ref: Handbook of Fractures, Kenneth Koval, 3/e p35.*
A pathologic fracture is one that occurs when the normal integrity and strength of bone have been compromised by destructive disease processes. Pathologic fractures may occur as a result ***of minimal trauma or even during normal activities***.
Causes include neoplasm, necrosis, metabolic disease, disuse, infection, metastatic disease, osteoporosis, iatrogenic causes (e.g., surgical defect), or primary bone tumor.
Osteoporosis is the most common cause of pathologic fractures in the elderly population.
Ref: Apley and Solomon's Concise System of Orthopedics and Trauma, 4/e p386,432,435
- ***Neck of femur fractures,***
- ***Intertrochanteric fractures and***
- ***Colle's fractures***

are common in older age group women who are suffering with ***post menopausal osteoporosis***. These fractures occurs due to trivial forces, hence are called pathological fractures.
The clavicle fractures are not pathological fractures, and they needs violent force.

3. **Ans. a. Posterior knee dislocation**
- Though the ***clavicle*** is close to vital structures, damage to the subclavian vessels and brachial plexus injuries are all very rare.
- Posterior ***knee*** dislocation: Popliteal artery damage occurs in nearly 20 per cent of patients and needs immediate repair.
- ***Supracondylar*** fracture: The great danger is injury to the brachial artery, the incidence is probably less than 1 percent.
- Posterior ***elbow*** dislocation: The brachial artery may be damaged. Absence of the radial pulse is a warning. If there are other signs of ischaemia, this should be treated as an emergency. Splints must be removed and the elbow should be straightened.

4. **Ans. a. Grade I.** *Ref: Maheshwari's Essential Orthopedics 4/e p21*
Type I (or Grade I) is – open fracture with clean wounds less than 1cm long.

5. **Ans. a. Debridement**

6. **Ans. c. Debdridement.** *Ref: Maheshwari's Essential Orthopedics 4/e p20–21*
A fracture is called ***open (or compound) fracture*** when there is a break in the overlying skin and soft tissues. Open fractures pose the following problems:
- Infection of the bone because of contamination of the wound by bacteria fro outside.
- We cannot use plaster cast or ORIF to manage these fractures
- Very difficult to achieve union.

The principles of treatment of open fracture is to convert it into a closed fracture by ***meticulous wound care.***
Campbell's Operative Orthopedics says: "As a general rule, however, all open fractures should be irrigated

and debrided thoroughly in the regular operating room with the patient under general or regional block anesthesia, and the patient should be admitted for observation and routine treatment with intravenous antibiotics."

7. **Ans. d. ORIF is used when closed reduction is impossible, inaccurate and difficult to maintain.**

Ref: Apley's System of Orthopedics and Fractures, 9/e p696

Open reduction of the fracture under direct vision is indicated:

- When closed reduction fails, either because of difficulty in controlling the fragments or
- Because soft tissues are interposed between them;
- When there is a large articular fragment that needs accurate positioning or
- For traction (avulsion) fractures in which the fragments are held apart.

8. **Ans. a. Consolidation.**

Campbell's Operative Orthopedics

The AO treatment guidelines for fracture treatment:

- Anatomical reduction of the fracture fragments,
- Stable internal fixation
- Preservation of blood supply to the injured area
- Active, pain-free mobilization of adjacent muscles and joints.

9. **Ans. c. Fracture neck of humerus.**

Ref: Apley's System of Orthopedics and fractures, 9/e p715, Maheshwari's Essential Orthopedics 4/e p47

Causes of Non-union:

- Inadequate (damage to) blood supply
- Soft tissue interposition
- Imperfect splintage
- Infection
- Inadequate immobilization
- Distraction at fracture site.

10. **Ans. a. Supracondylar fracture of the humerus** *Ref: Maheshwari's Essential Orthopedics 4/e p98*

Volkmann's Ischemic Contracture:

It is a late complication of ***supracondylar fracture of humerus***. The ishaemic muscles are replaced by fibrous tissues, the end result is contracture of forearm, wrist and hand.

Clinically,

- Atrophy of forearm
- Flexion deformity of wrist and fingers

Volkmann's sign:

It is possible to extend the fingers fully at interphalangeal joints only when the wrist is flexed.

On extending the wrist, the fingers get flexed at the inter-phalangeal joints.

Treatment:

Mild deformities: corrected by turn-buckle splint ***(Volkmann's splint).***

Moderate deformities: Release of flexor muscles from their origin at medial epicondyle. ***(Maxpage operation)***

11. **Ans. a. Anterior** *Ref: Maheshwari's Essential Orthopedics, 4/e p86*

Shoulder is the commonest joint in the body to dislocate.

Anterior dislocation is much more common than posterior dislocation.

Anterior Shoulder Dislocation: head of humerus lies anteriorly.

In the anterior location, the head comes below the coracoid process. ***(Subcoraoid type)***

12. **Ans. b. Abduction-External Rotation** *Ref: Maheshwari's Essential Orthopedics, 4/e p86*

Anterior *shoulder dislocation* Results from *ABDUCTION and EXTERNAL ROTATION.*

Posterior *shoulder dislocation: Result from direct blow on front of shoulder, or* ***electric shock, convulsions.***

13. **Ans. b. Hill-Sachs lesion** *Ref: Maheshwari's Essential Orthopedics, 4/e p87, fig 13.5*

Pathological changes of Anterior shoulder dislocation:

- Bankart lesion: Stripping of anterior glenoid labrum.
- Hill-Sachs lesion: a depression of postero-lateral quadrant of humeral head.

14. Ans. b. Posterior dislocation of shoulder *Ref: Apley's System of Orthopedics and fractures, 9/e p742, fig 24.13*

Posterior shoulder dislocation is very rare.

This happens most commonly during a convulsion, or with an electric shock.

The arm is held in ***internal rotation***.

In the AP x ray:

Because of internal rotation, humeral head looks like shape of ***electric light bulb.***

The glenoid fossa is empty: ***empty glenoid sign***

15. Ans. b. Flexion, adduction, internal rotation.

Deformities of Hip:

- Posterior Hip Dislocation: Flexion, adduction, internal rotation, Shortening
- Anterior Hip Dislocation: Flexion, Abduction, External Rotation, Shortening.
- Fracture of neck femur: External Rotation and shortening.

16. Ans. b. Flexion, Abduction and External rotation

17. Ans. a. McMurray's osteotomy *Ref: Maheshwari's Essential Orthopedics, 4/e p133, Flow chart 18.1*

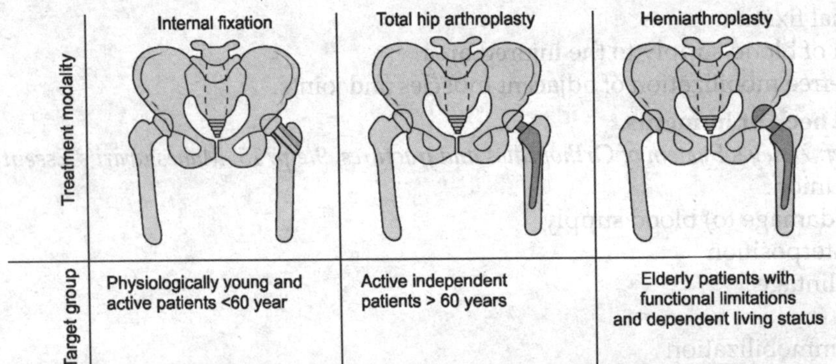

Fig. 19.67: Neck of femur fracture - treatment modality

In cases presenting late (more than 2-3weeks)

> 60 yrs of age: Hemiarthroplasty or Total Hip replacement

< 60 yrs of age: If the femoral head is vascular à Mc Murray or Pauwel's osteotomy

If the femoral head is avascular à Bipolar arthroplasty.

18. Ans. a. Kuntscher nail *Ref: Maheshwari's Essential Orthopedics, 4/e p137*

Treatment of fracture shaft of femur:

Conservative methods:

- In children: Skin Traction, Hip spica cast
- In adult: Pin (skeletal) traction using Steinmann pin

Operative Methods:

- Interlocked Nailing,
- Kuntscher's clover leaf Nail
- Plating.

19. Ans. a. 5 deg. *Ref: Kenneth J. Koval's Handbook of Fractures, 3/e p394*

Acceptable Reduction in Tibial shaft fractures:

- Less than 5 degrees of varus/valgus angulation
- Less than 10 degrees of anterior/posterior angulation
- Less than 10 degrees of rotational deformity
  – (external rotation better tolerated than internal rotation)
- Less than 1 cm of shortening
- More than 50% cortical contact.

20. b. Barton's fracture *Ref: Maheshwari's Essential Orthopedics, 4/e p11*

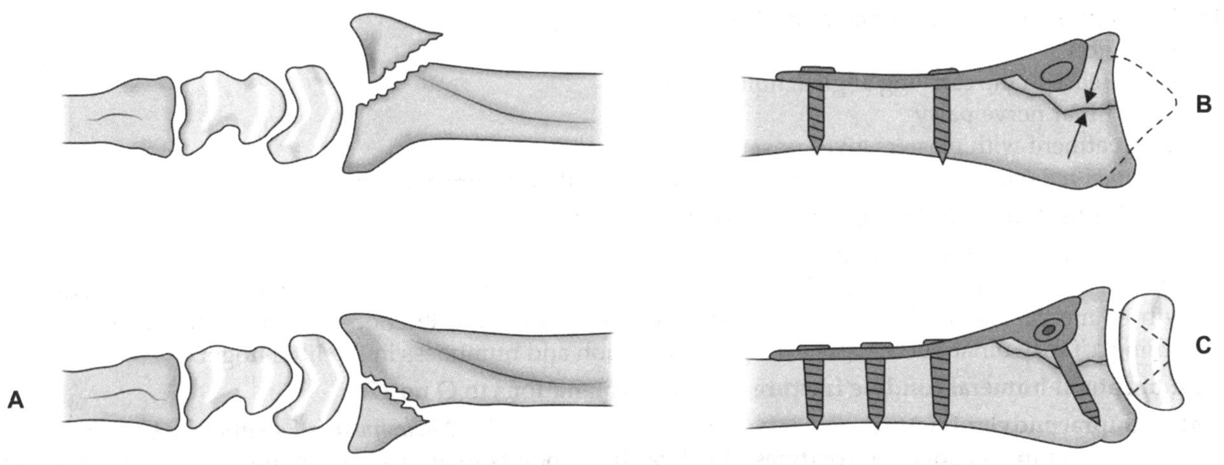

Fig. 19.68: Volar/Dorsal Barton's fracture, Treated by Buttress Plate

Barton's fracture is an intra-articular fracture of distal radius.
Depending upon the displacement:
- Anterior type is Volar Barton
- Posterior type is Dorsal Barton

Treatment is open reduction and internal fixation with plate.

21. **Ans. a. Junction of middle and outer 1/3rd**
Ref: Maheshwari's Essential Orthopedics, 4/e p85
The junction of the middle and outer third of the clavicle is the commonest site of fractures.

22. **Ans. d. Wrist drop.**
Ref: Maheshwari's Essential Orthopedics, 4/e p110
Complications of Colle's fracture (seen when treated with plaster):
- Stiffness of shoulder / wrist / elbow
- Malunion – most common late complication
- Subluxation of distal radio ulnar joint
- Carpal tunnel syndrome – Median N compression
- Sudeck's osteodystrophy
- Rupture of extensor pollicis longus tendon – very rare. Extension of thumb becomes weak.

Wrist drop: is caused by radial nerve injury at or above elbow.

23. **Ans. a. Rupture of extensor pollicis longus tendon (See the explanation of Q no 12)**

24. **Ans. b. Nonunion (See the explanations of Question No 12)**

25. **Ans. d. Fracture neck of femur** *Ref: Maheshwari's Essential Orthopedics, 4/e p130*
Neck of femur is often seen in the ***elderly*** with h/o ***slipping on the floor*** and inability to move the limb.
Clinically
- External rotation of lower limb
- Shortening
- Tenderness in the groin
- Active straight leg raising is not possible.

26. **Ans. b. Bennet's fracture** *Ref: Maheshwari's Essential Orthopedics, 4/e p112*
Bennett's fracture is an ***oblique intra-articular fracture of base of first metacarpal*** with subluxation of the metacarpal.
Treated with ***closed reduction and percutaneous K wire fixation.***

27. **Ans. c. Lateral condylar fracture of humerus** *Ref: Maheshwari's Essential Orthopedics, 4/e p99*
Lateral Condyle of Fracture of Humerus
Results from a varus injury to elbow
Displacement is common due to pull of the common extensor muscles which take origin from the lateral epicondyle.

This fracture is well-known for complications such as
- Nonunion
- An increase in the carrying angle (cubitus valgus),
- Tardy ulnar nerve palsy

Closed treatment with plasters gives unsatisfactory results.
Hence, ***open reduction and internal fixation is necessary ('a fracture of necessity'.)***

28. Ans. a. Valgus deformity. (See the explanation to Q no 17.)

29. Ans. b. Fracture of lateral condyle.

Fracture of lateral humeral condyle à Non union à Growth Disturbances on lateral humerus and Unopposed growth of medial humeral condyle à Cubital valgus deformiry à Friction neuritis of ulnar nerve due to stretching à Tardy ulnar nerve palsy à Tingling sensation and numbness in the little finger.

30. Ans. b. Lateral humeral condyle fracture (See the explanations to Q no 17)

31. Ans. c. Supracondylar fracture *Ref: Maheshwari's Essential Orthopedics, 4/e p94*

"Since the fracture is above the condyles, the three bony points relationship is maintained as in the normal elbow."

32. Ans. b. Supracondylar fracture.

Malunion is the ***commonest*** complication of supracondylar fracture.
This malunion results in ***cubitus varus*** deformity and ***Hyperextension*** of elbow joint.
The cubitus varus may be sometimes termed as ***Gunstock deformity.***

33. Ans. d. Baumann's angle *Ref: Apley's System of Orthopedics and fractures, 9/e p758 -759, fig 24.30*

The supracondylar fracture of humerus is seen ***clearly in the lateral view.***
Lateral view: In undisplaced fracture, look for the ***'fat pad sign'***
- There is a triangular lucency in front of the distal humerus, due to the fat pad being pushed forwards by a haematoma.

AP view: The fracture line is difficult to make out. In this case, measurement of ***Baumann's angle*** is helpful.

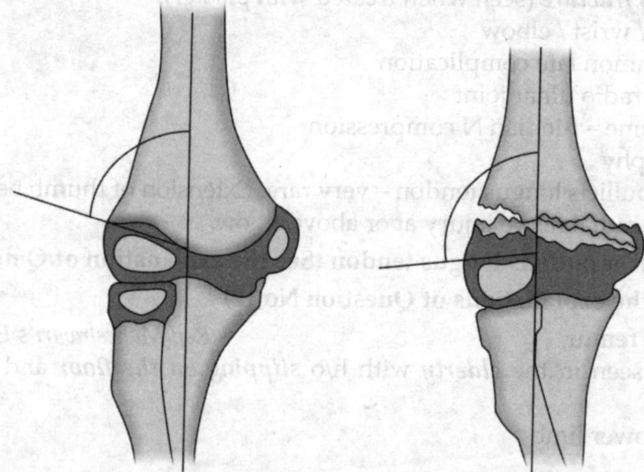

Fig. 19.69: Baumann's angle

BAUMANN'S ANGLE: This angle produced by lines, one by the longitudinal axis of the humeral shaft and a line through the coronal axis of the capitellar physis.
- Normally this angle is ***less than 80 degrees.***
- If the angle is more, cubitus varus deformity is the most likely result.

34. Ans. c. Fracture of proximal 1/3 of ulna with dislocation of proximal radioulnar joint.

Ref: Maheshwari's Essential Orthopedics, 4/e p106

Monteggia fracture: this is a fracture of upper third of ulna with dislocation of head of radius (proximal radio ulnar joint)
It is caused by fall on outstretched hand.

35. Ans. a. Scapula *Ref: Maheshwari's Essential Orthopedics, 4/e*

- Page 111. Blood supply of scaphoid is precarious. In fractures through the waist, there is high probability of the ***proximal fragment*** becoming avascular necrosis.
- Page 160. Talus: because of poor blood supply, after a fracture through the neck, the ***body of talus*** becomes avascular necrosis.
- Page 134. Femur: After a fracture through the neck, all the blood supply to the head are cut off. Because of this, ***avascular necrosis of femoral head*** occurs.

(It is femoral neck fracture that causes AVN of femoral head)

36. Ans. b. Median nerve *Ref: Apley's System of Orthopedics and Fractures, 9/e p288*

Common entrapment neuropathies:

- Carpal tunnel syndrome : Median nerve
- Pronator syndrome : Median nerve
- Ulnar Tunnel Syndrome (Guyon canal) : Ulnar nerve at wrist
- Cubital tunnel syndrome : Ulnar nerve at elbow
- Thoracic outlet syndrome : C8 and T1 roots
- Tarsal Tunnel Syndrome : Tibial nerve
- Meralgia pareasthetica : Lateral cutaneous nerve of thigh
- Chiralgia parasthetica : Superficial radial nerve
- Piriformis syndrome : Sciatic nerve

37. Ans. d. Tuberculosis *Ref: Apley's System of Orthopedics and Fractures, 9/e p288*

In the normal carpal tunnel there is barely room for all the tendons and the median nerve; consequently, any swelling is likely to result in compression and ischaemia of the nerve. The carpal tunnel syndrome is, common at the ***menopause, in rheumatoid arthritis, pregnancy and myxoedema.***

38. Ans. b. Anterior interosseous nerve *Ref: Pediatric Orthpaedic Secrets, 3/e p176*

Any of the three major nerves (median n, radial n, ulnar n) may be injured in supracondylar fractures. Among them, the ***anterior interosseus nerve*** (a branch of median nerve) is probably the most commonly injured nerve. This branch of median nerve stimulates muscles that flex interphalangeal joints of index finger and thumb. (When the index finger fails to flex, it is called ***Pointing index***)

39. Ans. b. Supracondylar fracture of humerus

Explanation: See the Ans. for Q no 3. *Ref: Maheshwari's Essential Orthpaedics, 4/e p65, see fig 10-7*

40. Ans. a. Radial nerve *Ref: Maheshwari's Essential Orthpaedics, 4/e p91*

The radial nerve is the most commonly injured nerve in a fracture of the shaft of humerus.

Generally, it is neuropraxia type only (means, very good recovery is expected)

The nerve injury can happen at the time of fracture, during manipulation or while the fracture heals by callus (nerve gets trapped by the callus).

The radial nerve injury results in ***paralysis of wrist/thumb/finger extensions.*** The brachioradialis and supinator may also be paralyzed.

41. Ans. b. Supracondylar fracture *Ref: Maheshwari's Essential Orthpaedics, 4/e p97, 101*

The median nerve is the most commonly injured nerve in supracondylar fractures. Elbow dislocation can also cause median nerve injury.

42. Ans. a. Axillary nerve

Ref: Apley's System of Orthopedics and Fractures, 9/e p743, 281

Inferior dislocation (*luxatio erecta*) is rare but it demands early recognition because the consequences are potentially very serious. Dislocation occurs with the arm in nearly full abduction/elevation. The humeral head is levered out of its socket and pokes into the axilla; the arm remains fixed in abduction.

The associated soft-tissue injury includes avulsion of the capsule and surrounding tendons, rupture of muscles, fractures of the glenoid or proximal humerus and ***damage to the brachial plexus and axillary artery.***

The axillary nerve (C5, 6) arises from the posterior cord of the brachial plexus and runs along subscapularis and across the axilla just inferior to the shoulder joint. The nerve is sometimes ruptured in a ***brachial plexus injury***. More often it is injured during ***shoulder dislocation or fractures of the humeral neck.***

43. Ans. b. Lateral cutaneous nerve of thigh

Ref: Maheshwari's Essential Orthpaedics, 4/e p296

In meralgia paresthetica, there is tingling/burning/numbness in the skin supplied by the lateral cutaneous nerve of thigh as it gets entrapped in the fascia just medial to anterior superior iliac spine.

44. Ans. b. Cubitus valgus

Ref: Maheshwari's Essential Orthpaedics, 4/e p100

Diminished growth of lateral humeral condyle results in cubitus valgus deformity. This may result in tardy ulnar nerve palsy.

45. Ans. d. Flexion and Rotation

Ref: Maheshwari's Essential Orthopedics 4/e p146

Mechanism of Meniscal Injury:

Injury happens when ***twisting a semi-flexed knee***. During this movement, ***rotation occurs between condyles of femur and tibia.***

Medial meniscus gets torn more often because it is ***less mobile*** as it is fixed to MCL.

46. Ans. a. Prepattellar bursa

47. Ans. c. Infrapatellar bursa

Ref: Apley's Sytem of Orthopedics and fractures, 9/e p578

48. Ans. is b. Anterior cruciate ligament tear

49. Ans. is c. Meniscal tear

Ref: Maheshwari's Essential Orthopedics 4/e p146

The presenting complaints are recurrent episodes of pain and locking of the knee.

LOCKING: It is of two types: True and pseudo-locking.

- **True locking:** rare, occurs when an intra-articular structure, loose body or meniscal tear interposes between the femoral condyle and tibial surface. Classically the patient loses terminal extension but is able to flex the knee.
- **Pseudo-locking**: more common, seen in patients with patellar disorders. Here, the knee extension is difficult because of pain, not because of mechanical block. Pseudolocking occurs after prolonged sitting or when coming downstairs, e.g ***chondromalacia of patella.***

50. Ans. d. Bucket handle tear of medial meniscus

Ref: Maheshwari's Essential Orthopedics 4/e p146

- ***Medial meniscus*** is ***more commonly injured***, as it is less mobile because of its attachment with medial collateral ligament.
- The meniscus is torn most commonly at its ***posterior horn,*** and then the tear extends anteriorly.
- ***Bucket-handle tear*** is the commonest type.

51. Ans. c. Lachman test.

Ref: Apley's Sytem of Orthopedics and fractures, 9/e p551

Anterior drawer test and Lachman's test are done to test ACL injury.

- Lachman's test is more sensitive than anterior drawer test.

More over, to perform anterior drawer test, knee flexion to 90 deg is needed; flexion to 90deg is very painful in freshly injured patients.

- In Lachman's test, flexion of about 15-30 deg is enough to perform this test, hence it is preferred.

52. Ans. a. Flexor tendon sheath infectious inflammation in hand

Ref: http://www.wheelessonline.com/ortho/kanavels_four_cardinal_signs.

Kanavel's Four Cardinal Signs: for diagnosing infectious ***tenosynovitis of flexor tendons***. (i.e acute suppurative tenosynovitis)

- Intense pain: accompanies any attempt to extend partly flexed finger
- Flexion posture: finger is held in flexion for comfort;
- Uniform swelling: involving entire finger in contrast to localized swelling in local inflammation
- Percussion tenderness: along the course of the tendon sheath.

53. Ans. d. All of the above. *Ref: Maheshwari's Essential Orthopedics 4/e p295*

Painful arc syndrome: is pain in the shoulder during the mid range of abduction of shoulder.

The common causes are:

- Minor tears of supraspinatous tendon
- Supraspinatous tendinitis
- Subacromial bursitis
- Fracture of greater tuberosity.

54. Ans. b. Avulsion of extensor tendon

Ref: Apley's Sytem of Orthopedics and fractures, 9/e p418

MALLET FINGER results from ***injury to the extensor tendon*** of the terminal phalanx.

It is treated by splintage with the ***DIP joint in extension*** for 6 weeks.

55. Ans. b. Tom Smith's arthritis

Ref: Adam's Outline of Orthopedics, 14/e p355

Pyogenic arthritis of infants is seen in children of less than one year of age with a known septic foci such as ***umbilical infection***. Clinically, the child becomes unwell and pyrexial.

Hip movements are restricted. Ultrasound scanning may show ***distention of the hip joint***. In late cases, head of femur (capital epiphysis) gets destroyed by the infectious process, so the xray will show ***absence of head of femur***.

56. Ans. d. Osteopenia

Ref: Maheswaris's Essential Orthopedics, 4/e p191.

Haziness (Osteopenia) around the hip is the earliest sign.

Reduction of joint space occurs because of destruction of cartilage.

57. Ans. d. TB of hip

Ref: Maheswaris's Essential Orthopedics, 4/e p191

Wandering acetabulum/Travelling acetabulum are seen in subluxation/dislocation stage of tuberculosis of hip joint.

In the Dislocation stage, the head of femur may be lying out of the acetabulum in a ***pseudo acetabulum*** (i.e wandering acetabulum) of the ilium.

In some cases, the acetabulum may simply gets enlarged and deepened; it gives a ***mortar and pestle appearance.***

58. Ans. c. Increased resistance to pathological fractures

Ref: Apley's System of Orthopedics and fractures, 9/e p137, 138

Osteomalacia: Changes common to almost all types of vitamin D related rickets and osteomalacia are

- Diminished levels of serum calcium and phosphate,
- Increased alkaline phosphatase
- Diminished urinary excretion of calcium.

In osteomalacia: There is ***spontaneous fractures*** of the ribs, pubic rami, femoral neck or the metaphyses above and below the knee.

59. Ans. C. Absence/rarity of pathological fractures *Ref: Apley's System of Orthopedics and fractures, 9/e p137, 138*

The classical lesion of *osteomalacia* is ***the Looser zone,*** a thin transverse band of rarefaction. These zones, are due to ***incomplete stress fractures*** which heal with callus lacking in calcium.

- Spine will show biconcave vertebrae (from disc pressure),
- Pelvis: lateral indentation of the acetabula produce a trefoil pelvis.
- Spontaneous (pathological) fractures of the ribs, pubic rami, femoral neck can occur.

60. Ans. d. Osteopetrosis *Ref: Maheshwari's Essential Orthopedics, 4/e p304, Table 37.4*

Conditions causing increased density of bone:

- Fluorosis
- Osteopetrosis
- Paget;s disease of bone
- Renal osteodystrophy
- Secondaries from Prostate malignancy
  - *Osteoporosis:* a decrease in bone mass
  - *Osteomalacia:* insufficient mineralization of bone.
  - Hyperparathyroidism increases bone resorption and thereby reduces the mass of the bone.

61. Ans. d. Osteopetrosis. (See previous Question 3's explanation.)

Osteopenia: Used to describe an ill-defined loss of radiographic density of bone. It can signify either osteomalacia/rickets or osteoporosis.

62. Ans. d. All of the above *Ref: Apley's System of Orthopedics and fractures, 9/e p136*

Some points about the Rickets:

- Thickening of the knees, ankles and wrists due to physeal overgrowth.
- Enlargement of the costochondral junctions ('rickety rosary')
- Lateral indentation of the chest (Harrison's sulcus)
- Thickening and widening of the growth plate, cupping of the metaphysis
- Diminished levels of serum calcium and phosphate
- Increased Alkaline Phosphatase and diminished urinary excretion of calcium

63. Ans. a. Interroseous membrane ossification *Ref: Maheshwari's Essential Orthopedics, 4/e p304*

Fluoride directly stimulates the osteoblastic activity and formation of fluorapatite crystals (which are resistant to osteoclastic resorption)

And thereby, it ***increases the bone density***.

Fluorosis: Results from excessive ingestion fluoride in drinking water. Excessive ***deposition of calcium occurs in bone and soft tissues.*** This results in calcifications of various ligaments. They are:

- Spine: Posterior longitudinal ligament
- Pelvis: Ischio-pubic and sacro-iliac ligaments
- Forearm: ***interosseus membrane***.

64. Ans. b. Congenital dislocation of hip *Ref: Adam's Outline of Orthopedics, 14/e p348. See fig. 17.15*

In CDH, moderate abduction and flexion of hips will reduce the dislocation. To maintain this position in children < 6 months of age, the following splints are used.

Von Rosen Splint: Old method, rigid.

Pavlik harness: New method, more flexible, adjustable, more frequently used.

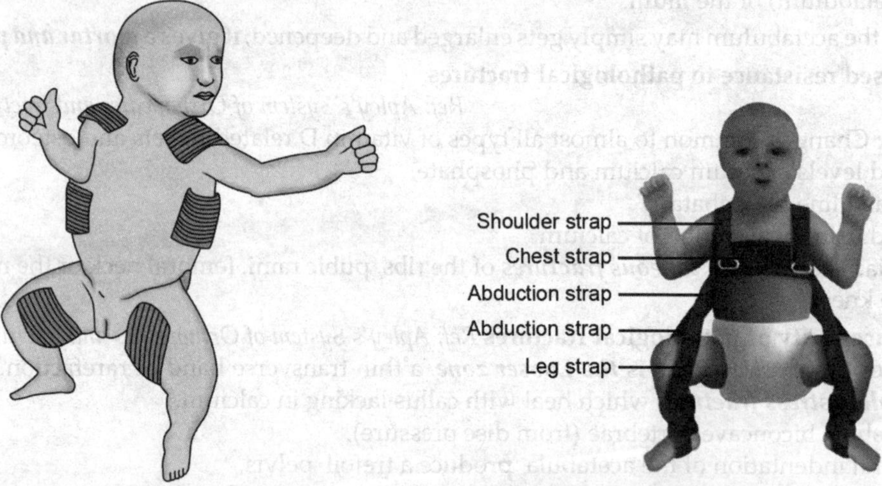

Figs 19.70 (A and B): A. Von Rosen splint; B. Pavlik harness

65. Ans. b. Thomas test *Ref: Adam's Outline of Orthopedics, 14/e p338. See fig 17.7*

Fixed flexion deformity of hip is determined by Thomas test.

If there is a fixed flexion deformity of hip joint, during lying down position, this deformity is masked by arching of spine and pelvis, i.e the deformity is hidden by lordosis of lumbar spine.

Thomas test will reveal this hidden deformity by flexing the normal hip.

66. Ans. b. Diagnozed radiologically at birth.

Ref: Adam's Outline of Orthopedics, 14/e p61; Apley's System of Orthopedics and Fractures, 9/e p163

Achondroplasia: an ***autosomal dominant*** inheritance. The length of the limbs are only half their normal length, where as the growth of ***spine (trunk) is only slightly affected***. Achondroplasia is ***apparent at birth.***

This is the commonest form of short stature.

Disproportionate shortening of the limb bones is ***detectable in utero by ultrasound scan.***

The abnormality is ***obvious in childhood.***

No mental retardation, the life span is usually normal.

67. Ans. a. Athlete's foot *Ref: Apley's System of Orthopedics and Fractures, 9/e p596, 597*

Flat Foot (Pes Planus): The longitudinal arch of the foot is reduced.

Two types:

- **Flexible flat foot:** Normal in children, women, and people with ligament laxity, obesity.
- **Rigid flat foot:** here, the deformity that cannot be corrected passively.
  - Congenital vertical talus
  - Tarsal coalition (peroneal spastic flat-foot)
  - Inflammatory arthritis
  - Neurological disorders
- Painful acquired flat-foot (tibialis posterior dysfunction)

Jack's test: to distinguish between flexible and rigid flat foot deformity.

Pes Cavus (High-Arched Feet):

The arch is higher than normal, and often there is also clawing of the toes. The causes are:

Muscular dystrophies	:	Duchenne, Becker
Neuropathies	:	HMSN I and II
Cord lesions	:	Poliomyelitis, syringomyelia, diastomatomyelia, tethered cord syndrome
Cerebral disorders	:	Cerebral palsy, Friedreich's ataxia

68. Ans. d. Peroneal muscles. *Ref: Maheshwari's Essential Orthopedics, 4/e p205, 206*

The following structures are tight in CTEV:

- Contracture of Achillis (producing equinus)
- Contracture of Tibialis posterior (producing Inversion)
- Plantar fascia.

Weakness of peroneal muscles (and/or Contracture of Tibialis posterior) ***will produce inversion.***

69. Ans. b. Gluteus medius. *Ref: Maheshwari's Essential Orthopedics, 4/e p348*

Trendlenberg's test is to examine the stability of abductor mechanism of the hip joint.

The following are the causes of weakening the abductor mechanism.

- Hip dislocation
- Loss of femoral head
- Neck of femur fracture
- Paralysis of abductor muscle – gluteus medius.

70. Ans. b. SCFE (Slipped Capital Femoral Epiphysis) *Ref: Maheshwari's Essential Orthopedics, 4/e p313*

Slipped Capital Femoral Epiphysis:

- Seen **more commonly in over weight children of 12-14 years of age.**
- **There may be a h/o trauma, pain in the groin.**
- **There** is limitation of abduction and internal rotation.

71. Ans. b. Blount's disease *Ref: A Practical Guide to Paediatric Emergency Medicine, Jamie Shandro, p486*

In Blount's disease, there is

- Varus deformity
- Limping
- Waddling gait
- Siffert-Katz sign: posteromedial instability of knee on mild flexion.

72. Ans. b. Manipulation and corrective splint *Ref: Adam's Outline of Orthopedics, 14/e p436*

Treatment of CTEV is by ***Ponseti technique***. The principles are

- To correct the deformity by manual pressure

- To hold / maintain the correction by plaster cast or by ***Denis Browne splint***.

If the casting and splintage fail to correct, then operative correction is carried out.

73. Ans. c. Increased dorsiflexion *Ref: Maheshwari's Essential Orthopedics, 4/e p205*

The components of CTEV are:
- Equinus (***Increased plantar flexion***)
- Inversion (the sole of the foot faces medially)
- Mid foot Cavus (showing excessive concavity)
- Forefoot is adducted
- Heel Varus (heel is tilted medially)

74. Ans. d. Osteogenesis Imperfecta *Ref: Apley's System of Orthopedics and Fractures, 9/e p172*

Osteogenesis Imperfecta (Brittle Bone Disease or Fragilitas Ossium)

Abnormal synthesis and structural defects of type I collagen result in abnormalities of:
- The bones
- Teeth
- Ligaments
- Sclerae and
- Skin.

The defining clinical features are:
- Osteopenia
- Liability to fracture
- Laxity of ligaments
- Blue coloration of the sclerae
- Dentinogenesis imperfecta ('crumbling teeth').

The most striking abnormality is ***the propensity to fracture***, generally after minor trauma.

X-rays:
- Generalized osteopenia
- Thinning of the long bones
- ***Fractures in various stages of healing***
- Vertebral compression and spinal deformity.
- The skull: may be enlarged and shows the presence of ***wormian bones – areas of vicarious ossification in the calvarium.***

75. Ans. b. Primitive neuroectodermal bone tumor *Ref: Campbell's Operative Orthopedics, 12/e p789*

Epiphyseal tumors:

In skeletally mature patient: giant cell tumor,

In a skeletally immature patient: chondroblastoma.

Diaphyseal tumors:

Ewing sarcoma,
Histiocytosis,
Lymphoma,
Fibrous dysplasia,
Adamantinoma (especially in the tibia).

Ewing's sarcoma is a primitive neuroectodermal tumor.

76. Ans. a. Metaphysis *Ref: Maheshwari's Essential Orthopedics, 4/e p241*

Osteochondroma arises from the growth plate and presents as a mass at ***metaphysis***.

It is a result of an aberration at the growth plate.

77. Ans. b. Osteoid osteoma *Ref: Apley's System of Orthopedics and Fractures, 9/e p196*

Osteoid osteoma:

Patients are usually under 30 years of age.

Most cases occur in the ***diaphysis of femur or tibia***.

Typically the pain is ***relieved by salicylates.***

X-ray shows a small radiolucent area, the so-called ***'nidus'***. This nidus is surrounded by dense sclerosis and cortical thickening;

The nidus can be seen only in fine cut ***CT scans.***

The only effective treatment is ***complete removal or destruction of the nidus***

78. Ans. a. Osteosarcoma *Ref: Campbell's Operative Orthopedics, 12/e p912 and 919*

Skip metastasis is metastasis within the same bone as the primary tumor or across the joint from primary tumor. The prognosis is same as that of distant metastasis. Skip ***(bone to bone)*** metastasis is seen in osteosarcoma. Skip metastasis is ***not reported*** in Ewing's sarcoma.

79. Ans. b. Giant cell tumor *Ref: Apley's System of Orthopedics and Fractures, 9/e p202*

Giant-cell tumor: is a lesion of uncertain origin

It appears in ***epiphysis*** of adult female,

Most commonly in the distal femur, proximal tibia and distal radius.

X-rays show a radiolucent ***eccentrically*** located lytic area with the cortex is thin and sometimes ballooned; this is seen as ***soap-bubble appearance.***

80. Ans. c. Myositis ossificans

Ref: Maheshwari's Essential Orthopedics, 4/e p51, Adam's Outline of Orthopedics, 14/e p156

Myositis ossificans (post traumatic ossification) is ossification of hematoma, resulting in formation of bone.

It is particularly common ***around the elbow joint.***

Massage is known to aggravate myositis.

It presents as a painful and tender ***lump in the muscle.***

CT will show rim of ***ossification at the peripheral zone*** of the lesion.

81. Ans. b. Ewing's sarcoma, c. Osteosarcoma *Ref: Campbell's Operative Orthopedics, 12/e p882*

Osteomyelitis can simulate tumors such as:

- Ewing sarcoma,
- Osteosarcoma,
- Osteoid osteoma,
- Eosinophilic granuloma.

82. Ans. b. Multiple enchondromas

Ref: Maheshwari's Essential Orthopedics, 4/e p241, Apley's System of Orthopedics and Fractures, 9/e p197

Maffucci syndrome is a hereditary disorder where ***multiple enchondromas and soft tissue hamagiomas*** occur together.

Risk of malignant change:

- Less than 2 per cent in single enchondroma
- 30 per cent in Ollier's disease (multiple enchondromas)
- Up to 100 per cent in Maffucci's syndrome.

83. Ans. c. Malignant cells with osteoid formation *Ref: Campbell's Operative Orthopedics, 12/e p909*

In osteosarcoma, the periosteal reaction may take the form of ***"Codman's triangle," or a "sunburst" or "hair on end"*** appearance.

Histologically, the osteosarcoma may be osteoblastic, fibroblastic, or chondroblastic; however, ***osteoid production from the tumor cells must be shown*** to confirm the diagnosis.

84. Ans. a. Aneurysmal bone cyst *Ref: Apley's System of Orthopedics and Fractures, 9/e p201-203*

Aneurysmal Bone Cyst:

Seen in young adults and in the long-bone ***metaphysis.***

X-rays show a well-defined radiolucent and ***eccentrically*** placed cyst.

With ***expanding lesions,*** patients may complain of pain.

Occasionally it causes ***marked ballooning*** of the bone end.

Well-defined radiolucent cyst, often eccentric within bone.

Marked ***'soap-bubble' expansion*** may be seen. *(A–Z of Musculoskeletal and Trauma Radiology, 2008/e p7, Rakesh R. Misra, Cambridge University Press)*

GIANT CELL TUMOR:

X-rays show a radiolucent area situated ***eccentrically*** at the end of a long bone ***(epiphysis)*** and bounded by the subchondral bone plate.

The centre sometimes has a ***soap-bubble appearance*** due to ridging of the surrounding bone.

- Soap-Bubble appearance: In epiphysis → Giant cell tumor
  In metaphysis → Aneurysmal bone cyst

85. Ans. b. Prostate.

Ref: Campbell's Operative Orthopedics, 12/e p930; Apley's System of Orthopedics and Fractures, 9/e p216

The radiographic appearance of metastatic carcinoma varies.

The lesions may be ***lytic, blastic, or mixed***.

Breast cancer and prostate cancer typically produce ***blastic*** lesions.

Kidney cancer and thyroid cancer usually are purely ***lytic lesions***.

Lung cancer may produce a mixed appearance.

The commonest source is carcinoma of the ***breast***; next in frequency are carcinomas of the ***prostate, kidney, lung, thyroid, bladder and gastrointestinal tract***. In about 10 per cent of cases no primary tumor is found.

The commonest sites for bone metastases are the ***vertebrae, pelvis, the proximal half of the femur and the humerus***. Spread is usually via the blood stream; occasionally, visceral tumors spread directly to adjacent bones (e.g. ***the pelvis or ribs***).

86. Ans. a. Ewing's sarcoma *Ref: Campbell's Operative Orthopedics, 12/e p798*

Most primary bone malignancies are relatively radioresistant.

The radiosensitive tumors are

- Multiple myeloma
- Lymphoma
- Ewing sarcoma.

87. Ans. d. All of the above *Ref: Apley's System of Orthopedics and Fractures, 9/e p91*

The cardinal radiographic signs of OA are:

- Asymmetrical loss of cartilage (narrowing of the 'joint space'),
- Sclerosis of the subchondral bone under the area of cartilage loss,
- Cysts close to the articular surface,
- Osteophytes at the margins of the joint
- Remodelling of the bone ends on either side of the joint.
- Late features may include joint displacement and bone destruction.

Microscopically, there is increase in water content of the cartilage and in later stage there is loss of proteoglycans. Progressive cartilage deformation and destruction is the primary feature. Loose bodies are also seen in osteoarthritis.

88. Ans. c. Ankylosis of small joints *Ref: Apley's System of Orthopedics and Fractures, 9/e p72*

The patterns of joint involvement in Psoriatic arthritis include:

- Arthritis of distal interphalangeal joints,
- Arthritis mutilans
- Asymmetrical large joint oligoarthritis
- Patterns mimicking rheumatoid arthritis or ankylosing spondylitis.

Arthritis mutilans: in psoriatic arthritis,the fingers and toes are severely deformed due to erosion and instability of the interphalangeal joints.

Sacroiliitis and spondylitis are seen in about one-third of patients, and occasionally this is the predominant change with a clinical picture resembling ankylosing spondylitis.

- Ankylosis of vertebrae and Telescoping of small joints are seen.

89. Ans. c. Ankylosing spondylitis *Ref: Apley's System of Orthopedics and Fractures, 9/e p68*

X-ray findings of ankylosing spondylitis:

Sacroiliac joints: The cardinal and the earliest changes are seen in sacroiliac joints: erosion à peri-articular sclerosis and finally à bony ankylosis.

Vertebrae:

- The earliest change is flattening of the normal anterior concavity of the vertebral body('squaring').
- Later, ossification of the ligaments around the intervertebral discs produces delicate bridges ***(syndesmophytes)*** between adjacent vertebrae.
- Bridging at several levels gives the appearance of a ***'bamboo spine'.***

90. Ans. c. Juxta articular osteosclerosis.

Ref: Maheshwari's Essential Orthopedics, 4/e p286; Apley's System of Orthopedics and Fractures, 9/e p92

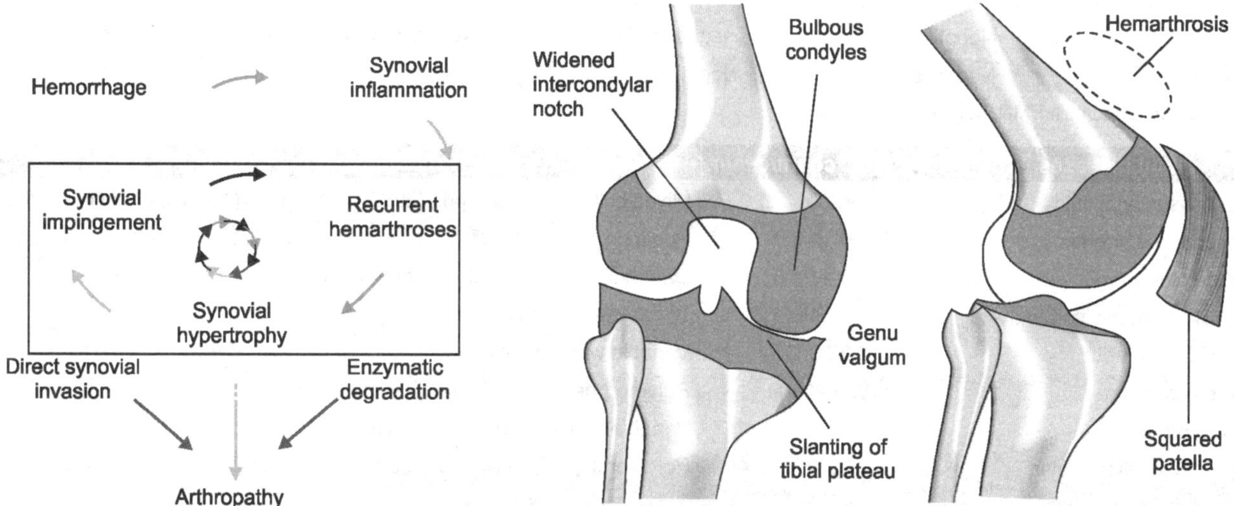

Fig. 19.71: Hemophilic arthropathy

Joints affected commonly are Knee, Elbow, Ankle, shoulder and hip. The changes are bone resorption, cyst formation, osteoporosis, and widening of intercondylar notch.

X-ray changes vary according to the stage of the disorder.

Stage I – soft-tissue swelling;

Stage II – osteoporosis and epiphyseal overgrowth;

Stage III – slight narrowing of the articular space and squaring of the bone ends;

Stage IV – marked narrowing of the articular space;

Stage V – joint disintegration.

Cysts and pseudotumors are rare complications.

91. Ans. a. Osteoarthritis *Ref: Maheshwari's Essential Orthopedics, 4/e p287 and 288*

OA occurs in elderly people.

Mostly major joints (hip in western population, Knee in Asians)of lower limbs are commonly affected.

Pain is the earliest symptom. ***Intermittent pain*** at the beginning and constant pain later stage of OA.

Coarse ***crepitus***, stiffness and swelling of the joints are seen in OA.

92. Ans. d. Neuropathic joint *Ref: Apley's System of Orthopedics and Fractures, 9/e p98*

The most common cause of neuropathic jointis ***diabetes mellitus***. The other causes are: ***tabes dorsalis, leprosy*** (affecting mainly the lower limb joints), ***syringomyelia*** (upper and lower limbs), ***multiple sclerosis, myelomeningocele, spinal cord compression.***

The patient complains of instability, swelling, laxity and progressive deformity of the joint: usually the ***tarsal or ankle joints*** are affected sin diabetics.

93. Ans. c. Granulomatous arthritis *Ref: Apley's System of Orthopedics and Fractures, 9/e p26*

Synovial fluid analysis				
Characteristic/Nature of arthropathy	Normal	Noninflammatory	Inflammatory	Septic
Volume	Low	High	High	High
Appearance	Clear	Clear	Cloudy	Cloudy
Viscosity	High	High	Low	Low (?)
WBC count (/μL)	<200	200-2000	2000-7500	>50,000
% PMN leukocytes	<25%	<50%	<75%	<90%
Crystals	Negative	Negative (?)	Negative/positive	Negative (?)
Culture	Negative	Negative	Negative	Positive
WBC, white blood cell, PMN, polymorphonuclear				

Joint diseases	Total WBC count/c mm	Predmominant cell type
Normal synovial fluid	<200	Mixed cell with polymorphs (20%), lymphocyte (15%) and monocyte (65%)
Rheumatoid arthritis	8500-14500	Polymorphs (65 to 80%)
Tubercular arthritis	5000-12000	Lymphocytes (60 to 80%) with monocytes
Chronic nonspecific Synovitis	500-12000	Variable from polymorphs and lymphocytes
Traumatic arthritis	200-2000	Variable with erythrocytes
Septic arthritis	14000-22000	Polymorphs (30 to 95%)
Osteoarthritis	350	Variable, polymorphs-lymphocytes
Pigmented villonodular synovitis	6500	Polymorphs (40%) with erythrocytes

94. Ans. D, Flexion, adduction, external rotation

Ref: Adam's Outline of Orthopedics, 14/e p361

In OA of hip joint, all hip movements are restricted.

Limitation of abduction, adduction and rotation is marked, whereas good range of flexion is preserved.

Fixed deformity: Flexion, Adduction and Lateral (external) rotation is common.

95. Ans. c. Calcium hydroxylapatite *Ref: Apley's System of Orthopedics and Fractures, 9/e p83, and fig 4.7*

Calcium hydroxyapatite is normal component of bone mineral, in the form of crystals. It also occurs abnormally in dead or damaged tissue.

Minute deposits in joints and periarticular tissues can give rise to either an acute reaction (synovitis or tendinitis) or a chronic, destructive arthropathy.

It affects most notably around the ***shoulder and knee joints.***

96. Ans. a. Lying supine. *Ref: Kineseology, http://www.pt.ntu.edu.tw/hmchai/Kines04/KINspine/Spine.htm*

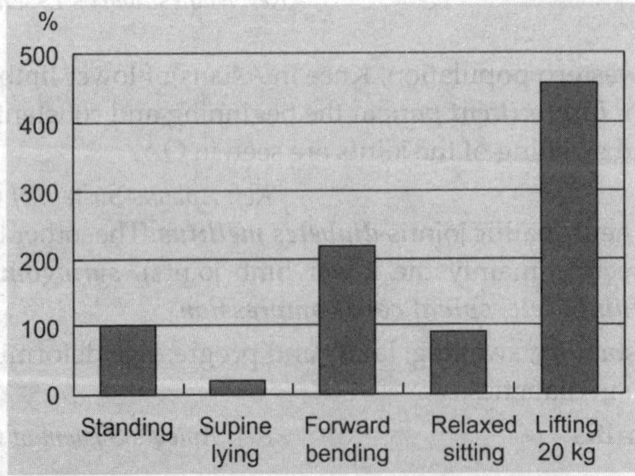

Fig. 19.72: Intradiscal pressure in different postures

97. Ans. a. Lumbar spine commonly involved. *Ref: Apley's System of Orthopedics and Fracture p820*

Whiplash injury: Soft-tissue sprains of the neck ***(Cervical spine)*** occurs due to low velocity ***rear-end collision*** while driving a car. Pain and stiffness of the neck usually appear within the next 12–48 hours. Neck muscles are tender and movements often restricted. Xray will be normal as there is no fracture seen in this condition.

98. Ans. c. Central cord syndrome *Ref: Lippincott Manual of Orthopedics, 7/e p255*

Central cord syndrome is commonly seen in ***hyperextension injury of cervical spine,*** particularly in the elderly age. There will be ***more loss of neurological functions in the upper limb*** than in the lower limbs. This has the best prognosis.

99. Ans. a. Fracture of C1 *Ref: Apley's System of Orthopedics and Fractures, p485*

Sudden severe load on the top of the head may cause a ***'bursting' force which fractures the ring of the atlas (C1)***. Usually, there is no neurological damage. The fracture is seen on the ***open-mouth view***. Treated with rigid cervical orthosis.

100. Ans. a. Defect of pars interarticularis *Ref: Maheshwari's Essential Orthopedics 4/e p217, 277*

Spondylolysis means there is a defect in the pars interarticularis, i.e a defect without slipping of the vertebra. Oblique view of xray shows Scottish dog wearing a collar.

A defect with slipping of vertebra is known as ***Spondylolisthesis,*** here the Scottish dog's neck looks broken in the xray.

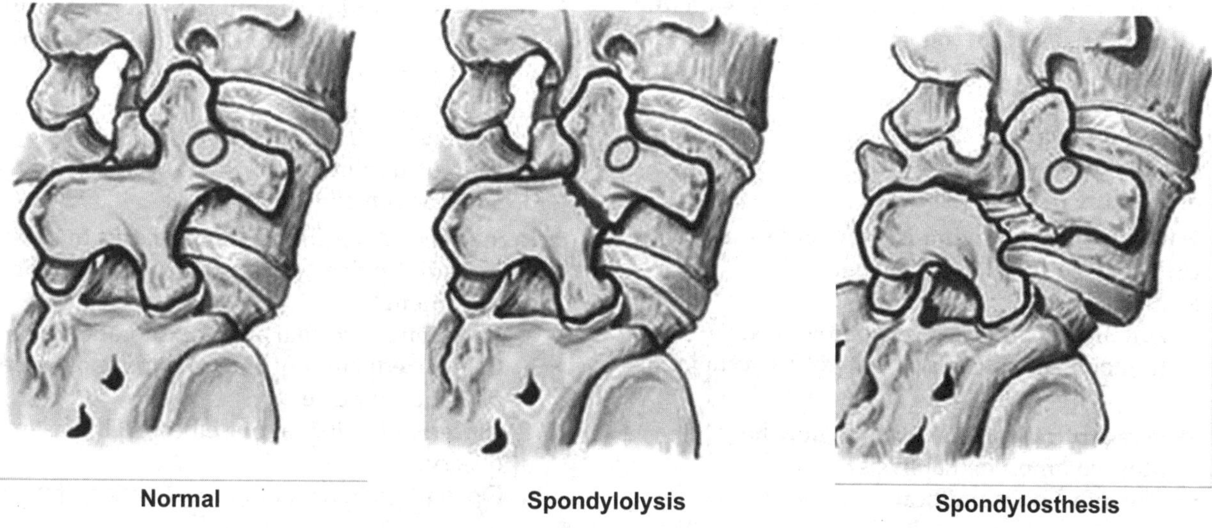

Fig. 19.73: Spondylolysis and spondylosthesis

101. Ans. c. L5 root *Ref: Maheshwari's Essential Orthopedics 4/e p247*

Level	Nerve root affected	Motor weakness
L_5-S_1	S_1 root	Weakness of plantar-flexors of the foot
L_4-L_5	L_5 root	Weakness of EHL* and dorsiflexors of the foot
L_3-L_4	L_4 root	Weakness of extensors of the knee
*EHL: Extensor hallucis longus		

The nerve root affected is usually the one which leaves the spinal canal ***below the next vertebra***. Thus, ***the nerve root affected in a disc prolapse between L4-L5 vertebrae is L5.*** The nerve root affected in Disc Prolapse of L5-S1 is S1.

QUESTIONS 2015

1. **A case of comminuted fracture of tibia presenting with severe pain in the calf on dorsiflexion of the foot. There is also numbness on the sole of foot. Distal pulses are present. What is the probable diagnosis?**
   a. Rupture of achilles tendon
   b. Gastronemius and Soleus muscle tear
   c. Compartment syndrome
   d. ?
2. **Trendelenburg gait is due to:**
   a. Superior gluteal nerve injury
   b. Inferior gluteal nerve injury
   c. Sciatic nerve injury
   d. Femoral nerve injury
3. **A child falls from a chair. Complains of pain in the mid leg. No visible deformity. The is unable to bear his weight on standing. What is the diagnosis?**
   a. Oblique fracture
   b. Spiral fracture
   c. Comminuted fracture
   d. Fracture of epiphysis
4. **Which of the following is true about fracture in children?**
   a. Brittle bone
   b. Angulation and rotation not tolerated
   c. Immobilization leads to fixity of adjacent joints
   d. ??
5. **True regarding osteomyelitis in new born?**
   a. Most common in diaphysis
   b. The infection is unifocal
   c. Organisms are derived from maternal genital tract
   d. ??
6. **Which of the following is true about osteosarcoma?**
   a. Sunburst appearance due to bony involvement
   b. Lung metastasis common
   c. Seen in epiphysis
   d. ??
7. **Which of the following is the investigation of choice for Perthes disease of the bone?**
   a. MRI
   b. CT
   c. X-ray
   d. USG
8. **Which of the following muscles seen on splitting tensor fascia lata during anterolateral approach before hip bone is exposed?**
   a. Gluteus maximus
   b. Gluteus medius
   c. Gluteus minimus
   d. Superor gemelli
9. **In Supracondylar fracture of humerus in children if the radial pulse is absent, what id next line of management?**
   a. Emergency brachial artery exploration
   b. Closed reduction of fracture and look of reappearance of pulse
   c. Closed reduction, above elbow slab plaster and observe
   d. Open reduction and internal fixation of fracture

ANSWERS AND EXPLANATIONS

1. **Ans. c. Compartment Syndrome** *Ref: Apley's System of Orthopedics and fractures, 9/e p713)*

Fractures of Elbow / Forearm / Leg (Tibia) can give rise to bleeding, oedema → **increases the pressure within the compartments** → there is reduced capillary flow → results in muscle ischaemia, further oedema → still greater pressure and more profound ischaemia –This vicious circle ends in **necrosis of nerve and muscle** within the compartment.

In compartment syndrome the ischaemia occurs at the capillary level, so **pulses may still be felt normally.**

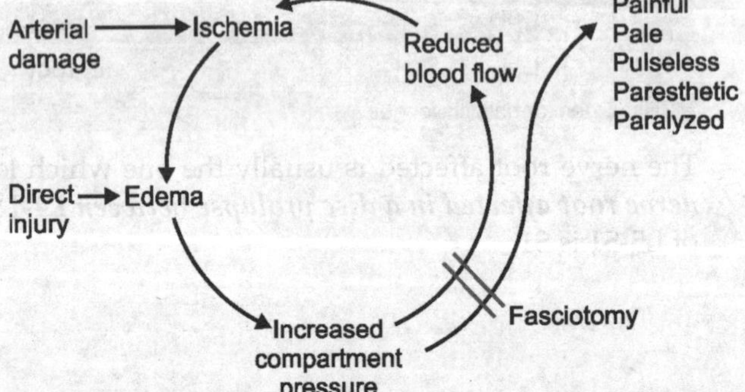

Ischaemic muscle is highly sensitive to stretch, so when the toes or fingers are passively stretched there will be severe pain in the calf or forearm. **(Stretch pain).**

Tibial nerve is affected by the compartment syndrome involving posterior compartment of the leg. When tibial nerve is compressed, it will result in **burning sensation or numbness of the sole.**

Volkmann's ischaemic contracture: Nerve is capable of regeneration but muscle, once infarcted, can never recover and is replaced by fibrous tissue. The end result of untreated compartment syndrome is Volkmann's contracture.

2. **Ans. a. Superior gluteal nerve injury** *Ref: Maheshwari's Essential Orthopedics, 4/e p349*

Trendelenberg gait pattern is seen in cases of weakness of abductor mechanism of the hip joint.

The abductor mechanism comprises:

- The Hip joint
- The Neck of femur
- The abductors of hip (Gluteus medius & minimus)

Disturbance on any one of the above structures such as

- **Hip dislocation**
- **Fracture of neck of femur**
- **Weakness of abductor (polio, nerve palsy)**

May end up in giving rise to a positive Trendelenberg test & gait.

As the gluteus medius & minimus are supplied by Superior Gluteal N, injury to superior gluteal nerve will result in Trendlenberg gait.

3. **Ans. b. Spiral fracture**

Childhood accidental spiral tibial (CAST) fractures are also called as **Toddler's fractures.**

It is named so because of common occurrence in toddlers (aged 9 months-3 years)

- Majority of cases, the fracture is found in the **middle and distal thirds of the tibia.**

Usually the fracture is an undisplaced spiral type of fracture.

- It occurs after **low-energy trauma** such as fall on the floor.

Symptoms include pain, refusing to walk or bear weight

Since the fracture is undiplaced, **deformity is absent.**

Treated by plaster cast.

4. **Ans. b. Angulation and rotation not tolerated** *Ref: Maheshwari's Essential Orthopedics, 4/e p55*

- Children's bones are more malleable, resilient, which allows bowing of the bone without fracture.
- The bones are weaker and can result can absorb more energy before breaking.
- The periosteum is thicker than in adults and usually remains intact on one side of the fracture. (Because of this, Greenstick fracture is common in children).
- This intact periosteum helps stabilize any reduction, decreases the amount of displacement.
- Though the remodeling potential is high in children, excessive varus or valgus angulation and rotational malalignment may not correct so readily.
- Significant angular deformity is cosmetically unacceptable, and it affects the function of the adjacent joints. For this reason, every effort should be made to correct varus or valgus angulation at the time of fracture.

5. **Ans. c. Organisms are derived from maternal genital tract.**

In infants with osteomyelitis, S. aureus is still a frequent causative organism, but group B streptococcus and gram-negative coliforms also are commonly found.

Majority will have **multifocal involvement.**

The **metaphysis** has relatively fewer phagocytic cells and presence tortuous **hairpin loop pattern** of vessels make metaphysis are the **favourite site** for hematogenous osteomyelitis.

The diaphysis rarely is involved in osteomyelitis.

6. **Ans. b. Lung metastasis common** *Ref: Apley's System of Orthopedics and fractures, 9/e p207, 208*

In Osteosarcoma, the **Sunburst effect** is due to streaks of new bone formation radiating outwards from the cortex.

It **most commonly involves the metaphyses** around the knee and at the proximal end of the humerus.

The **lung is the most common sites of metastases.**

7. Ans. a. MRI *Ref: Maheshwari's Essential Orthopedics, 4/e p308, 309*

Perthes' Disease is an osteochondritis of femoral head.

The underlying pathology is **avascular necrosis of head of femur.**

Commonly occurs in boys of 5-10 years of age.

X-ray shows collapse and sclerosis of femoral head.

MRI is the best modality for early diagnosis of avascular necrosis.

8. Ans. b. Gluteus medius *Ref: Campbell's Operative Orthopedics, 12/e*

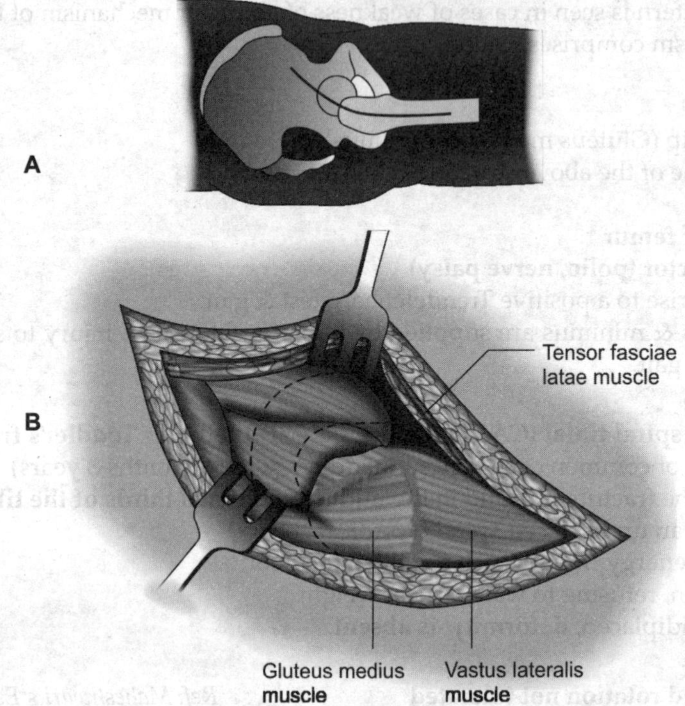

Figs 19.74 (A and B): Gluteus medius and Vastus lateralis

During anterolateral and lateral approach to the hip joint, after splitting the tensor fascia lata, two muscles are seen underneath.

Proximally gluteus medius and distally vastus lateralis.

9. Ans. b. Closed reduction of fracture and look of reappearance of pulse

Ref: Maheshwari's Essential Orthopedics, 4/e p97 flow chart

Supracondylar fracture with suspected vascular injury:

Radial pulse absent → immediate closed reduction.

- If the pulse returns within I hour → maintain with Plaster → Treat routinely viz CRIF with K wires
- If the pulse does not return → with poor circulation → Exploration of vessels and Internal fixation of fracture.

SOME ADDITIONAL POINTS

Eponymous Fractures

- Aviator's Fracture : Fracture of neck of talus
- Barton's Fracture : Intra-articular fracture of distal articular surface of radius
- Bennett's Fracture Dislocation : Oblique intra-articular fracture of first metacarpal with trapezio-metacarpal joint dislocation

- Boer's Fracture : Ventrally displaced fracture through neck of fifth metacarpal
- Bumper Fracture : Comminuted depressed Fracture of lateral tibial condyle
- Buttonhole Fracture : A fracture with loss of bone as in gunshot wound
- Chauffer's Fracture : Oblique radial styloid fracture
- Chance Fracture : Horizontal fracture through vertebra (body, pedicles, laminae) due to sudden deceleration with lap-only seatbelt; usually at L1 or L2
- Clay Shoveller's Fracture : A fracture of spinous process of T1 vertebra
- Colle's Fracture : Fracture occurring in adults at the corticocalcaneal junction of the distal radioulnar joint
- Cough Fracture : Rib (Fifth or seventh) caused by coughing
- Cotton's Fracture : Trimalleolar ankle fracture
- Curbstone Fracture : This avulsion fracture off the posterior tibia is produced by a tripping mechanism.
- Galeazzi Fracture : Fracture of distal third of radius with dislocation of distal radioulnar joint. (synonyms : Reverse Monteggia fracture, piedmont fracture and fracture of necessity)
- Monteggia Fracture : Fracture of proximal third of ulna with anterior dislocation of proximal radioulnar joint.
- Night Stick Fracture : Isolated fracture shaft of ulna
- Gosselin's Fracture : V shaped fracture of distal end of tibia
- Green Stick Fracture : Also called Hickory stick or Willow Fracture. Bending of a bone with incomplete Fracture.
- Jefferson's Fracture : Burst fracture of the Atlas (CI)
- Jone's Fracture : Avulsion fracture of base of fifth metatarsal
- Hangman's Fracture : Traumatic spondylolisthesis of C2 over C3
- March Fracture : Stress fracture of shaft of second of second or third metatarsal
- Pond Fracture : Depressed skull fracture in infants
- Pott's Fracture : Bimalleolar ankle fracture
- Rolando's Fracture : Comminuted intra articular Fracture across the base of the first metacarpal bone.
- Smith's Fracture : Reverse of Colle's fracture
- Tripod Fracture : Trimalar fracture involving the inferior the inferior orbital rim, ateral orbital wall and fracture/dislocation of zygomatic arch.
- Le-Fort-Wagstaffe Fracture : Anterior fibular tubercle avulsion fracture by the anterior tibiofibular ligament, usually associated with Lauge-Hansen SER type fracture patterns
- Malgaigne's Fracture : Sacroiliac disruption with pubic rami fractures
- Maisonneuve Fracture : Fracture of the proximal third of the fibula with an ext ernal rotation type injury.
- Seymour Fracture : Distal phalangeal growth plate fracture.
- Segond Fracture : Seen on AP X-ray (lateral capsular sign) is a capsular avulsion from the lateral tibial metaphysic that is highly associated with ACL disruption.
- Tillaux-Chaput Fracture : Avulsion of anterior tibial margin by the anterior tibiofibular ligament; tibital counterpart of LeForte-Wagstaff fracture.

Condition	Refers to
Forestier's disease	Diffuse idiopathic skeletal hyperostosis (DISH)
Marie-Strumpell disease	Ankylosing Spondylitis
Milwaukee shoulder	Chronic destructive arthritis (calcium hydroxyapatite deposition disorder)
Frozen shoulder	Adhesive Capsulitis, Periarthritis of shoulder.
Otto pelvis	Protrusio acetabuli (arthrokatadysis)
Gorham disease,	Massive osteolysis (disappearing bone disease)
Blount disease	Tibia vara
Genu valgum	Knock knee
Genu varum	Bow leg
Adolescent coxa vara	Slipped capital femoral epiphysis
Housemaid's knee.	Prepatellar Bursitis
Clergyman's knee	Infrapatellar Bursitis

Tests/Signs	Positive in
Yergason test and Speed's test:	Bicep Tendinitis
Popeye sign	Bicep Tendon Rupture
Neer Test, Hawkins Test	Supraspinatus tendinitis (impingement syndrome)
Drop-Arm Test	Rotator cuff (supraspinatus) tear
Belly -press test, Gerber lift-off test	Subscapularis tendinitis
"OK" sign	Anterior interosseous syndrome (due to FPL and FDP of index finger weakness)
Sulcus test	Inferior glenohumeral instability
Light bulb sign	Posterior shoulder dislocation
Adson's test, Wright's test, Roos' test	Thoracic outlet syndrome
Apprehension Test	Recurrent shoulder/patellar dislocation
Phalen's test (wrist flexion test), Durkan carpal compression test, and Tinel's sign	Carpal Tunnel Syndrome
Finkelstein's test	De Quervain's Tenosynovitis
Watson's test	Scapholunate instability
McMurray's test and Apley's test	Meniscal tears
FABER or Patrick test	Sacroiliac joint pathology
Trendelenburg test	Hip abductor mechanism disturbances (hip dislocation, neck of femur fracture, gluteus medius weakness, coxa vara)
Anterior Drawer Test, Lachman Test and Pivot shift test	Anterior cruciate ligament tear
Posterior Drawer Test and Posterior lag test	Posterior cruciate ligament tear
Valgus/Varus Stress Test	Medial/Lateral collateral ligament tears
Ober's Test	Iliotibial band contracture
Thompson's Test (calf muscle squeeze test)	Achilles tendon rupture
Straight-leg raising test	Sciatica
Reverse straight-leg raising test.	Femoral stretch test
Waddell's Signs	Nonorganic etiology of low back pain
Schober test	To assess lumbar flexion (used in ankylosing spondylitis)

Tests/Signs	Positive in
Looser's zones OR milkman's lines OR pseudo-fracture	Osteomalacia
White line of Frankel, Weinberger's line	Scurvy
"too many toes" sign	Pes planus (flat foot)
Terry Thomas sign	Scaphlunate dissociation
Crescent sign	Osteonecrosis of femoral head
Gage sign and Sagging rope sign	Perthes disease

TRACTION METHODS

Name	Usage
Gallow's traction and 90-90 traction	Treatment of fracture shaft of femur in children
Russell's traction	Fracture/dislocation around hip joint
Buck's traction	Other name for skin traction
Dunlop traction and Smith traction	Supracondylar fracture of humerus
Cruchfield traction and Gardner-Wells traction	For cervical spine injury. Applied at the skull bone.
Halo-pelvic traction	Non-operative correction of idiopathic scoliosis (curve <30 deg)

ORTHOSIS (SPLINTS and BRACES)

Name	Usage
von Rosen splint and Pavlik harness	Congenital dislocation of hip (CDH)
Denis-Brown splint	CTEV
Cock-up splint	Wrist drop
Knuckle-bender splint	Claw hand
Thomas splint	For temporary immobilization of fracture of shaft of femur bone.
Airplane splint	Brachial plexus injury
SOMI brace, Philadelphia collar, Four post collar	Cervical spine injury
Taylor's brace	Immobilization of dorsal spine in fracture, TB. etc
ASHE (Anterior Spinal Hyper Extension) brace	Dorsolumbar spinal injury
Milwaukee brace and Boston brace	Nonoperative correction of idiopathic scoliosis
Mermaid splint	For treatment of rickets

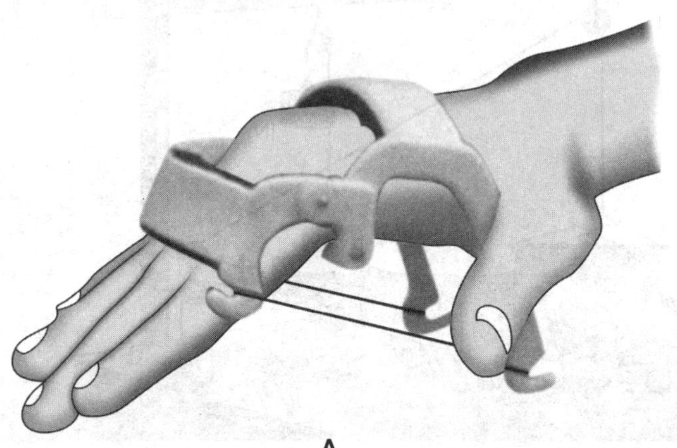

A

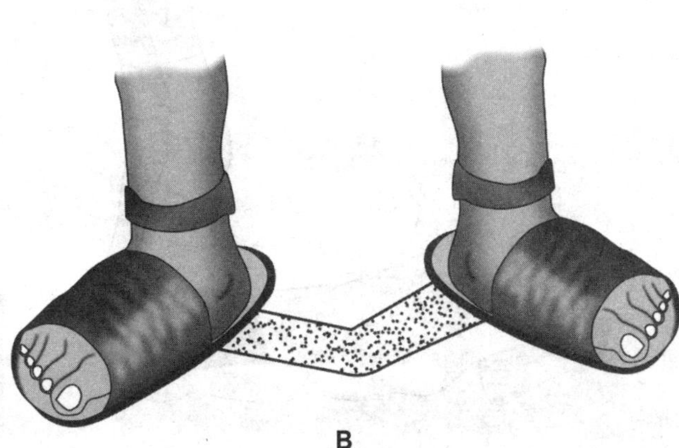

B

Contd...

Contd...

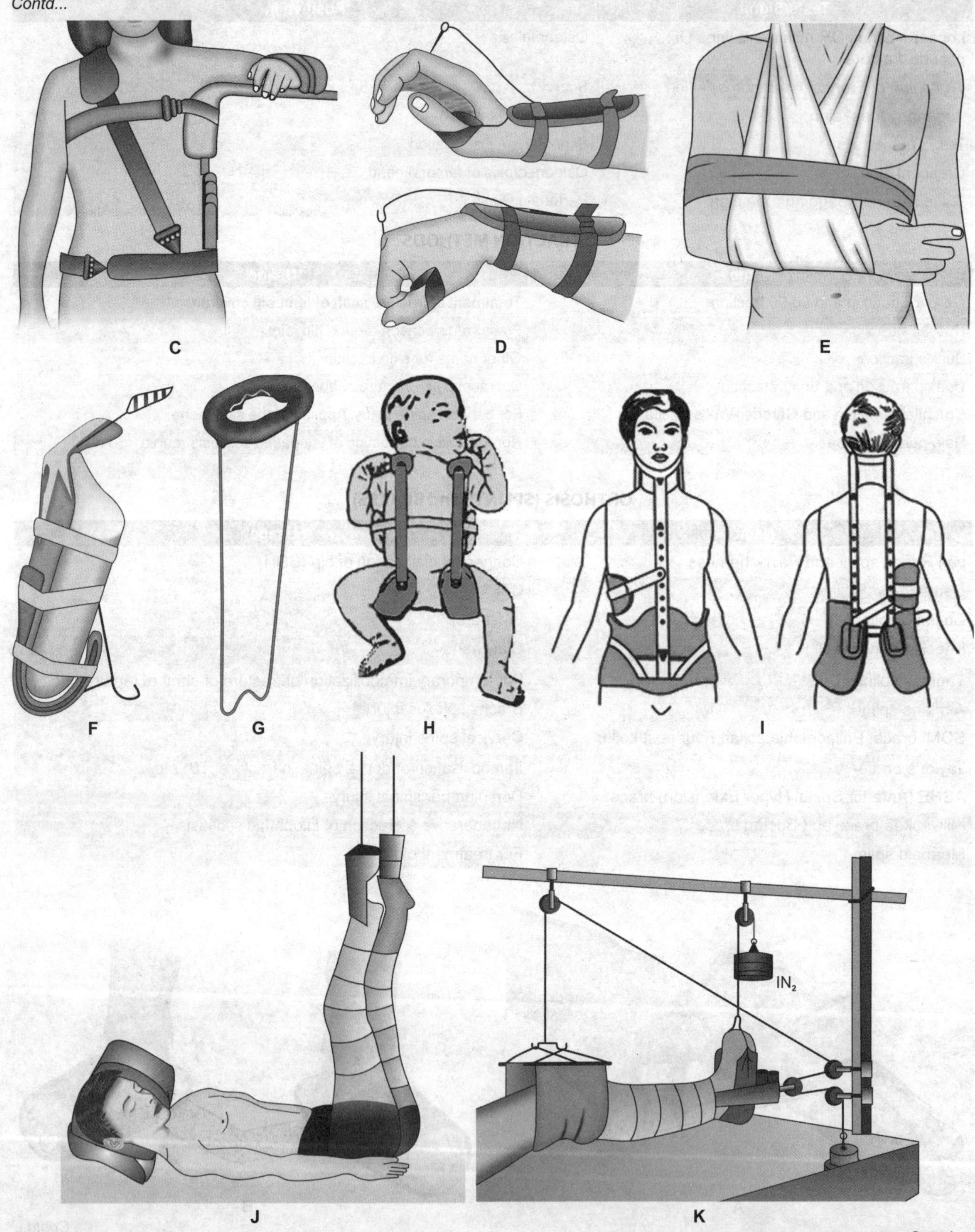

Contd...

Contd...

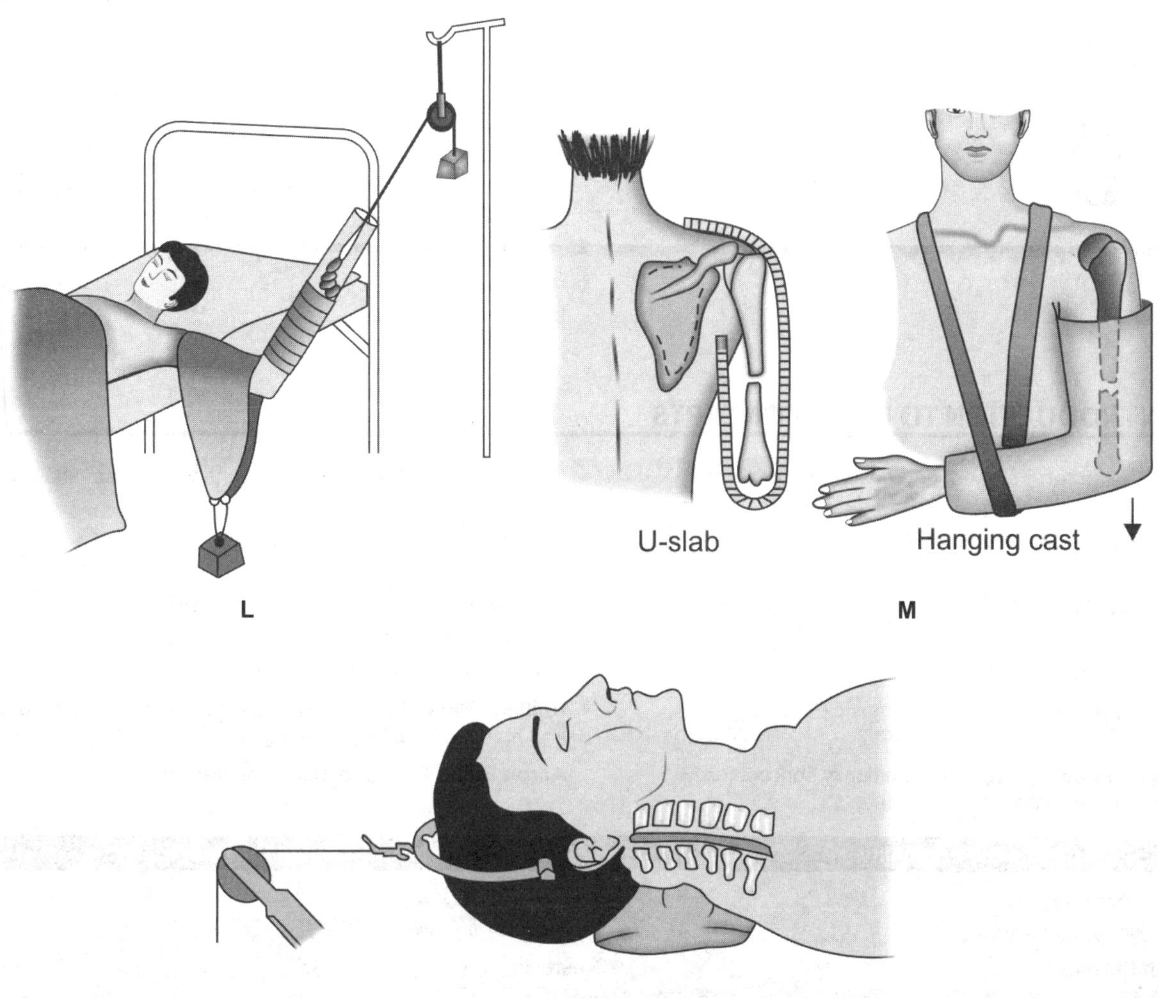

Figs 19.75 (A to N): Orthosis/traction

Name of Orthosis/Traction		Useful conditions
a.	Knuckle bender splint	Claw hand
b.	Dennis-Brown bar	CTEV
c.	Airplane splint	Brachial plexus palsy
d.	Cock-up splint	Wrist drop
e.	Sling and swath	Shoulder immobilization for fracture/dislocation around shoulder
f.	'U' slab	Humeral shaft fracture
g.	Thomas splint	Temporary immobilization of femoral shaft fracture
h.	von Rosen splint	Congenital dislocation of hip
i.	Milwaukee brace	Scoliosis
j.	Gallow's traction	Femoral shaft fracture in children (<2 yrs)
k.	Russell's traction	Immobilization for injury around hip joint
l.	Dunlop traction	Elbow and forearm fracture
m.	U-Slab and Hanging cast	Humeral shaft fracture
n.	Gardner-Wells-tong	Cervical spine injury

Chapter

20 Psychiatry

K Raman

INTRODUCTION TO BASIC CONCEPTS

Franz Alexander: Father of psychosomatic medicine	**Sigmud Freud:** Father of psychoanalysis, dream analysis, and structural model of mind
Franz Jospeh Gall: Founder of phrenology	**Wilhelm Griesinger:** Founder of the specialty of neuropsychiatry
Carl Gustav Jung: Founder of the school of analytical psychology	**Adolf Meyer:** Founder of psychobiology
Benjamin Rush: Father of American psychiatry	**John Broadus Watson:** Founder of behaviorism
Isaac Ray: Father of American forensic psychiatry	**Philippe Pinel:** Abandoned forceful restraints, proposed morale and humane Rx of the mentally ill
Jones Maxwell: Therapeutic community concept for rehabilitation of patients	**Aaron Beck:** Cognitive triad of depression

Personality	Coined the term
Eugen Bleuler	Schizophrenia
James Braid	Hypnosis
William Cullen	Neurosis
Dendy Walter Cooper	Psychotherapy
Karl Kahlbaum	Catatonia, cyclothymia
Jean Esquirol	Hallucination
Ernst von Feuchtersleben	Psychosis
Gockel	Psychology
Reil Johan Christian	Coined the term 'psychiatry' Johann Weyer is known as the Father of Modern Psychiatry
Ewald Hecker	Hebephrenia
Emil Kraeplin	Dementia precox
Sigmund Freud	Free association, Oedipus complex, penis envy, repression, psychoanalysis

Definitions

- **Hallucination:** A false sensory perception occurring in the absence of any external stimulus.
- **Illusion:** Misinterpretation of an external stimulus.
- **Delusion:** False belief, based on incorrect inference about external reality, not consistent with a patient's intelligence and cultural background which cannot be corrected by reasoning. It is a disorder of content of thought.

- **Impulse:** It is a disposition to act to decrease heightened tension caused by the build-up of instinctual drives or by diminished ego defenses against the drive.
- **Obsession:** Recurrent and persistent thought intrudes into conscious awareness, recognized as one's own idea but is ego-alien (foreign to one's personality). He attempts to ignore or suppress it, but is **unable to do**.
- **Compulsion:** Irresistible, repetitive behavior. Failure to resist the acts **aimed at** preventing or reducing the distress, thus leading to marked distress.
- **Depersonalization:** Feeling of detachment from oneself (an individual describes 'as if' experiences) seen in seizures, panic disorder, dissociative disorders, etc.

Disorders of Perception

Types	Features
Hallucination	Perception without stimulus
Illusion/misinterpretation	Misinterpretation of stimuli
Somatic passivity phenomenon	Presence of some external agency with patient being a passive recipient
Depersonalization	Feeling by the person as if the sense of self is strange and unreal
Derealization	Perception of objects in the external world as strange and unreal

Differences between various sensory deceptions:

Hallucination	Pseudohallucination	Imagery
Objective space	Subjective space	Subjective space
Clear, vivid	Not vivid	Not clear
Constant	Inconstant	Inconstant
Life like quality—Present	Absent	Absent
Independent of will	Independent of will	Dependent on will
No insight	Partial insight	Preserved insight

Disorders of Thought

Psychopathology	Thought disorder
Obsession	Egodystonic and ego alien ideas (disorder of possession of thought)
Phobia	Irrational fear
Delusion	False unshakable beliefs (disorder of content of thought)
Schizophrenia	Ideas/delusion of persecution Tangentiality, loosening of association (form of thought)
Mania	Ideas/delusion of grandeur Flight of ideas (form of thought)
Depression	Nihilistic ideas Poverty of thought (stream of thought)
Hypochondriasis	Preoccupied with thought of illness (overvalued idea)

Catatonia

- The concept of catatonia was formulated and named by the German clinician Karl Kahlbaum.
- Catatonia is a *syndrome of specific motor abnormalities.*
- Can occur in *major depressive disorder, schizophrenia.* Catatonia can also be caused by a variety of *medical conditions.*

Main features of catatonia

- Mutism
- Stupor

- Negativism
- Posturing
- Waxy flexibility
- Excitement

Stereotypy: *Nongoal-directed, repetitive motor behavior*. The repetition of phrases and sentences in an automatic fashion, similar to a scratched record, termed *verbigeration*, is a *verbal stereotypy*.

Automatic obedience: Despite instructions to the contrary, the patient permits the examiner's light pressure to move his limbs into a new position.

Ambitendency: The patient appears 'stuck' in an indecisive, hesitant movement.

Echophenomena: Includes echolalia, in which the patient repeats the examiner's utterances, and echopraxia, in which the patient spontaneously copies the examiner's movements.

Mannerisms: Odd, purposeful movements, such as saluting the passersby.

Differences between ICD-10 and DSM-IV

ICD-10	DSM-IV
Alphanumerical coding system	Numerical coding for disorders
Codes for all disorders including mental illness (chapter 5 and code F)	Codes are only for mental illness
Operational and clinical criteria	Operational criteria used for research purposes
Available in various languages and multiple versions such as primary care version, for research, etc.	Available as a single document in English

DSM-V Changes in terminology

- Mental retardation is replaced by intellectual disability
- OCD and stress-related disorders (PTSD) are separated from anxiety disorders
- Pervasive developmental disorder (Autism) is replaced by autism spectrum disroders
- Depression and bipolar disorders are given separate categories rather under mood disorders.

Duration criteria for mental illnesses

- Schizophrenia: 1 month (ICD-10) and 6 months (DSM-5).
- Acute and transient psychosis: <2 weeks (ICD-10); Brief reactive psychosis–1 month (DSM).
- Delusionsal disorder: 3 months
- Major depression: 2 weeks; Dysthymia: 2 years
- Mania: 1 week
- OCD: 2 weeks
- Acute stress reaction: within hours of stressful event and lasts for 2–3 days
- Adjustment disorder: onset of symptoms within 1 month of life event
- PTSD: onset within 6 months of trauma.

Differences between Psychosis and Neurosis

Features	Psychosis	Neurosis
Judgment, insight personality, contact with reality	Lacking or impaired	Present
Delusions/hallucinations	Common	Usually not present

Examples	• Schizophrenia
	• Delusional disorder
	• Mood disorder
	  – Mania
	  – Depression
	  – Dipolar disorder
		• Phobia
		• Dissociative disorder
		• Conversion/somatoform disorder
		• OCD (Obsession-compulsive Disorder)
		• Anxiety: generalized anxiety and panic disorder

Insight: It is defined as the patient's degree of awareness and understanding about being ill. There are 6 grades of insight from denial (grade 1) to intellectual (grade 5) and true emotional insight (grade 6).

Special Investigations in Psychiatry

EEG in delirium: Diffuse slowing except in delirium tremens (normal EEG)

Polysomnography: Includes EEG, EOG, EMG, ECG, respiratory monitoring, pulse oximetry, actigraphy, penile tumescence. It is used to assess nocturnal behaviors, vocalization and snoring during sleep.

Polygraph: Lie detector analyzes pulse rate, BP and galvanic skin changes when a series of questions were asked.

Dexamethasone suppression test: Research tool in depression in the past. If plasma cortisol is more than 5 mg/100 ml following administration of dexamethasone, it indicates nonsuppression.

Pentothal interview: 5% solution of sodium amobarbital (amytal) or thiopentone sodium (pentothal), i.e. 500 mg dissolved in 10 cc of normal saline infused at 1 cc/min. Maximum of 3–7 cc is enough for this procedure (abreaction). **Useful in** hysteria, mute patient, catatonia, differentiate organic from psychogenic stupor.

Lactate provocation test: Sodium lactate infusion provokes a panic attack.

Chromosomal regions in specific disorders

- **Schizophrenia**: Strong evidence for 22q, 5q, 8p, 13q linkage sites. Candidate genes include alpha 7 nicotinic receptor, COMT, mutation of genes dystrobrevin and neureglin.
- **Bipolar disorder:** Chromosome 18, 21q and 22q Alzheimer's dementia–chromosome 1, 14 and 21.
- **Autism:** Chromosome 2, 4, 7q (childhood onset schizophrenia), 15.
- **Tourette's disorder:** Chromosome 13.
- **Narcolepsy**: Chromosome 6.
- **ADHD**: 10q, 12q and 16p.
- **Anticipation**: It is described in schizophrenia and bipolar disorder.

PSYCHIC STRUCTURES

Structural theory of mind: Id (pleasure principle/primary process thinking), ego (reality priniciple/secondary process thinking) and superego (establishes individual's moral conscience based on values internalized from parents). Superego consists of ego ideal (rules and standards for good behaviors) and conscience (information about things that are viewed as bad by parents and society).

Topographical model of mind: Conscious, unconscious and preconscious.

Id: Drives (instincts) present at birth. There are only two drives—sex and aggression.

Ego: Defense mechanisms, judgment, relation to reality, object relationships, developed shortly after birth.

Superego: Conscience, formed during latency period.

Defense Mechanisms

The ways and means by which the **ego** wards off anxiety and controls instinctive urges and unpleasant effects (emotions). Defense mechanisms are—unconscious (except suppression), discrete, dynamic and irreversible, and adaptive and maladaptive.

Defenses used in Various Mental Illnesses

- Psychosis: projection
- Depression: anger turned inside
- Obsessive-compulsive disorder: undoing, isolation and reaction formation
- Phobia: displacement

Commonly used Ego Defense Mechanisms

Defense mechanism	Definition	Examples
• Primary – Repression	Unconscious exclusion from conscious awareness of anxiety-provoking ideas	Forgetting Seen in hysteria or dissociative states
• Psychotic – Regression	Reversion to psychological modes of earlier life stage, especially childhood	Dreams, regression in the service of ego
– Denial	Involuntary exclusion of unpleasant reality from conscious awareness	Grief in 3–6 years-aged children Denial of illness can be seen in psychotic individuals and alcoholics
– Projection	Unconscious attribution of one's own attitude and urges to others	Universal phenomenon Can be seen in psychosis (to explain delusions)
– Distortion	Unconscious gross reshaping of external reality to satisfy inner needs	
• Neurotic/immature – Conversion	Forbidden thought is kept out of awareness and expressed in the form of somatic disturbance	Hysteria
– Dissociation	Involuntary splitting or suppression of a mental function in a manner that allows expression of forbidden unconscious impulse without having responsibility for actions	Multiple personality disorder
– Displacement	Unconscious shifting of emotions to a less threatening object	Normal day-to-day reflection of anger seen in phobia
– Isolation	Separation of the idea of an unconscious impulse from its effect	Grief
– Reaction formation	Unconscious transformation of unacceptable impulse into exactly opposite attitudes	OCD
– Undoing	Unconsciously motivated acts that counteract unacceptable thoughts	Compulsive rituals
– Rationalization	Providing logical explanation	
– Intellectualization	Excessive use of intellectual processes (logic)	
– Acting out	Expression of an unconscious impulse, through action, thereby gratifying the impulse	Impulse control disorders
– Hypochondriasis	Unconscious transformation of unacceptable impulses to inappropriate somatic concern	
Others: inhibition, schizoid fantasy, turning against self, introjections, compensation, splitting		
• Mature – Sublimation	Channelization of unacceptable impulses into personally satisfying and socially valuable behavior patterns	
– Suppression (voluntary)	Voluntary postponement of focusing of attention on an impulse of conscious awareness	
Others: Anticipation, Humor, Altruism		

Stages of Cognitive Development (Jean Piaget)

Piaget believed that intelligence was an extension of biologic adaptation and had a logical structure. His theory was based on how children and adolescents think and acquire knowledge.

Stage 1: Sensorimotor Stage (birth to 2 years)

Infants begin to learn through sensory observation and gain control of their motor functions through activity, exploration, and manipulation of the environment. Object permanence is achieved.

Stage 2: Preoperational Stage (2 to 7 years)

Child uses symbols and language more extensively. Children are **egocentric, use animistic thinking** and have a sense of immanent justice. Death is reversible. Lack the law of conservation.

Stage 3: Concrete Operations Stage (7 to 11 years)

Egocentricity is replaced by operational thought; therefore, they can see things in other's perspective. Have the law of conservation; death is irreversible at the age of 10.

Stage 4: Formal Operations Stage (11 years to the end of adolescence)

Ability to think abstractly, reason deductively, and define concepts. Characterized by hypothetical thinking and deductive reasoning.

Psychosexual Stages (Sigmund Freud)

Freud believed that children were influenced by sexual drives. He noted that infants were capable of sexual activity from birth, the initial stages being nongenital.

Stage 1. Oral Stage (birth to 18 months)

The mouth is the main site of gratification and is manifested by chewing, biting, and sucking.

Stage 2. Anal Stage (1 to 3 years)

The anus and the surrounding areas are the main site of gratification. Primarily involved in bowel functions and bladder control. Harsh toilet training may become **anally fixated (obsessive-compulsive personality disorder)**.

Stage 3. Phallic Stage (3 to 5 years)

The genital area is the main site of gratification. Penis envy and fear of castration are evident during this stage. Increase in genital masturbation with fantasies involving the opposite-sex parent, 'oedipal complex.'

Stage 4. Latency Stage (5 to 11–13 years)

Formation of the supergo, resolution of the oedipal complex. Sexual interests during this period are believed to be quiescent. Sublimation of sexual energy into energetic learning and play activities.

Stage 5. Genital Stage (11–13 years to adulthood)

Capacity for true intimacy.

SCHIZOPHRENIA

Schneider's first-rank symptoms	Schneider's second-rank symptoms	Bleuler's '4–A'
• Hallucination – Audible thoughts – Voices head arguing – Voices commenting on one's action • Delusional perception • Thoughts alienation phenomena – Thoughts withdrawal – Thoughts insertion – Thoughts diffusion/broadcasting • Passivity phenomena – Made feeling (affect) – Made impulses – Made volition or act – Somatic passivity	• Other disorders of perception • Sudden delusional ideas • Perplexity • Depressive and euphoric mood changes • Feelings of emotional impoverishment • Several others as well	• Ambivalence (confusion) • Autism (withdrawal into self) • Affect disturbance • Association disturbance (loosening of association)

DSM–IV Criteria for Diagnosis of Schizophrenia

Two (or more) of the following, each present for a significant portion of time during a 1-month period (or less if successfully treated)

- Delusions
- Hallucinations
- Disorganized speech (e.g. frequent derailment or incoherence)
- Negative symptoms, i.e. affective flattening, alogia or avolition

Only one criterion symptom is required if delusions are bizarre or hallucinations consist of a voice keeping up a running commentary on the person's behavior or thoughts, or two or more voices conversing with each other.

Continuous signs of disturbance persist for at least 6 months.

- This **6-month period must include at least 1 month** of symptoms .
- Autism and not automatism is included in '4A'.
- The delusions included in 1st rank symptoms of schizophrenia are primary delusions, also called **autochthonous delusions**. These are characteristic of schizophrenia.

Genetics

Risk of schizophrenia if:

- One parent has schizophrenia: 10–12%
- Both parents: 40%
- Monozygotic twins: 46%
- Dizygotic twins: 14%

Types of Schizophrenia

- Commonest type: paranoid
- Amphetamine included: paranoid
- Early onset and bad prognosis: hebephrenic
- Late onset and best prognosis: catatonic
- Very late (3rd, 4th decades): paranoid (late onset schizophrenia is after 45 years, also called as paraphrenia predominantly characterized by positive symptoms)
- Worst prognosis and most difficult to diagnose: simple
- Associated with mental retardation: Pfropf

DSM-IV-TR Diagnostic Criteria for Schizophrenia Subtypes

Paranoid Type

- Preoccupation with one or more delusions or frequent auditory hallucinations
- Absence of disorganized speech, disorganized or catatonic behavior, or flat or inappropriate affect.

Disorganized Type (Hebephrenic)

- Prominence of disorganized speech, disorganized behavior and flat or inappropriate affect.

Catatonic Type

- Catalepsy (including waxy flexibility) or stupor
- Excessive motor activity (purposeless and not influenced by external stimuli)
- Negativism or mutism
- Automatic obedience
- Psychological pillow
- Peculiarities of posturing (voluntary assumption of inappropriate or bizarre postures), stereotyped movements, prominent mannerisms, or prominent grimacing
- Echolalia or echopraxia.

Types of catatonic schizophrenia

Excited Catatonic

- Increased psychomotor activity
- Death may occur. Also known as acute lethal catatonia or pernicious catatonia.

Retarded (Stupor) Catatonic

- Decreased psychomotor activity, mutism, rigidity, waxy flexibility, stupor, negativism, echolalia, echopraxia, mannerism and grimacing, automatic obedience.

Undifferentiated Type

Symptom clusters from all other types.

Residual Type

Absence of prominent delusions, hallucinations, disorganized speech and grossly disorganized or catatonic behavior. There is continuing evidence of the disturbance as indicated by the presence of negative symptoms or two or more symptoms listed in criterion A for schizophrenia, present in an attenuated form (e.g. odd beliefs, unusual perceptual experiences).

Schizophreniform disorder: patients who meet the symptom requirements but not the duration (between 1 and 6 months)

Schizoaffective disorder: manifest symptoms of schizophrenia and independent periods of mood disturbance.

Other Subtypes

- Bouffée délirante (acute delusional psychosis), latent schizophrenia, oneiroid state pseudoneurotic schizophrenia, deficit schizophrenia, early onset schizophrenia (onset between 5 and 13 years), late onset schizophrenia or paraphrenia (>45 years of age—commonest type paranoid)

Schizophrenia-like syndrome may be seen in:

- **Amphetamine use**, Mescaline, Phencyclidine abuse, LSD abuse
- Huntington's chorea, Homocystinuria, Hemochromatosis, Wilson's disease
- Acute intermittent porphyria

MOOD DISORDERS

- **Mania, depression and bipolar disorder are mood disorders.**
- Comprises of recurrent manic episodes or recurrent episodes of depression and mania (Bipolar–I)/hypomania (Bipolar–II).
- In the intervening period, patient is normal.

Classification of Mood Disorders

- Major depressive disorder: unipolar depression, without manic episodes.
- Depressive specifiers include atypical features, melancholic, postpartum onset and catatonic features. Omega sign and Otto Veraguth fold are signs in depression.
- **Dysthymia is chronic low mood lasting for 2 years.** Does not fulfill the criteria for major depression. When a depressive episode occurs in the presence of dysthymia, it is called double depression.
- **2 week duration is essential to diagnose depression.**
- **Pseudodementia and nihilistic delusions**: seen in depression
- **Grief is a form of adjustment disorder in response to loss**: stages of grief were given by Kubler Ross (denial, anger, bargaining, depression, acceptance).
- **SSRIs are the drug of choice for major depressive disorder.**

Bipolar mood disorder/mania depressive psychosis (MDP): unpredictable swings in mood from mania to depression at different times and in the intervening period, patient may be normal.

- Chromosomal regions linked to Bipolar disorder–18, 21, 22.
- Duration required for mania to be diagnosed is 1 week.

Bipolar-1 disorder—recurrent manic episodes with or without depression

Bipolar-2 disorder—presence of one or more depressive episodes with atleast one hypomanic episode

Rapid cycling bipolar disorder—episodes of mania, hypomania and depression (atleast 4 episodes in a year).

Cyclothymia—condition of persistent unstable mood with frequent mood swings of mild depression and mild elation without functional impairment lasting for 2 years' duration.

DELIRIUM (ACUTE CONFUSIONAL STATE/ORGANIC BRAIN SYNDROME)

- Acute onset of fluctuating cognitive impairment and a disturbance of consciousness.
- Delirum is associated with the acute failure of the brain.
- Classically, delirium has a sudden onset (hours or days), a brief and fluctuating course, and rapid improvement when the causative factor is identified and eliminated.

Etiology

- Seen in approximately 10 to 30% of medically ill patients who are hospitalized.
- **Common in general hospital setting.**
- The highest rate in terminally ill patients (80%) and postcardiotomy (ICU-tertiary care) patients (90%).
- Of nursing home residents over age 75, 60% have repeated episodes of delirium.
- Other predisposing factors—preexisting brain damage (e.g. dementia, cerebrovascular disease, tumor), a history of delirium, alcohol dependence, diabetes, cancer, sensory impairment (e.g. blindness), male gender and malnutrition.
- Systemic disease secondarily affecting the brain.
- Primary intracranial disease.
- Exogenous toxic agent.
- Withdrawal from substances of abuse.

Clinical Features

- **Common psychiatric symptoms**: abnormalities of mood, perception and behavior.
- **Common neurological symptoms**: tremor, asterixis, nystagmus, incoordination and urinary incontinence.
- Alteration in attention associated with disturbed consciousness and cognition.
- Fluctuating course. Symptoms are ever-changing.
- The patient's mental status varies from time to time.
- Sleep disturbance (reversal of sleep-wake cycle) and decreased consciousness
- Delirium may first present as sundowning with day-time drowsiness and night-time insomnia with confusion.
- When a psychiatric illness causes symptoms of delirium, patients are said to have a pseudodelirium.

Feature	Dementia	Delirium
Onset	Slow	Rapid
Duration	Months to years	Hours to weeks
Attention	Preserved	Fluctures
Memory	Impaired remote memory	Impaired recent and immediate memory
Speech	Word-finding difficulty	Incoherent (slow or rapid)
Sleep-wake cycle	Fragmented sleep	Frequent disruption (e.g. day and night reversal)
Thoughts	Impoverished	Disorganized
Awareness	Unchanged	Reduced
Alertness	Usually normal	Hypervigilant or reduced vigilance

- Delirium can occur in older patients wearing eye-patches after cataract surgery **(black-patch delirium/black-patch disease)**

DSM-IV-TR Classification of Delirium

- Delirium due to a general medical condition
- Substance intoxication delirium
- Substance withdrawal delirium
- Delirium due to multiple etiologies
- Delirium not otherwise specified

Treatment

- The two major symptoms that require treatment are psychosis and insomnia.
- Primary goal—treat the underlying cause.
- If underlying condition is anticholinergic toxicity—use of physostigmine salicylate.
- The other important goal is to provide physical, sensory and environmental support.
- **Commonly used drug to reduce psychomotor agitation—haloperidol.**

Points to remember about dementia

Dementia is diagnosed when there is memory impairment with one of the following cognitive disturbances—aphasia, agnosis, apraxia, and disturbances in executive functioning. **Catastrophic reaction and sundowners syndrome are common in dementia individuals.**

Alzheimer's dementia: most common type, Chromosome 21, Apo E lipoprotein, MMSE (Mini Mental State Examination) score less than 20

Vascular dementia: multiinfarct dementia, vascular risk factors, step wise deterioration, Hachinskis score to delineate vascular or alzhiemers type

Lewy body dementia: fluctuating sensorium, visual hallucinations, parkinsonian features, sensitivity to neuroleptics.

Picks' dementia: frontotemporal dementia; personality change is evident before memory loss.

CJD dementia: rapid progression, cerebellar symptoms, extrapyramidal symptoms (myoclonic jerks), EEG changes (periodic spikes against low–voltage background).

Punch drunk syndrome–seen in boxers called dementia pugilistica.

Drug of choice for dementia: acetyl cholinesterase inhibitors (Donepezil, Rivastigmine, Galantamine) and Memantine (Glutamate antagonists).

Memory Types

- *Explicit memory*—Factual information, e.g. (words, definitions, names, dates, faces, events, concepts, and ideas).
- *Implicit memory*—Memory for actions, skills, e.g. (riding a bike, typing, and tying one's shoes).

Amnesia: The amnestic disorders are characterized by a disturbance in memory alone. These disorders should not be diagnosed if the memory deficit is a feature of a dissociative disorder, is associated with dementia, or occurs in the presence of clouded sensorium, as in delirium. Anterograde amnesia is common following road traffic accident. Other causes of amnesia include transient global amnesia, BZD abuse, following ECT, etc.

SUBSTANCE USE DISORDERS

Alcohol withdrawal syndrome: hangover is the most common symptom.

- **Alcoholic hallucinations**
  - Hallucination (usually auditory) occurring in clear consciousness during abstinence, following regular intake.
- **Alcoholic seizures (rum fits)**
  - Multiple seizure (GTCS) occurring during abstinence usually 12–48 hours after heavy bout of drinking.

- **Delirium tremens**
  - Occurs within 3 days of complete or significant abstinence from heavy alcohol drinking. Recovery occurring within 7–10 days.
  - Characteristic features are clouding of consciousness, disorientation, hallucinations (mostly visual and auditory), illusion, autonomic disturbance, agitation and insomnia.
  - Death can occur in 5–10% of patients and is often due to cardiovascular collapse, infection, hyperthermia or self-inflicted injury.

Chronic Use Syndrome

- **Wernicke's encephalopathy**
  - Acute reactions to severe thiamine deficiency mostly due to chronic alcoholism
  - Characterized by global confusion, ophthalmoplegia, B/L external rectus palsy (6th nerve), papillary irregularities, nystagmus, papilledema, retinal hemorrhage, ataxia, apathy, etc.
- **Korsakoff's psychosis**
  - Delayed complication usually following Wernicke's encephalopathy
  - Characterized by amnesia and confabulation
  - Area of brain involved—mamillary body
- **Marchiafava-Bignami disease**
  - Characterized by ataxia, dysarthria, disorientation, epilepsy, hallucinations, spastic limb paralysis, etc.

Blood alcohol concentration (BAC)	Behavior
25–100 mg%	Excitement
80 mg%	Legal limit for driving (UK)
100–200 mg%	Serious intoxication, slurred speech, in coordination, nystagmus
200–300 mg%	Dangerous
300–350 mg%	Hypothermia, dysarthria, cold sweats
350–400 mg%	Coma, respiratory depression
>400 mg%	Death may occur

Urinary alcohol concentration	Diagnostic use	Equivalent BAC
>120 mg%	Suggestive	80 mg%
>200 mg%	Diagnostic	150 mg%

Screening tests for alcoholism—MAST (Michigan Alcoholism Screening Test), CAGE questionnaire test.

Cage Questionnaire

- Ever had to Cut down the amount of alcohol
- Been Annoyed by people's criticism of alcoholism
- Felt Guilty of drinking
- Need of an Eye opener

Terminologies in Substance Abuse

Amphetamine: speed; **Amyl nitrite**–gold rush, poppers, **Barbiturates**: idiot pills, **Cocaine**: crack, rock, coke, snow, **Heroin**: smack, brown sugar, **Phencyclidine**: angel dust, **White heroin**: china white.

Psychiatric Manifestations

Substance	Characteristic feature
Cocaine	Magnus symptom, (cocaine bugs/tactile hallucinations), formication, delusional parasitosis (Ekbom syndrome)

Contd...

Contd...

Substance	Characteristic feature
Cannabis	Run amok, amotivation syndrome, flashbacks, Hemp insanity Intoxication causes increased appetite (munchies) and conjunctival injection
Alcohol	Mc Evan's sign, Morbid jealousy
LSD	Bad trips, Flashbacks
Amphetamine	Paranoid hallucinatory syndrome (like paranoid schizophrenia)
Phencyclidine (angel dust)	Dissociative anesthesia

No withdrawal symptoms with LSD and cannabis

TREATMENT

Drug of choice for:

- Alcohol withdrawl: benzodiazepines (chlordiazepoxide) detoxification agent
- Alcohol dependence: disulfiram (deterrent agent), acamprosate (anticraving agent)
- Nicotine dependence: bupropion, varenicline tartrate
- Opioid dependence: overdose (naloxone), withdrawl (clonidine), maintenance (methadone)
- Cocaine dependence: amantadine
- Cannabis dependence: bupropion, N-acetyl cysteine

ANXIETY DISORDERS

Types of Anxiety Disorders (DSM-IV-TR)

- Panic disorder with or without agoraphobia
- Agoraphobia with or without panic disorder
- Specific phobia
- Social phobia
- Obsessive-compulsive disorder (OCD)
- Post-traumatic stress disorder (PTSD)
- Acute stress disorder
- Generalized anxiety disorder

DSM 5 has separated OCD and stress-related disorders into a separate category

Symptoms of Anxiety

- The experience of anxiety has two components:
  - Somatic—awareness of the physiological sensations (e.g. palpitations and sweating)
  - Psychological—awareness of being nervous or frightened
- A feeling of shame may increase anxiety.
- In addition to motor and visceral effects, anxiety affects thinking, perception, and learning.
- It tends to produce confusion and distortions of perception.
- These distortions can interfere with learning by lowering concentration, reducing recall, and impairing the ability to relate one item to another, that is, to make associations.

Panic disorder (Episodic paroxysmal anxiety attacks which are spontaneous, crescendo-decrescendo pattern of anxiety, catastrophic cognition or fear of impending doom at the peak of anxiety followed by anticipatory anxiety about the attack).

Phobia: Irrational fear with anxiety and avoidance

- **Insight is present**

Types

• **Agoraphobia:** fear of open places, crowded places or any place from where there is no escape to safe place	• **Claustrophobia:** fear of closed spaces
• **Acrophobia:** fear of high places	• **Algophobia:** fear of pain
• **Arachnophobia:** fear of spiders	• **Xeno phobia:** fear of strangers
• **Zoophobia:** fear of animals	• **Sitophobia:** fear of eating
• **Thanatophobia:** fear of death	• **Social phobia:** fear of social activities and interactions
• **Shy:** bladder: fear of urinating in public lavatory	• **Cynophobia:** fear of dogs
• **Mysophobia:** fear of dirt and germs	• **Pyrophobia:** fear of blushing

Generalised anxiety disorder: Free-floating anxiety, worries about day-to-day events, inability to relax, frequent headaches and sleep disturbances.

Obsessive Compulsive Disorder

Most common obsession is contamination and most common compulsion is washing/cleaning.
Defense mechanisms that operate in OCD include isolation, undoing and reaction formation.
Drug of choice for OCD is fluoxetine. Tricyclic that is approved for OCD is clomipramine. Behavioral therapy of choice is Exposure Response Prevention (ERP).

Post-traumatic Stress Disorder (PTSD)

- PTSD arises as a delayed/protracted response to an exceptionally stressful or catastrophic life event or situation which is likely to cause pervasive distress in almost any person (e.g. disaster, war, rape, torture, serious accident). **Total duration of the disturbance is more than 1 month. Onset within 6 months of traumatic event.**
- PTSD is characterized recurrent or intrusive recollections of the stressful event either in flashbacks (image, thoughts or perceptions) and/or in dreams and hyperarousal symptoms, such as startle reactions and nightmares.
- There is marked avoidance of the events or situations that arouse recollections of the stressful event.
- Alexithymia, characterized by the inability to identify and articulate feelings.
- EMDR (Eye Movement Desensitization Reprocessing) is proven therapy.

Note: Flashbacks are also common in cannabis poisoning and LSD abuse.

SOMATOFORM DISORDERS

Characters of the seven types of somatoform disorders as listed in DSM-IV-TR **(listed under somatic syndrome disorder in DSM 5)**:

- **Somatization disorder (Briquet's syndrome or hysteria):** Many physical complaints affecting many organ syetems (4 pain symptoms; 2 gastrointestinal symptoms; 1 sexual and 1 pseudoneurological symptom); Polysurgical, younger age with familial pattern.
- Conversion disorder: One or two neurological complaints (motor or sensory) associated with primary and secondary gain. Unconscious conflict is transformed into a physical symptom, such as paralysis or blindness. La Belle indifference (indifferent attitude towards her symptom by the patient) and astasia abasia (unsteady gait while standing or walking) are commoner.
- **Hypochondriasis:** Concern or preoccupation with a specific disease which amplifies symptoms (doctor shopping is common).
- **Body dysmorphic disorder:** A false belief or exaggerated perception that a body part is defective.
- **Pain disorder:** Symptoms of pain either solely related to, or exacerbated by, psychological factors.
- **Undifferentiated somatoform disorder:** It includes somatoform disorders not otherwise described that have been present for 6 months or longer.
- **Somatoform disorder not otherwise specified:** This is the category for somatoform symptoms that do not meet any of the somatoform disorder diagnoses mentioned herewith.

Somatoform autonomic dysfunction: symptoms of an organ system that is under autonomic control: heart (palpitations), upper GI (hiccough), lower GI (IBS), respiratory (hyperventilation), genitourinary (dysuria).

Dissociative Disorders

- Acute or gradual, transient or persistent, disruption of consciousness, perception, memory or awareness, not associated with physical disease or organic brain dysfunction, and severe enough to cause distress or impairment.
- Four types are described in DSM-IV, and there is a miscellaneous fifth group.

Types of Dissociative Disorders

- Dissociative amnesia, dissociative fugue, dissociative identity disorder
- Depersonalization disorder
- Dissociative disorder not otherwise specified:
  - Dissociative hallucinosis
  - Dissociation following torture or political indoctrination
  - Somnambulism
  - 'Out-of-body' experiences
  - Dissociative trances that are culturally sanctioned
  - Culture-bound 'possession' states
  - **Ganser syndrome (hysterical pseudodementia): approximate answers or vorbeireden.**

Types of Dissociative Amnesia

- **Localized amnesia (M/C form):** failure to recall all events occurring during a circumscribed period of time
- **Selective amnesia**: failure to recall some but not all of the events during a circumscribed period of time
- **Generalized amnesia**: failure of recall for important personal information that encompasses the person's life. This form most commonly presents to the police or in hospital emergency rooms
- **Continuous amnesia**: recall for events subsequent to a specific time up to and including the present is impaired
- **Systematized amnesia**: a loss of memory for specific categories of information, such as all memories relating to one's family or a particular person.

Factitious disorder: conscious feigning of symptoms to seek attention, more common in paramedical professionals and single women. They are called hospital addicts.

Malingering: conscious feigning of symptoms for external gain, such as compensation benefit, property, escape from punishment, etc.

Culture-bound Syndromes

Dhat syndrome → fear of losing semen	**Amok** → sudden, unprovoked episode of rage
Koro → strong belief that his penis is shrinking	Whitigo (wendigo) → belief that he has been transformed to a cannibal
Pibloktoq → **arctic hysteria** → eskimos, extereme excitement of as long as 30 minutes' duration and frequently followed by convulsive seizures and coma lasting as long as 12 hours	Latah → presence of automatic obedience, echolalia and echopraxia
Suchi-bai → purity mania	**Hwa-Byung/Wool-Hwa-Byung** → Korean folk syndrome [anger syndrome] and is attributed to the suppression of anger
Latah → hypersensitivity to sudden fright, often with echopraxia, echolalia, command obedience, and dissociative or trance-like behavior	**Locura** → Severe form of chronic psychosis [inherited vulnerability, the effect of multiple life difficulties, or a combination of both factors]
Mal de ojo → evil eye	**Ideas of nerves/Nervios** → General state of vulnerability to stressful life experiences and to a syndrome brought on by difficult life circumstances

DISORDERS OF PERSONALITY AND BEHAVIOR

Five-factor model of personality Ocean (Openness, Conscientiousness, Extraversion, Agreeableness, Neuroticism).
Novelty-seeking, persistence, reward dependence, harm avoidance are the temperamental traits.
'Temperament' is the term used to describe character logical traits of an individual before 18 years of age. Four character traits which describe temperament include harm avoidance, novelty-seeking, reward-dependence and persistence.
Type A personality: time urgency, competitiveness and hostility (risk for CAD)
Type B personality: relaxed, unhurried, less vigorous attempts to achieve a goal
Type C personality: competitive, perfectionistic
Type D personality: low drive, dysthymic (risk for depression and CAD).

Types of Personality Disorders

- **Cluster A (paranoid, schizoid, schizotypal)**, which includes individuals who are odd or eccentric.
- **Cluster B (antisocial, borderline, histrionic, narcissistic),** which includes individuals with dramatic, acting-out behaviors and who have problems with empathy.
- **Cluster C (avoidant, dependent, obsessive-compulsive),** which includes personality styles marked by prominent anxiety and novelty avoidance.

Sleep Disorders

- Narcolepsy is the most common cause of hypersomnia. Tetrad includes sleep attacks, hypnogogic/hypnopompic hallucinations, sleep paralysis and cataplexy (sudden loss of muscle tone). The drug of choice is Modafinil.
  Hypocretin system plays a critical role in narcolepsy
  Drug of choice for restless leg syndrome is Ropinirole.

Nightmares occur in REM sleep. Night terrors, somnambulism, bruxism, sleep talking, enuresis all occur during NREM sleep.

Ramelteon: It targets the Melatonin (MT1 and MT2) receptors; half life is 1–2.6 hours. Indicated for treatment of insomnia.

Impulse Control Disorders

- *Urge to commit certain acts* that are often illogical or harmful. The disorders included are trichotillomania, pathological gambling, pyromania, and kleptomania.

Eating Disorders

- Occur more common in females and adolescents
- Due to intense fear of becoming obese
- There is a body image disturbance
- **Russell's sign** is seen in bulimia nervosa (incisor marks on the dorsum of phalanx)

Features	Anorexia nervosa	Bulimia nervosa
Symptoms	Refusal to maintain body weight above a minimal normal (BMI <17.5 kg/m^2) Patients believe that their body as a whole or some part of their body is too fat	Irresistible craving for food with episodes of overeating in less time
Method of weight control	Very less eating Restrictive type is commoner	Attempts to counteract the effects of overeating by self-induced vomiting, purgative abuse, appetite suppressants, periods of starvation
Weight	Markedly decreased	Usually normal
Binge eating	25–50%	Required for diagnosis
Amenorrhea	100%	50%
Complications/ comorbidity	Ritualized exercise, decreased vitals, hypothermia, skin changes. OCD is a common comorbid condition	Dental caries are frequent. Antisocial behavior and drug abuse are common. Bipolar disorder and borderline personality are common comorbid conditions

Sexual disorders: Drug of choice for premature ejaculation is Dapoxetine (SSRI); Start-stop technique and squeeze technique are effective.

Impulse control disorders include intermittent explosive disorder, kleptomania, trichotillomania, pyromania and pathological gambling.

Syndromes

- Othello syndrome: jealousy (infidelity) involving the spouse [conjugal paranoia or morbid jealousy]
- De Clerambult's syndrome or erotomania: erotic delusions
- Capgras syndrome: syndrome of doubles
- Ganser's syndrome: approximate answers, common in prison inmates (vorbeireden/paralogia)
- Folie à deux: shared delusional disorder
- Alice in Wonderland syndrome: disturbance of one's view of self
- Couvades syndrome: experiencing the symptoms of pregnancy in males
- Ekbom syndrome: restless leg syndrome
- Gelinau syndrome: narcolepsy
- Strauss syndrome: ADHD
- **Blocq's disease**: also known as astasia-abasia. This is the inability to walk or stand in a normal manner. The gait is bizarre and is not suggestive of any organic lesion. It is a dissociative motor disorder in ICD–10.
- **Charles Bonnet syndrome**: this is a syndrome of visual hallucinations without any other psychotic features or any evidence of psychiatric disorder. It is associated with visual impairment.

CHILD PSYCHIATRY

ADHD: Onset of symptoms before 7 years of age (extended to 12 years of age as in DSM 5). Inattention and hyperactivity/impulsivity are the cardinal features. Most common comorbidities are learning disability and conduct disorder. Drug of choice is Methyl phenidate. Other drugs used are clonidine, Atomoxetine, Imipramine.

Autism: Onset of symptoms before 3 years of age. Triad of impairments includes deficits in social interaction, communication, restricted stereotyped pattern of behaviors. Common comorbid condition is mental retardation. Treatment is sensory integration therapy, applied behavioral analysis-based therapy, occupational therapy and speech therapy.

Mental retardation: Replaced by intellectual disability in DSM 5. The 1910 definition of mental retardation by American Association on Mental Retardation required the presence of a mental defect and an inability to manage ordinary affairs (corresponding to today's impairment in cognitive capacity and adaptive behavior) and inclusion of the classification of idiots (IQ 0–25) (mental age of 2 years or younger), imbeciles (IQ 26–50) (mental age of 2–7 years) and morons (IQ 51–70) (mental age of 7–12 years).

Severity of MR: mild (50–70) educable group, moderate (35–49) trainable group, severe (20–34) dependent group, profound (less than 20).

The Persons with Disabilities Act provides disability benefits for people with mental retardation and mental illness.

Learning disability is diagnosed if the child has a normal IQ, has normal hearing and visual acuity and is being provided adequate environment for education. Remedial teaching is effective (dyslexia–reading difficulty, dysgraphia: writing difficulty; dyscalculia: difficulty in mathematical calculations).

PSYCHOPHARMACOLOGY

Antidepressants (Mechanism of Action)

The tricyclics block the reuptake pumps for both serotonin and norepinephrine.

Other three actions: Blockade of muscarinic cholinergic receptors, blockade of H1 histamine receptors, and blockade of Alpha 1 adrenergic receptors.

Blockade of **Alpha 1 adrenergic receptors** causes orthostatic hypotension and dizziness.

Anticholinergic actions of **muscarinic cholinergic receptors** cause dry mouth, blurred vision, urinary retention, and constipation.

Blockade of **H1 histamine receptors** causes sedation and weight gain.

Overdosage of TCAs

Tricyclic antidepressants (TCAs) also block sodium channels in the heart and brain, which can cause cardiac arrhythmias in overdosage, as well as seizures.

Side Effects of SSRIs

All the side effects of SSRIs can be understood as undesirable actions of serotonin in undesirable pathways, at undesirable places and at undesirable receptor subtypes:

- Nausea or vomiting (stimulation of serotonin 3 receptors in the hypothalamus)
- Gastrointestinal cramps and diarrhea (stimulation of serotonin 3 and 4 receptors in the gastrointestinal tract)
- Sexual dysfunction (stimulation of serotonin 2A receptors in the spinal cord may inhibit the spinal reflexes of orgasm and ejaculation)
- Anxiety (stimulation of serotonin 2A and 2C receptors in the projection from raphe to limbic cortex)
- Akathisia, or even mild parkinsonism and dystonic movements (stimulation of 2A receptors in the basal ganglia).

Serotonin syndrome, also known as **serotonin toxicity**, is caused by excessive levels of circulating serotonin in the central nervous system (CNS) and the periphery. The syndrome is characterized by mental status changes, autonomic hyperactivity, and neuromuscular abnormalities that may range in severity from almost imperceptible to lethal.

Classification

Cyclic antidepressants	Tricyclic tertiary amines		Imipramine, amitriptyline, doxepine, tri-imipramine, clomipramine, dothiepin (dosulepin)
	Tricyclic secondary amines		Nortriptyline, protriptyline, desipramine
	Tetracyclic		Mianserin, maprotiline, amoxapine (antidepressant with antipsychotic metabolite)
	Bicyclic		Viloxazine
Selective serotonin reuptake inhibitors (SSRIs)			Fluoxetine, paroxetine, fluvoxamine, sertraline, citalopram, escitalopram, dapoxetine (approved for premature ejaculation)
Serotonin norepinephrine reuptake inhibitors (SNRIs)			Venlafaxine, desvenlafaxine, duloxetine, milnacipran
Norepinephrine serotonin reuptake enhancers (NSRE's)			Tianeptine
Noradrenergic and specific serotonergic antidepressants (NaSSAs)			Mirtazepine, mianserin
Norepinephrine dopamine reuptake inhibitors (NDRIs)			Bupropion
Serotonin antagonists and reuptake inhibitors (SARIs)			Trazadone (causes priapism), nefazodone
Noradrenergic reuptake inhibitors (NARIs)			Reboxetine, atomoxetine
MAO inhibitors	Irreversible		
	Reversible MAOI-A	MAOI-B	Selegiline
		Moclobemide	

Antipsychotics: block dopamine (D2 receptors); atypical antipsychotics block 5HT 2A and D2 receptors (serotonin dopamine antagonists).

Acts on dopamine receptors in four pathways—mesocortical (negative symptoms), mesolimbic (positive symptoms), nigrostriatal (EPS), tuberoinfundibular (hyperprolactinemia).

Clozapine

- Most potent with least extrapyramidal side effect and least antiemetic property; doesn't cause hyperprolactinemia.
- Most important side effect is agranulocytosis. Can also cause dose-dependent seizures, myocarditis and anti-cholinergic side effects.
- Has weak D2-blocking action and D4 specific.
- Reserve drug for resistant schizophrenia.
- Effective in treating negative symptoms and reducing suicidal risk.

Antipsychotics

Least extrapyramidal side effect: Clozopine (almost no extrapyramidal side effects) and thioridazine (causes retinitis pigmentosa)	Depot antipsychotics: Fluphenazine (2–4 weeks), penfluridol (1 week) Haloperidol deconoate Risperidone long-acting Paliperidone
Least potent: Chlorpromazine High potency: Haloperidol Third-generation antipsychotic: Aripiprazole (longer t½)	**With antidepressant action:** Flupenthixol **Sublingual antipsychotic:** Asenapine
More emetic potential: Clozapine/Olanzapine/Risperidone/Molindone	**Newer antipsychotics:** Blonanserin, Iloperidone,

Side Effects of Typical Antipsychotics

Dystonia: The symptoms include, abnormal positioning of the head and neck (e.g. torticollis); spasm of jaw muscles (e.g. trismus); impaired swallowing; slurred speech; tongue protrusion; deviated eyes in any direction (e.g. oculogyric crisis); and abnormal positioning of limbs or trunk (e.g. opisthotonos).

Akathisia: Greek meaning 'never to sit down'; The patient will complain of an inner sense of restlessness. fidgeting, pacing, lifting the feet as if marching in place, crossing and uncrossing the legs when sitting, *the inability to sit or stand in one place.*

Treatment of akathisia: β-blockers (e.g. propranolol) have been found to be the efficacious drugs for akathisia. Antipsychotic dosage reduction should also be done.

Tardive dyskinesia: The symptoms include involuntary movements of the tongue (e.g. twisting, protrusion), jaw (e.g. chewing), lips (e.g. smacking), cheeks (e.g. puffing) trunk, or extremities. Symptoms of tardive dyskinesia should develop after at least 2 months of exposure to a dopamine-blocking agent (or 1 month if the patient is 60 years or older).

Risk factors for tardive dyskinesia: Increasing age, preexisting parkinsonism, previous brain damage, antipsychotic treatment duration, and exposure to first-generation antipsychotics.

Neuroleptic malignant syndrome: Typical symptoms of neuroleptic malignant syndrome (NMS) are *muscle rigidity* and *elevated temperature* in a patient on antipsychotic medication.

Other symptoms: Diaphoresis, tachycardia, elevated or labile blood pressure, tremor, changes in the level of consciousness, ranging from confusion to coma, mutism, leukocytosis, laboratory evidence of muscle injury.

Risk factors for NMS: Dehydration, high potency first generation antipsychotics (e.G., Haloperidol), concurrent lithium treatment, high doses of an antipsychotic.

Treatment for NMS: Intravenous hydration, amantadine, bromocriptine, levodopa, benzodiazepines, electroconvulsive therapy, dantrolene.

Lithium

- Discovered in 1817 by John August Arfwedson, first used in the Rx of gout and salt replacement in cardiac disease, withdrawn due to fatal toxicity.
- Starting dose for acute mania: 900–2100 mg/day lithium carbonate.
- 300 mg of lithium is contained in 1,597 mg of lithium carbonate (Li_2CO_3).

Blood lithium levels

- Therapeutic levels [for Rx of acute mania]: 0.6–1.2 mEq/L
- Prophylactic levels [for relapse prevention in bipolar disorder]: 0.6–1.0 mEq/L
- Toxic levels: > 1.5 mEq/L
- Mild to moderate intoxication (lithium level = 1.5 to 2.0 mEq/L)
- Moderate to severe intoxication (lithium level = 2.0 to 2.5 mEq/L)
- Severe lithium intoxication (lithium level > 2.5 mEq/L)
  - Generalized convulsions
  - Oliguria and renal failure
  - Death
  - Treatment of lithium toxicity is hemodialysis.

Drug of choice for: Acute manic episode, prophylaxis of MDP.

Effects

- Most affected organ is kidney > thyroid, least affected organ is liver.
- Most common side effect are tremors. Lithium is contraindicated in sick sinus syndrome.
- Secreted in breast milk and, hence, contraindicated in pregnancy and lactation. Causes Ebstein's anomaly if given during pregnancy.
- Reduces thyroxine synthesis and leads to goiter and hypothyroidism.
- Leucocyte count is increased; hence used in Rx of chemotherapy-induced leucopenia and agranulocytosis.
- Inhibits ADH action on distal tube. So, used in case of SIADH.

Lithium toxicity: Lithium intoxication is primarily a *neurotoxicity* (often cerebellar as characterized by dysarthric speech and tremor). Severe toxicity occurs when the serum lithium level is above the therapeutic range of 0.5 to 1.5 mEq/L. Early clinical manifestations include gastrointestinal upset, dysarthria, ataxia, and coarse tremor. Ominous findings include *impaired consciousness, neuromuscular irritability* (fasciculations) and *seizures*.

Hemodialysis is the treatment of choice for severe intoxication.

Drugs used in prophylaxis of bipolar disorder (mood stabilizers):

Established	New
• Lithium • Carbamazepine • Valproate • Oxcarbazepine (doesn't produce side effect of CBZ but causes hyponatremia)	• Lamotrigine (causes Stevens-Johnson syndrome) • Levothyroxine (T3) • Calcium channel blockers • Clonazepam • Gabapentin • Topiramate

Drug effective for bipolar mania: Lithium plus atypical antipsychotics
Drug effective for bipolar depression: Lithium and lamotrigine

Treatment of Obsessive-compulsive Disorder

Treatment of choice:

Behavior therapy (exposure and response prevention (1st), systematic desensitization (2nd)

Medical treatment:

- Fluoxetine (drug of choice) and other SSRIs
- Fluvoxamine: Specific antiobsession actions
- Clomipramine (this TCA is most selective for serotonin reuptake) (drug of 2nd choice)

Clomipramine is the 2nd preferred drug after fluoxetine for treatment of OCD.

BEHAVIOR THERAPY

Type of BT	Based on	Used in
Systemic desensitization	Reciprocal inhibition	Phobias, OCD
Aversion therapy	Punishment Pairing of pleasant stimulus with an unpleasant response, e.g. pairing alcohol with electric shock When the unpleasant stimulus is given through verbal mode, it is called Covert sensitization	Drug abuse Sexual deviations
Flooding or implosion Graded exposure	Direct exposure to phobic object/situation but escape not possible Exposure to feared objects in a graded manner	Phobias
Exposure response prevention	Behavioral therapy	OCD
Operant conditioning for increasing a behavior	Positive reinforcement Negative reinforcement Modeling	For augmenting an adaptive behavior
Operant conditioning for decreasing a behavior	Time-out Punishment Satiation (negative practice procedure)	For decreasing maladaptive behavior

Desensitization is useful in:

- Phobias (treatment of choice)
- OCD (treatment of choice)
- Psychosexual dysfuntions

Motivational model *[for behavior change]*: Proposed by Prochaska.

- Precontemplation phase (does not even have a thought about change)
- Contemplation phase (thinks about a change but is ambivalent)
- Preparation phase (a decision has been made to change the behavior)
- Action phase (the behavior is changing)
- Maintenance phase (maintaining the behavioral change)

Psychological tests

Bender-Gestalt Test is a test for organic brain syndrome.

Rorschach Test and thematic apperception test are projective tests.

Binet Kamat Test, Weschler scale, Raven's progressive matrices are intelligence tests.

Electroconvulsive Therapy

Developed by Cerletti and Bini in 1938 as electroshock therapy; Prior to this, insulin coma therapy and camphor-induced seizures were used.

Types

- Direct ECT (unmodified): ECT given without muscle relaxants and anesthesia. Direct ECT causes decreased intraocular tension and fracture of vertebra.
- Modified ECT: ECT given with drug-induced muscle relaxation and anesthesia.

Indications

- **Major depression with suicidal risk is the first and most important indication of ECT.**
- ECT is treatment of choice for severe major depression, severe catatonia (functional), and severe psychosis (schizophrenia, mania) with:

- Suicidal risk, stupor, somatic syndrome, severe psychomotor retardation, psychotic features (e.g. delusional depression), intolerance to drug, drugs are contraindicated, not responding to drugs, poor intake.

Complications

- ECT-Direct: Most common side effect is fracture of T4-T8 vertebra.
- Modified ECT: Most common is retrograde amnesia.
  In modified ECT: Both retro- and antegrade amnesia are found but retrograde amnesia is more common.

Contraindications

- Absolute: Raised intracranial tension (fear of brain herniation).
  - Relative: Cerebrovascular accident (CVA), MI, severe hypertension, pheochromocytoma, severe pulmonary disease, retinal detachment.
- MC complication of modified ECT is amnesia (anterograde and retrograde that recovers within 1–6 months).
- MC complication of unmodified ECT is fractured spine (T4–T8 vertebra).

Transcranial magnetic stimulation: Noninvasive technique Efficacy shown in depression, OCD, PTSD.

Vagal nerve stimulation: Stimulation of left vagus through pulse generator. Efficacious in depression.

Deep brain stimulation: Creating a small hole and inserting a fine wire with pacemaker device to excite the brain areas. Usefulness demonstrated in Parkinson's disease.

QUESTIONS

1. **According to ICD–10, which letter is used to denote mental illness? (2014)**
   a. Q
   b. B
   c. G
   d. F
2. **The term 'psychiatry' was coined by: (2014)**
   a. Pinel
   b. Johann Christian Reil
   c. Sigmund Freud
   d. Benjamin Rush
3. **A patient who is alert but not giving response is best categorized as: (2014)**
   a. Stupor
   b. Coma
   c. Hysteria
   d. Delirium
4. **Cataplexy is: (2013)**
   a. Sudden loss of muscle tone
   b. Short-term muscle relaxation
   c. Sudden muscle rigidity
   d. Short period of loss of consciousness
5. **Which is not true regarding 'affect' in a psychiatric interview? (2012)**
   a. It has objective component
   b. It has subjective component
   c. It has a cross-sectional manifestation of emotion
   d. It has a persistent tone of feeling for a period of time
6. **Sigmund Freud's primary process of thinking is: (2011)**
   a. Absent in dreams
   b. Illogical and primitive
   c. Illogical and conscious
   d. Rational
7. **Ability to form a concept and generalize it is called: (2011)**
   a. Concrete thinking
   b. Abstract thinking
   c. Intellectualization
   d. Delusional thinking
8. **True statement about explicit memory is: (2010)**
   a. Consciously present
   b. Form of working memory
   c. Type of sensory memory
   d. Stored in striatum
9. **Deja vu phenomenon means: (2007)**
   a. Feeling that familiar things look unfamiliar
   b. Feeling that unfamiliar things look familiar
   c. Unable to recall the familiar name
   d. Feeling detached from one's own body
10. **Paranoid schizophrenia is caused by intake of: (2011)**
    a. Amphetamine
    b. Heroin
    c. Cannabis
    d. Cocaine

11. **Sudden onset of delusions de novo in a 35-year-old man with no previous symptom should prompt the physician to think of: (2011)**
    a. Substance abuse
    b. Schizophrenia
    c. Delusional disorder
    d. Depression
12. **In a patient with strikingly abnormal behavior, the most likely diagnosis is: (2009)**
    a. Paranoid schizophrenia
    b. Catatonic schizophrenia
    c. Hebephrenic schizophrenia
    d. Simple schizophrenia
13. **Which of the following is a first-rank symptom in schizophrenia? (2007)**
    a. Delusions
    b. Thought insertion
    c. Perceptional hallucinations
    d. Word salad
14. **Good prognostic factor in schizophrenia is:**
    a. Insidious onset **(2007)**
    b. Positive symptoms
    c. Disorganized subtype
    d. Absence of depression
15. **Catatonia is most commonly seen in: (2006)**
    a. Dementia
    b. Schizophrenia
    c. Depression
    d. Dissociative disorder
16. **Auditory hallucinations are seen except in:**
    a. Schizophrenia **(2006)**
    b. Acute and transient psychotic disorder
    c. Delirium tremens
    d. Panic disorder
17. **A patient has chronic low-grade depression for 2 years. What is the probable diagnosis? (2014)**
    a. Cyclothymia
    b. Dysthymia
    c. Minor depression
    d. Dysthymic personality disorder
18. **Which is the true statement? (2013)**
    a. Depression with suicidal tendencies will required ECT
    b. Chronic depression will require ECT
    c. Reactive depression responds to ECT better
    d. ECT is the treatment of choice for atypical depression
19. **Which of the following is a classical symptom of depression? (2007)**
    a. Altered sleep pattern
    b. Weight loss
    c. Guilt
    d. Decreased appetite
20. **Nihilistic delusions are seen in: (2006)**
    a. Depression
    b. Mania
    c. Schizophrenia
    d. OCD
21. **All the following are used in the treatment of bipolar disorder except:**
    a. Gabapentin
    b. Valproate
    c. Lithium
    d. Carbamazepine
22. **The mini-mental state examination is used in the diagnosis of: (2014)**
    a. Delirium
    b. Mania
    c. Depression
    d. Dementia
23. **All the following conditions regarding delirium are true except:**
    a. Acute onset **(2012, 2008)**
    b. Sleep disturbance
    c. Myoclonus
    d. Normal consciousness
24. **Which of the following is true regarding delirium? (2010)**
    a. Irreversible
    b. Insidious onset
    c. Behavioral change due to alteration in cerebral metabolism
    d. Clear consciousness
25. **The following drugs are used in Alzheimer's disease except: (2010)**
    a. Rivastigmine
    b. Memantine
    c. Donapezil
    d. Clonidine
26. **Reversible dementia is a feature of: (2007)**
    a. Alzheimer's disease
    b. Pick's disease
    c. Multi-infarct dementia
    d. Hypothyroidism
27. **Wernicke's encephalopathy occurs due to the deficiency of: (2010, 2009, 2008)**
    a. Thiamine
    b. Riboflavin
    c. Folate
    d. Vitamin B12

28. All the following are true regarding cocaine toxicity except: **(2010)**
a. Seizures
b. Myocardial infarction
c. Amantidine is the drug of choice
d. Mania symptoms

29. Morbid jealousy is seen in: **(2009)**
a. Alcoholism
b. Persons who are isolated from society
c. Social phobia
d. Depression

30. Which of the following is not seen in Korsakoff's syndrome? **(2007)**
a. Clear consciousness
b. Inability to learn new things
c. Hallucinations
d. Confabulation

31. Tactile hallucinations are seen in all except:
a. Delirium tremens **(2007)**
b. Amphetamine abuse
c. Opioid withdrawal
d. Frontal lobe tumor

32. True about post-traumatic stress disorder is:
a. Nightmares **(2013)**
b. Recollection of events
c. Depression
d. Increased sexual desire

33. The following conditions regarding anxiety are true except: **(2010)**
a. Adaptive response
b. Alert signal
c. Autonomic hyperactivity
d. Always pathological

34. Anxiety is different from fear in that it is: **(2006)**
a. Known
b. External
c. Vague
d. Nonconflictual

35. Brooding followed by homicidal tendency:
a. Amok **(2013)**
b. Dhat syndrome
c. Koro
d. Latah

36. True characteristic regarding Ganser's syndrome is: **(2009, 2006)**
a. Involuntary
b. Psychotic symptoms absent
c. Memory symptoms absent
d. Approximate answers

37. False regarding kleptomania is: **(2013)**
a. Fear before stealing
b. Stealing costly objects
c. Common in females
d. Irresistible desire to steal

38. Intense self-elation and feeling of self-importance and exploitation are seen with:
a. Narcissistic personality disorder **(2012)**
b. Schizoid personality disorder
c. Paranoid personality disorder
d. Schizotypal personality disorder

39. EEG changes are seen in which of the following disorders? **(2011)**
a. Intermittent explosive disorder
b. Panic disorder
c. Anxiety disorder
d. Somatoform disorder

40. Which of the following psychiatric illnesses is common in a patient with stroke? **(2011)**
a. Schizophrenia
b. Depression
c. Bipolar disorder
d. Psychosis

41. Impulsivity, angry outbursts, unstable relationships, deliberate self-harm and suicidal tendencies are characteristic of: **(2008)**
a. Narcissistic personality disorder
b. Schizoid personality disorder
c. Borderline personality disorder
d. Schizotypal personality disorder

42. Which of the following is not seen in a case of borderline personality disorder? **(2007)**
a. Identity crisis
b. Dissociative events
c. Risk-taking behavior
d. Strong interpersonal relationships

43. All the following are done in cognitive behavioral therapy except: **(2012)**
a. Maintenance
b. Consolidation
c. Contemplation
d. Precontemplation

44. Systematic desensitization as a form of therapy is done in: **(2009)**
a. Phobia
b. Obsessive-compulsive disorder
c. Generalized anxiety disorder
d. Hypochondriasis

45. **Electroconvulsive therapy is not useful except in case of: (2009)**
a. Delirium
b. Seizures
c. Depression
d. Panic attacks

46. **Neuroleptic malignant syndrome is treated with: (2008)**
a. Dantrolene
b. Corticosteroids
c. Diazepam
d. Hemodialysis

47. **Contraindication for electroconvulsive therapy: (2008)**
a. Second trimester pregnancy
b. Elderly
c. Raised ICT
d. Catatonia

48. **The following has least anticholinergic side effects: (2006)**
a. Clomipramine
b. Desipramine
c. Imipramine
d. Trimipramine

49. **Systematic desensitization is: (2006)**
a. Passive avoidance
b. Active avoidance
c. Sudden exposure
d. Graded exposure

50. **Infantile autism is seen in: (2009)**
a. Dysthmic personality disorder
b. Personality disorder
c. Paranoid personality disorder
d. Behavioral disorder

51. **The type of treatment which can be used for mental retardation is: (2007)**
a. Psychoanalysis
b. Family therapy
c. Transaction analysis
d. Rapid emotive treatment and response

52. **Regarding etiology of autism, all the following are true except: (2006)**
a. Fragile X syndrome
a. Tuberous sclerosis
b. Down's syndrome
d. Phenylketonuria

ANSWERS AND EXPLANATIONS

1. **Ans. d. F** *Ref: A Short Textbook of Psychiatry by Niraj Ahuja, 7/e p2*
There are two major systems of diagnostic classification in psychiatry (ICD-10 and DSM-5). ICD-10 (International Classification of Diseases, 10th Revision, 1992) is WHO's classification for all diseases and related health problems (and not only psychiatric disorders). Chapter F classifies psychiatric disorders as mental and behavioral disorders and codes them on an alphanumeric system from F00 to F99.

2. **Ans. b. Johann Christian Reil** *Ref: A Short Textbook of Psychiatry by Niraj Ahuja, 7/e p244*
He coined the term 'psychiatry'. He also founded the first psychiatric journal.

3. **Ans. a. Stupor** *Ref: Comprehensive Textbook of Psychiatry by Kaplan and Sadock, 9/e p928*
State of decreased reactivity to stimuli and less than full awareness of one, surroundings; as a disturbance of consciousness, it indicates a condition of partial coma or semicoma. In psychiatry, it is used synonymously with mutism and does not necessarily imply a disturbance of consciousness; in catatonic stupor, patients are ordinarily aware of their surroundings.

4. **Ans. a. Sudden loss of muscle tone** *Ref: Comprehensive Textbook of Psychiatry by Kaplan and Sadock, 9/e p921*
Temporary sudden loss of muscle tone causing weakness and immobilization; can be precipitated by a variety of emotional states and is often followed by sleep. Commonly seen in narcolepsy. Other features of narcolepsy includes sleep attacks, hypnogogic/hypnopompic hallucinations and sleep paralysis.

5. **Ans. d. It has a persistent tone of feeling for a period of time**
Ref: Comprehensive Textbook of Psychiatry by Kaplan and sadock, 9/e p920
The subjective and immediate experiences of emotion attached to ideas or mental representations of objects. Affect has outward manifestations that may be classified as restricted, blunted, flattened, broad, labile, appropriate or inappropriate whereas mood is pervasive and sustained feeling that is experienced internally and that, in the extreme, can markedly influence all aspects of a person's behavior and perception of the world.

6. **Ans. b. Illogical and primitive** *Ref: Comprehensive Textbook of Psychiatry by Kaplan and Sadock, 9/e p927*
In psychoanalysis, the mental activity is directly related to the functions of the id and characteristic of unconscious mental processes; marked by primitive, prelogical thinking and by the tendency to seek immediate discharge and gratification of instinctual demands. It includes thinking that is dereistic, illogical, magical: normally found in dreams, abnormally in psychosis: whereas secondary process thinking is logical, organized, reality-oriented and influenced by the demands of the environment; characterizes the mental activity of the ego.

7. **Ans. b. Abstract thinking** *Ref: Comprehensive Textbook of Psychiatry by Kaplan and Sadock, 9/e p897*
It is the ability to shift back and forth between general concepts and specific examples. Having the patient identify similarities between like objects or concepts as well as interpreting proverbs can be useful in assessing one's ability to abstract.

8. **Ans. a. Consciously present** *Ref: Synopsis of Psychiatry by Kaplan and Sadock, 10/e p87*
Explicit memory is called declarative memory whereas implicit memory is called nondeclarative memory. Explicit memory has two types called episodic memory and semantic memory. Episodic memory gives a record of personal experiences and medial temporal lobes are the primary structures involved. Semantic memory is an ability to remember facts and information. Procedural memory and priming are the types of implicit memory and basal ganglia is the structure implicated. Working memory is a type of short-term memory. It incorporates both immediate memory and recent memory.

9. **Ans. b. Feeling that unfamiliar things look familiar**
Ref: Comprehensive Textbook of Psychiatry by Kaplan and Sadock, 9/e p922
Illusion of visual recognition in which a new situation (unfamiliar) is incorrectly regarded as a repetition of a previous thought (familiar). Déjà enténdu is an illusion that what one is hearing one has heard previously; Déjà pensé is a condition in which a thought never entertained before is incorrectly regarded as a repetition of a previous thought.

10. **Ans. a. Amphetamine** *Ref: Synopsis of Psychiatry by Kaplan and Sadock, 10/e p410*
The clinical similarity of amphetamine-induced psychosis to paranoid schizophrenia has triggered extensive research. The hallmark feature of amphetamine-induced psychosis is paranoia. It is differentiated by the presence of visual hallucination, appropriate affect, hyperactivity, hypersexuality, confusion and incoherence.

11. **Ans. a. Substance abuse** *Ref: Synopsis of Psychiatry by Kaplan and Sadock, 10/e p512*
A wide range of nonpsychiatric medical conditions and a variety of substances can induce symptoms of psychosis in particular delusional disorder. Sudden onset of delusions without any precipitating factor should lead to ruling out of medical causes, such as neurodegenerative disorders, vascular causes, infectious causes and substances, such as amphetamines, alcohol, cocaine, cannabis, etc.

12. **Ans. b. Catatonic schizophrenia** *Ref: Synopsis of Psychiatry by Kaplan and Sadock, 10/e p477*
The classic feature of catatonic type is a marked disturbance in motor function, which may involve stupor, negativism, rigidity, excitement or posturing. The abnormal motor behavior will make this subtype to be diagnosed easily compared to other subtypes where thought and behavior require detailed evaluation, whereas other subtypes, such as paranoid depends on presence of delusions and hallucinations, hebephrenic subtype focuses on bizarre behavior and simple subtype on negative symptoms.

13. **Ans. b. Thought insertion** *Ref: Synopsis of Psychiatry by Kaplan and Sadock, 10/e p468, Table 13-1*
First-rank symptoms include audible thoughts, voices arguing or discussing or both, voices commenting, somatic passivity, thought withdrawl, thought insertion, thought broadcasting, delusional perception, all other experiences involving volition made affects and made impulses.

14. **Ans. b. Positive symptoms** *Ref: Synopsis of Psychiatry by Kaplan and Sadock, 10/e p476, Table 13-6*
Late onset, presence of precipitating factors, acute onset, good premorbid personality, mood disorder symptoms, family history of mood disorders, good support system, positive symptoms are features towards good prognosis.

15. **Ans. b. Schizophrenia** *Ref: Synopsis of Psychiatry by Kaplan and Sadock, 10/e p541*
As a symptom, catatonia can be present in several mental disorders, most commonly schizophrenia and mood disorders. Originally, catatonia was believed to be a type of schizophrenia, but more recent studies found

that more than one quarter of patients with mania and 20 percent of individuals with depression experience symptoms of catatonia. The presence of catatonic features in patients with mood disorders may have prognostic and treatment significance.

16. **Ans. d. Panic disorder** *Ref: Synopsis of Psychiatry by Kaplan and Sadock, 10/e p399*
Auditory hallucination is a psychotic symptom and is present in psychotic conditions, such as schizophrenia and acute and transient psychosis. The essential feature of delirium in delirium tremens is occurrence of symptoms within 1 week of stopping alcohol use characterized by autonomic hyperactivity, perceptual distortions most frequently visual or tactile hallucinations; fluctuating levels of psychomotor activity. Panic disorder is a type of neurotic condition characterized by anxiety attacks with autonomic arousal symptoms.

17. **Ans. b. Dysthymia** *Ref: Synopsis of Psychiatry by Kaplan and Sadock, 10/e p563*
Depressed mood for most of the day, for more days than not, as indicated by subjective account or observation by others for atleast 2 years. Presence of two or more of the following: poor appetite or overeating, insomnia or hypersomnia, low energy or fatigue, low self-esteem, poor concentration or difficulty making decisions, feeling of hopelessness. Classified as early onset if before 21 years and late onset if more than 21 years.

18. **Ans. a. Depression with suicidal tendencies requires ECT**
Ref: Synopsis of Psychiatry by Kaplan and Sadock, 10/e p1119
The most common indication for ECT is major depressive disorder for which ECT is the most effective therapy. It should be considered in patients who have failed medication trials, have not tolerated medications, have severe depression with psychotic symptoms, are acutely suicidal or homicidal or have marked symptoms of agitation or stupor.

19. **Ans. a. Altered sleep pattern** *Ref: Synopsis of Psychiatry by Kaplan and Sadock, 10/e p543*
A depressed mood and a loss of interest or pleasure are the key symptoms of depression. Almost all depressed patients (97%) complain about reduced energy; have less motivation and 80% of patients complain of trouble sleeping, especially early morning awakening (terminal insomnia). Anxiety, a common symptom of depression, affects as many as 90% of depressed patients.

20. **Ans. a. Depression** *Ref: Synopsis of Psychiatry by Kaplan and Sadock, 10/e p510*
In the 19th century, French Psychiatrist Jules Cotard described several patients who suffered from a syndrome called nihilistic delusional disorder or cotard syndrome. Patients complain of having lost not only possessions, status and strength, but also their heart, blood, and intestines. This relatively rare syndrome is usually considered a precursor to depressive episode.

21. **Ans. a. Gabapentin** *Ref: Synopsis of Psychiatry by Kaplan and Sadock, 10/e p560*
The drugs that are approved by USFDA for the treatment of bipolar disorder include lithium, divalproaex, carbamazepine, olanzapine, risperidone, quitiapine, and lamotrigine (for bipolar depression).

22. **Ans. d. Dementia** *Ref: Synopsis of Psychiatry by Kaplan and Sadock, 10/e p187*
MMSE is a screening test that can be used during a patient's clinical examination. It is a practical test to track the changes in a patient's cognitive state. Of the possible 30 points, a score below 30 suggests possible impairment, and a score below 20 indicates definite cognitive impairment of dementia. It encompasses orientation, attention and concentration, registration and recall, comprehension, reading, writing, repetition, etc.

23. **Ans. d. Normal consciousness** *Ref: Synopsis of Psychiatry by Kaplan and Sadock, 10/e p325 326*
The core features of delirium include altered consciousness, such as decreased level of consciousness, altered attention, impairment in other realms of cognitive functions which can manifest as disorientation, relatively rapid onset, brief duration, unpredictable fluctuations during the course of day, sometimes worse at night (sundowning). Others include illusions, hallucinations, psychomotor hyper/hypo activity, mood alterations, autonomic hyperactivity, myoclonic jerks, etc.

24. **Ans. c. Behavioral changes due to alteration in cerebral metabolism**
Ref: Postgraduate Textbook of Psychiatry by Niraj Ahuja, 2/e p47
Engel and Romano's classic study, involving EEG recordings, point to a general reduction in cerebral oxidative metabolism as the cause for delirium. This deficit in cerebral oxidative metabolism results in a reduction in acetylcholine synthesis leading to delirium. An imbalance between central cholinergic and adrenergic mechanisms is also responsible for producing delirious states.

25. Ans. d. Clonidine *Ref: Synopsis of Psychiatry by Kaplan and Sadock, 10/e p343*

Donepezil, rivastigmine, galantamine and tacrine are cholinesterase inhibitors used to treat mild to moderate cognitive impairment in Alzheimer's disease. They reduce the inactivation of the neurotransmitter acetylcholine and thus potentiate the cholinergic neurotransmitter, which, in turn, produces a modest improvement in memory and goal-directed thought. Memantine protects neurons from excessive amounts of glutamate, which may be neurotoxic.

26. Ans. d. Hypothyroidism *Ref: Synopsis of Psychiatry by Kaplan and Sadock, 10/e p330*

Many types of dementia evaluated in clinical settings can be attributable to reversible causes, such as metabolic abnormalities (e.g. hypothyroidism), nutritional deficiencies (vitamin B12 or folate) or dementia syndrome caused by depression.

27. Ans. d. Vitamin B12 *Ref: Synopsis of Psychiatry by Kaplan and Sadock, 10/e p400*

The classical names for alcohol-induced persisting amnestic disorder are Wernicke's encephalopathy and Korsakoff's syndrome. Whereas Wernicke's is completely reversible with treatment, only 20% of patients with Korsakoff's syndrome recover. Wernicke's is also called alcoholic encephalopathy characterized by ataxia, vestibular dysfunction, confusion and a variety of ocular motility abnormalities. In the early stages, Wernicke's encephalopathy responds rapidly to large doses of parenteral thiamine. The dosage is 100 mg orally two to three times daily continued for 1–2 weeks.

28. Ans. c. Amantadine is the drug of choice *Ref: Textbook of Postgraduate Psychiatry, Niraj Ahuja, 2/e p107*

Acute intoxication with high doses of cocaine is characterized by rambling speech, headache, paranoid ideation, auditory hallucination, tactile hallucination, tachycardia, hypertension, coronary vasospasm, mood changes like agitation, irritability, sexual behavior, aggression, emotional lability and possible symptoms of mania. Common medical complications are cardiovascular (arrhythmias and MI), respiratory (respiratory failure), neurological (seizures and headache), GI (nausea and abdominal pain).

29. Ans. a. Alcoholism *Ref: Postgraduate Textbook of Psychiatry, Niraj Ahuja, 2/e p105*

Patients with chronic alcohol use suspect their spouses of infidelity and the belief is morbid enough to influence various aspects of personal and social life. It is less common than a nondelusional suspicious attitude to the spouse. It is also called Othello syndrome or conjugal paranoia.

30. Ans. c. Hallucinations *Ref: Kaplan and Sadock's Synopsis of Psychiatry, p401*

Korsakoff syndrome is the chronic amnestic syndrome that can follow Wernicke's encephalopathy and the cardinal features are impaired mental syndrome (recent memory) and anterograde amnesia with confabulation. It is labeled under alcohol-induced persisting amnestic disorder. Treatment is thiamine given 100 mg orally two to three times daily for 3–12 months.

31. Ans. d. Frontal lobe tumor *Ref: Synopsis of Psychiatry by Kaplan and Sadock, 10/e p411*

The essential features of delirium include autonomic hyperactivity, perceptual distortions, most frequently visual or tactile hallucinations and fluctuating levels of psychomotor activity. Cocaine-induced tactile hallucination is called cocaine bugs or magnus symptom. Amphetamine as with cocaine can induce tactile hallucinations during intoxication

32. Ans. b. Recollection of events *Ref: Synopsis of Psychiatry by Kaplan and Sadock, 10/e p615*

The principal clinical features of PTSD are painful re-experiences of the event, a pattern of avoidance and emotional numbing and fairly constant hyperarousal. Patient may also describe dissociative states and panic attacks, illusions and hallucinations may be present. The onset is within 6 months of the traumatic event. Associated symptoms may include aggression, violence, poor impulse control, depression and substance related disorders.

33. Ans. d. Always pathological *Ref: Postgraduate Textbook of Psychiatry, Niraj Ahuja, 2/e p250*

Anxiety is commonly experienced by all humans. It is an alerting signal, warns of threat, external or internal, initiates a patient to take necessary steps to prevent the threat, and life-saving. Pathological anxiety is an inappropriate response to a given stimulus by virtue of its duration or intensity. It is associated with somatic and physical symptoms of autonomic arousal.

34. Ans. c. Vague *Ref: Synopsis of Psychiatry by Kaplan and Sadock, 10/e p579*

Anxiety and fear are both alerting signals. Anxiety can be conceptualized as a normal and adaptive response accompanied by somatic and autonomic activity. It warns of impending danger and enables a person to take measures to deal with a threat. Fear is a response to a known, external, definite, or nonconflictual threat. Anxiety is a response to a threat that is unknown, internal, vague or conflictual.

35. Ans. a. Amok *Ref: Synopsis of Psychiatry, Kaplan and Sadock, 10/e p522*

A dissociative episode characterized by a period of brooding followed by an outburst of violent, aggressive or homicidal behavior directed at persons and objects. It is precipitated by a perceived slight or insult and seems to be common among men. It is accompanied by persecutory idea, automatism, amnesia, exhaustion and a return to premorbid state following the episode.

36. Ans. d. Approximate answers *Ref: A Short Textbook of Psychiatry by Niraj Ahuja, p102*

Ganser's syndrome (hysterical pseudodementia) is commonly found in prison inmates. The characteristic feature is vorbireden, which is also called approximate answers. A clouding of consciousness also occurs, manifests by disorientation, amnesias, loss of personal information, visual and auditory hallucinations. Neurological examination may reveal hysterical stigmata, e.g. a non-neurological analgesia or shifting hyperalgesia.

37. Ans. b. Stealing costly objects *Ref: Synopsis of Psychiatry, Kaplan and Sadock, 10/e p776*

The essential feature is a recurrent failure to resist impulse to steal objects not needed for personal use or for monetary value. The objects taken are often given away, returned surreptitiously or kept and hidden. They feel guilty, ashamed, and embarrassed about their behavior. There is pleasure, gratification or relief at the time of committing the theft. Male to female ratio is 1 : 3. There are recurrent intrusive, irresistible urges or impulses to steal unneeded objects and may also be distressed about the possibility of being apprehended.

38. Ans. a. Narcissistic personality *Ref: Synopsis of Psychiatry, Kaplan and Sadock, 10/e p803*

They have a grandiose sense of self-importance; they consider themselves special and expect special treatment. They handle criticisms poorly and become enraged when someone dares to criticize them. Their relationships are fragile and interpersonal exploitiveness is commonplace. They cannot show empathy and they feign sympathy to achieve their selfish ends.

39. Ans. a. Intermittent explosive disorder *Ref: Synopsis of Psychiatry, Kaplan and Sadock, 10/e p775*

Persons with this disorder have a high incidence of soft neurological signs (e.g. reflex asymmetries), nonspecific EEG findings, abnormal neuropsychological testing results (e.g. letter reversal difficulties), and accident susceptibility. MRI may reveal changes in the prefrontal cortex which is associated with loss of impulse control. It is characterized by episodes of loss of control associated with aggressive outbursts out of proportion to precipitating psychosocial stressors.

40. Ans. b. Depression *Ref: Postgraduate Textbook of Psychiatry, Niraj Ahuja, 2/e p440*

A number of psychiatric syndromes are associated with stroke depending on the anatomical site involved and include depression, mania, anxiety, OC symptoms, personality alterations (apathetic or disinhibited), Kluver-Bucy syndrome, hallucinations and psychosis.

41. Ans. c. Borderline personality *Ref: Synopsis of Psychiatry, Kaplan and Sadock, 10/e p800*

Persons with BPD appear to be in a state of crisis. Mood swings are common. They can have shortlived psychotic episodes (called 'micropsychosis') and their behavior is highly unpredictable. The painful nature of their lives is reflected in repetitive self-destructive acts. They have tumultuous interpersonal relationships. They distort their relationships by considering each person to be either all good or all bad. They also complain about chronic feelings of emptiness and boredom and lack a consistent sense of identity.

42. Ans. d. Strong interpersonal relationships *Ref: Synopsis of Psychiatry, Kaplan and Sadock, 10/e p800*

Persons with BPD appear to be in a state of crisis. Mood swings are common. They can have shortlived psychotic episodes (called 'micropsychosis') and their behavior is highly unpredictable. The painful nature of their lives is reflected in repetitive self-destructive acts. They have tumultuous interpersonal relationships. They distort their relationships by considering each person to be either all good or all bad. They also complain about chronic feelings of emptiness and boredom and lack a consistent sense of identity.

43. Ans. b. Consolidation *Ref: Psychiatry by Allan Tasman, 2nd edition*

Prochaska and DiClemente have described a transtheoretical model of how people change addictive behaviors with or without formal treatment. In a transtheoretical perspective, individuals move through a series of stages of change as they progress in modifying problem behaviors. This concept of stages is important in understanding change. Each stage requires certain tasks to be accomplished and certain processes to be used in order to achieve change. Six separate stages have been identified in this model.

Individuals who are not considering change in their problem behavior are described as being in precontemplation.

The contemplation stage entails the person's beginning to consider both the existence of a problem and the feasibility and costs of changing the problem behavior.

As this individual progresses, he or she moves on to the determination stage, where the decision is made to take action and change.

Once the individual begins to modify the problem behavior, he or she enters the action stage, which normally continues for 3–6 months.

After successfully negotiating the action stage, the individual moves to maintenance or sustained change. If these efforts fail, a relapse occurs, and the individual begins another cycle.

44. Ans. a. Phobia *Ref: A Short Textbook of Psychiatry by Niraj Ahuja, p214*

It is based on the principle of reciprocal inhibition as described by Wolpe. It consists of relaxation training, hierarchy construction and systematic desensitsation proper. It is based on the principle that if a response incompatible with anxiety is made to occur at the same time as an anxiety-provoking stimulus, anxiety is reduced by reciprocal inhibition. It is the treatment of choice in phobias and OCD.

45. Ans. a. Depression *Ref: A Short Textbook of Psychiatry by Niraj Ahuja, p199*

The major indications for ECT are severe depression with suicidal risk, with stupor, with poor food intake, with melancholic features, with psychotic features, severe catatonia, severe psychosis and unresponsive to medications.

46. Ans. a. Dantrolene *Ref: Synopsis of Psychiatry, Kaplan and Sadock, 10/e p996*

NMS is a life-threatening complication characterized by muscular rigidity and dystonia, high fever, sweating, increase blood pressure, increased WBC count, and increased levels of CPK. The symptoms evolve over 24–72 hours and untreated syndrome lasts 10–14 days. In addition to supportive treatment, the most commonly used medications are dantrolene (1 mg/kg/day for 8 days) and bromocriptine, although amantadine is sometimes used.

47. Ans. c. Raised ICT *Ref: Synopsis of Psychiatry, Kaplan and Sadock, 10/e p1123*

ECT has no absolute contraindications, only situations in which a patient is at increased risk and has an increased need for close monitoring. Relative contraindications include raised ICT, aneurysm, retinal detachment, and recent MI. The mortality rate with ECT is about 0.002% per treatment.

48. Ans. b. Desipramine *Ref: Synopsis of Psychiatry, Kaplan and Sadock, 10/e p1109, Table 36.34–2*

Anticholinergic effects among tricyclics is less with desipramine and more with amitryptiline and trimipramine. Among tetracyclics, it is less with maprotiline. Sedation is less with desipramine and amoxapine. Orthostatic hypotension is the least with nortriptyline and amoxapine. Seizures are less with secondary amines. Conduction abnormalities are less with doxepin and amoxapine.

49. Ans. d. Graded exposure *Ref: A Short Textbook of Psychiatry by Niraj Ahuja, p214*

It is based on the principle of reciprocal inhibition as described by Wolpe. It consists of relaxation training, hierarchy construction and systematic desensitization proper. It is based on the principle that if a response incompatible with anxiety is made to occur at the same time as an anxiety-provoking stimulus, anxiety is reduced by reciprocal inhibition. It is the treatment of choice in phobias and OCD.

50. Ans. d. Behavioral disorder:

Autistic disorder is characterized by:

A. Qualitative impairment in social interaction (absence of eye-to-eye contact, failure to develop peer relationship, and lack of emotional reciprocity).

B. Qualitative impairment in communication (language delay, repetitive use of idiosyncratic language, and lack of social imitative play).

C. Restricted, repetitive and stereotyped patterns of behavior, interests and activities.

Delays or abnormal functioning in atleast one of the following areas, with onset prior to age 3 years: 1. social interaction; 2. language as used in social communication; or 3. symbolic or imaginative play.

51. Ans. b. Family therapy

Ref: Counselors' Manual for Family Intervention in Mental Retardation by Dr. Sathish Girimaji p40–42

One of the most important areas that a clinician can address is educating the family of a mentally retarded child about ways to enhance competence and self-esteem while maintaining realistic expectations for the patient. But ideally, behavioral therapy is essential to teach adaptive skills and decrease maladaptive behaviors. Basic skills, such as dressing, continence, and feeding require more of behavioral approach based on rewards and reinforcement to be taught to a mentally retarded child. Rewards are extremely useful to develop and strengthen new skills in children. Rewards which are given contingent on a particular desired behavior are the principle of contingency management. For example, a child who tries to learn feeding her/himself, should be rewarded with a praise contingent with every attempt that the child makes to complete the act (starting from picking up the spoon in hand, scooping some food onto the spoon, bringing hand towards mouth, etc).

52. Ans. b. Down's syndrome *Ref: Synopsis of Psychiatry, Kaplan and Sadock, 10/e p1192*

Linkage analyses have demonstrated that regions of chromosomes 7, 2, 4, 15 and 19 are likely to contribute to the genetic basis of autism. Approximately 1% of children with autistic disorder also have fragile X syndrome. Up to 2% of children with autism may also have tuberous sclerosis. It is also associated with neurological conditions, such as congential rubella and phenylketonuria.

HIGH-YIELD POINTS

1. Hallucination and illusion are disorders of perception
2. Delusion is a disorder of thought content
3. Eugen Bleuler coined the term 'schizophrenia'
4. Sigmund Freud is the father of psychoanalysis
5. First-rank symptoms of schizophrenia were given by Schneider
6. Delusion of persecution and reference are seen in schizophrenia
7. Delusion of grandiosity is seen in mania
8. Delusion of guilt and nihilism are seen in depression
9. Four As of schizophrenia include Autism, Ambivalence, Affective flattening, and Loosening of Association
10. Good prognostic factors in schizophrenia—late age of onset, positive symptoms, paranoid subtype, and normal imaging
11. Waxy flexibility and posturing are features of catatonic schizophrenia
12. Loosening of association is a formal thought disorder in schizophrenia
13. Flight of ideas and pressure of speech are features of mania
14. Core features of depression include pervasive sadness, anhedonia and anergia
15. Cognitive triad of depression (hopelessness, helplessness and worthlessness) was given by Aaron Temkin Beck
16. Delusion of persecution and delusional parasitosis are seen with cocaine abuse
17. Tactile hallucinations or formication or magnus symptoms are seen with cocaine abuse
18. Run amok is seen with cannabis abuse
19. CAGE questionnaire is a screening questionnaire for alcohol dependence
20. Delirium is also known as acute confusional state
21. Sundowning, sleep-wake cycle reversal are seen in delirium
22. Mini Mental State Examination is a screening tool for dementia
23. Step ladder pattern of memory decline is seen with vascular dementia
24. Myoclonus, Triphasic EEG abnormalities are commonly reported in Cruetzfeldt Jacob type of dementia
25. Pseudodementia is depressive dementia and is reversible
26. Spontaneous anxiety attacks with anticipatory anxiety are features of panic disorder

27. Unconscious conflicts presenting as physical symptoms: Conversion disorder
28. Conscious feigning of symptoms to assume sick role or attention: Factitious disorder
29. Conscious feigning of symptoms for external gain/benefit: Malingering
30. Drug of choice for OCD is fluoxetine
31. Drug of choice for alcohol withdrawl is chlordiazepoxide (benzodiazepine)
32. Drug of choice for bipolar disorder is Lithium
33. Therapeutic serum lithium level is 0.8–1.2 meq/L
34. Drug of choice for treatment resistant schizophrenia: Clozapine
35. Treatment of choice for severe depression with suicidal risk: Electroconvulsive therapy
36. Drug of choice for nocturnal enuresis: Imipramine
37. Drug of choice for ADHD: Methylphenidate
38. Drug of choice for neuroleptic malignant syndrome: Dantrolene
39. Drug-induced extrapyramidal symptoms include dystonia, akathisia, pseudoparkinsonism, tardive dyskinesia
40. Exposure response prevention is the behavior therapy for OCD

Important Dates to Remember

World Mental Health Day: October 10th every year (theme for year 2015–Dignity in Mental Health)
International Day against Drug Abuse and Trafficking: June 26th every year
International Suicide Prevention Day: September 10th of every year
World Schizophrenia Day: May 24th.

QUESTIONS 2015

1. **Lack of pleasure in previously enjoyed activities is termed as:**
   a. Alexithymia
   b. Abulia
   c. Anhedonia
   d. Affect

2. **Mutism and akinesia in an awake patient is called:**
   a. Stupor
   b. Dystonia
   c. Dyskinesia
   d. Akathisia

ANSWERS AND EXPLANATIONS

1. **Ans. a. Anhedonia** *Ref: Kaplan and Sadock's Synopsis of Psychiatry, 10/e 273–274.*
   Anhedonia—It is the loss of interest in, and withdrawal from, all regular and pleasurable activities. Often associated with depression, Alexithymia is inability or difficulty in describing or being aware of one's emotions or moods; elaboration of fantasies associated with depression, substance abuse, and post-traumatic stress disorder. Abulia is reduced impulse to act and think, associated with indifference about consequences of action. Occurs as a result of neurologic deficit, depression and schizophrenia. Affect is the subjective and immediate experience of emotion attached to ideas or mental representations of objects.
2. **Ans. a. Stupor** *Ref: Kaplan and Sadock's Synopsis of Psychiatry, 10/e 273, 282.*
   Stupor is a state of decreased reactivity to stimuli and less than full awareness of one's surroundings; as a disturbance of consciousness, it indicates a condition of partial or semicoma. In psychiatry, it is used synonymously with mutism and doesn't imply a disturbance of consciousness; in catatonic stupor, patients are ordinarily aware of their surroundings. Akinesia is lack of physical movement as in the extreme immobility of catatonic schizophrenia.